Nephrology

Nephrology

Edited by

Rex L. Jamison
Professor of Medicine
Division of Nephrology
Department of Medicine
Stanford University School of Medicine
Veterans Affairs Palo Alto Health Care System
Palo Alto
California
USA

and

Robert Wilkinson
Consultant Nephrologist and Professor of Renal Medicine
University of Newcastle upon Tyne
Freeman Hospital
Newcastle upon Tyne
UK

CHAPMAN & HALL
London · Weinheim · New York · Tokyo · Melbourne · Madras

Published by Chapman & Hall, 2–6 Boundary Row, London SE1 8HN, UK

Chapman & Hall, 2–6 Boundary Row, London SE1 8HN, UK

Chapman & Hall GmbH, Pappelallee 3, 69469 Weinheim, Germany

Chapman & Hall USA, 115 Fifth Avenue, New York, NY 10003, USA

Chapman & Hall Japan, ITP-Japan, Kyowa Building, 3F, 2-2-1 Hirakawacho, Chiyoda-ku, Tokyo 102, Japan

Chapman & Hall Australia, 102 Dodds Street, South Melbourne, Victoria 3205, Australia

Chapman & Hall India, R. Seshadri, 32 Second Main Road, CIT East, Madras 600035, India

First edition 1997

© 1997 Chapman and Hall

Typeset in 9/11.5pt Stone Serif by Best-set Typesetter Ltd., Hong Kong

Printed in Spain

ISBN 0 412 60930 4

A catalogue record for this book is available from the British Library

Library of Congress Catalog Card Number: 97-69676

Dedication

To: Dennis S. Parsons   George A. Smoot
      Alexander Leaf   John A. Luetsher
     Robert W. Berliner   David N.S. Kerr
"... and gladly woulde he learne and gladly teche ...:
(from Canterbury Tales by Geoffrey Chaucer, 1342–1400)

Contents

Preface

The publication of a new textbook of nephrology today is a bold undertaking. There is already an array of good nephrology textbooks in bookstores, offices and libraries. In this age of the computer, access to new information is increasingly easy to obtain, often within weeks of original discovery. This latter circumstance is, in part, what led to this book. In our view, the encyclopedic text is at risk of becoming less useful. It is expensive and heavy to carry around. At the other extreme, the small practical manual is relatively inexpensive and easy to put in one's pocket. What it lacks is the narrative explanation that weaves facts together to facilitate understanding and retention. One purpose of this book is to strike the right balance between the tome and the manual. The book can be readily carried between office and home and complemented by access to the computer network.

A second purpose is to provide an international perspective about issues in nephrology. Written by authors primarily from North America and Europe, the chapters reflect for the most part a world-wide consensus about the principles and practice of nephrology. The editors hope the reader will, after a few hours of study, understand the basic principles of a given renal function or disorder, learn a logical approach to prevention and treatment, and want to keep abreast of any uncertainty or controversy. In other words, we hope this book proves to be a reliable assistant to continuous self-instruction.

We endeavored to assure a readable text by our choice of authors and careful – even aggressive – editing. As Brooks Atkinson, the late drama critic for the *New Yorker*, once wrote, 'There is no good writing that is not clear. There is no clear writing that is not good.'

We wish to express our profound appeciation to our authors. The success of the book is attributable to them; the deficiencies are our responsibility. We invite the reader to inform us of inaccuracies, omissions and questionable assertions. We are very grateful to Dr Peter Altman of Chapman & Hall for his enduring patience and good will, to our wives for their forbearance and to our colleagues for their help.

We hope this book becomes a valued companion to those entering the world of nephrology. It is a unique discipline in medicine. There is probably no doctor who sees his or her patients more frequently over a longer time. To be a nephrologist is to experience inspiration along with a large dose of humility.

Rex L. Jamison
Stanford

Robert Wilkinson
Newcastle upon Tyne

Contributors

Rajiv Agarwal MD
Veteran Affairs Medical Center IIIN, 1481 West Tenth Street, Indianapolis, IN 46202, USA

Edward J. Alfrey MD
Division of Transplantation, Department of Surgery, Stanford University School of Medicine, Stanford, CA 94305, USA

Anders Alvestrand MD
Department of Clinical Sciences, Division of Renal Medicine, Karolinska Institute, Huddinge University Hospital, S-14186 Stockholm, Sweden

Jeffrey K. Aronson MA, MBChB, DPhil, FRCP
University Department of Clinical Pharmacology, Radcliffe Infirmary, Woodstock Road, Oxford OX2 6HE, UK

Francis W. Ballardie PhD, FRCP
Department of Nephrology, Manchester Royal Infirmary, Manchester M13 9WL, UK

David Bates MA, FRCP
Department of Neurology, Royal Victoria Infirmary, Newcastle upon Tyne NE1 4LP, UK

Chris Baylis PhD
Department of Physiology, Robert C. Byrd Health Sciences Center, West Virginia University, Morgantown, WV 26506-9229, USA

Ariela Benigni Biol.SCI.d
Mario Negri Institute for Pharmacological Research, Via Gavazzeni 11, 24125 Bergamo, Italy

Joseph V. Bonventre MD, PhD
Medical Services, Massachusetts General Hospital, Department of Medicine, Harvard Medical School, Charlestown, MA 02129, USA

Alison L. Brown MA, MD, MRCP
Department of Nephrology, Freeman Hospital, Newcastle upon Tyne NE7 7DN, UK

David J. Burn MD, MA, MRCP
Department of Neurology, Royal Victoria Infirmary, Newcastle upon Tyne NE1 4LP, UK

Kevin D. Burns MD, FRCP
Division of Nephrology, Department of Medicine, University of Ottawa, Ottawa, Ontario, Canada K1H 8L6

David A. Bushinsky MD
Nephrology Unit, Strong Memorial Hospital, University of Rochester School of Medicine and Dentistry, 601 Elmwood Avenue, Box 675, Rochester, NY 14642, USA

Carlo Catalano MD
Unità Operativa di Nefrologia e Dialisi, ULSS 17, Via Marconi 19, 35043 Monselice (Padova), Italy

G.A. Coles MD, FRCP
Institute of Nephrology, University of Wales College of Medicine, Cardiff Royal Infirmary, Newport Road, Cardiff CF2 1SZ, UK

John A. Cotterill MD, FRCP
Mid Yorkshire Nuffield Hospital, Outwood Lane, Horsforth, Leeds LS18 4HP, UK

Theodore Craig PhD
Nephrology Research Unit, Mayo Clinic/Foundation Rochester, MN 55905, USA

Donald C. Dafoe MD
Division of Transplantation, Department of Surgery, Stanford University School of Medicine, Stanford, CA 94305, USA

William H. Dantzler MD, PhD
Department of Physiology, College of Medicine, University of Arizona, Tucson, AZ 85724, USA

Alex M. Davison MD, FRCPE, FRCP
Department of Renal Medicine, St James's University Hospital NHS Trust, Leeds LS9 7TF, UK

John M. Davison MD, BS, MSc, FRCOG
Department of Obstetrics and Gynaecology, Royal Victoria Hospital, Newcastle upon Tyne NE1 4LP, UK

John B. Eastwood MD, FRCP
St George's Hospital Medical School, Cranmer Terrace, London SW17 0RE, UK

A. Meguid El Nahas PhD, FRCP
Sheffield Kidney Institute, Northern General Hospital Trust, Herries Road, Sheffield S5 7AU, UK

K. Farrington MD, FRCP
Renal Unit, Lister Hospital, Coreyes Hill Lane, Stevenage, Herts SG1 4AB, UK

John Feehally MA, DM, FRCP
Department of Nephrology, Leicester General Hospital, Gwendolen Road, Leicester LE5 9RT, UK

Fernando C. Fervenza MD
Division of Nephrology, Stanford University, School of Medicine and Veterans Affairs Palo Alto Health Care System, Palo Alto, CA 94304, USA

Gerald W. Friedland MD, FRCPE, FRCR
Department of Radiology, Stanford University School of Medicine, 790 Center Drive, Palo Alto, CA 94301, USA

R. Gokal MD, FRCP
Department of Renal Medicine, Manchester Royal Infirmary, Oxford Road, Manchester M13 9WL, UK

Timothy H.J. Goodship MD, FRCP
Department of Nephrology, Royal Victoria Infirmary, Newcastle upon Tyne NE1 4LP, UK

P.E. Gower MD, FRCP
Charing Cross Hospital, Fulham Palace Road, London W6 8RF, UK

R.N. Greenwood MD, FRCP
Renal Unit, Lister Hospital, Coreyes Hill Lane, Stevenage, Herts SG1 4AB, UK

R.R. Hall MS, FRCS
Department of Urology, Freeman Hospital, Newcastle upon Tyne NE7 7DN, UK

Kevin P.G. Harris MA, MD, FRCP
Department of Nephrology, Leicester General Hospital, Leicester LE4 5PW, UK

John Harty MD
Department of Renal Medicine, Manchester Royal Infirmary, Oxford Road, Manchester M13 9WL, UK

A.M. Heagerty MD, FRCP
Manchester Royal Infirmary, Oxford Road, Manchester M13 9WL, UK

Nicholas Andrew Hoenich PhD
Department of Medicine, Medical School, Framlington Place, Newcastle upon Tyne NE2 4HH, UK

Barry I. Hoffbrand MA, FRCP
Department of Nephrology, Whittington Hospital, Highgate Hill, London N19 5NF, UK

Alastair J. Hutchison MBChB, MRCP, MD
Department of Renal Medicine, Manchester Royal Infirmary, Oxford Road, Manchester M13 9WL, UK

Rex L. Jamison MD
Division of Nephrology, Department of Medicine, Stanford University School of Medicine, Veterans Affairs Palo Alto Health Care System, Palo Alto, CA 94304, USA

R. Brooke Jeffrey Jr MD
Department of Radiology, H-1307, Stanford University School of Medicine, Stanford, CA 94305-5105, USA

John N. Kabalin MD, FACS
Department of Urology, Stanford University School of Medicine, Veterans Affairs Palo Alto Health Care System, Palo Alto, CA 94305, USA

Michael Kashgarian MD
Department of Pathology and Biology, Yale University School of Medicine, 310 Cedar Street, New Haven, CT 06520-8023, USA

George A. Kaysen MD, PhD
Renal Biochemistry Laboratory, Division of Nephrology, Department of Medicine, University of California at Davis School of Medicine, Davis, CA 95616, USA

David N.S. Kerr MSc, FRCP
Department of Renal Medicine, Royal Postgraduate Medical School, Du Cane Road, London W12, UK

Raymond T. Krediet MD, PhD
Renal Unit F4-215, Academic Medical Centre, Meibergdreef 9, 1105 AZ Amsterdam, The Netherlands

Alan M. Krensky MD
Department of Pediatrics, Stanford University School of Medicine, Stanford, CA 94305, USA

Rajiv Kumar MBBS, FACP
Department of Medicine, Mayo Clinic and Foundation, Mayo Medical School, Rochester, MN 55905, USA

Paul C. Kuo MD
Department of Surgery, University of Maryland School of Medicine, Baltimore, MD 21201, USA

Richard A. Lafayette MD
Division of Nephrology, Stanford University School of Medicine, Stanford, CA 94305, USA

Kevin V. Lemley MD, PhD
Department of Pediatrics, Stanford University School of Medicine, Stanford, CA 94305, USA

Andrew S. Levey MD
Division of Nephrology, Tufts University School of Medicine, New England Medical Center, 750 Washington Street, Boston, MA 02111, USA

David Z. Levine MD, FRCP
Division of Nephrology, Department of Medicine, University of Ottawa, Ottawa, Ontario, Canada K1H 8L6

J.B. Levy MA, MRCP
Renal Unit, Department of Medicine, Royal Postgraduate Medical School, Hammersmith Hospital, Du Cane Road, London W12 0NN, UK

Clare M. Lloyd PhD
Renal Unit, United Medical and Dental Schools of Guy's and St Thomas's Hospitals, Guy's Campus, London SE1 9RT, UK

C.M. Lockwood FRCP, FRCPath
University of Cambridge, Department of Medicine and Pathology, Addenbrooke's Hospital, Hills Road, Cambridge, CB2 2QQ, UK

Ashutosh S. Lohe MBBS, MD
Department of Nephrology, Knox County Hospital, 321 High Street, Barbourville, KY 40906, USA

Christopher J. Lote PhD
Department of Renal Physiology, University of Birmingham Medical School, Birmingham B15 2TT, UK

G.S. Lucas MD, FRCP, FRCPath
Manchester Royal Infirmary, Oxford Road, Manchester M13 9WL, UK

N.P. Mallick MBChB, FRCP
Manchester Royal Infirmary, Oxford Road, Manchester M13 9WL, UK

Derek Manas MBBCh, FCS(SA)
Freeman Hospital, High Heaton, Newcastle upon Tyne NE7 7DN, UK

Paul Mead BMedsci, MRCP
Department of Nephrology, Freeman Hospital, Newcastle upon Tyne NE7 7DN, UK

Timothy Meyer MD
Division of Nephrology, Stanford University School of Medicine, Veterans Affairs Palo Alto Health Care System, Palo Alto, CA 94304, USA

W.E. Mitch MD
Renal Division, Emory University, School of Medicine Atlanta, GA 30322-0001, USA

Adrian R. Morley MD, FRCPath
Department of Pathology, Royal Victoria Hospital, Newcastle upon Tyne NE1 4LP, UK

Brian D. Myers MD
Division of Nephrology, Stanford University School of Medicine, Stanford, CA 94305, USA

Guy Neild MD, FRCP
Institute of Urology and Nephrology, Division of Nephrology, Middlesex Hospital, London W1N 8AA, UK

Marina Noris PharmD
Mario Negri Institute for Pharmacological Research, Via Gavazzeni 11, 24125 Bergamo, Italy

Donal J. O'Donoghue MBChB, FRCP
Department of Renal Medicine, Salford Royal Hospitals NHS Trust, Salford M6 8HD, UK

Kofi Oppong BM, MRCP
Department of Medicine, University of Newcastle upon Tyne, Queen Victoria Road, Newcastle upon Tyne NE1 4LP, UK

Charles Y.C. Pak MD
University of Texas Southwestern Medical Center, Department of Internal Medicine, Dallas, TX 75235-8885, USA

James M. Pattison BM, BCh, MRCP
Renal Unit, Guy's Hospital, London SE1 9RT, UK

Michael Pazianas MD
University of Pennsylvania, Chestnut Street, Philadelphia, PA 19104, USA

D.S. Peat MRCPath
University of Cambridge Department of Medicine and Pathology, Addenbrooke's Hospital, Hills Road, Cambridge CB2 2QQ, UK

Norberto Perico MD
Mario Negri Institute for Pharmacological Research, Via Gavazzeni 11, 24125 Bergamo, Italy

Jeffrey Petersen MD, FRCP
Division of Nephrology, Stanford University School of Medicine, Stanford, CA 94305, USA

Stephen H. Powis PhD, MRCP
Centre for Nephrology, Royal Free Hospital School of Medicine, Rowland Hill Street, Hampstead, London NW3 2PF, UK

C.D. Pusey MSc, FRCP
Renal Unit, Department of Medicine, Royal Postgraduate Medical School, Hammersmith Hospital, Du Cane Road, London W12 0NN, UK

Ralph Rabkin MD
Division of Nephrology, Stanford University School of Medicine, Veterans Affairs Palo Alto Health Care System, Palo Alto, CA 94304, USA

Anthony E.G. Raine MD, FRCP (deceased)
Department of Nephrology, St Bartholomew's Hospital, West Smithfield, London EC1, UK

Peter J. Ratcliffe MD, FRCP
Section of Nephrology, Institute of Molecular Medicine, John Radcliffe Hospital, Headington, Oxford OX3 9DU, UK

D. Reaich MD
Department of Medicine/Nephrology, South Cleveland Hospital, Marton Road, Middlesbrough, Cleveland TS4 3BW, UK

Christopher Record DPhil, FRCP
Royal Victoria Infirmary, Newcastle upon Tyne NE1 4LP, UK

Giuseppe Remuzzi MD
Mario Negri Institute for Pharmacological Research, Via Gavazzeni 11, 24125 Bergamo, Italy

Mark Roberts MB, ChB, MRCOG
Department of Obstetrics and Gynaecology, Royal Victoria Infirmary, Newcastle upon Tyne NE1 4LP, UK

R. Stuart C. Rodger MB, FRCP
The Renal Unit, Western Infirmary, Glasgow G11 6NT, UK

Lisa A. Ruml MD
Department of Internal Medicine, University of Texas, Southwestern Medical School, Dallas, TX 75235-8885, USA

Peter Rutherford BMedSci, MRCP, PhD
Department of Nephrology, Maelor Hospital, Clwyd LL13 7TD, UK

Steven H. Sacks PhD, FRCP
Department of Nephrology, United Medical and Dental Schools of Guy's and St Thomas's, St Thomas Street, London SE1 9RT, UK

John D. Scandling MD
Division of Nephrology, Stanford University School of Medicine, Stanford, CA 94305, USA

George Segall MD
Department of Radiology, Stanford University School of Medicine, Veterans Affairs Palo Alto Health Care System, Palo Alto, CA 94305-5105, USA

K.C. Siamopoulos MSc, MD
Department of Internal Medicine, Medical School, University of Ioannina, GR 451 10 Ioannina, Greece

F. Graham Sommer MD
Department of Radiology, H-1307, Stanford University School of Medicine, Stanford, CA 94305-5105, USA

Mitra Sorooshian MD
Division of Nephrology, Stanford University School of Medicine, Veterans Affairs Palo Alto Health Care System, Palo Alto, CA 94304, USA

G.P. Spickett MA, BM, BCh, DPhil, MRCPath, FRCP
Regional Department of Immunology, Royal Victoria Infirmary, Newcastle upon Tyne NE1 4LP, UK

Peter Stenvinkel MD
Department of Clinical Sciences, Division of Renal Medicine, Karolinska Institute, Huddinge University Hospital, S-14186 Stockholm, Sweden

N.P. Stephens BSc
Manchester Royal Infirmary, Oxford Road, Manchester M13 9WL, UK

J.H. Stewart MB, ChB, FRACP, FRCP (Lond)
Department of Medicine, University of Otago, Dunedin Hospital, Dunedin, New Zealand

M. Sussman PhD, FIBiol, FRCPath
Department of Microbiology, Medical School, Newcastle upon Tyne NE2 4HH, UK

David Talbot MBBS, MD, FRCS
Freeman Hospital, High Heaton, Newcastle upon Tyne NE7 7DN, UK

J.E. Tattersall MD, MRCP
Renal Unit, Lister Hospital, Coreyes Hill Lane, Stevenage, Herts SG1 4AB, UK

Roberto Trevisan MD, PhD
Divisione Malattie del Ricambio, Instituto di Medicina Clinica, Universita di Padova, Padova, Italy

Linda Uttley RGN
Department of Renal Medicine, Manchester Royal Infirmary, Oxford Road, Manchester M13, 9WL, UK

Joseph G. Verbalis MD
Division of Endocrinology and Metabolism, Georgetown University Medical Center, 4000 Reservoir Road NW, Washington, DC 20007, USA

GianCarlo Viberti MD, FRCP
Unit for Metabolic Medicine, United Medical and Dental Schools of Guy's and St Thomas's, St Thomas Street, London SE1 9RT, UK

R. Kasi Visweswaran MD, DM, MNAMS
Department of Nephrology, Medical College Kottayam-686008, Kerala, India

James D. Walker MD, MRCP
Department of Diabetes, Royal Infirmary of Edinburgh, Lauriston Place, Edinburgh, UK

John Walls MB, ChB, FRCP
Department of Nephrology, Leicester General Hospital, Leicester LE4 5PW, UK

Richard P. Wedeen MD
The New Jersey Medical School, University of Medicine and Dentistry of New Jersey, Veterans Affairs Medical Center, 385 Tremont Avenue, East Orange, NJ 07018-1095, USA

I. David Weiner MD
Division of Nephrology, Hypertension and Transplantation, University of Florida College of Medicine, Gainesville, FL 32610-0224, USA

Martin Wilkie MD, MRCP
Sheffield Kidney Institute, Northern General Hospital Trust, Herries Road, Sheffield S5 7AU UK

Robert Wilkinson BSc, MD, FRCP
Department of Medicine (Nephrology), Freeman Hospital, Newcastle upon Tyne NE7 7DN, UK

J.D. Williams MD, FRCP
Institute of Nephrology, University of Wales College of Medicine, Cardiff Royal Infirmary, Newport Road, Cardiff CF2 1SZ, UK

Charles S. Wingo MD
Division of Nephrology, Hypertension and Transplantation, University of Florida College of Medicine, Gainesville, FL 32610-0224, USA

Stephen H. Wright PhD
Department of Physiology, College of Medicine, University of Arizona, Tucson, AZ 85724, USA

Acknowledgements

We are grateful to Lord Walton of Detchant and to Dr John Moll who suggested the need for this book and put us in touch with the publishers. We would like to thank the chapter authors for their dedication in producing excellent chapters. We are grateful to the staff of the publishers in particular, Dr Peter Altman, Ms Tausi Seremba and Ms Lara Wilson for steering the book to completion. We are especially grateful to our secretaries Sheila Davidson and Robyn Kaiser for their hard work in preparing our own chapters but also in dealing with the work arising from editing the other chapters.

Finally we are grateful to our wives who have put up with the increased loneliness over the past several years during which we have worked on the book.

Rex L. Jamison
Robert Wilkinson

I

Normal Structure and Function

Section 1
Structure

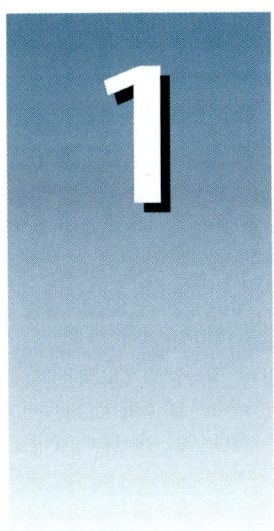

The structure of the kidney

Adrian R. Morley

A considerable body of information on renal structure and function is based on the study of rodent kidneys. The prominent single papilla that enables the high urinary concentrating ability in these animals means that there are significant structural and microanatomical differences between the rodent and the multipapillary human kidney. This chapter is based as far as possible on the normal human kidney.

General anatomy and macroscopic structure

Anatomical relationships

The kidneys are paired organs of 120–170 g in the male, approximately 5% smaller in the female. The size is related to body mass and surface area and the left kidney is somewhat larger than the right. In children the size is closely related to age and percentile growth charts are available [1]. With age the kidneys decrease in size. Physiological effects such as high urinary flow [2] may increase the size. The kidneys are situated on either side of the vertebral column extending from the twelfth thoracic to the third lumbar vertebrae with the right lower than the left. With respiration the kidneys move some 1–2 cm. Lying in the retroperitoneal space (Figure 1.1) the kidneys are surrounded by fat contained in the anterior and posterior perirenal fascia. Bridging septa between these fasciae may limit the spread of infection and sepsis [3]. Spread of infection from the retroperitoneal space to the renal pelvis is rare. Dissection has demonstrated that the ante-

rior and posterior renal fasciae fuse together inferiorly to form a multilamellar membrane which serves as an effective barrier [4]. The capsule which covers the kidney is thin, uniform, and easily removed in the absence of disease.

General attributes

The lateral aspects of the kidney are convex, whereas the medial surface is broken by an oval opening, the renal sinus. The convex surface often shows regular depressions representing the underlying lobular structure (fetal lobulation) which frequently persists into adult life (Figure 1.2). The lobules and pyramids fuse together at the poles to form compound papillae whereas those in the midzone fuse less completely leaving single papillae with their lobules separated by cortical tissue, known as the columns of Bertin. Within the renal sinus are the pelvis, calyces, arteries, veins and nerves with fibrous sheaths [5] and variable amounts of fat. The sinus points inward and anteriorly in line with the vascular connections to aorta and vena cava.

The pelvicalyceal system

The pelvis is a conical structure composed of two layers of smooth muscle lined by urothelium, extending from the inner aspect of the renal sinus and narrowing to become the ureter at the pelviureteric junction (Figure 1.3). Two or three major calyces arise from the pelvis dividing to form nine minor calyces. It has been sug-

Nephrology, Edited by Rex L. Jamison and Robert Wilkinson.
Published in 1997 by Chapman & Hall, London. ISBN 0 412 60930 4

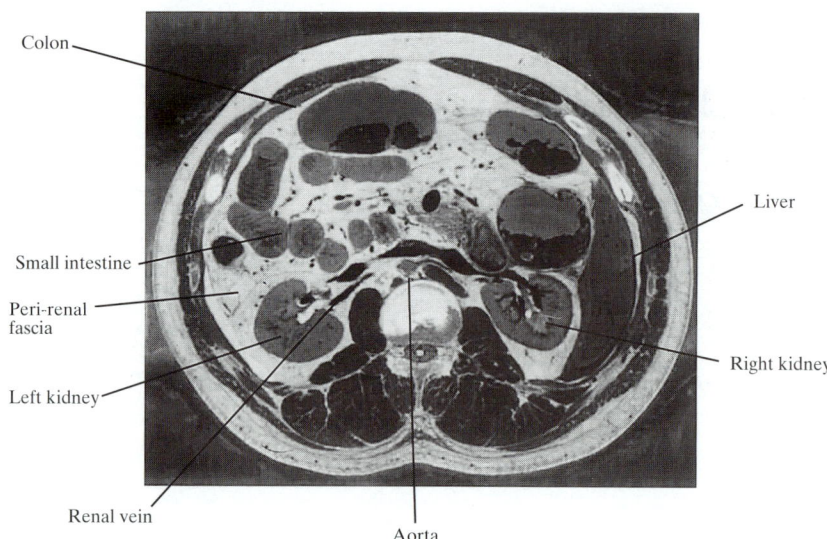

Colon

Small intestine

Peri-renal
fascia

Left kidney

Renal vein

Aorta

Liver

Right kidney

Figure 1.1 Cross-section of the human body showing the kidneys and main structures. The left and right kidneys are surrounded by the renal fascia. The Ileo-psoas muscles are posteromedial. In this section the right renal artery and both renal veins are seen as well as the aorta. Laterally on the right is the liver and the spleen on the left (not seen) The small and large intestine are seen anteriorly. (Acknowledgements: The visible man project. Dr Michael J. Ackerman, National Library of Medicine.)

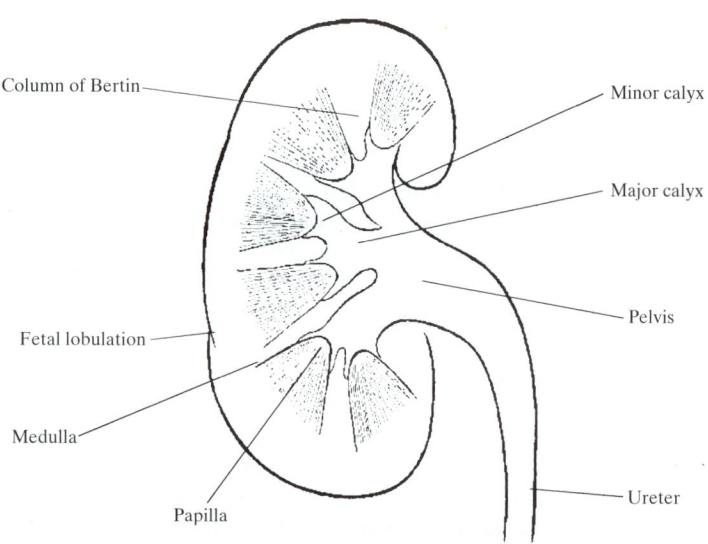

Column of Bertin

Fetal lobulation

Medulla

Papilla

Minor calyx

Major calyx

Pelvis

Ureter

Figure 1.2 Diagram to show the main features of the kidney. The fetal lobules relate to segmental structure and vary in their expression. The renal papillae project into the minor calyces. The calyces, major and minor, drain into the pelvis. The columns of Bertin are composed of cortical tissue. The medullary tubules run radially, perpendicular to the cortical surface.

gested that this complex system allows considerable surface area for back diffusion [6]. One or more renal papillae open into the cup-like calyces some of which receive compound or multiple papillae. The latter are more common at the renal poles. It has been demonstrated that reflux may occur in the wide open compound papillae and that the slit-like openings of simple papillae have a valvular function (Figure 1.4) [7].

Interconnections with the urinary tract

The ureter is lined by urothelium similar to that of the pelvis. There is a single muscle coat which extends through the pelvis as far as the minor calyces. A second layer of smooth muscle of similar appearance but lacking

non-specific cholinesterase covers the minor calyces and extends as an inner layer to the level of the pelvicalyceal junction. It has been suggested that this layer might act as a pacemaker for the initiation of contractions beginning at the minor calyces [8]. The structure of the pelvi-ureteric junction is of interest because of the frequency of pelviureteric obstruction associated with hydronephrosis and the suggestion [9] that abnormality of the muscle lining may be responsible.

Arteries and veins

The renal arteries

The right renal artery arises slightly below the left renal artery, and both proceed laterally and downward towards

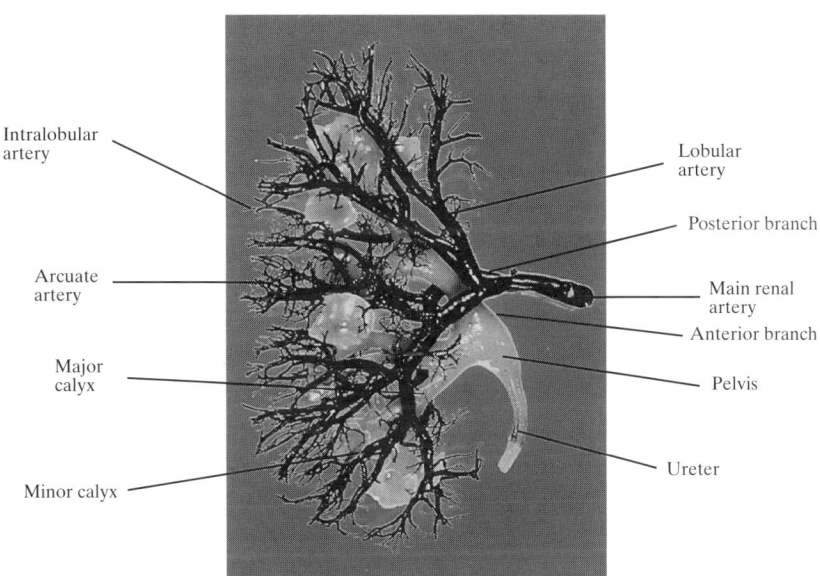

Intralobular artery

Arcuate artery

Major calyx

Minor calyx

Lobular artery

Posterior branch

Main renal artery

Anterior branch

Pelvis

Ureter

Figure 1.3 The arterial and urinary structures of kidney. A plastic cast of the arterial tree, ureter pelvis and calyces. The glomeruli and peripheral intralobular arterial branches have been removed for clarity. Note the relationship of the anterior and posterior branches of the main renal artery to the major upper pole calyx. The pelvis opens into the major calyces which subdivide into the minor calyces related to the renal papillae. (Courtesy of The Department of Anatomy, The Medical School, Newcastle upon Tyne.)

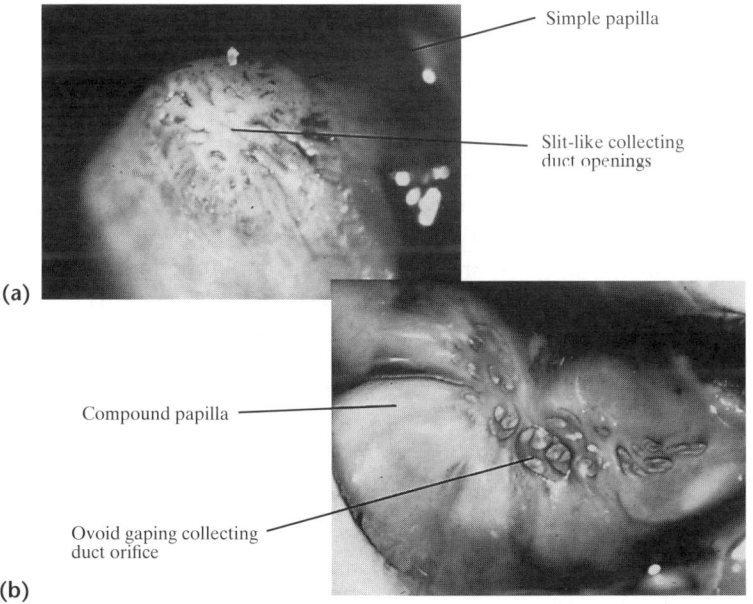

Simple papilla

Slit-like collecting duct openings

(a)

Compound papilla

Ovoid gaping collecting duct orifice

(b)

Figure 1.4 The renal papillae showing the narrow openings at the apex of the single renal papilla (a) compared with the gaping openings of the collecting ducts in the concave surface of the compound papilla (b). (Courtesy of Professor A. Risdon, Department of Pathology, Great Ormond Street Hospital, London.)

the kidneys. The main arteries commonly divide into anterior and posterior branches (Figure 1.3). The anterior branch sends segmental arteries to the poles and to the upper and lower zones of the large middle section anteriorly. The posterior branch sends segmental branches to the middle section posteriorly. There is considerable variation and, in particular, accessory polar arteries may arise from the aorta or renal artery to supply much of the polar zones. There are no significant connections across segmental boundaries. In the renal sinus interlobar branches enter the renal parenchyma between the pyramids.

There is considerable variation in the disposition of

the renal arteries, which is a matter of concern in transplant surgery. A recent study of 266 kidneys from 133 patients showed a single hilar artery in 53%, a hilar artery and superior pole extrahilar artery in 14%, two hilar arteries in 8%, and three hilar arteries in 2%. A superior pole artery was present in 7% and an inferior pole artery in 5%; the remainder had other variations [10].

Interlobar veins

These follow the arteries but interconnect through anastomotic channels around the calyces. These form a number of channels anterior to the pelvis which join in the renal sinus to form the main renal vein lying anterior to the artery [11]. Angiographic studies have revealed considerable variation in the disposition of the renal veins with a retroaortic left renal vein in 7%, a circumaortic left renal vein in 5% and multiple right renal veins in 8%. The inferior vena cava was reduplicated in 0.7% [12]. Additional renal veins are not infrequent, a second renal vein being present in 26% on the right side and 2.6% on the left side. Three renal veins were present in 5% on the right [13].

Nerves and lymphatics

Nerve supply

The autonomic nerves enter the kidney around the arteries and spread around the blood vessels up to the juxtaglomerular apparatus. The efferent sympathetic nerves extend to all parts of the vascular tree, but much less frequently to the nephron. The afferent sympathetic nerves are largely confined to the renal pelvis, the major blood vessels and the connective tissue of the periarterial sheath in the corticomedullary region [14].

Lymphatics

Capsular and parenchymal lymphatics form four or five trunks in the renal sinus which flow into the lateral aortic lymph nodes.

Cortex and medulla

The cortex

About 70% of the renal volume is cortex. This covers the base of the medullary pyramids and is 1–1.5 cm thick (Figure 1.2). The cortex reaches down between separate papillae to the renal sinus forming the columns of Bertin. Within the cortex two main zones can be distinguished: (1) the cortical labyrinth, composed of the glomeruli, convoluted tubules and associated vessels; and (2) the medullary rays composed of parallel groups of the straight segments of proximal tubule (pars recta) and thick ascending (distal) tubules as well as collecting ducts. The rays are perpendicular to the capsular surface with tubules from the more superficial glomeruli in the centre.

The medulla

The outer medulla can be divided into an outer (juxtacortical) stripe and an inner stripe. The outer stripe contains the proximal straight tubule and the medullary thick descending limb. The inner stripe contains the thin segments of the descending limb tubule and the thick ascending limb (loop of Henle). The vascular bundles consist of descending and ascending vasa recta sur-

rounded by the pars recta, the descending limb and the thick ascending limb. Further away are the collecting tubules. More complex arrangements are seen in species capable of high urinary concentration, particularly rodents.

The inner medulla contains the thin limbs of long loops (of Henle), both ascending and descending. The collecting ducts run through the above zones. The vascular bundles of vasa recta diminish in number as the bundle approaches the renal papilla. The interstitial space is prominent and contains lipid-filled interstitial cells.

Microanatomical structure

The basic unit: the nephron

The nephron is the basic structural unit of which there are about one million in each human kidney (Figure 1.5). Each nephron consists of a renal corpuscle, comprising Bowman's capsule, the glomerular capillary tuft and a renal tubule. Each Bowman's capsule communicates with the tubule and then the renal calyx via the collecting tubule and duct. The separation of the renal tubule and the collecting duct is significant since the former is derived from the metanephric cap and the latter from the ureteric bud. There is considerable debate about the exact site of this junction. Recent studies have suggested that it may be as proximal as the end of the cortical thick ascending limb at the macula densa [15]. The tubular segments are structurally, cytologically and functionally distinct. The renal tubule extends into or towards the medulla and loops (the loop of Henle) back to its own renal corpuscle before draining into a collecting tubule. The loops may be long or short. The short loop of Henle turns at the junction of outer and inner medulla and delineates a thin dividing line. The long loops extend into the inner medulla. A few loops may remain within the cortex. There is considerable species variation in the proportion of long and short loops. In humans the ratio is approximately 1:6 [16].

Bowman's capsule

The renal corpuscle is the term properly used to describe Bowman's capsule and the capillary tuft (the glomerulus). The elegance of this usage has escaped many workers so that the term 'glomerulus' is now used in most clinical situations and publications. Bowman's capsule consists of parietal epithelial cells and a basement membrane (Figure 1.6) which is reflected onto the glomerulus becoming continuous with the glomerular basement membrane in the point of entry of the afferent and efferent arterioles (the vascular pole) (see Figure 1.7). Bowman's capsule invests the glomerulus and is continuous with the proximal tubule at the tubular orifice (pole) which is found opposite the vascular pole but with considerable varia-

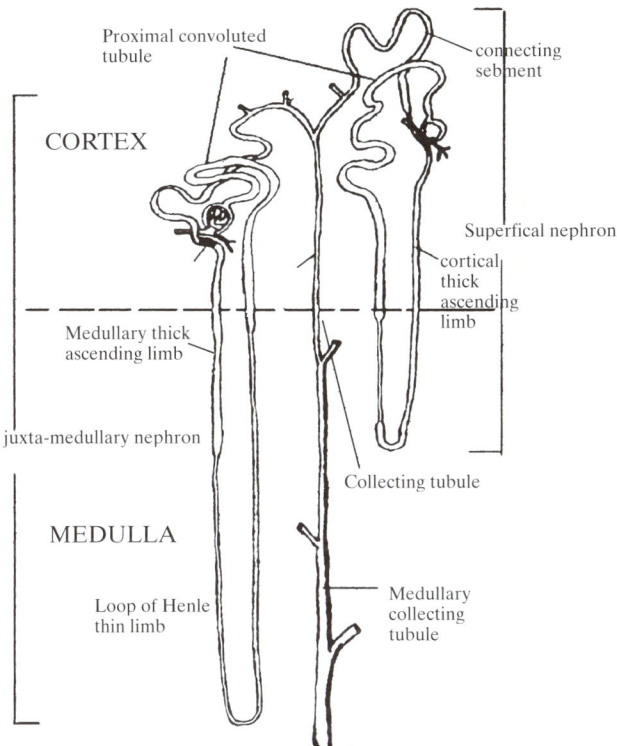

Figure 1.5 The general structure of the nephron. The proximal tubule arises from Bowman's capsule and descends via the thick descending limb into the outer stripe. Nephrons with long loops then develop into thin loops, while short nephrons continue to the boundary of the inner medulla before turning back and forming an ascending thin loop. The medullary thick ascending limb appears at the junction of inner and outer medulla. Note the close relationship of the distal convoluted tubule to the glomerulus. Beyond the glomerulus the connecting duct arises draining into the collecting ducts. (Modified from K.M. Madsen and B.M. Brenner, Fig. 21–1, p. 662, Chap. 21, *Renal Pathology*, Vol. 1, ed. C. Craig Tisher and Barry M. Brenner, pub. Lippincott.)

tion. It is lined with a layer of flattened epithelium, the parietal podocytes, which shows considerable variation in appearance (Figure 1.8). Filtrate from the glomerular tuft passes from Bowman's capsule into the renal tubule. The intriguing finding of podocyte foot-processes on the capsular surface suggests that Bowman's capsule may be more than a passive barrier [17]. The integrity of Bowman's capsule preventing the ingress of fibroblasts is an important factor in determining whether fibrous crescents develop in crescentic glomerulonephritis [18].

The glomerulus

The glomerular capillary tuft arises from the afferent arteriole which separates into 6–8 divisions each of which subdivides to form a lobule within which capillaries anas-

tomose (Figure 1.6). The capillary loops are lined with an endothelium that has a highly specialized basement membrane and visceral epithelial podocytes. The capillaries then recombine to form the efferent arteriole. The capillary loops within each lobule are supported by the mesangium which is composed of a basement membrane-like matrix in which are embedded mesangial cells. At the vascular pole mesangial cells are frequent and form part of the juxtaglomerular apparatus.

The juxtaglomerular apparatus (JGA)

The JGA is largely concerned with blood pressure and circulating fluid volume control (Figure 1.9). The components are (1) the terminal portion of the afferent arteriole and efferent arteriole, (2) the macula densa, a specialized segment of the distal tubule, (3) the extraglomerular mesangial (lacis) cells at the vascular pole, and (4) the sympathetic nerve supply. The recently described glomerular peripolar (Ryan) cells (Figure 1.10) are potential components whose function is as yet unknown [19]. Recent studies in hypertension (for example) have shown no relation between renin cells and peripolar cells [20]. In addition to normal smooth muscle cells there are groups of four or five myo-epithelioid granular cells in the afferent arteriole which have renin-containing granules and protogranules (Figure 1.9). The efferent arteriole has a contiguous relationship to the distal convoluted tubule, the two structures running parallel for a short distance.

The macula densa consists of a small patch of cells, of columnar cuboidal type with apical nuclei. The cells differ considerably from those of the adjacent distal convoluted tubule. In particular, the cells lack Tamm–Horsefall protein and have only weak sodium/potassium ATPase activity. The basement membrane on which the cells of the macula densa sit is perforated. Furthermore, the lateral membranes do not interdigitate (as in the remaining distal tubule), but are connected by desmosomes. Thus there is a ready extracellular channel between the lacis cells and the distal tubule. There is evidence that particulate material and IgA follow this route normally and in disease states [21].

The mesangial cells at the vascular pole (lacis cells) form a pyramid based on the macula densa and bounded laterally by the arterioles. They are embedded in basement membrane-like matrix, in contact with each other and cells of the afferent arteriole. Various regulatory functions have been suggested [22]. In particular there is evidence of tubuloglomerular feedback controlling glomerular vascular tone and renin production. The composition of tubular fluid may initiate signals from the macula densa via the extraglomerular mesangium. Recent studies suggest that nitric oxide produced in the macula densa may act as a mediator [23].

Nerves reach the JGA via the arterioles sending axonal branches to the myoepithelioid and smooth muscle cells.

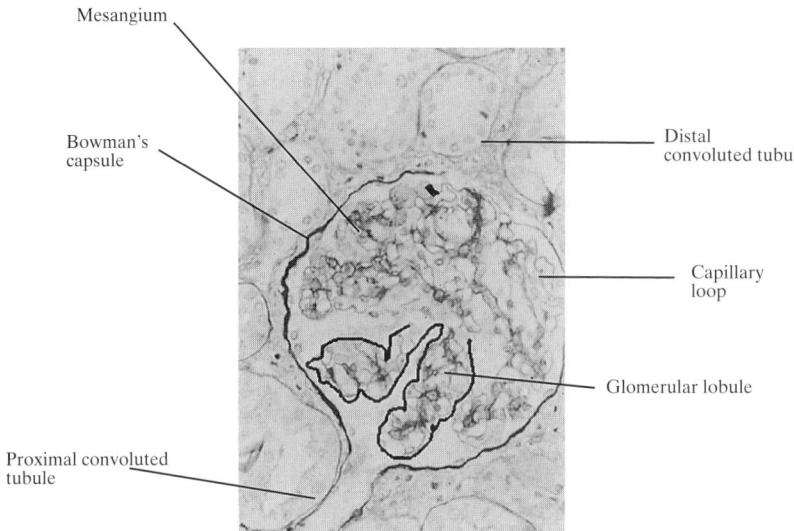

Mesangium

Bowman's capsule

Distal convoluted tubule

Capillary loop

Glomerular lobule

Proximal convoluted tubule

Figure 1.6 The glomerulus consists of capillary loops branching from the afferent arteriole and dividing into 6–8 lobules before rejoining and forming the efferent arteriole. Bowman's capsule is continuous with the proximal tubular basement membrane and reflects onto the glomerular tuft. The basement membranes of the glomerular capillary loops are continuous with the supporting mesangial matrix. (Periodicacid–Schiff; ×100.)

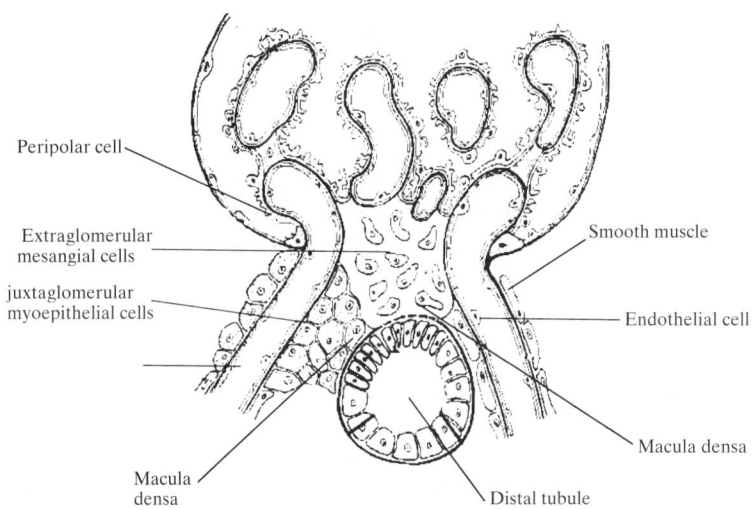

Peripolar cell

Extraglomerular mesangial cells

juxtaglomerular myoepithelial cells

Smooth muscle

Endothelial cell

Macula densa

Macula densa

Distal tubule

Figure 1.7 The juxtaglomerular apparatus. In this diagrammatic representation the close relationship between the macula densa of the distal tubule and the extra- glomerular mesangial cells (lacis) cells is apparent. The myoepithelial cells of the afferent arteriole are also closely situated to the macula densa. (Modified from W. Kriz and B. Kaissling Fig. 27, p. 731, Chap. 23. *The Kidney, Physiology and Pathophysiology*, ed. D.W. Seldin and G. Giesbach, 1992, Raven Press.)

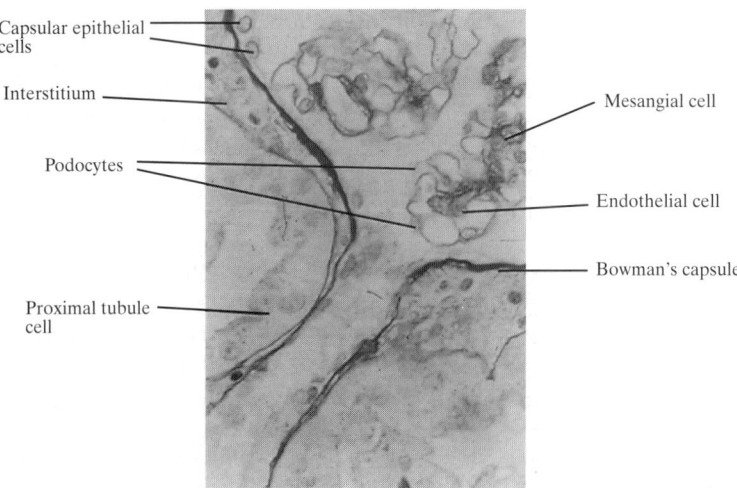

Capsular epithelial cells

Interstitium

Podocytes

Proximal tubule cell

Mesangial cell

Endothelial cell

Bowman's capsule

Figure 1.8 Bowman's capsule and orifice of the proximal convoluted tubule. Flattened capsular epithelial cells rest on the basement membrane of Bowman's capsule. Podocytes (visceral epithelial cells) rest on the glomerular basement membrane and fill the potential space. Mesangial cells are inconspicuous, lodged within the mesangial matrix. Endothelial cell nuclei are often found adjacent to the mesangial side of the capillary loop. (Periodic acid–Schiff; ×250.)

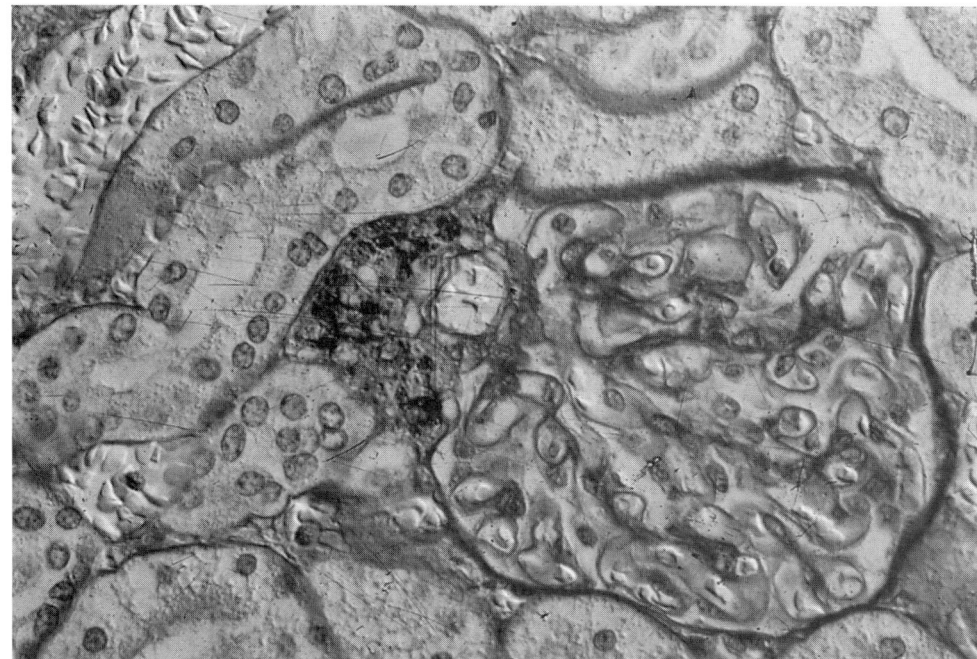

Figure 1.9 The Juxta-glomerular apparatus demonstrating renin (immunoperoxidase) in the wall of the afferent arteriole. Periodic acid–Schiff; ×200. (Courtesy of Dr G.B.M. Lindop, Western Infirmary, Glasgow.)

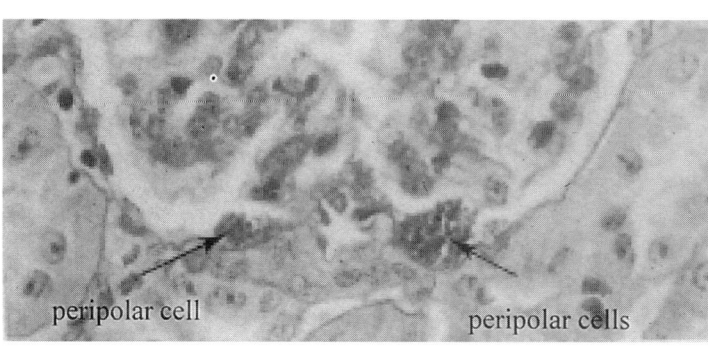

peripolar cell   peripolar cells

Figure 1.10 Peripolar cells adjacent to the reflection of Bowman's capsule onto the glomerular capillary tuft. Granular bodies fill much of the cytoplasm. (Immuno-histochemical identification of plasma proteins in different mammalian species, J.F. Trahair and O.B. Ryan, *J. Anat.*, 1988, **160**, pp. 109–115.)

Nerve fibers have not been observed among the lacis cells.

The tubules

The tubules comprise the following segments in order from the glomerulus (Figures 1.11 and 1.12):

1 the proximal tubule (convoluted section), the proximal tubule (straight part), also known as the pars recta;
2 the descending thin limb of Henle's loop (in long-loop nephrons only);
3 the medullary thick ascending limb of Henle's loop;
4 the cortical thick ascending limb of Henle's loop;
5 the distal convoluted tubule (Figure 1.5).

The proximal tubule

The convoluted part begins at the opening from Bowman's capsule, and cells of similar type may be seen within the Bowman's capsule. The convolutions are arranged randomly around their own glomerulus. The straight part of the proximal tubule (pars recta) along with other tubules comprises the medullary ray and descends into the outer stripe of the outer medulla.

The loop of Henle

The loops of Henle begin at the boundary of the inner and outer stripes of the outer medulla. The short loops remain in the outer medulla, turning at the junction with the inner medulla. The long loops descend into the inner medulla before turning to form the ascending thin loops. At the junction of the inner medulla and inner stripe of the outer medulla the medullary thick ascending limb is formed from the thin descending limb of the short loop or the thin ascending limb of the long loop.

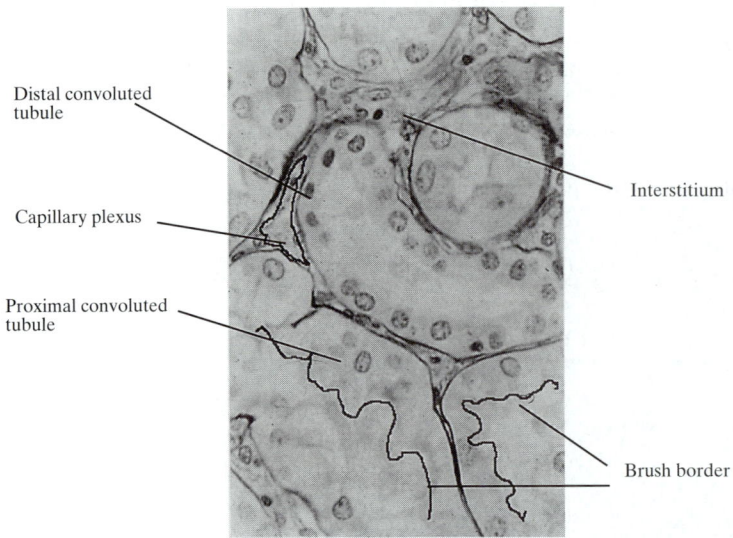

Distal convoluted
tubule

Capillary plexus

Proximal convoluted
tubule

Interstitium

Brush border

Figure 1.11 The cortical tubules. Tall columnar tubules of the proximal convoluted tubules with basal nuclei and a luminal brush border. The distal tubular epithelium is cuboidal, has central nuclei and lacks a brush border. Capillaries largely fill the interstitium. (Periodic acid–silver methenamine; ×250.)

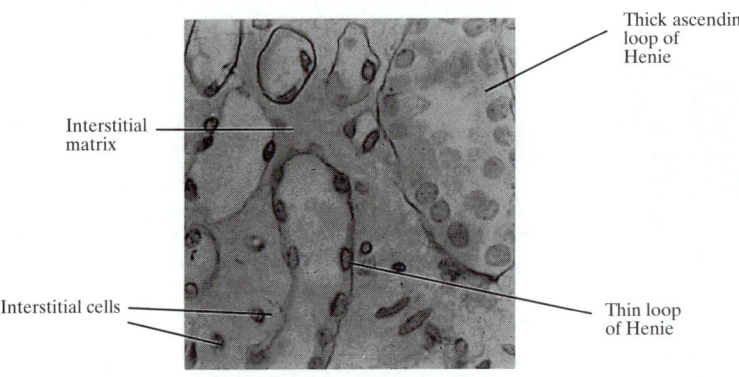

Thick ascending
loop of
Henle

Interstitial
matrix

Interstitial cells

Thin loop
of Henle

Figure 1.12 The medullary tubules. Thick and thin loops of Henle are widely separated by the interstitium in which interstitial cells are present, often orientated perpendicular to the tubules. (Periodic acid; ×250.)

The thick ascending limb

The thick ascending limb contrasts with the ascending thin limb of the loop of Henle from which it arises. It extends to the corticomedullary junction where it becomes the cortical thick ascending limb. The cortical thick ascending limb extends to the region of the vascular pole where it becomes the distal convoluted tubule and runs parallel to the efferent arteriole. The specialized structure of the macula densa and the JGA of the distal convoluted tubule is described above. The distal convoluted tubule drains into the connecting tubule.

The collecting ducts and connecting tubule

The collecting duct system begins with the connecting tubule. This segment, which is poorly defined in the

human kidney, resembles the distal convoluted tubule but differs in its cellular lining particularly in the rabbit. It is this region that represents the embryonic junction between the metanephric cap and the ureteric bud. At this junction staining for Tamm–Horsfall protein found throughout the distal tubule ends [15].

There is considerable interspecies variation in the drainage of the connecting duct. In general, deep nephrons drain individually into a collecting duct. In humans superficial nephrons also drain singly. In the rat and rabbit superficial nephrons drains into an arcade before entering a collecting duct [24].

The connecting tubule drains into the cortical collecting duct, which passes from the cortex into the outer medulla. On reaching the inner medulla paired fusions of collecting ducts occur approximately eight times, forming the inner medullary collecting ducts which drain into the renal papillae. It has been calculated that an average of 44 duct openings appear on the eight papillae of each kidney.

The renal papillae

The collecting ducts open into the calyces at the renal papillae which form the apices of the renal pyramids. In single papillae the apex is sharply convex and the ductal openings form narrow slits. At the renal poles compound papillae are flattered or concave with widely open orifices (Figure 1.4). These differences are thought to make intrarenal reflux more likely [25].

Arteries and arterioles, veins and venules

The lobar arteries extend along the edges of the calyces to penetrate the cortical tissue of the columns of Bertin. As the arcuate arteries these advance along the margin between the cortex and outer medulla sending interlobular arteries (Figure 1.14) toward the cortical surface. The interlobular arteries branch and sprout afferent arterioles at regular intervals. Adjacent arcuate arteries do not anastomose so that the intervening zone is a particular risk of ischemia. Smaller numbers of afferent arterioles arise from arcuate and interlobar arteries.

It is notable that the medulla has no direct arterial supply. The blood is supplied by the afferent arterioles of the juxtamedullary glomeruli. Descending vasa recta arise from the efferent arterioles of the juxtamedullary glomeruli and divide in the outer stripe. They course down through the medulla periodically forming capillary plexuses [26]. Ascending vasa recta arise from these plexuses and return to the cortex by one of two pathways. They either rejoin the vascular bundle to run along the descending vasa recta or they remain in the outer medulla and ascend in the interbundle region directly to the cortex.

The veins originate in stellate veins from the cortical surface which drain into the interlobular veins running with the respective arteries. The main source of blood is from the peritubular plexus which drains via thin-walled venules. The interlobular veins connect to the arcuate veins which, in contrast to the arteries, freely anastomose across lobular boundaries and have medullary branches.

Cellular and connective tissues

Parietal and visceral podocytes

The parietal (capsular) epithelial cells cover the inside of Bowan's capsule (Figures 1.14 and 1.15). Typically these are flattened cells with a few microvilli and a central cilium. The function of the cilium is uncertain but cilia are found in proximal tubular cells. The adhesion molecule V-CAM has been demonstrated on some parietal podocytes [27]. Recent studies have shown that cells of podocyte morphology, i.e. with pedicels and foot-processes, are present at the vascular pole.

The basement membrane of Bowman's capsule is a multilayered structure which is continuous with the glomerular basement membrane at the vascular pole and with the basement membrane of the proximal tubule. The membrane is composed of collagen type 4 and appears to contain the Goodpasture antigen. Amyloid P substance is also present in the normal glomerular basement membrane possibly reflecting its association elsewhere in the body with collagen type 4 [28]. The collagen fibers show a structured arrangement [29]. The visceral podocytes, the glomerular basement membrane and the endothelial cell lining together function as a complex filter [30] (Figure 1.16).

The podocytes are responsible for formation of the glomerular basement membrane. The podocytes have a large cell body projecting from the surface of the capillary loops. The cytoplasmic organelles, such as Golgi

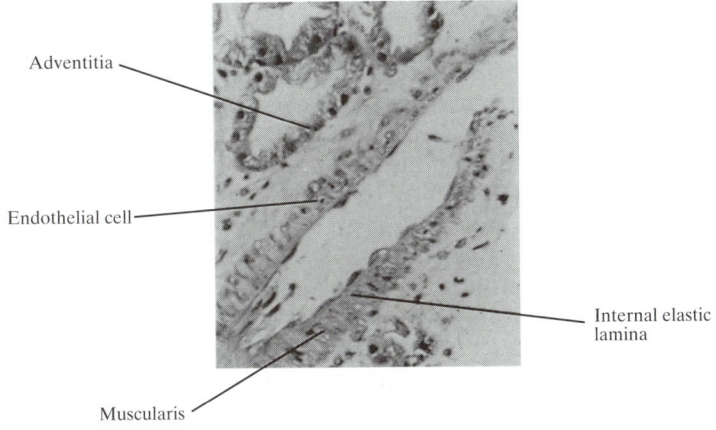

Adventitia

Endothelial cell

Internal elastic lamina

Muscularis

Figure 1.13 The structure of a small (interlobular) artery. In this sample from a young patient the endothelial cell appears to lie on the internal elastic lamina, and the muscularis contains no collagen. (Periodic acid; ×200.)

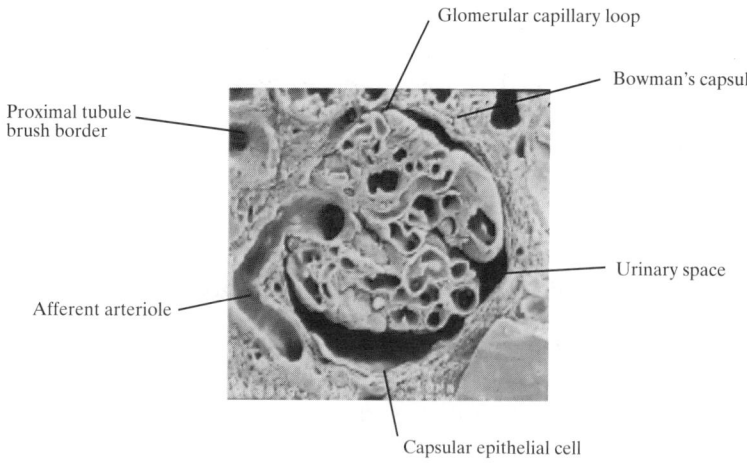

Proximal tubule brush border

Glomerular capillary loop

Bowman's capsule

Afferent arteriole

Urinary space

Capsular epithelial cell

Figure 1.14 The glomerulus, and Bowman's capsule. The flattened capsular epithelial cells of Bowman's capsule are seen. The urinary space is probably artefactual. (Scanning electron micrograph; ×100.) (Courtesy of Dr G.B.M. Lindop, Western Infirmary, Glasgow.)

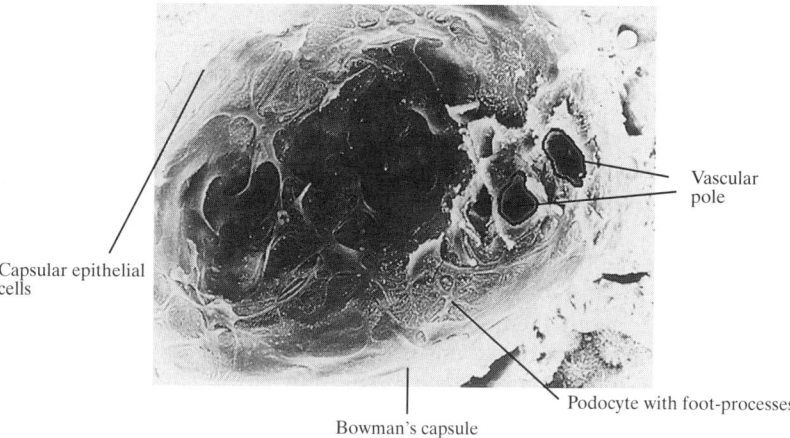

Capsular epithelial cells

Vascular pole

Bowman's capsule

Podocyte with foot-processes

Figure 1.15 Inside Bowman's capsule. After removal of the glomerular capillary tuft the openings of the arterioles can be seen. The inner surface of Bowman's capsule is lined by flattened epithelial cells as well as cells with the structure of visceral podocytes, i.e. with foot-processes. (Scanning electron micrograph; ×80.) (Courtesy of Dr G.B.M. Lindop, Western Infirmary, Glasgow.)

apparatus, smooth and rough endoplasmic reticulum and lysosomes, are inconspicuous, but become prominent with glomerular damage and proteinuria. Microtubules, actin and clathrin-coated pits are present, but in the adult cytokeratins are not demonstrable.

The cell body of the podocyte has a number of wide processes which embrace the capillary (Figures 1.16 and 1.17). The pedicels arise from the subdivisions of these processes. The podocytes are arranged with great regularity on the glomerular basement membrane perpendicular to the capillary axis. The pedicels from adjacent podocytes are arranged alternately (Figure 1.18). Immunoelectron microscope studies show β_1-integrins concentrated on the basal and lateral aspects of the pedicels suggesting an adhesive or 'anchoring' function [31]. In transverse section the pedicels appear to be embedded in the lamina rara externa (Figure 1.16). Actin fibers are present in the pedicels [32]. Contraction of these cells has been observed *in vitro*. Coated vesicles contain the brush border antigen gp330 [33].

The filtration slit diaphragm separates adjacent pedicels. It has a central line with regular alternating processes at right angles. It is 40 nm wide and is lined with negative polyanions. It is considered to be the site of ultrafiltration [34].

The glomerular basement membrane (GBM) is composed of three distinct layers: the central lamina densa and on either side less dense zones, the lamina interna rara and lamina externa rara. The GBM is 240–350 nm thick, thinner in females and children. Its main structural component is collagen type 4 which is tightly packed in the lamina densa, and has a looser arrangement in the laminae interna and externa. Importantly, collagen type 4 contains a non-collagenous domain in which is found the Goodpasture antigen [35]. Other adhesion molecules, such as laminin, fibronectin and indictin, are also present as is amyloid P substance [12] and the negatively charged heparan sulfate proteoglycan. The lamina externa has a net negative charge from numerous polyanionic sites.

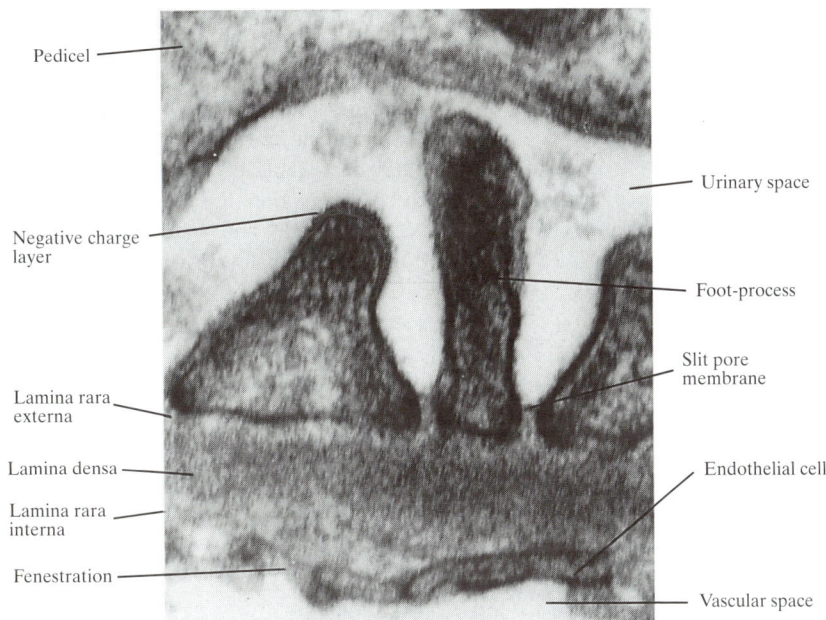

Pedicel

Negative charge layer

Lamina rara externa

Lamina densa

Lamina rara interna

Fenestration

Urinary space

Foot-process

Slit pore membrane

Endothelial cell

Vascular space

Figure 1.16 The glomerular basement membrane and foot-processes. The podocytes appear embedded in the urinary surface of the glomerular basement membrane with the slit pore membrane lying between them. An electron dense layer covers the podocytes and corresponds to a layer of negatively charged molecules. (Osmic acid–uranyl acetate; ×20 000.)

Glomerular endothelium

The glomerular capillaries are lined by endothelial cells. The cell nucleus is situated towards the mesangium and the attenuated cytoplasm (40 nm thick) covers the lamina rara interna. β_1-integrins are present but are distributed uniformly around the cell. The lack of polarization suggests functions other than adhesion [28]. Proteoglycans, produced by the endothelial cells, control the production of transforming growth factor-beta-1 (TGF-β_1), and may stimulate the formation of increased matrix in disease [36]. The cytoplasm is perforated by numerous fenestrations each up to 100 nm wide. In disease of the glomerulus, immunoglobulins and other proteins accumulate between the endothelium and the GMB. The body of the endothelial cell is in close contact with mesangial cell processes [37]. There is evidence that the glomerular endothelial cell has an important modulating role in intraglomerular coagulation and immune reactions [38]. It has also been demonstrated that endothelin-1 produced by glomerular endothelial cells may influence adjacent mesangial cells [39], which in glomerular disease may extend beneath the endothelium (mesangial interposition). The role of cytokines in angiogenesis has been reviewed [40].

The glomerular mesangium is analogous to the intestinal mesentery. It provides support for the glomerular capillary loops (Figure 1.17). The presence of mesangial cells was not finally settled until the development of the electron microscope [41]. The components of the mesangial matrix are produced by the mesangial cells. On the periphery of the mesangium are the capillary loops and on the interior a wrinkled glomerular basement membrane and associated podocytes. Mesangial tissue contains collagen types 4 and 6 as well as proteoglycans.

Mesangial cells are of two types. About 10% are of monocyte origin, containing Ia antigens. These cells may not be permanent residents but rather in transit. Their numbers increase greatly in some forms of glomerulonephritis. The remaining (intrinsic) mesangial cells have extensive cytoplasmic processes ramifying throughout the mesangial matrix. The presence of actin and myosin in these cells indicates a contractile function, which has been observed in cell culture *in vitro*. Mesangial processes attach to the glomerular basement membrane at the point where the capillary GBM transforms to the mesangial GBM (the mesangial angles). Contraction of the mesangium may influence glomerular capillary flow and filtration [42]. Mesangial cell contraction may depend on the balance between the release of endothelium-derived relaxing factor (EDRF), which is nitric oxide (NO) and endothelin-1, by endothelial cells [36]. Mesangial cells and lacis cells are connected by gap junctions and desmosomes. In a variety of glomerulonephritides involving proliferation, mesangial cells respond by secretion of mesangial matrix. The ability of these cells to produce fibronectin following thromboxane stimulation contributes to the development of sclerosis in renal disease [43]. Mediators of inflammation not only affect mesangial cells but are also produced by them. Receptors for serotonin (5-hydroxytryptamine), a mitogen, are present on mesangial cells which link them to

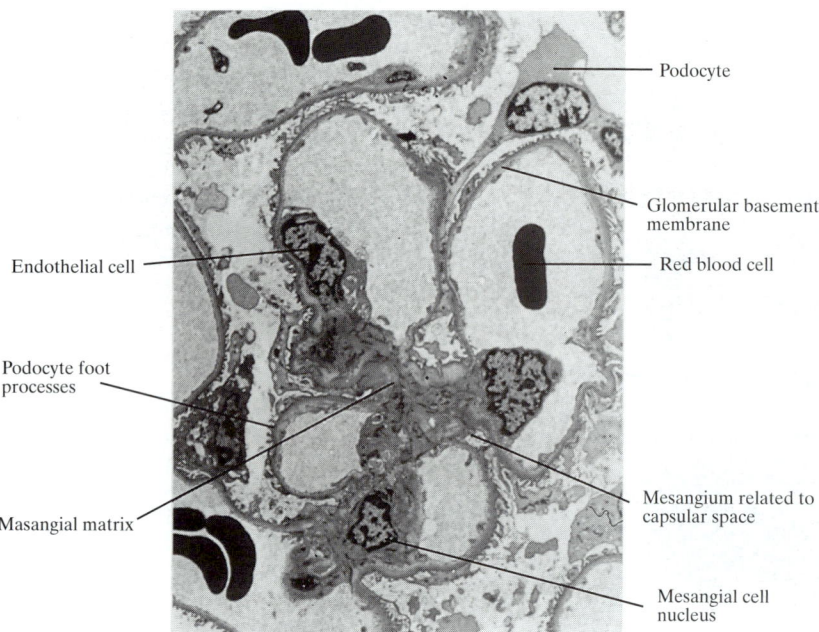

Podocyte

Glomerular basement membrane

Red blood cell

Endothelial cell

Podocyte foot processes

Masangial matrix

Mesangium related to capsular space

Mesangial cell nucleus

Figure 1.17 The glomerulus. Podocyte foot-processes are regularly disposed along the urinary surface of the glomerular basement membrane. Endothelial nuclei are seen on the mesangial aspect of the glomerular capillary. Mesangial cells are embedded within the mesangial matrix. Red blood cells and an oc-casional neutrophil are normally present. (Transmission electron micrograph; osmic acid–uranyl acetate; ×1000.)

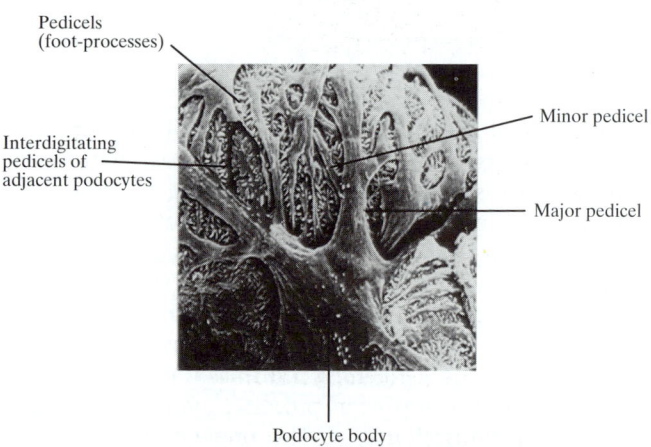

Pedicels (foot-processes)

Interdigitating pedicels of adjacent podocytes

Minor pedicel

Major pedicel

Podocyte body

Figure 1.18 The glomerular capillary and podocytes. Viewed from the urinary space the glomerular capillary loops are covered by the podocyte processes. Note the complex and regular interdigitation of foot-processes from adjacent podocytes. (Scanning electron micrograph; ×800.) (Courtesy of Dr G.B.M Lindop, Western Infirmary, Glasgow.)

an array of autocrine and paracrine signaling pathways [44]. Platelet-derived growth factor (PDGF) messenger RNA is expressed by mesangial cells [45]. They also ingest a wide range of proteins, immunoglobulins and small particulate matter, passing them from cell to cell to the vascular pole. Mesangial cells express a plasminogen activator receptor [46]. The demonstration of an ecto-enzyme alkaline phosphodiesterase-1 on the cell surface has led to the suggestion that DNA trapped in the mesangial space may be processed extracellularly [47].

The mesangial matrix, composed of collagen types 4 and 6, proteoglycan and fibronectin, is produced by mesangial cells [48].

Structural stabilization of the renal corpuscle

Recently Kriz has brought together evidence that the glomerular cells and glomerular basement membranes acting together produce stabilizing forces that balance the expansile forces of the pressure gradients within the glomerular tuft [49]. Mesangial cells develop an inwardly directed force opposing hydrostatic pressure, whereas the contractile elements of the foot-processes stabilize small areas of the glomerular basement membranes. Podocytes may also stabilize the folded pattern of the glomerular capillary tuft by connecting adjacent loops.

The Ryan cells (peripolar cells)

The peripolar cells are located at the junction of the glomerular capillary tuft and Bowman's capsule [17, 50] (Figure 1.9). The cells lie within Bowman's capsule and the cytoplasm contains prominent electron-dense granules. These have been shown to contain all the principal plasma proteins except IgM, as well as the amyloid-associated protein, transthyretin (pre-albumin) [51], and

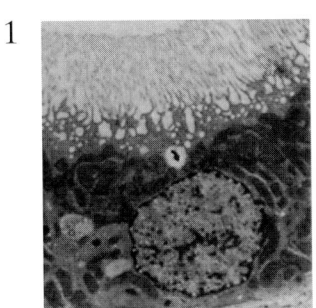
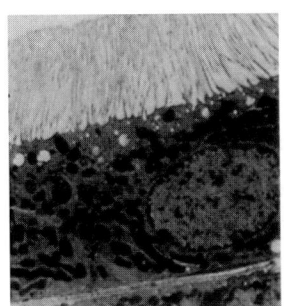
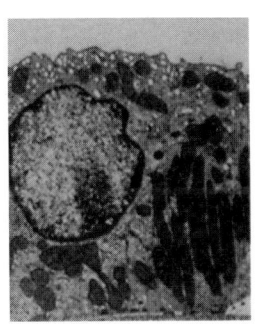
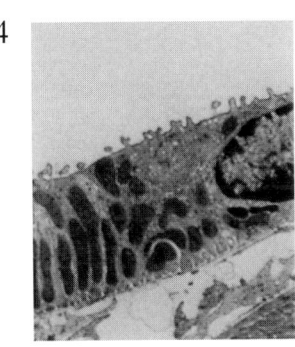
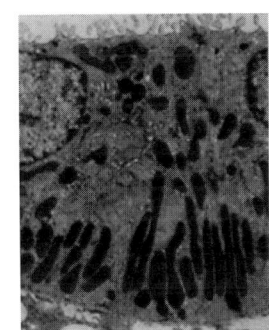

Figure 1.19 Electron microscopic structure of the rat nephron.
(a) Proximal tubule (pars convoluta) showing a high brush border, prominent pinocytosis and scattered lysosomes. There is marked infolding of the basolateral membranes.
(b) Proximal tubule (pars recta). Their is a tall brush border, prominent lysosomes and infrequent basolateral infoldings.
(c) The medullary thick ascending limb of the loop of Henle. Elongated mitochondria are seen close to the simple basolateral membrane.
(d) The cortical thick ascending limb of the loop of Henle. The epithelium is lower than in the medulla, and shows short microvilli.
(e) The distal convoluted tubules. The cells are tall with many mitochondria, prominent basolateral folds and short microvilli.
(Modified from K.M. Madsen and B.M. Brenner, Figs 21–2, 21–4, 21–12, 21–13, 21–15, Chap. 21, *Renal Pathology*, ed. C. Craig Tisher and Barry M. Brenner, pub. Lippincott.)

the cytoskeletal protein vimentin [19, 52–54]. Peripolar cells may participate in sodium and water control [55]. The suggestion has been made that the peripolar cell is part of the JGA [56], but the same workers have found no relation between the numbers of JGA cells and peripolar cells [57]. An association between the number of peripolar cells and the number of JGA cells has been noted in the hyperplasia of the JGA cells induced experimentally by hypocalcemia [58] (Figure 1.9).

Proximal tubular cells

The cells of the proximal tubule vary in structure corresponding to the convoluted segment, a transition zone, and the straight part. The appearances have received considerable study in rodents but less in the human kidney (Figure 1.19).

A typical proximal tubular cell is columnar with a basal nucleus. The luminal surface has closely packed microvilli (brush border) on the surface which amplifies the luminal absorptive area 40 times (Figures 1.19 and 1.20) [59]. The brush-border stains strongly with periodic acid–Schiff (PAS) and contains numerous enzymes related to its transport function. Some cells have a single cilium with a terminal bulb.

Between the microvilli there are numerous pinocytotic vesicles and clathrin-coated pits which contain gp330, a glycoprotein antigen associated with Heyman nephritis

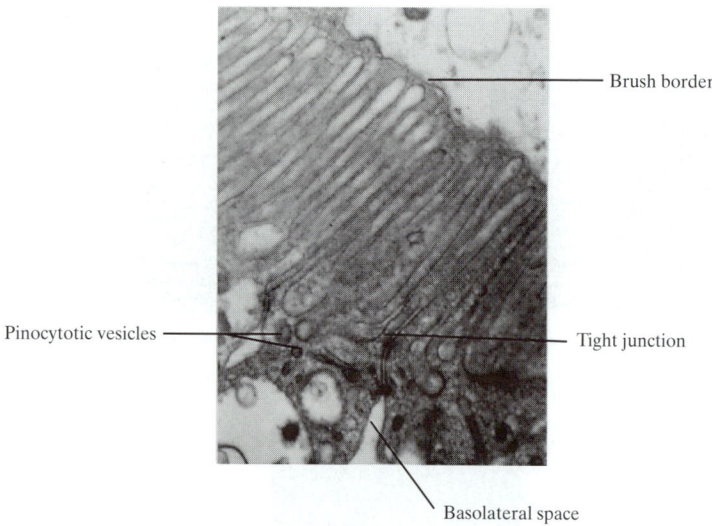

Brush border

Pinocytotic vesicles

Tight junction

Basolateral space

Figure 1.20 Brush border of the proximal tubule. The microvilli of the brush border form a parallel array with pinocytotic vesicles at the junction with cell cytoplasm. The basolateral space is sealed by the tight junction at the base of the brush border. (Osmic acid–uranyl acetate; ×15 000.)

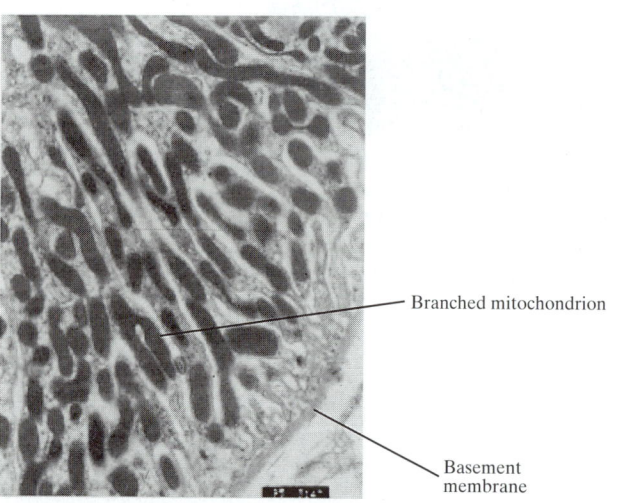

Branched mitochondrion

Basement membrane

Figure 1.21 The mitochondria of the proximal convoluted tubule. The basolateral membrane is folded, and partly encloses the elongated mitochondria. (Osmic acid–uranyl acetate; ×15 000.)

(an animal model of membranous glomerulonephritis). It is clear that in these cells that there is a continuous process of endocytosis, fusion of vesicles with lysosomes and excretion of phagolysosomes back into the lumen [60]. Cylindrical mitochondria are prominent throughout the cell (Figure 1.21). The base of the cell shows a complex infolding of the cell membrane (Figure 1.22). In injury of the cell absorption of protein and colloids accelerates the process of endocytosis with corresponding cytoplasmic changes.

In the transitional and straight parts of the proximal tubule there is progressive diminution in the complexity of cell structure with shorter microvilli, and less elaborate basolateral folds. The number of peroxisomes and secondary lysosomes, however, appears to increase.

There is a high degree of interdigitation between the basolateral margins of adjacent cells which form secondary and tertiary divisions. These basolateral folds increase the surface area. The basolateral membranes also contain $Na^+K^+ATPase$. Specialized elongated mitochondria are present in the cytoplasm of the basolateral folds. The basement membrane of the tubule forms a continuous sheet beneath these folds.

The basement membrane of the tubule forms a continuous sheet beneath these folds.

The loop of Henle

The structure of this segment has been extensively studied in kidney of the rat and other rodents but less so in the human kidney. How human loops differ is uncertain.

In the thin loop of Henle, in animals with a high urinary concentrating ability such as the rat and hamster, four segments with different types of epithelium have

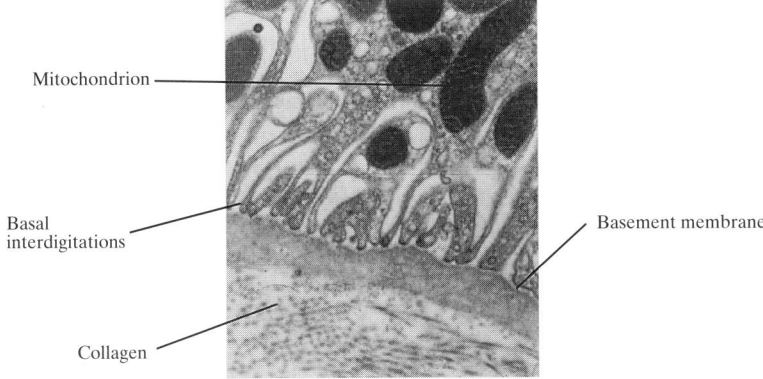

Mitochondrion

Basal
interdigitations

Collagen

Basement membrane

Figure 1.22 The basolateral membrane of the proximal convoluted tubule. The infolding of the basolateral membrane increases the surface area. Note the amorphous appearance of the tubular basement membrane (collagen 4) compared with the fibrillary structure of the interstitial collagen 1. (Osmic acid–uranyl acetate; ×15 000.)

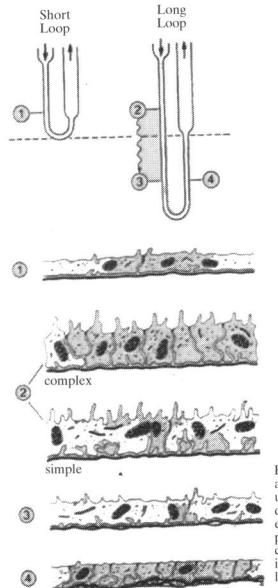

Short
Loop

Long
Loop

① complex

simple

Faudepcil

Figure 1.23 Cell types of the thin loops of Henle. Four types of cell structure are seen in the thin segments of the loops of Henle. The short loops show a single simple pattern. The long loops show patterns of varying complexity involving the luminal microvilli, and basolateral infoldings. There is considerable species variation. (W. Kriz and B. Kaissling Fig. 44, p. 749 Chap. 23, *The Kidney, Physiology and Pathophysiology* ed. D.W. Seldin and G. Giesbach, 1992, Raven Press.)

been described [61, 62] (Figure 1.23). At the end of the straight part of the proximal tubule in short loops there is a sharp transition to a flattened epithelium (type 1) with few microvilli and interdigitating cell borders. In the long loops, the epithelium may be of simple type 1 or a more complex interdigitating type 2. The degree of interdigitation between cells (type 3 cells) is lost as the thin

descending loop enters the inner medulla. The degree of interdigitation is regained in the ascending thin limb by the type 4 cells.

In short loops the descending limb type 1 cells have a simple non-interdigitating cell border and remain within the bounds of the outer medulla. The simple epithelium is thin with numerous junctional connections thought to be poorly permeable to solutes. The more complex type 2 and type 3 cells are thicker, contain more microvilli and the junctions suggest permeability. These cells show more cell organelles and sodium pump membrane-bound enzymes. The ascending thin loops are flattened but show considerable interdigitation.

The ascending thick limb (distal straight tubule) arises from the ascending thin limb at the junction of the inner and outer medulla. In humans this transition is gradual but in the majority of species there is an abrupt change in cell type. The epithelial cell borders interdigitate at the base. As in the proximal tubules elongated mitochondria are present in the basolateral folds. There are two cell types, one with short microvilli and the other with a smooth luminal surface. The cells are rich in ATPase and secrete Tamm–Horsfall protein [55, 63]. The cortical thick ascending tubule terminates a little beyond the macula densa.

The distal convoluted tubule arises just after the macula densa and terminates at the connecting tubule which subsequently opens into the cortical collecting duct. Unfortunately both these junctions are not well demarcated. The distal convoluted tubule contains a characteristic cell, the distal convoluted tubule cell (DCTC). There is an immediate increase in cell height at the start of the convoluted tubule. The cells have extensive lateral interdigitations containing parallel mitochondria. The nucleus is in the apical part of the cell. Short microvilli are present. There is marked ATPase activity. These cells are also an important site for mineralocorticoid activity [64]. Tamm–Horsfall protein is also present [55].

Type A cell

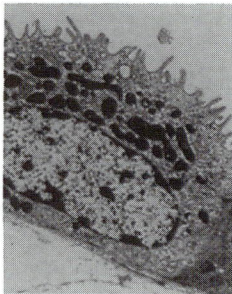

Type B cell

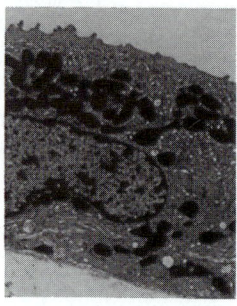

Figure 1.24 Electron micrographs of the intercalated cells of the distal convoluted tubule and collecting ducts (type A and type B cells). The type A cell has complex microplicae on the luminal surface, and numerous vesicles in the adjacent cytoplasm. A proton pump has been demonstrated at the apical surface. The type B cell has scattered short microvilli on the luminal surface and vesicular structures throughout the cytoplasm. Bicarbonate is secreted at the basal membrane. (Modified from K.M. Madsen and B.M. Brenner, Figs 21–19, 21–20, Chap. 21, *Renal Pathology*, ed. C. Craig Tisher and Barry M. Brenner, pub. Lippincott.)

The distal part of the convoluted tubule and connecting tubule contain another cell type, the intercalated cell (Figure 1.24).

The intercalated cell is present in the connecting tubule and collecting duct system. These cells have a simple polygonal outline and are readily observed by electron microscopy because of the dark staining caused by dense mitochondria. The cell surface shows a complex folded pattern (microplicae) which is negatively charged. Recent studies have shown that two types of intercalated cell can be distinguished on the basis of the position of a proton pump. This is situated in the microvesicles which are a prominent feature beneath the cytoplasmic membranes of the cells. The type A cell has a proton pump on the apical surface, whereas in the type B (beta) cell the pump is at the basolateral membrane and secretes $-HCO_3$. The appearance of these cells varies with their activity. It is suggested that the beta-intercalated cell is the precursor of both the type A intercalated cell and the principal cell (see below) [65].

Collecting ducts

Collecting ducts are composed of a mixture of intercalated cells and principal (collecting duct) cells. The main feature of the polygonal principal cell is the numerous regular infoldings (basal labyrinth) of the basal cell membrane. Mitochondrial are few, and the luminal surface has scanty microvilli. Lateral cell folds interlock with adjacent cells. Tight junctions and desmosomes are present. Within the papillae these features are lost and the cells become larger, columnar and lose the basal labyrinth. Despite this apparent structural homogeneity, histochemistry and electron microscopy reveal a mixed cell population, some containing intercalated cell markers [66].

The interstitium

In the cortex the interstitium is delineated by the tiny angular spaces between tubules and capillaries (Figure 1.11). These spaces become greatly expanded by eedema in inflammatory conditions and are the site of interstitial fibrosis in many chronic forms of renal disease. Inconspicuous fibroblasts are scattered throughout the cortex. In the medulla the main cell is normally a stellate fibroblast-like cell [5]. It is attached by cell processes to the loops of Henle and vasa recta. The cytoplasm contains lipid-filled vacuoles and endoplasmic reticulum. These cells are the source of intrarenal prostaglandin secretion [67]. Prostaglandin endoperoxide synthase has been demonstrated in collecting duct cells and interstitial cells [68].

A second population of mononuclear lymphocyte-like cells can be distinguished in the interstitium by the presence of MHC class II antigens [69]. A third cell with the distribution of a vascular pericyte has been described in the interstitium [70]. Fibers of collagen types 1, 3 and 4 are present in small numbers. The tubular and vascular components in the medulla are widely separated by an amorphous matrix (Figure 1.12) rich in proteoglycans.

The urothelium or transitional epithelium covers the renal papillae extending over the surfaces of the calyces and pelvis and down the ureter. The smooth white epithelium appears to be five or six cells thick, and the surface cells are large and polyhedral. Since all cells are attached to the basal layer by delicate processes this is a pseudostratified epithelium. This arrangement allows the expansion necessary for normal function.

References

1. Coppoletta, J.M. and Wolbach, S.B. (1993) Body length and organ weights in infants and children. *Am. J. Pathol.*, **9**, 55.
2. Hodson, C. (1961) Physiological changes in size in the human kidney. *Clin. Radiol.*, **12**, 91.

3. Kunin, M. (1986) Bridging septa of the perinephric space, anatomical, pathologic, and diagnostic considerations. *Radiology*, **158**, 361.

4. Raptopoulos, V., Lei, Q.F., Touliopoulos, P. *et al.* (1995) Why perirenal disease does not extend into the pelvis: the importance of closure of the cone of the renal fasciae. *Am. J. Roentgenol.*, **164**, 1179.

5. Swann, H. and Norman, R. (1970) The periarterial spaces of the kidney. *Tex. Rep. Biol. Med.*, **28**, 317.

6. Pfeiffer, E. (1968) Comparative anatomical observations of the mammalian renal pelvis and medulla. *J. Anat.*, **102**, 321.

7. Ransley, P. and Risdon, R. (1975) Renal papillary morphology and intrarenal reflux in the young pig. *Urol. Res.*, **3**, 105.

8. Gosling, J.A., Dixon, J.S. and Humpherson, J.R. (1982) The microscopic anatomy of the ureter, renal calyces and pelvis, in *Functional Anatomy of the Urinary Tract, An Integrated Text and Colour Atlas*. University Park Press, Baltimore, p. 2.

9. Gosling, J.A. and Dixon, J.S. (1982) The structure of the normal and hydronephrotic upper urinary tract, in *Idiopathic Hydronephrosis* (eds O'Reilly, P.H. and Gosling, J.S.), Springer-Verlag, London, p. 1.

10. Sampaio, F.J.B. and Passos, M.A.R.F. (1992) Renal arteries: anatomic study for surgical and radiological practice. *Surg. Radiol. Anat.*, **14**, 113.

11. Graves, F.T. (1986) *Anatomical Studies for Renal and Intrarenal Surgery*. Wright, Bristol.

12. Kaufman, J.A., Waltman, A.C., Rivitz, S.M. and Geller, S.C. (1995) Anatomical observations on the renal veins and inferior vena cava at magnetic resonance angiography. *CardioVasc. Intervent. Radiol.*, **18**, 153.

13. Satyapal, K.S., Rambiritch, V. and Pillai, G. (1995) Additional renal veins: incidence and morphometry. *Clin. Anat.*, **8**, 51.

14. Barajas, L., Liu, L. and Powers, K. (1992) Anatomy of the renal innervation: intrarenal aspects and ganglia of origin. *Can. J. Physiol. Pharmacol.*, **70**, 735.

15. Howie, A.J. and Rollason, T.P. (1993) Reconsideration of the development of the distal tubule of the human kidney. *J. Anat.*, **183**, 141.

16. Jamieson, R.L. and Kriz, W. (1982) *Urinary Concentrating Mechanism: Structure and Function*. Oxford University Press, New York.

17. Gibson, I.W., Downie, I., Downie, T.T. *et al.* (1992) The parietal podocyte: a study of the vascular pole of the human glomerulus. *Kidney Int.*, **41**, 211.

18. Silva, F. and Verani, R. (1984) Crescentic glomerulonephritis: relationship of the stage of crescent formation to gaps in Bowman's capsule. (South west Paediatric nephrology group). *Kidney Int.* **25**, 266A.

19. Gall, J.A., Alcorn, D., Burkus, A. *et al.* (1986) Distribution of glomerular peripolar cells in different mammalian species. *Cell Tissue Res.*, **244**, 203.

20. Gardiner, D.S., Jackson, R. and Lindop, G.B.M. (1992) The renin-secreting cell and the glomerular peripolar cell in renal artery stenosis and Addison's disease. *Virchows Archiv – A*, **420**, 533.

21. Veis, J., Yamashita, W., Lui, Y.J. and Ooi, B.S. (1990) The biology of mesangial cells in glomerulonephritis. *Proc. Soc. Exp. Biol. Med.*, 160.

22. Kriz, W.T.S. and Hosser, H. (1988) Morphological aspects of glomerular function, in *Xth International Congress of Nephrology* (ed. J.M. Davidson) Ballière Tindall, London, p. 2.

23. Wilcox, C.S., Welsh, W.J., Murad, F., Gross, S.S., Taylor, G., Levi, R. and Schmidt, H.H.W. Nitric oxide synthase in macula densa regulates glomerular capillary pressure. *Proc. Natl. Acad. Sci. USA*, **89**, 11993–7.

24. Jamison, R.L. and Kriz, W. (1982) The urinary concentrating mechanism, structure and function, Ch. 14, Distal convoluted tubule and collecting duct system, pp. 189–217.

25. Ransley, P.G. and Risdon, R.A. (1979) The pathogenesis of reflux nephropathy. *Contrib. Nephrol.*, **16**, 90–97.

26. Ljunguist, A. and Lagergren, C. (1962) Normal intrarenal arterial pattern in adult and aging human kidney: a microangiographical and histological study. *J. Anat.*, **96**, 285.

27. Seron, D., Cameron, J.S. and Haskard, D.O. (1991) Expression of VCAM-1 in the normal and diseased kidney. *Nephrol. Dial. Transplant.*, **6**, 917.

28. Dyck, R.F., Lockwood, C.M., Kershaw, M. *et al.* (1980) Amyloid P is a constituent of normal glomerular basement membrane. *J. Exp. Med.*, **152**, 1162.

29. Mbassa, G., Elger, M. and Kriz, W. (1988) The ultrastructural organisation of the basement membrane of Bowman's capsule in the rat renal corpuscle. *Cell Tissue Res.*, **253**, 151–63.

30. Batsford, S.R., Rohrbach, R. and Vogt, A. (1987) Size restriction in the glomerular capillary wall, importance of lamina densa. *Kidney Int.*, **31**, 710.

31. Baraldi, A., Zambruno, G., Furci, L. *et al.* (1994) Beta-1 integrins in the normal human glomerular capillary wall: an immunoelectron microscopy study. *Nephron*, 295.

32. Andrews, P.M. and Coffey, A.K. (1983) Cytoplasmic contractile elements in glomerular cells. *Fed. Proc.*, **42**, 3046.

33. Kerjaschki, G. and Farquahar, M. (1983) Immunocytochemical localisation of the Heymann antigen gp330. *J. Exp. Med.*, **157**, 667–86.

34. Shikata, K., Ichiyasu, A., Makino H. and Ota. Z. (1990) Three dimensional ultrastructure of the GBM revealed by chemical treatment. *XIth international Congress of Nephrology*, p. 365.

35. Pusey, C.D., Dash, A., Kershaw, M.J. *et al.* (1987) A single autoantigen in Goodpasture's syndrome identified by a monoclonal antibody to human glomerular basement membrane. *Lab. Invest.*, **56**, 23.

36. Kasinath, B.S. (1993) Glomerular endothelial cell proteoglycans – regulation by TGF-betal. *Arch. Biochem. Biophys.*, **305**, 370.

37. Akai, T. and Kriz, W. (1987) The structural relationship between mesangial cells and the basement membrane of the renal glomerulus. *Anat. Embryol.*, **176**, 373.

38. Savage, C. (1994) The biology of the glomerulus: endothelial cells. *Kidney Int.*, **35**, 314.
39. Ballermann, B.J. and Marsden, P.A. (1991) Endothelium-derived vasoactive mediators and renal glomerular function. *Clin. Invest. Med.*, **249**, 508.
40. Neild, G.H. and Brown, Z. (1991) Endothelium and glomerular growth. *Am. J. Kidney Dis.*, **17**, 670.
41. Latta, H., Maunsbach, A. and Madden, S.C. (1960) The centrilobular region of the renal glomerulus studied by electron microscopy. *J. Ultrastruct. Res.* **4**, 455.
42. Kreisberg, J., Venkatachalam, M. and Troyer, D. (1985) Contractile properties of cultured glomerular mesangial cells. *Am. J. Physiol.*, **249**, 999.
43. Studer, R.K., Craven, P.A. and Derubertis, F.R. (1994) Thromboxane stimulation of mesangial cell fibronectin synthesis is signalled by protein kinase C and modulated by cGMP. *Kidney Int.*, **46**, 1074.
44. Nebigil, C.G., Garnovskaya, M.N., Spurney, R.F. and Raymond, J.R. (1995) Identification of a rat glomerular mesangial cell mitogenic 5-HT (2A) receptor. *Am. J. Physiol.*, **268**, F122.
45. Bhandari, B., Wenzel, U.O., Marra, F. and Abboud, H.E. (1995) A nuclear protein in mesangial cells that binds to the promoter region of the platelet-derived growth factor-A chain gene: induction by phorbol ester. *J. Biol. Chem.*, **270**, 5541.
46. Nguyen, G., Li, X.M., Peraldi, M.N. *et al.* (1994) Receptor binding and degradation of urokinase-type plasminogen activator by human mesangial cells. *Kidney Int.*, **46**, 208.
47. Stefanovic, V., Vlahovic, P. and Ardaillou, R. (1995) Characterization and control of expression of cell surface alkaline phosphodiesterase I activity in rat mesangial glomerular cells. *Renal Physiol. Biochem.*, **18**, 12.
48. Michael, A.F., Keane, W.F., Rajii, L. and Vernier, R.L. (1980) The glomerular mesangium. *Kidney Int.*, **17**, 141.
49. Kriz, W., Elger, M., Mundel, P. and Lemley, K.V. (1995) Structure-stabilizing forces in the glomerular tuft. *J. Am. Soc. Nephrol.*, **5**, 1731.
50. Ryan, G.J.B.C. and Scoggins, B. (1979) The granulated peripolar epithelial cell: a potential secretory component of the renal juxta-glomerular complex. *Nature*, **277**, 655.
51. Hollywell, C.A., Jaworowski, A., Thumwood, C. *et al.* (1992) Immunohistochemical localization of transthyretin in glomerular peripolar cells of newborn sheep. *Cell Tissue Res.*, **267**, 193.
52. Gardiner, D.S. and Lindop, G.B.M. (1992) The glomerular peripolar cell. An immunohistochemical study. *APMIS*, **100**, 107.
53. Alcorn, D. and Ryan, G.B. (1993) The glomerular peripolar cell. *Kidney Int. Suppl.* **42**, S-35.
54. Gardiner, D.S. and Lindop G.B.M. (1985) The granular peripolar cell of the human glomerulus: a new component of the juxtaglomerular apparatus? *Histopathology*, **9**, 675.
55. Gardiner, D.S., Downie, I., Gibson, I.W. *et al.* (1991) The glomerular peripolar cell: a review. *Histol. Histopathol.*, **6**, 567.
56. Sikri, K.L., Foster, C.L., MacHugh, N. and Marshall, R.D. (1981) Localisation of Tamm–Horsfall glycoprotein in the human kidney using immunofluorescent and immunoelectron microscopical techniques. *J. Anat.*, **132**, 597.
57. Gibson, I.W., Gardiner, D.S., Downie, I. *et al.* (1994) A comparative study of the glomerular peripolar cell and the renin-secreting cell in twelve mammalian species. *Cell Tissue Res.*, **277**, 385.
58. Yamaguchi, H., Kaku, H., Onodera, T. *et al.* (1994) Peripolar cells in guinea pigs under experimental hyperplasia of juxtaglomerular cells induced by long-term, low-dose calcium condition. *Exp. Toxicol. Pathol.*, **46**, 283.
59. Wellings, A.W. and Wellings, D.J. (1976) Shape of epithelial cells and extracelluar channels in the rabbit proximal nephron. *Kidney Int.*, **8**, 343.
60. Van Deurs, B. and Christenson, E. (1984) Endocytosis in kidney proximal tubular cells and cultured fibroblasts: a review of the structural aspects of membrane recycling between the plasma membranes and endocytotic vesicles. *Eur. J. Cell Biol.*, **33**, 163.
61. Bachmann, S. and Kriz, W. (1982) Histotopography and ultrastructure of thin limbs of henle in the hamster. *Cell Tissue Res.*, **225**, 111.
62. Schwartz, M.M. and Venkatachalam, M.A. (1974) Structural differences in thin limbs of Henle: physiological implications. *Kidney Int.*, **6**, 193.
63. Tamm, I. and Horsfall, F.L. (1952) A mucoprotein derived from human urine which reacts with influenza, mumps and Newcastle disease virus. *J. Exp. Med.*, **95**, 71.
64. Fejestoth, A. and Fejestoth, G. (1995) Expression cloning of the aldosterone target cell-specific 11 beta-hydroxysteroid dehydrogenase from rabbit collecting duct cells. *Endocrinology*, **136**, 2579.
65. Fejestoth, G. and Narayfejestoth, A. (1992) Differentiation of renal beta-intercalated cells to alpha-intercalated and principal cells in culture. *Proc. Natl. Acad. Sci. USA*, **89**, 5487.
66. Kloth, S., Aigner, J., Brandt, E. *et al.* (1993) Histochemical markers reveal an unexpected heterogeneous composition of the renal collecting duct epithelium. *Kidney Int.*, **44**, 527.
67. Zusman, R.M. and Keiser, H.R. (1977) Prostaglandin biosynthesis by rabbit renomedullary interstitial cells in tissue culture stimulation by angiotensin 11, bradykinin and arginine vasopressin. *J. Clin. Invest.*, **60**, 215.
68. Govindarajan, S., Nast, C.C., Smith, W.L. *et al.* (1987) Immunohistochemical distribution of renal prostaglandin endoperoxide synthase and prostaglandin synthase: diminished endoperoxide synthase in the hepato-renal syndrome. *Hepatology*, **7**, 654–9.

69. Bohman, S.O., Sundelin, B., Forsum, U. and Tribukait, B. (1988) Experimental depletion of different renal interstitial cell populations. *Am. J. Med. Sci.*, **295**, 252.

70. Bohman, S-O. (1974) The ultrastructure of the rat renal medulla as observed after improved fixation methods. *J. Ultrastruct. Res.*, **47**, 329.

I

Normal Structure and Function

Section 2
Renal Physiology

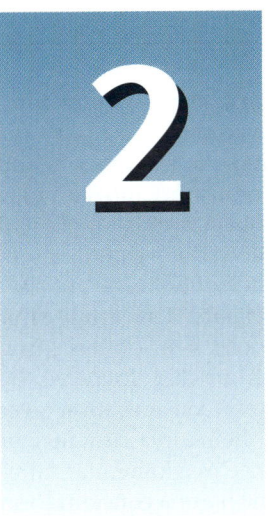

Glomerular filtration

Chris Baylis and Kevin V. Lemley

Introduction

Filtration of the aqueous component of the blood, at the glomerulus, provides the first step in urine formation. Glomerular filtration rate (GFR) is thus crucial to all functions of the kidney and GFR is normally closely regulated by multiple mechanisms which co-operate in the maintenance of a constant, high value of GFR.

History of glomerular function

The description of the structure of the glomerulus by Malpighi (1666) and the anatomical arrangements between glomerulus and tubule, by Bowman (1832), laid the framework for our current understanding of glomerular filtration. In 1842, Ludwig suggested that a protein-free filtrate was forced out of the glomerular capillaries into the tubule by the hydrostatic pressure of the blood, and in 1899 Starling described the importance of the colloid osmotic pressure of the plasma proteins and their role in transcapillary fluid movement. In 1924 Wearn and Richards published their landmark study, using the renal micropuncture technique, in which they reported that the glomerular filtrate in Bowman's space is a protein-free, ultrafiltrate of plasma [1, 2]. With the development of the urinary clearance methods by Homer Smith and colleagues it became possible to measure GFR accurately in a range of species, including man [2]. The development of the servonull pressure measuring device and the availability of the Munich Wistar rat, a mutant strain which possesses glomerular capillaries on the subcapsular surface of the kidney, gave rise to the studies by Brenner,

Deen, Robertson and others which were begun in the 1970s and continue today. The combination of direct measurements and mathematical modeling have led to a detailed description of the dynamic determinants of glomerular filtration and the many physiologic and pathophysiologic events that can influence GFR [3].

Composition of the glomerular filtrate

The glomerular wall functions as a sieve, restricting the passage of circulating cells and large molecules (see below) and allowing passage to water and small solutes. As a result the fluid in Bowman's space is an **ultrafiltrate** of plasma, containing only trace quantities of protein. Uncharged small solutes such as urea and glucose are present in Bowman's space fluid in the same concentrations as in plasma. There is a slight difference in the distribution of charged solutes due to the Donnan effect; the non-filterable plasma proteins are anionic and in order to maintain electrical balance across the glomerular wall, the concentration of anions (e.g. Cl^-, HCO_3^-) is slightly higher and the concentration of cations (e.g. Na^+) is slightly lower in Bowman's space fluid than in plasma.

Values of glomerular filtration rate

In normal humans the rate at which fluid is filtered across the glomeruli of both kidneys ranges from 80 to 200 ml/min; equivalent to ~100–300 l of plasma water filtered every day. The plasma volume is ~3–5 l; thus, this

Nephrology, Edited by Rex L. Jamison and Robert Wilkinson.
Published in 1997 by Chapman & Hall, London. ISBN 0 412 60930 4

very high rate of GFR is consistent with the primary role of the kidney, which is to monitor and control the volume and composition of the body fluids.

Both among and within species, GFR is roughly proportional to body size. In animal studies, GFR is often expressed in terms of kidney or body weight but in humans, GFR is most frequently corrected to $1.73 \, m^2$ body surface area (SA). This is an arbitrary value which approximates the average surface area of a normal sized adult male.

Measurement of GFR

Clearance method

A renal clearance is the volume of plasma that is completely cleared of a particular substance in a given time period, usually 1 min, by the kidneys. In practice, all the plasma flowing through the kidney will be partly cleared of a given substance in unit time, thus, a clearance is a virtual rather than a real volume. The clearance (C) of a substance (x) can be calculated as shown in equation (2.1):

$$\left(U_x \cdot V\right)/P_x = C_x \qquad (2.1)$$

where U_x and P_x are the urine and plasma concentrations of x, and V is urine flow rate. As indicated by Smith, the clearance of a substance that is freely filtered at the glomerulus but once within the tubule, is neither reabsorbed nor secreted, can be used as a marker for measurement of GFR. The sugar inulin obeys these criteria and has been used for many years to measure GFR, providing the 'gold standard' [2]. More recently, other radiolabeled substances such as iothalamate and ^{51}Cr-labeled edetate have also been used. In order to measure the renal clearance of inulin, which is foreign to the body, a priming dose followed by a constant infusion of inulin are given intravenously to establish a steady-state plasma concentration. Consecutive, timed urine collections are then made so that the excretion rate of inulin can be calculated ($U_{IN}V$) and divided by the steady-state plasma inulin concentration (P_{IN}), to give the inulin clearance (C_{IN}). Both steady-state plasma concentrations and complete urine collections are essential in order to obtain reliable clearance measurements. In animal experiments the bladder can be catheterized and irrigated to ensure complete collection of urine. In humans, an alternative is to establish a high rate of urine flow by creating a water diuresis to reduce dead space errors.

Alternative techniques for measuring GFR

In circumstances in which an accurate urine collection is difficult or impossible (oliguria, voiding dysfunction, in children), reliable alternatives to inulin clearance have been developed. The **constant infusion method** is based on the principle that in the steady state the rate of urinary excretion of inulin is equal to the rate of infusion. Thus, $C_{IN} = (U_{IN}V) / P_{IN}$ is replaced by $C = (I_{IN}R) / P_{IN}$, where I_{IN} is the inulin concentration of the infusate and R is the infusion rate. Constant ambulatory infusion may be achieved by means of a subcutaneous implanted pump. Adequate time must be allowed for equilibration, usually 3–4 h, but it may be considerably longer for very young children or edematous patients. The **single shot** or **plasma clearance method** consists of a bolus intravenous injection of a filtration marker followed by repeated determinations of plasma concentration over time. The method as-sumes that the plasma clearance of the marker is equal to the clearance by glomerular filtration and usually requires fitting the plasma concentration time course to a (two-compartment) model. It may require extended sampling to establish a clearance curve in patients with decreased renal function or edema. Although both the constant infusion and single shot methods slightly overestimate GFR, they are more reproducible than classic urinary clearances, when done simultaneously in patients [4].

Endogenous creatinine as a measure of GFR

Creatinine is a waste product of muscle metabolism that is freely filtered and is not reabsorbed within the renal tubule, although in some species, including humans, there is limited tubular secretion of creatinine. Since the quantity of creatinine excreted in the urine exceeds the quantity delivered into the tubule system by filtration, the creatinine clearance overestimates the GFR, although this tends to be balanced by an overestimate of plasma creatinine, measured by the Jaffe reaction, which tends to underestimate C_{cr}. The 24 h creatinine clearance (obtained by collection of a complete 24 h urine) is widely used as a measure of GFR although incomplete urine collections and analytical problems for creatinine (see below) can lead to great variability in this measurement. In a normal non-pregnant adult the rate of creatinine excreted by the kidneys is equal to the rate of creatinine produced by muscle metabolism; thus, plasma creatinine concentration (P_{cr}) remains constant. When renal function begins to deteriorate, the excretion of creatinine falls, leading to an increase in P_{cr}, which in turn increases the filtration of creatinine until a new steady state is reached between creatinine production rate and creatinine excretion rate by the kidneys. Figure 2.1(a) shows that with mild to moderate levels of renal impairment only small increases occur in P_{cr}, but with severe renal disease P_{cr} changes markedly and, thus, the plasma/serum creatinine value is widely used as a clinical index of GFR [5]. The reciprocal or logarithm of plasma/serum creatinine also provides an index of the rate of progression towards end stage for an individual patient with renal parenchymal disease (Figure 2.1b) [6].

There are many potential errors in the P_{cr} (or serum creatinine, S_{cr}) and C_{cr} measurements. These include ana-

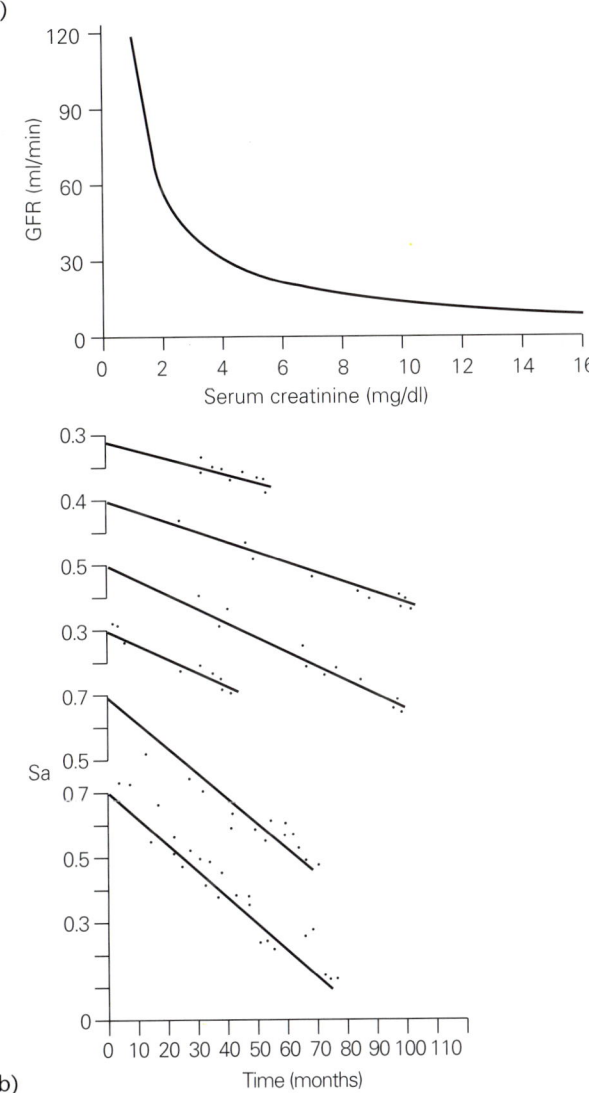

(a)

(b)

Figure 2.1 (a) The ideal relationship between GFR and plasma or serum creatinine (S_{cr}). In the normal individual GFR ~120 ml/min and S_{cr} ~1 mg/dl. As renal function declines (falls by half), S_{cr} increases (doubles) in proportion. (b) The relationship between the reciprocal of the serum creatinine concentration vs time in six patients with progressive renal failure. Each patient is progressing towards endstage (when $1/S_{cr} = 0$) at a rate defined by the slope of the line. PN = pyelonephritis; GN = glomerulonephritis; MCD = medullary cystic disease. (Reproduced, with permission, from Mitch *et al.* (1976), ref. 6, with permission.)

lytical problems with substances interfering with determinations of P_{cr} and variable extrarenal removal and renal tubular secretion of creatinine. The creatinine production is influenced by age, sex, body size and composition. Despite these limitations, S_{cr} and C_{cr} remain the most widely used clinical indices of GFR [5].

Determinants of glomerular filtration rate

The GFR is determined by the number of functioning glomeruli and by the filtration rate at each single glomerulus (single nephron GFR, SNGFR). The number of glomeruli per kidney is proportional to the size of the kidney. The rat possesses ~30 000 glomeruli per kidney, the dog ~400 000 glomeruli per kidney and in humans there are ~1 000 000 glomeruli per kidney [2]. About 90% of these glomeruli are located in the outer two-thirds of the cortex (the cortical glomeruli) and are relatively homogeneous with regard both to structure and function. The remaining 10% of glomeruli lie deep within the cortex at the border with the medulla (the juxtamedullary glomeruli), are larger and have a higher SNGFR than cortical glomeruli. It is generally accepted that in the absence of glomerular injury all glomeruli are functioning all of the time. Thus, the physiologic regulation of GFR is by control of SNGFR.

The rate of movement of fluid across the wall of the glomerular capillary is described by the Starling relationship, given below (equations 2.2 and 2.3):

$$\text{SNGFR} = \left[\left(P_{GC} - P_{BS} \right) - \left(\pi_{GC} - \pi_{BS} \right) \right] \cdot k \cdot S \qquad (2.2)$$

$$\text{SNGFR} = \left(\Delta P - \Delta \pi \right) \cdot K_f \qquad (2.3)$$

where SNGFR is the rate of fluid flux across the entire glomerular capillary/minute; P_{GC} is the pressure of the blood in the glomerular capillary, P_{BS} is the hydrostatic pressure of the fluid in Bowman's space and the transglomerular hydrostatic pressure difference is ΔP (= $P_{GC} - P_{BS}$); π_{GC} is the colloid osmotic pressure within the glomerular capillary and since the plasma proteins are not filtered at the glomerulus, π_{BS}, the colloid osmotic pressure in the Bowman's space fluid can be neglected. The k and S values are the intrinsic intraglomerular characteristics of water permeability and filtration surface area, respectively, and are frequently combined as a single value, the glomerular ultrafiltration coefficient K_f. Thus, SNGFR is regulated by control of ΔP, $\Delta \pi$ and K_f.

Filtration fraction (FF) is that fraction of the plasma arriving at the glomerulus (renal plasma flow, RPF) which is filtered during plasma flow through the glomerular network and is derived as follows:

$$\text{FF} = \text{GFR/RPF} \qquad (2.4)$$

This can be rearranged to give equations (2.5) and (2.6):

$$\text{GFR} = \text{RPF} \times \text{FF} \qquad (2.5)$$

$$\text{SNGFR} = Q_A \times \text{SNFF} \qquad (2.6)$$

According to this formulation, SNGFR is determined by the plasma flow to a single glomerulus (Q_A) and the single nephron FF (SNFF) which is itself controlled by ΔP, K_f and by the colloid osmotic pressure of the blood arriving at the glomerulus, π_A. Using the glomerular micropuncture technique it has been possible, in animals, to directly measure SNGFR and its four primary determinants, Q_A, ΔP, K_f and π_A, in the glomerular microcirculation [3, 7] and information derived from such studies is summarized below.

Relative importance of the determinants of SNGFR/GFR

The mathematical model of Deen, Robertson and Brenner [7a] allows prediction of the importance of the individual Starling determinants of SNGFR. Generally, experimental observations have agreed with these predictions, as discussed below.

Plasma flow, Q_A

Plasma flow is the single most important physiologic determinant of GFR and yet a plasma flow term does not appear in the Starling relationship (equations 2.2 and 2.3). How then does plasma flow control GFR? Figure 2.2 shows the transcapillary hydrostatic and colloid osmotic pressure profiles ΔP and $\Delta \pi$) along an idealized glomerular capillary. The $\Delta \pi$ profile increases exponentially as blood travels along the glomerulus. This results from the hemoconcentration of plasma proteins secondary to removal of plasma water by filtration. The difference between the ΔP and $\Delta \pi$ curves gives the mean net filtration pressure (FP) which provides the driving pressure for

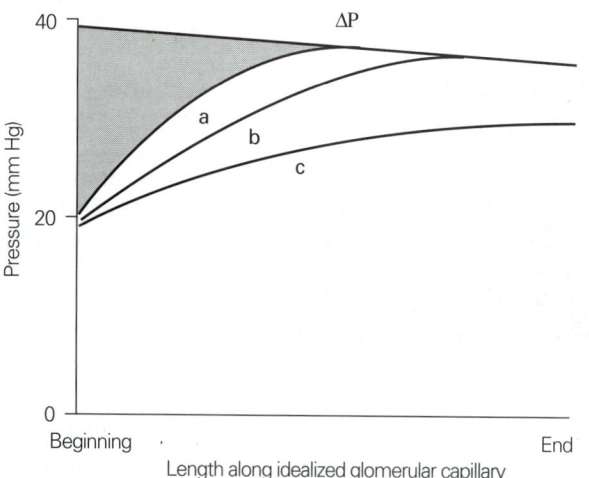

Figure 2.2 The transcapillary hydrostatic pressure difference (ΔP) and several possible oncotic pressure differences ($\Delta \pi$) along an idealized glomerular capillary. The net ultrafiltration pressure is the difference between the ΔP and $\Delta \pi$ curve averaged over the length of the glomerulus and is given by the shaded area for the ΔP and $\Delta \pi$ curve a. Curve a represents a low plasma flow state and curve b represents an intermediate plasma flow state, and the glomerulus is at filtration pressure equilibrium (i.e. no net filtration pressure by the end of the glomerulus) under both conditions. Curve c represents a high plasma flow state, when the glomerulus is at filtration pressure disequilibrium (i.e. positive filtration pressure at the end of the glomerulus).

filtration. An increase in plasma flow directly increases the filtration pressure by attenuating the rise in the $\Delta \pi$ curve. As plasma flow increases and the $\Delta \pi$ curve is shifted from curve a to curve b (Figure 2.2), a proportional increase in SNGFR is produced, thus FF remains unchanged. In this situation, filtration pressure equilibrium persists, that is, the filtration pressure is zero by the end of the glomerular capillary. With further increases in plasma flow the rise in $\Delta \pi$ is further attenuated, the available filtration surface area is exhausted and a positive filtration pressure persists at the end of the glomerular capillary. This situation is known as filtration pressure disequilibrium and is represented by a shift in the curve b to curve c (Figure 2.2). In this situation the increase in plasma flow evokes a proportionally smaller increase in SNGFR, thus filtration fraction falls. The predicted relationship between plasma flow (Q_A) and SNGFR based on mathematical modeling is shown in Figure 2.3(A), and animal studies in which Q_A was varied while the other determinants of SNGFR were maintained relatively constant have confirmed this relationship [7].

Glomerular plasma flow is determined by the axial pressure gradient across the vasculature of the kidney and by the resistance to flow of the renal blood vessels. As discussed in more detail in Chapter 3, the vascular anatomy of the kidney is complex and both preglomerular (R_A) and efferent arteriolar (R_E) resistances can control the rate of plasma flow. When either or both R_A and R_E relax, plasma flow through the kidney will increase. Since R_A provides the majority of the resistance to flow, a reduction in R_A will have a large impact to increase Q_A.

Transcapillary hydrostatic pressure gradient (ΔP)

The ΔP is another important physiologic determinant of GFR. ΔP is regulated by control of P_{GC}, which is determined by systemic blood pressure (BP) and the relative tone of R_A and R_E. As shown in Figure 2.3(b), increases in P_{GC} and thus ΔP (above a threshold which exceeds π_A) are predicted to increase SNGFR in a curvilinear fashion; this non-linearity results from the concomitant, smaller increase in $\Delta \pi$, produced by the increase in filtration associated with increased ΔP. Direct measurements have confirmed this relationship [3, 7]. Because of the presence of resistance vessels both before and after the glomerulus, P_{GC} may be 'fine tuned' and controlled independently of BP, thus alterations in R_A and R_E can have complex effects on ΔP, Q_A and, therefore, SNGFR. A selective change in R_A produces directionally similar effects on Q_A and ΔP; for example when R_A falls, plasma flow increases and ΔP also increases, due to an increased P_{GC}. When both R_A and R_E change in parallel the predominant effect is on plasma flow with little change in ΔP, and when a selective change occurs in R_E the effects on plasma flow and ΔP are directionally opposite, e.g. a fall in R_E leads to increased plasma flow and at the same time to a reduction in ΔP, via a fall in P_{GC}.

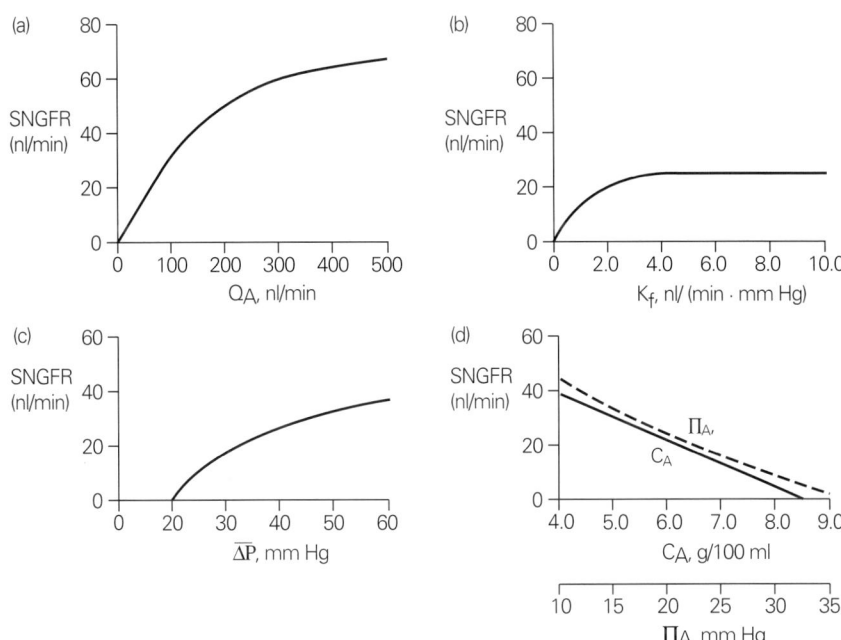

Figure 2.3 The predicted effects on SNGFR of selective alterations in glomerular plasma flow, Q_A (a); the transglomerular hydrostatic pressure gradient, ΔP (b); the glomerular capillary ultrafiltration coefficient, K_f (c); the systemic plasma protein concentration, C_A, or the colloid osmotic pressure due to the systemic plasma proteins, π_A (d). (Reproduced, with permission, from Brenner, B.M., Deen, Wm, and Robertson, C.R. (1976) Glomerular filtration in *The Kidney* (eds Brenner, B.M. and Rector, F.C. Jr), W.B. Saunders Co., Philadelphia.)

As indicated in Figure 2.2 the axial drop in P_{GC} (and ΔP) as blood flows through the glomerulus is very small, and both direct and indirect measurements in rats indicate that P_{GC} is ~45–55 mmHg (i.e. about half the systemic BP). Since the fluid pressure in Bowman's space is ~10–15 mmHg (and this value is relatively constant under physiologic conditions), ΔP is normally ~35–45 mmHg.

Glomerular capillary ultrafiltration coefficient (K_f)

There are also situations in which variations in K_f control SNGFR. As shown in Figure 2.3(c), the relationship between SNGFR and K_f is complex. At low values of K_f the animal is at filtration pressure disequilibrium, and in this situation alterations in K_f will have a major impact on the value of SNGFR. When K_f increases above a 'threshold' value, however, filtration pressure equilibrium occurs and at this point further increases in K_f have no further impact on SNGFR. The reasoning behind this is complex and is discussed in more detail elsewhere [3, 7]. In practice, this means that agents which increase K_f above normal have little effect on SNGFR whereas agents which reduce K_f may cause falls in SNGFR. Theoretically, K_f can be controlled either by changes in glomerular water permeability (k) and/or by regulation of filtration surface area. In general, most investigation of dynamic control of K_f is focused on control of surface area by the contractile glomerular mesangial cell. Glomerular mesangial cells contain many hormone receptors and are also capable of synthesizing a large range of vasoactive substances [3]. *In vitro*, cultured glomerular mesangial cells contract in response to a range of vasoconstrictor agonists such as angiotensin II and endothelin. Precontracted mesangial cells relax in the presence of vasodilatory agents such as prostacyclin and nitric oxide. Whether hormones and autocoids also control K_f by influence of k is uncertain; Savin and Terreros [8], using an *in vitro* glomerulus preparation, have indicated that k is fairly constant between species and that differences in K_f are a function of surface area.

Oncotic pressure of the blood arriving at the glomerulus (π_A)

According to equations (2.2) and (2.3) and Figures 2.2 and 2.3(d), changes in systemic protein concentration (C_A), and therefore π_A, should be inversely related to SNGFR, via an impact on the filtration pressure. However, *in vivo* micropuncture evidence suggests that the situation is more complicated since changes in π_A also produce directionally similar changes in K_f. For example, a fall in π_A should increase SNGFR via an increase in filtration pressure; however, this is offset by the SNGFR-reducing effect of a concomitant fall in K_f. In practice, small changes in π_A within the physiologic range have little impact on SNGFR, particularly since under normal circumstances the systemic plasma protein concentration (and thus π_A) change little [7]. Therefore, π_A is not a physiologic determinant of SNGFR.

In summary, the most important dynamic determinants of SNGFR are Q_A, ΔP and K_f and these determinants are themselves controlled by the contractile tone in the vascular smooth muscle in preglomerular and efferent arterioles (controlling Q_A and P_{GC}), and tone in the glomerular mesangial cells, which determines K_f, via regulation of glomerular filtration surface area. In practice, glomerular filtration is regulated by the tone of contractile cells within the kidney.

Indirect estimates in humans of determinants of glomerular filtration using dextran sieving curves

Naturally, invasive glomerular micropuncture measurements are not feasible in man but indirect estimates of glomerular hemodynamics have been made using modeling assumptions and measured GFR, RPF, π_A and dextran sieving curves. Dextran sieving curves are most often useful in assessing the glomerular permeability to large molecules (see below); however, values of ΔP and K_f can also be estimated since glomerular hemodynamics influence the transmembrane flux of dextrans. This analysis is based on a heteroporous model of the glomerular wall permeability to dextrans and uses a 'best fit' approach to estimate ΔP from the observed dextran sieving coefficients, GFR and FF. Once an optimal ΔP has been selected, K_f is calculated as described by Myers *et al.* [9]. This approach suggests that in normal man ΔP is ~35–40 mmHg and, based on the estimated value of π_{GC} at the efferent end of the glomerulus, this suggests that man is normally operating around the transition point between filtration pressure equilibrium and disequilibrium, a situation which allows maximum flexibility in control of glomerular hemodynamics. However, it is important to note that this analysis is based on assumptions that are not directly testable in man, thus this method provides only a 'guestimate' of the actual values in humans.

Individual regulatory systems

Since GFR is essentially controlled by the level of tone in R_A, R_E and the glomerular mesangial cells, vasoactive control systems provide the majority of regulation of GFR. These are described in detail in Chapter 3 on the renal circulation and are considered below briefly in terms of their specific effect on SNGFR and its determinants.

Renal nerves and catecholamines

In normal unstressed human, efferent renal sympathetic nerve activity is so low that it does not influence renal hemodynamics. In rats, stimulation of the renal nerve leads to frequency-dependent increases in R_A and R_E and falls in K_f presumably due to mesangial contraction. The increased R_A and R_E lower plasma flow, which together with a fall in K_f produces reductions in SNGFR. The effect of renal nerve stimulation of P_{GC} and ΔP is variable and apparently has little functional impact in the normal individual [10]. During high-frequency sympathetic discharge or in the presence of high levels of vasoconstrictor catecholamines, intense renal vasoconstriction can result in cessation of renal blood flow. Dopamine is a vasodilatory catecholamine which is clinically very useful since it selectively vasodilates the kidney when infused in low doses.

Vasoconstrictor hormones

In normal, unstressed individuals the activity of the renal renin–angiotensin system (RAS) is very low and is not controlling renal hemodynamics [11]. When the renin–angiotensin system is activated, however, for example by volume depletion, the potent vasoconstrictor angiotensin II (AII) has complex effects on glomerular hemodynamics. At the whole kidney level AII infusion produces falls in RPF with increases in filtration fraction and little net change in GFR. *In vivo* and *in vitro* studies have suggested that in the cortical microcirculation, although AII vasoconstricts both R_A and R_E its actions are preferential on R_E, leading therefore to a large increase in P_{GC} which offsets the fall in plasma flow. In addition, AII promotes reductions in K_f probably by mesangial cell contraction [3, 7]. Therefore, the actions of AII on glomerular function are complex and, depending on the level of AII, will result in either little change, or falls in GFR.

Endothelin (ET) is another potent vasoconstrictor which has similar complex effects on the glomerular microcirculation to AII. ET infusion produces falls in SNGFR due to reduction in plasma flow (both R_A and R_E increase) and mesangial cell constriction, leading to falls in K_f. It is not known whether ET has a physiologic role, but recent studies using ET receptor antagonists suggest that endogenous ET exerts a tonic **vasodilatory** action on R_A. These unexpected findings suggest that ET is acting via a vasodilatory system (possibly nitric oxide or prostacyclin) in the preglomerular resistance vessel [12]. The physiologic significance of these findings remains to be determined.

Arginine vasopressin (AVP) is a potent vasoconstrictor hormone which, when infused, causes increases in ΔP **without influencing** P_{GC}; this is an unusual situation where ΔP is increased due to falls in Bowman's space fluid pressure. In addition, AVP contracts the *in vitro* glomerular mesangial cell and *in vivo* leads to falls in K_f. Physiologic levels of AVP are too low, however, to have any effect on glomerular hemodynamics.

There are several vasoconstrictor arachidonic acid products such as thromboxane AII (TXA_2) and leukotrienes (LT) which produce increases in R_A and R_E and variable effects on K_f but are usually associated with reductions in GFR [3, 7]. However, the consensus is that under normal circumstances these systems are not activated and are not controlling glomerular hemodynamics although they may play a substantial role in some forms of renal disease.

Vasodilator systems

Atrial natriuretic peptide (ANP) increases GFR by an unusual combination of actions. In the normal kidney ANP has little effect on plasma flow since, although R_A dilates, ANP also leads to increases in R_E. Thus, ANP has oppositely directed actions on the segmental arterioles at the glomerulus. The net effect of the fall in R_A and an increase in R_E is to produce a marked elevation in glomerular blood pressure and this is responsible for the increase in SNGFR; K_f is relatively unaffected [3]. When the kidney vasculature is precontracted, ANP exerts a more prominent renal vasodilatory action and ANP infusions may be useful in vascoconstricted states of acute renal failure. It seems unlikely, however, that physiologic levels of ANP have any effect on glomerular hemodynamics.

Interpretation of animal studies in which various vasodilatory prostaglandins are infused have been complicated. In some settings prostacyclin (PGI_2) and prostaglandin E_2 (PGE_2) infusions, in the rat, produce renal vasoconstriction which can be prevented by concomitant AII inhibition. In other species the vasodilatory response predominates. The vasodilatory prostaglandins PGE and PGI_2 are made in substantial quantities by the mammalian kidney but do not apparently control glomerular hemodynamics under physiologic conditions, since the non-steroidal anti-inflammatory agents which block PG production have little effect on glomerular hemodynamics in the normal state. It is likely that under some pathophysiologic conditions where the cyclo-oxygenase system is activated in the kidney these vasodilatory cyclo-oxygenase products contribute to maintenance of adequate renal perfusion and GFR.

Nitric oxide is an extremely important, physiologic vasodilator. It vasodilates via activation of its second messenger cGMP and is produced by many cell types, including the vascular endothelium and nervous system. There is considerable evidence that tonically produced NO relaxes R_A and the glomerular mesangial cell under normal circumstances, since local intrarenal inhibition of NO leads to constriction of R_A and falls in K_f with consequent reductions in SNGFR [12]. When NO is blocked systemically as well as intrarenally, increases in R_E also occur, thus P_{GC} rises and the effect of NO blockade to lower SNGFR is blunted. The mechanism by which systemic NO blockade elicits an increase in R_E is currently unknown. When NO is chronically blocked the kidney remains persistently vasoconstricted with maintained systemic and glomerular hypertension, leading eventually to glomerular injury. Based on the importance of NO as a physiologic regulatory substance it seems likely that NO production controls GFR in the normal baseline state and that declines in GFR in some diseases may be associated with a deficit of NO [12].

Physiologic regulation of GFR

In practice GFR changes little in the normal adult, due to a range of compensatory and offsetting mechanisms. There are small postural effects, with GFR falling ~10% on the assumption of the upright position and a diurnal variation (~15%) in GFR, with the highest values in the afternoon and the lowest in the early morning. This probably reflects variations in renal plasma flow. During mild exercise there is little effect on GFR, but during severe exercise significant falls in GFR have been reported which last for the duration of the exercise. This is associated with vasoconstriction of the kidney, at least partly secondary to increased renal nerve activity [13].

Volume status is a potentially important determinant of GFR, with volume-expanded states being associated with increased GFR and volume-contracted states being associated with falls in GFR. These changes in GFR in response to changes in volume status are generally secondary to changes in renal plasma flow. The protein content of the diet is also an important determinant of GFR. Acutely, a meal high in protein produces a dose-dependent increase in GFR and maintenance on a high protein intake leads to chronically elevated GFR. The mechanism is thought to be via renal vasodilation predominantly of R_A, thus GFR increases due to increased plasma flow and increased glomerular blood pressure. There is no evidence that high protein intake causes any long-term damaging effects to the normal kidney, i.e. in the absence of underlying injury, but when underlying glomerular injury is present high protein feeding exacerbates the rate of development of glomerular damage, probably via increased glomerular blood pressure [3].

Although GFR remains nearly constant in healthy adults, GFR increases during maturational growth and pregnancy and decreases with advancing age. The increase in SNGFR during maturational growth is due to a combination of increases in plasma flow and increases in K_f, the latter most likely secondary to increased glomerular surface area [3]. There is no change in the number of functioning glomeruli since these are established at birth; however, when glomerular number is abnormally low, as in growth-retarded infants, this may predispose to later glomerular damage [14]. During pregnancy, marked increases occur in GFR which are sustained throughout most of the gestational period. Micropuncture studies in rats have indicated an even vasodilation of both R_A and R_E, such that GFR increases due entirely to an increase in plasma flow. With advancing age there is a gradual decline in the GFR both because the kidney tends to vasoconstrict and also due to loss of functioning glomeruli secondary to glomerular sclerosis. These subjects are discussed in more detail elsewhere in this book.

Autoregulation and tubuloglomerular feedback (TGF)

GFR is maintained relatively constant (autoregulated) over a wide range of values of BP by a combination of autoregulation of RPF (see Chapter 3) and ΔP, the latter achieved by maintenance of a near constant P_{GC}. Constancy of ΔP is achieved by reciprocal variations in tone of R_A and R_E [7]. Renal autoregulation is the product of the myogenic effect (see Chapter 3) and the activity of the tubuloglomerular feedback (TGF) system. The basis

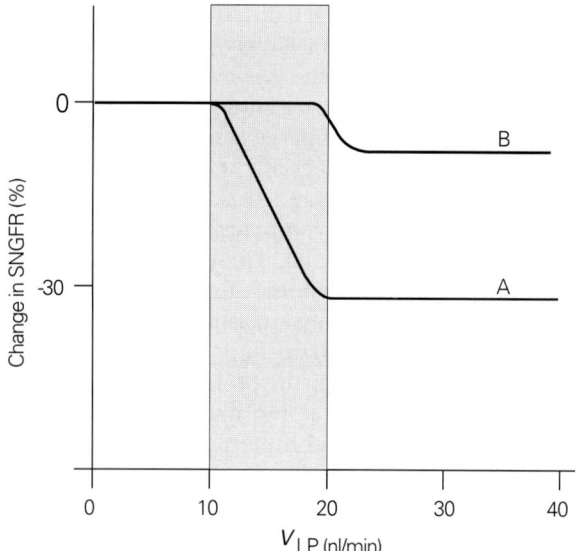

Figure 2.4 The relationship between SNGFR and the rate of fluid delivery through the loop of Henle (V_{LP}) to the macula densa in a normal animal with intact tubuloglomerular feedback, TGF (curve A) and in a volume-expanded animal with suppressed TGF (curve B). The shaded area denotes the normal operating range of the TGF.

of TGF is that fluid arriving at the early distal tubule is 'sensed' at the macula densa and that delivery of fluid to the macula densa is regulated at a 'set point', by control of filtration rate, via control of R_A. As shown in Figure 2.4, the TGF system has little impact on SNGFR when tubular flow is very low but in the normal operating range of tubular flow (shaded area) a small increase produces a marked fall in SNGFR, as shown by curve A. The maximum reduction in SNGFR due to activation of TGF is obtained in the physiologic flow range, thus supernormal values of tubular flow have no further impact on SNGFR under normal conditions (curve A). The TGF-mediated reduction in SNGFR results both from falls in Q_A and ΔP, secondary to increases in R_A. The reduction in SNGFR serves to lower tubule flow rate to the 'set point' of the macula densa.

Clearly, TGF is a volume regulatory system which serves to conserve fluid by regulation of filtered load, in the normal animal. In states of volume expansion, the TGF system is suppressed (curve B, Figure 2.4), which enables maintenance of SNGFR during increased intubule flow, thereby allowing filtration and excretion of the excess volume.

Control of TGF is extremely complex, involving many vasoactive hormones. The precise nature of the signal at the macula densa and the effector mechanism by which alteration in R_A are achieved remain uncertain but TGF is clearly an important physiologic regulatory mechanism both for autoregulation and volume homeostasis [15].

Permselectivity

The unique structure of the glomerular capillary wall allows a high rate of fluid filtration without significant filtration of the larger plasma proteins. There is at present no consensus on the principal site of restriction to the passage of macromolecules; there is evidence for a series of restrictive structures across the entire glomerular wall, from the lamina rara internal to the filtration slit diaphragm. The increasing restriction to filtration with increasing molecular size, from very high permeability to small molecules (water, electrolytes, glucose) to the virtual exclusion of large plasma proteins, is termed **permselectivity**. Molecular size is usually expressed as the Stokes–Einstein radius (SER in Å), the radius of a rigid sphere which would encounter the same frictional resistance to movement through water as the macromolecule. For linear molecules such as dextrans, restricted glomerular filtration relative to water begins at molecular sizes between 15 and 20 Å, about 60 kDa molecular weight. Serum albumin has an SER of 36 Å and its fractional filtration (relative to inulin with an SER of about 14 Å) is <0.001.

Although plasma proteins are the obvious molecules of interest in the study of renal disease, tubular and glomerular epithelial cell reabsorption complicates the interpretation of urinary protein excretion as an index of glomerular protein filtration. Therefore, glomerular permselectivity is studied experimentally by means of the fractional clearance of test macromolecules (dextrans, polyvinylpyrrolidone, etc.) which are filtered at the

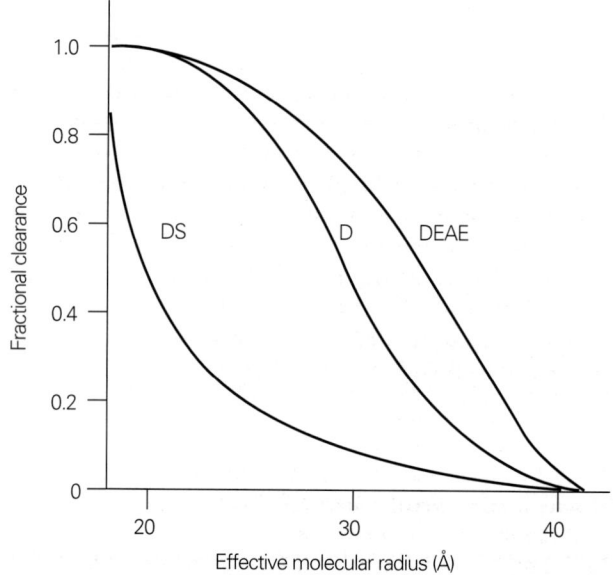

Figure 2.5 The relationship between fractional clearance of dextran (D) (i.e. clearance of dextran/clearance of inulin) over a range of molecular sizes, expressed as the Stokes–Einstein radius, for neutral, anionic (dextran sulfate, DS) and cationic (DEAE) dextrans, in the normal rat.

glomerulus and are neither secreted nor reabsorbed in the tubule. Examples of the fractional clearance profile (or sieving curve) for three species of dextrans, neutral, anionic and cationic, over a range of molecular size, are given in Figure 2.5. Although the data shown in Figure 2.5 were obtained in rats, fractional clearances for test molecules (sieving coefficients) are similar in humans and dogs.

Passage of macromolecules through the glomerular capillary wall results from both **convective** and **diffusive** movement. Convective transport (solvent drag) is proportional to the plasma concentration of the molecule and the water filtration rate. The diffusive component is the usual quantity described by the Fick equation, in which flux is proportional to the transmembrane concentration gradient and a membrane permeability/diffusion coefficient. Transcapillary flux is thus influenced by hemodynamic factors (inasmuch as they control GFR) as well as the intrinsic permeability of the capillary wall to the macromolecule.

Filtration is also influenced by other characteristics of the macromolecule in addition to its molecular size, i.e. shape, flexibility and charge. Albumin (a polyanion in physiologic solution) is much more restricted than Ficoll® (a neutral, globular polysaccharide) of equivalent SER and Ficoll® is less permeant than an equivalent mol-

ecular weight, branch-chain dextran. Positively and negatively charged dextrans have, respectively, greater and lesser fractional clearances than neutral dextran of the same SER (Figure 2.5). Such **charge selectivity** has been attributed to the presence of fixed negative charges in glomerular basement membrane (GBM), and both pore size (permeability) and fixed charges alter in some forms of renal disease, contributing to the development of proteinuria [16].

Mathematical models of the process of macromole filtration have been useful adjuncts in understanding the physical basis for proteinuria. Models have been developed of hindered transport of macromolecules through a porous membrane, most recently describing several **heteroporous** models including the log-normal pore size distribution and the isoporous plus shunt model. In the latter, flux of water and smaller molecules through the capillary wall is predominantly through a large population of pores of equal radius with a small fraction (<<1%) of the filtrate – but much of the flux of large molecules – passing through non-selective **shunts**. Most studies using this model have found that the majority of the increased macromolecule filtration in proteinuric diseases can be attributed to increases in the shunt [17]. Ultrastructurally, however, neither shunts nor pores have been identified in the GBM.

References

1. Gottschalk, C. (1992) Introduction: a history of renal physiology of 1950, in *The Kidney. Physiology and Pathophysiology*, 2nd edn (eds D.W. Seldin and G. Giebisch), Raven Press, New York, pp. 1–29.
2. Smith, H.W. (1951) *The Kidney: Structure and Function in Health and Disease*. Oxford University Press, New York.
3. Dworkin, L.D. and Brenner, B.M. (1992) Biophysical basis of glomerular filtration, in *The Kidney. Physiology and Pathophysiology*, 2nd edn (eds D.W. Seldin and G. Giebisch), Raven Press, New York, pp. 979–1016.
4. Florijn, K.W., Barendregt, J.N.M., Lentjes, E.G.W.M *et al.* (1994) Glomerular filtration rate measurement by 'single-shot' injection of inulin. *Kidney Int.*, **46**, 252–9.
5. Cameron, J.S. (1992) Renal function testing, in *Oxford Textbook of Clinical Nephrology* (eds J.S. Cameron, A.M. Davison, J.P. Grunfeld *et al.*), Oxford University Press, Oxford, New York, pp. 24–49.
6. Mitch, W.E., Walser, M., Buffington, G.A. and Lemann, J. Jr (1976) A simple method of estimating progression of chronic renal failure. *Lancet*, **ii**, 1326–8.
7. Baylis, C. (1986) Glomerular filtration dynamics, in *Advances in Renal Physiology* (ed. C.J. Lote), Grune & Stratton, London, pp. 33–83.
7a. Deen, W.M., Robertson, C.R. and Brenner, B.M. (1972) A model of glomerular ultrafiltration in the rat. *Am. J. Physiol.*, **223**, 1178–83.
8. Savin, V.J. and Terreros, D.A. (1981) A study of filtration in single isolated mammalian glomeruli. *Kidney Int.*, **20**, 188–97.
9. Myers, B.D., Peterson, C., Milona, C. *et al.* (1988) Role of

cardiac atria in the human renal response to changing plasma volume. *Am. J. Physiol.*, **254**, F562–73.
10. Kopp, U.C. and DiBona, G.F. (1992) The neural control of renal function, in *The Kidney. Physiology and Pathophysiology*, 2nd edn (eds D.W. Seldin and G. Giebisch), Raven Press, New York, pp. 1157–204.
11. Baylis, C. (1993) Renal responses to acute angiotensin II (AII) inhibition and administered AII in the ageing, conscious chronically catheterized rat. *Am. J. Kidney Dis.*, **22**, 842–50.
12. Raij, L. and Baylis, C. (1995) Glomerular actions of nitric oxide. Editorial review for *Kidney Int.* **48**, 20–32.
13. O'Connor, W.J. (1982) *Normal Renal Function*, Croom Helm, London.
14. Brenner, B.M. and Chertow, G.M. (1994) Congenital oligonephropathy and the etiology of adult hypertension and progressive renal injury. *Am. J. Kidney Dis.*, **23**, 171–5.
15. Schnermann, J. and Briggs, J.P. (1992) Function of the juxtaglomerular apparatus: control of glomerular hemodynamics and renin secretion, in *The Kidney. Physiology and Pathophysiology,* 2nd edn (eds D.W. Seldin and G. Giebisch), Raven Press, New York, pp. 1249–90.
16. Gausch, A., Deen, W.M. and Myers, B.D. (1993) Charge selectivity of the glomerular filtration barrier in healthy and nephrotic humans. *J. Clin. Invest.*, **92**, 2274–82.
17. Deen, W.M., Bridges, C.R., Brenner, B.M. and Myers, B.D. (1985) Heteroporous model of glomerular size selectivity: application to normal and nephrotic humans. *Am. J. Physiol.*, **249**, F374–89.

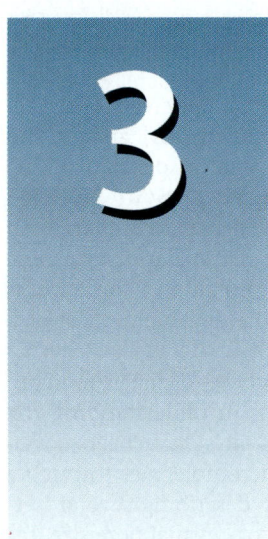

3

The renal circulation

Kevin V. Lemley and Chris Baylis

Introduction

The renal circulation is unique. The vasculature of the kidney contains two capillary networks in series, each preceded by an arteriole, and there are marked differences in vascular organization and blood flow between cortex and medulla. The renal perfusion rate is very high, about one-fifth of the cardiac output, even though the kidneys together comprise less than 0.5% of the total body mass.

There are many regulatory systems which influence renal blood flow. One important feature of this regulation is the ability of the kidney to maintain a nearly constant rate of perfusion, despite changes in systemic or renal perfusion pressures (autoregulation). The renal circulation supports glomerular filtration and tubular secretion and, in addition, supplies the cells of the kidney with oxygen and substrates. Virtually all tubule transport in the kidney is linked to the reabsorption of sodium, which is tightly correlated to O_2 consumption. Since normally >99% of the filtered sodium is reabsorbed, a change in renal blood flow will result in parallel changes in O_2 consumption. As a result the arteriovenous difference in O_2 tension remains remarkably constant. It is this characteristic that is essential for the regulation of erythropoietin production, another important function of the kidney. In addition, renal blood flow is an important factor in the control of systemic blood pressure through the renin–angiotensin system and in water balance by way of its effects on the concentration of the urine.

Vascular structure

The renal artery originates from the aorta and branches into two or three main divisions just before entering the kidney which then give rise to the **interlobar** arteries. In the renal parenchyma these in turn give rise to the **arcuate** arteries which follow a curved course parallel to the cortical surface. The **interlobular** arteries (also called **cortical radial** arteries) branch off of the arcuate arteries as a series of small muscular vessels which ascend through the cortex and supply the **afferent arterioles**. These are resistance vessels, although in the segment closest to the glomerulus, granular (renin-containing) cells replace the vascular smooth muscle cells. The glomerulus is an unusual, spherical or 'basket-like' capillary structure and the cortical glomeruli (located in the outer two-thirds of the cortex) are smaller than the inner cortical or juxtamedullary glomeruli. The **efferent arteriole**, leading from the glomerulus, lacks granular cells and the muscle layer of the efferent arteriole becomes increasingly incomplete and sparse along its course.

The efferent arterioles divide into the **peritubular capillaries** (in the outer cortex) and the juxtamedullary efferent arterioles give rise to **vasa recta** capillaries. The peritubular capillaries comprise an anastomotic network which forms a dense plexus surrounding the tubules. The vasa recta descend as relatively straight vessels to various depths within the renal medulla. Many of the **descending** vasa recta traverse the outer medulla within discrete **vascular bundles** and form a countercurrent array with

Nephrology, Edited by Rex L. Jamison and Robert Wilkinson.
Published in 1997 by Chapman & Hall, London. ISBN 0 412 60930 4

the thinner-walled **ascending** vasa recta from the inner medulla. Only a sparse plexus interconnects ascending and descending vessels within the inner medulla. Blood leaves the kidney via a system of veins which accompany the corresponding arteries.

Methods of measurement

Advances in our understanding of the various functions of the renal circulation have often followed improvements in techniques to quantitate renal perfusion. Over the last century, such techniques have evolved from unreliable and clinically inapplicable invasive methodologies (e.g. plethysmography) to repeatable and clinically applicable, non-invasive techniques (e.g. *p*-aminohippurate (PAH) clearance). The development of methods to measure urinary clearances of phenol red, diodrast and various derivatives of hippuric acid (e.g. PAH) in the 1930s by Van Slyke, Shannon, Goldring, Smith and their colleagues enabled renal plasma flow (RPF) and renal blood flow (RBF) to be measured reliably in humans. Using these techniques, RBF responses to many stimuli (renal denervation, water diuresis, pain, ingested protein, changes in perfusion pressure, and infusions of epinephrine, renin and other substances) were examined in the 1930s and 1940s. More recently, classical clearances as well as flow probe telemetry have been used to determine RBF in conscious, chronically instrumented experimental animals, an approach which avoids the confounding effects of anesthesia and surgical trauma.

The first methods (late 1950s and early 1960s) allowing estimation of regional blood flows used dye transit times and ^{133}Xe/^{85}Kr and H_2 washouts. These techniques were used for comparison of medullary and cortical blood flows in conditions such as hypotensive hemorrhage as well as to investigate the relationship of medullary perfusion to urine concentration. Because of difficulties in interpretation, these techniques have largely been abandoned; recently, more reliable imaging methods capable of measuring regional blood flows have become available. Other experimental techniques used to measure total and regional blood flow in the kidney have included various accumulation techniques (using markers such as ^{86}Rb, radiolabeled erythrocytes, microspheres and albumin), electromagnetic flow probes, and techniques for the determination of both single capillary and local blood flows (two-slit videophotometric and laser Doppler, respectively). Unfortunately, inherent limitations affect most of these techniques [1].

In the last 10–15 years, cell biological, molecular biological and morphological techniques have been used to analyze components of renal vascular regulatory processes: *in situ* videophotometric determination of changes in microvessel diameters in response to various agents; probes of vascular mRNA expression of many regulatory enzymes, hormones and receptors; specific pharmacologic inhibitors of a large number of mediator systems; and vascular cell culture, to name just a few.

Clinical measurement of renal perfusion

Assessment of renal perfusion is not necessary for most renal patients; it may, however, be important in the evaluation of hypertension and renal vascular disease, transplant dysfunction (e.g. in distinguishing acute rejection from obstruction), arterial or venous thrombosis and acute renal failure. Both quantitative and qualitative methods for determining RBF have been developed.

Quantitative methods currently find their application for the most part in clinical research. The most frequently used quantitative technique has been the PAH clearance. This method is based on the Fick principle, namely that the rate of removal of PAH from the renal circulation is equal to its rate of urinary excretion:

$$\text{RPF}_{ra} \times [\text{PAH}]_{ra} - \text{RPF}_{rv} \times [\text{PAH}]_{rv} = V \times [\text{PAH}]_u \qquad (3.1)$$

In practice, several simplifying assumptions and approximations are made: renal arterial plasma flow (RPF_{ra}) is equal to renal venous plasma flow (RPF_{rv}), the renal arterial PAH concentration ($[\text{PAH}]_{ra}$) is equal to the systemic plasma concentration $[\text{PAH}]_p$ and the renal extraction ratio, $E = ([\text{PAH}]_{ra} - [\text{PAH}]_{rv})/[\text{PAH}]_{ra}$, is constant. Thus, if the renal clearance of PAH, C_{PAH}, is given by

$$C_{PAH} = V \times [\text{PAH}]_u / [\text{PAH}]_p \qquad (3.2)$$

where V = urine flow rate and $[\text{PAH}]_u$ = urinary concentration of PAH, then

$$\text{RPF} = C_{PAH}/E \qquad (3.3)$$

Finally, renal blood flow is related to RPF by

$$\text{RBF} = \text{RPF}/(1 - \text{Hct}) \qquad (3.4)$$

where Hct is the hematocrit.

PAH is cleared by the kidney both by glomerular filtration and by active uptake from the peritubular capillary blood in the pars recta of the proximal tubule with subsequent secretion. When plasma PAH concentration is below the proximal tubular transport maximum, renal extraction of PAH is a constant proportion of renal plasma flow (~85–90%). Plasma PAH is not cleared completely because a small portion of the total renal blood flow perfuses the inner medulla which lacks the pars recta segment of the tubule, leading to incomplete extraction of PAH. When uncorrected for PAH extraction, C_{PAH} is referred to as the effective renal plasma flow (ERPF). It is important to be aware that renal PAH extraction may be less than the normal value of ~90%, especially in renal or cardiac disease [2]. A potential endogenous marker of renal perfusion has been described recently: 5-hydroxyindole acetic acid (5-HIAA), a major metabolite of serotonin [3]. The morning fasting plasma concentration of 5-HIAA varies inversely with C_{PAH} in both renal patients and healthy controls. The metabolite is an endogenous product and is eliminated in large part by glomerular filtration and tubular secretion. Therefore, the plasma concentration of 5-HIAA provides a rough index of RBF, much as the serum creatinine concentration does for GFR, without requiring an infusion or clearance study.

Doppler ultrasonography has been used to quantify blood flow in the main renal arteries, although it tends to overestimate RBF (due to overestimating vessel cross-sectional area). Intrarenal vascular resistivity has been examined by Doppler waveform analysis, and comparison of left and right kidney indices provides a sensitive and specific method for detecting severe (>60%) grades of unilateral renal artery stenosis. The reliability of these techniques is dependent on the skill of the operator. Newer methods based on imaging (such as cine ultrafast computed tomography (CT) and phase-contrast cine magnetic resonance imaging (MRI) – see Chapter 21) have recently been developed. Traditionally, imaging methods such as angiography, MRI and CT have been used to identify regions of stenosis in the renal arterial tree, although this morphologic assessment may not indicate the actual physiologic significance of the stenosis. This has motivated the development of functional imaging systems. These techniques provide a measure of perfusion **per unit tissue volume**, as well as the possibility of regional perfusion assessment. With MRI, excellent agreement with C_{PAH} may be achieved when the effects of respiratory motion are controlled [4]. Despite ongoing advances, these new methods have not yet been fully validated and an accurate, non-invasive method applicable to everyday clinical practice is still not available.

The most commonly used approaches of assessing renal perfusion in clinical settings are **semiquantitative and qualitative** methods. Traditionally, first phase intravenous pyelography (IVP) has been used. More recently, nuclear renography with ^{99m}Tc-DTPA (diethylene triamine penta-acetic acid) or MAG_3 (mercapto-acetyl-triglycine) and qualitative Doppler ultrasonography have gained acceptance (see Chapter 21).

Renal blood flow values

Renal perfusion comprises about 20% of the resting cardiac output, about $1000\,ml/min/1.73\,m^2$ body surface area (BSA). There are significant differences in RBF between men and women: 1209 ± 256 SD $ml/min/1.73$ m^2 BSA for men (RPF $654 \pm 163\,ml/min/1.73\,m^2$) vs. $982 \pm 184\,ml/min/1.73\,m^2$ BSA for women (RPF $592 \pm 153\,ml/min/1.73\,m^2$). Note that even allowing for differences in body size, gender differences in renal perfusion remain. Values of RBF also show rather wide variation even among healthy individuals. On average, total renal perfusion is about $4\,ml/min/g$ tissue weight in man and in other mammals, which is about four times the perfu-

sion rate of exercising muscle and eight times that of the brain. The approximate regional distribution of renal blood flow is 90% cortical and 10% medullary, with ~1% to the inner medulla (or papilla). Cortical perfusion is also greater (~8×) than medullary perfusion on a tissue volume basis, in normal humans and dogs, when measured using ultrafast cine CT with a rapid contrast bolus [5].

Effects of age

Renal blood flow changes significantly with age. Renal perfusion is low in the fetus (1–$2\,ml/min/g$ at 20 weeks) and there is a rapid increase in ERPF in newborns from $80\,ml/min/1.73\,m^2$ BSA at term, to $300\,ml/min/1.73\,m^2$ during the first three months of life. This is followed by a more gradual increase until 'adult' levels (normalized for BSA) are reached by 12–24 months of age. These changes are due mostly to falling renal vascular resistance, although increases in cardiac output and systemic blood pressure also play a role. There is also an increase in the extraction ratio for PAH (from 60% to 95%) between the neonatal period and five months of age, which results in an increase in C_{PAH} in excess of the actual increase in RPF. With advancing age, after maturity, there is a decrease in renal blood flow of about 10% per decade from the fourth decade onward, in men. Age-dependent decrements in renal hemodynamics are delayed in women (see Chapter 15).

Segmental vascular resistances and physical factors

Although the main sites of the total renal vascular resistance (RVR) have traditionally been ascribed to the pre- and postglomerular arterioles, there is evidence for substantial pressure drops in the pre-arteriolar vessels in the superficial cortical circuits of the rat. It is unclear whether or not this occurs in larger animals and man [6] (Figure 3.1). There is now considerable evidence from animal studies that the level of tone in the preglomerular and postglomerular arterioles can be independently regulated. This has relevance to the control of glomerular filtration, as discussed in Chapter 2. Unlike smaller animals such as the rat, the postarteriolar venous vessels may account for a substantial amount of total renal vascular resistance in man [7]. The perfusion of each region of the kidney is determined by the arteriovenous blood pressure gradient and the total segmental resistance of that region. There is no evidence that an alteration in vascular resistance in one part of the kidney directly affects perfusion of any other part. Medullary blood flow, for example, seems in many cases to be regulated independently of cortical blood flow. Therefore, as Aukland pointed out over 20 years ago, the phrase 'redistribution of renal blood flow' (implying the partition of some fixed quantity of total renal blood flow) should be abandoned.

In the phenomenon of **plasma skimming**, the axial

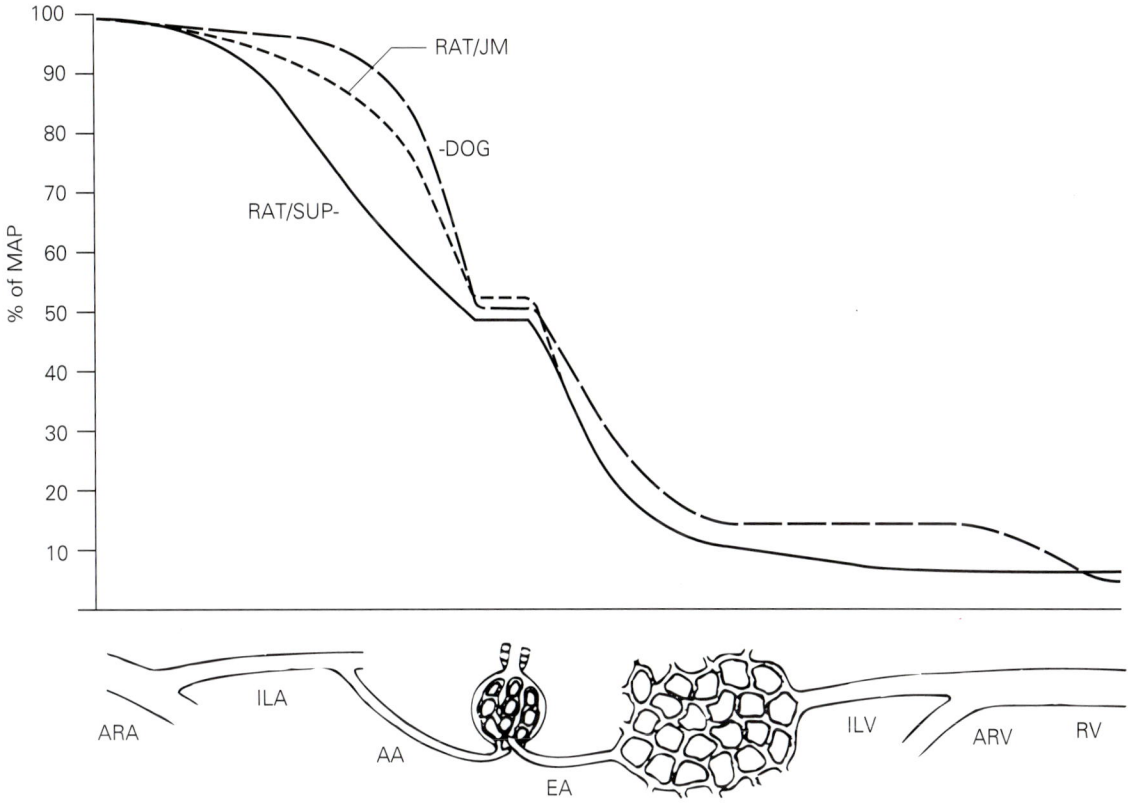

Figure 3.1 Pressure profile along the renal vasculature in dog and rat in both superficial cortical (SUP) and juxtamedullary (JM) glomeruli and associated vessels. MAP, mean arterial pressure; ARA, arcuate artery; ILA, interlobular artery; AA, afferent arteriole; EA, efferent arteriole; ILV, interlobular vein; ARV, arcuate vein; RV, renal vein. (Reproduced, with permission, from ref. 6.)

flow of erythrocytes in the interlobular (cortical radial) arteries and the acute (>90°) angle made by many juxtamedullary afferent arterioles branching from these arteries lead to the delivery of relatively low-hematocrit blood to the medullary circuits. A low hematocrit protects against 'sludging' of erythrocytes in the high osmolality environment of the medulla, but may also contribute to the low oxygen tension in that region [9]. The geometry of the renal vascular tree also influences blood rheology and shear forces at the vessel wall. Stagnation points and regions of flow separation (formation of local eddies or backflow, e.g. at vessel branch points) may be areas of increased residence time for platelets and leukocytes, allowing increased interaction with the endothelium. As in other parts of the circulation, platelet–endothelium interactions are shear-rate dependent [9]. Shear forces, those forces by which the flow of a viscous fluid exerts traction on the walls of a vessel, have a major impact on vascular endothelial cells. These endothelial responses to shear include rearrangement of the actin cytoskeletons [10]; shear stress-dependent gene expression of many proteins, including intercellular adhesion molecule-1 (ICAM-1), platelet-derived growth factor-B (PDGF-B) and nitric oxide synthase [9, 11]; and enhanced tonic release of

nitric oxide and prostacyclin, which in turn mediates flow-dependent vasodilation, as in post-stenotic vasodilation. Increased endothelial shear forces can result both from increases in the rate of blood flow and from reductions in vessel diameter [6, 9].

Regulation of renal blood flow

The circulation of the kidney is regulated by a variety of neural, humoral, endothelial and autocoid systems which play a role in control of several different renal functions. These systems may act independently or may interact at the level of second messengers (cAMP, cGMP), intracellular enzyme cascades (phospholipases, phosphokinases) or final intracellular effectors ($[Ca]_i$). Cellular mechanisms and second messengers are considered in detail in Chapter 13. In addition, several vascular regulatory systems also act on the tubule, including atrial natriuretic peptide, prostaglandins, angiotensin II, neural, and dopaminergic systems. Below, we consider the vascular actions of some of these systems in the kidney. Specific actions influencing glomerular filtration are considered in Chapter 2.

Autoregulation

The maintenance of tissue perfusion at optimal levels depends on both central and local control systems which regulate cardiac function, vascular tone and blood volume. The rapid (30–45 s), autonomous adjustment of vascular resistance in an organ or tissue, which results in a nearly constant perfusion rate and tissue blood pressure, is known as autoregulation (Figure 3.2). The adjustments in local vascular resistance are independent of neural or humoral signals from the rest of the body. Under basal conditions, the renin–angiotensin system (RAS) does not seem to have a pivotal role in RBF autoregulation, though it may be important for regulation of medullary blood flow. Two distinct autoregulatory systems are involved in RBF autoregulation: the **myogenic mechanism** [12] and **tubuloglomerular feedback** (TGF) [13]. The latter regulatory system is unique to the kidney.

With the **myogenic** mechanism, blood flow itself is not directly regulated but rather resistance vessel wall tension, which is the product of the transmural hydrostatic pressure difference and the vessel radius. In response to increased intraluminal pressure, the vessel constricts in order to maintain a constant wall tension. This raises segmental vascular resistance and attenuates the downstream transmission of the elevated pressure. Blood flow autoregulation results from the return to normal intravascular pressures at some point in the arterial tree, leading to a normal blood pressure gradient and thus flow rate from that point onward. Myogenic responses are present in the afferent arteriole and the pre-

arteriolar arteries of the kidney. If these resistance vessels function as series-coupled independent effectors, vascular radius adjustment should propagate just far enough downstream to fully attenuate the proximal pressure increment [12]. This restricts the upper and lower limits of myogenic autoregulation in shorter, juxtamedullary circuits [6].

In the **TGF** system, the tone of the preglomerular arteriole is controlled by solute delivery to the early distal tubule, sensed by the macula densa (see Chapter 2). The myogenic and TGF systems assure that acute changes in renal perfusion pressure within the autoregulatory range lead to compensatory adjustments in preglomerular arterial/arteriolar resistance to maintain constant blood flow. Postglomerular resistance changes little in these circumstances. There is evidence that the RBF autoregulatory system can be reset, acutely, by hormonal mediators and extracellular fluid volume status. TGF may also be chronically reset by 'work hypertrophy' of the thick ascending limb of Henle's loop (decreasing distal delivery of NaCl for the same filtered load). Details of GFR autoregulation have been considered in Chapter 2.

Although blood flow to the cortex is efficiently autoregulated, there is evidence that autoregulation of medullary blood flow is limited [14] (Figure 3.2). Studies in the rat show that vasa recta (papillary) blood flow autoregulation is greatly attenuated compared to cortical blood flow (and total RBF, not shown). In addition, unlike the cortical peritubular microcirculation, hydrostatic pressures within the vasa recta of the inner medulla are not autoregulated. Increased vasa recta pressure and flow during acute increases in renal perfusion pressure probably results in increased medullary and cortical interstitial hydrostatic pressures. This in turn leads to reduced tubular sodium reabsorption at several sites, and thence increased urinary sodium excretion. This may be the basis for the phenomenon of pressure natriuresis (Figure 3.3). In several forms of hypertension, the medullary resistance vessels are constricted and therefore attenuate increases in renal interstitial hydrostatic pressure in response to increased perfusion pressure. This shifts the pressure natriuresis curve (the plot of urinary sodium excretion against renal perfusion pressure, Figure 3.3) to the right and may play a role in the development and/or maintenance of the hypertension [14].

Renal nerves

In general, the nervous system plays only a minor physiologic role in regulating RBF although the renal vasculature receives extensive adrenergic innervation. Receptors are mostly α_1-type, but α_2, β_1, and dopaminergic (DA$_1$ and DA$_2$, and possibly other subtypes) have been reported as well as receptors for serotonin, neuropeptide Y, vasoactive intestinal peptide and substance P. Stimulation of the various receptors leads both to vasodilatory (DA$_1$, β_1) and vasoconstrictor (α_1, serotonergic) actions. Dopamine acts as a vasodilator at low concentrations (<10 µg/kg/min, an

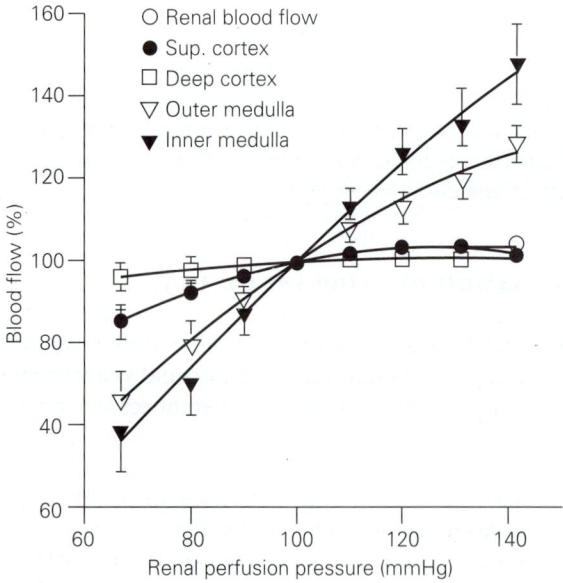

Figure 3.2 Autoregulation of whole kidney blood flow and regional blood flows in superficial and deep cortex, outer and inner medulla of the volume-expanded rat. Regional blood flows were measured using implanted fiber-optic probes and laser-Doppler flowmetry. (Reproduced, with permission, from ref. 14.)

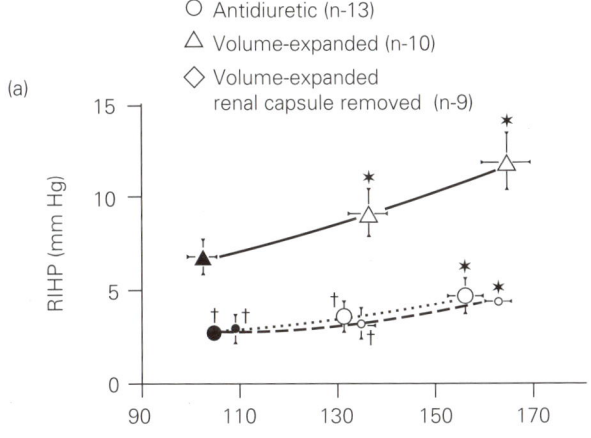

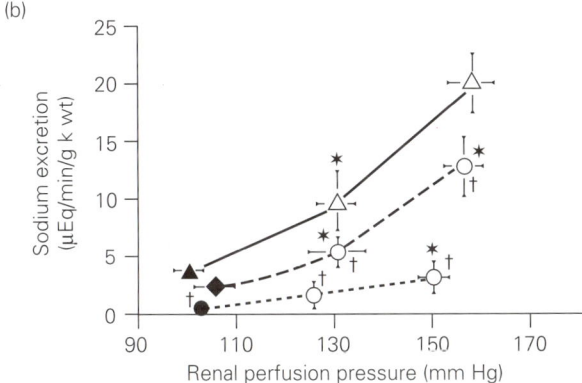

Figure 3.3 The relationship between renal perfusion pressure and (a) the renal excretion of sodium and (b) renal interstitial hydrostatic pressure (RIHP), in the antidiuretic and volume-expanded rat, with and without the renal capsule intact. In antidiuresis (○) the slopes of the pressure natriuresis relationship and the increase in RIHP with increasing renal perfusion pressure are both less steep than in the volume-expanded rat (△). After removal of the renal capsule (◇), the increases in RIHP and sodium excretion, with volume expansion, are attenuated. (Reproduced, with permission, from ref. 14.)

effect due to DA_1 receptor occupancy) and predominantly as a vasoconstrictor at higher concentrations (due to α-adrenoceptor occupancy and β-adrenoceptor-mediated renin release) [15].

Renal nerve stimulation above a threshold frequency leads to renal arteriolar constriction; the site of action is the preglomerular resistance vessels, and to a lesser extent the proximal efferent arteriole. Renal nerve activity seems to be responsible for the variation in renal blood flow with different levels of normal activity in conscious, unrestrained rats [16]. Neural mechanisms may also underlie increases in renal vascular resistance in humans in response to physical and mental stress, exercise and assumption of the upright posture [17]. With these exceptions, however, renal nerve activity has little direct physiologic role in the control of RBF: for example, basal renal vascular resistance is not altered following renal dener-

vation. Interactions with other regulatory systems are important; β_1 agonists stimulate renin release, and norepinephrine release from nerve terminals is enhanced by angiotensin II whereas dopamine (via DA_2 receptors) is inhibitory.

Vasoactive hormones and autocoids

Atrial natriuretic peptide (ANP) is a 28-amino acid vasoactive and natriuretic peptide released from cardiac atrial myocytes under the influence of stretch, as part of the low-pressure baroreceptor system [18]. The majority of its receptors in the kidney are C-type clearance receptors, giving ANP a short (3-minute) half-life in the circulation. The biologically active receptor on the larger renal vessels is part of a transmembrane (particulate) guanyl cyclase of the non-G protein type. This makes ANP unique as a peptide, endothelium-independent vasodilator with cGMP as a second messenger. The vascular actions of ANP in the kidney are complex since in the precontracted kidney ANP is vasodilatory, whereas in the basal state ANP has a mild vasoconstrictor action. There is evidence that ANP functions as a vasoconstrictor of cortical efferent arterioles, since ANP increases GFR via an elevation in glomerular capillary pressure even when total RPF changes little. Administration of ANP *in vivo* often leads to only a transient increase in renal blood flow, possibly due to the systemic hemodynamic (depressor) effects of the peptide. The medullary circulation seems to be more sensitive to the vasodilatory actions of ANP than that of the cortex.

The **renin–angiotensin system (RAS)** has many renal and systemic actions. We consider here some of the intrarenal vascular actions of the RAS. Renin release from granular cells of the juxtaglomerular portion of the afferent arteriole is influenced by numerous stimuli; it is decreased by stimuli which lead to increases in intracellular calcium concentration ($[Ca]_i$) and may be increased by cAMP-induced declines in $[Ca]_i$. In general, vasoconstrictors (angiotensin II, AVP, ET, α-agonists, substance P) inhibit renin release, as does adenosine. Vasodilators (PGI_2, β-agonists, bradykinin) for the most part stimulate renin release. On the other hand, the vasodilators ANP and possibly nitric oxide inhibit renin release and generally act as counterregulatory systems to the RAS in the kidney. Renin release is also stimulated by decreased afferent perfusion pressure and a decreased delivery of NaCl to the macula densa. These latter stimuli, together with β-adrenergic activation, represent the typical physiologic concomitants to volume depletion. The RAS itself modulates other vasoregulatory systems: angiotensin II (AII) leads to activation of the central sympathetic nervous system, increases release and decreases re-uptake of norepinephrine (NE) at adrenergic nerve terminals, and in subpressor doses enhances the reactivity of vascular smooth muslce to low concentrations of NE.

The final RAS product, AII, is a potent vasoconstrictor

of the renal vasculature and also a potent stimulant of vascular smooth muslce hypertrophy and hyperplasia, as well as extracellular matrix production. AII receptors (primarily AII_1) are widely distributed through the blood vessels of the kidney. There are some questions with respect to the relative sensitivities of the afferent and efferent arterioles to AII. In isolated vessel preparations and glomerular micropuncture studies, the afferent arteriole is less responsive than the efferent arteriole to exogenous AII. In other studies, a predominantly afferent or a balanced afferent/efferent site of action of AII has been suggested. In addition, the presence of an intact connection of the afferent arteriole to the glomerulus seems to be necessary for afferent constriction [19]. Since AII administration in the conscious animal or man invariably leads to decreased RPF and increased filtration fraction (and thus preservation of GFR), a predominant efferent arteriolar action of AII is indicated in these situations.

Studies of the actions of the RAS on the renal circulation must be interpreted carefully in light of several considerations. (1) The RAS has tubular actions in addition to its direct vascular effects; the former may influence RBF via their effects on TGF. (2) The vascular distribution of AII produced endogenously (i.e. within the periarterial lymphatic sheath) may differ substantially from that resulting from systemic or even intrarenal arterial administration of exogenous AII [20]. (3) Studies using inhibitors of angiotensin converting enzyme (ACE) may reflect, in part, the actions of increased levels of bradykinin, inasmuch as ACE is the bradykinin-degrading enzyme kininase II. Based on studies of AII inhibition in man, it seems that in normal, sodium-replete individuals the RAS system is not activated and does not substantially control either systemic or renal hemodynamics [9]. In states of volume depletion, during activation of the sympathetic nervous system and in some renal diseases, on the other hand, the RAS does contribute to basal renal and extrarenal vascular tone.

The **eicosanoids** are autocoids derived from arachidonic acid by the action of at least three different enzymes: (1) cyclo-oxygenase (prostaglandins (PG) and thromboxanes (TX)), (2) lipoxygenase (leukotrienes (LT), lipoxins (LX), hydroxyeicosatetraenoic acid (HETE)) and (3) P_{450}-NADPH oxidases (EET, HETE). The eicosanoids are synthesized by most renal cell types and the medullary production of PG per gram of tissue mass greatly exceeds cortical production. The principal prostaglandins in the kidney are PGE_2, $PGF_{2\alpha}$ and PGI_2. G-protein coupled receptors for various prostaglandins have recently been described, linked to several second messenger systems. Understanding the actions of the PG on the renal vasculature has been complicated by significant species differences.

In man, intravenous PGI_2 causes a decrease in RVR, whereas the PGE_1 analog misoprostol increases RVR, possibly due to PG-stimulated renin release [21]. It has been proposed that PG play a minimal role in maintaining RBF under basal conditions inasmuch as PG synthesis inhibition has no effect on blood flow or RBF autoregulation. This concept may need to be revised in light of studies which suggest a balanced vasoconstrictor (PGE) and vasodilator (PGI_2) effect on the renal vasculature. Many interactions exist with other vasoregulatory systems in the kidney. For example, PGI_2 and PGE both stimulate renin release. PG synthesis is stimulated by both vasodilatory (bradykinin) and vasoconstrictor (AII, AVP, ET, α-agonists) agents. In general, PGs act as counterregulatory vasodilators in the kidney, protecting the renal vasculature from excessive vasoconstriction. In settings of increased circulating levels of these vasopressor hormones, as in compensated congestive heart failure or in the fetus or neonate, inhibition of prostaglandin synthesis can lead to substantial decrements in renal perfusion. The role of PG in urine concentration and medullary blood flow regulation is considered in Chapter 6.

Actions of TX, LT, LX and HETE are less well understood. Although a role for the vasoconstrictor TXA_2 has been suggested in the action of AII, for the most part these vasoconstrictor and pro-inflammatory eicosanoids seem to have little or no role in the kidney under physiologic conditions.

Bradykinin (BK) is a nonapeptide autocoid with many effects in the kidney. It is released from its precursor kallidin by the enzyme kallikrein. Kallikrein mRNA is found at the vascular pole of the glomerulus and in the distal tubule. Vasodilatory B_1 and B_2 receptor subtypes have been described. Most high-affinity receptors are found within the renal medulla. Receptor activation leads to increased eicosanoid synthesis, resulting in vasodilation. Kinins in the bloodstream encounter the endothelium rather than vascular smooth muscle directly and may in fact bring about their primary vasoactive effects by stimulating endothelial synthesis of nitric oxide and PGI_2. There are species differences in primary sites of action. There are also interactions with other regulatory systems, including bradykinin-stimulated renin release and PG synthesis.

Nitric oxide (NO) is a free radical, enzymatically synthesized from L-arginine, which causes vasodilation via the production of cGMP. Basal and cytokine-stimulated NO synthesis have been reported throughout the kidney. Because of the short half-life of NO, the location of NO generation is a major determinant of its site of action. Within the cortical renal circulation, NO generated by the constitutive endothelial NO synthase participates in the regulation of the glomerular microcirculation via its actions on the preglomerular vasculature and on mesangial cells. In addition, NO generated by the macula densa and vascular smooth muscle cells in the afferent arteriole influences glomerular hemodynamics via TGF and by modulating renin release. When systemic NO production is blocked acutely, arterial blood pressure rises and both the preglomerular and postglomerular resistance vessels contract, even though the postglomerular resistance is not normally under tonic NO control. This implies the action of a secondary mechanism (currently unknown). Chronic NO blockade produces sustained hypertension and renal vasoconstriction, with the eventual development of glomerular damage and proteinuria. There is some evidence that NO deficiency may be causally involved in the genesis of salt-dependent hypertension. In addition to the effects of NO on the cortical circulation, NO is important in maintenance of medullary perfusion and NO inhibition impairs pressure natriuresis, without however significantly attenuating the autoregulatory ability of the kidney. Increased NO production may be involved in the early hemodynamic changes in diabetes, some forms of glomerulonephritis and in the physiologic hemodynamic responses to normal pregnancy [9].

Endothelin (ET) is a 21-amino acid peptide hormone made in vascular and tubular structures within the kidney [22]. It is an extremely potent vasoconstrictor which produces prolonged renal vasoconstriction after an initial and short-lived (NO-mediated) vasodilation. ET exists in three isoforms (ET-1, ET-2, and ET-3) and acts on different receptor subtypes ET_A, ET_B and possibly ET_C. Within the cortical microcirculation, ET constricts the mesangial cell and both preglomerular and postglomerular resistance vessels. As with AII, the relative potency of ET on the segmental arterioles is somewhat controversial. ET exerts its vasoconstrictor effects by triggering the phosphoinositide system and promoting calcium entry. It may also interact with other vasoregulatory systems, including the eicosanoids. In the peripheral vasculature, the vasoconstrictor actions of ET are mainly mediated by stimulation of the ET_A receptor, with ET_B stimulation providing the initial vasodilatory response via NO release. In the kidney, however, both vasoconstrictor and vasodilator responses to ET are predominantly mediated by ET_B receptors, at least in some species. There is increasing evidence that ET plays a pathogenic role in several types of renal injury, including cyclosporin- and ischemia-induced renal damage as well as some glomerular inflammatory states. Whether ET plays a physiologic role in control of renal function is not clear, although recent observations suggest that endogenous ET exerts a tonic vasodilatory action on the preglomerular vessels, presumably via NO- or eicosanoid-mediated effects [23]. A

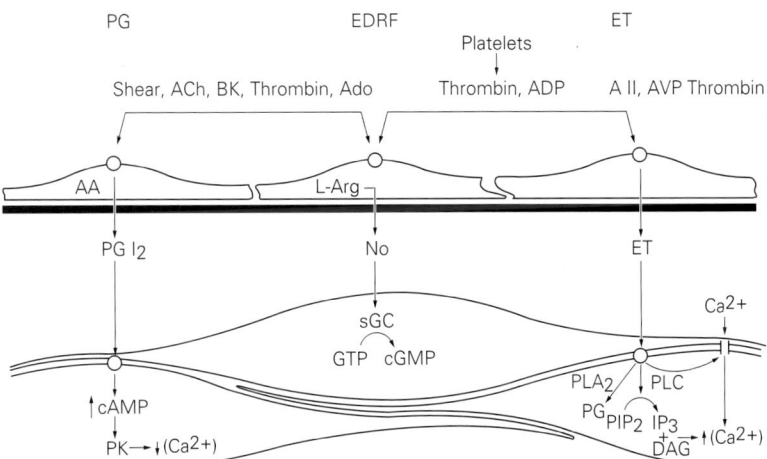

Figure 3.4 Simplified schematic representation of some of the endothelial systems controlling vascular smooth muscle cell contractility. The prostaglandins (PG) are represented by prostacyclin (PGI_2), formed from arachidonic acid (AA) which is released from membrane phospholipids by the action of phospholipase A_2 (PLA_2). In vascular smooth muscle, PGI_2 stimulates cAMP production which then activates a cascade involving protein kinase A (PK) resulting in decreased intracellular Ca^{2+}. Endothelium-derived relaxing factor (EDRF) is a non-eicosanoid vasodilator, now known to be nitric oxide (NO). NO derived from endothelial L-arginine diffuses to adjacent vascular smooth muscle where it activates cGMP formation by a soluble guanylate cyclase (sGC), leading to dephosphorylation of myosin light chains (MLC). NO also directly hyperpolarizes the cell via activation of a Ca^{2+}-dependent K^+ channel (not shown). Endothelin (ET) is a vasoconstrictor peptide made within endothelial cells. ET binds to receptors on the endothelium and causes release of NO (not shown), as well as PG synthesis via activation of PLA_2, phosphoinositol hydrolysis via phospholipase C (PLC) yielding 1,4,5-inositol trisphosphate (IP_3) and diacylglycerol (DAG), which in turn leads to release of Ca^{2+} from intracellular stores and activation of Ca^{2+} channels. Not all mediators are represented nor are all actions shown. (Reproduced with permission from ref. 4.)

summary of endothelium-based vasoregulatory systems is given in Figure 3.4.

There are a large number of other substances which also affect RBF although the physiologic significance of many is not apparent as yet. **Platelet activating factor** and **calcitonin gene-related peptide** produce renal vasodilation and **adenosine** has a biphasic action on RBF, pos-sibly reflecting different ligand affinities for the A_1 (vasoconstrictor) and A_2 (vasodilator) receptor types. **Arginine vasopressin** (AVP) is a nonapeptide hormone with vasoconstrictor (V_1) and antidiuretic (V_2) actions in the kidney. The ability of AVP to constrict afferent arterioles depends on synergism with AII in mobilizing intracellular calcium, and under physiologic conditions AVP has little influence on total or cortical RBF. Medullary blood flow is normally influenced by both V_1 and V_2 effects (both decrease blood flow). The vasoconstrictor action of AVP in the kidney is counteracted in large part (under physiologic conditions) by AVP-stimulated synthesis of vasodilatory PG.

Dietary protein and infused amino acids result in transient renal hyperemia. The acute phenomenon probably involves a complex mechanism in which DA_2 dopaminergic receptors, glucagon, hepatorenal neural efferents, NO and PG have all been suggested to participate. Chronic increases in RBF with high dietary protein intakes are associated with resetting of TGF. Alterations in RBF occur in normal pregnancy, aging and in response to sex hormones. These effects are discussed in Chapters 41 and 15.

Exogenous substances generally affect RBF by their effects on one of the above-mentioned physiologic regulatory systems. Cyclosporin A, for example, probably owes its vasoconstrictor effects to increased ET and decreased NO and PG synthesis, as a result of endothelial damage. It may also enhance adrenergic activity by decreasing NE re-uptake.

Functions of renal blood flow

The influence of renal blood flow on the process of glomerular filtration is considered in Chapter 2. Regulation of systemic blood pressure by the renin–angiotensin system of the kidney is considered in Chapter 13. Several other functions of renal perfusion will be considered briefly here.

Peritubular capillary circulation and proximal reabsorption

The peritubular capillaries return water and solutes reabsorbed by the tubules into the systemic circulation. Uptake of fluid by the peritubular capillaries is governed by Starling pressures: the gradients of oncotic and hydrostatic pressures across the capillary wall which act as the driving forces for transcapillary fluid movement. The Starling pressures within the cortical peritubular microcircu-

lation are determined in part by the filtration fraction. Filtration fraction determines the degree of hemoconcentration and thus the increase in the oncotic pressure of the blood due to the process of glomerular filtration. In addition, peritubular capillaries are controlled by the upstream and downstream vascular resistances, which determine the hydrostatic pressure within the peritubular capillaries. It was originally thought that the high oncotic pressure and low hydrostatic pressure of the postglomerular blood was the rate-limiting step in isotonic fluid reabsorption from the proximal nephron and that **glomerulotubular balance**, the matching of proximal tubule reabsorption to filtration, was a consequence of glomerular filtration and proximal fluid reabsorption being determined by the same physical forces. It is now clear, however, that peritubular capillary uptake of proximal tubular reabsorbate is not rate limiting for isotonic fluid reabsorption [24]. Rather, peritubular capillary Starling pressures exert their influence on proximal fluid reabsorption indirectly, by virtue of their effects on cortical interstitial oncotic and hydrostatic pressures. It is these **interstitial** Starling pressures which directly affect proximal fluid reabsorption, influencing rates of both transport and backleak, e.g. increases in interstitial hydrostatic pressure are associated with increased sodium excretion. The interstitial hydrostatic pressure is also influenced by events in the medullary circulation (see p. 39). The influence of peritubular capillary fluid reabsorption in the

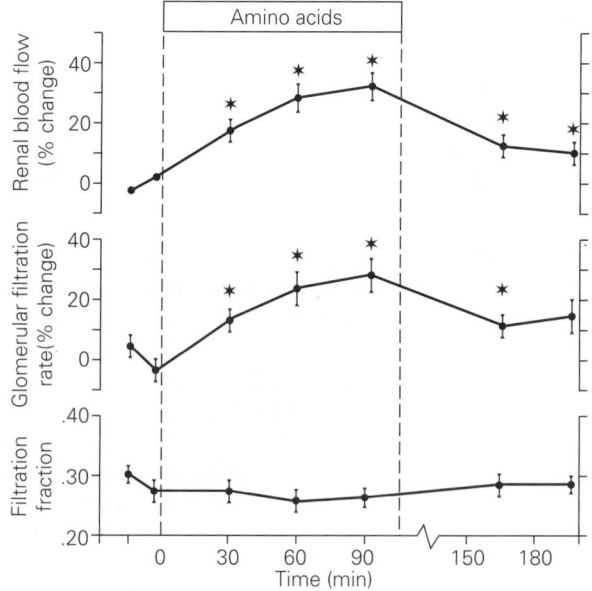

Figure 3.5 Effects of an intravenous infusion of mixed amino acids, 0.075 mmol/kg/min (equivalent to the amino acids present in a 10 g/kg meal of lean beef), in the normal, anesthetized dog, on renal blood flow, GFR and filtration fraction. (Reproduced, with permission, from Woods, L.L., Mizelle, H.L., Montani, J.P. and Hall, J.E. (1986) Mechanisms controlling renal hemodynamics and electrolyte excretion during amino acids. *Am. J. Physiol.*, **251**, F303–12.)

renal medulla on the process of urine concentration is considered in Chapter 6.

Another function of RBF is to sense and regulate the circulating red cell mass. Erythropoietin is synthesized by interstitial cells of the renal cortex. It is appropriate that a sensing system for arterial oxygenation should reside in a tissue with a blood supply so large that the local oxygen tension reflects systemic arterial pO_2 alone and not the effects of organ metabolism.

Peritubular blood flow supports tubular secretion of organic anions and cations, and of various drugs as well as supporting uptake and catabolism of several peptide hormones (insulin, glucagon, parathyroid hormone).

References

1. Pallone, T.L., Robertson, C.R. and Jamison, R.L. (1990) Renal medullary microcirculation. *Physiol. Rev.*, **70**, 885–920.

2. Battilana, C., Zhang, H., Olshen, R.A. *et al.* (1991) PAH extraction and estimation of plasma flow in diseased human kidneys. *Am. J. Physiol.*, **261**, F726–33.

3. Hannadouche, T., Laude, D., Déchaux, M. *et al.* (1989) Plasma 5-hydroxyindoleacetic acid as an endogenous index of renal plasma flow. *Kidney Int.*, **35**, 95–8.

4. Debatin, J.F., Ting, R.H., Wegmüller, H. *et al.* (1994) Renal artery blood flow: quantitation with phase-contrast MR imaging with and without breath holding. *Radiology*, **190**, 371–8.

5. Blomley, M.J.K., Kormano, M., Coulden, R. *et al.* (1994) Renal perfusion quantified with contrast-enhanced computed tomography. *Invest. Radiol.*, **29**(Suppl 2), S232–3.

6. Lemley, K.V. and Kriz, W. (1994) Structure and function of the renal vasculature, in *Renal Pathology: With Clinical and Functional Correlations*, 2nd edn (eds C.C. Tisher and B.M. Brenner), J.B. Lippincott Co., Philadelphia.

7. Willassen, Y. and Ofstad, J. (1979) Postglomerular vascular hydrostatic and oncotic pressures during acute saline volume expansion in normotensive man. *Scand. J. Clin. Lab. Invest.*, **39**, 707–15.

8. Brezis, M., Rosen, S., Silva, P. and Epstein, F.H. (1984) Renal ischemia: a new perspective. *Kidney Int.*, **26**, 375–83.

9. Raij, L. and Baylis, C. (1995) Glomerular actions of nitric oxide. *Kidney Int.*, **48**, 20–32.

10. Mulvany, M.J. and Aalkjær, C. (1990) Structure and function of small arteries. *Physiol. Rev.*, **70**, 921–61.

11. Nagel, T., Resnick, N., Atkinson, W.J. *et al.* (1994) Shear stress selectively upregulates intercellular adhesion molecule-1 expression in cultured human vascular endothelial cells. *J. Clin. Invest.*, **94**, 885–91.

12. Johnson, P.C. (1986) Autoregulation of blood flow. *Circ. Res.*, **59**, 483–95.

13. Schnermann, J. and Briggs, J.P. (1992) Function of the juxtaglomerular apparatus: control of glomerular hemodynamics and renin secretion, in *The Kidney: Physiology and Pathophysiology* (eds D.W. Seldin and G. Giebisch), Raven Press, New York, pp. 1249–89.

14. Roman, R.J. and Zou, A.-P. (1993) Influence of the renal medullary circulation on the control of sodium excretion. *Am. J. Physiol.*, **265**, R963–73.

15. Kopp, U.C. and DiBona, G.F. (1992) The neural control of renal function, in *The Kidney: Physiology and Pathophysiology* (eds D.W. Seldin and G. Giebisch), Raven Press, New York, pp. 1157–1204.

16. Grady, H.C. and Bullivant, E.M.A. (1992) Renal blood flow varies during normal activity in conscious unrestrained rats. *Am. J. Physiol.*, **262**, R926–32.

17. Tidgren, B., Hjemdahl, P., Theodorsson, E. and Nussberger, J. (1991) Renal neurohormonal and vascular responses to dynamic exercise in humans. *J. Appl. Physiol.*, **70**, 2279–86.

18. Wilkins, M.R. and Needleman, P. (1992) Effect of pharmacological manipulation of endogenous atriopeptin activity on renal function. *Am. J. Physiol.*, **262**, F161–7.

19. Weihprecht, H., Lorenz, J.N., Briggs, J.P. and Schnermann, J. (1991) Vasoconstrictor effect of angiotensin and vasopressin in isolated rabbit afferent arterioles. *Am. J. Physiol.*, **261**, F273–82.

20. Lemley, K.V. and Kriz, W. (1992) Intrarenal distribution pathways of the renin–angiotensin system, in *The Renin–Angiotensin System* (eds J.I.S. Robertson and M.G. Nicholls), Gower Medical Publishing, London.

21. Natov, S., Schmitt, F., Ikeni, A. *et al.* (1994) Opposite renal effects of a PGE_1 analog and prostacyclin in humans. *Kidney Int.*, **45**, 1457–64.

22. Simonson, M.S. and Dunn, M.J. (1993) Endothelin peptides and the kidney. *Annu. Rev. Physiol.*, **55**, 249–65.

23. Qiu, C., Samsell, L. and Baylis, C. (1994) Actions of endogenous endothelin (ET) on renal hemodynamics in the normal rat. *J. Am. Soc. Nephrol.*, **5**, 610A.

24. Wilcox, C.S., Baylis, C. and Wingo, C.S. (1992) Glomerular-tubular balance and proximal regulation, in *The Kidney: Physiology and Pathophysiology* (eds D.W. Seldin and G. Giebisch), Raven Press, New York, pp. 1807–41.

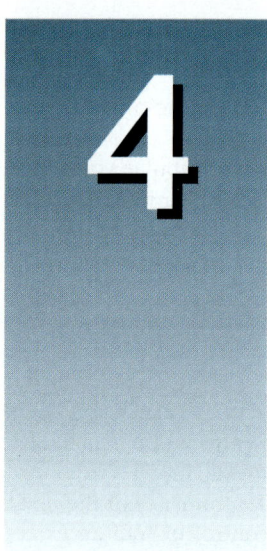

4

Ion transport by the renal tubule

Charles S. Wingo and I. David Weiner

Basic principles of ion transport

The kidney regulates body fluid and ion composition by the separate processes of glomerular filtration and renal tubular reabsorption and secretion. Many inorganic ions depend critically on renal tubular transport to maintain normal homeostasis. This chapter reviews the basic mechanisms of inorganic ion reabsorption and secretion along the nephron.

Ion transport may be active or passive. Passive transport between two compartments can occur due to differences of chemical concentration* or electrical potential (voltage). In the former case a chemical concentration gradient drives passive diffusion. In the latter case the electrical potential, or voltage, is the driving force. When two compartments differ in both chemical concentration and electrical potential the net passive movement of an ion will be determined by the electrochemical gradient, which vectorially sums each force to determine the net driving force for ion transport.

Transepithelial ion transport can be either paracellular or transcellular. Paracellular transport refers to the movement of ions through the tight junctions connecting adjacent cells. The paracellular pathway can, depending on the tissue, preferentially transport either cations or anions, and transport via this pathway is usually passive. Transcellular transport refers to the movement of ions across both the apical and basolateral membranes. Most transcellular ion transport requires the interaction of an ion with one or more membrane proteins, which may be generally classified as channels, pumps and transporters (Figure 4.1). These membrane proteins either facilitate ion movement down an electrochemical gradient (facilitated diffusion), use energy directly, generally from adenosine triphosphate (ATP) hydrolysis (primary active transport), or use the electrochemical gradient (or the chemical gradient for electroneutral transporters) for one molecule to move a second ion (secondary active transport). Transporters can be further subdivided into those that move two or more ions in the same direction, which are referred to as co-transporters or symporters, and those that move ions in opposite directions, which are referred to as exchangers or antiporters.

*Strictly speaking, it is the 'activity' and not the 'concentration' of an ion that determines the force for diffusion.

Nephrology, Edited by Rex L. Jamison and Robert Wilkinson.
Published in 1997 by Chapman & Hall, London. ISBN 0 412 60930 4

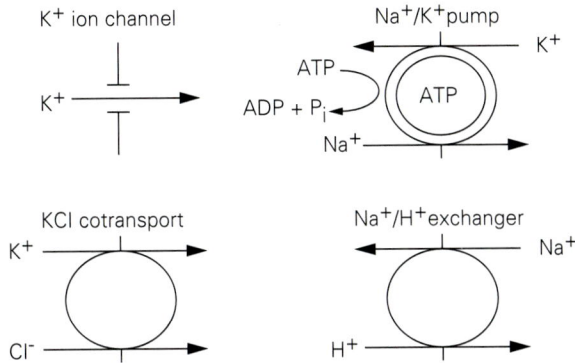

Figure 4.1 Examples of various mechanisms of ion transport.

Sodium and chloride transport along the nephron

Introduction

Na^+ and Cl^- represent the major extracellular cation and anion, respectively, and are the principal determinants of extracellular fluid (ECF) volume. Disturbances of NaCl balance predominantly result in disturbances in ECF volume. In contrast, disturbances in water balance are largely reflected in states of cellular dehydration (hypernatremia) or overhydration (hyponatremia). The kidney primarily regulates NaCl excretion, which is a major determinant, along with intake, of NaCl balance. Renal NaCl excretion, in turn, is determined by glomerular filtration rate (GFR) and the rate of tubular reabsorption. The kidney adjusts the rate of NaCl excretion largely in response to changes in the state of intravascular volume and not Na ion concentration $[Na^+]$, or Cl ion concentration $[Cl^-]$.

Proximal tubule

Under euvolemic conditions the proximal tubule reabsorbs ~60% of the glomerular ultrafiltrate. This segment is heterogeneous and consists of three anatomically defined regions referred to as S_1, S_2 and S_3 [1]. Accordingly, the mechanisms of volume reabsorption are qualitatively heterogeneous within the proximal tubule, and can be divided into those characteristic of the early proximal tubule and those characteristic of the late proximal tubule.

Early proximal tubule NaCl transport

The early proximal tubule exhibits some of the largest rates of Na, Cl and fluid reabsorption along the nephron. Fluid absorption in the proximal tubule is largely isotonic, but the magnitude of NaCl reabsorption in the early proximal tubule is exceeded by the even greater rates of $NaHCO_3$ reabsorption. Although there is no change in the luminal $[Na^+]$ along the proximal tubule, there is a significant increase in the luminal $[Cl^-]$, which reflects preferential reabsorption of $NaHCO_3$ in the early

proximal tubule. This results in an outward Cl gradient which allows passive Cl reabsorption in the late proximal tubule. The mechanism of Na reabsorption in the early proximal tubule is illustrated in Figure 4.2. A ouabain-sensitive basolateral Na^+,K^+-ATPase drives the primary active transport of Na^+ from the cytoplasm to the peritubular fluid and the intracellular accumulation of K^+. The outward leak of K^+ from the cell creates a cell interior which is more negative than the tubular lumen. The decrease in intracellular $[Na^+]$ and the intracellular negativity result in a large electrochemical gradient for passive Na^+ entry at the apical membrane. This combined electrochemical gradient provides a powerful force driving Na^+ from the lumen into the cell and drives the absorption or secretion of a variety of solutes by secondary active transport. These include glucose absorption (Na-glucose co-transport), inorganic phosphate (P_i) absorption (Na-P_i co-transport), Na-dependent amino acid transport, and proton secretion (Na–H exchange). In addition, the early proximal convoluted tubule exhibits

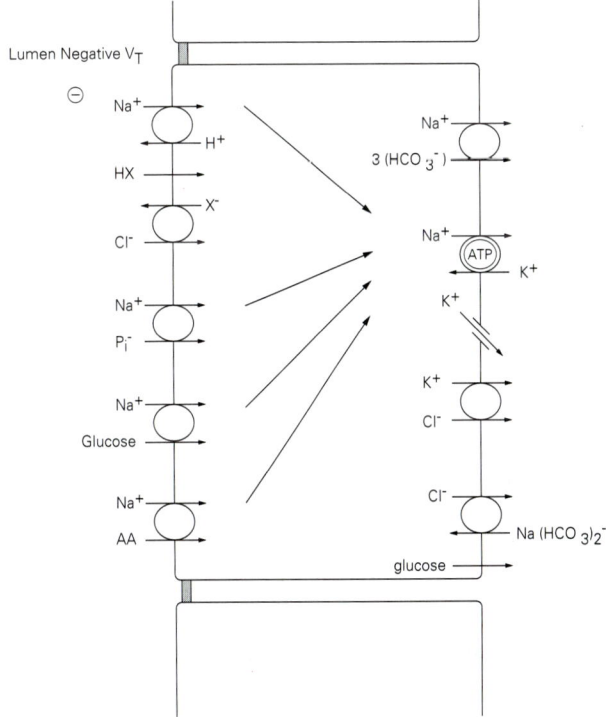

Figure 4.2 Mechanism of Na^+ reabsorption in the early proximal tubule. A ouabain-sensitive basolateral Na^+,K^+-ATPase drives the primary active transport of Na^+ from the cytoplasm to the peritubular fluid and the intracellular accumulation of K^+. The outward leak of K^+ from the cell creates a cell interior which is more negative than the tubular lumen. The favorable chemical and electrical gradients for passive apical Na^+ entry are additive and result in a large electrochemical gradient for Na^+ uptake across the apical membrane. This electrochemical gradient provides a powerful force that drives Na^+ from the lumen into the cell and the secondary active absorption or secretion of a variety of solutes. (AA = amino acids.)

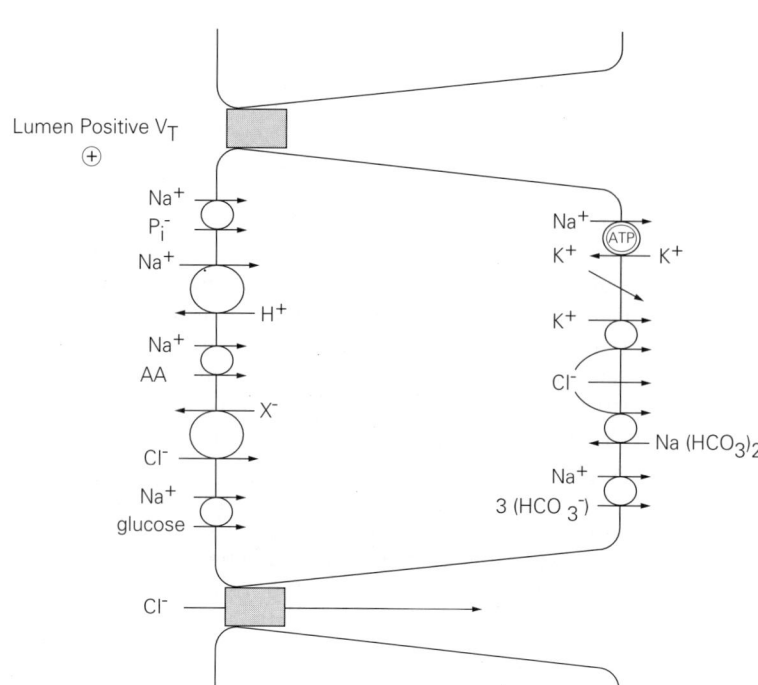

Figure 4.3 Mechanism of NaCl absorption in the late proximal tubule. Most Na^+ absorption is with Cl^- and proceeds via both transcellular and paracellular pathways. Paracellular Cl^- absorption occurs due to preferential $NaHCO_3$ absorption in the early proximal tubule.

active Cl^- absorption. This may reflect either secondary active absorption (NaCl co-transport) or tertiary active transport (parallel Na-H and Cl-base exchangers).

Late proximal tubule NaCl transport

NaCl transport in the late proximal tubule involves both active (transcellular) and passive (paracellular) components. The mechanisms of NaCl reabsorption are illustrated in Figure 4.3. This process is ultimately driven by basolateral Na^+,K^+-ATPase. NaCl movement across the apical membrane has been attributed to the parallel operation of apical Na-H and Cl-base exchangers. The base species involved in this coupled transport may represent either hydroxyl, formate, oxalate or bicarbonate (HCO_3^-).

Late proximal tubule: mechanisms of active transport

Apical Na–H exchange occurs, at least in part, via the NHE3-isoform of the Na–H family of exchangers. Apical Na–H exchange is relatively resistant to the action of amiloride, and high concentrations, approximately 4 mM, are required for full inhibition in the proximal tubule. Cl^- absorption occurs across the apical membrane in part via transport by Cl-formate (HCO_2) exchange [2].

Basolateral NaCl transport requires Cl^- exit coupled to Na^+ extrusion by the Na,K pump which is regulated by basolateral K^+ channels and cytoplasmic ATP concentrations. The mechanisms of Cl^- exit include Na-dependent $Cl–HCO_3$ exchange, KCl co-transport, and conductive Cl^- exit. Although basolateral Cl^- channels have been reported, which would allow for conductive Cl^- exit, changes in basolateral membrane voltage fail to affect

basolateral Cl^- exit which suggests that Cl^- extrusion is largely electroneutral [3]. The authors concluded that Na-dependent Cl^-/HCO_3^- exchange ($Na/HCO_3/Cl$) was more important for basolateral Cl^- exit than KCl co-transport. Since Na-dependent, $Cl–HCO_3$ exchange would result in cellular HCO_3^- uptake, net $NaHCO_3$ absorption requires the parallel operation of this exchanger with an electrogenic $Na(HCO_3)_3$ symporter.

Late proximal tubule: mechanism of passive transport

When active transport is inhibited by a variety of maneuvers, including a reduction in temperature, removal of bath K^+, or addition of ouabain or cyanide, NaCl and fluid reabsorption is reduced 30–60%, but substantial passive ion flux remains. These observations suggest a significant contribution of passive paracellular NaCl absorption to overall vectorial NaCl absorption. The greater rate of $NaHCO_3$ absorption compared with NaCl absorption in the early proximal tubule alters the composition of the tubular fluid, and results in a high luminal Cl^- concentration [Cl^-], a reduced HCO_3^- concentration, [HCO_3^-], and a favorable gradient for Cl^- absorption. Because $NaHCO_3$ possesses a greater reflection coefficient* than

*The reflection coefficient was introduced to explain why solutes often do not exert their full osmotic effect across a membrane due to the penetration of the membrane by the solute. The deviation can be defined as the ratio of the experimentally observed osmolality to the value calculated from the van't Hoff relation, $\Delta\pi = RT\Delta C$, where $\Delta\pi$ is the transmembrane difference in osmotic pressure due to ΔC, the transmembrane difference in solute concentration, R is the gas constant and T is the absolute temperature. The reflection coefficient, σ, modifies $\Delta\pi$ such that $\sigma\Delta\pi$ is the effective transmembrane osmotic pressure exerted by the solute. σ has a range of $0 \leq \sigma \leq 1$.

does NaCl across the proximal tubule and thus exerts a greater osmotic pressure across the epithelium, there is an effective osmotic driving force for fluid absorption. In addition, Na$^+$ moves down its electrical gradient by the lumen-positive transepithelial voltage (V_T) present in late proximal tubule.

Loop of Henle

The loop of Henle is a heterogeneous structure composed of the pars recta of the proximal tubule, the thin descending limb (tdl), the thin ascending limb (tal), and the thick ascending limb of Henle (TALH).

Thin descending limb

The thin descending limb (tdl) is morphologically heterogeneous. The upper portion of long-loop nephrons have a more complex architecture with abundant microvilli and mitochondria, whereas the deeper portions of long-looped nephrons and short-looped thin descending limbs have a simpler structure suggesting less active transport. Studies in isolated perfused tubules provide little evidence for active transport in the tdl. This segment has a large water permeability but in general a small solute permeability which allows passive water absorption from the lumen to the peritubular fluid and thence into the ascending vasa recta. Thus, the overall affect of these permeability differences allows the removal of water, concentration of the remaining solute, and only small amounts of solute addition to a thin descending limb.

Thin ascending limb

The thin ascending limb (tal) of Henle begins shortly beyond the bend of the loop of Henle of long-loop nephrons. This segment is not present in short-loop nephrons. The tal has one of the highest reported NaCl permeabilities, and a moderate urea permeability, but is largely water impermeable. These properties allow the rapid diffusion of solute without commensurate water absorption and results in dilution of the luminal fluid osmolality. Anion exchange inhibitors such as disulfonic stilbenes, phloretin, and furosemide inhibit tal Cl$^-$ permeability, and Cl$^-$ transport is not directly coupled to Na$^+$, K$^+$ or HCO$_3^-$, but is affected by pH and Ca^{2+}. It has been concluded that the Cl$^-$ transport by the tal is consistent with facilitated Cl$^-$ diffusion, and a model proposed for passive Cl$^-$ efflux by Cl$^-$ channels which are pH and Ca^{2+} sensitive [4].

Thick ascending limb

Approximately 25–30% of the filtered load of NaCl is reabsorbed by the thick ascending limb of loop of Henle (TALH) which exhibits a high solute but low water permeability. For this reason, the active transport of NaCl from lumen to bath is not accompanied by a significant rate of volume or water flux (J_v). This segment is hetero-

geneous and may be subdivided into the medullary TALH (mTALH) and the cortical TALH (cTALH).

The mTALH is thicker than the cTALH and has abundant mitochondria located adjacent to a highly invaginated basolateral membrane. Functionally, the mTALH represents a high-capacity segment for net NaCl transport (J_{NaCl}) which exceeds that of most other segments. However, this segment has a limited capacity to establish transepithelial concentration gradients [5]. The cTALH has a smaller rate of NaCl reabsorption [5], but can generate approximately twice the maximum gradient of the mTALH. These characteristics allow the cTALH to generate a hypotonic luminal fluid which is essential for the excretion of solute-free water.

Despite the quantitative differences in transport capacities of these two segments, the overall mechanism of solute transport in the cTALH and the mTALH is similar. Basolateral Na$^+$,K$^+$-ATPase drives secondary active Cl$^-$ absorption at the apical membrane coupled to Na$^+$ and potassium ion (K$^+$) entry, via a co-transporter that has a stoichiometry of 1Na : 1K : 2Cl. The K$^+$ that enters apically is largely recycled at the apical membrane through an apical K$^+$ conductance. Na$^+$ exits via the Na,K-pump, and Cl$^-$ exits through both an electroneutral basolateral KCl co-transporter and conductively through a basolateral Cl channel.

Apical NaCl entry

Apical membrane NaCl absorption proceeds via two mechanisms (Figure 4.4). The principal mechanism of NaCl movement transport across the apical membrane is by a bumetanide- and furosemide-sensitive 1Na : 1K : 2Cl co-transporter which effects the electroneutral movement of two cations and two anions as part of its reaction cycle [6, 7]. The inward solute flux is driven by the product of the Na$^+$ concentration gradient and the Cl$^-$ concentration gradient. This results in the energetically unfavorable or 'uphill' movement of K$^+$ against its concentration gradient. The Na-K-2Cl co-transporter is pH-sensitive and acidosis significantly inhibits co-transport activity and net Cl$^-$ transport. This co-transporter has a high affinity for Na$^+$ ($K_m = 1$ mM) and K$^+$ ($K_m = 3$ mM), but its affinity for Cl$^-$ is substantially less ($K_m = 50$ mM). Recent studies have identified cDNAs for Na-K-2Cl cotransport [8].

Some studies have reported that NaCl transport in the medullary thick ascending limb is K-independent [9]. Specifically, in rabbit mTALH cells furosemide-sensitive co-transport of Na with Cl and Cl with Na was observed that was independent of extracellular [K$^+$]. However, antidiuretic hormone (ADH) alters the mode of apical Cl entry from Na-Cl to Na-K-2Cl [10]. When operating in the NaCl mode, Na reabsorption is exclusively transcellular, but in the Na-K-2Cl mode approximately 50% of Na reabsorption is paracellular, driven by V_T.

Apical Na-H exchange

In some species (rat) but not others (rabbit), an apical Na-H exchanger effects net bicarbonate absorption (J_{tco2}) in

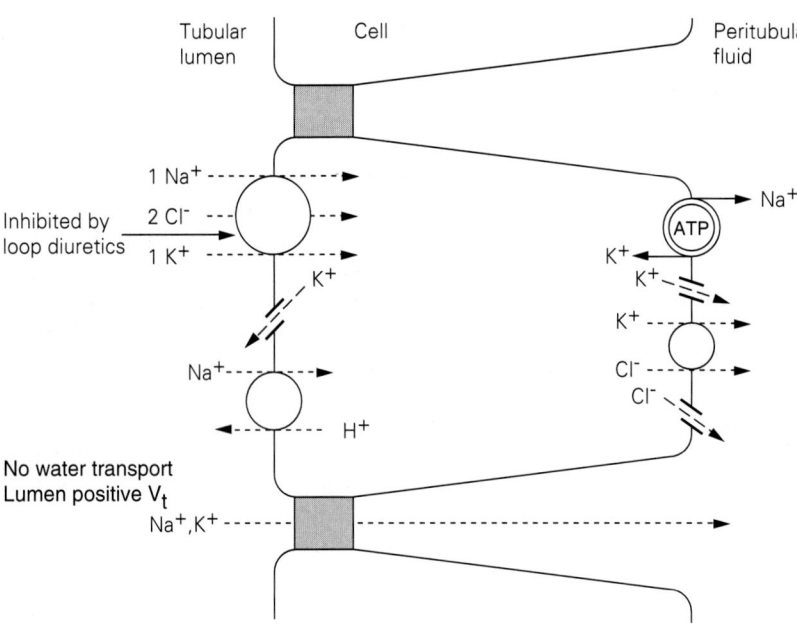

Figure 4.4 Mechanism of NaCl absorption in the thick ascending limb of Henle. (Slightly modified by permission from Valtin, H. and Schafer, J.A. (1995) *Renal Function*, 3rd edn, Little, Brown, Boston, pp. 244–5.)

the cTALH and mTALH. In the mouse cTALH, NaCl absorption is enhanced in the presence of CO_2/HCO_3^-, but this effect is not apparent in the mTALH.

Apical K conductance

The TALH apical membrane is largely K-selective, and luminal K removal inhibits NaCl absorption. The combination of K removal and barium addition largely abolishes NaCl absorption [7]. Moreover, net K absorption is only a fraction of Na or Cl absorption in the mTALH [11]. These facts indicate that substantial K recycling occurs at the apical membrane of the TALH which may occur through either of two types of apical K channels [12]. The requirement of luminal K for maximal rates of NaCl absorption is consistent with micropuncture data that demonstrate impairment in solute transport in the loop of Henle during K^+ depletion.

Basolateral NaCl exit

Extrusion of NaCl at the basolateral membrane involves the action of the Na-K pump, basolateral Cl conductances, and basolateral KCl co-transport system [7]. Ouabain-sensitive cellular Na efflux occurs via the basolateral Na^+, K^+-ATPase and the K which is taken up by the pump appears to exit largely by an electroneutral mechanism, although some studies suggest both conductive and electroneutral K exit mechanisms exist in separate cells [13]. The principal conductance of the basolateral membrane is to Cl^- [7]. This Cl^- conductance appears to vary considerably, and is affected by intracellular Cl activity (a_{Cl}). A reduction in a_{Cl} from 20 to 7 mM reduces basolateral membrane conductance by approximately 50%.

Paracellular transport

The V_T in both the mTALH and cTALH is lumen-positive, which drives substantial rates of paracellular cation flux. As noted previously, a significant portion of Na flux may be paracellular in the presence of ADH. Other cations, such as Ca^{2+}, Mg^{2+}, K^+ and ammonium, are absorbed in part paracellularly. Paracellular cation reabsorption is also favored by the permselectivity of the paracellular pathway which is cation-selective.

Distal convolution

The distal convolution refers to a region of the nephron originally defined from micropuncture studies of surface distal nephrons. The structure begins at the macula densa and continues to the first branch point of the cortical collecting duct (CCD). This segment is both anatomically and physiologically heterogeneous and is composed of four discrete epithelia: (1) a segment of the cTALH; (2) the distal convoluted tubule (DCT); (3) the connecting segment; and (4) the initial cortical collecting duct (iCCD) which represents the beginning of the collecting duct (CD). The distinction between these four anatomically discrete regions varies between species. For example, in the rabbit, discrete transitions can be appreciated for the cTALH, the DCT and the connecting segment, whereas these transitions are gradual in the rat.

Distal convoluted tubule

The DCT is lined by a tall cuboidal epithelium, which is morphologically homogeneous, possesses numerous mitochondria, and there is extensive infolding of the basolateral membrane. This segment possesses the greatest Na$^+$,K$^+$-ATPase activity of any renal tubule segment; it consists of a single cell population, the distal convoluted tubule cell. There appear to be differences in the mechanism of NaCl transport in the rat, studied by *in vivo* microperfusion, and in the rabbit, studied by *in vitro* microperfusion. Thiazide diuretics inhibit NaCl transport in the former [14], but not in the latter [15], and immunohistochemical studies localize NaCl co-transporter immunoreactivity to the rat DCT [16].

NaCl exit at the basolateral membrane is dependent on basolateral Na$^+$,K$^+$-ATPase for Na extrusion, but the Cl exit mechanism is not clear. Greger and Velazquez [17] have proposed that Cl exit in the early DCT is via KCl co-transport because of the small magnitude of the basolateral K conductance relative to the rates of absorptive NaCl flux.

Connecting tubule

In the rabbit, but not in the rat, an anatomically discrete segment, termed the connecting tubule, has been defined which connects the DCT to the iCCD. The connecting segment is a heterogeneous structure, consisting of both intercalated cells and connecting tubule cells. The connecting segment of the rabbit possesses three distinct transport mechanisms at the luminal membrane: an amiloride-sensitive Na conductance; a simple NaCl co-transporter which is distinct from the Na-K-2Cl co-transporter present in the TALH; and parallel antiporters for Na-H and Cl-HCO$_3$. Qualitatively, this last mechanism appears to be the least important [15].

Collecting duct

The collecting duct (CD) reabsorbs approximately 2–3% of the filtered Na load normally and changes in dietary Na intake are first reflected in this segment, but with more severe degrees of Na depletion Na reabsorption is enhanced in more proximal portions of the nephron. The CD of the cortex (CCD), the outer medulla (OMCD), and the initial portion of the inner medulla possess two cell types, referred to as principal cells and intercalated cells, whereas the middle and terminal portions of the inner medullary collecting duct (IMCD) possess one cell type, referred to as the IMCD cell. Principal cells make up approximately two-thirds of the cell types in the CCD and OMCD. Intercalated cells comprise approximately 35–40% of the cells in the CCD, and the outer stripe of OMCD (OMCD$_o$). The percentage of intercalated cells decreases progressively more distally [1]. Thus, in the rat intercalated cells comprise only 10% of the cells of the initial IMCD.

The principal cells of the CD are involved in Na$^+$ absorption and K$^+$ secretion. Under selected conditions, Cl$^-$ secretion occurs through this cell type. Intercalated cells, on the other hand, are involved primarily in proton secretion, HCO$_3^-$ secretion, and active K$^+$ absorption. The intercalated cells of the cortex can be subdivided into two distinct cell populations, A-type intercalated cells and B-type intercalated cells [18].

Cortical collecting duct

The CCD responds dramatically to changes in dietary Na, Cl and K composition. Diets rich in Na and poor in K are associated with small rates of Na absorption and K secretion. The V_T may be slightly lumen-negative to lumen-positive. When Na is removed from the diet and K content increased, the rates of Na absorption and K secretion increase dramatically and V_T may exceed $-60 \, \text{mV}$.

A model of the three cell types of the CCD is illustrated in Figure 4.5. NaCl reabsorption is largely via principal cells of the CCD where active basolateral Na$^+$ extrusion by the Na$^+$,K$^+$-ATPase allows passive apical entry of Na$^+$ to proceed by an amiloride-sensitive Na channel [19]. The frequency of apical Na channels is regulated by mineralocorticoid activity. Molecular characterization of this channel demonstrates that it is composed of three subunits [20].

Electrogenic Na$^+$ reabsorption results in the depolarization of the apical membrane and the development of the significant lumen-negative V_T which drives a portion of Cl$^-$ absorption passively via the paracellular pathway. Electrophysiological studies [21] demonstrate that the apical membrane of the principal cell of the CD possesses a Cl$^-$ transport pathway which may represent a Cl channel [22] or a KCl co-transporter [23].

Under conditions of dietary K loading, the CCD is capable of active Cl$^-$ secretion. This Cl$^-$ secretion is a form of secondary active Cl$^-$ secretion which is co-dependent on K$^+$ secretion and can be inhibited by blocking the basolateral Na,K pump [23]. Active Cl$^-$ secretion is also present under conditions of electrogenic NaCl absorption. However, under these conditions the predominant Cl flux is absorptive, via the paracellular pathway, which masks the Cl$^-$ component of KCl secretion. Reduction in luminal Cl$^-$ concentration augments K$^+$ secretion via a stimulation of KCl secretion [23]. These results suggest the presence of an apical KCl co-transport mechanism. In the rat, a thiazide-sensitive Na and Cl transport system has been described.

Basolateral NaCl exit occurs via active Na$^+$ extrusion by the Na,K pump and conductive Cl$^-$ exit. The basolateral membrane has a K$^+$ conductance which is responsible for K recycling associated with the turnover of the Na,K pump.

Outer medullary collecting duct

The outer medullary collecting duct (OMCD) is composed of the portion in the outer stripe (OMCD$_o$) and the portion in the inner stripe (OMCD$_i$). The OMCD$_o$ generally has smaller rates of Na absorption and K secretion than the CCD [24] and is generally considered a transition region with properties that are intermediate between the properties of the CCD in the OMCD$_i$. The OMCD$_i$ pos-

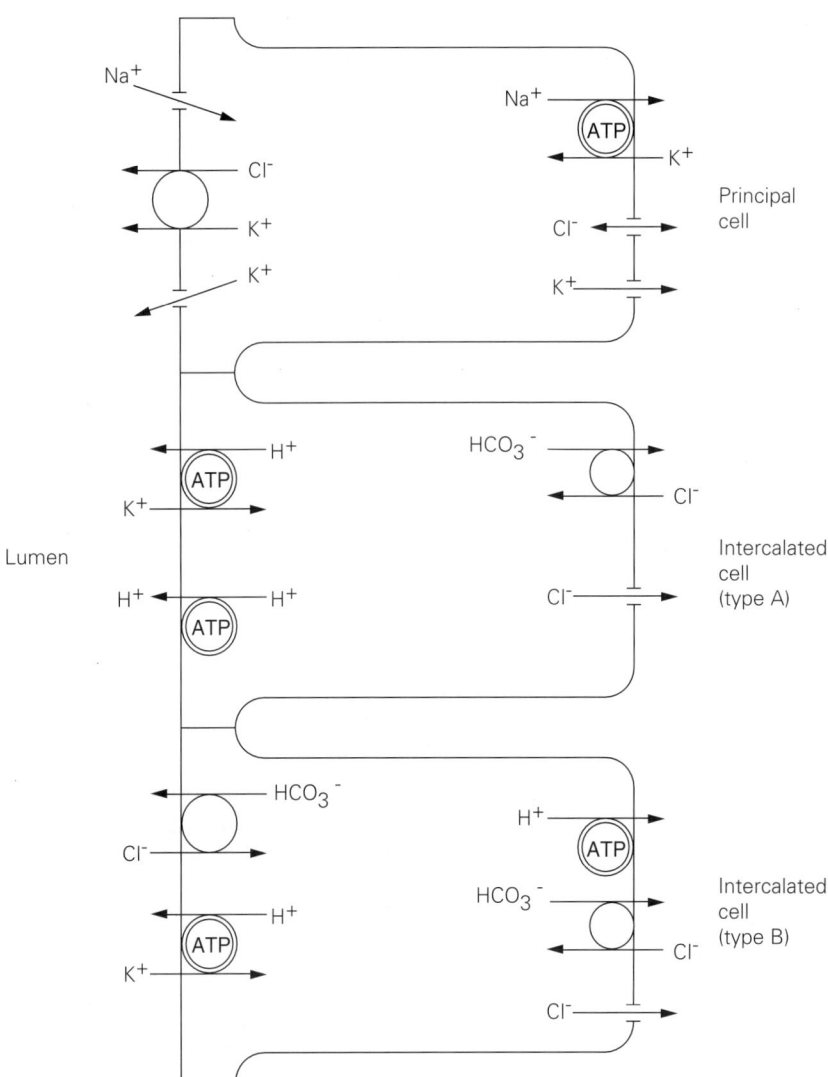

Figure 4.5 Model of the three cell types of the cortical collecting duct.

sesses only small rates of Na absorption and K secretion [24] and the V_T is typically lumen-positive. The mechanism of Na transport has not been systematically studied.

Inner medullary collecting duct

The inner medullary collecting duct (IMCD) is composed of three sections, the initial, middle and terminal portions, referred to, respectively, as $IMCD_1$, $IMCD_2$, $IMCD_3$. Only the $IMCD_1$ of the rat possesses intercalated cells. The major cell type of the IMCD is referred to as the IMCD cell, which differs from principal cells of the CCD and OMCD in several attributes. The IMCD cell is taller than principal cells of the OMCD and CCD and lacks a central cilium. Figure 4.6 illustrates a model of Na transport in the IMCD [25]. The V_T is slightly lumen-negative and the apical membrane contains an amiloride-sensitive Na channel. Na^+ extrusion is via basolateral Na^+,K^+-ATPase and the basolateral membrane also possesses conductances for K^+ and HCO_3^-, although HCO_3^- exit also occurs via $Cl^--HCO_3^-$ exchange.

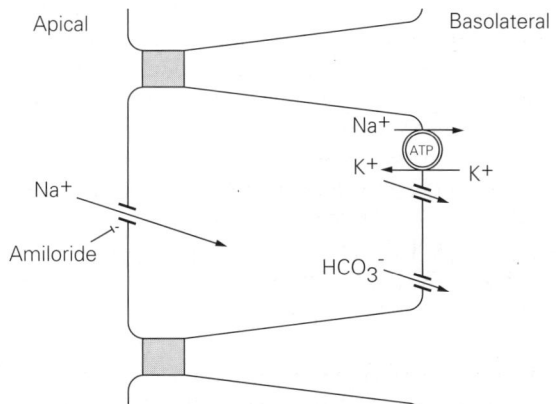

Figure 4.6 Model of Na transport in the inner medullary collecting duct. (Reproduced, with permission, from ref. 25.)

Potassium transport along the nephron

Introduction

K+ is the major intracellular cation and is vital for normal cellular function. The majority of cells have K+ conductances that regulate plasma membrane voltage and electrical excitability. Cellular K+ uptake is an energetically unfavorable process and requires active transport, primarily by Na+,K+-ATPase or co-transport with Na+ and Cl− (Na-K-2Cl co-transporter). The vast majority of K+ is contained within the intracellular fluid and only approximately 2% is extracellular. Extracellular fluid [K+] is regulated by hormones that stimulate cellular K+ uptake. These hormones include insulin, beta-adrenergic catecholamines and aldosterone. Extrarenal K+ homeostasis via cellular uptake is important in preventing acute changes in extracellular [K+]. Long-term K+ homeostasis is regulated by the kidney, which accounts for 90% of the excretion of K+ intake. The majority of the remainder of K+ excretion is via the colon, which has a more limited capacity to secrete K+.

Renal handling of potassium

Figure 4.7 illustrates the renal handling of K. Potassium (K) is freely filtered at the glomerulus and, under normal circumstances, approximately 15–30% of the filtered load of K is excreted depending on dietary intake and the individual's degree of renal function. K is largely reabsorbed (~90%), regardless of dietary K intake, in the proximal tubule and loop of Henle. Urinary K excretion is principally due to active secretion of K in the CD, primarily the iCCD and the CCD, and this mechanism of K transport is highly regulated. The CD also possesses the capacity for active K absorption during K deprivation.

Proximal tubule

K filtered at the glomerulus is reabsorbed largely in proportion to fluid and volume reabsorption (~60%) in the proximal tubule. Thus, luminal K ion concentration, $[K^+]_l$, changes little along the length of the proximal tubule. The mechanism of K absorption in the proximal tubule is illustrated in Figure 4.8.

The nature of K transport in the proximal tubule is not fully clarified. Because proximal tubule cellular K activity (a_K) remains above electrochemical equilibrium [26], K absorption must occur either by an active apical absorptive mechanism or by passive entrainment and diffusion via the paracellular pathway. A model of proximal tubule K transport [27] suggests that movement of K against an electrochemical gradient can occur by active K cellular uptake via laterally located Na+,K+-ATPase. According to this model active K absorption from the lateral intercellular space allows paracellular K absorption by entrainment and passive diffusion. Osmotic diuretics retard fluid

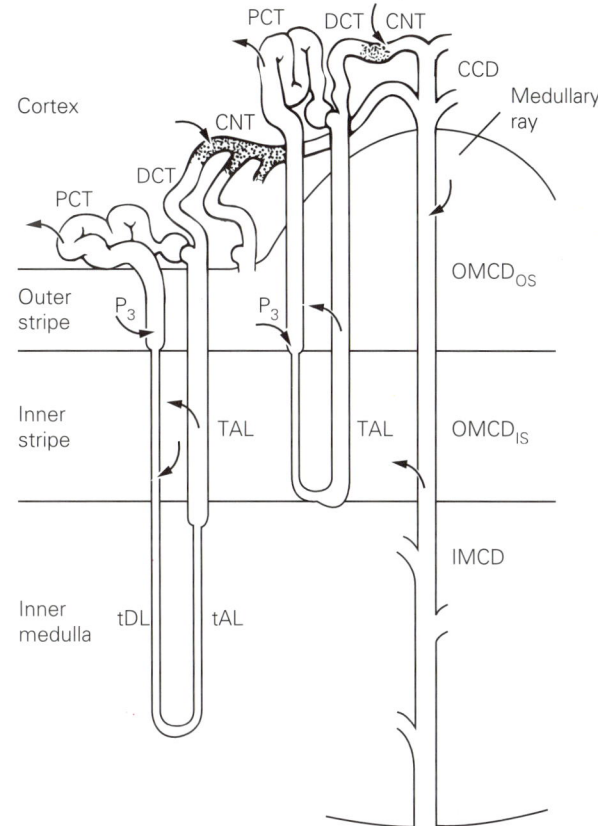

Figure 4.7 Overview of renal K transport. K is reabsorbed in the superficial proximal tubule and ascending limb of the loop of Henle. Distal secretion, largely in the iCCD and CCD, are principally responsible for renal K excretion, but some of the distally secreted K is reabsorbed in the OMCD and IMCD, a proportion of which enters the descending limb of the loop of Henle. K loading enhances CD K secretion, whereas K deprivation enhances CD K reabsorption. (Reproduced, with permssion, from Jamison, R.L. (1987) Potassium recycling. *Kidney Int.*, **3**, 695–703.)

reabsorption in the proximal tubule and decrease proximal tubule K reabsorption, which suggests that a significant component of K movement is by paracellular transport.

Loop of Henle

Approximately 20–30% of filtered load of K is reabsorbed within the loop of Henle. Fluid that exits the proximal tubule undergoes passive water absorption in the thin descending limb (tdl) of the loop of Henle. Micropuncture studies demonstrate that the fractional excretion of K (FE_K) in the tdl of juxtamedullary nephrons can exceed the filtered K load, which provides clear evidence for K secretion by more proximal segments. K loading significantly increases the filtered load of K to the tdl of juxtamedullary nephrons [28]; whereas administration of amiloride results in a sharp decrease in the delivery of K

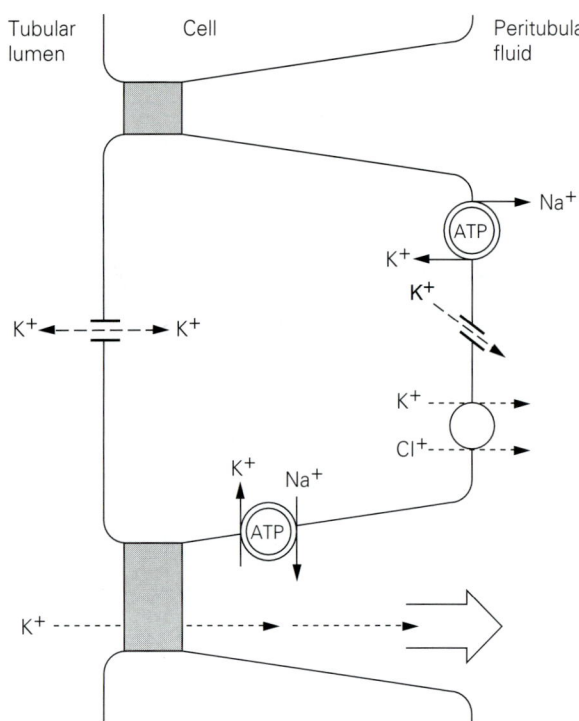

Tubular lumen | Cell | Peritubular fluid

Figure 4.8 Model of K transport by the proximal tubule. (Slightly modified by permission from Valtin, H. and Schafer, J.A. (1995) *Renal Function*, 3rd edn, Little, Brown, Boston, pp. 244–5.)

to the terminal tdl [28, 29]. These observations suggest that a portion of K which is secreted in the CD is reabsorbed into the medullary interstitium and thence secreted into tdl of the juxtamedullary nephrons.

The mechanism for K entry into the luminal fluid of the tdl has not been extensively studied. However, active, ouabain-sensitive K secretion has been reported in the rabbit pars recta of the proximal tubule [30]. Although the rates of K secretion were modest and were reduced by perfusing with a solution that simulated the composition present in the late proximal tubule, the magnitude of K secretion could be markedly increased by a small (5 mM) bath-to-lumen K gradient. Thus, a component of K secretion in the pars recta is active, transcellular and dependent on basolateral Na^+,K^+-ATPase.

Thick ascending limb

The transport mechanisms of the TALH have been extensively studied. The basic transport mechanisms are similar in both the cTALH and mTALH, although in some species ADH stimulates solute transport in the mTALH, and CO_2/HCO_3^- stimulates solute absorption in the cTALH. This segment reasorbs NaCl (J_{NaCl}) in the absence of appreciable water flux, serving to dilute the luminal fluid. When studied *in vitro* in the absence of ion gradients, only small rates of K transport have been observed in the rabbit mTALH [11], or the mouse cTALH [31]. However,

modest ion gradients from bath-to-lumen or lumen-to-bath result in appreciable K secretion or reabsorption, respectively. The mTALH exhibits significant rectification suggesting that a significant component of this flux is transcellular [11]. Interestingly, glucagon substantially stimulates Ca absorption in the mouse cTALH without affecting K transport [31].

The mechanism of K transport in the TALH is illustrated in Figure 4.4. Apical K absorption is mediated by electroneutral transport with one Na^+ and two Cl^- and driven by the chemical Na and Cl concentration gradients from lumen to cell. The majority of K absorbed at the apical membrane recycles by an apical K channel [7]. Cl absorbed by the apical Na-K-2Cl co-transporter exits the basolateral membrane, both conductively through a Cl channel and through a KCl co-transporter. Na is reabsorbed both via transcellular and paracellular pathways. Paracellular transport is driven by the lumen-positive V_T and the cation selectivity of the paracellular pathway. In the mouse mTALH, ADH enhances NaCl absorption by increasing the activity of the Na-K-2Cl co-transporter [6]. ADH also alters the mode of transport from a K-independent NaCl absorptive mechanism to a K-dependent NaCl absorptive mechanism which serves to transport NaCl more efficiently by increasing the efficiency of paracellular voltage-mediated Na absorption as K is recycled at the apical membrane [10].

K absorbed via the Na-K-2Cl cotransporter exits through apical K channels. Two such channels have been identified at the apical membrane of the thick ascending limb [12]. Both channels exhibit high open probability, are sensitive to barium (Ba), and inhibited by acidosis and ATP. The effect of pH on apical K channel activity helps to explain the effects of acidosis on transport in the cTALH.

Distal convolution

Distal convoluted tubule

Limited information is available for this segment in the rabbit because of the difficulty of dissection and the short length of this segment. In the rat the early distal convolution, which includes the DCT, possesses smaller rates of K secretion than does the late distal convolution, which includes the connecting segment and iCCD [32, 33].

Connecting segment and initial cortical collecting duct

The connecting segment of the rabbit is an anatomically discrete nephron segment, and amiloride inhibits V_T and Na absorption [15]. Neither Na nor Cl transport is affected by furosemide, but trichlormethiazide inhibits Na and Cl transport [15].

The iCCD represents the major site within the distal convolution for K secretion [32, 33]. Both luminal flow rate and Na delivery appear to stimulate K secretion, but luminal flow rate appears to be quantitatively of greater importance [34]. These findings indicate a substantial apical K permeability of this region. K secretion is also stimulated by reduction of luminal [Cl⁻] [33]. Since this effect is not blocked by luminal Ba, K secretion in the iCCD appears to occur in part by KCl co-transport [35]. Dietary K content clearly affects K secretion in this segment, with large rates of K secretion in K-loaded animals, whereas K secretion is virtually abolished and there is a tendency toward K absorption during K depletion.

Collecting duct

Cortical collecting duct K secretion

Of the two cell types, principal cells are involved in K secretion whereas intercalated cells are responsible for K absorption. The mechanisms of K transport in the CCD are illustrated in Figure 4.9. K secretion by the principal cell depends on the basolateral Na⁺,K⁺-ATPase and requires Na absorption at the apical membrane via an amiloride-sensitive Na channel for turnover of the Na,K-ATPase and basolateral K uptake. K exits apically both conductively and via co-transport with Cl. The apical membrane of the CCD possesses several K channels which could be responsible for K secretion. Initially, a large-conductance K channel was proposed as a candidate K channel for K secretion. However, the pharmacological profile and single channel characteristics of this channel suggest that it does not normally participate in K secretion. More recently, a small-conductance, voltage-insensitive K channel with a high open probability and external Ba sensitivity has been identified at the CCD apical membrane [36] and is a plausible candidate for a K channel responsible K secretion.

KCl secretion

The nature of Cl transport with K is more complex. Electrogenic Na absorption and the resulting lumen-negative V_T drives passive Cl absorption via the paracellular pathway. However, under appropriate circumstances, the CCD can actively secrete Cl [23]. The precise mechanism for this Cl secretion is not fully established but represents either KCl co-transport or parallel apical conductive K and Cl channels [22, 23]. As noted previously, evidence in the rat iCCD suggests that K secretion occurs by an apical co-transporter [33]. During K loading a component of K secretion occurs coupled to Cl [23], and the coupled secretion of K with Cl helps to explain why conditions associated with a low luminal [Cl⁻] promote K wasting [33].

Cortical collecting duct K absorption

As shown in Figure 4.9, the intercalated cells of the CCD possess a mechanism of K absorption coupled to proton

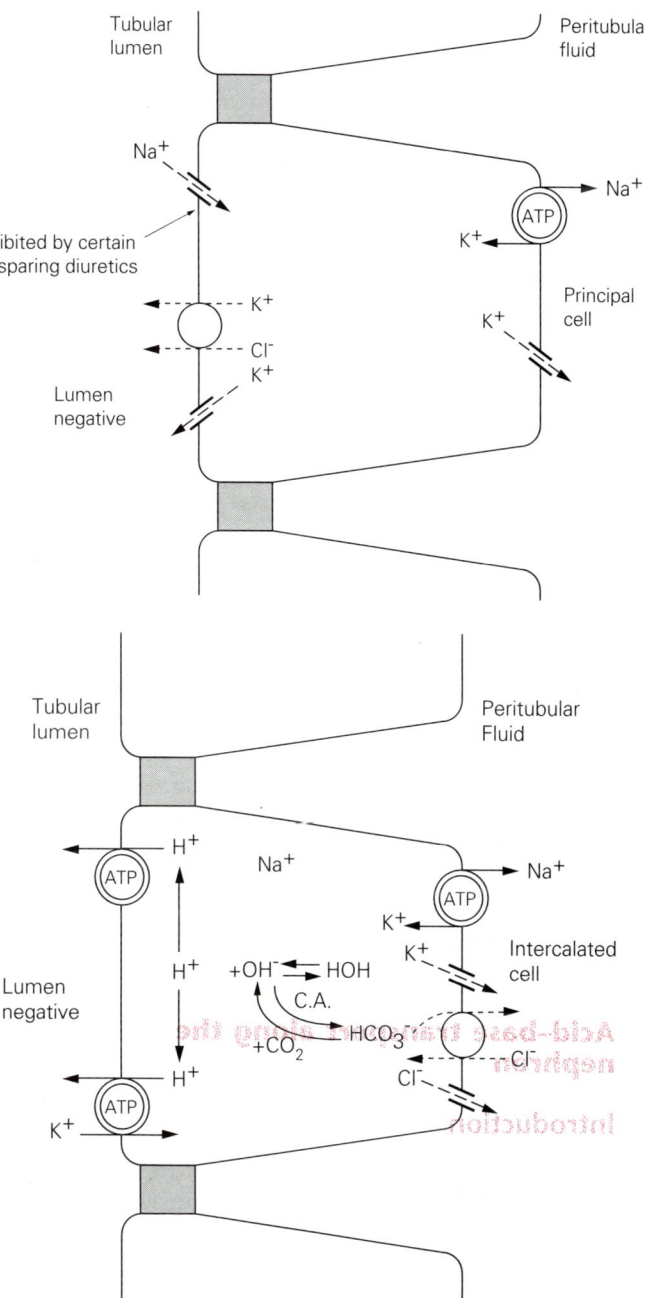

Figure 4.9 Mechanism of K transport in the CCD. K secretion occurs via principal cells. K absorption occurs via intercalated cells. (Slightly modified by permission from Valtin, H. and Schafer, J.A. (1995) *Renal Function*, 3rd edn, Little, Brown Boston, pp. 244–5.)

secretion and mediated via a luminal H⁺,K⁺-ATPase [37]. Luminal K is absorbed against its electrochemical gradient via this primary active P-type proton pump in exchange for cytosolic protons. During K restriction K exits basolaterally via a Ba-sensitive pathway, whereas during K repletion K is recycled across the apical membrane. In both situations acute increases in $p\mathrm{CO_2}$ stimulate H⁺,K⁺-ATPase activity [37].

Outer medullary collecting duct K transport

The OMCD possesses limited capacity to secrete K during K loading, but is a major site of K reabsorption during K deprivation [38]. Studies in the rat demonstrate intense hypertrophy of the cells of the $OMCD_i$ in response to K depletion [39, 40]. The mechanism of K absorption in the OMCD is similar to that present in the type A intercalated cell of the CCD (Figure 4.9). Presently, little is known about the regulation of this transport process.

Inner medullary collecting duct K transport

Little net K transport occurs in the IMCD under normal dietary K intake [41], but with severe K loading this segment can contribute substantially to K excretion [42]. On the other hand, during severe K depletion the rat IMCD reabsorbs ~90% of the K delivered to this segment [41]. Thus, the IMCD, similar to the CCD, possess the capacity for bidirectional K transport. As with the more proximal CD segments, K absorption probably involves the action of an apical H,K-ATPase and a basolateral K channel since this segment possesses H,K-ATPase activity [37] and a K conductance at the basolateral membrane [25]. The mechanism of K secretion is not well characterized but may reflect the activity of a non-selective cation channel that has been identified at the apical membrane of the IMCD [43].

Acid–base transport along the nephron

Introduction

The kidney must both reabsorb filtered HCO_3^- and generate 'new' HCO_3^- to replace that consumed by the titration of endogenous or exogenous acid sources. The renal contribution to acid–base homeostasis has three components. These are reabsorption of filtered HCO_3, generation and secretion of ammonia, and excretion of titratable acids. The kidney must also secrete HCO_3 under some circumstances, such as metabolic alkalosis.

Bicarbonate absorption

Reabsorption of the ~4320 mEq per day of filtered HCO_3 (120 ml/min, 24 mEq/l, 1440 min/day) occurs throughout the nephron. Figure 4.10 summarizes the contribution of various nephron segments to this process. The mechanism of HCO_3 transport differs along the nephron, and each segment is considered separately.

The proximal tubule reabsorbs ~80% of filtered HCO_3 [44]. An apical Na^+/H^+ exchanger is the primary mechanism of proton secretion. Luminal Na concentration is

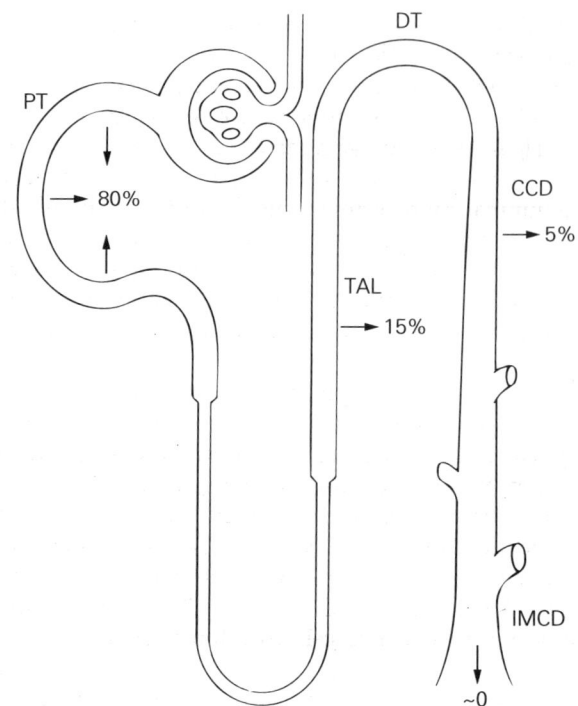

Figure 4.10 Contribution of various nephron segments to HCO_3 absorption. (Reproduced with permission, from Koeppen, B.M. and Stanton, B.A. (1997) *Renal Physiology*, 2nd edn, Mosby Year Book, St Louis, p. 139.)

similar to plasma, whereas intracellular Na is low, providing a gradient for Na entry and proton secretion. An apical H^+-ATPase also secretes protons, although at only half the rate of the apical Na^+/H^+ exchange [44]. The secreted protons react with luminal bicarbonate forming carbonic acid (H_2CO_3), which dissociates to water (H_2O) and carbon dioxide (CO_2). Carbon dioxide can diffuse into the cell, where it reacts with intracellular water forming carbonic acid, dissociating into protons and bicarbonate and replenishing the secreted protons. Basolateral $Na^+(HCO_3)_{n>1}$ co-transport transports HCO_3 across the basolateral membrane [44]. The net effect is bicarbonate transport from the luminal to the peritubular space, where it enters the peritubular capillaries, is transferred to the renal vein and returns to the systemic circulation. Because the majority of proximal tubule proton secretion is linked to Na reabsorption, factors that alter proximal tubule Na reabsorption frequently have similar effects on bicarbonate reabsorption.

The loop of Henle reabsorbs ~10–15% of filtered HCO_3 [45]. The descending limb of the loop of Henle does not significantly reabsorb HCO_3, but instead water abstraction, due to interstitial hypertonicity and a significant permeability to water, increases the luminal HCO_3 concentration [45]. The medullary and cortical TALH secrete protons and reabsorb luminal HCO_3 by mechanisms similar to the proximal tubule [46].

Reabsorption of the remaining filtered HCO_3^- occurs in the distal tubule and the collecting duct (CD). In the cortical CD (CCD) and the outer medullary CD from the outer stripe (OMCD$_o$) only a subset of CD cells, the intercalated cells, secretes protons and reabsorb HCO$_3^-$ [47, 48]. At least two intercalated subtypes are present (see Figure 4.5). An acid-secreting, A-type, intercalated cell is believed to reabsorb filtered HCO$_3^-$ and acidify the luminal fluid (urine), whereas a B-type intercalated cell is generally modeled to secrete HCO$_3$ (see below) [47]. Both intercalated cells and non-intercalated cells reabsorb HCO$_3^-$ in the outer medullary CD from the inner stripe (OMCD$_i$) and the inner medullary CD (IMCD) [48, 49].

Bicarbonate reabsorption in the distal tubule and collecting duct has several differences from more proximal segments. First, an apical H$^+$-ATPase and H$^+$,K$^+$-ATPase, but not Na$^+$/H$^+$ exchange, secrete protons [37, 47, 50]. Second, basolateral HCO$_3^-$ transport occurs via an Na-independent Cl$^-$/HCO$_3^-$ exchanger [47]. Cl$^-$ which enters via this transporter recycles via a basolateral Cl$^-$ channel. Figure 4.5 shows a schematic of H$^+$/HCO$_3^-$ transport by the A-type intercalated cell. Non-intercalated cells in the OMCD$_i$ and the IMCD probably secrete protons and reabsorb HCO$_3$ via mechanisms similar to the A cell [38, 47, 49, 51].

Recent studies indicate that the CCD B-type intercalated cell possesses both apical H$^+$,K$^+$-ATPase and a basolateral Cl$^-$/HCO$_3^+$ exchanger [52]. These observations suggest that this cell may also secrete protons and reabsorb HCO$_3^-$. Furthermore, the apical H$^+$,K$^+$-ATPase is stimulated by *in vivo* metabolic acidosis and *in vitro* respiratory acidosis [37].

The CD is able to secrete protons despite a steep electrochemical gradient, decreasing luminal pH to as low as 4.4. Luminal acidification is important for both ammonium secretion and excretion of titratable acids, as discussed below.

Secretion of HCO$_3$

Besides reabsorption of filtered bicarbonate, the CCD can secrete bicarbonate during metabolic alkalosis. Most evidence indicates that the B-type intercalated cell (B cell) secretes bicarbonate via an apical Cl$^-$/HCO$_3^-$ exchanger [47]. Without delivered (luminal) Cl$^-$, HCO$_3$ secretion does not occur. Intracellular protons exit the basolateral membrane probably via an H$^+$-ATPase [48, 52]. Figure 4.5 shows a schematic of HCO$_3$ secretion by the B-type intercalated cell. Cytoplasmic carbonic anhydrase catalyzes bicarbonate formation from OH$^-$ and water, providing a source for continued bicarbonate secretion [53].

Ammonium transport

The second component of acid–base homeostasis is generation of 'new' bicarbonate through excretion of ammonium (NH$_4^+$). Ammonium excretion results from the co-ordinated actions of proximal tubule ammonium production, reabsorption into the medullary ammonium

concentration by the loop of Henle, and 'trapping' of ammonium by the CD.

Ammonium is produced by proximal tubule glutamine metabolism, which results in formation of two ammonium molecules and two 'new' bicarbonate molecules [54]. Bicarbonate exits via the basolateral Na$^+$(HCO$_3$)$_{n>1}$ co-transporter, enters the peritubular capillaries and is returned to the systemic circulation. Ammonium is secreted preferentially into the luminal fluid via substitution for H$^+$ on the proximal tubule apical Na$^+$/H$^+$ exchanger [55, 56], although some NH$_4^+$ absorption can occur in the late proximal tubule.

The ascending limb of the loop of Henle reabsorbs luminal ammonium, resulting in its concentration in the medullary interstitium. The primary mechanism for ammonium reabsorption appears to be substitution for potassium on the apical Na$^+$-K$^+$-2Cl$^-$ co-transporter [57]. Because of the large gradients for Na and chloride entry, ammonium can be transported against its electrochemical gradient by this transporter. The mechanism of basolateral ammonium exit is not completely defined. The net effect is ammonium reabsorption and concentration in the medullary interstitium [56, 58]. Because ammonium and potassium compete for the same binding site on the apical Na$^+$-K$^+$-2Cl$^-$ co-transporter, increased potassium levels can decrease ammonium reabsorption.

Finally, ammonium is transported from the medullary interstitium into CD cells and secreted into the luminal fluid. The rate-limiting step for net ammonium secretion appears to be ammonia diffusion from the interstitium into the luminal fluid [59]. Two factors regulate the rate of CD ammonia diffusion: (1) the medullary ammonia concentration; and (2) the CD luminal fluid pH. Medullary interstitial ammonia concentration results from proximal tubule ammonium production and loop of Henle ammonium reabsorption. Since ammonium and ammonia are in equilibrium, a higher medullary ammonium concentration results in a higher ammonia concentration. The pH of the luminal fluid of the CD results from proton secretion, as described above, combined with a small paracellular proton permeability. A lower luminal pH shifts the reaction, H$^+$ + NH$_3$ $\rightleftharpoons$ NH$_4^+$, to the right, increasing total luminal ammonium content while decreasing the ammonia concentration, thus maintaining a gradient for ammonia diffusion. This process is termed diffusion trapping.

Approximately 50% of ammonium produced in the proximal tubule is not excreted, but is returned to the peritubular capillaries and thence to the systemic circulation. The liver metabolizes ammonium to urea in a reaction that consumes equimolar bicarbonate and ammonium [54]. Thus, an ammonium molecule produced in the proximal tubule but returned to the systemic circulation results in production of one bicarbonate in the proximal tubule and consumption of one bicarbonate in the liver, and no net bicarbonate generation. As noted above, both the medullary interstitium ammonium concentration and the luminal fluid pH of the CD largely determine the proportion that is returned to the systemic circulation. Ammonium not reabsorbed in the loop of Henle is subject to reabsorption in the distal convoluted and connecting tubules, where it can enter the peritubular capillaries, return to the systemic circulation, and is metabolized by the liver.

Titratable acid transport

Besides reabsorption of filtered bicarbonate and secretion of ammonium, the kidney excretes protons via the excretion of titratable acids, which reversibly bind protons and prevent changes in luminal fluid pH. The major buffer systems include inorganic phosphate, creatinine, uric acid and citrate, although phosphate is quantitatively the most import titratable acid [60].

Calcium transport along the nephron

Introduction

In contrast to monovalent ions, 35–40% of plasma calcium is bound to proteins, and only 60–65% is filtered by the glomerulus. Of the filtered calcium, ~10% is complexed with bicarbonate, phosphate, sulfate and citrate. Reabsorption of the remaining filtered calcium occurs in many segments of the tubule, as summarized in Figure 4.11.

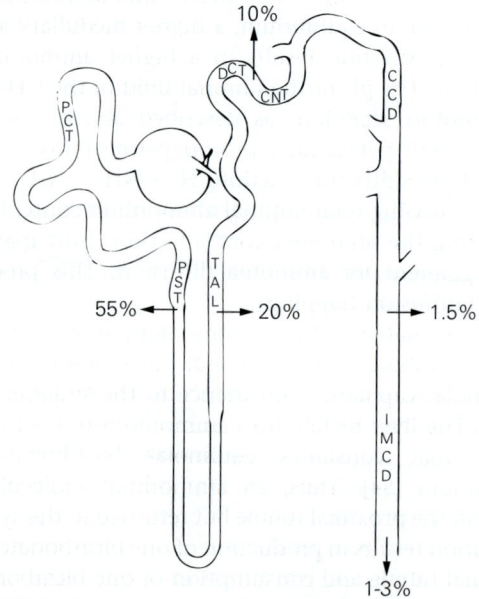

Figure 4.11 Contribution of various nephron segments to Ca absorption. (Reproduced, with permission, from ref. 61.)

Segmental analysis

Most filtered calcium is reabsorbed in the proximal tubule via the paracellular pathway. The lumen-positive voltage occurring from chloride reabsorption, with a relatively high paracellular calcium permeability, allows for rapid calcium reabsorption in this segment of the nephron. A small amount of transcellular calcium reabsorption is present probably, but the exact mechanisms are unclear [61].

The loop of Henle reabsorbs approximately 20% of filtered calcium. The medullary and cortical thick ascending limbs are responsible for essentially all of the calcium transport in the loop of Henle. In these segments approximately 50% of calcium reabsorption is paracellular, driven by the lumen-positive voltage [61]. The magnitude of the lumen-positive voltage is determined by the rate of chloride reabsorption. Thus, conditions that inhibit chloride reabsorption, such as volume expansion or loop diuretics, inhibit paracellular calcium reabsorption, whereas states that increase chloride reabsorption, such as volume depletion, increase calcium reabsorption [61].

In contrast to the proximal tubule, transcellular calcium reabsorption is a significant component of loop of Henle calcium reabsorption. The exact mechanisms of loop of Henle transcellular calcium transport are unknown, but in the mouse cTALH several hormones, including parathyroid hormone calcitonin, glucagon and ADH, stimulate calcium absorption without significant changes in V_T, which suggest a component of calcium absorption is active [31, 61, 62].

The distal convoluted tubule and the connecting tubule reabsorb ~10% of filtered calcium. In these segments and the CD, see below, paracellular calcium transport is small, and essentially all calcium transport occurs via transcellular mechanisms. Most evidence suggests that calcium enters the cell from the luminal fluid via an apical calcium channel [61]. Intracellular electronegativity and the low intracellular ionized calcium concentration (≤100 nM) result in a steep electrochemical gradient for calcium entry. There is a general consensus that basolateral calcium transport is active, mediated by a Ca^{2+}-ATPase and a Na^+/Ca^{2+} exchanger [61, 63].

The CD reabsorb ~1–3% of filtered Ca^{2+} [64]. The exact mechanisms are unknown, but generally believed to be similar to those in the distal convoluted tubule.

Phosphate transport along the nephron

Introduction

Phosphate plays an important role as a titratable acid in acid–base homeostasis and is essential for formation of ATP from ADP. Although organic phosphorus comprises most of total body phosphorus, inorganic phosphorus

(P_i) is present in plasma, is filtered by the glomerulus and is excreted by the kidney. Inorganic phosphorus in plasma exists in two forms, the monobasic and the dibasic form, $H_2PO_4^-$ and HPO_4^{2-}, respectively, and the transport of these differs. The relative amount of each is determined by the equilibrium reaction, $H^+ + HPO_4^{2-} \rightleftharpoons H_2PO_4^-$, where the p$Ka'$ for the reaction is 6.8. At a plasma pH of 7.40 approximately 80% of phosphate is present as HPO_4^{2-}.

Segmental analysis

Most phosphate reabsorption occurs in the proximal tubule. Since intracellular phosphate is present at concentrations that exceed its electrochemical equilibrium the apical uptake step must be active, whereas the basolateral exit step can be passive. An apical Na/P_i co-transporter, transporting 2 Na^+ per phosphate, is the primary mechanism of apical phosphate uptake [65]. Dibasic HPO_4^{2-} is transported more rapidly than monobasic $H_2PO_4^-$. An Na^+-independent, electrogenic phosphate transporter is the primary basolateral exit mechanism [65]. Intracellular electronegativity provides the electrochemical gradient for phosphate exit via this transporter. Small components of basolateral phosphate transport are mediated by an Na^+-independent, electroneutral anion exchanger [65] and a basolateral Na^+-dependent, electrogenic co-transporter [65]. Figure 4.12 shows a schematic of proximal tubule phosphate transport.

The relative amount of phosphate transport in the loop of Henle and more distal segments of the nephron is less clear. Although some studies suggest the presence of small amounts of phosphate transport in the loop of Henle [66], most evidence suggests little to no phosphate transport in this region [67]. Even less is known about the CD, but at least IMCD has the capacity to reabsorb phosphate under some circumstances. In this segment phos-

phate transport appears to be Na-independent [66]. The cellular mechanisms are otherwise unknown.

Magnesium transport along the nephron

Introduction

Magnesium (Mg) is predominantly contained intracellularly, where it is second only to K^+ as the most abundant cation in the intracellular space. Only 1% of total body Mg stores is extracellular, and the skeleton contains the majority of body Mg stores (~60%) with the muscles containing the second largest pool (~20–30%). Normal Mg intake is ~20–50 mEq (240–1200 mg), and Mg balance is regulated by the gastrointestinal tract, the skeleton and the kidney. Only about one-third of Mg intake is excreted by the kidney, which normally conserves Mg efficiently and can maintain Mg balance when Mg intake is reduced to ~1 mEq/24 h.

Segmental analysis

Approximately 97% of Mg filtered is reabsorbed, with the majority of reabsorption (~65%) occurring in the loop of Henle. The proximal tubule reabsorbs ~30% and the remainder (~5%) is reabsorbed by the distal convolution and the CD. Proximal tubule Mg reabsorption is thought to be passive although some studies have suggested that an active, transcellular mechanism is also present [68].

The loop of Henle is the major site of Mg reabsorption, and this region reabsorbs ~50–60% of the filtered Mg load [68]. Although transport in the tdl or the tal has not been studied directly, the TALH appears to be the major site within the loop of Henle responsible for Mg reabsorption since reabsorption by the pars recta is only ~5% of the fil-

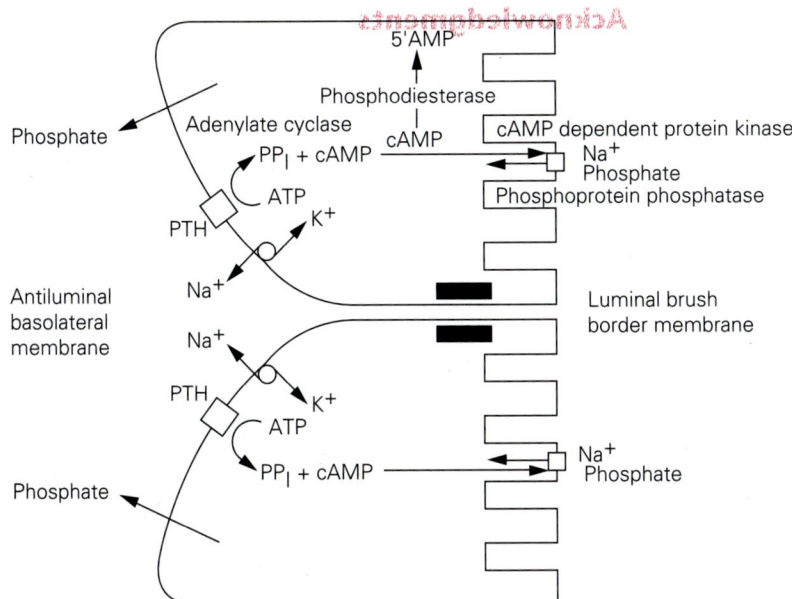

Figure 4.12 Mechanism of phosphate transport by the proximal tubule. (Reproduced, with permission, from ref. 65.)

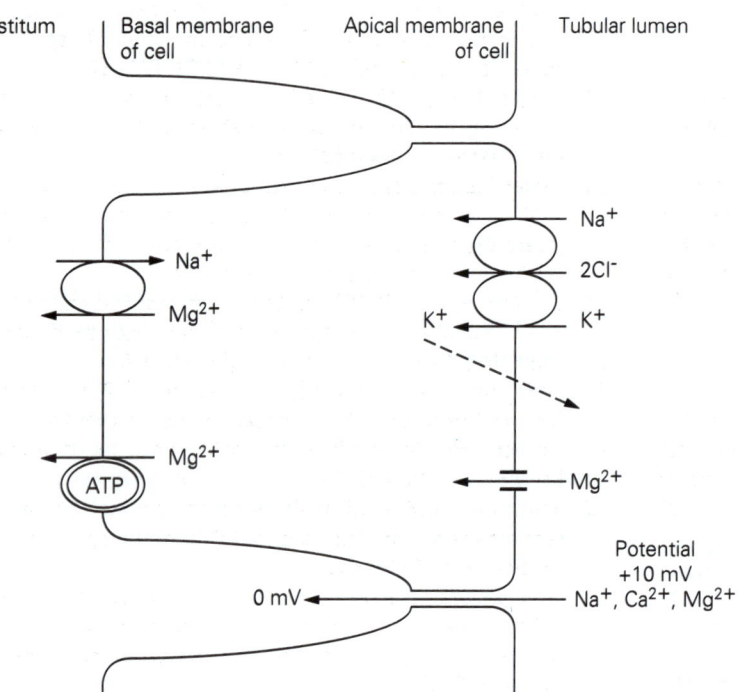

Interstitum | Basal membrane of cell | Apical membrane of cell | Tubular lumen

Figure 4.13 Mechanism of Mg transport by the thick ascending limb of Henle.

tered load and micropuncture studies reveal little absorption of Mg along the tdl or tal [69]. Mg transport in the loop of Henle increases proportional to luminal [Mg] up to 5 mM, but is dramatically suppressed by hypermagnesemia [68]. In the isolated cTALH increasing luminal [Mg] increases Mg absorption whereas increasing peritubular [Mg] suppresses absorption [70].

The mechanism of Mg absorption by the TALH is illustrated in Figure 4.13. Mg absorption increases in proportion to the lumen-positive transepithelial voltage (V_T) and decreases with furosemide administration and volume expansion [70]. The linear increase in Mg absorption with load and the effect of diuretics that inhibit V_T on Mg absorption have led most investigators to conclude that Mg transport in the TALH can be explained on the basis of passive, voltage-driven flux via the paracellular pathway. However, in the cTALH of the mouse glucagon, ADH, parathyroid hormone and calcitonin increase Mg absorption with only small effects on V_T which suggests that some of Mg absorption is active [31, 62, 71, 72].

Micropuncture studies have examined Mg transport in the distal convolution and demonstrate that this region is capable of reabsorbing ~2–5% of the filtered Mg load [73] against a lumen-negative V_T which suggests that active transport is present in this region. The cellular mechanisms for active Mg transport are unclear at the time of writing.

The transport capacity of the CD is small, ~1–3% of the filtered load. Studies of the rabbit CCD [74] or the rat IMCD [75] provide little evidence for active absorption.

Acknowledgments

The excellent secretarial assistance of Ms Gina Cowsert is gratefully acknowledged. This work was supported in part by funds from the Merit Review Program of the Department of Veteran Affairs and by R01-DK49750 and R29-45788 from the National Institutes of Health.

References

1. Tisher, C.C. and Madsen K.M. (1996) Anatomy of the Kidney in *The Kidney* (ed B.M. Brenner), 5th edn. W.B. Saunders, Philadelphia, pp. 3–71.
2. Schild, L., Giebisch, G., Karniski, L.P. and Aronson, P.S. (1987) Effect of formate on volume reabsorption in the rabbit proximal tubule. *J. Clin. Invest.*, **79**, 32–8.
3. Ishibashi, K., Rector, F.C. Jr and Berry, C.A. (1993) Role of Na-dependent Cl/HCO₃ exchange in basolateral Cl transport of rabbit proximal tubules. *Am. J. Physiol.*, **264**, F251–8.
4. Yoshitomi, K., Kondo, Y. and Imai, M. (1988) Evidence for conductive Cl⁻ pathways across the cell membranes of the thin ascending limb of Henle's loop. *J. Clin. Invest.*, **82**, 866–71.
5. Burg, M.B. and Green, N. (1973) Function of the thick ascending limb of Henle's loop. *Am. J. Physiol.*, **224**, 659–68.
6. Molony, D.A., Reeves, W.B., Hebert, S.C. and Andreoli,

T.E. (1987) ADH increases apical Na^+, K^+, $2Cl^-$ entry in mouse medullary thick ascending limbs of Henle. *Am. J. Physiol.*, **252**, F177–87.

7. Greger, R. (1985) Ion transport mechanisms in thick ascending limb of Henle's loop of mammalian nephron. *Physiol. Rev.*, **65**, 760–97.

8. Gamba, G., Miyanoshita, A., Lombardi, M. *et al.* (1994) Molecular cloning, primary structure, and characterization of two members of the mammalian electroneutral sodium-(potassium)-chloride cotransporter family expressed in kidney. *J. Biol. Chem.*, **269**, 17713–22.

9. Eveloff, J.L. and Warnock, D.G. (1987) Activation of ion transport systems during cell volume regulation. *Am. J. Physiol.*, **252**, F1–10.

10. Sun, A., Grossman, E.B., Lombardi, M. and Hebert, S.C. (1991) Vasopressin alters the mechanism of apical Cl^- entry from $Na^+:Cl^-$ to $Na^+:K^+:2Cl^-$ cotransport in mouse medullary thick ascending limb. *J. Membr. Biol.*, **120**, 83–94.

11. Stokes, J.B. (1982) Consequences of potassium recycling in the renal medulla. Effects of ion transport by the medullary thick ascending limb of Henle's loop. *J. Clin. Invest.*, **70**, 219–29.

12. Wang, W.H. (1994) Two types of K^+ channel in thick ascending limb of rat kidney. *Am. J. Physiol.*, **267**, F599–605.

13. Guggino, W.B. (1986) Functional heterogeneity in the early distal tubule of the Amphiuma kidney: evidence for two modes of Cl^- and K^+ transport across the basolateral cell membrane. *Am. J. Physiol.*, **250**, F430–40.

14. Costanzo, L.S. Localization of diuretic action in microperfused rat distal tubules: Ca and Na transport. *Am. J. Physiol.*, **248**, F527–35.

15. Shimizu, T., Yoshitomi, K., Nakamura, M. and Imai, M. (1988) Site and mechanism of action of trichlormethiazide in rabbit distal nephron segments perfused in vitro. *J. Clin. Invest.*, **82**, 721–30.

16. Plotkin, M.D., Kaplan, M.R., Verlander, J.W. *et al.* (1996) Localization of the thiazide sensitive Na-Cl contransporter, rTSC1, in the rat kidney. *Kidney Int.*, **50**, 174–83.

17. Greger, R. and Velazquez, H. (1987) The cortical thick ascending limb and early distal convoluted tubule in the urinary concentrating mechanism. *Kidney Int.*, **31**, 590–6.

18. Verlander, J.W., Madsen, K.M. and Tisher, C.C. (1987) Effect of acute respiratory acidosis on two populations of intercalated cells in the rat cortical collecting duct. *Am. J. Physiol.*, **253**, F1142–56.

19. Ling, B.N., Hinton, C.F. and Eaton, D.C. (1991) Amiloride-sensitive sodium channels in rabbit cortical collecting tubule primary cultures. *Am. J. Physiol.*, **261**, F933–44.

20. Canessa, C.M., Schild, L., Buell, G. *et al.* (1994) Amiloride-sensitive epithelial Na^+ channel is made of three homologous subunits. *Nature*, **367**, 463–7.

21. Muto, S., Yasoshima, K., Yoshitomi, K. *et al.* (1990) Electrophysiological identification of α- and β-intercalated cells and their distribution along the rabbit distal nephron segments. *J. Clin. Invest.*, **86**, 1829–39.

22. Ling, BN., Kokko, K.E. and Eaton, D.C. (1994) Prostaglandin E_2 activates clusters of apical Cl^- channels in principal cells via a cyclic adenosine monophosphate-dependent pathway. *J. Clin. Invest.*, **93**, 829–37.

23. Wingo, C.S. (1989) Potassium secretion by the cortical collecting tubule: effects of ouabain and Cl gradients. *Am. J. Physiol.*, **256**, F306–13.

24. Stokes, J.B., Ingram, M.J., Williams, A.D. and Ingram, D. (1981) Heterogeneity of the rabbit collecting tubule: localization of mineralocorticoid hormone action to the cortical portion. *Kidney Int.*, **20**, 340–7.

25. Stanton, B.A. (1989) Characterization of apical and basolateral membrane conductances of rat inner medullary collecting duct. *Am. J. Physiol.*, **256**, F862–8.

26. Koeppen, B.M., Giebisch, G. and Biagi, B.A. (1983) Electrophysiology of mammalian renal tubules: inferences from intracellular microelectrode studies. *Annu. Rev. Physiol.*, **45**, 497–517.

27. Weinstein, A.M. (1988) Modeling the proximal tubule: complications of the paracellular pathway. *Am. J. Physiol.*, **254**, F297–305.

28. Jamison, R.L., Lacey, F.B., Pennell, J.P. and Sanjana, V.M. (1976) Potassium secretion by the descending limb or pars recta of the juxtamedullary nephron *in vivo*. *Kidney Int.*, **9**, 323–32.

29. Battilana, C.A., Dobyan, D.C., Lacey, F.B. *et al.* (1978) Effect of chronic potassium loading on potassium secretion by the pars recta or descending limb of the juxtamedullary nephron in the rat. *J. Clin. Invest.*, **62**, 1093–103.

30. Wasserstein, A.G. and Agus, Z.S. (1983) Potassium secretion in the rabbit proximal straight tubule. *Am. J. Physiol.*, **245**, F167–74.

31. Di Stefano, A., Wittner, M., Nitschke, R. *et al.* (1989) Effects of glucagon on Na^+, Cl^-, K^+, Mg^{2+} and Ca^{2+} transports in cortical and medullary thick ascending limbs of mouse kidney. *Pflugers Arch.*, **414**, 640–6.

32. Stanton, B.A., Biemesderfer, D., Wade, J.B. and Giebisch, G. (1981) Structural and functional study of the rat distal nephron: effects of potassium adaptation and depletion. *Kidney Int.*, **19**, 36–48.

33. Velazquez, H., Ellison, D.H. and Wright, F.S. (1987) Chloride-dependent potassium secretion in early and late renal distal tubules. *Am. J. Physiol.*, **253**, F555–62.

34. Good, D.W. and Wright, F.S. (1979) Luminal influences on potassium secretion: sodium concentration and luminal flow rate. *Am. J. Physiol.*, **236**, F192–205.

35. Ellison, D.H., Velazquez, H. and Wright, F.S. (1985) Stimulation of distal potassium secretion by low luminal chloride in the presence of barium. *Am. J. Physiol.*, **248**, F638–49.

36. Wang, W., Sackin, H. and Giebisch, C. (1992) Renal potassium channels and their regulation. *Annu. Rev. Physiol.*, **54**, 81–96.

37. Wingo, C.S. and Smolka, A. (1995) Function and structure of H,K-ATPase in the kidney. *Am. J. Physiol.*, **269**, F1–16.

38. Wingo, C.S. and Cain, B.D. (1993) The renal H-K-ATPase: physiological significance and role in potassium homeostasis. *Annu. Rev. Physiol.*, **55**, 323–47.

39. Elger, M., Bankir, L. and Kriz, W. (1992) Morphometric analysis of kidney hypertrophy in rats after chronic

potassium depletion. *Am. J. Physiol.*, **262**, F656–67.

40. Hansen, G.T., Tisher, C.C. and Robinson, R.R. (1980) Response of the collecting duct ot disturbances of acid base and potassium balance. *Kidney Int.*, **17**, 326–37.

41. Backman, K.A. and Hayslett, J.P. (1983) Role of the medullary collecting duct in potassium conservation. *Pflugers Arch.*, **396**, 297–300.

42. Schon, D.A., Backman, K.A. and Hayslett, J.P. (1981) Role of the medullary collecting duct in potassium excretion in potassium-adapted animals. *Kidney Int.*, **20**, 655–62.

43. Light, D.B., McCann, F.V., Keller, T.M. and Stanton, B.A. (1988) Amiloride-sensitive cation channel in apical membrane of inner medullary collecting duct. *Am. J. Physiol.*, **255**, F278–86.

44. Moe, O.W., Preisig, P.A. and Alpern, R.J. (1990) Cellular model of proximal tubule NaCl and $NaHCO_3$ absorption. *Kidney Int.*, **38**, 605–11.

45. Buerkert, J., Martin, D. and Trigg, D. (1982) Segmental analysis of the renal tubule in buffer production and net acid formation. *Am. J. Physiol.*, **244**, F442–54.

46. Good, D.S. (1985) Sodium-dependent bicarbonate absorption by cortical thick ascending limb of rat kidney. *Am. J. Physiol.*, **248**, F821–9.

47. Hamm, L.L. and Hering-Smith, K.S. (1993) Acid–base transport in the collecting duct. *Semin. Nephrol.*, **13**, 246–55.

48. Verlander, J.W., Madsen, K.M. and Tisher, C.C. (1991) Structural and functional features of proton and bicarbonate transport in the rat collecting duct. *Semin. Nephrol.*, **11**, 465–77.

49. Weiner, I.D., Wingo, C.S. and Hamm, L.L. (1993) Regulation of intracellular pH in two cell populations of inner stripe of rabbit outer medullary collecting duct. *Am. J. Physiol.*, **265**, F406–15.

50. Weill, A.E., Tisher, C.C., Conde, M.F. and Weiner, I.D. (1994) Mechanisms of bicarbonate transport by cultured rabbit inner medullary collecting duct cells. *Am. J. Physiol.*, **35**, F466–76.

51. Wall, S.M. and Knepper, M.A. (1990) Acid–base transport in the inner medullary collecting duct. *Semin. Nephrol.*, **10**, 148–58.

52. Weiner, I.D. and Milton, A.E. (1996) H^+-K^+-ATPase in rabbit cortical collecting duct B-type intercalated cell. *Am. J. Physiol.*, **270**, F518–30.

53. Madsen, K.M. and Tisher, C.C. (1986) Structural–functional relationships along the distal nephron. *Am. J. Physiol.*, **250**, F1–15.

54. Halperin, M.L., Kamel, K.S., Ethier, J.H. *et al.* (1992) Biochemistry and physiology of ammonium excretion, in *The Kidney: Physiology and Pathophysiology* (eds D.W. Seldin and G. Giebisch), Raven Press, New York, pp. 2645–79.

55. Kinsella, J.L. and Aronson, P.S. (1981) Interaction of NH_4^+ and Li^+ with the renal microvillus membrane Na^+-H^+ exchanger. *Am. J. Physiol.*, **241**, C220–6.

56. Knepper, M.A. (1991) NH_4^+ transport in the kidney. *Kidney Int. Suppl.*, **33**, S95–102.

57. Good, D.W. (1988) Active absorption of NH_4^+ by rat medullary thick ascending limb: inhibition by potas-

sium. *Am. J. Physiol.*, **255**, F78–87.

58. Good, D.W. and DuBose, T.D.J. (1988) Concentrations of NH_3 in cortex and medulla of rat kidney. *Contrib. Nephrol.*, **63**, 16–20.

59. Good, D.W. and Knepper, M.A. (1990) Mechanisms of ammonium excretion: role of the renal medulla. *Semin. Nephrol.*, **10**, 166–73.

60. Hamm, L.L. and Simon, E.E. (1987) Roles and mechanisms of urinary buffer excretion. *Am. J. Physiol.*, **253**, F595–605.

61. Friedman, P.A. and Gesek, F.A. (1993) Calcium transport in renal epithelial cells. *Am. J. Physiol.*, **264**, F181–98.

62. Di Stefano, A., Wittner, M., Nitschke, R. *et al.* (1990) Effects of parathyroid hormone and calcitonin on Na^+, Cl^-, K^+, Mg^{2+} and Ca^{2+} transport in cortical and medullary thick ascending limbs of mouse kidney. *Pflugers Arch.*, **417**(2), 161–7.

63. Bourdeau, J.E. Mechanisms and regulation of calcium transport in the nephron. *Semin. Nephrol.*, **13**, 191–201.

64. Sutton, R.A.L. and Dirks, J.H. (1975) The renal excretion of calcium: a review of micropuncture data. *Can. J. Physiol. Pharmacol.*, **53**, 979–88.

65. Hammerman, M.R. (1986) Phosphate transport across renal proximal tubular cell membranes. *Am. J. Physiol.*, **251**, F385–98.

66. Elalouf, J.M., Roinel, N. and de-Rouffignac, C. (1984) ADH-like effects of calcitonin on electrolyte transport by Henle's loop of rat kidney. *Am. J. Physiol.*, **256**, F213–20.

67. Jamison, R.L. and Arrascue, J.F. (1980) Calcium and phosphorous reabsorption by the loop of Henle. *Miner. Electrolyte Metab.*, **4**, 97–105.

68. Quamme, G.A. and Dirks, J.H. (1980) Magnesium transport in the nephron. *Am. J. Physiol.*, **239**, F393–401.

69. Roy, D.R. (1987) Magnesium reabsorption in the juxtamedullary loop of Henle: effect of magnesium deprivation. *Can. J. Physiol. Pharmacol.*, **65**, 1918–22.

70. Quamme, G.A. (1989) Control of magnesium transport in the thick ascending limb. *Am. J. Physiol.*, **256**, F197–210.

71. Wittner, M. and Di Stefano, A. (1990) Effects of antidiuretic hormone, parathyroid hormone and glucagon on transepithelial voltage and resistance of the cortical and medullary thick ascending limb of Henle's loop of the mouse nephron. *Pflugers Arch.*, **415**, 707–12.

72. Wittner, M., Di Stefano, A., Wangemann, P. *et al.* (1988) Differential effects of ADH on sodium, chloride, potassium, calcium and magnesium transport in cortical and medullary thick ascending limbs of mouse nephron. *Pflugers Arch.*, **412**, 516–23.

73. Quamme, G.A. and Dirks, J.H. (1980) Intraluminal and contraluminal magnesium on magnesium and calcium transfer in the rat nephron. *Am. J. Physiol.*, **283**, F187–98.

74. Shareghi, G.R. and Agus Z.S (1982) Phosphate transport in the light segment of the rabbit cortical collecting tubule. *Am. J. Physiol.*, **242**, F379–84.

75. Bengele, H.H., Alexander, E.A. and Lechene, C.P. (1980) Calcium and magnesium transport along the inner medullary collecting duct of the rat. *Am. J. Physiol.*, **239**, F24–9.

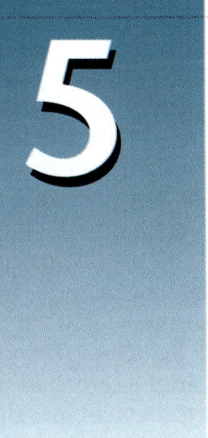

5

Organic solute transport

William H. Dantzler, Stephen H. Wright and Christopher J. Lote

Introduction

This chapter is concerned with the transport of organic solutes by the renal tubules. However, it is limited to the transport of glucose, amino acids and oligopeptides, organic anions, urate and organic cations. Even within these categories, only the major transport processes are considered. The common features of the basic processes within categories and between categories are emphasized. This is done to provide an up-to-date framework for understanding the regulation of body levels of both endogenous and exogenous substances in these categories.

Glucose transport

Studies with whole animal and whole organ clearance techniques have shown that glucose is freely filtered at the glomerulus and then is effectively completely reabsorbed from the tubular filtrate. Subsequent studies employing micropuncture, microperfusion and indicator-dilution techniques showed that the proximal tubule is the site for the net reabsorption of D-glucose [1]. The proximal tubule is also the site for reabsorption of other sugars and competitive inhibition studies support the presence, in addition to transporters specific for D-glucose and related structures, of distinct transport pathways for (1) mannose and D-fructose and (2) *myo*-inositol. However, the cellular processes involved in the transepithelial transport of glucose have been the center of attention [1], including in recent years the cloning of the

several transporters responsible for active tubular transport [2], and the results of these studies will be the focus of the following discussion.

Figure 5.1 presents a schematic representation of the individual transport events involved in the net reabsorptive flux of glucose in the proximal tubule. The movement of glucose from the filtrate into the proximal cell, across the luminal membrane, is a secondary active transport process and involves the co-transport of glucose with Na^+. The electrochemical gradient for Na^+ is directed into the cell, i.e. from the luminal fluid to the cytoplasm of proximal cells. By coupling the inward flux of glucose to that of Na^+ moving down its electrochemical gradient, net movement of glucose into the cell can occur against a substantial concentration gradient (as discussed in more detail below). The glucose flux across the peritubular (basolateral) membrane is limited to carrier-mediated facilitated diffusion. However, because the intracellular concentration of glucose is larger than that in the blood (as a consequence of the active transport step in the luminal membrane), there is a net efflux of glucose from the proximal cell. Thus, the concerted activity of distinct transporters arrayed 'in series' in the luminal and peritubular membranes results in a net reabsorptive flux of glucose (Figure 5.1).

As noted above, the inwardly directed electrochemical gradient for Na^+ is the immediate source of energy for the active transport of glucose. This gradient is maintained through the active extrusion of Na^+ from the cell. This occurs through the activity of the Na^+,K^+-ATPase, a primary active transport process that uses the energy

Nephrology, Edited by Rex L. Jamison and Robert Wilkinson.
Published in 1997 by Chapman & Hall, London. ISBN 0 412 60930 4

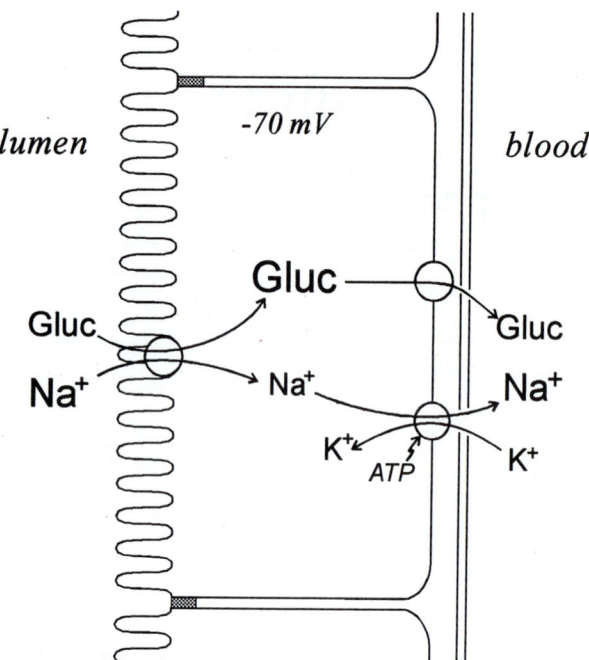

lumen

−70 mV

blood

Gluc

Gluc

Na⁺

Gluc

Na⁺

Na⁺

K⁺

ATP

K⁺

Figure 5.1 Model of glucose (Gluc) reabsorption by cells of proximal renal tubules. In this and the remaining figures, circles and arrows indicate the direction of net, carrier-mediated solute transport arising as a consequence of the electrochemical driving forces that predominate in the proximal tubule. Note that the primary transport of Na⁺ by Na⁺,K⁺-ATPase at the basolateral membrane establishes the Na⁺ gradient that accounts for all other transport steps.

obtained from the hydrolysis of ATP as the immediate source of energy for the movement of solute (i.e. Na⁺ and K⁺) against electrochemical gradients. Significantly, because the Na⁺,K⁺-ATPase is located in the basolateral membrane of proximal tubule cells, the reabsorption of glucose also results in the net reabsorption of Na⁺ (Figure 5.1). Indeed, the coupling of Na⁺ to the reabsorption of a wide variety of solutes probably accounts for ~50% of the total reabsorption of Na⁺ that occurs in the proximal tubule [3].

There are at least two distinct luminal Na⁺-glucose transport proteins distributed along the length of the nephron [1]. The luminal membrane of the S1 and S2 regions of the proximal tubule contains a transporter that has a relatively low affinity for glucose. However, the total transport capacity of this pathway is high and it is responsible for the reabsorption of most of the glucose filtered at the glomerulus. The gene product responsible for glucose transport in the early proximal tubule is referred to as SGLT2 (for sodium-glucose luminal transporter 2; [4]). The S3 region of the proximal tubule is characterized by having a different Na⁺-glucose co-transporter. This transporter has a much higher affinity for glucose and so is able to bind to glucose at the very low concentrations of glucose left in the filtrate in the S3 region of the proximal tubule. Also, unlike SGLT2, this transporter (called

SGLT1; [4]), couples two (rather than one) Na⁺ to the flux of every glucose molecule. Consequently, net transport of glucose in the S3 region can occur against much larger concentration gradients than those found in the earlier regions of the tubule and, therefore, can succeed in effectively clearing glucose from the tubular filtrate [4].

There is also axial heterogeneity in the distribution of the basolateral glucose transporters that catalyze the exit of glucose from proximal cells. All the basolateral transporters are members of the GLUT ('glucose transporter') family of glucose transporters [5]. In the early part of the proximal tubule GLUT1 (the erythrocyter-type glucose transporter) and GLUT2 (the liver-type glucose transporter) appear to be expressed. However, in the late, S3 region of proximal tubule, where transcellular glucose flux is low, only GLUT1 appears to be expressed.

The luminal (SGLT) glucose transporters show a marked specificity for D-glucose, D-galactose, α-methyl-D-glucopyranoside, 2-deoxy-D-glucose, D-fructose, and *myo*-inositol, as well as a profound sensitivity to the drug phlorizin [1]. The basolateral (GLUT) transporters, in addition to handling D-glucose, D-galactose, D-fructose, 2-deoxy-D-glucose, and *myo*-inositol, also transport 3-*O*-methyl-D-glucose, D-mannose, D-xylose and L-arabinose. Also, the GLUT family of transporters are sensitive to the drugs phloretin and cytochalasin, rather than to phlorizin.

Renal glycosuria (Types A and B) is probably a consequence of genetic defects in the SGLT2 glucose transporter [4], resulting in significant decreases either in the transport capacity (i.e. decreases in turnover of the transporter; Type A) or in the apparent affinity of the transporters for glucose (Type B). Interestingly, defects in SGLT1 result in a mild glycosuria, because of the resulting inability to clear glucose from the low concentrations of this compound found in the late proximal tubule. However, because SGLT1 is the predominant active glucose transporter in the intestine, these patients suffer from glucose–galactose malabsorption syndrome.

Amino acid transport

Amino acids are typically reabsorbed by the kidney. Although reabsorption of amino acids is not as efficient as for glucose, on average only about 1.1% of the filtered load of amino acid is excreted (for specific amino acids this can vary from <0.5% to >5%; [6]). Early stop-flow experiments suggested that the proximal tubule is the site for amino acid reabsorption. Although recent studies still implicate the early part of the proximal tubule as the primary site for amino acid reabsorption, it is now evident that distal components of the nephron, particularly the loop of Henle, also play an important role in the reabsorption of some of the more slowly transported amino acids (e.g. glycine and taurine) [6].

At the cellular level, the transport steps associated with reabsorption of zwitterionic (neutral) amino acids show a marked similarity to those associated with reabsorption of glucose. The entry of amino acid from the filtrate into the cell across the luminal membrane typically involves an Na^+-co-transport process which can move the amino acid against its electrochemical gradient (Figure 5.2). The relatively large intracellular concentration of amino acids developed by these processes then favors their downhill efflux across the peritubular membrane via an Na^+-independent, facilitated diffusion process. The continued net reabsorption of amino acids requires the maintenance of the Na^+ electrochemical gradient via the basolateral Na^+,K^+-ATPase.

Although most of the luminal reabsorptive transport processes described to date involve a coupling of (one or more) Na^+ ions with amino acid, other inorganic ions, including, K^+, H^+ and Cl^-, have been found to influence the transport of some amino acids [6]. Most notably, the cycle of events associated with the influx of anionic (acidic) amino acids (glutamate and aspartate) across the luminal membrane involves a co-transport with two Na^+ ions and a countertransport with one K^+ ion, illustrated for glutamate in Figure 5.3. Thus, transport of dibasic amino acids is coupled to both the inwardly-directed Na^+-gradient and the outwardly-directed K^+-gradient. The transluminal transport of the zwitterionic amino acid taurine also involves the co-transport of one Cl^- ion along with two Na^+ ions and one taurine molecule. Finally, the reabsorptive flux of some amino acids (e.g. proline) is driven by the inwardly directed electrochemical gradient for H^+, rather than Na^+ (Figure 5.3). Whereas these examples represent variations of a similar strategy for driving

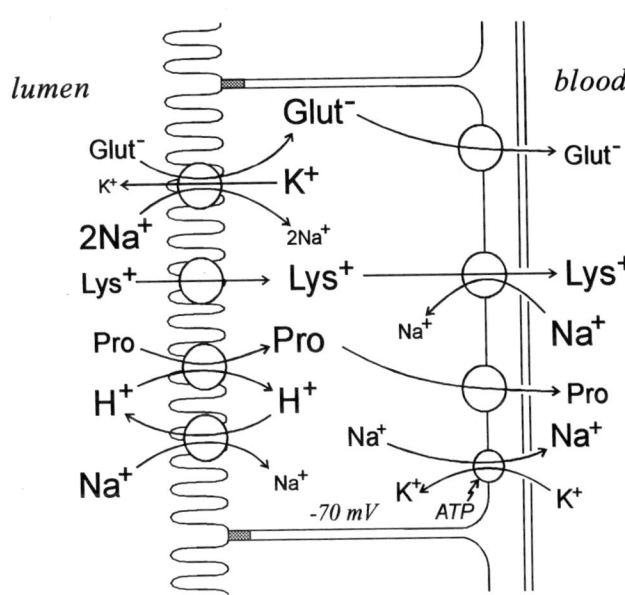

Figure 5.3 Model for reabsorption of three specific amino acids (glutamate, $Glut^-$; lysine, Lys^+; and proline, Pro) that do not fit the general model shown in Figure 5.2. Other symbols and role of Na^+,K^+-ATPase are as in Figure 5.1.

the reabsorptive flux of anionic and zwitterionic amino acids, reabsorption of cationic (dibasic) amino acids may involve a very different set of processes (Figure 5.3). Lysine transport across the luminal membrane occurs by Na^+-independent, electrogenic facilitated diffusion, driven by the inside-negative membrane potential of the proximal tubule cell. Efflux of the cationic substrate appears to involve the carrier-mediated, electroneutral exchange of lysine for Na^+. Thus, the active step in net reabsorption for lysine resides in the basolateral membrane, driven by the inwardly directed chemical gradient for Na^+.

The basolateral exit of amino acids typically involves facilitated diffusion. However, Na^+-amino acid co-transporters have also been found in the basolateral membrane of some tubular cells, particularly in the late proximal tubule and postproximal regions of the nephron where luminal delivery of amino acids is slight. It is likely that these processes are required by cells of the late proximal and postproximal region for nutritive purposes, to provide substrate for protein synthesis, gluconeogenesis, ammoniagenesis, glutamine and arginine synthesis, and so forth.

The chemical class of compounds referred to collectively as 'amino acids' includes a diverse array of molecular structures, as implied by the preceding discussion. It is not surprising, therefore, that transport of amino acids across each pole of proximal tubule cells involves the concerted activity of a number of distinct transport processes displaying varying degrees of overlap in their structural specificity [7]. The actual number of distinct transport processes present in, for example, renal proximal cells remains the subject of extensive study. Nevertheless,

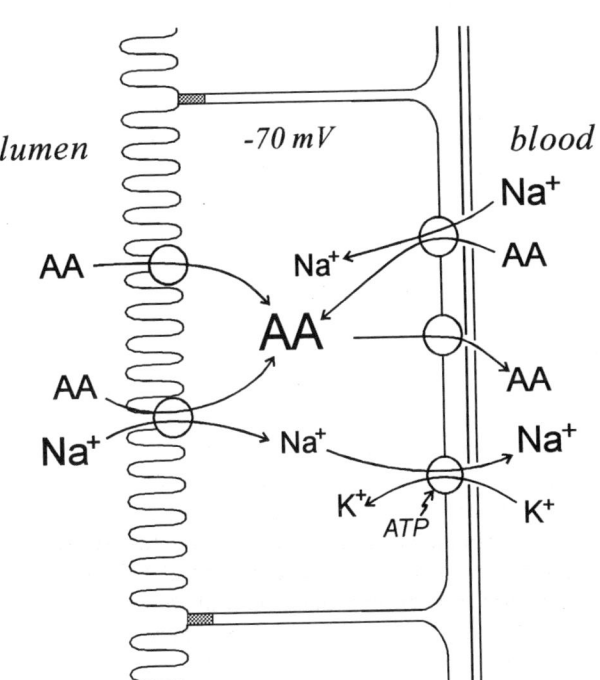

Figure 5.2 General model for amino acid (AA) reabsorption by cells of proximal renal tubule. Other symbols and role of Na^+,K^+-ATPase are as in Figure 5.1.

when the results of experimental studies are compared to known defects in amino acid absorption observed in patients (e.g. Fanconi syndrome, cystinuria and Hartrup disease), the presence of several unique transport processes can be inferred [8]. These include pathways for (1) anionic amino acids (e.g. aspartate and glutamate); (2) cationic amino acids (e.g. L-lysine and L-arginine); and the zwitterionic substrates (3) L-cystine and L-cysteine; (4) glycine; (5) taurine (a non-protein, sulfur-containing β-zwitterionic amino acid); (6) citrulline (a non-protein, α-zwitterionic amino acid); and (7) 'imino' acids (e.g. proline). In addition, there are at least two pathways displaying broad, overlapping specificity for α-zwitterionic amino acids (e.g. phenylalanine, alanine, serine, leucine, etc.). In general, the naturally occurring L-isomers are reabsorbed to a much greater extent than are the D-isomers of these compounds, although the stereoselectivity is not as extreme as that noted for the reabsorption of glucose. In contrast to this general rule, however, is the observation that D- and L-aspartate are handled fairly similarly by the acidic amino acid transport pathway.

All of the many low-molecular-weight oligopeptides present in plasma (e.g. vasopressin, angiotensin I and II, kinins, atrial naturetic peptides, glucagon, oxytocin) are freely filterable. The kidney contains four major routes for transport of such molecules [6]: (1) reabsorption of a filtered peptide/protein via endocytosis with subsequent intracellular degradation; (2) luminal hydrolysis of the filtered peptide with subsequent reabsorption of the released amino acids; (3) carrier-mediated reabsorption of small intact peptides; and (4) peritubular uptake of peptides. A discussion of processes 1 and 4 is beyond the scope of this chapter [7].

The luminal membrane contains several oligopeptidases capable of the rapid hydrolysis of filtered oligopeptides resulting in the liberation of the constituent amino acids which are subsequently cleared from the filtrate by the various amino acid transporters. For example, filtered angiotensin II is almost completely degraded in the proximal tubule with subsequent reabsorption of the constituent amino acids. Similar results have been observed for angiotensin I, kinins and a variety of di-, tri- and tetrapeptides. Even rather large peptides, e.g. the linear peptide glucagon, can be almost completely hydrolyzed in the lumen of the proximal tubule. Significantly, luminal degradation of insulin is quite limited, probably due to the presence in this molecule of a number of disulfide bridges. Instead, insulin appears to undergo endocytotic uptake followed by lysosomal degradation.

The uptake of intact oligopeptides across the apical membrane of kidney tubule cells is mediated by at least two distinct transport processes [9–11]. One is a high-affinity/low-capacity oligopeptide transporter which only operates in the presence of an inwardly directed H^+ gradient (i.e. filtrate-to-cell). The second process is a low-affinity/high-capacity transporter which does not require a pH gradient for its operation [12]. Recently, the high-affinity/low-capacity oligopeptide transporter from rabbit small intestine has been cloned and functionally characterized [13]. This transporter has been denoted PepT1. The mRNA for PepT1 is also present in the kidney so it is likely that the same protein is involved in renal oligopeptide transport. This transporter has a very broad substrate specificity. The optimum number of amino acids in oligopeptides transported by PepT1 is two (assessed using glycine peptides), and oligopeptides of more than five amino acids are not transported by this process. Although the affinity of PepT1 for different dipeptides varies, it seems that any dipeptide can serve as a substrate, whether containing anionic, cationic or hydrophobic amino acid residues.

The renal transport of the tripeptide glutathione is believed to play an important role in the overall cycle of detoxification and elimination from the body of xenobiotic agents [6]. The brush border membrane contains the degradative enzyme, γ-glutamyltranspeptidase. The main physiological substrates of this enzyme are glutathione and its S-conjugated derivatives, the latter arising primarily in the liver during the process of hepatic detoxification of xenobiotic compounds. Hydrolysis of the γ-glutamyl group of glutathione results in the production of glutamate and the dipeptide, cysteinyl-glycine, which is hydrolyzed, in turn, by a rather non-specific aminopeptidase. The constituent amino acids, i.e. glutamate, cysteine and glycine, are rapidly reabsorbed in the tubule.

Certain dipeptides (e.g. carnosine) are resistant to the attack of luminal peptidases. They are, nevertheless, reabsorbed by the kidney via one or more carrier-mediated processes [6]. Active transport of intact dipeptides does not appear to be coupled to a co-transport of Na^+ but, instead, to a co-transport with H^+. Because the inwardly directed H^+ gradient that drives dipeptide transport is itself a product of a secondary active transporter (i.e. the luminal Na^+-H^+ exchanger) that relies on a primary active pump (the Na^+,K^+-ATPase) to maintain the Na^+-gradient, H^+-dipeptide co-transport can be referred to as a tertiary active transport process.

Organic anion transport

A major system for secretion of a wide range of hydrophobic organic anions exists in the renal proximal tubules. Although the system is capable of secreting a number of endogenous compounds, it very effectively removes numerous exogenous compounds, including many drugs, environmental xenobiotics, and plant and animal toxins from the body. It also secretes the toxic metabolic breakdown products of numerous exogenous and some endogenous compounds. Some examples of excreted compounds are shown in Table 5.1. The primary function of this system is to remove such compounds from the body as effectively as possible.

Table 5.1 Examples of organic anions and cations secreted by the renal tubules

Organic anions	Organic cations
Chlorothiazide	Amiloride
Diodrast	Cimetidine
Ester glucuronides	Isoproterenol
Ether glucuronides	N'-methylnicotinamide (NMN)
Furosemide	Morphine
Para-aminohippurate (PAH)	Procainamide
Penicillins	Procaine
Pyrazinoate	Quinidine
Saccharin	Quinine
Salicylates	Tetraethylammonium (TEA)

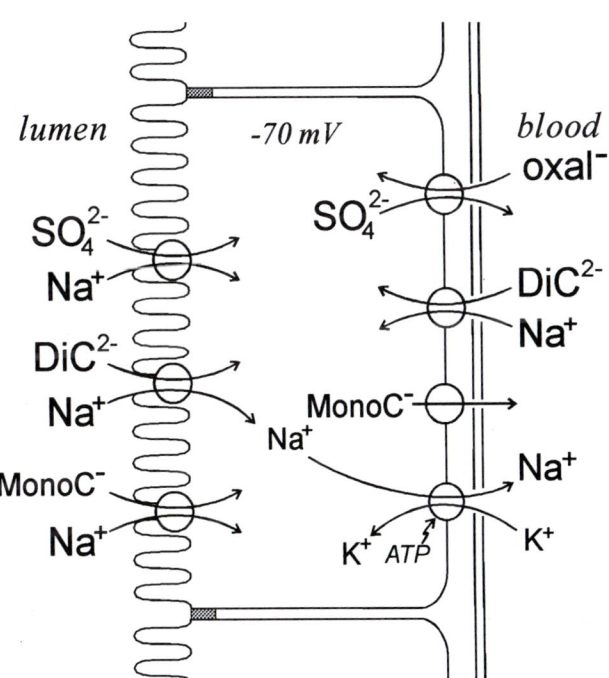

Figure 5.4 Model of known transport pathways for specific organic anions at the luminal and basolateral membranes of cells of proximal renal tubules. DiC^{2-}, dicarboxylate; $MonoC^-$, monocarboxylate; $oxal^-$, oxalate. Other symbols and role of Na^+,K^+-ATPase are as in Figure 5.1.

Although this chapter concentrates only on this major system for secreting a very wide range of organic anions, there are a number of other systems for transporting specific types of anions into the cells at the basolateral membrane (secretory direction) and the luminal membrane (reabsorptive direction) [14, 15]. Some of these are illustrated in Figure 5.4. For example, at the basolateral membrane, there are an exchange system for oxalate uptake and sulfate exit, an Na^+-dependent co-transport system for dicarboxylates (such as α-ketoglutarate and succinate), and a transport system for some small monocarboxylates (such as lactate). At the luminal membrane, there are an Na^+-dependent transport system for sulfate, an Na^+-dependent co-transport system for dicarboxylates (again including α-ketoglutarate and succinate, but also citrate), an Na^+-dependent transport system for some small monocarboxylates (such as lactate) and an anion-exchange transport system for urate. Except for the transport system for urate, which will be discussed separately below, these other systems will only be mentioned as they relate to the general system for the secretion of organic anions.

The organic anions secreted by this general organic anion system, the prototype of which is para-aminohippurate (PAH), do not move passively across the epithelium. Instead, they are transported into the cells across the basolateral membrane against an electrochemical gradient and then move down an electrochemical gradient into the lumen across luminal membrane (Figure 5.5). This net secretion takes place primarily in the S2 segment of the proximal renal tubule.

The affinity of the basolateral 'PAH transporter' for

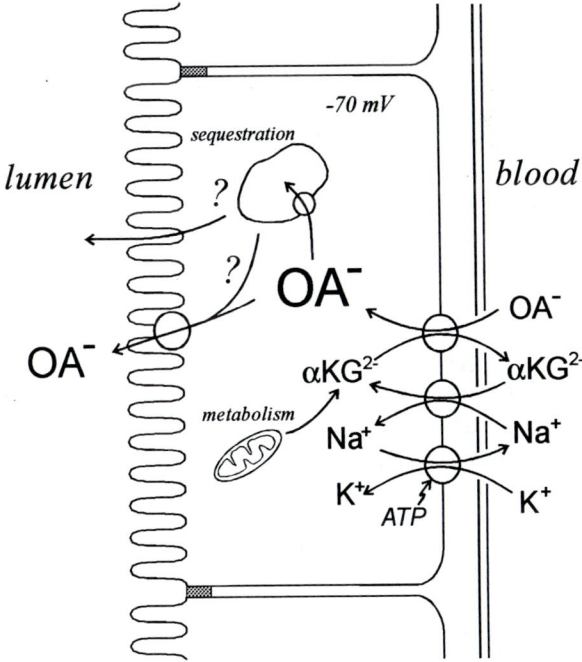

Figure 5.5 Model of the general pathway for secretion of organic anions (OA^-) by cells of proximal renal tubules. Note that the outwardly directed gradient for α-ketoglutarate ($αKG^{2-}$) can be maintained by both intracellular metabolism and by transport into the cells via the Na^+-dicarboxylate co-transporter. Also note that sequestration of OA^- in intracellular vesicles may play some role in the transepithelial transport process. Other symbols and role of Na^+,K^+-ATPase are as in Figure 5.1.

various substrates is determined by the charge, charge placement and the hydrophobicity of the molecule [15]. This transporter accepts monovalent hydrophobic anions with a negative or partial negative charge. The minimum length of the hydrophobic region for effective binding to the transporter is 4 Å. It also accepts divalent compounds with two negative or partially negative charges, optimally 6–7 Å apart. These can apparently include some zwitterions. Because the hydrophobic domain in these divalent compounds can have a length up to 10 Å, it may be located at least partially outside a direct line between the charges. Unfortunately, despite numerous attempts, the basolateral PAH transporter has yet to be isolated and its molecular structure characterized.

Although the basolateral transporter has yet to be characterized, the basic steps in the transport process have now been well characterized (Figure 5.5). Transport into the cells of PAH (and other organic anions that share this system) is a tertiary active process, the final step in which is the countertransport of PAH against its electrochemical gradient for an intracellular dicarboxylate (physiologically α-ketoglutarate, αKG) moving down its electrochemical gradient (Figure 5.5). The intracellular concentration of αKG is maintained above the extracellular concentration by metabolism and by transport into the cells via the Na$^+$-dicarboxylate co-transport system at the basolateral and, possibly, the luminal membrane (Figures 5.4 and 5.5). The inwardly directed Na$^+$ gradient that drives dicarboxylate entry is maintained, in turn, by the primary energy-requiring step in this tertiary process, the transport of Na$^+$ out of the cells via Na$^+$,K$^+$-ATPase at the basolateral membrane (Figure 5.5). These steps in the basolateral transport process, delineated initially with isolated basolateral membranes [16, 17] have been documented in intact renal tubules [18]. Finally, the basolateral transport step appears to be rate limiting for transepithelial secretion [19].

The transport step for PAH from the cells into the lumen is much less well understood than the transport step at the basolateral membrane. It is a carrier-mediated step down an electrochemical gradient, illustrated for organic ions as a class in Figure 5.5. However, the nature of the mediated step is unknown. It may involve some form of anion exchange. Indeed, in some species, probably including humans, PAH can be exchanged for urate. However, as discussed below, this exchanger appears poised primarily to reabsorb urate and PAH is probably much less likely than other anions to be exchanged for urate.

Finally, organic anions, such as PAH, transported into the cells at the basolateral membrane may not simply diffuse through the cytoplasm from the basolateral pole to the luminal pole as generally supposed. Recent studies on tissues from non-mammalian vertebrates have suggested that the anion may be sequestered in vesicles that move across the cells (Figure 5.5) [20]. Intracellular movement within vesicles could prevent the development of high concentrations of toxic substances free within the cytoplasm [20]. This possibility has yet to be demonstrated for mammalian renal tubules.

Urate transport

Transepithelial urate transport occurs in the proximal tubule. However, determining the mechanism of such transport has proven difficult, because most species exhibit both reabsorption and secretion and the predominance of net secretion or net reabsorption varies among species. Among the mammals, humans, chimpanzees, rats and mongrel dogs exhibit net tubular reabsorption whereas others studied generally show net tubular secretion. Despite the difficulties, studies on tissues from rats and dogs, species in which urate transport appears similar to that in humans, have partially elucidated reabsorptive steps that may reflect those in humans [20, 21].

As noted above, luminal membranes isolated from proximal tubules of rats and dogs exhibit an anion exchanger that can transport both urate and PAH (Figure 5.6). This exchanger appears poised to reabsorb urate by moving it against its electrochemical gradient in exchange for another anion moving down its electrochemical gradient (Figure 5.6) [21]. The cell-to-lumen electrochemical gradient for these other anions can be produced by the inwardly directed Na$^+$ gradient established by Na$^+$,K$^+$-ATPase on the basolateral membrane. Thus, as in the case of PAH transport into the cells at the basolateral membrane, urate transport into the cells at the

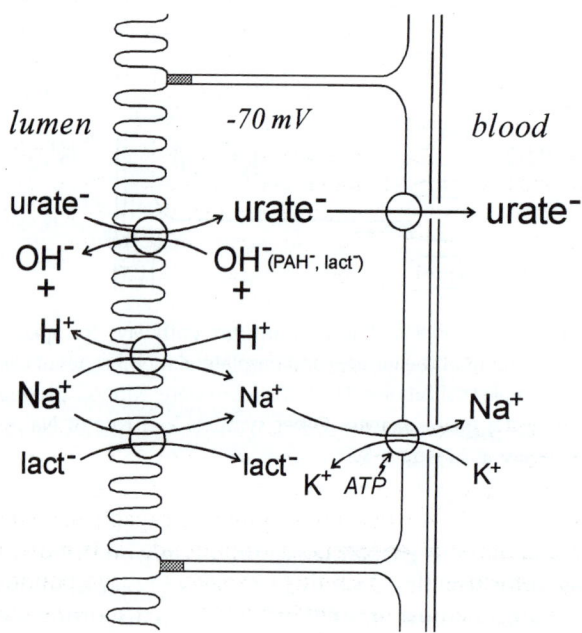

Figure 5.6 Model for urate (urate$^-$) reabsorption by cells of proximal renal tubule. Other symbols are: PAH$^-$, *para*-aminohippurate; and lact$^-$, lactate. Other symbols and role of Na$^+$,K$^+$-ATPase are as in Figure 5.1.

luminal membrane may be a tertiary active transport system. This luminal exchanger for urate is shared by a number of organic and inorganic anions (OH^-, Cl^-, HCO_3^-, lactate and some dicarboxylates), some of which could countertransport urate into the cells as they move down electrochemical gradients established by coupling to the Na^+ gradient. For example, the transport of protons out of the cells into the lumen by the luminal Na^+-H^+ countertransport system would help maintain a cell-to-lumen OH^- gradient to drive urate countertransport (Figure 5.6). Also, Na^+-coupled co-transport of substances such as lactate into the cells across the luminal membrane could establish a cell-to-lumen lactate gradient to drive urate countertransport (Figure 5.6). As discussed above, organic anions, such as PAH, transported into the cells across the basolateral membrane could move down their electrochemical gradients into the lumen via this exchanger and countertransport urate into the cells (Figure 5.6). Finally, a uricosuric dicarboxylate like pyrazinoate that can share this system may produce its effect by blocking the binding of urate to the transporter on the luminal side.

Less is known about the exit step for urate at the basolateral membrane during the reabsorptive process than about the entry step at the luminal membrane. Studies with rat basolateral membrane vesicles indicate that urate exit occurs down an electrochemical gradient by a carrier-mediated process that can be driven by the inside-negative membrane potential (Figure 5.6) [22]. In addition, this exit step may be capable of being driven by anion countertransport, although PAH does not serve as a countertransported substrate [20]. Pyrazinoate may also interact with this carrier [20]. Finally, some studies, which remain controversial, suggest that the enzyme uricase is involved in the transport step at this membrane [23].

Even less is known about the transepithelial secretion of urate in humans or other species that generally demonstrate net transepithelial reabsorption. Studies in normal humans and with rat basolateral membrane vesicles indicate that the step at the basolateral membrane is separate from that for PAH [22, 24]. Moreover, this basolateral step can be inhibited by probenecid and DIDS [22].

Organic cation transport

As in the case of the organic anions, a major system for the secretion of a wide range of hydrophobic organic cations exists in the renal proximal tubules. Although this system, like the organic anion system, is capable of secreting a number of endogenous compounds, it is particularly effective in secreting exogenous compounds, including many drugs, environmental xenobiotics and plant and animal toxins. It also secretes the toxic metabolic breakdown products of numerous exogenous and some endogenous compounds. Examples of excreted compounds are given in Table 5.1. The primary function of this system, like the organic anion system, is to remove such compounds from the body as effectively as possible. Because a very large number of therapeutic agents exist as organic cations or are converted into organic cations in the body, this system plays a particularly important role in determining the concentrations of these substances in the body. Moreover, because many common drugs are organic cations that are substrates for this general system, competition for the transporter and, thus, for excretion could play an important role in observed drug interactions. In addition, because some endogenous metabolites share this transport system with exogenous compounds, the extent of metabolic production of such metabolites may also influence the excretion of drugs.

Although net secretion predominates for most organic cations, some reabsorptive transport probably occurs in humans and other mammals as well. Net reabsorption is significant, however, primarily for the important endogenous organic cation, choline, and this chapter will consider reabsorption only for this substance.

Most organic cations do not move readily across the entire tubule epithelium by passive diffusion. Instead, they move across the basolateral and luminal membranes in series, as in the case of organic anions. In contrast to organic anions, organic cations enter the cells down an electrochemical gradient at the basolateral membrane and exit the cells against an electrochemical gradient at the luminal membrane (Figure 5.7). Along the proximal tubule, net secretion is highest in the S1 segment, less in the S2 segment, and least in the S3 segment.

Studies *in vivo* and *in vitro* indicate that, in general, the affinity of the transporter at the basolateral membrane for substrates increases as their hydrophobicity and charge (or pK_a) increase [15, 20, 25]. However, whereas these general rules hold within a homologous series of compounds, a number of individual compounds (e.g. cimetidine) do not fit this pattern. Thus, a number of other factors may influence the binding of various molecules to the carrier. In addition, an increasing body of evidence suggests that the rate of transport via this basolateral carrier varies inversely with its affinity for the substrate [25].

Organic cation entry into the cells across the basolateral membrane can involve carrier-mediated flux driven by both the inside-negative membrane potential and organic cation/organic cation exchange (Figure 5.7) [20]. Both types of entry appear to be different modes of the same basic transport process. However, because there appear to be few intracellular organic cations that would normally be exchanged for extracellular cations, the exchange process is probably significant only for the reabsorption of choline (see below). A carrier with the apparent characteristics of the basolateral organic cation transporter has been cloned and sequenced from rat kidney [26].

Organic cation exit from the cells against an electrochemical gradient at the luminal membrane during the secretory process involves electroneutral countertrans-

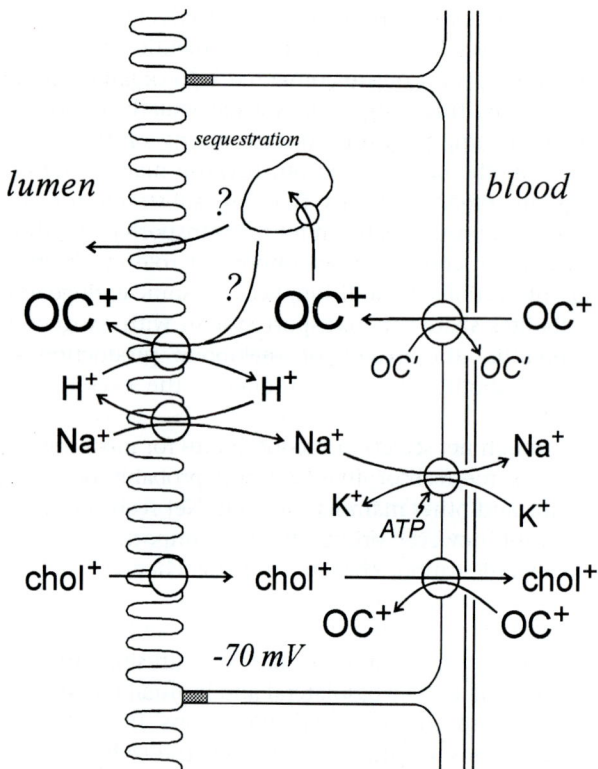

Figure 5.7 Model for secretion of organic cations (OC⁺) and reabsorption of choline (chol⁺) by cells of proximal renal tubules. Note that sequestration of OC⁺ in intracellular vesicles may play some role in transepithelial transport process. Other symbols and role of Na⁺,K⁺-ATPase are as in Figure 5.1.

port for protons moving down their electrochemical gradient (Figure 5.7). This has been confirmed in studies with isolated luminal membranes, intact renal tubules, and proximal tubule cell lines [20]. The inwardly directed proton gradient necessary for this transport step is established by the Na⁺-H⁺ countertransport system on the luminal membrane in which protons are transported from the cells to the lumen in exchange for Na⁺ ions moving into the cells down their electrochemical gradient (Figure 5.7). The inwardly directed Na⁺ gradient is maintained, in turn, by transport of sodium out of the cells at the basolateral membrane via Na⁺,K⁺-ATPase (Figure 5.7). Therefore, transport of organic cations out of the cells at the luminal membrane, like transport of PAH and urate into the cells at the basolateral and luminal membranes, respectively, can be viewed as a tertiary active transport step (Figures 5.5, 5.6 and 5.7).

The affinity of the luminal organic cation-proton countertransporter for organic cations, like that of the basolateral transporter, increases with their hydrophobicity [27]. Other characteristics of the substrates also appear to influence their binding to this transporter. For example, the hydrophobic portion oriented at right angles to the longitudinal axis of the compound may reduce steric hindrance and increase binding [27].

Although no mechanism for basolateral transport of organic cations into renal tubule cells against an electrochemical gradient has been identified, the steady-state concentration measured in isolated mammalian tubules during the net secretory process generally exceeds that predicted for passive distribution at electrochemical equilibrium [20, 28]. These conflicting observations have suggested that organic cations may be sequestered within the cells during the transepithelial transport process. Such sequestration could involve binding to cytosolic proteins [29] or accumulation within intracellular vesicular organelles (e.g. endosomes) [20]. However, although uptake of organic cations by endosomes isolated from renal tubules has been described, this process has yet to be shown to account for the high intracellular concentrations observed in intact tubules.

Although the endogenous organic cation, choline, can undergo net secretion when the plasma levels are high enough, it undergoes net reabsorption at normal plasma levels. The net secretory process is apparently the same as that just described (Figure 5.7), but the affinity of choline for the luminal membrane organic cation-proton countertransporter is very low [30]. Moreover, in addition to this transporter, there exists a separate luminal transporter with a very high affinity for choline but not for other commonly secreted organic cations (Figure 5.7) [30]. Choline at the low concentrations normally present in the glomerular filtrate can readily bind to this carrier and enter the cells from the lumen via carrier-mediated diffusion driven by the inside-negative membrane potential (Figure 5.7). Although choline is rapidly metabolized to betaine within the cells, some of it undergoes net transepithelial reabsorption. In this process, the basolateral step out of the cells against an electrochemical gradient could involve countertransport for other organic cations entering down an electrochemical gradient, as mentioned above (Figure 5.7) [31]. This reabsorptive process helps to conserve an organic cation important for membrane repair and formation and for the synthesis of numerous essential compounds (e.g. acetylcholine).

Conclusion

The basic mechanisms for the transepithelial transport of a broad range of organic solutes by the renal tubules have been described. For all compounds, transepithelial transport involves movement across the two cell membranes, luminal and basolateral, arranged in series. The order in which these membranes are crossed depends on whether the compound is undergoing reabsorption or secretion. Transport of all of these compounds across each membrane is carrier-mediated and, at one membrane, involves transport against an electrochemical gradient. However, such uphill transport always involves coupling to the movement of another substance down its electrochemical gradient in the same or opposite direction as the compound of interest. In all cases, the energy for these coupled processes ultimately resides in the inwardly directed Na^+ gradient maintained by the action of Na^+,K^+-ATPase at the basolateral membrane, the only point in the overall process at which metabolic energy is used directly in transport.

Acknowledgments

The personal research included and the writing of this manuscript were supported in part by NIH Program Project Grant PO1 DK41006 and RO1 ES06757.

References

1. Silverman, M. and Turner, R.J. (1992) Glucose transport in the renal proximal tubule, in *Handbook of Physiology. Sec. 8. Renal Physiology*, Vol. II (ed. E.E. Windhager), Oxford University Press, New York, pp. 2017–38.
2. Hediger, M.A. and Rhoads, D.B. (1994) Molecular physiology of sodium-glucose cotransporters. *Annu. Rev. Physiol.*, **74**, 993–1026.
3. Berry, C.A. and Rector, F.C., Jr (1980) Active and passive sodium transport in the proximal tubule. *Miner. Elect. Metab.*, **4**, 149–60.
4. Desjeux, J.-F., Turk, E. and Wright, E. (1995) Congenital selective Na^+ D-glucose cotransport defects leading to renal glycosuria and congenital selective intestinal malabsorption of glucose and galactose, in *Basis of Inherited Disease* (ed. C.R. Scriver), McGraw-Hill, Baltimore.
5. Gould, G.W. and Bell, G.I. (1990) Facilitative glucose transporters: an expanding family. *Trends Biochem. Sei.*, **15**, 18–23.
6. Silbernagl, S. (1992) Tubular transport of amino acids and small peptides, in *Handbook of Physiology. Sec. 8. Renal Physiology*, Vol. II (ed. E.E. Windhager), Oxford University Press, New York, pp. 1937–76.
7. Silbernagl, S. (1988) The renal handling of amino acids and oligopeptides. *Physiol. Rev.*, **68**, 911–1007.
8. Scriver, C.R. and Tenenhouse, H.S. (1992) Mendelian phenotypes as 'probes' of renal transport systems for amino acids and phosphate, in *Handbook of Physiology*, Sec. 8. Renal Physiology, Vol. II (ed. E.E. Windhager), Oxford University Press, New York, pp. 1977–2016.
9. Daniel, H., Morse, E.L. and Adibi, S.A. (1991) The high and low affinity transport systems for dipeptides in kidney brush border membrane respond differently to alternations in pH gradient and membrane potential. *J. Biol. Chem.*, **26**, 19917–24.
10. Silbernagl, S., Ganapathy, V. and Leibach, F.H. (1987) H^+-gradient-driven dipeptide reabsorption in proximal tubule of rat kidney: studies *in vivo* and *in vitro*. *Am. J. Physiol.*, **253**, F448–57.
11. Skopicki, H., Fisher, A.K., Zikos, D. *et al.* (1991) Multiple carriers for dipeptide transport: carrier-mediated transport of glycyl-L-proline in renal BBMV. *Am. J. Physiol.*, **261**, F670–8.
12. Zelikovic, I. and Chesney, R.W. (1989) Sodium-coupled amino acid transport in renal tubule. *Kidney Int.*, **36**, 351–9.
13. Fei, Y.-J., Kanai, Y., Nussberger, S. *et al.* (1994) Expression cloning of a mammalian proton-coupled oligopeptide transporter. *Nature*, **368**, 563–6.
14. Murer, H., Manganel, M. and Roch-Ramel, F. (1992) Tubular transport of monocarboxylates, Krebs cycle intermediates, and inorganic sulfate, in *Handbook of Physiology*, Sec. 8. Renal Physiology, Vol. II (ed. E.E. Windhager), Oxford University Press, New York, pp. 2165–88.
15. Ullrich, K.J., Rumrich, G. and Fritzsch, G. (1992) Substrate specificity of the organic anion and organic cation transport systems in the proximal renal tubule, in *Progress in Cell Research* (eds E. Bamberg and H. Passow), Elsevier, Amsterdam, pp. 315–21.
16. Pritchard, J.B. (1988) Coupled transport of p-aminohippurate by rat kidney basolateral membrane vesicles. *Am. J. Physiol.*, **255**, F597–604.
17. Shimada, H., Moewes, B. and Burckhardt, G. (1987) Indirect coupling to Na^+ of p-aminohippuric acid uptake into rat renal basolateral membrane vesicles. *Am. J. Physiol.*, **253**, F795–801.
18. Chatsudthipong, V. and Dantzler, W.H. (1992) PAH/a-KG countertransport stimulates PAH uptake and net secretion in isolated rabbit renal tubules. *Am. J. Physiol.*, **263**, F384–91.
19. Dantzler, W.H., Evans, K.K. and Wright, S.H. (1995) Kinetics of interactions of para-aminohippurate, probenecid, cysteine conjugates, and N-acetyl cysteine conjugates with basolateral organic anion transporter in isolated rabbit proximal renal tubules. *J. Pharmacol. Exp. Ther.* **272**, 663–72.
20. Pritchard, J.B. and Miller, D.S. (1993) Mechanisms mediating renal secretion of organic anions and cations. *Physiol. Rev.*, **73**, 765–96.
21. Aronson, P.S. (1989) The renal proximal tubule: a model for diversity of anion exchangers and stilbene-sensitive anion transporters. *Annu. Rev. Physiol.*, **51**, 419–41.
22. Polkowski, C.A. and Grassl, S.M. (1993) Uric acid transport in rat renal basolateral vesicles. *Biochim. Biophys. Acta* **1146**, 145–52.
23. Pordy, W.T., Lipkowitz, M.S. and Abramson, R.G. (1987) Evidence for the transport function of uricase, an oxidative enzyme. *Am. J. Physiol.*, **253**, F702–11.
24. Boner, G. and Steele, T.H. (1973) Relationship of urate and p-aminohippurate secretion in man. *Am. J. Physiol.*, **225**, 100–4.
25. Groves, C.E., Evans, K., Dantzler, W.H. and Wright, S.H. (1994) Peritubular organic cation transport in isolated rabbit proximal tubules. *Am. J. Physiol.*, **266**, F450–8.
26. Gründemann, D., Gorboulev, V., Gambarian, S. and Koepsell, H. (1995) Cloning of an organic cation transporter which mediates renal and hepatic excretion of multiple drugs. *Nature*, **372**, 549–52.
27. Wright, S.H., Wunz, T.M. and Wunz, T.P. (1995) Structure and interaction of inhibitors with the TEA/H^+

exchanger of rabbit renal brush border membranes. *Pflugers Arch.* **429**, 313–24.

28. Schäli, C., Schild, L., Overney, J. and Roch-Ramel, F. (1983) Secretion of tetraethylammonium by proximal tubules of rabbit kidneys. *Am. J. Physiol.*, **245**, F238–46.

29. Berndt, W.O. (1981) Organic base transport: a comparative study. *Pharmacology*, **22**, 251–62.

30. Wright, S.H., Wunz, T.M. and Wunz, T.P. (1992) A choline transporter in renal brush-border membrane vesicles: energetics and structural specificity. *J. Membr. Biol.*, **126**, 51–65.

31. Dantzler, W.H., Wright, S.H., Chatsudthipong, V. and Brokl, O. (1991) Basolateral tetraethylammonium transport in intact tubules: specificity and *trans*-stimulation. *Am. J. Physiol.*, **261**, F386–92.

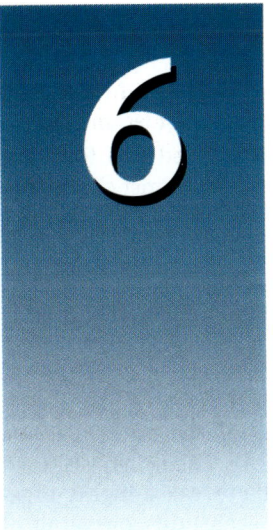

6

The urinary concentrating mechanism

Rex L. Jamison

Introduction

The purpose of this chapter is to describe the urinary concentrating mechanism. The reader is referred to other publications for a description of early contributions [1–3]. Although 'urinary concentrating mechanism' is commonly used, a more precise description is the capacity of the kidney to alter urinary flow and total solute excretion independently of each other over a wide range. Urine flow in the human can range from 400 to 20 000 ml daily; usually it varies between 1000 and 2000 ml. Urinary osmolality can vary from 50 to 1400 mosmol/kg H_2O; normally it is between 500 and 1000 mosmol/kg H_2O. If urine osmolality (U_{osm}) is less than plasma osmolality (P_{osm}), the urine is 'dilute'; if $U_{osm} = P_{osm}$, it is 'isosthenuric'; if $U_{osm} > P_{osm}$, it is 'concentrated'. Most of the chapter will be devoted to explaining how urine is concentrated. Urinary dilution will also be briefly described.

The modern era in this field was launched by Wirz, Hargitay and Kühn in 1951 [4]. In the kidney of the dehydrated rat they showed that the renal cortical tissue was isotonic to plasma, there was a moderate rise in osmolality in the outer medulla, and an exponential increase in the osmolality of the inner medulla to a value in the papilla ten times higher than that of the cortex (Figure 6.1). A mathematical treatise by Hargitay and Kühn [5], published at the same time, modified and advanced the original countercurrent multiplier theory of Kühn and

Ryffel in 1942 [6] which had been largely ignored. Experiments in the 1950s and 1960s confirmed several predictions of the theory. The contents of all structures in the medulla – loop of Henle, collecting duct and vasa recta – of the antidiuretic animal were similarly hypertonic; fluid emerging from the ascending limb of Henle was always dilute, and in the presence of arginine vasopressin (AVP) the final urine was concentrated by osmotic equilibration in the collecting duct with the hypertonic medulla. In the absence of AVP, the tubule fluid remained dilute from the ascending limb throughout the remainder of the renal tubule. In the 1970s and 1980s the *in vitro* perfusion technique devised by Burg and Green [7] enabled individual segments of the tubule to be examined. Several surprises resulted. The thick ascending limb (TAL) contained a transporter in the apical membrane that required Na^+, K^+ and $2Cl^-$ ions to operate. The urea permeability of the collecting duct (CD) was increased by AVP, but only in the inner medulla; in contrast, the water permeability of the entire collecting duct was increased by AVP. A major unexpected finding was that the thin descending limb of Henle (tdl) of the rabbit was very permeable to water but impermeable to NaCl and urea; the rabbit thin ascending limb (tal) was extremely permeable to NaCl, moderately permeable to urea and impermeable to water. Try as they might, investigators could not demonstrate active transcellular transport of Na (or any other solute) in the thin ascending limb, in contrast to the vigorous Na pump in

Nephrology, Edited by Rex L. Jamison and Robert Wilkinson.
Published in 1997 by Chapman & Hall, London. ISBN 0 412 60930 4

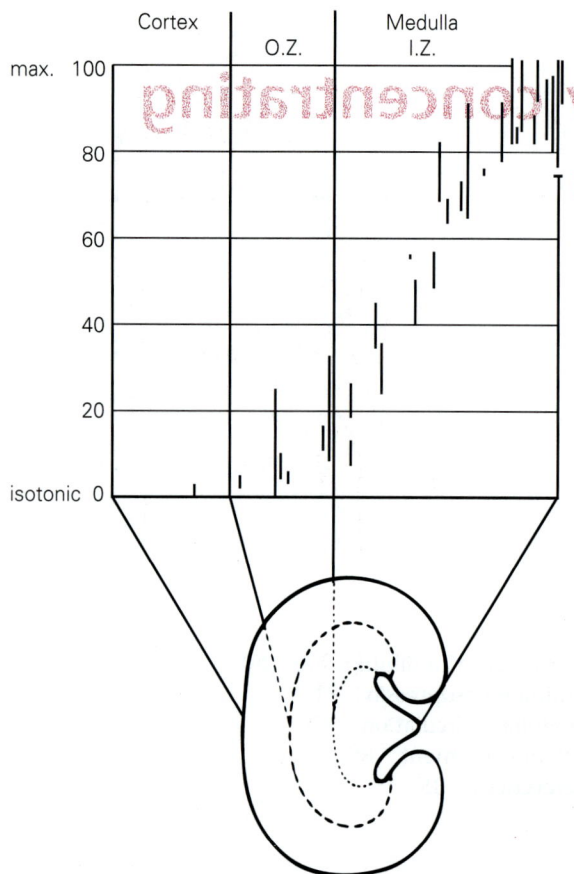

Figure 6.1 Variation of osmolality in cortical and medullary kidney slices of five hydropenic rats. Ordinate: osmolality of renal tissue as percentage of maximum osmolality at the tip of the renal papilla. O.Z., outer zone (outer medulla); I.Z., inner zone (inner medulla). (Reproduced, with permission, from ref. 4.)

the thick ascending limb. These findings led to revisions of the Kühn theory by Stephenson [8] and Kokko and Rector [9] (abbreviated SKR) that became known as the 'passive models'. The SKR models stimulated many experimental and theoretical studies. The effect of these studies was to show that a purely passive concentrating mechanism does not account for the rise in osmolality in the inner medulla. In retrospect, the failure of the SKR theory was attributable to two groups of experiments. First, studies of the thin descending limb from animals other than the rabbit revealed that it had different permeability properties. It was highly permeable to urea and, in certain parts, moderately permeable to NaCl. Second, incorporation of the experimentally determined transport characteristics into computer simulations enabled the passive hypotheses to be tested appropriately – and they were unable to generate the characteristic axial hypertonicity in the inner medulla.

Studies of the permeability properties of the collecting duct led to new insights about how AVP acts. Development of video cameras and techniques to determine permeability properties of vasa recta capillaries in the

medulla contributed to a clearer understanding of their role in countercurrent exchange [10]. A new class of molecules, the osmolytes, was discovered and found to protect medullary cells and other cells against changes in cell volume [11].

Architecture of the renal medulla

The mammalian medulla consists of three regions (Figure 6.2), the outer and inner stripes of the outer medulla (OM) and the inner medulla (IM) [1, 12]. Kriz has shown that a cross-section of the medulla reveals a highly organized pattern of adjacent units, each unit consisting of vasa recta, Henle's loops and collecting tubules. At the center of a unit is the vascular bundle that extends from the corticomedullary junction into the inner medulla. The bundle is composed of descending vasa recta (DVR) formed from juxtamedullary efferent arterioles and ascending vasa recta (AVR) originating from a capillary network at varying levels of the inner medulla. In the outer medulla, the pars recta is immediately adjacent to the vascular bundle with the collecting ducts in the outermost ring.

In the inner stripe of the outer medulla, the vascular bundles dominate the topography. In the section of inner stripe nearest the outer stripe, short-loop nephrons give rise to thin descending limbs that are located within the periphery of the bundles. (In highly concentrating species, thin descending limbs are distributed throughout the vascular bundle; in humans they are excluded from the bundle.) Outside but adjacent to the bundles are thick ascending limbs of long-loop nephrons. The thin descending limbs of long-loop nephrons are located in the interbundle region amid thick ascending limbs of short-loop nephrons. The collecting duct is far from the bundle in the outer layer of the unit.

In the inner medulla, loops of Henle, vasa recta and collecting ducts rapidly decline in number toward the papillary tip. The bundle disappears. The collecting duct is spatially separated from descending vasa recta and closer to thin ascending limbs and ascending vasa recta.

In the outer medulla the interstitium within the bundle is very narrow and separates ascending vasa recta from descending vasa recta. The interstitium of the interbundle region has a larger volume and contains capillaries in a lateral array which form a plexus. In the inner medulla, the interstitium in which interstitial cells are interspersed has a gelatinous matrix of mucopolysaccharides devoid of capillary plexuses or laterally flowing capillaries. The interstitium of the inner medulla would greatly retard lateral dispersion of water and solutes. Note that the inner medulla is devoid of lymphatics.

The morphology of the thin descending limb epithelium varies along the length of the long-loop nephrons. The upper segment has relatively tall and extensively

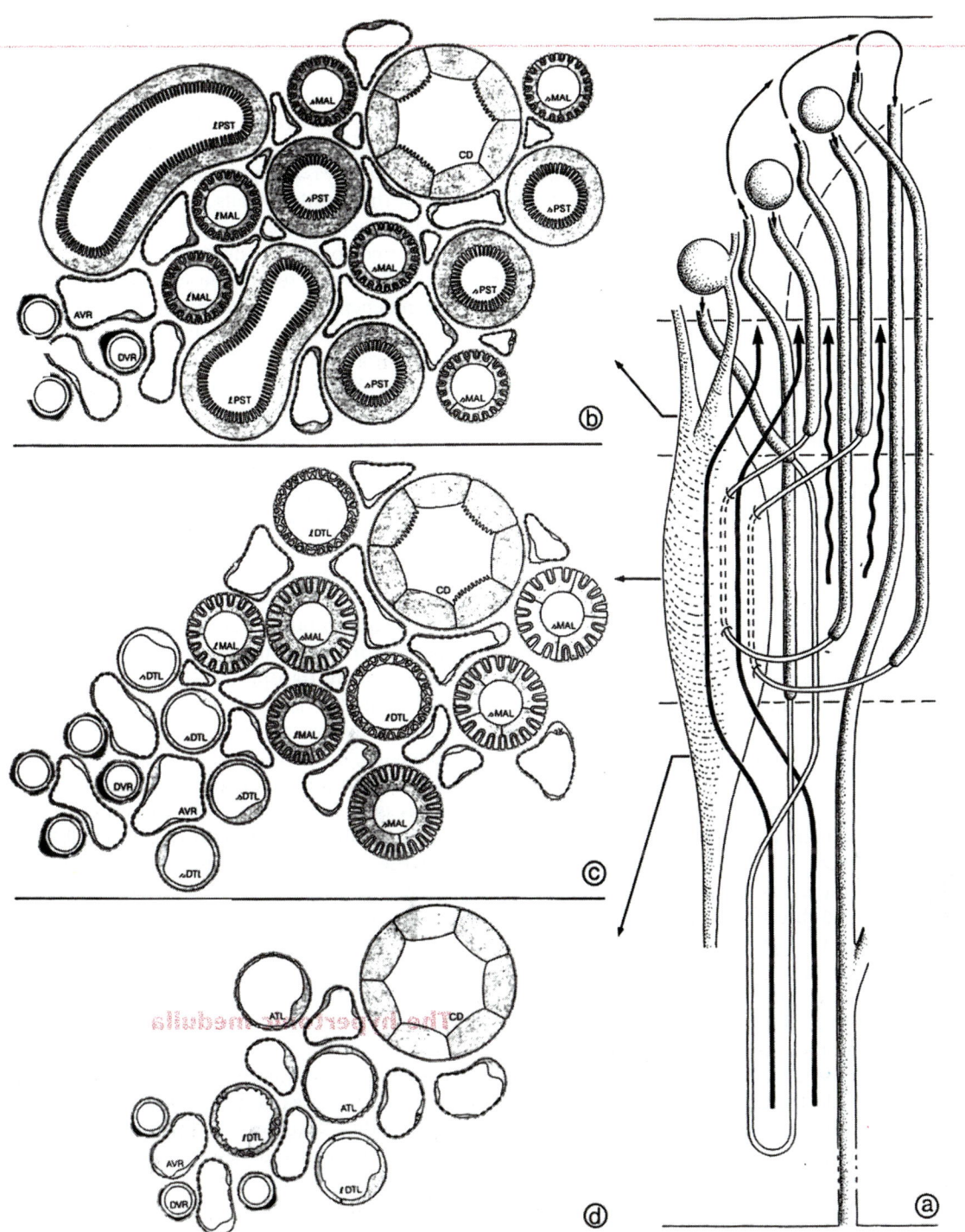

Figure 6.2 Architectural organization of rat renal medulla in schematic longitudinal section (a) and cross sections through the outer stripe (b) and inner stripe (c) of the outer medulla, and the inner medulla (d). (a) One long and two short loops of Henle, collecting duct and vascular bundle. Individual vessels are not shown in the bundle; rather, an attempt at its 'three-dimensional solid form' is shown. The vascular bundle contains ascending vasa recta coming from the inner medulla (thick arrows), descending vasa recta, and thin descending limbs of short loop nephrons. Ascending vasa recta originating in the inner stripe (thick wavy arrows) ascend directly within inner bundle region. (b–d) Topographical relationships of four short and two long Henle's loops shown with collecting duct and vasa recta. In the outer stripe (b), the proximal straight tubule (PST) and medullary thick ascending limb (MAL) of long loops (l) among ascending vasa recta (AVR) are near the vascular bundle. Displaced from the bundle are the collecting duct (CD) and PST and MAL of short loops (s), surrounded by ascending vasa recta originating from the inner stripe and capillaries. These capillaries form a plexus, which are smaller than vasa recta. In the inner stripe (c), the core of the vascular bundle contains ascending vasa recta and descending vasa recta (DVR), whereas now, the short descending thin limbs (DTL) are found in the periphery among ascending vasa recta coming from inner medulla. In the inner bundle region, long DTL and collecting duct run together with the thick ascending limb of the short loop. Thick ascending limbs of long loops border the vascular bundle. In the upper inner medulla (d), the vascular bundle is still discernible, but ascending vasa recta are distributed uniformly throughout the cross-section. Note that the collecting duct is distant from the vascular bundle, and between the collecting ducts are the DTL and ascending thin limb (ATL) of long loops. (Reproduced, with permission, from ref. 12.)

interdigitated epithelial cells with short microvilli on the luminal surface. The cytoplasm is rich in filamentous material and contains mitochondria. By contrast, the lower segment has a relatively flat non-interdigitating epithelium that lacks mitochondria. It resembles the thin descending limb of short-loop nephrons. Among highly concentrating species, the longer the thin descending limb, the greater the depth in the inner medulla that the thin descending limb is lined by upper segment epithelium.

Efferent arterioles of juxtamedullary glomeruli descend into the outer stripe of the outer medulla where they provide small branches to the capillary plexus of the outer stripe and divide into as many as 30 descending vasa recta. The descending vasa recta travel straight down the medulla intermixed with ascending vasa recta within the vascular bundles. As a descending vas rectus descends it peels off to supply the capillary plexus. The smooth muscle in the wall of the efferent arteriole is replaced in the descending vasa recta by pericytes or myoid cells, which have a contractile capacity. The pericytes disappear gradually after the descending vasa recta reach the inner medulla. The descending vasa recta have a non-fenestrated endothelium. Sympathetic innervation has been identified along the course of the descending vasa recta until the disappearance of the myoid cells.

Ascending vasa recta follow two distinct pathways in the medulla (Figure 6.2). Those originating in the inner medulla travel within the bundle until they reach the cortex. Some ascending vasa recta that originate in the outer medulla ascend directly in the interbundle region to the cortex without being incorporated into a bundle. Quantitative methods have revealed that the ascending vasa recta outnumber the descending vasa recta by approximately 2.3 to 1. The ascending vasa recta serve to remove water reabsorbed from the collecting duct into the medulla. The position of a major portion of ascending vasa recta outside the bundle and not consistently adjacent to a counterflow channel suggests that these interbundle ascending vasa recta serve as channels to carry reabsorbed fluid out of the medulla. The endothelium of the ascending vasa recta is fenestrated like that of the glomerular capillary.

The above description and inspection of Figure 6.2 show that several intramedullary pathways for solute and water exist. When paired with an adjacent channel in which flow is countercurrent, that channel will serve to retard axillary transfer of a solute, provided the linings of both countercurrent channels are permeable to that solute. On the other hand, if the wall of a channel is impermeable to a given solute, then the channel will serve as a conduit for the axial movement of that solute. The vascular bundle facilitates countercurrent exchange between descending vasa recta and ascending vasa recta. The flow of fluid entering the medulla in the descending vasa recta is reduced as water is shunted from descending vasa recta to ascending vasa recta and returned to the

cortex. The flow of solute leaving the medulla in the ascending vasa recta within the vascular bundle is reduced as solute is shunted from ascending vasa recta to descending vasa recta and returned to the papilla, provided the capillary walls are permeable to the solute, as previously mentioned. There are other countercurrent exchange pairs besides the descending vasa recta–ascending vasa recta. The extent of exchange between them depends on the permeability properties of the walls lining both channels. Exchange can occur between the ascending vasa recta and thin descending limb of short-loop nephrons. In the interbundle region of the outer medulla, the pars recta or thin descending limb (down channel) and ascending vasa recta (up channel) are likely the site of countercurrent exchange, as are the pars recta or thin descending limb (down) and thick ascending limb (up). For those solutes added to the medulla – NaCl by reabsorption from the thin and thick ascending limb and urea by reabsorption primarily from the terminal inner medullary collecting duct – these countercurrent exchangers hinder their escape from the medulla, i.e. trap them in the medulla. When lateral movement is facilitated by transporters such as the urea transporter, the exchange is most effective. On the other hand, water added to the medulla by reabsorption from the collecting duct would dilute the concentrated medullary interstitium. Thus the ideal arrangement in antidiuresis is to have as much of the water in the collecting tubules reabsorbed in the cortex as possible before reaching the medulla. That diversion of fluid is facilitated because the cortical collecting duct is lined by an epithelium whose water permeability is enhanced by arginine vasopressin.

The hypertonic medulla

The cryoscopic findings of Wirz *et al.* (Figure 6.1) were confirmed and extended by Thomas and his colleagues who studied sequential changes in content and concentration of water and solute in the rat kidney during the transition between antidiuresis and water diuresis (references cited in [1]). The inner medulla of the rat kidney in antidiuresis is hypertonic because its solute content is higher and its water content is lower, respectively, than in water diuresis. In most animals, the principal added solute is urea but there is a rise in NaCl content, too. In *Psammomys obesus* (the sand rat), however, whose diet is low in protein, NaCl is the major solute in the inner medulla [1]. Analysis of solute concentrations of individual structures in the inner medulla with the electron probe disclosed that the concentrations of NaCl, urea and K are approximately the same in fluid in the thin limbs, vasa recta and interstitium, but much higher than in the extracellular fluid elsewhere. The osmolality of epithelial cells in the medulla accounted for by the sum of the concentrations of their intracellular Na^+ and K^+ together with their anions is less than the osmolality of the surrounding extracellular fluid due to Na$^+$ and K$^+$ and their anions. Since the cells are at osmotic equilibrium with their surroundings, this argues for the presence of other solutes in the cells. This is of fundamental importance because these other solutes play a vital role in protecting medullary cells against the wide and sometimes rapid changes in extracellular fluid osmolality.

Osmolytes

Most cells including those of the renal medulla respond to changes in the effective osmolality of the surrounding extracellular fluid by swelling or shrinking, which activate processes that return their volume to normal. Regulation of cell volume occurs by gain or loss of osmotically active solutes, either inorganic ions (principally Na$^+$, K$^+$ and Cl$^-$) or small organic molecules called organic osmolytes [11, 13–15]. A regulatory volume increase in response to hypertonicity-induced cell volume shrinkage is mediated first by the uptake of electrolytes (minutes) followed by the accumulation of organic osmolytes (hours). Immediately after the shift to a hypertonic medium, the high cell K$^+$ perturbs the 'exquisitely coordinated metabolic and functional networks' that exist at the normal cell K concentration. 'In a striking example of convergent evolution, a variety of cells and organisms exposed to increased tonicity maintain intracellular potassium concentration at the same level as in isotonic cells, balancing extracellular hypertonicity by accumulating small organic solutes (osmolytes) that do not perturb function' [15]. A regulatory volume decrease in response to the swelling induced by exposure to a hypotonic medium, on the other hand, occurs by the rapid loss of both inorganic electrolytes and organic osmolytes in minutes.

Organic osmolytes are present in the cytosol of all organisms from bacteria to primates, including humans. There are three classes of organic osmolytes: polyhydric alcohols such as sorbitol, *myo*-inositol and glycerol; amino acids and their derivatives, like taurine, alanine and proline; and methylamines, for example, glycerophosphorylcholine (GPC) and betaine [11, 14]. These osmolytes are 'compatible' or 'non-perturbing' solutes, so called because their unique biophysical and biochemical characteristics enable them to accumulate to reach high concentrations in cells without injuring the cytoskeleton or impairing cell function. High intracellular concentrations of inorganic ions can denature cell proteins. Accumulation of osmolytes allows medullary cells to survive in an extremely hypertonic medium while maintaining their Na$^+$ and K$^+$ concentrations approximately the same as those, respectively, of cells in an isotonic environment. In contrast, the concentration of urea inside medullary cells is much higher than that in cells in the renal cortex or elsewhere in the body. Urea is also a 'perturbing solute' because it destabilizes the molecular structure of proteins, rendering them inactive. Methylamines stabilize the

structure and activate the function of proteins (as measured by enzyme kinetics). When combined with urea at a ratio of 1 methylamine to 2 urea molecules, the destabilizing action of high concentration of urea is prevented.

In the antidiuretic rat, organic osmolytes account for 20% of intracellular osmolality and offset 60% of extracellular osmolality due to Na$^+$, K$^+$ and Cl$^-$ (Figure 6.3). With the exception of inositol, whose concentration is greatest in the outer medulla, the concentration of osmolytes rises towards the papillary tip. The osmolytes accumulate in the medulla by one of three mechanisms: increased synthesis (sorbitol), transport into cells (*myo*-inositol and betaine) or decreased degradation (GPC).

Sorbitol is synthesized from glucose by aldose reductase. The induction of aldose reductase activity is mediated by a change in mRNA stimulated by a rise in medullary interstitial osmolality [16]. This induces an increase in ionic strength of the cell interior, which is the primary signal rather than a fall in cell volume. In water diuresis, medullary hypertonicity falls and the permeability of the medullary cell to sorbitol increases sharply, allowing sorbitol to escape.

Myo-inositol is transported into kidney cells by an Na co-transporter against a high concentration gradient, suggesting that the transporter is coupled to two Na$^+$ ions. The transporter weighs 78 000 daltons and has 12 membrane-spanning domains. Betaine is taken up by an NaCl–betaine co-transporter. The transporter has a molecular weight of 69 000 daltons, and 12 membrane-

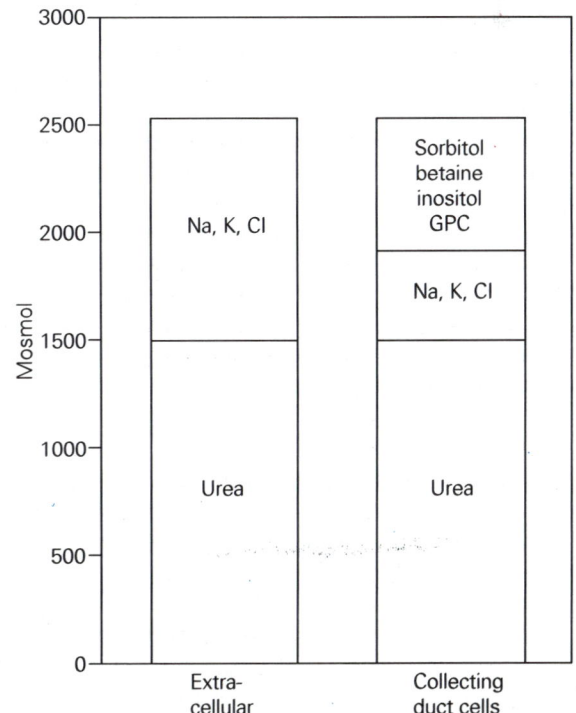

Figure 6.3 Osmolytes in renal medullary cells and extracellular fluid of antidiuretic rat. (Reproduced, with permission, from ref. 13.)

spanning domains. It is thought that a high K concentration triggers enhanced transcription of mRNA for both transporters. Hypo-osmolality reduces the transport rate of these osmolytes.

An intermediate in the catabolism of phosphatidylcholine, GPC is synthesized by phospholipases and metabolized by a pathway involving GPC-choline diesterase (GPC-C-D). In hypertonicity, phospholipase activity is suppressed. Indirect evidence suggests that accumulation of GPC is mediated by a decrease in activity of GPC-C-D. Accumulation of GPC is stimulated by a rise in either NaCl or urea concentration. With no AVP, GPC-C-D activity rises and GPC leaks out of the cells.

In summary the osmolytes protect the cells in the renal medulla against changes in medullary interstitial hypertonicity. There is no evidence they play a role in the generation of the hypertonicity.

Countercurrent theory

In 1942, Kühn and Ryffel [6] proposed that the loop of Henle functions as a countercurrent 'multiplier' (more precisely, 'augmenter') in which a small transverse difference in osmotic pressure (the 'single effect') is augmented by countercurrent flow. The augmentation results in a large axial difference in osmotic pressure between cortex and papilla. Kühn was an engineer; to test his hypothesis, he constructed an apparatus schematically illustrated in Figure 6.4. Channels 1 and 2 were connected at one end to provide continuous countercurrent flow as in Henle's loop. Channel 3 was not analogous to any kidney structure; its purpose was to supply energy. Initially, the contents of all three channels were isosmotic. Channels 1 and 2 contained 0.1 M sucrose solution; channel 3, a 0.1 M phenol solution. A cupric ferrocyanate membrane permeable to water but not to sucrose or phenol separated channels 1 and 2; a rubber membrane, permeable to phenol but not to water or sucrose, separated channels 2 and 3. In operation, phenol permeated the rubber membrane to enter channel 2, raising the osmotic pressure, causing water withdrawal from channel 1 until the osmotic pressures of channels 1 and 2 were equal. Continuing flow brought the concentrated sucrose solution from channel 1 to channel 2, where entry of phenol further raised its osmotic pressure and the cycle was repeated. Operation of the apparatus increased the sucrose concentration 3.5 times at the end of channel 1.

The apparatus illustrates Kühn's fundamental requirements for countercurrent multiplication: (1) countercurrent flow, (2) a source of energy (free energy was generated by dilution of the phenol solution to concentrate the sucrose solution), and (3) differing membrane permeabilities. These three requirements became guideposts for subsequent theory. They are satisfied by the loops of Henle in the outer medulla, but not in the inner medulla. A source of energy for the single effect has not been identified in the inner medulla.

In 1951, Hargitay and Kühn [5] described more fully the countercurrent multiplication hypothesis. The driving force for the single effect was assumed to be hydrostatic pressure (HP). Subsequent calculations indicated the magnitude of HP required was unrealistic. An alternative energy source, active transport of salt from ascending to descending limb was incorporated into a revised model by Kühn and Ramel. The solution in the descending limb was concentrated by solute addition rather than water removal; the contents of the ascending limb were dilute relative to fluid in the descending limb. The model was attractive because of later evidence for active reabsorption of NaCl from the thick ascending limb. All models now incorporate active salt transport as the single effect in the outer medulla.

Kühn and Ramel's model, however, failed to explain fully the concentrating mechanism. Its inadequacies reveal the necessary (if not sufficient) conditions to be fulfilled by a successful model.

1 A driving force (energy source) for the single effect must be identified in the inner medulla.
2 The role of urea must be explained. In most species, urea reaches high concentrations in the inner medullary collecting duct where reabsorption serves to enrich the inner medulla. Urea administration enhances maximum urinary concentration in protein-deprived animals and humans.
3 The medullary circulation must be incorporated.

Models of the concentrating mechanism

In this section, only a few models will be described. Please see recent reviews for more extensive descriptions [3, 17–19].

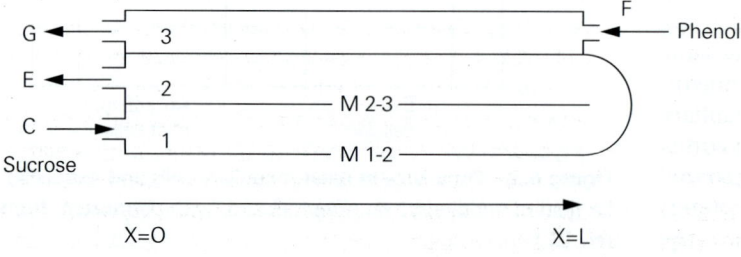

Figure 6.4 Model of Kühn and Ryffel [6]. The sucrose solution enters channel 1 at C and exits from channel 2 at E. Phenol solution enters channel 3 at F and exits at G. Membrane 1–2 is permeable to water, but not to sucrose or phenol. Membrane 2–3 is permeable to phenol but not to water or sucrose. See text for further description.

SKR model

As noted above the models by Stephenson and by Kokko and Rector (SKR) [8, 9] attempted to show how the inner medulla is concentrated without an energy source generated within the inner medulla. As summarized in Figure 6.5, active salt reabsorption in the thick ascending limb dilutes the tubule fluid and increases the NaCl concentration in the interstitium of the outer medulla (1 in Figure 6.5). The urea concentration is increased by urea-free water reabsorption in the cortical collecting duct (under the influence of AVP) and the outer medullary collecting duct by water reabsorption across the transepithelial gradient established by NaCl deposition in the outer medulla by the thick ascending limb (2 in Figure 6.5). When tubule fluid enters the inner medullary collecting duct, urea is further concentrated by water reabsorption until it reaches the terminal inner medullary collecting duct, where, in the presence of AVP, it diffuses into the interstitium (3 in Figure 6.5), is trapped by countercurrent exchange (see below) between ascending vasa recta and descending vasa recta and accumulates in the medulla.

Urea in the inner medulla extracts water from the thin descending limb (4 in Figure 6.5). Since the urea concentration in thin descending limb fluid is low and the osmolality of the medullary interstitium is composed of about equal contributions of NaCl and urea, the NaCl concentration of thin descending limb fluid exceeds that of the interstitium. As thin descending limb fluid enters the thin ascending limb, NaCl passively diffuses from the thin ascending limb (5 in Figure 6.5) thereby elevating

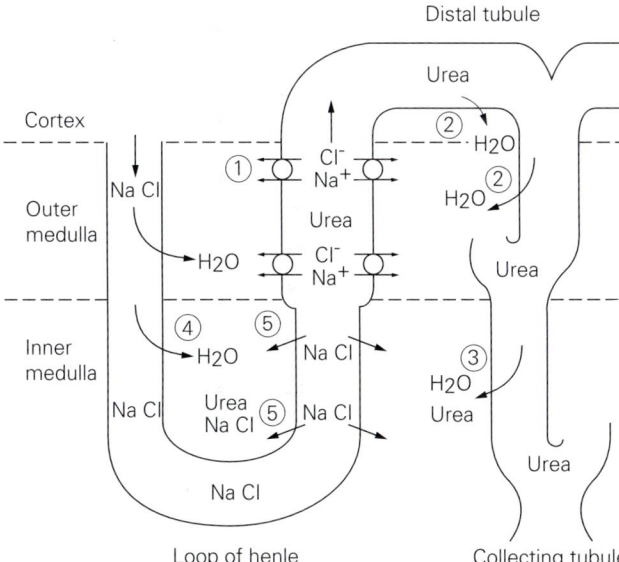

Figure 6.5 Passive model of Kokko and Rector of the concentrating mechanism in the inner medulla [9]. See text for description of the mechanism of action. Arrows indicate movements of water, NaCl, and urea between tubule and the interstitium. In the vasa recta, it is assumed there is perfect exchange between the two limbs. (Reproduced, with permission, from ref. 1.)

the NaCl concentration of the inner medulla and further enhancing extraction of water from the collecting duct. Urea permeates the thin ascending limb at a slower rate than NaCl diffuses out, and since the thin ascending limb is impermeable to water, the result is that fluid in the thin ascending limb becomes hypotonic to the interstitium – the essential separation of solute and water, i.e. the single effect. If there is active transport of NaCl or other solute in the thin ascending limb or active secretion of NaCl or other solute in the thin descending limb, this mechanism would act to enhance the latter effect.

The SKR models provided an explanation for the role of urea in the concentrating mechanism. Computer simulations using a variety of assumptions, numerical methods, and transport parameters, however, have consistently been unable to generate an axial osmotic gradient in the inner medulla, provided they employ the experimentally determined urea permeabilities of the long loops of Henle. The essential reason why the simulations fail is that urea enters the thin descending limb. This reduces the NaCl gradient available to drive passive NaCl reabsorption from the thin ascending limb to dilute the luminal fluid in the thin ascending limb (single effect).

Recent models of the concentrating mechanism

Recent models incorporate the quantitative features of the medullary architecture and experimentally determined permeabilities and transport capabilities of tubules and solute composition of the contents of Henle's loops, collecting ducts and vasa recta. They differ from each other in key assumptions. The model by Hamada *et al.* [18] assumes that the thin ascending limb preferentially interacts with the inner medullary collecting duct and the reflection coefficient (σ) for urea (σ_{urea}) of the inner medullary collecting duct is less than σ_{Na}.

The σ is a characteristic property of a membrane with respect to a specific solute. It indicates the osmotic effectiveness of a solute. Given a concentration difference, ΔC_X, for a solute, x, across a membrane, σ expresses the effective difference in osmolality, $\Delta\pi_X$, generated by the solute relative to the maximum theoretical osmolality defined by Van't Hoff's equation ($\pi_X = RTC_X$), that is:

$$\Delta\pi_X = \sigma RT\Delta C_X$$

where R is the gas constant and T the absolute temperature. Generally, $0 \leq \sigma \leq 1$. A solute with $\sigma = 0$, would be osmotically ineffective, as if the solute was not there. A solute with $\sigma = 1$ would generate its full osmotic effect, i.e. $\pi_X = RTC_X$.

In the inner medulla, the composition of the medullary interstitium is such that about two-thirds of the total osmolality is due to NaCl and one-third due to urea. The urine in the inner medullary collecting duct has very little NaCl; a least two-thirds of its osmolality is due to urea. As pointed out by Hamada *et al.* [18] if σ_{urea} of the inner medullary collecting duct is less than σ_{Na}, this would explain why water is reabsorbed across the inner medullary collecting duct, despite equal total osmolalites of inner medullary collecting duct fluid and medullary interstitium. (The reabsorbed fluid would dilute the NaCl in the inner medulla interstitum and create a gradient for reabsorption of NaCl from the thin ascending limb.) However, there is a controversy whether σ_{urea} of the inner medullary collecting duct is actually less than σ_{Na}. Recent experimental evidence suggests that $\sigma_{urea} = \sigma_{Na}$.

Wexler *et al.* [17] assume thin ascending limbs preferentially interact with collecting ducts and that the outer medullary collecting duct has a very low hydraulic water permeability (L_p) and the thin descending limb is spatially separated from inner medullary collecting duct. Neither of the last assumptions, however, was verified when examined.

Layton and Davies [20] represented the decreasing population of Henle's thin limbs in the inner medulla in a dynamic model employing an explicit method to solve the numerical equations. The method avoids the instability inherent in many models when tested by the use of the computer. It also incorporates permeabilities of the chinchilla thin limbs. The model failed to generate an axial gradient in the inner medulla, however.

Kriz and Knepper and Stephenson (see [3]) have suggested the thin ascending limb is not the site of the single effect since it lacks an active transport mechanism and the passive single effect it could generate is too small. They seek but have not yet found a means to generate a hypertonic fluid within the thin descending limb. Their proposal resembles Kühn's original apparatus, except that it was the ascending limb which was made hyperosmotic (by addition of phenol).

One point to keep in mind is that the experimental conditions in which the permeability properties (*in vitro* experiments) and composition of the contents of various medullary structures (*in vivo*) are determined may be deficient in some key factor. For example, to study directly the tubules and vessels in the medulla *in vivo*, it is necessary to remove the ureter overlying the tip of the papilla. Excision of the ureter always reduces inner medulla hypertonicity by 30–40% [21]. Why this occurs is not clear. It has been suggested that urea in the pelvic urine re-enters the papilla to enrich the inner medulla interstitium. Besides the fact that pelvic recycling of urea appears to be a perpetual motion machine (urea from a concentrated urine re-enters the interstitium to concentrate the urine), the evidence is inconsistent with the theory, since the epithelium lining the pelvis has a very low urea permeability.

Figure 6.6 incorporates recent findings into a current view of the medullary concentrating mechanism.

Renal tubule

Descending limb

The initial studies of the rabbit thin descending limb led to formulation of the passive model in which urea extracted water from but did not enter the thin descending limb. Micropuncture studies of rodents, however, showed the urea concentration in the end of the thin descending limb was very high from transepithelial entry of urea upstream in the thin descending limb and possibly pars recta. In *Psammomys*, transepithelial NaCl entry also occurred. The discrepancy between the *in vitro* studies of the rabbit thin descending limb and *in vivo* studies of rat, hamster and *Psammomys* was resolved by the recognition that the epithelium of the long-loop thin descending limb has functionally three distinct segments [22]. The thin descending limb segment of short loops located in the outer medulla (type 1) has a high hydraulic water permeability (L_p), a low permeability to urea (P_u), and a low permeability to sodium (P_{Na}). The proximal segment of the long-loop thin descending limb (type 2) has a high L_p, a low P_u, and a high P_{Na}. The distal segment of the long-loop thin descending limb (type 3) has a moderate L_p, a high P_u, and a variable P_{Na}. The distal-most segment of the chinchilla long-loop thin descending limb, which appears to be unique, has a very low L_p and very high P_u and P_{Na}.

In summary, the thin descending limb of the long-loop has a segment-dependent P_u and for the most part a high P_{Na}. These characteristics are inconsistent with the assumptions of the passive models.

Thin ascending limb

The permeabilities of the thin ascending limb are similar among species. The thin ascending limb has a very low L_p and very high P_{Na} and permeability to chloride (P_{Cl}). P_u, although less than P_{Na}, is still 10 times higher than the P_u in type 1 thin descending limb. The initial segment of thin ascending limb of the chinchilla has an extremely high P_u. The passive models of SKR required a high transepithelial NaCl concentration difference (lumen > interstitium), ca 400 mM, and a high transepithelial urea concentration difference of a similar magnitude in the opposite direction (lumen < interstitium). The transepithelial differences *in vivo* have been found to be in the required direction but an order of magnitude lower (37–60 mmol/l) for NaCl (rat) and 125–145 mmol/l) for urea (hamster). Given the permeabilities to NaCl and urea, a passive single effect would be limited to the first 0.1 mm of thin ascending limb.

Thick ascending limb

Within the two segments of thick ascending limb (medullary thick ascending limb and cortical thick ascending limb), 30% of the filtered NaCl is reabsorbed.

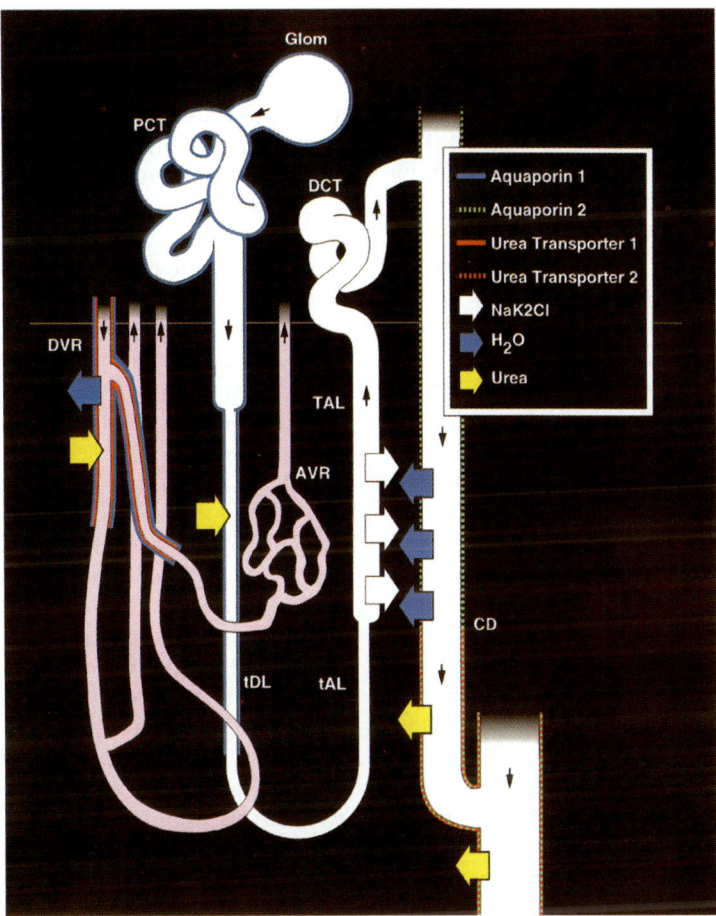

Figure 6.6 Flow of urea, NaCl and water along cortical–medullary axis and perpendicular to axis. The histotopographical proximity of vessel, nephron and collecting duct is distorted by the two-dimensional depiction and the widening of the interstitial space for clarity. The thin horizontal line represents the junction of cortex and outer medulla. The vertical small black arrows indicate the direction of fluid flow within capillary and renal tubule. The horizontal arrows indicate the movement of urea, NaCl and water across capillary and tubule as defined in the inset. A portion of the descending vasa recta endothelium in the outer medulla has Aquaporin-1 (AQP-1) and a urea transporter. The entire collecting duct is lined by AQP-2; the medullary collecting duct, particularly the inner medullary collecting duct, is lined also by a urea transporter. Water is extracted from the descending vasa recta by the higher concentration of NaCl in the interstitium, which exerts a small osmotic force across the descending vasa recta endothelium because σNaCl > 0. The water movement is facilitated by AQP-1 channels. This concentrates the plasma proteins within the descending vasa recta lumen. In ascending vasa recta, the transendothelial Starling forces (net transendothelial hydrostatic pressure difference minus net transendothelial oncotic pressure difference) drives water uptake across the capillary endothelium, which is so porous it does not require water channels.

Urea reabsorbed from the terminal inner medullary collecting duct enters ascending vasa recta. In the outer medulla some of it leaves the ascending vasa recta and enters the descending vasa recta. In this way urea is trapped and accumulates in the medulla, particularly in the inner medulla, to reach a high concentration. Urea transport from the collecting duct and into the descending vasa recta is facilitated by urea transporters. Some urea enters the thin descending limb and thin ascending limb of Henle's loop and probably leaves the thick ascending limb (not shown).

NaCl is reabsorbed from the thick ascending limb and thin ascending limb and enters descending vasa recta, circulates and leaves ascending vasa recta to re-enter descending vasa recta. The reabsorption from the thick ascending limb occurs by way of the apical membrane Na^+-K^+-2Cl^- transporter, with energy supplied by the basolateral Na^+-K^+-ATPase. In this way NaCl is trapped and accumulates in the medulla, particularly in the inner medulla, to reach a high concentration. There is no evidence that NaCl transport is facilitated by a carrier in the vasa recta. The end result of the highly concentrated inner medulla interstitium is the reabsorption of water from the collecting duct. Arginine vasopressin (AVP) stimulates the insertion of AQP-2 water channels into the collecting duct which facilitates the bulk reabsorption of water from the cortical collecting duct (not shown) and the maximum possible removal of the small amount of water remaining in the inner medullary collecting duct. It is thought that AVP also stimulates the formation of the urea transporter in the outer medullary collecting duct. Abbreviations: AVR, ascending vasa recta; CD, collecting duct; DCT, distal convoluted tubule; DVR, descending vasa recta; Glom, glomerulus; PCT, proximal convoluted tubule; TAL, thick ascending limb; tAL, thin ascending limb; tDL, thin descending limb.

Because of the very low L_P of the thick ascending limb, active NaCl reabsorption dilutes the tubule fluid and is the engine for generating a concentrated or dilute urine. The thicker, mitochondria-packed medullary thick ascending limb has a high NaCl transport rate that enriches the medulla with NaCl and establishes a transepithelial NaCl concentration difference (single effect) of 60 mM. The thinner, less mitochondria-laden cortical thick ascending limb has a lower NaCl transport rate, but can create a twofold greater transepithelial concentration difference and is principally responsible for the dilution of tubule fluid and final urine. Other ions, notably Ca^{2+}, Mg^{2+}, NH_4^+, K^+, HCO_3^- and H^+, are also transported by these two segments. In the basolateral membrane, Na^+,K^+-ATPase makes the cell interior low in Na^+ and high in K^+. Outward diffusion of K^+ renders the cell interior electrically negative to the lumen as well as to the blood side. The apical membrane contains a transporter that requires 1Na:1K:2Cl. The apical transmembrane electrical-chemical gradient for Na^+ provides the driving force for the transport of all three ions to the cell interior.

Among factors that regulate transport in the thick ascending limb [23], four are important with regard to the concentrating mechanism: the flow of luminal NaCl reaching the medullary thick ascending limb, AVP, β-adrenergic agonists and renal sympathetic nerves. All stimulate NaCl reabsorption by the 1Na:1K:2Cl transporter. Aldosterone is necessary for full expression of NaCl transport. In contrast, prostaglandins and an increase in Ca^{2+} or K^+ on the basolateral side inhibit NaCl reabsorption. Loop diuretics inhibit reabsorption by interfering with the Cl^- binding site of the apical transporter.

Collecting duct

As discussed above, in the presence of AVP, the cortical collecting duct, outer medullary collecting duct and inner medullary collecting duct become very permeable to water but not to urea – except for the terminal inner medullary collecting duct in which P_U is also increased. As a result, the urea concentration increases an order of magnitude as most of the remaining tubule fluid is reabsorbed during its journey through the collecting duct. In the terminal inner medullary collecting duct, AVP increases the already high P_u by stimulation of a urea transporter of the inner medullary collecting duct, thus ensuring that a urea-laden reabsorbate is delivered to enrich the inner medulla interstitium. The cortical and medullary collecting duct actively reabsorb NaCl. This contributes to urinary dilution, but is probably of no importance to the generation of the hypertonic medulla in antidiuresis. Normally ≤1% of the filtered NaCl is reabsorbed in the medullary collecting duct and in any case, reabsorption of NaCl lowers the solute concentration of the concentrated urine.

Formation of a dilute urine

The architecture of the kidney and the topographical relationships and the transport and permeability properties of the tubules and vessels are constituted to form a dilute urine in the absence of circulating AVP. Fluid leaving the proximal tubule is isosmotic. Along the pars recta and descending limb of Henle, osmolality of tubule fluid rises with that of the interstitium. Fluid at the end of the thin descending limb is always hypertonic, whether the urine is concentrated or not. Fluid at the earliest accessible DT is always dilute. In the absence of AVP urine osmolality is even lower than the osmolality of distal tubule fluid, despite the fact that water is reabsorbed along the collecting duct. These observations establish several important features of urinary dilution [1, 2].

1   The site of urinary dilution is not just the thick ascending limb, although that is quantitatively the most important; the collecting duct also participates in urinary dilution.
2   Even though the water permeability of the collecting duct is very low in the absence of AVP, water is reabsorbed, particularly in the terminal collecting duct, because of the large osmotic gradient between the dilute luminal fluid and the hypertonic interstitium. Reabsorption of this water causes an increase of medullary blood flow and medullary washout of solute.
3   Sodium reabsorption in the thick ascending limb, which provides the driving force for the hypertonic medulla and elaboration of a concentrated urine, is also responsible for diluting the renal tubule fluid and the final urine. This is a beautiful illustration of biologic economy. The only difference between formation of a concentrated and a dilute urine is whether AVP is present. Its presence is necessary to concentrate the urine; its absence is necessary to dilute it.

Urinary dilution has been investigated in humans and other species indirectly by clearance techniques. Urine is considered to consist of two parts:

$$V = C_{osm} + C_{H_2O}$$

where V is urinary flow, C_{H_2O} is free water clearance, and C_{osm} is osmolar clearance = $V \cdot [U_{osm}/P_{osm}]$, and U_{osm} and P_{osm} represent the osmolality of urine and plasma, respectively. C_{H_2O} represents the extent to which at a given urine flow urine osmolality is reduced below that of plasma. Although C_{H_2O} is a useful approximation of urinary diluting ability there are a number of assumptions involved in its interpretation which are erroneous, and therefore render it at best a rough approximation.

The same limitations apply to $T^c_{H_2O}$, which has been used as a measure of the absorption of water free of solute ('free' water) when the urine is concentrated.

$$T^c_{H_2O} = -C_{H_2O} = C_{osm} - V$$

Although $T^c_{H_2O}$ and C_{H_2O} are still used, for example in studies of human kidney function, their usefulness as a research tool is diminishing [1].

Arginine vasopressin

Arginine vasopressin (AVP) is an octapeptide with a molecular weight slightly in excess of 1000 which serves as the antidiuretic hormone in all mammals except the pig and hippopotamus [1]. The volume and tonicity of total body water are regulated by the thirst center and AVP through its action in the kidney. Thirst regulates water drinking (intake) and AVP controls the urinary flow and osmolality (output). Those unfortunate to have a hereditary lack of AVP (central diabetes insipidus) excrete 10–20 l of urine each day if not treated. Inappropriate secretion of AVP as occurs, for example, in association with certain cancers, leads to pathological water retention and a fall in the serum Na^+ concentration to levels as low as 100 mEq/l. AVP is synthesized in magnocellular neurons in the supraoptic and paraventricular regions of the hypothalamus. Its primary function is to regulate the flow and osmolality of the urine. It is released into the systemic circulation from nerve terminals in the posterior pituitary in response to stimulation of osmoreceptors in the hypothalamus by a rise in the serum sodium concentration. These cells are also stimulated by a fall in 'effective' circulating blood volume and input from the cerebral cortex. The principal destination of AVP is the kidney, where it increases the osmotic water permeability (hydraulic conductivity) (L_p) of the entire collecting duct and the urea permeability (P_u) of the inner medullary collecting duct (IMCD) [1, 3]. The result is a fall in urinary flow (V) and rise in U_{osm}. Except for a transient decrease in urinary excretion of urea, total solute excretion remains unchanged. The resulting conservation of water, together with the increased fluid intake in response to the concomitant sensation of thirst, increase total body water. The serum sodium and circulating blood volume are restored to normal. The increase in urea reabsorption helps maintain the high solute concentration of the medulla.

Two classes of receptors for AVP have been identified. The V_1 receptor acts through phosphatidylinositol hydrolysis and is believed to mediate the action of AVP on medullary blood vessels, for example. The second messenger released on stimulation of the V_2 receptor is cyclic adenosine monophosphate (cAMP) formed by the hydrolysis of ATP by adenylcyclase. The V_2 receptor mediates the water-conserving actions of AVP on the collecting duct.

Aquaporins

A new group of water channel proteins, the aquaporins, have been discovered [24]. Four aquaporins have been identified in the kidney that are distinct in molecular structure, renal tubular location and behavior. The prototype was identified by Nielsen *et al.* [25], originally named the channel forming integral membrane protein, and now renamed **aquaporin-1** (AQP-1). As its original name implies, its configuration in the cell membrane resembles a channel that facilitates the selective rapid passage of water molecules. AQP-1 is present in the apical and basolateral cell membranes of the proximal tubule and thin descending limb. **Aquaporin-2** (AQP-2) was found in the cytoplasm and apical membrane of the principal cell of the collecting duct but not in the intercalated cell [26]. AVP stimulates the insertion of AQP-2 into the apical membrane, an action that is pivotal to the rapid increase in water permeability of the collecting duct. **Aquaporin 3** (AQP-3) is confined to the basolateral membrane of the principal cell [24]. AVP promotes the synthesis of both AQP-2 and AQP-3, which enhances the long-term response to the hormone. **Aquaporin-4** (AQP-4), like AQP-3, is in the basolateral membrane of the principal cell [24]. Neither AQP-1 nor AQP-4 are affected by AVP. The thin and thick ascending limb and distal tubule lack aquaporins. These segments have a low L_p that is not increased by AVP, and together form the 'diluting segment'.

The water channel proteins are not limited to the kidney. They are members of a family of membrane intrinsic proteins (MIPs) which are distributed throughout the body [27]. Their function is to facilitate transmembrane water movement in a variety of tissues. One of the most intriguing sites is the supraoptic and paraventricular neurons in the hypothalamus, the osmoreceptors that secrete AVP. Their cell membranes contain AQP-4 [28] and a cation-selective channel sensitive to membrane tension [29]. *In vitro* studies of cells of the supraoptic nuclei from the rat hypothalamus have demonstrated that these cation channels respond to changes in cell volume induced by changes in the tonicity of the bathing fluid [29]. Aquaporins appear to play an essential role in both afferent and efferent arcs of the regulation of water balance.

AVP increases the P_u of the inner medullary collecting duct, particularly the terminal portion [3]. A urea transporter protein has been identified in the inner medullary collecting duct that likely mediates the AVP effect, though this remains to be established [3]. Of great interest is the discovery that the endothelium of the vasa recta in the outer medulla also contains a urea transporter [30]. Urea transport is enhanced in two ways. First, AVP crosses over reabsorption of urea by the terminal inner medullary collecting duct. The reabsorbed urea has four alternative pathways: enter the thin ascending limb or thin descending limb of Henle's loop, the ascending vasa recta (AVR) or descending vasa recta (DVR). Second, urea diffuses out of ascending vasa recta and is captured and crosses over into the descending vasa recta in the outer medulla, facilitated by the urea transporter in the outer medullary descending vasa recta. In this way urea is trapped in the medulla. Urea comprises one-third to one-half of the total solute in the inner medulla. AVP enhances accumulation of osmolytes in the collecting duct cell. The potential adverse effects of the high intracellular urea concentration to the structure and function of cells in the inner medulla is prevented by the organic osmolytes (methylamines) as previously described [15, 16].

AVP has other actions besides those on the collecting duct. It reduces the filtration coefficient (K_f) of the glomerulus [1]. Normally this would cause the GFR to fall, but resistance to tubule fluid flow is reduced by the AVP-enhanced reabsorption of water downstream in the collecting duct which reduces hydrostatic pressure in the proximal tubule (PT). The transglomerular difference in pressure between the glomerular capillary (P_{GC}) and proximal tubule is thereby increased, which offsets the fall in K_f and maintains GFR constant.

AVP stimulates NaCl reabsorption by the thick ascending limb [2], which further dilutes the tubule fluid. The mechanism of stimulation is believed to be an AVP-induced increase in assembly of Na-K-2Cl transporters in the luminal membrane. Separation of water from solute drives both concentration and dilution, by enhancing the 'single effect'. A secondary effect is to stimulate potassium secretion in the distal tubule. The stimulation of NaCl reabsorption and potassium secretion is probably not important to the regulation of excretion of these ions.

AVP reduces medullary blood flow in the vasa recta [10], by two mechanisms. It reduces blood flow directly by causing vasoconstriction of juxtamedullary efferent arterioles and outer medullary descending vasa recta, an effect mediated through the vasopressin V_1 receptor. This effect may also be indirectly transmitted through interstitial cells in the medulla which have been recently shown to have contractile properties. AVP reduces blood flow indirectly by greatly enhancing water reabsorption by the cortical collecting duct. Delivery of water to the medullary collecting duct is reduced sufficiently such that the volume of water reabsorbed in the inner medullary collecting duct is less in antidiuresis than in water diuresis, even though the L_p of the inner medullary collecting duct is much higher.

In summary, AVP facilitates the creation of the hypertonicity of the renal medulla by enhancing the single effect in the thick ascending limb and urea reabsorption from the medullary collecting duct and accumulation in the medulla, and reducing the volume of water delivered to the medullary collecting duct to be concentrated. It increases the water permeability of the collecting duct to permit the urine to become as concentrated as the hypertonic medulla. It facilitates trapping of urea by the medullary circulation. These actions enhance urinary concentration without affecting GFR or excretion of total solute.

Medullary circulation

Besides supplying energy and removing wastes, the medullary circulation has two other functions [10]. The counterflow arrangement of vasa recta in the medulla, analogous to that of Henle's loops, minimizes dissipation of the medullary osmotic gradient that would otherwise occur with a flow-through circulation. Ascending vasa recta remove water reabsorbed from the collecting duct to concentrate the urine. Another feature of the medullary circulation is that all blood perfusing the medulla has first passed through afferent arterioles, glomeruli and efferent arterioles of juxtamedullary cortex. Despite this fact, the medullary circulation can be altered independently of the cortical circulation. The three sections that follow describe countercurrent exchange, medullary blood flow and regulation of the medullary circulation.

Countercurrent exchange

The idea that vascular bundles of descending vasa recta and ascending vasa recta in the medulla subserve countercurrent (cc) exchange originated with Kühn, Wirz and their colleagues. Berliner et al. in 1958 [31] published a classic description. Solutes smaller than protein and supplied to the medulla by reabsorption from the ascending limb (NaCl) and collecting duct (urea) diffuse out of ascending vasa recta into descending vasa recta and are thereby trapped in the medulla. Water entering the medulla in descending vasa recta is shunted into ascending vasa recta, reducing descending vasa recta blood flow which would otherwise wash out the hypertonic medulla. Water shunting and small solute trapping maintain the hypertonic medullary interstitium generated by cc multiplication by Henle's loops. The essential differences between a multiplier and an exchanger are that the exchanger does not require different permeabilities of the walls of its two channels or a source of energy. The theory did not explain, however, how water reabsorbed from medullary collecting ducts returned to the cortex, since it ought to be trapped in the medulla. To explain water removal, the theory was modified by introducing 'Starling' forces – the differences in transcapillary oncotic pressure ($\Delta\pi_p$) between plasma and interstitial protein (mainly albumin) and differences in transcapillary hydraulic pressure (ΔP). The revised 'cc-Starling' theory assumes that for small solutes (ss) descending vasa recta endothelium has a finite reflection coefficient ($\sigma_{ss} > 0$). This explains how the rising axial gradient of small solutes in the medullary interstitium generates a transcapillary difference in osmotic pressure due to small solutes, $\Delta\pi_{ss}$, that exceeds that due to protein, $\Delta\pi_p$, and extracts water and concentrates plasma protein in the descending vasa recta. In blood entering the initial ascending vasa recta, $\Delta\pi_p$ is now sufficient to draw enough water into the ascending vasa recta to account for the water removed from the descending vasa recta and that reabsorbed from the medullary collecting duct.

Recent experiments have confirmed the revised cc-Starling theory [10, 21, 30, 32] (Figure 6.6).

1 Transcapillary $\Delta\pi_{ss}$ influences transcapillary fluid movement in descending vasa recta (see point 4 below). Plasma protein concentration in descending vasa recta rises due to volume efflux from descending vasa recta.

2 Water movement across the descending vasa recta endothelium is determined by transcapillary Starling forces ($\Delta\pi_{ss}$, $\Delta\pi_p$, and differences in hydraulic pressure, ΔP) of about 20 mmHg. Descending vasa recta hydraulic conductivity (L_p) is $\geq 1.4 \times 10^6$ cm/s/mmHg, about 10 times greater than muscle capillary L_p, but less than glomerular capillary L_p (41×10^6 cm/s/mmHg). The minimum value for the L_p (a unique value could not be determined) indicates descending vasa recta are sufficiently water conductive to enable $\Delta\pi_{ss}$, $\Delta\pi_p$ and ΔP to determine transcapillary water movement.

3 Ascending vasa recta are more than twice as numerous as descending vasa recta, as noted previously, and have a higher L_p than descending vasa recta. That means they have the required capacity for water removal from the medulla. Ascending vasa recta L_p = 12–19 × 10^6 cm/s/mmHg, higher than descending vasa recta L_p but less than glomerular L_p.

4 The transcapillary differences in osmolality due to differences in NaCl concentration, $\Delta\pi_{NaCl}$, induce water movement across the endothelium of descending vasa recta. Sodium permeability (P_{Na}) = 60×10^{-5} cm/s, and the NaCl reflection coefficient, σ_{NaCl}, ranges from 0.02 to 0.05. A finite value for σ_{NaCl} means that, despite the high value for P_{Na}, transcapillary $\Delta\pi_{NaCl}$ is an effective force for transcapillary volume flux.

5 Ascending vasa recta are highly permeable to Na^+, and transcapillary $\Delta\pi_{NaCl}$ does not generate a driving force for water movement in ascending vasa recta. This is a key observation: ascending vasa recta segments were perfused *in vivo* with varying concentrations of NaCl in an attempt to induce transcapillary water movement across ascending vasa recta. P_{Na} = 113×10^{-5} cm/s, twice as high as descending vasa recta P_{Na}. Water transport was not affected. Thus $\Delta\pi_p$ and ΔP, but not $\Delta\pi_{NaCl}$, determine water movement across ascending vasa recta.

6 At normal vasa recta blood flows, transcapillary movement of albumin is zero, a finding consistent with its role in generating a driving force, $\Delta\pi_p$, for transcapillary water flow. At high vasa recta blood flows, however, there is transcapillary transport of albumin across ascending vasa recta – albumin permeates by solvent drag. Since the inner medulla lacks lymphatics and $\Delta\pi_p$ is assumed to be an important driving force for transcapillary water movement, several questions arise: Does the interstitium contain protein and, if so, how much? How did it get there and how does it get out of the medulla? Individual descending vasa recta or ascending vasa recta were perfused *in vivo* with ^{125}I-labeled albumin. At low perfusion rates, there was no albumin loss (i.e. no transcapillary diffusion); at high perfusion rates, albumin loss occurred. The $\sigma_{albumin}$ was 0.78, indicating that it is transported by solvent drag. The medullary interstitial protein was 5 g/100 ml, a high value. The protein may be supplied to the medulla by terminal branches of descending vasa recta, since albumin slowly leaks from descending vasa recta. Albumin is thus removed from the medulla by the ascending vasa recta.

7 Transcapillary transport of urea and Na^+ in outer medullary descending vasa recta differs strikingly: Na moves by diffusion; urea transport is carrier-mediated by a urea transporter across the descending vasa recta endothelium. The urea transporter in outer medullary descending vasa recta is similar to that in inner medullary collecting duct (Figure 6.6). Both urea transporters are ideally placed to facilitate urea trapping in the medulla by hastening entry into the descending vasa recta of urea reabsorbed from ascending vasa recta and inner medullary collecting ducts. (The highly permeable ascending vasa recta would not need a urea transporter.)

Medullary blood flow

The many different methods employed to measure medullary blood flow are testimony to the fact that the ideal method does not exist [10, 33]. Each one has advantages and disadvantages. One disadvantage of the methods employing tracers is the assumption regarding the renal extraction of a tracer introduced into the renal circulation. The assumption that PAH is extracted entirely from the cortex, but not in the medulla, for example, is not correct. The method employing rubidium or other radiolabeled cations has the disadvantage that it is an acute experiment requiring sacrifice of the animal. The albumin accumulation technique is probably nearest to a quantitative measure of papillary blood flow but it is also an acute experiment. Microspheres depend on the assumption that they are distributed equally throughout the glomeruli in the renal cortex. Recent evidence indicates that is not the case.

Laser Doppler and video microscopy are both methods of direct observation of renal blood flow. With both methods, multiple measurements of blood flow in the same region are possible and they do not require invasion of medullary tissue. On the other hand, excision of the ureter is necessary, a maneuver that causes an increase in the medullary blood flow and it is difficult to relate directly the signal to tissue blood flow. Laser Doppler measures inner medullary blood flow only. Video microscopy enables determination of individual capillary blood flow. To convert vasa recta flow into overall medullary blood flow required determining the number of vasa recta in the medulla, a difficult task.

Combining the results from various methods has shown that, in terms of ml/min/g of kidney tissue, values for medullary blood flow vary from 1.2 to 3.2 in the outer medulla and from 0.2 to 2.4 in the inner medulla. For comparison the cortical flow values range from 2.6 to 7.3. These values are widely scattered. As a rule of thumb, in the normal kidney, the respective blood flows for cortex, outer medulla and inner medulla are 5, 2 and 0.7 ml/min/g, respectively.

Regulation of medullary blood flow

For maximum urinary concentrating capacity, the optimum value for medullary blood flow is as low as possible, as long as sufficient oxygen and other forms of energy reach the medulla and water and waste products are not allowed to accumulate in the medulla. Assuming that a low value represents the normal state of medullary blood flow, anything that increases medullary blood flow reduces the efficiency of countercurrent exchange, decreases medullary hypertonicity (medullary washout) and impairs maximum urine concentration. A reduction in blood flow below normal might temporarily increase urine concentratrating ability, but the effect would be short-lived. The effect of autoregulation, and extrinsic regulation by the adrenergic nervous system, hormones and autocoids on urinary concentration is therefore complex and somewhat speculative. The importance of maintaining an optimal balance may explain why there are so many regulators of medullary blood flow.

Autoregulation

Total blood flow to the kidney is relatively constant despite wide changes in arterial pressure, a phenomenon known as autoregulation [10, 34]. Early studies of medullary blood flow suggested it is not autoregulated. Since then several studies have either supported or failed to support the concept of autoregulation in the medulla. In a recent investigation in dogs using computed tomography, only inner medullary blood flow decreased with reduced renal perfusion pressure. Takenaka et al. demonstrated autoregulation of blood flow to afferent arterioles of juxtamedullary glomeruli using video microscopy and a partially infarcted kidney to gain access to the medulla [35]. As pressure was lowered, medullary blood flow fell before total renal blood flow decreased.

In summary, it appears that medullary blood flow is autoregulated within a range of changes in pressure which are narrower than those for cortical blood flow, and inner medullary blood flow is autoregulated within a narrower range of pressure changes than medullary blood flow as a whole.

External regulation

Innervation of the kidney is exclusively adrenergic and the principal effect of renal nerve stimulation is a reduction in total renal blood flow [36, 37]. Renal vasoconstriction appears to be mediated by the α_1-adrenoceptor, but the roles of the α_1-adrenoceptor and β-receptor are not well established. There is no functional evidence for the existence of vasodilator-mediated neural effects. The neural effect on the medullary circulation appears to be similar to that on the cortical circulation.

Vasoactive peptides, hormones and autocoids (see also Chapter 13)

Angiotensin II reduces medullary blood flow. It acts on both afferent and efferent arteriole of juxtamedullary nephron to cause vasoconstriction; inhibitors of angiotensin II action increase medullary blood flow [10, 31, 35]. An infusion of angiotensin II reduces medullary blood flow in dogs. The location of angiotensin II receptors in the medulla has been controversial. They have been found on glomeruli, vascular bundles and on afferent arterioles. Pallone, in an elegant study of perfusion of outer medullary descending vasa recta in vitro, showed that application of angiotensin II to the outside of the vessels caused constriction, whereas angiotensin II applied to the luminal side had no effect [38]. Angiotensin II receptors have been localized to interstitial cells in vascular bundles, so it is possible they mediate angiotensin II-induced vasoconstriction of outer medullary descending vasa recta.

Atrial natriuretic peptide (ANP) increases glomerular blood flow by dilation of the afferent and constriction of the efferent arterioles [10, 39]. ANP-receptors are present in the afferent and efferent arteriole, glomeruli and vascular bundles, but they are mostly clearance receptors. Video microscopy has shown that ANP increases inner medullary blood flow. The rise in sodium excretion following ANP occurs before and at lower doses of ANP than the increase in medullary blood flow, so it seems unlikely that a change in the medullary circulation mediates the natriuresis.

Arginine vasopressin (see above) reduces medullary blood flow directly, via the V_1 receptor, and indirectly, by reducing fluid uptake, an effect mediated by V_2 receptor [10].

Endothelin has several forms – ETI, ETII, and ETIII [40]. Infusion of ETI causes vasodilatation followed by vasoconstriction and reduction in renal blood flow. This is mediated by greater vasoconstriction in the efferent than in the afferent arteriole. The peptides have two receptors. Receptor A has a high affinity for ETI and ETII and a low affinity for ETIII. Receptor B binds equally to all three endothelins. In preliminary studies, Sildorff et al. [41] showed in outer medullary descending vasa recta that all three forms of ET cause vasoconstriction, particularly ETI and ETII. These data suggest that outer medullary descending vasa recta have both receptors, and that ET reduces medullary blood flow. The effect would be to enhance urinary concentration.

Adenosine is a ubiquitous nucleoside that causes vasodilatation in regional vascular beds [10]. Studies of its effect on renal hemodynamics have yielded conflicting results. Aortic infusion of adenosine caused a decrease followed by an increase in renal blood flow. When it was administered directly into the renal artery of the rat, inner medullary blood flow nearly doubled. At lower doses, a marked diuresis and natriuresis were apparent before a detectable effect on vasa recta blood flow. As in the case of ANF, adenosine causes increase in vasa recta blood flow, but this effect does not mediate the natriuresis and diuresis. On the other hand it would impair urinary concentration.

It is likely that **nitric oxide** (NO) (or endothelial-derived relaxing factor) is an autocoid, i.e. it exerts its action within the cell in which it is produced (autocrine) or on a neighboring cell (paracrine) [42]. NO appears to increase renal blood flow in general and medullary blood flow in particular. If an inhibitor of NO is given, medullary blood flow falls sooner and to a greater extent than cortical blood flow. Nakanishi *et al.* [43] have proposed that this is an important step in the development of systemic hypertension that follows the use of an NO inhibitor. It was suggested that NO is continuously released to maintain dilatation of afferent and efferent arterioles of juxtamedullary nephrons. If so, this would accord an important regulatory role to NO. This hypothesis remains to be established. Brezis and Rosen [44] have

shown that inhibition of prostaglandin and NO coupled with administration of a nephrotoxic agent results in acute tubular necrosis.

Prostaglandins (PGE_2; PGF_{2a}, thromboxane) are synthesized by the medulla [1, 2, 10]. Stimulation of prostaglandin biosynthesis is associated with an increase in blood flow to the renal medulla; inhibition reduces medullary blood flow. Pallone [38] found that prostaglandin E_2 (PGE_2) reversibly dilated outer medullary descending vasa recta preconstricted by angiotensin II. It seems likely that prostaglandins play an important role, perhaps as paracrines, in regulation of the renal medullary circulation.

Acknowledgment

I wish to thank Roger Green for his constructive criticism of this chapter.

References

1. Jamison, R.L. and Kriz, W. (1982) *Urinary Concentrating Mechanism: Structure and Function.* Oxford University Press, New York, 340 pp.
2. Jamison, R.L. and Gehrig, J.J. (1992) Urinary concentration and dilution: physiology, in *Handbook of Physiology*, Section 8, Renal Physiology (ed. E. Windhager), Oxford University Press, New York, pp. 1219–79.
3. Chou, C-L., Knepper, M.A. and Layton, H.E. (1993) Urinary concentrating mechanism: the role of the inner medulla. *Semin. Nephrol*, **13**, 168–81.
4. Wirz, H., Hargitay, B. and Kühn, W. (1951) Lokalisation des konzentrierungs-prozesses in der Niere durch direkte kryoskopie. *Helv. Physiol. Pharmacol Acta*, **9**, 196–207.
5. Hargitay, B. and Kühn, W. (1951) Das Multiplikationsprinzip als Grandlage der Harnkonzentrierung in der Niere. *Z. Elektrochem.*, **55**, 539–58.
6. Kühn, W. and Ryffel, K. (1942) Herstellung konzentrierter Lösungen aus verdünnen durch blosse Membranwirkung. *Hoppe-Seylers Z. Physiol. Chem.*, **276**, 145–78.
7. Burg, M. and Green, N. (1973) Function of the thick ascending limb of Henle's loop. *Am. J. Physiol.*, **224**, 659–68.
8. Stephenson, J.L. (1972) Central core model of the renal counterflow system. *Kidney Int.*, **2**, 85–94.
9. Kokko, J. and Rector, F. (1972) Countercurrent multiplication system without active transport in inner medulla. *Kidney Int.*, **2**, 214–23.
10. Pallone, T.L., Robertson, C.R. and Jamison, R.L. (1990) Renal medullary microcirculation. *Physiol. Rev.*, **70**, 885–920.
11. Garcia-Perez, A. and Burg, M. (1991) Renal medullary organic osmolytes, *Physiol. Rev.*, **71**, 1081–115.
12. Lemley, K. and Kriz, W. (1987) Cycles and separations: the histotopography of the urinary concentrating process. *Kidney Int.*, **31**, 538–48.
13. Garcia-Perez, A. and Burg, M. (1990) Importance of

organic osmolytes for osmoregulation by renal medullary cells. *Hypertension*, **16**, 595–602.
14. McManus, M.D., Churchwell, K.B. and Strange, K. (1995) Mechanisms of disease: regulation of cell volume in health and disease. *N. Engl. J. Med.*, **333**, 1260–6.
15. Handler, J.S. and Kwon, H.M. (1993) Regulation of renal cell organic osmolyte transport by tonicity. *Am. J. Physiol.*, **265**, C1449–55.
16. Cowley, B.D. Jr, Ferraris, J.D., Carper, D. *et al.* (1990) *In vivo* osmoregulation of aldose reductase mRNA, protein and sorbitol in renal medulla. *Am. J. Physiol.*, **258**, F154–61.
17. Wexler, A.S., Kalaba, R.E. and Marsh, D.J. (1991) Three-dimensional anatomy and renal concentrating mechanism. I. Modeling results. *Am. J. Physiol.*, **260**, F368–83.
18. Hamada, Y., Taniguchi, J. and Imai, M. (1993) The urinary concentrating mechanism: the countercurrent multiplication between thin ascending limb and inner medullary collecting duct, in *Vasopressin* (eds P. Gross, D. Richter and G.L. Robertson), John Libbey Eurotest, Paris, pp. 407–17.
19. Stephenson, J.L., Jen, J.F., Wang H. *et al.* (1995) Convective uphill transport of NaCl from ascending limb of loop of Henle. *Am. J. Physiol.*, **268**, F680–92.
20. Layton, H.E. and Davies, J.M. (1993) Distributed solute and water reabsorption in a central core model of the renal concentration mechanism. *Math. Biosci.*, **116**, 169.
21. Pallone, T.L. and Jamison, R.L. (1988) Effect of ureteral excision on the corticomedullary solute gradients in the rat. *Am. J. Physiol.*, **255**, F1225–9.
22. Chou, C-L., Nielsen, S. and Knepper, M.A. (1993) Structural–functional correlation in chinchilla long loop of Henle thin limbs: a novel papillary subsegment. *Am. J. Physiol.*, **265**, F863–74.
23. Sun, A.M., Kikeri, D. and Hebert, S. (1992) Vasopressin

regulates apical and basolateral Na(+)-K(+) antiporters in mouse medullary thick ascending limbs. *Am. J. Physiol.*, **262**, F241–7.

24. Knepper, M.A., Wade, J.B., Terris, J., Ecelbarger, C.A., Marples, D., Mandon, B., Chou, C.-L., Kishore, B.K. and Nielsen, S. (1996) Renal aquaporins. *Kidney Int.*, **49**, 1712–17.

25. Nielsen, S. and Agre, P. (1995) The aquaporin family of water channels in kidney. *Kidney Int.*, **48**, 1057–68.

26. Sasaki, S., Fushimi, F., Saito, H., Saito, F., Uchida, S., Ishibashi, K., Kuwahara, M., Ikeuchi, T., Inui, K., Nakajima, R., Watanabe, X. and Marumo, F. (1994) Cloning, characterization and chromosomal mapping of human aquaporin of collecting duct. *J. Clin. Invest.*, **93**, 1250–6.

27. Verkman, A.S., Shi, L.-B., Frigeri, A., Hasegawa, H., Farinase, J., Mitra, A., Skach, W., Brown, D., van Hoek, A.N. and Ma, T. (1995) Structure and function of kidney water channels. *Kidney Int.*, **48**, 1069–81.

28. Jung, J.S., Bhat, R.V., Preston, G.M., Guggino, W.B., Baraban, J.M. and Agre, P. (1994) Molecular characterization of an aquaporin cDNA from brain: candidate osmoreceptor and regulator of water balance. *Proc. Natl. Acad. Sci. USA*, **91**, 13052–6.

29. Ollet, S.H.R. and Bourque, C.S. (1993) Mechanosensitive channels transduce osmosensitivity in supraoptic neurons. *Nature*, **364**, 341–3.

30. Pallone, T.L. (1994) Characterization of the urea transporter in outer medullary descending vasa. *Am. J. Physiol.*, **267**, R260–7.

31. Berliner, R.W., Levinsky, N.G., Davidson, D.B. *et al.* (1958) Dilution and concentration of the urine and the action of antidiuretic hormone. *Am. J. Med.*, **24**, 730–44.

32. Pallone, T.L., Work, J., Myers, R.L. *et al.* (1994) Transport of sodium and urea in outer medullary descending vasa recta. *J. Clin. Invest.*, **93**, 212–22.

33. Chou, S.Y., Porush, J.G. and Faubert, R.T. (1990) Renal medullary circulation: hormonal control. *Kidney Int.*, **37**, 1–13.

34. Holstein-Rathlou, N.H. and Marsh, D.J. (1994) Renal blood flow regulation and arterial pressure fluctuations: a case study in nonlinear dynamics. *Physiol. Rev.*, **74**, 637–81.

35. Takenaka, T., Harrison-Bernard, L.M., Inscho, E.W. *et al.* (1994) Autoregulation of afferent arteriolar blood flow in juxtamedullary nephrons. *Am. J. Physiol.*, **267**, F879–87.

36. Kopp, U.C. and DiBona, G. (1992) The neural control of renal function, in *The Kidney: Physiology and Pathophysiology* (eds D.W. Seldin and G. Giebisch), Raven Press, New York, pp. 1157–204.

37. Kriz, W. and Kaissling, B. (1992) Structural organization of the mammalian kidney, in *The Kidney: Physiology and Pathophysiology* (eds D.W. Seldin and G. Giebisch), Raven Press, New York, pp. 707–78.

38. Pallone, T.L. (1994) Vasoconstriction of outer medullary vasa recta by angiotensin II is modulated by prostaglandin E_2. *Am. J. Physiol.*, **266**, F850–7.

39. Jamison, R.L., Canaan-Kühl, S. and Pratt, R. (1992) The natriuretic peptides and their receptors. *Am. J. Kidney Dis.*, **20**, 519–30.

40. Simonson, M.S. and Dunn, M.J. (1992) The molecular mechanisms of cardiovascular and renal regulation by endothelin peptides. *J. Lab. Clin. Med.*, **119**, 622–39.

41. Sildorff, E.P., Yang, S. and Pallone, T.L. (1994) Constriction of outer medullary descending vasa recta (OMDVR) by endothelins (ET): modulation by PGE_2. *J. Am. Soc. Nephrol.*, **5**, 592.

42. Moncada, S. and Higgs, A. (1993) The L-arginine–nitric oxide pathway. *N. Engl. J. Med.*, **329**, 2002–12.

43. Nakanishi, K., Mattson, D.L. and Cowley, A.W., Jr (1995) Role of renal medullary blood flow in development of L-NAME hypertension in rats. *Am. J. Physiol.*, **268**, R310–16.

44. Brezis, M. and Rosen, S. (1995) Hypoxia of the renal medulla – its implications for disease. *N. Engl. J. Med.*, **332**, 647–55.

Section 3
Renal Regulation of
Volume and
Composition of
Body Fluids

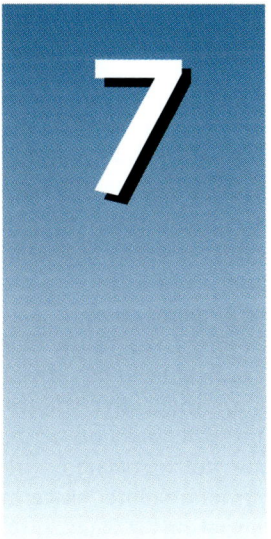

7

Body water and osmolality

Joseph G. Verbalis

Introduction

Disorders of body fluids are among the most commonly encountered problems in the practice of clinical medicine. This is in large part because many different disease states can potentially disrupt the finely balanced mechanisms that control the intake and output of water and solute. Consequently, a detailed working knowledge of the regulatory mechanisms underlying water and sodium metabolism, the two major determinants of body fluid homeostasis, is essential for understanding both the pathogenesis and the therapy of disorders of body fluids.

The two major variables that are regulated to maintain body fluid homeostasis are the composition and the volume of the various body fluid compartments. The first chapter of this section will consider the osmotic composition of body fluids, which is largely a function of the amount of body water, and the second chapter will address the volume of the extracellular fluid, which is largely a function of the amount of body sodium. Although such a separation represents an oversimplification of complicated interactions between water and sodium metabolism, it is nonetheless of practical utility in understanding how body fluids are regulated.

Body fluid compartments

Water constitutes approximately 55–65% of body weight, varying somewhat with age, sex and amount of body fat, and therefore constitutes the largest single constituent of the body. Total body water (TBW) is distributed between the intracellular fluid (ICF) and the extracellular fluid (ECF) compartments. Estimates of the relative sizes of these two important pools differ significantly depending on the tracer used to measure the ECF volume, but most studies in animals and humans have suggested that 55–65% (or just under two-thirds) of TBW resides in the ICF and 35–45% (or slightly more than one-third) is in the ECF. Approximately three-quarters of the ECF compartment is interstitial fluid and one-quarter is intravascular fluid (blood volume). Figure 7.1 summarizes the estimated body fluid spaces of an average-weight adult. The solute composition of the ICF and ECF differ considerably, since membrane-bound Na^+/K^+ pumps maintain Na^+ in a primarily extracellular location and K^+ in a primarily intracellular location. Nonetheless, it is important to remember that the osmotic pressure, which is a function of the concentrations of all the solutes in a fluid compartment, must always be equivalent in the ICF and ECF because most biological membranes are semipermeable (i.e. freely permeable to water but not to aqueous solutes). Thus, water will flow across membranes into a compartment with a higher solute concentration until a steady-state is reached where the osmotic pressures have equalized on both sides of the cell membrane. An important consequence of this thermodynamic law is that the volume of distribution of body Na^+ and K^+ is actually the TBW rather than just the ECF or ICF volume, respectively. For example, any increase in ECF $[Na^+]$ will cause water to shift from the ICF to the ECF until the ICF and ECF

Nephrology, Edited by Rex L. Jamison and Robert Wilkinson.
Published in 1997 by Chapman & Hall, London. ISBN 0 412 60930

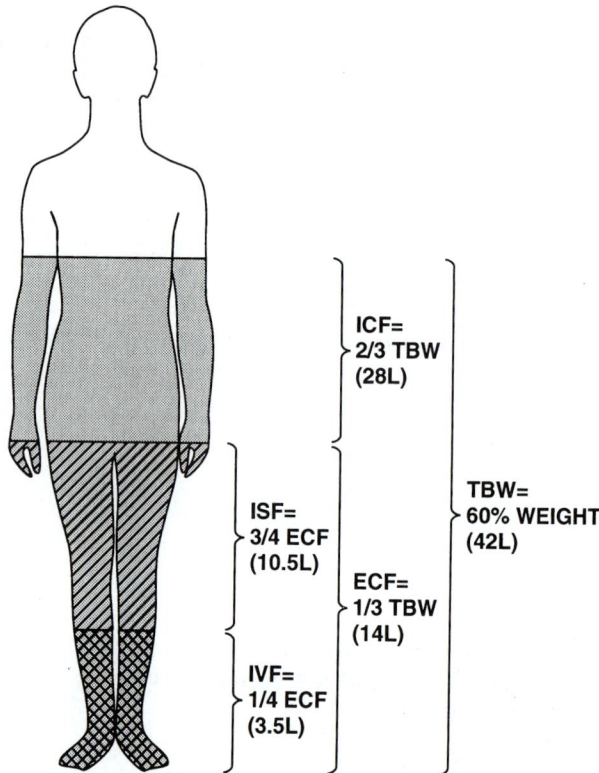

ICF=
2/3 TBW
(28L)

ISF=
3/4 ECF
(10.5L)

TBW=
60% WEIGHT
(42L)

ECF=
1/3 TBW
(14L)

IVF=
1/4 ECF
(3.5L)

Figure 7.1 Schematic representation of body fluid compartments in man. The shaded areas depict the approximate size of each compartment as a function of body weight. The figures indicate the relative sizes of the various fluid compartments and the approximate absolute volumes of the compartments (in liters) in a 70 kg adult. Abbreviations: TBW = total body water; ICF = intracellular fluid; ECF = extracellular fluid; ISF = interstitial fluid; IVF = intravascular fluid.

osmotic pressures are equal, thereby in effect distributing the Na^+ across both extracellular and intracellular water.

Total and effective osmolality

Osmolality is defined as the concentration of all of the solutes in a given weight of water. Plasma osmolality can be measured directly (via determination of freezing point depression or vapor pressure, since each of these are colligative properties of the number of free solute particles in a given volume of plasma), or estimated as:

$$P_{osm}(\text{mosmol/kg H}_2\text{O}) = 2 \times \text{plasma}[Na^+](\text{mEq/l})$$
$$+ \text{glucose}(\text{mg/dl})/18$$
$$+ \text{BUN}(\text{mg/dl})/2.8$$

Both methods produce comparable results under most conditions, as will simply doubling the plasma sodium concentration ($[Na^+]$) since sodium and its accompanying anions are by far the predominant solutes present in plasma. However, the total osmolality of plasma is not

always equivalent to the 'effective' osmolality (sometimes referred to as the 'tonicity' of the plasma), because the latter is a function of the relative solute permeability properties of the membranes separating the two compartments. Solutes that are impermeable to cell membranes (Na^+, mannitol) are restricted to the ECF compartment and are effective solutes, since they create osmotic pressure gradients across cell membranes leading to osmotic movement of water from the ICF to the ECF compartments. Solutes that are permeable to cell membranes (urea, ethanol, methanol) are ineffective solutes, since they do not create osmotic pressure gradients across cell membranes and therefore are not associated with such water shifts. Glucose is a unique solute, since at normal physiologic plasma concentrations it is taken up by cells via active transport mechanisms and therefore acts as an ineffective solute, but under conditions of impaired cellular uptake (e.g. insulin deficiency) it becomes an effective extracellular solute.

The importance of this distinction between total and effective osmolality lies with the fact that only the effective solutes in plasma are determinants of whether clinically significant hyperosmolality or hypoosmolality is present. An example of this is uremia: a patient with a urea concentration that has increased by 30 mM/l will have a corresponding 30 mosmol/kg H_2O elevation in plasma osmolality, but the effective osmolality will remain normal since the increased urea is proportionally distributed across both the ECF and ICF. In contrast, a patient whose plasma $[Na^+]$ has increased by 15 mEq/l will also have a 30 mosmol/kg H_2O elevation of plasma osmolality, since the increased cation must be balanced by an equivalent increase in plasma anions, but in this case the effective osmolality will also be elevated by 30 mosmol/kg H_2O since the Na^+ and accompanying anions will largely remain restricted to the ECF due to the relative impermeability of cell membranes to Na^+ and other univalent ions. Thus, elevations of solutes such as urea, unlike elevations in plasma $[Na^+]$, do not cause cellular dehydration, and consequently do not activate mechanisms that defend body fluid homeostasis by acting to increase body water stores.

Water metabolism

Water metabolism represents a balance between the intake and excretion of water. Each side of this balance equation can be considered to consist of a 'regulated' and an 'unregulated' component, the magnitudes of which can vary quite markedly under different physiological and pathophysiological conditions. The unregulated component of water intake consists of the intrinsic water content of ingested foods, the consumption of beverages primarily for reasons of palatability or desired secondary effects (e.g. caffeine), or for social or habitual reasons (e.g. alcoholic beverages), whereas the regulated component of water intake consists of fluids consumed in response to a perceived sensation of thirst. Similarly, the unregulated component of water excretion occurs via insensible water losses from a variety of sources (cutaneous losses from sweating, evaporative losses in exhaled air, gastrointestinal losses) as well as the obligate amount of water that the kidneys must excrete to eliminate solutes generated by body metabolism, whereas the regulated component of water excretion is composed of the renal excretion of free water in excess of the obligate amount necessary to excrete metabolic solutes. In effect, the regulated components are those that act to maintain water balance by compensating for whatever perturbations result from unregulated water losses or gains. Within this framework, it is clear that the two major mechanisms responsible for regulating water metabolism are thirst and pituitary secretion of the hormone arginine vasopressin.

Thirst

Thirst is the body's defense mechanism to increase water consumption in response to perceived deficits of body fluids. Thirst can be stimulated in animals and humans either by intracellular dehydration caused by increases in the effective osmolality of the ECF, or by intravascular hypovolemia caused by losses of ECF. Substantial evidence to date has supported mediation of the former by osmoreceptors located in the anterior hypothalamus of the brain, whereas the latter appears to be stimulated primarily via activation of low- and/or high-pressure baroreceptors, with a likely contribution from circulating angiotensin II during more severe degrees of intravascular hypovolemia and hypotension. Controlled studies in animals have consistently reported thresholds for osmotically induced drinking ranging from 1% to 4% increases in plasma osmolality above basal levels, and analogous studies in humans using quantitative estimates of subjective symptoms of thirst have confirmed that increases in plasma osmolality of similar magnitudes are necessary to produce an unequivocal sensation described as 'thirst'.

Conversely, the threshold for producing hypovolemic, or extracellular, thirst is significantly greater in both animals and humans. Studies in several species have shown that sustained decreases in plasma volume or blood pressure of at least 4–8%, and in some species 10–15%, are necessary to consistently stimulate drinking. In humans, it has been difficult to demonstrate any effects of mild to moderate hypovolemia to stimulate thirst independently of osmotic changes occurring with dehydration. This blunted sensitivity to changes in extracellular fluid volume or blood pressure in humans probably represents an adaptation that occurred as a result of the erect posture of primates, which predisposes them to wide fluctuations in blood and atrial filling pressures as a result of orthostatic pooling of blood in the lower body; stimulation of thirst (and vasopressin secretion) by such transient postural changes in blood pressure might lead

to overdrinking and inappropriate antidiuresis in situations where the ECF volume was actually normal but only transiently maldistributed. Consistent with a blunted response to baroreceptor activation, recent studies have also shown that systemic infusion of angiotensin II to pharmacological levels is a much less potent stimulus to thirst in humans than in animals. Nonetheless, this response is not completely absent in humans, as demonstrated by rare cases of polydipsia in patients with pathological causes of hyperreninemia.

Although osmotic changes clearly are more effective stimulants of thirst than are volume changes in humans, it is not clear whether relatively small changes in plasma osmolality are responsible for day-to-day fluid intakes. Most humans consume the majority of their ingested water as a result of the unregulated components of fluid intake discussed previously, and generally ingest volumes in excess of what can be considered to be actual 'need'. Consistent with this observation is the fact that under most conditions plasma osmolalities in man remain within 1–2% of basal levels, and these relatively small changes in plasma osmolality are generally below the threshold levels that have been found to stimulate thirst in most individuals. This suggests that despite the obvious vital importance of thirst during pathological situations of hyperosmolality and hypovolemia, under normal physiological conditions water balance in man is accomplished more by regulated free water excretion than by regulated water intake.

Arginine vasopressin secretion

The prime determinant of free water excretion in animals and man is the regulation of urinary flow by circulating levels of arginine vasopressin (AVP) in plasma. Before AVP was biochemically characterized, early studies of antidiuresis used the term 'antidiuretic hormone' (ADH) to describe this substance. Now that its structure and function as the only naturally occurring antidiuretic substance are known, it is more appropriate to refer to it by its real name. AVP is a nine-amino acid peptide that is synthesized in specialized (magnocellular) neural cells located in two discrete areas of the hypothalamus, the supraoptic (SON) and paraventricular (PVN) nuclei. The synthesized peptide is enzymatically cleaved from its prohormone and is transported to the posterior pituitary where it is stored within neurosecretory granules until specific stimuli cause secretion of AVP into the bloodstream. Antidiuresis then occurs via interaction of the circulating hormone with V_2 AVP receptors in the kidney, which results in increased water permeability of the collecting duct through the insertion of water channels into the apical membranes of tubular epithelial cells (see Chapter 6). The importance of AVP for maintaining water balance is underscored by the fact that the normal pituitary stores of this hormone are very large, allowing more than a week's supply of hormone for maximal antidiuresis under conditions of sustained dehydration. Knowledge of the different conditions that stimulate pituitary AVP release in man is therefore essential for understanding water metabolism.

Osmotic regulation

The primary renal response to AVP is an increase in water permeability of the collecting tubule (see Chapter 6). Although an increase in solute reabsorption (primarily urea) occurs as well, the total solute reabsorption is proportionally much less than water. Consequently, a decrease in urine flow and an increase in urine osmolality occur as secondary responses to the increased net water reabsorption. With refinement of radioimmunoassays for AVP, the unique sensitivity of this hormone to small changes in osmolality, as well as the corresponding sensitivity of the kidney to small changes in plasma AVP levels, have become apparent. Although there is still some debate with regard to the exact pattern of osmotically stimulated AVP secretion, most studies to date have supported the concept of a discrete osmotic threshold for AVP secretion above which a linear relationship between plasma osmolality and AVP levels occurs (Figure 7.2). The slope of the regression line relating AVP to plasma osmolality can vary significantly across individual human subjects, in part because of genetic factors. In general, each 1 mosmol/kg H_2O increase in plasma osmolality causes an increase in plasma AVP level from 0.4 to 0.8 pg/ml. The renal response to circulating AVP is similarly linear, with urinary concentration that is directly proportional to AVP levels from 0.5 to 4–5 pg/ml, after which urinary osmo-

lality is maximal and cannot increase further despite additional increases in AVP levels. Thus, changes of 1% or less in plasma osmolality are sufficient to cause significant increases in plasma AVP levels with proportional increases in urine concentration, and maximal antidiuresis is achieved after increases in plasma osmolality of only 5–10 mosmol/kg H_2O (2–4%) above the threshold for AVP secretion.

However, even this analysis underestimates the sensitivity of this system to regulate free water excretion for the following reason. Urinary osmolality is directly proportional to plasma AVP levels as a consequence of the fall in urine flow induced by the AVP, but urine volume is inversely related to urine osmolality (Figure 7.3; the actual relation between urine osmolality and urine volume is more complex, since AVP induces urea as well as water reabsorption from the medullary collecting duct, see Chapter 6). Thus, an increase in plasma AVP concentration from 0.5 to 2 pg/ml has a much greater relative effect to decrease urine flow than does a subsequent increase in AVP concentration from 2 to 5 pg/ml, thereby further magnifying the physiological effects of small initial changes in plasma AVP levels. The net result of these relations is a finely tuned regulatory system that adjusts the rate of free water excretion accurately to the ambient plasma osmolality via changes in pituitary AVP secretion. Furthermore, the rapid response of pituitary AVP secretion to changes in plasma osmolality coupled with the short half-life (10–20 min) of AVP in human plasma enables this regulatory system to adjust renal water excretion to changes in plasma osmolality on a minute-to-minute basis.

Volemic regulation

As in the case of thirst, hypovolemia is also a stimulus for AVP secretion in man; an appropriate physiological response to volume depletion should include urinary concentration and renal water conservation. But similar to thirst, AVP secretion is much less sensitive to small changes in blood volume and blood pressure than to changes in osmolality; some have even suggested that the AVP response to decreases in blood volume is absent in man, though most likely this is simply a manifestation of the significantly higher threshold for AVP secretion to volemic stimuli. Such marked differences in AVP responses represent additional corroborative evidence that osmolality represents a more sensitive regulatory system for water balance than does blood or ECF volume.

Nonetheless, modest changes in blood volume and pressure influence AVP secretion indirectly, even though they are weak stimuli by themselves. This occurs via shifting the sensitivity of AVP secretion to osmotic stimuli so that a given increase in osmolality will cause a greater secretion of AVP during hypovolemic conditions than during euvolemic states (Figure 7.4). Although this effect has been demonstrated in human as well as in animal studies, it has only been shown convincingly with sub-

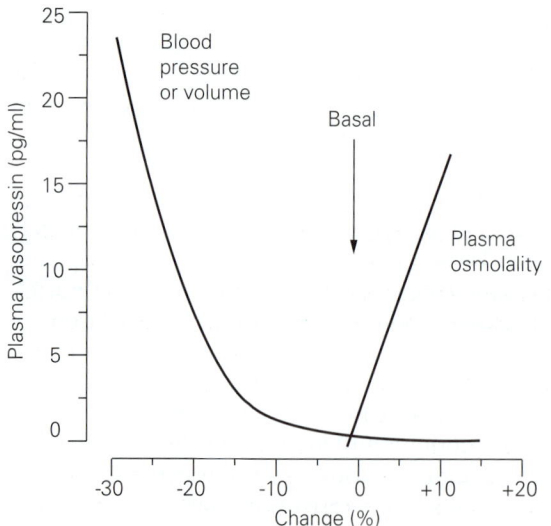

Figure 7.2 Comparative sensitivity of AVP secretion in response to increases in plasma osmolality versus decreases in blood volume or blood pressure in human subjects. The arrow indicates the low plasma AVP concentrations found at basal plasma osmolality. (Modified, with permission, from Robertson, 1995.)

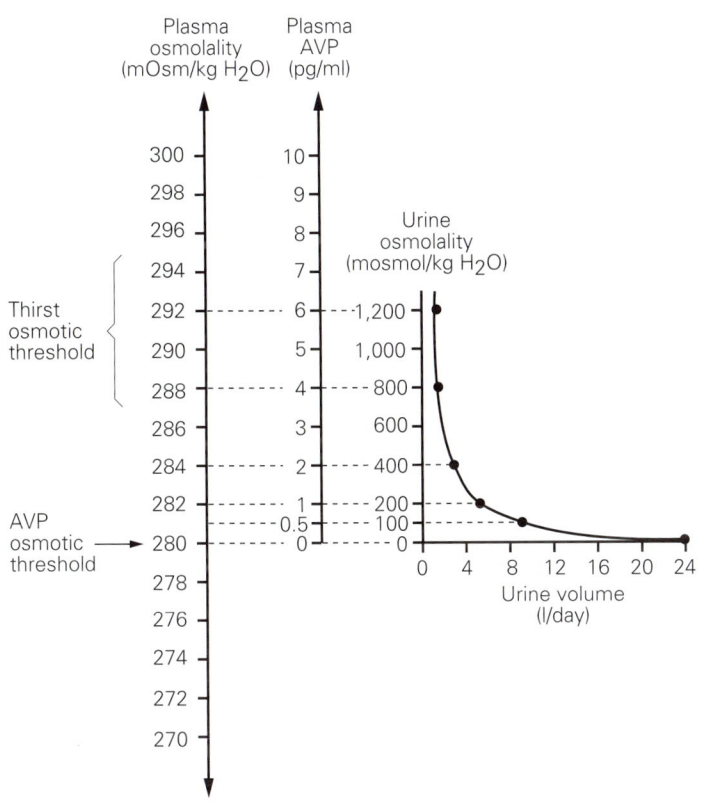

Figure 7.3 Schematic representation of normal physiological relationships among plasma osmolality, plasma AVP concentrations, urine osmolality and urine volume in humans. Note particularly the inverse nature of the relation between urine osmolality and urine volume, resulting in disproportionate effects of small changes in plasma AVP concentrations on urine volume at lower AVP levels. (Modified with permission from Robinson, A.G. (1985) Disorders of antidiuretic hormone secretion. *Clin. Endocrinol. Metab.*, **14**, 55–88.)

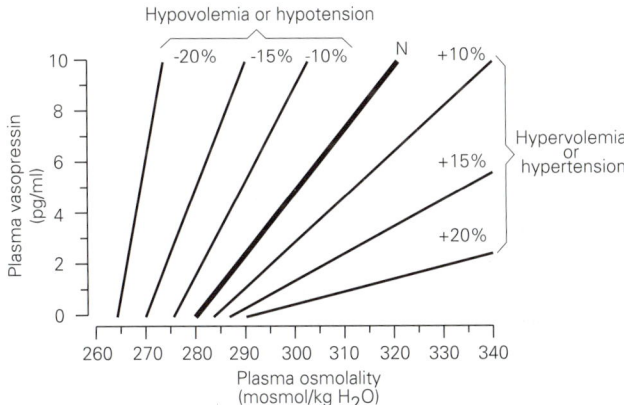

Figure 7.4 Relation between plasma AVP concentrations and plasma osmolality under conditions of varying blood volume and pressure. The line labeled 'N' depicts the linear regression line associating these variables in euvolemic normotensive adult subjects. The lines to the left depict the changes in this regression line with progressive decreases in blood volume and/or pressure and the lines to the right depict the opposite changes with progressive increases in blood volume and/or pressure (in each case the numbers at the ends of the lines indicate the relative percentage changes in blood volume and/or blood pressure associated with each regression line). (Modified, with permission, from Robertson, 1995).

stantial degrees of hypovolemia, and the magnitude of this effect during mild degrees of volume depletion remains conjectural. Consequently, it is reasonable to conclude that the major effect of moderate degrees of hypovolemia on both AVP secretion and thirst is to modulate the gain of the osmoregulatory responses, with direct effects on thirst and AVP secretion occurring only during more severe degrees of hypovolemia (e.g. ≥10% reductions in blood volume).

Other stimuli

Several other non-osmotic stimuli to AVP secretion have been described in man. Most prominent among these is nausea. The sensation of nausea, with or without vomiting, is by far the most potent stimulus to AVP secretion known in man. Although a 20% increase in osmolality will typically elevate plasma AVP levels to the range of 5–20% pg/ml, and a 20% decrease in blood pressure raise them to 10–100 pg/ml, nausea has been described to cause increases in AVP in excess of 200–400 pg/ml. The reason for this profound stimulation is not known (although it has been speculated that the AVP response assists evacuation of stomach contents via contraction of gastric smooth muscle, AVP is not necessary for vomiting to occur), but it is probably responsible for the intense vasoconstriction which produces the pallor often associated with this state. Hypoglycemia also stimulates AVP release in man, but to relatively low levels which are not consistent among individuals. As will be discussed in the chapter on clinical disorders, a variety of drugs also stimulate AVP secretion, including nicotine. However, despite the importance of these stimuli during pathological conditions, none of them is a significant determinant of physiological regulation of AVP secretion in man.

Integration of thirst and AVP secretion

A synthesis of what is presently known about the regulation of thirst and AVP secretion in humans leads to a relatively simple but elegant system to maintain water balance. Under normal physiological conditions, the sensitivity of the osmoregulatory system for AVP secretion accounts for maintenance of plasma osmolality within narrow limits by adjusting renal water excretion to small changes in osmolality. Stimulated thirst does not represent a major regulatory mechanism under these conditions, and unregulated fluid ingestion supplies adequate water in excess of true 'need', which is then excreted in relation to osmoregulated pituitary AVP secretion. However, when unregulated water intake cannot adequately supply body needs in the presence of plasma AVP levels sufficient to produce maximal antidiuresis, then plasma osmolality rises to levels that stimulate thirst and produce water intake proportional to the elevation of osmolality above this threshold. In such a system, thirst essentially represents a backup mechanism called into play when pituitary and renal mechanisms prove insufficient to maintain plasma osmolality within a few percentage points of basal levels. This arrangement has the advantage of freeing humans from frequent episodes of thirst that would require a diversion of activities toward behavior oriented to seeking water when water deficiency is sufficiently mild to be compensated for by renal water conservation, but would stimulate water ingestion once water deficiency reaches potentially harmful levels. Stimulation of AVP secretion at plasma osmolalities below the threshold for subjective thirst acts to maintain an excess of body water sufficient to eliminate the need to drink whenever slight elevations in plasma osmolality occur.

This system of differential effective thresholds for thirst and AVP secretion therefore nicely complements many studies which have demonstrated excess unregulated, or 'need-free', drinking in both humans and animals.

Despite the intrinsic appeal of this theory and a substantial body of data in support of it, a recent study has found that when human subjects are allowed to differentiate between basal degrees of thirst rather than assuming that thirst is absent under conditions of *ad libitum* fluid intake, then the thresholds for thirst and AVP secretion are quite similar. This raises an important question concerning neural regulation of water ingestion, namely, whether central pathways that stimulate fluid intake are activated in response to small changes in osmolality even before the subjective sensation of thirst occurs. Arguing against this interpretation is the observation that basal plasma osmolality in man and animals is maintained at levels associated with easily measurable plasma AVP concentrations and moderately concentrated urine, indicating that the threshold for AVP secretion must be below the threshold for stimulation of thirst. Although increases in basal plasma osmolality of only 1–4% are necessary for stimulation of thirst, the threshold for AVP secretion must lie below basal plasma osmolality because basal urine osmolalities in man and animals under conditions of *ad libitum* fluid intake are typically concentrated above isotonicity rather than maximally dilute. Consequently, although the magnitude of the difference in effective osmotic set points for thirst and AVP secretion remains debatable and is clearly subject to substantial individual variability, the bulk of experimental results to date support the concept of a higher effective osmotic threshold for thirst than for AVP secretion in man.

Therefore, in summary, during normal day-to-day conditions body water homeostasis appears to be maintained primarily by *ad libitum*, or unregulated, fluid intake in association with AVP-regulated changes in urine flow, most of which occur before the threshold is reached for osmotically stimulated, or regulated, thirst. But when these mechanisms become inadequate to maintain body fluid homeostasis, then thirst-induced regulated fluid intake becomes the predominant defense mechanism for the prevention of dehydration.

Further reading

Baylis, P.H. and Thompson, C.J. (1988) Osmoregulation of vasopressin secretion and thirst in health and disease. *Clin. Endocrinol.*, **29**, 549–76.

Booth, D.B. and Ramsay, D.J. (1991) *Thirst – Physiological and Psychological Aspects*. Springer-Verlag, Berlin.

Fanestil, D.D. and Moore, F.D. (1994) Compartmentalization of body water, in *Cinical Disorders of Fluid and Electrolyte Metabolism* (ed. R.G. Narins), McGraw-Hill, New York, pp. 3–20.

Fitzsimons, J.T. (1979) *The Physiology of Thirst and Sodium Appetite*. Cambridge University Press, Cambridge.

Ramsay, D.J. (1985) Osmoreceptors subserving vasopressin secretion and drinking – an overview, in *Vasopressin* (ed. R.W. Schrier), Raven Press, New York, pp. 291–8.

Robertson, G.L. (1995) Posterior pituitary, in *Endocrinology and Metabolism* (eds P. Felig, J.D. Baxter and L.A. Frohman), McGraw-Hill, New York, pp. 385–432.

Robinson, A.G. (1985) Disorders of antidiuretic hormone secretion. *Clin. Endocrinol. Metab.*, **14**, 55–88.

Verbalis, J.G. (1990) Clinical aspects of body fluid homeostasis in humans, in *Handbook of Behavioral Neurobiology* (ed. E.M. Stricker), Plenum Press, New York, pp. 421–62.

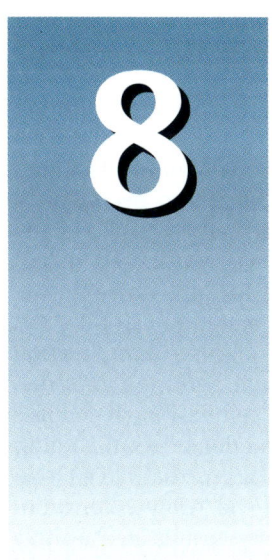

8

Body sodium and extracellular fluid volume

Joseph G. Verbalis

Introduction

As discussed in Chapter 7, most biological membranes are freely permeable to water, so water will distribute along osmotic gradients between intracellular (ICF) and extracellular (ECF) fluid until the osmotic pressure is equivalent between these two compartments. Their relative volumes will therefore be a function of the number of free solute particles on either side of cell membranes. In mammals, the activity of ATP-dependent membrane Na^+-K^+ pumps maintains K^+ primarily within cells and Na^+ primarily outside cells. As a result of this active partitioning of Na^+ and K^+ across cell membranes, the volume of the ICF is largely a function of the amount of body K^+ along with other intracellular inorganic (Mg^{2+}, Ca^{2+}, PO_4^{2-}, SO_4^{2-}, HCO_3^-) and organic solutes. Correspondingly, the volume of the ECF is predominantly determined by the amount of body Na^+ along with its attendant anions (Cl^- and HCO_3^-), since non-Na^+ cell membrane-impermeable cations comprise only a small proportion (<5%) of all ECF solutes.

ECF and plasma volume

As summarized in Chapter 7, approximately 35–45% of total body water (TBW) resides in the ECF. The exact proportion is uncertain because different markers used to estimate the volume of this compartment yield varying results. The lower percentages were found in studies using disaccharide markers such as inulin and mannitol, but these compounds are larger and less able to penetrate into some of the extracellular spaces of denser connective tissues such as bone. Somewhat higher values are obtained using chloride and sodium volumes of distribution, though some intracellular entry of these ions occurs. Nonetheless, from the arguments presented above it follows that the ratio of ECF volume to ICF volume should be roughly equal to the ratio of exchangeable Na^+:K^+, which in adults has been found to be 41%:59%. The amount of intravascular ECF, or plasma volume, can be quantified more accurately using ^{125}I-labeled albumin or ^{51}Cr-tagged red blood cells, and averages 7–8% of TBW in adults; thus, approximately one-fifth of the ECF resides intravascularly.

The distribution of fluid between intravascular and interstitial compartments is determined by a balance between hydrostatic pressure and colloid osmotic (oncotic) pressure. The high hydrostatic pressure of intravascular fluid is maintained as a result of cardiac pumping and arteriolar vasoconstriction in order to circulate oxygen and other blood-borne nutrients throughout the body. If no additional forces were present, the resulting transcapillary hydrostatic pressure gradient would force water out of capillaries until intravascular and interstitial pressures were equal. This does not occur because of the opposing osmotic pressure contributed by plasma proteins that are primarily confined within the vascular space, since the permeability of capillary membranes to large proteins is low. Although these proteins contribute little to overall plasma osmolality (generally <1–2%), they exert a pressure differential of approxi-

Nephrology, Edited by Rex L. Jamison and Robert Wilkinson.
Published in 1997 by Chapman & Hall, London. ISBN 0 412 60930 4

mately 15–20 mmHg higher in the intravascular than in the interstitial fluid, which is called the colloid osmotic, or oncotic, pressure. Figure 8.1 summarizes the Starling forces governing transcapillary fluid transfer. At the arteriolar end of the capillary the difference between the intravascular hydrostatic pressure (P_c) and the interstitial hydrostatic pressure (P_i) exceeds the opposite difference between the intravascular oncotic pressure (π_c) and the interstitial oncotic pressure (π_i); the resultant pressure gradient drives capillary fluid into the interstitial space. As fluid leaves the capillary, P_c decreases due to fluid loss and π_c increases due to hemoconcentration. Consequently, at more distal capillary sites closer to the venous circulation the net oncotic pressure exceeds the net hydrostatic forces, thereby pulling interstitial fluid back into the intravascular space. Thus, at any given site of the capillary the net fluid flow (J_v) can be described by the following equation (where K_f = the ultrafiltration coefficient of the capillary, $\Delta P = P_c - P_i$, and $\Delta\pi = \pi_c - \pi_i$):

$$J_v = K_f\left(\Delta P - \Delta\pi\right)$$

This mechanism promotes efficient fluid transfer between the two compartments while preserving intravascular volume and pressure. However, as a backup any excess fluid not reabsorbed back into the intravascular space is returned later via the lymphatic system. The consequences of a low plasma protein concentration in certain disease states (e.g. nephrotic syndrome, liver dysfunction) are readily apparent from the increased interstitial fluid

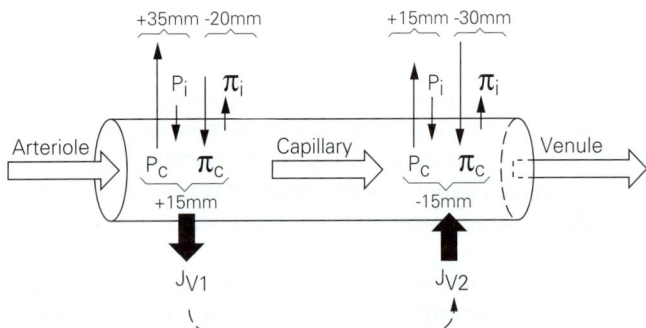

Figure 8.1 Starling forces governing transcapillary fluid transfer. At the arteriolar end of the capillary the difference between intravascular hydrostatic pressure (P_c) and the interstitial hydrostatic pressure (P_i) exceeds the opposite difference between the intravascular oncotic pressure (π_c) and the interstitial oncotic pressure (π_i); the resultant pressure gradient drives capillary fluid into the interstitial space (solid arrow, J_{v1}). As fluid leaves the capillary, P_c decreases due to fluid loss and π_c increases due to hemoconcentration. Consequently, at more distal capillary sites closer to the venous circulation the net oncotic pressure exceeds the net hydrostatic forces, thereby pulling interstitial fluid back into the intravascular space (solid arrow, J_{v2}). The numerical values indicate the approximate net pressure differences between the intravascular and interstitial spaces in mmHg.

volume (edema) and relative hypotension often found in such patients.

In view of the importance of maintaining ECF and plasma volume at optimal levels, it is also necessary to understand how ECF volume is actually sensed. For the most part this is accomplished via specialized neural stretch receptors located in the cardiac atria (low-pressure baroreceptors), and in the aortic arch and carotid sinus (high-pressure baroreceptors). In addition, experimental data have demonstrated that renal perfusion pressure, brain sodium receptors, and even compositional changes in the interstitial fluid can all modulate renal sodium excretion in response to manipulations that alter blood volume. Attempting to decipher the relative contributions of these various ECF volume sensing mechanisms during different physiological and pathophysiological conditions has been difficult, with seemingly conflicting reports. This undoubtedly reflects the fact that multiple systems are responsible for monitoring this important parameter; such redundancy of control mechanisms is commonplace in the nervous system, and ensures that vital functions are preserved even after malfunction of some of the regulatory components. Regardless of which mechanisms actually monitor ECF volume, it is clear that it is not the absolute volume that is recognized, but rather the volume relative to the potential capacity of the intravascular system, which is often called the effective ECF volume. Recent studies have suggested that arterial blood flow is the major determinant of effective ECF volume in many pathological conditions, and this will be discussed further in Chapter 24. Although this remains a controversial concept which has defied quantitative characterization, there is little doubt about the importance of effective ECF volume for volume homeostasis. Examples of marked alterations of renal function despite the absence of any changes in absolute ECF volume are numerous (e.g. cold-induced diuresis as a result of peripheral vasoconstriction thereby reducing the capacitance of the vascular system; orthostatic antidiuresis and antinatriuresis as a result of lower extremity pooling of blood; the diuresis and natriuresis accompanying water immersion as a result of increased negative intrathoracic pressure causing atrial distension, etc.).

Sodium metabolism

Maintenance of sodium homeostasis requires a simple balance between intake and excretion of Na$^+$. As in the case of water metabolism, it is possible to define regulated and unregulated components of both Na$^+$ intake and Na$^+$ excretion. Unlike water intake, however, there is little evidence in humans to support a significant role for regulated Na$^+$ intake, with the possible exception of some pathological conditions. Consequently, there is an even greater dependence on mechanisms for regulated renal excretion of sodium than is the case for excretion of water. Whether for this reason or not, the mechanisms for renal excretion of sodium are more numerous and substantially more complex than the relatively simple, albeit quite efficient, system for AVP-regualted excretion of water.

Salt appetite

The only solute for which any specific appetite has been clearly demonstrated in humans is sodium (as with animals, this is generally expressed as an appetite for the chloride salt of sodium, so it is usually called NaCl, or salt, appetite). Because of the importance of Na^+ for ensuring maintenance of the ECF volume, which in turn directly supports blood volume and pressure, its uniqueness insofar as meriting a specific mechanism for regulated intake seems appropriate. However, despite abundant evidence in many different species demonstrating a salt appetite that is proportionately related to Na^+ losses, there is only one pathological condition in which a specific stimulated sodium appetite has been unequivocally observed in humans, namely Addison's disease caused by adrenal insufficiency. Since the initial discovery of this disorder, salt craving has remained one of the well-known manifestations of Addison's disease. A robust salt appetite also occurs prominently in adrenalectomized animals, and appears to be related in part to the high plasma levels of adrenocorticotropin (ACTH) produced as a result of the loss of cortisol feedback on the pituitary. However, despite the presence of Na^+ deficiency in most patients with untreated Addison's disease, only 15–20% of such patients manifest salt-seeking behavior. Even more striking is the apparent absence of salt appetite during a variety of other disorders causing severe Na^+ and ECF volume depletion in humans (patients with hemorrhagic blood loss, diuretic-induced hypovolemia, or hypotension of any etiology become thirsty when intravascular deficits are marked, but almost never express a pronounced desire for salty foods or fluids). Yet, as with thirst, the possibility of subclinical activation of neural mechanisms stimulating salt intake without a conscious subjective sensation of salt 'hunger' must-be entertained. However, this possibility cannot be supported either, because many such patients actually become hyponatremic as a result of continued ingestion of only water or osmotically dilute fluids in response to their volume depletion. It is also noteworthy that athletes must be instructed to ingest sodium as NaCl tablets or electrolyte solutions during periods of sodium losses from profuse sweating since they fail to develop a salt appetite, which would be protective under these circumstances. As a corollary to the infrequency of stimulated salt appetite in humans, there is also no evidence to support inhibition of sodium intake under conditions of Na^+ and ECF excess, as demonstrated by the difficulty in maintaining even moderate degrees of sodium restriction in patients with edema-forming diseases such as congestive heart failure.

The absence of a prominent sodium appetite in man is not unique, however, and appears to be characteristic of carnivores in general. This has been hypothesized to reflect an evolutionary adaptation in response to the naturally occurring high sodium intake of flesh-eating animals, as opposed to the low salt intake of herbivores, possibly accounting for the preservation of specific mechanisms to seek sodium in the latter group. Nonetheless, the fact that pathological conditions such as adrenal insufficiency are associated with sodium appetite even in carnivores indicates basic regulatory mechanisms for body fluid homeostasis are common to all mammalian species, but their relative importance and utilization can vary markedly as a result of prior evolutionary pressures.

Renal sodium excretion

Although specific mechanisms exist for regulated renal excretion of all major electrolytes, none is as numerous or as complex as those controlling Na^+ excretion, which is not surprising in view of the fact that maintenance of ECF volume is crucial to normal health and function. The most important of these mechanisms are discussed below.

Glomerular filtration rate

Glomerular filtration rate (GFR) is one of two classical mechanisms known to regulate renal Na^+ excretion. Multiple factors influence GFR, including the glomerular plasma flow, the glomerular capillary surface area, the hydrostatic pressure gradient between the glomerular capillaries and Bowman's capsule, and the oncotic pressure produced by the proteins in glomerular capillaries. The same formula described earlier for calculating fluid transfer across capillary walls also applies to glomerular filtration; however, in the glomerular capillaries K_f, the ultrafiltration coefficient, is markedly larger (by 1–2 orders of magnitude) than in systemic capillaries, thereby enabling much greater rates of fluid transfer (J_v) into the nephron as glomerular filtrate.

Because the amount of Na^+ filtered through the kidney is huge (approximately 25 000 mmol/day in healthy adults), relatively small changes in GFR can potentially have large effects on filtered Na^+. However, changes in filtered load of Na^+ are compensated for by concomitant changes in proximal tubular sodium reabsorption via a process known as glomerular-tubular balance. As the filtered Na^+ load increases, Na^+ absorption in the proximal tubule also increases, largely compensating for the increased filtered load. Although the mechanism(s) responsible for glomerular-tubular balance are not completely understood, one important factor appears to be changes in peritubular capillary forces, analogous to the Starling forces in the systemic capillaries. An increase in filtered fluid at the glomerulus decreases the hydrostatic pressure and increases the oncotic pressure of the non-filtered fluid delivered to the peritubular capillaries, thereby increasing the pressure gradient for reabsorbing the Na⁺ which is actively transported from the proximal tubular epithelial cells into the extracellular fluid surrounding the proximal tubule (Figure 8.2). Although this mechanism dampens the effects of alterations in GFR on renal Na⁺ excretion and prevents large changes in urine Na⁺ excretion in response to minor changes in GFR, nonetheless many experimental results indicate that sustained alterations of GFR can significantly modulate renal Na⁺ excretion.

Aldosterone

The second major factor long known to influence renal Na⁺ excretion is adrenal aldosterone secretion, which increases Na⁺ resorption in the distal nephron by inducing synthesis of a protein that affects sodium–potassium exchange in tubular epithelial cells. The importance of this hormone for Na⁺ homeostasis is best illustrated by the well-known renal Na⁺ wasting of patients with primary adrenal insufficiency. Multiple factors stimulate adrenal mineralocorticoid secretion. Most prominent of these is angiotensin II, which is formed as the end result of renin secretion from the juxtaglomerular apparatus in response to renal hypoperfusion. High plasma K⁺ concentrations also stimulate aldosterone secretion, thereby

increasing urinary K⁺ excretion at the expense of Na⁺ retention. More recently two inhibitors of aldosterone secretion have been described: atrial natriuretic peptide (ANP) and hyperosomolality; both of these stimuli appear to be sufficiently potent to completely block stimulated aldosterone secretion. Although aldosterone clearly plays an important role in sodium homeostasis, its effects to stimulate Na⁺ resorption in the distal tubule can be overridden by other natriuretic factors. This is evident in the phenomenon of renal 'escape' from mineralocorticoids, in which experimental animals and man re-establish sodium balance after an initial period of Na⁺ retention and ECF volume expansion. Potential mechanisms responsible for this phenomenon are discussed below.

Intrarenal hemodynamic and peritubular factors

Although GFR and aldosterone effects can account for much of the observed variation in renal Na⁺ excretion, it has long been known that they cannot completely explain the natriuresis that occurs in the absence of measurable changes in GFR or aldosterone secretion during isotonic saline volume expansion. This led to the postulation of the existence of a 'third factor', or factors, regu-

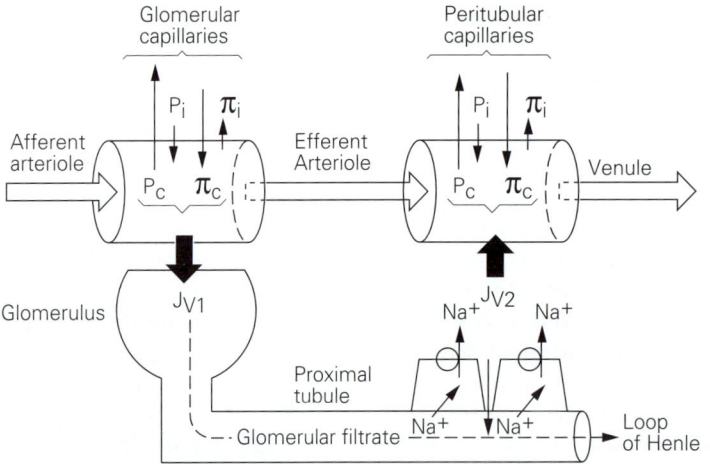

Figure 8.2 Peritubular mechanisms responsible for glomerulotubular balance. A proximal nephron segment has been superimposed on the capillary shown in Figure 8.1; the arteriolar side of the capillary now represents the glomerular capillary and the venous side the peritubular capillary. As the glomerular filtrate moves through the proximal tubule, Na⁺ is passively reabsorbed from the lumen due to the large concentration gradient between the lumen and the intracellular fluid, and then actively secreted into the peritubular interstitial space. The extent to which this Na⁺ is then reabsorbed into the peritubular capillary, or leaks back into the tubule, will depend on the net Starling forces between the intravascular and interstitial fluid, just as for capillary tissue exchange. When the filtration fraction and GFR are increased, peritubular P_c will be lower and π_c will be higher, thus increasing tubular Na⁺ reabsorption and preventing large increases in excreted sodium.

lating Na$^+$ excretion. Intrarenal hemodynamic factors are now known to be important in this regard, particularly changes in renal perfusion pressure. This is illustrated by aldosterone escape described above, which appears to be mediated primarily by increased renal perfusion pressure with subsequent increased fractional sodium excretion. In effect this represents a 'safety-valve' mechanism; when renal artery pressure rises as a result of volume expansion, the increase in filtered load of Na$^+$ is sufficient to overwhelm the aldosterone-mediated distal sodium resorption. Note that the term 'escape' is somewhat of a misnomer, since aldosterone effects are still present but a new steady-state of volume expansion has been reached in which no additional sodium retention occurs due to activation of compensatory mechanisms for sodium excretion. Although sodium balance is re-established, nonetheless a substantial degree of volume expansion persists confirming the presence of continued systemic mineralocorticoid effects (Figure 8.3).

Humoral factors

Several humoral factors in addition to aldosterone have also been found to influence renal sodium excretion. It is now apparent that angiotensin II itself, independently of its effects on aldosterone secretion, can exert potent anti-natriuretic effects at physiological plasma concentrations by its actions to stimulate proximal tubular NaHCO$_3$

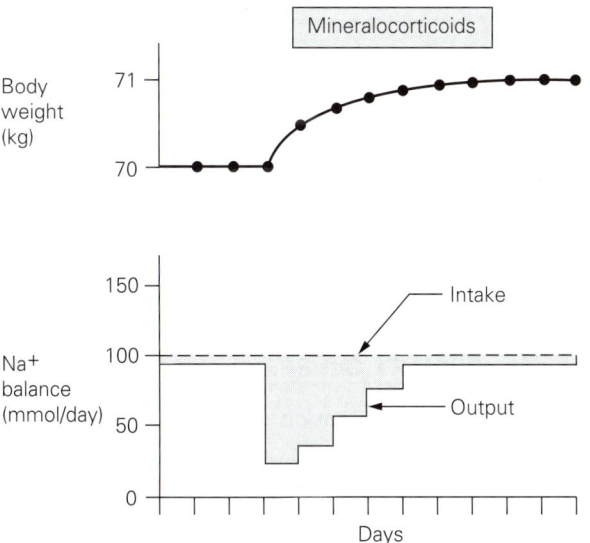

Figure 8.3 Schematic summary of aldosterone escape. Sodium is retained in response to elevated mineralocorticoid levels, resulting in a positive sodium balance and progressive weight gain. However, after several days urine Na$^+$ excretion increases sufficiently to balance Na$^+$ intake, thereby preventing continued fluid retention and weight gain. Consequently, a new steady state is reached in which continued aldosterone-mediated effects to conserve Na$^+$ are offset by natriuretic effects produced by the Na$^+$-induced volume expansion.

resorption, and to constrict efferent arterioles, which sustains GFR despite decreases in glomerular plasma flow. Arginine vasopressin (AVP) weakly stimulates natriuresis, presumably via receptor-mediated mechanisms similar to those by which both AVP and oxytocin stimulate Na$^+$ excretion in animals. However, the physiological conditions in which AVP-induced natriuresis might be expected to play a significant role are quite limited, since plasma AVP levels are elevated during states of volume deficiency when Na$^+$ retention is the appropriate response. More suitable candidates for volume-induced natriuresis are peptides of the atrial natriuretic family (ANP), which are secreted from the atria of the heart in direct proportion to increases in atrial stretch, whether in response to true volume expansion or to stimuli causing increased atrial pressure. ANP stimulates natriuresis by its actions to increase glomerular filtration rate, block Na$^+$ reabsorption in the collecting tubules, and inhibit adrenal aldosterone secretion. Early studies of ANP-induced natriuresis in animals and man utilized supraphysiological doses of this peptide, but more recent studies using much lower infusion rates that reproduce plasma ANP concentrations within physiological ranges have also succeeded in demonstrating increases in renal Na$^+$ and water excretion. Unfortunately, the magnitude of stimulated natriuresis at more physiological levels appears to be insufficient to account for the Na$^+$ excretion observed in response to stimuli such as isotonic volume expansion. Nonetheless, ANP remains attractive as a humoral regulator of Na$^+$ excretion in view of its spectrum of potential activities in conjunction with its pattern of release in response to appropriate stimuli such as volume expansion. Future studies with an effective specific antagonist of ANP receptors, when this becomes available, will finally define the true role of ANP both in physiological and pathophysiological situations.

Renal nerve activity, dopamine

Many studies have implicated neural input to the kidney in the regulation of sodium excretion: increased sympathetic activity is generally associated with a reduction in urine Na$^+$ excretion and renal denervation tends to increase urine Na$^+$ excretion. However, many of these effects have proven to be somewhat inconsistent, particularly the denervation studies, and may be due to indirect effects on renal hemodynamic factors. Both β-adrenergic and α-adrenergic mechanisms play a role in sympathetic effects on Na$^+$ excretion, and more recent studies have suggested that dopamine antagonists blunt the natriuresis stimulated by volume loading in both animals and man. It therefore seems clear that both renal sympathetic nerve activity and intrarenal dopamine modulate urinary Na$^+$ excretion primarily by attenuating or enhancing the natriuresis stimulated by other factors, although neither appears to be essential for maintaining normal sodium balance.

Prostaglandins

Several studies have demonstrated natriuretic effects of several prostaglandins, primarily PGE_2, PGI_2 and $PGF_{2\alpha}$, infused into the renal arteries. Whether this is a direct effect of prostaglandins on Na^+ transport mechanisms or is secondary to prostaglandin-mediated vasodilatory effects remains uncertain. Similarly, prostaglandin synthase inhibitors have been shown to blunt natriuresis in response to volume expansion but do not appear to affect basal Na^+ excretion. Consequently, an unequivocal physiological role for renal prostaglandins to modulate sodium excretion has yet to be demonstrated.

Integration

A consideration of what is presently known about the regulation of sodium appetite and renal sodium excretion leads to the conclusion that sodium homeostasis in humans is achieved almost exclusively by regulation of sodium excretion. A normal dietary intake ensures ingestion of excess amounts of Na^+, and the multiple regulatory mechanisms of Na^+ excretion acting at different sites in the nephron adjust the appropriate amount to be retained depending on physiological conditions. Virtu-

ally all the regulators of sodium excretion in man are responsive to changes in effective ECF volume and blood pressure and are relatively insensitive to changes in ECF osmolality, except for aldosterone secretion and AVP release under some conditions. The ability of the kidney to reduce Na^+ excretion virtually to zero allows preservation of sodium homeostasis even during periods of prolonged sodium deprivation. The relative absence of a specific sodium appetite, however, leaves humans vulnerable to severe degrees of volume depletion in pathological states of ECF Na^+ and fluid losses. Although to some extent this is compensated for by thirst-induced water consumption, water is a relatively ineffective mechanism to expand plasma and ECF volume because of its distribution throughout all body fluid compartments.

Synthesis of osmotic and volume homeostasis

This chapter and Chapter 7 have summarized the various mechanisms by which water and Na^+ balances are maintained in humans. Understanding the physiology of body fluids also requires knowledge of how these two regula-

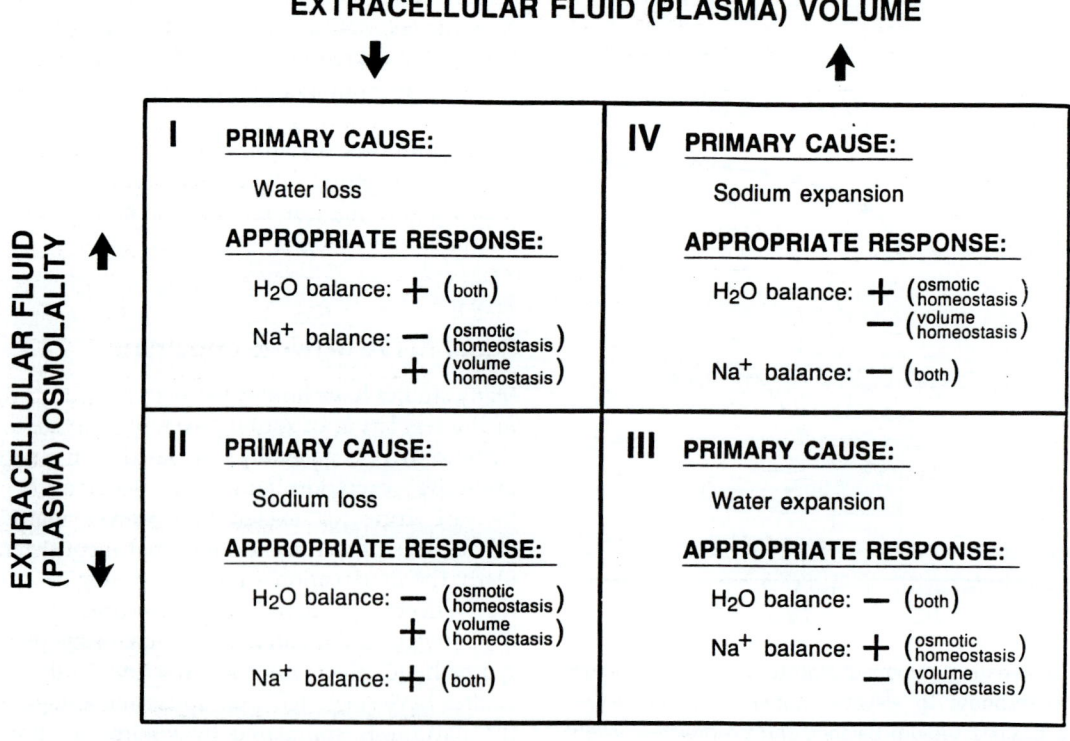

Figure 8.4 Summary of the potential combinations of derangements in both ECF (or plasma) osmolality and volume. For each category is shown the predominant clinical disorder responsible for that pattern of altered ECF osmolality and volume, and the effects on water and sodium balance predicted in response to the derangement under normal physiological conditions. Note that within each category some opposite responses for water or sodium balance are predicted depending on whether regulatory mechanisms for maintenance of osmotic homeostasis or volume homeostasis prevail. (Reproduced, with permission, from Verbalis (1990).)

tory processes interact to achieve homeostasis of all body fluids. Body fluid homeostasis is directed at achieving stability of the two major functions of body fluids: (1) maintenance of body osmolality within narrow limits, or osmotic homeostasis, and (2) maintenance of ECF and plasma volume at adequate levels, or volume homeostasis. Osmotic homeostasis is important to prevent large osmotic shifts of water into and out of cells, which would interfere with normal cell function, whereas volume homeostasis is important to allow normal cardiovascular and circulatory function. The previous analyses have suggested that in man water balance is more finely regulated by changes in osmolality whereas sodium balance is regulated to a greater degree by changes in effective ECF volume. Although this is an oversimplification of complex regulatory processes, nonetheless under most conditions it represents an accurate summary of normal homeostatic mechanisms and provides a useful framework for understanding body fluid homeostasis during normal physiological conditions and in pathological disorders.

Specific pathological disorders of body fluid homeostasis will be discussed in Chapters 23 and 24. In general, these can be divided into disorders of osmotic homeo-

stasis, which for the most part are caused by abnormalities of water balance, and disorders of volume homeostasis, which largely result from abnormalities of sodium balance. It is apparent, however, that multiple interactions between osmotic and volume homeostasis must be considered for each individual disorder. When requirements for water and sodium intake and excretion are complementary, both homeostatic systems act in concert to regulate body fluids. Other occasions arise clinically in which requirements for osmotic and volume homeostasis conflict, and these cases are particularly useful for understanding the overall integration of the many different controls of body fluid homeostasis. Figure 8.4 illustrates the four possible pathological states arising from derangements of ECF osmolality and/or ECF volume. For each category, the theoretical effects on water and Na^+ balances that would be predicted to occur for maintenance of osmotic and volume homeostasis are shown. As various disorders of fluid and electrolyte balance are considered it will be useful to refer to this diagrammatic summary to consider what is known about how such regulatory conflicts are resolved in humans and the implications that this entails for overall body fluid homeostasis in each situation.

Further reading

Burg, M.B. (1986) Renal handling of sodium, chloride, water, amino acids, and glucose, in *The Kidney* (eds B.M. Brenner and F.C. Rector Jr), W.B. Saunders, Philadelphia, pp. 145–75.

Edelman, I.S. and Leibman, J. (1959) Anatomy of body water and electrolytes. *Am. J. Med.*, **27**, 256.

Fanestil, D.D. and Moore, F.D. (1994) Compartmentalization of body water, in *Clinical Disorders of Fluid and Electrolyte Metabolism* (ed. R.G. Narins), McGraw-Hill, New York, pp. 3–20.

Fitzsimons, J.T. (1992) Physiology and pathophysiology of thirst and sodium appetite, in *The Kidney, Physiology and Pathophysiology* (eds D.W. Seldin and G. Giebisch), Raven Press, New York, pp. 1615–48.

Gunning, M.E. and Brenner, B.M. (1992) Natriuretic peptides and the kidney: current concepts. *Kidney Int.*, **42**, S-127–33.

Hall, J.E., Granger, J.P., Smith, M.J. Jr and Premen, A.J. (1984) Role of renal hemodynamics and arterial pressure in aldosterone 'escape'. *Hypertension*, **6**, 183–92.

Kirchner, K.A. and Stein, J.H. (1994) Sodium metabolism, in *Cinical Disorders of Fluid and Electrolyte Metabolism* (ed. R.G. Narins), McGraw-Hill, New York, pp. 45–80.

Schneider, E.G., Radke, K.J., Ulderich, D. and Taylor, R. Jr (1985) Effect of osmolality on aldosterone secretion. *Endocrinology*, **116**, 1621–6.

Seldin, D.W. (1975) Sodium and water balance, in *The Sea Within Us* (ed. N.S. Bricker), Science and Medicine, New York, pp. 5–14.

Verbalis, J.G. (1990) Clinical aspects of body fluid homeostasis in humans, in *Handbook of Behavioral Neurobiology* (ed. E.M. Stricker), Plenum Press, New York, pp. 421–62.

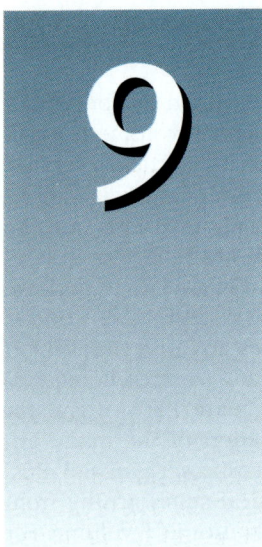

9

Potassium

Rex L. Jamison

Introduction

It can be said that potassium is the stuff of life itself. It is the most prevalent ion in animal cells and the most important in generating the resting potential difference across the plasma membrane of cardiac neuromuscular and polarized epithelial cells. Changes of a mere 1 or 2 mEq/l from the normal range of its serum concentration may go unnoticed – until suddenly and without warning, the situation becomes perilous. Studies by Wirz, Berliner, and Mudge and their colleagues in the 1940s and 1950s led to the proposal that K$^+$ undergoes simultaneous reabsorption and secretion by the renal tubule, the first time the theory of bidirectional transport of a solute by the renal tubule was proposed [1]. Within a few years, the theory was confirmed by Giebisch and Windhager and their coworkers, using the micropuncture technique [1, 2]. Different cells in the collecting duct were identified as either potassium secretory or reabsorptive. It was discovered that potassium, like urea, is recycled in the renal medulla [3].

This chapter considers the physiological role, distribution in the body and renal excretion of potassium and its regulation.

Physiological role of K$^+$

The cell concentration of K$^+$ is about 140 mEq/l, whereas the extracellular fluid K$^+$ concentration is 3.5–5.0 mEq/l – the mirror image of Na$^+$ distribution. The high cell con-

centration of K$^+$ is required for cell growth, enzyme activity, and regulation of cell volume and pH. The low extracellular fluid concentration of K$^+$ creates the high transmembrane K$^+$ concentration difference, a key determinant of the transmembrane electical potential necessary for the function of the excitable tissues, nerve and muscle. The enzyme Na$^+$,K$^+$-ATPase in cell membranes is responsible for the asymmetry of Na$^+$ and K$^+$. The K$^+$ asymmetry is the major determinant of the resting electrical potential difference, E_M, across cell membranes and conforms to the Goldman equation:

$$E_M = -61\log\frac{\left[K^+\right]_c + \alpha\left[Na^+\right]_c}{\left[K^+\right]_e + \alpha\left[Na^+\right]_e} \tag{9.1}$$

where $[K^+]_c$ and $[Na^+]_c$ are the cell concentrations and $[K^+]_e$ and $[Na^+]_e$ are the extracellular concentrations of K$^+$ and Na$^+$, respectively, and α is the relative permeability of the membrane, Na$^+$ to K$^+$. At the normal concentrations of Na$^+$ and K$^+$ in cells and extracellular fluid (in mEq/l), and the experimentally determined $\alpha = 0.01$,

$$E_M = -61\log\frac{\left[140\right]_c + 0.01\left[12\right]_c}{\left[4.0\right]_e + 0.01\left[140\right]_e} = -86\,\text{mV} \tag{9.2}$$

The resting membrane potential difference (E_M) is vital to the function of a wide variety of cells. In excitable tissue, the E_M is the precondition for membrane depolarization, i.e. the generation of the action potential. Changes in the transmembrane K$^+$ ratio alter the E_M and thereby alter the likelihood of an action potential (cell excitability). From

Nephrology, Edited by Rex L. Jamison and Robert Wilkinson.
Published in 1997 by Chapman & Hall, London. ISBN 0 412 60930 4

equation (9.2) it can be seen that a fall in extracellular K^+ (hypokalemia) increases E_M (cell interior more electronegative) and decreases excitability. A rise (hyperkalemia) has the reverse result. Hypokalemia impairs nerve and neuromuscular transmission, cardiac conduction and muscular (skeletal, smooth, cardiac) contraction. Muscular weakness, ileus of the intestine and U waves in the electrocardiogram are typical clinical manifestations. Hyperkalemia renders conducting tissue and muscle more unstable. The most important consequence of hyperkalemia is a cardiac arrhythmia that can be fatal. The E_M also influences transcellular ion movement in epithelial tissue, e.g. gastrointestinal and renal epithelia. Potassium homeostasis requires the maintenance of a high cell K^+ concentration and a low extracellular K^+ concentration simultaneously [3]. The high cell K^+ depends on cell membrane Na^+,K^+-ATPase. Physiological conditions which directly regulate the distribution of K^+ do so by influencing cell uptake of K^+. These are summarized in Table 9.1.

Table 9.1 Physiological conditions that regulate potassium distribution

Acute: physiological and pathological conditions that directly influence cell K^+ uptake

Increase cell uptake	Decrease cell uptake or enhanced cell loss
Insulin	Lack of insulin
β-catecholamines	β-Adrenergic receptor blockers
	α-Catecholamines
Alkalosis (primarily metabolic)	Acidosis (primarily respiratory)
High ECF K^+ concentration	Low ECF K^+ concentration
Increased ECF osmolality	Reduced ECF osmolality
	Cell injury

Chronic: physiological and pathological conditions that influence cell membrane density of Na^+,K^+-ATPase

Increase Na^+,K^+-ATPase density	Decrease Na^+,K^+-ATPase density
Increased thyroid hormone	Decreased thyroid hormone
Increased adrenal steroids	Decreased adrenal steroids
Exercise	Diabetes mellitus
Growth	K^+ deficiency
	Chronic renal insufficiency

ECF = extracellular fluid.
Adapted from Giebich and Wang [2].

Regulation of K^+ distribution

Approximately 98% of total body K^+ is within cells (Figure 9.1). Because of its tissue mass, skeletal muscle contains approximately two-thirds of total body K^+ (Figure 9.2). Total body K^+ is less in females, owing to a smaller fraction of body mass that is water, and steadily declines in adult men and women as a function of age.

In view of the small amount of K^+ in the extracellular fluid (ECF), ingestion of K^+ could cause a dangerous rise in serum K^+, were it not for mechanisms that influence K^+ distribution between ECF and intracellular fluid (ICF). These are summarized in Table 9.1 and considered further in Chapter 25. Some of the ingested K^+ temporarily enters the cells. Eventually, the excess K^+ is excreted – primarily (>90%) by the kidney. The remainder is excreted in the stool. Normally, no K^+ is lost by the sweat glands; in states of excessive perspiration, as much as 10 mEq of K^+ can be lost in a day. The ECF K^+ concentration and pH, insulin and epinephrine (via the β_2-adrenergic receptor) all influence K^+ distribution.

ECF K^+ concentration

A rise in ECF K^+ stimulates cell K^+ uptake via the activity of Na^+,K^+-ATPase.

Acid–base balance

When ECF pH falls, K^+ leaves cells in exchange for H^+. A greater change in ECF K^+ occurs during 'mineral' metabolic acidoses (hyperchloremic acidosis, as in uremia) than in 'organic' metabolic acidoses (ketosis, lactic acidosis) [4] because the organic anions, unlike the inorganic ions, accompany the entry of hydrogen ions rather than exchange with the exit of K^+. Respiratory acidosis has less of an effect on K^+ distribution than metabolic acidosis.

Insulin

Insulin increases cell uptake of K^+ by stimulating Na^+,K^+-ATPase in the cell membrane. De Fronzo et al. [5] and others have shown that the infusion of insulin decreases serum K^+. Patients with diabetes who lack insulin (insulin-dependent diabetes) have impaired regulation of cell K^+ uptake.

Catecholamines

K^+ uptake is enhanced by β_2-adrenergic agonists and diminished by β_2-adrenergic receptor blocking agents and α-adrenergic agonists [6]. The second messenger stimulates cell membrane Na^+,K^+-ATPase.

Extracellular fluid osmolality

When cells are exposed to a reduced ECF osmolality, water enters the cell causing cell swelling, causes Ca^+-

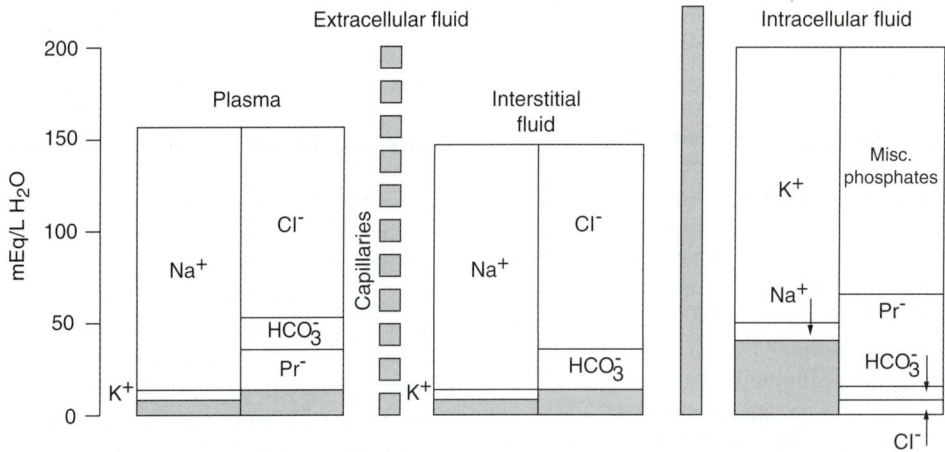

Figure 9.1 Principal constituents of the plasma, interstitial and intracellular fluid, expressed in units of concentration. Cross-hatched areas refer to minor constituents. Pr⁻, anionic proteins. (Reproduced, with permission, from Johnson, L.R. (1992) *Essential Medical Physiology*, Lippincott-Raven, Philadelphia, p. 5.)

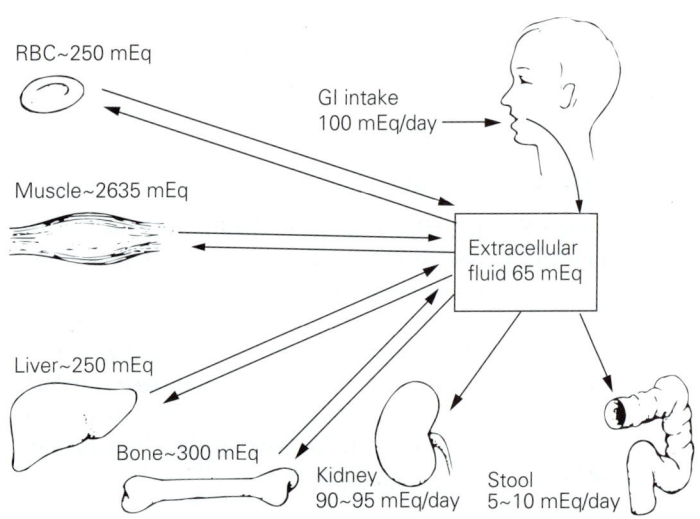

Figure 9.2 Potassium balance in humans. (Reproduced, with permission, from Smith, J.D., Bia, M. and DeFronzo, R.A. (1985) Clinical disorders of potassium metabolism, in *Fluid, Electrolyte and Acid–Base Disorders* (eds A. Arieff and R.A. DeFronzo), Churchill Livingsone, New York, pp. 413–509.)

mediated increase in K⁺ and Cl⁻ channels and loss of KCl. Conversely hyperosmolality results in cell shrinkage. The response of the cell to regain its volume is the uptake of Na⁺ and K⁺, accompanied by Cl⁻ [7].

The conditions that influence cell membrane density of Na⁺,K⁺-ATPase are considered in Chapter 25.

Renal excretion of K⁺

Overview

K⁺ is freely filtered in the glomerulus (Figure 9.3). At a normal GFR of 180 l/day and a serum K⁺ of 4.5 mEq/l, the daily filtered load of K⁺ in the adult human, 810 mEq,

exceeds the usual daily K⁺ intake of 100–150 mEq. The main source of K⁺ in the urine normally is not filtered K⁺ remaining unreabsorbed by the nephron, but K⁺ secreted in the distal nephron (mainly the collecting tubule) [1]. It is important to understand K⁺ transport along the entire nephron in order to comprehend how physiologic and pharmacological factors alter urinary K⁺ excretion. In the proximal convoluted tubule and loop of Henle of the superficial nephron, net reabsorption of K⁺ occurs, approximately proportional to and driven by Na⁺ reabsorption (Figure 9.3). In the pars recta, it is probable that some K⁺ secretion occurs, at least under certain circumstances, based on analogy to findings in the juxtamedullary nephron (see below). *In vitro* studies of the isolated perfused pars recta have shown K⁺ secretion in about half the segments perfused under normal condi-

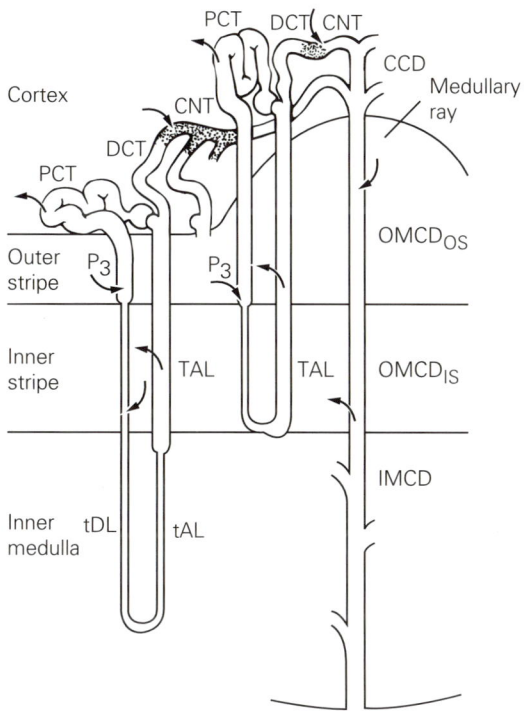

Figure 9.3 Transport of potassium in the renal tubule. The arrows indicate net transepithelial movement of potassium under normal conditions in which excess dietary potassium is excreted. Abbreviations: PCT, proximal convoluted tubule; P₃, third or straight segment of the proximal tubule (also called the pars recta); tDL, thin descending limb; tAL, thin ascending limb; TAL, thick ascending limb; DCT, distal convoluted tubule; CNT, connecting tubule (stippled regions); CCD, cortical collecting duct; OMCD$_{OS}$, outer medullary collecting duct, outer stripe; OMCD$_{IS}$, outer medullary collecting duct, inner stripe; and IMCD, inner medullary collecting duct. (Adapted from ref. 3.)

tions. About 60–70% of filtered K⁺ is reabsorbed by the proximal tubule; 20–30% by the loop of Henle. Transport of K⁺ in the juxtamedullary nephron (JM) probably resembles that in the superficial nephron, except in the long loop of Henle. As described below, there is substantial net entry (secretion) of K⁺ into the JM pars recta or thin descending limb. Transport of K⁺ in the connecting tubule and collecting duct, primarily the cortical collecting duct (CCD), determines the urinary excretion rate. Usually K⁺ is secreted in the CCD, increasing the K⁺ in the tubule fluid to an amount equivalent to 15–20% of the filtered load of K⁺. In circumstances of K⁺ deprivation, K⁺ secretion is inhibited and K⁺ reabsorption reduces urinary K⁺ excretion to less than 5% of the filtered load.

Transport of K⁺ by renal tubule segment

There is a basic pump–leak system common to the epithelial cells lining the renal tubule [8, 9]. Na⁺,K⁺-ATPase is

located on the lateral and blood-facing (basal) cell membrane only, i.e. not on the tubule lumen-facing (apical) membrane. The basolateral Na⁺,K⁺-ATPase drives 3 Na⁺ out and 2 K⁺ in, creating a cell interior low in Na⁺, high in K⁺ and electrically negative with respect to the tubule fluid on the apical side and to the ECF on the basolateral side. The basolateral membrane is permeable to K⁺ (i.e. 'leaks' K⁺) but not to Na⁺. Among the different tubule segments, while only a few changes are superimposed on the pump–leak system in the basolateral membrane, the permeability and transport characteristics of the apical membrane vary sharply from segment to segment [10].

Proximal convoluted tubule and straight tubule (pars recta)

Potassium is reabsorbed through the cells via a K⁺ transporter in the apical membrane and between cells through a paracellular pathway (Figure 9.4). Reabsorption of K⁺ is dependent on fluid reabsorption driven by Na⁺ reabsorption in the proximal tubule. As fluid is reabsorbed, the K⁺ concentration in the tubule fluid rises, creating a favorable transmembrane electrical chemical gradient for K⁺ to be transported into the cell interior and a favorable transmembrane chemical gradient for K⁺ paracellular movement, abetted by solvent drag. A diuretic like acetazolamide that blocks NaHCO₃ and water reabsorption would increase urinary K⁺ excretion little or not at all, because the increase in K⁺ remaining at the end of the proximal tubule would be reabsorbed by the tubule downstream. In the portion of pars recta (PR) of all nephron that dips into the outer medulla, the interstitial K⁺ concentration may be higher than in the tubule fluid and reverse the direction of K⁺ transport from reabsorption to secretion.

Thin loop of Henle

The movement of K⁺ into the lumen is passive. The K⁺ concentration rises until the amount of K⁺ remaining at the end of the thin descending limb (tdl) of the juxtamedullary nephron (Figure 9.3) normally equals or even exceeds the filtered load of K⁺. This finding and others established that K⁺ is secreted in either the PR or tDL (or both) [3]. In the thin ascending limb (tAL), the direction of transepithelial movement of K⁺ is uncertain.

Thick ascending limb of Henle (TAL)

Potassium movement is along two routes – through the cells and between cells (Figure 9.4). The apical membrane has a coupled co-transport mechanism, a carrier that requires 1Na⁺, 2Cl⁻ and 1K⁺. Inhibition of this co-transporter by the 'loop' diuretics increases K⁺ excretion, primarily because of the increased delivery of Na⁺ to the collecting duct, since the co-transporter has little effect on the luminal K⁺ concentration because of K⁺ back-leak. The electrochemical gradient from lumen to cell interior for Na⁺, established by the Na⁺,K⁺-ATPase on the basolat-

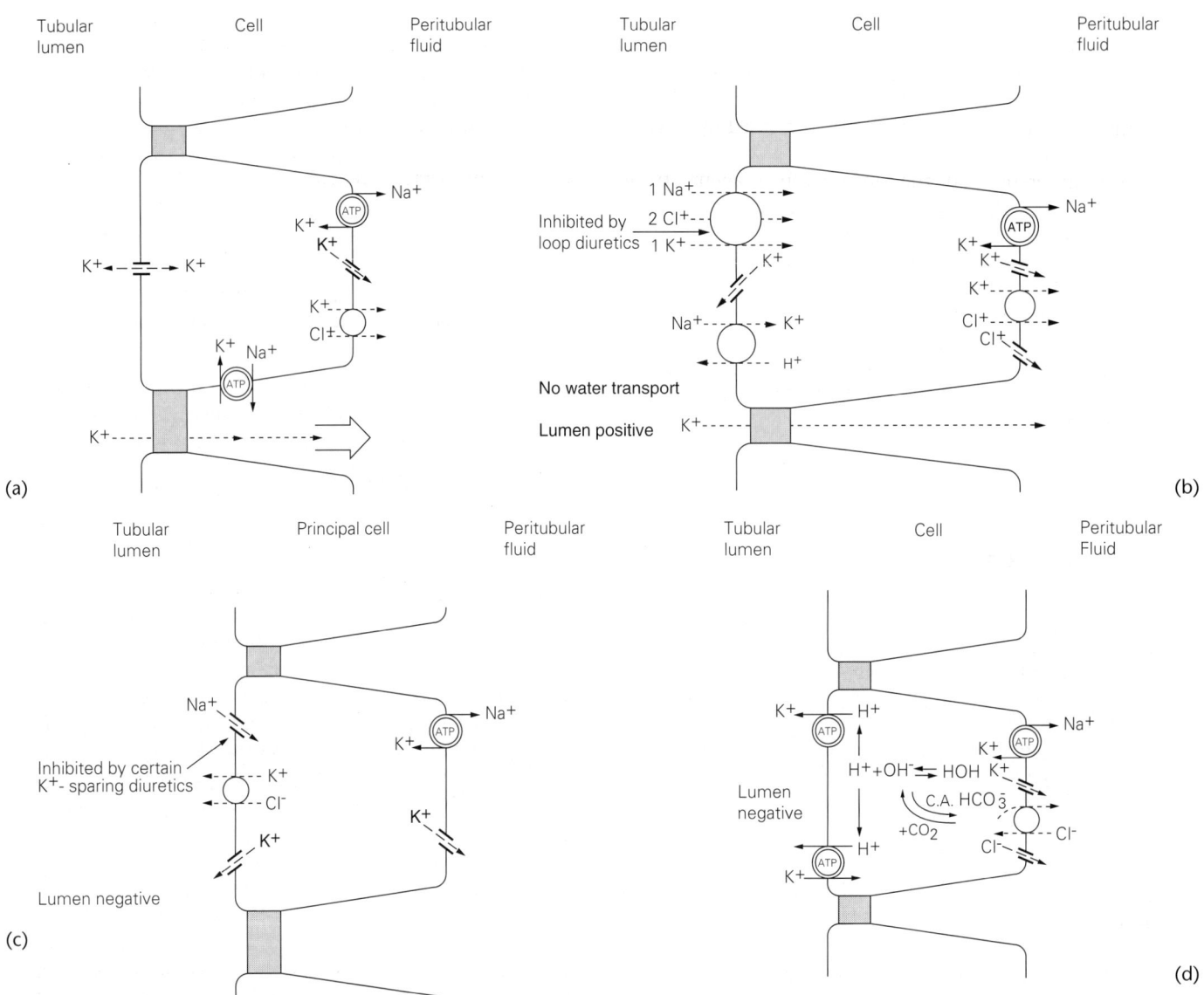

Figure 9.4 Transport of K$^+$ by the major segments of the tubule. (a) Proximal tubule. The circle labeled ATP represents the enzyme Na$^+$,K$^+$-ATPase that actively extrudes Na$^+$ and pumps in K$^+$. The other circle stands for a protein carrier that mediates passive transport, in this case the outward co-transport of K$^+$ and Cl$^-$. The parallel bars indicate a membrane channel. The large open arrow indicates fluid movement which carries K$^+$ by solvent drag. Solid lines with arrows, active transport; dotted or dashed lines with arrows, passive transport. (b) Thick ascending limb. The open circle with three arrows is the Na$^+$2Cl$^-$K$^+$ co-transporter. Another open circle indicates a protein that mediates the oppositely directed passive transport of Na$^+$ in and H$^+$ out (called an 'antiporter'). Otherwise, symbols are as for (a). Note that there is no water transport across the TAL. (c) Principal cell of the collecting duct. Although this cell is distributed to a varying degree in the connecting tubule, and cortical and medullary collecting duct, the processes depicted here occur primarily in the cortical CD. Symbols are as for (a). (d) α-Intercalated cell of the collecting duct. C.A. = carbonic anhyrdase. Otherwise, symbols are as for (a). (Slightly modified from ref. [7], with permission).

eral cell membrane, is the driving force for passive inward movement of the co-transporter. The apical membrane is also permeable to K$^+$. The basolateral cell membrane has K$^+$ and Cl$^-$ passive transporters. This permits the passive outward movement of K$^+$ from cell interior and accomplishes the final step of the net reabsorption of K$^+$ in this segment. It should be noted that NH$_4^+$ can substitute for K$^+$ in the 1Na$^+$ 2Cl$^-$ 1K$^+$ co-transporter.

Cortical collecting duct

The cortical collecting duct (CCD) is the primary site at which urinary excretion of K$^+$ is regulated. There are two types of cells in the epithelium (Figure 9.4). The principal cell secretes K$^+$. Its apical membrane has a K$^+$ channel that responds to changes in electrochemical gradient. Increased Na$^+$ reabsorption depolarizes the cell, increasing K$^+$ secretion through the open K$^+$ channels. K$^+$ is also co-secreted with Cl$^-$. K$^+$ permeability is increased by increased pH in the luminal fluid, and aldosterone and arginine vasopressin (AVP), on the basolateral side. Somehow apical K$^+$ permeability is increased by a rise in ECF K$^+$. The 'potassium-sparing diuretics' like amiloride and triamterene and the antimicrobial agent, trimethoprim [11], directly block the apical Na$^+$ channel. Spironolactone, on the other hand, blocks the aldosterone receptor, which closes the Na$^+$ channel.

The α intercalated cell (Figure 9.4) reabsorbs K$^+$. Its apical membrane, which is not permeable to K$^+$, has a K$^+$ reabsorptive pump coupled to H$^+$ secretion.

These permeability and transport characteristics mediate the action of several factors that regulate urinary K$^+$ excretion.

Regulation of K$^+$ excretion

Potassium concentration in the ECF

Acute changes in ECF K$^+$ concentration directly affect K$^+$ movement in the collecting duct, primarily the CCD. In adrenalectomized animals, acute changes in plasma K$^+$ simulate the effects of aldosterone on the principal cells (see below). A rise in ECF K$^+$ concentration increases apical membrane permeability to K$^+$ and Na$^+$ and stimulates the activity of basolateral Na$^+$,K$^+$-ATPase [9]. If animals are chronically fed a high K$^+$ diet, urinary excretion of K$^+$ increases in efficiency in response to a superimposed acute load of K$^+$, even in the absence of aldosterone (although it is a much more effective response if the adrenal gland is intact). This phenomenon is known as potassium tolerance and becomes important if kidney function is permanently impaired.

Aldosterone

Along with ECF K$^+$ concentration, the renin–angiotensin–aldosterone axis plays a major role in regulating K$^+$ excretion [12]. Aldosterone secretion by the adrenal cortex is very sensitive to the plasma K$^+$ concentration; a change in the plasma K$^+$ concentration of 0.2 mEq/l alters the secretory rate [13]. Aldosterone secretion is also stimulated by angiotensin II. Aldosterone stimulates K$^+$ secretion and Na$^+$ reabsorption in the principal cells, primarily in the CCD, by increasing basolateral Na$^+$,K$^+$-ATPase activity and apical membrane permeability to Na$^+$ and K$^+$.

Fluid flow rate in the distal tubule

A rise in fluid flow rate in the distal and collecting tubule stimulates K$^+$ secretion, if the ECF K$^+$ concentration is not below normal, and especially if aldosterone levels are high. The effect of the flow rate is thought to be in part

due to the reciprocal change in the luminal K$^+$ concentration. Normally the K$^+$ concentration in fluid entering the distal tubule is 1–2 mEq/l. In antidiuresis, arginine vasopressin (AVP) enhances water reabsorption in the CCD, causing the K$^+$ concentration to rise. In water diuresis, or other conditions which cause enhanced distal flow, the K$^+$ concentration remains low, so that the transtubular concentration gradient for K$^+$ favors continued K$^+$ secretion.

Sodium delivery to the distal tubule

Under circumstances of increased fluid flow entering the distal and collecting tubule, the delivery of Na$^+$ also rises, which also stimulates K$^+$ secretion. The electrical potential difference across the apical membrane is reduced ('shorted') by the Na$^+$ entry, allowing more K$^+$ to enter the tubule lumen from the cell, basolateral Na$^+$,K$^+$-ATPase is stimulated by the rise in cell Na$^+$ and basolateral cell uptake of K$^+$ increases.

Potassium recycling

Like the CCD, the outer medullary collecting duct (OMCD) is lined by principal and intercalated cells. In contrast to the CCD, however, the OMCD appears to be a site of K$^+$ reabsorption only, with little evidence of K$^+$ secretion [14]. Some of the reabsorbed K$^+$ supplied re-enters the nephron by secretion in the PR or tDL, i.e. it recycles (Figure 9.3). The physiological role of K$^+$ recycling is uncertain. The high interstitial K$^+$ concentration resulting from medullary recycling may decrease backleak of K$^+$ from the medullary collecting duct and thereby influence urinary K$^+$ excretion. Potassium recycling may inhibit Na$^+$ reabsorption in the thick ascending limb [15], delivering more Na$^+$ to the CCD which in turn promotes K$^+$ secretion.

Elucidation of this phenomenon awaits further studies.

Other factors

Arginine vasopressin (AVP) stimulates K$^+$ secretion by increasing apical K$^+$ permeability [16]. Its primary action is to increase water reabsorption by enhancing water permeability of the collecting duct (as mentioned above), which would increase the K$^+$ concentration in the luminal fluid and thereby reduce the transmembrane gradient favoring K$^+$ secretion. The action of AVP to increase K$^+$ permeability appears to offset this effect and assures that regulation of K$^+$ excretion is independent of regulation of urinary water excretion. An exception to this independence of K$^+$ excretion and urine flow occurs if the urinary flow drops to very low levels (oliguria), in which case K$^+$ excretion is impaired.

Summary

In summary, the various influences that increase K^+ secretion (an opposite change would decrease K^+ secretion) are as follows.

1   Luminal fluid:
   (a)   increased Na^+ delivery to the CCD;
   (b)   increaseed flow of fluid;
   (c)   decreased K^+ concentration;
   (d)   increased pH;
   (e)   decreased Cl^- concentration below 10 mEq/l. (In this last circumstance, other less permeant anions substitute for Cl^-; Na^+ reabsorption with these anions increases cell negativity and enhances K^+ secretion [17]);
   (f) Na^+ channel blocking drugs, e.g. amiloride and trimethoprim [11].
2   Basolateral interstitial fluid (plasma):
   (a)   increased K^+ concentration;
   (b)   aldosterone;
   (c)   AVP;
   (d)   increased pH.

References

1. Giebisch, G., Malnic, G. and Berliner, R.W. (1991) Renal transport and control of potassium excretion, in *The Kidney* (eds B.M. Brenner and F.W. Rector, Jr), Saunders, Philadelphia, pp. 283–317.
2. Giebisch, G. and Wang, W. (1996) Potassium transport: from clearance to channels and pumps. *Kidney Int.*, **49**, 1624–31.
3. Jamison, R.L. (1978) Potassium recycling. *Kidney Int.*, **3**, 695–703.
4. Fulop, M. (1979) Serum potassium in lactic acidosis and ketoacidosis. *N. Engl. J. Med.*, **300**, 1087.
5. DeFronzo, R.A., Sherwin, R.T., S. Dilingham, M. *et al.* (1978) Influence of basal insulin and glucagon secretion on potassium and sodium metabolism. *J. Clin. Invest.*, **61**, 472–9.
6. Rosa, R.M., Silva, P., Young, J.B. *et al.* (1980) Adrenergic modulation of extrarenal potassium disposal. *N. Engl. J. Med.*, **302**, 431–4.
7. McManus, M.L., Churchwell, K.B. and Strange, K. (1995) Regulation of cell volume in health and disease. *N. Engl. J. Med.*, **333**, 1260–6.
8. Valtin, H. and Schafer, J.A. (1995) *Renal Function*, 3rd edn, Little, Brown, Boston, pp. 235–57.
9. Bertorella, A.M. and Katz, A.I. (1993) Short-term regulation of renal Na-K-ATPase activity: physiological relevance and cellular mechanisms. *Am. J. Physiol.*, **265**, F743–55.

10. Wang, W., Sackin, H. and Giebisch, G. (1992) Renal potassium channels and their regulation. *Annu. Rev. Physiol.*, **54**, 81–96.
11. Velazquez, H., Perzaella, M.A., Wright, F.S. and Ellison, D.H. (1993) Renal mechanism of trimethoprim-induced hyperkalemia. *Ann. Intern. Med.*, **119**, 296–301.
12. Young, D.B. (1988) Quantitative analysis of aldosterone's role in potassium regulation. *Am. J. Physiol.*, **255**.
13. Himathongam, T., Dluhy, R. and Williams, G.H. (1975) Potassium–aldosterone–renin interrelationships. *J. Clin. Endocrinol. Metab.*, **41**.
14. Stokes, J.B. (1982) Na and K transport across the cortical and outer medullary collecting tubule of the rabbit: evidence for diffusion across the outer medullary portion. *Am. J. Physiol.*, **242**.
15. Milanes, C.L. and Jamison, R.L. (1985) Effect of acute potassium load on reabsorption in Henle's loop in chronic renal failure in the rat. *Kidney Int.*, **27**, 919–27.
16. Cassola, A.C., Giebisch, G. and Wang, W. (1993) Vasopressin increases density of apical low-conductance K^+ channels in rat CCD. *Am. J. Physiol.*, **264**, F502–9.
17. Velazquez, H., Ellison, D.H. and Wright, F.S. (1992) Luminal influences on potassium secretion: chloride, sodium and thiazide diuretics. *Am. J. Physiol.*, **262**, F1076–82.

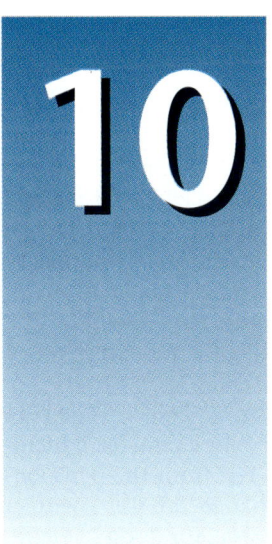

Divalent ions

Christopher J. Lote

Introduction

The main divalent cations which the kidney handles, and which are the focus of this chapter, are calcium and magnesium. Although there are similarities in the ways that these are transported in the nephron segments, there are also major differences. These are summarized in the conclusion of the chapter.

Calcium

Calcium excretion by the kidney is a function of glomerular filtration, and subsequent reabsorption of most of the filtered load. The total calcium concentration in plasma is 2.5 mmol/l (5 mEq/l). Approximately 60% of this is ultrafilterable and the remainder is protein-bound, primarily to albumin. The ultrafilterable fraction consists of free ionized calcium, Ca^{2+} 1.25 mmol/l (2.5 mEq/l), and complexed calcium (0.1 mmol/l 0.2 mEq/l, 4% of the total plasma calcium concentration), attached to polyvalent anions such as phosphate, citrate, bicarbonate and sulfate [1]. Calcium homeostasis depends on the balance of intestinal absorption, bone resorption and deposition and urinary excretion (Figure 10.1).

Tubular reabsorption of calcium
(Table 10.1)

In a normal individual with a plasma calcium concentration of 2.5 mmol/l (5 mEq/l) the filtered calcium is 200–250 mmol/24 h. Some 95–99% of this is reabsorbed along the nephron, with only 1–5% being excreted. Reabsorption is by two main mechanisms: paracellular (passive) transport predominates in the proximal tubule and thick ascending limb of Henle's loop and transcellular (active) transport occurs in the distal tubule.

Reabsorption of calcium in the proximal tubule (S1, S2, S3 segments)

About 65% of the filtered calcium is reabsorbed in the proximal tubule. Generally calcium reabsorption parallels sodium and fluid reabsorption in the proximal tubule, and the tubular fluid:ultrafiltrate calcium ratio [(TF/UF)Ca] remains close to one [2–4]. Only a minor component of the reabsorption of calcium in the proximal tubule is active, and most of the reabsorption occurs by passive, paracellular mechanisms driven by the concentration gradients set up by Na^+ and fluid reabsorption. *In vivo* microperfusion and microinjection experiments in Munich–Wistar rats have shown a high Ca^{2+} permeability in the proximal tubule, with the unidirectional efflux (lumen to serosa) being about threefold greater than net efflux, i.e. there is a high backflux. Bomsztyk and Wright [5] have suggested that calcium absorption is dependent on water movement, as a consequence of three mechanisms: (1) water absorption raising the intratubular Ca^{2+} concentration to create a transepithelial Ca^{2+} concentration gradient; (2) water absorption raising the Ca^{2+} concentration in a microscopic unstirred layer of fluid

Nephrology, Edited by Rex L. Jamison and Robert Wilkinson.
Published in 1997 by Chapman & Hall, London. ISBN 0 412 60930 4

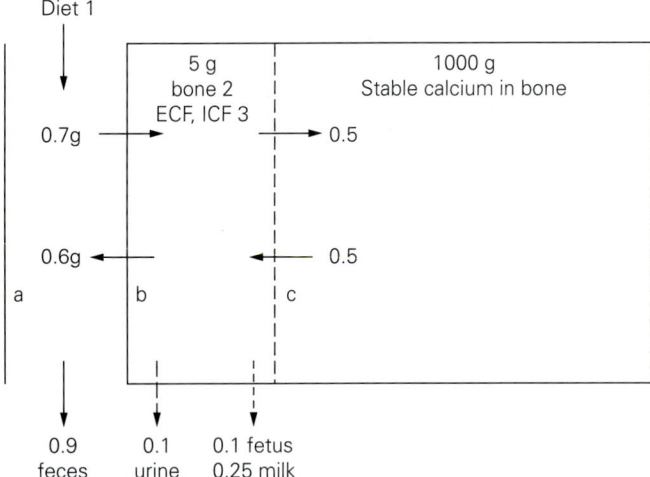

Diet 1

| | 5 g bone 2 ECF, ICF 3 | 1000 g Stable calcium in bone |

0.7g → 0.5

0.6g ← ← 0.5

a   b   c

0.9 feces   0.1 urine   0.1 fetus 0.25 milk

Figure 10.1 Daily calcium intake and output. All numerical values in the diagram are grams. Functionally the calcium in the body can be divided into three pools, labeled a, b, c. (a) The gut: this normally receives 1 g (25 mmol) of which about 700 mg (17.5 mmol) is absorbed. However, net reabsorption is only 100 mg (2.5 mmol), since 600 mg (15 mmol) re-enters the gut. Thus the feces contain 900 mg (22.5 mmol) calcium. During pregnancy and lactation there are additional requirements for calcium, and net gut absorption increases. (b) The 'pool' of exchangeable calcium: about 5 g calcium in the body is 'exchangeable' on bone surfaces (2 g, 50 mmol) and in body fluids (3 g, 75 mmol). Exchanges occur between this pool and the gut, and also between this pool and the 'stable calcium' in bone. (c) Stable calcium in bone: of the 1000 g (25 mol) total only 0.5 g (12.5 mmol) exchanges each day with the 'exchangeable' calcium pool. Losses of calcium from the exchangeable pool occur normally in the urine. (Reproduced, with permission, from Lote, C.J. (1994) *Principles of Renal Physiology*. Chapman & Hall, London.)

immediately adjacent to the luminal membrane; and (3) solvent drag.

However, recently Zhang and O'Neil [6] have identified an L-type calcium channel (voltage activated) in the apical membranes of cultured proximal tubule cells from the rabbit, and have suggested that such channels, which are activated by membrane depolarization, may participate in calcium reabsorption during periods of enhanced sodium reabsorption.

There is still controversy regarding the nature and importance of the active component of Ca^{2+} reabsorption on the basolateral membrane of the proximal tubule (Figure 10.2). The proximal tubule epithelial cell membrane is permeable to calcium, with calcium permeability 23×10^{-5} cm/s [7], very similar to sodium permeability, 24.7×10^{-5} cm/s [8]. The epithelial permeability, coupled with a very low cytosolic Ca^{2+} concentration (10^{-7} M) and the negative intracellular electrical potential drives calcium into the cells. Several mechanisms of calcium extrusion across the basolateral membrane have been

proposed, but there have been relatively few investigations. Doucet and Katz [9] suggested that the high affinity Ca^{2+},Mg^{2+}-ATPase, present in all segments of the nephron, may act as the calcium pump at the basolateral membrane. However, the role of Ca^{2+},Mg^{2+}-ATPase has not yet been clearly defined. It is a high-affinity, low-capacity calmodulin-dependent enzyme, with an apparent K_m of 100–200 nmol for Ca^{2+}. It appears to resemble the Ca^{2+},Mg^{2+}-ATPase in other tissues (with the exception of the liver).

An alternative mechanism could involve sodium–calcium antiport at the basolateral cell membrane. According to this scheme, Na^+ from the peritubular space enters the cell in exchange for Ca^{2+}, with a stoichiometry of approximately $3Na^+$ for 1 Ca^{2+} (Figure 10.2). The concentrations of Na^+ and Ca^{2+} in the two compartments, however, make it unlikely that Na^+–Ca^{2+} exchange constitutes a significant fraction of the overall Ca^{2+} reabsorption in the proximal tubule [10].

For the pars recta of the proximal tubule, there is no direct *in vivo* information about calcium transport. The mechanisms of calcium transport in this segment are similar to those of the proximal convoluted tubule, with paracellular transport being the route of calcium absorption [11].

Calcium transport in the loops of Henle

The thin descending and thin ascending limbs of Henle's loop have a very low permeability to calcium [12], and contribute little to overall calcium reabsorption. In contrast, the cortical thick ascending limb (TALH) is a quantitatively important site of calcium transport, accounting for reabsorption of 20% of the filtered calcium [13]. Much of this reabsorption is by passive paracellular transport driven by the lumen-positive voltage of this segment [14]. There is also evidence for an active transcellular transport

Table 10.1 Fractional Ca^{2+} and Mg^{2+} reabsorption along the nephron

	Filtered load reabsorbed (%)	
	Ca^{2+}	Mg^{2+}
Proximal tubule (pars convoluta)	60	15
Proximal tubule (pars recta)	10	15
Thick ascending limb of Henle	20–25	60
Distal convoluted tubule	5–10	2–5
Collecting tubule system	<0.5	<0.5

Reproduced, with permission, from Lote, C.J. (1994) *Principles of Renal Physiology*. Chapman & Hall, London.

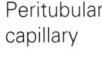

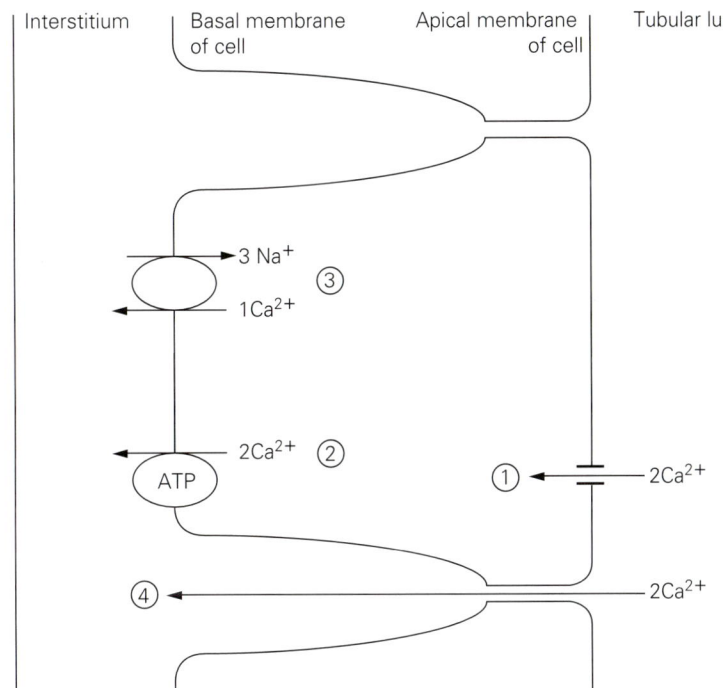

| Peritubular capillary | Interstitium | Basal membrane of cell | Apical membrane of cell | Tubular lumen |

Figure 10.2 Proximal tubular calcium reabsorption. 1. PTH-induced calcium channels in the apical membrane. 2. High-affinity calmodulin-sensitive Ca^{2+}-ATPase on the basal membrane. This is present in other nephron segments but its highest levels are in the distal convoluted tubules. 3. Sodium–calcium exchange.

process [15] in the cortical TALH. The proportion of calcium reabsorbed in the TALH is greater than that of water, so the tubular fluid calcium concentration falls along the TALH to values lower than that in plasma.

Calcium transport in the medullary TALH (mTALH) is controversial. Many reports show no significant net reabsorption of calcium in the mTALH, whether or not hormones such as PTH are present [e.g. 14]. Friedman and Gesek [15], however, claim that there is transcellular calcium transport in both cTALH and mTALH, and that the transport is stimulated by PTH. The most recent evidence, obtained in mouse kidneys, indicates that calcium is not reabsorbed in the mTALH, and that the passive permeability of this nephron segment to divalent cations is very low [16].

Calcium transport in the distal tubule and collecting tubule (distal nephron)

The distal (convoluted) tubule (the segment between the macula densa and the merger of two distal tubules to form a collecting tubule) is responsible for reabsorption of about 10% of the filtered calcium. The calcium concentration in fluid entering the distal tubule is lower than that of plasma, and continues to fall along the distal tubule [17]: this fact, together with the lumen-negative transepithelial potential, indicates active calcium transport at this site [18].

The distal nephron is the main site of hormonal regulation of calcium reabsorption. The initial step in calcium reabsorption in the distal nephron is passive influx of

luminal Ca^{2+}, via a carrier-mediated process or a Ca^{2+} channel. Recent studies suggest it is unlikely that a Ca^{2+}/H^+ exchanger in the apical membrane is involved; more likely a voltage-independent Ca^{2+} channel exists which is insensitive to Ca^{2+} blockers, but inhibited by apical acidification [19].

Calcitriol ($1\alpha,25$-dihydroxy vitamin D_3) plays an important role in calcium homeostasis. It acts in the kidney mainly by genomic mechanisms, mediated by the vitamin D receptor (VDR), which acts as a transcription factor to increase the expression of genes for calbindin D_{28k}, calbindin D_{9k}, and the VDR itself [20–22].

The exit of calcium from the cells of the distal nephron across the basal membrane is thought to be mediated by Ca^{2+},Mg^{2+}-ATPase or Na^+–Ca^{2+} exchange [10]; the former is more likely, however, as the electrical and concentration gradients for the exchange mechanism may favor Ca^{2+} entry into the cells, rather than efflux across the basolateral cell membranes [23].

Hormonal control of renal calcium excretion

Many hormones have been shown to affect the renal handling of calcium, the most intensively investigated being parathyroid hormone (PTH), vitamin D_3 and calcitonin. It is important, however, not to lose sight of the fact that adjustments in renal calcium excretion that occur in response to hormonal activity play only a minor role in calcium homeostasis.

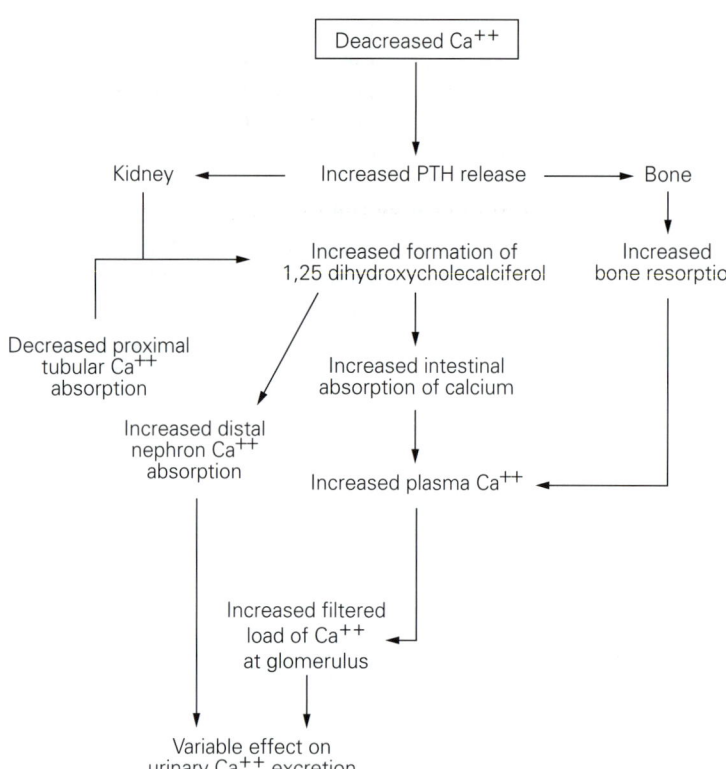

Figure 10.3 The effects of changes in PTH release on urinary Ca^{2+} excretion. (Reproduced, with permission, from Lote, C.J. (1994) *Principles of Renal Physiology*, Chapman & Hall, London.)

Parathyroid hormone

Most accounts of the renal actions of PTH stress its role in promoting tubular calcium reabsorption, and ignore the fact that PTH has a very minor effect to reduce calcium excretion, and may even increase it. The reason for this is that, although PTH does enhance renal calcium reabsorption, particularly in the distal nephron, its main effect is to promote bone resorption, and to enhance intestinal calcium absorption. These last two actions increase the plasma calcium concentration, and hence the filtered load of calcium, which can lead to increased calcium excretion notwithstanding the increased reabsorption (Figure 10.3). Consequently, hyperparathyroidism is generally associated with increased urinary calcium excretion, and hypoparathyroidism with decreased calcium excretion.

The effects of PTH on renal tubular cells occur via cyclic AMP (cAMP), primarily in the cTALH [14, 10] and distal tubule [15, 10]. The effect of PTH in the proximal tubule is variable depending on the animal species investigated. In the dog, PTH administration inhibits calcium (and phosphate) reabsorption [10], whereas in the hamster PTH enhances calcium reabsorption in the proximal tubule [1].

Calcitonin

The effects of calcitonin on calcium excretion are not clear. Reports in the literature are inconsistent; although enhancement of tubular calcium reabsorption has been reported, calcitonin has a primarily hypocalcemic action, but this is due to its effects on bone deposition (enhancing it), not its renal action. In fact, like PTH, calcitonin increases nephron calcium reabsorption and hence has a renal calcium-conserving effect [24].

Vitamin D

The renal effects of $1\alpha,25$-dihydroxycholecalciferol ($1\alpha25(OH)_2D_3$) remain controversial. Vitamin D is not essential for the renal conservation of calcium; indeed large doses of vitamin D are hypercalciuric in humans, an effect probably attributable to increased filtered calcium load [1].

Magnesium

Whereas the intestine and bone play a more important role in regulating plasma calcium than does the kidney, for magnesium balance the kidney is the primary regulatory organ [25].

Tubular reabsorption of magnesium (Table 10.1)

The plasma magnesium concentration is about 0.9 mmol/l (1.8 mEq/l) and 70–80% of this is ultrafilterable. Hence magnesium enters the proximal tubules at a concentration of approximately 0.8 mmol/l. Most of this magnesium (70–80%) is free Mg^{2+}, the remainder being complexed to filterable anions such as citrate, phosphate and oxalate [26].

Proximal tubular handling of magnesium

Unlike calcium, the concentration of which changes little along the proximal tubule, magnesium concentration in the proximal tubular lumen increases progressively as a consequence of water reabsorption. Only about 15% of filtered magnesium is reabsorbed in the proximal tubule in the adult, but studies on young rats (age two weeks) show higher levels of absorption (50–60%), with fractional reabsorption decreasing with age [27]. This has been attributed to decreasing permeability to Mg^{2+} of the paracellular pathway (tight junction) with increasing maturity. The permeability coefficient for magnesium in the proximal tubule is 1.1×10^{-5} cm/s, less than one-twentieth of that for Ca^{2+} or Na^+ [28]. The pars recta of the proximal tubule also has a low permeability to magnesium and appears to have essentially identical properties in relation to magnesium as the pars convoluta [28].

Consequently, the concentration of magnesium in the fluid entering the loops of Henle is 1–1.5 mmol/l.

Magnesium transport in the loops of Henle

Most of the filtered magnesium (60%) is reabsorbed in the loop of Henle. *In vitro* experiments using isolated tubule segments of mice and rats indicate unequivocally that, like calcium, magnesium is reabsorbed in the cortical thick ascending limb of Henle (cTALH), but not in the (rat) medullary thick ascending limb (mTALH) [16].

The mechanism of magnesium transport in the cTALH has been the subject of intensive investigation. Shareghi and Agus [29] used rabbit cTALH, and showed that magnesium reabsorption is passive, and likely to be paracel-

lular (Figure 10.4). Similar findings have been obtained in the mouse [30], and indicate close similarity between magnesium reabsorption and calcium reabsorption in this nephron segment. However, there may be a small active component of magnesium transport in the cTALH [31].

The question of how the cTALH can be permeable to magnesium (and calcium) but not to water has recently been addressed [32], but remains controversial.

Magnesium transport in the distal tubule and connecting tubule and collecting duct

About 5% of the filtered magnesium is reabsorbed in the distal tubule and connecting tubule by a load-dependent mechanism, i.e. increased magnesium delivery to this site increases magnesium reabsorption [33, 34]. There is little net magnesium transport in the collecting ducts and reabsorption here accounts for only about 1% of the filtered load [35].

Regulation of magnesium excretion

The magnesium intake from food is normally about 300 mg/day, although this can be increased considerably in subjects who ingest antacids such as magnesium hydroxide. About 40% of the ingested magnesium is absorbed by the intestine, predominantly the small intestine although there is some absorption by the colon.

The excretion of magnesium in the urine reflects dietary magnesium intake and absorption. For the kidney as a whole, magnesium behaves as if there is a tubular maximum (T_m) for magnesium reabsorption, with the normal tubular reabsorption being very close to the T_m. This means that a small increase in plasma magnesium, thereby increasing the filtered load, will automatically increase magnesium excretion (i.e. fractional reabsorption decreases). In rat micropuncture studies, magnesium loading led to a fall in the fractional reabsorption of

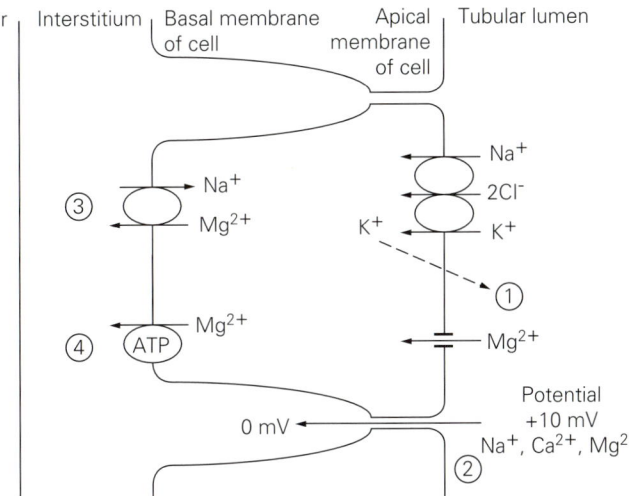

Figure 10.4 Magnesium absorption in the (cortical) thick ascending limb of the loop of Henle. The $Na^+ : K^+ : 2Cl^-$ co-transporter in the apical membrane, with back-leak of some K^+, (1), establishes a lumen-positive potential which drives Mg^{2+} absorption by the paracellular route (2). Ca^{2+} and Na^+ are also absorbed in this way. There is also some $Na^+ : Mg^{2+}$ antiport (3) across the basal membrane, as well as Mg^{2+}-ATPase (4).

Table 10.2 Comparison of the major features of Ca^{2+} and Mg^{2+} homeostasis and renal handling

Ca^{2+} (ionized calcium)	Mg^{2+} (ionized magnesium)
1. Predominantly an extracellular ion. Plasma concentration of Ca^{2+}, 1.25 mM approx. Intracellular concentration typically 10^{-7}M[a]	Even distribution in intracellular and extracellular fluid. Plasma Mg^{2+} approx 0.8 mM, intracellular concentration 0.5–1 mM[a]
2. Plasma concentration controlled by extrarenal mechanisms. Kidneys play minor role.	Plasma concentration controlled primarily by kidneys. T_m for Mg^{2+} reabsorption is close to normal filtered load.
3. Proximal tubular reabsorption parallels Na$^+$ and H$_2$O reabsorption. Little change in tubular fluid Ca^{2+} concentration. 60% of filtered load absorbed proximally.	Proximal tubular reabsorption is only 15% of filtered load. Mg^{2+} concentration increases along proximal tubule.

[a] For both calcium and magnesium intracellular total concentrations are higher than ionized concentrations because some calcium and magnesium is present in chelated form.

magnesium, from an initial value of 92%, to 44%. The main site at which the reduction in absorption occurred was the loop of Henle. Quamme and colleagues have argued that the peritubular magnesium concentration determines the extent of reabsorption of magnesium in the loop of Henle (i.e. elevated plasma and peritubular magnesium decreases reabsorption) and that this explains the apparent T_m for magnesium [25, 36], since changes in magnesium transport in the loop of Henle elicit similar changes in urinary magnesium excretion. If dietary magnesium intake is curtailed, the urinary magnesium excretion decreases to values close to zero as a consequence of enhanced loop of Henle magnesium reabsorption [37, 38].

Hormonal effects on magnesium excretion

The main hormones which have been shown to affect the renal handling of magnesium are parathyroid hormone (PTH), calcitonin, vasopressin (ADH) and glucagon. None of these hormones has any effect on magnesium reabsorption in the proximal tubule [25], and their effects in the thin segments of the loop of Henle have not been investigated (although neither glucagon nor PTH alters magnesium delivery to the tips of the long loops). In the thick ascending limb of the loop of Henle (TALH), the above hormones all increase the adenylate cyclase activity (of the cortical TALH), and increase magnesium absorption. The direct cause of this increase is a rise in the transepithelial lumen-positive voltage of this segment, and an increase in magnesium permeability,

probably of the paracellular pathway (these data are from the mouse). That paracellular ionic permeability can be controlled by hormones has been suggested for a number of transporting epithelia [39]. It seems likely that in the cTALH, hormones which increase cAMP concentration phosphorylate proteins in the tight junctions of the paracellular pathways.

Summary

For both calcium and magnesium, the details of the nephron transport processes show some species differences. Since the techniques used to investigate the transport mechanisms are in general not applicable in humans, there remains uncertainty over the applicability of findings from other species to humans. However, it is clear that, although there are similarities between renal calcium handling and magnesium handing, there are also important differences. These are summarized in Table 10.2.

The major differences between the two ions are in the extent to which the plasma concentration is controlled by the kidneys. For magnesium, the kidneys are the major regulatory organ. For calcium, the kidneys play a minor regulatory role, with bone reabsorption/deposition and intestinal absorption being of greater importance.

There is a close relationship between calcium homeostasis and magnesium homeostasis – each depends to some extend on the other. This interrelationship is discussed more fully in Chapter 27.

References

1. Buck, A.C. and Lote, C.J. (1990) The renal handling of calcium, in *Renal Tract Stone* (eds J.E.A. Wickham and A.C. Buck), Churchill Livingstone, Edinburgh, pp. 165–82.

2. Lassiter, W.E., Gottschalk, C.W. and Mylle, M. (1963) Micropuncture study of renal tubular reabsorption of calcium in normal rodents. *Am. J. Physiol.*, **204**, 771–5.

3. Edwards, B.R., Baer, P.G., Sutton, R.A. and Dirks, J.H. (1973) Micropuncture study of diuretic effects on sodium and calcium reabsorption in the dog nephron. *J. Clin. Invest.*, **52**, 2418–27.

4. Agus, Z.S., Gardner, L.B., Beck, L.H. and Goldberg, M. (1973) Effects of parathyroid hormone on renal tubular reabsorption of calcium, sodium and phosphate. *Am. J. Physiol.*, **224**, 1143–8.

5. Bomsztyk, K. and Wright, F.S. (1986) Dependence of ion fluxes on fluid transport by rat proximal tubule. *Am. J. Physiol.*, **250**, F680–9.

6. Zhang, M.I.N., O'Neil, R.G. (1996) An L-type calcium channel in renal epithelial cells. *J. Membr. Biol.*, **154**, 259–66.

7. Ullrich, K.J., Rumrich, G. and Kloss, S. (1976) Active Ca reabsorption in the proximal tubule of the rat kidney. *Pflugers Archiv.*, **364**, 223–8.

8. Bomsztyk, K., George, J.P. and Wright, F.S. (1984) Effects of luminal fluid arions on calcium transport by proximal tubule. *Am J. Physiol.*, **246**, F600–8.

9. Doucet, A. and Katz, A.I. (1982) High affinity Ca-Mg-ATPase along the rabbit nephron. *Am. J. Physiol.*, **242**, F346–52.

10. Ullrich, K.J. (1973) Permeability characteristics of the mammalian nephron, in *Handbook of Physiology*, Section 8, *Renal Physiology* (eds J. Orloff and R.W. Berliner), American Physiological Society, pp. 377–414.

11. Sacks, P. and Bourdeau, J.E. (1989) Ca^{2+} absorption in the parts recta of cortical S2 rabbit proximal tubules: role of diffusion. *Am. J. Physiol.*, **257**, F262–7.

12. Rouse, D., Ng, R.C. and Suki, W.N. (1980) Calcium transport in the pars recta and thin descending limb of Henle of the rabbit, perfused *in vitro*. *J. Clin. Invest.*, **65**, 37–42.

13. Greger, R. (1985) Ion transport mechanisms in thick ascending limb of Henle's loop of mammalian nephron. *Physiol. Rev.*, **65**, 760–97.

14. Suki, W.N., Rouse, D., Ng, R.C.K. and Kokko, J.P. (1980) Calcium transport in the thick ascending limb of Henle. Heterogeneity of function in the medullary and cortical segments. *J. Clin. Invest.*, **66**, 1004–8.

15. Friedman, P.A. and Gesek, F.A. (1993) Calcium transport in renal epithelial cells. *Am. J. Physiol.*, **264**, F181–98.

16. Wittner, M., Desfleurs, E., Pajaud, S., Moine, G., De Rouffignac, C. and DiStefano, A. (1996) Calcium and magnesium – low passive permeability and tubular secretion in the mouse medullary thick ascending limb of Henle's loop (mTAL). *J. Membr. Biol.*, **153**, 27–35.

17. Costanzo, L.S. and Windhager, E.E. (1978) Calcium and sodium transport by the distal convoluted tubule of the rat. *Am. J. Physiol.*, **235**, F492–506.

18. Wright, F.S. (1971) Increasing magnitude of electrical potential along the renal distal tubule. *Am. J. Physiol.*, **220**, 624–38.

19. Bindels, R.J.M., Hartog, A., Abrahamse, S.L. and Van Os, C.H. (1994) Effects of pH on apical calcium entry and archive calcium transport in rabbit cortical collecting system. *Am. J. Physiol.*, **266**, F620–7.

20. Kumar, R., Schaefer, J., Grande, J.P. and Roche, P.C. (1994) Immunolocalization of calcitriol receptor, 24 hydroxylase cytochrome P450, and calbindin D_{28k} in human kidney. *Am. J. Physiol.*, **266**, F477–85.

21. Liu, L., Khastir, A., McCauley, J.M., Dunn, S.T., Morrissey, J.H., Christakos, S., Hughes, M.R. and Bourdeau, J.E. (1996) RT-PCR microlocalization of mRNA for calbindin D_{28} and vitamin D receptor in the murine nephron. *Am. J. Physiol.*, **270**, F677–81.

22. Van Baal, J., Yu, A., Hartog, A., Fransen, J.A.M., Fransen, P.H., Willems, G.H., Lytton, J. and Bindels, R.J.M. (1996) Localization and regulation by vitamin D of calcium transport proteins in rabbit cortical collecting system. *Am. J. Physiol.*, **271**, F985–93.

23. Bindels, R.J.M., Ramakers, P.L.M., Dempster, J.A. *et al.* (1992) Role of Na^+–Ca^{2+} exchange in transcellular Ca^{2+} transport across primary cultures of rabbit kidney collecting system. *Pflugers Arch.*, **420**, 566–72.

24. Carney, S.L. (1995) Acute effects of endogenous calcitonin on rat renal function. *Mineral Electrolyte Metab.*, **21**, 411–16.

25. Costanzo, L.S. and Windhager, E.E. (1992) Renal regulation of calcium balance, in *The Kidney: Physiology and Pathophysiology*, 2nd edn (eds D.W. Seldin and G. Giebisch), Raven Press, New York, pp. 2375–93.

26. Walser, M. (1973) Divalent cations: physicochemical state in glomerular filtrate and urine and renal extraction, in *Handbook of Physiology*. Section 8, *Renal Physiology* (eds J. Orloff and R.W. Berliner), American Physiological Society, pp. 555–86.

27. Lelievre-Pegorier, M., Merlet-Benichou, C., Roinel, N. and De Rouffignac, C. (1983) Developmental pattern of water and electrolyte transport in rat superficial nephron. *Am. J. Physiol.*, **245**, F15–21.

28. Quamme, G.A. and Smith, C. (1984) Magnesium transport in the proximal straight tubule of the rabbit. *Am. J. Physiol.*, **246**, 544–50.

29. Shareghi, G.R. and Agus, Z.S. (1982) Magnesium transport in the cortical thick ascending limb of Henle's loop of the rabbit. *J. Clin. Invest.*, **69**, 759–69.

30. Di Stefano, A., Roinel, N., De Rouffignac, C. and Wittner, M. (1993) Transepithelial Ca^{2+} and Mg^{2+} transport in the cortical thick ascending limb of Henle's loop of the mouse is a voltage-dependent process. *Renal Physiol. Biochem.*, **16**, 157–66.

31. Wittner, M. and Di Stefano, A. (1990) PTH and glucagon on the cortical and medullary thick ascending limb of Henle's loop of the mouse nephron. *Pflugers Arch.*, **415**, 707–12.

32. De Rouffignac, C. (1995) Multihormonal regulation of nephron epithelia – achieved through combinational mode. *Am. J. Physiol.*, **269**, R739–48.

33. Quamme, G.A. (1989) Effect of furosemide on calcium and magnesium transport in the rat nephron. *Am. J. Physiol.*, **241**, F340–7.

34. Quamme, G.A. and Dirks, J.H. (1980) Effect of intraluminal and contraluminal magnesium on magnesium and calcium transfer in the rat nephron. *Am. J. Physiol.*, **238**, F187–98.

35. Brunette, M.G., Vigneault, N. and Carrier, S. (1975) Magnesium handling by the papilla of the young rat. *Pflugers Arch.*, **373**, 229–35.

36. De Rouffignac, C. and Quamme, G. (1994) Renal magnesium handling and its hormonal control. *Physiol. Rev.*, **74**, 305–22.

37. Quamme, G.A. (1992) Magnesium: cellular and renal exchanges, in *The Kidney, Physiology and Pathophysiology*, 2nd edn (eds D.W. Seldin and G. Giebish), Raven Press, New York, pp. 2339–55.

38. Roy, D.R. (1987) Magnesium absorption in the juxtamedullary loop of Henle. Effect of magnesium deprivation. *Can. J. Physiol. Pharmacol.*, **65**, 1918–27.

39. Madara, J.L. and Pappenheimer, J.R. (1987) Structural basis for physiological regulation of paracellular pathways in intestinal epithelia. *J. Membr. Biol.*, **100**, 149–64.

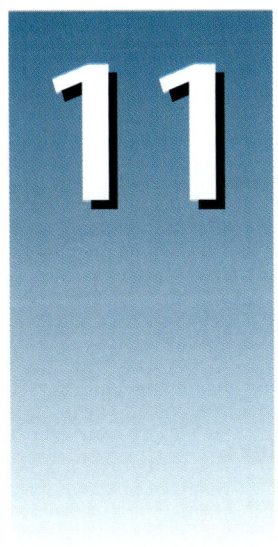

Acid–base balance

Kevin D. Burns and David Z. Levine

Introduction

The purpose of this chapter is not only to present basic information enabling the reader to diagnose acid–base disturbances, but to also provide an up-to-date survey of how nephron segments transport HCO_3^- and H^+. Since fundamental principles regarding blood buffers and the renal and respiratory compensatory responses to acid–base stimuli have been well described in recent texts [1–3], these areas are reviewed only briefly. In contrast, with exciting new insights revealing regulation of renal tubular epithelial cell function, the focus is on how single nephron segments, cells and their constituent transporters may contribute to net acid excretion. Within the confines of this short chapter, the intent is to provide a progressive analysis, segment by segment, of cell types, and of different transport proteins. It is hoped this will equip the reader to join us in pondering a single overriding question when confronted with the patients described in Chapter 26: what change in cellular function might account for the abnormality in systemic acid–base balance, or urine acidification, in the individual presenting with kidney disease?

The bicarbonate (HCO_3^-) buffering system

Three principal mechanisms are involved in body acid–base balance. First, an H^+ load is delivered daily, derived mainly from oxidation of fuels. Second, buffering of this H^+ load must occur to prevent major deviations in the $[H^+]$. Finally, there must be excretion of the H^+.

Buffers minimize the change in extracellular fluid $[H^+]$ when an acid or alkali is added. A buffer system is a pair of substances that can donate or accept H^+ in a way that blunts changes in $[H^+]$. All buffers depend on a simple equilibrium determined by the unique dissociation constant (K_d or pK) of the buffer. A buffer is most effective at a concentration identical to the concentration of its conjugate base or acid. Several intracellular and extracellular (ECF) buffer systems exist, including proteins and bone buffers. However, the HCO_3^- buffer system is the most important of these. Although buffers are effective in preventing major changes in $[H^+]$, the amount of available buffer is finite. Ultimately, the offending acid or base must be removed to restore acid–base balance.

The HCO_3^- buffer system is utilized as a first defense against acid loads. Because CO_2 is freely diffusible, alveolar CO_2 tension establishes CO_2 tension throughout the arterial system, normally set at 40 mmHg (arterial PCO_2 = $PaCO_2$). CO_2 can be reversibly hydrated to carbonic acid (H_2CO_3):

$$CO_2 + H_2O = H_2CO_3 = H^+ + HCO_3^- \qquad (11.1)$$

This reaction reaches equilibrium more rapidly in the presence of the enzyme carbonic anhydrase (CA). Once equilibrium has been reached, the $[H_2CO_3]$ is proportional to CO_2 tension. When acid is added to the ECF, the

Nephrology, Edited by Rex L. Jamison and Robert Wilkinson.
Published in 1997 by Chapman & Hall, London. ISBN 0 412 60930 4

[H⁺] rises, shifting the reaction to produce more CO_2 initially. The H^+ stimulates the respiratory center, however, and alveolar ventilation increases, resulting finally in a decrease in Pa_{CO_2}.

The metabolism of fats and carbohydrates normally generates ~15 000 mmol of CO_2 per day. In contrast to fats and carbohydrates, proteins cannot be entirely metabolized to CO_2 and H_2O, and produce non-volatile 'fixed acids'. Sulfur-containing amino acids such as cystine and methionine yield sulfuric acid; phospholipids yield phosphoric acid; and a small quantity of organic acid is formed endogenously but not metabolized. Each day these processes yield, with a typical adult diet, 60–70 mmol of H^+ (~1 mmol/kg body weight), all destined for renal excretion. This excretion is dependent on renal H^+ secretion, found to occur in the cells of all tubule segments studied. Since the major extracellular buffering system is the HCO_3^- buffer system, the addition of H^+ to the ECF is physiologically equivalent to the destruction of an equal amount of HCO_3^-:

$$H^+ + HCO_3^- = H_2O + CO_2 \tag{11.2}$$

When an HCO_3^- is consumed by H^+ addition to the ECF, the CO_2 that is generated is quantitatively negligible compared to the huge amounts produced metabolically. The continual release of endogenously produced H^+ would soon bankrupt the supply of HCO_3^-, were it not for the ability of the kidneys to excrete acid.

Evaluation of acid–base balance

Acid–base status is evaluated by examining the $[H^+]$, $[HCO_3^-]$, and Pa_{CO_2} in the blood. As noted above,

$$H^+ + HCO_3^- \rightleftharpoons H_2CO_3 \rightleftharpoons H_2O + CO_2$$

The $[H^+]$ in the ECF is usually reported as its negative log, the pH. The Henderson–Hasselbalch equation relates the three parameters, $[H^+]$, Pa_{CO_2}, and $[HCO_3^-]$:

$$pH = 6.1 + \log[HCO_3^-]/0.03 \times Pa_{CO_2}, \tag{11.3}$$

where $[HCO_3^-]$ is in mM, and Pa_{CO_2} is in mmHg.

A simple approximation of this equation is of practical value in bedside evaluation of all acid–base disorders.

$$[H^+] = 24 \times Pa_{CO_2}/[HCO_3^-] \tag{11.4}$$

At pH 7.25–7.50, this equation is useful in determining any one of these parameters, once the other two are known, and in determining internal consistency in these values in arterial blood gas measurements. At the University of Ottawa, we use a formula that is applicable over a wider range of pH values: the $[H^+]$ (and, therefore, the pH) can be related to the ratio $Pa_{CO_2}:[HCO_3^-]$ in a simplified, approximate fashion.

For example, when

$$pH = 6.90([H^+] = 120 \, nEq/l), Pa_{CO_2} = 5 \times [HCO_3^-];$$

$$pH = 7.00([H^+] = 100 \, nEq/l), Pa_{CO_2} = 4 \times [HCO_3^-];$$

$$pH = 7.20([H^+] = 64 \, nEq/l), Pa_{CO_2} = 2.5 \times [HCO_3^-]$$

$$pH = 7.30([H^+] = 51 \, nEq/l), Pa_{CO_2} = 2 \times [HCO_3^-];$$

$$pH = 7.60([H^+] = 24 \, nEq/l), Pa_{CO_2} = [HCO_3^-].$$

Primary acid–base disorders

There are four primary acid–base disorders.

1   Metabolic acidosis: a reduction in plasma $[HCO_3^-]$, and an increased $[H^+]$.
2   Metabolic alkalosis: an increase in plasma $[HCO_3^-]$, and a reduced $[H^+]$.
3   Respiratory acidosis: a primary increase in Pa_{CO_2}, and an increased $[H^+]$.
4   Respiratory alkalosis: a primary decrease in Pa_{CO_2}, and a reduced $[H^+]$.

It is important to emphasize that the terms acidosis and alkalosis refer to physiological processes which, when present alone, refers to changes in blood $[H^+]$ (acidemia or alkalemia, respectively).

Metabolic acidosis

Metabolic acidosis results whenever HCO_3^- is consumed by $[H^+]$, whether from acid ingestion or endogenous production, as in renal impairment that prevents excretion of the endogenous load. The amount of H^+ generated per day is 10^5-fold greater than the quantity in the ECF. If H^+ is added to the ECF faster than the kidneys excrete it, HCO_3^- destroyed in the buffering process is not completely regenerated, and metabolic acidosis ensures. Metabolic acidosis may also follow significant losses of HCO_3^--rich solutions, such as diarrheal fluids, pancreatic juices, or duodenal drainage. Loss of HCO_3^- reduces the ratio of HCO_3^- to H_2CO_3 and shifts the equilibrium in the direction of higher blood $[H^+]$ (lower pH).

Classification

Metabolic acidosis is subdivided into those presentations in which the anion gap ($Na^+ - [Cl^- + HCO_3^-]$) is increased, and those in which the anion gap remains normal (Table 11.1). The anion gap is normally 12 ± 2 mEq/l, and consists principally of negative charges on proteins, phosphates, sulfates and organic anions. In metabolic acidosis with an elevation of the anion gap, there are two possible clinical scenarios. Either there is overproduction of an organic acid, or underexcretion, due to renal failure. In the former, the addition of a strong acid other than HCl causes the measurable chloride to be replaced by some

Table 11.1 Differential diagnosis of metabolic acidosis

Increased anion gap	Normal anion gap
Diabetic ketoacidosis	Direct loss of HCO_3^-
Lactic acidosis	Gastrointestinal losses:
Alcoholic ketoacidosis	Diarrhea, pancreatic drainage
Starvation	Ileal conduit
Toxins:	Urinary losses:
Salicylates	Proximal renal tubular acidosis
Methanol	Use of acetazolamide
Ethylene glycol	Indirect loss of HCO_3^-
Paraldehyde	Failure of renal new HCO_3^- generation:
Renal failure	low distal nephron H^+ secretion
D-lactic acidosis	low renal NH_4^+ excretion (low GFR,
	hyperkalemia, hypoaldosteronism)
	Recovery phase of diabetic ketoacidosis

unmeasured anion (e.g. lactate, β-hydroxybutyrate). In renal failure, phosphate, sulfate and salts of organic acids cannot be excreted adequately because of diminished glomerular filtration rate. These contribute to the increased anion gap. However, the cause of the acidosis is not overproduction of acid, but rather diminished tubular excretion of acid.

In metabolic acidosis associated with a normal anion gap, there is usually evidence for losses of HCO_3^-. Direct losses of HCO_3^- may occur in the urine (e.g. proximal renal tubular acidosis (RTA)) or from the gastrointestinal tract (e.g. diarrhea). Indirect losses of HCO_3^- occur due to failure of the kidneys to excrete sufficient NH_4^+, and to generate new HCO_3^- (e.g. distal RTA).

Respiratory compensation in metabolic acidosis

When HCO_3^- is lost, the resulting acidemia causes an increase in the depth and, sometimes, the rate of respiration, which removes the trivial quantity of CO_2 produced by the buffering process. This reduces Pa_{CO_2}, tending to restore blood pH towards, but never to, normal. Table 11.2 shows the 95% confidence intervals for Pa_{CO_2} adjustments in humans with uremic metabolic acidosis [4]. For each 1 mM reduction in plasma $[HCO_3^-]$ below 25 mM, expect a reduction in arterial Pa_{CO_2} of 0.6–1.5 mmHg. When the HCO_3^- deficit is severe, Pa_{CO_2} may be reduced to as low as 10 mmHg. Reductions below this level are unusual, since further ventilatory effort increases CO_2 production more than its elimination.

Metabolic alkalosis

Metabolic alkalosis is present when the $[HCO_3^-]$ rises and the $[H^+]$ declines in the ECF. The acute alkalemia that occurs with H^+ losses or HCO_3^- loads will be sustained if there is impaired renal excretion of HCO_3^-. The causes of

Table 11.2 Significance bands for arterial blood P_{CO_2} and hydrogen ion concentration during chronic metabolic acidosis due to uremia

$[HCO_3^-]$ (mEq/l)	Pa_{CO_2} (mmHg[a])	[Hydrogen ion] (nM)	pH
10	18.7–27.3	44.7–65.3	7.35–7.19
11	20.0–28.5	43.4–61.9	7.36–7.21
12	21.2–29.7	42.2–59.1	7.37–7.23
13	22.4–30.9	41.3–56.7	7.38–7.25
14	23.7–32.1	40.4–54.7	7.39–7.26
15	24.9–33.3	39.7–53.0	7.40–7.28
16	26.1–34.5	39.0–51.5	7.41–7.29
17	27.3–35.7	38.4–50.2	7.42–7.30
18	28.5–36.9	37.9–49.0	7.42–7.31
19	29.8–38.1	37.4–48.0	7.43–7.32
20	30.9–39.4	37.0–47.0	7.43–7.33
21	32.1–40.6	36.6–46.2	7.44–7.34

Reprinted, with permission, from ref. 4 courtesy of S. Karger AG, Basel.
[a] 1 mm Hg = ~7 kPascals.

metabolic alkalosis are divided into two groups, based on the mechanisms responsible for maintaining the alkalosis (Table 11.3). In the first group, there is evidence for Cl^- depletion (ECF volume contraction). These disorders are typified by gastric losses of H^+ (as HCl, as in vomiting) or diuretics, and are characterized by low rates of urinary excretion of Cl^- (<10 mM), when diuretics are not acting. Repair of the alkalosis occurs with administration of either NaCl or KCl; non-Cl^--containing supplements are usually ineffective in these patients. In fact, with repair of Cl^- depletion, bicarbonaturia is evident. At least three mechanisms account for this: (1) there is a decrease

Table 11.3   Major causes of metabolic alkalosis

1. Chloride depletion (saline-responsive; ECF volume contraction: urine [Cl⁻] < 10 mM)
   Loss of gastric fluids
   Diuretics
2. Saline-unresponsive (often ECF volume expansion: urine [Cl⁻] > 20 mM)
   Exogenous mineralocorticoids
   Cushing's syndrome
   Primary hyperaldosteronism
   Renal artery stenosis

in glomerular filtration rate with ECF volume contraction, resulting in a decreased filtered load of HCO_3^-; (2) Cl^- depletion increases absolute reabsorption of HCO_3^-; (3) secondary hyperaldosteronism occurs due to volume contraction, resulting in enhanced distal nephron acid excretion. The mechanisms mediating these effects at the tubular cell level are discussed in more detail below.

The second set of disorders maintaining metabolic alkalosis is uncommon, and is often characterized by ECF volume expansion, high urinary [Cl⁻] (>30 mM) and endocrine excess states (usually hyperaldosteronism). Within this group, patients with renovascular disease, Conn's syndrome, or Cushing's syndrome present with hypertension. The maintenance of alkalosis in these disorders is due to mineralocorticoid-induced stimulation of distal nephron acidification, which is partly dependent on sufficient distal Na⁺ delivery. Accordingly, NaCl is ineffective in the treatment of these forms of alkalosis: therapy is directed at the underlying cause. It must be noted that in end-stage renal disease, metabolic alkalosis can be severe: since there is little capacity for renal HCO_3^- excretion, the addition of HCO_3^- to the ECF by ingestion, infusion or endogenous production (vomiting) can result in sustained metabolic alkalosis, with plasma [HCO_3^-] as high as 40 mM.

Respiratory compensation in metabolic alkalosis

Alkalemia inhibits the central respiratory drive. However, the rise in the Pa_{CO_2} is usually modest, because of respiratory stimulation by hypoxia. In metabolic alkalosis, for every 1 mM increase in the plasma [HCO_3^-], expect a 0.6 mmHg increase in Pa_{CO_2}, although the response is variable.

Respiratory acidosis

When blood Pa_{CO_2} rises, H_2CO_3 is formed and buffered by carboxyhemoglobin and plasma proteins. The buffering process results in an increase in the plasma [HCO_3^-], attenuating the fall in blood pH. Nevertheless, in acute respiratory acidosis, of minutes to a few hours duration,

the rise in plasma [HCO_3^-] is small, and blood pH may fall precipitously. However, in chronic respiratory acidosis, HCO_3^- generation by the kidneys is brisk, and blood pH is better defended. Accordingly, in a patient with stable long-standing chronic obstructive pulmonary disease, a Pa_{CO_2} of 70 mmHg might be associated with a plasma [HCO_3^-] of 35 mM, and a blood pH of 7.30. However, the trauma victim, brought to the emergency room with airway obstruction and the same Pa_{CO_2}, may have a plasma [HCO_3^-] of only 28 mM, and therefore a more acidic blood pH of 7.20. Indeed, as shown in Tables 11.4, 11.5 and 11.6, there are experimental human data describing plasma [HCO_3^-] adjustments to respiratory acidosis and alkalosis [5–7]. In acute respiratory acidosis, expect a 1 mM increase in [HCO_3^-] for every 10 mmHg increase in Pa_{CO_2}. In chronic respiratory acidosis the response is more variable. Expect a 3–7 mM increase in [HCO_3^-] for every 10 mmHg rise in Pa_{CO_2}.

Respiratory alkalosis

Respiratory alkalosis is characterized by a low Pa_{CO_2}, which results in an increase in blood pH. The physico-

Table 11.4   Significance bands for plasma hydrogen ion and bicarbonate concentrations during acute hypercapnia in normal humans

Pa_{CO_2} (mmHg (kPa))	[Hydrogen ion] (nM)	pH	[HCO_3^-] (mEq/l)
40 (5.4)	35.7–41.9	7.45–7.38	22.8–26.8
50 (6.8)	43.5–49.5	7.36–7.31	24.1–27.5
60 (8.1)	51.4–57.2	7.29–7.24	25.1–27.9
70 (9.5)	58.8–65.0	7.23–7.19	25.7–28.5
80 (10.8)	66.2–73.0	7.18–7.14	26.2–28.9
90 (12.2)	73.6–81.2	7.13–7.09	26.5–29.2

Reprinted, with permission, from ref. 6.

Table 11.5   Significance bands for plasma hydrogen ion activity and bicarbonate concentrations during chronic hypercapnia in humans

Pa_{CO_2} (mmHg (kPa))	[Hydrogen ion] (nM)	pH	[HCO_3^-] (mEq/l)
40 (5.4)	31–43	7.51–7.37	30.9–22.4
50 (6.8)	34–45	7.47–7.35	35.3–26.8
60 (8.1)	36–47	7.44–7.35	39.5–30.7
70 (9.5)	38–50	7.42–7.30	44.0–33.4
80 (10.8)	41–52	7.39–7.28	47.0–36.5
100 (13.5)	45–58	7.35–7.24	53.5–41.6

Reprinted, with permission, from ref. 7.

Table 11.6 Significance bands for plasma hydrogen ion activities and bicarbonate concentration during acute hypocapnia in humans

Pa_{CO_2} (mmHg (kPa))	[Hydrogen ion] (nM)	pH	[HCO₃⁻] (mEq/l)
45 (6.1)	40.4–46.7	7.39–7.33	24.1–27.9
40 (5.4)	36.7–43.0	7.44–7.37	23.3–27.3
35 (4.7)	33.1–39.4	7.48–7.40	22.2–26.5
30 (4.1)	29.4–35.7	7.53–7.45	21.0–25.6
25 (3.4)	25.7–32.0	7.59–7.49	19.6–24.4
20 (2.7)	22.0–28.3	7.66–7.55	17.7–22.8
15 (2.0)	18.3–24.6	7.74–7.61	15.3–20.5

Reprinted, with permission, from ref. 5.

chemical response is a reduction in plasma [HCO₃⁻]. As with respiratory acidosis, the change in plasma [HCO₃⁻] is modest in acute disorders (for every 10 mmHg reduction in Pa_{CO_2}, expect a 1–3 mM decrease in [HCO₃⁻]), and more significant in chronic disturbances (for every 10 mmHg reduction in Pa_{CO_2}, expect a 5 mM reduction in [HCO₃⁻]), due to renal compensatory mechanisms.

Mixed acid–base disorders

The presence of one acid–base disturbance does not prevent a patient from having another, and, indeed, it is possible to have all four disturbances simultaneously. It should be noted that the adaptive response to a simple acid–base disorder is not a component of a mixed disorder. Rational therapy in such situations requires dissecting the disturbance into its components, determining the etiology of each component, and using this information to decide how much of the correction will occur spontaneously, and how much will require therapeutic intervention.

Diagnosis requires knowledge of appropriate compensation for each uncomplicated disturbance. If the patient exhibits compensation that is inappropriate for the uncomplicated disturbance, the presence of a second acid–base disorder can be inferred. It is apparent that in uncomplicated acid–base disturbances, plasma [HCO₃⁻] and Pa_{CO_2} always move in the same direction.

The magnitude of the compensation that is appropriate for a disorder of a given severity derives from experimental data. Two examples illustrate the use of data shown in Tables 11.2 and 11.5, the former derived from patients with uremic acidosis [4]. First, if a patient has a metabolic acidosis with a plasma [HCO₃⁻] of 15 mM, the finding of a Pa_{CO_2} of 40 mmHg would establish the presence of a superimposed respiratory acidosis (Table 11.2): the finding of a normal Pa_{CO_2} implies the inability to hyperventilate appropriately. Secondly, in a patient with

uncomplicated chronic respiratory acidosis, and a Pa_{CO_2} of 60 mmHg, experimental observations indicate the [HCO₃⁻] concentration should be ~34 mM (range 30.7–39.5 mM). The finding of a plasma [HCO₃⁻] of 42 mM would imply that a metabolic alkalosis is also present.

Renal regulation of acid–base balance

Overview

It has been stressed that the immediate defense against the daily load of non-volatile acid is largely achieved by the extracellular HCO₃⁻ buffer system. It is the kidneys, however, that eliminate this acid in order to maintain acid–base balance. Recent arguments have proposed that the liver, not the kidneys, is the regulator of whole body acid–base balance, based, in part, on observations that amino acid catabolism generates ammonium (NH₄⁺) and HCO₃⁻ in equal amounts, and that hepatic ureagenesis is required to dispose of the HCO₃⁻, whereas the kidney 'passively' eliminates the NH₄⁺, instead of primarily excreting H⁺ [8]. We believe this to be unlikely, since renal metabolism of glutamine to NH₄⁺ leads to a 1:1 generation of new HCO₃⁻ (see below). Furthermore, as detailed in Chapter 26 many clinical disorders, accompanied by impaired renal ammoniagenesis and tubular dysfunction without liver disease, are associated with metabolic acidosis.

The kidneys influence acid–base balance by regulating two processes: (1) tubular reabsorption of filtered HCO₃⁻; and (2) generation of new HCO₃⁻. The net excretion of H⁺ depends on two separate mechanisms. First, H⁺ can be excreted in combination with fixed urinary buffers, as titratable acids. Phosphate is the major buffer of this category. Buffering of urinary phosphate contributes importantly to net acid excretion, but is somewhat limited since, (1) phosphate excretion cannot be substantially increased, and (2) the pKa of phosphate is 6.8, and, therefore, 90% of its buffer capacity is consumed before the urine pH decreases to 5.7. A second, and more important, mechanism for H⁺ excretion is the renal production and excretion of NH₄⁺. This accounts for most net acid excretion by the kidneys, defined as the sum of titratable acid plus NH₄⁺, minus the small amount of HCO₃⁻ that escapes into the urine. Our discussion begins with mechanisms and regulation of renal ammoniagenesis, followed by a segment-by-segment analysis of HCO₃⁻ handling along the nephron.

Renal ammoniagenesis and excretion

Physiology

In the past decade, exciting developments from the laboratories of Halperin [9], Knepper [10], Tannen [11], and others have defined the mechanisms and regulation of renal NH_4^+ transport. Circulating levels of NH_4^+ are extremely low. Most NH_4^+ in final urine is derived from synthesis in the proximal tubule as a result of metabolism of amino acids, mainly glutamine. Entry of blood-derived glutamine into mitochondria of proximal tubule cells is the critical rate-determining step in the renal production of NH_4^+ [11]. Within mitochondria, glutamine is deamidated by the enzyme phosphate-dependent glutaminase and then deaminated by glutamate deaminase, resulting in net production of two NH_4^+ ions and the divalent anion, α-ketoglutarate. Generation of HCO_3^- occurs when α-ketoglutarate is metabolized in the citric acid cycle or utilized in gluconeogenesis. If the synthesized NH_4^+ were not excreted into the urine, no net change in acid–base balance would ensue, since NH_4^+ would enter the circulation, and release H^+ within the liver during ureagenesis. HCO_3^- consumed by buffering of H^+ would equal the amount of newly generated renal HCO_3^-, resulting in a zero net gain [9].

How does NH_4^+ exit the proximal tubule cell? Elegant studies indicate that NH_4^+ can replace H^+ on the apical membrane Na^+-H^+ exchanger and leave the cell in exchange for Na^+ entry [12]. Alternatively, if transmembrane concentration gradients and permeability are sufficient, ammonia (NH_3) may leave the cell by nonionic diffusion, combining with H^+ in the lumen. NH_4^+ secreted into the lumen is carried to the thick ascending limb of the loop of Henle (TAL), where it is reabsorbed actively. It substitutes for K^+ on the apical membrane Na^+-K^+-$2Cl^-$ co-transporter. In addition, NH_4^+ may enter TAL cells through apical K^+ channels or a paracellular pathway, driven by the lumen-positive potential [10]. NH_4^+ reabsorbed in the TAL leaves cells at the basolateral membrane and accumulates in the interstitium of the medulla.

A corticomedullary gradient exists for NH_4^+, with high concentrations in the medulla, and NH_4^+ accumulates in the medulla by countercurrent multiplication between the two limbs of Henle's loop, similar to the process for medullary accumulation of NaCl. This requires that NH_4^+ be actively reabsorbed by the TAL, and enter the thin descending limb of the loop of Henle, thus creating a cycling pathway between both limbs [10] (Figure 11.1). Parallel H^+ and NH_3 secretion account for NH_4^+ movement into thin descending limbs. NH_4^+ in the medulla is transformed into NH_3 because of the relatively alkaline milieu of the interstitium, where HCO_3^- is concentrated and CO_2 is shunted away. Accordingly, at the medullary tip, NH_4^+ readily becomes NH_3 after deprotonation, and is poised to diffuse into collecting ducts. If collecting duct H^+ secretion is active, i.e. if H^+ transporters (H^+-ATPase, H^+,K^+-ATPase, Cl^-/HCO_3^- exchanger) are intact and functioning to raise luminal H^+ concentration, creating an acid 'sink', NH_3 will continue to diffuse into collecting duct urine, allowing the excretion of large amounts of NH_4^+, and, hence, net acid. Indeed, the handling of renal transport

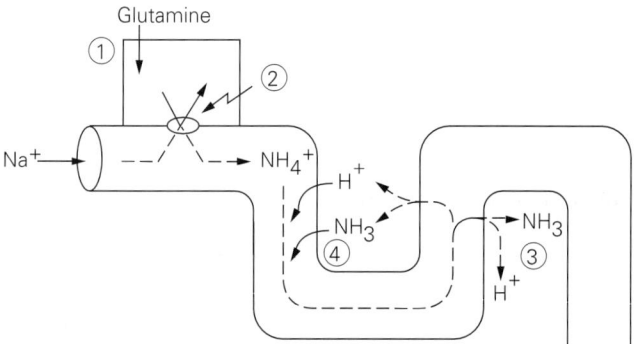

Figure 11.1 Generation of high $[NH_3]$ in the medullary interstitium. There are four steps: (1) production of NH_4^+ in proximal tubule cells; (2) secretion of NH_4^+ into the lumen of the proximal tubule via the Na^+-H^+ antiporter (replacing H^+); (3) reabsorption of NH_4^+ in the thick ascending limb of the loop of Henle via the Na^+-K^+-$2Cl^-$ co-transporter (NH_4^+ replaces K^+); and (4) secretion of NH_4^+ into the descending limb of the loop of Henle together with the operation of a countercurrent system. All these events lead to trapping of NH_3 in the medulla. (Reproduced, with permission, from ref. 3.)

of NH_4^+ represents a remarkable advance in our understanding of renal acid–base balance.

Regulation

This section briefly reviews the major physiological and pathophysiological conditions known to modulate NH_4^+ excretion.

Proximal tubular flow rate

Nagami and Kurokawa [13] have shown that increases in luminal flow rate are associated with enhanced NH_3 production. The mechanism for this is unknown, but may be important in adaptive increases in NH_3 generation in chronic renal failure, in which surviving nephrons have high flow rates.

Acute acidosis

Acute (<2 h) metabolic or respiratory acidosis increases proximal tubule NH_3 production. A low pH *in vitro*, whether produced by changes in $[HCO_3^-]$ or in $P\text{a}CO_2$, increases NH_3 production. It appears that the stimulatory effect of acidosis is mediated by a reduction in intracellular pH in proximal tubule cells. There are three mechanisms for enhanced NH_3 formation: (1) low pH stimulates glutamine transport into submitochondrial particles; (2) flux through the glutamate deaminase pathway to α-ketoglutarate is increased at low pH [11]; and (3) the severity of acidosis is also important; in LLC-PK$_1$ cells at pH 6.8, increased flux through mitochondrial phosphate-dependent glutaminase contributes to stimulation of NH_3 synthesis [14].

Chronic acidosis

In chronic metabolic acidosis, proximal tubule NH_3 production is stimulated, due to increased renal glutamine extraction, transport and activity of phosphate-dependent glutaminase. In chronic respiratory acidosis, increases in urinary NH_4^+ excretion occur in dogs [15]. In contrast, Tannen and colleagues were unable to demonstrate an increase in renal capacity to augment NH_3 production in rats with chronic respiratory acidosis [16]. These investigators suggest that respiratory acidosis stimulates NH_4^+ excretion by a direct effect of low pH on ammoniagenesis. When plasma $[HCO_3^-]$ has increased to a new steady state (i.e. the chronic phase), increased renal acid excretion is not required to sustain a stable $[HCO_3^-]$. Instead, proximal tubule ammoniagenesis returns to basal levels due to maintenance of intracellular pH by the increased filtered load of HCO_3^- and resultant stimulation of luminal Na^+-H^+ exchange.

In rats subjected to dietary acid loads or to water deprivation, the corticomedullary NH_4^+ gradient increases, consistent with expected changes in urinary NH_4^+ concentrations, supporting the important role for countercurrent multiplication of NH_4^+ in acid excretion [17].

Alkalosis

In experimental animals, HCO_3^- infusion or acute respiratory alkalosis reduces renal NH_3 generation. This effect is not simply the converse of the immediate stimulatory effect of acute acidosis; a lag phase of ~45 min is required.

K^+ balance

In chronic metabolic alkalosis, the effects of hypokalemia on ammoniagenesis must be considered in the compensatory response. Proximal tubule NH_3 production is stimulated by K^+ deficiency, and proximal tubule segments *in vitro* significantly increase NH_3 formation in the presence of low extracellular K^+ [18]. Thus, the effect of K^+ deficiency may be mediated directly by K^+ ion, although it is postulated that development of low intracellular pH plays a dominant role.

In conditions of decreases in glomerular filtration rate, aldosterone levels, or extracellular buffering capacity, hyperkalemia may contribute to development of metabolic acidosis via inhibition of renal NH_3 synthesis. This may contribute to the acidosis of hyporeninemic hypoaldosteronism. In addition, hyperkalemia may impair renal NH_4^+ excretion by increasing K^+ levels in the lumen of the loop of Henle, with competition for transport on the apical Na^+-K^+-$2Cl^-$ co-transporter. It is of interest that patients with chronic respiratory acidosis who develop hyperkalemia are unable to generate the expected increase in plasma $[HCO_3^-]$ [19].

Hormones/cellular signaling pathways

Hormones which increase cellular cAMP levels (e.g. parathyroid hormone (PTH)) stimulate proximal tubule ammoniagenesis. Insulin and growth hormone also increase NH_3 production. Interestingly, angiotensin II stimulates proximal ammoniagenesis in a calcium-calmodulin-dependent fashion. In contrast, physiological concentrations of angiotensin II inhibit net luminal secretion of NH_3.

Prostaglandins (PGs) are negative feedback modulators of renal NH_3 formation. Acute metabolic and acute respiratory acidosis are associated with enhanced urinary excretion of PGE_2 and $PGF_{2\alpha}$. In the isolated perfused rat kidney, renal cortical tubules, and LLC-PK_1 renal epithelial cells, $PGF_{2\alpha}$ has been implicated as an inhibitor of the ammoniagenic response to acidosis [11].

Renal ammoniagenesis and NH_4^+ excretion are impaired in adrenal insufficiency, as is renal net acid excretion in adrenalectomized rats. Furthermore, administration of glucocorticoids or aldosterone to intact animals increases NH_4^+ excretion. However, in adrenalectomized animals, the adaptive increase in ammoniagenesis in reponse to metabolic acidosis is still observed, indicating that adrenal hormones 'permit' rather than directly stimulate renal NH_3 production. It has been postulated that corticosteroids increase NH_3 formation by inhibiting renal prostaglandin synthesis [11].

Nephron loss

In chronic renal failure, as nephrons are progressively lost, surviving nephrons adapt by increasing ammoniagenesis. The stimulus for increased nephron NH_3 production is unclear, but may be directly related to dietary protein intake. As a consequence, acid excretion per nephron is increased, until glomerular filtration rate is severely decreased, when individual proximal tubular cells can no longer augment NH_3 synthesis to maintain normal acid–base balance. Metabolic acidosis ensues, further stimulating NH_3 generation per nephron. There is also evidence that metabolic pathways for NH_3 synthesis are impaired: in patients with chronic renal failure, oral glutamine loading does not enhance urinary NH_4^+ excretion, as it does in normal subjects with or without metabolic acidosis.

It is interesting that in rats with remnant kidneys, dietary administration of $NaHCO_3$ blunts the development of renal tubulointerstitial injury and decreases urinary NH_4^+ excretion [20]. Since NH_4^+ can activate the alternate pathway for complement, it has been postulated that increased renal NH_4^+ concentrations might mediate accelerated tubulointerstitial injury in chronic renal disease.

Proximal tubule reabsorption of HCO₃⁻

Overview

In addition to its vital role in renal ammoniagenesis, the proximal tubule also begins the process of reclamation of the ~4500 mmol of HCO₃⁻ normally filtered daily. Here (mainly in the proximal convoluted segment) bulk HCO₃⁻ transport occurs, which accounts for 70–85% of reabsorption of filtered HCO₃⁻. Remarkably, this large movement of HCO₃⁻ is tightly regulated in response to systemic acid–base, electrolyte and renal disturbances. Regulation involves changes in the kinetics and numbers of ion transporters mediating net HCO₃⁻ movement. Defects in the function of one or more of these transporters may be responsible for disorders of proximal RTA (see below), characterized by inadequate HCO₃⁻ reabsorption by this segment, and metabolic acidosis.

The proximal tubule is a leaky epithelium with very low paracellular electrical resistance, implying that tight junctions between cells are highly permeable to ions. Indeed, the transepithelial membrane potential does not contribute importantly to net H⁺ movement in this segment. Ion transporters on either apical or basolateral membranes mediate net HCO₃⁻ reabsorption. Of these, three are of critical importance to H⁺/HCO₃⁻ transport: (1) the apical Na⁺-H⁺ exchanger; (2) the apical vacuolar-type H⁺-ATPase (H⁺ pump); and (3) the basolateral Na⁺-3HCO₃⁻ co-transporter. The apical Na⁺-H⁺ exchanger, accounting for 65% of net HCO₃⁻ reabsorption, operates via secondary active transport. The energy required for H⁺ secretion into the tubular lumen is derived from the activity of the basolateral membrane Na⁺,K⁺-ATPase, which utilizes ATP to maintain a low intracellular Na⁺ concentration necessary for transcellular Na⁺ transport. A proximal tubule apical H⁺-ATPase pumps H⁺ into the lumen (primary active transport), accounting for most of the remaining 35% of proximal HCO₃⁻ reabsorption. Once HCO₃⁻ is reclaimed within the proximal tubule cell, it exits to the blood side, along with Na⁺, via the basolateral Na⁺-3HCO₃⁻ co-transporter.

Carbonic anhydrase (CA) is an enzyme which catalyzes the rapid conversion of carbonic acid (H_2CO_3) into CO_2 and water or of HCO₃⁻ into OH⁻ and CO_2. In the proximal tubule, an isoenzyme that functions in the presence of chloride, CA type IV, is present on the apical and basolateral membranes, and has functional contact with luminal fluid. The cytoplasm contains CA type II isoenzyme, also found in erythrocytes. Proximal HCO₃⁻ reabsorption is diminished in the presence of CA inhibitors. H⁺ is secreted into the proximal tubule lumen, where it is titrated by luminal HCO₃⁻, followed by conversion to CO_2 and water by luminal CA. CO_2 then passively enters the cell, where it combines with OH⁻ (generated by extrusion of H⁺ at the apical membrane) and is converted into HCO₃⁻ in the presence of cytosolic CA. HCO₃⁻ then exits the cell on the basolateral side (Figure 11.2). Recently, the

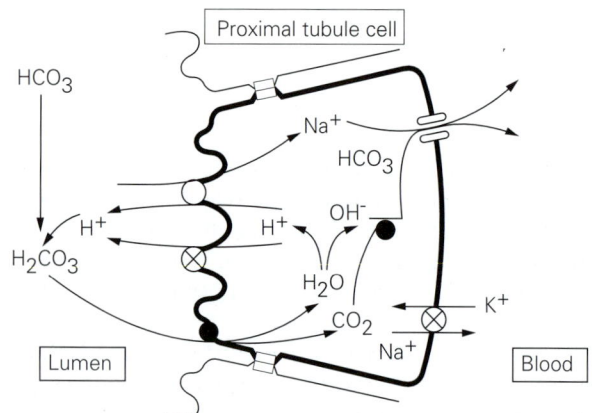

Figure 11.2 Proximal tubule acidification mechanisms. A model of a proximal tubule cell is shown in which H⁺ are secreted into the lumen by apical Na⁺-H⁺ exchanger and H⁺-ATPase. In the luminal fluid, filtered HCO₃⁻ is titrated with the secreted H⁺, forming H_2CO_3. Membrane-bound carbonic anhydrase (CA) catalyzes formation of CO_2 and H_2O. The CO_2 diffuses into the cell, where HCO₃⁻ is reconstituted for transport across the basolateral membrane via the Na⁺-3HCO₃⁻ co-transporter. An electrochemical gradient for Na⁺ entry at the luminal membrane is maintained by action of the basolateral Na⁺,K⁺-ATPase.

activities of both proximal tubule CA II and CA IV were shown to be increased in rabbits with chronic metabolic acidosis [21]. Finally, it is important to note that HCO₃⁻ is not directly reabsorbed at the apical membrane; rather, H⁺ secretion accounts for net HCO₃⁻ transport. The function and regulation of the three ion transporters accounting for most of transcellular transport of HCO₃⁻ in proximal tubule (apical Na⁺-H⁺ exchanger, apical H⁺-ATPase, and basolateral Na⁺-3HCO₃⁻ co-transporter) will be reviewed in the following sections, with emphasis on the Na⁺-H⁺ exchanger.

Apical Na⁺-H⁺ exchange

The proximal tubule apical membrane contains an electroneutral Na⁺-H⁺ exchanger, which permits one Na⁺ ion to enter the cell for every H⁺ secreted into the lumen (Figure 11.2). Although most mammalian cells possess a growth factor-activated Na⁺-H⁺ exchanger in the plasma membrane which serves to maintain intracellular pH and cell volume (a 'housekeeping' function), the apical Na⁺-H⁺ exchanger differs from this ubiquitous antiporter in several respects. Recent cloning of mammalian Na⁺-H⁺ exchangers reveals that at least four isoforms exist, referred to as NHE-1, NHE-2, NHE-3, and NHE-4 [22]. These single-chain polypeptide proteins have 10 hydrophobic transmembrane spanning domains, with significant amino acid homology, and long cytoplasmic tails that may serve as regulatory regions. By immunofluorescence, it has been shown that the 'housekeeping' antiporter (NHE-1), a protein of 95–110 kDa, is present in abundance within the rabbit kidney on basolateral membranes of proximal tubule, thick ascending limb, and distal convoluted tubule cells [23]. It is noteworthy that functional basolateral Na^+-H^+ exchange activity is largely absent in proximal tubule, except in the S3 segment, but is present in the S1 and S2 segments of juxtamedullary nephrons. In contrast, proximal tubule brush border membranes stain intensely for the 80 kDa NHE-3 isoform [24]. In contrast to the amiloride-sensitive NHE-1, the NHE-3 isoform is found only in kidney and intestine, both sites of Na^+ reabsorption, and is relatively resistant to inhibition by amiloride ($K_i \sim 10$–$50 \mu M$). This suggests that NHE-3 represents the apical Na^+-H^+ exchanger of proximal tubule. However, more than one isoform may exist on the apical surface.

Among properties of the apical Na^+-H^+ exchanger, the most important is that it is capable of operating as an Na^+-Na^+, Li^+-H^+ or Na^+-NH_4^+ exchanger. As noted above, this is a critical mechanism for NH_4^+ secretion by the proximal tubule. Although the exchanger can function in the reverse direction (Na^+ out/H^+ in), the gradients in physiological conditions ensure that it operates to carry an Na^+ ion into the cell in exchange for H^+. Consequently, this antiporter accounts for the majority of both Na^+ and HCO_3^- transport into the proximal tubule cell.

Regulators of proximal Na^+-H^+ exchange

Load dependence

The early proximal tubule readily increases HCO_3^- reabsorption in response to an increased filtered load of HCO_3^- ($FL_{HCO_3^-}$). The reverse is true with reductions in $FL_{HCO_3^-}$. Load dependence has been postulated to explain these changes in proximal HCO_3^- reabsorption. As noted below, however, these conditions may alter the number of apical Na^+-H^+ exchangers present in the apical membrane, independent of $FL_{HCO_3^-}$.

pH and osmolality

The activity of apical Na^+-H^+ exchange is highly sensitive to changes in intracellular pH. A site on the cytoplasmic face is allosterically modified by H^+, such that intracellular acidosis activates antiporter activity to a greater extent than an increased H^+ transmembrane concentration gradient alone [25]. The degree to which this mechanism regulates Na^+-H^+ exchange activity during states of acute or chronic acidosis is unclear. In metabolic acidosis, the reduction in $FL_{HCO_3^-}$ is likely to offset the rise in HCO_3^- reabsorption due to any activation of the exchanger by cytoplasmic H^+. Reduction in cytoplasmic H^+ with HCO_3^- loads, however, may facilitate urinary HCO_3^- excretion in the face of increased $FL_{HCO_3^-}$, by reducing Na^+-H^+ exchanger-mediated HCO_3^- retrieval.

It is noteworthy that whereas NHE-1 activity is stimulated by osmotic cell shrinkage, a provocative *in vitro* study indicated that NHE-3 activity in proximal tubule cells was decreased by exposure to increased osmolality (510 mosmol/l), induced by mannitol or NaCl [26]. Although the proximal tubule is not normally exposed to this elevated osmolality *in vivo*, it is interesting to speculate that this unique feature of NHE-3 might contribute to the impaired urinary acidification in advanced renal failure or with elevations of blood glucose concentration, where there are increases in luminal urea and glucose concentrations.

Hormones and intracellular second messengers

Various hormones, including angiotensin II, glucocorticoids, thyroid hormone, catecholamines and endothelin, activate apical Na^+-H^+ exchange, via binding to receptors on proximal tubule cells [27]. Angiotensin II may exert the strongest regulatory effect. The proximal tubule is capable of endogenous angiotensin II synthesis, with nanomolar levels reported in proximal tubular fluid. It is estimated from *in vivo* microperfusion studies that angiotensin II could modulate 15–30% of all Na^+ and HCO_3^- handling by the proximal tubule [28].

Several hormones appear to activate the exchanger by decreasing intracellular cAMP, causing a reduction in cAMP-dependent protein kinase-induced inhibition of the antiporter. Activation of protein kinase C has been reported to either inhibit or stimulate the antiporter [27]. In contrast, PTH exerts a potent inhibitory effect on apical Na^+-H^+ exchange, mediated at least in part by increases in cellular cAMP levels.

Pathophysiologic states: adaptive responses

Acid–base status   Acute respiratory acidosis, associated with Pa_{CO_2} as high as 120 mmHg, has no effect on absolute net reabsorption of HCO_3^- in rat proximal tubule, without HCO_3^- loading. In contrast, several studies have shown that chronic acid feeding or chronic respiratory acidosis enhances HCO_3^- reabsorption by the proximal tubule [29–31], due to an increase in the number of apical Na^+-H^+ exchangers (increased V_{max} of transport). Chronic alkalosis reduces proximal HCO_3^- reabsorption. Incubation of proximal tubule cell lines in culture in acid medium (either by increase in P_{CO_2} or decrease in HCO_3^-) increases apical Na^+-H^+ exchange activity, and messenger RNA (mRNA) expression of the NHE-3 isoform [27]. In contrast, metabolic, but not respiratory acidosis increases mRNA levels for the 'housekeeping' NHE-1 isoform [32]. The cellular mechanisms mediating these adaptive changes are poorly understood: long-term activation of protein kinase C may be involved in chronic metabolic acidosis, and glucocorticoids have been implicated in inducing the increase in Na^+-H^+ exchange in chronic respiratory acidosis.

Chronic hyperfiltration (uninephrectomy, nephron ablation, protein feeding, diabetes mellitus) With increases in glomerular filtration rate, the filtered load of HCO_3^- increases, and tubular reabsorption of HCO_3^- must increase to prevent bicarbonaturia. Independent of $FL_{HCO_3^-}$, luminal flow appears to augment HCO_3^- reabsorption. In addition to load-dependent increases in HCO_3^- reabsorption, apical Na^+-H^+ exchange activity is enhanced, via an increase in antiporter V_{max}. These adaptive changes accompany the proximal tubule hypertrophy that occurs in remnant kidney studies.

K+ depletion In K^+-depleted rats, KCl infusions do not alter absolute proximal tubule HCO_3^- reabsorption, indicating that K^+ itself does not alter HCO_3^- transport [33]. However, experimental K^+ depletion is associated with enhanced activity of proximal brush border Na^+-H^+ exchange. The mediators of this response are unknown. Although intracellular pH may decline with K^+ depletion, this does not account for the increase in antiporter V_{max} in this situation.

ATP depletion and phosphate deficiency Cellular ATP depletion or inorganic phosphate deficiency causes dramatic reductions in apical Na^+-H^+ exchange, due to decreased V_{max}. The contribution of this effect to the metabolic acidosis in states of ischemic/toxic tubular damage is unknown.

Apical H+-ATPase

Besides the Na^+-H^+ exchanger, the proximal tubule apical membrane also contains a vacuolar type H^+-ATPase pump, sensitive to inhibition by the macrolide antibiotic, bafilomycin A1. The subunit composition of the proximal tubule H^+-ATPase may differ from that in distal nephron segments. Luminal H^+ secretion by this pump contributes up to ~20–35% of proximal tubule HCO_3^- reabsorption, and utilizes a considerable fraction of cell energy stores.

The regulation of this H^+-ATPase in pathophysiological states is incompletely understood. In rats with chronic metabolic acidosis, an adaptive increase in proximal tubule H^+-ATPase activity has been reported [34].

Basolateral Na+-3HCO3− co-transporter

The remarkable amounts of HCO_3^- transported into the proximal tubule cell leave it by passive transport mechanisms, mainly via an Na^+-$3HCO_3^-$ co-transporter on the basolateral membrane. *In vitro* assays in proximal tubule cells reveal that this transporter is electrogenic: it transfers three bicarbonate ions for every sodium ion, resulting in a net transfer of two negative charges. It is sensitive to inhibition by disulfonic stilbene derivatives (e.g. 4′-isothiocyanostilbene-2,2′-disulfonic acid, 4,4′-diisothiocyanostilbene-2,2′-disulfonic acid). The transporter also accepts a divalent carbonate anion (CO_3^{2-}) as substrate.

Regulation of the Na^+-$3HCO_3^-$ co-transporter is complex. The pH sensitivity has been studied: optimal transport occurs at pH 7.00–7.40, with less activity at lower or higher pH [34]. The pH sensitivity appears to reside on the cytoplasmic side of the protein.

Angiotensin II stimulates the co-transporter, which accounts for the transcellular movement of HCO_3^- mediated by this hormone. Although the cellular regulatory signals are unclear, one study revealed that decreases in intracellular cAMP, induced by adenosine, stimulated basolateral Na^+-$3HCO_3^-$ co-transport [35].

Chronic acid feeding and chronic respiratory acidosis enhance co-transporter activity. This effect may be mediated by insertion of co-transporters into the basolateral membrane. Interestingly, incubation of rabbit proximal tubules at acidic pH increases the V_{max} of Na^+-$3HCO_3^-$ co-transport [31]. As with apical Na^+-H^+ exchange, increased activity of basolateral Na^+-HCO_3^- co-transport occurs with glomerular hyperfiltration and K^+ depletion.

Other transporters in proximal tubule acidification

The three ion transporters described above account for most transcellular HCO_3^- movement in the proximal tubule. The apical membrane also contains Cl-OH and Cl-formate exchangers, and the basolateral membrane has Na^+-dependent and -independent Cl^-/HCO_3^- exchangers. These transporters likely contribute to transcellular NaCl reabsorption, rather than to acid–base balance. A theoretical role exists for tertiary active H^+ extrusion into the lumen, mediated by apical Na^+-anion co-transporters.

Loop of Henle

The role of the loop of Henle in acid–base balance has been firmly established by micropuncture studies [36]. Approximately 15% of filtered HCO_3^- is reabsorbed in this segment, mainly via a carbonic anhydrase-sensitive mechanism of apical Na^+-H^+ exchange. There is also evidence for electrogenic H^+ secretion by an H^+-ATPase. As in the proximal tubule, a basolateral Na^+-$3HCO_3^-$ co-transporter is present. In addition to reabsorption of HCO_3^-, the loop of Henle plays an important role in reabsorption of NH_4^+, via the apical Na^+-K^+-$2Cl^-$ cotransporter.

HCO_3^- reabsorption in the loop of Henle is regulated by several factors. Acute and chronic metabolic acidosis increase HCO_3^- transport, whereas acute metabolic alkalosis reduces HCO_3^- reabsorption [37]. Angiotensin II, glucocorticoids, and aldosterone all stimulate HCO_3^- transport in the loop of Henle. In contrast, increases in dietary sodium intake increase HCO_3^- reabsorption in the thick ascending limb [37]. This may represent an adaptive response, since angiotensin II and aldosterone are reduced by high sodium intake, which would lead to decreased reabsorption of HCO_3^- by the proximal tubule and Henle's loop, and decreased H^+ secretion in the cortical collecting duct. The thick ascending limb is stimulated under these conditions to reabsorb the HCO_3^- that escaped reabsorption by the proximal tubule.

Distal tubule and collecting tubule

Overview

Final regulation of acid–base balance occurs in the distal tubule and collecting tubule (DT-CT). HCO_3^- which has escaped reabsorption proximally (normally delivered to the distal tubule at concentrations of 5–7 mM) is reabsorbed in this segment. In addition, net H^+ secretion occurs; indeed, distal tubule H^+ secretion exceeds the amount of filtered HCO_3^-. H^+ is titrated mainly by tubular fluid phosphate and NH_3, and the process restores HCO_3^- that has been consumed by daily metabolic acid generation. Recent technological advances have led to more precise definition of acidification disorders in this part of the nephron, based on molecular identification of specific transporters. The most important of these is the H^+-ATPase, which accounts for most, if not all, of distal H^+ secretion [38].

The DT-CT is composed of several morphologically distinct segments, which differ in their capacities for net H^+ secretion. The DT-CT consists of a 'tight' epithelial barrier, capable of generating steep pH (urine pH < 4.5 vs blood pH 7.4) and electrical gradients. This feature, as well as the capacity for precise regulation of H^+ secretion, accounts for the overall importance of the DT-CT in acid–base balance. The first part of the DT-CT, the distal tubule, is composed of the distal convoluted tubule (DCT), the connecting segment, and the initial collecting tubule. In early distal tubule, apical Na^+-H^+ exchange appears to mediate most HCO_3^- reabsorption. Studies indicate that the DCT may account for up to 10% of renal HCO_3^- reabsorption under physiologic conditions; this segment may also mediate net HCO_3^- secretion, depending on dietary intake. The cortical collecting tubule (CCT) begins where individual connecting tubules join to form a collecting tubule, and is also capable of HCO_3^- reabsorption and secretion. In contrast, the final segments, the outer medullary collecting tubule (OMCT) and papillary (inner medullary) collecting tubule (IMCT), are only able to reabsorb HCO_3^-.

Renal tubule cells involved in distal HCO_3^- transport

Intercalated cells, constituting 40% of the cells in the DT-CT, are rich in carbonic anhydrase, and mediate transcellular HCO_3^- transport (Figure 11.3). In the connecting tubule and cortical collecting tubule, there are two func-

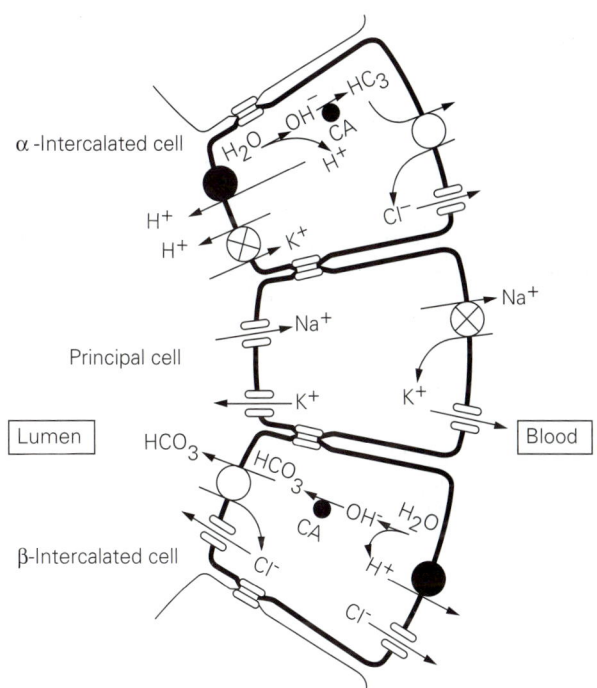

Figure 11.3 Acidification in the distal tubule. The three cell types of the distal tubule are shown. The apical surface of the α-intercalated cell contains the H^+-ATPase pump, and the basolateral surface has the Cl^-/HCO_3^- (band 3) exchanger. The dissociation of H_2O provides an H^+ that is pumped into the distal lumen by H^+-ATPase. Cytosolic carbonic anhydrase (CA) combines CO_2 with the remaining OH^- to form HCO_3^-, which exits the cell via basolateral band 3. β-intercalated cells function similarly, but in the reverse direction. Both cell types have basolateral Cl^- channels for recirculation of Cl^-: α-intercalated cells have apical H^+,K^+-ATPase pumps for secretion of H^+ in exchange for K^+ entry. In principal cells, the basolateral Na^+,K^+-ATPase provides the driving force for luminal Na^+ entry through amiloride-sensitive Na^+ channels. Na^+ transport produces a negative luminal voltage, which favors H^+ secretion by the α-intercalated cells. (Adapted, with permission, from ref. 39.)

tionally distinct types of intercalated cells. The α-intercalated cells have H^+ pumps located primarily in the luminal membrane or in subapical vesicles. Luminal membrane insertion of these pumps mediates H^+ secretion into the urine. This generates intracellular HCO_3^-, followed by HCO_3^- exit via a basolateral Cl^-/HCO_3^- exchanger. The latter is similar in structure and function to the erythrocyte band 3 anion exchanger, and is sensitive to stilbene derivatives. Thus, this cell stains with antibodies to H^+-ATPase on the luminal membrane, and with antibodies for band 3 protein on the basolateral membrane (Figure 11.4). The α-intercalated cell mediates HCO_3^- reabsorption.

β-Intercalated cells constitute the remaining 60% of intercalated cells in DT-CT, and are poised for HCO_3^- secretion. H^+ pumps are found predominantly in the cyto-

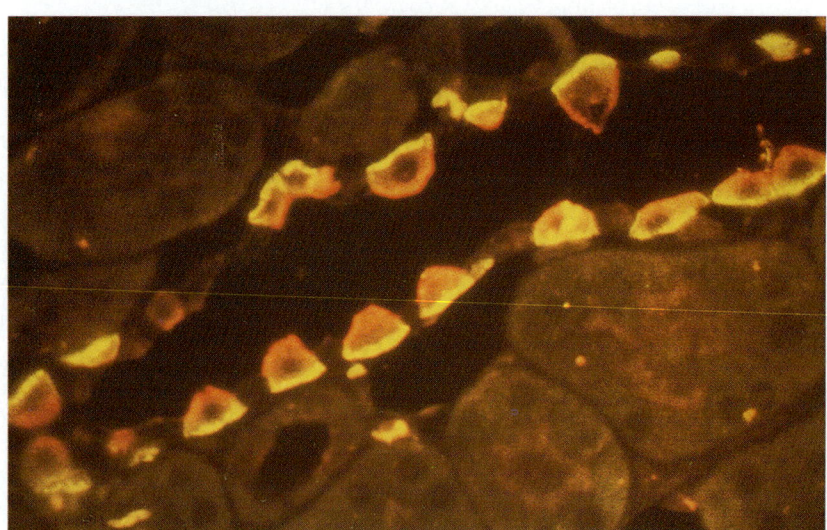

Figure 11.4 Double antibody labeling of rat medullary collecting duct α-intercalated cells. H+-ATPase labeled with rhodamine (orange), band 3 labeled with fluorescein (yellow). Photograph courtesy of Drs D. Brown, S. Gluck, and S. Alper.

plasm or basolateral membrane, and a Cl^-/HCO_3^- exchanger is present on the luminal surface. H^+ pumping across the basolateral membrane generates intracellular HCO_3^-, which is secreted into the urine in exchange for Cl^- at the apical membrane. In contrast to the basolateral Cl^-/HCO_3^- exchanger of α-intercalated cells, the luminal Cl^-/HCO_3^- exchanger in β-cells is antigenically different from the band 3 protein of erythrocytes, and is not inhibited by stilbenes. Thus, the β-intercalated cell is morphologically and functionally the reverse of the α-intercalated cell. In *in vivo* animal studies, net HCO_3^- secretion can be demonstrated with alkali loading, and is inhibited with low luminal chloride [40].

The OMCT has the highest H^+ secretory capacity of any DT-CT segment. This segment has α-intercalated cells but lacks β-intercalated cells. The papillary collecting tubule has intercalated cells only in its proximal one-third. In this segment, HCO_3^- reabsorption occurs via an apical H^+-ATPase [38].

The DT-CT also contains principal cells, primarily involved in Na^+ and water reabsorption and K^+ secretion. Principal cells are not directly involved in acid–base balance. The basolateral Na^+,K^+-ATPase in these cells provides a driving force for apical Na^+ influx, however, which generates a lumen-negative voltage that favors H^+ secretion by H^+ pumps of α-intercalated cells. Inhibitors of Na^+ transport (e.g. amiloride, triamterene, lithium) or deficiency of aldosterone may inhibit H^+ secretion by preventing development of this lumen-negative voltage.

Distal acid–base transporters

H+-ATPase

Pioneering studies by Gluck [41], Brown [42], and others have revealed the importance of the kidney H^+-ATPase in acid–base balance. This section focuses on recent developments on the properties and regulation of this transporter.

Properties

A large (~580 kDa), vacuolar H^+-ATPase, inhibited by *N*-ethylmaleimide (NEM) and bafilomycin A1, has been isolated from the bovine renal medulla [41]. This enzyme is closely related to the vacuolar H^+-ATPases mediating acidification of intracellular vesicles and lysosomes.

Like other vacuolar H^+-ATPases, it is a multimeric protein, with 10 subunits. The genes encoding several of these subunits have been cloned and sequenced. The 31-, 56- and 70-kDa subunits are located on the cytoplasmic surface of the cell membrane, where they form a stud-like structure that projects ~10 nm from the plasma membrane (Figure 11.5). It has been proposed that the 56- and 70-kDa subunits are attached to the plasma membrane via a 31-kDa subunit, that links them to a 16-kDa transmembrane subunit, which is the putative H^+-conducting channel. The 70-kDa subunit appears to be the site of ATP binding and hydrolysis.

By immunohistochemistry, vacuolar H^+-ATPase has been detected in the proximal tubule, thick ascending limb, connecting tubule, and cortical and medullary collecting tubules. cDNA cloning has revealed two isoforms of the 56-kDa subunit, encoded by different genes. One isoform is found in the brain, the other in the kidney, in intercalated cells only.

Regulation of H+-ATPase

Acid–base disturbances Metabolic acidosis induces changes in the number of H^+-ATPases in the apical membrane of α-intercalated cells. These cells have a reserve of vesicles which contain H^+-ATPase: an increase in H^+ pumps in the luminal membrane occurs by insertion of new membrane. In rat cortical and medullary collecting ducts, chronic acid loading leads to a redistribution of H^+-ATPase from the cytoplasmic vesicles to the apical membrane [43]. Alkali loading results in changes in the opposite direction. Increases in ambient P_{CO_2} stimulate

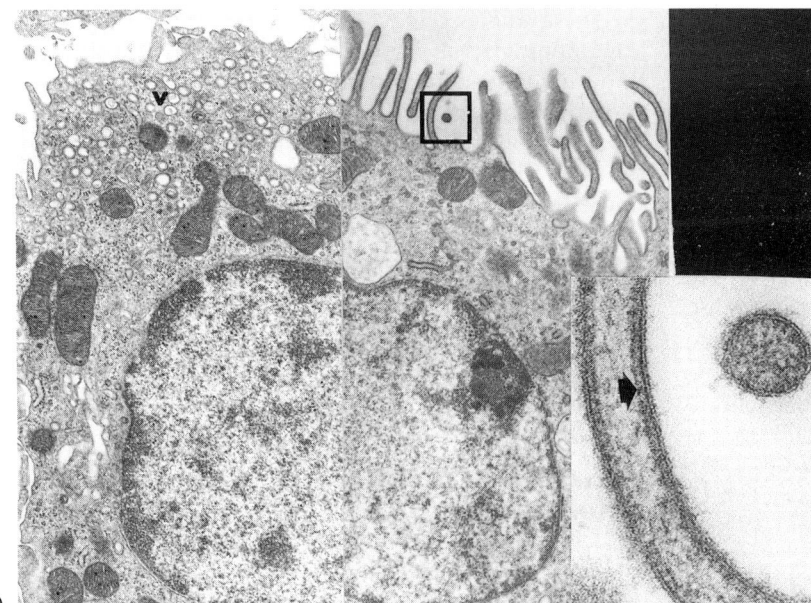

Figure 11.5 (A) Electron micrograph of the H$^+$-ATPase of the α-intercalated cell. An inactive α-intercalated cell is shown on the left, containing few microvilli and many subapical vesicles. On the right is shown an active α-intercalated cell, with dense microvillae and apical studs, representing H$^+$-ATPase (inset). (B) Model of the H$^+$-ATPase from mammalian kidney. The enzymatic part of the H$^+$-ATPase protrudes into the cytoplasm as a spherical head consisting of tightly packed globular subunits. The 70-kDa subunits appear to include the binding sites where hydrolysis of ATP creates the electrochemical gradient for expulsion of H$^+$ through the pump's membranous domain. (Part B is reproduced, with permission, from ref. 38.)

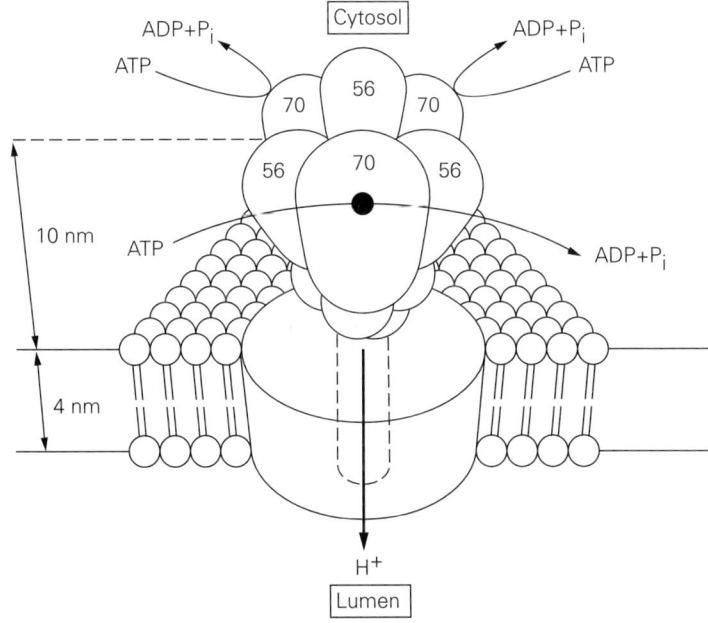

exocytotic fusion of these vesicles to the luminal membrane, thus increasing H$^+$ secretion.

Regulation may be mediated by effects of changes in intracellular pH [38] on enzyme activity, since ATP hydrolysis by isolated kidney H$^+$-ATPase increases with decreasing pH. Regulation of H$^+$ pump activity may involve other cellular proteins. In this regard, a cytosolic heat-labile specific inhibitor [44] and a heat-stable activator [45] of H$^+$-ATPase activity have recently been isolated from the mammalian kidney.

In rats with chronic metabolic acidosis, enhanced net H$^+$ secretion by the IMCT persists despite discontinuation of the acid load or development of alkalosis [46]. This contrasts with the effects of acute respiratory alkalosis in control rats, in which net acid secretion by the IMCT is completely suppressed. Thus, it appears that shuttling of cytosolic H$^+$-ATPase-containing vesicles to the luminal plasma membrane provides a new set point in response to acid–base disturbances, and maintains a long-term, adaptive 'memory' effect.

Luminal factors As noted above, factors that increase luminal negativity enhance H$^+$ secretion. These include Na$^+$ delivery, Na$^+$ reabsorption (largely controlled by aldosterone), drugs inhibiting Na$^+$ entry or non-permeant anions (e.g. bicarbonate, and drugs such as ticarcillin and carbenicillin). Aldosterone also directly increases H$^+$-ATPase activity [38]. The availability to NH$_3$ and phosphate to buffer secreted H$^+$ is also critical, since further H$^+$ secretion would come to a halt in their absence.

The Cl⁻/HCO₃⁻ exchanger

The erythrocyte Cl^-/HCO_3^- exchanger, red cell band 3 (AE-1), is the prototypic member of the anion exchanger gene family, which includes the genes AE-2 and AE-3 [47]. The band 3 exchanger is a protein of molecular weight 100 kDa, and has 14 putative hydrophobic membrane-spanning domains. Within the kidney, AE-1 expression is restricted to the basolateral surface of α-intercalated cells, as detected by immunohistochemistry. The mRNA transcripts encode a protein identical to erythroid band 3, differing from erythroid band 3 mRNA in the 5′ upstream sequence only. The nature of the apical Cl^-/HCO_3^- exchanger of β-intercalated cells is unclear. Biochemical studies have localized AE-1 and AE-2 proteins to the epithelial cell apical plasma membrane [47]. However, the apical Cl^-/HCO_3^- exchanger of the β-intercalated cells does not immunostain with antibodies to band 3, indicating that it may be antigenically distinct.

Studies of the regulation of kidney Cl^-/HCO_3^- exchange are in their infancy. In preliminary studies, acute acid loading leads to increased immunostaining of AE-1 in α-intercalated cells, whereas 6-h alkali loading reduces levels [48]. Chronic respiratory acidosis in rats increases kidney AE-1 mRNA levels [49]. Of course, if basolateral AE-1 in α-intercalated cells is up-regulated, this will increase apical H^+ secretion, due to diminished cytoplasmic [HCO_3^-].

In rabbits fed $NaHCO_3$, net HCO_3^- secretion is observed in the isolated cortical collecting tubule [50]. In fed rats, at high chloride loads, distal tubules secrete HCO_3^- *in vivo*. Distal tubules from fasted rats reabsorb HCO_3^- at normal tubular flow rates. The stimulus evoked by feeding is unknown. However, release of hormones (e.g. vasoactive intestinal peptide), which signal via activation of adenylate cyclase, could be important. In this regard, in β-intercalated cells, increases in cyclic AMP stimulate the luminal Cl^-/HCO_3^- exchanger, resulting in increased HCO_3^- secretion [51].

Kidney H⁺,K⁺-ATPase

In the stomach, an H^+,K^+-ATPase exchanger mediates electroneutral H^+ extrusion, in exchange for K^+. Wingo and Cain [52] demonstrated the presence of an antigenically similar membrane-spanning H^+,K^+-ATPase in α-intercalated cells of the kidney. Preliminary studies have localized mRNA for this ATPase to the intercalated cells and principal cells of the connecting segment, cortical and medullary collecting ducts of the outer and inner medulla, by *in situ* hybridization [53]. The mRNA for another H^+,K^+-ATPase species, an isoform found in the colon, has recently been localized to whole kidney [54]. Functional studies have localized H^+,K^+-ATPase activity to cortical and inner medullary collecting duct cells. In animal models, inhibition of the renal H^+,K^+-ATPase decreases urinary acid secretion and K^+ reabsorption [52].

These studies suggest that the renal H^+,K^+-ATPase has an important role in distal acidification. Recent work indicates that expression of the colonic-type H^+,K^+-ATPase isoform found in cortical collecting tubule is up-regulated by metabolic alkalosis [55]. In chronic K^+ depletion, mRNA for the gastric-type H^+,K^+-ATPase isoform is increased in both outer and inner renal medulla of rats [56]. This suggests a role for this transporter in maintenance of metabolic alkalosis associated with hypokalemia. Further work will undoubtedly soon uncover the regulation and relative contribution of this transporter to maintenance and repair of acute and chronic acid–base disturbances.

Renal adaptation to acid–base disorders

This section reviews the adaptive responses in nephron segments during primary acid–base disturbances, and provides an approach to understanding possible defects in the patient with kidney disease who has an acid–base disorder.

Metabolic acidosis

In acute and chronic metabolic acidosis, an increase in renal ammoniagenesis is critical to the adaptive response. Proximal tubule synthesis of NH_3 is enhanced and increases the interstitium-to-lumen gradient of NH_3. More NH_3 diffuses into the lumen to form NH_4^+, which is excreted.

The filtered load of HCO_3^- is reduced in metabolic acidosis because of the reduction in plasma [HCO_3^-], so that despite vigorous retrieval of HCO_3^- by the proximal tubule, H^+ secretion is lower than normal. The proximal tubule is 'primed' for enhanced H^+ secretion, due to increased synthesis of apical Na^+-H^+ exchangers, and enhanced activity of the basolateral Na^+-$3HCO_3^-$ cotransporter. When the filtered load in acidotic rats is increased by systemic alkali infusions, the rate of HCO_3^- reabsorption increases above that in normal rats with similar alkali loads.

In the loop of Henle, HCO_3^- reabsorption is enhanced: it is likely that enhanced apical Na^+-H^+ exchange and H^+-ATPase mediate this response. Glucocorticoids and mineralocorticoids may stimulate HCO_3^- transport. In the DT-CT, HCO_3^- reabsorptive capacity is markedly increased, due to increased insertion of H^+-ATPases into the luminal membrane of α-intercalated cells. AE-1 may also be up-regulated. Acid secretion in the inner medullary collecting duct is also enhanced. It is important to note, however, that adaptive increases in HCO_3^- reabsorption have little impact on correction of the acidosis, unless the HCO_3^- load is also increased. Stimulation of NH_3 synthesis in the proximal tubule and diffusion of NH_3 into the collecting duct lumen is required to generate new HCO_3^-.

Metabolic alkalosis

The renal mechanisms for maintenance and repair of chronic metabolic alkalosis have been a source of controversy for many years. We have noted that renal ammoniagenesis is inhibited by HCO_3^- infusion. It has been emphasized that the decrease in filtered load of HCO_3^-, induced by ECF volume contraction, maintains elevation of plasma $[HCO_3^-]$ in metabolic alkalosis, rather than the stimulation of HCO_3^- reabsorption [57]. Of course, there is also evidence of enhanced rates of proximal, loop of Henle, and distal HCO_3^- reabsorption [58]. Deficits of Cl^- stimulate nephron segments to reabsorb HCO_3^-, and, at one or more distal segments, provision of Cl^- is likely to cause bicarbonaturia and repair of the alkalosis. Levine *et al.* [40] have demonstrated that luminal Cl^- is an important modulator *in vivo*: its availability might permit luminal HCO_3^- secretion by β-intercalated cells.

Respiratory acidosis and alkalosis

As noted above, HCO_3^- reabsorption by the proximal tubule is not increased in acute respiratory acidosis, in the absence of HCO_3^- loading. The increase in plasma $[HCO_3^-]$ in acute respiratory acidosis can be accounted for, instead, by extrarenal buffering.

In chronic respiratory acidosis, enhanced proximal tubule HCO_3^- reabsorption occurs, and persists for hours after $PaCO_2$ has returned to normal. Proximal tubule apical Na^+-H^+ exchange and basolateral Na^+-$3HCO_3^-$ co-transport are increased in chronic respiratory acidosis: in contrast, proximal ammoniagenesis has not been shown to increase. In the DT-CT, insertion of H^+-ATPase into the luminal membrane and renal AE-1 mRNA levels are stimulated by respiratory acidosis.

The adaptive changes with respiratory alkalosis are likely, for the most part, to be the opposite of those for respiratory acidosis.

Molecular basis of renal tubular acidosis

With this wealth of new information on renal acidification, we can now approach RTA from a molecular standpoint. RTA comprises a group of conditions in which the renal capacity to maintain acid–base balance is impaired. Patients have a normal anion gap metabolic acidosis. The defect may be located in the proximal tubule or DT-CT, hence the separation into 'proximal' or 'distal' RTA. Both varieties are characterized by impaired renal NH_4^+ excretion.

Proximal RTA is due to a defect in the reabsorption of filtered HCO_3^- by the proximal tubule. Proximal H^+ secretion is impaired. The H^+ secretory defect may be isolated or associated with other defects (e.g. in transport of urate, glucose, phosphate, amino acids), resulting in Fanconi's syndrome.

It is clear that the defect in H^+ secretion is due to decreased activities of apical Na^+-H^+ exchange, proximal H^+-ATPase, or basolateral Na^+-$3HCO_3^-$ co-transport. However, the molecular basis for the disorder remains unknown. One unifying hypothesis suggests there is alkalinization of the proximal tubule cell [3]. This would explain the low reabsorption of HCO_3^-, and the low proximal tubular production of NH_3 despite chronic metabolic acidosis.

In distal RTA, NH_4^+ excretion and DT-CT H^+ secretion are impaired. Traditionally, studies of these disorders have

Table 11.7   Acidification defects in renal tubular acidosis

Cell type	Possible defect	Manifestation
Proximal tubule cell	Defective Na^+-H^+ exchange, H^+-ATPase, or Na^+-$3HCO_3^-$ co-transport	Proximal RTA: defect in HCO_3^- reabsorption
α-intercalated cell	Absent or defective H^+-ATPase, Decreased number of H^+-ATPase pumps, Defect in H^+,K^+-ATPase Defect in basolateral Cl^-/HCO_3^- exchange	Classic distal RTA, Sjogren's syndrome Mild renal transplant rejection Unknown Unknown
β-intercalated cell	Increased luminal Cl^-/HCO_3^- exchange, or basolateral H^+-ATPase activity	Increased HCO_3^- secretion (increased dietary ash or alkali)
Principal cell	Decreased Na^+ reabsorption	Voltage defect-distal RTA (e.g. drugs such as amiloride, triamterene, trimethoprim)
α-intercalated and principal cells	Back diffusion of H^+ out of the lumen Decreased number of nephrons and aldosterone deficiency or resistance	Gradient-distal RTA (e.g. amphotericin B) Voltage and secretory defects Hyporeninemic hypoaldosteronism (diabetes), obstructive uropathy

relied on indirect evidence derived from clearance measurements. With the increasing availability of molecular probes, it is now possible to classify these disorders more precisely [39] (Table 11.7). An isolated defect in the H^+-ATPase of the α-intercalated cell will result in an inability to acidify the urine normally (urine pH > 5.5). Even if HCO_3^- reabsorption and NH_3 production are normal, this defect will reduce NH_4^+ excretion (by the decrease in the urinary acid 'sink'), but net acid excretion by the kidney may be only mildly impaired. On the other hand, aldosterone deficiency or resistance to aldosterone will result in several defects in α-intercalated cells and principal cells: (1) diminished H^+ secretion by the luminal H^+-ATPase; (2) decreased distal reabsorption of sodium, leading to a 'voltage' defect (i.e. associated with a lumen-positive charge) impairing H^+ secretion; and (3) decreased ammoniagenesis due to hyperkalemia.

The purpose of this chapter was to challenge the reader to begin to view acid–base balance from a molecular basis, with attention to specific transporters that could be defective in a patient with a disorder of acid–base. In Chapter 26, recent exciting developments are reviewed that have uncovered specific molecular defects present in the syndromes of RTA associated with interstitial renal disease and obstructive uropathy.

References

1. Alpern, R.J., Stone, D.K. and Rector, F.C. Jr (1991) Renal acidification mechanisms, in *The Kidney* (eds B.M. Brenner and F.C. Rector, Jr), W.B. Saunders, Philadelphia.
2. Cogan, M.G. and Rector, F.C. Jr (1991) Acid–base disorders, in *The Kidney* (eds B.M. Brenner and F.C. Rector, Jr), W.B. Saunders, Philadelphia.
3. Halperin, M.L. and Goldstein, M.B. (1994) in *Fluid, Electrolyte and Acid–base Physiology. A Problem-based Approach.* W.B. Saunders, Philadelphia.
4. Van Ypersele de Strihou, Ch. and Frans, S. (1970) The pattern of respiratory compensation in chronic uremic acidosis: the influence of dialysis. *Nephron*, 7, 37–50.
5. Arbus, G.S. (1969) Characterization and clinical application of the 'significance band' for acute respiratory alkalosis. *N. Engl. J. Med.*, 280, 117–23.
6. Brackett, N.C. Jr (1965) Carbon dioxide titration curve of normal man. *N. Engl. J. Med.*, 272, 6–12.
7. Brackett, N.C. Jr (1969) Acid–base response to chronic hypercapnia in man. *N. Engl. J. Med.*, 280, 124–30.
8. Atkinson, D.E. and Bourke, E. (1987) Metabolic aspects of the regulation of systemic pH. *Am. J. Physiol.*, 252, F947–56.
9. Halperin, M.L. (1989) How much 'new' bicarbonate is formed in the distal nephron in the process of net acid excretion? *Kidney Int.*, 35, 1277–81.
10. Knepper, M.A. (1991) NH_4^+ transport in the kidney. *Kidney Int.*, 40, S95–102.
11. Tannen, R.L. and Sahai, A. (1990) Biochemical pathways and modulators of renal ammoniagenesis. *Miner. Electrolyte Metab.*, 16, 249–58.
12. Nagami, G.T. (1988) Luminal secretion of ammonia in the mouse proximal tubule perfused *in vitro*. *J. Clin. Invest.*, 81, 159–64.
13. Nagami, G.T. and Kurokawa, K. (1985) Regulation of ammonia production by mouse proximal tubules *in vitro*. *J. Clin. Invest.*, 75, 844–9.
14. Nissim, I., Sahai, A., Sandler, R.S. *et al.* (1994) The intensity of acidosis differentially alters the pathways of ammoniagenesis in LLC-PK_1 cells. *Kidney Int.*, 45, 1014–19.
15. Schwartz, W.B., Brackett, N.C. and Cohen, J.J. (1965) The response of extracellular hydrogen ion concentration to graded degrees of chronic hypercapnia: the physiologic limits of the defense of pH. *J. Clin. Invest.*, 44, 291–302.
16. Rodriguez-Nichols, F., Laughrey, E. and Tannen, R.L. (1984) Response of renal NH_3 production to chronic respiratory acidosis. *Am. J. Physiol.*, 247, F896–903.
17. Packer, R.K., Desai, S.S., Hornbuckle, K. *et al.* (1991) Role of countercurrent multiplication in renal ammonium handling: regulation of medullary ammonium accumulation. *J. Am. Soc. Nephrol.*, 2, 77–83.
18. Nagami, G.T. (1990) Effect of bath and luminal potassium concentration on ammonia production and secretion by mouse proximal tubules perfused *in vitro*. *J. Clin. Invest.*, 86, 32–9.
19. Krapf, R. and Cogan, M.G. (1989) Hyperkalemia suppresses the renal adaptation to chronic respiratory acidosis. *Am. J. Kidney Dis.*, 14, 158–60.
20. Nath, K.A., Hostetter, M.K. and Hostetter, T.H. (1985) Pathophysiology of chronic tubulo-interstitial disease in rats. Interactions of dietary acid load, ammonia and complement component C3. *J. Clin. Invest.*, 97, 667–75.
21. Briton, L.P., Zavilowitz, B.J., Suarez, C. *et al.* (1994) Metabolic acidosis stimulates carbonic anhydrase activity in rabbit proximal tubule and medullary collecting duct. *Am. J. Physiol.*, 266, F185–95.
22. Tse, M., Levine, S., Yun, C. *et al.* (1993) Structure/function studies of the epithelial isoforms of the mammalian Na^+/H^+ exchanger gene family. *J. Membr. Biol.*, 135, 93–108.
23. Biemesderfer, D., Reilly, R.F., Exner, M. *et al.* (1992) Immunocytochemical characterization of Na^+-H^+ exchanger isoform NHE-1 in rabbit kidney. *Am. J. Physiol.*, 263, F833–40.
24. Biemesderfer, D., Pizzonia, J., Abu-Alfa, A. *et al.* (1993) NHE3: a Na^+/H^+ exchanger isoform of renal brush border. *Am. J. Physiol*, 265, F736–42.
25. Aronson, P.S., Nee, J. and Suhm, M.A. (1982) Modifier role of internal H^+ in activating the Na^+-H^+ exchanger in renal microvillus membrane vesicles. *Nature (Lond.)*, 299, 161–3.
26. Soleimani, M., Bookstein, C., McAteer, J.A. *et al.* (1994) Effect of high osmolality on Na^+/H^+ exchange in renal proximal tubule cells. *J. Biol. Chem.*, 269, 15613–18.

27. Murer, H., Krapf, R. and Helmle-Kolb, C. (1994) Regulation of renal proximal tubular Na/H-exchange: a tissue culture approach. *Kidney Int.*, **45**, S23–31.

28. Cogan, M.G. (1990) Regulation and control of bicarbonate reabsorption in the proximal tubule. *Semin. Nephrol.*, **10**, 115–21.

29. Santella, R.N., Gennari, F.J. and Maddox, D.A. (1989) Metabolic acidosis stimulates bicarbonate reabsorption in the early proximal tubule. *Am. J. Physiol.*, **257**, F35–42.

30. Santella, R.N., Maddox, D.A. and Gennari, F.J. (1991) Delivery dependence of early proximal bicarbonate reabsorption in the rat in respiratory acidosis and alkalosis. *J. Clin. Invest.*, **87**, 631–8.

31. Soleimani, M., Bizal, G.L., McKinney, T.D. *et al.* (1992) Effect of *in vitro* metabolic acidosis on luminal Na^+/H^+ exchange and basolateral $Na^+:HCO_3^-$ co-transport in rabbit kidney proximal tubules. *J. Clin. Invest.*, **90**, 211–18.

32. Krapf, R., Pearce, D., Lynch, C. *et al.* (1991) Expression of rat renal Na/H-antiporter mRNA levels in response to respiratory and metabolic acidosis. *J. Clin. Invest.*, **87**, 747–51.

33. Levine, D.Z., Walker, T. and Nash, L. (1973) Effects of KCl infusions on proximal tubular functions in normal and K-depleted rats. *Kidney Int.*, **4**, 318–25.

34. Chambrey, R., Paillard, M. and Podevin, R.A. (1994) Enzymatic and functional evidence for adaptation of the vacuolar H(+)-ATPase in proximal tubule apical membranes from rats with chronic metabolic acidosis. *J. Biol. Chem.*, **269**, 3243–50.

34. Soleimani, M., Hattabaugh, Y.J. and Bizal, G.L. (1992) pH sensitivity of the $Na^+:HCO_3^-$ co-transporter in basolateral membrane vesicles isolated from rabbit kidney cortex. *J. Biol. Chem.*, **267**, 18349–55.

35. Takeda, M., Yoshitomi, K. and Imai, M. (1993) Regulation of $Na(+)$-$3HCO_3^-$ cotransport in rabbit proximal convoluted tubule via adenosine A_1 receptor. *Am. J. Physiol.*, **265**, F511–19.

36. Good, D.W. (1993) The thick ascending limb as a site of renal bicarbonate reabsorption. *Semin. Nephrol.*, **13**, 225–35.

37. Capasso, G., Unwin, R., Ciani, F. *et al.* (1994) Bicarbonate transport along the loop of Henle II: effects of acid–base, dietary, and neurohumoral determinants. *J. Clin. Invest.*, **94**, 830–8.

38. Gluck, S.L. (1989) Cellular and molecular aspects of renal H^+ transport. *Hosp. Pract.*, **24**, 149–66.

39. Arruda, J.A.L. and Cowell, G. (1994) Distal renal tubular acidosis: molecular and clinical aspects. *Hosp. Pract.*, **29**, 75–88.

40. Levine, D.Z., VanDorpe, D. and Iacovitti, M. (1990) Distal tubule (DT) bidirectional HCO_3^- flux *in vivo*: effect of luminal chloride. *J. Clin. Invest.*, **85**, 1793–8.

41. Gluck, S. and Al-Awqati, Q. (1984) An electrogenic proton-translocating adenosine triphosphatase from bovine kidney medulla. *J. Clin. Invest.*, **73**, 1704–10.

42. Brown, D., Hirsch, S. and Gluck, S. (1988) An H^+-ATPase is present in opposite plasma membrane domains in subpopulations of kidney epithelial cells. *Nature (Lond.)*, **331**, 622–4.

43. Bastani, B., Purcell, H., Hemken, P. *et al.* (1991) Expression and distribution of renal vacuolar proton-translocating adenosine triphosphatase in response to chronic acid and alkali loads in the rat. *J. Clin. Invest.*, **88**, 126–36.

44. Zhang, K., Wang, Z.-Q. and Gluck, S. (1992) A cytosolic inhibitor of vacuolar H^+-ATPases from mammalian kidney. *J. Biol. Chem.*, **267**, 14539–42.

45. Zhang, K., Wang, Z.-Q. and Gluck, S. (1992) Identification and partial purification of a cytosolic activator of vacuolar H^+-ATPases from mammalian kidney. *J. Biol. Chem.*, **267**, 9701–5.

46. Bastani, B., McEnaney, S., Yang, L. *et al.* (1994) Adaptation of inner medullary collecting duct H-adenosine triphosphatase to chronic acid or alkali loads in the rat. *Exp. Nephrol.*, **2**, 171–5.

47. Alper, S.L. (1994) The band 3-related AE anion exchanger gene family. *Cell Physiol. Biochem.*, **4**, 265–81.

48. Alper, S.L., Sabolic, I., Tyszkowski, R. *et al.* (1991) Metabolic acidosis and alkalosis modulate anion exchanger (AE1) expression in kidney collecting ducts. *J. Am. Soc. Nephrol.*, **2**, 693 (abstr.).

49. Texeira da Silva, J.C.J., Perrone, R.D., Johns, C.A. *et al.* (1991) Rat kidney band 3 mRNA modulation in chronic respiratory acidosis. *Am. J. Physiol.*, **260**, F204–9.

50. McKinney, T.D. and Burg, M.B. (1977) Bicarbonate transport by rabbit cortical collecting tubules. *J. Clin. Invest.*, **60**, 766–8.

51. Schuster, V.L. (1993) Function and regulation of collecting duct intercalated cells. *Annu. Rev. Physiol.*, **55**, 267–88.

52. Wingo, C.S. and Cain, B.D. (1993) The renal H-K-ATPase: physiological significance and role in potassium homeostasis. *Annu. Rev. Physiol.*, **55**, 323.

53. Campbell-Thompson, M.L., Verlander, J.W., Curran, K.A. *et al.* (1994) H,K-ATPase β-subunit mRNA localization in rat and rabbit collecting duct. *J. Am. Soc. Nephrol.*, **5**, 249 (abstr.).

54. DuBose, T.D., Burges, A. and Pressley, T.A. (1994) Rat whole kidney expresses mRNA for H^+,K^+-ATPase. *J. Am. Soc. Nephrol.*, **5**, 251 (abstr.).

55. Naray-Fejes-Toth, A. and Fejes-Toth, G. (1994) Opposite regulation of 31 Kd H-ATPase and colonic H-K-ATPase expression by metabolic acidosis and alkalosis in the cortical collecting duct (CCD). *J. Am. Soc. Nephrol.*, **5**, 257 (abstr.).

56. Ahn, K.Y., Madsen, K.M. and Kone, B.C. (1994) Cellular expression of mRNA encoding the 'gastric' isoform of the H/K ATPase α subunit in kidneys of normal and potassium (K)-depleted rats. *J. Am. Soc. Nephrol.* **5**, 281 (abstr.).

57. Cogan, M.G. and Liu, F.Y. (1983) Metabolic alkalosis in the rat. Evidence that reduced glomerular filtration rather than enhanced tubular bicarbonate reabsorption is responsible for maintaining the alkalotic state. *J. Clin. Invest.*, **71**, 1141–60.

58. Maddox, D.A. and Gennari, F.J. (1986) Load dependence of proximal tubular bicarbonate reabsorption in chronic metabolic alkalosis in the rat. *J. Clin. Invest.*, **77**, 709–16.

I

Normal Structure and Function

Section 4
Blood Pressure and Renal Function

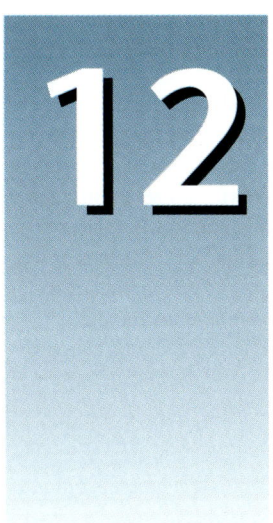

12

The sympathetic nervous system in regulation of blood pressure

A.M. Heagerty and N.P. Stephens

Introduction

Meticulous histological and neuroanatomical studies have gradually unveiled the central location of the control areas that initiate and modulate autonomic nervous function and how vascular tone is controlled. Therefore an intricate system that can influence blood pressure has been defined and clinical observations suggest that abnormalities of it may underlie essential hypertension and are certainly present in renal disease. This chapter seeks to summarize what is known about the sympathetic nervous system and the evidence that when it is dysfunctional blood pressure may rise.

Central origin of sympathetic tone

Sympathetic premotor neurons

It is generally accepted that basal sympathetic nerve activity originates from sites located within the medulla oblongata of the brain [1]. The application of inhibitory pharmacological agents to the ventral surface of the medulla, or electrolytic lesions within the ventrolateral medulla, caused a profound fall in blood pressure similar in magnitude to that caused by spinal transection. As a result, much attention has been focused on the rostral ventrolateral medulla (RVLM) as a site containing neurons which are essential for the maintenance of basal

arterial blood pressure. Localized electrical stimulation of areas within the RVLM, or microinjection of excitatory amino acids into the RVLM, elicit an elevation in blood pressure. Conversely, lesions of neuron groups within the RVLM, or microinjection into the RVLM of agents which abolish neuronal discharge, reduce blood pressure to the level observed after spinal transection, demonstrating that the tonic discharge of neurons located within the RVLM is essential for maintaining arterial blood pressure [2].

Analysis of precise anatomical locations has revealed that several sites within the RVLM may underlie tonic sympathoexcitatory drive (Figure 12.1). In particular, it has been suggested that neurons of the paragigantocellular lateralis (PGL) and the C1 area may be important. Although the RVLM has been studied most thoroughly with regard to its role in the generation of basal vasomotor tone, it is probably not exclusive. Other areas of the medulla, including the caudal raphe nuclei, rostral ventromedial medulla and paraventricular nucleus of the hypothalamus, have also been implicated but their precise role as premotor neurons remains to be established [1]. Furthermore, noradrenergic cell groups have been ascribed a role in cardiovascular regulation. The so-called A5 noradrenergic cell group in the caudal ventrolateral pons provides a substantial innervation to sympathetic preganglionic neurons in the spinal cord [1]. Stimulation of A5 cells produces an increase in peripheral sympathetic nerve activity, but it has been suggested that these cells provide more than an excitatory

Nephrology, Edited by Rex L. Jamison and Robert Wilkinson.
Published in 1997 by Chapman & Hall, London. ISBN 0 412 60930 4

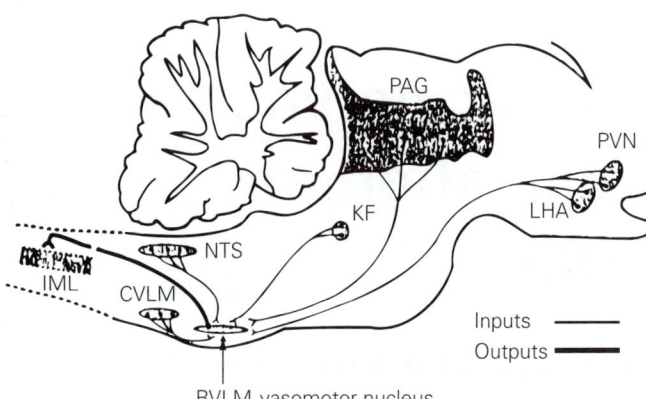

Figure 12.1 Major afferent and efferent connections of rostral ventrolateral medulla (RVLM) region containing presympathetic vasomotor neurons, as revealed by anatomic studies in rat, rabbit and cat. CVLM, caudal ventrolateral medulla; IML, intermediolateral cell column; KF, Kölliker-Fuse nucleus; LHA, lateral hypothalamic area; NTS, nucleus of solitary tract; PAG, periaqueductal gray; PVN, paraventricular nucleus. (Reproduced, with permission, from ref. 1.)

input to sympathetic preganglionic neurons. It is hypothesized that A5 cells influence integrated cardiovascular responses via widespread projections to various cardiovascular nuclei. The role of noradrenergic nuclei in cardiovascular regulation has led to assessment of cerebral norepinephrine spillover (that is overflow from tissue to plasma), as an index of central excitatory sympathetic drive, and this methodology has been used to investigate central abnormalities which may underlie increased sympathetic firing in hypertension (see Sympathetic nervous system and hypertension).

The mechanism which generates the tonic neuronal discharge underlying basal activity in sympathetic premotor neurons has not been determined, but several hypotheses have been proposed. First, it has been suggested that neurons in the RVLM are chemosensitive to pH, P_{O_2} and P_{CO_2} within the normal range, so that they are tonically excited [1]. Second, neurons have been identified in the RVLM which exhibit spontaneous, regular discharge in the absence of synaptic input and, thus, have been described as possessing intrinsic pacemaker activity. Such activity is not observed in all RVLM cells and, in particular, C1 adrenergic neurons appear to be devoid of spontaneous activity. These are a group of catecholamine cells containing epinephrine-synthesizing enzymes [1]. Although it has been suggested that the pacemaker cells within the RVLM may be largely responsible for generating basal sympathetic vasomotor tone, they are unlikely to be the sole source since clonidine, to which pacemaker cells are insensitive, markedly reduces blood pressure when injected into the RVLM. A third proposal suggests that there is a 'network oscillator' in the brain stem, comprising an ensemble of neurons interconnected to generate rhythmic activity. This hypothesis is based upon the 2–6 Hz rhythm which is ubiquitous to sympathetic activity, is independent of baroreceptors and is abolished by spinal transection. Single neurons, located in the RVLM, caudal raphe nuclei and lateral tegmental field, have been identified with spontaneous discharges that synchronize with activity recorded in peripheral sympathetic nerves, suggesting that central firing in these regions determines peripheral activity. Analysis of the time courses of dis-

charge indicates that the lateral tegmental field neurons fire before the RVLM and caudal raphe nuclei neurons, onto which they project, suggesting that the lateral tegmental neurons may trigger discharge in the latter. The irregular discharge pattern of these neurons suggests that network ineractions, rather than endogenous activity, are responsible for the 2–6 Hz rhythm underlying basal sympathetic nerve activity. The precise role of each of the proposed mechanisms in generating tonic activity in sympathetic premotor neurons remains inconclusive. At present, it is not clear which of these mechanisms or to what extent each may be responsible for the generation of basal sympathetic nerve activity originating in the medulla oblongata [1].

Sympathetic preganglionic neurons

The cell bodies of sympathetic preganglionic neurons (SPNs), whose axons project to sympathetic ganglia and the adrenal medulla, are located predominantly in the intermediolateral column (IML) and the adjacent lateral funiculus of the spinal cord, in the thoracic and upper lumbar segments of the spinal cord. It is clear from neuroanatomical and electrophysiological studies that neurons within the RVLM project directly to the IML of the spinal cord [1]. However, other neuron groups implicated in the genesis of vasomotor tone have also been shown to project to the IML and transneuronal retrograde labeling has identified five cell groups which innervate SPNs in the spinal column; these comprise the rostral ventrolateral medulla, rostral ventromedial medulla, caudal raphe nuclei, A5 noradrenergic group and paraventricular nucleus in the hypothalamus.

Sympathetic preganglionic neurons represent the final central site for integration of sympathetic nerve activity emanating from the central nervous system. Measurement of electrical activity in SPNs indicates that 10–30% exhibit ongoing discharge, with a low firing rate predominantly less than 2 Hz. The activity takes the form of subthreshold excitatory postsynaptic potentials (EPSPs), which bombard SPNs and summate to initiate action potentials, but inhibitory postsynaptic potentials (IPSPs) are rarely observed suggesting that inhibition of SPNs may occur by reduction in the frequency of EPSPs. There is no evidence for ongoing depolarization or pacemaker-type potentials in SPNs [1], but the dependency of their activity on supraspinal input and spinal afferent nerves, or possibly intrinsic activity, is not fully resolved. Certainly, spinal transection reduces total sympathetic nerve activity and blood pressure, favoring a predominant role for supraspinal input. Although there is some evidence that SPNs exhibit regular, spontaneous firing in the absence of supraspinal input, the role of this in the physiological regulation of vasomotor tone is not clear.

Differentiation of sympathetic outflow

The idea that the sympathetic nervous system functions as a homogeneous system which responds en masse, to trigger uniform sympathetic outflow in postganglionic nerve bundles, is no longer accepted. It is clear that central circuits are capable of formulating complex and highly differentiated response patterns to different target organs. There is now evidence that subpopulations of neurons within the RVLM are able to control sympathetic outflow to different vascular beds, selectively [1]. Microinjection of excitatory amino acids elicits different blood flow responses in muscle, renal or splanchnic circulations depending on the exact site of injection. A topographical scheme for sympathetic neurons located within the PGL of the ventrolateral medulla has been proposed, such that they are arranged in separate, overlapping pools each controlling individual vascular beds. Electrophysiological measurement of sympathetic outflow in postganglionic sympathetic nerves has confirmed this view. Dampney and McAllen [3] stimulated subpopulations of neurons within the RVLM and simultaneously measured sympathetic nerve activity in postganglionic fibers supplying muscle and skin vasculature. Muscle or skin fibers were selectively activated depending on the exact site of injection of glutamate, indicating that this region of the RVLM is topographically organized and specific cell groups are dedicated to the regulation of particular vascular tissues. Differentiation of sympathetic outflow to vascular beds is also clear from other experiments in which the general pattern of sympathetic outflow, at rest and during afferent receptor stimulation, is shown to vary considerably in vasoconstrictor fibers supplying muscle, skin and viscera (see below).

Basal sympathetic nerve activity

A microneurographic technique for measuring sympathetic activity in human peripheral nerves was first described by Hagbarth and Vallbo [4]. Nerve fascicles are impaled with microelectrodes and, as such, recordings are generally confined to sympathetic nerves of the extremities, most commonly those supplying skeletal muscle and skin. In human skin sympathetic nerves, spontaneous discharges occur at irregular intervals separated by periods of quiescence, and this pattern of activity is similar to that first observed in sympathetic nerves in animals. At rest, the average firing rate does not exceed 15 impulses/min (0.25 Hz) and some sympathetic units are completely silent. However, during mental activation or other maneuvers, the discharge rate increased with a maximum instantaneous frequency of up to 35 Hz, which is much higher than previously supposed on the basis of average values.

In human skin nerves, random bursts of sympathetic activity show no correlation to cardiac rhythm. The general pattern of activity in sympathetic nerves supplying skeletal muscle is similar to skin, in that irregular discharge bursts are separated by periods of inactivity, except that muscle sympathetic nerve activity is locked into the cardiac rhythm. Thus, muscle nerve activity is synchronous with variation in blood pressure during the cardiac cycle and this pattern of activity is thought to be mediated via the baroreceptor mechanism. Bursts of sympathetic activity are preceded by reductions in blood pressure, and neural silence follows elevations in pressure, so that there is an inverse relation between blood pressure and sympathetic nerve activity with a constant time delay of 1–1.5 s. Diastolic blood pressure is the major determinant of sympathetic activity and exerts a directional influence on sympathetic nerve activity; at a given diastolic blood pressure, sympathetic nerve activity is greater if pressure is falling rather than rising. The burst incidence of muscle sympathetic nerve activity varies considerably between individuals at rest, but is remarkably similar when measured within subjects on different occasions. Thus, individuals appear to have characteristic levels of basal sympathetic nerve activity. Furthermore, there was a striking similarity between nerve activity recorded in two separate muscle, or skin, nerve fascicles, so that recordings were almost superimposable, indicating the homogeneity of sympathetic output to a particular region.

Thus, measurement of sympathetic nerve activity in humans indicates that the pattern of sympathetic outflow to vascular beds varies with different functions. The irregular pattern of sympathetic discharge may have important functional significance since it is clear that both neurotransmitter release and effector organ response are produced more effectively by irregular than regular nerve impulses. In isolated segments of small mesenteric artery, stimulation, effected using microneurographic recordings of human sympathetic nerve activity, was markedly more effective at eliciting contraction than regular stimulation at the same mean frequency [5]. Also, direct visualization of rat gastric submucosal microvessels revealed that intermittent high-frequency bursts of stimulation produced greater constriction than continuous stimulation at the same mean frequency.

The vascular sympathetic neuroeffector junction

Postganglionic sympathetic nerves

Postganglionic sympathetic fibers form a neuronal network extending through the adventitia of blood vessels. This can be divided into two layers: an outer, primary plexus, which is made up of a bundle of nerve axons which are non-varicose and ultimately destined for more distal sites, and an inner, ground plexus, which consists of single or smaller bundles of non-myelinated axons which are varicose and directly innervate the smooth muscle below. Sympathetic neurons generally terminate at the adventitia–media border and only rarely penetrate into the media layer. Nerve plexuses can be observed directly using histological techniques to induce fluorescence of adrenergic neurons, and such methods demonstrate that the density of innervation may vary widely between species, vascular bed and position along the arterial tree. In a study of sympathetic innervation at different sections of the vascular tree, nerve density was shown to be relatively sparse in the aorta and superior mesenteric artery but much greater in the more distal mesenteric arteries [6], and it was possible to correlate the functional response to nerve stimulation with the observed pattern of innervation. The magnitude of the neurogenic response, expressed as a percentage of that to exogenous norepinephrine, was greatest in small mesenteric arteries but became progressively less in the superior mesenteric artery and aorta. In addition, the rate of development of contraction was slowest in the aorta and much more rapid in the small mesenteric arteries, and this was borne out by the response to a single nerve impulse which was seen in the smaller vessels only [6]. In a study of the entire mesenteric bed, it was shown that the principal arteries, small arteries and terminal arterioles constricted to nerve stimulation, but the smallest precapillary arterioles (diameter <18 µm) did not respond. Thus, the very smallest precapillary vessels in the rat mesentery appear to be devoid of direct neurogenic control, but this is not the case in all vascular beds; in rat skeletal muscle vasculature neurogenic constriction may be elicited right down to the precapillary resistance arterioles.

Areas of intense fluorescence reflect the high concentrations of norepinephrine located at varicosities along the axon length, and these are considered to be the active site for neurotransmission, which occurs via a diffuse network of such varicose terminals which in most vessels is located at the medioadventitial border (Figure 12.2). Varicosities are surrounded by Schwann cells, apart from the membrane surface facing the smooth muscle where

neurotransmitter is released. Electron microscopy identifies two or three types of vesicle present in the varicosity: small granular vesicles (35–60 µm) which store norepinephrine, larger granular vesicles (60–120 µm) and sometimes agranular vesicles which may contain acetylcholine. The region between the presynaptic axon membrane and the postsynaptic smooth muscle cell is termed the synaptic cleft, and its width may vary considerably with vascular bed and artery size. In some cases, the basal lamina of the nerve axon actually fuses with the smooth muscle cell; here the synaptic cleft is <100 nm, and may be as small as 15–25 nm, and true neuroeffector junctions are considered to have formed. Such neuroeffector junctions have been observed in rat mesenteric arterioles and guinea-pig ileum submucosal arterioles [7], but only a small proportion of varicosities (4–12%) form these tight junctions. In guinea-pig submucosal arteries, specialization of the perjunctional membrane has been observed at some neuroeffector junctions, characterized by electron-dense areas on the axon membrane towards which vesicles appear to cluster [8]. Examination of a number of vessels (basilar, carotid, mesenteric, renal, femoral and aorta) from several species (rat, rabbit and guinea-pig) revealed that neuroeffector junctions were generally present in muscular arteries but absent from elastic arteries, although exceptions were noted [8]. In general, the frequency of neuroeffector junctions was inversely proportional to vessel diameter, and it has been suggested that the frequency of neuroeffector junctions may provide a good index of innervation density, as these structures are directly relevant to neurotransmitter release [8].

Neurotransmitter synthesis, storage and release

Norepinephrine is the principal transmitter contained within sympathetic neurons, and its synthesis in nerves innervating blood vessels has been well documented. Terminal axons are considered to be the important site for norepinephrine synthesis, where L-tyrosine is taken up into the neuron and converted into 3,4-dihydroxyphenylalanine (DOPA) in the axoplasm, via the enzyme tyrosine hydroxylase. This is the rate-limiting step in the synthesis pathway and is subject to regulatory influences. For example, norepinephrine present in the axoplasm, which is in equilibrium with stored norepinephrine, exerts negative feedback inhibition of tyrosine hydroxylase, so that synthesis can be switched off when stores are adequate. DOPA is rapidly converted into dopamine, via DOPA decarboxylase which is free within the axoplasm. Following active uptake of dopamine into storage vesicles, it is bound and converted into norepinephrine via dopamine-β-hydroxylase. Norepinephrine is stored in vesicles in two forms, cytoplasmic and bound, along with ATP which is present in a ratio of 1:4 with the catecholamine. Water-soluble proteins, called chromogranins, are also contained within the vesicles and are

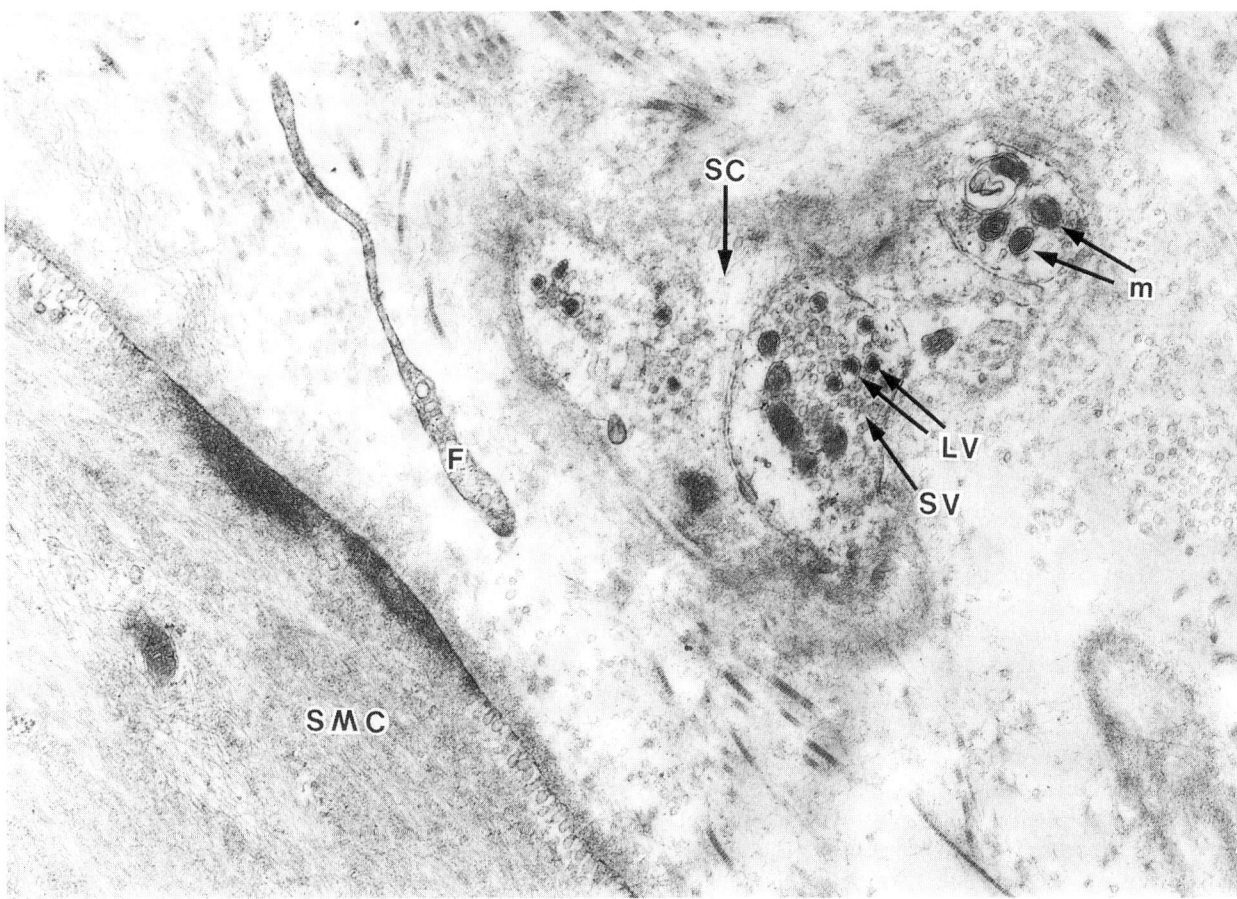

Figure 12.2 Electron micrograph of a human omental artery showing a cross-section through a sympathetic nerve adjacent to a smooth muscle cell (SMC). A fibroblast (F) can be seen in between. The nerve contains three varicosities surrounded by a Schwann cell (SC). Both large dense-cored vesicles (LV) and smaller dense-cored vesicles (SV) can be seen within the same varicosity whereas another contains mostly mitochondria (m). (×99 000.) (This electron micrograph was kindly provided by Dr Jonathan Tulip, Department of Pathology, University of Leicester.)

thought to be involved in the binding of norepinephrine. Stimulation of sympathetic nerves results in the release of norepinephrine, along with ATP, dopamine-β-hydroxylase and chromogranins in the proportions that they were present in storage vesicles. The mechanism of transmitter release has not been elucidated fully, but influx of extracellular calcium into the varicosity after neuronal depolarization is thought to trigger the process. Storage vesicles may move to the prejunctional membrane, possibly involving the microtubule system, fuse with the axonal membrane and release their contents, probably by exocytosis.

The nature of transmitter release in sympathetically innervated tissue was first studied by comparing the overflow of transmitter from vasoconstrictor nerves with the total tissue norepinephrine content. It was hypothesized that a single impulse would release 1/1000 of the tissue norepinephrine content; if each nerve varicosity contained 1000 vesicles and each impulse released one quantum of norepinephrine, this is equivalent to the con-

tents of a vesicle. In practice, one nerve impulse released approximately 1/50 000 of the tissue norepinephrine content. Thus, two explanations were proposed: that each impulse releases transmitter from every varicosity, but only 2% of the contents of a vesicle are released (nonintermittent hypothesis) or that the entire contents of a vesicle are released, but each varicosity responds to only 1 in 50 nerve impulses (intermittent hypothesis). In order to distinguish between these two possibilities, it is necessary to determine transmitter release from individual varicosities.

Electrophysiological measurements of excitatory junction potentials (EJPs), which are elicited by transmitter released onto postjunctional membranes, have been used to address this issue. Due to the multiple innervation and electrical coupling of smooth muscle cells, measurement of EJPs will reflect transmitter released from more than one nerve varicosity. However, electrically evoked EJPs may have fast components reflecting transmitter released from close varicosities and slower components reflecting release from more distant varicosities. Blakeley and Cunnane [9] used this principle to identify single varicosities in an attempt to elucidate the nature of neurotransmitter release. They identified different components of a compound EJP, which they termed discrete events (DEs). These occurred at several fixed latencies after the nerve impulse, and each latency was thought to reflect the release of transmitter from a single varicosity. It was possible to identify spontaneous EJPs and electrically evoked EJPs which had identical amplitudes and time courses, suggesting that they reflected the same underlying event, that is the release of a single quantum from an individual varicosity. In addition, the amplitude of discrete events at a given latency varies in a stepwise rather than graded fashion, presumably reflecting the release of transmitter as multiples of quanta [9] or single quanta released from sites so close that they can not be distinguished. Frequently, nerve stimulation failed to elicit a discrete event at a given latency after each impulse. Therefore, the release of transmitter was described as intermittent and the probability of release from an individual varicosity was estimated to be in the range 0.5–0.02 [9] or 0.03–0.002. Similar findings have been reported in mesenteric arterioles [10], in which very short sections of arteriole were studied to diminish the problem of multiple innervation and electrical coupling of cells. The amplitude of spontaneous EJPs corresponded to that of the smallest evoked EJPs, suggesting that both responded from the release of single quanta. In addition, fewer quanta were released per impulse than the estimated number of varicosities in the preparation, indicating that the probability of release was low. Extracellular measurement of excitatory junction currents (EJCs), which mirror the EJPs and also allow simultaneous measurement of nerve action potentials, have confirmed that transmitter release is quantal and intermittent in sympathetically innervated tissues including arteries. The low probability of transmitter release never resulted from failure of an action potential to invade a nerve varicosity, suggesting that ineffective depolarization–secretion coupling is responsible for the intermittent nature of sympathetic neurotransmitter release.

Regulation of transmitter release

The presence of a great variety of presynaptic receptors on nerve terminal membranes, which regulate neurotransmitter release, is now well recognized (Figure 12.3). These include α- and β-adrenergic receptors, as well as those for acetylcholine, angiotensin II, dopamine, purines, prostaglandins, serotonin and various peptides. It was the role of presynaptic adrenoceptors that was first recognized, when several groups reported that the α-adrenoceptor antagonist, phenoxybenzamine, increased the overflow into the circulation of norepinephrine at concentrations which did not block neuronal amine uptake. Enhancement of norepinephrine overflow with α-adrenoceptor antagonists was observed regardless of

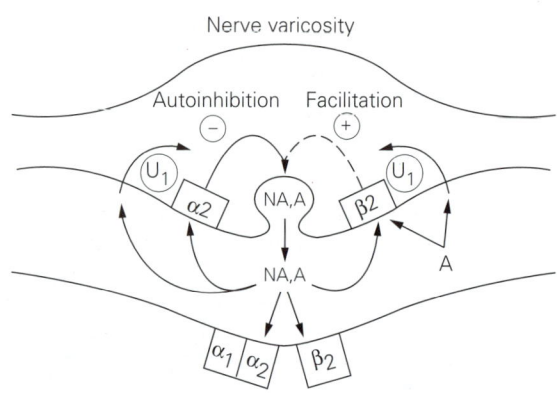

Figure 12.3 Diagram indicating the release of adrenergic transmitters (NA, norepinephrine; A, epinephrine) and prejunctional adrenergic receptors at the sympathetic vascular neuroeffector junction. Circulating epinephrine is taken up into the nerve terminal via neuronal amine uptake (U_1) and subsequently coreleased with norepinephrine. Facilitatory prejunctional β2-adrenoceptors, which enhance the overflow of neurotransmitters, are activated by both circulating and coreleased epinephrine. Norepinephrine is the endogenous agonist for inhibitory prejunctional α2-adrenoceptors which reduce neurotransmitter overflow. In addition, the concentration of norepinephrine in the synaptic cleft is influenced by neuronal amine uptake which pumps norepinephrine back into the varicosity. On the postjunctional smooth muscle cell, vasoconstriction may be elicited via α1- and α2-adrenoceptors and vasodilation via β2-adrenoceptors. (Reproduced, with permission, from ref. 19.)

whether the postjunctional receptor was the α- or β-adrenoceptor subtype, suggesting that there was no relation between the postjunctional receptor on the effector organ and the increased transmitter release. Thus, these data prompted the hypothesis that α-adrenoceptors exist on the presynaptic nerve terminal membrane and inhibit neurotransmitter release via a negative feedback mechanism [11]. Support for the hypothesis was provided by numerous observations that α-adrenoceptor agonists inhibited norepinephrine overflow and α-adrenoceptor antagonists enhanced overflow, in a variety of preparations. The physiological significance of α-adrenoceptor-mediated inhibition has been assessed by studying the postjunctional effector response following interruption of the negative feedback mechanism. In guinea-pig atria, the α-adrenoceptor antagonist, phentolamine, increased the rate of contraction as well as norepinephrine overflow, indicating that presynaptic α-adrenoceptors normally modulate the neuroeffector response [11]. There have been many examples which indicate that interruption of α-adrenoceptor feedback inhibition results in a potentiation of effector organ response suggesting that these receptors play a physiological role in neurotransmission.

Differing potencies of agonists and antagonists at prejunctional and postjunctional α-adrenoceptors indicated that the receptor populations were not homogeneous but that two subtypes may exist, which were termed α$_1$- and α$_2$-adrenoceptors. Presynaptic α-adrenoceptors are generally classified as the α$_2$-subtype, although the existence of presynaptic α$_1$-adrenoceptors has been proposed in a minority of preparations.

Since presynaptic α-adrenoceptors appear to be activated by endogenously released norepinephrine, which inhibits its own subsequent release, they have been described as 'autoreceptors' and the process of negative feedback as 'autoinhibition'. The autoreceptor hypothesis predicts that a threshold concentration of norepinephrine must be reached in the biophase in order to activate presynaptic α-adrenoceptors. Thus, autoinhibition would not be expected to operate during transmitter release evoked by a single nerve impulse, and several studies support this. In guinea-pig atria, α-adrenoceptor antagonists were ineffective during single nerve impulses or trains of four impulses, but phentolamine increased both norepinephrine overflow and rate of contraction during longer stimulations of 16 pulses. Similarly, in rabbit ear artery, norepinephrine overflow evoked by 100 nerve impulses, but not that evoked by 10 pulses, was markedly enhanced by α-adrenoceptor inhibition. Electrophysiological measurement of postjunctional events confirms these findings. α-Adrenoceptor antagonists increase the amplitude of EJPs and EJCs during nerve stimulation which reflect an increase in neurotransmitter overflow, but only after five or so impulses [9]. However, incubation of the tissue in the neuronal amine uptake inhibitor, desipramine, increased the effectiveness of α-adrenoceptor antagonists during the initial (1–5) pulses [9], presumably by potentiating the norepinephrine concentration in the biophase. Therefore, the data suggest that autoinhibition fails to operate during single or short trains of impulses, but that longer trains allowing accumulation of norepinephrine in the synaptic cleft are required.

However, the autoreceptor hypothesis has not gone unchallenged. Kalsner cites a number of observations, which do not appear to fit with the hypothesis, and thus there are strong views both in favor and against [12]. In addition, Kalsner [13] questions whether presynaptic α-adrenoceptors respond to transmitter released from their own varicosity, and therefore could be termed autoreceptors, or whether they respond to transmitter released from nearly varicosities, in which case the term homoreceptor may be more appropriate. In view of the intermittent nature of transmitter release from sympathetic nerve varicosities (see Neurotransmitter synthesis, storage and release) it seems unlikely that transmitter release could modulate subsequent release from the same varicosity. Therefore, it has been suggested that transmitter released from a varicosity modulates release from adjacent varicosities, a mechanism of 'lateral' rather than 'local' inhibition.

The presence of presynaptic β-adrenoceptors on sympathetic nerve terminals, which facilitate the release of norepinephrine upon nerve stimulation, was first proposed by Langer and Enero [14], and there is now considerable evidence that β-adrenoceptor agonists increase transmitter spillover in a number of sympathetically innervated preparations including human blood vessels [15]. Although the effect of β-adrenoceptor activation is readily blocked by β-adrenoceptor antagonists, it is not always possible to demonstrate a reduction in transmitter overflow following exposure to a β-adrenoceptor antagonist alone, suggesting that noradrenergic transmission does not basally stimulate presynaptic β-adrenoceptors [15]. Indeed, the endogenous agonist for β-adrenoceptors is considered to be epinephrine, which certainly has a higher affinity for this receptor subtype than norepinephrine. When noradrenergic nerve terminals are loaded with epinephrine, β-adrenoceptor antagonists become more effective in reducing transmitter release.

Epinephrine may influence presynaptic β-adrenoceptors directly as a circulating hormone, although its short plasma half-life means that its effects will be short lived. However, there is now considerable evidence that epinephrine is taken up into sympathetic nerve terminals, via neuronal amine uptake, and co-released with norepinephrine upon subsequent nerve stimulation. In this way, the influence of epinephrine on neurotransmitter overflow is greatly prolonged, and may last for up to 24 h. Although the capacity of presynaptic β-adrenoceptors to regulate neurotransmission is thought to be less than that of α-adrenoceptors, there is considerable interest in the role of epinephrine acting as a cotransmitter in the facilitation of neurotransmission via presynaptic β-adrenoceptors and its possible role in the pathogenesis of hypertension (see Sympathetic nervous system and hypertension).

Postjunctional responses

Release of neurotransmitter from sympathetic nerve varicosities results in electrical and mechanical postjunctional, vascular smooth muscle responses. Nerve stimulation elicits small, rapid depolarizations of the postjunctional membrane, EJPs, in many mammalian arteries. Although individual EJPs cause insufficient depolarization to activate arterial calcium channels, the sum of EJPs during a train of nerve impulses may give rise to a greater depolarization which reaches threshold for calcium channel activation. In arterioles, action potentials may result from calcium influx, but these are generally not seen in larger arteries.

EJPs are abolished by inhibitors of neurotransmission, such as tetrodotoxin and guanethidine, but are completely resistant to α-adrenoceptor antagonists. Two hypotheses have been proposed to explain this finding: first, that norepinephrine elicits EJPs via low-affinity γ-adrenoceptors, or, second, that a cotransmitter, adenosine triphosphate (ATP), mediates these electrical events. In support of the first theory, Hirst and Neild [10] reported that iontophoretic application of norepinephrine elicits rapid depolarizations which are resistant to α-adrenoceptor antagonists. The depolarizations were detected only when very high norepinephrine concentrations were applied at sites close to the nerve plexus [10]. Furthermore, the response to norepinephrine was enhanced by neuronal amine uptake blockade, which would increase norepinephrine concentration close to the nerve varicosity. In contrast, the second hypothesis suggests that a cotransmitter, ATP, initiates EJPs in vascular smooth muscle. Iontophoretic application of ATP elicits rapid depolarizations similar in profile to EJPs. After reserpine-induced depletion of norepinephrine from sympathetic nerves, both ATP release [16] and EJPs persist during nerve stimulation. Furthermore, α,β-methylene ATP which desensitizes P2-purinoceptors abolishes EJPs elicited by nerve stimulation, indicating that ATP may mediate these events. Furthermore, the persistence of EJPs after norepinephrine depletion from sympathetic nerves, and their abolition by purinergic blockade, favors a role for a transmitter other than norepinephrine in these events.

Sympathetic nerve stimulation results in a biphasic contraction in many arteries. An initial rapid constriction lasting several seconds is followed by a slower sustained contraction lasting the duration of the stimulation [17]. Although nerve-mediated contraction is abolished by inhibitors of neurotransmission, it is also partially resistant to α-adrenoceptor antagonists in many preparations. The residual, non-adrenergic component is sensitive to α,β-methylene ATP, implicating ATP and P2-purinoceptors in the constrictor response [17]. Invariably, the combination of adrenergic and purinergic blockade abolishes neurogenic constriction [17]. However, the relative contribution of the adrenergic and purinergic component depends on the stimulation parameters used. Purinergic transmission is favored by low frequency and short bursts of stimulation whereas adrenergic transmission predominates as frequency and duration of stimulation increase [17].

The adrenergic component of vasoconstriction has been shown to be mediated by postjunctional α₂-adrenoceptors, as well as α₁-adrenoceptors, in various human vascular preparations. Infusion of α₂-adrenoceptor antagonists into human forearm elicits a vasodilator response, comparable to that produced by an α₁-adrenoceptor antagonist, and indicates that these postjunctional receptors contribute substantially to basal vasoconstrictor tone. The observation that the response to infused norepinephrine was preferentially blocked by an α₂-adrenoceptor antagonist, whereas the response to neurally released norepinephrine, evoked by lower body negative pressure (LBNP), was preferentially blocked by an α₁-adrenoceptor antagonist, led to the proposal that the two α-adrenoceptor subtypes are topographically organized in human forearm. They suggest that α₁-adrenoceptors are located intrasynaptically and are a target for

norepinephrine released as a neurotransmitter, whereas α₂-adrenoceptors are located extrasynaptically and respond predominantly to circulating catecholamines. In isolated segments of human subcutaneous arteries, the role of α₁- and α₂-adrenoceptors in vasoconstriction elicited by exogenous norepinephrine has been confirmed. Furthermore, both α-adrenoceptor subtypes mediated vasoconstriction to neurally released norepinephrine, evoked by electrical field stimulation [18], suggesting that the topographical classification of α-adrenoceptors is not accurate for all vascular beds in humans.

Sympathetic nervous system and essential hypertension

Studies on animal models of genetic hypertension provide a wealth of evidence to implicate the sympathetic nervous system in the genesis of hypertension [19]. For example, sympathetic nerve activity measured using microneurography is elevated in renal nerves in spontaneously hypertensive rats (SHR), and the level of activity correlates with blood pressure in the sixth generation normotensive back-cross rats genetically related to SHR. Sympathectomy from birth in young SHR, suing a combination of guanethidine and antinerve growth factor, strongly attenuates the development of hypertension. Furthermore, it is clear that the peripheral vasculature of SHR displays a hyperinnervation, which results in an elevated neurotransmitter overflow and pressor response following nerve stimulation. The following discussion concentrates on the evidence for an abnormality in the sympathetic nervous system in the development of human hypertension.

Hemodynamic studies

A role for the sympathetic nervous system in the pathophysiology of hypertension is clear, from hemodynamic profiles, at the very earliest stages of the disease. In young patients with borderline hypertension, cardiac output is elevated as a result of both an increased heart rate and stroke volume, and this characteristic state has been termed hyperkinetic borderline hypertension [20]. Oxygen consumption is elevated at the same time as cardiac output. Such a profile could be explained in terms of an increased sympathetic drive to the heart and vasculature. Indeed, autonomic blockade of the heart, using propranolol and atropine, normalizes cardiac output, indicating that the abnormality arises from both an increased sympathetic and a decreased parasympathetic drive. The data suggest that the elevation of cardiac output in borderline hypertension is entirely neurogenic.

Epidemiological evidence suggests that tachycardia in youth, independent of blood pressure, is a predictor of hypertension in later life, although not all hyperkinetic borderline hypertensives go on to develop the full condition [20]. In patients in which hypertension does become established, the hemodynamic profile alters; cardiac output tends to normalize and peripheral vascular resistance rises further. The actual transition has been tracked in few longitudinal studies, but has been documented by Lund-Johansen [21] in a 20-year follow-up study of patients with hyperkinetic borderline hypertension. The most likely mechanism for the hemodynamic transition is thought to be a change in cardiovascular responsiveness, as a consequence of the enhanced sympathetic drive to the heart and blood vessels [20]. Thus, the normalization of cardiac output may occur as a result of functional down-regulation of myocyte β-adrenoceptors and decreased cardiac compliance [20]. The origin of the increased peripheral vascular resistance remains unresolved, but may result from an increased adrenergic vasoconstrictor tone, due to increased sympathetic drive or increased blood vessel responsiveness to constrictor influences.

Evidence for sympathetic overactivity

Apart from hemodynamic studies, evidence for sympathetic overactivity in hypertension has been derived from biochemical assessment of norepinephrine, and its metabolites, in urine and plasma [22]. Plasma norepinephrine concentration has been used extensively as a marker for sympathetic nerve activity, even though it depends on norepinephrine clearance as well as release [23]. Although such studies provide a relatively crude index of the sympathetic nerve activity, they do suggest that norepinephrine release is elevated in essential hypertension. A review of this literature [24] indicates that plasma norepinephrine is elevated in essential hypertension, by an average of 55 pg/ml, in 80% of studies published, but the increased norepinephrine concentration in patients compared to controls was only statistically significant in 40% of studies published. However, a strong age-related trend was observed; significantly elevated plasma norepinephrine levels were much more common in studies of younger hypertensive subjects than studies of older patients [24]. These findings have been confirmed in a study of hypertensives spanning a wide age range (22–74 years), in which plasma norepinephrine concentration was significantly raised in patients less than 40 years of age, but not in two groups of older patients (40–59 years, 60–79 years).

A more refined assessment of norepinephrine release from sympathetic nerves can be derived from the measurement of norepinephrine spillover into the circulation, using radioisotope dilution methodology, in which the plasma clearance of norepinephrine can also be determined. Using this technique, total norepinephrine spillover into plasma has been shown to be elevated in essential hypertensives [24], but this may in part be due

to a reduced neuronal reuptake of norepinephrine. Investigation of the kinetics of norepinephrine in different vascular beds has identified the regional pattern of norepinephrine spillover which underlies the increased total plasma spillover. These studies indicate that norepinephrine spillover is enhanced predominantly in the cardiac and renal beds, with little contribution from the pulmonary vasculature or hepatomesenteric circulation [23, 25]. Thus, sympathetic overactivity appears to be restricted to specific vascular beds, rather than being a global phenomenon. It is also clear from these studies that augmented total and renal norepinephrine spillover is more readily apparent in younger hypertensives, than in older patients in whom norepinephrine spillover tends to normalize [23].

Microneurography has been used to assess sympathetic nerve activity directly, in patients with hypertension, but can only be applied to superficial sites (see Basal sympathetic nerve activity). The earliest studies using this technique provided little evidence for abnormality in the characteristic pattern of sympathetic discharge in hypertensive patients. There was a tendency for increased sympathetic burst incidence in patients with hypertension, but this may reflect the age difference between the patients and controls (hypertensives were older) since sympathetic nerve activity was also shown to correlate positively with age. Although these data suggest that muscle sympathetic nerve activity is not a major determinant of blood pressure in established hypertension, they may not reflect sympathetic outflow to other vascular beds, nor do they exclude sympathetic overactivity as a pathogenetic factor during the early stages of hypertension. In this respect, more recent data indicate that muscle sympathetic nerve activity is elevated in considerably younger patients (approximate mean age, 25 years) with borderline hypertension [26] (Figure 12.4). This patient group is more likely to reflect the developing stages of the disease, and supports the existence of elevated sympathetic drive at this time. Yamada et al. [27] reported that muscle sympathetic nerve activity is elevated not only in young patients, but also in middle-aged and older patients with established hypertension. Thus, although both studies [26, 27] support the existence of sympathetic overactivity in early hypertension, the precise relation with the time course of the disease remains to be resolved.

The pharmacological, biochemical and electrophysiological techniques described above indicate that peripheral sympathetic nerve activity may be raised in patients with hypertension, particularly in the earliest stages of the disease. More recently, studies have extended to the investigation of norepinephrine turnover within the central nervous system, in order to determine a central basis for sympathetic overactivity. Norepinephrine is one of the transmitters involved in sympathoexcitatory pathways which control blood pressure regulation (see Sympathetic premotor neurons), and measurement of its spillover from the brain may provide an insight into the

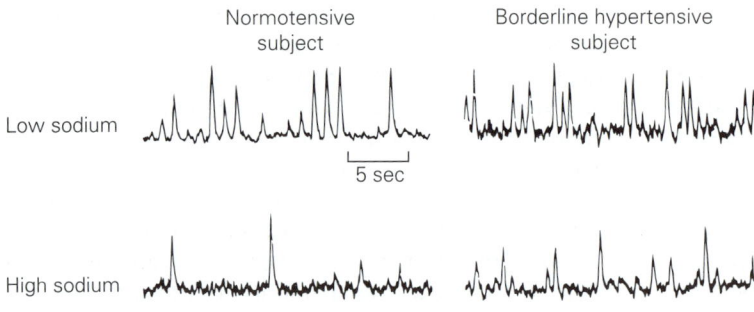

Figure 12.4 Neurogram of muscle sympathetic nerve activity in a normotensive subject and in a borderline hypertensive subject on both high and low sodium diets. Spikes indicate bursts of muscle sympathetic nerve activity. Muscle sympathetic nerve activity, which declined from low to high sodium diets, was consistently higher in the borderline hypertensive subject. (Reproduced, with permission, from ref. 26.)

activity of these pathways in hypertension. Overflow of endogenous norepinephrine into the jugular venous system, assessed using a radioisotope dilution, was uninfluenced by sympathetic ganglion blockade and in patients with idiopathic peripheral autonomic insufficiency, suggesting that it originated from brain neurons rather than cerebrovascular sympathetic nerves. Cerebral norepinephrine spillover was significantly elevated in patients with essential hypertension, compared to healthy subjects, indicating that there is an increased norepinephrine release within the brain, which may reflect an enhanced noradrenergic sympathoexcitatory drive in patients with hypertension.

Psychosomatic link

The precise cause of the increased sympathetic and decreased parasympathetic drive in hypertension is unknown. The reciprocal nature of these changes suggests that it originates in the medulla oblongata which integrates the basal output to both branches of the autonomic nervous system. Psychosomatic factors may play a role in abnormal autonomic control of the circulation in borderline hypertension, since the observed hemodynamic pattern is representative of that induced during the 'defense response' [28]. Psychometric tests indicate that certain personality traits, such as submissiveness, hostility and inability to express anger, are associated with borderline hypertension [29], whereas mild hypertensives and normotensive offspring of hypertensives show larger than normal blood pressure responses to mental stress [30]. However, it is still unclear whether such behavioral patterns could represent the mechanism of development of hypertension since it has never been proved experimentally that hypertension may develop through the summation of repeated, emotionally induced pressor episodes.

Epinephrine and modulation of transmitter release

In addition to an enhanced centrally mediated sympathetic drive, peripheral factors may contribute to enhanced neurotransmission in hypertension. At the neuroeffector junction, where sympathetic postgan-

glionic fibers terminate onto vascular smooth muscle, a number of mechanisms are present which regulate neurotransmitter overflow. These include presynaptic α- and β-adrenoceptors, which inhibit and facilitate transmitter release, respectively (see Regulation of transmitter release). It has been hypothesized that epinephrine may play a role in the pathogenesis of hypertension via its facilitatory action at presynaptic β-adrenoceptors to increase norepinephrine overflow and subsequently potentiate vasoconstriction. Infusion of epinephrine, into normotensive healthy subjects, results in an increase in blood pressure, which is sustained for up to 18 h after infusion has ceased and plasma epinephrine levels have returned to normal. This delayed pressor response was specific to epinephrine and not produced by norepinephrine infusion. In support of facilitation of transmitter release, plasma norepinephrine levels were also shown to increase after epinephrine infusion. The epinephrine-induced elevation in blood pressure and plasma norepinephrine could be prevented by coadministration of the β-adrenoceptor antagonist, propranolol, confirming that the action of epinephrine was via β-adrenoceptors.

The fact that the effect of epinephrine was sustained, long after plasma levels returned to normal, supports the hypothesis that epinephrine is accumulated into sympathetic nerve terminals, stored, and co-released during subsequent neurotransmission. In this case, the delayed pressor response elicited by β-adrenoceptor agonists should depend critically on neuronal amine uptake. This has been tested in humans using the β-adrenoceptor agonist, isoprenaline, which is not a substrate for neuronal amine uptake [31], and the neuronal amine uptake blocker, desipramine [32]. Epinephrine, but not isoprenaline, caused an increase in sympathetic vasoconstriction evoked by lower body negative pressure (LBNP), up to 30 min after epinephrine infusion had ceased [31], and the effect of epinephrine could be prevented by desipramine [32]. These data confirm the requirement for neuronal amine uptake of β-adrenoceptor agonists, in order to produce sustained facilitation of sympathetic neurotransmission, thereby supporting the proposed mechanism of action of epinephrine in a delayed pressor effect.

When responses to epinephrine infusion have been

compared in hypertensive patients and normal control subjects, plasma norepinephrine levels and vasoconstriction elicited by LBNP [33] were elevated to the same extent in both groups. This indicates that the response elicited by epinephrine, and presumably presynaptic β-adrenoceptor function *per se*, is not deranged in hypertension. However, identification of the β-adrenoceptor mechanism in humans, which facilitates sympathetic neurotransmission and results in a sustained pressor response, raises the possibility that an increased concentration of circulating epinephrine in patients with hypertension may contribute to the elevation in blood pressure via this mechanism. Thus, epinephrine may play a role in the development and maintenance of hypertension, particularly if borderline hypertensive subjects have more frequent or exaggerated surges of epinephrine in response to psychological or physiological stimuli.

The sympathetic nervous system and renal disease

Experiments in animals have indicated that the kidney is a sensory organ which contains nerve fibers which can be stimulated by both mechanical and chemical signals. These could conceivably be involved in the pathogenesis of hypertension by inducing reflex activation of the sympathetic nervous system [34]. Furthermore, in the kidney, sympathetic activity itself stimulates renin release, sodium and water reabsorption and renal artery vasoconstriction. The latter action will raise blood pressure and cause further sodium retention. Stimulation of renal afferent nerves with the intrarenal administration of urea or adenosine reflexly increases efferent sympathetic nervous system activity and blood pressure. Denervation reduces sympathetic overactivity and blood pressure in experimental renovascular hypertension. In consequence, elevated sympathetic nervous system activity and blood pressure in some patients with end-stage renal disease may be caused in part by uremic toxins acting on excitatory renal afference in the failing kidney. This mechanism can be eliminated by bilateral nephrectomy [35]. In humans, enhanced sympathetic nervous system activity has been reported in patients with renal artery stenosis with higher concentrations of catecholamines in the ischemic kidney. Also sympathetic overactivity has been implicated in patients with nephrotic syndrome: the secretion rate of plasma norepinephrine was quantified by radionucleide tracer techniques and found to be increased. In rats, the turnover rates of norepinephrine and the posterior and lateral hypothalamic nuclei are increased in renal failure. Whether the enhanced sympathetic nervous activity is the cause of the nephrogenic hypertension or renal failure is still open to debate. It is

probably more likely to be due to increased stimulation of the renin–angiotensin cascade in response to renal ischemia but once autonomic overactivity has been triggered, there is no question that it will contribute to the hypertension observed. As indicated above, there is no doubt that a mechanism can be shown whereby the failure to clear toxins such as urea could raise blood pressure by stimulation of renal afferent sympathetic fibers. The work of Di Bona [36] is especially important in this context. He demonstrated that, in rats, renal sympathetic nervous system activity could cause renal vasoconstriction as well as the enhanced release of renin and sodium reabsorption and water from the renal tubules at relatively low frequencies of renal nerve stimulation that do not affect renal blood flow or glomular filtration. Therefore, low levels of renal sympathetic nervous system activity can alter the pressure natriuresis curve and facilitate the maintenance of hypertension by interfering with the ability of the kidney to compensate for changes upward in blood pressure via the expected pressure natriuresis.

In summary, in renal disease it is likely that the mechanism by which some patients develop hypertension rests on renal sympathetic nervous system stimulation and a derangement in the usual compensatory mechanisms. In some respects, the same abnormalities may be important for the genesis of essential hypertension as a result of similar disordering of the compensatory mechanisms such as pressure natriuresis, but of course in this context the stimulus would come from the central nervous system modulation of sympathetic nervous system activity, whereas in renal disease it will come from local afferent provocation.

Summary

Our knowledge of the anatomical control of the autonomic nervous system remains incomplete but the picture is becoming clearer. Sympathetic overactivity has been demonstrated in patients with essential hypertension. Sympathetic nervous activity in skeletal muscle is enhanced and cardiac output is increased in young patients with essential hypertension. The cause may reside in a functional abnormality of the integrative brain centers such as the hypothalamus, RVLM and the baroreflex. Autoregressive spectral analyses have shown that the sympathetic component of blood pressure regulation is enhanced in hypertensive patients and that baroreflex sensitivity declines as the sympathetic component rises. Disturbances of autonomic function in renal disease are probably secondary to the disease process rather than causative.

References

1. Dampney, R.A. (1994) Functional organisation of central pathways regulating the cardiovascular system. *Physiol. Rev.*, **74**, 323–64.

2. Dean, C. and Coote, J.H. (1986) A ventromedullary relay involved in the hypothalamic and chemoreceptor activation of sympathetic postganglionic neurones to skeletal muscle, kidney and splanchnic area. *Brain Res.*, **377**, 279–85.

3. Dampney, R.A.L. and McAllen, R.M. (1988) Differential control of sympathetic fibres supplying hindlimb skin and muscle by subretrofacial neurones in the cat. *J. Physiol.*, **395**, 41–56.

4. Hagbarth, K.E. and Vallbo, A.B. (1968) Pulse and respiratory grouping of sympathetic impulses in human muscle nerves. *Acta Physiol. Scand.*, **74**, 96–108.

5. Nilsson, H., Lung, B., Sjoblom, N. and Wallin, B.G. (1985) The influence of the sympathetic impulse pattern on contractile responses of rat mesenteric arteries and veins. *Acta Physiol. Scand.*, **123**, 303–9.

6. Nilsson, H., Goldstein, M. and Nilsson, O. (1986) Adrenergic innervation and neurogenic response in large and small arteries and veins from the rat. *Acta Physiol. Scand.*, **126**, 121–33.

7. Luff, S.E., McLachlan, E.M. and Hirst, G.D.S. (1987) An ultrastructural analysis of the sympathetic neuromuscular junctions on arterioles of the submusoca of the guinea-pig ileum. *J. Comp. Neurol.*, **257**, 578–94.

8. Luff, S.E. and McLachlan, E.M. (1989) Frequency of neuromuscular junctions on arteries of different dimensions in the rabbit, guinea-pig and rat. *Blood Vessels*, **26**, 95–106.

9. Blakeley, A.G.H. and Cunane, T.C. (1979) The packaged release of transmitter from the sympathetic nerves of the guinea-pig vas deferens: an electrophysiological study. *J. Physiol.*, **296**, 85–96.

10. Hirst, G.D.S. and Neild, T.O. (1981) Localization of specialized noradrenaline receptors at neuromuscular junctions on arterioles of the guinea-pig. *J. Physiol.*, **313**, 343–50.

11. Langer, S.Z. (1977) Presynaptic receptors and their role in the regulation of transmitter release. *Br. J. Pharmocal.*, **60**, 481–97.

12. Kalsner, S. (1984) Limitations of presynaptic theory: no support for feedback control of autonomic effectors. *Fed. Proc.*, **43**, 1358–64.

13. Kalsner, S. (1990) Heteroreceptors, autoreceptors and other terminal sites. *Ann. NY Acad. Sci.*, **604**, 1–6.

14. Langer, S.Z. and Enero, M.A. (1974) The potentiation of responses to adrenergic nerve stimulation in the presence of cocaine: its relationship to the metabolic fate of released noradrenaline. *J. Pharmocal. Exp. Ther.*, **191**, 431–43.

15. Stjarne, L. and Brundin, J. (1975) Dual adrenoceptor mediated control of noradrenaline secretion from human vasoconstrictor nerves: facilitation by β-receptors and inhibition by α-receptors. *Acta Physiol. Scand.*, **94**, 139–41.

16. Kirkpatrick, K. and Burnstock, G. (1987) Sympathetic nerve-mediated release of ATP from the guinea-pig vas deferens is unaffected by reserpine. *Eur. J. Pharmacol.*, **138**, 207.

17. Burnstock, G. and Warland, J.J.I. (1987) A pharmacological study of the rabbit saphenous artery *in vitro*: a vessel with a large purinergic contractile response to sympathetic nerve stimulation. *Br. J. Pharmacol.*, **90**, 111–20.

18. Stephens, N., Bund, S.J., Faragher, E.B. and Heagerty, A.M. (1992) Neurotransmission in human resistance arteries: contribution of α_1- and α_2-adrenoceptors but not P2-purinoceptors. *J. Vasc. Res.*, **29**, 347–52.

19. Stephens, N. and Heagerty, A.M. (1994) The sympathetic nervous system and small artery neuroeffector function in hypertension. *Vasc. Med. Rev.*, **5**, 73–91.

20. Julius, S. (1990) Changing role of the autonomic nervous system in human hypertension. *J. Hypertens.*, **8**, S59–65.

21. Lund-Johansen, P. (1989) Central hemodynamics in essential hypertension at rest and during exercise: a 20 year follow-up study. *J. Hypertens.*, **7**(suppl 6), S52–5.

22. Esler, M., Eisenhofer, G., Chu, J. *et al.* (1991) Release of adrenaline from the human sympathetic nervous system. *Clin. Autonom. Res.*, **1**, 103–8.

23. Esler, M., Jennings, G., Korner, P. *et al.* (1988) Assessment of human sympathetic nervous activity from measurements of norepinephrine turnover. *Hypertension*, **11**, 3–20.

24. Goldstein, D.S. (1983) Plasma catecholamines and essential hypertension: an analytical review. *Hypertension*, **5**, 86–99.

25. Esler, M., Jennings, G., Biviano, B. *et al.* (1986) Mechanism of elevated plasma noradrenaline in the course of essential hypertension. *J. Cardiovasc. Pharmacol.*, **8**(suppl 5), S39–43.

26. Anderson, E.A., Sinkey, C.A., Lawton, W.J. and Mark, A.L. (1989) Elevated sympathetic nerve activity in borderline hypertensive humans: evidence from direct intraneural recordings. *Hypertension*, **14**, 177–83.

27. Yamada, Y., Miyajima, E., Tochikubo, O. *et al.* (1989) Age-related changes in muscle sympathetic nerve activity in essential hypertension. *Hypertension*, **13**, 870–7.

28. Julius, S. (1993) Sympathetic hyperactivity and coronary risk in hypertension. *Hypertension*, **21**, 886–93.

29. Esler, M., Julius, S., Zweifter, A. *et al.* (1977) Mild high-renin essential hypertension: a neurogenic human hypertension. *N. Engl. J. Med.*, **296**, 405–11.

30. Falkner, B., Onesti, G., Angelakos, E.T. *et al.* (1979) Cardiovascular response to mental stress in normal adolescents with hypertensive parents. *Hypertension*, **1**, 23–30.

31. Floras, J.S., Aylward, D.E., Victor, R.G. *et al.* (1988) Epinephrine facilitates neurogenic vasoconstriction in humans. *J. Clin. Invest.*, **81**, 1265–74.

32. Floras, J.S., Aylward, D.E., Mark, A.L. and Abboud, F.M. (1990) Adrenaline facilitates neurogenic vasoconstriction in borderline hypertensives. *J. Hypertens.*, **8**, 443–8.

33. Floras, J.S., Sole, M.J. and Morris, B.L. (1990) Desipramine blocks augmented neurogenic vasoconstriction to epinephrine. *Hypertension*, **15**, 132–9.

34. DiBona, G.F. (1982) The functions of the renal nerves. *Rev. Physiol. Biochem. Pharmacol.*, **94**, 76–181.

35. Converse, R.L. Jr, Tage, N., Jacobsen, T.N. *et al.* (1992) Sympathetic overactivity in patients with chronic renal failure. *N. Engl. J. Med.*, **327**, 1912–18.

36. DiBona, G.F. (1989) Sympathetic nervous system: influence on the kidney, role in hypertension. *Am. J. Hypertens.*, **2**, 119S–24S.

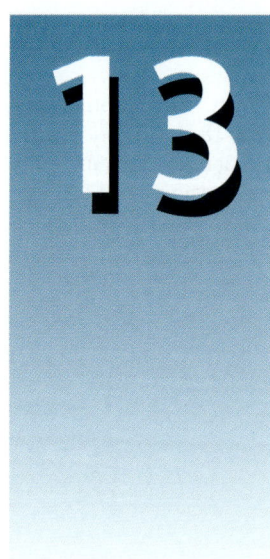

Vasoactive mediators in blood pressure control and the regulation of renal function

Norberto Perico, Ariela Benigni, Marina Noris and Giuseppe Remuzzi

Introduction

The vascular endothelium responds to a variety of mechanical and neurohumoral stimuli by modulating the tone of underlying smooth muscle cells. This has been attributed to the presence on the cell surface of binding sites specific for circulatory vasoactive hormones, such as bradykinin and angiotensin II, or to the release of vasoactive substances that may control vascular tone through their vasodilatory or vasoconstrictory actions. The important role of the kallikrein–kinin system and renin–angiotensin system in the regulation of blood pressure has now been clearly established. There is also renewed interest in the contribution of these hormonal systems and in the role of recently discovered vasoactive mediators in the control of cardiovascular and renal functions. Here we shall provide the reader with an overview of the role of kallikrein–kinin components in blood pressure regulation, the physiological actions of the renin–angiotensin system with special emphasis on the involvement of different angiotensin II receptor subtypes, and the latest findings related to the extrarenal and renal actions of atrial natriuretic peptide, endothelin and nitric oxide.

The kallikrein–kinin system

Plasma and renal kallikrein–kinin

The kallikrein–kinin system participates in circulatory homeostasis by generating the peptide bradykinin, a potent vasodilator [1]. Kinins generated within the kidney do not gain access to the systemic circulation, so the systemic and renal kallikrein–kinin systems act in two separate compartments. Kallikreins are enzymes which release kinin from the precursor glycoprotein kininogens (Figure 13.1). The enzymatic activity of these proteases depends on a serine residue at their catalytic site.

There are two distinct enzymes in this family, plasma and glandular kallikrein, with different molecular weights, immunoreactivity, *in vivo* localization and sites at which they cleave their substrate kininogen. High (HMW) and low (LMW) molecular weight kininogens are synthesized in the liver and are substrates for plasma kallikrein; LMW kininogen is probably a substrate for glandular kallikrein as well but its site of synthesis is unknown. Plasma kallikrein acts on its substrate to release the nonapeptide, bradykinin, whereas glandular kallikrein cleaves kininogens to generate the decapeptide lys-bradykinin, kallidin, which is converted into bradykinin by an aminopeptidase.

Several serine protease inhibitors, including aprotinin and α_1-antitrypsin, block the enzymatic activity of kallikrein. Bradykinin, the vasoactive peptide of the kininogen–kallikrein system, is rapidly inactivated by kininase I and II (angiotensin I converting enzyme) by hydrolysis of the C-terminal arginine or the dipeptide phenylalanine-arginine, respectively.

Vasoactive properties

Combining high-performance liquid chromatography and N-terminal and C-terminal kinin radioimmunoassay,

Nephrology, Edited by Rex L. Jamison and Robert Wilkinson.
Published in 1997 by Chapman & Hall, London. ISBN 0 412 60930 4

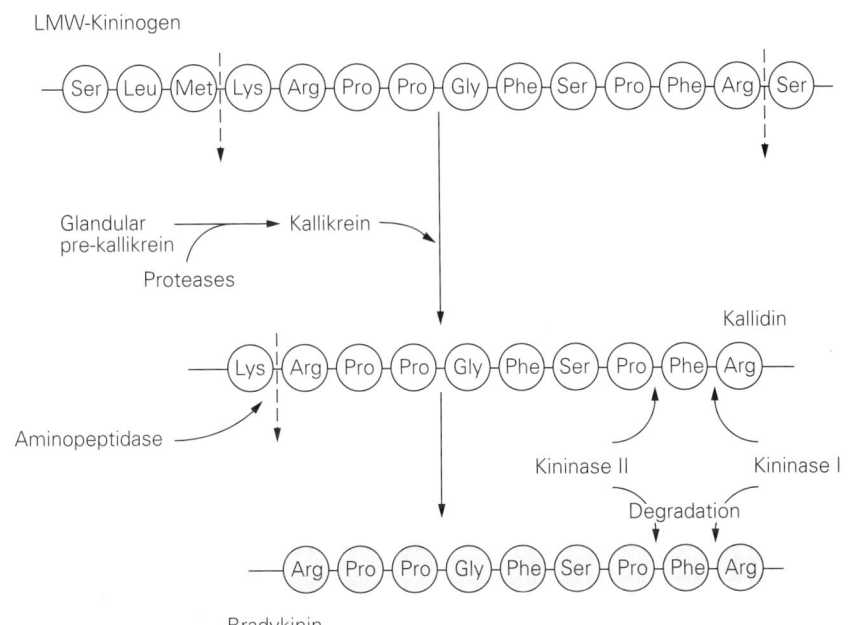

LMW-Kininogen

Figure 13.1 Pathways involved in the synthesis and degradation of glandular kinins. LMW, low molecular weight.

Campbell *et al.* [2] have measured individual kinins in tissue and blood. In the rat, the wall of the aorta contained the highest level of kinins, mostly the bradykinin-(1–9) peptide (340 fmol/g), which was approximately three times higher than in kidney, adrenal and lung. Tissue bradykinin levels were much higher than blood levels, indicating that the peptide is formed locally. That kinins are generated in vessels is supported by recent evidence that exposure of preconstricted isolated canine coronary artery rings to kallikrein induced an endothelium-dependent relaxation, which was inhibited by aprotinin and potentiated by coincubation with a converting enzyme inhibitor [3]. Thus local kinins may be generated from vascular kininogen and have vasoactive properties.

Bradykinin vasorelaxation requires an intact endothelium. *In vitro* experiments suggest that cyclic guanosine monophosphate (cGMP) acts as a second messenger induced by bradykinin binding to its receptor, as documented by the increased concentration of cyclic GMP in the perfusion bath. Since vessel relaxation in response to bradykinin is prevented by the nitric oxide (NO) synthase inhibitor, L-NAME, which also completely abolished the bradykinin-induced increase in cGMP, it has been proposed that NO actually mediates bradykinin-induced endothelium-dependent vasorelaxation [4]. Besides NO, hyperpolarizing factor(s) released by the endothelial cells on exposure to bradykinin have been suggested as playing a role in its vasorelaxing activity. This possibility rests on the observation that endothelium-dependent hyperpolarization of vascular smooth muscle cells and the consequent vasodilation did not change in the presence of L-NAME, but increased on challenge with the converting enzyme inhibitor captopril [4]. It has been well documented *in vivo* that inhibition of converting enzyme,

which also blocks the main pathway of kinin degradation, enhances the vasoactive properties of bradykinin [3]. Thus the vasodepressor effect of both endogenous and exogenous bradykinin is potentiated in animals given angiotensin converting enzyme (ACE) inhibitors. However, *in vitro* experiments have given contradictory results [3]. In isolated mesenteric arteries preconstricted with phenylephrine, bradykinin induced a dose-related decrease in perfusion pressure. In the presence of captopril, vasorelaxation was followed by vasoconstriction. This biphasic response was abolished and prolonged vasorelaxation was observed when the arteries were treated with indomethacin, suggesting that vasoconstriction might be due to the release of vasoconstrictor prostanoids. In other experiments perindopril, cilazapril and to a lower extent captopril potentiated the bradykinin-induced relaxation of porcine femoral arterial rings and canine coronary artery preconstricted with prostaglandin $F_{2\alpha}$. Inconsistencies in the effect of converting enzyme inhibition have also been reported in preparations of femoral artery rings or perfused arterial segments, with potentiation of bradykinin-induced relaxation observed only in the latter. This has been explained by assuming that converting enzyme is only distributed on the endothelial surface of the vessels, so that only in the perfused segments could it contribute to kinin metabolism. However, not all vascular segments behave in the same way in this respect.

In vitro bradykinin can contract porcine femoral artery rings by an endothelium-independent pathway, but this does not apply to its actions in all tissues. The contractile response is probably mediated by activation of B1-type receptors on smooth muscle cells, to the extent that contraction induced by the selective B1-kinin receptor agonist, des-Arg^9-bradykinin, is selectively inhibited by a

B1-receptor antagonist. Responses of rabbit aorta were largely dependent on the influx of extracellular calcium, whereas the rabbit jugular vein required both external calcium and mobilization of calcium from intracellular stores. Moreover bradykinin-induced contractions in jugular vein but not in aorta appeared to involve activation of protein kinase C, indicating coupling with different second messengers.

Blood pressure control in normal conditions

There is still considerable uncertainty about the physiological role of the plasma kallikrein–kinin system in cardiovascular homeostasis. Hypotensive episodes in patients given plasma protein fractions containing high concentrations of the active fragment of factor XII were originally considered related to activation of the plasma kallikrein–kinin system. This was supported by the demonstration that in normal rats purified human factor XII induced a dose-dependent drop in blood pressure, which was significantly enhanced by pretreatment with captopril. This finding and data in rats showing that a bradykinin antagonist prevented the hypotensive effect of factor XII indicated that bradykinin can reach a high enough concentration in the circulation to exert a hemodynamic effect. In conscious normotensive rats, however, bradykinin antagonists did not change blood pressure either with a functionally intact ACE or after captopril.

These last observations argue against a major role for circulating bradykinin in the control of blood pressure in normotensive rats. There are recent data that in anesthetized normotensive rats the intravenous infusion of a specific active site-directed inhibitor of endopeptidase-24.15, a neutral metalloenzyme that cleaves bradykinin, caused a dose-dependent, immediate but short-lived drop in blood pressure [3]. This hypotensive effect was almost completely attenuated by a B_2-kinin receptor antagonist. These findings suggest that the enzyme is directly involved in the control of blood pressure and, at variance with previous observations, that endogenous kinins are involved in the control of normal blood pressure.

In transgenic mice overexpressing human tissue kallikrein, high levels of the immunoreactive enzyme were detected in the circulation and blood pressure was significantly lower than in control mice. Administration of aprotinin, a potent tissue kallikrein inhibitor, restored the blood pressure of the transgenic mice but had no effect on control littermates, raising the possibility that tissue kallikrein is also implicated in regulation of pressure.

Endogenous bradykinin may participate indirectly in the regulation of cardiovascular homeostasis by virtue of its ability to blunt the activity of vasopressors [5]. This is suggested by the further rise in blood pressure when normal rats, previously infused with angiotensin II or lysine-vasopressin, were given a bradykinin-antagonist.

The blood pressure effect of bradykinin also depends on sodium balance. In normotensive rats given a single injection of furosemide, a bradykinin antagonist raised blood pressure more than in vehicle-treated animals.

Role in the development of hypertension

In 1934 Elliott and Nazum [6] showed that patients with hypertension excreted in the urine a depressor substance they identified as the 'kallikrein of Frey and Kraut', suggesting for the first time that kallikrein might be related to hypertensive diseases. The role of the kallikrein–kinin system in hypertension, however, remains unclear. Spontaneously hypertensive rats and rats with deoxycorticosterone acetate (DOCA)–salt hypertension had lower urinary kallikrein excretion than normotensive Wistar controls [3]. Spontaneously hypertensive Okamoto–Aoki rats (SHR) on a normal sodium diet had lower urinary kallikrein than normotensive Wistar–Kyoto (WKY) rats on the same diet. Because kinins increase the excretion of sodium and water, a reduced activity of the renal kallikrein–kinin system in young SHR may predispose to salt retention and hypertension. However, the above observation was made at 4 weeks of age when systolic blood pressure was already significantly higher than in controls. Thus the precise role of kinins in the development of chronic hypertension in these animals remains unclear. Interestingly, the abnormality in kallikrein excretion showed no tendency to increase with age or with the development of hypertension, so it may indeed be an inherited defect.

In Brown–Norway rats that are congenitally deficient in HMW and LMW kininogens, DOCA–salt treatment at 5 weeks of age [3] did not raise blood pressure compared to normal rats of the same strain. Uninephrectomy at 7 weeks of age and weekly injections of DOCA salt induced a rapid increase in blood pressure in kininogen-deficient rats, whereas normal rats only gradually developed hypertension. After six weeks of treatment blood pressure was similar in the two groups. These findings suggested that the kallikrein–kinin system may contribute to lowering systolic blood pressure in the development of this form of hypertension. The suppressive role of kinins in the initial increase of blood pressure in DOCA–salt rats is borne out by the observation that aprotinin, an inhibitor of plasma and glandular kallikrein, continuously infused to Brown–Norway rats increased the rate of blood pressure rise induced by DOCA–salt treatment [3].

In SHR rats, abnormalities in fluid balance may precede the development of hypertension. Plante et al. [7] showed that in SHR rats at 4 weeks of age, when they were still normotensive, the renal content of Evans-Blue-bound-albumin, a marker of vascular permeability, was higher than in aged-matched WKY rats. At 8, 12 and 16 weeks SHR rats had high blood pressure and a further increase in vascular permeability. Administration of a B_2-kinin receptor antagonist to young SHR rats reduced the accumulation of renal tissue albumin to a level comparable to that in WKY rats. Thus kinins may contribute to renal vascular permeability in SHR rats, increasing the total extracellular fluid volume associated with the development of hypertension in this model.

The role of the kallikrein–kinin system in blood pressure control in humans is not known. Since the first report early this century, the area has been neglected for 40 years although patients with various forms of hypertension have been studied. Most studies agree that in essential hypertension urinary excretion of kallikrein is reduced compared to that in age-matched normotensive controls. The same abnormality is found in normotensive subjects with a family history of essential hypertension. These findings are consistent with the suggestion of a genetically determined decrease in renal kallikrein activity that may contribute to the development of hypertension. This is in line with data indicating a familial tendency for kallikrein excretion, with 51% of the total variance attributable to a single gene. The expression of this gene separates individuals into groups with different relative risks of a history of parental hypertension.

Kinins and the antihypertensive activity of ACE inhibitors

The antihypertensive effect of ACE inhibitors is mainly due to diminished formation of angiotensin II, but reduced degradation of kinins may also play a role. The acute antihypertensive effect of ACE inhibitors is in fact attenuated by antikinin antibodies or kinin antagonists in rat models of renin-dependent hypertension [3]. Infusion of a B_2-kinin antagonist, although not modifying basal blood pressure, attenuated the hypotensive effects of acute captopril and ramipril in SHR rats. Whether this also applies to chronic ACE inhibition has been investigated in two-kidney, one-clip hypertensive Wistar rats. In these animals chronic kinin receptor blockade with the bradykinin B_2-receptor antagonist HOE 140 attenuated the antihypertensive effect of ramipril.

Atrial natriuretic peptide

Atrial natriuretic factor

Mammalian cardiac atria synthesize and store a peptide hormone that is secreted in response to atrial distension and was originally known by a variety of names, including atriopeptin, cardionatrin, cardiodilatin, or auriculin. It is now termed atrial natriuretic peptide (ANP) [8]. Soon after the discovery of ANP in 1981 when it was shown that crude extracts of rat atria contained a potent diuretic and natriuretic substance, this peptide and its precursors were purified, their gene sequence was determined and radioimmunoassays were developed.

In addition to contractile elements, the atrial muscle contains myoendocrine cells that synthesize ANP as a 151-amino acid 'prepro-ANP' precursor [8]. This is processed to a 126-amino acid 'pro ANP', which is temporarily stored in secretory granules. The prohormone is probably converted into the final 28-amino acid peptide ANP as part of the secretory process by a cleavage enzyme. ANP with one disulfide bond is the carboxy-terminus of pro-ANP (sequence 99 through 126) and is the major biologically active form released in the circulation, although some pro-ANP may reach the bloodstream intact. The amino acid sequence of ANP is well preserved between animal species as documented by the fact that the peptide in the human and the dog differs by only one amino acid from that in the rat, mouse and rabbit.

Physiological perturbations associated with a rise in atrial pressure, including head-out water immersion and blood volume expansion, lead to a two- to threefold increase in plasma levels of immunoreactive ANP [8]. This has been attributed to an intrinsic stretch–secretion coupling mechanism as a consequence of atrial distension, since in isolated rat atria, ANP is released in direct proportion to the mechanical load.

Although ANP was first recognized as an atrial hormone, recent evidence shows that the ANP gene is expressed in the ventricles of adult hearts as well as in embryonic ventricles. In the rat both distal and proximal ANP gene regulatory domains are crucial for cardiac ANP gene expression [9], whereas in humans an additional 64-base pair (bp) element has been found to confer cardiac-specific expression to the ANP gene [9]. Studies in cultured neonatal ventricular cells have shown that activation of this gene, reported during cardiac hypertrophy, occurs either through a protein kinase C-dependent transcriptional mechanism or through an increase in the cytoplasmic calcium concentration independent of protein kinase C activity [9].

Vasoactive and renal properties

Once released in the circulation ANP reaches target tissue and organs where it exerts vasoactive, natriuretic and diuretic effects through binding to its receptors. Two major classes of ANP receptor have been identified with distinct biochemical characteristics and functional properties [10]. The guanylate cyclase (GC) receptors mediate the end-organ effects of ANP and contain the enzyme as a part of the cytoplasmic domain of the receptor molecule. At least two subtypes of GC receptors have been characterized, A and B [10]. The cytoplasmic domain of the GC_A and GC_B receptors is identical, but they differ in the extracellular domain. This leads to different ligand specificities, as documented by a very low affinity for ANP of the GC_B receptors, which thus cannot function as true receptors of ANP, and high affinity of the GC_A receptors. Besides the GC sequence, the cytoplasmic domain of these receptors contains a protein-kinase sequence that inhibits the activation of GC.

The other major class of ANP receptors does not mediate any of the known effects of ANP in the target tissues but participates in removal of ANP from the circulation; they are therefore known as clearance receptors (C-ANP) [10]. These are homodimers of approximately 120 kDa, with a very short cytoplasmic domain, as for other clearance receptors, and a large extracellular tail which shows high homology, hence similar affinity, to GC_A-ANP receptors. Unlike other polypeptide hormone receptors, GC_A-ANP receptors do not require G-proteins for receptor–enzyme coupling, but directly activate GC after ligand binding, leading to generation of guanosine 3',5'-cyclic monophosphate (cGMP), the second messenger of most of ANP's effects. This is supported by findings of increased cGMP in target tissues and plasma after ANP challenge in all studies reported, together with the observation that cGMP analogues mimic the vasorelaxant and some of the renal actions of ANP.

The poor correlation found between the ability of ANP analogues to increase cGMP in rat aortic smooth muscle cells in culture and their vasorelaxant effect in preconstricted strips of rat aorta has been attributed to differences in the type of receptors in cultured cells and intact aorta, GC_B-ANP and C-ANP being the major receptors in smooth muscle cells, and GC_A-ANP in the aorta. Similarly, the difference noted between the affinity (kDa) of binding and the ED_{50} of the cGMP generating effect of ANP has been explained by temperatures at which experiments have been done (i.e. below or at 37°C).

The view of increased cGMP generation as a primary event in the cellular action of ANP has been challenged by some investigators who consider inhibition of cAMP production as the intracellular pathway that mediates the vascular, adrenal and renal effects of ANP. This is based on the demonstration that ANP, at a very low concentration, inhibited the enzyme adenylate cyclase through activation of a pertussis toxin-sensitive G_1 protein in many preparations including vessels, glomeruli, and some nephron segments. C-ANP has been suggested as the receptor for this effect. However, these findings have not been confirmed, and further work is required to clarify this still controversial issue.

The intracellular mechanisms by which cGMP mediates the actions of ANP are not well defined (Figure 13.2). It has been suggested that some of these mechanisms involve the activation of Ca^{2+}-ATPase, leading to a decrease in cytosolic Ca^{2+}; the stimulation of furosemide-sensitive Na-2Cl-K co-transporter; the inhibition of amiloride-sensitive sodium or cation channels; and the inhibition of thiazide-sensitive neutral NaCl co-transport [10]. Although these events may explain the major vascular, adrenal and renal effects of ANP, evidence in support of these intracellular pathways remains descriptive in nature and does not allow any clear interpretation of the known cellular actions of ANP or a demonstration of common pathways in the different cell targets.

ANP has multiple actions that reflect the distribution of specific receptors in tissues and organs, including vas-culature, kidney, adrenal, lung, intestine and brain [8, 10]. In the vascular system ANP strongly antagonizes vasoconstriction and may even have weak agonist action *per se*. The cardiovascular effects include a reduction in cardiac output as a result of a shift of fluid from the intravascular compartment to the interstitium that ultimately reduces plasma volume. In the kidney, ANP modulates renal hemodynamics and tubular function in such a way as to increase fluid and sodium excretion. It affects endocrine function by inhibiting the renin–angiotensin–aldosterone system, a property that may substantially contribute to the cardiovascular and renal effects of the peptide and to the regulation of plasma volume and blood pressure.

Regulation of blood pressure

Much experimental work has focused on the potential association between ANP and blood pressure control [11]. This rests on the observation that several actions of ANP may specifically antagonize the postulated mechanisms involved in the development of hypertension. Among these, the smooth muscle relaxing properties of ANP may counteract enhanced arteriolar vasoconstriction induced by norepinephrine and angiotensin II. Moreover, the diuretic and natriuretic actions of ANP may overwhelm the defect in sodium excretion in hypertension, and thus influence the pressure/natriuresis set point.

Together, these major effects of ANP operate in concert to antagonize the elevation of blood pressure. This implies that ANP may be associated with the pathophysiology of hypertension, but definite proof is still lacking. If this were the case, some changes in plasma ANP levels would be expected in hypertension. In healthy humans specific radioimmunoassays of plasma ANP yield values in the range 10–80 pg/ml [11]. In hypertensive patients the earliest reports found that plasma ANP was significantly higher than normal, but more recent studies have not confirmed the findings [10]. A meta-analysis of 37 studies including 1367 hypertensive and 1371 normal subjects showed a weighted mean difference in plasma ANP concentration of 16 ± 39 pg/ml, with the hypertensives higher than normal [11]. These studies included all stages of essential hypertension, without controlling for age or sodium intake. The difference, however, was reduced to 5 ± 19 pg/ml in reports which were controlled for age and sodium intake and had a careful definition of hypertension with no evidence of end-organ damage. Overall, the difference may be inappropriately low given the increase in atrial filling pressures associated with hypertension. This observation suggests that inadequate secretion of ANP in response to a volume/pressure stimulus may account for persistent elevation of blood pressure in these patients. This would be in line with some animal studies that have documented a reduced secretory ANP response to volume stimuli in SHR rats [11]. Additional experiments suggest that this is only transient and occurs in young, prehypertensive but not

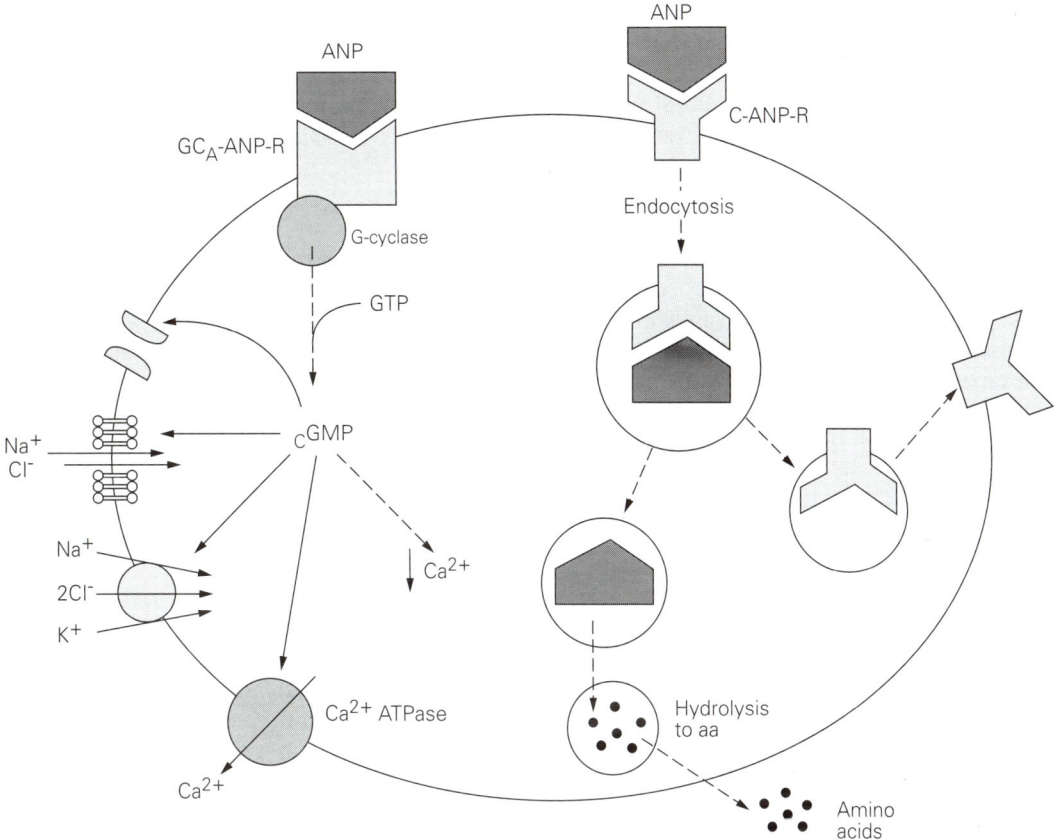

Figure 13.2 Schematic representation of the intracellular events that follow ANP binding to its guanylate cyclase and clearance receptors. Guanylate cyclase receptors (GCA-ANP-R) mediate the effects of ANP, while clearance receptors (C-ANP-R) participate in the removal of ANP from the circulation. G-cyclase, guanylate cyclase; Na^+, amiloride-sensitive sodium or cation channels; Na^+Cl^-, thiazide-sensitive neutral NaCl co-transport; $Na^+ - 2Cl^- - K^+$, furosemide $Na^+ - 2Cl^- - K^+$ co-transport.

adult SHR rats. Sodium loading caused a smaller rise in plasma ANP levels in the normotensive offspring of hypertensive patients than in age-matched offspring of normal rats.

Independently of plasma ANP concentrations, evidence of resistance to the actions of ANP in experimental animal models and in patients with essential hypertension suggests a connection between ANP and hypertension. This may reflect failure of ANP to elicit a vasodilatory response, as in SHR rats, or a reduced ability of the peptide to suppress renin and aldosterone secretion, but so far data are conflicting [11]. A lower than normal inhibition of sympathetic nervous system activity by ANP has been reported in hypertensive rats; whether this also applies in hypertensive humans has yet to be established.

Enhanced ANP clearance has also been considered in hypertension, but renal clearance is normal or somewhat reduced in essential and in renovascular hypertension, and the plasma half-life of exogenous ANP is normal or slightly prolonged in hypertensive patients [11]. Overall, in the absence of clear defects in its plasma levels, secretory response and actions in hypertension, it is difficult

to assign to ANP a pathophysiological role in essential hypertension. It appears more as a compensatory than a causative hormone in hypertension and its part in the control of systemic blood pressure remains to be demonstrated.

Regulation of renal function

When given by bolus injection or infusion, ANP markedly increases renal salt and water excretion [12]. Although the maximal natriuresis induced by ANP is much less than that attained by high doses of furosemide, approximately 1000 times more furosemide is required on a molar basis to induce the same natriuretic effect as ANP. ANP is one of the most potent endogenous natriuretic and diuretic substances known. The intrarenal mechanism(s) whereby it induces natriuresis and diuresis have been a matter of debate. Its excretory effects may be caused by elevation of the glomerular filtration rate (GFR) and by alterations of tubular NaCl transport. In most animal species, as well as in humans, bolus administration or continuous infusion of atrial extracts or synthetic ANP consistently increase GFR [8, 12]. By contrast, renal plasma flow only occasionally and transiently rises in response to ANP, resulting, in most instances, in a substantial rise in filtration fraction.

Micropuncture studies show that ANP infusion increases single nephron GFR and filtration fraction as a consequence of a rise in glomerular capillary hydraulic pressure. This change in pressure, in turn, is due to afferent arteriolar vasodilatation and a concurrent rise in efferent arteriolar tone [12]. These modifications were independent of endogenous angiotensin II activity and ANP-induced reduction in renal perfusion pressure.

It has therefore been proposed that the higher GFR might account entirely for the enhanced natriuresis and diuresis evoked by ANP, possibly by increasing salt delivery to the distal portion of the nephron. Delivery of sodium chloride may also be increased by medullary washout, which reduces passive movement of sodium out of the papillary thin ascending limb of Henle's loop [8, 12]. The increased delivery of salt and water to distal tubules may overwhelm their reabsorptive capacity and thus account fully for the ANP-induced natriuresis. However, micropuncture studies have shown that solute and fluid delivery to the last accessible portion of the distal tubule increased only two- to threefold with ANP, far less than the 10- to 50-fold increases in final urinary sodium excretion that commonly occur. Therefore, some investigators argued against the assumption that ANP-induced natriuresis results solely from increments in GFR and from the increased sodium chloride delivery, suggesting it must be due in large part to actions at other sites along the nephron [8, 12]. This was borne out by early micropuncture studies with atrial tissue extracts, and more recent microcatheterization experiments with synthetic ANP in rats, that documented decreased reabsorption of sodium chloride in the medullary collecting duct system. The finding that synthetic ANP stimulates cGMP accumulation in cultured papillary collecting duct cells *in vitro*, and enhances bath-to-lumen NaCl permeability in isolated rat papillary collecting ducts perfused *in vitro*, and that ANP inhibits sodium entry-dependent oxygen consumption in a suspension of rabbit papillary collecting duct cells *in vitro* further supports the concept that ANP acts on terminal nephron segments [12].

All these data, however, have been obtained with exogenous ANP. Information on the physiological significance of endogenous circulating ANP in the regulation of renal function was scarce until the discovery of inhibitors of the ANP-degrading enzyme, neutral endopeptidase 24.11, and the availability of ANP receptor antagonists [13]. In experimental animals under normal physiological conditions the administration of neutral endopeptidase inhibitors increases sodium excretion with a minimal or no increment in GFR. That these natriuretic actions of neutral endopeptidase inhibition are linked with changes in ANP metabolism is supported by the fact that most studies found parallel increases in plasma ANP and urinary ANP immunoreactivity, consistent with decreased renal degradation, as well as enhanced urinary cGMP excretion.

The neutral endopeptidase inhibitor sinorphan, given to healthy normotensive subjects on a normal-sodium diet, induced distal tubular natriuresis and a transient increase in GFR. Although neutral endopeptidase is not specific for ANP catabolism and may also interfere with the degradation of bradykinin and urodilatin (a natriuretic peptide synthesized by the kidney), which are also vasoactive and natriuretic, the effects of sinorphan mimics changes found when plasma ANP increases. Earlier studies showed that the natriuretic and diuretic responses to volume expansion may be blocked by specific anti-ANP antiserum [12], but a pharmacological blocker of natriuretic peptide receptors provides a more precise tool for elucidating the contribution of endogenous ANP.

Recently HS-142-1, a polysaccharide fermentation product, was found to compete for binding sites at the guanylyl cyclase-linked ANP receptors, and to inhibit the production of cyclic GMP by ANP. In anesthetized rats pretreatment with HS-142-1 prevented the increase in urine flow and urinary sodium excretion elicited by ANP [14]. More importantly, acute administration of HS-142-1 markedly blunted the natriuretic and diuretic responses to acute saline loading in euvolemic rats, by blocking both the increase in filtered load and the decreased tubular reabsorption of sodium [14]. These observations suggest ANP plays a major role in the regulation of salt and body fluid homeostasis by affecting sodium handling along the nephron.

The renin–angiotensin system

The renin–angiotensin system (RAS) is a phylogenetically old system for control of systemic blood pressure, fluid and electrolyte homeostasis that involves multiple organ systems. Renin, a glycoprotein synthesized in the juxtaglomerular apparatus of the kidney, converts its substrate, the α_2-globulin angiotensinogen synthesized and released by the liver cells, to the decapeptide angiotensin I (AI). This is believed to take place in the plasma. Then angiotensin converting enzyme (ACE), a non-specific dipeptidyl carboxypeptidase present primarily on endothelial cells, acts on AI by cleaving the octapeptide angiotensin II (AII) from its carboxy-terminal dipeptide.

The major effector of the system is actually AII, whose actions include vasoconstriction, stimulation of aldosterone secretion, increased sodium reabsorption by the macula densa, stimulation of thirst by interacting with sympathetic nerve transmission in the central nervous system, and direct inhibition of renin release in the kidney.

The availability of specific inhibitors and antagonists of AII receptors has recently helped in defining the concept that not all the actions of endogenous AII are carried out by the circulating form of the peptide. ACE inhibitors control blood pressure for periods of time that greatly exceed their plasma half-lives [15]. There is also a discrepancy between the antihypertensive effect of ACE inhibitors and plasma ACE activity.

These observations prompted investigators to look for the possible local form of the renin–angiotensin system (RAS), in addition to the systemic form. The finding that bilateral nephrectomy virtually eliminated plasma renin activity without reducing arterial wall renin concentrations in normotensive and hypertensive rats suggested the arterial renin concentration was independent of renal renin [15]. Moreover, isolated and perfused vascular tissues generate AII, which could be taken to indicate that all components of the cascade are present in vascular tissues [15].

Molecular biology tenchniques allowed cloning and DNA sequencing of all the components of the RAS, including renin, angiotensin, ACE, and the AII receptors [16]. Renin is expressed in various tissues/organs in the mouse and rat, including vascular tissue, brain, testes, heart, the submandibular gland and kidney. Angiotensinogen mRNA is present in the heart and vascular tissue, and angiotensinogen expression has been detected in the vascular smooth muscle cells of the aorta. *In vivo* autoradiography methods and mRNA have located ACE in the heart, with higher signals in the atria than in ventricles. These studies confirmed earlier immunocytochemical observations that ACE activity can be detected in the endothelial cell layer, and further indicate the importance of an intact endothelium for the local generation of AII in the vascular wall.

Vasoactive and renal properties

Circulating and locally produced AII exerts its effects by binding to specific receptors. Recently two subtypes of AII receptors have been described in various tissues, based on their affinity for recently developed AII antagonists, namely the non-peptide biphenylimidazoles, typified by losartan, and the tetrahydroimidapyridines (PD), typified by PD 123177 and PD 121981, or CGP 42112A, a modified peptide analog of AII [17, 18]. Inhibition by losartan characterizes the AT_1 subtype, whereas the PD compounds and CGP 42112A identify the AT_2 subtype receptor. Using inhibitors of these subtypes, it has been shown that the AT_1 receptor is the predominant receptor subtype in the vasculature, liver and kidney of adult rats, but expression of mRNA for AT_1 receptor has also been found in adrenal gland and lung. AT_2 receptors have been detected mainly in adrenal medulla, brain, uterus and ovary. cDNA clones for AT_1 receptors have been isolated from rabbits, humans and mice, and show a high degree of homology with the original rat clone. These nucleotide sequences encode for a 359 amino acid protein that has the seven hydrophobic transmembrane domains typical of G protein-coupled receptors. The rat and mouse have a second form of AT_1 receptor, now identified as AT_{1B}

receptor, with 96% amino acid homology with the original rat AT_1 receptor, now designated as AT_{1A}. These receptor subtypes are very similar in ligand specificity and signal transduction mechanisms. Vascular smooth muscle and lung express primarily the AT_{1A} mRNA, the adrenal and pituitary glands express mainly AT_{1B} and kidney expresses both. These two receptor isoforms may differ more in the regulation of their expression than in their functional properties. This is supported by findings that in ovariectomized rats treated with estrogens, the expression of AT_{1B} but not AT_{1A} mRNA was suppressed in the pituitary gland. So far, these two forms of the AT_1 receptor have only been detected in rodents.

Binding of AII to the AT_1 receptor activates a number of different signal transduction pathways, which include stimulation of phospholipase C and, as a consequence, activation of phosphoinositide turnover and calcium mobilization, and inhibition of adenylate cyclase activity [17, 18].

Unlike other receptor systems, such as α-adrenergic receptors or vasopressin receptors, the AT_1 receptor is coupled to multiple signal transduction pathways through different G proteins (Gq or Gi). This has been shown in Chinese hamster ovary cells expressing the recombinant rat AT_{1A} receptor, in cells from rat anterior pituitary tumors, in bovine adrenal glomerulosa cells, in human astrocytes and in rat vascular smooth muscle. Much less is known about the signaling mechanism(s) coupled to the AT_2 receptor. However, this receptor does not appear to operate through the classical signal transduction pathways and in most tissues is not coupled to G proteins. Based on studies of activation of the AT_2 receptor in membrane preparations from rat adrenal glomerulosa cells, it has been suggested that AII, through the AT_2 receptor, activates a phosphotyrosine phosphatase that may regulate ATP binding to the kinase domain of particulate GC. This view has recently been challenged by the observation that in cells permanently transfected with a plasmid harboring the AT_2 complementary DNA, activation of this receptor is linked to the inhibition of protein phosphotyrosine phosphatase activity. In some cells AT_2 receptors have been shown to inhibit guanylyl cyclase [18]. Additional studies will be required to clarify the signal transduction mechanisms involved in the action of AT_2 receptors.

Role of angiotensin II in the regulation of vascular tone and function

The renin–angiotensin axis, through its effector AII, is thought to be central in the regulation of systemic blood pressure. This is achieved either by binding of circulating AII to its receptors on vascular smooth muscle cells or by locally generated AII which exerts tonic effects on the vessel wall. Although the vasoconstrictor activity of AII is well known, it is now becoming clear that this hormone may play an equally important role in numerous physiological processes, including vascular remodeling and smooth muscle cell growth [15]. Structural changes in the vasculature are in fact consistent features of hypertension, and may involve local tissue renin–angiotensin systems.

Although the data are to some extent conflicting, it has been shown that AII increases smooth muscle cell growth, through either hyperplasia or hypertrophy [15]. Most studies have indicated that these changes result from hypertrophy, rather than hyperplasia, although a number have found hyperplastic changes. These apparent inconsistencies may have been related to species differences in culture conditions but all results point to an important role for AII in the growth of smooth muscle cells. Coupled with the finding of local vascular generation of AII and expression of all the components of the RAS in the vascular wall, it is obvious that local AII is important in vascular smooth muscle cell growth in hypertension.

Role of angiotensin II in regulation of renal function

AII is a potent vasoconstrictor of the renal vascular bed with potential targets to regulate the glomerular microcirculation, i.e. the afferent and efferent arterioles as well as mesangial cells, which dictate glomerular size and filtration area through their contractile properties. *In vivo* studies have shown that AII contracts both afferent and efferent arterioles, modulating intraglomerular capillary pressure and ultimately glomerular filtration.

How AII contributes to the regulation of renal perfusion and glomerular filtration has been clarified by pharmacological manipulations that interfere with the renin–angiotensin axis. In animals and humans – particularly in conditions of activation of the RAS – inhibition of ACE normally increases renal plasma flow but does not change GFR [19]. It thus appears that AII is a predominant vasoconstrictor of efferent arteriole [19]. Besides their effect on the RAS, converting enzyme inhibitors inhibit the hydrolysis of other peptides, including bradykinin. This contributes to enhancing renal vasodilation. The fact that converting enzyme catalyzes the formation of both AII and bradykinin limits the actual contribution of AII to renal hemodynamics.

AII receptor antagonists have been used to define the role of endogenous AII in modulating glomerular microcirculation [17, 18]. In the isolated perfused rat kidney preparation, AII receptor blockade with losartan completely prevented the increase in renal vascular resistance induced by AII. Using the hydronephrotic rabbit kidney model that enables direct access to renal microvessels, AII receptor antagonists fully block the effect of the peptide on both the afferent and efferent arterioles. In normotensive rats short-term AII receptor blockade does not change GFR, but in most cases increases RPF [18]. This was also observed in dogs given the AT_1 receptor antagonist losartan; there was a selective increase in renal blood flow or a combined increase of RPF and GFR depending on whether animals were normotensive or hypertensive, respectively. There have been few studies in humans to assess the effect of AII receptor blockade on renal function. In normotensive subjects on a low- or high-sodium diet, losartan did not change renal flow or GFR [18]. However, AII receptor blockade enhanced RPF but not GFR in hypertensive patients with moderate chronic renal failure. AT_1 receptor blocking agents were used in all these studies, thus providing evidence of the renal vascular and glomerular effect of AII through its AT_1 receptor. The effects of AT_2 receptor antagonists have also been examined but in most cases no changes in renal hemodynamics were found [17], thus excluding a major role of these receptors in the control of glomerular function.

In addition to its effects on the glomerular microcirculation, AII appears to play a part in the control of glomerular sieving properties to macromolecules. The glomerular capillary wall imposes a permeability barrier with selectivity to the size and charge of macromolecules. Initial studies attributed the proteinuric effect of AII solely to its ability to raise glomerular capillary hydraulic pressure and the plasma concentrations of macromolecules within the glomerular capillary tuft [20]. However, more recent evidence suggests that AII regulates sieving function independently from its hemodynamic effects, possibly by modifying the F-actin fiber assembly of the podocytes and/or modulating the matrix network of the glomerular basement membrane.

In addition to its vascular effects, AII participates in the regulation of urinary sodium excretion [17, 20]. Increasing evidence suggests that AII controls renal sodium excretion not only by affecting renal hemodynamics and aldosterone biosynthesis but also by directly regulating epithelial sodium transport. AII acts predominantly in the S1 subsegment of the proximal convoluted tubule to reduce intracellular cAMP and hence increase Na^+/H^+ antiport activity. Both the basolateral and luminal membranes have AII receptors, which have a biphasic effect on sodium transport. Thus both *in vitro* and *in vivo* experiments have shown that at low concentrations ($\sim 10^{-12}$–10^{-10} M) AII stimulates Na^+ and water reabsorption, whereas at higher concentrations ($\sim 10^{-8}$–10^{-6} M) it inhibits Na^+ transport in the microperfused subcortical rabbit proximal convoluted tubule. A reduction in AII concentration also reduces sodium transport both in the loop of Henle due to vasodilation of the medullary circulation, and in the cortical collecting tubule secondary to a reduction in plasma aldosterone levels.

The receptor subtypes involved in the complex and unique mechanism of action of AII on the proximal tubule have not been clearly established, although AT_1 receptors appear to play a role. However, in sodium-depleted anesthetized dogs the AT_2 receptor antagonist PD123319 increased urine volume and free water clearance in a dose-dependent manner without affecting renal hemodynamics. Since PD123319 did not affect circulating vasopressin, a direct tubular effect mediated by the AT_2 has been suggested [17].

In addition to the direct effect mediated by AII binding to proximal tubule receptors, proximal tubule transport may also be indirectly regulated by AII. Thus proximal tubular cells are intensively innervated by sympathetic nerves through binding to presynaptic receptors. Denervation of the proximal tubule resulted in marked attenuation of the stimulatory effect of AII on sodium reabsorption.

There is now convincing evidence that AII is a hypertrophogenic hormone that participates in the regulation of renal cell growth [21]. Tubular hypertrophy is an important factor in the adaptive response of the kidney to various physiological and pathological stimuli. The important observation that activation of the intrarenal RAS is altered in situations associated with renal growth, and the fact that ACE inhibitors block compensatory renal hypertrophy in many models, provided a basis for establishing the influence of AII on the growth of various renal cell lines. AII had no effect on the growth of murine fibroblasts isolated from the interstitium, but induced proliferation of a murine mesangial cell line and induced cellular enlargement in proximal tubular cells after several days. Other investigators found evidence of AII-mediated hypertrophy in primary cultures of rabbit proximal tubules. These stimulatory effects were transduced through AT_1 receptors since losartan abolished the AII-induced hypertrophy.

AII-induced hypertrophy in proximal tubular cells is characterized by elevated secretion of collagen type IV, but not type I. Since type IV collagen is an integral part of the basement membrane, an increase in its biosynthesis looks like an appropriate consequence of cellular enlargement to accommodate the increased cellular mass. The *in vitro* hypertrophogenic activity of AII has been confirmed by the *in vivo* observation in rats that infusion of AII into the renal artery led to a significant increase in the renal expression of *c-fos* and *Egr-1*, the immediate early genes, which was blocked by saralasin, and was independent of blood pressure. Although this AII-receptor mediated induction suggests a direct cellular effect of AII on the expression of these early genes, the effect of AII may be through the induction of ischemia, which is also associated with an increase in immediate early genes.

Endothelins

Endothelins are extremely potent vasoconstrictor peptides implicated in the control of renal function and blood pressure. The first member of the family, ET-1, was isolated from the culture supernatant of porcine aortic endothelial cells by Yanagisawa *et al.* in 1988 [22]. Within a year, two further endothelin isoforms, ET-2 and ET-3, were described, the former differing from ET-1 by two amino acids, the latter by six. Mouse–rat ET-2 was originally thought to be a novel endothelin isoform (vasoactive intestinal contractor), but it was later found, by Southern blot analysis, that it is most likely the mouse–rat analogue of human ET-2. All endothelin isopeptides have 21 amino acids and share a common structure consisting of two intrachain disulfide bonds forming a hairpin loop and a hydrophobic carboxy-COOH-terminal tail, His^{16}-Trp^{21}; the latter is essential as the loop configuration for bioactivity.

Endothelin isopeptides derive from proteolytic processing of isopeptide-specific prohormones (~200 amino acids) encoded by three separate genes, preproendothelin-1, -2 and -3 being mapped on chromosomes 6, 1 and 20, respectively. Endopeptidases that recognize paired basic amino acids (Arg-Arg or Lys-Arg) process preproendothelins into Big-endothelin, which is then converted into the mature peptide by cleavage of the Trp^{21}-Val^{22} bond by a highly specific endothelin-converting enzyme, a phosphoramidon-sensitive membrane-bound metalloprotease (Figure 13.3).

Endothelins act as local hormones

Several lines of evidence suggest that endothelins act primarily as local hormones. First, plasma ET-1 levels in healthy subjects (1–5 pmol/l) are well below the concentrations required to activate ET-1 receptors. In rats infused with radiolabeled ET-1 the peptide was rapidly cleared from the circulation, with more than 60% being removed in the first minute mainly through the lung, kidney and liver. The observation that more than 80% of the total ET-1 released by endothelial and epithelial cells is directed abluminally toward the underlying smooth muscle confirms the view of ET-1 as a local hormone. Finally, in some conditions, tissue levels of ET-1 are much higher than blood levels, indicating that the peptide is formed locally.

Sites and modulation of endothelin synthesis

Endothelin synthesis was originally believed to be confined to vascular endothelium, but it has been shown to occur in other tissues and organs also. Immunohistochemistry and *in situ* hybridization techniques helped show that endothelin is synthesized in the central nervous system, particularly brain and spinal cord, and in the lung, liver, gut, heart and kidney. In addition, cultured cells as well as transformed cell lines from human tumor explants secrete endothelin peptides. Circulating cells also secrete ET-1 and macrophages are probably the best example. Neutrophils, on the other hand, can convert exogenous proendothelin into bioactive endothelin that serves to raise the local concentration of the hormone at the site of inflammation. Endothelial cells secrete ET-1, but not ET-3.

Prepro-ET-1 mRNA expression and the rate of peptide

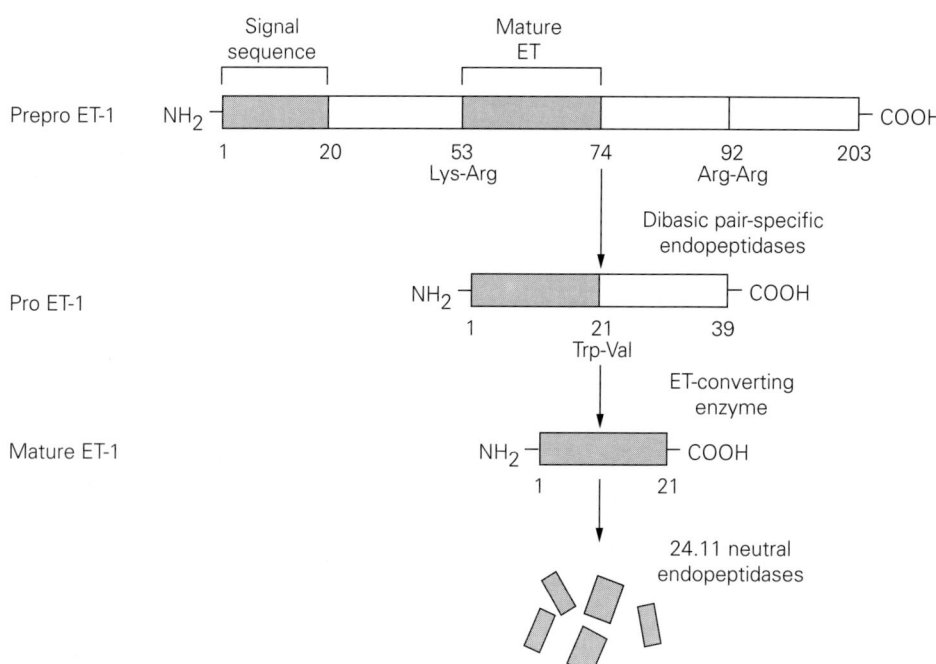

Figure 13.3 Pathway of endothelin biosynthesis and degradation.

release in cultured endothelial cells are enhanced by a variety of agents including thrombin, transforming growth factor β (TGF-β), tumor necrosis factor, AII and oxygen radicals [23]. Endothelial cell ET-1 production is inhibited by oxidized low-density lipoproteins, atrial and brain natriuretic peptides and nitrates. Shear stress forces and mechanical stretching also regulate ET-1 synthesis and release.

Experiments in renal cell cultures showed that ET-1 is produced by numerous cells within the kidney. Glomerular capillary endothelial cells release ET-1 in a time-dependent fashion and its secretion is stimulated by bradykinin. Resting rat and human mesangial cells in culture as well as glomerular epithelial cells constitutively express prepro-ET-1 mRNA, whose transcripts are up-regulated by thrombin and TGF-β. Findings in primary epithelial cell cultures derived from different nephron segments suggest that renal tubules secrete mainly ET-1 and smaller amounts of ET-3. ET-1 secretion in tubules is present in inner medullary collecting ducts > medullary ascending limb > cortical collecting duct >> proximal tubules.

Localization of endothelin receptors in the kidney and heart

In 1990 two distinct seven-transmembrane-spanning endothelin receptor subtypes belonging to the superfamily of G-protein-linked receptors were cloned from cDNA libraries in bovine and rat lines and called ET_A and ET_B. Radioligand binding studies indicated that ET_A binds ET-1 and ET-2 with higher affinity than ET-3. ET_B has similar affinity for all three ET isopeptides. In vessels ET_A receptors reside in smooth muscle cells and mediate vasocon-

striction and smooth muscle cell proliferation. ET_B receptors are present on endothelial cells, where they mediate a vasodilatory effect through nitric oxide (NO), and smooth muscle cells where they appear to mediate vasoconstriction.

Subtype B receptors with 'super-high' affinity sites have been identified in rat brain and cardiac atrium. Whether the super-high-affinity ET_B receptors are related to the vasodilatory property of ET, and the high-affinity receptor to the vasoconstrictory action of the peptide, is open to speculation. Several reports show that ET_B receptors on smooth muscle mediate vasoconstriction if challenged with low concentrations of ET. A recent preliminary observation suggested that ET-1 autoinduction of its own gene expression and peptide elaboration is mediated by the ET_B receptor. Renal tissue expresses mRNA for both ET_A and ET_B receptors, the former being expressed mainly in afferent and efferent arterioles and in glomeruli, the latter on the surface of glomerular endothelial, mesangial cells, epithelial podocytes and vasa recta bundles. Both subtypes are present in inner medullary collecting ducts.

A different distribution of ET_A and ET_B receptors in human and rat kidney has been proposed. The human kidney has at least twice as much of the ET_B subtype as ET_A. Whereas ET_A is confined to vascular structures, ET_B is not present on vascular smooth muscle, but is at least partly expressed on epithelial cells. It is likely that in humans (and also in the dog) vasoconstriction is ET_A-mediated, whereas in the rat ET_B seems to be the vasoconstrictor receptor.

Two ET receptor subtypes have been detected in chick heart and bovine atrium, but only ET_A receptors are present in rat atrium. Both subtypes are found in human atrial and ventricular myocardium, the atrioventricular conducting system and endocardial cells. Quantitative autoradiography showed a higher proportion of ET_B in the conducting system than in myocardium. ET_A receptors are dominant in the myocardium, particularly in myocytes, where they account for 91% of the total population of endothelin receptors.

Renal actions of endothelin

Renal vessels are particularly sensitive to the vasoconstrictive effect of ET-1. Infusion of ET-1 into the renal artery increases renal vascular resistance with a consequent decrease in renal blood flow. As in the systemic circulation, renal vasoconstriction follows a transient phase of vasodilation due to induction of endothelium-derived vasodilators through ET_B receptors on endothelial cells. By binding to the ET_A receptor, ET-1 contracts afferent and efferent arterioles and increases the tone of the arcuate and interlobular arteries, giving rise to a long-lasting vasoconstriction [24]. The effect of pharmacological doses of ET-1 on renal hemodynamics has been clearly defined by systemic infusion studies, but the effects of physiological concentrations of ET-1 have not yet been determined. This will only be clarified by experiments with specific receptor antagonists or by studies on transgenic animals. In addition to pre- and postglomerular vessel vasoconstriction, ET-1 also affects mesangial cell function, stimulating mitogenesis and up-regulating mesangial matrix protein gene expression, as documented by increased levels of mRNA for collagen types I, III and IV, and for laminin in rat mesangial cells exposed to ET-1. ET-1 also activates mesangial cell phospholipase A_2 and promotes arachidonate release from membrane phospholipids leading to excessive formation of thromboxane A_2, a potent stimulus for extracellular matrix protein synthesis, altogether this *in vitro* evidence indicates that ET-1 might be responsible for renal damage *in vivo*.

ET-1 has complex direct effects on sodium homeostasis and water balance which add to those mediated by other hormones including AII, aldosterone and ANP. In experimental animals low-dose systemic ET-1 has a natriuretic effect despite a fall in GFR and renal blood flow. Natriuresis may be due to stimulation of ANP or secondary to higher blood pressure during endothelin infusion. In the isolated perfused kidney, sodium excretion also increases after ET-1 administration. Unlike in the rat, systemic infusion of high doses of ET-1 in dogs reduced sodium excretion because of a decrease in filtered load and/or renin–angiotensin stimulation.

In humans, systemic administration of ET-1 at concentrations comparable to those measured in physiological conditions, such as during upright tilt, causes renal sodium retention. However, higher dosages of ET-1, like those found in pathological conditions such as heart failure, hepatorenal syndrome and renal failure, cause strong sodium retention and in addition, renal vasocon-

striction. Calcium channel blockers protect against these effects. Since sodium retention continues after discontinuation of low-dosage ET-1 in the absence of changes in renal hemodynamics, it has been suggested that ET-1 may directly stimulate tubular sodium reabsorption.

Role of endothelin-1 in renal disease progression

Evidence that ET-1 participates in the process of progressive renal injury has been provided in rats with renal mass ablation, a model of chronic renal disease characterized by compensatory glomerular hemodynamic alterations and progressive glomerulosclerosis. Preliminary studies have shown that although plasma ET-1 levels remained unchanged, urinary excretion of the peptide, which very likely reflects ET-1 renal synthesis, increased significantly in rats with reduced renal mass compared to sham-operated rats. In the same model, subsequent experiments showed a parallel increase with time of renal prepro-ET-1 gene expression and urinary excretion of the mature peptide [25]. Urinary excretion correlated with urinary proteins and with the severity of glomerulosclerosis.

The recent availability of endothelin receptor antagonists has helped clarify whether ET-1 is at least partly involved in mediating progressive renal damage in this model. A selective antagonist for the ET_A receptor, FR139317, given chronically to rats with a remnant kidney, normalized blood pressure, reduced the abnormal glomerular permeability to proteins and prevented renal function deterioration [26]. The most striking finding of this study was the drug's protective effect on glomerular structural damage, as reflected by almost no mesangial hypercellularity and a very low average frequency of segmental glomerulosclerosis (Figure 13.4). The ET_A receptor antagonist suppressed renal expression of c-fos proto-oncogene, an early marker of cell proliferation, which was up-regulated in untreated remnant kidney animals. These findings suggested that progressive renal damage is mediated by ET_A but did not exclude a contributory role of the ET_B receptor.

The observation that the renal ET_B receptor mRNA increased in a time-dependent manner in rats with remnant kidney has led to investigation of the *in vivo* relevance of this finding. Bosentan, an orally active ET_A/ ET_B receptor antagonist, was given daily to rats from days 7 to 45 after the surgical procedure. Preliminary results suggest that the antagonist reduced blood pressure and partially prevented the increase in urinary protein excretion.

Few data are available in humans on the role of ET-1 in progressive renal disease. Urinary excretion of ET-1 is increased in patients with chronic progressive nephropathies. It has also been found that urinary ET-1 is significantly higher in patients with unilateral nephrectomy than after adrenalectomy. However, there is no evidence of a cause and effect relationship between

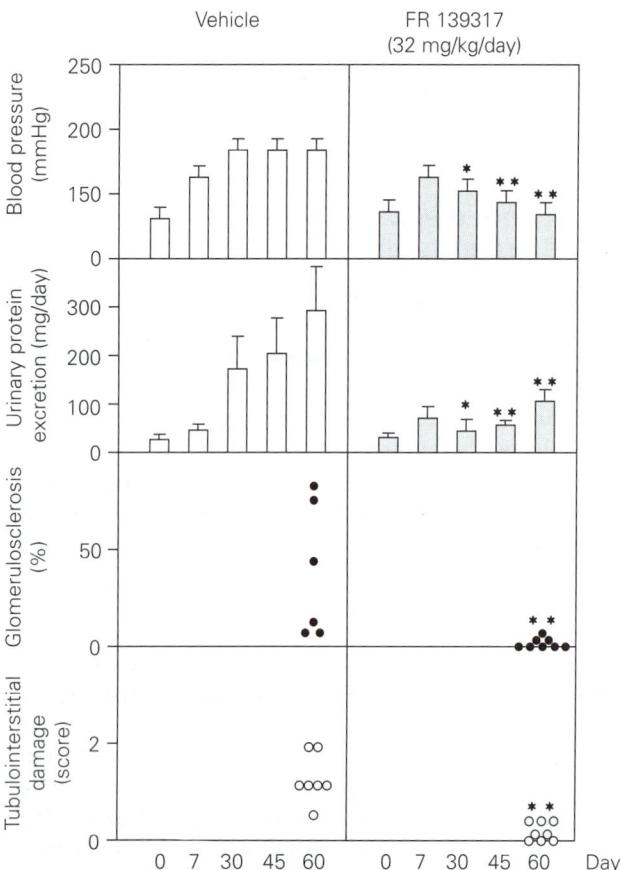

Figure 13.4 Effect of chronic administration of a selective ET_A receptor antagonist or its vehicle (saline) on blood pressure, urinary protein excretion and renal damage in rats after renal mass ablation. Treatment started seven days after surgery. *P < 0.05, **P < 0.01 vehicle at corresponding time.

abnormal ET generation and development of sclerotic lesions in humans. Specific ET receptor antagonists, now entering phase I evaluation, will, it is hoped, help clarify the role of ET in the progressive deteriorating renal function associated with most human nephropathies.

Action of endothelin on blood pressure

ET-1 was originally characterized by its action on blood pressure. Intravenous infusion in experimental animals first induces a depressor response due to stimulation of the endothelial vasodilator NO and prostacyclin. Mean arterial pressure then steadily rises because of an increase in total peripheral resistance and an increase in cardiac output, the latter as a consequence of a direct inotropic effect on cardiac atria. Neither blocking the α-adrenergic, β-adrenergic, serotonergic and histaminergic receptors nor inhibiting prostaglandin synthesis prevented the increase in cardiac output induced by ET-1. Unlike other vasoactive peptides such as AII, the inotropic effect of ET develops slowly but is long-lasting, and is mediated by activation of inositol-specific phospholipase

C, so far the best-characterized effector coupled to the endothelin receptor in cardiac myocytes. By specifically binding to cardiac receptors, ET-1 increases cytosolic Ca^{2+} in myocytes by releasing Ca^{2+} from intracellular stores.

ET-1 induces vasoconstriction through a direct effect on vascular smooth muscle cells and is reversed by NO. There is, thus, a fine interplay between the two hormones in the control of vascular tone. A complex interaction between ET-1 and many other vasoactive mediators, mainly endogenous vasodilators, may also limit the peptide constrictor effect. Probably through direct action on cardiac atria, EF-1 infusion raises plasma ANP in experimental animals. Since ET-1 and ANP have opposite effects on peripheral vascular resistance and blood pressure, ANP may possibly be a physiological modulator of the effects of ET-1 on the systemic circulation. ET-1 inhibits renin release in isolated juxtaglomerular cells, while by stimulating ACE it could theoretically raise the level of AII.

In contrast with the marked vasoconstriction in animals, systemic infusion of ET-1 in humans results in only a modest increase in blood pressure and a decrease in pulse rate. This limited effect on blood pressure may possibly be the result of ET-1 reducing cardiac output despite the increase in total peripheral resistance. Plasma concentrations of vasoactive mediators, including ANP, AII, aldosterone and vasopressin, were not influenced by infused ET-1. There are few data on local vascular effects of ET-1 in humans. The first report showed that ET-1 induced potent and long-lasting vasoconstriction of the forearm resistance vessels of the dorsal hand veins. Subsequently a dual action of the peptide was found on human resistance vessels, leading to an increase in forearm blood flow after infusion of a low dose of ET-1, but lasting vasoconstriction after a high dose.

Endogenous ET-1 appears to be involved in the maintenance of peripheral vascular tone. Brachial artery infusions of phosphoramidon, an inhibitor of endothelin converting enzyme, or a selective ET_A receptor antagonist BQ 123, caused progressive vasodilation, with blood flow increasing 37% and 64%, respectively.

Role of endothelin in hypertension and heart failure

Hypertension is characterized by an increase in peripheral vascular resistance and is frequently associated with cardiovascular complications including chronic heart failure and myocardial infarction. Several humoral candidates responsible for these diseases have been studied, particularly the RAS and catecholamines, although no definitive answer has been found. The involvement of endothelin in hypertension and its complications has been studied [27].

Conflicting results have been reported so far on ET-1 circulating levels in rat experimental and human essential hypertension. Plasma ET-1 appears to be decreased in genetically hypertensive rats and unaltered in rats with DOCA-salt hypertension despite increased vascular reactivity to ET-1 in both models, suggesting it is involved in some but not all forms of experimental hypertension. In humans, some studies described normal, but others reported increased circulating levels of the peptide. Patients with pulmonary hypertension invariably have higher plasma levels of ET-1 than normal subjects, possibly because of decreased lung extraction of the peptide.

The presence of endothelial cell dysfunction in some pathological conditions associated with hypertension, including atherosclerosis, heart failure and renal insufficiency, would lead to increased circulating levels of the peptide. One study has shown that high levels of plasma ET, primarily due to elevated circulating 'Big ET-1', are characteristic of late severe chronic renal failure but not of asymptomatic left ventricular dysfunction, and correlate with the magnitude of alterations in cardiac hemodynamics. Since elevated plasma ET-1 levels persisted after cardiac transplantation despite restoration of normal cardiac function, increased plasma ET-1 in chronic renal failure might be related to endothelial cell derangement rather than to ventricular dysfunction.

ET-1 may have a role in acute myocardial infarction. High plasma and cardiac ET-1 concentrations were found in a model of left coronary artery ligation in which the infarction size was reduced by an anti-ET-1 antibody. In humans, a significant rise in plasma ET-1 has been reported during acute ischemia and elevated plasma levels of the peptide are thought to be an indicator of unfavorable prognosis of patients after myocardial infarction. The conflicting results on plasma ET-1 levels in hypertension together with the high local levels of ET-1 despite normal plasma levels of the peptide have suggested that the plasma concentration does not reflect vascular ET-1 production. ET-1 most likely acts in a paracrine fashion, predominantly regulating vascular smooth muscle cells. Since ET-1 secretion is clearly directed towards the underlying smooth muscle cells, plasma ET-1 may possibly reflect an overflow of local production; large increases in local concentration might produce only small increases in the periphery. Methodological problems, particularly related to the cross-reactivity of ET-1 antibodies with isoforms and its precursor or other unrelated peptides, could also contribute to the conflicting and confusing results.

In summary, overproduction of ET-1 is a feature of some but not all forms of hypertension. However, elevation of plasma ET-1 has been consistently documented in heart diseases with endothelial cell dysfunction, possibly as a marker of endothelial cell damage.

Nitric oxide

The discovery of endothelium-derived relaxing factor (EDRF) by Furchgott and Zawadski [28] in 1980 cast fresh light on the concept that blood pressure reflects the net contribution of vasodilator and vasoconstrictor influences. In these classic experiments, preconstricted arterial ring preparations with an intact endothelium relaxed when stimulated with acetylcholine *ex vivo*. However, acetylcholine did not dilate preconstricted arterial rings whose adjacent endothelium had been removed by mechanical or chemical means. EDFR has subsequently been characterized as nitric oxide (NO) or an endogenously produced NO-generating compound.

The synthesis of NO by vascular endothelium is responsible for vasodilator tone, essential for the regulation of blood pressure. In the central nervous system, NO is a neurotransmitter that underpins several functions, including the formation of memory. In the periphery, there is a widespread network of nerves, previously recognized as non-adrenergic and non-cholinergic, that operate through an NO-dependent mechanism to mediate some forms of neurogenic vasodilatation and regulate various gastrointestinal, respiratory and genitourinary tract functions [29]. Nitric oxide also contributes to the control of platelet aggregation and the regulation of cardiac contractility. These actions are mediated by the activation of soluble guanylate cyclase and the consequent increase in the concentration of cyclic guanosine monophosphate (GMP) in target cells.

In addition, NO is produced in large quantities during host defense and immune reactions. Because it has cytotoxic properties and is generated by activated macrophages, NO is a potential modulator of immune cell defenses. Furthermore, NO is involved in the pathogenesis of conditions such as septic shock and perhaps also in the hyperdynamic state of cirrhosis and in inflammation.

Nitric oxide acts as a local hormone

Given the exquisite reactivity and metabolism of this radical, its predominant biological effect appears to relate to the amount present and the site of production. For example, NO produced by macrophages has mainly a cytotoxic role, whereas NO produced in the arterial wall results primarily in vasorelaxation. NO can combine with superoxide anion to form peroxynitrite (ONOO), a potent oxidant that under certain conditions, such as reperfusion after anoxia, is produced in sufficient quantities to cause tissue damage. NO can induce dose-dependent breaks in DNA *in vitro* by nitrosation of amines on guanine and adenine. Another cytotoxic effect of NO is nitrosation and inactivation of iron-containing enzymes of the mitochondrial electron-transport chain. NO oxidizes the iron atom in heme-containing proteins such as hemoglobin to yield methemoglobin. Because of this reaction and the rapid oxidation of NO if it appears in the arterial lumen, NO serves as a paracrine or autocrine factor in vasodilatation.

Regulation of nitric oxide synthesis

NO is made by NO synthase (NOS) in an unusual reaction that converts arginine and oxygen into citrulline and NO [30]. The mechanism of NO synthesis is not completely understood, but it involves the transfer of electrons between various cofactors, including flavin adenine dinucleotide, flavin mononucleotide, nicotinamide adenine dinucleotide phosphate (NADPH), tetrahydrobiopterin and heme. Finally, one atom of oxygen binds with the terminal guanidine nitrogen from arginine to form NO.

Although several NOS isoforms have been isolated, all are homologous and divided into two categories with different regulation and activities. The constitutive isoforms in neuronal or endothelial cells are always present. These NOS isoforms are inactive until intracellular calcium levels rise, the calcium-binding protein calmodulin binds to calcium, and the calcium–calmodulin complex binds and activates NOS. The constitutive NOS isoforms then synthesize small amounts of NO until calcium levels decrease. The intermittent production of small amounts of NO transmits signals.

In contrast, the inducible NOS isoform is normally absent from macrophages and hepatocytes, but when these cells are activated by specific cytokines, an inducible NOS enzyme is produced which synthesizes large amounts of NO. Inducible NOS is regulated at the transcriptional level. The continuous production of large amounts of NO kills or inhibits pathogens.

Alternative mechanisms also operate in regulating NOS enzymes. Neuronal NOS can be phosphorylated by protein kinases to reduce its activity. The subcellular location of NOS in endothelial cells can be changed by its phosphorylation. The constitutive isoforms are regulated by calcium, and the inducible isoforms also appear to bind calmodulin, although calcium has little effect on their activity. The role of calmodulin in inducible NOS function is not known.

Nitric oxide synthesis in the kidney

In the glomerulus, NO may be synthesized by NOS in intrinsic glomerular cells or by infiltrating inflammatory cells, particularly macrophages, neutrophils or lymphocytes. There is a calcium-dependent form of NOS in the normal glomerulus; mRNA for endothelial NOS has been demonstrated by reverse transcription polymerase chain reaction (RT-PCR) in the glomerulus and afferent and efferent arterioles [31]. Endothelial NOS has been studied immunohistochemically and was found in glomerular endothelium; efferent arteriolar endothelium showed stronger staining than afferent. Immunohistochemistry and *in situ* hybridization showed that the macula densa is the major site of neuronal NOS in the kidney. These two forms of NOS – endothelial and neuronal – are impor-

tant in the control of renal blood flow and glomerulotubular feedback respectively.

The rat, bovine and human mesangial cell expressed inducible NOS after cytokine stimulation. In rat mesangial cells, inducible NOS is induced by interleukin-1β (IL-1β), tumor necrosis factor-α (TNF-α) and lipopolysaccharide (LPS). Forskolin, an activator of adenyl cyclase, interacts tumor necrosis factor with cytokines to increase inducible NOS in mesangial cells, indicating that cAMP stimulates an independent pathway of induction. Further evidence of two separate pathways of stimulation is provided by the fact that pyrrolidine dithiocarbamate, a potent inhibitor of nuclear factor κB, inhibits IL-1β-stimulated but not cAMP-stimulated nitrite production.

In human mesangial cells inducible NOS is induced by IL-1β and interferon-γ (IFN-γ) in combination; the effect is enhanced by TNF-α. NO synthesis by mesangial cells leads to increased cGMP both within stimulated mesangial cells themselves and in untreated control cells.

Using the PCR technique on mRNA extracted from control and cytokine-stimulated human proximal tubular cells, McLay *et al.* [32] found a NOS product with >97% homology with human hepatocyte-inducible NOS. This study found that proximal tubular cells also can produce NO in response to an immune challenge through the induction of NOS.

Renal action of nitric oxide

Intrarenal administration of *N*-monomethyl-L-arginine (L-NMMA) in doses with no or only minimum systemic effects results in increased renal vascular resistance accompanied by a decrease in renal blood flow with preservation of the GFR. Tolins and Raij [33] suggested that part of the intrarenal hemodynamic effects of inhibiting NO synthesis might be due to unmasking the effect of intrarenal AII. Indeed, concomitant administration of L-NMMA with an AII receptor blocker attenuated the hemodynamic effect of inhibition of NO synthesis. Ito *et al.* [34], in elegant preparations of isolated glomeruli, have shown that NO modulates the effects of AII on the afferent arteriole. De Nicola *et al.* [35] have shown in micropuncture studies that inhibition of NO synthesis results in glomerular arteriolar vasoconstriction, a lower glomerular ultrafiltration coefficient, and reduced single-nephron glomerular filtration rate. They also showed that these changes could be prevented to a great extent by simultaneous administration of an AII receptor antagonist. Baylis *et al.* [36] reported that in rats chronic administration of an inhibitor of NO synthesis resulted in sustained systemic and glomerular hypertension accompanied by glomerular injury.

Besides its vasodilatory function, NO inhibits mesangial cell proliferation induced by serum and by platelet-derived growth factor (PDGF). Nitric oxide may participate in a paracrine fashion in the modulation of growth-related events in vessels as well as in glomeruli.

It appears that, within the kidney, NO, ANP and vasodilatory prostanoids are the natural antagonists of vasoconstrictive agents such as AII and ET-1. It is likely that NO, ANP, PGI_2 and AII continuously interact in the kidney modulating renal hemodynamics and, to a certain extent, sodium excretion. The interaction between NO and ET-1 may be more important in pathological situations that result in renal ischemia. Endothelium-dependent relaxation in response to NO agonists is impaired in kidneys with post-ischemic acute renal failure. At the same time intrarenal synthesis of ET-1 is markedly and persistently increased after ischemia.

In studies using kidney slices, stimulation of NO synthesis and release with NO agonists reduced renin release. Henrich et al. [37] have shown that the inhibitory effect of NO on renin release is mediated by cGMP. Other agents that increase cGMP accumulation, such as sodium nitroprusside and 8-bromo-cGMP, also inhibit renin release. Furthermore, inhibition of guanylate cyclase with methylene blue blocks the inhibition of renin release as well as the increase of cGMP induced by ANP and sodium nitroprusside.

Experimental evidence suggests that NO induces natriuresis by antagonizing the effect of AII on sodium reabsorption in proximal tubules and by directly inhibiting sodium reabsorption in proximal tubular cells. The latter effect appears to be mediated by increases in cellular cGMP.

Nitric oxide and prostaglandins may interact closely in the regulation of sodium excretion. The blockade of sodium excretion resulting from inhibition of NO synthesis is greatly magnified if prostanoid synthesis is concomitantly stopped by cyclo-oxygenase inhibitors. Further studies may clarify whether and to what extent alterations in NO synthesis or release or both are responsible for salt-sensitive hypertension. NO may also participate in renal blood flow autoregulation and the intrarenal distribution of blood flow [38].

Nitric oxide and glomerulonephritis

Apart from its beneficial role on renal hemodynamics, NO has potential harmful effects, possibly by direct toxicity or indirectly by interacting with leukocyte-derived oxygen radicals. Cattel and coworkers [39] first demonstrated increased activity of the L-arginine–NO pathway in experimental glomerulonephritis. Glomeruli from rats with nephrotoxic nephritis synthesized increased amounts of nitrite, the stable end product of NO, in culture, and this could be prevented by the NOS inhibitor L-NMMA. Nitrite generation was seen in glomeruli isolated at 4 h after the induction of glomerulonephritis, was maximal by 24 h but persisted for up to three weeks. Normal glomeruli do not synthesize nitrite under these conditions. The inducible NOS message was just detectable in normal glomeruli and was increased several

hundredfold 6 h after induction of glomerulonephritis with high levels persisting for seven days.

It has also been shown that there is nitrite production from glomeruli as well as increased inducible NOS gene expression in other experimental models of glomerulonephritis, including in situ immune complex glomerulonephritis, membranous glomerulonephritis and mesangial proliferative glomerulonephritis induced by an antibody to the mesangial cell antigen Thy-1. In these models the levels of nitrite generation correlated with glomerular macrophage infiltration and in active Heymann nephritis nitrite synthesis was reduced by whole body irradiation which suppressed macrophage infiltration, implying that macrophages are of vital importance in glomerular NO synthesis. Inhibition by dexamethasone suggested that NO synthesis occurred through the induction of inducible NOS.

What role does enhanced NO synthesis play in glomerulonephritis? Analogy with injury at other sites and knowledge of the action of NO in the kidney suggest a range of possible effects. Beneficial effects could include maintenance of renal blood flow and glomerular filtration rate, inhibition of thrombosis (as has been shown for glomeruli after endotoxin administration), superoxide scavenging with reduction of adhesion molecule expression, down-regulation of the expression of pro-inflammatory cytokines, and inhibition of mesangial cell proliferation. Detrimental effects might include toxicity to intrinsic glomerular cells, either directly or through the formation of peroxynitrite with subsequent peroxidative damage. NO may also activate cyclo-oxygenase to stimulate glomerular prostaglandin production.

There is a major obstacle to establishing the role of NO in glomerulonephritis since it is difficult with available inhibitors of NOS to achieve inhibition of inducible NOS without also inhibiting endothelial NOS, thus causing systemic hypertension which itself tends to exacerbate the course of glomerulonephritis. A second problem in some experimental models is that of separating the local effects of NO synthesis in the glomerulus from the effect of systemic NOS inhibition on the generation of the immune response.

Weinberg et al. [40] studied the role of NO in MRL-lpr/lpr mice which spontaneously develop an autoimmune disease characterized by autoantibody production, glomerulonephritis, vasculitis and arthritis, all of which mimic human systemic lupus erythematosus. During the course of the disease there was an increase in urinary excretion of the NO products, nitrite and nitrate, and an increased expression of mRNA for inducible NOS in kidney and spleen. Over the period from 8 to 18 weeks of age, mice developed arthritis and proteinuria and the histological changes of glomerulonephritis. Treatment with L-NMMA in the drinking water over this period prevented the development of proteinuria and markedly improved the histological changes of glomerulonephritis and arthritis. The levels of circulating antidouble-stranded DNA antibody did not differ in the treatment and control groups, suggesting that this is not due to an effect on the immune mechanism.

There is a preliminary report of a beneficial effect of short-term NOS inhibition in a model of mesangial proliferative glomerulonephritis. Rats were given a single dose of L-NMMA 1 h before antithymocyte serum (ATS). Mesangial cell lysis was 90% prevented by NOS inhibition as was subsequent accumulation of extracellular matrix. Although there was a transient rise in blood pressure with L-NMMA treatment there was no difference in glomerular binding of ATS.

A protective effect has been suggested for NO in the early phase of nephrotoxic nephritis from a preliminary study in which the NOS inhibitor N^G-nitro-L-arginine methyl ester (L-NAME) was given, but the treated rats were hypertensive. A deleterious effect of NOS inhibition has also been reported in Heymann nephritis, a model of chronic membranous glomerulonephritis, in which L-NAME aggravated proteinuria and increased interstitial infiltration of mononuclear cells. However, the effects could be reversed by restoring normal blood pressure with captopril, suggesting that they may be due to the hypertensive effect of L-NAME.

In summary, in glomerulonephritis there is clear evidence of induction of inducible NOS in glomeruli and an increased capacity for NO synthesis. The major source of NO appears to be macrophages but inducible NOS from mesangial cells may contribute. The role of NO remains to be elucidated. However, there is evidence of both beneficial and detrimental effects depending on the model of glomerulonephritis, the timing of NOS inhibition and the agents used to inhibit NO synthesis.

Nitric oxide in hypertension

Intravenous infusion of L-NMMA produces a rapid and concentration-dependent increase in blood pressure in humans and other mammals; this increase is reduced by intravenous L-arginine. L-NMMA reduces blood flow to a variety of arterial beds including the renal, mesenteric and internal carotid arteries. Chronic oral treatment with arginine analogs, including L-NMMA and L-NAME, produces sustained increases in blood pressure in rats. Changes compatible with malignant nephrosclerosis occurred in rats after prolonged exposure to high concentrations of these analogs. Infusion of acetylcholine, which stimulates release of NO by endothelial cells, caused a concentration-dependent decrease in blood pressure and increase in urinary cGMP excretion. In that study, urinary cGMP, an index of NO production *in vivo*, correlated inversely with blood pressure. These studies show that NO is an important factor in resting arteriolar tone and modulates blood pressure *in vivo*.

The L-arginine–NO pathways appear to be altered in certain experimental animal models of hypertension. First, the *Dahl/Rapp* strains of rat have been genetically manipulated through inbreeding either to develop hypertension (salt-sensitive, SS/Jr strain) or remain normoten-

sive (salt-resistant, SR/Jr strain), when placed on a high-salt diet. Untreated SS/Jr rats rapidly develop severe renal failure and display morphological features in the kidney identical to the arterial and glomerular changes of malignant nephrosclerosis in humans. SR/Jr rats and Sprague–Dawley rats increased their production of NO in response to an increase in dietary salt, whereas SS/Jr rats did not. In SS/Jr rats on a high-salt diet, L-arginine, the metabolic precursor of NO, increased NO production and completely prevented hypertension, as well as the associated renal failure. Renal morphology in arginine-treated SS/Jr rats was normal and identical to that in SR/Jr rats on the same high-salt diet. These findings suggest that hypertension in the SS/Jr strain is due to a genetic defect in the endogenous nitrovasodilator pathway; addition of L-arginine corrects the deficient NO production induced by a high-salt diet. Experiments to clarify the mechanism(s) of this derangement and establish which L-arginine–NO pathway is involved are under way.

Concomitant administration of dexamethasone, an inhibitor of inducible NOS expression, prevented the antihypertensive effect of L-arginine in SS/Jr rats on a high-salt diet. Dexamethasone also prevents the increase in urinary excretion of cGMP and nitrate seen ordinarily in arginine-treated SS/Jr rats on a high-salt diet. These studies suggest a primary role of inducible NOS in prevention of salt-sensitive hypertension in these rats.

In another genetic model of hypertension, the spontaneously hypertensive rat (SHR), L-arginine neither prevents nor corrects hypertension. Instead of defective production of NO, Nakazono *et al.* [41] suggested that there is excessive NO consumption related to overproduction of superoxide radicals by xanthine oxidase; infusion of oxypurinol lowered blood pressure in these rats. Certainly, alteration of the L-arginine–NO pathways is not responsible for all forms of hypertension. For example, L-arginine does not reduce blood pressure in the DOCA–salt model of hypertension.

Intravenous infusion of L-arginine does lower blood pressure in patients with essential hypertension and in normal volunteers. The blood pressure falls more in the hypertensive patients. L-Arginine concomitantly raises the plasma concentration of cGMP and urinary nitrate, supporting the precursor role of this amino acid in NO production in humans. Patients with essential hypertension have a defect in endothelium-dependent vasodilation, though endothelium-independent vasodilation is preserved. Because hypertension itself reduces endothelium-dependent vasodilation, establishing a cause and effect relationship in humans is difficult. However, studies using prehypertensive Dahl/Rapp rats suggest that the defect in NO production is responsible for salt-sensitive hypertension.

A form of acquired low-renin salt-sensitive hypertension occurs in patients receiving cyclosporin. Cyclosporin damages vascular endothelium and produces intense vasoconstriction, especially in the renal vasculature. Recently, Xuan *et al.* [42] found that cyclosporin inhibited endothelium-dependent vasorelaxation but did not affect relaxation to an exogenous nitrovasodilator; loss of endogenous nitrovasodilator activity from endothelial damage potentially contributes not only to hypertension but also to renal failure.

In summary, certain types of hypertension are due to altered nitrovasodilator activity, either exogenously produced by cyclosporin therapy or accumulation of arginine analogs that inhibit NO synthases, or due to hereditary defect [43].

Nitric oxide in hypotension

Some hypotensive conditions are associated with stimulation of the inducible L-arginine–NO pathway. NO has been implicated in the hypotension from endotoxic shock. Lipopolysaccharide induces the calcium-independent NOS in the arterial wall. L-NMMA, 20 mg/kg, reverses endotoxin-induced hypotension in dogs, whereas L-arginine, 400 mg/kg, returns blood pressure to the original low levels. In a rat model of endotoxic shock, an intravenous bolus of 3 mg/kg L-NMMA did not reverse hypotension; an intermediate dose, 30 mg/kg, restored normotension; and a high dose, 300 mg/kg, aggravated

the hypotension to the extent that all rats died. These authors suggested that high doses of L-NMMA, by inhibiting both inducible and constitutive NO synthases, block NO production in all vascular beds, producing tissue hypoperfusion and death.

Whether NOS inhibitors are useful clinically is uncertain. Anecdotal experience in two patients with septic shock reports an improvement in blood pressure and hemodynamic profile after acute administration of L-NMMA. Platelet count fell in both patients. The authors were unable to establish whether L-NMMA produced this side effect, but certainly NO plays an important role in platelet function.

A variety of cytokines affect NO production. IFN-γ, TNF-α, interleukin-1 (IL-1), and interleukin-2 (IL-2) stimulate NO production from L-arginine in humans and other mammals. As expected, NO plays a central role in hypotension associated with cytokine infusion. Kilbourn *et al.* injected TNF-α into dogs and produced hypotension that was corrected with a single bolus of L-NMMA, 4.4 mg/kg. Other cytokines, such as IL-10 and TGF-β, inhibit NO production.

The potential role of cytokines in the pathogenesis of hypertension remains to be explored.

References

1. Carretero, D.A., Cabrini, L.A. and Scicli, A.G. (1993) The molecular biology of the kallikrein–kinin system: I. General description, nomenclature and the mouse gene family. *J. Hypertens.*, **7**, 693–7.
2. Campbell, D.J., Kladis, A. and Duncan, A-M. (1993) Bradykinin peptides in kidney, blood, and other tissues of the rat. *Hypertension*, **21**, 155–65.
3. Fitzgibbon, W.R., Ploth, D.W. and Margolius, H.S. (1993) Kinins as vasoactive peptides. *Curr. Opin. Nephrol. Hypertens.*, **2**, 283–90.
4. Mombouli, J-V., Illiano, S., Nagao, T. *et al.* (1992) Potentiation of endothelium-dependent relaxations to bradykinin by angiotensin I converting enzyme inhibitors in canine coronary artery involves both endothelium-derived relaxing and hyperpolarizing factors. *Circ. Res.*, **71**, 137–44.
5. Waeber, B., Aubert, J-F., Fluckiger, J-P. *et al.* (1988) Role of endogenous bradykinin in blood pressure control of conscious rats. *Kidney Int.*, **34**(Suppl 26), S63–8.
6. Elliott, A.H. and Nazum, F.R. (1934) Urinary excretion of a depressor substance (Kallikrein of Frey and Kraut) in arterial hypertension. *Endocrinology*, **18**, 462–74.
7. Plante, G.E., Bissonnette, M., Sirois, M.G. *et al.* (1992) Renal permeability alteration precedes hypertension and involves bradykinin in the spontaneously hypertensive rat. *J. Clin. Invest.*, **89**, 2030–2.
8. Trippodo, N.C., Cole, F.E., Macphee, A.A. and Pegram, B.L. (1987) Biologic mechanisms of atrial natriuretic factor. *J. Lab. Clin. Med.*, **109**, 112–19.
9. Nakao, K., Itoh H., Suga, S-I. *et al.* (1993) The natriuretic peptide family. *Curr. Opin. Nephrol. Hypertens.*, **2**, 45–50.
10. Maack, T., Okolicany, J., Koh, G.Y. and Price, D.A. (1993) Functional properties of atrial natriuretic factor receptors. *Semin. Nephrol.*, **13**, 50–60.
11. Hollister, A.S. and Inagami, T. (1991) Atrial natriuretic factor and hypertension. *Am. J. Hypertens.*, **4**, 850–65.
12. Brenner, B.M., Ballermann, B.J. and Gunning, M.E. *et al.* (1990) Diverse biological actions of atrial natriuretic peptide. *Physiol. Rev.*, **70**, 665–99.
13. Margulies, K.B. and Burnett, J.C. Jr (1993) Neutral endopeptidase 24.11: a modulator of natriuretic petides. *Semin. Nephrol.*, **13**, 71–7.
14. Zhang, P.L., Mackenzie, H.S., Troy, J.L. and Brenner, B.M. (1994) Effects of natriuretic peptide receptor inhibition on remnant kidney function in rats. *Kidney Int.*, **46**, 414–20.
15. Naftilan, A.J. (1994) Role of the tissue renin–angiotensin system in vascular remodeling and smooth muscle cell growth. *Curr. Opin. Nephrol. Hypertens.*, **3**, 218–27.
16. Dzau, V.J., Burt, D.W. and Pratt, R.E. (1988) Molecular biology of the renin-angiotensin system. *Am. J. Physiol.*, **255**, F563–73.
17. Edwards, R.M. and Aiyar, N. (1993) Angiotensin II receptor subtypes in the kidney. *J. Am. Soc. Nephrol.*, **3**, 1643–52.
18. Burnier, M. and Bruuner, H.R. (1994) Angiotensin II receptor antagonists and the kidney. *Curr. Opin. Nephrol. Hypertens.*, **3**, 537–45.

19. Brunner, H.R. (1992) ACE inhibitors in renal diseases. *Kidney Int.*, **42**, 463–79.

20. Burns, K.D., Homma, T. and Harris, R.C. (1993) The intrarenal renin–angiotensin system. *Semin. Nephrol.*, **13**, 13–30.

21. Wolf, G. and Neilson, E.G. (1993) Angiotensin II as a hypertrophogenic cytokine for proximal tubular cells. *Kidney Int.*, **43**(Suppl 39), S100–7.

22. Yanagisawa, M., Kurihara, H., Kimura, S. *et al.* (1988) A novel potent vasoconstrictor peptide produced by vascular endothelial cells. *Nature*, **332**, 411–15.

23. Simonson, M.S. and Dunn, M.J. (1992) The molecular mechanisms of cardiovascular and renal regulation by endothelin peptides. *J. Lab. Clin. Med.*, **119**, 622–39.

24. Remuzzi, G. and Benigni, A. (1993) Endothelins in the control of cardiovascular and renal function. *Lancet*, **342**, 589–93.

25. Orisio, S., Benigni, A., Bruzzi, I. *et al.* (1993) Renal endothelin gene expression is increased in remnant kidney and correlates with disease progression. *Kidney Int.*, **43**, 354–8.

26. Benigni, A., Zoja, C., Corna, D. *et al.* (1993) A specific endothelin subtype A receptor antagonist protects against injury in renal disease progression. *Kidney Int.*, **44**, 440–4.

27. Luscher, T.F., Seo, B. and Buhler, F. (1993) Potential role of endothelin in hypertension – controversy on endothelin in hypertension. *Hypertension*, **21**, 752–7.

28. Furchgott, R.F. and Zawadski, J.V. (1980) The obligatory role of endothelial cells in the relaxation of smooth muscle by acetylcholine. *Nature*, **288**, 373–6.

29. Schmidt, H.H.H.W. and Walter, U. (1994) NO at work. *Cell*, **78**, 919–25.

30. Marletta, M.A. (1994) Nitric oxide synthase: aspects concerning structure and catalysis. *Cell*, **78**, 927–30.

31. Ujrie, K., Yuen, J., Hogarth, L. *et al.* (1994) Localization and regulation of endothelial NO synthase mRNA expression in rat kidney. *Am. J. Physiol.*, **267**, F296–302.

32. McLay, J.S., Chatterjee, P., Graham Nicolson, A. *et al.* (1994) Nitric oxide production by human proximal tubular cells: a novel immunomodulatory mechanism? *Kidney Int.*, **46**, 1043–9.

33. Tolins, J.P. and Raij, L. (1991) Effects of aminoacid infusion on renal hemodynamics: Role of endothelium-derived relaxing factor. *Hypertension*, **17**, 1045–51.

34. Ito S. (1995) Nitric oxide in the kidney. *Curr. Opin. Nephrol. Hypertens.*, **4**, 23–30.

35. De Nicola, L., Blantz, R.C. and Gabbai, F.B. (1992) Nitric oxide and angiotensin II glomerular and tubular interaction in the rat. *J. Clin. Invest.*, **89**, 1248–56.

36. Baylis, C., Mitruka, B. and Deng, A. (1992) Chronic blockade of nitric oxide synthesis in the rat produces systemic hypertension and glomerular damage. *J. Clin. Invest.*, **90**, 278–81.

37. Henrich, W.L., McAllister, E.A., Smith, P.B. and Campbell, W.B. (1988) Guanosine 3′,5′-cyclic monophosphate as a mediator of inhibition of renin release. *Am. J. Physiol.*, **255**, F474–8.

38. Luscher, T.F., Bock, H.A., Yang, Z. and Diederich, D. (1991) Endothelium-derived relaxing and contracting factors: perspectives in nephrology. *Kidney. Int.*, **39**, 575–90.

39. Cattel, V., Cook, T. and Moncada, S. (1990) Glomeruli synthesize nitrite in experimental nephrotoxic nephritis. *Kidney. Int.*, **38**, 1056–60.

40. Weinberg, J.B., Granger, D.L. Pisetsky, D.S. *et al.* (1994) The role of nitric oxide in the pathogenesis of spontaneous murine autoimmune disease: increased nitric oxide production and nitric oxide synthase expression in MRL-lpr/lpr mice, and reduction of spontaneous glomerulonephritis and arthritis by orally administered NG-monomethyl-L-arginine. *J. Exp. Med.*, **179**, 651–60.

41. Nakazano, K., Watanabe, N., Matsuno, K., Sasaki, J., Sato, T. and Inove, M. (1991) Does superoxide underlie the pathogenesis of hypertension? *Proc. Natl. Acad. Sci. USA*, **88**, 10045–8.

42. Xuan, A.T.D., Fan, T.P.D., Higenbottam, T.W. and Wallwork, J. (1990) Cyclosporine in vitro reduces endothelium-dependent relaxation to acetylcholine but does not affect relaxation to nitrovasodilators. *Transplant. Proc.*, **22**, 1723–25.

43. Moncada, S. and Higgs, A. (1993) The L-arginine–nitric oxide pathway. *N. Engl. J. Med.*, **329**, 2002–12.

I

Normal Structure and Function

Section 5
Renal Biology

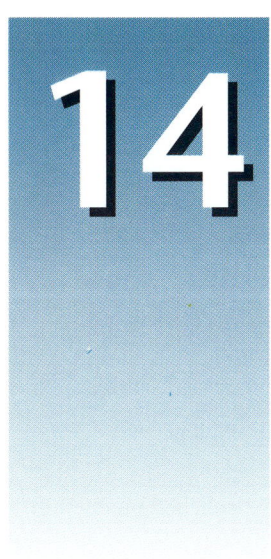

14

Growth factors in kidney development and disease

Ralph Rabkin and Fernando C. Fervenza

Introduction

The kidney is a complex organ consisting of an intricate vascular system and an array of cell types with a variety of specialized functions organized into functional units known as nephrons. Development of this complex organ is under the influence of an array of growth factors which together regulate the transformation of three early embryonic kidneys into the functioning mature kidney [1, 2]. The term growth factors refers to polypeptides that have as a major property the ability to influence cell pro-liferation, differentiation or hypertrophy. Although growth factors are essential for normal embryogenesis [1, 3] and though there is experimental evidence suggesting that perturbations in renal growth factor balance may lead to hypoplastic and dysplastic nephropathies, equiv-alent human disorders have not as yet been described [4]. Abnormalities of local growth factor production and sen-sitivity may, however, contribute to cyst formation in polycystic disease of the kidney.

Essential for embryonic development, growth factors also have important functions in the mature kidney espe-cially in response to stressful situations that require regeneration, repair or compensatory growth as occurs after acute or chronic injury to the kidney. If the insult is acute and non-sustained, injury is usually followed by repair and resolution with return of the activated growth factor systems to basal levels [5]. If injury is sustained then driving forces may be set into motion that provoke persistent secretion of growth factors that contribute to the progression of kidney disease [6].

Factors affecting renal growth may be derived from the circulation or from within the kidney. Circulating factors include growth hormone (GH), insulin-like growth factor -I (IGF-I) and hepatocyte growth factor (HGF), whereas kidney-derived factors include IGF-I, HGF, epidermal growth factor (EGF), transforming growth factor-β (TGF-β), heparin-binding epidermal growth factor (HB-EGF) and platelet-derived growth factor (PDGF). Key features of the major renal growth factors are summarized in Table 14.1.

Local factors are produced by intrinsic cells of the glomeruli, tubules and interstitium. Growth factors are also released by cells infiltrating the kidney. Among the growth factors released in response to injury are a sub-class known as cytokines. These factors, which include interleukins, tumor necrosis factor-α and chemokines such as RANTES, regulate a broader range of cellular processes including chemotaxis and immune regulation. Locally produced growth factors may act in a paracrine manner on nearby cells or in an autocrine manner on the same cells that produce the growth factor. Growth factors bind to their specific receptors situated on the plasma membrane and this activates a complex signal transduc-tion system commonly involving tyrosine kinase enzyme activity [7].

A common feature of growth factors is their multi-functional actions, as they may induce actions other than

Nephrology, Edited by Rex L. Jamison and Robert Wilkinson.
Published in 1997 by Chapman & Hall, London. ISBN 0 412 60930 4

Table 14.1   Major renal growth factors

Factor	Source	Major targets	Predominant action
IGF-I	Circulation TALH	Blood vessels Glomeruli Tubules	Increases RBF, GFR and proliferation Inhibits apoptosis Increases phosphate transport
EGF	TALH Platelets	Tubules	Increases proliferation, inhibits apoptosis Decreases RBF and GFR
HGF	Circulation Interstitium	Tubules	Increases proliferation, migration and tubulogenesis
PDGF	Glomeruli Tubules Interstitial fibroblasts Platelets	Mesangium vsmc	Increases proliferation, chemotaxis and collagen production
TGF-α	Tubules	Tubules	Increases proliferation
TGF-β	Glomeruli Tubules	Tubules Glomeruli	Inhibits proliferation, induces hypertrophy Increases matrix synthesis, decreases matrix degradation
HB-EGF	Glomeruli Tubules	Mesangium Tubules vsmc	Increases proliferation
GH	Circulation	TALH	Stimulates IGF-I production Metabolic effects

TALH: thick ascending limb of Henlé's loop; vsmc: vascular smooth muscle cells.

growth promotion (Table 14.1). Thus for example IGF-I not only promotes kidney growth but it directly increases renal blood flow (RBF) and glomerular filtration rate (GFR) and enhances sodium and phosphate reabsorption [8]. Other factors such as TGF-β_1 have potent effects on extracellular matrix turnover [9]. In respect to their growth-promoting actions some growth factors not only promote proliferation or hypertrophy but may stimulate cell differentiation and migration and even prolong cell survival by inhibiting programmed cell death (apoptosis) [8]. Examples are given later.

Growth factors in the development of the embryonic kidney

During the growth of the embryo to maturity three anatomically and temporally distinct excretory organs arise from the mesoderm. The earlier and transient organs are known as the pronephros and mesonephros whereas the permanent organ is known as the metanephros. This permanent embryonic kidney is invaded by the ureteric bud and together these structures grow and develop into the final mature kidney [10] (Figure 14.1). The ureteric bud, which is an epithelial structure, originates from the pronephros and mesonephros through a complex process

of growth and degeneration. This key structure has the property of inducing the undifferentiated mesenchymal cells of the metanephros to differentiate into the cells comprising the glomeruli, proximal and distal tubules and the loops of Henle. The ureteric bud in turn undergoes branching and differentiates into the collecting ducts, calyces, pelvis and ureters. Vascularization of the kidney occurs through vessels arising from the aorta. This complex development process is described in detail in several recent reviews [1, 11, 12].

The factors that mediate the transformation of mesodermal cells, or mesenchyme, into tubular epithelium and lead to the formation of the glomerular vasculature are incompletely defined. Included among these factors are extracellular matrix components, extracellular proteases, cell adhesion molecules and polypeptide growth factors. It appears that growth factors and their receptors are synthesized in the embryonic renal tissue in a sequential manner and serve to guide the development and maturation of the embryonic kidney. Since most of our knowledge is derived from *in vitro* studies, their relevance to the situation *in vivo* remains to be established.

Growth factors implicated in renal development include IGF-I and IGF-II, EGF and TGF-α, TGF-β, PDGF, HGF, nerve growth factor, angiotensin II, vascular endothelial growth factor (VEGF) and fibroblastic growth

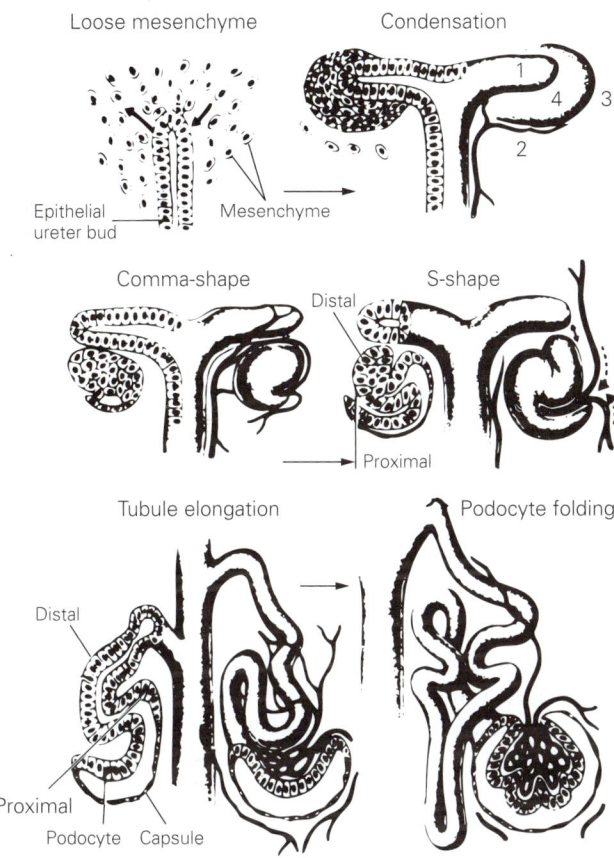

Loose mesenchyme   Condensation

Epithelial ureter bud   Mesenchyme

Comma-shape   S-shape

Distal

Proximal

Tubule elongation   Podocyte folding

Distal

Proximal

Podocyte   Capsule

Figure 14.1 Embryonic development of the nephron. This figure outlines the branching of the ureter, ingrowth of blood vessels and differentiation of the mesenchyme into epithelium. To begin with the ureteric bud grows into the loose mesenchyme inducing differentiation and condensation of mesenchymal cells. At this stage four different cell lineages are seen: (1) ureter, (2) ingrowing blood vessels derived from the aorta, (3) uninduced mesenchyme and (4) induced mesenchyme. The mesenchymal condensate takes on a comma shape and then an S-shape structure. The tubules elongate and there is folding of podocytes in the glomeruli. The S-shaped body, which originates from the condensed mesenchymal cells, differentiates into proximal and distal tubules whereas the ureteric bud forms the collecting ducts and pyelocalyceal system. (Reproduced, with permission, from ref. 10.)

factor (FGF) [1, 3]. In general, these growth factors, to a greater or lesser extent, promote cell proliferation, differentiation, migration and tubulogenesis. They may also influence the production and modeling of extracellular matrix. Individual growth factors are characterized by their special actions or by the prominence of an action which is common to other growth factors. Thus for example EGF and perhaps IGF-I have the property of preventing programmed cell death, whereas HGF is a powerful promoter of tubulogenesis. PDGF likely promotes the acquisition and proliferation of mesangial cells; VEGF, basic FGF and IGF-I are potent angiogenic factors. Based on *in vitro* studies it appears that TGF-β may provide inhibitory control of tubulogenesis and that IGF-II and IGF-I are required for the growth and development of the metanephros, but as with the other growth factors their precise roles in nephrogenesis *in vivo* is unclear.

Thus, although it is apparent that growth factors are important in embryonic nephrogenesis, how they interact with other modulators of kidney growth and development such as extracellular matrix components, adhesion molecules and as yet undiscovered inducers of growth and differentiation remains to be elucidated. When this knowledge is finally acquired the role played by disorders of growth factors in developmental disease will be more readily understood. This should provide the opportunity to develop novel therapeutic strategies to prevent or correct developmental abnormalities of the kidney.

Role of growth factors in recovery from acute tubular necrosis

Severe acute injury to renal tubular epithelium, whether induced by ischemia or nephrotoxins, is followed by exfoliation of necrotic cells and then regeneration of damaged nephron segments. Repair involves regain of polarity and cell–cell contact by damaged cells, proliferation, differentiation and migration of intact cells into denuded areas. Growth factors appear to play an important role in initiating and promoting the regenerative process [5, 13]. Of the several growth factors that are generally involved in tissue repair, there is evidence that TGF-α, TGF-β, HGF, IGF-I, EGF and heparin-binding EGF-like growth factor (HB-EGF) participate in the proliferative repair of damaged renal tubular epithelium (Figure 14.2). IGF-I may also promote an increase in RBF and GFR.

Growth factors promoting repair may be derived from the circulation, as occurs with HGF and IGF-I, or they may originate locally in the kidney. Thus, for example after renal injury there is increased production of HGF by endothelial cells and interstitial macrophages within the kidney and also HGF-producing cells in distant organs such as the liver, lung and spleen. Circulating HGF levels rise and the renal exposure to HGF is increased. In contrast, serum IGF-I levels are unchanged following acute tubular necrosis. Locally produced growth factors are synthesized by tubular cells and infiltrating inflammatory cells. Tubular cells produce EGF, IGF-I and TGF-α and -β whereas infiltrating monocyte/macrophages are a source of EGF, IGF-I, TGF-α and HGF.

After acute injury there is a decrease in IGF-I and EGF gene expression in the thick ascending loop of Henle, and total kidney IGF-I and EGF content falls [14–16]. Concomitantly there is transient expression of IGF-I in regenerating proximal tubule cells, a site where it is not normally produced. Bioavailable EGF peptide increases due to more efficient precursor processing, and there is

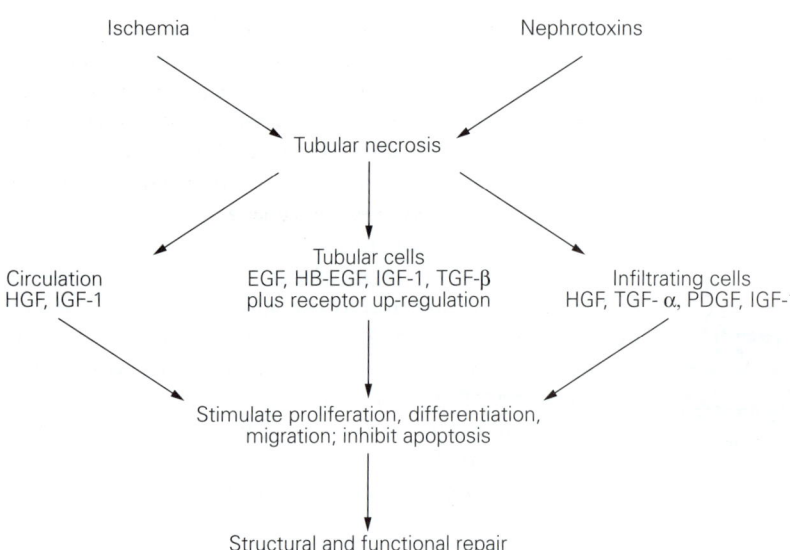

Figure 14.2 Source and action of local growth factors that may mediate regeneration after renal injury. Up-regulation of IGF-I and EGF receptors also favors recovery. Administration of selected recombinant growth factors may accelerate recovery.

increased expression of HB-EGF in distal tubular structures. HB-EGF is a member of the EGF family which interacts with the EGF receptor. There is also an increase in IGF-I and EGF receptor number and activity, a response that will enhance the renal responsiveness to these growth factors [15, 16].

Of considerable potential clinical relevance is the growing body of evidence demonstrating that administration of selected recombinant growth factors including EGF, IGF-I and HGF promotes regeneration and enhances recovery from experimental acute ischemic or nephrotoxic acute renal failure [8, 17–19]. Taking all this information together there is compelling evidence indicating that endogenous growth factors play an important role in the natural regenerative process.

Role of growth factors in glomerular and tubulointerstitial disease of the kidney

Following a renal insult, irrespective of the cause, the expression of several local growth factors, including cytokines, increase in the kidney. Given the broad range of actions exhibited by growth factors it can readily be appreciated that if produced in excess, they may play a prominent role in the functional and structural changes that follow injury. By promoting cellular proliferation and hypertrophy, accumulation of extracellular matrix components, attracting inflammatory cells and affecting vascular tone, growth factors contribute to the structural and functional changes that occur in acute and chronic glomerular and interstitial disease [6, 20, 21]. In addition to these effects of overproduced growth factors, underproduction of a growth factor, as occurs with VEGF, may also lead to altered structure or function.

The growth factors involved in glomerular and tubu-

lointerstitial kidney disease are produced within the affected glomeruli, tubules or interstitium by their constituent cells and by infiltrating inflammatory cells and platelets [22, 23]. Although an array of growth factors may be overexpressed in glomerular and tubulointerstitial disease, several studies have implicated TGF-β_1 and PDGF as being the most prominent growth factors involved in the disease processes [9, 24, 25]. In a seminal study Border *et al.* [26] provided compelling evidence indicating that TGF-β_1 is a mediator of pathologic changes in a rat model of acute mesangioproliferative glomerulonephritis. They showed an early increase in TGF-β_1 levels before the appearance of acute mesangial matrix expansion. More importantly they demonstrated that the pathologic changes could be blocked by reducing TGF-β_1 bioavailability [27]. This was achieved by the pre-emptive administration of a specific TGF-β_1 antibody or the proteoglycan decorin, both of which bind free TGF-β_1.

Overexpression of TGF-β_1 occurs in a variety of experimental chronic renal diseases including progressive diffuse glomerulosclerosis, focal glomerulosclerosis, antiglomerular basement membrane nephritis, tubulointerstitial nephritis and diabetic nephropathy [9, 28]. Since transfection of the TGF-β_1 gene into the normal rat kidney leads to mesangial expansion and glomerulosclerosis, it is likely that TGF-β_1 plays a key role in the pathogenesis of progressive sclerosis. This factor may also be an important mediator of progressive sclerosis in certain human kidney disease. Increased TGF-β production has been noted in glomeruli from patients with diabetic nephropathy, IGA nephropathy, mesangioproliferative glomerulonephritis and idiopathic focal sclerosis but not in idiopathic membranous nephropathy or minimal change disease [9].

Platelet-derived growth factor, which is the most potent mesangial cell mitogen known, also appears to be an important factor in the genesis of acute experimental

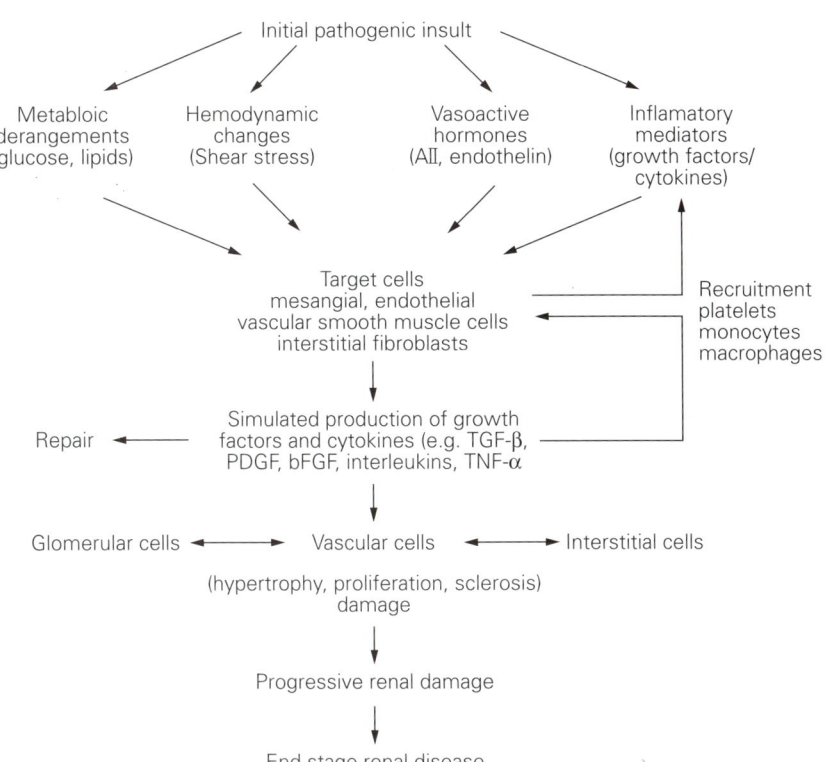

Figure 14.3 Growth factors in progressive renal disease. This hypothetical scheme outlines the stimuli for overproduction of growth factors following an insult to the kidney. This in turn may lead to repair or, if secondary stimuli persist, to progressive damage.

mesangioproliferative glomerulonephritis [29]. In this condition there is increased glomerular expression of PDGF and its receptor. Unlike TGF-β it appears to induce mesangial cell proliferation rather than matrix expansion. Indeed infusion of PDGF or glomerular transfection with the PDGF gene leads to mesangial cell proliferation with only mild extracellular matrix expansion. Enhanced PDGF and/or PDGF receptor gene expression also occurs in chronic progressive experimental kidney diseases such as Heymann's nephritis, lupus nephritis and chemically induced focal glomerulosclerosis, diabetes and interstitial nephritis [24, 29, 30]. This growth factor and its receptor are also overexpressed in a variety of human kidney diseases [24], including proliferative glomerulonephritis, transplant rejection and lupus nephritis.

A common factor driving the expression of both TGF-β and PDGF in chronic kidney disease appears to be the vasoactive peptide angiotensin II. It now appears that apart from its deleterious vasoconstrictor effects on the glomerular circulation, angiotensin II may cause glomerulosclerosis by directly stimulating the overproduction of TGF-β and PDGF in the kidney [25]. This interplay between peptide factors may not end here, for the released PDGF may stimulate even more TGF-β produc-

tion. Ultimately these interactions promote progressive sclerosis.

Although the focus in this chapter has been on a few prominent growth factors, the true situation is far more complicated. Other growth factors such as growth hormone, basic fibroblastic factor and a host of cytokines including interleukins, colony-stimulating factors, TNF-α and chemokines such as RANTES also appear to contribute to the pathogenesis of chronic progressive glomerular and tubulointerstitial disease of the kidney [31, 32] (Figure 14.3). Furthermore, the contribution of individual factors may vary over time and in the different structures of the kidney. However, at this stage of our knowledge it appears that TGF-β and PDGF are the most important players. Together with an array of supporting characters these key factors lead to glomerular enlargement and proliferation of mesangial cells and interstitial fibroblasts and extracellular matrix expansion. This all eventually leads to glomerulosclerosis and interstitial fibrosis. As our understanding of these processes improves it may be possible to develop therapeutic interventions targeted to block the unwanted effects of growth factors and thus treat chronic renal disease, even after the initiating insult has abated.

References

1. Hammermann, M.R. (1995) Growth factors in renal development. *Semin. Nephrol.*, **15**, 291–9.

2. Fouser, L. and Avner, E.D. (1993) Normal and abnormal nephrogenesis. *Am. J. Kidney Dis.*, **21**, 64–70.

3. Clapp, W.L. and Abrahamson, D.R. (1993) Regulation of kidney organogenesis: homeobox genes, growth factors, and Wilms tumor. *Curr. Opin. Nephrol. Hypertens.*, **2**, 419–29.

4. Woolf, A.S. (1995) Clinical impact and biologic basis of renal malformations. *Semin. Nephrol.*, **15**, 361–72.

5. Shigang, L. and Humes D.H. (1994) Cellular and molecular basis of renal repair in acute renal failure. *J. Lab. Clin. Med.*, **12**, 749–54.

6. Fogo, A. (1993) Growth factors promoting progression in renal failure, in *Experimental and Genetic Rat Models of Chronic Renal Failure* (eds N. Gretz and M. Strauch), Karger, Basel, pp. 184–201.

7. Margolis, B. and Skolnik, E.Y. (1994) Activation of Ras by receptor tyrosine kinase. *J. Am. Soc. Nephrol.*, **5**, 1288–99.

8. Rabkin, R. (1995) Insulin-like growth factor-I treatment of acute renal failure. *J. Lab. Clin. Med.*, **125**, 684–5.

9. Sharma, K. and Ziyadeh, F.N. (1994) The emerging role of transforming growth factor-β in kidney diseases. *Am. J. Physiol.*, **266**, F829–42.

10. Mugrauer, G., Alt, F.W. and Ekblom, P. (1988) N-myc proto-oncogene expression during organogenesis in the developing mouse as revealed by *in situ* hybridization. *J. Cell Biol.*, **107**, 1325–35.

11. Stuart, R.O., Barros, E.J.G., Ribeiro, E. and Nigam, S.K. (1995) Epithelial tubulogenesis through branching morphogenesis: relevance to collecting system development. *J. Am. Soc. Nephrol.*, **6**, 1151–9.

12. Hyink, D.P. and Abrahamson, D.R. (1995) Origin of the glomerular vasculature in the developing kidney. *Semin. Nephrol.*, **15**, 327–40.

13. Humes, H.D., Lake, E.W. and Lui, S. (1995) Renal tubule cell repair following acute renal injury. *Miner. Electrolyte Metab.*, **21**, 353–65.

14. Verstrepen, W.A., Nouwen, E.J. and De Broe, M.E. (1994) Renal epidermal growth factor and insulin-like growth factor I in acute renal failure. *Nephrol. Dial. Transplant.*, **9**(suppl 4), 57–68.

15. Tsao, T., Wang, J., Fervenza, F.C. *et al.* (1995) Renal growth hormone–insulin-like growth factor-I system in acute renal failure. *Kidney Int.*, **47**, 1658–68.

16. Saferstein, R., Price, P.M., Saggi, S.J. and Harris, R.C. (1990) Changes in gene expression after temporary renal ischemia. *Kidney Int.*, **37**, 1515–21.

17. Hammerman, M.R. and Miller, S.B. (1994) Therapeutic use of growth factors in renal failure. *J. Am. Soc. Nephrol.*, **5**, 1–11.

18. O'Shea, M., Miller, S.B., Finkel, K. and Hammerman, M.R. (1993) Roles of growth hormone and growth factors in the pathogenesis and treatment of kidney disease. *Curr. Opin. Nephrol. Hypertens.*, **2**, 67–72.

19. Lake, E.W. and Humes, H.D. (1994) Acute renal failure: directed therapy to enhance renal tubular regeneration. *Semin. Nephrol.*, **14**, 83–97.

20. Fogo, A. (1994) Internephron heterogeneity of growth factors and sclerosis. *Kidney Int.*, **45**, S24–6.

21. Couser, W.G. and Johnson, R.J. (1994) Mechanisms of progressive renal disease in glomerulonephritis. *Am. J. Kidney Dis.*, **23**, 193–8.

22. Ong, A.C.M. and Fine, L.G. (1994) Tubular-derived growth factors and cytokines in the pathogenesis of tubulointerstitial fibrosis: Implication for human renal disease progression. *Am. J Kidney Dis.*, **23**, 205–9.

23. Eddy, A.A. (1994) Experimental insights into the tubulointerstitial disease accompanying primary glomerular lesions. *J. Am. Soc. Nephrol.*, **5**, 1273–87.

24. Abboud, H.E. (1995) Role of platelet-derived growth factor in renal injury. *Annu. Rev. Physiol.*, **57**, 297–309.

25. Ketteler, M., Noble, N.A. and Border, W.A. (1995) Transforming growth factor-β and angiotensin II: the missing link from glomerular hyperfiltration to glomerulosclerosis? *Annu. Rev. Physiol.*, **57**, 279–95.

26. Border, W.A., Okuda, S., Languino, L.R., Sporn, M.B. and Ruoslahti, E. (1990) Suppression of experimental glomerulonephritis by antiserum against transforming growth factor β1. *Nature*, **346**, 371–4.

27. Border, W.A., Noble, N.A. and Ketteler, M. (1995) TGF-β: a cytokine mediator of glomerulosclerosis and a target for therapeutic intervention. *Kidney Int.*, **47**, S59–61.

28. Coimbra, T., Wiggins, R., Noh, J.W. and Phan, S.H. (1991) Transforming growth factor β production in anti-glomerular basement membrane disease in the rabbit. *Am. J. Pathol.*, **138**, 223–34.

29. Iida, H., Seifert, R., Alpers, C.E. *et al.* (1991) Platelet-derived growth factor (PDGF) and PDGF receptor are induced in mesangial proliferative nephritis in the rat. *Proc. Natl. Acad. Sci. USA*, **88**, 6560–4.

30. Isaka, Y., Fujiwara, Y., Ueda, N. *et al.* (1993) Glomerulosclerosis induced by *in vivo* transfection of transforming growth factor-β or platelet-derived growth factor gene into the rat kidney. *J. Clin. Invest.*, **92**, 2597–601.

31. Floege, J. and Gröne, H.-J. (1995) Progression of renal failure: what is the role of cytokines? *Nephrol. Dial. Transplant.*, **10**, 1575–86.

32. Wenzel, U.O. and Abboud, H.E. (1995) Chemokines and renal disease. *Am. J. Kidney Dis.*, **26**, 982–94.

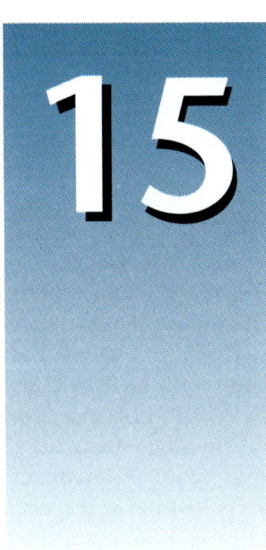

15

The aging kidney

Chris Baylis

Introduction

From young adulthood to middle age, renal function remains constant but with further advances in age, a slow deterioration occurs in many of the functions of the kidney. These functional declines include: a slow progressive reduction in glomerular filtration rate (GFR); reduced ability to conserve and excrete sodium; declines in the ability of the kidney to produce a concentrated urine and to excrete an acid load. In addition, the aging kidney exhibits structural alterations which include the appearance of damage in various parts of the renal vasculature. Fortunately, these age-dependent changes proceed slowly, so that even in the very old kidney, function remains adequate for survival when other disease or injury processes are absent. When hypertension, renal disease, diabetes or other diseases or acute insults such as systemic hemorrhage are present, however, the aging kidney becomes particularly vulnerable to development of severe dysfunction and/or failure. In addition, the aging kidney is increasingly susceptible to drug toxicity due to alterations which occur in renal handling of drugs and their metabolites and this must be considered when prescribing drugs for the elderly.

Renal vasculature: function and structure

Glomerular filtration rate

Many clinical studies have reported a slow decline in GFR after the third to the fourth decade of life, at the rate of approximately 1% per year. Age-dependent falls in GFR have been measured using both the 24 h urinary creatinine clearance and inulin clearances. Most of these studies have been cross-sectional, although age-dependent declines in GFR have also been observed in longitudinal studies [1]. Although an average decline in GFR was seen in this total population studied longitudinally, approximately one-third of the subjects showed no age-dependent reduction in GFR and one-third showed accelerated declines. A recent longitudinal report in the very old indicated that renal function is stable (over a 3-year period) in the majority of the ~500 subjects studied [2]. Thus, as shown in Figure 15.1, which reports data derived from the Baltimore Longitudinal Study of Aging, the effect of age on GFR is quite variable and the reasons for this variability are not yet clear.

There is a marked sexual dimorphism in the renal

Nephrology, Edited by Rex L. Jamison and Robert Wilkinson.
Published in 1997 by Chapman & Hall, London. ISBN 0 412 60930 4

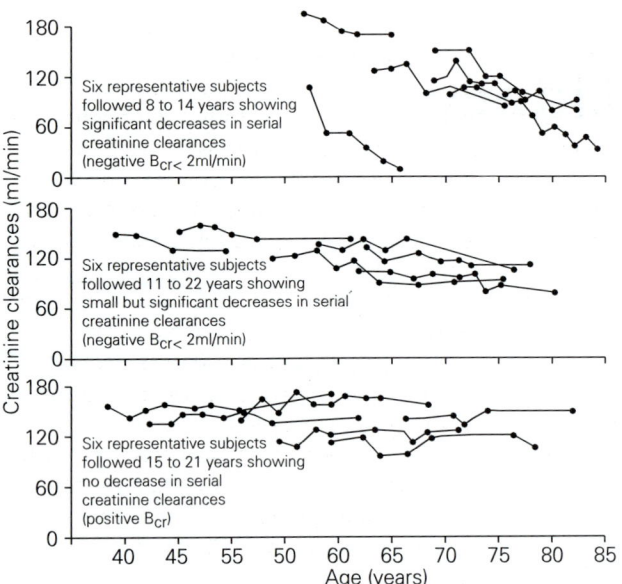

Figure 15.1 Longitudinal individual measurements of serial 24h creatinine clearance in three groups of subjects; one group shows a marked decline in GFR (measured as 24h creatinine clearance) with advancing age (top panel); one group shows a slight decline in GFR with age (middle panel) and one group shows no age-dependent decrement in GFR (lower panel). (Reproduced, with permission, from ref. 1.)

responses to aging, with women being protected from both the decline in GFR and structural damage which occurs. In young adults, GFR is higher in males than in females, and this sex difference gradually disappears with advancing age due to the more rapid reduction in GFR in the male [3]. This sex difference has also been documented in animal studies; it is particularly marked in the rat, and in this species age-dependent deterioration in kidney function results in substantial mortality in the male, due directly to renal failure [4, 5].

Despite the falls in GFR that occur in the aged, serum creatinine concentration does not usually increase because of a concomitant reduction in creatinine production secondary to decreasing muscle mass. In order to gain an estimate of the GFR from the serum creatinine concentration, the patient's age, weight and sex must be taken into account, using the formula given below:

$$C_{cr}(\text{ml/min}) = \frac{140 - \text{age}\,(\text{years})}{\text{serum creatinine}\,(\text{mg/dl})}$$
$$\times \frac{\text{Body weight}\,(\text{kg})}{72}$$

In women, the value is multiplied by 0.85 [6]. It is extremely important to recognize that the majority of aging individuals will experience some decline in glomerular function and that serum creatinine values must be corrected in order to be interpreted accurately.

When determining drug doses for the elderly, an accurate assessment of renal function is particularly important.

Renal/glomerular hemodynamics

Some of the decline in GFR with aging results from structural damage to the kidney (see below) and some is due to alterations in renal/glomerular hemodynamics. There is considerable evidence to suggest that renal blood flow (RBF) diminishes with advancing age and, as with GFR, the age-dependent decline in RBF and renal plasma flow (RPF) is particularly pronounced in the male. Reductions in RBF result from increasing renal vascular resistance due, in part, to functional alterations in the renal blood vessels (see below). The decline in RBF is more marked in the cortex than medulla [3, 6, 7]. The RPF declines to a greater extent than the GFR, thus the filtration fraction rises. An increase in filtration fraction may result from an increase in glomerular blood pressure, although it is quite possible for an increase in FF to occur due exclusively to a reduction in RPF when the individual is at or close to a state of filtration pressure disequilibrium as probably occurs in the young adult (see Chapter 2 for further discussion). Micropuncture studies in the rat have demonstrated that glomerular blood pressure does not rise until late in the aging process [5]. Figure 15.2 shows that glomerular blood pressure remains unchanged up to 20 months of age in intact male rats, and also in intact females and castrated rats of both sexes. In the intact

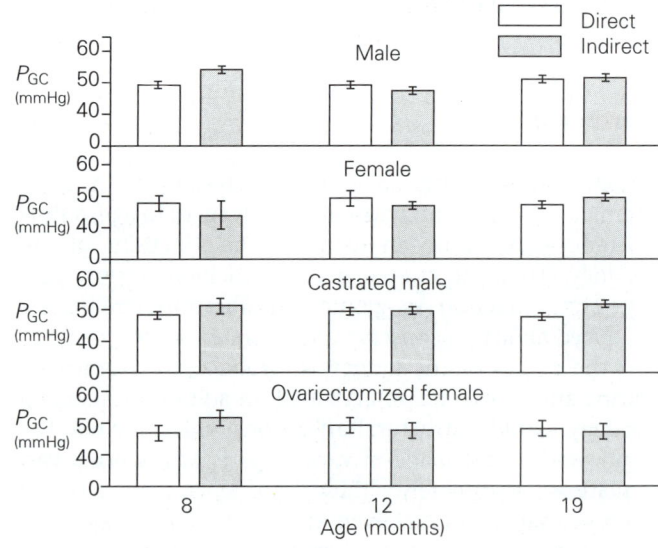

Figure 15.2 Glomerular blood pressure (P_{GC}) measured by direct puncture in superficial glomeruli and by the indirect stop flow method sampling from deeper cortical glomeruli, in rats at 8, 12 and 19 months of age. Data are given as mean ± SE for intact male (upper panel), intact female (second panel), castrated male (third panel) and ovariectomized female (bottom panel) and as shown there is no tendency for P_{GC} to increase over this period of life. (Reproduced, with permission, from ref. 5.)

male rat both afferent and efferent arteriolar resistances (R_A and R_E) increase in parallel with age, leading to reductions in glomerular plasma flow and accounting for the constancy of glomerular blood pressure. The female kidney is vasoconstricted compared to that of the male in the young adult and, as reported by us previously, this is partly due to the presence of the ovarian hormones [4]. With advancing age in females, both R_A and R_E relax, such that by 18–20 months there are no differences in R_A and R_E between the sexes. In addition to plasma flow and glomerular blood pressure, the glomerular capillary ultrafiltration coefficient (K_f) is also a physiologically important determinant of glomerular filtration rate (see Chapter 2). In the aging male and female rat, this value remains unchanged with advancing age, despite progressive increases in glomerular tuft volume, which are particularly pronounced in the male [5]. Presumably this increase in filtration surface area is offset by a reduction in glomerular water permeability, secondary to the well-documented thickening of the glomerular basement membrane seen with aging [3, 7]. Thus, the functional component of the age-related decline in GFR is the result of renal vasoconstriction and thus reduced RPF.

Control of the renal vascular resistance

Vasoconstrictor influences

There are major alterations in the autonomic control of the cardiovascular system with advancing age which include blunted responsiveness to α_2- and β-vascular adrenoceptors, and a blunting of the arterial baroreflex [8]. Increased renal sympathetic nerve activity results from the age-dependent impairment in the arterial baroreflex, which tends to increase both renal vascular resistance and the sensitivity of the kidney to other vasoconstrictor agents [9]. This increased renal nerve activity may play a role in the defective pressure natriuretic response of the old kidney (see below).

The renin–angiotensin system alters with advancing age. Falls in plasma renin activity are seen in most species, including humans, although recent preliminary studies in the aging rat have suggested that plasma angiotensin II (AII) levels do not fall in parallel, and in fact, that AII production may increase with advancing age [10]. Dissociation between plasma renin and AII levels has also been reported in aging humans [11]. Studies in humans and rats have shown that the renal vascular response to administered AII does not change with advancing age [12, 13]. In contrast, the activity of the endogenous intrarenal AII system is enhanced in aging since acute converting enzyme inhibition (CEI) produces an enhanced renal vasodilation in old subjects on both normal and low salt diets [14]. Similar findings have been reported in the rat using the more selective AII AT_1 receptor antagonist losartan [13]. Chronic administration of CEI in the normal rat

may produce renal vasodilation, although this is controversial [15, 16]. It is clear that chronic CEI in aging rats leads to reduced arterial and glomerular blood pressure and, although GFR and RPF show persistent age-dependent declines, the proteinuria is reduced substantially and glomerular structure is preserved [15, 16]. Of particular note, in rats with genetic hypertension and established glomerular injury, CEI is antiproteinuric and may actually reverse some of the glomerulopathy [17, 18]. AII is a mitogen on the glomerular mesangial cell, therefore chronic CEI is probably antimitotic – an action which may be associated with protection against the age-dependent deterioration in glomerular structure, afforded by chronic AII inhibition (see below).

Endothelin (ET) is a potent vasoconstrictor synthesized in several locations including vascular endothelial cells and which is normally present in extremely low concentrations in the plasma. Plasma ET levels increase in aging men and ET synthesis is increased due to elevated mRNA expression in cultured vascular endothelial cells from old compared to young individuals [19]. *In vitro* studies show that the sensitivity of vascular smooth muscle to the direct vasoconstrictor actions of ET diminishes with advancing age, although the potentiating effects of ET to enhance the vasoconstrictor actions of other agents is enhanced [20]. ET is a mitogen of the glomerular mesangial cell and may produce a direct damaging action at the glomerulus (see below). The only study to date on renal vascular actions of ET in aging reports an enhanced renal vasconstrictor but similar pressor response to ET in moderately old versus young animals [21].

Vasodilators

It is well established that with advancing age there is a widespread reduction in vascular endothelial prostacyclin (PGI_2) synthesis. Thromboxane (TXA_2) levels remain unchanged or rise, leading to a reduction in the PGI_2/TXA_2 ratio, a maladaptation which is atherogenic [22]. The ratio of urinary prostacyclin to thromboxane decreases in old subjects [23] and the PGI_2/TXA_2 ratio is reduced in glomeruli and inner and outer medulla of old rat kidneys [24]. In the normal adult kidney, eicosinoids play little overall role in control of renal function, thus non-steroidal anti-inflammatory agents such as aspirin do not reduce kidney function. In the old, however, renal hemodynamics become dependent on vasodilatory prostaglandins and non-steroidal anti-inflammatory agents can decrease GFR and renal blood flow and produce renal failure [25]. In addition to the potent vascular actions of these agents, PGI_2 inhibits and TXA_2 enhances mesangial cell growth, thus these eicosinoids can directly regulate glomerular structure (see below).

Atrial natriuretic peptide (ANP) has a depressor action but variable effects on the microcirculation. ANP lowers BP due to declines in cardiac output secondary to venous dilation [8]. ANP dilates the resistance vessels in a number of vascular beds, and in the skin microcirculation the response is more marked in elderly vs young individuals [26]. In contrast, *in vitro* studies in vascular tissues from animals suggest that ANP-induced vascular relaxation is attenuated by aging in several locations including both rat and monkey renal arteries [27, 28]. The effect of administered ANP on the renal vasculature depends on the pre-existing level of vascular tone, i.e. in stressed or precontracted renal vessels ANP is vasodilatory, whereas in the relaxed basal state ANP can increase RVR due to efferent arteriole vasoconstriction. In the conscious rat, a mildly depressor dose of ANP has no effect on renal hemodynamics but does have a potent and selective natriuretic effect on the old kidney [29]. Basal and stimulated circulating levels of ANP are elevated with aging in man and animals [30–32] at least in part due to a decreased renal clearance of ANP from the plasma in elderly [32], although age-related increases in BP may contribute to increased ANP release.

The nitric oxide (NO) system is a very important controller of BP and kidney function in man and animals [33–35]. NO is tonically released by vascular endothelium and maintains BP at the normal low value [34, 35] both by actively vasodilating and by opposing vasoconstrictor influences. There is some *in vitro* evidence from animal studies that the peripheral vasculature has a diminished ability to produce NO with advancing age [36, 37] and the vascular response to administered nitrodilators is impaired in some blood vessels with aging [8]. In addition, in the rat, 24 h excretion of urinary $NO_2 + NO_3$ (the stable oxidation products of NO) are markedly reduced with aging, suggesting overall reduction of systemic NO production, possibly related to reduced substrate (L-arginine) availability since plasma L-arginine levels also fall markedly [38, 39]. An early report suggested that the NO responsiveness of the kidney vasculature also becomes impaired with age since RBF (measured by the unpredictable xenon washout) became refractory to the actions of acetylcholine in old subjects [12]. In the old rat, however, several recent reports have suggested that NO is important in control of renal vascular tone, since both acute and chronic NO blockade in the rat cause similar or exaggerated renal vasoconstriction in old animals [21, 40, 41]. This suggests that basal NO tone is high in the old rat kidney, which would provide a counterregulatory influence of the activated intrarenal AII. In addition, renal vasodilation due to stimulated NO, either produced by acetylcholine or L-arginine infusion, leads to unblunted responses in old rat kidneys [42]. In contrast, the renal vasodilatory response to acute infusion of the amino acid glycine and to chronic high protein feeding (thought to be mediated in part by NO) are blunted with advancing age in the rat [43, 44] but not in humans [45]. Further, the enhanced susceptibility of the old rat kidney to ischemic acute renal failure is associated with superoxide-mediated quenching of intrarenal NO [46],

thus the importance of NO in maintaining renal perfusion in aging remains uncertain.

In addition to their vasodilatory actions, both ANP and NO inhibit hypertrophic and proliferative growth of vascular smooth muscle and glomerular mesangial cells. As discussed below, growth and extracellular matrix production by glomerular mesangial cells probably play a crucial role in the development of glomerular injury, and alterations in activity of the various vasoactive systems will also influence mesangial cell growth and extracellular matrix production.

Structural changes in the aging kidney

The weight of the kidney diminishes with age and this loss of renal mass is confined mainly to the cortex. The larger blood vessels of the kidney show an increased and variable amount of sclerosis. The incidence of focal and segmental glomerular sclerosis and hyalinization increases with advancing age. This process of sclerosis extends to the entire glomerulus with increasing frequency during aging, leading to glomerular obsolescence. In juxtamedullary glomeruli, shunts develop between the afferent and efferent arterioles which bypass the glomerulus and also lead to loss of functioning glomeruli. Therefore, there is a significant decline in glomerular number with advancing age. Other glomerular alterations include expansion of the glomerular mesangial cells as well as marked thickening of the glomerular basement membrane [3, 6, 7]. In the rat, age-dependent glomerular injury develops at a variable rate, depending on gender, strain and caloric/protein intake [47, 48].

It is not clear what causes the progressive development of glomerular injury with advancing age. A large number of factors have been implicated in the pathogenesis of progressive glomerular disease, one of which is the presence of glomerular capillary hypertension, suggested to cause age-dependent glomerular damage [47]. Long-term, low protein feeding has a protective effect on glomerular architecture in the aging rat, although exactly how much of the protection is due to caloric rather than protein restriction is not clear [47–49].

Chronic CEI also attenuates glomerular injury and, since the glomeruloprotective actions of both low protein feeding and CEI are partly hemodynamically mediated, these observations have been interpreted as indicating a primary role of increased glomerular blood pressure in development of age-dependent glomerulopathy. However, as discussed above, glomerular structural injury in intact male Munich Wistar rats precedes increased glomerular blood pressure; in fact glomerular blood pressure is similar in males (who develop injury) and in females and castrated rats of both sexes who are protected from glomerular injury [5]. By 24 months of age, glomerular blood pressure is elevated in male Munich

Wistar rats [16] presumably as a secondary, compensatory response to glomerular damage. Although dietary protein restriction and CEI may evoke some beneficial effects by lowering glomerular blood pressure to subnormal values, it is likely that they also act via other, non-hemodynamic mechanisms (see below).

In the Sprague–Dawley rat, glomerular injury develops at an accelerated pace vs Munich Wistars [50] and in this strain small increases in glomerular blood pressure have been reported at 13–18 months of age [40, 51], although not at 20–22 months [52], which could contribute to the increased tendency of this strain to develop glomerular injury. This, together with the wealth of evidence suggesting that systemic hypertension worsens age-dependent glomerular injury [7, 47, 48], implies that when increases in glomerular blood pressure do occur, they will exacerbate the underlying development of age-dependent glomerular injury.

It has been suggested that hypertrophy of the glomerular tuft provides a separate risk factor for development of glomerular injury by increased intramural tension [53, 54]. In the castrated male rat, however, glomerular volume increases as in intact males, but is not associated with the development of injury in castrated rats [5]. Thus, whereas it is clear that both glomerular hypertension and glomerular hypertrophy can produce glomerular injury in some situations, neither of these risk factors provides the primary mechanisms for the development of age-dependent glomerulopathy in intact male rats.

Gender is an important determinant of the rate at which glomeruli are damaged with age. Female rats aged over a similar time period to males do not develop comparable glomerular damage or proteinuria and clinical studies suggest that female human kidneys are protected against glomerular injury in a number of glomerulopathies including age-dependent injury [5, 55]. Ovarian hormones are widely recognized to be protective of the cardiovascular system but, surprisingly, ovariectomy does not alter the protected status of the intact female rat, with regard to age-dependent glomerular damage [5]. In view of this finding, and since castration of the male is protective, it seems that either directly or indirectly the presence of androgens, rather than the absence of ovarian hormones, promotes age-dependent glomerular damage, at least in rats.

The cause of age-dependent glomerular damage has not yet been determined. There is, however, evidence to suggest that mesangial cell expansion and mesangial matrix accumulation play a pathogenic role in some forms of primary glomerular injury including aging. Mesangial lesions and mesangial expansion precede development of focal glomerular sclerosis due to aging and increases in mesangial matrix products have been reported in aging male but not female Wistar rats. In the Wistar/Lou strain, no age-dependent glomerular injury develops and morphometric studies show no increase in mesangial matrix or mesangial cellularity in males up to 36 months of age and females up to 42 months of age. The increased susceptibility of the male rat to develop glomerular sclerosis after subtotal nephrectomy correlates with mesangial expansion and higher levels of glomerular procollagen mRNA levels vs female kidneys, suggesting that androgens increase collagen synthesis [5]. Mesangial matrix products can also accumulate because of reduced rates of degradation. Indeed, activity of a glomerular metalloprotease, which is responsible for degradation of mesangial matrix products, is inversely related to age-dependent injury, being low in intact males but raised in females and castrated rats of both sexes, who are protected from damage [56]. Glomerular extracellular matrix production by the glomerular mesangial cells is regulated by many paracrine and autocrine factors including cytokines, eicosinoids, NO, AII and other vasoactive substances [57]. In addition elevated lipids increased oxidants, and advanced glycosylated end products, all of which accumulate in normal aging, have been implicated in glomerular injury, possibly by enhancing extracellular matrix expression [57–59]. There is also a strong correlation between glomerulosclerosis and atherosclerosis in the aged [7].

Glomerular permeability is not markedly altered in aging humans since frank proteinuria is not seen in the absence of glomerular disease. Microalbuminuria does occur with increasing frequency and is associated with a general increase in cardiovascular morbidity, as is also the case in younger patients [60].

The elderly are susceptible to a similar range of glomerular diseases to younger patients although the incidence is different; proliferative or necrotizing glomerulonephritis, membranous glomerulopathy, glomerulosclerosis and crescentic glomerulonephritis are more frequently seen in older patients. Arterionephrosclerosis is also seen in old patients, both alone and superimposed on other glomerulopathies [61]. When renal disease progresses to end stage the elderly adapt quite well to hemodialysis and peritoneal dialysis although the rate of complications increases. Renal transplantation is also reasonably successful in old patients and rejection problems are actually diminished, although the limited availability of donor organs provides practical and ethical barriers to widespread transplantation in the elderly [62].

Changes – renal aspects of sodium, potassium and acid–base balance

Sodium

Sodium balance

Under optimal circumstances, sodium balance is effectively regulated in the old, and plasma volume does not change due to advancing age alone although total exchangeable sodium increases with advancing age. There are impairments in sodium homeostatic mechanisms with age, such that both sodium conservation in salt restriction, and sodium excretion in salt overloaded states, are significantly impaired. These maladaptations, together with the reduced urinary concentrating and diluting ability, characteristic of aging (see below), account for the high incidence of disordered water and sodium balance seen in the elderly [63].

Sodium conservation

In response to sodium deprivation, renal conservation of sodium is clearly impaired with aging. Based on clearance studies in man, it seems that the site of diminution in sodium reabsorption is in the thick ascending limb of the loop of Henle. In addition, circulating aldosterone levels are reduced in the old, in the basal state, and particularly in response to sodium deprivation, which contributed to blunted reabsorption in more distal nephron sites [3, 7]. The defective aldosterone response is generalized since in addition to sodium restriction, furosemide and assumption of the upright posture are also associated with a diminished aldosterone response in the aged. Chronic adaptation to a low salt intake is also impaired in the old, and the combination of high sodium excretion together with sodium depletion is frequently found in geriatric patients [3].

Natriuretic capacity

Although there is some disagreement in the literature, most studies indicate a diminished natriuretic response to acute sodium loading. This is unlikely to be due to alterations in atrial natriuretic peptide (ANP), since circulating ANP actually increases with advancing age, and an enhanced natriuretic response to administered ANP occurs in the aging rat [29], possibly due to reduction in renal degradation of ANP, secondary to diminished proximal tubular proteolytic enzyme activity [64]. Increased renal vasoconstriction tends to be antinatriuretic and both intrarenal AII and efferent renal sympathetic nerve activity are increased with advancing age (see above). Although the precise mechanism is unknown, it is clear that a blunted natriuretic response can lead to dangerous volume overloading in geriatric patients receiving intravenous saline [3]. In addition to an absolute reduction in natriuretic capacity of the old kidney, the circadian rhythm is also altered, with more sodium being excreted at night in the elderly (which may account for nocturia).

Hypertension: role of salt sensitivity

The incidence of both isolated systolic and diastolic hypertension increases substantially with advancing age [65, 66]. There are many factors involved, one of which is the increased sodium sensitivity of the aging population. According to Guyton et al. [67], the long-term regulation of blood pressure is highly dependent on the ability of the kidney to produce a natriuretic response to a rise in blood pressure – so called pressure natriuresis. When pressure natriuresis is defective in an individual who eats a high salt diet, blood pressure must increase in order to maintain sodium balance, leading to a salt-sensitive (salt-dependent) hypertension [67]. It is noteworthy that several groups have demonstrated that the incidence of salt-sensitive hypertension rises substantially with increasing age [68–70]. Therefore, high dietary salt intake is more likely to lead to hypertension, and dietary salt restriction is more likely to provide an effective antihypertensive treatment, in older subjects. Studies in the aging rat have shown that the pressure natriuretic response is markedly blunted and shifted to the right in the old versus the young rat, partly due to increased renal nerve activity [71]; most likely the increased intrarenal AII activity, discussed above, also contributes. As shown in Figure 15.3, when the pressure natriuresis curve is shifted to the right and the gain is reduced, a salt-dependent hypertension will result [67].

Alterations in the NO system may also be associated with the increased sodium sensitivity of aging. In the normal animal, an increased dietary salt intake leads to increased NO production, and chronic blockade of NO together with a high dietary salt intake causes volume-dependent hypertension [72, 73]. In addition, the hypertension that develops in the Dahl genetically salt-sensitive rat when on a high salt intake is associated with a defective NO production [74] as well as with a rightward shift of the pressure natriuresis curve [75]. Thus, based on animal studies, it is likely that the increased incidence of sodium sensitivity and salt-dependent hypertension with advancing age is due both to a defective pressure natriuretic response as well as to the reduction which occurs in systemic NO activity (see above).

Potassium balance

The total body potassium content is lower in old than in young individuals, although plasma potassium concentration is similar. The cause of the reduced total body potassium content in the old is probably multifactorial, and whether any renal mechanisms are involved is unclear since the data are conflicting [3, 7]. Studies in rats suggest that the kaliuretic response to acute potassium loading is intact on a normal potassium intake, but is impaired in rats whose potassium intake is chronically elevated. In addition, the aging kidney has a reduced ability to conserve potassium since, although absolute potassium excretion falls with age, potassium intake also goes down and the fractional excretion of potassium increases [3]. It therefore seems that the aging kidney has a reduced ability to maintain potassium balance when potassium homeostasis is impaired due either to changes

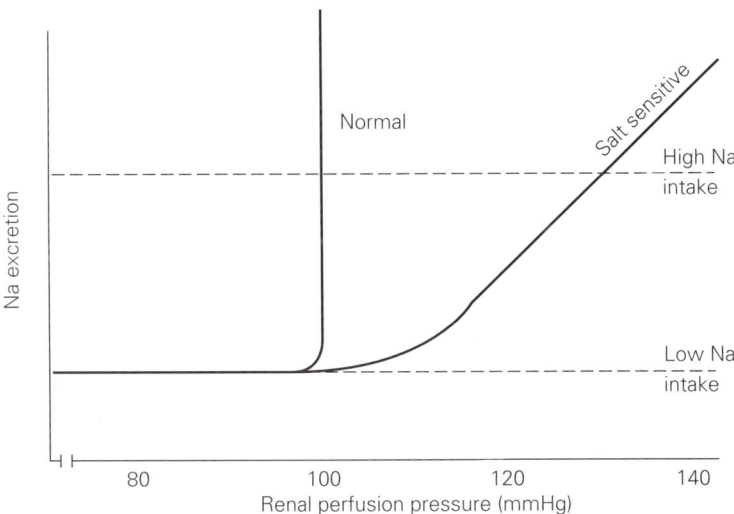

Figure 15.3 The relationship between renal perfusion pressure and renal sodium excretion (the pressure natriuresis relationship) in normal and salt sensitive individuals. As shown when an individual with a normal pressure natriuresis moves from a low to a high salt intake, they remain in sodium balance without a marked change in BP because of the high gain pressure natriuresis slope. In contrast, when a salt sensitive individual increases their salt intake, BP must rise to maintain salt balance, because the pressure natriuresis slope is blunted and shifted to the right.

in intake and/or alterations in the extrarenal mechanisms that control potassium distribution in the body.

Water balance

Water balance is controlled by control of intake (regulated by the thirst mechanism) and renal excretion of water and aging is associated with alterations in both intake and output regulation. Fluid intake diminishes with advancing age and there is a marked diminution in the thirst mechanism in the elderly. Normally the total body water content is slightly reduced with aging, probably due to the reduction in lean body mass that occurs with age.

Urine concentration

It is well established that the maximum renal concentrating capacity declines with advancing age. Clinical studies suggest that this blunted concentrating ability is due to a reduced medullary interstitial concentration gradient, probably secondary to the decrease in sodium chloride reabsorption which occurs in the thick ascending limb with advancing age [3, 7]. Whether alterations in the antidiuretic hormone system are also involved is unclear. The osmotic release of AVP (the primary physiologic stimulus) is actually enhanced in old people, although non-osmotic AVP release (in response to volume depletion) is blunted, an effect also seen in the aged rat. Studies in the rat have also indicated that the cellular action of AVP in the collecting duct is impaired with aging [76].

Urinary dilution

The ability to produce a dilute urine is also blunted with aging, and the minimum urine osmolality and free water clearance are reduced in old subjects undergoing a maximal water diuresis. The reduction in urinary dilut-

ing capacity in the old kidney has been attributed to the impairment in sodium chloride transport in the thick ascending limb, as well as the reductions in GFR, although this subject has not been widely investigated.

Use of diuretics

As discussed above, there are widespread deficiencies in the ability of the old kidney to maintain sodium, potassium, and water balance. Not surprisingly therefore, the response to diuretics in the elderly tends to be somewhat unpredictable. Diuretics are the first-line drug of choice for treatment of isolated systolic hypertension in the elderly, but may produce exaggerated effects leading to volume depletion, hyponatremia, as well as hypokalemia. Administration of potassium supplementation or potassium-sparing diuretics may lead to hyperkalemia. Over-diuresis leads to severe volume depletion and hypernatremia and the frequency of these side effects is increased in the elderly due to the alterations which occur in the renal handing of drugs [3, 7, 66].

Acid-base balance

In the normal aged population, acid–base balance is well maintained, but when challenged with an acid load the immediate buffering response is diminished, as is the long-term compensatory excretion of the acid load via the kidneys. Most clinical studies suggest that the defect resides in a blunted, slower excretion of ammonium by the old kidney [3, 7].

Mineral metabolism

Alterations occur in calcium and phosphate balance with advancing age, due predominantly to extrarenal causes. There are alterations in renal function, however, which also influence mineral metabolism. Renal tubular calcium handling is apparently normal but reductions occur in renal tubular reabsorption of phosphate with advancing age, although animal studies suggest that this is not related to the increasing levels of parathyroid hormones which occur with aging. Reductions in intestinal calcium and phosphate absorption, resulting from impaired 1,25-dihydroxy-vitamin D production within the kidney [77], together with the phosphaturia secondary to reduced renal phosphate reabsorption, are factors in the increased incidence of osteoporosis seen in the aging population.

Summary

Multiple defects develop in the aging kidney leading to declines in GFR, structural injury, alterations in the renal disposition of drugs and impairment in the renal aspects of sodium, potassium, water and acid–base balance. Together these decremental changes render the aging kidney more vulnerable to a range of insults, including ischemic, nephrotoxic and primary glomerular diseases as well as derangements in volume control produced by events such as dehydration, increased salt intake, administration of diuretics or i.v. fluids.

References

1. Lindeman, R.D., Tobin, J. and Shock, N.W. (1985) Longitudinal studies on the rate of decline in renal function with age. *J. Am. Geriatr. Soc.*, **33**, 278–85.
2. Feinfeld, D.A., Guzik, H., Carvounis, C.P. *et al.* (1995) Sequential changes in renal function tests in the old: Results from the Bronx longitudinal aging study. *J. Am. Geriatr. Soc.*, **43**, 412–14.
3. Macias-Nunez, J.F. and Cameron, J.S. (1992) Renal function in the elderly, in *Oxford Textbook of Clinical Nephrology* (eds S. Cameron, A.M. Davison, J.P. Grunfeld *et al.*), Oxford University Press, Oxford, pp. 56–70.
4. Munger, K.A. and Baylis, C. (1988) Sex differences in renal hemodynamic in rats. *Am. J. Physiol.*, **254**, F223–31.
5. Baylis, C. (1994) Age-dependent glomerular damage in the rat: dissociation between glomerular injury and both glomerular hypertension and hypertrophy. Male gender as a primary risk factor. *J. Clin. Invest.*, **94**, 1823–9.
6. Chou, S.Y. and Lindeman, R.D. (1995) Structural and functional changes in the aging kidney, in *The Principles and Practice of Nephrology*, 2nd edn (eds H.R. Jacobson, G.E. Striker and S. Klahr), Mosby, St Louis, pp. 510–14.
7. Levi, M. and Rowe, J.W. (1992) Renal function and dysfunction in aging, in *The Kidney: Physiology and Pathophysiology* (eds D.W. Seldin and G. Giebisch), Raven Press, New York, pp. 3433–56.
8. Docherty, J.R. (1990) Cardiovascular responses in ageing: a review. *Pharmacol. Rev.*, **42**, 103–25.
9. Hajduczok, G. and Chapleau, M.W. (1991) Increase in sympathetic activity with age I. Role of impairment of arterial baroreflexes. *Am. J. Physiol.*, **260**, H1113–20.
10. Baylis, C., Engels, K., Hymel, A. and Navar, L.G. (1995) Age dependent alterations in the metabolic clearance rate (MCR) of angiotensin II (AII) in the rat. *J. Am. Soc. Nephrol.*, **6**, 731.
11. Lubran, M.M. (1995) Renal function in the elderly. *Ann. Clin. Lab. Sci.*, **25**, 122–33.
12. Hollenberg, N.K., Adams, D.F., Solomon, H.S. *et al.* (1974) Senescence and the renal vasculature in normal man. *Circ. Res.*, **34**, 309–16.
13. Baylis, C. (1993) Renal responses to acute angiotensin II (AII) inhibition and administered AII in the ageing, conscious chronically catheterized rat. *Am. J. Kidney Dis.*, **22**, 842–50.
14. Hollenberg, N.K. and Moore, T.J. (1994) Age and the renal blood supply: renal vascular responses to Angiotensin converting enzyme inhibition in healthy humans. *J. Am. Geriatr. Soc.*, **42**, 805–8.
15. Heudes, D., Michel, O., Chevalier, J. *et al.* (1994) Effect of chronic ANG I-converting enzyme inhibition on aging processes. I. Kidney structure and function. *Am. J. Physiol.*, **266**, R1038–51.
16. Anderson, S., Rennke, H.G. and Zatz, R. (1994) Glomerular adaptations with normal aging and with long-term converting enzyme inhibition in rats. *Am. J. Physiol.*, **267**, F35–43.
17. Komatsu, K., Frohlich, E.D., Ono, H. *et al.* (1995) Glomerular dynamics and morphology of aged spontaneously hypertensive rats. Effects of angiotensin-converting enzyme inhibition. *Hypertension*, **25**, 207–13.
18. Vienet, R., Grognet, J.M., Ezan, E. *et al.* (1994) Effect of chronic converting-enzyme inhibition on kidney function of senescent hypertensive rats. *J. Cardiovasc. Pharmacol.*, **23**, S19–25.
19. Kumazaki, T., Fujii, T., Kobayashi, M. and Mitsui, Y. (1994) Aging- and growth-dependent modulation of endothelin-1 gene expression in human vascular endothelial cells. *Exp. Cell Res.*, **211**, 6–11.
20. Dohi, Y. and Luscher, T. (1990) Aging differentially affects direct and indirect actions of endothelin-1 in perfused mesenteric arteries of the rat. *Br. J. Pharmacol.*, **100**, 889–93.
21. Tank, J.E. and Vora, J.P. (1994) Altered renal vascular responses in the aging rat kidney. *Am. J. Physiol.*, **266**, F942–8.
22. Menconi, M., Taylor, L., Martin, B. and Polgar, P. (1987) A review: prostaglandins, aging, and blood vessels. *Geriatr Biosci.*, **35**, 239–47.
23. Hornych, A., Forette, F., Bariety, J. *et al.* (1991) The influence of age on renal prostaglandin synthesis in man. *Prostaglandins Leukot. Essent. Fatty Acids*, **43**, 191–5.
24. Rathaus, M., Greenfeld, Z., Podjarny, E. *et al.* (1993) Sodium loading and renal prostaglandins in old rats. *Prostaglandins Leukot. Essent. Fatty Acids*, **49**, 815–19.
25. Johnson, A.G. and Day, R.O. (1991) The problems and pitfalls of NSAID therapy in the elderly (Part 1). *Drugs Aging*, **1**, 130–43.

26. Jansen, T.L., Tan, A.C., Wollersheim, H. *et al.* (1991) Age-dependent vasodilation of the skin microcirculation by atrial natriuretic factor. *J. Cardiovasc. Pharmacol.*, **18**, 622–30.

27. Kawai, Y. and Ohhashi, T. (1990) Age-related changes in relaxant response of vascular smooth muscles to atrial natriuretic peptide. *J. Pharmacol. Exp. Ther.*, **252**, 1234–9.

28. Moritoki, H., Yoshikawa, T., Hisayama, T. and Takeuchi, S. (1992) Possible mechanisms of age-associated reduction of vascular relaxation caused by atrial natriuretic peptide. *Eur. J. Pharmacol.*, **210**, 61–8.

29. DePriest, D., Zimmermann, C. and Baylis, C. (1990) Renal-effects of administered atrial natriuretic peptide in the conscious, aging rat. *Life Sci.*, **46**, 785–92.

30. Ohashi, M., Fujio, N., Nawata, H. *et al.* (1987) High plasma concentrations of human atrial natriuretic polypeptide in aged men. *J. Clin. Endocrinol. Metab.*, **64**, 81–5.

31. Haller, B., Zust, H., Shaw, S. *et al.* (1987) Effects of posture and ageing on circulating atrial natriuretic peptide levels in man. *J. Hypertens.*, **5**, 551–6.

32. Tan, A.C., Jansen, T.L., Termond, E.F.S. *et al.* (1992) Kinetics of atrial natriuretic peptide in young and elderly subjects. *Eur. J. Clin. Pharmacol.*, **42**, 449–52.

33. Haynes, W.G., Noon, J.P., Walker, B.R. and Webb, D.J. (1993) Inhibition of nitric oxide synthesis increases blood pressure in healthy humans. *J. Hypertens.*, **11**, 1375–80.

34. Moncada, S., Palmer, R.M.J. and Higgs, E.A. (1991) Nitric oxide: physiology, pathophysiology, and pharmacology. *Pharmacol. Rev.*, **43**, 109–41.

35. Baylis, C., Harton, P. and Engels, K. (1990) Endothelial derived relaxing factor (EDRF) controls renal hemodynamics in the normal rat kidney. *J. Am. Soc. Nephrol.*, **1**, 875–81.

36. Tominaga, M., Fujii, K., Abe, I. *et al.* (1994) Hypertension and ageing impair acetylcholine-induced vasodilation in rats. *J. Hypertens.*, **12**, 259–68.

37. Dohi, Y., Thiel, M.A., Buhler, F.R. and Luscher, T.F. (1990) Activation of endothelial L-arginine pathway in resistance arteries. *Hypertension*, **15**, 170–9.

38. Sonaka, I., Futami, Y. and Maki, T. (1994) L-Arginine–nitric oxide pathway and chronic nephropathy in aged rats. *J. Gerontol. Biol. Sci.*, **49**, B157–61.

39. Reckelhoff, J.F., Kellum, J.A., Blanchard, E.J. *et al.* (1994) Changes in nitric oxide precursor, L-arginine, and metabolites, nitrate and nitrite, with aging. *Life Sci.*, **55**, 1895–902.

40. Reckelhoff, J.F. and Manning, R.D. Jr (1993) Role of endothelium-derived nitric oxide in control of renal microvasculature in aging male rats. *Am. J. Physiol.*, **265**, R1126–31.

41. Hill, C., Engels, K. and Baylis, C. (1993) Endothelial derived relaxing factor (EDRF) and the ageing rat kidney. *FASEB J.*, **7**, A771 (Abstract no. 4452).

42. Hill, C., Engels, K. and Baylis, C. (1993) The old rat kidney has a normal response to vasodilatory agents acting via nitric oxide (NO) production. *J. Am. Soc. Nephrol.*, **4**, 554A.

43. Baylis, C., Fredericks, M., Wilson, C. *et al.* (1990) Renal vasodilatory response to IV glycine in the ageing rat kidney. *Am. J. Kidney Dis.*, **15**, 244–51.

44. Corman, B., Chami-Khazraji, S., Schaeverbeke, J. and Michel, J.B. (1988) Effect of feeding on glomerular filtration rate and proteinuria in conscious aging rats. *Am. J. Physiol.*, **255**, F250–6.

45. Fliser, D., Zeier, M., Nowack, R. and Ritz, E. (1993) Renal functional reserve in healthy elderly subjects. *J. Am. Soc. Nephrol.*, **3**, 1371–7.

46. Sabbatini, M., Sansone, G., Uccello, F. *et al.* (1994) Functional versus structural changes in the pathophysiology of acute ischemic renal failure in aging rats. *Kidney Int.*, **45**, 1355–61.

47. Anderson, S. and Brenner, B.M. (1986) Effects of aging on the renal glomerulus. *Am. J. Med.*, **80**, 435–42.

48. Goldstein, R.S., Tarloff, J.B. and Hook, J.B. (1988) Age-related nephropathy in laboratory rats. *FASEB J.*, **2**, 2241–51.

49. Masoro, E.J. and Yu, B.P. (1989) Editorial. Diet and nephropathy. *Lab. Invest.*, **60**, 165–7.

50. Gray, J.E., Van Zwieten, M.J. and Hollandes, C.F. (1982) Early light microscopic changes of chronic progressive nephrosis in several strains of aging laboratory rats. *J. Gerontol.*, **37**, 142–50.

51. Fujihara, C.K., Limongi, D.M.Z.P., DeOliveira, H.C.F. and Zatz, R. (1992) Absence of focal glomerulosclerosis in aging analbuminemic rats. *Am. J. Physiol.*, **262**, R947–54.

52. Reckelhoff, J.F., Samsell, L., Racusen, L. *et al.* (1992) The effect of ageing on glomerular hemodynamics in the Sprague–Dawley rat. *Am. J. Kidney Dis.*, **20**, 70–5.

53. Yoshida, Y., Fogo, A. and Ichikawa, I. (1989) Glomerular hemodynamic changes vs hypertrophy in experimental glomerular sclerosis. *Kidney Int.*, **35**, 654–60.

54. Daniels, B.S. and Hostetter, T.H. (1990) Adverse effects of growth in the glomerular microcirculation. *Am. J. Physiol.*, **258**, F1409–16.

55. Silbiger, S.R. and Neugarten, J. (1995) The impact of gender on the progression of chronic renal disease. *Am. J. Kidney Dis.*, **25**, 515–33.

56. Reckelhoff, J.F. and Baylis, C. (1993) Glomerular metalloprotease activity is suppressed by androgens in the ageing kidney. *J. Am. Soc. Nephrol.*, **3**, 1835–8.

57. Sterzel, R.B., Schulze-Lohoff, E., Weber, M. and Goodman, S.L. (1992) Interactions between glomerular mesangial cells, cytokines, and extracellular matrix. *J. Am. Soc. Nephrol.*, **2**, S126–31.

58. Kasiske, B.L. (1988) Treatment of hyperlipidemia reduces glomerular injury in obese Zucker rats. *Kidney Int.*, **33**, 667–72.

59. Doi, T., Vlassara, H., Kirstein, M. *et al.* (1992) Receptor specific increased mesangial cell extracellular matrix production is mediated by PDGF. *Proc. Natl Acad Sci USA*, **89**, 2873–7.

60. Metcalf, P., Baker, J., Scott, A. *et al.* (1992) Albuminuria in people at least 40 years old: effect of obesity, hypertension and hyperlipidemia. *Clin. Chem.*, **38**, 1802–8.

61. Falk, R.J. and Jennette, J.C. (1995) Glomerular disease in the elderly, in *The Principles and Practice of Nephrology*,

2nd edn (eds H.R. Jacobson, G.E. Striker and S. Klahr), Mosby, St Louis, pp. 518–24.

62. Shapiro, W.B. (1995) Renal replacement therapy in the elderly, in *The Principles nad Practice of Nephrology*, 2nd edn (eds H.R. Jacobson, G.E. Striker and S. Klahr), Mosby, St Louis, pp. 533–41.

63. Faubert, P.F. and Porush, J.G. (1995) Disorders of water, sodium and divalent ion metabolism, in *The Principles and Practice of Nephrology*, 2nd edn (eds H.R. Jacobson, G.E. Striker and S. Klahr), Mosby, St Louis, pp. 515–18.

64. Reckelhoff, J.F. and Baylis, C. (1992) Proximal tubular metalloprotease activity is decreased in the senescent rat kidney. *Life Sci.*, **50**, 959–63.

65. National High Blood Pressure Education Program Working Group (1994) National high blood pressure education program working group report on hypertension in the elderly. *Hypertension*, **23**, 275–85.

66. Spitalewitz, S. and Hollenberg, N.K. (1995) Hypertension in the elderly, in *The Principles and Practice of Nephrology*, 2nd edn (eds H.R. Jacobson, G.E. Striker and S. Klahr), Mosby, St Louis, pp. 524–30.

67. Guyton, A.C., Coleman, T.G., Cowley, A.W. *et al.* (1972) Arterial pressure regulation: overriding dominance of the kidneys in long term regulation and in hypertension. *Am. J. Med.*, **52**, 584–94.

68. Luft, F.C., Weinberger, M.H., Fineberg, N.S. *et al.* (1987) Effects of age on renal sodium homeostasis and its relevance to sodium sensitivity. *Am. J. Med.*, **82**(Suppl 1B), 9–15.

69. Nestel, P.J., Clifton, P.M., Noakes, M. *et al.* (1993) Enhanced blood pressure response to dietary salt in elderly women, especially those with small waist:hip ratio. *J. Hypertens.*, **11**, 1387–94.

70. Ishibashi, K., Oshima, T., Matsuura, H. *et al.* (1994) Effects of age and sex on sodium chloride sensitivity: association with plasma renin activity. *Clin. Nephrol.*, **42**, 376–80.

71. Masilamani, S. and Baylis, C. (1993) Defective pressure natriuresis in the ageing kidney. *J. Am. Soc. Nephrol.*, **4**, 516A.

72. Shultz, P.J. and Tolins, J.P. (1993) Adaptation to increased dietary salt intake in the rat. Role of endogenous nitric oxide. *J. Clin. Invest.*, **91**, 642–50.

73. Salazar, F.J., Alberola, A., Pinilla, J.M. *et al.* (1993) Salt-induced increase in arterial pressure during NOS inhibition. *Hypertension*, **22**, 49–55.

74. Chen, P.Y. and Sanders, P.W. (1991) L-Arginine abrogates salt-sensitive hypertension in Dahl/Rapp rats. *J. Clin. Invest.*, **88**, 1559–67.

75. Roman, R.J. (1986) Abnormal renal hemodynamics and pressure natriuresis relationship in Dahl salt sensitive rats. *Am. J. Physiol.*, **251**, F57–65.

76. Geelen, G. and Corman, B. (1992) Relationship between vasopressin and renal concentrating ability in aging rats. *Am. J. Physiol.*, **262**, R826–33.

77. Armbrecht, H.J., Forte, L.R. and Halloran, B.P. (1984) Effect of age and dietary calcium on renal 1,25(OH)2D, and PTH. *Am. J. Physiol.*, **246**, E266–70.

16

Renal biology of erythropoietin

Peter J. Ratcliffe

Introduction

The existence of a factor in anemic plasma which could stimulate erythropoiesis was first proposed at the beginning of this century by Carnot and Deflandre. Nevertheless, the contrary view, that anemia had a direct effect on the marrow, prevailed for nearly 50 years. In the 1950s, Reissman's classic experiments using parabiotic rats, and Erslev's plasma transfer experiments, provided convincing evidence for hormonal control of erythropoiesis by erythropoietin [1, 2]. In 1957, Jacobsen and colleagues demonstrated, in rats subject to hemorrhagic anemia, that nephrectomy abolished erythropoietin production, thereby implicating the kidneys as necessary for the response [3]. Doubt remained as to whether the kidneys were the site of *de novo* synthesis or whether they activated a factor produced at another site. Kidney perfusion experiments, and immunoassay of tissue homogenates, favored *de novo* renal synthesis and following cloning of the gene this was finally proven by the demonstration of erythropoietin mRNA in kidney. It is now established that erythropoietin is a glycoprotein hormone which stimulates erythropoiesis by interaction with a specific receptor, and so forms part of a feedback loop controlling red cell production. Both hormone and receptor bear structural and functional homologies with a large family of hematopoietic growth factors. Among the hematopoietic growth factors erythropoietin is unusual in two ways: first, in its operation as a bloodstream hormone, and second, in its specificity for the erythroid lineage. In contrast with other components of hematopoiesis, it has proved possible to gain an important insight into the physiology of the system from plasma assays.

The hormonal operation of erythropoietin

Basal production of erythropoietin maintains a low plasma level of the hormone which is essential for erythropoiesis. In most individuals this baseline level of erythropoietin is rather constant, though in some studies a small diurnal variation has been reported, with an increase around midnight. Between individuals there is greater variability and the range of plasma levels in normal individuals is rather wide (e.g. 4–26 mU/ml [4]). This range is independent of gender, and beyond the neonatal period it is independent of age.

In addition to anemia, reduction in arterial Po_2 and increased hemoglobin oxygen affinity also increase plasma erythropoietin, indicating that the major stimulus for production is tissue hypoxia arising from reduced blood oxygen availability. Regulation of the circulating level of erythropoietin is achieved through changes in the rate of production and there is no evidence for regulation of erythropoietin clearance. In acutely hypoxic rodents erythropoietin mRNA increases in the kidneys within 1 h, and peak plasma levels of erythropoietin are attained within 24 h.

Nephrology, Edited by Rex L. Jamison and Robert Wilkinson.
Published in 1997 by Chapman & Hall, London. ISBN 0 412 60930 4

Though there is a wide scatter in the values, in anemic patients without renal disease there is an inverse relationship between the hematocrit and the logarithm of the erythropoietin level (Figure 16.1), with levels up to 1000-fold above baseline in the most severely anemic cases. In renal disease this relationship is not evident and erythropoietin levels are inappropriately low for the degree of anemia [5]. Less dramatic reduction in the response of erythropoietin to anemia occurs in a number of other conditions. These include anorexia and starvation, certain endocrine deficiencies (thyroid, pituitary, adrenal), systemic inflammatory and malignant disease, acidosis and the use of angiotensin converting enzyme inhibitors. For some conditions (e.g. starvation or hypothyroidism) it has been proposed that the effect arises from reduced oxygen demand. Acidosis reduces hemoglobin oxygen affinity, thus increasing tissue oxygen delivery, though this may not be the only reason for the reduced erythropoietin production. In inflammatory disease it has been proposed that increased levels of particular cytokines act to reduce erythropoietin production. Evidence for this is provided by the reduction in erythropoietin production by recombinant cytokines such as interleukin-1 (α or β) and tumor necrosis factor (TFN)-α (for review: [4, 6, 7]).

In addition to the massive increases in erythropoietin which are caused by severe stimulation, there is also evidence that small changes in hematocrit can be sensed and lead to altered erythropoietin production. For instance, serial plasma estimations following donation of a unit of blood demonstrate a rise in erythropoietin, albeit within the normal range. Since this blood loss is effectively replaced, it is also likely that small variations in levels of erythropoietin near the normal range have important effects on erythropoiesis. In clinical nephrology, evidence of this is seen in the effect of nephrectomy on the plasma erythropoietin in dialysis patients; after nephrectomy a small reduction in erythropoietin is associated with a large reduction in erythropoiesis. Thus it appears that the feedback loop is functioning in the dynamic control of erythropoiesis near the normal range as well as producing a large erythropoietic response to severe stimulation. In keeping with this, erythropoietin levels are usually suppressed below the normal range in hypertransfused animals and in patients with polycythemia rubra vera.

Erythropoietin and the control of erythropoiesis

The human erythropoietin gene encodes a 193-amino acid polypeptide [8, 9]. A 27-amino acid leader sequence is cleaved during secretion, and removal of the C-terminal arginine residue results in a 165-amino acid mature polypeptide. Structural predictions based on this sequence are consistent with the formation of four antiparallel helices in an arrangement similar to that which has been determined for growth hormone. Erythropoietin is heavily glycosylated and comparison of the measured molecular weight of human erythropoietin (30.4 kDa) with that of the polypeptide indicates a 40% carbohydrate content. Glycosylation is important for cellular processing, structural stability and *in vivo* metabolism, but some deglycosylated forms retain full activity *in vitro*.

Stimulation of erythropoiesis by erythropoietin involves interaction with a specific receptor. The gene encoding the erythropoietin binding component of the receptor has been cloned and in man it encodes a 508-amino acid polypeptide. The N-terminal region of this molecule is extracellular and contains the erythropoietin-binding domain. The receptor polypeptide also contains a single transmembrane domain and an intracellular C-terminal which possesses properties required for signal transduction (for review: [10]). Analysis of the sequence shows homologies with other growth factor receptors; not only receptors for other hematopoietic cytokines, but also receptors for other growth-related molecules such as

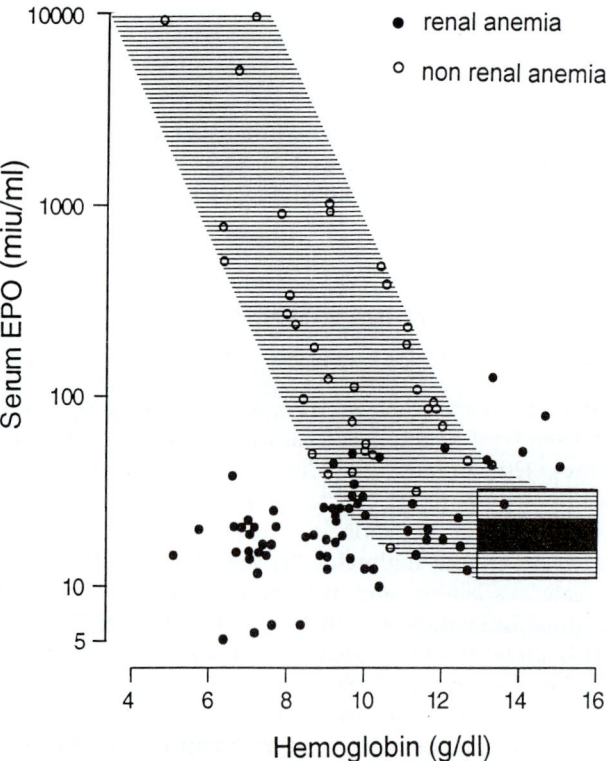

Figure 16.1 Relationship between immunoreactive erythropoietin levels and hemoglobin concentrations in patients with non-renal anemias (o) and in patients with chronic renal failure (•) (excluding polycystic kidney disease). The rectangle depicts the interquartile range (solid box) and 95% confidence interval (stippled) for erythropoietin levels in non-anemic healthy adults. (Reproduced, with permission, from ref. 33.)

growth hormone and prolactin. In the receptor complex, the erythropoietin binding polypeptide is non-covalently linked with other polypeptides. The binding of erythropoietin is followed rapidly by receptor internalization and a series of molecular events which include calcium entry and tyrosine phosphorylation. Activation of tyrosine kinase is a common event in growth-promoting systems. Functional interaction of the erythropoietin receptor with common intracellular components is demonstrated by the fact that transfection of a variety of non-erythroid cells with the erythropoietin binding polypeptide alone confers erythropoietin-dependent growth, indicating that all the necessary interacting factors are already present in the transfectants. The specific dependence of erythropoiesis on erythropoietin is therefore dependent on the controlled expression of the erythropoietin receptor. Early erythroid progenitors first express the erythropoietin receptor in conjunction with receptors for other hematopoietic growth factors. Later progenitors lose their responsiveness to other growth factors, express larger numbers of erythropoietin receptors, and are absolutely dependent on erythropoietin for several cell cycles. Withdrawal of erythropoietin from such cells is followed rapidly by apoptosis which allows the level of erythro-

A   Normal erythropoietin

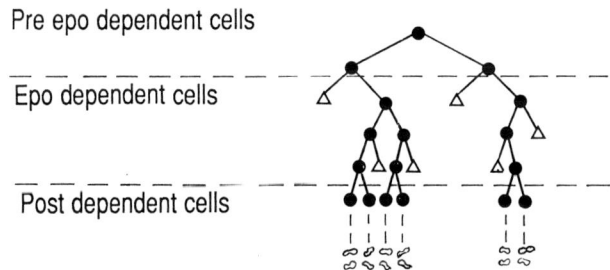

B   Increased erythropoietin

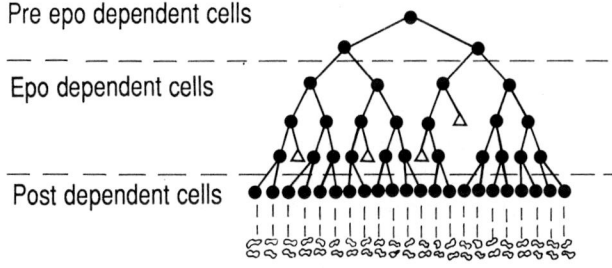

C   Decreased erythropoietin

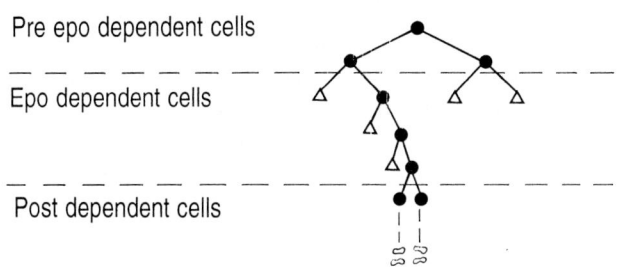

Figure 16.2   Model of erythropoiesis based on erythropoietin suppression of programmed cell death (apoptosis). Erythroid progenitor cells enter a period of development in which they are dependent on erythropoietin (Epo) for survival. Cells surviving transit through this period can complete maturation into reticulocytes without erythropoietin and ultimately become red cells. •, Surviving viable cells; △, cells undergoing programmed cell death owing to insufficient erythropoietin. (Reproduced, with modification, from ref. 11.)

poietin to control erythropoiesis by regulating the number of progenitors able to cross this critical phase (Figure 16.2) (for review: [11]). In some systems erythropoietin also exerts a mitogenic action. *In vivo*, the precise interplay between such processes is not yet clear but the net result of erythropoietin action is increased reticulocyte production, which, with maximal stimulation, can be increased about 15-fold over normal. Erythropoietin also acts to promote early release of reticulocytes from the marrow.

In inflammatory diseases the response to erythropoietin is commonly reduced; particular cytokines (e.g. TNF) can suppress erythropoiesis, either directly or indirectly though stimulation of β interferon. The mechanism of the interaction with erythropoietin remains unclear, though, both *in vivo* and with cultured marrow cells, large doses of erythropoietin can sometimes overcome inhibition (for review: [7]).

Source of erythropoietin

The kidneys are the principal site of erythropoietin synthesis in adults. In contrast, in fetal and neonatal animals the liver is the principal source. The switch from hepatic to renal production occurs perinataly at slightly different times in different species. Even in adult life, however, the liver retains significant potential for erythropoietin synthesis, the exact contribution of the liver to total erythropoietin production being dependent on the severity of stimulation and varying between species. In severely stimulated adult rats up to 30–40% of total erythropoietin mRNA is in the liver. Though the liver accounts for the vast majority of extrarenal production, small amounts of erythropoietin mRNA are also detectable in other organs such as brain and testis; the physiological significance is unknown.

In kidney, *in situ* mRNA hybridization studies indicated that erythropoietin is produced by a population of peritubular cells lying within the renal interstitium of the cortex and outer stripe of outer medulla [12, 13]. Within the cortex these cells are more frequent within the cortical labyrinth than in the medullary rays. The renal erythropoietin-producing cells have been shown to be fibroblastoid (type 1) interstitial cells [14, 15]. In liver two cell populations are capable of erythropoietin production: a subpopulation of hepatocytes [16] and the fibroblastoid fat-storing cells, termed Ito cells [17].

There are a number of phenotypic similarities between the type I interstitial cells of the kidney and the Ito cells of the liver. They both possess extensive fine processes and are closely apposed to parenchymal and endothelial cells. In each organ, they are the major connective tissue-producing cells, and they proliferate in response to injury. Both cell populations express immunoreactive 5'-ectonucleotidase (5'-NT), an enzyme located in the cell membrane which promotes adenosine formation from adenosine monophosphate. In both cell types expression

of this enzyme is also inducible by anemia. Although this has led to the suggestion that adenosine formation could be involved in the regulation of erythropoietin, differences in the temporal and spatial patterns of 5'-NT and erythropoietin expression indicate that a causal relationship is unlikely.

In response to hypoxic stimuli, the increase in hormone production parallels the increase in erythropoietin mRNA, and *in situ* hybridization studies have shown that increases in mRNA are largely achieved through an increase in the number of cells expressing erythropoietin mRNA, with individual cells expressing the gene in a near all-or-none fashion. In the unstimulated state, just a few cells are observed in deep cortex but with progressively more severe stimulation cells are recruited to produce erythropoietin at progressively more superficial sites (Figure 16.3). It is probable that this distribution is partly determined by local renal tissue oxygenation. There is as yet no direct proof of this, however, since there have been no concurrent measurements of renal oxygen tensions during progressive anemia. Furthermore, since the inner medulla does not contain erythropoietin-producing cells despite having the lowest oxygen tensions [18], it is clear that oxygen gradients cannot be the only determinant of the cellular distribution of erythropoietin synthesis within kidney.

In liver, erythropoietin-producing cells are present in all lobes, but within lobules erythropoietin gene expression is zonal. For both liver cell populations with the potential for erythropoietin expression (hepatocytes and Ito cells), positive cells are clustered around the central veins [16, 17]. With increasingly severe hypoxic stimulation, the region containing positive cells extends periportally. Such a distribution is consistent with the sinusoidal oxygen gradients, which run from relatively high periportal oxygen tensions to lower pericentral oxygen tensions.

There have been many attempts to obtain regulated erythropoietin production in primary cultures and cell lines derived from kidney and liver. Surprisingly there are no erythropoietin-producing cell lines derived from type 1 renal interstitial fibroblasts or Ito cells. In contrast, primary cultures of hepatocytes and certain hepatoma cell lines produce erythropoietin in an oxygen-regulated manner in tissue culture indicating that oxygen sensing and erythropoietin production can take place in the same cell [19]. Both erythropoietin-producing cell lines (HepG2 and Hep3B) were derived from hepatomas, and erythropoietin production sufficient to cause erythrocytosis is a known complication of these tumors. It is notable that erythropoietin production is also a well recognized feature of renal cell carcinomas. *In situ* hybridization studies have clearly demonstrated that in these tumors erythropoietin mRNA is localized in the epithelial cells [20]. This observation, together with the occurrence of erythropoietin mRNA in hepatocytes as well as Ito cells in liver, has led some to argue that renal tubular cells may also contribute to erythropoietin production in normal

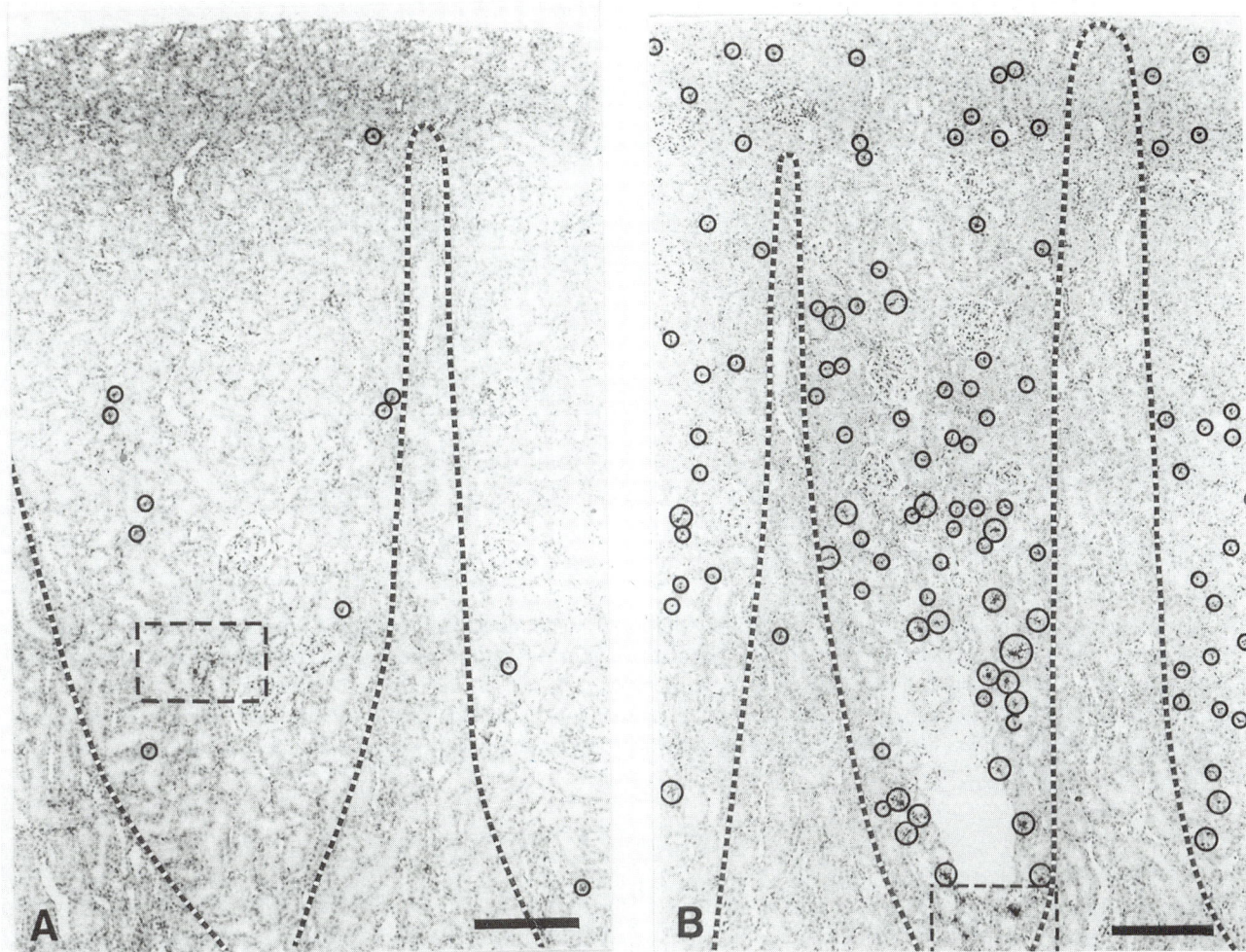

Figure 16.3 Photomicrographs of *in situ* autoradiograms showing the distribution of cells producing erythropoietin mRNA in the renal cortex of rats exposed (a) to mild hypoxia (11.5% O_2 for 8 h) and (b) more severe hypoxia (9% O_2 for 8 h). Single cells or clusters of a few cells covered with silver grains were identified at high magnification and are marked on the photomicrographs with circles. Dotted lines indicate the border between the cortical labyrinth and the medullary rays. Bar = 200 µm. (Reproduced, with permission, from ref. 35.)

kidney. However, there is no convincing evidence that this is the case.

Regulation of erythropoietin gene expression

The large increases in plasma erythropoietin after hypoxic stimulation are achieved by *de novo* synthesis and reflect rapid increases in erythropoietin mRNA levels. Increases in mRNA level could arise either from an increase in gene transcription or increased stability of the mRNA. Hypoxia induces a large increase in the rate of erythropoietin gene transcription, though it is likely that the effect is magnified by additional effects on mRNA stability [21].

Control of gene transcription is achieved by multiple interactions between DNA sequences in the vicinity of the gene termed *cis*-acting sequences, and nuclear pro-

teins termed transcription factors. These transcription factors provide an activating influence on the general transcriptional apparatus associated with the RNA polymerase (for general review: [22]). Bending of DNA allows interactions between proteins bound at distant sites. Inducing stimuli activate transcription by modifying transcription factors to allow or promote DNA binding, or by increasing the activating power of factors which are already bound to DNA. Definition of *cis*-acting DNA sequences and the transcription factors which bind them thus provides important insights into the mechanisms controlling gene expression.

Transfection studies in erythropoietin-producing hepatoma cell lines (Hep3B and HepG2) have been used to locate the DNA sequences which mediate hypoxia-inducible expression. The most clearly defined of these sequences lies just 3' to the erythropoietin gene, and is termed the erythropoietin 3' enhancer (Figure 16.4) (for

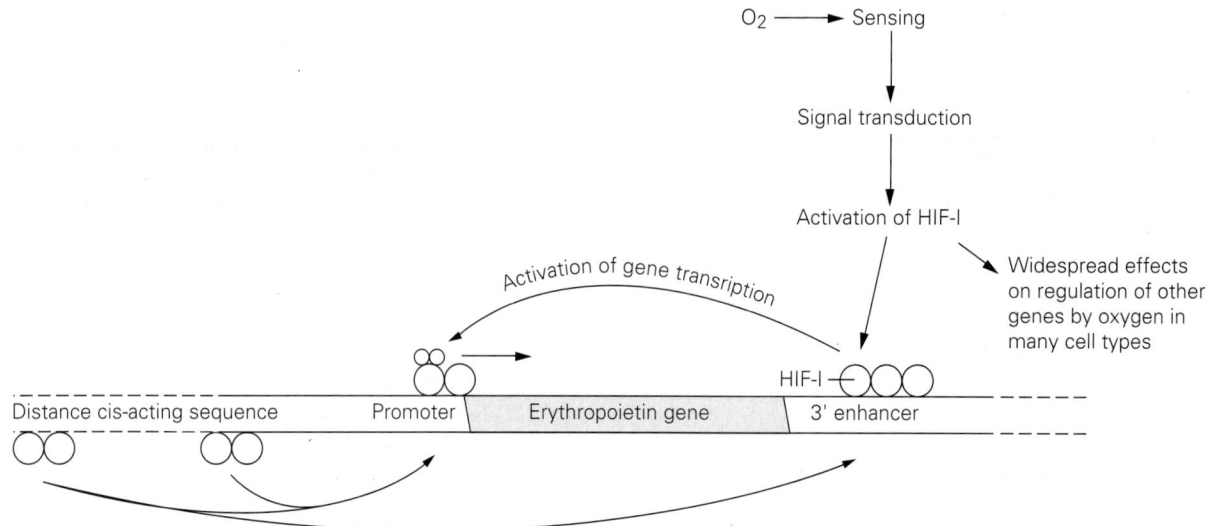

Multiple sequences constrain expression
of the erythropoietin

Figure 16.4 Diagram illustrating some aspects of erythropoietin gene regulation by hypoxia. Interaction of oxygen with the sensing mechanism (possibly a heme protein) generates a signal which is transduced to control the binding of transcription factors such as HIF-1. In the case of the erythropoietin gene, HIF-1 binds to the 3′ enhancer and activates gene transcription. HIF-1 is controlled in this way in all cells; transcriptional activation of the erythropoietin gene is subject to additional controls by tissue-specific transcription factors which limit erythropoietin expression to hepatocytes, Ito cells and renal interstitial fibroblasts.

review: [23]). This DNA sequence will confer hypoxically inducible responses when linked to heterologous genes, and, as is usual for such transcriptional enhancers, its operation is independent of orientation and (up to several kilobases) independent of distance from the heterologous gene. Analysis has shown that the hypoxia-inducible function of the enhancer is critically dependent on the binding of an inducible nuclear protein termed hypoxia-inducible factor (HIF-1) [24]. It is not yet known, however, how hypoxia regulates the inducible DNA binding of this protein.

Studies of the erythropoietin 3′ enhancer have also indicated that regulation of erythropoietin expression by hypoxia forms part of a widespread system of mammalian gene regulation by oxygen. The first evidence of this was obtained when it was found that this sequence would operate in a hypoxia-inducible way when transfected into a wide variety of non-erythropoietin-producing cells, implying that all these cells contained a similar oxygen-sensing, signal transduction and transcriptional activation system which could operate on other genes [25]. In keeping with this, HIF-1 binding elements have been defined in control sequences which regulate the expression of other genes such as those encoding hypoxia-inducible glycolytic enzymes [26].

That unrelated genes, such as those encoding glycolytic enzymes and erythropoietin, share a common regulatory mechanism indicates that the mechanism is probably widely conserved among mammalian genes which are regulated by oxygen, and indeed may have a counterpart in more primitive organisms. Functional similarities have also been described between the regulation of erythropoietin by hypoxia and a number of genes encoding vascular growth factors, and analysis of cis-acting sequence has demonstrated the involvement of HIF-1.

If HIF-1 and the oxygen-sensing mechanism are ubiquitous in mammalian cells, how is erythropoietin expression constrained to certain cells within kidney and liver? The answer most probably lies in the operation of tissue-specific transcription factors which bind the DNA at other sites and determine the chromatin structure at the erythropoietin locus and thus whether the inducible control sequences are available for interactions with factors such as HIF-1 [for general review: [27]]. Control of tissue-specific expression is commonly analyzed by determining the expression pattern of different lengths of sequence from the gene locus under study in transgenic mice. Such studies show that interactions with multiple distant DNA sequences are required for correct cell-specific expression of the erythropoietin gene; in particular a sequence several kilobases 5′ to the gene is required for renal expression [28]. The sequences necessary for hepatocyte gene expression differ from those required for renal and liver Ito cell expression, and it is likely that the developmental shift in expression from liver to kidney is dependent on developmental expression of factors which interact with these sequences.

Mechanism of oxygen sensing

An important feature of erythropoietin regulation is that in cultured cells, perfused kidneys and whole animals the effect of hypoxia cannot be mimicked by cyanide or other inhibitors of mitochondrial respiration. Neither is erythropoietin induced by heat shock or glucose starvation. It therefore appears that the sensing mechanism is rather specific for hypoxia, and distinct from known cell stress responses.

Certain transition metal ions, Co^{2+}, Ni^{2+} and M^{2+}, can stimulate erythropoietin gene expression. In the hepatoma tissue culture cells carbon monoxide (a heme liganding molecule) reduces the hypoxic stimulation. (Note this response differs from carbon monoxide poisoning *in vivo*, where the increase in hemoglobin oxygen affinity produced by much lower concentrations of carbon monoxide is a powerful stimulus for erythropoietin production.) Based on the responses in hepatoma cells, Goldberg *et al.* [19] have proposed a model in which the oxygen-dependent signal is generated by the reversible binding of dioxygen to a hemoglobin-like molecule which undergoes a ligand-dependent conformational change; the action of the transition metals was explained by substitution of these ions for a ferrous ion in the sensor; since such substituted porphyrins do not bind oxygen it was proposed that the sensor would adopt a deoxy conformation constitutively.

Another possible mechanism of oxygen sensing arises from the involvement of oxygen as the terminal electron acceptor in many types of redox reaction. For instance, many members of the cytochrome P_{450} superfamily use oxygen as a substrate, operate in an oxygen-dependent manner and, like erythropoietin regulation, are not sensitive to cyanide. In such a system the signal could be generated by a redox-dependent conformational change of any of the coupled components. Alternatively, the production of partially reduced oxygen species such as superoxide ions and hydrogen peroxide could provide a potential oxygen-sensing mechanism. These molecules are produced in an oxygen-dependent manner by such electron transport systems and have been proposed as intracellular signaling molecules (for review: [29]).

It has been shown that acute exposure to desferrioxamine and other iron chelating agents markedly induces erythropoietin expression [30]. It is not yet clear how these results can be accommodated by the above hypotheses as heme iron is not chelatable. One possible explanation is that the sensing mechanism involves a multicomponent system in which both a labile (and chelatable) non-heme iron moiety and a heme moiety are involved. Such multicomponent systems, with different types of redox active center, are observed in many electron transport chains.

The physiology of renal oxygenation

In contrast to the massive induction of erythropoietin production by severe anemia or severe arterial hypoxemia, the response of erythropoietin to reduction in renal perfusion is small or absent. For instance, during exercise, profound changes occur in renal blood flow but erythropoietin production is barely altered. Disturbance of erythropoietin regulation is not a prominent feature of renal artery stenosis. How can these surprising findings be explained? One possible explanation is that the sensing of oxygen takes place mainly at extrarenal sites and a further neural or humoral signal is then transmitted to the kidneys. To date, no such signal has been convincingly demonstrated. Furthermore, in the short term, isolated perfused kidneys can show an oxygen-regulated induction of erythropoietin mRNA which is similar to that which is achieved *in vivo*. An alternative explanation for the low reponse of erythropoietin to reduced renal perfusion could lie in the unusual physiology of renal oxygenation. Transport of sodium accounts for the majority of renal oxygen consumption. Since in the region of 99% of the filtered load of sodium is reabsorbed, it follows that renal oxygen consumption should be closely determined by the glomerular filtration rate. Thus, parallel changes in renal blood flow and glomerular filtration rate which arise in the setting of reduced renal perfusion might not disturb the balance of oxygen consumption and supply greatly.

Another important but complex feature of intrarenal oxygenation arises from the countercurrent arrangement of renal blood vessels which allows for the shunt diffusion of oxygen direct from arterial to venous limbs. This countercurrent exchange of oxygen is most marked in the renal medulla where renal tissue oxygen tension is lowest (for review: [18]). However, countercurrent exchange of oxygen also occurs between adjacent arterial and venous vessels in the renal cortex [31] and creates tissue PO_2 levels which are still well below those observed in the renal veins. Though the operation of such a system in the organ principally responsible for sensing blood oxygen availability is intriguing, the exact role is unclear. Mathematical modeling of a countercurrent exchange of oxygen can demonstrate ways in which blood oxygen-carrying capacity could exert more profound effects on tissue oxygenation than blood flow rate or oxygen tension, but whether this actually happens requires more experimental measurements of intrarenal oxygen tensions.

Erythropoietin production in renal disease

Failure of diseased kidneys to respond to anemia with an appropriate increase in erythropoietin production is an important component of the anemia of renal disease (for review: [32]). A further contribution is made by reduced red cell survival. Although 'uremic' inhibitors of marrow responsiveness have been demonstrated *in vitro*, their role *in vivo* remains controversial.

In chronic renal disease severity of anemia increases with severity of the disease. However, the relationship is rather imprecise. It does not appear to depend on the type of renal disease, with the exception of polycystic kidney disease, where hematocrit is relatively preserved and erythropoietin levels are somewhat higher. It is not easy to define the point at which hematocrit is first reduced and it is probable that almost all chronic renal disease is associated with some impairment of the erythropoietin response to hypoxic stimulation. Measurement of erythropoietin in patients with varying severity of chronic renal failure, and serial measurements in patients showing progression, show levels which stay generally within the normal range as anemia progresses; thus there is no relation between the serum erythropoietin level and either hematocrit or glomerular filtration rate. In acute renal failure, anemia often develops rapidly because of blood loss or hemolysis. As in chronic renal failure erythropoietin levels generally remain within the normal range, and are therefore inappropriately low for the level of anemia. This relative deficiency of erythropoietin is observed in acute renal failure from both glomerular and tubular disease and in obstructive nephropathy. Although the response of erythropoietin to hypoxic stimulation is reduced in all these situations it is by no means absent; with severe stimulation plasma levels can be elevated several times above normal, and if these levels were maintained, they would be more than enough to sustain a normal level of erythropoiesis. In rodent models, analysis of erythropoietin mRNA has indicated that the potential for increased erythropoietin production resides in both the liver and the diseased kidneys. In dialysis patients subject to intercurrent hypoxic stress, considerable elevations of erythropoietin have been observed; such responses have also been reported in anephric patients. It therefore appears that the deficiency of erythropoietin in renal disease arises from altered sensitivity to stimulation rather than an absolute inability to produce sufficient hormone (for review: [33]). Following renal transplantation, anemia is corrected by the production of erythropoietin by the functioning graft. Erythropoietin production by the native kidneys may also persist and dysregulated native kidney erythropoietin production is the usual reason for the erythrocytosis which is observed at some stage in 5–10% of transplanted patients.

Glomerular, tubular and obstructive renal diseases are all associated with interstitial abnormalities. However, since the renal interstitial fibroblasts generally proliferate in response to organ injury, it is not clear why production of erythropoietin should be reduced. Both type 1 interstitial cells, and the hepatic Ito cells, adopt a more myofibroblastoid phenotype following injury, with the expression of contractile proteins. This change appears to be associated with a reduced potential for erythropoietin gene expression though the changes are not necessarily linked causally. Disturbance of the vascular anatomy, or reduced oxygen consumption following reduced tubular transport work, could lead to altered intrarenal oxygenation. Alternatively other mechanisms such as local production of antagonistic cytokines, or derangement of some necessary intercellular interaction, could underlie impairment of erythropoietin production. Some support for this last possibility comes from the lack of erythropoietin production by hypoxically stimulated outgrowths of renal fibroblasts in tissue culture. The reasons for the relatively preserved erythropoietin production in inherited polycystic kidney disease are unclear. Relatively high erythropoietin production is also a feature of end-stage kidneys which develop acquired cystic disease, and elevated levels are often found in the fluid from simple cysts. In polycystic kidney disease, *in situ* hybridization studies have shown erythropoietin mRNA in fibroblast-like stromal cells within the cyst wall [34]. Erythropoietin levels in cyst fluid can be very high, high levels being particularly common in cysts with a high sodium content which are believed to be of proximal tubular origin. This implies that some form of interaction with proximal tubular epithelium could be involved. Again, the nature of any such interaction is unclear, but the phenomenon provides more evidence that the capacity for erythropoietin production is not entirely destroyed in renal disease.

References

1. Reissmann, K.R., Nomura, T., Gunn, R.W. and Brosius, F. (1960) Erythropoietic response to anaemia or Epo injection in uraemic rats with or without functioning renal tissue. *Blood*, **16**, 1411–22.
2. Erslev, A.J. (1953) Humoral regulation of red cell production. *Blood*, **8**, 349–57.
3. Jacobson, L.O., Goldwasser, E., Fried, W. and Plzak, L. (1957) Role of the kidney in erythropoiesis. *Nature*, **179**, 633–4.
4. Cotes, P.M. and Spivak, J.L. (1991) Erythropoietin in health and disease, in *Erythropoietin: Molecular, Cellular and Clinical Biology* (eds A.J. Erslev, J.W. Adamson, J.W. Eschbach and C.G. Winearls). Johns Hopkins University Press, Baltimore and London, pp. 184–207.
5. Caro, J., Brown, S., Miller, O. *et al.* (1979) Erythropoietin levels in uremic nephric and anephric patients. *J. Lab. Clin. Med.*, **93**, 449–58.
6. Jelkmann, W. (1992) Erythropoietin: structure, control of production, and function. *Physiol. Rev.*, **72**, 449–89.
7. Means, R.T. and Krantz, S.B. (1992) Progress in under-

standing the pathogenesis of the anemia of chronic disease. *Blood*, **80**, 1639–47.

8. Lin, F.-K., Suggs, S., Lin, C.-H. *et al.* (1985) Cloning and expression of the human erythropoietin gene. *Proc. Natl. Acad. Sci. USA*, **82**, 7580–4.

9. Jacobs, K., Shoemaker, C., Rudersdorf, R. *et al.* (1985) Isolation and characterization of genomic and cDNA clones of human erythropoietin. *Nature*, **313**, 806–10.

10. D'Andrea, A.D. and Zon, L.I. (1990) Erythropoietin receptor. Subunit structure and activation. *J. Clin. Invest.*, **86**, 681–7.

11. Koury, M.J. and Bondurant, M.C. (1992) The molecular mechanism of erythropoietin action. *Eur. J. Biochem.*, **210**, 649–63.

12. Lacombe, C., Da Silva, J.-L., Bruneval, P. *et al.* (1988) Peritubular cells are the site of erythropoietin synthesis in the murine hypoxic kidney. *J. Clin. Invest.*, **81**, 620–3.

13. Koury, S.T., Bondurant, M.C. and Koury, M.J. (1988) Localization of erythropoietin synthesizing cells in murine kidneys by *in situ* hybridization. *Blood*, **71**, 524–7.

14. Maxwell, P.H., Osmond, M.K., Pugh, C.W. *et al.* (1993) Identification of the renal erythropoietin-producing cells using transgenic mice. *Kidney Int.*, **44**, 1149–62.

15. Bachmann, S., Le Hir, M. and Eckardt, K.-U. (1993) Co-localization of erythropoietin messenger RNA and ecto-5'-nucleotidase immunoreactivity in peritubular cells of rat renal cortex indicates that fibroblasts produce erythropoietin. *J. Histochem. Cytochem.*, **41**, 335–41.

16. Koury, S.T., Bondurant, M.C., Koury, M.J. and Semenza, G.L. (1991) Localization of cells producing erythropoietin in murine liver by *in situ* hybridization. *Blood*, **77**, 2497–503.

17. Maxwell, P.H., Ferguson, D.J.P., Osmond, M.K. *et al.* (1994) Expression of a homologously recombined erythropoietin-SV40 T antigen fusion gene in mouse liver: evidence for erythropoietin production by Ito cells. *Blood*, **84**, 1823–30.

18. Brezis, M., Rosen, S., Silva, P. and Epstein, F.H. (1984) Renal ischemia: a new perspective. *Kidney Int.*, **26**, 375–83.

19. Goldberg, M.A., Dunning, S.P. and Bunn, H.F. (1988) Regulation of the erythropoietin gene: evidence that the oxygen sensor is a heme protein. *Science*, **242**, 1412–15.

20. Da Silva, J.L., Lacombe, C. Bruneval, P. *et al.* (1990) Tumour cells are the site of erythropoietin synthesis in human renal cancers associated with polycythemia. *Blood*, **75**, 577–82.

21. Goldberg, M.A., Gaut, C.C. and Bunn, H.F. (1991) Erythropoietin mRNA levels are governed by both the rate of gene transcription and posttranscriptional events. *Blood*, **77**, 271–7.

22. Tjian, R. and Maniatis, T. (1994) Transcriptional activation: a complex puzzle with few easy pieces. *Cell*, **77**, 5–8.

23. Ratcliffe, P.J. (1993) Molecular biology of erythropoietin. *Kidney Int.*, **44**, 887–904.

24. Semenza, G.L. and Wang, G.L. (1992) A nuclear factor induced by hypoxia via de novo protein synthesis binds to the human erythropoietin gene enhancer at a site required for transcriptional activation. *Mol. Cell. Biol.*, **12**, 5447–54.

25. Maxwell, P.H., Pugh, C.W. and Ratcliffe, P.J. (1993) Inducible operation of the erythropoietin 3' enhancer in multiple cell lines: evidence for a widespread oxygen sensing mechanism. *Proc. Natl. Acad. Sci. USA*, **90**, 2423–7.

26. Firth, J.D., Ebert, B.L., Pugh, C.W. and Ratcliffe, P.J. (1994) Oxygen-regulated control elements in the phosphoglycerate kinase 1 and lactate dehydrogenase A genes: similarities with the erythropoietin 3' enhancer. *Proc. Natl. Acad. Sci. USA*, **91**, 6496–500.

27. Felsenfeld, G. (1992) Chromatin as an essential part of the transcriptional mechanism. *Nature*, **355**, 219–24.

28. Semenza, G.L., Koury, S.T., Nejfelt, M.K. *et al.* (1991) Cell type-specific and hypoxia-inducible expression of the human erythropoietin gene in transgenic mice. *Proc. Natl. Acad. Sci. USA*, **88**, 8725–9.

29. Schreck, R. and Baeuerle, P.A. (1991) A role for oxygen radicals as second messengers. *Trends Cell Biol.*, **1**, 39–42.

30. Wang, G.L. and Semenza, G.L. (1993) Desferrioxamine induces erythropoietin gene expression and hypoxia-inducible factor 1 DNA-binding activity: implications for models of hypoxia signal transduction. *Blood*, **82**, 3610–15.

31. Schurek, H.J., Jost, U., Baumgartl, H. *et al.* (1990) Evidence for a preglomerular oxygen diffusion shunt in rat renal cortex. *Am. J. Physiol.*, **259**, F910–15.

32. Eschbach, J.W. (1989) The anemia of chronic renal failure: pathophysiology and the effects of recombinant erythropoietin. *Kidney Int.*, **35**, 134–48.

33. Eckardt, K.-U. (1994) Erythropoietin: oxygen-dependent control of erythropoiesis and its failure in renal disease. *Nephron*, **67**, 7–23.

34. Eckardt, K.-U., Möllmann, M., Neumann, R. *et al.* (1989) Erythropoietin in polycystic kidneys. *J. Clin. Invest.*, **84**, 1160–6.

35. Eckardt, K.-U., Koury, S.T., Tan, C.C. *et al.* (1993) Distribution of erythropoietin producing cells in rat kidneys during hypoxic hypoxia. *Kidney Int.*, **43**, 815–23.

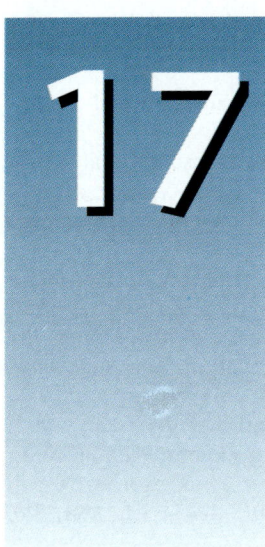

17

Arachidonic acid metabolism

Joseph V. Bonventre

Overview of arachidonic acid metabolism

Arachidonic acid can be taken into the body in the diet or synthesized from the essential dietary fatty acid, linoleic acid ($18:2\omega6$) (Figure 17.1). Arachidonic acid is in large part esterified to the sn-2 position of phospholipids, although some is also present in triglycerides. It can be enzymatically released from either site. There is evidence that arachidonic acid delivered to cells in the form of cholesterol esters of phospholipids of low-density lipoproteins can be utilized for production of prostaglandins. Arachidonic acid can be released in response to physiological and pathophysiological stimuli. The lipid origin of arachidonic acid varies depending on the cell type and the agonist used to stimulate release. In most systems phospholipase A_2 (PLA_2), which acts at the sn-2 position of phospholipids, is believed to be the primary effector enzyme for arachidonate release. The levels of free arachidonic acid are influenced, not only by these release mechanisms, but also by very efficient reacylation processes.

Arachidonic acid can be metabolized to a large number of compounds via three primary enzymatic pathways – the prostaglandin endoperoxide (PGH) synthase/cyclooxygenase (Figure 17.2), lipoxygenase and P450 mixed function oxidase pathways as well as non-enzymatic pathways. The PGH synthase pathway leads to the production of prostaglandins and thromboxanes. PGH synthase is a protein with two enzymatic functions: a cyclooxygenase component which catalyzes the insertion

of two molecules of oxygen into arachidonic acid to form prostaglandin G_2 (PGG_2), and a hydroperoxidase-induced two-electron reduction of the 15-hydroperoxy group of PGG_2 to yield prostaglandin H_2 (PGH_2). This is an O_2-consuming process and results in the generation of reactive oxygen species which may, under certain circumstances, be toxic to the cell. PGH_2 is then converted into the biologically active prostaglandins, PGE_2, PGD_2, $PGF_{2\alpha}$, PGI_2 (prostacyclin) and thromboxane A_2 (TxA_2). Non-steroidal anti-inflammatory agents inhibit the cyclooxygenase component of PGH_2 synthase, and hence the production of various prostaglandins and thromboxanes. There are also non-enzymatic pathways for generation of prostaglandins. Isoprostanes are compounds generated by the free radical-induced oxidation of unsaturated fatty acids in membrane phospholipids.

The diverse intrarenal effect of prostaglandins is mediated by a number of distinct receptors. Most of these receptors are localized to the cell plasma membrane and signal via guanine nucleotide binding proteins (G proteins). Intranuclear receptors have also been identified.

A second pathway for arachidonate metabolism is the lipoxygenase pathway. Lipoxygenases catalyze a dioxygenase reduction resulting in the formation of 5-, 8-, 12- or 15-HPETEs (hydroperoxyeicosatetraenoic acids). The leukotrienes are products of further metabolism of 5-HPETE and the hydroxyeicosatetraenoic acids (HETEs) are products of 8-, 12- or 15-HPETE. The combined action of more than one lipoxygenase can lead to the production of lipoxins.

The cytochrome P450 monooxygenase results in the

Nephrology, Edited by Rex L. Jamison and Robert Wilkinson.
Published in 1997 by Chapman & Hall, London. ISBN 0 412 60930 4

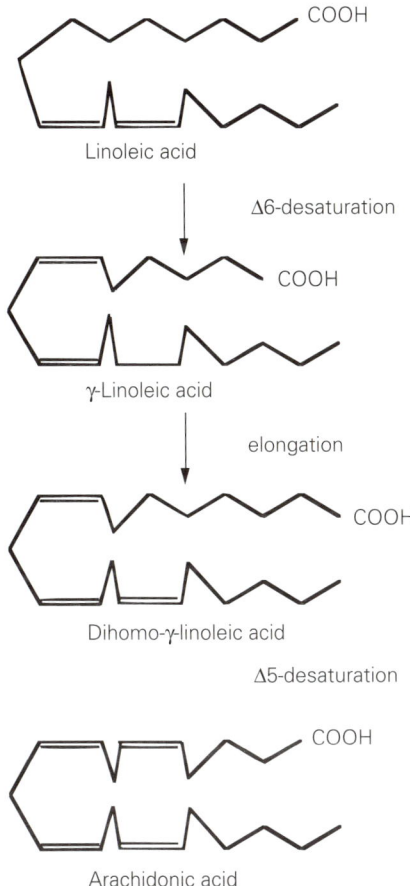

Figure 17.1 Metabolic pathways for the production of arachidonic acid from dietary linoleic acid.

oxidative transformation of a number of endogenous and exogenous substrates including saturated fatty acids, leukotrienes, prostaglandins, steroids and hydrocarbons.

Acylhydrolases

The first step in the generation of prostaglandins, lipoxygenase or P450 products is the generation of arachidonic acid by the action of acylhydrolases on lipids, primarily phospholipids. The primary acylhydrolases involved in arachidonic acid release are the phospholipases A_2 (PLA$_2$s). PLA$_2$s comprise a family of enzymes which act on phospholipids to generate a free fatty acid and lysophospholipid. If the substrate lipid is a 1-*O*-alkyl, 2-acyl phospholipid the lysophospholipid produced by PLA$_2$ can then be acetylated at the *sn*-2 position to form platelet activating factor (PAF). PAF can be released from a variety of cells, including platelets, macrophages, endothelial cells and polymorphonuclear leukocytes, and has been implicated in a number of inflammatory processes,

including graft rejection, sepsis, anaphylaxis and glomerulonephritis as well as ischemic acute renal failure. PAF is a potent vasoconstrictor and chemotactic agent. It activates neutrophils and enhances neutrophil–endothelial interactions. It increases vascular permeability, constricts smooth muscle and increases the activity of PLA$_2$ resulting in more arachidonic acid metabolites being formed.

PLA$_2$s are ubiquitous enzymes, which exist in both secretory and intracellular forms. Secretory and membrane-associated (mol. wt ~12 000–18 000 Da) calcium-dependent and independent forms of the enzyme have been implicated in inflammatory processes. There are also larger molecular weight intracellular cytosolic forms of PLA$_2$ that can be activated at much lower calcium concentrations and some that are not dependent on calcium at all for their activity.

Other forms of acylhydrolase that may be important for arachidonic acid release are diacylglycerol and triglyceride lipases, although these enzymes are not likely to be of the importance of the PLA$_2$s. Triglyceride lipases may be of particular importance in inner medullary interstitial cells which have large lipid droplets and are believed to

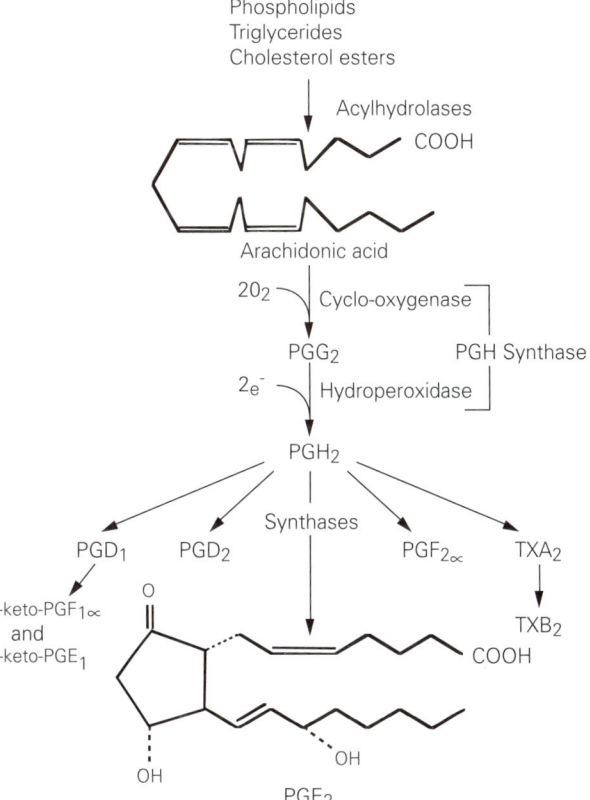

Figure 17.2 Synthetic pathways for the generation of prostaglandins and thromboxanes. Note that PGH synthase is a bifunctional enzyme with cyclooxygenase and hydroperoxide activity.

be important in the generation of medullary prostaglandins.

Prostaglandin H synthase products

Characteristics of the enzyme

There are two PGH synthase isozymes: PGH synthase-1 and -2, also referred to as cyclooxygenase 1 (COX-1) and cyclooxygenase 2 (COX-2). Both isozymes are inhibited by non-steroidal anti-inflammatory agents. PGH synthase-1 is constitutively expressed in many organs including the kidney and is the principal enzyme involved in production of prostaglandins for normal kidney function. PGH synthase-2, by contrast, is inducible in response to cytokines, growth factors and other mediators of inflammation. Expression of PGH synthase-2 is inhibited by glucocorticoids and is also distinguishable from PGH synthase-1 in that it is inhibited by transforming growth factor $\beta 1$ and interleukin 10.

Production within the kidney

Most prostaglandin synthase activity in the kidney is found in the microsomal fraction. With the exception of PGI_2, prostaglandin synthesis is greater in the renal medulla than it is in the cortex. Cortical prostaglandin production occurs primarily in the glomerulus, vasculature and cortical collecting duct. Mesangial cells and glomerular epithelial cells produce prostaglandins, with the mesangial cell producing greater amounts. Proximal tubule prostaglandin production is low. Prostaglandin E_2 (PGE_2) synthesis increases when moving from the branched connecting tubule to the cortical and medullary collecting tubules.

Most medullary production of prostaglandins derives from the medullary collecting tubule, the interstitial cells and thick ascending limb. The contribution of the thin descending limb to prostaglandin production remains controversial. In every tubular segment where prostaglandin synthesis has been noted, PGE_2 is the primary prostaglandin produced. $PGF_{2\alpha}$ synthesis is 50–100 times lower than that of PGE_2 in each segment except for the glomerulus, where they are approximately equivalent. Synthesis of 6-keto-$PGF_{1\alpha}$ is extensive in the glomerulus and medullary collecting duct. Medullary interstitial cells produce PGE_2 and $PGF_{2\alpha}$ *in vitro* and likely contribute in an important way to the papillary prostaglandin production *in vivo*. In human kidneys PGH synthase is present in the collecting duct, thin ascending limb epithelial cells and possibly mesangial cells. Prostacyclin synthase is localized to the peritubular capillaries, renal interstitial cells and glomerular mesangial cells. The normal kidney synthesizes little thromboxane.

Effects of PGH synthase products on renal function

Renal blood flow and glomerular filtration rate

In general PGI_2, PGF_2 and PGA_2 are vasodilatory and exogenous TxA_2 is a vasoconstrictor in the kidney. Under normal conditions prostaglandins likely play a minimal role in blood flow regulation, as reflected by the fact that systemic treatment with non-steroidal anti-inflammatory agents has little effect on renal blood flow or glomerular filtration rate (GFR).

By contrast to the minimal role of PGH synthase/cyclo-oxygenase products in normal regulation of renal blood flow and GFR, these metabolites play a very important role when the circulation is compromised, as occurs with hemorrhage, congestive heart failure or cirrhosis. In these conditions inhibition of PGH synthase causes marked decreases in renal blood flow and GFR. This is presumed to be due to inhibition of the production of vasodilatory prostaglandins. Prostaglandins act to counteract the vasoconstrictive influences of angiotensin II, vasopression and the stimulated sympathetic nervous system, even when the renin–angiotensin system has been suppressed. Prostaglandins are produced by mesangial cells and may affect GFR via their action to inhibit mesangial cell contraction and efferent arteriolar constriction that occurs secondary to arginine vasopressin (AVP) and angiotensin II (AII).

In addition to its effects to vasoconstrict blood vessels, thromboxane A_2 is a potent aggregator of platelets and hence can contribute to thrombosis. Thromboxane A_2 may also mediate the vasoconstrictor actions of PAF. The thromboxane A_2 receptor, or a closely related receptor, mediates the vasoconstrictive actions of isoprostane PG F_2-like compounds which are products of the non-enzymatic oxidation of arachidonic acid and are produced at high levels in pathophysiological states characterized by high levels of reactive oxygen species.

Renin secretion

Prostaglandins of the I and E class are potent stimuli of renal renin release whereas thromboxanes inhibit renin release. Arachidonic acid infusion into the kidney results in enhanced renin production that is inhibited by indomethacin. PGI_2, PGE_2 and PGE_1 release renin from rabbit cortical slices with PGI_2 and PGE_1 being the most effective agents. PGI_2 is most effective in stimulating renin release from isolated glomeruli.

Prostaglandins are also important for the renin release which occurs secondary to changes in macula densa NaCl delivery. The ability to increase renin production as a result of a steep decrease in NaCl concentration at the macula densa requires a functional PGH synthase enzyme.

Sodium excretion

When PGE_2 is infused intravenously or directly into the renal artery of animals that are salt replete, there is a marked natriuresis. This natriuresis is likely due in part to the above described effects on renal blood flow but, in addition, is likely also related to direct effects of PGE_2 on tubular sodium transport. Since cyclo-oxygenase inhibitors markedly reduce the natriuresis associated with volume expansion, prostaglandins have been implicated in the natriuresis observed with volume expansion.

PGE_2 alters sodium transport characteristics in the thick ascending limb and collecting duct and possibly in the proximal tubule. PGE_2 inhibits NaCl reabsorption from the AVP- or steroid-stimulated ascending limb. Furosemide, ethacrynic acid and bumetanide significantly increase PGE_2 production in the thick ascending limb and the effects of PGE_2 on this nephron segment may facilitate the natriuretic action of these diuretics.

In the collecting duct PGE_2 and PGI_2 inhibit sodium reabsorption. Whether PGE_2 acts directly to inhibit apical Na^+ entry into the cells or indirectly by affecting the activity of the Na^+,K^+-ATPase is not clear at present.

Water excretion

Prostaglandins alter the concentrating ability of the kidney in a number of ways. Since prostaglandins alter thick ascending limb Na^+ reabsorption they would be expected to alter the medullary concentration gradient and hence free water reabsorption. Enhanced medullary blood flow mediated by local prostaglandin synthesis results in partial wash-out of the medullary solute gradient. Agents which inhibit prostaglandin synthesis decrease vasa recta blood flow. Vasopressin increases cortical collecting duct prostaglandin production and the prostaglandins inhibit the antidiuretic action of vasopressin. This inhibition occurs, at least in part, because of prostanglandin-induced inhibition of the generation of cAMP by AVP. Thus, AVP, by promoting the formation of prostaglandins, inhibits its own action on water permeability. Bradykinin also enhances PGE_2 synthesis in cortical and medullary collecting tubules and inhibits the hydro-osmotic effect of vasopressin via a prostaglandin-dependent mechanism. Prostaglandins also reduce urea reabsorption from the collecting duct and this effect may interfere with 'urea recycling', which is important for maintenance of medullary solute concentrations. Non-steroidal anti-inflammatory agents, which inhibit prostaglandin production, increase concentrating ability. In addition to these effects of prostaglandins on free water reabsorption these agents would be expected to inhibit free water excretion also due to their inhibition of thick ascending limb Na^+ reabsorption and consequent decrease in medullary concentration gradient.

Renal disease secondary to non-steroidal anti-inflammatory agents (NSAIDs)

NSAIDs are commonly used drugs, accounting for a large percentage of over-the-counter drug use as well as prescription drug use. Important side effects of these drugs can be explained by their action to inhibit the cyclo-oxygenase component of PGH synthase and hence block prostaglandin production in the kidney. Blocking this pathway of arachidonic acid metabolism also has the effect of increasing the availability of arachidonic acid for the lipoxygenase and P450 metabolic pathways.

Because of the natriuretic effects of renal prostaglandins, it is not surprising that NSAIDs can lead to volume retention, particularly in patients with congestive heart failure or cirrhosis who can least afford this increase in volume. This effect may also interfere with the actions of antihypertensive drugs. NSAIDs also affect potassium homeostasis. The stimulation of renin production by prostaglandins explains why NSAIDs are associated with hyporeninemia, hypoaldosteronism and hyperkalemia with type IV renal tubular acidosis. Renal toxicity occurs most commonly from hemodynamic effects in patients in whom the circulation is compromised in such a way that renal perfusion and GFR are maintained at normal levels by the production of cyclooxygenase products. For example, the vasoconstrictive actions of catecholamines and angiotensin II on the afferent and efferent arterioles are counterbalanced by the vasodilatory actions of PGI_2 and PGE_2. Administration of NSAIDs to these individuals can therefore result in unopposed efferent vasoconstriction with acute reductions in renal blood flow and GFR and can result in ischemic acute renal failure. The long-term effects of NSAIDs on the kidney are discussed in Chapter 57.

PGH synthase products and kidney disease

Hypertension

Prostaglandin synthase activity is greater in adult spontaneously hypertensive rats (SHR) than in the control rats. There is enhanced microsomal phospholipase A_2 (PLA_2) activity in SHR animals. This activity increases with age (and blood pressure) in the SHR animals but not in controls.

Tubulointerstitial disease

Arachidonic acid and its metabolites may be involved in tubulointerstitial inflammatory processes in a number of different ways. Interstitial cell infiltration is an almost invariant essential component of tubulointerstitial disease. Most of the mononuclear cells in the interstitium are T cells and many have the appearance and carry markers of activated lymphocytes. In acute interstitial nephritis of various etiologies there are abundant numbers of T_4+ (T helper cells) and T_8+ (suppressor/cytotoxic cells) lymphocytes with various ratios of cell populations reported. In the rejecting kidney allograft there is a heavy infiltrate of cells bearing the T_8 phenotype of cytotoxic T cells. As rejection becomes more severe there is a marked infiltration of macrophages. Increased levels of interleukin-1 or arachidonic acid itself, via its activation of protein kinase C in T cells, stimulate the T cell to generate interleukin-2 (IL-2). IL-2 results in clonal proliferation and continued viability of activated T cells. It stimulates phospholipid turnover and arachidonate release from IL-2-dependent cell lines and its lipoxygenase products may play a central role in γ-interferon production. Gamma-interferon up-regulates MHC class II antigens, which are expressed on proximal tubular cells in various inflammatory states.

Nitric oxide production is increased in many inflammatory states; the inducible nitric oxide synthase isoform is expressed in response to tumor necrosis factor-α (TNF-α), *Escherichia coli* lipopolysaccharide and IL-1β, in a number of cell types. It has recently been demonstrated that nitric oxide activates cyclo-oxygenases by a non-cGMP mechanism, increasing the production of PGE_2. This formation of PGE_2 may contribute to the inflammatory response.

Prostaglandins may also be anti-inflammatory. Prostaglandin E_1 has been found to be immunosuppressive in a murine model of interstitial nephritis. This suppressive effect was associated with a reduction in spleen cell product-induced effector Lyt2+ T cells. Prostaglandins may also affect macrophage function and hence alter the inflammatory response. TNF-α, also called cachectin, is a polypeptide cytokine produced primarily by monocytes and macrophages in response to endotoxin or other immune and inflammatory stimuli. PGE_2 reduces TNF production by stimulated macrophages by an action at the level of TNF-gene transcription.

Urinary tract obstruction

Hydronephrosis results in renal tubulointerstitial inflammation and is characterized by marked stimulation of renal arachidonate metabolism. There is enhanced cyclo-oxygenase and thromboxane synthase activity. Infiltrating macrophages play an important role in the altered arachidonic acid metabolism. In addition to generating eicosanoids themselves, the macrophages produce nitric oxide which can have a paracrine action on other cells to enhance cyclooxygenase activity and prostaglandin production. The released prostaglandins may contribute to the natriuresis and decreased concentrating ability of the hydronephrotic kidney and may play a role in the inflammatory response.

Hepatorenal syndrome

Although PGH synthase staining is comparable to normal kidneys in renal tissue from patients with acute tubular necrosis, tubulointerstitial nephritis, or liver disease without the hepatorenal syndrome, staining is markedly suppressed in kidneys from patients with hepatorenal syndrome. The investigators who reported these findings suggested that the reduced medullary PGH synthase activity may explain the reduced prostaglandin E_2 excretion observed with the hepatorenal syndrome which may relate in an important way to the pathophysiology of the syndrome.

Diabetes mellitus

In experimental diabetes in the rat there are glomerular hyperfiltration and kidney hypertrophy, just as there are in patients with diabetes mellitus. Hyperfiltration and hypertrophy are associated with an increased glomerular production of PGE_2, 6-keto-$PGF_{1\alpha}$ and TXB_2, related to an increased availability of arachidonic acid in the diabetic glomerulus. The net effect of NSAIDs is to mitigate the glomerular hyperfiltration of diabetes, consistent with a net vasodilatory effect of the combination of eicosanoids produced. The administration of thromboxane synthesis inhibitors to patients reduces urinary protein excretion but whether this has any effect on the progression of the underlying renal disease is not clear.

Sepsis

With various infectious processes there is enhanced renal blood flow and natriuresis. These changes in renal blood flow and sodium excretion may be mediated by prostaglandins. Many of the physiological changes associated with infection are believed to be secondary to interleukin-1 (IL-1). This cytokine, when injected into the rat, causes a marked natriuresis and associated enhanced PGE_2 excretion, likely due to an effect of IL-1 on the papillary collecting duct. Indomethacin abolishes the IL-1-induced natriuresis.

In addition to these potential roles for prostaglandins in vasodilatory responses to sepsis, PGH synthase/cyclooxygenase products may also be important intrarenal vasoconstrictors in sepsis. Endotoxin is a potent stimulus for thromboxane A_2 synthesis in the renal cortex.

Effects of prostaglandin synthase-2 gene disruption on the kidney

Given the multiple effects of prostaglandins on the kidney it is not surprising that disruption of the PGH synthase genes by homologous recombination might have important consequences for the kidney. Mice have been produced with selective deletion of either PGH synthase-1 or -2. In the animals where PGH synthase-1 is no longer produced there were minimal renal abnormalities in animals up to five months of age, suggesting that the absence of this enzyme is not deleterious under normal physiological condition. The situation was quite different in animals in which the PGH synthase-1 gene was disrupted. These animals develop severe nephropathy and are prone to develop peritonitis. There is normal renal histology at three days of life but severe abnormalities in mice aged six weeks or more. At six weeks the primary lesions appear to be those of nephron hypoplasia, reduced number of glomeruli, cortical atrophy and regeneration. At eight weeks and later there is interstitial fibrosis that was not present at younger ages. It was proposed that the kidney pathology may be a result of arrest of postnatal kidney maturation in the subcapsular nephrogenic zone.

Lipoxygenase products

Characteristics of the enzymes

Arachidonic acid can be oxidized by 5-, 8-, 12- and 15-lipoxygenases leading to the formation of hydroperoxy- and hydroxyeicosatetraenoic acids (HPETEs and HETEs) (Figure 17.3). In the case of the 5-lipoxygenase, the products can be converted to leukotriene B_4 (LTB_4) or undergo enzymatic adduction of glutathione forming sulfidopeptide leukotrienes, LTC_4, LTD_4 or LTE_4. Five-lipoxygenase activating protein (FLAP) is a membrane protein which is important for leukotriene synthesis in intact cells.

Production within the kidney

To date there is no evidence for 5-lipoxygenase activity and subsequent leukotriene production by renal cells, with the possible exception of normal resident glomerular macrophages. By contrast, 12- and 15-lipoxygenase activity is found in the cortex of the normal rat kidney. 12-HETE is produced by isolated glomeruli, glomerular epithelial and mesangial cells in culture, and cortical tubules, although it was not clear whether this cortical tubule activity was due to cortical epithelial cells, glomeruli or vascular structures which contaminated the tubule preparation. 15-HETE is produced by mesangial cells in culture.

Effects on kidney function

Renal blood flow and GFR

Leukotrienes LTC_4 and LTD_4 are vasoconstrictive in the kidney. LTD_4 causes postglomerular arteriolar vasoconstriction and a decrease in the glomerular capillary ultrafiltration coefficient, possibly related to its effect to contract mesangial cells. LTB_4 and 12(R)-HETE are vasodilatory for the renal vasculature. In the normal

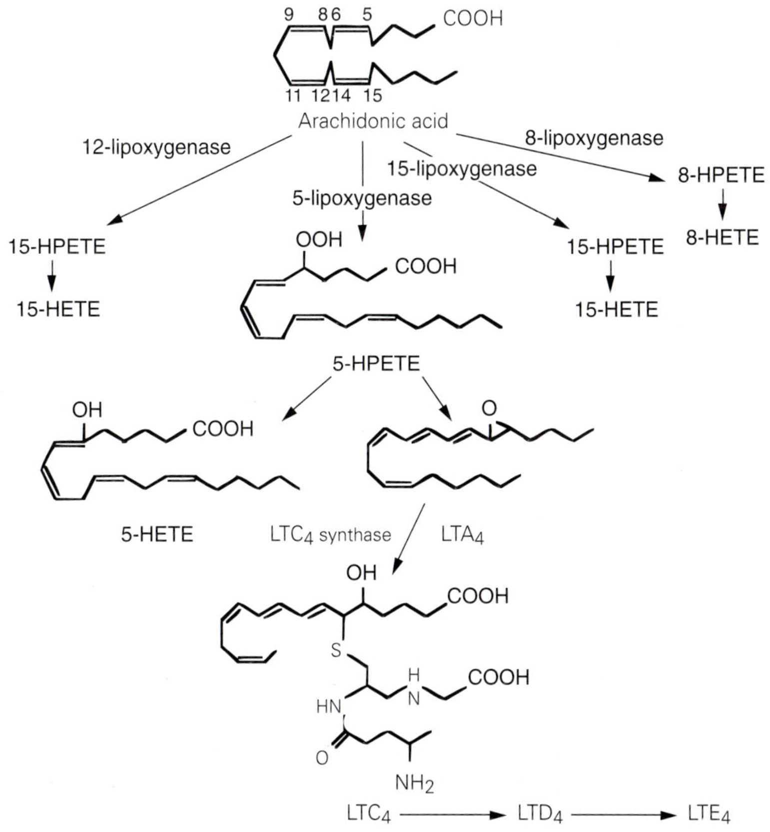

Figure 17.3 Lipoxygenase pathways of arachidonic acid metabolism. Lipoxins, not depicted on this figure, are the products of more than one of the lipoxygenases. HPETE, hydroperoxyeicosatetraenoic acid; HETE, hydroxyeicosatetraenoic acid; LT, leukotriene.

kidney, lipoxin A_4, a trihydroxyeicosatetraenoic acid produced by lipoxygenase metabolism of a di-HPETE, is vasodilatory, increases renal blood flow via an effect on the preglomerular vasculature and enhances GFR. These effects are mediated by vasodilatory prostaglandins, not by the direct effect of the lipoxin itself.

Renin secretion

The 12- and 15-HPETEs and their corresponding HETEs inhibit renin release from the kidney. The products of 12-lipoxygenase are believed to mediate angiotensin II-induced inhibition of renin release. Products of 5-lipoxygenase do not affect renin production in the kidney.

Sodium excretion

Lipoxygenase products may affect transmembrane transport by mediating the effects of G protein subunits on sodium and potassium channel activation.

Lipoxygenase products and kidney disease

Glomerular disease

There are increased levels of leukotrienes in various disease models associated with inflammation of the glomerulus. Inhibition of LTD_4 action by receptor antagonists leads to higher GFRs in nephritic animals. Elevated glomerular levels of LTB_4 are observed only during the early phase of nephritis in experimental models. Nevertheless, inhibition of production of leukotrienes early on can lead to marked mitigation of proteinuria two weeks later.

15(S)-HETE decreases the production of and antagonizes many of the actions of LTB_4 in the inflamed glomerulus. Lipoxin A_4 inhibits LTD_4-mediated adhesion of polymorphonuclear leukocytes to mesangial cells and this effect may be anti-inflammatory *in vivo*.

Urinary tract obstruction

Glomeruli isolated from hydronephrotic animals generate more LTB_4 than control glomeruli. This increase in leukotriene synthesis can be mitigated by prevention of leukocyte infiltration into the glomerulus. Furthermore, the decrease in GFR and renal blood flow in hydronephrosis can be prevented by inhibiting either leukocyte infiltration or 5-lipoxygenase activity. Thus leukotrienes have been proposed to mediate the hemodynamic changes in the glomerulus observed with urinary tract obstruction. Whereas the inflammatory cell agonist *N*-formyl-L-methionyl-L-leucil-L-phenylalanine (fMLP) has no effect on leukotriene synthesis in the normal kidney, it enhances leukotrienes B_4 and C_4 in the hydronephrotic kidney, presumably by acting on an increased number of monocytes present in the kidney.

Tubulointerstitial disease

Leukotrienes have been implicated as mediators of tubulointerstitial renal disease. Leukotriene B_4 increases TNF levels and TNF stimulates IL-1 production by macrophages, increases neutrophil-mediated antibody-dependent cytotoxicity, phagocytosis, superoxide production and class II antigen expression.

The cortex, but not medulla, of canine kidney undergoing rejection, synthesizes significantly greater quantities of 12-HETE and LTB_4 than normal or auto-transplanted control renal cortices. The histologic appearance of tissue destruction and cellular infiltration correlate with the amount of 12-HETE found in the allograft. The dual cyclooxygenase/lipoxygenase inhibitor (BW 755C) reduced levels of 12-HETE and LTB_4 as well as cellular infiltration and tissue damage in rejecting renal allografts. Selective cyclo-oxygenase inhibition with indomethacin did not improve allograft function. Thus lipoxygenase products may be important for allograft rejection. It is not clear from these studies, however, whether all the lipoxygenase products were derived from infiltrating cells or whether some were made by renal cells themselves. Lipoxygenase products may also affect other components of arachidonate metabolism. In the platelet and neutrophil the monoHETEs inhibit PLA_2 activity.

Sepsis

Endotoxin releases leukotrienes from leukocytes and inhibits biliary elimination of these compounds. There is evidence that at least some of the intrarenal vasoconstriction associated with endotoxin is mediated via leukotrienes.

Cytochrome P450 mono-oxygenase products

Characteristics of the enzymes

Cytochrome P450 monooxygenases comprise a family of enzymes. Mixed function oxidase activity involves the hemoprotein, cytochrome P450, together with a flavoprotein reductase (NADPH cytochrome P450 reductase) and phosphatidylcholine. This enzyme system results in the generation of HETEs, a number of different epoxy-eicosatrienoic acids (EETs) which can then be rapidly converted into dihydroxyeicosatrienoic acid (DHETs), and ω and ω-1 hydroxylation products (Figure 17.4).

Production within the kidney

In the kidney, P450 products are made in the medullary thick ascending limb of Henle, the S_1 segment of the proximal tubule and the cortical collecting duct. These products can be acted on by cyclooxygenase to generate

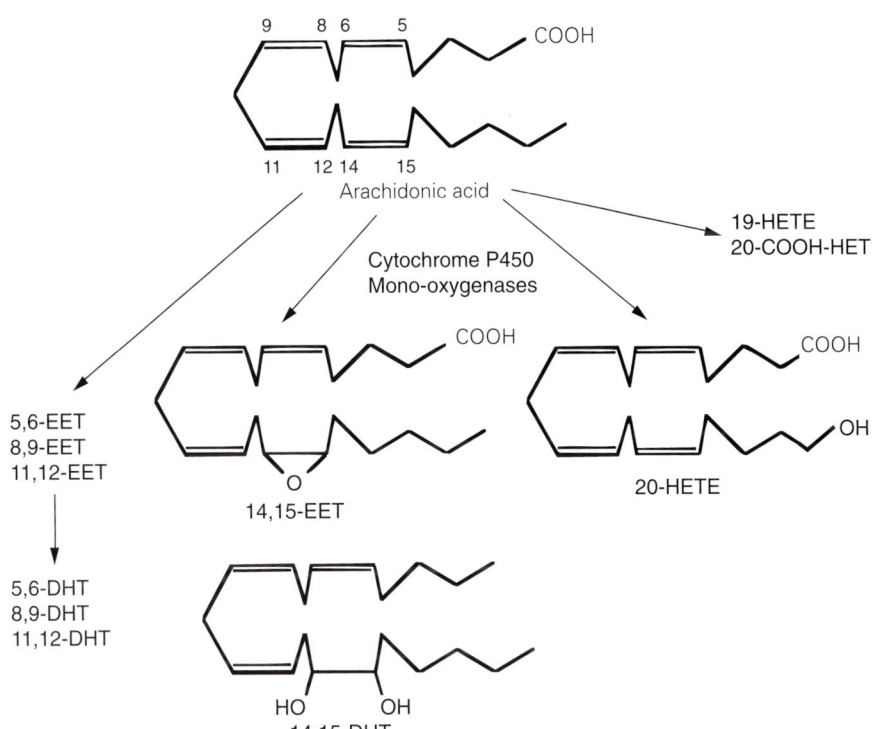

other biologically important derivatives. EETs and HETEs are present in human urine.

Effects on kidney function

Renal blood flow

Like the cyclooxygenase products the vasoactive effects of P450 products depend in part on the animal species and vascular bed studied. The most potent vasoactive compounds are 20-HETE and 5,6-EET, both of which appear to exert their vascular effects after metabolism by cyclooxygenase. Other EETs are vasoactive to a varying extent, also depending on species and vascular bed studied. 5,6-EET and 20- and 19-HETE dilate the renal vasculature of rabbits but constrict the vasculature of the rat kidney. In both cases, these effects are inhibited by cyclooxygenase inhibition. In canine vasculature 20-HETE also is vasoconstrictive and it is believed to be important in the myogenic vasoconstrictive response to the elevation of blood pressure, and hence may play an important role in the autoregulation of renal blood flow.

Renin secretion

Renin production is reduced by 12(R)-HETE in the kidney.

Sodium excretion

Renal cortical epoxygenase activity is increased after administration of high salt diets to animals. P450 prod-

ucts, 19- and 20-HETE and 20-COOH-arachidonic acid, generated by the medullary thick ascending limb are potent inhibitors of the $Na^+,K^+,2Cl^-$ transporter and inhibit sodium reabsorption. It has been proposed that 5,6-EET mediates the increased sodium excretion which occurs in response to AII action on the tubule.

Water excretion

Given the effects of the P450 products to inhibit sodium reabsorption in the medullary thick ascending limb, it is not surprising that these agents increase water excretion. In addition to this effect on the medullary thick ascending limb, however, all four EETs inhibit the hydroosmotic effect of vasopressin in the cortical collecting duct, providing another mechanism of enhanced water excretion.

Cytochrome P450 monooxygenase products and kidney disease

Hypertension

As indicated above, high salt intake leads to the induction of kidney epoxygenase activity. This has led to the proposal that deficient P450 activity may play a role in salt-sensitive hypertension. In support of this hypothesis is the observation that production of epoxygenase products from renal cortical microsomes is lower in prehypertensive Dahl salt-sensitive rats than control salt-resistant animals on low or high salt diets.

Renal disease

There is little information regarding the role of P450 products in renal glomerular or tubulointerstitial disease. Antagonists of the P450 system markedly inhibit mesangial cell proliferation and mRNA levels of the immediate early genes, *Egr-1* and *c-fos*. These data suggest a role for P450 products of arachidonic acid in the regulation of mesangial cell growth with the potential for involvement in disease states characterized by enhanced mesangial cell proliferation.

Summary

The three pathways of arachidonic acid metabolism are involved in many facets of renal function in health and disease. The many metabolic products modulate vascular reactivity, GFR, renin secretion, sodium and water excretion. They are implicated in many diseases of the kidney, including hypertension, glomerulonephritis, tubulointerstitial diseases of various etiologies, urinary tract obstruction, hepatorenal syndrome, diabetic nephropathy and sepsis. Many of the products are counterregulatory, with the proper balance of production being necessary to maintain normal function, especially under conditions of physiological or pathological stress. Products of one enzymatic pathway may serve as substrates for another. Intracellular effects of the metabolites are poorly understood and likely underestimated. There is recent evidence that prostaglandin synthesis can be compartmentalized within the nucleus where prostaglandin recepters also exist. A role for prostaglandins in regulation of gene expression has been demonstrated. Elucidation of the multiple effects of the various metabolites and implications of the complex interrelationships among the metabolites will take many more years of intense investigation but likely will yield important insight into normal and abnormal renal function.

Acknowledgments

The author is supported by National Institutes of Health grants DK39773, DK38452, DK38165, DK39902 and NS 10828.

Further reading

Bonventre, J.V. (1992) Phospholipase A_2 and signal transduction. *J. Am. Soc. Nephrol.*, **3**, 128–50.

Bonventre, J.V. and Nemenoff, R. (1991) Renal tubular arachidonic acid metabolism. *Kidney Int.*, **39**, 438–49.

Breyer, M.D. and Badr, K.F. (1996) Arachidonic acid metabolites and the kidney, in *The kidney* 5th edn (ed. B.M. Brenner), Saunders, Philadelphia, pp. 755–788.

Breyer, M.D., Jacobson, H.R. and Breyer, R.M. (1996) Functional and molecular aspects of renal prostaglandin receptors. *J. Am. Soc Nephrol.*, **7**, 8–17.

Carroll, M.A., Balazy, M., Margiotta, P. *et al.* (1993) Renal vasodilator activity of 5,6-epoxyeicosatrienoic acid depends upon conversions by cyclooxygenase and release of prostaglandins. *J. Biol. Chem.*, **268**, 12260–6.

DeRubertis, F.R. and Craven, P.A. (1993) Eicosanoids in the pathogenesis of the functional and structural alterations of the kidney in diabetes. *Am. J. Kidney Dis.*, **22**, 727–35.

Katoh, T., Takahashi, K., DeBoer, D.K. *et al.* (1992) Renal hemodynamic actions of lipoxins in rats: a comparative physiological study. *Am. J. Physiol.*, **263**, F436–42.

Ma, Y.-H., Schwartzman, M.L. and Roman, R.J. (1994) Altered renal P-450 metabolism of arachidonic acid in Dahl salt-sensitive rats. *Am. J. Physiol.*, **267**, R579–89.

McGiff, J.C., Quilley, C.P. and Carroll, M.A. (1993) The contribution of cytochrome P450-dependent arachidonate metabolites to integrated renal function. *Steroids*, **58**, 573–9.

Mené, P. and Dunn, M.J. (1992) Vascular, glomerular, and tubular effects of angiotensin II, kinins, and prostaglandins, in *The Kidney: Physiology and Pathophysiology* (eds D.W. Seldin and G. Giebisch), Raven Press, New York, pp. 1205–48.

Morham, S.G., Langenbach, R., Loftin, C.D. *et al.* (1995) Prostaglandin synthase 2 gene disruption causes severe renal pathology in the mouse. *Cell*, **83**, 473–82.

Murray, M.D. and Brater, D.C. (1993) Renal toxicity of the nonsteroidal anti-inflammatory drugs. *Annu. Rev. Pharmacol. Toxicol.*, **33**, 435–65.

Roman, R.J. and Harder, D.R. (1993) Cellular and ionic signal transduction mechanisms for the mechanical activation of renal arterial vascular smooth muscle. *J. Am. Soc. Nephrol.*, **4**, 986–96.

Salvemini, D., Misko, T.P., Masferrer, J.L. *et al.* (1993) Nitric oxide activates cyclooxygenase enzymes. *Proc. Natl. Acad. Sci. USA*, **90**, 7240–4.

Sellmayer, A., Uedelhoven, W.M., Weber, P.C. and Bonventre, J.V. (1991) Endogenous non-cyclooxygenase metabolites of arachidonic acid modulate growth and mRNA levels of Immediate-Early response genes in rat mesangial cells. *J. Biol. Chem.*, **266**, 3800–7.

Simon, L.S. (1994) Actions and toxic effects of the nonsteroidal anti-inflammatory drugs. *Curr. Opin. Rheumatol.*, **6**, 238–51.

Smith, W.L. (1992) Prostanoid biosynthesis and mechanisms of action. *Am. J. Physiol.*, **263**, F181–91.

Takahashi, K. and Badr, K.F. (1993) Lipoxygenase products as mediators in immune-mediated glomerular injury. *Semin. Nephrol.*, **13**, 129–36.

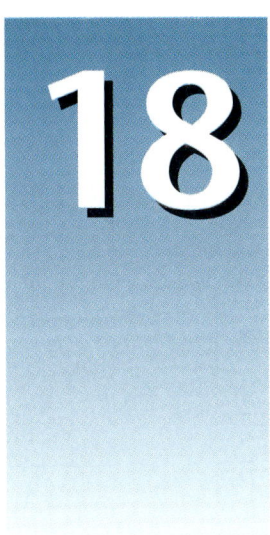

18

Vitamin D metabolism

Rajiv Kumar and Theodore Craig

Introduction

The vitamin D–endocrine system plays a major role in the control of calcium and phosphorus balance. Significant abnormalities occur in the system in patients with renal failure and end-stage renal disease and in patients with some types of nephrolithiasis. An understanding of the metabolism of vitamin D and interactions among vitamin D, parathyroid hormone and calcitonin is vital to understanding the pathogenesis and the treatment of these disorders.

Calcium and phosphorus balance and the role of vitamin D

The amounts of calcium and phosphorus absorbed and secreted by the intestine and the amounts excreted by the kidney are shown in Figures 18.1 and 18.2. Vitamin D via its active metabolite, 1,25-dihydroxyvitamin D, plays a central role in controlling the efficiency of calcium and phosphorus absorption in the intestine and, to a lesser extent, in the kidney. Calcium absorption in the intestine occurs by active and passive processes. Passive calcium transport occurs at high luminal calcium concentrations via a paracellular mechanism and does not require the

expenditure of energy. Calcium absorption by active mechanisms is a transcellular phenomenon that occurs at low luminal calcium concentrations and requires sodium and the expenditure of energy. It is the process of active calcium absorption that is influenced by vitamin D. In normal humans, both active and passive processes contribute to the absorption of calcium from the intestine.

It is not commonly appreciated that vitamin D also increases the efficiency of phosphorus absorption in the intestine and, to some extent, in the kidney as well. The absorption of phosphorus occurs by a mechanism distinct from that of the absorption of calcium.

Vitamin D nomenclature

The term vitamin D refers to both vitamin D_3 and vitamin D_2. These substances are equipotent and are metabolized in a similar manner in humans and other mammalian species. In birds, however, vitamin D_2 is considerably less active than vitamin D_3. In this chapter the term vitamin D will be used when referring to both vitamin D_3 and vitamin D_2. When necessary the individual types of the vitamin will be referred to in the text. The structures of vitamin D_2, vitamin D_3 and other vitamin D metabolites and analogs are shown in Figure 18.3. Some of these

Nephrology, Edited by Rex L. Jamison and Robert Wilkinson.
Published in 1997 by Chapman & Hall, London. ISBN 0 412 60930 4

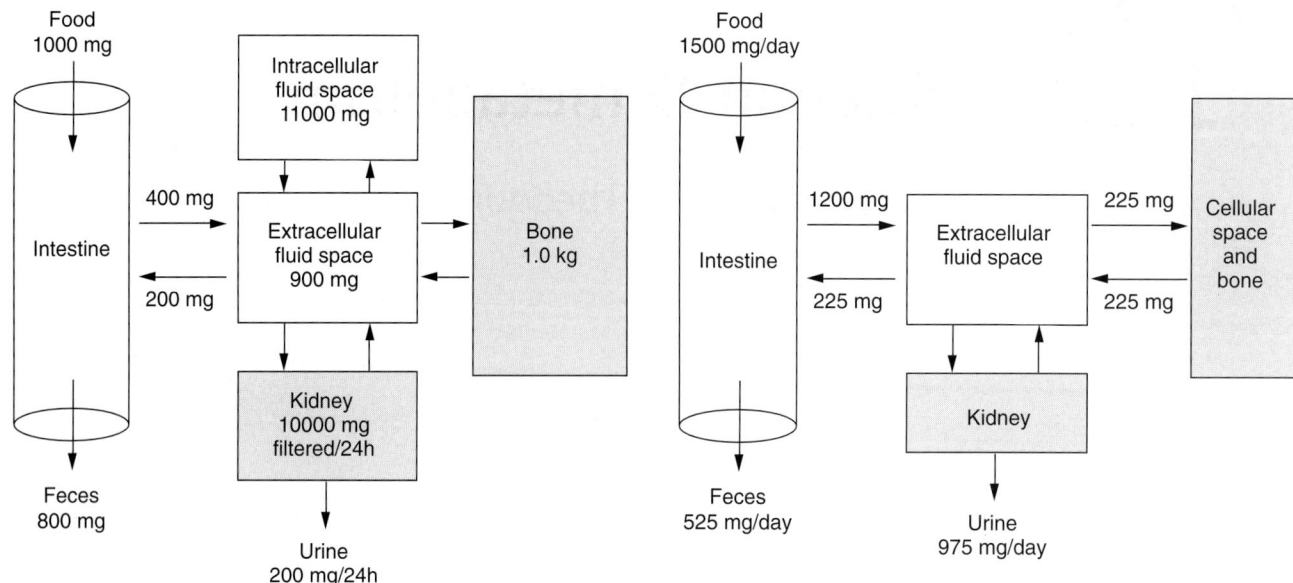

Figure 18.1 Calcium balance in normal human subjects.

Figure 18.2 Phosphorus balance in normal human subjects.

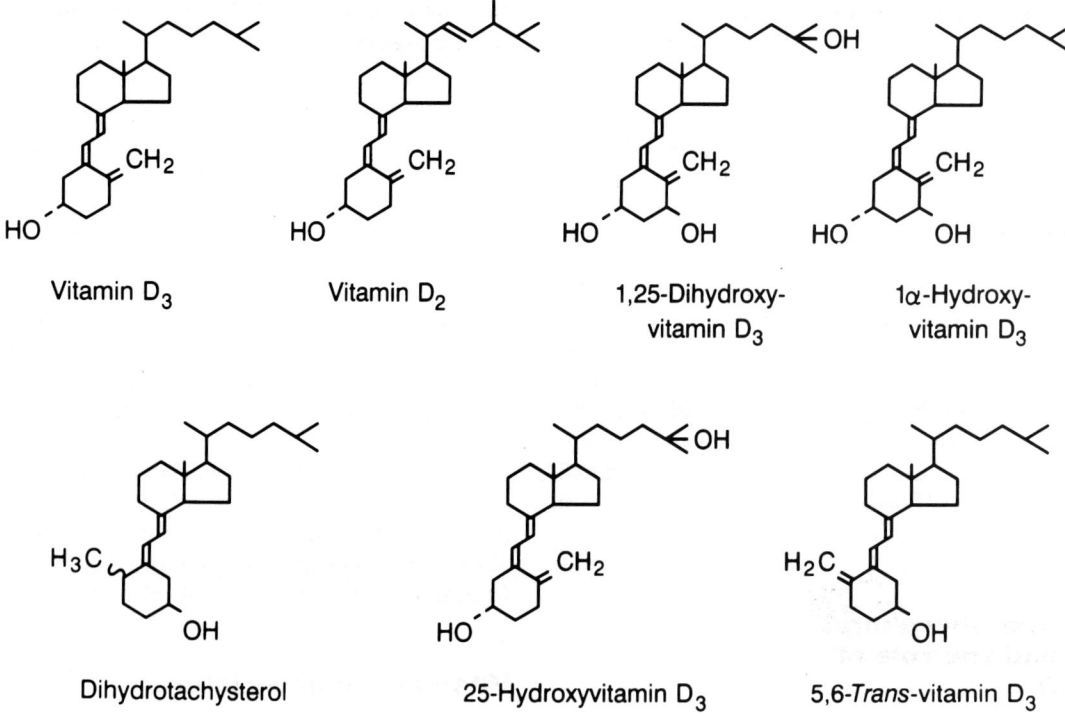

Figure 18.3 Chemical structures of vitamin D metabolites and analogs. (Reproduced, with permission, from Kumar, R. (1990) *J. Am. Soc. Nephrol.*, **1**, 30–42.)

metabolites and analogs such as 1α,25-dihydroxyvitamin D$_3$, 1α-hydroxyvitamin D$_3$ and dihydrotachysterol are used therapeutically in patients with renal osteodystrophy and calcium malabsorption associated with renal failure.

Sources of vitamin D and vitamin D synthesis in the skin

Vitamin D$_2$ and D$_3$ are both present in food products. Milk and dairy products in the USA are fortified with vitamin D; however, fortification of milk is not practiced in the UK. The extent of fortification of milk is quite variable and sometimes the amounts of vitamin D in dairy products are considerably lower than stated on food product labels. Vitamin D present in the diet is absorbed, like other fat-soluble substances, in the chylomicron fraction and enters the circulation via the thoracic duct. Malabsorption syndromes are often associated with decreased absorption of the vitamin from the intestine. Vitamin D_2 is exclusively of dietary origin, whereas vitamin D_3 is also synthesized endogenously in the skin.

Steenbock and Black showed that ultraviolet irradiation of skin and foods was associated with the formation of antirachitic substances. Earlier, Saomes and Goldblatt had demonstrated that the irradiation of rachitic rat livers conferred antirachitic properties on them. The work of Steenbock and Black explained the earlier observations of Huldshinsky and Chick who showed that exposure to sunlight cured rickets in children. It also laid the basis for the subsequent work of Askew and Windaus on the chemical structure of vitamin D_2 and vitamin D_3.

It is now well established that vitamin D_3 is formed in the skin from a precursor molecule, 7-dehydrocholesterol, in the presence of ultraviolet light (Figure 18.4). Ultraviolet light of a wavelength 254–300 nm is effective in carrying out the photolysis of the B-ring of 7-dehydrocholesterol to form an intermediary substance, previtamin D_3. Previtamin D_3 undergoes thermal isomerization to vitamin D_3. These reactions also occur in human skin. The amount of vitamin D_3 formed is influenced by the spectral properties of the incident light, the duration of exposure to light, the presence of melanin in the skin and perhaps the presence of other substances that may interfere with the photolytic cleavage of the B-ring of 7-dehydrocholesterol. Other sterol by-products such as tachysterol and lumisterol are formed in the photolytic reaction. The amount of previtamin D_3 formed during the photolysis reaction can be increased by carrying out sequential irradiation, first at 254 nm and subsequently at 300 nm. A reaction similar to that for 7-dehydrocholesterol occurs with ergosterol, a plant sterol. Irradiation of ergosterol results in the formation of previtamin D_2, the thermal isomerization of which results in the formation of vitamin D_2. Vitamin D_2 formation does not occur in the skin of animals and man.

Thus, it is clear that vitamin D is not a vitamin in the sense that it is not an essential exogenous micronutrient. Rather it has become one, as the amount of sunlight exposure that a normal human receives is limited and insufficient to generate adequate amounts of the vitamin in the skin.

Once vitamin D_3 is formed in the skin it is transported out of this organ associated with vitamin D-binding protein. It has been suggested that the affinity of vitamin D_3 for vitamin D-binding protein is severalfold greater than the affinity of previtamin D_3 for the protein. This allows the preferential movement of vitamin D_3 out of the skin and allows the reaction to proceed to the right by removing the final product of the reaction.

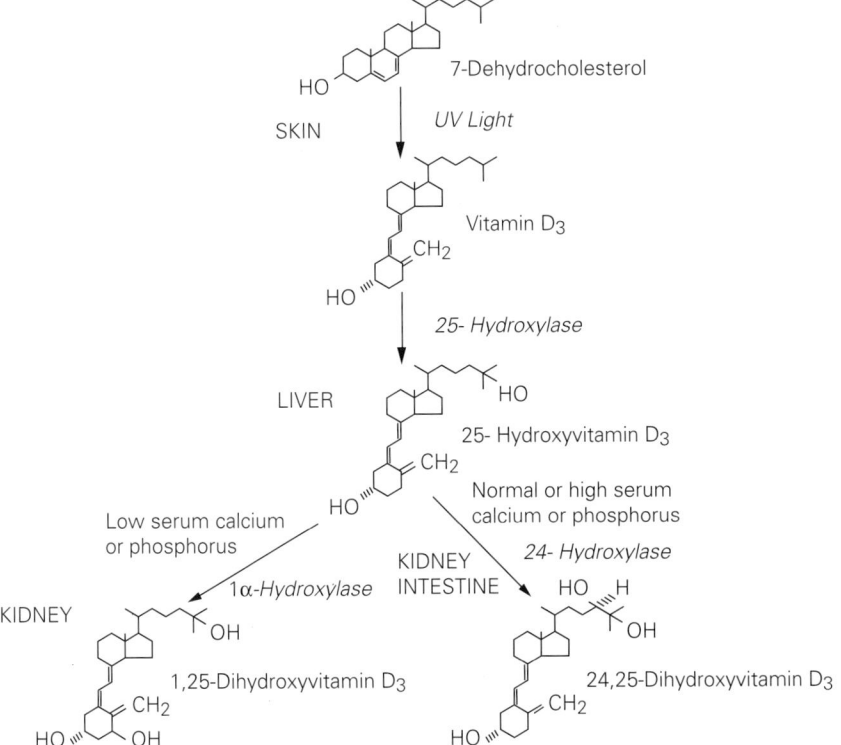

Figure 18.4 The metabolism of vitamin D_3. (Reproduced, with permission, from Kumar, R. (1990) *J. Am. Soc. Nephrol.*, **1**, 30–42.)

Metabolism of vitamin D in the liver

Vitamin D_3 is metabolized in the liver to 25-hydroxy-vitamin D_3 by the action of vitamin D_3 25-hydroxylase (Figure 18.4). There are two enzymes that catalyze this reaction: a microsomal hydroxylase that is probably the physiologically relevant enzyme and a mitochondrial hydroxylase that is operative at pharmacological concentrations of the substrate. The microsomal enzyme has a lower K_m than the mitochondrial enzyme and is regulated by the concentration of 25-hydroxyvitamin D or vitamin D. The mitochondrial enzyme, however, is not regulated by the product and, therefore, the ingestion of large amounts of vitamin D is associated with high concentrations of 25-hydroxyvitamin D in the circulation. The microsomal enzyme contains cytochrome P450. It is inhibited by drugs such as isoniazid and ketoconazole. Inducers of other cytochrome P450 enzymes such as phenobarbital and phenytoin (dilantin) on occasion, cause the conversion of vitamin D_3 into other inactive metabolites. 25-Hydroxyvitamin D is biologically inert in the amounts that normally circulate in plasma. It remains inactive in anephric animals unless it is administered in pharmacological amounts. In the latter circumstance it is active, in part, as a result of conversion into 5,6-*trans*-25-hydroxyvitamin D_3 and, in part, as a result of the binding of large amounts of the naturally occurring form, 5,6-*cis*-25-hydroxyvitamin D_3 to the 1,25-dihydroxyvitamin D receptor.

The further metabolism of 25-hydroxyvitamin D₃

As noted above, 25-hydroxyvitamin D_3 is biologically inactive in the anephric state in amounts that normally circulate in plasma. 25-Hydroxyvitamin D_3 circulates in plasma bound to a vitamin D-binding protein – an α-globulin related to α-fetoprotein. Vitamin D-binding protein also binds 1,25-dihydroxyvitamin D_3, but with a lesser affinity than that with which it binds 25-hydroxyvitamin D_3. 25-Hydroxyvitamin D_3 must be further metabolized to 1,25-dihydroxyvitamin D_3 in the kidney by 25-hydroxyvitamin D_3 1α-hydroxylase (Figure 18.4). This enzyme is a multicomponent enzyme composed of ferredoxin, a ferredoxin reductase and a cytochrome P450. In physiological circumstances, it is present in the mitochondria of proximal tubules of the kidney. The enzyme is regulated by several factors which

Table 18.1 Factors altering the plasma concentration of 1,25-dihydroxyvitamin D or the 25-hydroxyvitamin D 1α-hydroxylase activity

Factor	Change in activity or amount of factor	Effect on 1,25(OH)₂D₃ 1α-hydroxylase
Parathyroid hormone	Increase	+
	Decrease	–
Serum inorganic phosphate	Increase	–
	Decrease	+
1,25-Dihydroxyvitamin D	Increase	–
	Decrease	+
Calcium (direct effect)	Increase	?
	Decrease	+
Calcitonin	Increase	Variable
	Decrease	?
Hydrogen ion	Increase	–
	Decrease	?
Sex steroids	Increase	+
	Decrease	?
Prolactin	Increase	+/0
	Decrease	?
Growth hormone	Increase	Variable
	Decrease	?
Glucocorticoids	Increase	–
	Decrease	?
Thyroid hormone	Increase	–
	Decrease	+
Pregnancy		+

+, increase in concentration or a stimulation of enzyme activity.
–, decrease in concentration or a decrease of enzyme activity.

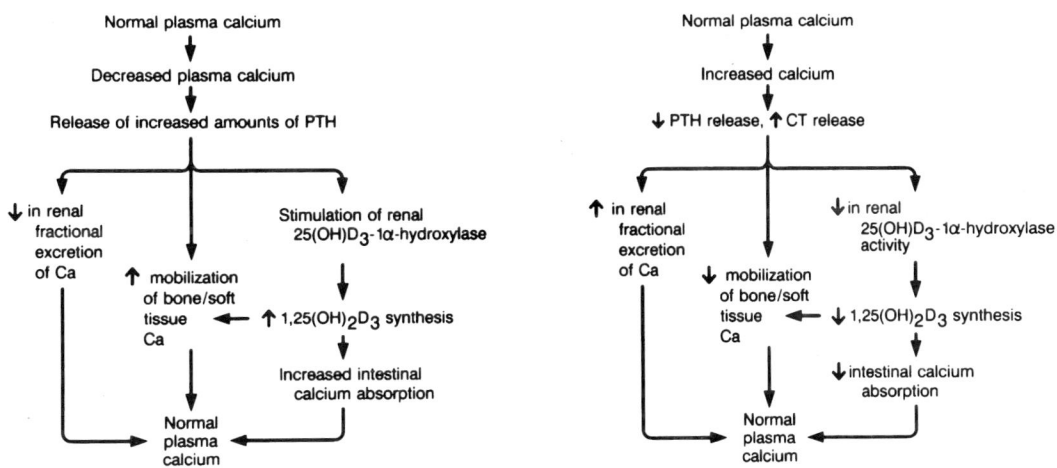

Figure 18.5 Physiological adaptations to (a) hypocalcemia and (b) hypercalcemia (From Kumar, R. (1991) *Kidney Int.*, **40**, 1177–89.)

are summarized in Table 18.1. The 25-hydroxyvitamin D_3 1α-hydroxylase is present, in certain situations, in other normal and abnormal tissues. During normal pregnancy the placenta expresses the enzyme and the rise in 1,25-dihydroxyvitamin D concentration during pregnancy is due to the presence of this enzyme in the placenta in addition to its presence in the kidney. The skin also expresses the enzyme in small amounts and it is believed that in the skin, 1,25-dihydroxyvitamin D is a paracrine factor that modulates keratinocyte cell growth. In granulomatous disorders such as sarcoidosis and tuberculosis and in certain lymphomas, the enzyme is present in macrophages and granulomatous cells or in lymphoid cells. The presence of the enzyme that functions in a disregulated fashion in these cells is responsible for the hypercalcemia that is occasionally seen in these disorders.

The major factors influencing the activity of the 25-hydroxyvitamin D_3 1α-hydroxylase are parathyroid hormone and the concentration of inorganic phosphate in the extracellular fluid. Parathyroid hormone plays an important role in increasing 25-hydroxyvitamin D_3 1α-hydroxylase activity in hypocalcemic conditions. Hypocalcemia results in the rapid release of parathyroid hormone from hormone secretory vesicles in parathyroid cells (Figure 18.5). Parathyroid hormone increases the mobilization of calcium from bone by increasing the activity of osteoclasts; it increases the efficiency of calcium absorption in the distal tubule of the kidney; and it increases the activity of the 25-hydroxyvitamin D_3 1α-hydroxylase in the proximal nephron. The precise manner in which parathyroid hormone increases 25-hydroxyvitamin D_3 1α-hydroxylase activity is not known although the various possibilities include the stimulation of protein kinase A and protein kinase C activities. An increase in 25-hydroxyvitamin D_3 1α-hydroxylase activity results in an increase in 1,25-dihydroxyvitamin D_3 synthesis and in the absorption of calcium from the intes-

tine. In this manner, serum calcium concentrations are restored to normal. Normal serum calcium concentrations decrease the release of parathyroid hormone from the parathyroid gland and parathyroid hormone concentrations return to normal. In addition to the inhibition of parathyroid hormone release by calcium, there is good evidence to indicate that 1,25-dihydroxyvitamin D_3 directly inhibits the synthesis of parathyroid hormone by associating with a negative regulatory element in the 5' region of the parathyroid hormone gene. The association of 1,25-dihydroxyvitamin D_3 with the vitamin D-regulatory element in the parathyroid hormone gene occurs after 1,25-dihydroxyvitamin D_3 binds to its receptor, the vitamin D receptor. In chronic renal failure, renal 1,25-dihydroxyvitamin D_3 synthesis is decreased due to decreased nephron mass and a suppression of 25-hydroxyvitamin D 1α-hydroxylase activity by hyperphosphatemia. Hypocalcemia occurs as a result of decreased intestinal calcium absorption. Secondary hyperparathyroidism results. Also the reduced 1,25-dihydroxyvitamin D_3 concentrations fail to directly inhibit parathyroid hormone synthesis. This is compounded by a loss of 1,25-dihydroxyvitamin D_3 receptor in the parathyroid gland in chronic renal failure. The net effect is that parathyroid hormone synthesis is not 'switched off'. In hypercalcemic states (Figure 18.5), parathyroid hormone release is inhibited. Fractional calcium excretion in the kidney is increased, bone calcium mobilization occurs at a reduced rate and 25-hydroxyvitamin D_3 1α-hydroxylase activity is diminished. A reduction in circulating 1,25-dihydroxyvitamin D concentrations results in a reduction in the efficiency of calcium absorption in the intestine. Normocalcemia is thus restored.

Serum phosphate plays an important role in altering the activity of the 25-hydroxyvitamin D_3 1α-hydroxylase enzyme. It does so independently of changes in the concentration of parathyroid hormone. There is evidence that the pituitary gland and growth hormone are required

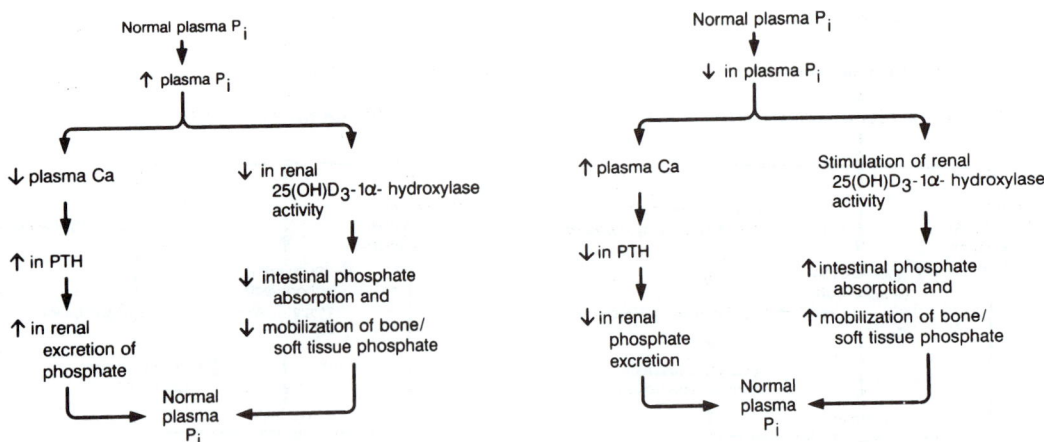

Figure 18.6 Physiological adaptations to (a) hypophosphatemia and (b) hyperphosphatemia. (Reproduced, with permission, from Kumar, R. (1991) *Kidney Int.*, **40**, 1177–89.)

to bring about the increase in 25-hydroxyvitamin D_3 1α-hydroxylase activity in response to a decrease in phosphate concentrations. In hypophosphatemic states (Figure 18.6) there is a secondary increase in serum calcium concentration due to mobilization of calcium on the basis of poorly understood biophysical phenomena. This results in a decrease in parathyroid hormone concentration and a decrease in the rejection of phosphate by the kidney. At the same time, and despite diminished parathyroid hormone concentrations, there is an increase in the activity of the 25-hydroxyvitamin D_3 1α-hydroxylase enzyme. This results in an increase in the concentration of 1,25-dihydroxyvitamin D_3 in plasma. An increase in the efficiency of phosphate absorption in the intestine occurs as a result of the increased 1,25-dihydroxyvitamin D_3 concentration. In hyperphosphatemia (Figure 18.6), serum calcium concentrations are decreased and the release of parathyroid hormone from the parathyroid gland is increased. This results in an increase in the rejection of phosphate by the kidney. At the same time, and despite the elevated concentrations of parathyroid hormone, 25-hydroxyvitamin D_3 1α-hydroxylase activity is diminished, resulting in decreased 1,25-dihydroxyvitamin D_3 concentrations in plasma and decreased phosphate absorption from the intestine. These factors normalize serum phosphate concentrations. The adaptations seen in hyperphosphatemia are particularly relevant to renal failure as transient- and later fixed-hyperphosphatemia occurs in chronic renal failure of all types. The resultant reduction in 25-hydroxyvitamin D_3 1α-hydroxylase activity and 1,25-dihydroxyvitamin D_3 concentrations contributes to the pathogenesis of calcium malabsorption in chronic renal failure.

When the synthesis of 1,25-dihydroxyvitamin D_3 is diminished, as occurs in normocalcemic or hypercalcemic states, or in normophosphatemic or hyperphosphatemic states, there is formation of another 25-hydroxyvitamin D_3 metabolite, 24,25-dihydroxyvitamin D_3 (Figure 18.4). Conversely, in hypocalcemic and hypophosphatemic states when the synthesis of 1,25-dihydroxyvitamin D_3 is high, 24,25-dihydroxyvitamin D_3 synthesis is diminished. The enzyme responsible for this biotransformation, 25-hydroxyvitamin D_3 24-hydroxylase, is present in the kidney, intestine, bone and other target tissues of 1,25-dihydroxyvitamin D_3. It also transforms 1,25-dihydroxyvitamin D_3 to 1,24,25-trihydroxyvitamin D_3 which is a biologically less potent form of the vitamin. Although there is some disagreement as to the biological role of 24,25-dihydroxyvitamin D_3, most investigators believe that it is a degradation product of the vitamin.

The mechanism of action of 1,25-dihydroxyvitamin D_3

1,25-Dihydroxyvitamin D_3 mediates the actions of vitamin D in target cells which are involved in the transport of calcium; these include the absorptive cells of the intestine, the cells of the distal tubule of the kidney and osteoblasts and osteoclasts. In addition, the hormone acts in cells that do not transport calcium such as keratinocytes, fibroblasts, tumor cells of various types and circulating lymphoid cells; in these cells the hormone modulates growth and differentiation.

In calcium-transporting and other cells the hormone acts after associating with an intracellular binding protein, the 1,25-dihydroxyvitamin D_3 receptor (VDR). Changes in protein synthesis brought about by the activation of relevant genes is necessary for the action of the sterol in cells. There is, however, mounting evidence for a non-genomic mechanism of action of 1,25-dihydroxyvitamin D_3 that involves changes in lipid composition of membranes and an opening of calcium channels in different parts of the cell membrane in response to the hormone. It is likely that both protein synthetic events and non-genomic events are necessary for vitamin D action in calcium-transporting cells. Following the association of 1,25-dihydroxyvitamin D_3 with its receptor, the receptor–hormone complex associates with other intracellular factors, such as the retinoic acid X-receptor, *c-fos* and *c-jun*, and the promoter regions of various vitamin D-responsive genes to increase or decrease the transcription of the latter genes. The VDR belongs to a family of steroid receptors which include those for glucocorticoids, progesterone, estrogen, thyroid hormone and retinoic acid. The VDR is most closely related to the retinoic acid and tri-iodothyronine receptors. It is a protein with a molecular weight of approximately 50 000 Da and is widely distributed among various vitamin D-responsive organs and cells. Like other steroid hormone receptors, VDR has a steroid binding domain in the carboxyl terminal portion of the molecule and a DNA binding domain in the amino terminal portion of the protein. The DNA binding domain of the VDR has an amino acid sequence pattern known as a 'zinc-finger' that enables the protein to bind to specific regulatory (or promoter) sequences in DNA. Nucleotide sequences present in promoter regions of genes regulated by 1,25-dihydroxyvitamin D_3 also have specific patterns. This enables the VDR to recognize and bind to these specific segments of DNA within genes that are regulated by the hormone. The VDR binds to the promoter elements in vitamin D-responsive genes either as a 'homo-dimer' where two molecules of the VDR associate with the promoter DNA, or as a 'hetero-dimer' where a single molecule of the VDR combines with a molecule of another protein (such as the retinoic acid–X-receptor) and the complex then binds to the appropriate DNA sequence. The important role of the VDR in mineral homeostasis is illustrated by the examination of biochemical and clinical abnormalities in patients with vitamin D-dependency rickets, type II. This is a rare disorder in which affected subjects have all the clinical and radiological features of rickets. Biochemical examination reveals the expected hypocalcemia, hypophosphatemia and secondary hyperparathyroidism. However, unlike subjects with nutritional vitamin D-deficiency rickets, these subjects have greatly increased serum concentrations of 1,25-dihydroxyvitamin D_3. An analysis of the VDRs in such individuals shows that the receptors are unable to bind to the hormone and that there are mutations in the receptor DNA or ligand-binding domains.

Several proteins are induced in the cell following the administration of 1,25-dihydroxyvitamin D_3 to experimental animals. Important among these are the vitamin D-dependent calcium-binding proteins and the plasma membrane calcium pump which play an important role in the transport of calcium across calcium-transporting epithelia (Tables 18.2 and 18.3). The vitamin D-dependent calcium-binding protein, the plasma membrane calcium pump and the vitamin D receptor all co-localize in calcium-transporting cells of the intestine, the distal tubule of the kidney and the ciliary body of the anterior segment of the eye. In the absence of 1,25-dihydroxyvitamin D_3, active calcium transport across calcium-transporting epithelia is low. Calcium movement across the apical membrane of the cell is lower than in the presence of 1,25-dihydroxyvitamin D_3. The concentration of vitamin D-dependent calcium-binding protein in the cell is low and this prevents the rapid diffusion of calcium across the cellular compartment. There is evidence that movement of calcium across the cell in vesicles is also diminished. Finally, in the absence of 1,25-dihydroxyvitamin D_3, the amount and activity of the plasma membrane calcium pump are greatly reduced, thus preventing the extrusion of calcium from the cell. When 1,25-dihydroxyvitamin D_3 is administered to a rachitic animal, the movement of calcium across the apical membrane of the cell is enhanced, the synthesis of calcium-binding protein is increased – thus facilitating the diffusion of calcium across the cell – and the activity and amount of the plasma membrane calcium pump are increased, thus enhancing the extrusion of calcium at the basolateral portion of the cell. A model for vitamin D-induced increases in calcium transport is shown in Figure 18.7.

In addition to its effects on the transport of calcium, 1,25-dihydroxyvitamin D_3 alters the growth and differentiation of cells. Keratinocyte proliferation is inhibited by high concentrations of 1,25-dihydroxyvitamin D_3. This property of the hormone has been exploited in the treatment of hyperproliferative skin disorders such as psoriasis. Tumor cell growth is inhibited by 1,25-dihydroxyvitamin D_3. Proliferation of other cell types is enhanced by the sterol. Formation of osteoclasts from precursor cells appears to be 1,25-dihydroxyvitamin D_3 dependent. 1,25-Dihydroxyvitamin D_3 alters lymphoid function *in vitro*. The manner in which the hormone influences cellular growth and differentiation is not known.

Table 18.2 Distribution of vitamin D-dependent calcium-binding proteins and their molecular weights

Tissue	Molecular weight (kDa)				
	Human	*Rat*	*Mouse*	*Pig*	*Chick*
Intestine	10,28	9	9	9	28
Kidney	28	28	9,25	9,25	28
Bone	ND	ND	ND	ND	28
Brain[a]	28	28	ND	ND	28
Pancreas	28	28	ND	12	28
Eye	28	28	ND	ND	ND

[a] Note calcium-binding protein in the brain is not vitamin D-dependent.
ND – not detected.

Table 18.3 Distribution of plasma membrane calcium pump in transporting epithelia as assessed by immunohistochemistry

Tissue	Source	Cell type	Location in cell
Kidney	Rat, human	Distal convoluted tubule, principal cell	Basolateral
Intestine	Rat, chick	Absorptive cell	Basolateral
Trophoblast	Rat, human	Syncytiotrophoblast	Basal
Choroid plexus of brain	Cat Human	Choroid plexus Secretory cell	Apical
Shell gland	Chick	Principal cell	Apical
Osteoblasts	Human	Osteoblasts	Not vectorially oriented
Osteoclast	Chick	Osteoclasts	Not vectorially oriented
Retina	Human, rat	Photoreceptors, ganglion cells, inner nuclear layer	Not vectorially oriented
Ciliary body, lens	Human, rat		Not vectorially oriented

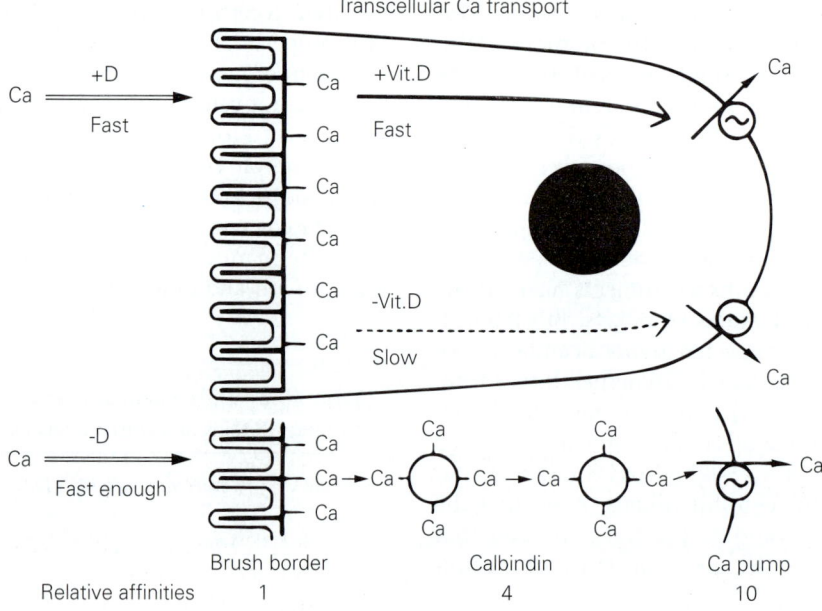

Figure 18.7 A model for vitamin D-induced calcium transport in an intestinal or distal tubular renal epithelial cell. In the absence of vitamin D (–D), the rate of calcium movement across the cell is slow due to diminished calbindin synthesis. The activity and amount of the basolateral membrane calcium pump are also low. In the presence of vitamin D movement of calcium across the cell is greatly enhanced by the synthesis of calbindin, synthesis of which is regulated by vitamin D. In addition, the amount of plasma membrane calcium as well as plasma membrane calcium pump activity is increased. In the lower panel the relative affinities of the brush border, calbindin and plasma membrane calcium pump and calcium are shown. (Reproduced, with permission, from Wasserman, R.H., Chandler, J.S., Meyer, S.A. *et al.* (1992) *J. Nutr.*, **122**, 662–71.)

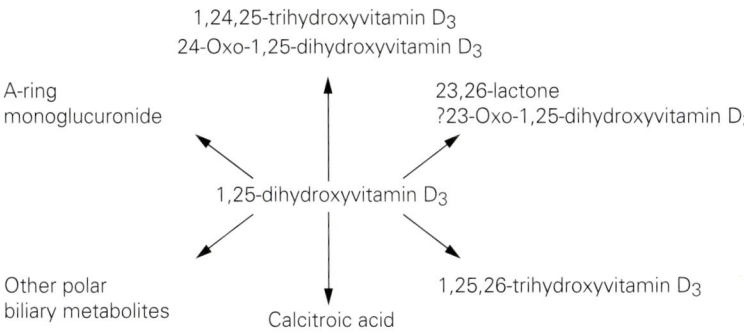

1,24,25-trihydroxyvitamin D₃
24-Oxo-1,25-dihydroxyvitamin D₃

A-ring
monoglucuronide

23,26-lactone
?23-Oxo-1,25-dihydroxyvitamin D₃

1,25-dihydroxyvitamin D₃

Other polar
biliary metabolites

Calcitroic acid

1,25,26-trihydroxyvitamin D₃

Figure 18.8 Metabolism of 1,25-dihydroxyvitamin D₃ to other metabolites of lesser biological potency. (Reproduced, with permission, from Kumar, R. (1990) *J. Am. Soc. Nephrol.*, **1**, 30–42.)

The metabolism of 1,25-dihydroxyvitamin D₃

Once 1,25-dihydroxyvitamin D₃ has brought about its various functions in cells it is metabolized to less active forms (Figures 18.8 and 18.9). Following administration of side-chain radiolabeled 1,25-dihydroxyvitamin D₃ to a human or animal, a majority of the radiolabel appears in the stool within a period of 5–7 days. This occurs as a result of the biliary excretion of various forms of 1,25-dihydroxyvitamin D₃. In general, biliary metabolites of 1,25-dihydroxyvitamin D₃ are more polar than the parent sterol and are charged or neutral molecules. Some of the secreted metabolites are monoglucuronides of 1,25-dihydroxyvitamin D₃; the biliary metabolites of the sterol undergo an enterohepatic circulation and are re-utilized. About 20–30% of the hormone is metabolized by side-chain oxidation in the liver and intestine to calcitroic acid, water and carbon dioxide. Other pathways of metabolism include 24-hydroxylation to 1,24,25-trihydroxyvitamin D₃. Lactonization of the side chain also occurs. It is important to remember that many of the

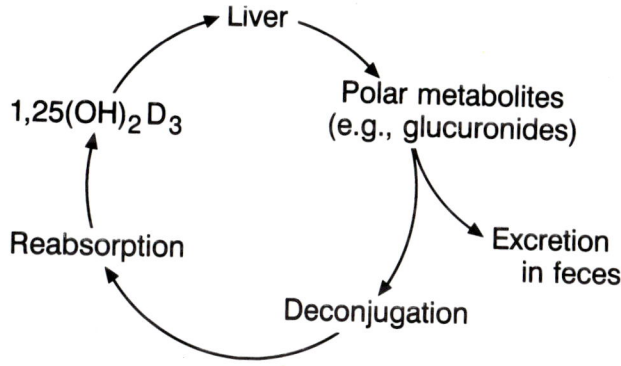

Liver

Polar metabolites
(e.g., glucuronides)

1,25(OH)₂D₃

Reabsorption

Excretion
in feces

Deconjugation

Figure 18.9 The enterohepatic recirculation of 1,25-dihydroxyvitamin D₃. (Reproduced, with permission, from Kumar, R. (1990) *J. Am. Soc. Nephrol.*, **1**, 30–42.)

metabolic processes that degrade 1,25-dihydroxyvitamin D₃ are induced by 1,25-dihydroxyvitamin D₃ itself. Thus, the amount of 1,25-dihydroxyvitamin D₃ in a target tissue is rapidly limited by the induction of degradative enzymes.

Further reading

Audran, M. and Kumar, R. (1985) The physiology and pathophysiology of vitamin D. *Mayo Clin. Proc.*, **60**, 851–66.

Audran, M., Gross, M. and Kumar, R. (1986) The physiology of the vitamin D endocrine system. *Semin. Nephrol.*, **6**, 4–20.

Darwish, H. and DeLuca, H.F. (1993) Vitamin D-regulated gene expression. *Crit. Rev. Eukaryot. Gene Expr.*, **3**, 89–116.

DeLuca, H.F. (1984) The metabolism, physiology, and function of vitamin D, in *Vitamin D. Basic and Clinical Aspects*. Martinus Nijhoff, Boston, pp. 1–68.

DeLuca, H.F. (1992) New concepts of vitamin D functions. *Ann. NY Acad. Sci.*, **669**, 59–68.

DeLuca, H.F., Krisinger, J. and Darwish, H. (1990) The vitamin D system: 1990. *Kidney Int.*, **29**, S2–8.

Gross, M. and Kumar, R. (1990) Physiology and biochemistry of vitamin D-dependent calcium binding proteins. *Am. J. Physiol.*, **259**, F195–209.

Johnson, J.A. and Kumar, R. (1994) Renal and intestinal calcium transport: roles of vitamin D and vitamin D-dependent calcium binding proteins. *Semin. Nephrol.*, **14**, 119–28.

Kumar, R. (1984) *Vitamin D. Basic and Clinical Aspects*. Martinus Nijhoff, Boston.

Kumar, R. (1990) Vitamin D metabolism and mechanisms of calcium transport. *J. Am. Soc. Nephrol.*, **1**, 30–42.

Kumar, R. (1991) Vitamin D and calcium transport. *Kidney Int.*, **40**, 1177–89.

Lowe, K.E., Maiyar, A.C. and Norman, A.W. (1992) Vitamin D-mediated gene expression. *Crit. Rev. Eukaryot. Gene Expr.*, **2**, 65–109.

Lowe, K.E. and Norman, A.W. (1992) Vitamin D and psoriasis. *Nutr. Rev.*, **50**, 138–42.

MacDonald, P.N., Dowd, D.R. and Haussler, M.R. (1994) New insight into the structure and functions of the vitamin D receptor. *Semin. Nephrol.*, **14**, 101–18.

McCarthy, J.T. and Kumar, R. (1986) Behavior of the vitamin D endocrine system in the development of renal osteodystrophy. *Semin. Nephrol.*, **6**, 21–30.

Norman, A.W. (1990) Intestinal calcium absorption: a vitamin D-hormone-mediated adaptive response. *Am. J. Clin. Nutr.*, **51**, 290–300.

Norman, A.W. (1992) Vitamin D research frontiers. *J. Cell. Biochem.*, **49**, 1–3.

Norman, A.W., Nemere, I., Zhou, L.X. *et al.* (1992) 1,25-(OH)2-vitamin D_3, a steroid hormone that produces biologic effects via both genomic and nongenomic pathways. *J. Steroid Biochem. Mol. Biol.*, **41**, 231–40.

Wasserman, R.H., Chandler, J.S., Meyer, S.A. *et al.* (1992) Intestinal calcium transport and calcium extrusion processes at the basolateral membrane. *J. Nutr.*, **122**, 662–71.

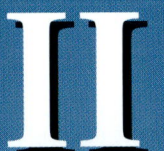

II

Impaired Renal Function

Section 1
Methods of
Assessment

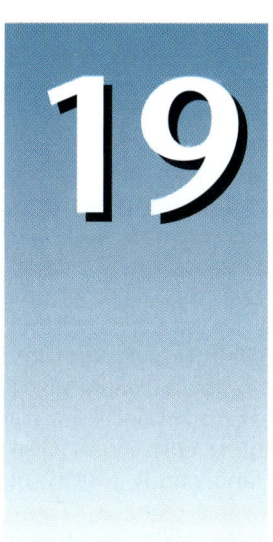

19

Initial investigation and general approach

David N.S. Kerr

Introduction

Experienced clinicians adopt rapid diagnostic pathways, relying on knowledge and experience to guide them quickly to the most relevant aspects of history and physical examination. Much of nephrology can be dealt with in this manner, e.g. the investigation of hematuria, nephrotic syndrome or renal calculi follows a fairly stereotyped pattern in which a full neurological examination seldom features.

However it is sometimes necessary to revert to the practices of internship when every patient merited a full history of current illness, a system review, family, drug and social history and a thorough examination of every body system. One of these occasions is the first encounter with a patient with impaired renal function. A comprehensive review is needed because future management will be influenced by the primary disease, the complications of chronic renal disease, coincidental disease, family support and social circumstances. Chapters 28–39 cover all the main body systems except the respiratory system and even this is often affected in chronic renal failure (CRF). More than half of all patients with CRF are diagnosed over the age of 60 [1] and in richer countries start dialysis after that age [2, 3]. Coincidental diseases such as chronic bronchitis, coronary artery disease, diverticulitis and arthritis are common at this age and may affect the choice of treatment and the prognosis. A growing proportion of patients starting dialysis are diabetics with multisystem disease – in the United States they contribute over a third of such patients [3]. These are cogent reasons

for preparing for the interview and allotting it sufficient time.

A full account of this first encounter, the follow-up visits and predialysis assessment is given elsewhere [4, 5]; this chapter focuses on the aspects of history and examination which help in assessing the degree of renal failure. The emphasis differs with different modes of presentation; two are discussed here: presentation with stable chronic renal impairment, and (briefly) presentation as an acute uremic emergency.

Presentation with stable/steadily progressive renal impairment

Introduction

Some patients with renal impairment attend the renal clinic because the referring doctor has found a slightly raised plasma urea and creatinine and seeks an explanation. It may prove to be functional (most commonly a side effect of diuretic therapy in the elderly) or evidence of chronic renal disease but in either case clinical features of chronic renal failure are typically absent. In Britain, many patients are sent later in their illness, for advice on the need for renal replacement therapy, typically with a glomerular filtration rate (GFR) of 30 ml/min or less, a stage at which symptoms of renal failure become prevalent. The following description addresses the latter group. The tasks of the nephrologist at this first visit are to:

Nephrology, Edited by Rex L. Jamison and Robert Wilkinson.
Published in 1997 by Chapman & Hall, London. ISBN 0 412 60930 4

1 Identify or confirm the primary disease and review its treatment;

2 Assess the patient's understanding of the disease and its prognosis;

3 Judge the degree of renal failure;

4 Detect and correct exacerbating factors;

5 Detect the complications of chronic renal impairment (Chapters 28–39);

6 Detect coincidental diseases;

7 Assess social circumstances;

8 Plan follow-up and management and explain these to the patient and relatives.

Before the consultation, all previous case records should be obtained and summarized in a draft problem list (Table 19.1). Patients are asked to bring with them all medications they are currently taking and their blood pressure record and other patient-held records, and warned that a urine sample will be requested on arrival. If they are known to be hypertensive or diabetic they should be warned that their pupils will be dilated and they should not drive home.

The history

Primary diagnosis

The history is directed first at the cause of chronic renal impairment if this has not been established. In some, the history will reveal a potential primary cause such as gout, renal stone disease, systemic lupus erythematosus (SLE), prostatic hyperplasia, cancer treated with nephrotoxic agents or abdominal irradiation, spinal injury or other neurological disease affecting bladder function, sickle cell disease or tuberculosis (the last particularly in the Asian community in Britain [6]). Clues that must be sought by direct questions include previous symptoms suggesting glomerulonephritis (hematuria, edema), urinary infection particularly in childhood, consumption of nephrotoxic drugs (e.g. analgesics, lithium, germanium, Chinese herbs), symptoms of bladder outflow obstruction, residence abroad in bilharzial areas and family history of renal disease in first or second degree relatives. If any form of inherited disease is suspected a family tree should be drawn and annotated to the limit of information available. Screening other members of the family is often informative but, where possible, a clinical geneticist should be consulted before embarking on it [7].

Assessing degree of renal impairment

The main measures of renal function during CRF employ biochemistry and nuclear medicine; these are discussed in Chapters 20 and 21. The days when patients had to earn a place on a dialysis program by enduring months of uremic symptoms have long passed; the aim is now to keep them free of symptoms and ensure that they start

---

Table 19.1 A problem list and brief case summary of a patient in chronic renal failure

Ms. A.T. Age 28

(Label showing hospital number, date of birth, address, telephone number and GP's address and telephone number)

1. Reflux nephropathy

    Urinary infections investigated age 2 at Hospital for Sick Children. Reflux and bilateral renal scarring on MCU and IVU. Recurrent UTI since – poor compliance with prophylactic co-trimoxazole. No subsequent imaging traced.

2. Chronic renal failure

    Serum creatinine normal until age 16 when lost to follow-up. Investigated for hypertension and proteinuria in pregnancy age 21; serum creatinine 140 µmol/l rising to 210 at delivery and climbing steadily since to 780 µmol/l 2 months ago.

3. Hypertension

    Persisted after pregnancy. Has taken antihypertensives since with erratic control. Currently controlled on captopril. ECG and chest Xray age 27 showed probably LVH (St Luke's Hospital, case number).

4. Allergic to sulphonamide

    Skin rash following co-trimoxazole age 15; skin tests suggested sulphonamide moiety responsible.

5. Social problems

    Single mother, unemployed, no support from father, on social security.

dialysis well nourished and with high morale. But a thorough review of symptoms at each visit is an essential safeguard because serum creatinine – much the most widely used measure of renal function – can seriously overestimate GFR, particularly in elderly and wasted patients. There is a remarkable paucity of published information on the incidence of symptoms and physical signs in patients approaching the need for dialysis in contrast to the plethora of information on symptoms during dialysis. The most comprehensive account is a retrospective study of the case records of 402 patients at the start of dialysis in Providence, RI, USA in 1969–83 [8]. There is no prospective study of symptoms at stages from mild chronic renal failure to end-stage disease so the following account is anecdotal, based on personal experience of patients in the predialysis clinic in Newcastle upon Tyne, 1963–83, and the renal clinic at Hammersmith Hospital 1984–96.

The symptoms have been divided into three groups: those that may occur early in CRF and are elicited to offer the patient reassurance and treatment; those that develop late in renal failure and alert the clinician to a more serious decline in GFR than the biochemistry suggests; and the 'red alert' symptoms which show that end stage is imminent and dialysis overdue. Table 19.2 summarizes the experience of Malangone *et al.* [8] and I comment where my own experience differs substantially from theirs.

Early symptoms

Muscle cramps are a very common complaint in patients on dialysis; the usual sites are the calves and insteps but they can affect other muscle groups, notably in the thighs, upper limbs and abdominal wall. They also occur earlier in CRF. Calf and foot cramps are common in the normal elderly population and are by no means rare in normal young adults but their first appearance during CRF is common enough to suggest a true association.

Raynaud's phenomenon is also common in CRF and in some of the primary diseases that cause it, e.g. hypertension, atherosclerosis, SLE and scleroderma. Doctors seeking evidence of peripheral neuropathy from CRF or causative diseases such as diabetes, amyloidosis and systemic vasculitis often ask 'do you get tingling in your fingers or toes?'. A positive response should lead to further questioning since it may indicate Raynaud's phenomenon, in which tingling is common particularly in the recovery phase, rather than neuropathy.

Later symptoms

Tiredness is one of the commonest complaints in CRF. It is often commented upon in retrospect when patients first start dialysis, because its insidious onset has escaped notice until it was partially relieved. Questioning should distinguish muscle weakness, breathlessness and lethargy which are sometimes confused by patients and may have

Table 19.2 Prevalence of symptoms and signs among patients starting dialysis in Providence, RI [8]

Symptom or sign	Prevalence (%)
Anorexia, nausea or vomiting	76
Fatigue, weakness	72
Pruritus	40
Lethargy	36
Peripheral edema	30
Dyspnea, orthopnea	26
Insomnia	14
Bleeding tendency	14
Pulmonary edema	13
Apathy, mental changes	12
Diarrhea	11
Asterixis, muscle twitching or cramps	11
Nocturia, polyuria	10
Dysgeusia	8
Headache	8
Visual abnormalities	4
Pericarditis	4
Fever	4
Cough	4
Constipation	3
Seizures	3
Hiccough	2
Restless legs syndrome	1

(Percentages have been rounded to nearest whole number).

different causes in CRF, though anemia may cause or exacerbate all three, as shown by their partial relief during treatment with erythropoietin [9, 10].

An important cause of tiredness which has been studied mainly in patients on dialysis is **sleep disturbance**. Diurnal sleepiness is particularly common and often associated with sleep apnea or disturbance of sleep by the restless legs syndrome [11, 12]. The spouse or partner should be asked specifically about snoring, apneic pauses, jerking and restless movements during sleep.

Restless legs syndrome is a characteristic feature of late CRF and a source of anxiety to patients who sometimes have difficulty in describing it; they may refer to it as discomfort or even pain in the legs. Articulate patients describe a peculiar sensation that builds up until it has to be relieved by moving the legs. In seriously uremic patients it can spread to involve the whole body, producing a state like bilateral hemiballismus; this was uncommon even in the days of late and inadequate dialysis and should never be seen now in a well run renal clinic. Restless legs syndrome has been much commoner in my experience than shown in Table 19.2 but often revealed only on direct questioning.

Myoclonic jerks often accompany the restless legs

syndrome, reawakening patients as they fall asleep. Both restless legs syndrome and myoclonic jerks are fairly common in the elderly with normal renal function, which limits their value as signs of uremia in this age group, but an increase in their severity should be taken seriously at any age.

Proximal muscle weakness, most noticeable when trying to climb stairs, step on to buses, or rise from the squatting position is a characteristic accompaniment of severe renal bone disease, whether osteomalacic, hyperparathyroid or aluminum-induced. All these diseases are preventable and it should be a rare symptom in the 1990s.

Pruritus is a common symptom in patients approaching end-stage renal failure and increases further after the start of dialysis [13]. Other common causes of itching, such as eczema and scabies [14], should be excluded. One of its causes is secondary hyperparathyroidism; itching may be centered on small calcium phosphate deposits in the skin which are palpable or visible but often affects skin of normal appearance, which also has a high concentration of calcium and magnesium phosphate [15]. A dramatic reduction in itching after parathyroidectomy has been reported [15, 16] but the effect is certainly not universal and itching is also common in the absence of severe hyperparathyroidism. It is frequently accompanied by a papular rash (Figure 19.1) excoriated by scratching (Figure 19.2). Other skin manifestations of renal failure are dryness (Figure 19.3), due to reduced sebum secretion; pigmentation in fair skinned races (Figure 19.4); and vitiligo. Pigmentation occurs late in chronic renal failure and affects only a small minority of patients if dialysis is started at the recommended time.

Growth retardation is almost universal in children with severe chronic renal failure and is greatest in those who develop renal failure below two years [17]. Height and weight charts are an essential part of the documentation of renal failure in childhood. A growth velocity chart is necessary to judge response to treatments such as calcitriol/alfacalcidiol or recombinant growth hormone.

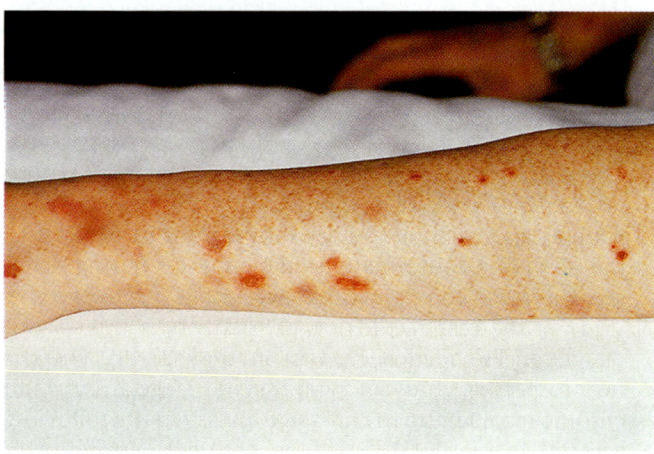

Figure 19.2 Excoriated papules with secondary infection in a woman with CRF who was a nasal *Staphylococcus aureus* carrier.

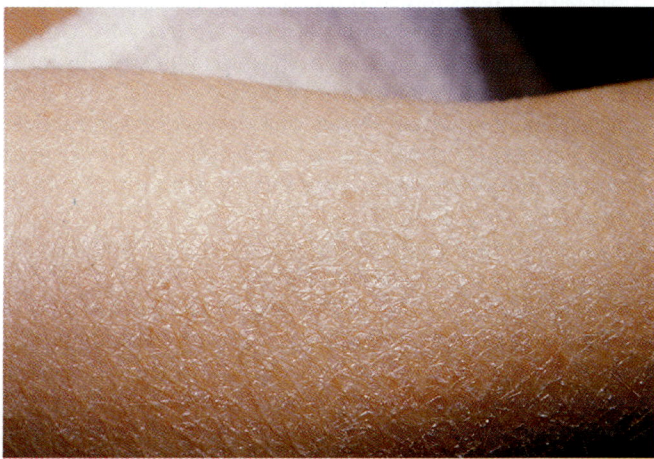

Figure 19.3 Dry scaly skin in CRF.

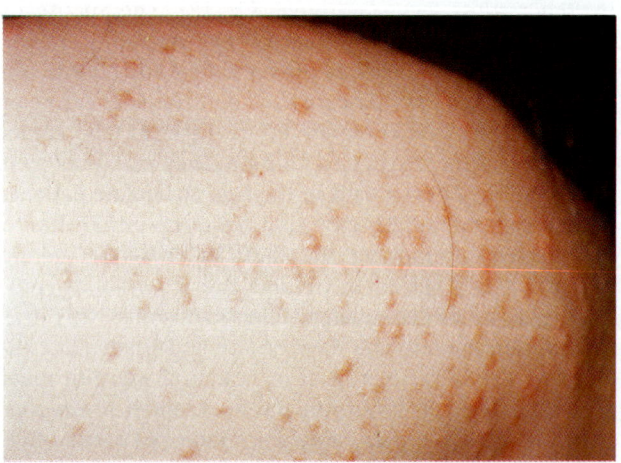

Figure 19.1 Papular rash on the shoulder of a man with CRF.

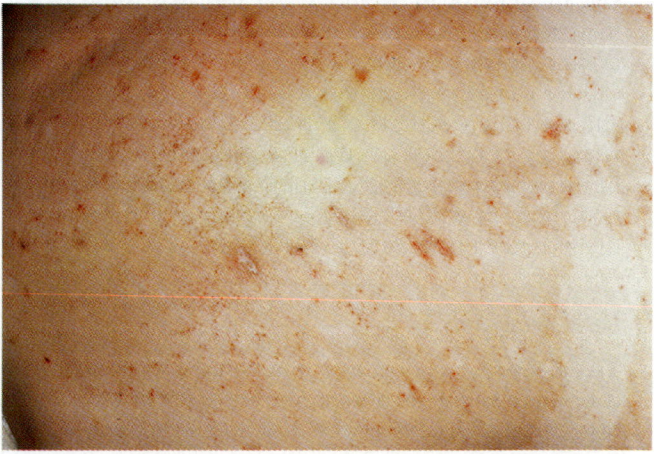

Figure 19.4 Pigmentation in light exposed areas of the back in a woman with CRF, also showing numerous scratch marks.

Bone age is retarded compared with chronological age and sexual maturation is delayed in children with CRF if it begins before puberty.

Sexual function in adults is disturbed very late in CRF. Patients seldom complain of it spontaneously which probably explains its absence from Table 19.2. Direct questioning is required at each visit in a tactful manner which does not precipitate psychological sexual dysfunction. Men complain of impotence and loss of libido. The former is nearly always organic and therefore accompanied by loss of spontaneous nocturnal erections. A review of drug therapy is essential since drugs which reduce potency are commonly given in CRF (e.g. beta-blockers, thiazides, methyl dopa, antidepressants, phenothiazines, cimetidine). Fertility is also depressed but not to the extent that it can be relied on as a contraceptive method. Loss of libido and potency are partly corrected by erythropoietin therapy so are presumably due in part to anemia [18]. In women fertility is reduced from quite early in CRF but conception has been reported in women with a GFR below 4 ml/min and on dialysis, so again it is not a substitute for contraceptive advice. Irregular periods, often anovulatory, are a feature of late CRF; this, coupled with the unreliability of urine tests for pregnancy in chronic renal failure, makes the early diagnosis of pregnancy difficult. Loss of libido is a common complaint which may again be partly due to anemia.

Fluid overload is an important complication of late CRF which, if not controlled by diet and diuretics, may precipitate the need for dialysis. The main complaints are ankle and leg edema and breathlessness. Blood pressure often rises with fluid retention.

Nocturia develops at varying levels of renal function depending on the primary disease; it is more prominent in diseases affecting the medulla such as reflux nephropathy than in glomerular disease but with substantial individual variation. Polyuria is often described as a feature of chronic renal failure but is in fact uncommon except when patients have been advised to drink extra fluid to help their renal disease; such advice is usually unwise except in calculous disease.

'Red alert' symptoms

Peripheral neuropathy, both sensory and motor, was described as a common feature of terminal renal failure and of inadequate dialysis in the 1960s; reduction of nerve conduction was used as a trigger for starting dialysis or increasing the 'dose'. Rapid progression of motor neuropathy to severe disability was well described but is now so rare that it is likely that in some of these cases drug toxicity was overlooked; nitrofurantoin was an important cause before the risk in patients with CRF was widely recognized. Although changes in nerve conduction and vibratory sensory perception can be detected in end-stage renal disease, symptoms and physical signs of neuropathy are now rare. When neuropathy occurs, sensory symptoms such as tingling usually precede muscle weakness. The development of clinical neuropathy, not explained by the primary disease or drug therapy, calls for an early start to intensive dialysis.

Autonomic neuropathy was also much studied in the 1960s and 1970s and regarded as a sensitive test for severity of uremia. Subclinical autonomic dysfunction can be detected by the Valsalva maneuver or ECG recordings but the symptoms are uncommon and difficult to disentangle from those of primary diseases such as diabetes and urinary obstruction and the other causes of sexual dysfunction. Consequently it is seldom useful as a 'red alert' symptom.

Cognitive impairment, confusion and coma were part of the terminal decline in the days before dialysis and transplantation. Deterioration in cognitive ability, judged by tests of verbal and performance IQ, is detectable in very late chronic renal failure and persists during dialysis [19], but seldom gives rise to spontaneous complaint. Direct questioning is necessary to elicit a history of reduced performance at work. Cognitive impairment is a particular problem in young children [20].

The onset of confusion calls for a review of drug therapy, particularly night time sedatives, the metabolites of which may cumulate to levels at which they can cause a sedative effect throughout the 24 h. Outbreaks and isolated cases of dialysis encephalopathy were described in the 1970s and early 1980s but have largely disappeared since aluminum was identified as the cause. Patients on conservative therapy can still be affected if they take aluminum hydroxide, particularly with other medications that enhance aluminum absorption such as sodium citrate [21]. The clinical features include dysarthria and dysphasia, apraxia, convulsions and progressive dementia. In the absence of these iatrogenic causes, confusion is an urgent indication for dialysis, which should be started slowly to avoid disequilibrium syndrome.

Anorexia, nausea and vomiting are among the best indicators that the time for dialysis is overdue, provided there is no other explanation, e.g. the peptic ulcer disease that is common in chronic renal failure. Taste disturbance is common in patients in CRF whether treated conservatively or by dialysis [22] and may contribute to anorexia. The taste threshold is raised for all four primary sensations (sweet, sour, bitter and salty); the threshold for salty is particularly high, which may explain why many patients with CRF have difficulty in sticking to a low salt diet.

Diarrhea due to uremic colitis was one of the terminal events in untreated CRF but is now rarely seen (my experience conflicts strongly with that in Table 19.2; perhaps the substantial differences between British and American diet are partly responsible). Many patients even in end-stage renal disease complain of constipation, made worse by medications such as calcium carbonate and aluminum hydroxide. If diarrhea develops suddenly other causes such as pseudomembranous colitis – endemic in some renal units – should be eliminated before blaming uremia.

Hiccough, often prolonged and exhausting, was a frequent occurrence in the last stages of untreated CRF. Its appearance today is an urgent reminder of the need to start dialysis.

Uremic pericarditis may present with pain, typically exacerbated by deep inspiration or movement and relieved by sitting forward, but is sometimes picked up by regular auscultation in asymptomatic patients. It is usually accompanied by an effusion which is readily detected by echocardiography but seldom diagnosed on physical signs until tamponade is imminent. A loud rub can coexist with a large effusion. Whenever pericarditis is suspected the patient should be tested for pulsus paradoxus. As the blood pressure is taken, the bag pressure is lowered very slowly across the appearance of the first Korotkoff sound while the patient is asked to breathe in and out. The pressures at which the sounds first appear only in expiration and first appear throughout the respiratory cycle are noted. The difference is referred to in jargon as 'X mm of paradox'; 5 mm of paradox is common in patients with a dilated left ventricle; 10 mm or more is strongly suggestive of tamponade.

Uremic pericarditis was known as the 'harbinger of death' since survival was measured in weeks after its onset. It is a sign that dialysis is well overdue and should be started with reduced heparin or by peritoneal dialysis because of the risk of hemorrhagic effusion.

Detecting exacerbating factors (acute-on-chronic renal failure)

These should be sought at the initial visit and at any subsequent stage when renal function falls faster than predicted by the reciprocal creatinine graph (see Chapter 20). The commonest are flare-ups in the primary disease, infections, uncontrolled hypertension, drugs and sodium and water depletion. Specific enquiry should be made about aspirin and other non-steroidal analgesics, diuretics, ACE inhibitors (which depress GFR in the presence of renal vascular disease or sodium depletion) and tetracyclines. Sodium and water overload is much commoner in CRF than depletion but the latter occurs in patients with a renal sodium leak or with diarrhea or vomiting. The first clue to its presence is normotension or hypotension with a postural drop in blood pressure which precedes the traditional signs of loss of tissue turgor, sunken orbits etc.

The duration of chronic renal failure

Knowing how long the patient has had chronic renal failure influences how far investigation should proceed to identify a primary cause. Knowing the primary disease is valuable even if it is not treatable since some diseases recur after renal transplant (Chapter 82) or call for family studies (Chapter 40). However, the hazards of renal biopsy increase, and the value of the information it provides decreases, when kidneys are scarred by long-standing disease (Chapter 22).

Clues that must be sought by direct questions include the results of blood pressure measurements and urine tests at previous medical examinations for life insurance, employment, military service, pregnancy, screening in general practice or hospital admissions. The onset of nocturia is a helpful clue though less valuable in the elderly and those with edema. Substantial growth retardation suggests prolonged chronic renal failure in children unless there is an alternative explanation such as corticosteroid therapy or psychosocial deprivation.

The physical examination

This should cover all body systems. The signs of primary diseases are discussed in other chapters. Points of special interest in CRF include the following.

General

Height and weight should be recorded along with weight before the illness. Height, weight and height velocity charts should be started for children.

Cardiovascular

Blood pressure should be measured supine and standing. Jugular venous pressure, presence of edema and crepitations at lung bases should be recorded. Site and nature of the apex beat should be noted since left ventricular hypertrophy adversely affects prognosis in CRF [23]. A mitral systolic murmur and less frequently an aortic diastolic murmur can develop in the presence of fluid overload and disappear after it is treated. All peripheral pulses should be palpated since peripheral vascular disease is another adverse prognostic feature and affects the siting of fistulas. Auscultation over the carotid, femoral and renal arteries should be performed.

Respiratory

Pulmonary edema and pleural effusions are common in end-stage renal failure if fluid balance and blood pressure are poorly controlled. If there is any history of asthma or bronchitis a peak flow measurement should be taken.

Abdominal

The kidney and liver are usually easily palpable in polycystic disease and enlarged kidneys may be felt in patients with obstruction. Signs of chronic liver disease should be sought in view of its high incidence in many countries and important influence on subsequent management. The scars of previous surgery and hernias should be noted as they may affect decisions about peritoneal dialysis.

Nervous system

Simple tests of cognitive function should be carried out if the history suggests a recent change. Hearing should be assessed clinically since it is affected by CRF and the changes are established before the start of dialysis [24]. Both low and high tones are affected [25] but the socially important range of 250–2000 Hz is relatively spared [24] so spontaneous complaint is uncommon. This mild deafness is independent of drug therapy since patients with a history of ototoxic drug therapy were excluded by Bazzi *et al.* [24] and Gatland *et al.* [25] found no association with drug therapy. However, all the cases of disabling deafness or/and vestibular damage arising during renal failure that I have encountered have dated from treatment with aminoglycosides, vancomycin or (rarely) erythromycin; a history of exposure to these and other ototoxic drugs should be recorded since their effects are cumulative.

In the peripheral nervous system touch, pain and position sense and reflexes should be recorded. A more sensitive measure of early neuropathy is vibratory sensory threshold but it requires equipment not routinely available in renal clinics so is not often used. Results should be compared with age-corrected norms since vibration sense deteriorates during aging. Proximal muscle strength should be tested. This is traditionally done by asking the patient to adopt the 'knees-full-bend' (squatting) position and stand up, three times. Even elderly subjects should be able to do this if they do not suffer from arthritis and are steadied by holding the observer's hands.

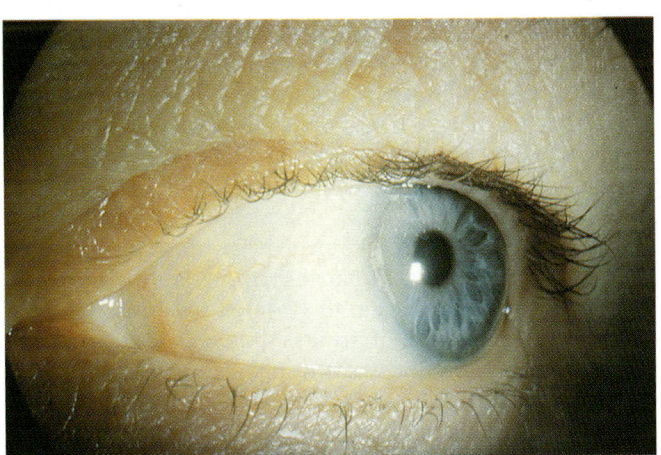

Figure 19.5 Corneal calcification, most pronounced (as usual) in the 3 and 9 o'clock positions in the limbus. White patches of conjunctival calcification can often be seen in patients with corneal calcification. Both are readily visualized with an ophthalmoscope using a +20 lens and approaching from the side or with a slit lamp. (Reproduced from Cassidy and Ter Wee (1997), with permission of authors and publisher.)

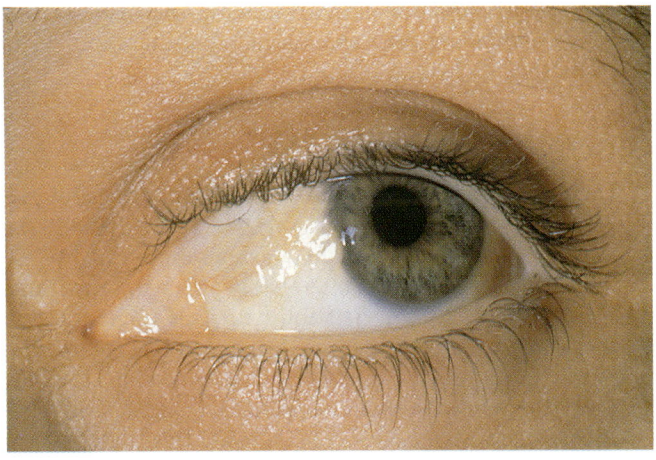

Figure 19.6 Pinguecula and surrounding increase in vascularity of the conjunctiva in a young man in CRF. (Reproduced from Cassidy and Ter Wee (1997), with permission of authors and publisher.)

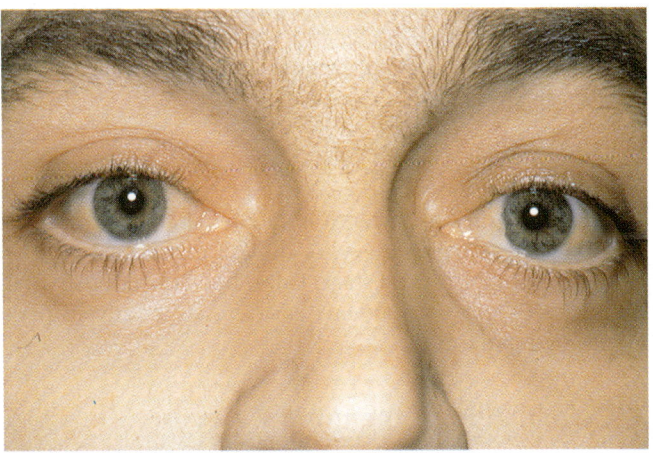

Figure 19.7 Uremic red eye caused by acute hypercalcemia in a patient in CRF. In this case hypercalcemia was caused by a combination of aluminum bone disease, vitamin D therapy, fracture and immobilization. (Reproduced from Cassidy and Ter Wee (1997), with permission of authors, publisher and patient.)

Eyes

Several of the eye signs in CRF are manifestations of secondary hyperparathyroidism and its treatment. They include corneal and conjunctival calcification (Figure 19.5), pingueculae (Figure 19.6) and uremic red eye (Figure 19.7) which is precipitated by acute hypercalcemia, usually due to vitamin D therapy. The lenses should be examined for cataract (usually coincidental or due to diabetes but occasionally complicating hypocalcemia in CRF) and posterior pole cataract caused by corticosteroid therapy for the primary disease. The fundi should be examined through dilated pupils; fundal examination through undilated pupils is unreliable, particularly in the elderly. The changes usually seen are those of hypertension, the primary disease (particularly diabetes) and aging (drusen, macular degeneration, glaucoma etc).

Skin and nails

The dry flaky skin, papular rash, scratch marks and pigmentation illustrated in Figures 19.1–19.4 should be sought. Changes are usually most pronounced on the forearms but the back is often badly affected. Brown nail arcs (Figure 19.8) and half-and-half nails (pigmentation spreading well down the nail bed) were once regarded as characteristic of CRF but are now seldom seen; like pigmentation elsewhere they were a feature of late and inadequate dialysis.

Endocrine system

Gynecomastia is another sign of CRF which is now rare. It was usually seen in the first few months of dialysis, possibly due to refeeding after the near starvation of conservative treatment in the 1960s and 1970s. Testicular size should be judged, preferably with an orchidometer. In children the signs of sexual maturation should be recorded.

Hematopoietic system

Anemia is almost universal in late renal failure [26] but a few patients with polycystic disease maintain a normal hemoglobin until end stage. Pallor has a notoriously high observer error until anemia is severe, especially in dark-skinned patients.

Examination of the urine

This is an extension of the physical examination. A fresh midstream urine sample is collected in a sterile disposable plastic or waxed cardboard container, and is divided into aliquots for dipstick testing, urine microscopy and culture. The more expensive dipsticks detect pH, specific gravity (SG), dextrose, ketones, protein, blood, bilirubin, urobilinogen, nitrite and leukocyte esterase. The functions of these tests in the context of CRF, and their important sources of error, are shown in Table 19.3. A more detailed account is given by Newall and Howell [27] and in promotional literature from suppliers of dipsticks. This is one of the most cost-effective laboratory tests but several precautions are needed and often overlooked.

Patients need careful instruction in **collecting midstream urine**. Uncircumcized males should retract the foreskin and wash the glans penis with a water or saline wipe (no antiseptic). Females should sit on the toilet with thighs widely abducted and flexed, should hold the labia apart with one hand and collect the urine sample with the other. It must be emphasized to both sexes that the sample is collected from a free flowing stream, not by stopping and restarting. The sample should be labeled with name, hospital number, date and time of collection; samples for culture should reach the laboratory within 2 h at room temperature. Patients sometimes bring samples from home in domestic containers (used jars, jugs etc., sterilized by boiling) which are too old for culture and produce a variety or artefacts on microscopy [28]. They are best discarded.

The test strips must be read at the times indicated on the bottle to avoid false negative or positive results. This is particularly important when testing for blood. Red–green colour-blind subjects should not be asked to read the strips.

Urine microscopy requires high standards of equipment and considerable skill. Minimum requirements are a good-quality binocular microscope with low (×10), medium (×20) and high (×40) objectives, variable illumination, a racking condenser and variable diaphragm. Highly desirable accessories are phase contrast and polarized light; the former needs expert maintenance. An oil-immersion (×80) lens is useful. Interference contrast microscopy, scanning electron microscopy and fluorescence microscopy of deposits stained with antibodies to components of casts, leukocytes and tubular cells are valuable research tools but rarely available in clinical practice. For a description of the equipment and these techniques see Birch *et al.* [28] and Fogazzi *et al.* [29]. With phase contrast a great deal of information can be obtained on an unstained urine deposit but if it is not available staining is strongly recommended. At Hammersmith Hospital we use the Kova system: a 10 ml aliquot of urine is spun at 3000 r.p.m. for about 5 min. A bulbous plastic pipette (the 'petter') is pushed down the tube to isolate the last 0.5 ml of urine and the supernatant is discarded. Two drops of Kova stain, resembling Sternheimer's, is added, the 20× concentrated urine and stain are mixed with the petter and run into the counting chambers of a disposable plastic slide with built-in coverslip and graduated area for quantitative counts. Its optic qualities are inferior to those of a glass slide and coverslip but its convenience more than compensates.

The main functions of urine microscopy, in the

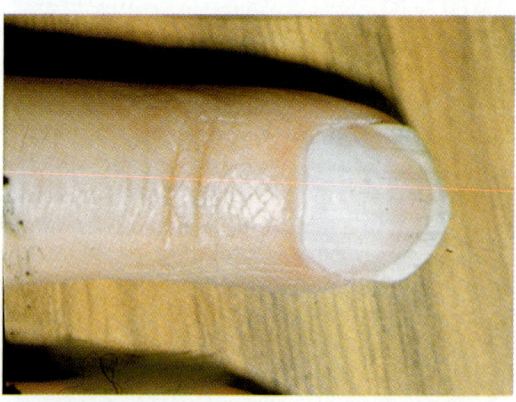

Figure 19.8 Brown nail arc in chronic renal failure.

Table 19.3 Relevance of urinalysis by dipstick to chronic renal failure

Test	Cautions	Importance in CRF
SG	Method actually measures ionic concentration but gives rough guide to SG[a]	Checking whether a sample is dilute or concentrated when interpreting other tests
pH	Requires fresh urine. Affected by highly concentrated urine[a]	Detecting infection by urea-splitting organisms. Monitoring compliance with low protein diet.
Protein	Does not detect light chains. False positive in alkaline urine	Rough quantification of proteinuria
Blood	Very sensitive. Positive with hemoglobinuria, myoglobinuria	Detecting hematuria
Dextrose	Also detects lactose, fructose and galactose	Detecting diabetes mellitus
Ketones		Detecting ketosis in diabetes and undernutrition
Bilirubin		Detecting coincidental liver disease
Urobilinogen	Difficult to read if bilirubin present	Detecting liver disease, hemolysis
Nitrite	Requires adequate nitrate excretion. Not all staphylococci give positive results. Therefore some false negatives	Detecting bacteriuria
Esterase	Positive if urine contaminated with vaginal leukocytes	Detecting pyuria

[a] Dipstick tests are not sufficiently accurate for testing urinary concentrating power or diagnosis of renal tubular acidosis.

context of CRF, are distinguishing between glomerular and subglomerular hematuria (Figures 19.9 and 19.10), establishing the cause of the CRF, following the activity of the disease and detecting urinary tract infection or the development of neoplasia, e.g. complicating analgesic nephropathy. The detailed procedure outlined above is required for all of these except the detection of urinary infection. Most nephrologists depend for this on the microscopy and culture performed in their microbiology laboratory. However, in symptomatic patients it is helpful to perform a very swift and simple urine microscopy in the clinic. A drop of uncentrifuged urine is examined under low power to detect vaginal squames (Figure 19.11) and other evidence of a poorly taken MSU and, with a coverslip, under high power to detect leukocytes and bacteria (Figure 19.12). In symptomatic infections both are usually visible in large numbers, making a confident diagnosis easy provided the MSU has been well collected. The presence of an epithelial tumor of the bladder, ureter or renal pelvis can be revealed by clumps of bizarre cells (Figure 19.13) but their absence does not exclude it. Triple early morning samples should be sent for cytology whenever there is a reason to suspect a neoplasm.

The main findings on microscopy that are useful in distinguishing between renal diseases are shown in Figures 19.14–19.20. The typical findings in some of the commoner causes of renal failure are summarized in Table 19.4. Much fuller accounts are given by Fogazzi et al. [29] and Birch et al. [28] which should be readily accessible wherever urine microscopy is performed. Even with the best available techniques, urine microscopy seldom provides a definitive diagnosis of the cause of CRF in the patient with stable CRF, small kidneys and modest proteinuria but it is particularly helpful in the uremic emergency discussed below.

Other investigations

The primary disease

A wide variety of tests may be required to identify the primary disease if it is not already known; these are discussed in other chapters. If the history, examination, urinalysis and microscopy have given no clear clues the starting point is often an ultrasound scan of the kidneys to show renal size, cortical thickness, local scars, high echogenicity indicating general scarring, stones, calcified papillae or obstruction (Chapter 21). If the kidneys are small and uniformly scarred and the disease is of long duration renal biopsy may be contraindicated or unhelpful and the diagnostic label 'chronic renal failure cause unknown' is attached.

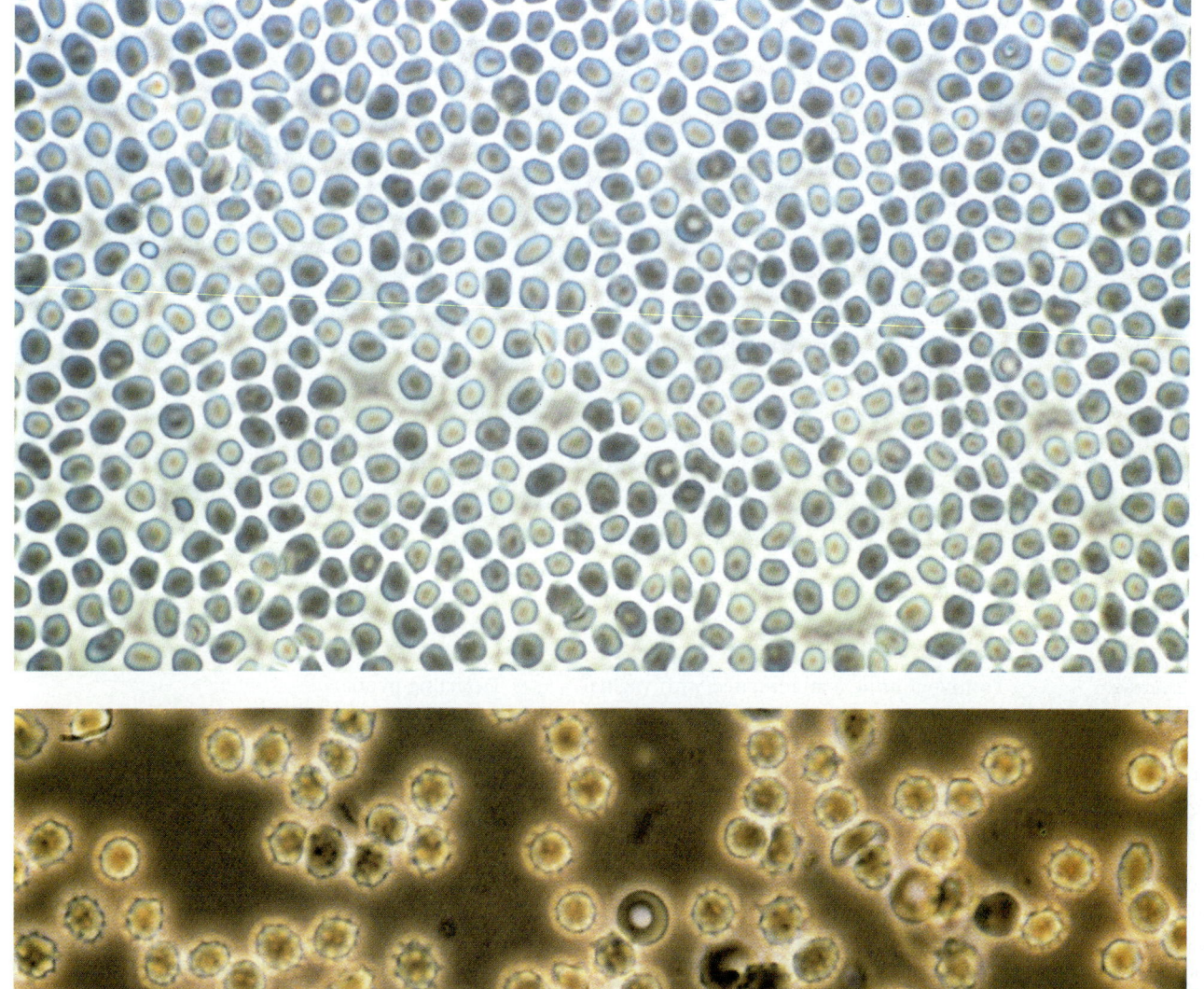

Figure 19.9 Two examples of non-glomerular hematuria: (a) uniform red cells of a single type; (b) uniform crenated hemoglobinized red cells with a few larger cells with less hemoglobin. (Phase contrast.) As red cells change shape or lyse, particularly in acid urine, two populations of cells may arise.

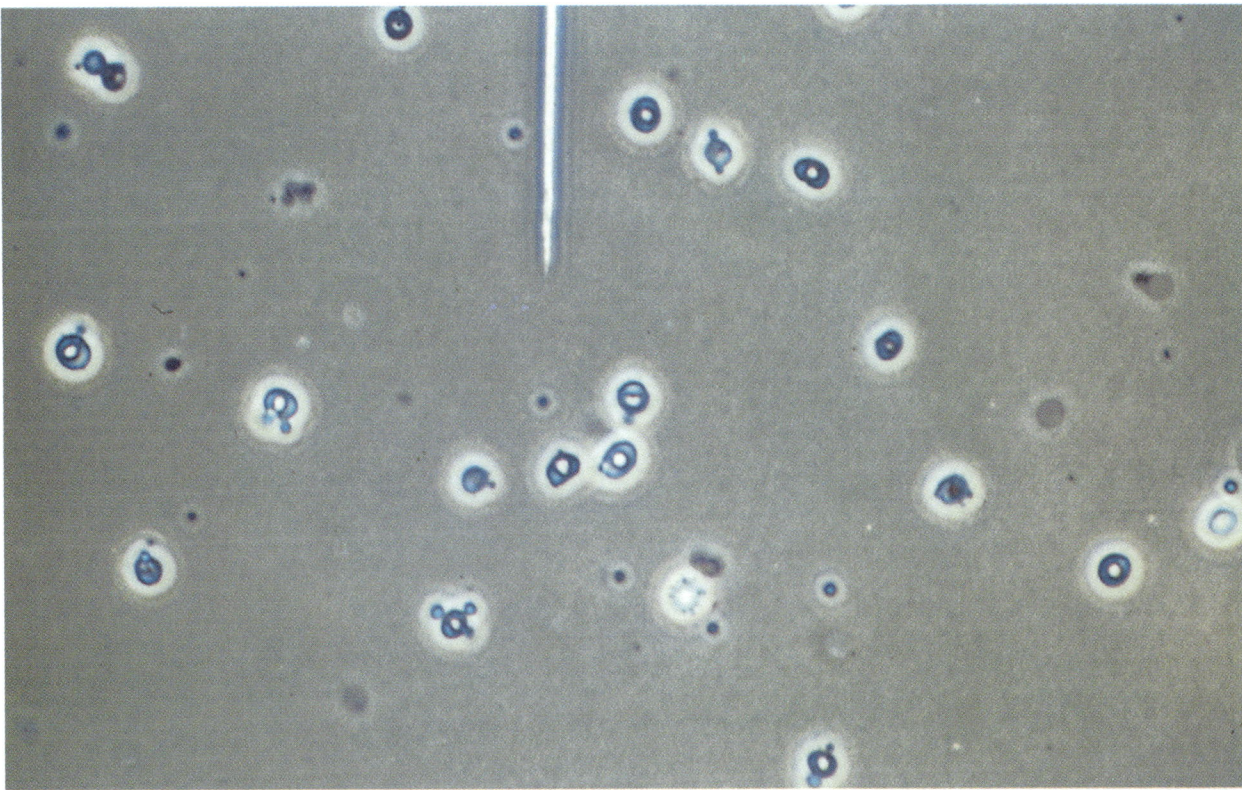

Figure 19.10 Glomerular hematuria. The variation in size and shape is brought out by phase contrast and much less obvious on bright field microscopy. Several different types of red cell are seen – normal hemoglobinized cells, cells with dense membranes (arrows), helmet cells and budding cells (acanthocytes); three or more types indicate glomerular hematuria.

Renal failure and its consequences

A fairly standard set of blood tests relevant to chronic renal failure is taken. The biochemical screen is usually carried out on a multichannel automatic analyzer. The tests are chosen for general hospital use but most of them are relevant to the patient with CRF; the Hammersmith screen is shown in Table 19.5. Additional blood tests that may be required include serum chloride (often slightly raised in early renal failure and helpful in assessing renal tubular acidosis), serum magnesium (usually normal or slightly raised in CRF but increased by medications containing magnesium or vitamin D therapy) and serum aluminum if aluminum-containing medications are taken (requires approved syringe, needle and tube to avoid contamination and should be sent to a laboratory expert in the analysis). Serum immunoreactive parathyroid hormone (iPTH) should be measured by a two-site (whole molecule) assay that is not affected by the accumulation of breakdown products of PTH. Serum prolactin should be measured if any of the drugs known to increase it is in use or if the patient complains of loss of libido or impotence or has gynecomastia; it is often raised in CRF. If malnutrition is suspected serum prealbumin and transferrin are useful adjuncts to serum albumin (Chapter 65).

Fasting serum total cholesterol, HDL cholesterol and triglycerides should be arranged at a subsequent visit if the patient has not come fasting.

If proteinuria beyond + is detected on dipstick a quantitative measure of proteinuria is required. This may be carried out on a 24 h collection in parallel with creatinine clearance (Chapter 20) or on an early morning sample on which the protein:creatinine ratio is measured (Chapter 28). The latter is more convenient for serial measurements. Urine should be sent for culture at the initial and subsequent visits if the patient has one of the diseases in which urinary tract infection is common, e.g. reflux nephropathy, analgesic nephropathy, calculous disease, polycystic kidneys and urinary obstruction. In other renal diseases culture is carried only in response to symptoms or findings on urine microscopy. Many laboratories carry out culture only if the microscopy is abnormal or culture is specifically requested by the clinician regardless of microscopy.

A full blood count is requested. The anemia of chronic renal failure is usually normochromic, normocytic and accompanied by a normal white cell count and differential leukocyte count and a normal or slightly reduced platelet count (Chapter 35); variations from this pattern call for further investigations (Table 19.6). Only moder-

Table 19.4 Typical findings on urine microscopy in major causes of progressive CRF or acute uremic emergency

Disease	RBCs	WBC	TC[a]			Casts		
			Hyaline	Granular	Tubule cell	Leukocyte	Red cell	Other
Acute tubular necrosis	+	+	++	++	+++			myoglobin/hemoglobin[c]
Crescentic nephritis[b]	++	++		++	++		++++	
SLE	++	+	++	++	++		occ–++	
IgA nephropathy	+++	+	++	++	+		occ–++	
Membranous GN	+	occ[d]	++	+++	occ		rarely	
Mesangioproliferative GN	++	+	++	+++	+		+–++	
Diabetic nephropathy	+	+	++	+++	occ		occ	
Reflux nephropathy	occ	++	+	+	occ	occ–+		
Obstructive uropathy	0	0	0	0	0	0		

[a] TC, tubular cells.
[b] Anti-GBM, Wegener's, systemic vasculitis etc.
[c] Hemoglobin casts indicate intravascular hemolysis, myoglobin casts, rhabdomyolysis.
[d] occ, occasional.
The pattern in each disease varies widely with the activity. This table assumes that there is no urinary infection and that obstruction is extrinsic.

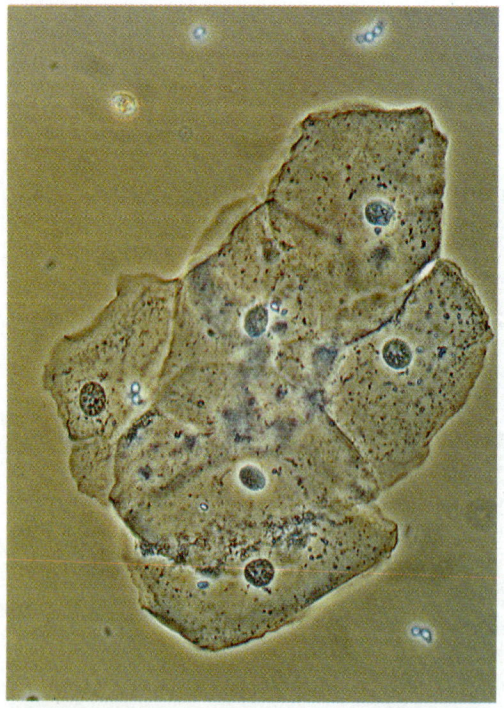

Figure 19.11 The number of squames in female urine varies with the menstrual cycle and is particularly high during pregnancy. Large numbers, accompanied by large bacilli and leukocytes suggest contamination with vaginal secretions.

ate doses of aluminum-containing medications are needed to cause a microcytic anemia [30] and resistance to erythropoietin therapy. Bleeding time is usually prolonged in late CRF but is measured only if there is a history of bleeding or easy bruising or if a procedure such as major surgery, renal or hepatic biopsy is required (Chapter 22). A coagulation screen is also carried out under these circumstances but more for medicolegal than clinical reasons since it is seldom abnormal. Blood is sent for grouping before renal biopsy and held ready for cross-matching until hematuria or other signs of bleeding have ceased.

Electrocardiography, chest radiography and echocardiography are usually carried out to assess left ventricular hypertrophy, systolic dysfunction, cardiac dilatation and coronary artery disease, all adverse prognostic features [23], in patients with hypertension or angina. Bone radiographs, initially of the hands, are taken if there is biochemical evidence of substantial hyperparathyroidism.

Tissue typing and identification of cytotoxic antibodies to HLA antigens are usually carried out during the predialysis work-up (Chapter 81).

Coincident disease

Blood should be tested for markers of hepatitis B and C and human immunodeficiency virus (HIV). For legal

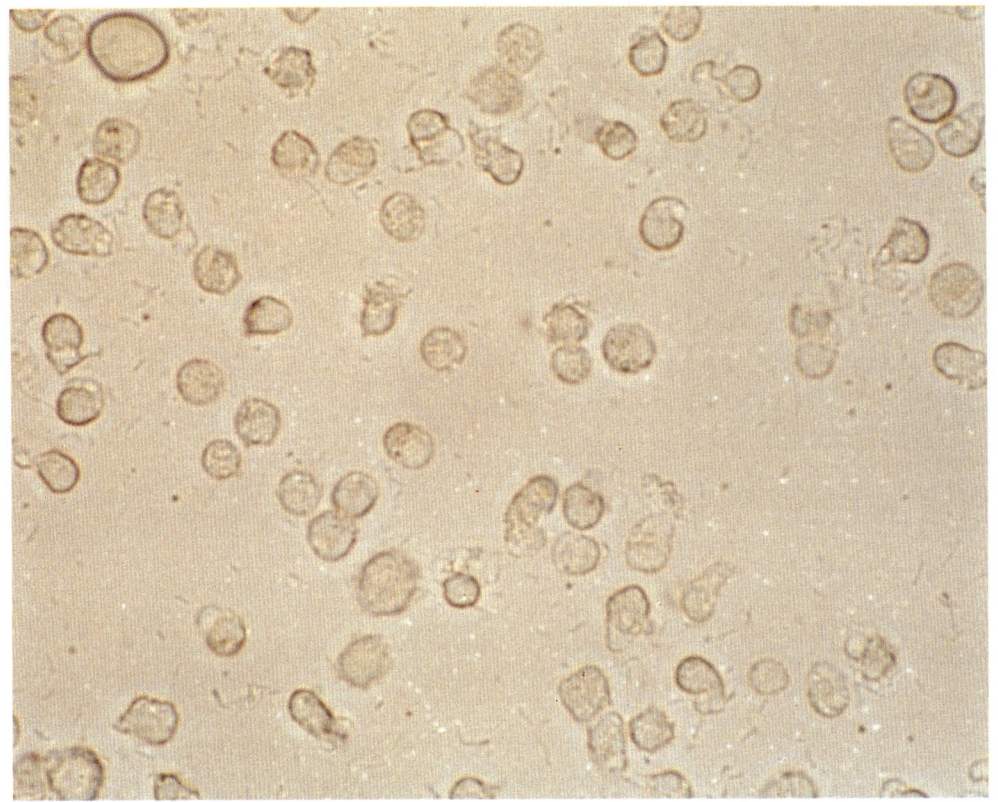

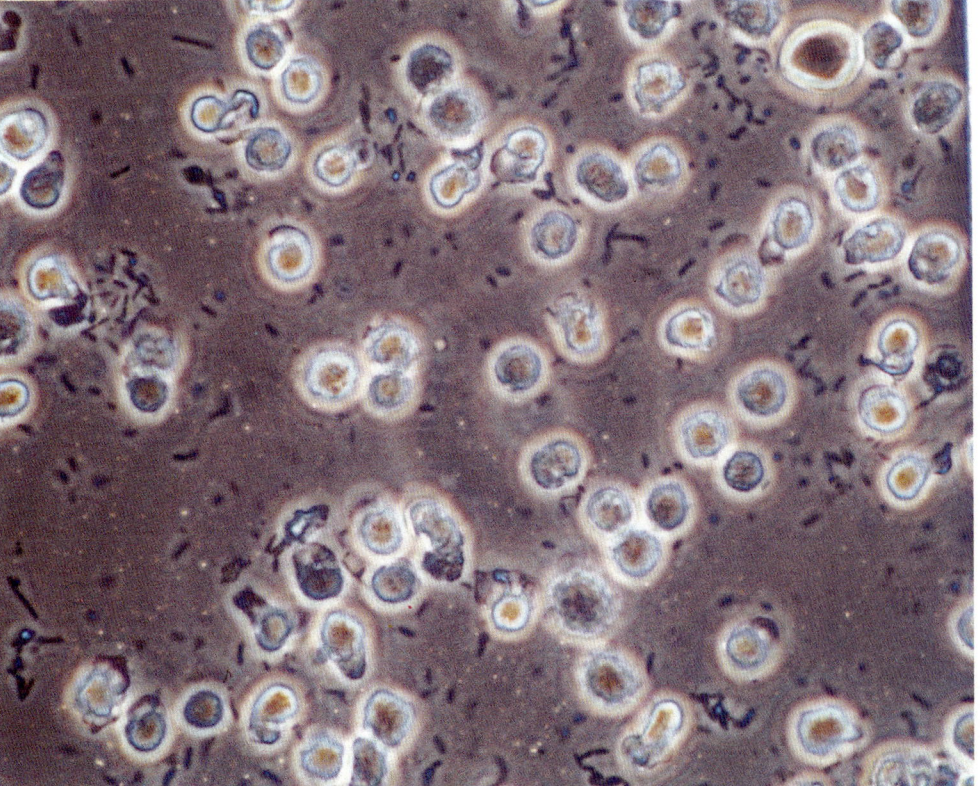

Figure 19.12   Urinary tract infection: leukocytes and bacilli seen faintly by bright field microscopy (a) and more distinctly by phase contrast (b).

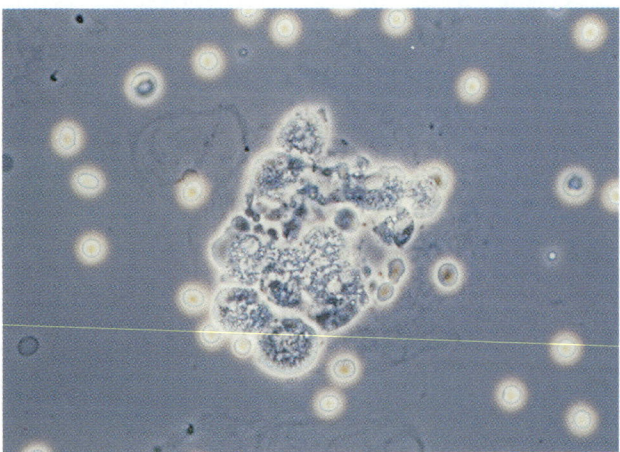

Figure 19.13 A clump of malignant cells in the urine deposit from a man with bladder epithelioma. Red blood cells are also visible. Phase contrast.

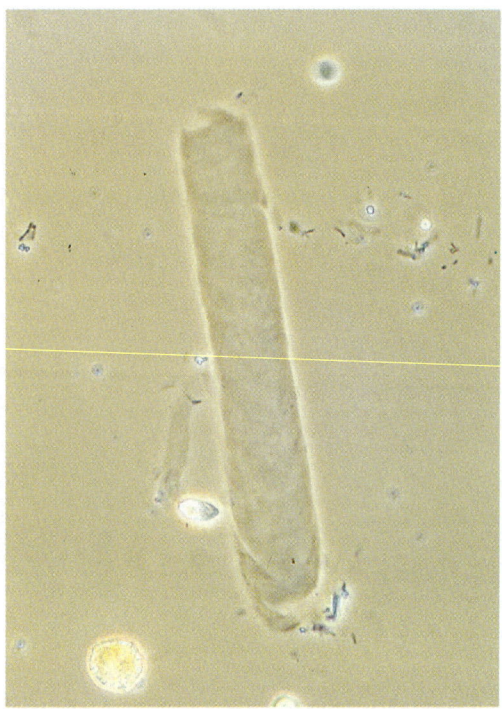

reasons patients must be counseled before these tests are carried out, though common sense might dictate otherwise in a country such as Britain where the carrier rate is about 1:1000 for HIV and 1 in 200 for hepatitis B or C. The minimum tests are HBsAg and HBsAb, a second-generation test for HCAb and a standard antibody test for HIV. Patients positive for HBsAg should also be tested for HBeAg and HBeAb and where possible those positive

Figure 19.14 A hyaline cast. Normal subjects excrete these is sufficient numbers to be seen on random microscopy after exercise or loop diuretics. They are common in essential hypertensives even after treatment and in many renal diseases.

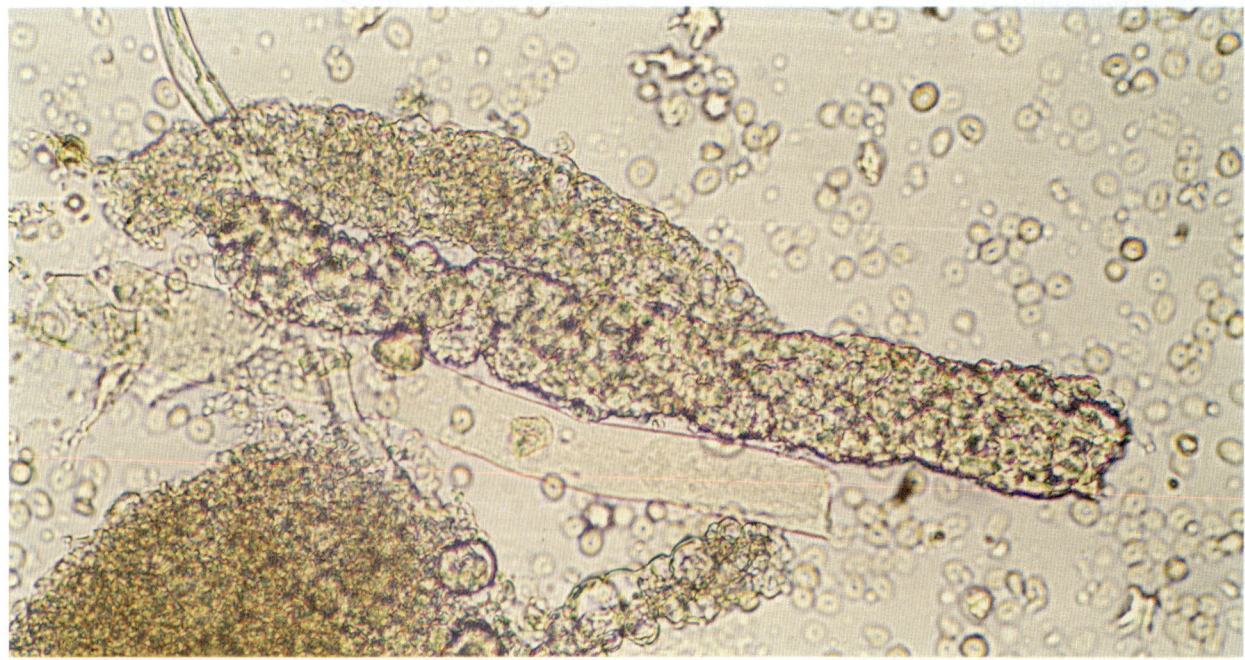

Figure 19.15 A finely granular cast (above), coarsely granular cast (middle) and waxy cast (below) with numerous red cells from a patient with mesangial IgA disease.

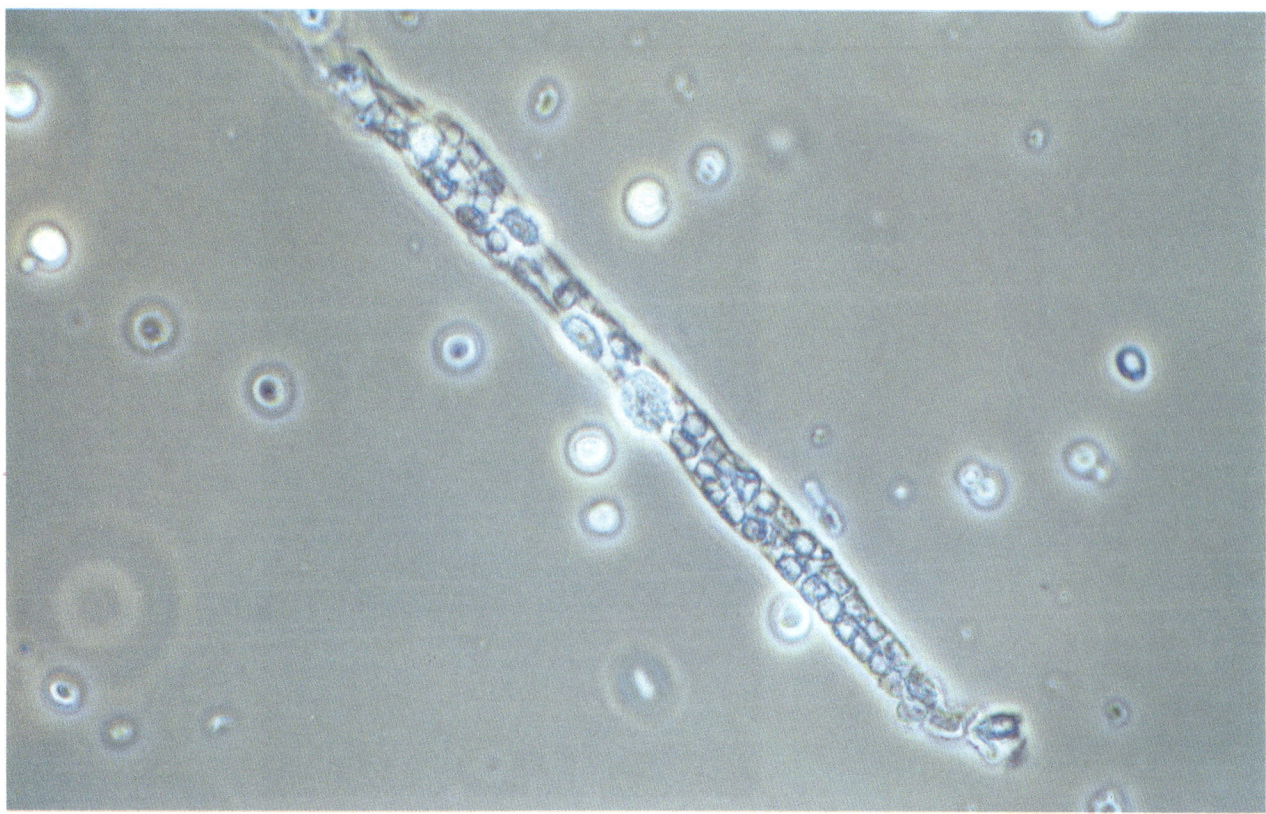

Figure 19.16 A long thin hyaline erythrocyte cast (red cell cast) under phase contrast. Red cell casts vary in size and the number of red cells entrapped and the matrix varies from scarcely visible to well defined, hyaline or granular.

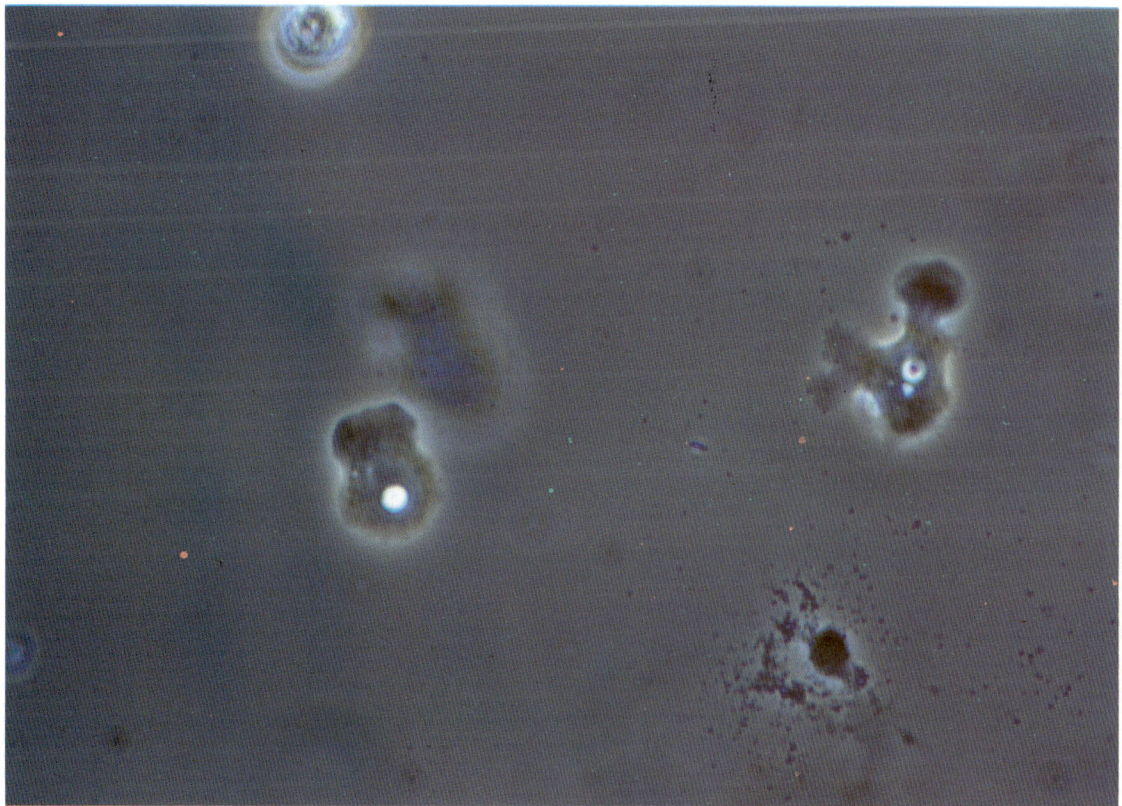

Figure 19.17 Polymorphonuclear leukocytes within a hyaline cast ('white cell cast'). White cell casts show the same variability as red cell casts. (Phase contrast ×1000.)

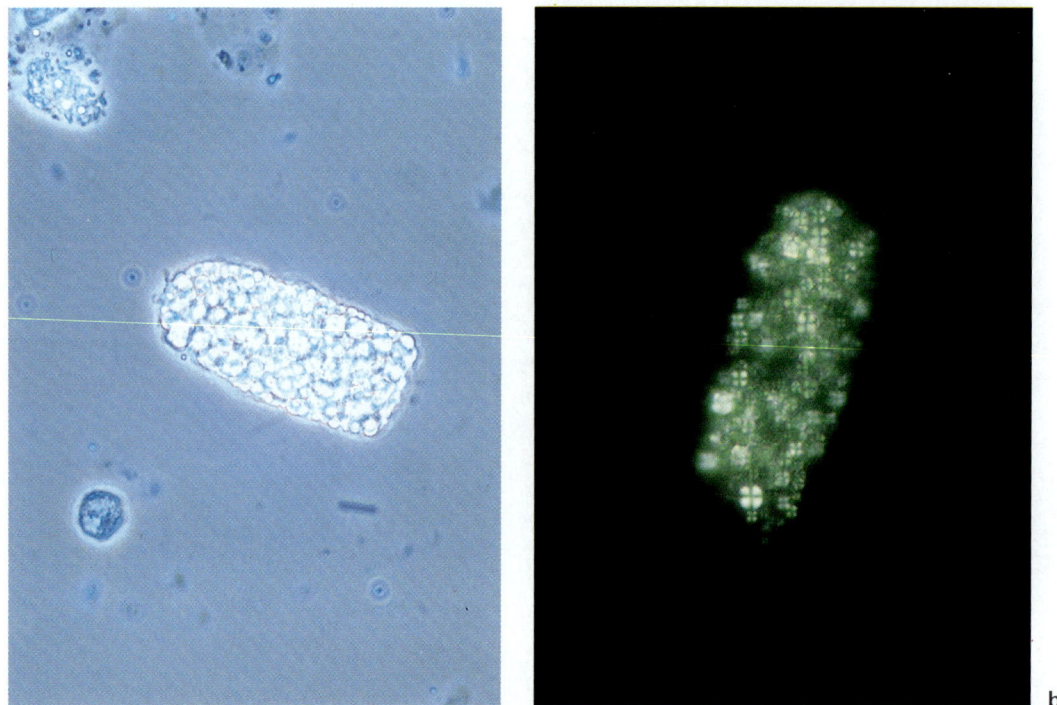

a   b

Figure 19.18 (a) Fatty cast (phase contrast ×400). (b) Under polarized light (×640), the fatty droplets are shown to contain cholesterol esters which give the Maltese cross appearance.

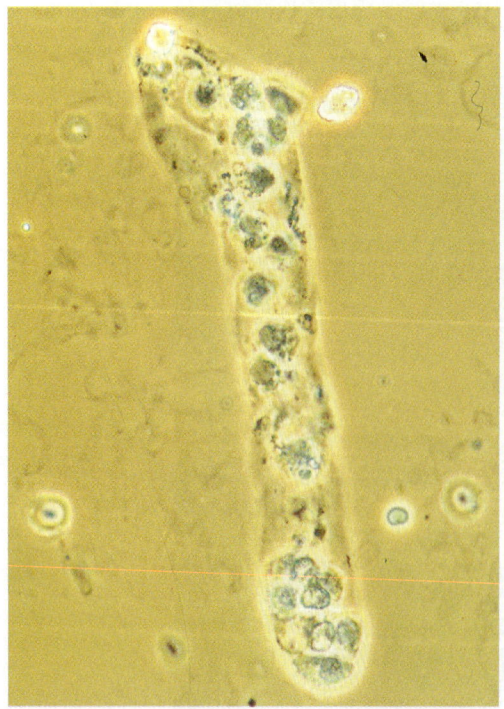

Figure 19.19 Hyaline cast with renal tubular cells ('cellular cast'). The tubular cells are often on the surface of the cast (shown by focusing up and down through the cast) in contrast to leukocyte casts. (Phase contrast ×400.)

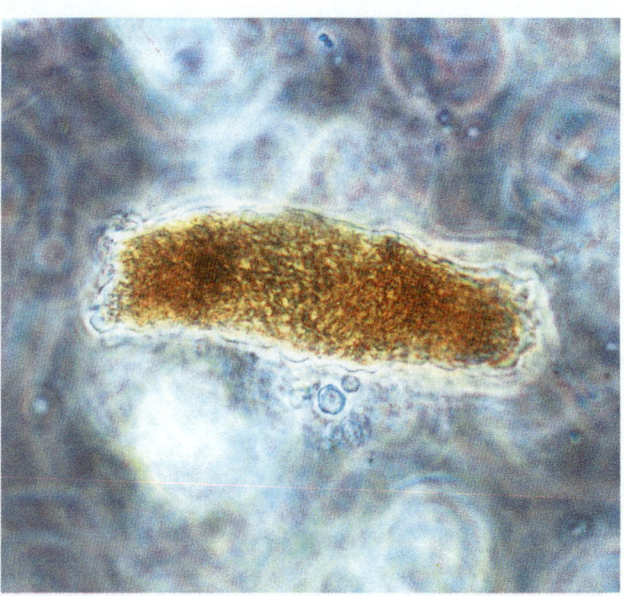

Figure 19.20 Myoglobin-stained granular casts may be seen in patients with acute tubular necrosis following rhabdomyolysis. The absence of dysmorphic erythrocytes in this sample was firm evidence against glomerulonephritis.

Table 19.5   Standard biochemical screen at Hammersmith Hospital. Relevance to CRF

Test	Relevance to CRF
Sodium	Usually normal. Changes reflect hydration/sodium balance
Potassium	Often raised in late CRF and earlier in CRF following stimuli such as high potassium intake, potassium-sparing diuretics, ACE inhibitors, transfusion, muscle relaxants and surgery
Bicarbonate	Falls during CRF, reflecting acidosis. Good measure of acidosis in absence of respiratory disease
Urea	Measure of renal failure and protein intake. Affected by fluid intake and liver disease
Creatinine	Standard measure of excretory function. Affected by muscle mass (and therefore by sex and age) and by increasing tubular secretion as CRF advances
Total protein	Difference from serum albumin gives rough measure of serum globulins
Albumin	Reflects urinary losses and protein intake. Falls in many chronic illnesses. Very strong predictor of prognosis in patients starting dialysis. Level affects binding of many drugs; important in a few, e.g. phenytoin, clofibrate
Calcium	Falls during CRF unless hyperparathyroidism becomes autonomous, when it may rise above normal
Phosphate	Usually normal in early CRF but rises through late CRF. Ca × P product is a guide to risk of metastatic calcification
Alkaline phosphatase (AP)	Normal in early CRF but may rise in late CRF due to an increase in intestinal AP, rising bone AP reflecting hyperparathyroidism or osteomalacia, or raised liver AP in liver disease. Reference range must be age related in under 18 year olds
Bilirubin	Detection of liver disease and hemolysis
Aspartate aminotransferase	Detection of liver disease
Urate	Moderately raised in CRF but seldom accompanied by gout

Statements about the usual behavior in CRF are based on refs 8 and 34.

Table 19.6   Further investigation of abnormalities in full blood count in chronic renal failure

Test	Abnormality	Further tests required
MCV and MCHC	Low	Serum iron, transferrin and ferritin for iron deficiency. If normal: serum aluminum, tests for abnormal Hb (thalassemia)
MCV	High	Reticulocytes and haptoglobins (for hemolysis). Serum folate and vitamin B_{12}
Platelets	Low	Look for other causes, e.g. drugs, hypersplenism, aplasia, before blaming uremia
WBC	Low	Look for other causes before blaming uremia
Platelets	High	Look first for iron deficiency, as above
WBC	High	If not due to corticosteroids, look for occult sepsis (CRP, gallium scan etc.)

for HCAb should be tested by polymerase chain reaction (PCR) for hepatitis C virus. Patients negative for HBsAg and HBsAb should be offered vaccination against hepatitis B and retested for HBsAb after the initial course of injections and, where necessary, additional injections and boosters. The results of these tests will influence subsequent treatment by dialysis and transplantation. Tests for antibodies to the cytomegalovirus (CMV) are usually taken closer to the start of dialysis since their main relevance is to transplantation.

Investigation of other coincidental diseases is carried out if not already completed before referral to the renal clinic.

Follow-up appointments

Division of labour and communication

Follow-up may be entirely at the renal clinic or shared with a general physician at a local hospital depending on geography and transport. In Britain all patients continue to receive care from their general practitioner (GP) who prescribes most of their drugs. In large cities individual specialties are increasingly concentrated in single hospitals so a renal patient may attend one hospital for renal disease and one or more others for special needs, e.g. the sickle cell clinic, ophthalmology, audiology or cardiac surgery. Good communication is essential but often lacking. Progress towards a national computerized database has been halted due to anxiety about confidentiality. Patient-held records are a partial solution and particularly helpful in the control of hypertension, providing a profile of recordings taken at various times of the day in relation to medication and with differing degrees of 'white coat hypertension' [31].

Interval between visits

This depends on the primary disease and the rate of decline of renal function, which are related. In a study of 80 patients at the Newcastle predialysis clinic the average rate of decline was 4–7 ml/min/year for patients with reflux nephropathy, polycystic disease and essential hypertension, 15 ml/min/year for glomerulonephritis but with a wide scatter in each disease (Figure 19.21). In view of this individual variation new patients should be followed at fairly close intervals initially until the rate of decline can be estimated. Thereafter, the most stable patients can be seen every three to six months, the interval widening even to one year after prolonged stability. If GFR is declining rapidly or unpredictably or if the treatment of hypertension, diabetes, fluid overload, renal bone disease etc. require close monitoring, monthly or more frequent visits are needed.

Symptoms, signs and tests

A duplicated check list of symptoms and signs recorded at each visit has been found to be very helpful. It includes the most important of the symptoms discussed above, e.g. tiredness, anorexia, nausea, vomiting, pruritus, restless legs, myoclonic jerks, chest pain, dyspnea, edema. Some parts of physical examination can also be included, e.g. weight, BP lying and standing, fundal examination, edema, jugular venous pressure (JVP), basal crepitations, heart sounds. If the check list form is generated in-house it can also include space for symptoms and signs relevant to the primary disease. A space for current medications is essential and should be filled in each time from the containers brought by the patient; changes generated by the patient, GP or others are common and frequently missed by questions such as 'Are your pills the same as last time?'

Tests may be required to monitor the primary disease, e.g. C3, C4 for SLE, C-reactive protein for systemic vas-

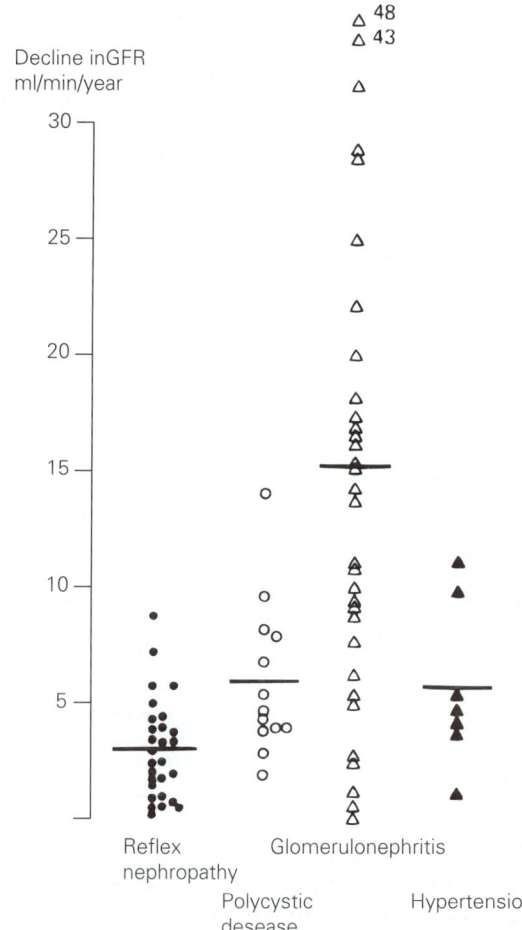

Figure 19.21 Rate of fall of GFR in ml/min/year (calculated from serial serum creatinine measurements) in patients followed in the Newcastle predialysis clinic. (Reproduced from ref. 35 with permission of the publisher.)

Table 19.7 Some primary diseases causing acute uremic emergencies which require urgent diagnosis and treatment: initial diagnostic pathways

Cause	Initial clues	Confirmatory tests
Urinary obstruction	Total anuria or 'benign' urinary deposit	Ultrasound of urinary tract
	Pelvic/rectal examination (for Ca cervix/rectum)	Straight radiograph for calculi
Retroperitoneal fibrosis	Backache, high ESR	Ultrasound for obstruction. CT scan for periaortitis
Goodpasture's syndrome	Urinary deposit	Serum anti-GBM antibodies
	Lung hemorrhage	Chest radiograph, CO diffusing capacity, sputum stain
Systemic vasculitis (including Wegener's/microscopic polyarteritis)	Urinary deposit	ANCA, chest radiograph, nasal biopsy
Accelerated hypertension	Fundal changes	Observe changes in urine deposit on lowering BP
Bilateral renal vascular disease	Age, atheroma elsewhere	Doppler ultrasound. Digital subtraction angiography
Acute pyelonephritis in diabetics, transplant recipients, patients with stones, analgesic nephropathy etc.	Urine deposit and culture	CT scan or MRI
Malakoplakia or xanthogranulomatous pyelonephritis (bilateral)	Urine deposit and culture	CT scan or MRI

Definitive confirmation of obstruction is usually by response to relief (nephrostomy, retrograde catheter, ureterolysis etc.). Final confirmation of most other conditions is renal biopsy once uremia has been corrected but treatment cannot always await the result.

culitis. For CRF the routine requirements are urinalysis with a dipstick; culture and quantitative proteinuria where indicated; standard biochemical screen and full blood count (Tables 19.5 and 19.6). Ideally serum iPTH should be measured regularly since it is a much more sensitive measure of hyperparathyroidism than is serum alkaline phosphatase, but expense and availability may limit its use. A 24h urinary urea excretion is measured to check compliance with a low protein diet, if prescribed.

Presentation as a uremic emergency

In some centers in inner cities a quarter or more patients with CRF present to the renal clinic in end-stage renal failure, often with no primary diagnosis. It may be necessary to initiate dialysis speedily and arrive at a primary diagnosis at leisure. However, it is essential to diagnose or exclude a few treatable causes of acute or rapid-onset renal failure for which treatment is only effective if started within hours or a few days. Some of these

are listed in Table 19.7 with the initial tests to establish or confirm the diagnosis after the thorough history, examination, urinalysis and microscopy outlined above.

A presumptive diagnosis of acute renal failure (ARF) can be made if there is an obvious cause such as recent trauma, crush injury, shock, antepartum hemorrhage, toxemia of pregnancy, exposure to nephrotoxic agents, etc. (Chapter 61). In the young and middle aged, return of renal function within four weeks is expected but in the elderly a substantial minority of patients with an initial diagnosis of ARF remain dialysis dependent [32]. Dialysis-dependent patients who present as uremic emergencies have a much higher mortality, particularly in the first three months, than those who are seen earlier in the illness. This higher mortality is partly explained by a number of risk factors associated with late presentation [33] but probably results in part from deprivation of proper management during renal failure. Late presentation at the renal clinic is sometimes unavoidable because patients present to their GP already in a terminal state; more often it is due to avoidable delays in the chain of referral.

References

1. Feest, T.G., Mistry, C.D., Grimes, D.S. and Mallick, N.P. (1990) Incidence of advanced renal failure and the need for renal replacement therapy. *Br. Med. J.*, **301**, 897–900.

2. Valderrábano, F., Jones, E.H.P. and Mallick, N.P. (1995) Report on management of renal failure in Europe, XXIV, 1993. *Nephrol. Dial. Transplant.*, **10**(suppl 5), 3.

3. USRDS (1995) *US Renal Data System Annual Data Report*. National Institutes of Health, Bethesda, p. 30.

4. Cassidy, M.J.D. and Kerr, D.N.S. (1992) The assessment of the patient with chronic renal insufficiency, in *Oxford Textbook of Clinical Nephrology* (eds S. Cameron, A.M. Davison, J-P. Grünfeld *et al.*), Oxford University Press, Oxford, pp. 1149–73.

5. Cassidy, M.J.D. and Ter Wee, P.M. (1997) The assessment and initial management of the patient with failing renal function, in *Oxford Textbook of Clinical Nephrology*, 2nd edn (eds J.S. Cameron, A.M. Davison, J-P. Grünfeld *et al.*), Oxford University Press, Oxford.

6. Lightstone, L., Rees, A.J., Tomson, C. *et al.* (1995) High incidence of end-stage renal disease in Indo-Asians in the UK. *Q. J. Med.*, **88**, 191–5.

7. Harris, R. and Williamson, P. (1996) Confidential enquiry into counselling for genetic disorders. A review of the aims and outcome. *J. R. Coll. Physicians Lond.*, **30**, 316–17.

8. Malangone, J.M., Abuelo, J.G., Pezzullo, J.C. *et al.* (1989) Clinical and laboratory features of patients with chronic renal disease at the start of dialysis. *Clin. Nephrol.*, **31**, 77–87.

9. Jacobs, C. (1995) Starting r-HuEPO in chronic renal failure: when, why, and how? *Nephrol. Dial. Transpl.*, **10**(suppl 2), 43–7.

10. Walls, J. (1995) Haemoglobin – is more better? *Nephrol. Dial. Transplant.*, **10**(suppl 2), 56–61.

11. Walker, S., Fine, A. and Kryger, M.H. (1995) Sleep complaints are common in a dialysis unit. *Am. J. Kidney Dis.*, **26**, 751–6.

12. Hallett, M., Burden, S., Stewart, D. *et al.* (1995) Sleep apnea in end-stage renal disease patients on hemodialysis and continuous ambulatory peritoneal dialysis. *Am. Soc. Artif. Intern. Organs. J.*, **41**, M435–4.

13. Ponticelli, C. and Bencini, P.L. (1992) Uremic pruritus: a review. *Nephron*, **60**, 1–5.

14. Lempert, K.D., Balts, P.S., Welton, W.A. and Whittier, F.C. (1985) Pseudo uremic pruritus: a scabies epidemic in a dialysis unit. *Am. J. Kidney Dis.*, **5**, 117–19.

15. Massry, S.G., Popovtzer, M.M., Cockburn, J.W. *et al.* (1968) Intractable pruritus as a manifestation of secondary hyperparathyroidism in uremia. Disappearance of itching after subtotal parathyroidectomy. *N. Engl. J. Med.*, **279**, 697–700.

16. Hampers, C.L., Katz, A.L., Wilson, R.E. and Merrill, J.P. (1968) Disappearance of uremic itching after subtotal parathyroidectomy. *N. Engl. J. Med.*, **279**, 695–7.

17. Karlberg, J., Schaefer, F., Hennicke, M. *et al.* and European Study Group for Nutritional Treatment of Chronic Renal Failure in Childhood (1996) Early age-dependent growth impairment in chronic renal failure. *Paediatr. Nephrol.*, **10**, 283–7.

18. Bommer, J., Kugel, M., Schwöbel, B. *et al.* (1990) Improved sexual function during recombinant human erythropoietin therapy. *Nephrol. Dial. Transplant.*, **5**, 204–7.

19. Baker, L.R.I., Brown, A.L., Byrne, J. *et al.* (1989) Head scan appearances and cognitive function in renal failure. *Clin. Nephrol.*, **32**, 242–8.

20. Hulstijn-Dirkmaat, G.M., Damhuis, I.H.W., Jetten, M.L.J. *et al.* (1995) The cognitive development of pre-school children treated for chronic renal failure. *Pediatr. Nephrol.*, **9**, 464–9.

21. Molitoris, B.A., Froment, D.H., MacKenzie, T.A. *et al.* (1989) Citrate: a major factor in the toxicity of orally administered aluminum compounds. *Kidney Int.*, **36**, 949–53.

22. Fornari, A.J. and Avram, M.M. (1978) Altered taste perception in uremia. *Trans. Am. Soc. Artif. Intern. Organs*, **29**, 385–7.

23. Harnett, J.D., Kew, G.M., Foley, R.P., Parfey, P.S. (1995) Cardiac function and hematocrit. *Am. J. Kidney Dis.*, **25**(suppl 1), 53–7.

24. Bazzi, C., Venturini, C.T., Pagani, G. and D'Amico, G. (1995) Hearing loss in short- and long-term haemodialysed patients. *Nephrol. Dial. Transplant.*, **10**, 1865–8.

25. Gatland, D., Tucker, B., Chalstrey, S. *et al.* (1991) Hearing loss in chronic renal failure: hearing threshold changes following haemodialysis. *J. R. Soc. Med.*, **84**, 587–9.

26. Kerr, D.N.S., Poon, T.F-H. and Rodger, R.S.C. (1983) The Lumleian Lecture: uraemia, in *Advanced Medicine*, vol. 19 (ed. K.B. Saunders), Pitman, Bath, pp. 384–411.

27. Newall, R.G. and Howell, R. (1990) *Clinical Urinalysis*. Ames Division, Miles Laboratories. (Available from Bayer Diagnostics.)

28. Birch, D.F., Fairley, K.F., Becker, G.J. and Kincaid-Smith, P. (1994) *A Colour Atlas of Urine Microscopy*. Chapman & Hall, London.

29. Fogazzi, G.B., Passerini, P., Ponticelli, C. and Ritz, E. (1994) *The Urinary Sediment. An Integrated View*. Chapman & Hall, London.

30. Lin, J-L., Kou, M-T. and Leu, M-L. (1996) Effect of long term low dose aluminium-containing agents on hemoglobin synthesis in patients with chronic renal insufficiency. *Nephron*, **74**, 33–8.

31. Ezedum, S. and Kerr, D.N.S. (1977) Collaborative care of hypertensives, using a shared record. *Br. Med. J.*, **2**, 1402–3.

32. Bhandari, S. and Turney, J.H. (1996) Survivors of acute renal failure who do not recover renal function. *Q. J. Med.*, **89**, 415–21.

33. Khan, I.H., Catto, G.R.D., Edward, N. and MacLeod, A.M. (1995) Death during the first 90 days of dialysis: a case control study. *Am. J. Kidney Dis.*, **25**, 276–80.

34. Kerr, D.N.S. (1979) Chronic renal failure, in *Cecil Textbook of Medicine*, 15th edn (eds P. Beeson, W. McDermott and J.P. Wyngaarden), W.B. Saunders Company, Philadelphia, pp. 1351–67.

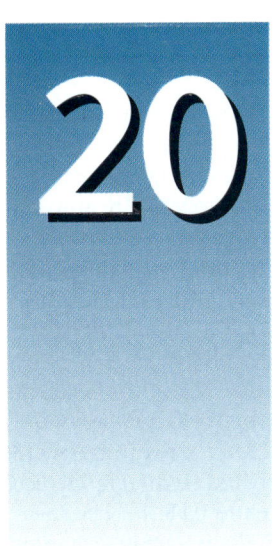

20

Laboratory evaluation of renal function

Richard A. Lafayette, Jeffrey Petersen and Andrew S. Levey

Introduction

The kidney plays a major role in the maintenance of homeostasis. It regulates extracellular fluid volume and composition, produces and catabolizes hormones and regulates acid–base balance. It has the capacity to adapt to wide variations in intake and extrarenal loss of fluid and electrolytes. In view of this central role of the kidney in health and disease, it is important to assess certain aspects of renal function. This chapter focuses on the laboratory evaluation of selected areas of renal function that are of greatest importance in the clinical practice of medicine.

Glomerular filtration

The clearance of inulin, a fructose polymer, remains the gold standard for the measurement of glomerular filtration rate (GFR) [1–4]. Inulin is an ideal filtration marker as it is: (1) freely filtered by the glomerulus; (2) neither secreted nor reabsorbed by the tubules; and (3) inert and does not affect kidney function. However, inulin is an exogenous substance which must be infused in order to achieve serum levels. This makes its routine use as a marker of filtration rather cumbersome. Therefore, the most popular methods in clinical practice for the assessment of GFR are steady-state plasma levels or renal clearance of endogenous compounds, such as creatinine or urea.

Normal GFR

The GFR is remarkably constant when measured repeatedly in a single individual but interindividual variation is quite large, and normal values show considerable spread. Values are typically adjusted for body size (surface area) and compared to normative values for age and gender [5]. A compilation of inulin clearance measurements in young adults (adjusted to a standard body surface area of $1.73\,m^2$) shows the mean value in men to be $131\,ml/min$ and in women $120\,ml/min$. An approximate age-related decline in GFR or $10\,ml/min/1.73\,m^2$ per decade occurs after the age of 30 years [6–7].

Creatinine clearance

The use of creatinine clearance (Ccr) as an index of GFR rests on the assumption that creatinine is an ideal filtration marker, hence Ccr equals GFR. Therefore,

$$GFR = Ccr = \frac{Ucr \times V}{Pcr} \qquad (20.1)$$

where Ucr is urinary creatinine concentration and V the urine flow rate, so that Ucr $\times$ V is the urinary excretion rate of creatinine, and Pcr is the plasma concentration. Ths use of serum (or plasma) creatinine as an index of GFR is based on the additional assumption that the creatinine generation rate (Gcr) is constant. Under these conditions, the serum level (Pcr) is inversely related to GFR, as follows:

Nephrology, Edited by Rex L. Jamison and Robert Wilkinson.
Published in 1997 by Chapman & Hall, London. ISBN 0 412 60930 4

$$Pcr = \frac{Gcr}{GFR} = \frac{Ucr \times V}{GFR} \qquad (20.2)$$

The normal level of GFR (range 80–140 ml/min) is sufficient to maintain a low concentration of creatinine in serum, approximately 0.8–1.2 mg/dl. A fall in GFR would be required to raise serum creatinine from the normal to the elevated range because of the above reciprocal relationship. This relationship can be described as a curve (Figure 20.1) in which each decrement in GFR is reflected by a proportionately greater increment in serum creatinine. Expression of the serum creatinine level as its reciprocal (1/Pcr) more clearly reflects the decline in GFR.

A more accurate expression of the relationship between Ccr and GFR takes into account tubular secretion of creatinine (TScr):

$$Ucr \times V = GFR \times Pcr + TScr \qquad (20.3)$$

Then GFR is as follows:

$$GFR = Ccr - \frac{TScr}{Pcr} \qquad (20.4)$$

where TScr/Pcr is the clearance of creatinine due to tubular secretion. Ccr therefore tends to exceed GFR by an amount equal to the excretion of creatinine due to tubular secretion. However, in the most widely used method for the measurement of plasma creatinine (the Jaffe reaction), non-creatinine chromogens are not distinguished from creatinine, leading to an overestimate of plasma creatinine and therefore an underestimate of GFR. These two errors tend to balance each other and it is only at low levels of GFR, when tubular secretion is increased, that Ccr significantly overestimates GFR.

In normal individuals, creatinine secretion accounts for 5–10% of excreted creatinine, hence Ccr exceeds GFR by approximately 10 ml/min/1.73 m^2. Creatinine secretion is enhanced in patients with reduced GFR, leading to a greater disparity between Ccr and GFR [8]. The mean difference between Ccr and GFR is greatest (about 35 ml/min/1.73 m^2) within the range of GFR from 40–80 ml/min/1.73 m^2. Other factors determining the magnitude of creatinine secretion are the type of renal disease and the quantity of dietary protein intake. Patients with polycystic kidney disease and tubulointerstitial diseases have less tubular secretion of creatinine than patients with glomerular and other renal diseases [9].

Several common medications, including cimetidine [10] and trimethoprim [11], competitively inhibit creatinine secretion, thereby reducing Ccr and raising the serum creatinine concentration, without changing GFR. A clue to inhibition of creatinine secretion is that urea clearance and blood urea nitrogen concentration remain normal despite a rise in serum creatinine. Creatinine may also be reabsorbed by the tubules when there is a very low urine flow rate [12–14]. Based on the clearance ratios observed in these studies, the maximum effect of creatinine reabsorption is a 5–10% decrease in Ccr.

The Ccr is generally calculated from a 24 h urine collection for creatinine and single measurement of serum creatinine, assuming a steady state. The most common strategies are to measure serum creatinine at the midpoint of the urine collection or at the beginning and end of the urine collection and average the results. The commonest error in calculating Ccr is undercollection of the 24 h specimen. Creatinine generation is proportional to muscle mass, which can be estimated from age, gender and body size. Walser [15] derived the following equations which can be used to verify the adequacy of the urine collection:

$$Ucr \times V = 28.2 - 0.172 \times age \; (men) \qquad (20.5)$$

$$Ucr \times V = 21.9 - 0.115 \times age \; (women) \qquad (20.6)$$

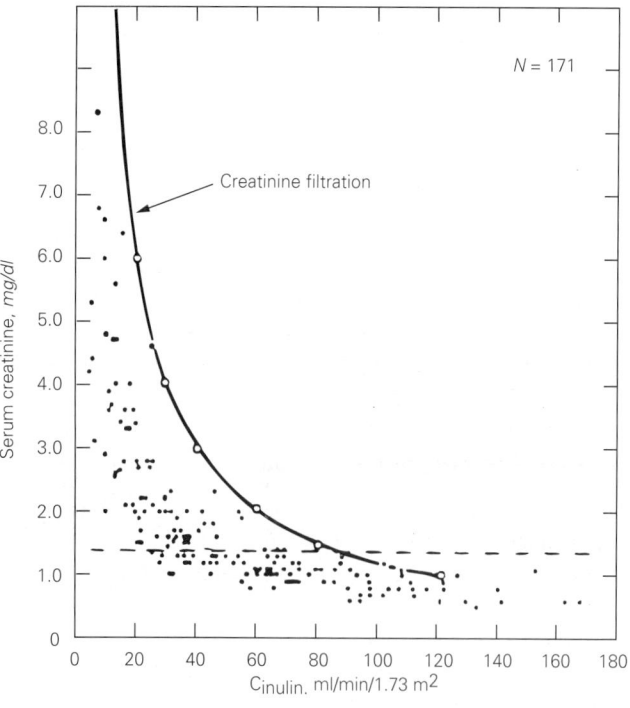

Figure 20.1 Serum creatinine levels vs GFR. The open circles joined by a continuous line represent the hypothetical relationship between GFR and serum creatinine. The broken horizontal line respresents the upper limit of normal for serum creatinine in our laboratory. Substantial numbers of patients have 'normal' values with abnormal GFRs. (Reprinted, with permission, from ref. 15.)

where creatinine excretion (mg/kg/day) is assumed to equal creatinine generation and age is given in years. These equations may not be accurate in patients with muscle wasting or in patients on a low protein diet. In addition, although extrarenal loss of creatinine is not detectable in normal individuals, it may account for up to two-thirds of daily creatinine excretion in patients with severe renal insufficiency [16–18].

Serum creatinine

Because of difficulties in obtaining accurately timed and complete urine collections, the serum creatinine concentration alone is commonly used to assess GFR. The true relationship between serum creatinine and GFR is considerably more complicated than expressed in (20.2). Expanding equation (20.4) by including consideration of extrarenal elimination of creatinine (Ecr) results in the following:

$$Pcr = \frac{(Gcr - Ecr - TScr)}{GFR} \qquad (20.7)$$

Thus, the serum creatinine concentration is indeed inversely proportional to GFR, but is also affected by the generation rate (Gcr), extrarenal elimination (Ecr) and tubular secretion of creatinine (TScr). None the less, an elevated serum creatinine usually indicates a reduced level of GFR. However, a normal serum creatinine does not exclude the possibility of a reduced GFR. The rate of creatinine generation is lower in women, children, the elderly, malnourished individuals, those with reduced muscle bulk due to conditions such as poliomyelitis, and those with restricted meat intake. Hence, at any given GFR, serum creatinine is lower in these groups and serum creatinine may remain within the normal range despite a reduction in GFR. Thus, in detecting a reduction in GFR, the serum creatinine is less sensitive than the Ccr. These relationships are shown in Figure 20.1. Some investigators have derived equations to predict Ccr from serum creatinine, age, gender and body size. The Cockcroft and Gault formula is easiest to use [19]:

$$Ccr = \frac{(140 - age) \times weight}{Pcr} \times 72 (men) \qquad (20.8)$$

$$Ccr = \frac{(140 - age) \times weight}{Pcr} \times 85 (women) \qquad (20.9)$$

where Ccr is in ml/min, age is in years, weight is in kilograms, and Pcr is in mg/dl. Because these formulas do not explicitly take into account nutritional status or protein intake, they are likely to overestimate Ccr in vegetarians and patients eating a low protein diet or in patients with malnutrition. This may be especially important in patients with chronic renal disease. Recent studies have sought equations to predict GFR, rather than Ccr, in patients with renal disease. These equations are more complicated than the Cockcroft–Gault formula [20]. Despite all the uncertainties surrounding the measurement of serum creatinine, men with serum creatinine concentrations greater than 1.8 mg/dl and women with creatinine concentrations greater than 1.4 mg/dl almost invariably have a reduced GFR [21]. If an accurate index

of GFR is desired in a patient whose serum creatinine concentration is borderline, a carefully performed isotope clearance [22, 23] or an inulin clearance should be performed.

The validity of assessing changes in GFR from changes in serum creatinine or the reciprocal of serum creatinine (1/Pcr) as a measure of GFR also remains a matter of debate [4, 24]. One recent analytic review concluded that the decline in renal function in patients with progressive renal failure, in fact, can be monitored accurately by serial measurement of the reciprocal of serum creatinine [24]. However, in a recent prospective study of dietary protein restriction, changes in Ccr and reciprocal of serum creatinine did not accurately reflect changes in GFR [9]. For practical purposes, large changes in serum creatinine reflect changes in GFR. However, small changes in serum creatinine may be due to changes in creatinine secretion, generation or possibly extrarenal excretion.

Blood urea nitrogen concentration and GFR

The blood urea nitrogen (BUN) is not as reliable an indicator of GFR as is serum creatinine. Its blood level is affected by four factors in addition to GFR: (1) reabsorption by the renal tubule; (2) dietary protein intake; (3) non-dietary protein (e.g. blood) in the gastrointestinal tract [25]; and (4) metabolism of protein to urea in the liver. Conversion of protein into urea increases in catabolic states such as febrile illnesses [26], acidosis and acute renal failure and when anabolism is inhibited by corticosteroids or tetracycline therapy [27, 28]. Conversely, urea synthesis is diminished in severe liver disease. In the kidney, the portion of filtered urea reabsorbed by the tubule is increased by vasopressin, so that in dehydration and other states associated with high plasma vasopressin, the BUN rises even though GFR is constant [29].

Patients with severe renal disease excrete a large fraction of the filtered urea regardless of urine flow rate. When GFR is less than 20% of normal, the clearance of urea increases to 70% or more of GFR. It is noteworthy that the underestimation of true GFR by urea clearance, coupled with the overestimation of GFR by Ccr, means that the average of the creatinine and urea clearances approximates the true GFR [30, 31].

Despite these limitations, the BUN concentration does have clinical value. A low BUN (less than 8–10 mg/dl) is usually associated with normal renal function, overhydration (as in the syndrome of inappropriate antidiuretic hormone (ADH) secretion) or liver failure. A BUN of 10–15 mg/dl almost always indicates normal GFR whereas a BUN in the range 50–150 mg/dl is beyond the level anticipated from variations in urine flow or nitrogen balance alone and implies impairment of glomerular filtration. Further, in patients with elevated BUN, the degree of azotemia strongly correlates with the presence of uremic symptoms [32].

In stable patients with intrinsic renal disease, the BUN concentration is normally approximately ten times the serum creatinine concentration when both are expressed in mg/dl. In patients with a reduction in GFR due to dehydration or urinary tract obstruction, the clearance of urea is reduced to a greater extent than the Ccr due to low rates of urine flow in the distal nephron. Thus, there may be a disproportionate increase in the BUN concentration, with values greater than 20 times higher than the serum creatinine concentration.

Alternative methods to measure GFR

Newer methods have been developed to circumvent the need for intravenous (i.v.) infusions or timed urine collections. These methods include the modified infusion technique, the single (bolus) i.v. injection, and even external isotopic counting which requires neither urine collections nor blood sampling. In the modified infusion technique, the marker substance (e.g. [125I]iothalamate) is given subcutaneously and is released slowly into the circulation, providing fairly constant plasma levels [33, 34]; GFR is calculated using the standard clearance formula. It has the advantage of not requiring an infusion and of avoiding the need for the difficult assay of inulin. The single (bolus) i.v. technique rests on the principle that the rate of disappearance of a substance (either inulin or newer isotopic markers) removed from the body exclusively by glomerular filtration is a direct function of the GFR [35, 36]. Timed urine samples can be collected (i.e. the GFR is calculated by standard renal clearance formula) or, alternatively, the GFR can be calculated from either the area under the disappearance curve or the terminal slope of the plasma disappearance plot. This method appears to underestimate GFR at high values and to overestimate GFR at low values [37]. In addition, it overestimates GFR in patients with moderate to severe edema probably due to the larger volume of distribution. External counting over the kidneys and bladder of an ingested isotopic marker substance can also be used [38]. The patient is given ^{99m}Tc-labeled diethylene triamine pentaacetic acid (DTPA), and the percentage renal (and bladder) uptake at a defined time after injection are determined by renal imaging and compared to simultaneously measured GFR by other techniques, e.g. ^{51}Cr-labeled EDTA.

Other new markers used include radiolabeled inulin (e.g. [carboxy-^{14}C] inulin), radiolabeled vitamin B_{12} (using cobalt-57 or cobalt-58), ^{125}I-labeled diatrizoate, ^{125}I-labeled iothalamate, ^{51}Cr-labeled EDTA and ^{99m}Tc-labeled DTPA. Studies of clearances using iothalamate and the metal chelates have demonstrated a high degree of correlation with simultaneous inulin clearances [39]. GFR also can be measured using non-radioisotopic contrast agents, e.g. iothalamate [40]. More recently, however, tubular secretion of iothalamate has been demonstrated [40] which results in an overestimation of GFR by at least 7%.

Renal blood flow

Renal blood flow (RBF) measurements are rarely used in clinical practice, which in part reflects the imprecision of current techniques of measurement. The urinary clearance of p-aminohippurate (PAH) is an excellent measure of RBF in the healthy kidney as it is almost completely extracted during a single pass [41]. However, in the presence of acute and chronic renal disease, the PAH transporter is impaired so that extraction is variably and unpredictably depressed [42]. Samples from the renal artery and vein are therefore required to determine the extraction ratio with accuracy. Coupled with the need for a constant infusion, this renders the method impractical for routine use. Similar problems occur with hippuran as it is handled by the same pathway. PAH or hippuran clearances or the fractional uptake of ^{131}I-labeled hippuran during isotopic scanning all underestimate RBF in the diseased kidney. More recent developments suffer from different problems. RBF can be calculated from a compartmental analysis of the disappearance of radiolabeled ammonia using positron emission tomography [43]. The need for frequent arterial samples and specialized expensive equipment limits the use of this novel technique. Doppler ultrasonography shows promise but is both operator and patient dependent [44]. Recently, phase-contrast cine-magnetic resonance imaging (MRI) has been used with reproducible results in both healthy and diseased kidneys [45].

Renal biopsy

The examination of renal tissue obtained by percutaneous biopsy can provide a precise diagnosis, determine the extent of disease activity and provide the basis for specific therapy [46]. The procedure is not without risk and the indications and contraindications should be carefully considered in each individual patient. The most common risk is excessive bleeding. It is our practice that prior to the biopsy, patients are screened for coagulopathy, blood is typed or self-donated and all platelet antagonists are withheld for at least one week. Absolute contraindications therefore include bleeding diathesis and the inability to co-operate. Relative contraindications include severe refractory hypertension or hypotension, renal abcesses, pyelonephritis, obstructive nephropathy or uncorrected anemia or uremia. There are several methods to visualize the kidney but it is our preference to use real-time ultrasound guidance. This method, coupled with the use of a spring loaded device, has been found to be both safe and efficacious [47]. We reserve open renal biopsy for high risk cases or those patients with a single functioning kidney. However, it may well be that the latter is only a relative contraindication to percutaneous renal biopsy as the risk of death from general anesthesia is compara-ble to the risk of nephrectomy following a closed biopsy. For a more detailed discussion about renal biopsy, refer to Chapter 24.

References

1. Smith, H.W. (1951) *The Kidney: Structure and Function in Health and Disease*, Oxford University Press, New York.
2. Perrone, R.D., Steinman, T.I., Beck, G.J. *et al.* (1990) Utility of radioisotopic filtration markers in chronic renal insufficiency: simultaneous comparison of ^{125}I-iothalamate, ^{169}Yb-DTPA, ^{99m}Tc-DTPA, and inulin. *Am. J. Kidney Dis.*, **26**, 224.
3. Richards, A.N., Westfall, B.B. and Bott, P.A. (1934) Renal excretion of inulin, creatinine and xylose in normal dogs. *Proc. Soc. Exp. Biol. Med.*, **32**, 73–4.
4. Levey, A.S. (1990) Nephrology Forum. Measurement of renal function in chronic renal disease. *Kidney Int.*, **38**, 167.
5. Macias-Nunez, J.F. and Cameron, J.S. (1987) *Renal Function and Disease in the Elderly*, Butterworth, London.
6. Wesson, L.G. (1969) *Physiology of the Human Kidney*, Grune & Stratton, New York.
7. Rowe, J.W., Andres, R., Tobin, J.D. *et al.* (1976) Age adjusted standards for creatinine clearance. *Ann. Intern. Med.*, **84**, 567.
8. Siersbaek-Nielson, K., Molholm Hansen, J.M., Kamp-mann, J. and Kristensen, M. (1971) Rapid evaluation of creatinine clearance. *Lancet*, **i**, 1133.
9. Modification of Diet in Renal Disease Study Group (Levey, A.S., Bosch, J.P., Coggins, C.H. *et al.*) (1997) Effects of diet and antihypertensive therapy on creati-nine clearance and serum creatinine in the Modification of Diet in Renal Disease Study. Submitted.
10. Dubb, J.W., Stote, R.M., Familiar, R.G. *et al.* (1978) Effect of cimetidine on renal function in normal man. *Clin. Pharmacol. Ther.*, **24**, 76.
11. Berglund, F., Killander, J. and Pompeius, R. (1975) Effect of trimethoprimsulfamethoxazole on the renal excretion of creatinine in man. *J. Urol.*, **114**, 802.
12. Chesley, L. (1938) Renal excretion at low urine volumes and the mechanism of oliguria. *J. Clin. Invest.*, **17**, 591.
13. Ladd, M., Liddle, L. and Gagnon, J.A. (1956) Renal excre-tion of inulin, creatinine and ferrocyanide, at normal and reduced clearance levels in the dog. *Am. J. Physiol.*, **184**, 505.
14. Levinsky, N.G. and Berliner, R.W. (1959) Changes in composition of the urine in ureter and bladder at low urine flow. *Am. J. Physiol.*, **196**, 549.
15. Walser, M. (1987) Creatinine excretion as a measure of protein nutrition in adults of varying age. *JPEN*, **11**, 73.
16. Jones, J.D. and Burnett, P.C. (1974) Creatinine metabo-lism in humans with decreased renal function: creatinine deficit. *Clin. Chem.*, **20**, 1204.
17. Hankins, D.A., Babb, A.L., Uvelli, D.A. and Scribner, B.H. (1981) Creatinine degradation I: the kinetics of creati-nine removal in patients with chronic kidney disease. *Int. J. Artif. Organs*, **4**, 35.
18. Mitch, W.E., Collier, V.U. and Walser, M. (1980) Creati-nine metabolism in chronic renal failure. *Clin. Sci.*, **58**, 327.
19. Cockcroft, D.W. and Gault, M.H. (1976) Prediction of creatinine clearance from serum creatinine. *Nephron*, **16**, 31.
20. Modification of Diet in Renal Disease Study Group (Bosch, J., Breyer, J. *et al.*) (1994) Predicting GFR from serum creatinine in the Modification of Diet in Renal Disease Study. Abstracts of the Seventh International Congress of Nutrition and Metabolism in Renal Disease. Stockholm, Sweden, p. 38.
21. Shemesh, O., Golbetz, H., Kriss, J.P. and Myers, B.D. (1985) Limitations of creatinine as a filtration marker in glomerulopathic patients. *Kidney Int.*, **28**, 830.
22. Brochner-Mortensen, J. (1978) Routine methods and their reliability for assessment of glomerular filtration rate in adults with special reference to total [^{51}Cr] EDTA plasma clearance. *Dan. Med. Bull.*, **25**, 181.
23. Chantler, C., Garnett, E.S., Parsons, V. and Veall, N. (1969) Glomerular filtration rate measurement in man by the single injection method using ^{51}Cr-EDTA. *Clin. Sci.*, **37**, 169.
24. Walser, M., Drew, H.H. and Guldan, J.L. (1993) Predic-tion of glomerular filtration rate from serum creatinine concentration in advanced renal failure. *Kidney Int.*, **44**, 1145.
25. Cohn, T.D., Lane, M., Zuckerman, S. *et al.* (1956) Induced azotemia in humans following massive protein and blood ingestion and the mechanism of azotemia in gastrointestinal hemorrhage. *Am. J. Med. Sci.*, **231**, 394.
26. Goldring, W. (1931) Studies on the kidney in acute infec-tion: III. Observations with the urine sediment count (Addis) and the urea clearance test in lobar pneumonia. *J. Clin. Invest.*, **10**, 355.
27. Long, C.N.H., Katzin, B. and Fry, E.G. (1940) Adrenal cortex and carbohydrate metabolism. *Endocrinology*, **26**, 309.
28. Shils, M.E. (1963) Renal disease and the metabolic effects of tetracycline. *Ann. Intern. Med.*, **58**, 389.
29. Walser, M. and Bodenlos, L.J. (1959) Urea metabolism in man. *J. Clin. Invest.*, **38**, 1617.
30. Lubowitz, H., Slatopolsky, E., Shankel, S. *et al.* (1967) Glomerular filtration rate: determination in patients with chronic renal disease. *JAMA*, **199**, 252.
31. Lavender, S., Hilton, P.J. and Jones, N.F. (1969) The mea-surement of glomerular filtration rate in renal disease. *Lancet*, **ii**, 1216.
32. Lowrie, E.G., Laird, N.M., Parker, T.F. and Sargent, J.A. (1981) The effect of hemodialysis prescription on patient morbidity: report from the National Cooperative Dialy-sis Study. *N. Engl. J. Med.*, **305**, 1176.

33. Israelit, A.H., Long, D.L., White, M.G. and Hull, A.R. (1973) Measurement of glomerular filtration rate utilizing a single subcutaneous injection of ^{125}I-iothalamate. *Kidney Int.*, **4**, 346.

34. Ott, N.T. and Wilson, D.M. (1975) A simple technique for estimating glomerular filtration rate with subcutaneous injection of [^{125}I]iothalamate. *Mayo Clin. Proc.*, **50**, 664.

35. Hall, J.E., Guyton, A.C. and Farr, B.M. (1977) A single-injection method for measuring glomerular filtration rate. *Am. J. Physiol.*, **232**(1), F72.

36. Balachandran, S., Toguri, A.G., Petrusick, T.W. and Abbott, L.C. (1981) Comparative evaluation of quantitative glomerular filtration rate measured by isotopic and nonisotopic methods. *Clin. Nucl. Med.*, **6**, 150.

37. La France, N.D., Drew, H.H. and Walser, M. (1988) Radioisotopic measurement of glomerular filtration rate in severe chronic renal failure. *J. Nucl. Med.*, **29**, 1927.

38. Chervu, L.R. and Blaufox, M.D. (1982) Renal radiopharmaceuticals – an update. *Semin. Nucl. Med.*, **12**, 224.

39. Perrone, R.D., Steinman, T.I., Beck, G.J. *et al.* (1990) Utility of radioisotopic filtration markers in chronic renal insufficiency: simultaneous comparison of ^{125}I-iothalamate, ^{169}Yb-DTPA, ^{99m}Tc-DTPA, and inulin. *Am. J. Kidney Dis.*, **26**, 224.

40. Almen, T., Bergquist, D., Frennby, B. *et al.* (1991) Use of urographic contrast media to determine glomerular filtration rate. Determining the glomerular filtration rate of each kidney with computed tomography and scintigraphy. *Invest. Radiol.*, **26**(Suppl 1), S72.

41. Myers, B. (1994) *Diagnosis and Evaluation of Renal Disease. Year Book of Nephrology*, Mosby, Year Book Inc., St Louis, MO.

42. Levinsky, N.G. and Levy, M. (1973) Clearance techniques, in *Renal Physiology* (eds J. Orloff and R.W. Berliner), American Physiology Society, Washington.

43. Nitzsche, E.U., Choi, Y., Killion, D. *et al.* (1993) Quantification and parametric imaging of renal cortical blood flow in vivo based on Patlak graphical analysis. *Kidney Int.*, **44**, 985–96.

44. Sturgiss, S.N., Martin, K., Whittingham, T.A. and Davison, J.M. (1992) Assessment of the renal circulation during pregnancy with color Doppler ultrasonography. *Am. J. Obstet. Gynecol.*, **167**, 1250–4.

45. Sommer, G., Noorbehesht, B., Pelc, N. *et al.* (1992) Normal renal blood flow measurement using phase-contrast cine magnetic resonance imaging. *Invest. Radiol.*, **27**, 465–70.

46. Madaio, M.P. (1990) Nephrology forum. Renal biopsy. *Kidney Int.*, **38**, 529–43.

47. Mahoney, M.C., Racadio, J.M., Merhar, G.L. and First, M.R. (1993) Safety and efficacy of kidney transplant biopsy: tru-cut needle vs sonographically guided biopty gun. *AJR*, **160**, 325–6.

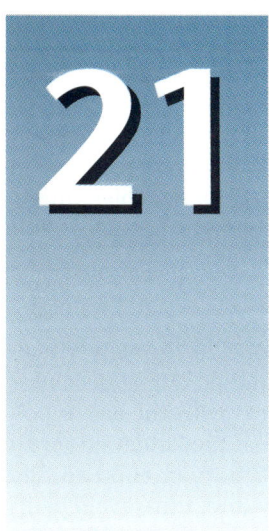

21

Diagnostic imaging

Gerald W. Friedland, F. Graham Sommer, George Segall and R. Brooke Jeffrey

Introduction

Although the following statements were written several years ago [1], the concepts they describe still hold true today:

> When requesting an imaging examination, the referring clinician should ask, What examination will involve the least radiation, the least likelihood of an adverse reaction to intravascular contrast materials and what examination will be the least invasive and least expensive – but will still yield the desired results? The answers to these questions depend upon a close interaction between the referring clinician and the radiologist, so that the radiologist knows at every step just what the referring clinician needs to know.

Results from any imaging examination are most dependent on the prior probability, that is, the probability that a given disorder exists before the examination is even performed, which is why it is vital to communicate clinical information about the patient to the radiologist. In addition, it is important for the referring clinician and radiologist to decide what performance characteristics, sensitivity or specificity, are most desirable. Principles are now firmly established for deciding this question:

1   If the prior probability is high, a sensitive imaging examination is needed

2   If the prior probability is low, a specific imaging examination is needed
3   If the consequences of missing a diagnosis are serious, a sensitive imaging examination is needed
4   If the consequences of missing the diagnosis are not serious, a specific imaging examination is needed.

Using these principles, a discussion of current imaging examinations follows. The discussion starts with a description of the ultrasound examination of the kidneys because most nephrologists request this examination more frequently than any other type of imaging examination.

Ultrasound examination of the kidneys

Introduction

Ultrasonography is widely used because it is non-invasive, safe, can be performed rapidly, and provides diagnostic information for a substantial range of disease processes. Additional features that make ultrasonography attractive include the following: it is relatively cheap (an important consideration in this era of cost containment), and the examiner does not need to inject contrast materials or expose the patient to ionizing radiation.

Nephrology, Edited by Rex L. Jamison and Robert Wilkinson.
Published in 1997 by Chapman & Hall, London. ISBN 0 412 60930 4

Ultrasonic image creation

Ultrasound technology has recently undergone substantial development, which has resulted in a variety of different forms of ultrasonic images and quantitative information [2]. By far the most common type of ultrasonic information used is the two-dimensional ultrasound image, or 'B-mode' image. The creation of these images with ultrasound relies on the pulse–echo technique in which an array of piezoelectric elements emit ultrasound which passes through the abdominal wall; when the high-frequency sound is either reflected or scattered back to the transducer array, the recorded signals are used to create two-dimensional images. An operator obtains the images of the kidney in real time. The velocity of sound in tissue is high enough so that images of kidneys are created at a frame rate of about 15 frames/s. This allows an operator to adjust the position and angulation of the ultrasound beam to obtain satisfactory renal images in a number of desired orientations and to examine the entire renal substance. The recorded ultrasonic examination generally consists of a number of frozen images of each kidney in longitudinal and transverse orientations.

Doppler ultrasonic imaging

In addition to B-mode images depicting the morphology of the kidney, a variety of Doppler information forms describe blood flow in renal arteries and veins [2]. All such information relies on the Doppler principle, in which a frequency shift is observed when there is relative motion of a radiant wave energy source and an observer. In renal Doppler ultrasound, blood cells moving in renal arteries and veins scatter sound causing an observable shift in the ultrasound backscattered to the interrogating transducer array. The observed Doppler frequency shift of the ultrasound returned to the transducer array may be displayed in the following forms: (1) as a graphical function of time for a region of interest in a renal vessel selected interactively with the aid of the real-time B-mode ultrasonic image (the duplex Doppler waveform tracing), and (2) in image format, superimposed on the standard B-mode image of the kidney. Many ultrasound machines have a color Doppler display which superimposes a color coding depicting the local frequency shifts due to blood flowing in renal arteries and veins. Using this sort of display, Doppler frequency shift may be either positive or negative depending on whether blood is flowing towards or away from the transducer array. The superimposed color display employs a scale which depicts both the direction of the Doppler frequency shift, as well as the magnitude of the shift.

Doppler power or energy imaging is an alternative form for depicting Doppler information in image format [3]. This alternative form superimposes a color depiction of the overall power in the Doppler frequency spectrum due to flowing blood on the conventional real-time ultrasonic image of the kidney. This type of color Doppler imaging is significantly more sensitive to Doppler information, and, thus, is more readily able to depict flow in small vessels than the standard color Doppler image. However, no flow directional encoding is possible.

Examination technique

Using real-time ultrasound, the operator usually visualizes the kidneys in partial right and left lateral decubitus positions, after positioning patients with the aid of bolsters. The operator usually examines the kidneys from an anterior and rather lateral approach in an effort to find an appropriate acoustical pathway, and, thus, avoid paths impeded by either the patient's ribs or gas within the bowel. These pathways generally involve both the layers of abdominal wall and the liver or spleen. It is often easier to image the right kidney with ultrasound, since the liver is a much larger homogeneous organ and provides a better acoustic window than the spleen.

Normal renal ultrasonic images

A B-mode frozen image of a normal right kidney is shown in Figure 21.1(a). It is possible in a real-time kidney examination to discern the imaging plane, showing the kidney in its greatest length, and to perform a measurement of the kidney long axis, as shown in Figure 21.1(a). The average length of an adult kidney measured with ultrasound is about 11 cm, and there are charts of maximal renal lengths, as determined on ultrasound, for both adult and pediatric kidneys for individuals of a given age and gender. It should be noted that renal length, as determined on sonography, is about 15% less than that determined with excretory urography. This is due to the radiographic magnification present in urograms.

The operator can sometimes distinguish medullary pyramids from the renal cortex because at least some medullary pyramids can look somewhat darker or less echogenic than the renal cortex (Figure 21.1a). The renal sinus, consisting of the renal collecting structures and associated fat, appears very brightly echogenic (Figure 21.1a). Normal blood vessels in the renal sinus can mimic hydronephrosis since both can produce dark regions or lucency within the renal sinus.

Information on various Doppler shifts in renal blood vessels is depicted in Figure 21.1(b–d). In Figure 21.1(b), a region of interest in an intrarenal artery allows creation of a duplex Doppler waveform tracing, which depicts the Doppler frequency shift for this vessel as a time function. Such Doppler waveform tracings are employed as the basis for a number of quantitative and semiquantitative measures of Doppler frequency shifts due to flow in renal arteries. Figure 21.1(c) is an image of the same kidney in color Doppler format. Here, intrarenal blood vessels are displayed in color as shown in the color bar at the left of the image. Velocity shifts for blood flowing in vessels toward the transducer are displayed in red; the flow of

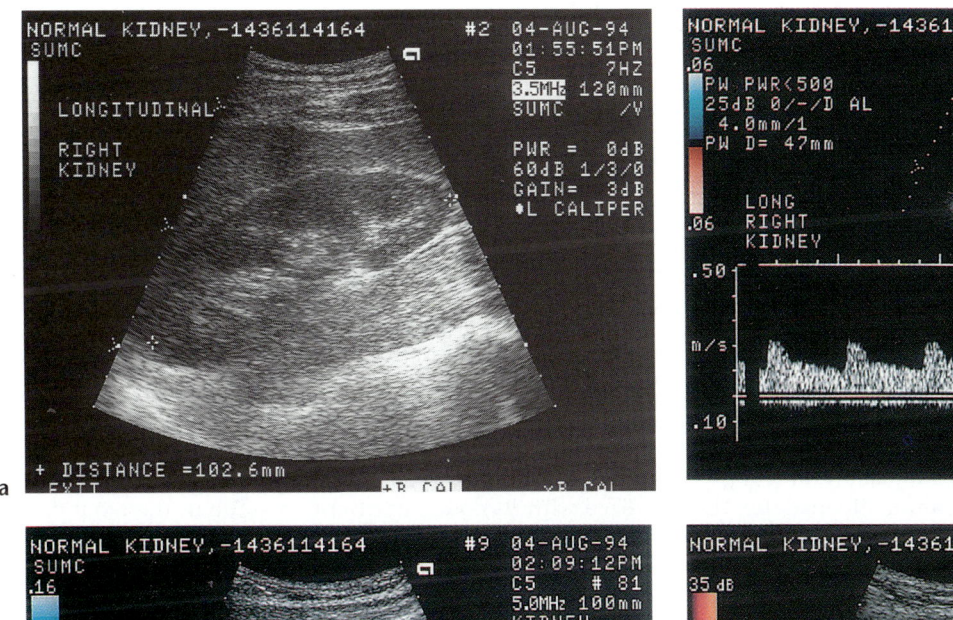
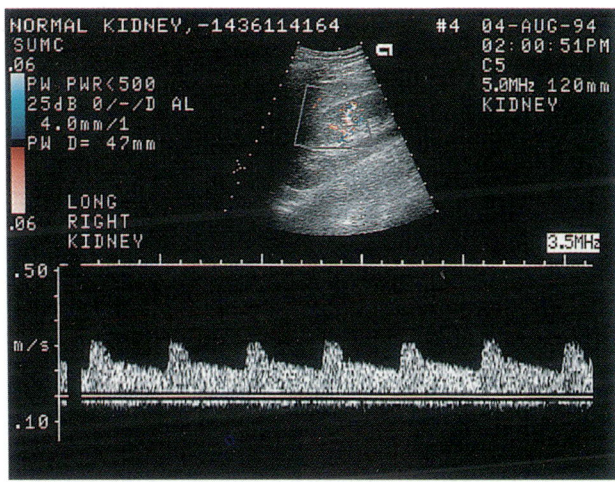
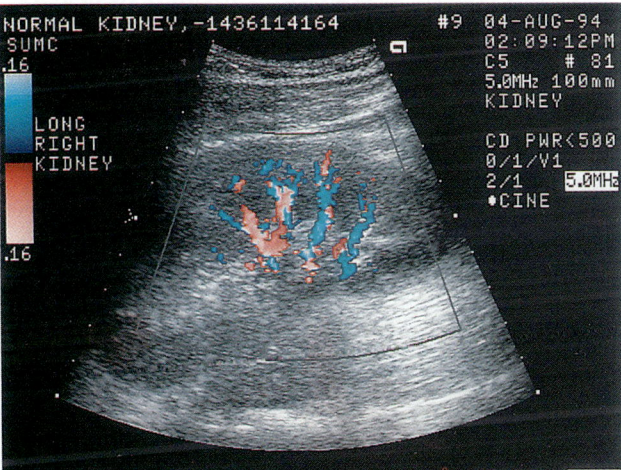
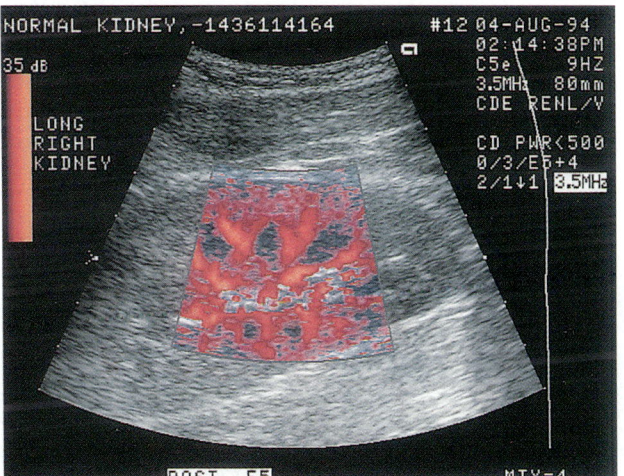

Figure 21.1 Longitudinal ultrasonic images of a normal right kidney: (a) B-mode image shows renal length of 11 cm. The renal sinus, containing the collecting structures and fat, appears as a group of bright echoes centrally. (b) Duplex Doppler tracing from a branch of the right renal artery. (c) Conventional color Doppler image in which flow in branches of the renal arteries and veins is depicted in a color overlay on the B-mode image. (d) Doppler power or energy image depicting flowing blood as dark red regions.

blood away from the transducer is depicted in blue, with higher velocities in both directions depicted in white. The pictorial display shows the distribution of the arteries and veins in the kidney and provides the direction of flow along with an indication of the velocity of the flowing blood. This is valuable for a number of purposes, including finding a renal artery or vein for performance of Doppler waveform analysis, as in Figure 21.1(b), and sometimes to differentiate renal blood vessels in the renal sinus from collecting structures distended with urine. Figure 21.1(d) depicts the overall power in the Doppler frequency spectrum due to flowing blood in a red color and is superimposed over the standard image of the same kidney. Due to the high sensitivity of flow with this type of imaging, often referred to as Doppler power or energy imaging, there is a more complete display of the intrarenal vasculature, but no information about the direction of blood flow is encoded.

Applications

Detection of hydronephrosis

By far the most common application of renal ultrasonography is the detection and characterization of the degree of renal obstruction [2]. The degree of dilatation of renal collecting structures, visualized as dark or anechoic areas in the region of the renal sinus, correlates well with the degree of hydronephrosis as imaged at excretory urography. To have a high sensitivity for obstruction with ultrasound, it is necessary to call any significant lucency in the renal sinus as being due to renal obstruction.

In order to maximize diagnostic specificity, two technical points are important. First, the color Doppler capability permits differentiation of blood in vessels in the renal sinus from distended collecting structures. Second, a full urinary bladder sometimes partially occludes the distal ureters, making the upper collecting structures appear somewhat dilated. Rescanning the kidneys after the patient has voided allows recognition of this source of possible false-positives. Figure 21.2(a) shows the typical appearance of moderate hydronephrosis in a patient with renal colic due to a stone at the right ureterovesical junction (Figure 21.2b).

In recent years, some investigators have made an effort to exploit renal arterial waveform data and color Doppler information to enhance the diagnostic capabilities of ultrasound for obstruction. In some studies, the authors have noted that in acutely obstructed kidneys there is a decrease in arterial diastolic flow for branch vessels within the kidney. These authors have proposed a 'resistive index' for the kidney, defined as the maximum Doppler frequency shift minus the minimum, divided by the maximum measured for a branch renal arterial waveform tracing. Some studies have shown this parameter to measure below 0.7 in normal kidneys and higher in cases of obstruction. Various studies have produced conflicting results, however, and the technique does not provide sufficiently useful or reliable ancillary information [4].

Another technique used for diagnosing ureteral obstruction is to examine the trigone region of the distended urinary bladder with color Doppler ultrasound to observe for the presence of urine flowing rapidly from the ureteral orifices. This phenomenon is referred to as ureteral jets. It has been shown that the presence of such jets is related to differences in the specific gravity of urine in the bladder and urine in the jets. The value of looking for ureteral jets is shown in Figure 21.2(c). The patient shown has right ureteral colic due to a right ureteral stone. There is a normal ureteral jet on the left, but the ureteral jet on the right is absent.

Renal calculi

Calculi within the renal collecting structures may be visualized with B-mode ultrasound. A stone in the renal collecting structures produces an echogenic or bright density which casts an acoustic shadow posteriorly, since it occludes a portion of the ultrasound beam. To detect renal calculi some authors compared the relative abilities of ultrasound and other modalities, including standard X-ray tomography. It appears at this time that, although ultrasound is quite sensitive to the detection of renal

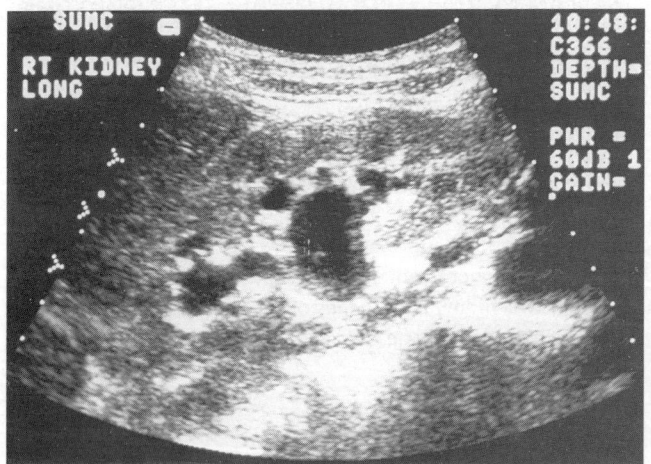

a

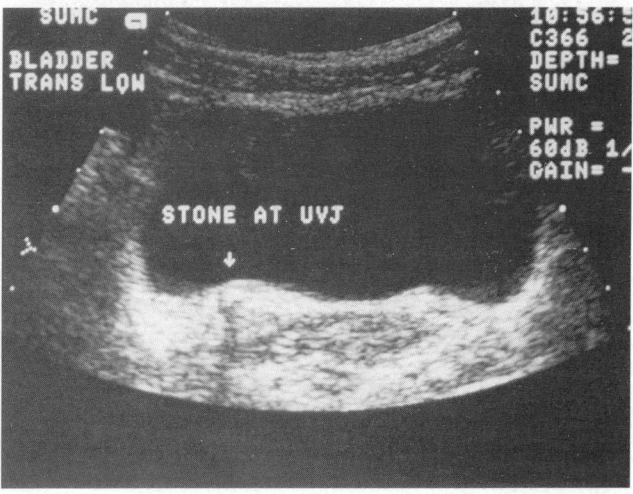

b

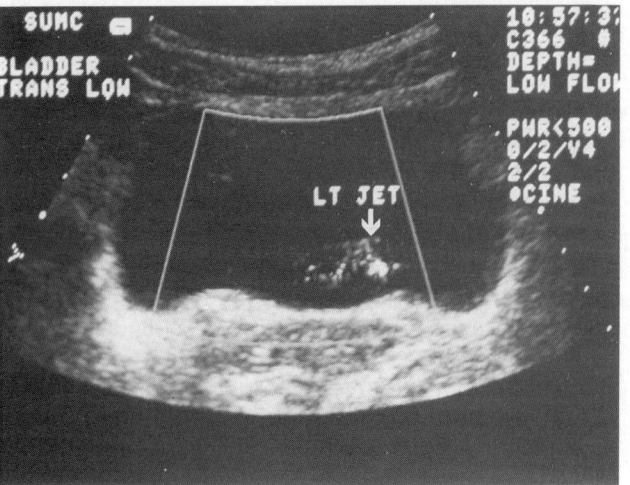

c

Figure 21.2 Ultrasonic images of a patient with right renal colic and hydronephrosis due to a stone at the right ureterovesical junction (UVJ). (a) Longitudinal image of the right kidney shows moderate hydronephrosis. (b) Transverse view of the bladder at the level of the trigone shows UVJs as slightly elevated regions posteriorly in the bladder. A bright, echogenic stone is seen at the right UVJ, casting a shadow posteriorly. (c) Color Doppler exam shows a left ureteral jet, but no right jet.

calculi, it is probably not as sensitive as X-ray tomography for the detection of very small renal stones.

A number of studies evaluated renal ultrasound as a technique for diagnosing renal colic. The differing results in these studies appear to be related to methodologic details [4, 5]. In studies where the renal ultrasound is preceded by an abdominal plain film (which serves to aid in the search for a calcified renal calculus) and in which the patient is adequately hydrated prior to the ultrasound, diagnostic sensitivity is equivalent to that of excretory urography [5]. Patient hydration appears important because the primary diagnostic feature is significant hydronephrosis on the affected side. The offending renal calculus is visible in only a minority of cases, most frequently at the ureterovesical junction. Figure 21.2(a–c) shows a patient who had right ureteral colic. The illustrations show hydronephrosis on the right side, a shadowing calculus at the right ureterovesical junction and asymmetrical ureteral jets with an absent jet on the right side.

Renal parenchymal disease

Diffuse renal diseases with a wide range of etiologies may appear, generally when in an advanced form, as rather bright or echogenic kidneys on diagnostic ultrasound [2]. The ultrasonic appearance appears to be related to the interstitial changes in the kidney and in most cases does not give specific information on the etiology of disease; specific diagnosis of etiology would require biopsy. An example of such an appearance on ultrasound is shown in Figure 21.3. Here the diffusely abnormal right kidney is shown to be significantly brighter than the liver, compared to a normal kidney which will generally by somewhat less bright than the liver. In patients with diffuse renal disease the corticomedullary differentiation also tends to be enhanced.

There is one exception to the rule that ultrasound lacks

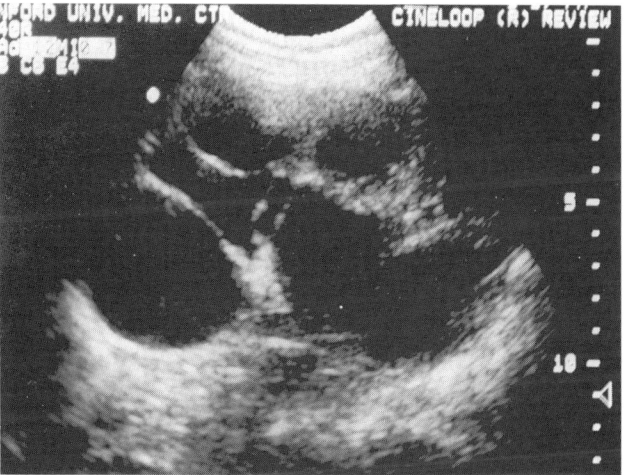

a

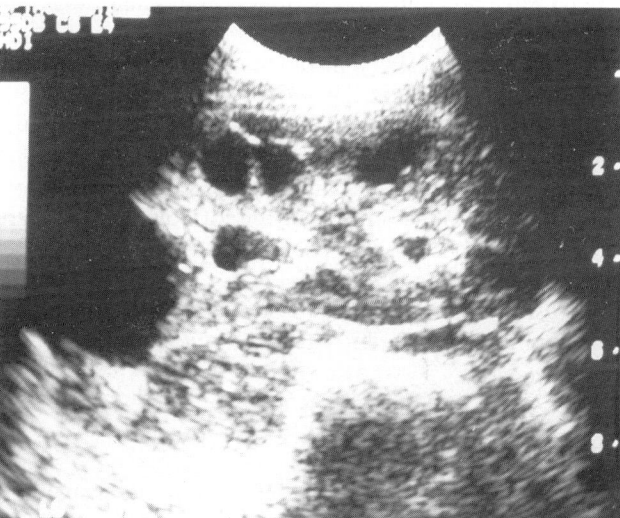

b

Figure 21.4 (a) Right kidney and (b) left kidney. Autosomal dominant polycystic kidney disease in a 30-year-old woman. There are a large number of cysts which have supplanted renal parenchyma and enlarged both kidneys.

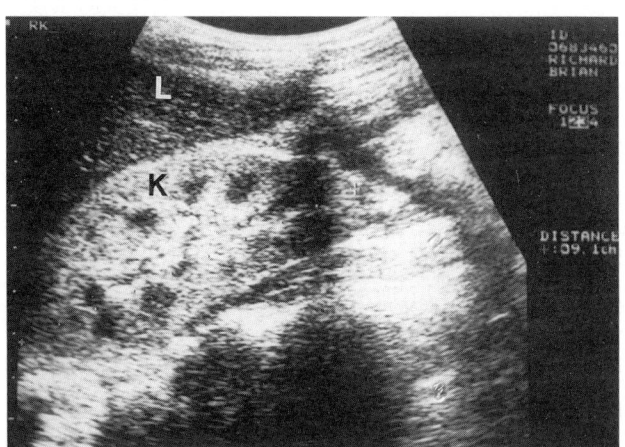

Figure 21.3 Chronic renal disease. The right kidney (K) is abnormally bright, being much brighter than the adjacent liver (L).

specificity in patients with diffuse renal diseases: adult type autosomal dominant polycystic kidney disease. Here ultrasound shows the kidneys supplanted by an abnormally large number of cysts, which enlarge the kidneys and eventually replace the functioning renal parenchyma. The same examination may also reveal accompanying liver cysts. The typical appearance of kidneys involved with adult-type polycystic kidney disease is shown in Figure 21.4. Ultrasound is the screening examination of choice for this disease entity; it may reveal cysts early in life – childhood or adolescence – in some affected individuals.

Renal infections

Ultrasound is a sensitive examination for detecting focal renal and perirenal abscesses and obstructed infected renal collecting systems (pyonephrosis). In some patients with pyonephrosis, a urine/debris level may exist in the obstructed infected kidney. In patients with chronic atrophic pyelonephritis, ultrasound may reveal small kidneys with renal scarring.

Renal vascular imaging

Ultrasound imaging and Doppler is of some value for diagnosing renal vein thrombosis or tumor thrombus extending into the veins from renal cell carcinoma. The operator can visualize thrombus in the real-time images, sometimes aided by the color Doppler format. A lack of Doppler flow on a duplex Doppler waveform examination indicates that renal vein thrombosis is present. In general, however, evaluation of the renal vessels with ultrasound is very difficult because overlying bowel gas frequently obscures the kidneys and there may be anatomic variations of the renal vessels.

A variety of efforts made to diagnose renal artery stenosis by ultrasound have indicated that ultrasound is not reliable enough. Direct visualization of the renal arteries is too difficult for technical reasons and, therefore, does not provide reliable results. Some investigators analyzing the waveforms from the intrarenal vasculature have reported that when renal arterial stenosis is present the duplex Doppler waveforms are abnormal, with decreased sharpness of the upstroke. Results have been conflicting, however, and the technique does not appear reliable.

Renal allograft imaging

Ultrasound is very useful in imaging transplanted kidneys, which are readily accessible for examination in the iliac fossa. The operator can easily detect and monitor perinephric fluid collections and hydronephrosis in trans-

plant recipients. Efforts have been made to diagnose renal transplant rejection by the features of the transplanted kidney on a B-mode exam and by the appearance of the Doppler arterial waveforms. The non-specificity of such findings seriously limits their utility, however, and ultrasound cannot limit the need for biopsy in cases of transplant dysfunction.

Another type of imaging examination that nephrologists frequently request is scintigraphy; a discussion of this follows.

Scintigraphic evaluation of the urinary system

Introduction

Scintigraphy provides less anatomic detail than radiography, computer-assisted tomography, or ultrasound. The lower limit of resolution is approximately 5–6 mm. Scintigraphy, however, excels at measuring blood flow and organ function. The information provided by scintigraphy is often unique and complementary to information provided by other imaging modalities. Other advantages of scintigraphy include low radiation exposure, the ability to quantitate blood flow and physiologic parameters, and the lack of nephrotoxicity or adverse reaction to contrast media.

Radiopharmaceuticals

Radiopharmaceuticals consist of a radioisotope attached to a non-radioactive carrier. The radioisotope emits gamma rays which produce the image and the non-radioactive carrier determines the distribution of the radiopharmaceutical. The radioisotope which is used

Table 21.1   Common radiopharmaceuticals used for imaging the urinary system

Radiopharmaceutical	Renal handling	Clinical applications
^{99m}Tc MAG3, ^{123}I Hippuran, ^{131}I Hippuran	1. Tubular secretion 2. Glomerular filtration	1. Measurement of ERPF 2. Diagnosis of renovascular disease, renal parenchymal disease, and obstructive uropathy
^{99m}Tc DTPA	Glomerular filtration	1. Measurement of GFR 2. Diagnosis of renovascular disease, renal parenchymal disease, and obstructive uropathy
^{99m}TC DMSA	1. Cortical tubular binding 2. Glomerular filtration	1. Differentiation of mass lesions from normal renal parenchyma 2. Measurement of renal size and mass
^{99m}TC gluceptate	1. Glomerular filtration 2. Tubular secretion 3. Cortical tubular binding	1. Diagnosis of renovascular disease, renal parenchymal disease, and obstructive uropathy 2. Differentiation of mass lesions from normal renal parenchyma

Abbreviations: MAG3, mercaptoacetyltriglycine; DMSA, dimercaptosuccinic acid; DTPA, diethylene triamine pentaacetic acid.

most often is technetium 99m (^{99m}Tc). ^{99m}Tc is a pure gamma emitter with a 140 keV photon and a 6 h half-life. These properties make it suitable for imaging. It is difficult, however, to link ^{99m}Tc chemically to some carriers. Other radioisotopes, most notably ^{123}I and ^{131}I, are used for this reason. The radiopharmaceuticals used for evaluation of the urinary system are listed in Table 21.1 [6].

Measurement of glomerular filtration rate and effective renal plasma flow

The radiopharmaceutical used most frequently to measure glomerular filtration rate (GFR) is ^{99m}Tc-labeled DTPA. ^{99m}Tc-labeled DTPA is a small compound which is freely filtered through the glomeruli and is neither secreted nor absorbed by the renal tubules. GFR measured with ^{99m}Tc-DTPA is slightly lower than the value obtained with inulin because 5–10% of the radiopharmaceutical is bound to plasma proteins [7].

Effective renal plasma flow (ERPF) is usually measured with hippuran labeled with ^{131}I or ^{123}I. Hippuran, or orthoiodohippuric acid, is chemically very similar to *p*-aminohippuric acid (PAH). Approximately 20% is excreted by glomerular filtration and 80% by tubular secretion. The term effective indicates the value is lower than true renal plasma flow because the compounds are not completely extracted in a single pass through the kidney. ERPF measured with hippuran is approximately 10–15% lower than the value obtained with PAH because of free iodine in the preparation as well as other factors. ERPF can also be measured with ^{99m}Tc-MAG3. The calculation, however, must use a factor to correct for decreased renal clearance secondary to a high level of protein binding.

GFR and ERPF measurements can be performed non-invasively by measuring renal uptake with a gamma camera 1–3 min after injection of the radiopharmaceutical. Renal uptake during this period is proportional to GFR and ERPF. The measurements, however, are not as accurate as techniques employing venous sampling [8–10]. The most accurate values are obtained by collecting multiple venous samples and fitting the plasma disappearance curve to a multicompartmental model [11]. Since this is laborious, a simpler calculation using one or two venous samples is used in clinical practice [11–13]. This method is based on the observation that the plasma concentration of the radiopharmaceutical is inversely related to the GFR or ERPF.

Renogram

A time–activity curve showing the uptake and excretion of a radiopharmaceutical by the kidneys is called a renogram (Figure 21.5). Serial 1–5 min images of the kidneys are obtained for up to 60 min beginning immediately after injection of the radiopharmaceutical.

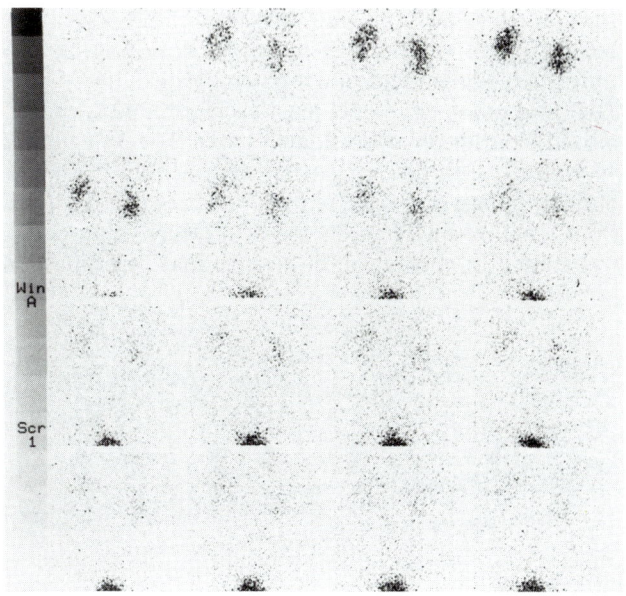

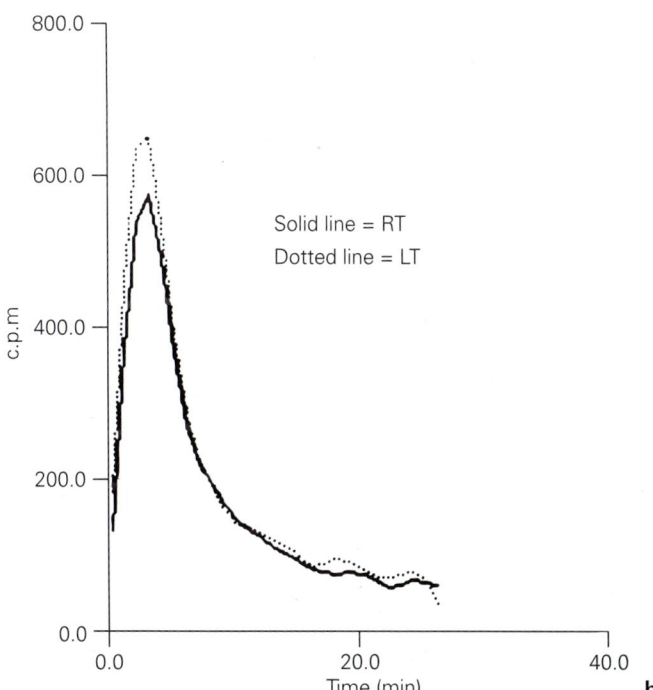

Figure 21.5 Normal renogram performed with [^{131}I] hippuran. (a) Serial 1-min posterior images obtained during the first 16 min of the study show symmetric and prompt uptake of the radiopharmaceutical with rapid excretion from both kidneys. The bladder is seen at the bottom of the frames. (b) Time–activity curves show rapid upslope with activity peaking at 4 min, followed by rapid downslope.

Regions of interest are drawn around each kidney and the number of counts is plotted as a function of time after correction for background activity.

The renogram consists of three phases. The first phase represents renal perfusion. It is rapidly upsloping and lasts less than 60 s following injection of the tracer. The second phase represents renal extraction. During this time the renogram typically reaches a plateau in 3–5 min. The third phase represents renal excretion and is characterized by a steeply downsloping curve. The renogram is very sensitive in detecting renal dysfunction. It may be difficult, however, to differentiate renovascular disorders from renal parenchyma disease or obstructive uropathy. Sometimes the etiology of the disorder may be established

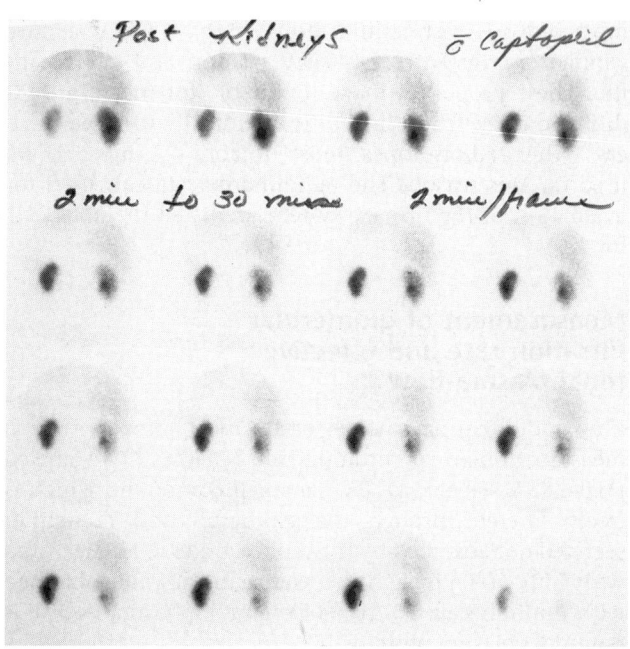

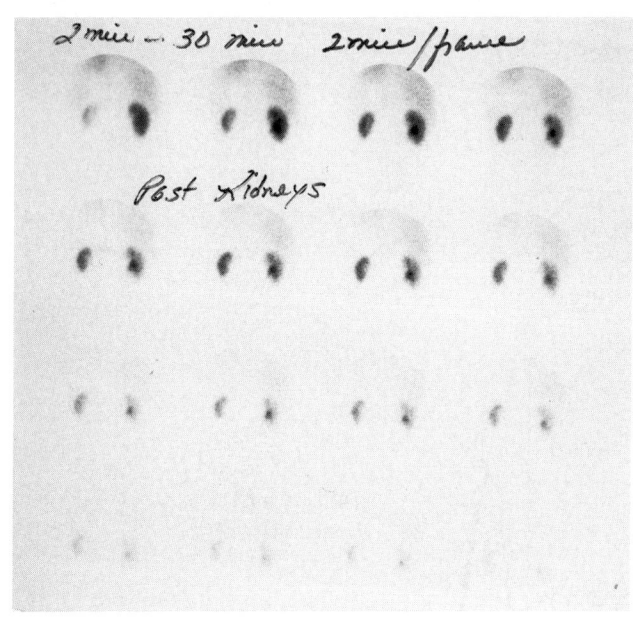

(a)

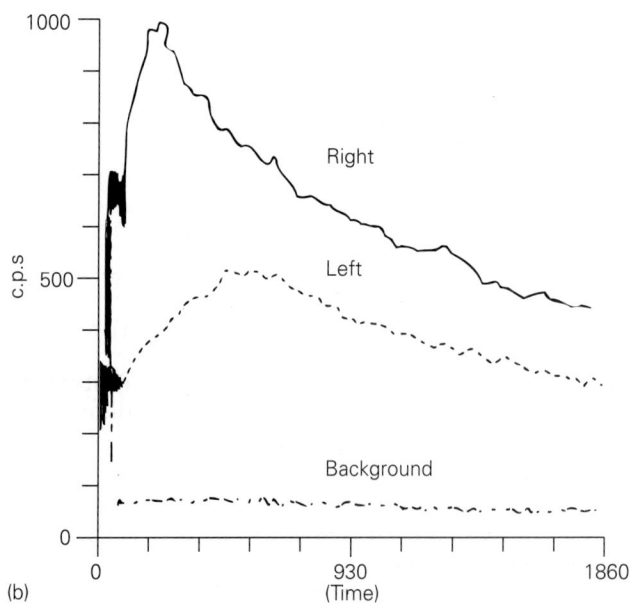

(b)

Figure 21.6   Baseline renogram performed with ^{99m}Tc-MAG3 in a man with renovascular hypertension. (a) Serial 2-min posterior images obtained during the first 32 min of the study show a small left kidney and normal right kidney. (b) Time–activity curves show normal kinetics on the right side with slow uptake, late peak, and normal excretion on the left side.

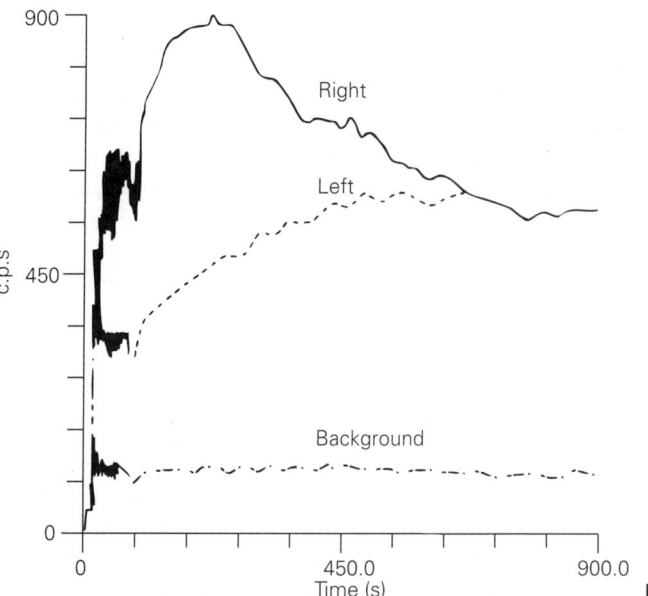

Figure 21.7   Captopril renogram performed with ^{99m}Tc-MAG3 in the same man shown in Figure 21.6. (a) Serial 2-min posterior images obtained during the first 32 min show marked retention of the radiopharmaceulical by the left kidney. (b) Time–activity curves show a marked change in renal kinetics on the left side with a persistently upsloping curve. The change following captopril is pathognomonic for renal artery stenosis.

with pharmacological intervention. A discussion appears below in greater detail.

Renovascular hypertension

Severe renal artery stenosis results in decreased upslope of phase 1 and 2 of the renogram, lower peak activity, and delay in peak activity with decreased downslope or even upslope in phase 3 (Figure 21.6). Although this pattern may be seen in other disorders, the unilateral presence of this finding in a young patient with hypertension and normal serum creatinine concentration is very specific. The renogram may be normal, however, when stenosis is less severe. Sensitivity of the renogram for hemodynamically significant renal artery stenosis may be increased by giving the patient an angiotensin converting enzyme (ACE) inhibitor such as captopril or enalapril immediately before the study [14–23]. ACE inhibitors interfere with compensatory vasoconstriction of the efferent glomerular arteriole which maintains hydrostatic pressure across the glomerulus. Vasodilatation of the efferent arteriole causes the glomerular filtration pressure to drop, the urine flow rate to decrease, and excretion of the radiopharmaceutical to decrease (Figure 21.7). If the renogram

is normal, hemodynamically significant renal artery stenosis is unlikely. If the renogram is abnormal, the study is usually repeated without an ACE inhibitor to exclude a coexisting abnormality mimicking renal artery stenosis.

Obstructive uropathy

The renogram is very useful in determining if pelvicalyceal dilatation is due to obstruction [24–26]. Pelvicalyceal dilatation causes prolongation of phase 3 of the renogram because the dilated collecting system takes longer to fill before emptying (Figure 21.8a, b). Obstruction can be differentiated from a non-obstructed system by administering furosemide during the study (Figure 21.8c). The standard dose is 0.5 mg/kg, which is

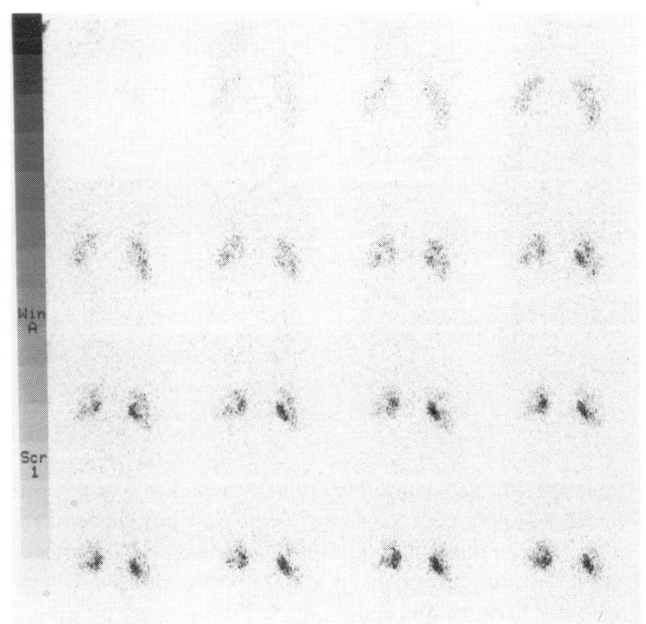

(a)

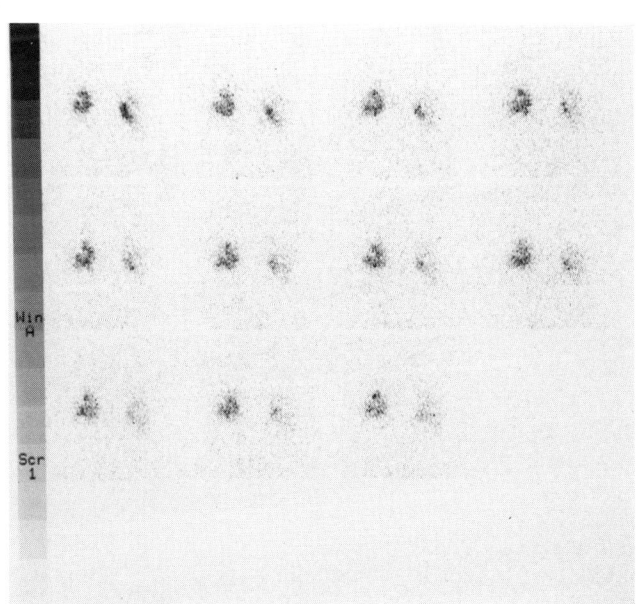

(b)

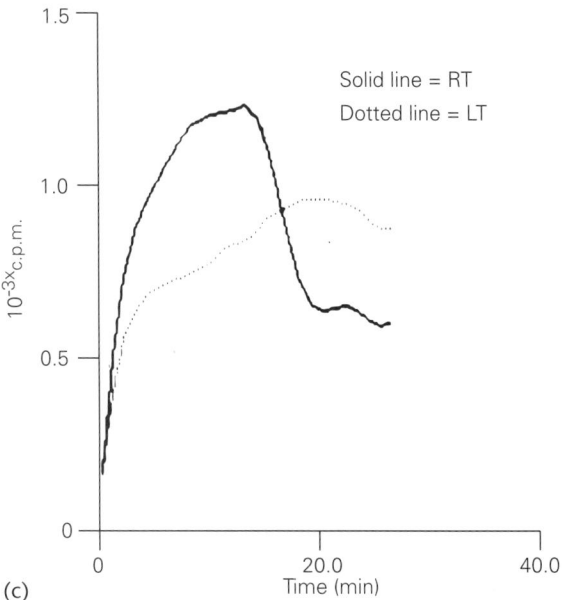

(c)

Figure 21.8 Diuretic renogram performed with [131I] hippuran in a man with a history of left pyeloplasty for ureteropelvic junction obstruction. (a) and (b) Serial 1-min posterior images obtained for 27 min show prompt uptake with pooling of the radiopharmaceutical in the collecting system of both kidneys prior to the intravenous administration of 40 mg of furosemide at 12 min. (c) Time–activity curves show prompt emptying of the right renal pelvis with little change on the left side after furosemide administration indicating recurrent left renal obstruction.

given intravenously during the study after the collecting system has filled. Increased urine flow will cause prompt washout of the radiopharmaceultical from the kidney if it is not obstructed. This is reflected in the renogram as a plateau followed by a rapid down slope. Furosemide has no effect on the renogram if the kidney is obstructed, although the renogram shows a greatly prolonged plateau.

Other applications

The renogram is useful in many other renal disorders, including renal vein thrombosis, infarction, pyelonephri-

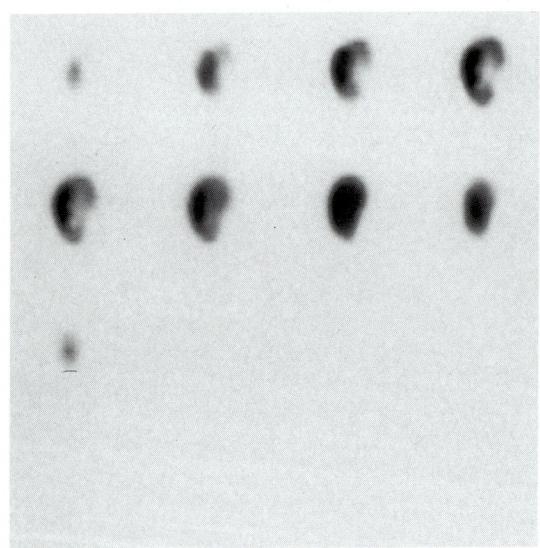

a

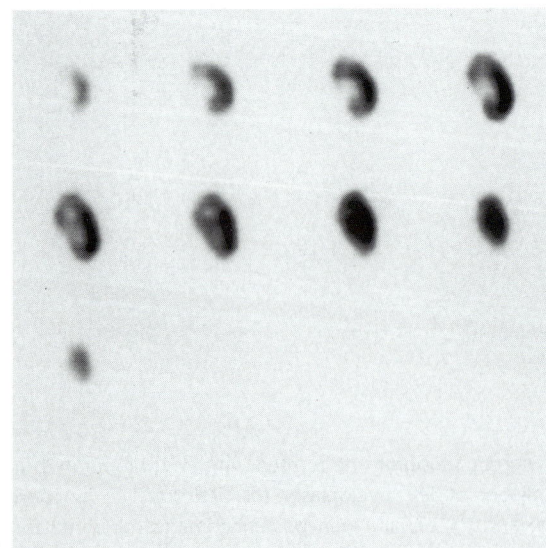

b

Figure 21.9 Tomographic images of the kidneys obtained 1 h after the injection of ^{99m}Tc-DMSA in a patient suspected of having a mass lesion in the left kidney on intravenous urogram. Coronal slices through the right (a) and left (b) kidney show normal cortical uptake of the radiopharmaceutical.

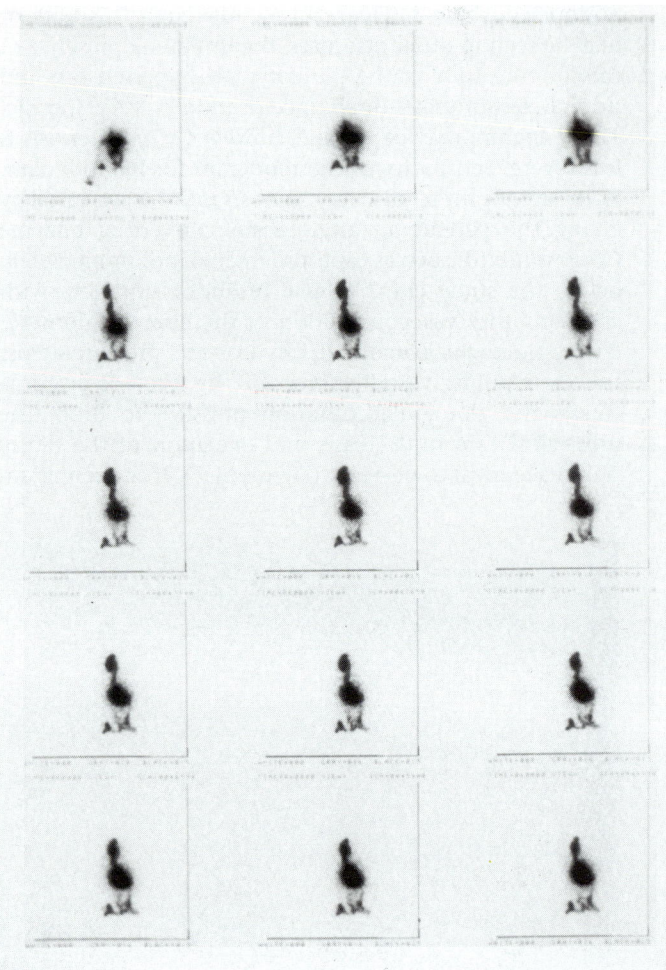

Figure 21.10 Radionuclide cystourethrogram in a child with recurrent urinary tract infections. Serial 30-s posterior images were obtained during filling of the bladder with [^{99m}Tc]pertechnetate. Vesicoureteral reflux up to the left renal pelvis is seen by the fourth frame of the study.

tis, glomerulonephritis, interstitial nephritis, acute tubular necrosis, renal trauma, radiation nephritis, and complications of transplantation. The renogram is usually used to track the course of the illness and evaluate response to therapy rather than as a primary test for diagnosis.

Renal scintigraphy and tomography

Radiopharmaceuticals, which are retained in the kidney for several hours, can generate static images which represent functioning renal parenchyma. Images may be acquired in a two-dimensional format analogous to plain film radiographs, or they may be acquired tomographically for greater detail (Figure 21.9). Renal scintigrams may be used to measure renal size and relative renal mass, and to detect pyelonephritis and reflux nephropathy [27–32].

Scintigraphy is also useful for differentiating normal renal parenchyma, such as dromedary humps and large septa of Bertin (cloisons), from neoplasms which appear as cold defects. However, ultrasound and computer-assisted tomography, which provide more anatomic detail, have largely supplanted scintigraphy.

Radionuclide voiding cystourethrography

Scintigraphy can be used to detect vesicoureteral reflux [27]. The same technique is used when the test is performed with contrast media. Low grades of reflux may not be detected because of interfering activity from the bladder. The radionuclide technique, however, may be more sensitive than contrast methods for detecting clinically significant reflux which reaches the renal pelvis (Figure 21.10). Radiation exposure is also lower than it is with contrast methods. This is particularly important for children with vesicoureteral reflux who require repeated evaluation.

Computed tomography of the kidneys

Introduction

Computed tomographic or CT scanning has a well-established role in modern-day renal imaging [33]. In addition, the spiral form of CT appears to be a useful test for patients suspected of having ureteral colic [34, 35]. Spiral CT angiography is a sensitive, relatively non-invasive test for diagnosing renal artery stenosis [36].

Technical details of CT imaging

Contemporary computed tomographic scanners utilize an X-ray tube source which rotates axially about the patient. Either a rotating or fixed array of detector elements detects X-rays transmitted through the patient at the opposite side. Computer algorithms use the digitized data from the transmitted X-ray beam to create, rapidly, axial CT scan images of the body (Figures 21.30a and 21.33a).

CT scanning has recently undergone a technical improvement called spiral CT [37, 38]. In conventional CT scanning, the scanner repetitively moves the patient linearly through a fixed distance, and performs axial scanning at fixed locations. In spiral CT, the scanner continuously moves the patient linearly at a constant rate while the X-ray source continuously rotates about the patient, producing a series of axial scan data through a selected cylindrical volume. Data are acquired from the entire region of the kidneys within one breathholding interval.

This represents a considerable advance over conventional CT methods which require multiple different breathholdings for acquisition of scan data through the region of the kidneys. A significant problem with this conventional approach is that patients typically suspend breathing at somewhat different levels with each breathhold, resulting in significant relative misregistration of the kidneys spatially on different breathholds. By using the spiral CT technique, which eliminates this spatial misregistration problem, the possibility of employing versatile reformatting techniques in a variety of planes and projections is realistic and permits the display of CT data in new and useful ways.

Applications

Renal imaging

CT scanning is widely used because it portrays retroperitoneal structures (such as the kidneys, adrenal glands and vessels) very well [39]. The excellent contrast differentiation of structures based on their X-ray density has several diagnostic advantages. With the high CT number of calcium, calcifications within the kidney (including calcifications in parenchyma or in neoplasms or renal calculi) are readily visible [39]. The ability to unequivocally define fat density on the basis of CT numbers allows the definitive diagnosis of renal angiomyolipoma with CT, since the presence of fat is virtually diagnostic of this neoplasm [39]. Perhaps the most common application of renal CT is for the diagnosis and staging of renal cell carcinoma, but there is wide application for the diagnosis of a variety of other processes including infectious and postinfectious conditions. In fact, CT is the best imaging technique for diagnosing acute pyelonephritis in an adult patient. CT is also commonly employed for imaging-assisted biopsy of the native kidney and adjacent structures, and for the assessment of living renal donors [40].

Renal and ureteral calculi

Spiral CT scanning without the use of contrast material is a rapid and effective test for the diagnosis of ureteral colic because it enables the examiner to visualize the high-density stone within the ureter. Figure 21.11(a, b) illustrates the capabilities for the display of reformatted CT data obtained in a breathholding interval; such reconstructions are not possible with conventional CT examination [34]. Figure 21.11(a) is an oblique coronal view showing both kidneys in a projection similar to that commonly seen with a conventional excretory urogram. The renal size discrepancy, left hydronephrosis and a lower pole left renal calculus are clearly visualized in this projection. Figure 21.11(b) is a sagittal reconstruction performed using a technique known as curved planar reformatting. Image data in which the course of the left ureter is visualized are interactively selected

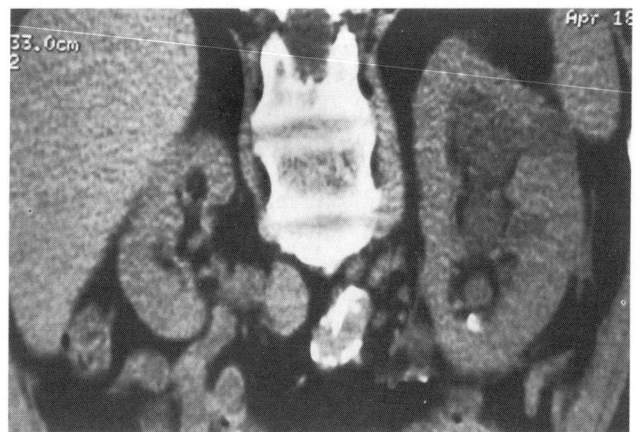

a

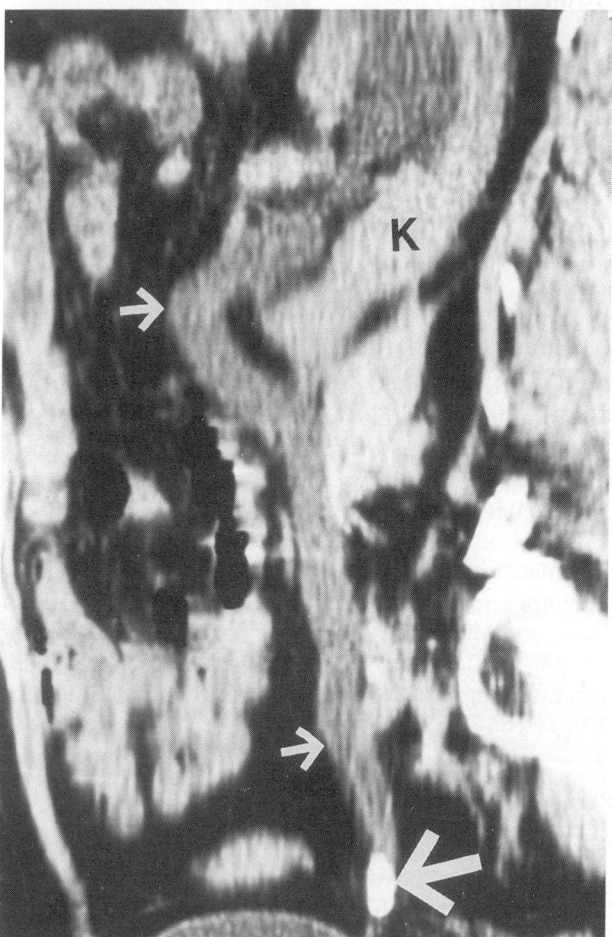

b

Figure 21.11 Reformatted spiral CT scan images of a patient with renal colic. (a) Oblique coronal view of the kidneys shows renal size discrepancy, hydronephrosis, a renal cyst and renal calculus on the left. (b) Sagittal curved planar reformatted image demonstrates left hydronephrosis and hydroureter (small arrows) proximal to a large distal ureteral stone (large arrow). K, kidney.

for various portions of the reconstruction. The observer can readily appreciate the hydronephrosis involving the left kidney as well as the dilated ureter passing down to the renal calculus near the ureterovesical junction; the appearance is similar to that seen on excretory urography.

Renal vascular imaging

Another innovative approach available with the spiral form of CT scanning is spiral CT angiography [36]. Data acquisition for a spiral CT angiogram of the renal vasculature, as shown in Figure 21.12, used a different technique from that used for conventional contrast CT of the kidneys. A test intravenous injection is given in order to time the passage of contrast from the injected vein to the renal arteries and to determine when the acquisition should begin. A higher injection rate than commonly

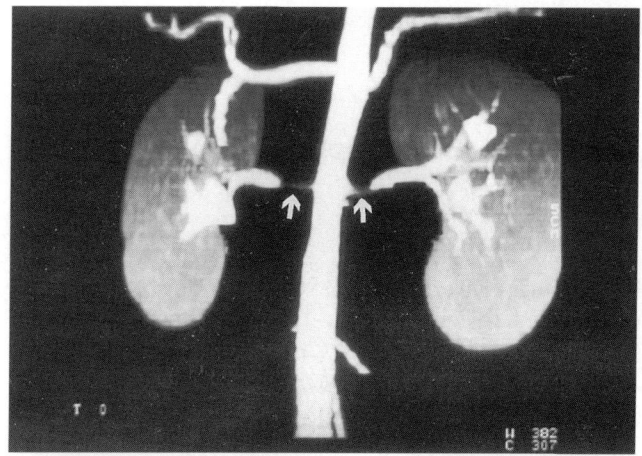

a

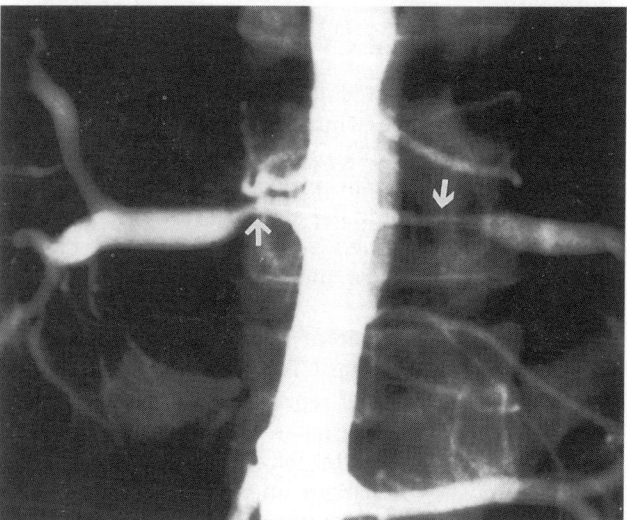

b

Figure 21.12 Young woman with Takayasu's arteritis and bilateral proximal renal artery stenosis. (a) Maximum intensity projection spiral CT angiogram, and (b) conventional arteriogram, showing the bilateral stenoses (arrows).

employed is used to obtain maximal opacification of the renal vasculature. A spiral CT acquisition volume is then set to encompass the region of both kidneys. Since the scan proceeds from superior to inferior, and contrast has not yet reached the kidneys early in the scans, the superior portions of the kidneys are not well opacified with contrast agent. The projection shown (Figure 21.12a) is called maximum intensity projection, which means that a projection or volume image is created which looks through the region of the kidneys and constructs a view consisting of the brightest point along each line through the selected imaging plane. Bilateral proximal renal artery stenoses are seen in a patient with Takayasu's arteritis and confirmed on the conventional arteriogram (Figure 21.12b). Studies comparing the capability of spiral CT angiography with standard angiographic techniques have confirmed the use of the spiral CT as a sensitive, relatively non-invasive tool for the evaluation of renal artery stenosis [41, 42].

Virtual endoscopy

CT virtual endoscopy [43, 44] can generate spectacular pictures of lesions involving the upper collecting system or bladder (Figure 21.13).

Plain radiography and urography are the oldest imaging examinations used for evaluating the urinary tract. The number of urographic examinations requested by clinicians in our institution has declined sharply in recent years because other examinations, especially ultrasonography, scintigraphy and CT, have rightfully replaced urography as the examination of choice for diagnosing a number of common disorders of the urinary tract. Many institutions throughout the world have noticed a similar decline. Nonetheless, we have not seen the complete demise of urography, the role of which is described below.

Plain radiography and urography

Plain radiography

Plain radiography is performed either alone or immediately before urography. The films, which must include the entire abdomen, provide a large amount of information about the bones, soft tissues and the position, size and shape of the kidneys. They are particularly important for showing stones and calcifications that contrast materials might obscure.

Plain film tomography is used to demonstrate stones and is also used prior to urography in patients with hematuria without proteinuria or casts.

Urography

Urography includes intravenous (excretory) urography, retrograde urography, cystography, voiding cystourethrography, retrograde urethrography, and special examinations of various surgically-created conduits. Figure 21.14 demonstrates the value of loopography for demonstrating a new transitional cell carcinoma in the upper collecting system in a patient who had a total cystectomy and ileal loop diversion for carcinoma of the bladder. Table 21.2 lists common indications for urography. Of these examinations, nephrologists most commonly request the intravenous urogram.

Intravenous (excretory) urography

Contrast materials

Modern contrast materials used for intravenous urography have either a higher or a low osmolality [45] and are excreted primarily by glomerular filtration [46]. The advantage of low-osmolality contrast materials is that, following intravenous injection, the prevalence of systemic reactions of all types is 3%, whereas it may be as high as 13% for high-osmolality contrast materials – although mild reactions account for about 98% of the latter [47]. For this reason, low-osmolality contrast materials are used almost exclusively outside the United States. Because of their high cost in the United States, some institutions use them selectively for high-risk patients. The definition of 'high-risk patient' varies from institution to institution.

Adverse reactions

Adverse reactions include systemic reactions and organ toxicity.

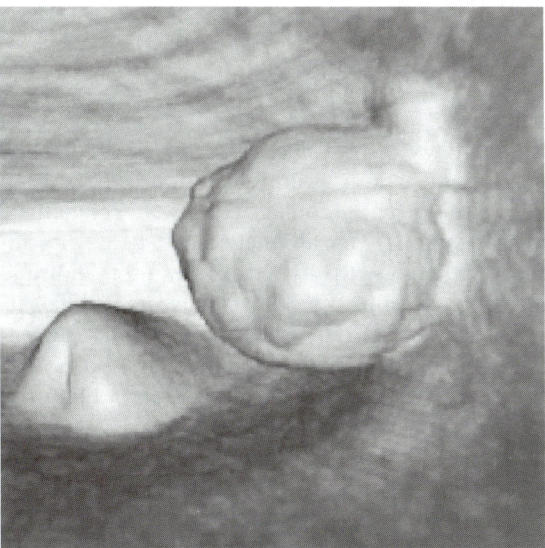

Figure 21.13 CT virtual endoscopy showing a polypoidal transitional cell carcinoma arising from the left lateral wall of the bladder. An enlarged prostate projects into the trigone.

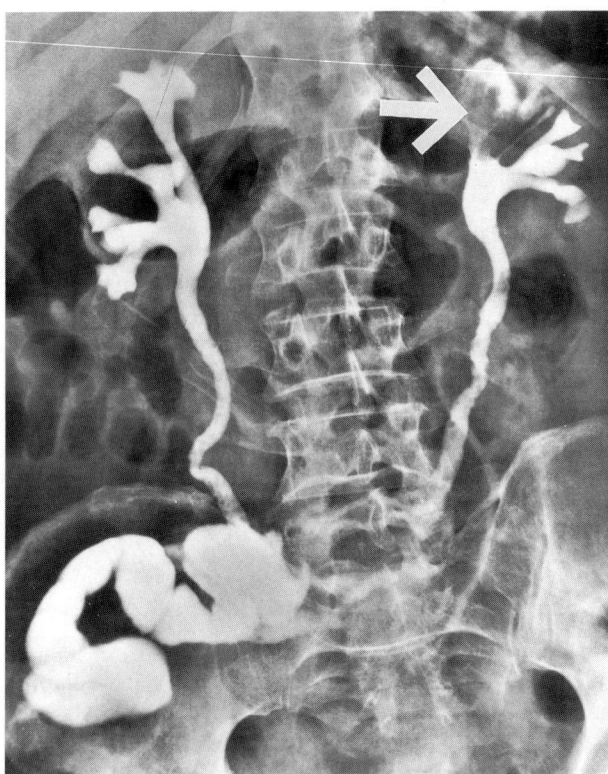

Figure 21.14 Loopogram illustrating bilateral ureteral reflux. A transitional cell carcinoma has produced a large filling defect in the infundibulum of the upper pole calyces of the left kidney (arrow). Ureteritis cystica accounts for the multiple ureteral filling defects (surgical proof). (Reproduced, with permission, from Friedland, G.W. *et al.* (1983) *Uroradiology: an Integrated Approach*, Churchill Livingstone, New York.)

Table 21.2   Common indications for urography

Examination	Common indications
Intravenous urography	1. Suspected papillary necrosis 2. Hematuria without proteinuria or casts 3. Persistent infections including? TB 4. Acute pain, ? arising from urinary tract 5. Hypertension in young adult females
Retrograde urography	1. Technically inadequate intravenous urogram in a patient in whom the clinicians suspect a ureteral lesion 2. To show ureteral leaks
Cystography	1. To show vesicoureteral reflux 2. To show bladder leaks
Voiding cystourethrogram	1. To show vesicoureteral reflux 2. To show urethral lesions
Retrograde urethrogram	1. To show lesions of the anterior urethra 2. Initial examination in patients with suspected urethral injury
Examination of surgically created conduits	1. To search of anastomotic leaks 2. To demonstrate dysfunction 3. To rule out upper tract obstruction (refluxing conduits) 4. To show recurrence of carcinoma

Non-idiosyncratic systemic reactions are usually mild. Idiosyncratic (anaphylactoid) systemic reactions vary in intensity, ranging from intermediate to severe to fatal. The risk of a severe reaction is 11 times higher in patients who have had a reaction to contrast materials, eight times higher in patients with a history of asthma, and four to five times higher in patients with a history of allergy to seafood or medications, hay fever, or other allergies [45, 48]. Most patients who develop idiosyncratic reactions, however, have no prior history of contrast reactions, asthma or allergies. Prophylaxis with adrenocorticosteroids, administered 12 and 2 h before examination, reduces the incidence of severe idiosyncratic systemic reactions in the general population [49, 50].

Organ toxicity usually involves either the kidney or the heart. The incidence of radiocontrast nephropathy depends on several risk factors, the best established of which are chronic renal insufficiency and diabetes mellitus. The risk of toxicity is directly related to the serum creatinine concentration in patients with renal disease.

Approximately 9% of patients, who have diabetic nephropathy and whose serum creatinine levels exceed 1.7 mg/dl, develop acute tubular necrosis after they have received intravenous contrast materials [51, 52]. In addition, in patients with hyperuricosuria or multiple myeloma, filtered contrast materials may precipitate sufficient uric acid crystals or abnormal proteins, respectively, to occlude the tubules. Adequate hydration, and in patients with hyperuricosuria, alkalinization of the urine as well, usually prevents such problems.

About 18% of patients with pre-existing heart disease, such as coronary artery disease, valvular disease and conduction disturbances, develop major cardiac arrhythmias or myocardial ischemia during administration of contrast materials [53]. Such patients should receive low-osmolality contrast materials, which should be administered slowly.

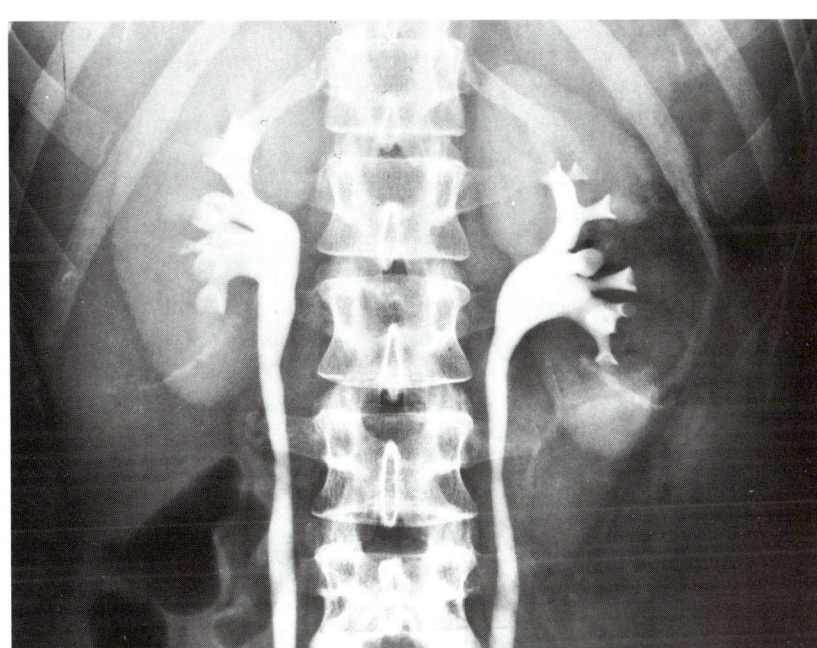

Figure 21.15 Intravenous urogram. Normal kidneys and upper urinary tracts. The only unusual – but not abnormal – feature is that the left kidney is lower than the right. (Reproduced, with permission, from Friedland, G.W. *et al.* (1983) *Uroradiology: An Integrated Approach*, Churchill Livingstone, New York.)

Interpretation

The kidneys

The examiner should study the urogram (Figure 21.15) and tomogram (Figure 21.16) and note the position, size and shape of the kidneys, the appearance of the renal papillae, as well as the nephrographic density.

Position

In 90% of people, the right kidney is lower than the left. The upper pole of the kidney is medial and posterior to the lower pole, and the posterior papillae and calyces are medial to the anterior papillae and calyces (the medial–posterior rule). The medial border is much more anterior than the lateral border, so that the kidney lies at an angle of about 30° from the horizontal. A kidney may lie in an abnormal position for several reasons: a mass has displaced it, it is unusually mobile (renal ptosis), a rotational anomaly is present, or it is congenitally in an abnormal location (ectopic).

Size and shape

There are several charts giving normal renal size on intravenous urography [53–57]. Equally important, however, is the evaluation of the renal parenchymal thickness [58], which involves sketching the interpapillary line uniting the tips of the outermost papillae and measuring the distance between this line and the renal outline (Figure 21.17). In any given individual, measurements made in similar places are nearly equal on both sides, and any dif-

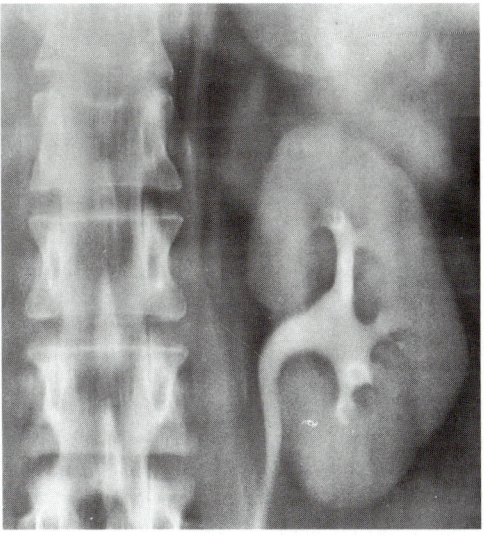

Figure 21.16 Nephrotomogram. Normal left kidney.

ference should lead the examiner to suspect that a lesion may exist.

A normal kidney can be large if its collecting system is duplicated or if it has undergone compensatory hypertrophy.

Common normal variations in shape include fetal lobations, the remnants of the divisions separating the fetal renal lobes, which are seen as sharp clefts located between calyces (Figure 21.18); the splenic impression, a smooth impression indenting the upper lateral margin

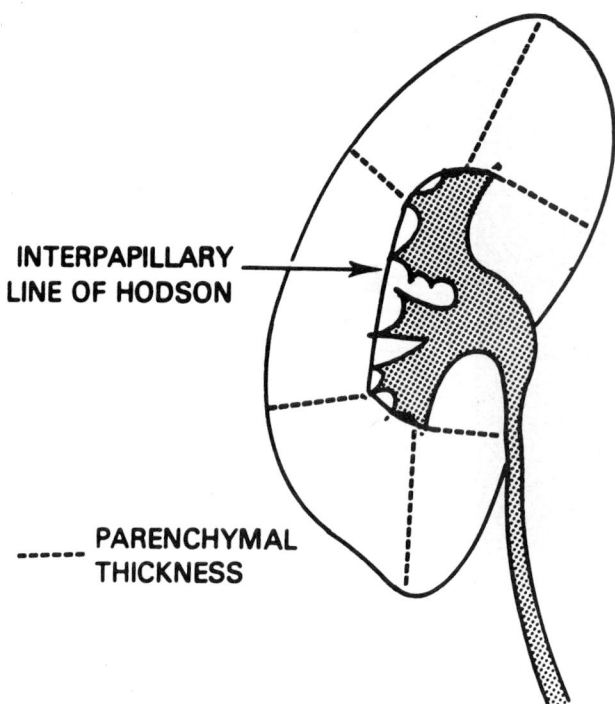

INTERPAPILLARY LINE OF HODSON

PARENCHYMAL THICKNESS

Figure 21.17 The interpapillary line of Hodson, actually first described by Pendergrass [58]. This line is used to measure the renal parenchymal thickness in multiple sites in each kidney. (Reproduced, with permission, from Friedland, G.W. (1984) Urography. *Monogr. Urol.*, **5**, 26–59.)

increases the size of the kidney. If such processes are diffuse, the kidney appears smooth in outline; if they are focal, the kidney appears lumpy.

Chronic processes that scar the kidney, significantly reduce the number of nephrons, or reduce the arterial supply, will generally produce a small kidney. Again, if the process is diffuse, the kidney will generally appear smooth in outline; if focal, then focal areas of parenchymal thinning result. The appearance of the associated papillae provides further evidence as to the possible pathology. For example, if the parenchyma overlying a normal-appearing calyx is thinned, a renal infarct is the most likely etiology (Figure 21.19), but if the calyx is clubbed, chronic pyelonephritis (Figure 21.20), tuberculosis or postobstructive atrophy due to prior stone are probable causes. Intravenous urography is useful in following children with chronic pyelonephritis to show the development and progression of clubbing and scarring (Figures 21.20 and 21.21) [60].

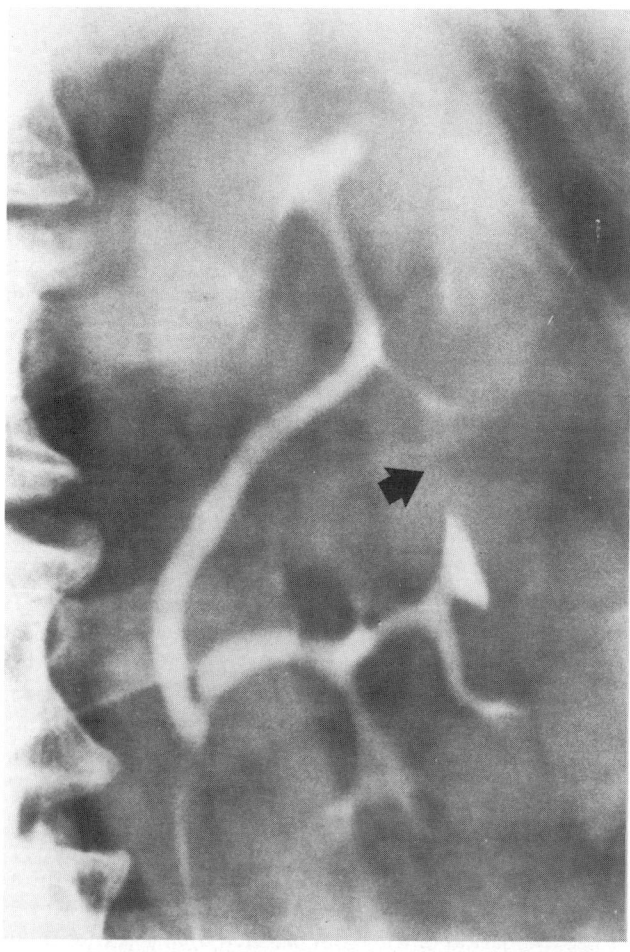

Figure 21.18 Fetal lobation, seen as a sharp cleft located between calyces (arrow). The renal pelvis is duplicated. (Reproduced, with permission, from Friedland, G.W. *et al.* (1984) *Uroradiology: an Integrated Approach*, Churchill Livingstone, New York.)

of the left kidney; the dromedary hump, normal renal tissue resembling a mass protruding from the lateral margin of the midzone of the left kidney, often located below the splenic impression, the parenchymal thickness of which is similar to the thickness of the midzone on the right; and a large septum of Bertin, a renal mass consisting of normally functioning nephrons, ranging from 2 to 6 cm in diameter, located between the upper pole and midzone in 93% of patients, which drains into unusual-looking calyces, and which is bilateral in 60% of cases [59].

A fused kidney, such as a horseshoe kidney, is a classic example of an abnormality in shape.

Diseased kidneys can vary in size from small to normal to large, as can their measured parenchymal thickness. They may be smooth or lobulated in outline. Abnormalities in size or shape or both may involve both kidneys, one kidney, or a part of one kidney. Using basic principles, the examiner can usually arrive at the most likely causes for a given appearance. Acute inflammatory processes, infiltration with cells or abnormal substances, increase in interstitial fluid, hemorrhage, cystic lesions, acute obstruction of the draining veins or the renal tubules or obstruction of the collecting system, usually

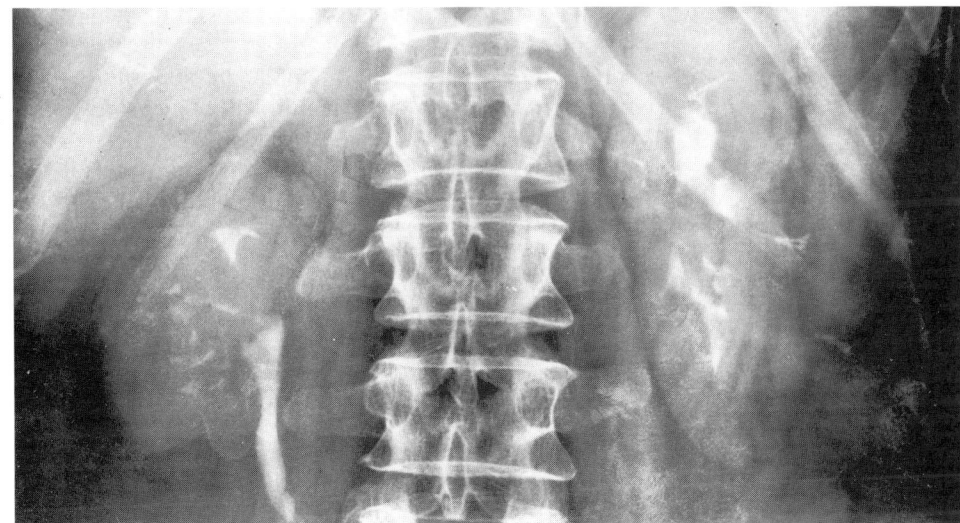

Figure 21.19 Multiple renal infarcts. There are multiple parenchymal scars overlying normal-appearing calyces. The patient had mitral stenosis and atrial fibrillation – the source of the renal emboli. (Reproduced, with permission, from Friedland. G.W. *et al.* (1983) *Uroradiology: an Integrated Approach*, Churchill Livingstone, New York.)

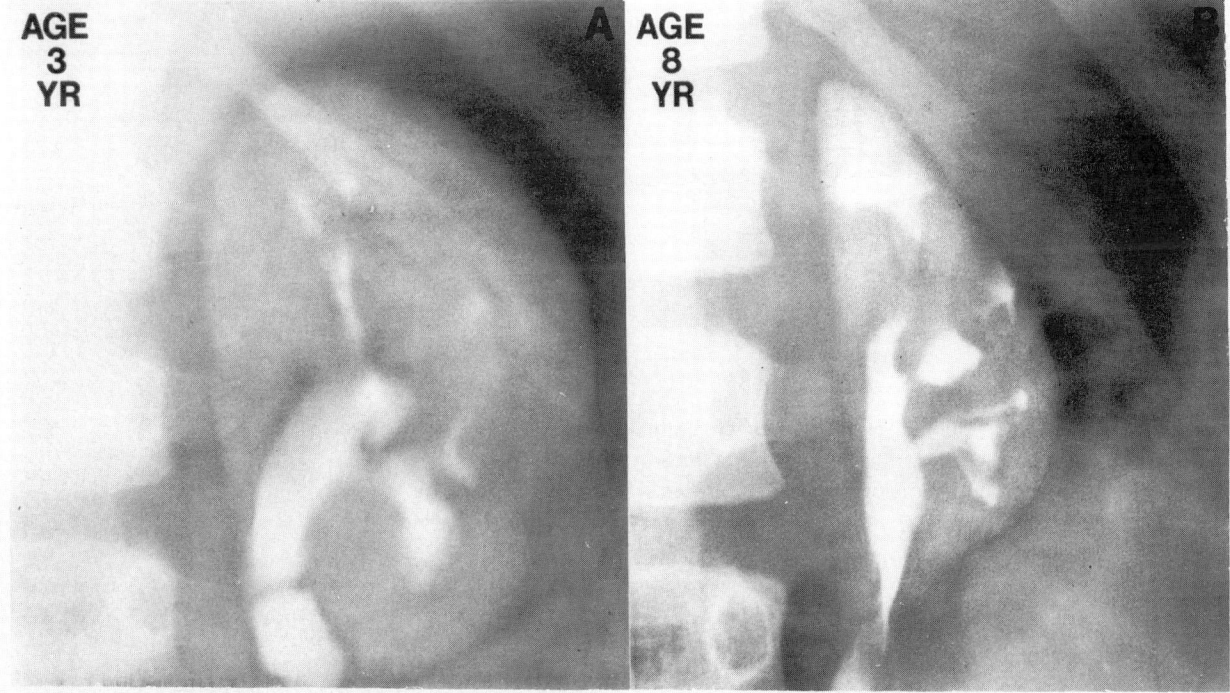

Figure 21.20 Chronic pyelonephritis involving the left kidney which has progressed from ages 3 to 8 years. Unlike the appearances seen in Figure 21.19, the calyces are clubbed. Between ages 3 and 8 years, the upper pole calyx has moved closer to the spine, the lower pole calyx has moved closer to the ureter, and the renal pelvis has become more vertical – all common findings when parenchymal scarring affects the medial aspect of the kidney. (Reproduced, with permission, from Friedland, G.W. *et al.* (1974) Distance of upper pole calyx to ureter as indicators of parenchymal loss in children. *Pediatr. Radiol.*, **2**, 29–38).

It is important to realize that intravenous urography is not the examination of choice for patients who might have some of the disease processes that alter renal size or shape (e.g. acute pyelonephritis; the acute glomerulonephritides), and that some such patients do not require imaging examinations for diagnosis at all.

Papillae

Renal papillae are the nipple-shaped projections of the renal medulla into the cup-shaped calyces of the collecting system. The term simple papilla describes a papilla that drains a single renal lobe. Some papillae, particularly

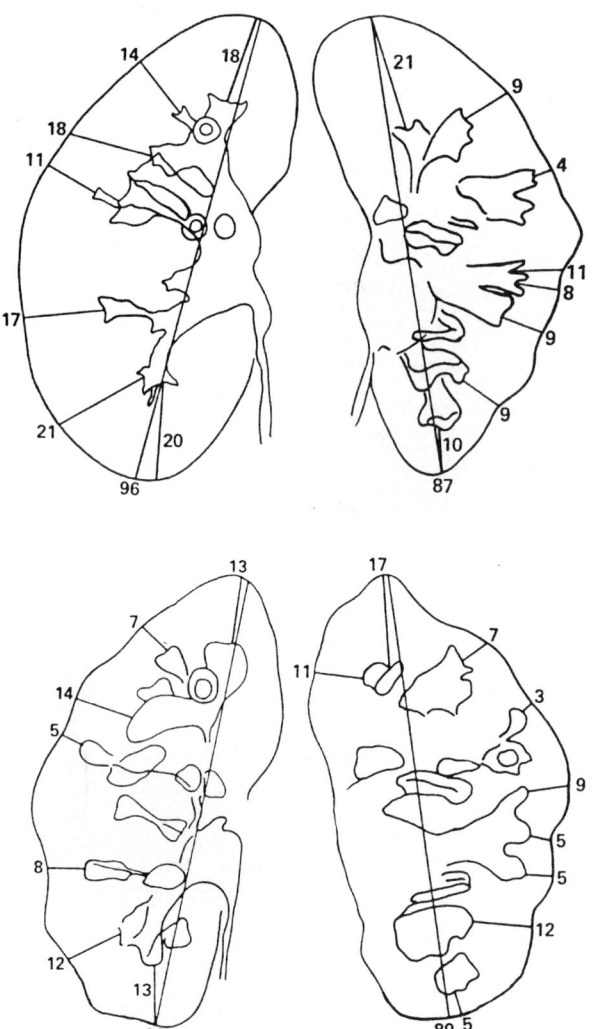

Figure 21.21 Progressive clubbing and scarring of both kidneys over a 3-year period. The scarring is detected by measuring the parenchymal thickness at multiple sites. (Reproduced, with permission, from reference [60].)

upper pole papillae, may fuse with adjacent papillae during their development, forming compound papillae, which are more likely to allow intrarenal reflux (retrograde flow into the tubules) (Figure 21.22) and which may resemble abnormal papillae on an intravenous urogram. Whether normal papillae are simple or compound, however, the fornices of their associated calyces should appear sharp.

Most papillary changes are due to hydrocalycosis, papillary necrosis, papillary scarring, medullary nephrocalcinosis or medullary sponge kidneys. With early hydrocalycosis, the fornix of the calyx becomes blunted and the papilla appears flattened. Later, the calyx may become club-shaped and the renal parenchyma thinned. When papillary necrosis is present, contrast material may flow into ragged cavities, extending either from the tip of the papilla or from one or both fornices

(Figure 21.23). As the disease advances, the cavities may become flame-shape, ring-shaped (contrast material surrounding the sloughed papilla) or butterfly-shaped. In patients with analgesic nephropathy, the papillae may calcify.

The presence of multiple punctate calcifications in the papillae suggest medullary nephrocalcinosis. If multiple linear streaks or rice-grain-sized opacities appear in one or more papillae during intravenous urography, the patient has medullary sponge kidneys (Figure 21.24).

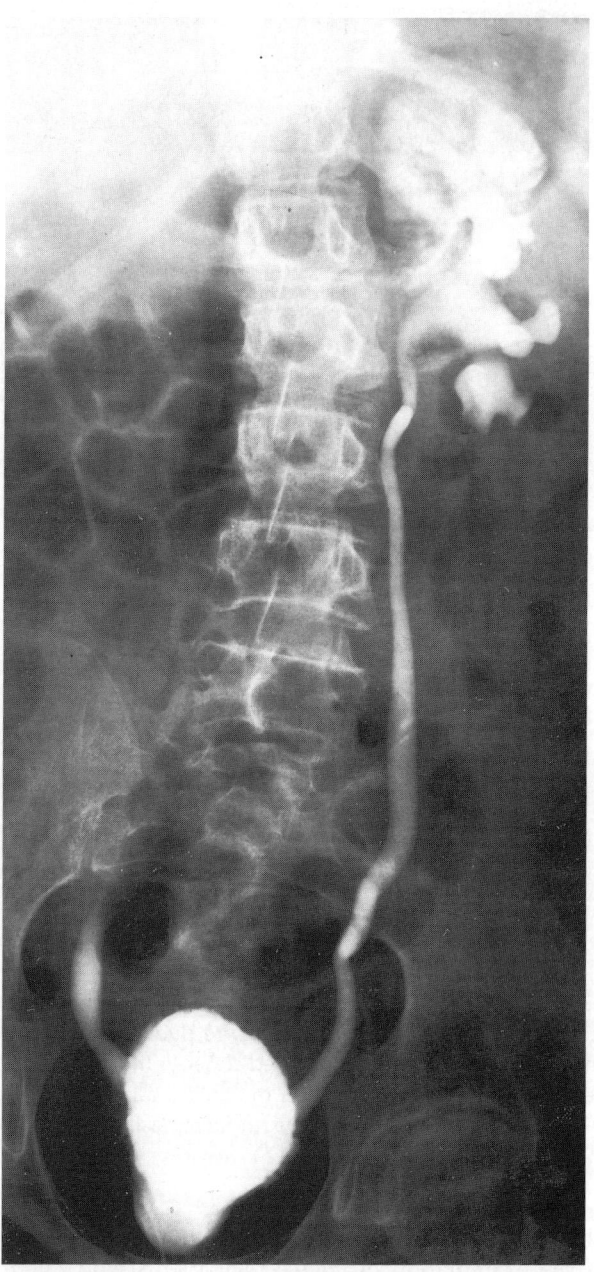

Figure 21.22 Cystogram. There is grade I reflux on the right, and grade II reflux on the left. Contrast material fills the renal tubules in the upper pole of the left kidney (intrarenal reflux).

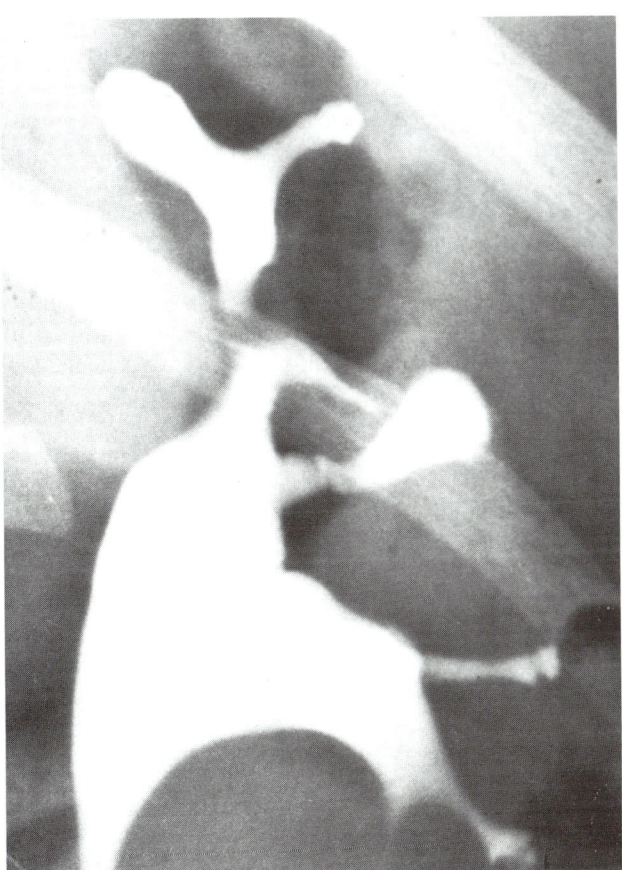

Figure 21.23 Papillary necrosis. (Reproduced, with permission, from Friedland, G.W. *et al.* (1983) *Uroradiology: an Integrated Approach*, Churchill Livingstone, New York.)

The nephrogram

Shortly after intravenous injection, contrast material opacifies the kidney. During this early vascular phase of the nephrogram, the cortex and septa of Bertin appear more opaque than the medulla because 80% of the blood flow is directed to the cortex and 20% to the medulla (Figure 21.25). At 1 min after intravenous injection, filtered contrast material fills the renal tubules, rendering normal kidneys uniformly opaque on a radiograph – the urographic nephrogram. By 2–2.5 min, contrast material appears in the calyces, after which the nephrogram gradually fades.

Table 21.3 lists nephrographic abnormalities and their common causes [47], although, at the present time, intravenous urography is not indicated for diagnosing all the entities marked with an asterisk. Figure 21.26 illustrates the typical dense nephrogram on the left, seen 1 h after injection of contrast material, in a patient with acute left ureteral obstruction due to a stone at the ureterovesical junction.

In some emergency situations, correct interpretation of the nephrographic abnormality may lead to kidney-saving intervention. In a patient with acute ureteral colic,

for example, an absent nephrogram on the painful side suggests acute arterial occlusion rather than a ureteral calculus.

Upper collecting system and bladder

Crossing vessels frequently indent the infundibula of the calyces, usually creating lucent defects with parallel margins. Most renal pelves are trumpet-shaped, with a convex upper margin and a concave lower margin. After leaving the ureteropelvic junction, the ureter crosses the psoas muscle and runs downward between the tips of the transverse processes and the bodies of the lumbar vertebrae. Upon entering the pelvis, the ureter usually curves laterally before sweeping medially and forward to enter the bladder posteriorly. Crossing vessels and the psoas muscle may notch the ureter.

The bladder has an oval or round configuration; the colon or uterus may indent its fundus.

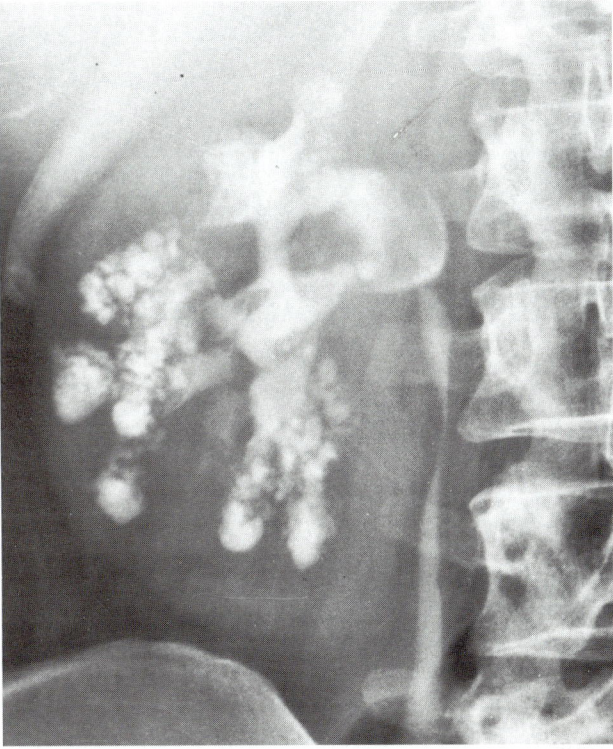

Figure 21.24 Intravenous urogram. The right kidney in a patient with bilateral medullary sponge kidneys is shown. The papillae contain multiple small cavities, which vary in size. The filling defect seen in the renal pelvis disappeared on a follow-up examination, and probably represented a blood clot. Nephrocalcinosis was visible on the preliminary radiograph. (Reproduced, with permission, from Friedland, G.W. *et al.* (1983) *Uroradiology: an Integrated Approach*, Churchill Livingstone, New York.)

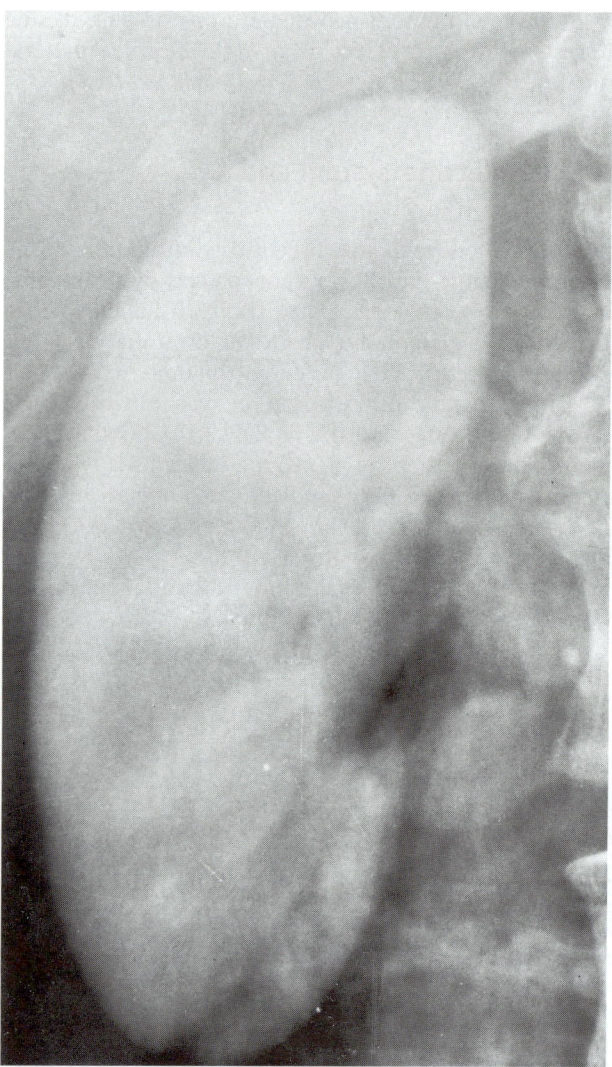

Figure 21.25 Vascular phase of the nephrogram. The medullary pyramids are visible as faint lucencies.

nical capabilities are continuing to expand. As a result, its role in renal imaging is not yet fully defined. The MRI images shown in this section may be obtained without ionizing radiation or, in most cases, intravenous contrast material.

MRI is useful for staging renal cell carcinoma in patients who cannot receive iodinated contrast materials. It shows clear potential for evaluating patients with renal vascular diseases. Although MRI can provide clinically helpful images in patients with renal failure or with a transplanted kidney, ultrasound is equally informative and considerably cheaper. MRI does not detect calcifications and calculi.

Important abnormalities involving the upper collecting system or the bladder include calculi (either opaque or non-opaque), filling defects due to neoplasms (Figure 21.27), calculi, sloughed papillae, fungus balls or blood clots, ureteral narrowing or obstruction due to intrinsic neoplasms, retroperitoneal fibrosis or abdominal or retroperitoneal masses, and the impressions of the bladder base in men due to an enlarged prostate.

Magnetic resonance imaging of the kidneys

Introduction

Renal magnetic resonance imaging (MRI) is still relatively new compared to other imaging modalities and its tech-

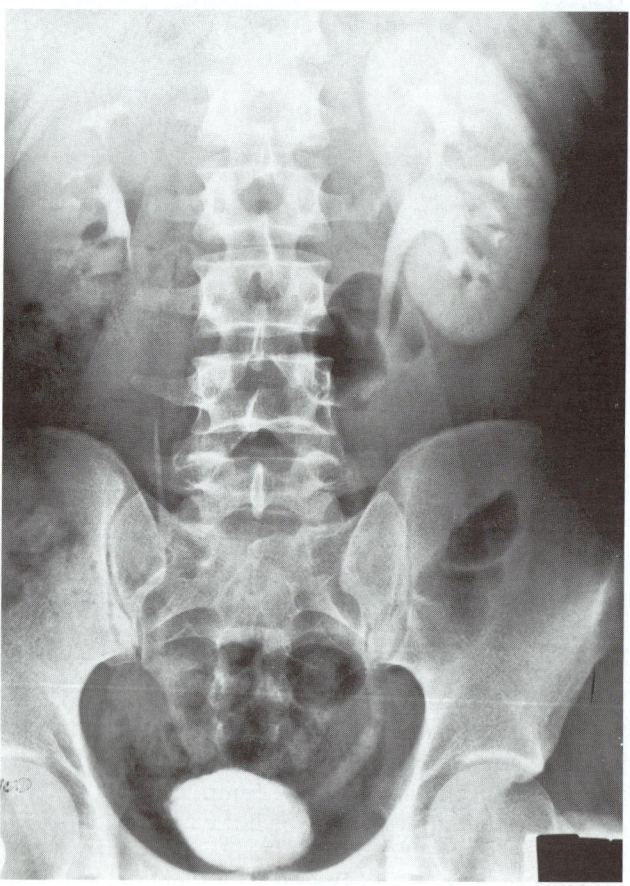

Figure 21.26 Obstructive nephrogram. The patient had a calculus obstructing the distal end of the left ureter. This radiography, exposed 1 h after contrast material was injected intravenously, shows a dense nephrogram on the left, and a mild left hydroureteronephrosis. Provided the patient is well hydrated, a plain film of the abdomen plus an ultrasound examination in the urinary tract (Figure 21.2) or a spiral CT examination (Figure 21.11) will produce an equally satisfactory diagnostic result, much faster, and with much less discomfort to the patient.

Table 21.3 Nephrographic abnormalities and their common causes

Nephrographic abnormality	Common causes

Absent	1. Acute arterial occlusion
	2. Severely diseased kidney
	  • unilateral
	  • bilateral*
	3. Absent kidney

Appears at 1 min, but is faint and persists for hours	1. Chronic glomerular disease* 2. Widespread microthromboembolic disease
Initially faint, but becomes increasingly dense over hours or days	1. Acute ureteral obstruction 2. Acute hypotension (bilateral) 3. Severe main renal artery stenosis (usually unilateral)* 4. Acute tubular necrosis* 5. Acute intratubular obstruction* 6. Acute renal vein thrombosis
Normal at 1 min, but persists or increases over hours or days	1. Acute tubular necrosis* 2. Acute bacterial nephritis*
Striated	1. Acute ureteral obstruction 2. Acute bacterial nephritis* 3. Acute pyelonephritis* 4. Autosomal recessive polycystic kidney disease*
Patchy	1. Obliterative diseases of the renal microvasculature

* Intravenous urography not the imaging examination of choice.

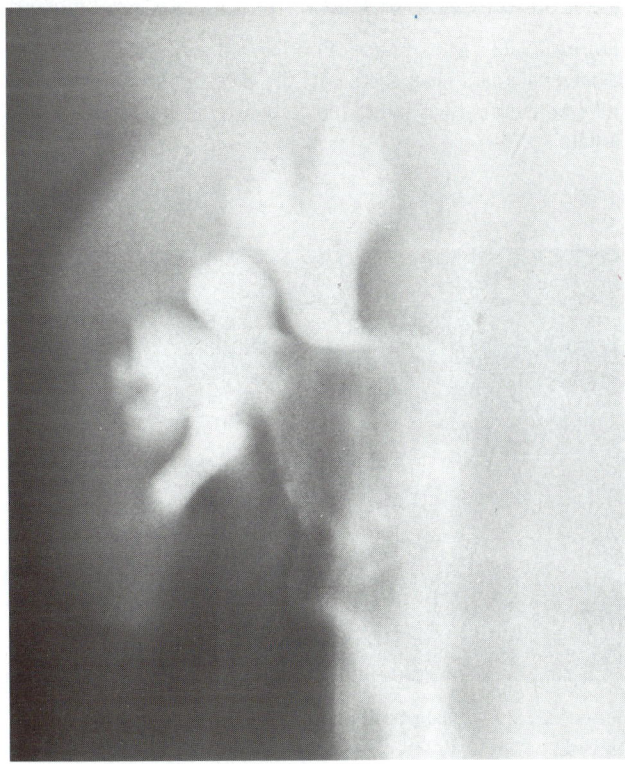

Figure 21.27 Nephrotomogram showing a large filling defect in the renal pelvis due to a transitional cell carcinoma (surgical proof). (Reproduced, with permission, from Friedland, G.W. *et al.* (1983) *Uroradiology: an Integrated Approach*, Churchill Livingstone, New York.)

MRI creation

In MRI, cross-sectional images in any desired plane may be created by exploiting the fact that, in a high magnetic field, water protons in the body may be induced to emit radiowave energy. This energy, which may be detected and localized, is ultimately displayed in image format [61]. The technique uses the inherent magnetization properties of water protons functioning as small magnets. Their overall magnetization, following appropriate per-turbation with a radio frequency field, is governed by two relaxation constants referred to as T1 and T2. It is important to know this general principle because mag-netic resonance images are generally produced to either reflect predominantly the T1 values of tissue, or the T2 values of tissues. A representative axial T1-weighted image and a T2-weighted coronal image of normal kidneys in two different patients are shown in Figure 21.28(a) and (b) respectively. In T1-weighted imaging, as shown, corticomedullary differentiation is possible since there is a significant difference between the T1 values of cortical and medullary renal tissue. Although T2-weighted images in many cases give superior image con-trast to T1-weighted images, and better demonstration of pathologic processes, corticomedullary differentiation is generally not readily evident, as in Figure 21.28(b).

Magnetic resonance contrast agents generally function similarly to those employed for X-ray CT scanning because, in T1-weighted imaging, materials with short T1 appear relatively bright. Intravenous gadolinium con-trast agent, widely used in MRI, causes substantial T1 shortening when the blood supply brings it to the kidney, providing the enhancement for T1-weighted images [61, 62].

Applications of renal MRI

General considerations

Renal vascular imaging is an area of particular interest and promise. The flow of blood can be exploited in MRI to create various classes of images, whereby blood is visu-alized due to its motion in the body [63]. One such class of images (termed phase-contrast images) uses the fact that protons moving within a magnetic field gradient acquire a phase shift which may be detected via a mag-netic resonance technique. An example of such an image is shown in Figure 21.29, which depicts the renal vessels of a normal subject. The lack of ionizing radiation and wealth of information available even without an intra-venous contrast agent injection are attractive features of the MRI technique.

There are limitations, nonetheless, to renal imaging with MRI, including the lack of ability to detect calcifi-cations or renal calculi as there are no mobile protons associated with such calcifications. MRI thus has no present or expected future role in evaluation of renal cal-cifications or calculi.

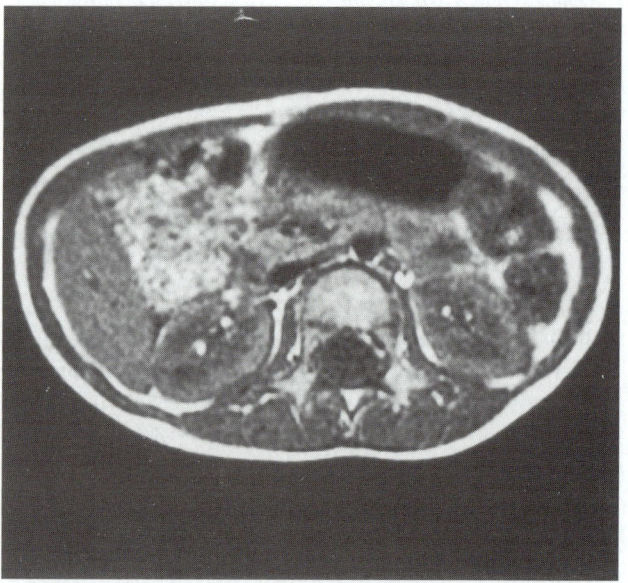

a

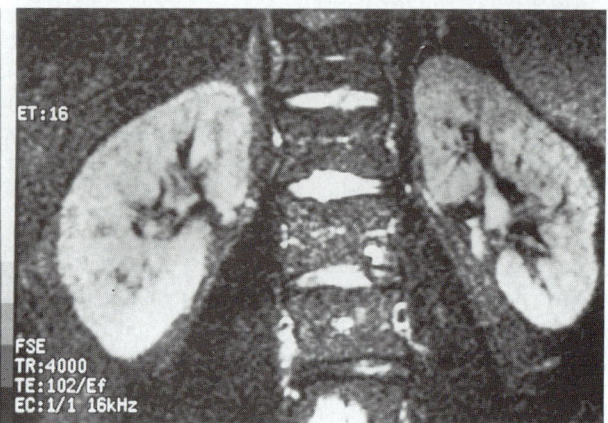

b

Figure 21.28   MRI images of normal kidneys. (a) T1-weighted axial renal images in a child; note the excellent corticomedullary differentiation; (b) T2-weighted coronal renal images in a young adult.

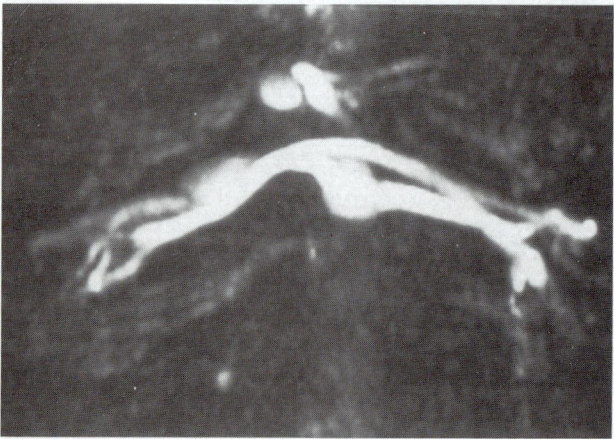

Figure 21.29   Axial phase-contrast MRI image of normal renal vessels.

Evaluation of renal masses

Most studies to date have concerned the evaluation of renal masses, including various forms of renal neoplasms and cystic diseases. A common practical use of MRI is in the staging of renal malignancies, particularly renal cell carcinoma, in patients for whom an intravenous injection of iodinated contrast material may be contraindicated. Without contrast, CT would not demonstrate intravascular extension of the neoplasm or differentiate vessels from enlarged lymph nodes [61–63]. In this application, MRI is particularly useful for the evaluation of venous extension of neoplasm due to the ease with which MR sequences may demonstrate renal vessels.

Renal failure

For common entities associated with renal failure, including renal obstruction, diffuse renal diseases and adult-type polycystic kidney disease, MRI provides images which are clearly diagnostic of these conditions. At present, MRI is not the method of choice for these evaluations, since competing tests, particularly diagnostic ultrasound, can diagnose these entities with equal effectiveness and at a substantially lower cost.

The transplanted kidney

Similarly, for the transplanted kidney, MRI is effective at demonstrating obstruction and perinephric fluid collections, but does not offer significant benefits over ultrasound. It was initially hoped that a loss of corticomedullary differentiation in T1-weighted images would prove a sign specific for transplant rejection, but this is a non-specific finding.

Vascular diseases of the kidney

An area in which MRI shows clear potential is in the evaluation of vascular diseases affecting the kidney [64–66]. The various forms of MRI available today permit visualization of the renal arteries and veins with image quality which allows diagnosis of some significant abnormalities affecting the arteries and veins. Renal vein thrombosis may readily be detected as a lack of flow and/or filling defect in a renal vein. In addition, phase-contrast MRI techniques may be adapted for quantitative measures of renal blood flow. This may prove valuable in the future for assessing flow to kidneys in which ischemia is suspected.

Significant arterial stenotic disease may also be detected with MRI techniques, often as a dark region or flow void related to turbulent flow distal to a region of stenosis in an artery. The current quality of MRI studies of the renal arteries, and ability of MRI to diagnose arterial stenoses, are inferior to that of conventional arteriography. Improvements in these techniques are needed if these methods are to become competitive for clinical use.

Renal angiography

Introduction

Selected renal angiography has been in clinical practice for over 30 years [67, 68]. It is the gold standard for renal vascular disorder diagnosis. The introduction of high resolution CT, ultrasound and MRI, however, has greatly diminished the need for invasive techniques such as renal arteriography. In combination with excretory urography these cross-sectional imaging techniques are now the imaging methods of choice to evaluate renal trauma, inflammatory disease, renal cysts and parenchymal masses [69, 70]. Nevertheless, renal angiography is still valuable to confirm the diagnosis of renal artery stenosis and to detect microangiopathic abnormalities such as vasculitis. In the past decade there has been increased utilization of angiography to guide renal vascular interventions. These include angioplasty, stent placement, and embolization of tumors and vascular lesions.

Technique

In most instances the radiologist can perform renal angiography on an outpatient basis. It is important that the radiologist observes the femoral artery puncture site for 6h after the procedure. After obtaining informed consent and using sterile technique, the radiologist catheterizes the femoral artery using the Seldinger method. A 5-French pigtail catheter is advanced to the level of the renal arteries and a midstream aortogram is performed. This preliminary study is essential in order to identify the number and location of the renal arteries and to evaluate the renal ostia prior to selective catheterization. The catheter for the midstream angiogram is then exchanged over a guidewire for a 5-French preshaped renal catheter for selective renal angiography. Most renal angiography is performed with 5-French catheters. Larger size catheters, however, may be used on occasion to improve torque control.

One important technical refinement is the increased use of digital subtraction angiography. The following principles are involved in conventional photographic subtraction: The radiologist obtains a scout radiograph of the area of interest, without contrast agent in the vessels. The radiologist then copies this radiograph on special film, which produces a photographic negative called the mask. The bones, which looked white on the original radiograph, appear black on the mask; similarly, the soft tissues, which looked off-white on the original radiograph, appear dark gray on the mask. Finally, the radiologist superimposes the mask on each subsequent radiograph of the same area obtained during contrast injection with the patient in the same position, and makes a copy (one set at a time) of each set of superimposed films. These copies are called the subtraction films. The black and dark gray images of the bones and soft tissues, respectively, present on the mask, cancel out the superimposed white and off-white images of these structures present on the films obtained during contrast injection, so that only the injected contrast agent, which was not present on the mask, is now visible on the subtraction films, without overlying bones and soft tissues. In digital subtraction angiography, the equipment performs the subtraction digitally, without the use of films. The advantages of the digital subtraction techniques are that they are very rapid and use lower volumes of contrast agents.

Indications for renal angiography

Current indications for renal arteriography include the following: (1) diagnosis of renal artery stenosis, (2) evaluation for suspected vasculitis such as polyarteritis nodosa, (3) guidance for renal vascular interventions including angioplasty stenting and embolization.

Cross-sectional imaging techniques such as CT, ultrasound and MRI cannot reliably demonstrate renal microaneurysms in vasculitis. Selective renal angiography with magnification views remains the diagnostic method of choice when vasculitis is a clinical consideration (Figure 21.30).

A variety of imaging techniques is used to screen for renovascular hypertension including renal scintigraphy, duplex Doppler sonography, MR angiography and, most recently, three-dimensional CT angiography. The reported sensitivity and specificity of the above techniques vary widely among institutions. Renal scintigraphy with angiotensin converting enzyme inhibitors may provide important functional information about renal blood flow. However, it is sometimes difficult to recognize bilateral stenosis.

Color Doppler sonography with spectral Doppler tracings can be used to evaluate the main renal arteries as well as obtaining spectral waveforms from intrarenal vessels. There is some controversy in the radiologic literature regarding the ultimate reliability of the technique in the diagnosis of renal artery stenosis. In many patients the origins of the renal arteries cannot be identified clearly due to overlying bowel gas. The Doppler waveform obtained from segmental renal vessels distal to a functionally significant renal artery stenosis may demonstrate blunting and loss of the early systolic peak of the arterial waveform (travus-parvus abnormality). More recent studies suggest this abnormality is not specific for renal artery stenosis.

In selected patients both MR angiography and three-dimensional CT angiography may provide excellent anatomic detail of the proximal main renal arteries [41, 66]. Initial preliminary studies suggest that with further development it is quite possible that one or both of these techniques may ultimately be the screening method of choice to evaluate patients with suspected renovascular hypertension. MR has two advantages over CT: (1) images are obtained without intravenous contrast and (2) blood

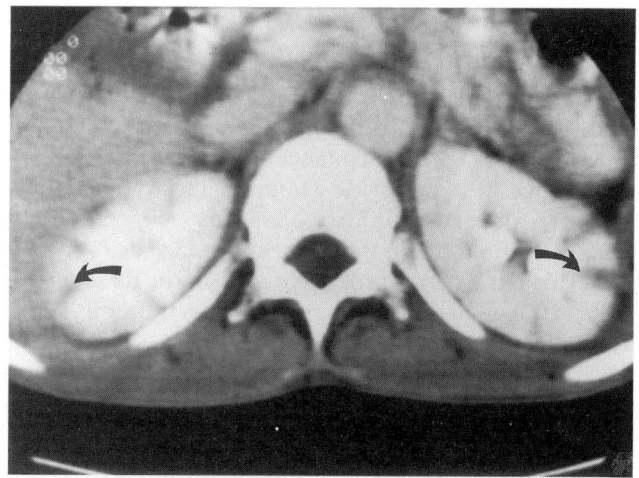

a

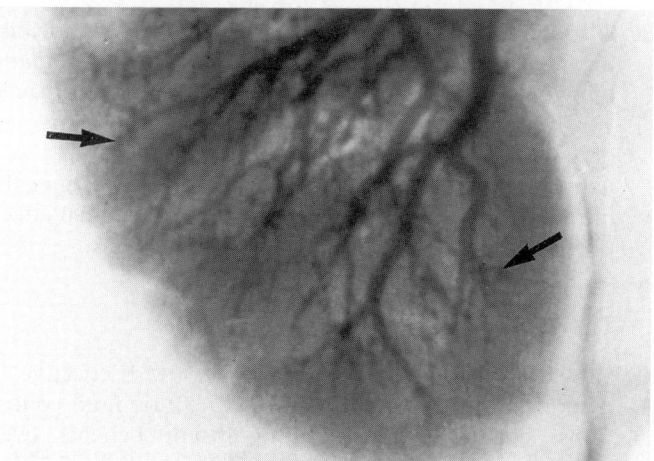

b

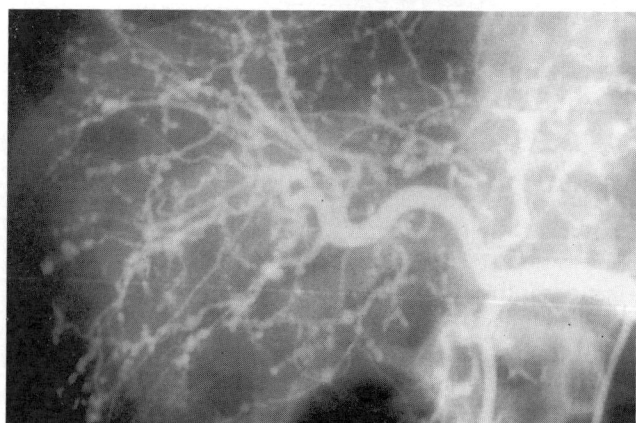

c

Figure 21.30 Angiographic diagnosis of polyarteritis nodosa. (a) A contrast-enhanced CT scan demonstrating only small peripheral cortical infarcts (arrows). No aneurysms were detected within the renal parenchyma. (b) A magnification subtraction angiogram of the right renal artery demonstrating numerous microaneurysms diagnostic of polyarteritis nodosa (arrows = microaneurysms). (c) A selective hepatic arteriogram demonstrating a myriad of microaneurysms in the hepatic arterial circulation.

flow to the renal artery and vein can be quantified with reasonable accuracy. Three-dimensional CT provides exquisite anatomic detail of the proximal renal arteries, but has the disadvantage of requiring intravenous contrast media. Quantitative flow measurements are not possible with CT. Unlike MR, however, CT can readily demonstrate arterial calcification.

Renal angiography remains the gold standard for diagnosis for renovascular hypertension. Because of its expense and invasive nature, it is not feasible to employ this as a screening technique.

Renovascular intervention

Although the use of diagnostic renal angiography has clearly diminished in the past decade, considerable progress has occurred using renovascular interventional procedures such as angioplasty, stent placement and embolization.

Renal angioplasty is a safe and effective treatment for many forms of renal arterial stenosis, particularly lesions secondary to fibromuscular dysplasia [71, 72], but long-term results are poor for ostial lesions. The recent development of expandable metallic stents shows promise for

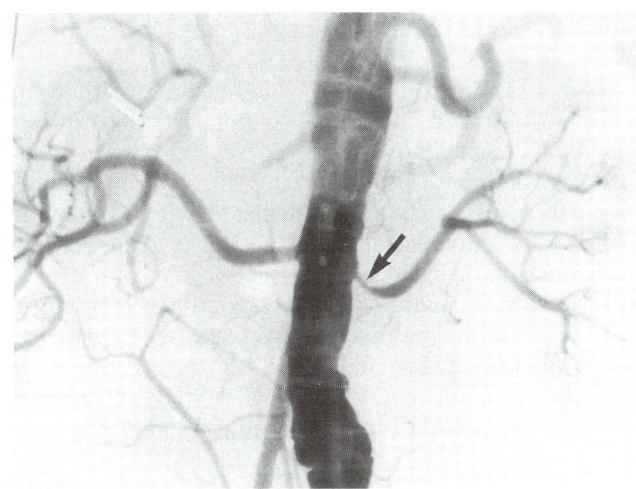

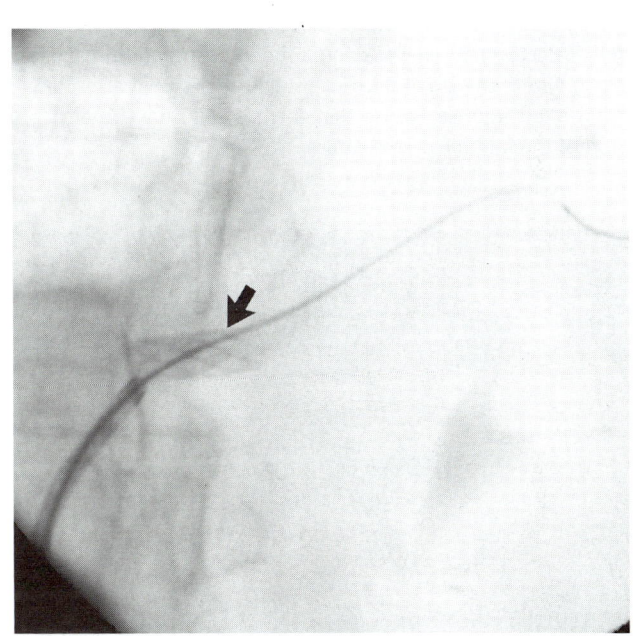

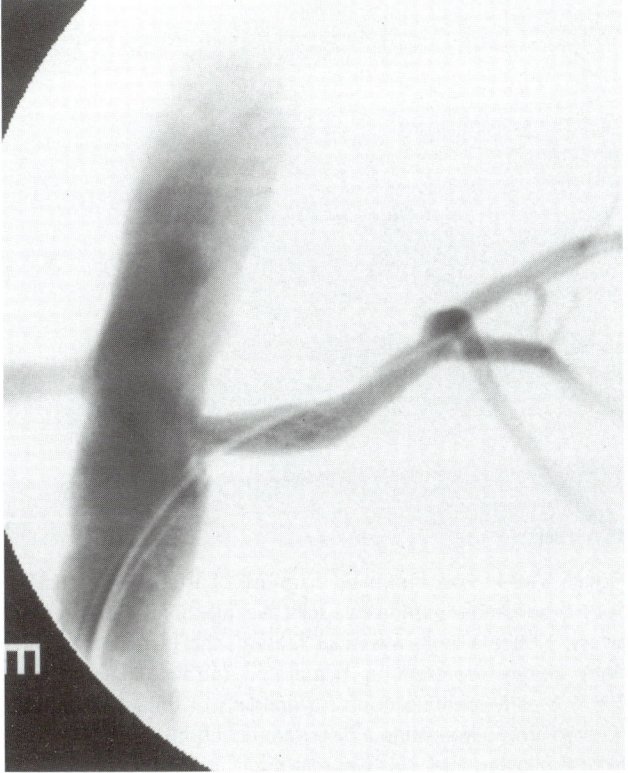

Figure 21.31 Renal artery stent placement for proximal renal artery stenosis. (a) A midstream aortogram demonstrating high-grade stenosis of the proximal left renal artery (arrow). Initial balloon angioplasty of the lesion was unsatisfactory. (b) Notice that a stent has been inflated into the proximal left renal artery (arrow = stent). (c) A repeat aortogram following renal artery stent placement demonstrating excellent patency of the left renal artery without residual stenosis.

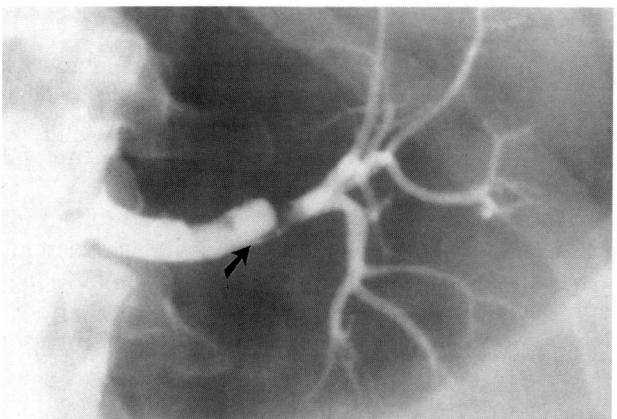

Figure 21.32 Traumatic intimal dissection of the left main renal artery. Selective left renal arteriogram demonstrates intimal flap (arrow) within the distal third of the left main renal artery following blunt trauma. Notice that there is still good distal perfusion of the intrarenal vasculature.

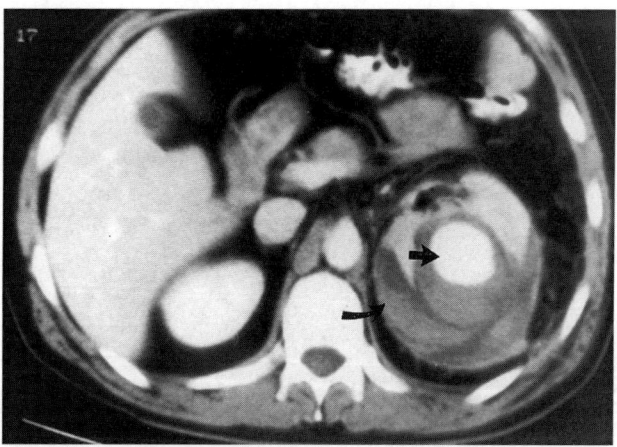

a

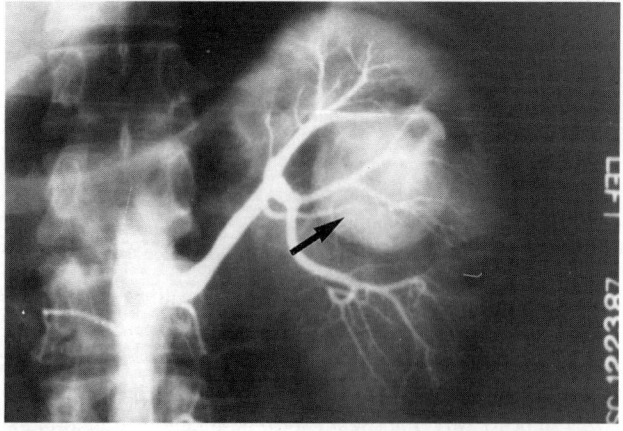

b

Figure 21.33 Post-traumatic left renal artery pseudoaneurysm. (a) Contrast-enhanced CT demonstrating a rounded pseudoaneurysm essentially within the parenchyma of the left kidney (arrow). Notice the large surrounding subcapsular hematoma (curved arrow). (b) Selective renal arteriogram confirming the pseudoaneurysm (arrow). This was selectively embolized with steel coils.

endoluminal therapy for ostial stenosis (Figure 21.31) [73]. The metallic stents are loaded over an expandable balloon. The stents are deployed by inflating a balloon to the appropriate diameter of the renal artery. Once the balloon has been expanded within the stenotic segment, the metallic stent prevents recoil and collapse of the lumen. Although initial results are promising, the development of intimal fibroplasia within the stent may lead to stent restenosis months or years later. The use of metallic stents at this time must be viewed as experimental since there are no large series evaluating 5 and 10 year patency rates.

Renal angioplasty may be performed in high-risk patients with acute renal failure to improve renal blood flow. Preliminary studies suggest stabilization of renal function can be achieved through successful angioplasty [74].

Contrast-enhanced CT is the imaging method of choice to evaluate blunt renal trauma. The diagnosis of traumatic renal artery occlusion can readily be established by CT due to the characteristic lack of enhancement and excretion of the affected kidney [69]. Traumatic intimal dissection of the main renal artery causes delay in perfusion and excretion compared to the contralateral normal kidney (Figure 21.32). Angiography is this setting may be useful in the preoperative planning for vascular reconstruction of the renal artery. Penetrating injuries to the flank may involve the colon or kidney. CT may be useful to assess trauma to these organs. Angiography may

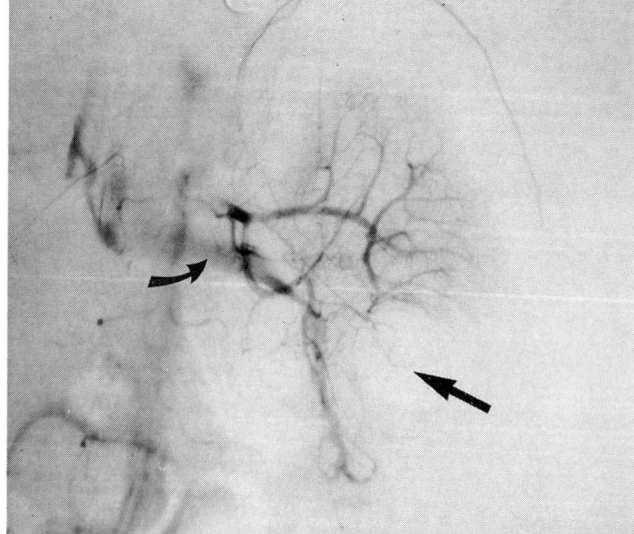

Figure 21.34 Post-traumatic diagnosis of arteriovenous fistula. Subtraction angiogram from a selective injection to the left renal artery. Notice a large avascular mass in the lower pole of the right kidney representing hematoma (arrow = hematoma). There is early identification of a draining of the left renal vein (curved arrow) indicating a direct arteriovenous communication from the lower pole. This was selectively embolized and treated without surgery.

then be used to diagnose and then embolize pseudo-aneurysms (Figure 21.33) or arteriovenous fistulas (Figure 21.34).

Complications of renal arteriography

Major complications of renal arteriography, although distinctly uncommon, do occur. Fatal complications include anaphylactic reactions to injected contrast media and massive retroperitoneal hemorrhage from rupture of the renal arteries. Renal artery thrombosis may occur, although rarely, as a result of subintimal contrast injection or arterial damage by a guidewire. If a thrombus forms at the catheter tip and then breaks loose, or if manipulation of the guidewire dislodges atheromatous debris, the resultant emboli may occlude smaller arteries downstream.

As with all arteriography procedures local complications at the puncture site may occur. These include hematoma, pseudoaneurysm formation and arteriovenous fistulas.

References

1. Friedland, G.W. (1989) Problem solving in radiology. *Dialog. Pediat. Urol.*, **12**, 10–2.
2. Rosenfield, A.T., Rigsby, C.M., Burns, P.N. *et al.* (1990) Ultrasonography of the urinary tract, in *Clinical Urography* (ed. H.M. Pollack), W.B. Saunders, Philadelphia, pp. 319–86.
3. Bude, R.O., Rubin, J.M. and Adler, R.S. (1994) Power versus conventional color Doppler sonography: comparison in the depiction of normal intrarenal vasculature. *Radiology*, **192**, 777–80.
4. Sommer, F.G. (1993) Sonographic evaluation of renal colic. *Kidney: A Current Survey of World Literature*, **2**, 129–30.
5. Haddad, M.C., Sharif, H.S., Shahed, M.S. *et al.* (1992) Renal colic: diagnosis and outcome. *Radiology*, **184**, 83–8.
6. Eshima, D. and Taylor, A., Jr (1992) Technetium-99m (^{99m}Tc) mercaptoacetyltriglycine: update on the new ^{99m}Tc renal tubular function agent. *Semin. Nucl. Med.*, **22**, 61–73.
7. Goates, J.J., Morton, K.A., Whooten, W.W. *et al.* (1990) Comparison of methods for calculating glomerular filtration rate: technetium-99m-DTPA scintigraphic analysis, protein-free and whole-plasma clearance of technetium-99m-DTPA and iodine-125-iothalamate clearance. *J. Nucl. Med.*, **31**, 424–9.
8. Cerino, M., Lette, J., Eybalin, M.C. *et al.* (1991) In vivo glomerular filtration rate measurement based solely on image processing. *Clin. Nucl. Med.*, **16**, 79–83.
9. Higa, T. and Nakatsu, M. (1993) A comparison of methods in measurement of effective renal plasma flow and glomerular filtration rate in clinical practice. *Clin. Nucl. Med.*, **18**, 873–7.
10. Milligan, J.S., Blue, P.W. and Hasbargen, J.A. (1990) Methods for measuring GFR with technetium-99m-DTPA: an analysis of several common methods. *J. Nucl. Med.*, **31**, 1211–19.
11. Russel, C.D. (1993) Optimum sample times for single-injection, multisample renal clearance method. *J. Nucl. Med.*, **34**, 1761–5.
12. Muller-Suur, R., Magnusson, G., Bois-Svensson, I. *et al.* (1991) Estimation of technetium 99m mercaptoacetyltrigylcine plasma clearance by use of one single plasma sample. *Eur J. Nucl. Med.*, **18**, 28–31.
13. Taylor, A., Jr, Corrigan, P., Eshima, D. *et al.* (1992) Prospective validation of a single sample technique to determine technetium-99m-MAG3 clearance. *J. Nucl. Med.*, **33**, 1620–2.
14. Dey, H.M., Hoffer, P.B., Lerner, E. *et al.* (1993) Quantitative analysis of the technetium-99m-DTPA captopril renogram: contribution of washout parameters to the diagnosis of renal artery stenosis. *J. Nucl. Med.*, **34**, 1416–19.
15. Erbas, B., Erbas, T.S.A. *et al.* (1993) Scintigraphic evaluation of functional renal reserve using angiotensin-converting enzyme inhibition in patients with type II diabetes mellitus. *Am. J. Nephrol.*, **13**, 203–9.
16. Itoh, K., Tsukamoto, E., Nagao, K. *et al.* (1993) Captopril renoscintigraphy with Tc-99m DTPA in patients with suspected renovascular hypertension. Prospective and restrospective evaluation. *Clin. Nucl. Med.*, **18**, 463–71.
17. Jensen, G., Moonen, M., Aurell, M. *et al.* (1993) Reliability of ACE inhibitor-enhanced 99m Tc-DTPA gamma camera renography in the detection of renovascular hypertension. *Nucl. Med. Commun.*, **14**, 169–75.
18. Lewis, D.H., Jacobson, A.F. and Graham, N.M. (1993) Renin-dependent renal parenchymatous hypertension detected by angiotensin-converting enzyme inhibitor renography. *Am. J. Nephrol.*, **13**, 281–5.
19. Meir, G.H., Sumpio, B., Setaro, J.F. *et al.* (1993) Captopril renal scintigraphy: a new standard for predicting outcome after renal revascularization. *J. Vasc. Surg.*, **17**, 280–5.
20. Shamlou, K.K., Drane, W.E., Hawkins, I.F. *et al.* (1994) Captopril renography and the hypertensive renal transplantation patient: a predictive test of therapeutic outcome. *Radiology*, **190**, 153–9.
21. Takata, M., Yoshida, K., Tomoda, F. *et al.* (1994) Diagnostic value of captopril test in hypertensive patients with renal artery stenosis. *Angiology*, **45**, 181–6.
22. Nally, J.V., Jr (1994) Provocative captopril testing in the diagnosis of renovascular hypertension. *Urol. Clin. North Am.*, **21**, 227–34.
23. Nally, J.V., Jr and Black, H.R. (1992) State of the art review: captopril renography – pathophyliological considerations and clinical observations. *Semin. Nucl. Med.*, **22**, 85–94.
24. Choong, K.K., Gruenewald, S.M., Hodson, E.M. *et al.* (1992) Volume expanded diuretic renography in the postnatal assessment of suspected uretero-pelvic junction obstruction. *J. Nucl. Med.*, **33**, 2094–8.

25. Neste, M.D., duCret, R.P. and Finlay, D.E. (1993) Postoperative diuresis renography and ultrasound in patients undergoing pyeloplasty. Predictors of surgical outcome. *Clin. Nucl. Med.*, **18**, 872–6.

26. Rossleigh, M.A., Leighton, D.M. and Farnsworth, R.H. (1993) Diuresis renography. The need for an additional view after gravity-assisted drainage. *Clin. Nucl. Med.*, **18**, 210–13.

27. Fox, C.W., Jr, Vaccaro, J.A., Kiesling, V.J., Jr *et al.* (1994) Determination of indwelling ureteral stent patency: comparison of standard contrast and nuclear cystography, and lasix renography. *Urology*, **43**, 442–5.

28. Groshar, D., Moskovitz, B., Gorenberg, M. *et al.* (1994) Quantitative SPECT of technetium-99m-DMSA uptake in the kidneys of normal children and in kidneys with vesicoureteral reflux: detection of unilateral kidney disease. *J. Nucl. Med.*, **35**, 445–9.

29. Ash, J.M. and McLorie, G.A. (1994) Can DMSA detect early renal injury in children with vesicoureteral reflux? [editorial]. *J. Nucl. Med.*, **35**, 449–50.

30. Conway, J.J. (1992) 'Well tempered' disuresis renography: its historical development, physiological and technical pitfalls, and standardized technique protocol. *Semin. Nucl. Med.*, **22**, 74–84.

31. Majd, M. and Rushton, H.G. (1992) Renal cortical scintigraphy in the diagnosis of acute pyelonephritis. *Semin. Nucl. Med.*, **22**, 98–112.

32. Rushton, H.G. and Majd, M. (1992) Dimercaptosuccinic acid renal scintigraphy for the evaluation of pyelonephritis and scarring: a review of experimental and clinical studies. *J. Urol.*, **148**, 1726–32.

33. Friedland, G.W. and Thurber, B.D. (1996) The birth of CT. *Am. J. Roentgenol.*, **167**, 1365–70.

34. Sommer, F.G., Jeffrey, R.B., Jr, Rubin, G.D. *et al.* (1995) Detection of ureteral calculi in patients with suspected renal colic: value of reformatted noncontrast helical CT. *Am. J. Roentgenol.*, **165**, 509–13.

35. Katz, D.S., Lane, M.J. and Sommer, F.G. (1996) Unenhanced helical CT of ureteral stones: incidence of associated urinary tract findings. *Am. J. Roentgenol.*, **166**, 1319–22.

36. Jeffrey, R.B., Jr (1994) Three-dimensional spiral computed tomographic angiography. *West. J. Med.*, **160**, 457–8.

37. Fishman, E.K. and Jeffrey, R.B., Jr (1994) *Spiral CT: Principles, Techniques and Clinical Applications*. Raven Press, New York.

38. Liao, J.R., Sommer, F.G., Herfkens, R.J. *et al.* (1995) Cine spiral imaging. *Magn. Reson. Med.*, **34**, 490–3.

39. Love, L. and Churchill, R.J. (1990) Computed tomography of the upper urinary tract, in *Clinical Urography* (ed. H.M. Pollack), W.B. Saunders, Philadelphia, pp. 387–406.

40. Rubin, G.D., Alfrey, E.J., Dake, M.D. *et al.* (1995) Assessment of living renal donors with spiral CT. *Radiology*, **195**, 457–62.

41. Costello, P. and Gaa, J. (1993) Spiral CT angiography of the abdominal aorta and its branches. *Eur. Radiol.*, **3**, 359–65.

42. Rubin, G.D., Dake, M.D., Napel, S. *et al.* (1994) Spiral CT of renal artery stenosis: comparison of three-dimensional rendering techniques. *Radiology*, **190**, 181–9.

43. Rubin, G.D., Beaulieu, C.F., Argiro, V. *et al.* (1996) Perspective volume rendering of CT and MR images: applications for endoscopic imaging. *Radiology*, **199**, 321–30.

44. Sommer, F.G., Olcott, E., Ch'en, I. *et al.* (1997) Volume rendering of CT data: applications to the genitourinary tract. *Am. J. Roentgenol.*, **168**, 132–9.

45. Katayama, H., Yamaguchi, K., Kozuka, T. *et al.* (1990) Adverse reactions to ionic and nonionic contrast media: a report from the Japanese committee on the safety of contrast media. *Radiology*, **175**, 621–8.

46. Cattell, W.R., Fry, I.K. and Spencer, A.G. (1967) Excretion urography. I: Factors affecting the excretion of Hypaque. *Br. J. Radiol.*, **40**, 561–71.

47. Davidson, A.J. and Hartman, D.S. (1994) *Radiology of the Kidney and Urinary Tract*, W.B. Saunders, Philadelphia.

48. Ansell, G., Tweedie, M.C.K., West, C.R. *et al.* (1980) The current status of reactions to intravenous contrast media. *Invest. Radiol. (Suppl.)*, **15**, S32–9.

49. Lasser, E.C., Berry, C.C., Mishkin, M.M. *et al.* (1994) Pretreatment with corticosteroids to prevent adverse reactions to nonionic contrast media. *Am. J. Roentgenol.*, **162**, 523–6.

50. Lasser, E.C. (1988) Pretreatment with corticosteroids to prevent reactions to IV contrast material: Overview and implications. *Am. J. Roentgenol.*, **150**, 257–9.

51. Parfrey, P.S., Griffiths, S.M., Barrett, B.J. *et al.* (1989) Contrast-induced renal failure in patients with diabetes mellitus, renal insufficiency or both: a prospective controlled study. *N. Engl. J. Med.*, **320**, 143–53.

52. Schwab, S.J., Hlatky, M.A., Peiper, K.S. *et al.* (1989) Contrast nephrotoxicity: A radiological controlled trial of a nonionic and an ionic radiographic contrast agent. *N. Engl. J. Med.*, **320**, 149–53.

53. Pfister, R.C. and Hutter, A.M.C. (1980) Cardiac alterations during intravenous urography. *Invest. Radiol. (Suppl.)*, **15**, S239–42.

54. Currarino, G., Williams, B. and Dana, K. (1984) Kidney length correlated with age: normal values in children. *Radiology*, **150**, 703–4.

55. Griffith, G.J., Cartwright, G. and McLachlan, M.S.F. (1975) Estimation of renal size from radiographs: is it worthwhile? *Clin. Radiol.*, **26**, 249–56.

56. Hodson, C.J., Davies, Z. and Prescod, A. (1975) Renal parenchymal radiographic measurements in infants and children. *Pediatr. Radiol.*, **3**, 16–19.

57. Moel, H. (1956) Size of normal kidneys. *Acta Radiol. (Diagn.)*, **46**, 640–5.

58. Pendegrass, E.P. (1943) Excretory urography as a test of urinary tract function. *Radiology*, **40**, 223–46.

59. Hodson, C.J. and Mariani, S. (1982) Large cloisons. *Am. J. Roentgenol.*, **139**, 327–32.

60. Filly, R., Friedland, G.W., Govan, D.E. *et al.* (1974) Development and progression of clubbing and scarring in children with recurrent urinary tract infections. *Radiology*, **113**, 145–53.

61. Kressel, H.Y. (1990) Magnetic resonance imaging, in *Clinical Urography* (ed. H.M. Pollack), W.B. Saunders, Philadelphia, pp. 433–55.

62. Baumgartner, B.R., Stafford, S.A., Stark, D.D. *et al.* (1992) Kidneys, in *Magnetic Resonance Imaging* (eds D.D. Stark

and W.G. Bradley), Mosby Yearbook, St Louis, pp. 1904–44.

63. Pelc, N.J., Sommer, F.G., Li, K.C. *et al.* (1994) Quantitative magnetic resonance flow imaging. *Magn. Reson. Q.,* **10**, 125–47.

64. Debatin, J.F., Ting, R.H., Wegmüller, H. *et al.* (1994) Renal artery blood flow: quantitation with phase-contrast MR imaging with and without breath holding. *Radiology,* **190**, 371–8.

65. Debatin, J.F. Spritzer, C.E., Grist, T.H. *et al.* (1991) Imaging of the renal arteries: value of MR angiography. *Am. J. Roentgenol.,* **157**, 981–90.

66. Koslin, D.B., Kenney, P.J., Keller, F.S. *et al.* (1988) Preoperative evaluation of abdominal aortic aneurysm by MR imaging with aortography correlation. *Cardiovasc. Intervent. Radiol.,* **11**, 329–35.

67. Edholm, P. and Seldinger, S.I. (1956) Percutaneous catheterization of the renal artery. *Acta Radiol.,* **45**, 15.

68. Edling, N.P.G. and Ovenfors, C.O. (1964) Risks in selective renal catheterization and arteriography. An experimental study in dogs. *Acta Radiol. [Diagn.],* **2**, 241.

69. Lang, E.K., Sullivan, J. and Frentz, G. (1985) Renal trauma: radiologic studies comparison of urography, computed tomography, angiography and radionuclide studies. *Radiology,* **154**, 1–6.

70. Jeffrey, R.B., Jr and Federle, M.P. (1983) CT and ultrasonography of acute renal abnormalities. *Radiol. Clin. North Am.,* **23**, 515–26.

71. Klinge, J., Mali, W.P.T.M., Puijlaert, C.B.A.J. *et al.* (1989) Percutaneous transluminal renal angioplasty: initial and long-term results. *Radiology,* **171**, 501.

72. Martin, L.G., Casarella, W.J., Alspaugh, J.P. *et al.* (1986) Renal artery angioplasty increased technical success and decreased complications in second 100 patients. *Radiology,* **1592**, 631.

73. Hennequin, L.M., Joffre, F.G., Rousseau, H.P. *et al.* (1994) Renal artery stent placement: long-term results with the Wallstent endoprosthesis. *Radiology,* **191**, 713–19.

74. Martin, L.G., Casarella, W.J. and M.G.G. (1988) Azotemia caused by renal artery stenosis: Treatment by percutaneous angioplasty. *Am. J. Roentgenol.,* **150**, 844.

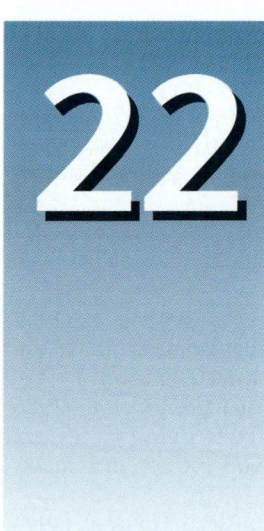

22

Methods and assessment of renal biopsy

Adrian R. Morley

Introduction

Needle biopsy is a major part of the diagnostic armamentarium of the nephrologist and is increasingly used for renal tumor diagnosis by oncologists and urologists [1]. Despite the development of non-invasive tests and imaging, biopsy remains central to both diagnosis and prognosis. The use of this technique by Iverson and Brun in 1951 [2] has resulted in the development of classifications of glomerular and tubular disorders based on morphology and immunological findings. In addition biopsy has a major role in the diagnosis and treatment of transplantation rejection. Renal biopsy is also being undertaken in an increasing range of clinical situations. In intensive care it has been suggested that needle biopsy has a role in the investigation of patients on ventilation with suspected pulmonary–renal syndromes [3]. The routine use of light and electron microscopy and immunological studies led to renal pathology becoming a distinct speciality with close clinical liaison with nephrology.

Technique

Renal biopsy

Open renal biopsy

Open renal biopsy was used to a limited extent before the advent of percutaneous biopsy and the technique has been described elsewhere [4]. It is occasionally used before renal transplantation. Removal of a wedge of cortex without compression artifact is difficult to achieve and, in addition, subcapsular changes, such as fibrosis and lymphoid infiltrate, may give an erroneous impression of the degree of parenchymal damage. The wedge also has the disadvantage of being confined to the cortex. For these reasons some have advocated the use of a biopsy needle even in open biopsies [5].

Percutaneous renal biopsy

This procedure is usually performed with local anesthetic and a conscious patient. A few may require sedation, and young children usually have a general anesthetic. The lower pole of the kidney is selected, since it avoids the renal pelvis and large vessels. Accidental biopsy of the liver, the spleen or pancreas occasionally occur but rarely cause problems. Ultrasonography is used both to locate the kidney and to visualize and guide the needle [6]. The movement of an exploring needle in contact with the kidney is easily seen. The Menghini needle has now been largely superseded by the Trucut needle, which requires some dexterity to ensure that the sample is taken into the needle. The Biopty gun or similar spring-activated mechanism is widely used combined with ultrasonography (Figure 22.1). This makes the actual tissue sampling largely automatic and has a high rate of success [7]. Since the introduction of needle biopsy there has been a trend towards smaller needle diameters (i.e. 14–18 gauge). The

Nephrology, Edited by Rex L. Jamison and Robert Wilkinson.
Published in 1997 by Chapman & Hall, London. ISBN 0 412 60930 4

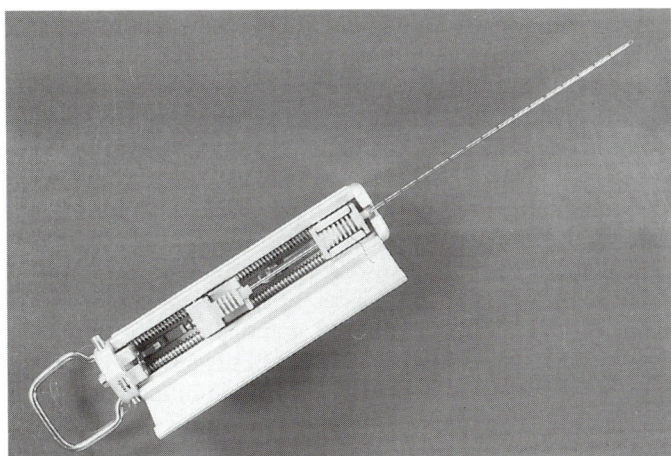

Fig. 22.1 Biopty needle. The Biopty gun by mechanizing the rapid advance and withdrawal of the biopsy needle, with the use of one hand and without the manual dexterity needed by previous biopsy needles, can produce a high rate of success. It should be recognized that this type of needle produces a somewhat shorter sample than older needles such as the Franklin variant of the Vim–Silverman needle and the Menghini.

complication rates between Trucut and spring-loaded types do not appear to differ [8]. Post-biopsy complications are less common with small needles [9] but this advantage has to be balanced against the disadvantage of a higher proportion of small non-diagnostic biopsies [10]. A recent study in renal transplant recipients [11] has shown that ultrasonography combined with immediate stereomicroscopic examination to confirm the presence of glomeruli in the sample achieves 100% success in obtaining adequate biopsy material. The use of ultrasonography has resulted in many renal biopsies now being undertaken by radiologists rather than nephrologists. In a recent study over one-third of these procedures were undertaken by radiologists [12]. An adverse aspect of this development is the loss of direct communication between the renal pathologist and the nephrologist at the time of biopsy.

Preparation and aftercare in renal biopsy

Confirmation that both kidneys are structurally normal and functioning, and the localization of cysts and masses, requires ultrasonography and in some cases isotope renogram or intravenous pyelography before biopsy. Blood pressure is reduced to 140 mmHg systolic and bleeding and coagulation abnormalities may need correction. In some cases transfusion of clotting factors will be necessary to produce a transient shortening of the clotting time sufficient to allow biopsy.

After biopsy there are considerable variations in aftercare. Examination for hematuria and checking the blood pressure and pulse rate at regular intervals is undertaken. Bed rest overnight is usually advised. However, recent studies have demonstrated that complication rates were

no higher in patients biopsied as outpatients [13, 14]. It has been suggested that there is a high rate of hemorrhage in biopsy samples which contain only medulla; limiting the tissue taken to superficial cortex has been advocated [15].

Transjugular renal biopsy

Recent reports of transjugular renal biopsy indicate that advances in technique are continuing [16]. An uncorrectable bleeding disorder is the main indication for this technique which eliminates the possibility of perinephric hematoma.

Preparation and staining of kidney tissue

The nephrologist's responsibility does not end with obtaining a biopsy. Examination with an inverted ocular or stereomicroscope will determine if the tissue obtained is renal cortex. Glomeruli protruding from the edges of the sample are easily recognized. Rapid transport to the laboratory in a suitable medium must be arranged. Buffered saline should only be used for short periods (5–10 min). Fixatives commonly used such as buffered formalin, formal–sublimate and Dubosq–Brasil all produce characteristic artifacts with which the pathologist needs to be familiar. Rapid processing including the use of sponges in biopsy cassettes [17] or of nylon bags can lead to pressure distortion of the tissue (Figure 22.2).

Light microscopy

The preparation of slides and the use of special stains contribute to the success or otherwise of the whole procedure. The baseline is hematoxylin and eosin, periodic acid–Schiff (PAS), and periodic acid–silver methenamine (PASM). Solez [18] emphasized the importance of the PAS staining of tubular basement membranes in the recognition of tubulitis in transplant rejection. In general a

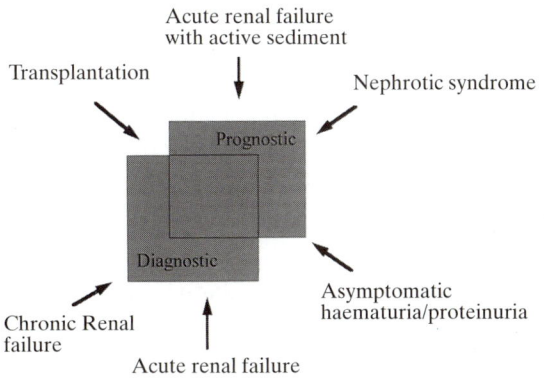

Fig. 22.2 Diagnostic categories of renal biopsy.

stronger stain is required than the routine mucin stain of many laboratories. The combination of a trichrome stain with PASM is also useful [19], and the routine use of a stain for amyloid is recommended. Sections need to be around 3–4 μm thick for optimum use of these stains. Thinner sections (1 μm) can be obtained by the use of methacrylate or other resin as embedding agents [20]. There is no doubt that both special stains and immunoperoxidase techniques can be undertaken in plastic-embedded material but in general paraffin wax remains the preferred embedding medium.

Glomerular lesions may be extremely focal and segmental, and in vascular kidney transplant rejection lesions may be similarly scattered. Renal biopsies are also small. Precious tissue is lost if technical staff cut into the tissue to any depth before taking sections for staining. The protocol shown in Table 22.1 has been found useful in minimizing waste. Ideally the first slide will be from the first face of the renal tissue. Spare, unstained slides should also be taken at the same time since any attempt to re-chuck the wax block later will lead to tissue loss.

Immunofluorescent/immunoperoxidase findings are vital parts of the diagnostic criteria in some diseases, may confirm the light microscopy findings, or be non-contributory. It is not possible to determine beforehand into which category a biopsy will fall. In about 10% of biopsy samples there will be medulla only or insufficient tissue for immunochemical study. Light microscopy or electron microscopy may then give sufficient information for a working diagnosis. These immunological techniques are, however, an integral part of the study of renal pathology especially in the context of findings by light and electron microscopy.

Any patient with rapidly developing renal failure with or without an active urinary sediment needs immunofluorescent examination at the same time as light microscopy. The differential diagnosis includes an acute immune complex glomerulonephritis, Goodpasture's syndrome, Wegener's granulomatosis and possibly Henoch–Schonlein disease or IgA glomerulonephritis. The chief distinction is between the linear antiglomerular basement membrane disorders and the granularity of acute immune complex diseases such as poststreptococcal nephritis. Large amounts of granular IgG, IgA, IgM and complement (C3) in the glomeruli suggest lupus erythematosus. Fibrin alone with traces of immunoglobulins indicates a pauci-immune glomerulonephritis associated with Wegener's granulomatosis or microscopic polyarteritis. In Henoch–Schonlein disease and mesangial IgA disease a predominantly mesangial deposition of IgA may be found but the more severe crescentic forms also have subendothelial deposits on the basement membranes.

In routine histopathology immunoperoxidase methods have largely taken over the role of immunofluorescent examination because of their ability to provide precise localization, thin sections and permanent preparation. This change to new methods has been slow in renal pathology because of the difficulty of demonstrating extracellular immune deposits without background, and the need for a rapid and robust method for the demonstration of linear deposits in potential cases of Goodpasture's syndrome. Immunoperoxidase methods are gaining ground, but the methods still require precise titration of the removal of plasma protein and enzyme digestion for success [21]. The use of the confocal microscope with potential double-labeling techniques and three-dimensional observations suggest a continuing role for immunofluorescent examination [22] (Figure 22.3).

The range of potential markers which can be applied to renal tissue is now enormous. A basic immunological staining screen includes IgG, IgA, IgM, C3, C4 and fibrinogen. C9 has been recommended as a robust marker of complement activation, and it has been suggested that this is of value in tubular–interstitial diseases [23]. The demonstration of glomerular kappa and lambda light chains in light chain disease frequently causes difficulty. T cell markers such as CD3 may be useful in the diagnosis of transplant rejection and in combination with Ki-67 (MIB1) can provide convincing evidence of cell activation in tubulitis (Figure 22.4). Immunoglobulin controls are valuable and the internal controls of IgA present in tubular casts and capillary fibrin should not be forgotten. The use of previous renal biopsies or nephrectomy samples for control staining is preferable to the frequently used lymphoid tissues.

Table 22.1 Protocol for preparing sections from renal biopsy material

Slide 1	Serial sections	numbers 1–5
Slide 2	Serial sections	numbers 6–10
Slide 3	Serial sections	numbers 11–15
Slide 4	Serial sections	numbers 16–20
	All stained hematoxylin and eosin	
Slide 5	Hematoxylin and eosin[a]	
Slides 6, 7, 8, 9	Hematoxylin and eosin, PAS[a], PASM[a], Sirius Red (amyloid). The addition of a trichrome stain such as Picro–Mallory, or Martius Scarlet–blue may be helpful in demonstrating protein deposits and fibrosis.	

[a] Special care is required to obtain thin sections 2–3 μm thick for these special stains which require examination with ×40–100 objectives.
PAS, periodic acid–Schiff; PASM, periodic acid – silver methenamine.

Electron microscopy

The use of the electron microscope is one of the methods of renal pathology which distinguishes it from most other

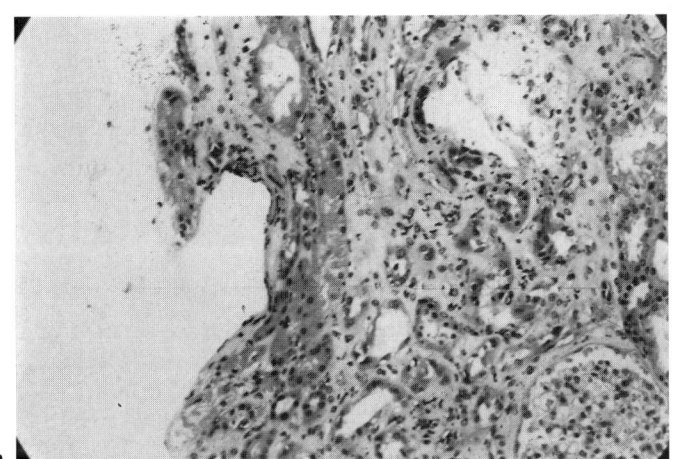

a

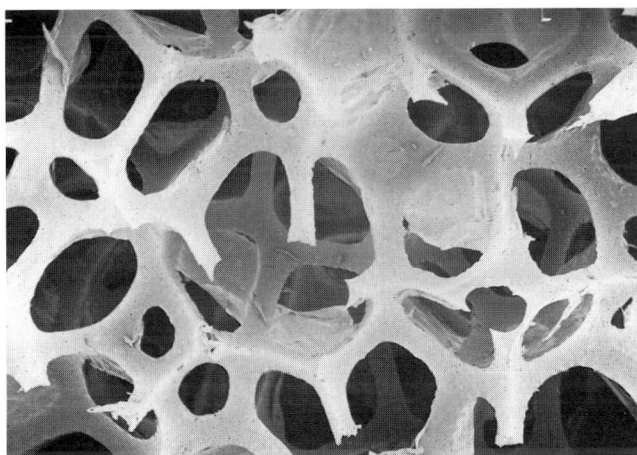

b

Fig. 22.3 Sponge artefact. Preparation can do much to enhance or detract from the value of renal biopsy – the sponge artefact is not seen with fixed tissues but may occur when rapid processing leads to unfixed tissue being compressed by sponges inserted into processing cassettes. (Hematoxylin and eosin, with scanning electron microscopy, ×200.)

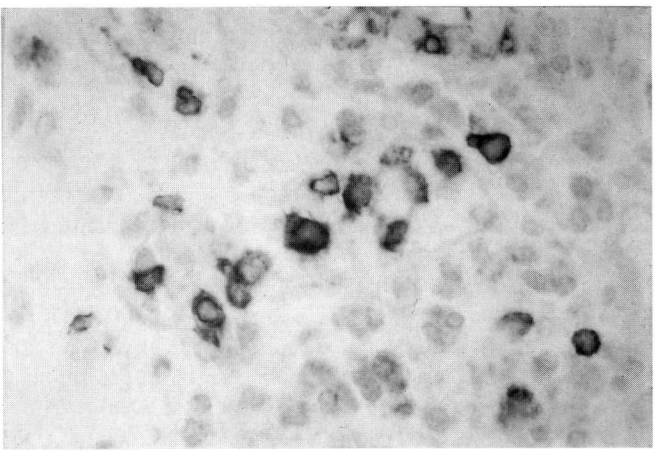

Fig. 22.4 Confocal microscopy of IgA. Technological advances may enhance the use of classical methods such as immunofluorescence. Thus double-labeling and three-dimensional reconstruction may give diagnostic insights. IgA deposits have a central core of IgA-C_{3c} and an outer coat of IgA alone. (Reproduced from Onetti-Muda *et al.*, *Journal of Pathology*, **177**, 201–208.)

branches of histopathology. The localization of diagnostic features to the glomerulus, and the existence of clinically important diseases in which definitive diagnosis requires electron microscopy, are convincing arguments for its use. The value of this is so widely accepted that there are few objective studies of its value. One study has demonstrated diagnostic value in some 75% of cases [24]. If electron microscopy is confined to those cases in which diagnosis remains in doubt after light microscopy and immunofluorescent examination then less than 50% are essential.

Ideally the renal pathologist should undertake electron microscopy but in reality this is not the case and increasingly technologists provide micrographs. Close liaison is required since the examination by the electron microscopist can only be of a tiny part of the sample. Routine electron micrographs should cover glomerular capillary loops, the mesangium, and Bowman's capsule at a magnification of ×5000–10 000. For measurement of basement membrane thickness in thin membrane disease

and diabetes, several electron micrographs at a standard magnification of ×20 000–30 000 are valuable [25]. Examination of specific structures such as the juxtaglomerular apparatus or infrequent segmental glomerular lesions can be extremely time consuming. Immunoperoxidase and other marker studies are possible but require special fixation and are to be regarded as research procedures.

There are some forms of glomerular lesion which cannot be diagnosed with certainty without the use of electron microscopy. **Alport's syndrome** shows characteristic splitting and fibrillation of the lamina densa combined with focal thinning of the glomerular basement membrane. **Thin glomerular basement membrane disease**, associated with asymptomatic hematuria, is an increasingly common diagnosis partly due to increasing awareness. Several methods have been devised for sampling and measurement of glomerular basement membrane width [26, 27]. **Membranous glomerulonephritis** before the development of basement membrane spikes requires electron micrscopy for the demonstration of immune deposits. **Mesangiocapillary glomerulonephritides** types I and II often need electron microscopy to demonstrate the exact siting of deposits.

Sometimes there is insufficient tissue for immunochemical studies and equivocal light microscopy results. Electron microscopy enables clinical and light microscopy suspicions to be confirmed or rejected. For example the presence of electron-dense mesangial deposits will favor a diagnosis of IgA glomerulonephritis. Atypical amyloid lacking the usual tinctorial characteristics or showing the unusual membranous pattern is readily identified by electron microscopy. Inherited lipoidoses such as Fabry's disease may show characteristic laminated inclusions. Clearly such conditions are unusual but the renal pathologist needs to be prepared and expe-

Table 22.2 The core features examined in a renal biopsy

Glomeruli	Number
	Number (%) obsolescent
	Number (%) Crescents
	Type of crescents
	cellular, fibrous, occlusive, exploding
	Rupture of Bowman's capsule
	Capsular adhesions
	Size and shape of capillary tuft
	Mesangial matrix and cellularity
	Cellular infiltrates, distribution and type
	Focal and segmental hyalinosis and
	necrosis
	Basement membrane thickening,
	deposits, spikes
Tubules	Tubular atrophy (% area)
	Basement membrane thickening
	Hypertrophy proximal tubules
	Epithelial cell changes
	vacuolation
	swelling, flattening
	nuclear pleomorphism
	necrosis
	Tubular lumen
	size, dilatation, diminished
	casts hyaline, red blood cells,
	mixed, debris
	crystals
Interstitium	Infiltrate, extent and cell type
	Fibrosis
	Crystal, amyloid
Blood vessels	Arteriosclerosis
	Hyalinization
	Arteritis
	Fibrin
	Proliferative endarteritis
	Vascular rejection

rienced in the whole range of potential disorders. Thus a case can be made for routine electron microscopy to confirm and amplify light microscopy observations.

Evaluation of the renal biopsy

The structure of the kidney as seen in a renal biopsy falls naturally into four main parts: (1) glomeruli; (2) tubules; (c) interstitium; and (4) blood vessels. Comprehensive lists of lesions and observations provide useful checklists [28]. Table 22.2 represents the core features to be examined and will be expanded on the basis of available clinical information. The extent to which these features require to be characterized and quantified depends much on clinical needs. It has been suggested that the

principles of the Banff classification for transplant rejection, in which histological assessment and clinical outcome are used to determine the value of histological observations, should become part of diagnostic renal pathology [18].

Indications for renal biopsy

General information obtained

The role of biopsy in the diagnosis of space-occupying lesions is growing with use of sophisticated imaging. Usually such patients will be under the care of a urologist. In nephrology the importance of biopsy is related to the high diagnostic and predictive value that small samples can provide in diffuse diseases. The pathologist and nephrologist must be aware that sampling errors are likely in diseases with a focal, localized pattern.

Before considering specific indications for biopsy it is worth looking at the kind of information that is obtained. This can be divided into two categories (Figure 22.5).

Diagnostic information

Biopsy findings place the renal disorder into a more or less well-recognized immunomorphological category. This information gives a guide to treatment and the probability of success, as well as general information about the natural history of the disease. Biopsy may also throw up totally unexpected findings guiding investigation and treatment into previously unconsidered paths.

Prognostic information

Biopsy findings also provide information about the degree of renal injury and enable estimates of acute and chronic functional deficits. Experience of the variability of human disease teaches caution, but the information is valuable in planning further treatment.

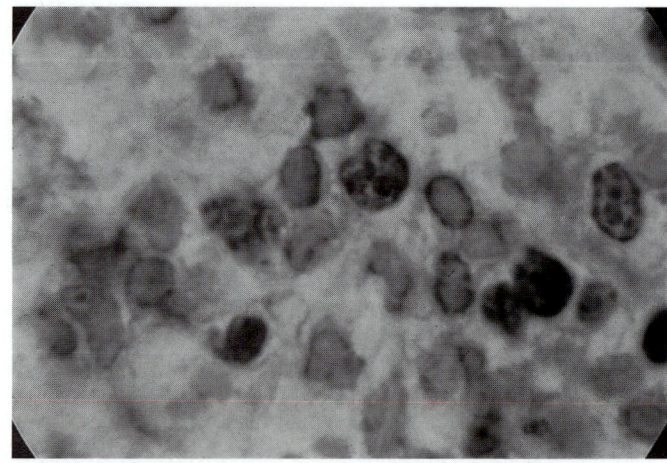

Fig. 22.5 Cells in tubulitis of transplant rejection to demonstrate both T cell (CD3) and proliferation (MIB 1) markers in the same cell.

For example, a linear IgG pattern on the glomerular basement membrane associated with crescentic glomerulonephritis and lung hemorrhage is consistent with Goodpasture's syndrome (a diagnostic category). If the crescents are large, occlusive and involve 100% of the glomeruli seen in an adequate sample (prognostic observations), there is little chance of recovery of function. Similarly it has been shown that in lupus erythematosus the prediction of clinical outcome based on race, age, sex and serum antibodies is enhanced by histological information, with cellular crescents and interstitial hemorrhage being particularly ominous [29].

The amount of information in each category varies enormously. Even when the diagnosis is known, the question of prognosis may justify biopsy.

Classification of renal biopsy findings

The need for standardization in the classification of biopsy findings is particularly acute in renal transplantation. This has been recognized by the recent production of the Banff classification of transplant rejection [18]. Annual Banff conferences are held to audit the use of the classification. Development and amendment of the criteria for histological rejection are important in a field in which treatment and clinical practice are rapidly changing.

In membranous glomeruloncphritis the classification of glomerular basement membrane lesions by Ehrenreich and Churg [30] is valuable. In lupus erythematosus the classification of morphological changes [31, 32] is also a useful guide to outcome and treatment. Such studies are needed to determine which morphological observations are associated with function or prognosis.

Specific indications

Nephrologists vary in the amount of information they require before initiating treatment, the extent to which they will go to establish a diagnosis and the frequency with which they undertake renal biopsy. The increasing emergence of treatable diseases emphasizes the need for accurate diagnosis before the use of potent drugs.

Acute nephritic syndrome

Few would question the need for biopsy in the situation of rapidly developing renal failure with an active urine sediment. Such patients may have acute crescentic glomerulonephritis, interstitial nephritis, vasculitis or systemic diseases such as lupus erythematosus or systemic sclerosis. It should be remembered that the urine sediment is not always active in these conditions. More rarely a coagulopathy or dysproteinemia will be present. In these circumstances a renal biopsy can establish the diagnosis, indicate appropriate therapy or show that therapy is unlikely to succeed. In the presence of recognized systemic disorders such as postinfectious glomerulonephritis, glomerulonephritis associated with endocarditis and

mixed cryoglobulinemia, biopsy may not be required unless prognostic information is needed for planning treatment. The development of rapid tests for antineutrophil cytoplasmic antibody and antiglomerular basement membrane antibody will facilitate rapid diagnosis, but it is unlikely that any non-invasive tests will supersede renal biopsy in the near future.

Idiopathic nephrotic syndrome

In children the nephrotic syndrome is usually the result of steroid-sensitive minimal change glomerulopathy. Many pediatric nephrologists would treat with steroids [33], reserving biopsy for patients who fail to respond and those with atypical features such as hypertension, unselective proteinuria or hematuria. In this group, focal/segmental glomerulosclerosis may be found. The glomerular tip lesion with adhesion of the glomerular tuft to the tubular opening from Bowman's capsule has raised wide interest, occurring as it does in a wide range of patients with nephrotic syndrome [34]. Less common causes of non-response to steroids in children are dense deposit disease and mesangiocapillary nephritis.

In adults, minimal change glomerulopathy is less common although it is the commonest cause in the 15–29 years age group. There is a wide range of potential causes of nephrotic syndrome including membranous glomerulonephritis, minimal change glomerulopathy, amyloid, lupus erythematosus, diabetes mellitus and all the conditions considered in childhood. The suggestion has been made that renal biopsy is not needed in patients with minimal change glomerulopathy or membranous glomerulonephritis. Even if other conditions could be excluded without biopsy it is not usually possible to distinguish between minimal change and membranous glomerulonephritis without biopsy and, since their management is quite different, biopsy is essential. In established systemic diseases such as diabetes mellitus, amyloidosis and multiple myeloma, diagnosis is often clear; renal biopsy then provides an indication of the extent and activity of the disease process. Several studies have shown that the clinical prediction of diagnosis needed alteration in half the cases after biopsy [35, 36]. Biopsy is therefore required in nearly all adults with nephrotic syndrome.

Acute renal failure of obscure origin

In acute renal failure the cause will be obvious in many instances associated with shock, trauma etc. The majority of these will recover with supportive treatment. Where anuria is prolonged to four to six weeks, renal biopsy may be useful to establish the diagnosis and indicate the likelihood of recovery.

Chronic renal failure

In chronic renal failure associated with small kidneys biopsy often fails to produce diagnostic information. The reasons include technical difficulty in producing an adequate sample as well as severe problems of interpretation of changes associated with end-stage renal disease, namely atrophy and scarring.

Asymptomatic hematuria

Perhaps the greatest variation in practice occurs in the investigation of asymptomatic hematuria and proteinuria. Some nephrologists do not biopsy on the grounds that biopsy for isolated hematuria rarely changes management decisions [37] unless there is evidence of renal impairment or hypertension. Others biopsy the majority of these patients to exclude serious treatable disease. Many of this group of patients will have mesangial IgA glomerulonephritis, others will have thin glomerular basement membrane disease or Alport's syndrome. Discovery of severe glomerular damage in this group may have prognostic value and a significant effect on employment, insurance or emigration prospects. The patient should play a major role in the decision on biopsy since social factors such as the necessity for life insurance may determine the need for biopsy.

Non-nephrotic proteinuria

Patients with isolated non-nephrotic proteinuria and normal renal function are not generally biopsied. A few patients will have early membranous glomerulonephritis but many will show non-specific changes loosely called focal glomerulosclerosis but lacking the poor prognosis of focal glomerulosclerosis of childhood. In older patients ischemic nephrosclerosis may be present.

Renal transplantation

Renal transplantation is a major source of renal biopsies in many centers. Patients may have several biopsies within months. The most common problem is rejection. In the early stages, infection and pathology related to vascularization may occur. Later recurrence of glomerulonephritis and cyclosporin A toxicity enter the diagnosis. In this field estimation of structural damage and potential function are important factors in determining future treatment.

Complications of renal biopsy

Bleeding

Bleeding problems are of two types – hematuria and perirenal hematoma.

Microscopic hematuria occurs in all patients and there is macroscopic hematuria in 10% of patients. The incidence of hematuria is greater in transplant kidneys than in native kidneys (9.9% vs 4.8%) [38]. Approximately one quarter of patients will develop a small perirenal hematoma, but less than 1% will develop a hematoma greater than 100 ml or palpable [7, 39]. Most of these hematomas resolve spontaneously over a few months. Rare complications are severe anemia following bleeding, diminution in renal function and the development of perirenal abscess. Exceptionally, interventional radiology or surgical intervention may be required to control bleeding.

Arteriovenous fistula can be demonstrated in about 15% of biopsies [40]. They rarely cause problems, and 75% of them spontaneously occlude. In the few cases causing high output failure or hypertension surgical intervention or occlusion by embolization may be needed [41, 42].

Pain

Pain in the loin occurs in the first 12 h in 4% of patients [43]. In children 7% report pain on micturition [7].

Mortality

Renal biopsy is a safe procedure with nephrectomy being needed for about 0.06% [44]. Deaths related to biopsy were 0.2% in one large series [43] but in another series no deaths were encountered in over 1500 procedures [45].

Special situations in which complications are more likely or more serious

Single kidney

A single orthotopic kidney is usually an absolute contraindication to biopsy; in such patients open renal biopsy with direct control of bleeding may be undertaken. A horseshoe kidney falls into this category. In patients with severe uremia, with a normal sized single kidney, the risks of closed biopsy are usually considered acceptable.

Renal masses

Renal masses such as cysts or tumors are not absolute contraindications, and there is increasing use of sonography-guided biopsy or aspiration cytology. The risk of tumor arising along the track of the biopsy is small and justified by the information gained.

Small kidneys

Kidneys less than 6 cm long in the adult, associated with chronic renal failure, are difficult to localize and biopsies have a high failure rate. In many cases the changes are too advanced for interpretation by the pathologist. Biopsy in this situation is accompanied by an increased risk of bleeding.

Coagulation defects and hypertension

Uncorrected coagulation disorders may lead to hemorrhage and perinephric hematoma. The combination of coagulation defect and hypertension is a potent cause of hemorrhage. Even when blood pressure is controlled arteriosclerosis may prevent vascular contraction. Patients with amyloid may have a coagulation disorder with factor X deficiency, but this rarely produces problems.

Renal transplantation

The acutely rejecting swollen kidney has an increased internal pressure and biopsy may lead to rupture of such kidneys, requiring nephrectomy. This is a rare complication and renal biopsy retains a central role in the diagnosis of rejection.

Renal or perinephric infection

The focal nature of such disease makes it unlikely that diagnostic tissue will be obtained, and biopsy is not performed in this situation.

The uncooperative patient

Sedation or anesthetic is generally used in renal biopsy of children. In adults mild sedation may be required. Explanation of the benefit to the patient and the need to know the nature of the disease process before treatment will usually allay the patient's disquiet. The risks of biopsy are greater in an uncooperative patient. Biopsy is a significant procedure for which the patient's informed consent is needed.

The future

Renal biopsy continues to play a central role in the management of renal diseases and renal transplantation. The increasing involvement of radiologists in renal biopsy should not obscure the need for nephrologists to maintain their expertise in this area. In particular, understanding of limitations due to sampling errors is needed. Bias is inevitable if the nephrologist attempts biopsy interpretation without the opinion of a well-trained renal pathologist. The development of a strong working relationship will do much to maximize the benefit to the patient.

References

1. Abe, M. and Saitoh, M. (1992) Selective renal tumour biopsy under ultrasonic guidance. *Br. J. Urol.*, **70**, 7.
2. Iverson, P. and Brunn, C. (1951) Aspiration biopsy of the Kidney. *Am. J. Nephrol.*, **11**, 324.
3. Conlon, P.J., Kovalik, E. and Schwab, S.J. (1995) Percutaneous renal biopsy of ventilated intensive care unit patients. *Clin. Nephrol.*, **43**, 309.
4. Ponticelli, C., Mihatsch, M.J. and Imbasciati, E. (1992) Renal Biopsy: performance and interpretation, in *Oxford Textbook of Clinical Nephrology*, 1st edn (eds S. Cameron, A.M. Davison, J.P. Grunfeld, D. Kerr and E. Ritz), Oxford University Press, Oxford, vol. 1, p. 141.
5. Kark, R.M. (1968) Renal biopsy. *JAMA*, **205**, 80.
6. Ohmori, H., Arimoto, K., Taki, M. *et al.* (1990) A new automated renal biopsy technique under ultrasound guidance. *XIth Int. Cong. Nephrol.*, p. 87.
7. Bohlin, A.B., Edstrom, S., Almgren, B. *et al.* (1995) Renal biopsy in children: indications, technique and efficacy in 119 consecutive cases. *Pediatr. Nephrol.*, **9**, 201.
8. Burstein, D.M., Korbet, S.M. and Schwartz, M.M. (1993) The use of the automatic core biopsy system in percutaneous renal biopsies: A comparative study. *Am. J. Kidney Dis.*, **22**, 545.
9. Gazelle, G.S., Haaga, J.R. and Rowland, D.Y. (1992) Effect of needle gauge, level of anticoagulation, and target organ on bleeding associated with aspiration biopsy: work in progress. *Radiology*, **183**, 509.
10. Rose, J.D.G., Geddy, P.M., England, S. *et al.* (1993) Renal biopsy: the effect of ultrasound guidance and needle size. *J. Intervent. Radiol.*, **7**, 177.
11. Beckingham, I.J., Nicholson, M.L., Kirk, G. *et al.* (1994) Comparison of three methods to obtain percutaneous needle core biopsies of a renal allograft. *Br. J. Surg.*, **81**, 898.
12. Levin, D.C., Flanders, S.J., Spettell, C.M. *et al.* (1995) Participation by radiologists and other specialists in percutaneous vascular and nonvascular interventions: findings from a seven-state database. *Radiology*, **196**, 51.
13. Fraser, I.R. and Fairley, K.F. (1995) Renal biopsy as an outpatient procedure. *Am. J. Kidney Dis.*, **25**, 876.
14. Maddux, F.W., Maddux, D.W., Starling, J.F. *et al.* (1992) Outpatient renal biopsy is a safe procedure in the community setting. *J. Am. Soc. Nephrol.*, **3**, 345.
15. Beckingham, I.J., Nicholson, M.L. and Bell, P.R.F. (1994) Analysis of factors associated with complications following renal transplant needle core biopsy. *Br. J. Urol.*, **73**, 13.
16. Mal, F., Meyrier, A., Callard, P. *et al.* (1992) The diagnostic yield of transjugular renal biopsy. Experience in 200 cases. *Kidney Int.*, **41**, 445.
17. Farrell, D.J., Thompson, P.A. and Morley, A.R. (1992) Tissue artefacts caused by sponges. *J. Clin. Pathol.*, **45**, 923.
18. Solez, K. (1994) International standardization in renal allograft biopsy reporting: A model for a new approach to renal pathology. *Nephrol. Dial. Transplant.*, **9**, 157.
19. Birchall, I.E. (1994) Evaluation of renal biopsies with the silver methenamine/Masson trichrome technique. *J. Histotechnol.*, **17**, 131.

20. Hoffmann, E.O. (1995) High-resolution light microscopy for interpretation of renal biopsies. *Pediatr. Nephrol.*, **9**, 763.

21. Furness, P.N. and Boyd, S. (1996) Electron microscopy and immunocytochemistry in the assessment of renal biopsy specimens: Actual and optimal practice. *J. Clin. Pathol.*, **49**, 233.

22. Onetti-Muda, A., Feriozzi, S., Rahimi, S. and Faraggiana, T. (1995) Spatial arrangement of IgA and C3 as a prognostic indicator of IgA nephropathy. *J. Pathol.*, **177**, 201.

23. Khan, T.N. and Sinniah, R. (1995) Role of complement in renal tubular damage. *Histopathology*, **26**, 351.

24. Pearson, J.M., Mcwilliam, L.J., Coyne, J.D. and Curry, A. (1994) Value of electron microscopy in diagnosis of renal disease. *J. Clin. Pathol.*, **47**, 126.

25. Steffes, M., Barbosa, J., Basgen, J.A. *et al.* (1983) Quantitative glomerular morphology of the normal human kidney. *Lab. Invest.*, **53**, 82.

26. Dische, F.E. (1992) Measurement of glomerular basement membrane thickness and its application to the diagnosis of thin-membrane nephropathy. *Arch. Pathol. Lab. Med.*, **116**, 43.

27. Mclay, A.L.C., Jackson, R., Meyboom, F. and Boulton-Jones, J.M. (1992) Glomerular basement membrane thinning in adults: Clinicopathological correlations of a new diagnostic approach. *Nephrol. Dial. Transplant.*, **7**, 191.

28. Ponticelli, C., Mihatsch, M.J. and Imbasciati, E. (1992) *Oxford Textbook of Clinical Nephrology*, 1st edn, Oxford Medical Publications, Oxford, vol 1, p. 141.

29. Austin, H.A.I.I.I., Boumpas, D.T., Vaughan, E.M. and Balow, J.E. (1994) Predicting renal outcomes in severe lupus nephritis: Contributions of clinical and histologic data. *Kidney Int.*, **45**, 544.

30. Ehrenreich, T. and Churg, J. (1968) Pathology of membranous glomerulopathy, in *Pathology Annual*, (ed. S.C. Sommer), Appleton–Century–Crofts, New York, p. 145.

31. McCluskey, R.T. (1975) Lupus nephritis 1, in *Kidney Pathology Decenal*, (ed. S.C. Sommer), Appleton–Century–Crofts, New York, p. 435.

32. Kashgarian, M. (1992) Clinical significance of renal biopsy in subacute lupus erythematosus. *Transfus. Sci.*, **13**, 135.

33. Habib, R., Levy, M. and Gubler, M.C. (1979) Clinicopathological correlations in the nephrotic syndrome. *Pediatrician*, **8**, 325.

34. Howie, A.J. and Brewer, D.B. (1988) The glomerular tip lesion; a distinct entity or not? *J. Pathol.*, **154**, 191.

35. Cohen, A.H., Nast, C.C, Adler, S.G. and Kopple, J.D. (1989) Clinical utility of renal biopsies in the diagnosis and management of renal disease. *Am. J. Nephrol.*, **9**, 309.

36. Turner, M.W., Hutchinson, T.A., Barre, P.E. *et al.* (1986) A prospective study on the impact of renal biopsy on clinical management. *Clin. Nephrol.*, **26**, 217.

37. Richards, N.T., Darby, S., Howie, A.J. *et al.* (1994) Knowledge of renal histology alters patient management in over 40% of cases. *Nephrol. Dial. Transplant.*, **9**, 1255.

38. Gainza, F.J., Minguela, I., Lopezvidaur, I. *et al.* (1995) Evaluation of complications due to percutaneous renal biopsy in allografts and native kidneys with color–coded Doppler sonography. *Clin. Nephrol.*, **43**, 303.

39. Meola, M., Barsotti, G., Cupisti, A. *et al.* (1994) Free-hand ultrasound-guided renal biopsy: Report of 650 consecutive cases. *Nephron*, **67**, 425.

40. Eklund, L. and Lindholm, T. (1971) Arteriovenous fistula following renal biopsy. *Acta Radiol.*, **11**, 38.

41. Wickre, C.G. and Golper, T.A. (1982) Complications of percutaneous needle biopsy of the kidney. *Am. J. Nephrol.*, **2**, 173.

42. Farrugia, M.M., Howlett, D.C. and Irvine, A.T. (1994) Percutaneous embolization of a hemodynamically significant post-biopsy arteriovenous fistula in a transplant renal allograft. *J. Intervent. Radiol.*, **9**, 179.

43. Parrish, A.E. (1992) Complications of percutaneous renal biopsy: a review of 37 years' experience. *Clin. Nephrol.*, **38**, 135.

44. Tisher, C.C. (1994) Clinical indications for renal biopsy, in *Renal Pathology, with Clinical and Functional Correlations*, 2nd edn (eds C.C. Tisher and B. Brenner), J.B. Lippincott, Philadelphia, p. 75.

45. Gault, M.H. and Muehrcke, R.C. (1983) Renal biopsy: current views and controversies. *Nephron*, **38**, 1.

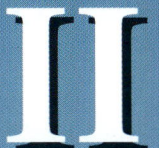

Impaired Renal Function

Section 2
Fluid and Electrolyte Disorders

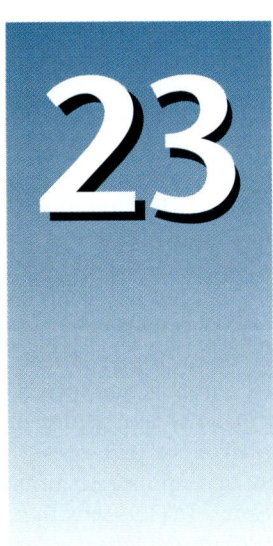

23

Disorders of water metabolism

Joseph G. Verbalis

Introduction

Abnormalities of water balance are the most common cause of fluid and electrolyte disorders in clinical practice. Since body water is the primary determinant of the osmolality of the extracellular fluid (ECF), disorders of water metabolism can be broadly divided into hypo-osmolar disorders, in which there is an excess of body water relative to body solute, and hyperosmolar disorders, in which there is a deficiency of body water relative to body solute. Because sodium is the main constituent of plasma osmolality, these disorders are typically characterized by hyponatremia and hypernatremia, respectively.

Hypo-osmolality and hyponatremia

Pathogenesis

Hypo-osmolality indicates excess water relative to solute in the ECF; because water moves freely between ECF and intracellular fluid (ICF), this also indicates an excess of total body water (TBW) relative to total body solute. Imbalances between body water and solute can be generated either by depletion of body solute more than body water, or by dilution of body solute from increases in body water more than body solute (Table 23.1). This represents an oversimplification, because most hypo-osmolar states include components of both solute depletion and water retention (e.g. isotonic solute losses, as occurs during an acute hemorrhage, do not produce hypo-osmolality until subsequent retention of ingested or infused hypotonic fluids causes a secondary dilution of the remaining ECF solute). Nonetheless, this concept has proven to be useful because it provides a simple framework for understanding the diagnosis and therapy of hypo-osmolar disorders.

Differential diagnosis

Evaluation of hypo-osmolar patients should include a careful history (especially concerning medications), clinical assessment of ECF volume, thorough neurological evaluation, plasma electrolytes, glucose, uric acid, blood urea nitrogen (BUN) and creatinine, calculated and/or directly measured plasma osmolality and simultaneous urine electrolytes and osmolality. Hyponatremia and hypo-osmolality are usually synonymous, with two exceptions. First, pseudohyponatremia can be produced by marked elevation of plasma lipids and/or proteins; although the concentration of Na^+/l of plasma water is unchanged, the concentration of Na^+/l of plasma is decreased because of the increased non-aqueous portion of the plasma occupied by lipid or protein. However, the directly measured plasma osmolality is not affected by increased lipids or proteins. Second, high concentrations of effective solutes other than Na^+, e.g. glucose, cause relative decreases in plasma sodium concentration ($[Na^+]$) despite an unchanged plasma osmolality. Misdiagnosis can be avoided by direct measurement of plasma osmolality, or in the case of hyperglycemia by correcting the plasma $[Na^+]$ by 1.6 mEq/l for each 100 mg/dl increase in the plasma glucose concentration above 100 mg/dl,

Nephrology, Edited by Rex L. Jamison and Robert Wilkinson.
Published in 1997 by Chapman & Hall, London. ISBN 0 412 60930 4

Table 23.1   Pathogenesis of hypo-osmolar disorders

Solute depletion (primary decreases in total body solute + secondary water retention)[a]
1. Renal solute loss
   Diuretic use
   Solute diuresis (glucose, mannitol)
   Salt wasting nephropathy
   Mineralocorticoid deficiency
2. Non-renal solute loss
   Gastrointestinal (diarrhea, vomiting, pancreatitis, bowel obstruction)
   Cutaneous (sweating, burns)
   Blood loss

Solute dilution (primary increases in total body water ± secondary solute depletion)[a]
1. Impaired renal free water excretion
   (a) Increased proximal nephron reabsorption
       Congestive heart failure
       Cirrhosis
       Nephrotic syndrome
       Hypothyroidism
   (b) Impaired distal nephron dilution
       Syndrome of inappropriate antidiuretic hormone secretion (SIADH)
       Glucocorticoid deficiency
2. Excess water intake
   Primary polydipsia

[a] Virtually all disorders of solute depletion are accompanied by some degree of secondary retention of water by the kidneys in response to the resulting intravascular hypovolemia; this mechanism can lead to hypo-osmolality even when the solute depletion occurs via hypotonic or isotonic body fluid losses. Disorders of water retention can cause hypo-osmolality in the absence of any solute losses, but often some secondary solute losses occur in response to the resulting intravascular hypervolemia and this can then further aggravate the dilutional hypo-osmolality.

which provides an estimate of the contribution of the glucose to the plasma osmolality. Definitive identification of the etiology of the hypo-osmolality is not always possible at the time of presentation, but categorization according to the patient's ECF volume status will allow determination of an appropriate initial therapy in the majority of cases (Figure 23.1).

Decreased ECF volume

Clinically detectable hypovolemia indicates some degree of solute depletion. Elevation of BUN is a useful laboratory correlate of decreased ECF volume. Even isotonic or hypotonic fluid losses can cause hypo-osmolality if water

or hypotonic fluids are subsequently ingested or infused. A low urine Na^+ concentration (U_{Na}) suggests a non-renal cause of solute depletion, whereas a high U_{Na} suggests renal causes of solute depletion (Table 23.1). Diuretic use is the most common cause of hypovolemic hypo-osmolality; thiazides are more commonly associated with severe hyponatremia than are loop diuretics such as furosemide. Although this is seemingly a simple example of solute depletion, the pathophysiological mechanisms underlying the hypo-osmolality are complex and include multiple components. Many such patients do not present with clinical evidence of hypovolemia, in part because ingested water has been retained in response to non–osmotically stimulated vasopressin (AVP) secretion, which occurs in all disorders of solute depletion as an attempt to maintain volume homeostasis (see Figure 8.4, Chapter 8). In addition, U_{Na} may be high or low depending on when the last diuretic dose was taken. Consequently, any suspicion of diuretic use mandates careful consideration of this diagnosis regardless of clinical or laboratory findings. Most other etiologies of solute losses causing hypovolemic hypo-osmolality will be clinically apparent, although some salt-wasting nephropathies (chronic interstitial nephropathy, polycystic kidney disease, obstructive uropathy or Bartter's syndrome) or mineralocorticoid deficiency (Addison's disease) may be challenging to diagnose during early phases of these diseases.

Normal ECF volume

Virtually any disorder causing hypo-osmolality can present with a volume status that appears normal by standard methods of clinical evaluation. Because clinical assessment of volume status is not very sensitive, the presence of normal or low BUN and uric acid concentrations are helpful laboratory correlates of relatively normal ECF volume. In these cases a low U_{Na} (<30 mEq/l) suggests depletional hypo-osmolality secondary to ECF losses with subsequent volume replacement by water or other hypotonic fluids; as discussed earlier, such patients may appear euvolemic by the usual clinical parameters used to assess hydrational status. Hypo-osmolar disorders caused primarily by dilution (Table 23.1) are less likely with a low U_{Na}, although this can occur in hypothyroidism or in the syndrome of inappropriate antidiuretic hormone secretion (SIADH) with superimposed volume depletion. A high U_{Na} (>30 mEq/l) generally indicates a dilutional hypo-osmolality such as SIADH, the most common cause of euvolemic hypo-osmolality. The clinical criteria necessary for a diagnosis of SIADH are as follows. First, ECF hypo-osmolality must be present and hyponatremia secondary to pseudohyponatremia or hyperglycemia excluded. Second, urinary osmolality must be inappropriate for plasma hypo-osmolality; this simply requires that the urine be less than maximally dilute (i.e. U_{osm} > 100 mosmol/kg H_2O). Furthermore, urine osmolality need not be inappropriately elevated at all levels of P_{osm} but

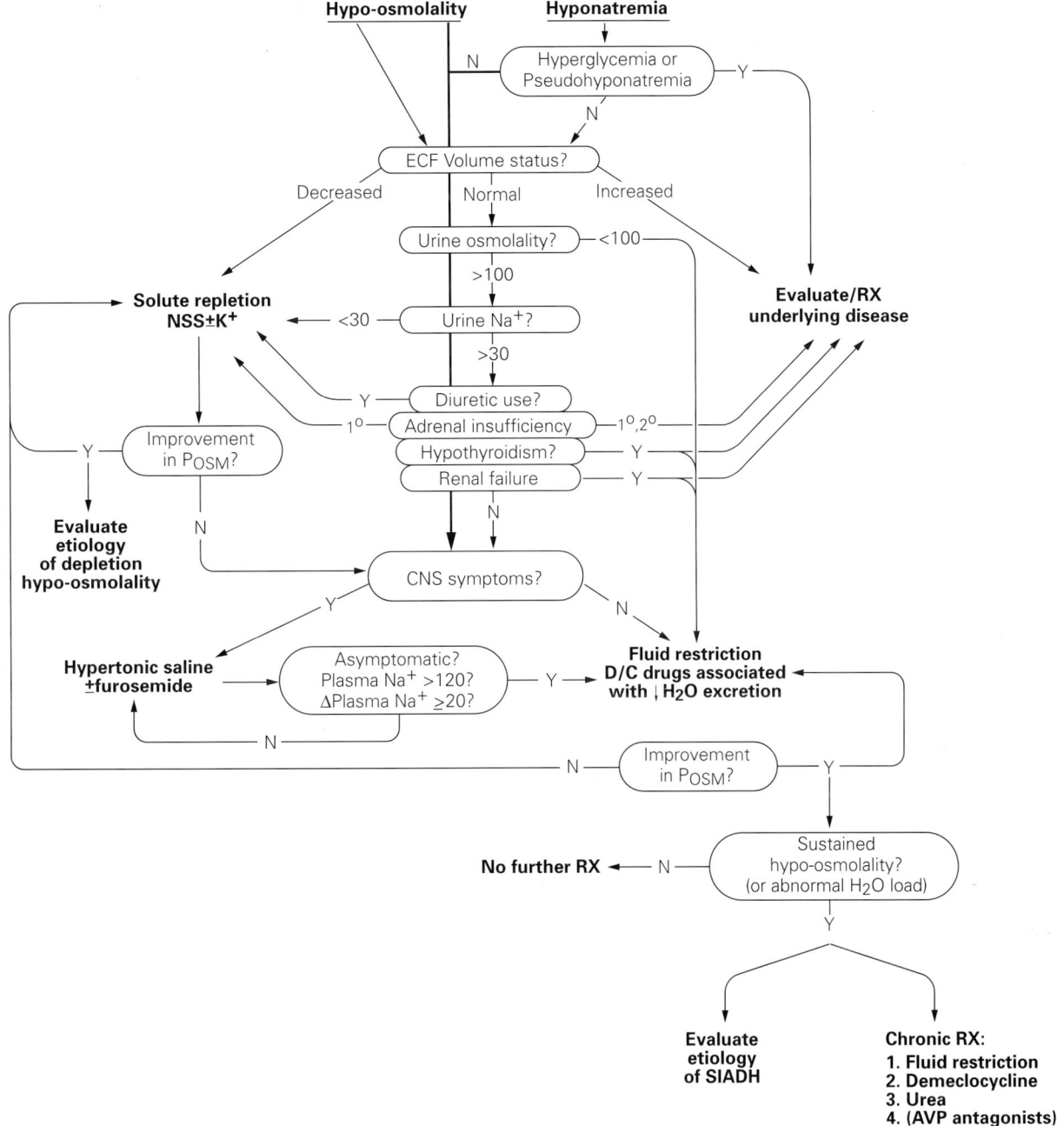

Figure 23.1 Schematic summary of the evaluation and therapy of hypo-osmolar patients. The dark arrow in the center emphasizes that the presence of CNS dysfunction due to hyponatremia should always be assessed immediately, so that appropriate therapy can be started as soon as possible in symptomatic patients while the outlined diagnostic evaluation is proceeding. Abbreviations: N = no; Y = yes; ECF = extracellular fluid volume; NSS = normal (isotonic) saline; RX = treat; 1° = primary; 2° = secondary; P_{OSM} = plasma osmolality; D/C = discontinue; SIADH = syndrome of inappropriate antidiuretic hormone secretion; numbers referring to osmolality are in mosmol/kg H_2O, numbers referring to Na^+ concentration are in mEq/l. (Modified with permission from Verbalis, 1995.)

simply at some level below 275 mosmol/kg H_2O, since in patients with a reset osmostat AVP secretion is suppressed at some lower level of plasma osmolality resulting in maximal urinary dilution and free water excretion at plasma osmolalities below this level. Third, clinical eu-

volemia must be present; this does not mean that patients with SIADH cannot become hypovolemic for other reasons, but in such cases it is impossible to make a diagnosis of SIADH until the patient is made euvolemic. The fourth criterion, an elevated U_{Na}, has caused much confusion; its importance lies in differentiating hypo-osmolality caused by decreased relative intravascular volume, in which renal Na^+ conservation occurs, from dilutional disorders, in which urinary Na^+ excretion is normal or increased due to ECF volume expansion. The continued excretion of ingested Na^+ by such patients reflects the importance of mechanisms for volume homeostasis, which in this case override osmotic homeostatic mechanisms that would favor Na^+ conservation (see Figure 8.4, Chapter 8). However, U_{Na} can also be high in renal causes of solute depletion such as diuretic use or Addison's disease, and conversely patients with SIADH can have a low urinary Na^+ excretion if they subsequently become hypovolemic or solute depleted. Consequently, although elevated urinary Na^+ excretion is the rule in most patients with SIADH, its presence does not confirm this diagnosis nor does its absence rule it out. Finally, SIADH is a diagnosis of exclusion, and other potential causes of hypo-osmolality must always be excluded (Figure 23.1). Glucocorticoid deficiency and SIADH can be especially difficult to distinguish, since hypocortisolism can cause elevated plasma AVP levels and impair maximal urinary dilution; no patient should be diagnosed as having SIADH without an evaluation of adrenal function, preferably via a rapid ACTH stimulation test. Although additional testing is generally not necessary to establish a diagnosis of SIADH, abnormal excretion (<80%) of a standard water load (20 ml/kg body weight) within 4 h can be helpful in confirming the diagnosis in difficult cases. However, water loading should be avoided in patients with more severe hypo-osmolality (plasma $[Na^+] < 125$ mEq/l), since abnormal retention of the ingested water can cause a significant (4–6 mEq/l) further decrease in plasma $[Na^+]$. Many different disorders have been associated with SIADH; these can be divided into four major etiologic groups: tumors, central nervous system (CNS) disorders, drug effects, and pulmonary diseases (Table 23.2).

Increased ECF volume

Clinically detectable hypervolemia indicates whole body sodium excess, and hypo-osmolality in these patients suggests a relatively decreased intravascular volume and/or pressure leading to water retention as a result of elevated plasma AVP levels and decreased distal delivery of glomerular filtrate. Such patients usually have a low U_{Na} because of secondary hyperaldosteronism, but under certain conditions the U_{Na} may be elevated (e.g. diuretic therapy). Hyponatremia generally does not occur until advanced stages of congestive heart failure, cirrhosis or nephrotic syndrome, so diagnosis is usually not difficult. Renal failure can also cause retention of both sodium and water, but in this case the factor limiting excretion of excess body fluid is not decreased effective circulating volume but rather decreased glomerular filtration. Although primary polydipsia can rarely cause hypo-osmolality, these patients rarely if ever manifest signs

Table 23.2 Common etiologies of SIADH

Tumors	Pulmonary/mediastinal (bronchogenic carcinoma; mesothelioma; thymoma)
	Non-chest (duodenal carcinoma; pancreatic carcinoma; ureteral/prostate carcinoma; uterine carcinoma; nasopharyngeal carcinoma; leukemia)
Central nervous system disorders	Mass lesions (tumors; brain abscesses; subdural hematoma)
	Inflammatory diseases (encephalitis; meningitis; systemic lupus)
	Degenerative/demyelinative diseases (Guillain–Barré; spinal cord lesions)
	Miscellaneous (subarachnoid hemorrhage; head trauma; acute psychosis; delirium tremens; pituitary stalk section)
Drug induced	Stimulated AVP release (nicotine; phenothiazines; tricyclics)
	Direct renal effects and/or potentiation of AVP effects (dDAVP; oxytocin; prostaglandin synthesis inhibitors)
	Mixed or uncertain actions (chlorpropamide; clofibrate; carbamazepine; cyclophosphamide; vincristine)
Pulmonary diseases	Infections (tuberculosis; aspergillosis; pneumonia; empyema)
	Mechanical/ventilatory (acute respiratory failure; COPD; positive pressure ventilation)

of hypervolemia since water retention alone without sodium excess does not cause significant volume expansion.

Clinical manifestations

The clinical manifestations of hyponatremia are largely neurological, and primarily reflect brain edema resulting from osmotic water shifts into the brain. These range from non-specific symptoms such as headache and confusion, to more severe manifestations such as decreased sensorium, coma, seizures and death. Significant CNS symptoms generally do not occur until plasma $[Na^+]$ falls below 125 mEq/l, and the severity of symptoms can be roughly correlated with the degree of hypo-osmolality. Individual variability is marked, and for any patient the level of plasma [Na$^+$] at which symptoms will appear cannot be predicted. Several factors other than the severity of the hypo-osmolality also affect the degree of neurological dysfunction. The most important is the time-course over which hypo-osmolality develops. Rapid development of severe hypo-osmolality frequently causes marked neurologic symptoms, whereas gradual development over several days or weeks is often associated with relatively mild symptomatology despite profound degrees of hypo-osmolality. This is because the brain counteracts osmotic swelling by extruding extracellular and intracellular solutes (including potassium and organic osmolytes). Since this is a time-dependent process, rapid development of hypo-osmolality can result in brain edema before this adaptation occurs, but with slower development of the same degree of hypo-osmolality brain cells can lose solute sufficiently rapidly to prevent cell swelling, brain edema, and neurological dysfunction. Underlying neurological disease also affects the level of hypo-osmolality at which CNS symptoms appear; moderate hypo-osmolality is of little concern in an otherwise healthy patient, but can cause morbidity in a patient with an underlying seizure disorder. Non-neurological metabolic disorders (hypoxia, hypercapnia, acidosis, hypercalcemia, etc.) similarly can affect the level of plasma osmolality at which CNS symptoms occur. Recent clinical studies have suggested that menstruating females and young children may be particularly susceptible to the development of neurological morbidity and mortality during hyponatremia, especially in the acute postoperative setting. The true clinical incidence as well as the underlying mechanisms responsible for these sometimes catastrophic cases remains to be determined.

Therapy

Despite continuing controversy concerning the optimal speed of correction of osmolality in hyponatremic patients, there is general consensus regarding appropriate therapy in most cases (Figure 23.1). If hypovolemia is present the patient should be considered to have a solute depletion-induced hypo-osmolality and treated with isotonic (0.9%) NaCl at a rate appropriate for the estimated volume depletion. If diuretic use is known or suspected, this should be supplemented with potassium (20–40 mEq/l) even if plasma [K$^+$] is not low because of the propensity of such patients to have total body potassium depletion. Most often the hypo-osmolar patient will be clinically euvolemic, but several situations will dictate reconsideration of potential solute depletion even in patients without clinically apparent hypovolemia: a decreased U$_{Na}$, a history of recent diuretic use and any suggestion of primary adrenal insufficiency. As a general rule, whenever a reasonable likelihood of depletional rather than dilutional hypo-osmolality exists it is appropriate to treat initially with a trial of isotonic NaCl. If the patient has SIADH no harm will have been done with a limited (1–2 l) saline infusion, since such patients will simply

excrete excess NaCl without significantly changing their P$_{osm}$. However, this therapy should be abandoned if plasma [Na$^+$] does not improve, since larger volumes of isotonic NaCl infusion can worsen the hyponatremia by virtue of gradual water retention. The treatment of euvolemic hypo-osmolar patients will vary depending on their presentation. A patient who has fulfilled all criteria for SIADH except that U$_{osm}$ is low should simply be observed since this may represent the spontaneous reversal of a transient form of SIADH. If there is suspicion of either primary or secondary adrenal insufficiency, glucocorticoid replacement should be started immediately after completion of a rapid ACTH stimulation test. Prompt water diuresis following glucocorticoid replacement strongly supports glucocorticoid deficiency, but the absence of a rapid response does not negate this diagnosis since several days of glucocorticoid treatment are sometimes required for normalization of P$_{osm}$. Hypervolemic hypo-osmolar patients are generally best treated initially by diuresis and other measures directed at their underlying disorder. Such patients rarely require specific therapy to increase plasma osmolality acutely, but often benefit from sodium and water restriction to reduce body fluid retention.

In a significantly hyponatremic patient the question of how quickly the plasma osmolality should be corrected must be addressed. Although hyponatremia is associated with a broad spectrum of neurological symptoms, sometimes leading to death in severe cases, too rapid correction of severe hyponatremia can produce pontine and extrapontine myelinolysis, a demyelinating disease that is associated with substantial neurological morbidity and mortality. Recent clinical and experimental results suggest that optimal treatment of hyponatremic patients entails balancing the risks of hyponatremia against the risks of correction for each patient individually. Several factors should be considered when making a treatment decision in hyponatremic patients: the severity of the hyponatremia, the duration of the hyponatremia, and the patient's symptoms. Neither sequelae from hyponatremia itself nor myelinolysis after therapy are very likely to occur in patients whose plasma [Na$^+$] remains ≥120 mEq/l, although on occasion significant symptoms can develop even at higher serum [Na$^+$] levels if the rate of fall of plasma osmolality has been very rapid (>0.5 mEq/l/h). The importance of duration and symptomatology relate to how well the brain has adapted to the hyponatremia (see above), and consequently the risk of demyelination with rapid correction. Cases of acute hyponatremia (≤48 h duration) are usually symptomatic if the hyponatremia is ≤120 mEq/l; these patients are at great risk from neurological complications from the hyponatremia and should be corrected to higher plasma [Na$^+$] levels promptly (Figure 23.1). Conversely, patients with more chronic hyponatremia (>48 h in duration) who have minimal neurological symptomatology are at little risk from hyponatremia, but can develop demyelination following rapid correction. There is no need to correct these patients rapidly, and they should be treated using slower-acting therapies such as fluid restriction.

Although these extremes have clear treatment indications, most hyponatremic patients will be of indeterminate duration and have varying degrees of milder neurological symptoms. This group is the most challenging to treat, since the hyponatremia will have been present long enough to allow some degree of brain volume regulation, but not to prevent some brain edema and neurological symptoms. Such patients should be treated promptly because of their symptoms, but using methods that allow a controlled and limited correction of their hyponatremia. Reasonable correction parameters consist of a maximal rate of correction of plasma [Na$^+$] in the range of 1–2 mEq/l/h as long as the total magnitude of correction does not exceed 25 mEq/l over the first 48 h. Some argue that these parameters should be even more conservative, with maximal correction rates of ≤0.5 mEq/l/h and magnitudes of correction that do not exceed 12 mEq/l in the first 24 h and 18 mEq/l in the first 48 h. Treatments for individual patients should be chosen within these limits depending on their symptoms: in patients who are only moderately symptomatic one should proceed at the lower recommended limits of ≤0.5 mEq/l/h, whereas in those who manifest more severe neurological symptoms an initial correction at a rate of 1–2 mEq/l/h is more appropriate. Controlled corrections are generally best accomplished with hypertonic (3%) NaCl solution given via continuous infusion. An initial infusion rate can be estimated by multiplying the patient's body weight in kg, by the desired rate of increase in plasma [Na$^+$] in mEq/l/h (e.g. in a 70 kg patient an infusion of 3% NaCl at 70 ml/h will increase plasma [Na$^+$] by approximately 1 mEq/l/h, whereas infusing 35 ml/h will increase plasma [Na$^+$] by approximately 0.5 mEq/l/h). Patients with diuretic-induced hyponatremia usually respond well to isotonic NaCl and do not require 3% NaCl. Regardless of the initial rate of correction chosen, acute treatment should be interrupted if any of three endpoints is reached: (1) the patient's symptoms are abolished; (2) a safe plasma [Na$^+$] (generally ≥120 mEq/l) is achieved; or (3) a total magnitude of correction of 20 mEq/l is achieved (Figure 23.1). Plasma [Na$^+$] levels must be carefully monitored at frequent intervals (at least every 4 h) during the active phases of treatment to adjust therapy so that the correction stays within these guidelines. It cannot be emphasized too strongly that it is only necessary to correct the plasma [Na$^+$] acutely to a safe range rather than completely to normonatremia. In some situations patients may spontaneously correct their hyponatremia via a water diuresis. If the hyponatremia is acute (e.g. psychogenic polydipsia with water intoxication) such patients are not at risk for subsequent demyelination; however, in cases where the hyponatremia has been chronic (e.g. hypocortisolism) intervention should be considered to limit the rate and magnitude of correction of plasma [Na$^+$] using the same endpoints as for active correction.

Chronic treatment of hyponatremia requires choosing among several suboptimal therapies. One important exception is patients with the reset osmostat syndrome; because the hyponatremia of such patients is not progressive but rather fluctuates around their reset level of plasma [Na$^+$], no therapy is generally effective or required. For most other cases of mild to moderate SIADH fluid restriction represents the least toxic therapy, and is the treatment of choice. This should always be tried as the initial therapy, with pharmacologic intervention reserved for refractory cases where the degree of fluid restriction required to avoid hypo-osmolality is so severe that the patient is unable, or unwilling, to maintain it. If pharmacologic treatment is necessary, the preferred drug at present is the tetracycline derivative demeclocycline, which causes nephrogenic diabetes insipidus, thereby decreasing urine concentration. The effective dose of demeclocycline ranges from 600 to 1200 mg/day; several days of therapy are necessary to achieve maximum effects, so one should wait three to four days before increasing the dose. Demeclocycline can cause reversible nephrotoxicity, especially in patients with cirrhosis or other edema-forming disorders; renal function should be monitored and the medication stopped if increasing azotemia occurs. Several other drugs decrease AVP hypersecretion in selected cases (diphenylhydantoin, opiates, ethanol), but responses are unpredictable. Currently an ideal therapeutic agent for chronic SIADH is not available, but this is likely to change in the near future with the development of specific antagonists to the AVP V$_2$ (antidiuretic) receptor. Such agents are likely to become the treatment of choice for SIADH in the future. However, their use to correct established hyponatremia will require judicious adherence to the same guidelines already established to prevent complications from demyelination.

Hyperosmolality and hypernatremia

Pathogenesis

Hyperosmolality indicates a deficiency of water relative to solute in the ECF. Because water moves freely between the ICF and ECF, this also indicates a deficiency of TBW relative to total body solute. Although hypernatremia can be caused by an excess of body sodium, the vast majority of cases are due to losses of body water in excess of body solutes, caused by either insufficient water intake or excessive water excretion. Consequently, most of the disorders causing hyperosmolality are those associated with inadequate water intake and/or deficient AVP secretion (Table 23.3). The best known of these is diabetes insipidus, in which AVP secretion or its renal effects is impaired without an abnormality of thirst. Much less common are disorders of osmoreceptor function resulting in abnormalities of both AVP secretion and thirst. Although hyperosmolality from inadequate water intake

Table 23.3   Pathogenesis of hyperosmolar disorders

Water depletion (decreases in total body water in excess of body solute)
1. Insufficient water intake
   Unavailability of water
   Hypodipsia (osmoreceptor dysfunction, age)
   Neurological deficits (cognitive dysfunction, motor impairments)
2. Hypotonic fluid loss[a]
   (a) Renal: diabetes insipidus (DI)
       Insufficient AVP secretion (central DI, osmoreceptor dysfunction)
       Insufficient AVP effect (nephrogenic DI)
   (b) Renal: other fluid loss
       Osmotic diuresis (hyperglycemia, mannitol)
       Diuretic drugs (furosemide, ethacrynic acid, thiazides)
       Postobstructive diuresis
       Diuretic phase of acute tubular necrosis
   (c) Non-renal fluid loss
       Gastrointestinal (vomiting, diarrhea, nasogastric suction)
       Cutaneous (sweating, burns)
       Pulmonary (hyperventilation)
       Peritoneal dialysis

Solute excess (increases in total body solute in excess of body water):
1. Sodium
   Excess Na^+ administration (NaCl, $NaHCO_3$)
   Sea water drowning
2. Other
   Hyperalimentation (intravenous, parenteral)

---

[a] Most hypotonic fluid losses will not produce hyperosmolality unless insufficient free water is ingested or infused to replace the ongoing losses, so these disorders also usually involve some component of insufficient water intake as well.

is seen frequently in clinical practice, this is usually not due to an underlying defect in thirst but rather results from a generalized incapacity to obtain and/or ingest fluids, often stemming from a depressed sensorium. An example is hyperosmolar coma caused by renal water losses from hyperglycemia-induced diuresis in elderly patients who eventually are unable to drink enough fluid to keep up with the ongoing osmotic diuresis.

Differential diagnosis

Evaluation of hyperosmolar patients should include a careful history, clinical assessment of ECF volume, a thorough neurological evaluation, plasma electrolytes, glucose, BUN and creatinine, calculated and/or directly measured plasma osmolality, simultaneous urine electrolytes and osmolality and urine glucose. Hypernatremia is always synonymous with hyperosmolality since Na^+ is the main constituent of plasma osmolality, but hyperosmolality can exist without hypernatremia when there is an excess of non-sodium solute. This occurs most often with marked elevations of plasma glucose, as in patients with non-ketotic hyperglycemic hyperosmolar coma. As for cases of artifactual hyponatremia caused by hyperglycemia, misdiagnosis can be avoided by direct measurement of plasma osmolality, or by correcting the plasma $[Na^+]$ by 1.6 mEq/l for each 100 mg/dl increase in plasma glucose concentration above 100 mg/dl. Evaluation of the patient's ECF volume status is important as a guide to fluid replacement therapy, but it is not as useful for differential diagnosis since most hyperosmolar patients will manifest some degree of hypovolemia. Rather, assessment of urinary concentrating ability provides the most useful data with regard to the type of disorder present. Using this approach, disorders of hyperosmolality can be categorized as those in which renal water conservation mechanisms are intact but are unable to compensate for inadequately replaced losses of hypotonic fluids from other sources, or those in which renal concentrating defects are a contributing factor to the deficiency of body water.

An appropriately concentrated urine in a hyperosmolar patient eliminates the possibility of a primary renal cause of the disorder in most cases. Maximum urine concentrating ability varies between individuals and decreases with age, but in general urine osmolalities above 800 mosmol/kg H_2O are considered sufficient to verify normal AVP secretion and renal response. Potential causes of non-renal fluid losses should be investigated, particularly gastrointestinal and cutaneous losses (although as discussed previously, subsequent ingestion of free water can produce hypo-osmolality in such patients as a result of AVP-induced water retention). In the absence of disorders causing fluid losses, primary disorders of thirst should be considered, especially in the elderly who have a decreased sensation of thirst and ingest lesser amounts of fluids in response to induced dehydration. Rarely a primary disorder of thirst may be present, as will be discussed below. One situation in which a normally concentrated urine may not completely eliminate the possibility of an underlying renal-concentrating defect is in patients with mild partial central diabetes insipidus, who can sometimes achieve maximally concentrated urine during extreme dehydration through a combination of severely limited GFR and stimulated AVP secretion at high plasma osmolalities, as will be discussed below. However, as plasma osmolality is corrected, these patients will demonstrate inappropriate dilution of their urine before reaching normal levels of plasma osmolality.

An inappropriately low urine osmolality (e.g. less than 800 mosmol/kg H_2O in a hyperosmolar patient) signifies the presence of a renal-concentrating defect. The urine should always be checked for glucose, since a solute diuresis will limit urine concentrating ability and urine osmolality can approach isotonicity at high rates of urine excretion. In the absence of glucosuria or any other cause of osmotic diuresis, inadequate urine concentration in a hyperosmolar patient generally indicates the presence of diabetes insipidus and further testing is then indicated to ascertain the etiology.

Diabetes insipidus

Diabetes insipidus (DI) can result from either inadequate AVP secretion (central or neurogenic) or inadequate renal response to AVP (nephrogenic) (Table 23.4). Central DI is caused by a variety of acquired or congenital anatomic lesions that disrupt the hypothalamic–posterior pituitary axis, including pituitary surgery, tumors, trauma, hemorrhage, thrombosis, infarction or granulomatous disease. Severe nephrogenic DI is most commonly congenital due to defects in the gene for the AVP V_2 receptor (X–linked recessive pattern of inheritance) or in the gene for the aquaporin-2 water channel (autosomal recessive pattern of inheritance), but relief of chronic urinary obstruction or therapy with drugs such as lithium can cause an acquired form sufficient to warrant treatment. Short-lived nephrogenic DI can result from hypokalemia or hypercalcemia, but the mild concentrating defect generally does not by itself cause hypertonicity and responds to correction of the underlying disorder. Regardless of the etiology of the DI, the end result is a free water diuresis due to an inability to concentrate urine appropriately. Because renal mechanisms for sodium conservation are unimpaired, there is no accompanying sodium deficiency. Although untreated DI can lead to both hyperosmolality and volume depletion, until the water losses become severe, volume depletion is minimized by osmotic shifts of water from the ICF to the more osmotically concentrated ECF. This phenomenon is not as evident following increases in ECF Na^+ concentration, since such osmotic shifts result in a slower increase in the plasma $[Na^+]$ than would otherwise occur. However, when non-sodium solutes such as mannitol are infused, this effect is more obvious due to the progressive dilutional decrease in plasma $[Na^+]$ caused by translocation of intracellular water to the ECF compartment.

Because patients with DI do not have impaired urine Na^+ conservation, the ECF volume is generally not markedly decreased and regulatory mechanisms for maintenance of osmotic homeostasis are primarily activated: stimulation of thirst and AVP secretion (to whatever degree the neurohypophysis is still able to secrete AVP). In cases where AVP secretion is totally absent (complete DI), patients are dependent entirely on water intake for maintenance of water balance. However, in cases where some residual capacity to secrete AVP remains (partial DI), plasma osmolality can eventually reach levels that allow moderate degrees of urinary concentration (cf. Figure 7.3, Chapter 7 that even small concentrations of AVP can

Table 23.4 · Common etiologies of polydipsia and hypotonic polyuria

Central (neurogenic) diabetes insipidus	Congenital (congenital malformations; autosomal dominant: AVP-neurophysin gene mutations)
	Drug/toxin-induced (ethanol; diphenylhydantoin; snake venom)
	Granulomatous (histiocytosis; sarcoidosis)
	Neoplastic (craniopharyngioma; meningioma; germinoma; pituitary tumor or metastases)
	Infectious (meningitis; encephalitis)
	Inflammatory/autoimmune (lymphocytic infundibuloneurohypophysitis)
	Trauma (neurosurgery; deceleration injury)
	Vascular (cerebral hemorrhage or infarction)
Nephrogenic diabetes insipidus	Congenital (X-linked recessive: AVP V_2 receptor gene mutations; autosomal recessive: aquaporin-2 water channel gene mutations)
	Drug-induced (demeclocycline; lithium; cisplatin; methoxyflurane)
	Hypercalcemia
	Hypokalemia
	Infiltrating lesions (sarcoidosis; amyloidosis)
	Vascular (sickle cell anemia)
Osmoreceptor dysfunction	Granulomatous (histiocytosis; sarcoidosis)
	Neoplastic (craniopharyngioma; pinealoma; meningioma; metastases)
	Vascular (anterior communicating artery aneurysm/ligation; intrahypothalamic hemorrhage)
	Other (hydrocephalus; ventricular/suprasellar cyst; trauma; degenerative diseases; idiopathic)
Increased AVP metabolism	Pregnancy
Primary polydipsia	Psychogenic (schizophrenia)
	Dipsogenic (downward resetting of thirst threshold: similar lesions as central DI)

have substantial effects to limit urine volume). As the plasma osmolality increases, some patients with partial DI can secrete enough AVP to achieve near maximal urine osmolalities (Figure 23.2). However, this should not cause confusion about the diagnosis of DI, since in such patients the urine osmolality will still be inappropriately low at plasma osmolalities within normal ranges, and they will respond to exogenous AVP administration with a further rise in urine osmolality.

Distinguishing between central and nephrogenic DI in a patient who is already hyperosmolar is straightforward, and consists simply of evaluating the response to administered AVP (5 units s.c.) or, preferably, desmopressin (1-deamino-8-D-arginine vasopressin; dDAVP; 1 μg s.c. or i.v.). A significant increase in urine osmolality within 1–2 h after injection indicates insufficient endogenous AVP secretion, and therefore central DI, whereas an absent response indicates renal resistance to AVP effects, and therefore nephrogenic DI (NDI). Although conceptually simple, interpretational difficulties often arise because the water diuresis produced by AVP deficiency produces a 'wash-out' of the renal medullary concentrating gradient so that increases in urine osmolality in response to administered AVP or dDAVP are not as great as would be expected. Generally, increases of ≥50% reliably indicate central DI and responses of ≤10% indicate NDI, but responses between 10% and 50% are less certain. For this reason, plasma AVP levels should be measured to aid in this distinction: hyperosmolar patients with NDI

will have clearly elevated AVP levels whereas those with central DI will have absent (complete) or blunted (partial) AVP responses relative to their plasma osmolality. Since it will not be known beforehand which patients will have diagnostic versus indeterminate responses to AVP or dDAVP, a plasma AVP level should be drawn before AVP or dDAVP administration in all patients. One drawback to using the AVP levels for diagnosis is the relatively long turnaround time (5–10 days in most laboratories) for results. An alternative in such cases is to continue dDAVP treatment for 1–2 days as a clinical trial; if central DI is present the medullary tonicity will gradually re-establish itself, and as it does so more pronounced responses to successive administered dDAVP doses will occur, thereby confirming the diagnosis.

Since patients with DI have intact thirst mechanisms, most often they do not present with hyperosmolality but rather with a normal plasma osmolality and [Na$^+$] and symptoms of polyuria and polydipsia. In these cases it is most appropriate to perform a water deprivation test. This entails following the patient's plasma [Na$^+$], urine volume and urine osmolality in the absence of fluid intake until the plasma [Na$^+$] is ≥146 mEq/l or the urine osmolality reaches a plateau (generally defined as three successive urine samples with less than 10% differences in osmolality) and the patient has lost at least 2% of body weight. At this point a plasma AVP level is drawn and the patient is given AVP or dDAVP (as discussed above for hyperosmolar patients). The same criteria are used to evaluate

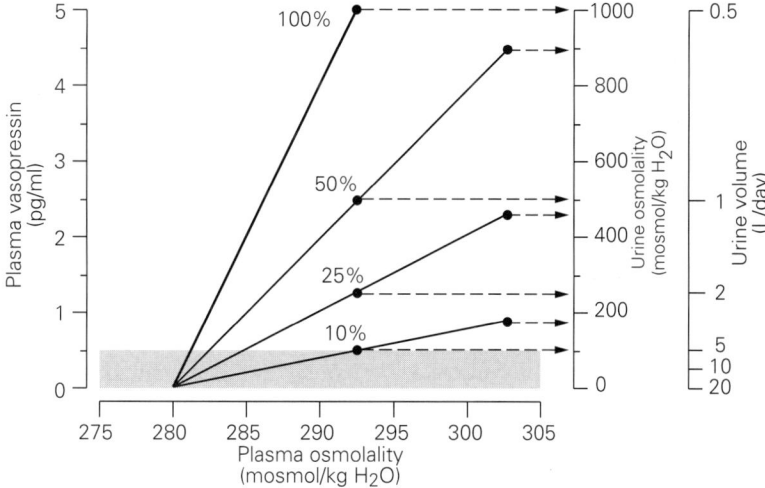

Figure 23.2 Relation between plasma AVP levels, urine osmolality, and plasma osmolality in subjects with normal pituitary function (100%) compared to patients with graded reductions in AVP-secreting neurons (to 50%, 25% and 10% of normal). Note that the patient with a 50% secretory capacity can only achieve half the plasma AVP level and half the urine osmolality of normal subjects at a plasma osmolality of 293 mosmol/kg H$_2$O, but with increasing plasma osmolality this patient can nonetheless eventually stimulate sufficient AVP secretion to reach a near maximal urine osmolality. In contrast, patients with more severe degrees of AVP-secreting neuron deficits are unable to reach maximal urine osmolalities at any levels of plasma osmolality. (Modified with permission from Robertson, 1995a.)

the etiology of the DI following this test, but one additional entity, primary polydipsia, must be considered in the differential diagnosis of normonatremic polyuria and polydipsia (Table 23.4). Primary polydipsia is usually a result of psychiatric disease. Such patients ingest large amounts of fluids for a variety of reasons, but generally not because of physiological sensations of thirst; this is referred to as psychogenic polydipsia. A smaller subset of patients with primary polydipsia have a true disorder of thirst regulation, usually manifested by a downward resetting of the osmotic threshold for stimulated thirst; this is sometimes called dipsogenic diabetes insipidus. Regardless of the cause of the excessive fluid intake, because the ensuing water diuresis can wash out the medullary concentration gradient, such patients may concentrate their urine subnormally in response to water deprivation and therefore can resemble partial central DI. In contrast to central DI, however, patients with primary polydipsia will concentrate their urine <10% in response to administered AVP or dDAVP and will have plasma AVP levels appropriate to their plasma osmolality. With use of the water deprivation test combined with plasma AVP determinations >90% of all cases of polyuria and polydipsia can be diagnosed appropriately; diagnoses in the remaining patients will generally become evident over time based on their responses to therapeutic clinical trials.

Osmoreceptor dysfunction

There is an extensive literature in animals indicating that the primary osmoreceptors that control AVP secretion and thirst are located in the anterior hypothalamus. Lesions of this region in animals cause hyperosmolality through a combination of impaired thirst and osmotically stimulated AVP secretion. Initial reports in humans described this syndrome as 'essential hypernatremia,' and subsequent studies used the term 'adipsic hypernatremia' in recognition of the profound thirst deficits found in most patients. All of these syndromes are grouped together as disorders of osmoreceptor function. Four major patterns of osmoreceptor dysfunction have been described as characterized by defects in thirst and/or AVP secretory responses: (1) upward resetting of the osmostat for both thirst and AVP secretion (normal AVP and thirst responses but at an abnormally high plasma osmolality; (2) partial osmoreceptor destruction (blunted AVP and thirst responses at all plasma osmolalities); (3) total osmoreceptor destruction (absent AVP secretion and thirst regardless of plasma osmolality); and (4) selective dysfunction of thirst osmoregulation with intact AVP secretion. Most of the cases reported to date have represented various degrees of osmoreceptor destruction associated with different brain lesions (Table 23.4). As opposed to lesions causing central DI, these lesions usually occur more anteriorly in the hypothalamus, consistent with the anterior hypothalamic location of the primary osmoreceptor cells. Whether some of these

patients also have an inability to suppress as well as stimulate AVP secretion, thereby leading to hypoosmolality in some situations, remains an interesting but incompletely evaluated possibility. For all cases of osmoreceptor dysfunction it is important to remember that afferent pathways from the brainstem to the hypothalamus remain intact; therefore, these patients will usually have normal AVP and renal concentrating responses to baroreceptor-mediated stimuli such as hypovolemia and hypotension. This often causes confusion, since at some times these patients appear to have DI yet at other times they can concentrate their urine quite normally.

Clinical manifestations

The clinical manifestations of hyperosmolar patients can be divided into those produced by dehydration, which are largely cardiovascular, those caused by the hyperosmolality itself, which are largely neurological and reflect brain dehydration as a result of osmotic water shifts out of the CNS, and those which are secondary to excessive renal water losses in patients with DI. Cardiovascular manifestations of hypertonic dehydration include hypotension, azotemia, acute tubular necrosis secondary to renal hypoperfusion or rhabdomyolysis and shock. Neurological manifestations range from non-specific symptoms such as irritability and decreased sensorium to more severe manifestations such as chorea, seizures, coma, focal neurological deficits and cerebral infarction. As with hypo-osmolality, the severity of symptoms can be roughly correlated with the degree of hyperosmolality, but individual variability is marked and for any single patient the level of plasma [Na+] at which symptoms will appear cannot be predicted. Also as with hypo-osmolar syndromes, the length of time over which hyperosmolality develops can markedly affect clinical symptomatology. Rapid development of severe hyperosmolality is frequently associated with marked neurologic symptoms, whereas gradual development over several days or weeks generally causes milder symptoms. In this case the brain counteracts osmotic shrinkage by increasing intracellular content of solutes. These include electrolytes such as potassium and a variety of organic osmolytes which previously had been called 'idiogenic osmoles' (for the most part these are the same organic osmolytes that are lost from the brain during adaptation to hypo-osmolality discussed previously). The net effect of this process is to protect the brain against excessive shrinkage during sustained hypertonicity. However, once the brain has adapted by increasing its solute content, rapid correction of the hyperosmolality can cause brain edema since it takes a finite time (24–48 h in animal studies) to dissipate the accumulated solutes, and until this process has been completed the brain will accumulate excess water as plasma osmolality is normalized. This effect is most often seen in dehydrated pediatric patients who can develop seizures with rapid rehydration, but has been described only rarely in adults, including the most severely hyperosmolar patients with non-ketotic hyperglycemic hyperosmolar coma.

The characteristic symptoms of DI are the polyuria and polydipsia which result from the underlying impairment of urinary concentrating mechanisms. Interestingly, patients with DI typically describe a craving for cold water which seems to quench their thirst better. Patients with central DI also typically describe a precipitous onset of their polyuria and polydipsia, which simply reflects the fact that urinary concentration can be maintained fairly well until the number of AVP-producing neurons in the hypothalamus decreases to 10–15% of normal, after which plasma AVP levels decrease to the range where urine output increases dramatically (see Figure 7.3 in Chapter 7).

Therapy

The general goals of treatment of all hyperosmolar disorders are: (1) correction of pre-existing water deficits and (2) reduction in ongoing excessive urinary water losses. The specific therapy required varies with the clinical situation. Awake ambulatory patients with DI and normal thirst have little body water deficit but benefit from relief of the polyuria and polydipsia that disrupt normal activities. In contrast, comatose patients with or without DI are unable to drink in response to thirst, and in these patients progressive hypertonicity may be life-threatening. The established water deficit may be estimated using the following formula:

$$\text{Water deficit} = 0.6 \times \text{premorbid weight}$$
$$\times \left[1 - 140/\text{plasma}\left[Na^+\right]\left(\text{mEq}/l\right)\right]$$

This formula is dependent on several assumptions (TBW is approximately 60% of body weight, no body solute is lost as hypertonicity developed, and the premorbid [Na^+] is 140 mEq/l), but nonetheless provides a valid estimate of the approximate TBW deficit. To reduce the risk of CNS injury from protracted exposure to severe hypertonicity, the serum osmolality should be lowered to the range of 330 mosmol/kg H_2O within the first 24 h of therapy. As noted previously, because the organic osmolytes accumulated in the brain during chronic hyperosmolality cannot be immediately dissipated, further correction to a normal osmolality should be spread over the subsequent 1–3 days to avoid producing cerebral edema during treatment, particularly in pediatric patients.

It should be remembered that formulae which estimate body water deficits do not take ongoing water losses into account. Consequently, frequent serum electrolyte determinations must be made, and the administration rate of oral water or intravenous 5% dextrose in water should be adjusted accordingly. For example, the estimated water deficit of a 70 kg patient whose plasma [Na^+] is 160 mEq/l would be 5.25 l. In such an individual, administration of water at a rate >200 ml/h would be required simply to correct the established deficit over 24 h, but additional fluid would be needed to keep up with any ongoing losses in a patient with DI until a response to treatment has occurred.

A variety of antidiuretic agents have been used to treat central DI, but dDAVP is the treatment of choice for this disorder. dDAVP was synthesized as a selective antagonist of AVP V_2 receptors, and it is particularly useful therapeutically because it has a much longer half-life than AVP and is devoid of the pressor activity of AVP at vascular V_1 receptors. Desmopressin is generally administered intranasally (5–20 µg every 8–24 h), but can be given parenterally in acute situations (1–2 µg i.v., i.m. or s.c.). For both the intranasal and parenteral preparations, increasing the administered dose generally has the effect of prolonging the duration of antidiuresis rather than increasing its magnitude; consequently, altering the dose can be useful to reduce the required frequency of administration. Synthetic AVP (Pitressin) can also be used to treat central DI, but its use is limited by a much shorter half-life necessitating more frequent dosing or a continuous infusion, and the production of pressor effects due to vasoconstriction. The sulfonylurea chlorpropamide potentiates the effect of AVP in the kidney and can be useful adjunctive therapy in selected cases of partial central DI. However, caution regarding the development of hypoglycemia, particularly in patients with anterior pituitary insufficiency, is necessary and several days of treatment are required before maximal effects are seen.

NDI is more difficult to treat since the kidney is resistant to all AVP-type agents. Limited responses can sometimes be achieved using thiazide diuretics (any drug of the thiazide class may be used with equal potential for benefit). Thiazides cause natriuresis by blocking sodium absorption in the cortical diluting site; when combined with dietary sodium restriction a modest hypovolemia results, which stimulates isotonic proximal tubular solute reabsorption and diminishes solute delivery to the distal parts of the nephron. Together, these effects diminish free water clearance independently of actions of AVP, thereby decreasing the polyuria of patients with NDI. Monitoring for hypokalemia is necessary and K^+ supplementation is occasionally required. Care must be exercised when treating patients taking lithium with diuretics, since the induced contraction of plasma volume may increase lithium concentrations by increasing proximal tubular absorption and worsen potential toxic effects of the therapy. Because prostaglandins increase renal medullary blood flow and diminish medullary solute concentration, effects that modestly decrease the interstitial gradient for water reabsorption, drugs that block renal prostaglandin synthesis (e.g. non-steroidal anti-inflammatory agents) can increase non-AVP-mediated water reabsorption and impair urinary dilution, thereby reducing free water clearance and urine output. Although these agents are somewhat effective in central DI, their main usefulness is as adjunctive therapy in NDI, in which more direct antidiuretic therapies are limited.

Further reading

Anderson, R.J., Chung, H-M., Kluge, R. *et al.* (1985) Hyponatremia: a prospective analysis of its epidemiology and the pathogenetic role of vasopressin. *Ann. Intern. Med.*, **102**, 164–8.

Arieff, A.I., Llach, F. and Massry, S.G. (1976) Neurological manifestations and morbidity of hyponatremia: correlation with brain water and electrolytes. *Medicine*, **55**, 121–9.

Ayus, J.C., Wheeler, J.M. and Arieff, A.I. (1992) Postoperative hyponatremic encephalopathy in menstruant women. *Ann. Intern. Med.*, **117**, 891–7.

Bartter, F.C. and Schwartz, W.B. (1967) The syndrome of inappropriate secretion of antidiuretic hormone. *Am. J. Med.*, **42**, 790–806.

Baylis, P.H. and Thompson, C.J. (1988) Osmoregulation of vasopressin secretion and thirst in health and disease. *Clin. Endocrinol.*, **29**, 549–76.

Berl, T. (1990) Treating hyponatremia: damned if we do and damned if we don't. *Kidney Int.*, **37**, 1006–18.

Fugiwara, T.M., Morgan, K. and Bichet, D.G. (1995) Molecular biology of diabetes insipidus. *Annu. Rev. Med.*, **46**, 331–43.

Gullans, S.R. and Verbalis, J.G. (1993) Control of brain volume during hyperosmolar and hypoosmolar conditions. *Annu. Rev. Med.*, **44**, 289–301.

Katz, M.A. (1973) Hyperglycemia-induced hyponatremia: calculation of expected serum sodium depression. *N. Engl. J. Med.*, **289**, 843.

Robertson, G.L., Aycinena, P. and Zerbe, R.L. (1982) Neurogenic disorders of osmoregulation. *Am. J. Med.*, **72**, 339–53.

Robertson, G.L. (1995a) Posterior pituitary, in *Endocrinology and Metabolism* (eds P. Felig and L.A. Frohman), McGraw-Hill, New York, pp. 385–42.

Robertson, G.L. (1995b) Diabetes insipidus. *Endocrinol. Metab. Clin. North Am.*, **24**, 549–72.

Robinson, A.G. (1985) Disorders of antidiuretic hormone secretion. *Clin. Endocrinol. Metab.*, **14**, 55–88.

Robinson, A.G. and DeRubertis, F.R. (1993) Disorders of sodium and water balance associated with adrenal, thyroid, and pituitary disease, in *Disease of the Kidney* (eds R.W. Schrier and C.W. Gottschalk), Little, Brown, Boston, pp. 2563–97.

Schrier, R.W. (1988) Pathogenesis of sodium and water retention in high-output and low-output cardiac failure, nephrotic syndrome, cirrhosis and pregnancy. *N. Engl. J. Med.*, **319**, 1065–72 and 1127–34.

Sterns, R.H. (1987) Severe symptomatic hyponatremia: treatment and outcome. *Ann. Intern. Med.*, **107**, 656–64.

Teitelbaum, I., Kelleher, S.P. and Berl, T. (1993) Diabetes insipidus and the syndrome of inappropriate antidiuretic hormone secretion, in *Diseases of the Kidney* (eds R.W. Schrier and C.W. Gottschalk), Little, Brown, Boston, pp. 2503–38.

Verbalis, J.G. (1995) Inappropriate antidiuresis and other hypoosmolar states, in *Principles and Practice of Endocrinology and Metabolism* (ed. K.G. Becker), J.B. Lippincott, Philadelphia, pp. 265–76.

Verbalis, J.G. (1990) Clinical aspects of body fluid homeostasis in humans, in *Handbook of Behavioral Neurobiology* (ed. E.M. Stricker), Plenum Press, New York, pp. 421–62.

Verbalis, J.G. (1993) Hyponatremia: epidemiology, pathophysiology, and therapy. *Curr. Opin. Nephrol. Hypertens.*, **2**, 636–52.

24

Disorders of sodium metabolism

Joseph G. Verbalis

Introduction

After disorders of water metabolism, abnormalities of sodium balance are the next most common cause of fluid and electrolyte disorders in clinical practice. Since body sodium is the primary determinant of the volume of the extracellular fluid (ECF), disorders of sodium metabolism can be broadly divided into hypovolemic disorders, in which there is a deficiency of ECF and plasma volume, and hypervolemic disorders, in which there is an excess of ECF and plasma volume. Depending on the relative balance between body sodium and water, these disorders can be associated with either hyponatremia or hypernatremia.

Hypovolemia

Pathogenesis

It is important to distinguish dehydration, which indicates a relative deficiency of body water, from hypovolemia, which indicates insufficient ECF to maintain blood volume within normal ranges and almost always requires a deficiency of body sodium. Since dehydration often occurs in association with hypovolemia, these terms are frequently used interchangeably but inappropriately. Although water loss or inadequate intake can also produce hypovolemia, to a large degree the ECF volume deficits will be reduced by osmotic water shifts from the intracellular fluid (ICF) space (Chapter 7). Indeed, the degrees of hyperosmolality that can be

achieved in dehydrated patients with relatively small effects on circulating blood volume and pressure are striking. Clinically significant hypovolemia develops much more quickly, and to a much more pathological degree, when water losses occur in conjunction with solute losses. In this case, sodium balance is critically important for maintenance of body fluid homeostasis. Because of the relative absence of regulated sodium intake in humans, renal sodium conservation represents the main defense for maintenance of volume homeostasis during hypovolemic conditions.

Differential diagnosis

As for patients with disorders of water metabolism, evaluation of hypovolemic patients should include a careful history, clinical assessment of ECF volume, neurological evaluation, plasma electrolytes, glucose, blood urea nitrogen (BUN) and creatinine, calculated and/or directly measured plasma osmolality, simultaneous urine electrolytes and osmolality and urine glucose. Hypovolemic states can be classified into those in which solute is lost from extrarenal causes but renal function is unimpaired, and those in which an impairment of renal sodium conservation mechanisms either causes or exacerbates the hypovolemia.

Solute losses by extrarenal pathways

The presence of a low urinary Na^+ (<10 mEq/l) in a patient with clinical manifestations of hypovolemia generally indicates an extrarenal cause. This can occur via a variety

Nephrology, Edited by Rex L. Jamison and Robert Wilkinson.
Published in 1997 by Chapman & Hall, London. ISBN 0 412 60930 4

of etiologies (Table 24.1). In most cases the source of the Na^+ and water losses (cutaneous, gastrointestinal, blood loss, etc.) will be readily apparent. In some patients the loss of water is disproportionately greater than the loss of sodium. When primarily water is lost, as in diabetes insipidus, then intracellular dehydration will be more marked than extracellular hypovolemia, as described earlier, and osmotic homeostatic mechanisms will be activated to a greater degree than the renal mechanisms subserving volume homeostasis. In contrast, isotonic hypovolemia, as produced by large amounts of blood loss from hemorrhage, represents a situation where the regulatory mechanisms for water and sodium balance activated will be primarily those subserving volume homeostasis without much contribution from osmotic regulatory systems. However, most body fluid losses, whether from excessive sweating, gastrointestinal excretions, or diuretic use, result in losses of both water and sodium, but the fluid lost in such situations is relatively hypotonic, generally in the range of 75 mm NaCl, or half-isotonic. As a result, both hypovolemia and hyperosmolality occur. Such cases for the most part fall into category I of Figure 8.4 (Chapter 8), and volume homeostatic mechanisms will be activated more than in cases of pure water losses such as diabetes insipidus. It is not surprising, therefore, that renal sodium conservation is so prominent in cases of hypovolemia in patients with normal renal function.

However, because both osmotic and volume homeostatic mechanisms are activated in most hypovolemic patients, and because osmoregulatory mechanisms are generally more sensitive to small increases in plasma osmolality than are volume regulatory mechanisms to small decreases in ECF volume, it might be predicted that very early in the process of ECF fluid loss sodium excretion might actually be increased in response to osmoregulatory mechanisms, and only during more advanced stages of hypovolemia would volume homeostatic mechanisms producing renal sodium conservation prevail. Although not yet well studied in humans, this sequence of events has long been known to occur in various animal species as the phenomenon of dehydration natriuresis. The physiological mechanisms underlying the osmotically induced natriuresis remain unclear at this time, but it is likely that osmotically stimulated secretion of arginine vasopressin (AVP), and in some species possibly oxytocin, plays a role in this response. Whatever the mechanism, the apparent paradox of natriuresis occurring during early phases of fluid loss can be more readily understood as being not really paradoxical at all by taking into account an analysis of the relative degrees of activation of osmotic versus volume homeostatic mechanisms at various times in the progression from mild to more severe degrees of hypovolemia.

Renal solute losses

The presence of an elevated urinary Na^+ concentration (i.e. ≥ 20 mEq/l) in a patient with clinical manifestations of hypovolemia generally indicates a renal cause of hypovolemia (Table 24.1).

Adrenal insufficiency (Addison's disease)

Addison's disease is caused by bilateral destruction of the adrenal glands, now more commonly on an autoimmune basis than from tuberculosis. Because the adrenal glands are the site of synthesis of aldosterone in addition to glucocorticoids, patients with Addison's disease have impaired renal Na^+ conservation. This leads to renal salt

Table 24.1 Pathogenesis of hypovolemic disorders

Extrarenal solute and water depletion	Renal solute and water depletion

1. Blood loss
    Hemorrhage
    Severe anemia
	1. Mineralocorticoid deficiency
	    Addison's disease

2. Gastrointestinal fluid losses
    Diarrhea
    Vomiting
    Nasogastric suctioning
    Pancreatitis
    Bowel obstruction
	2. Salt-wasting nephropathy
	    Chronic interstitial nephropathy
	    Polycystic kidney disease
	    Medullary cystic disease
	    Obstructive uropathy
	    Bartter's syndrome
	    Drugs

3. Cutaneous fluid losses
    Sweating
    Burns
	3. Diuretic agents

	4. Solute diuresis
	    Glucose
	    Mannitol

wasting in excess of the Na$^+$ losses observed with various other forms of hypovolemia, resulting in both hypo-osmolality and hypovolemia. As shown in Figure 8.4 (Chapter 8) (category II), the net effect on sodium balance will be to activate mechanisms for both sodium intake and renal sodium conservation. However, because aldosterone acts on the distal nephron, the more proximal sodium-conserving mechanisms cannot adequately compensate for the salt wasting in this case. Although responses producing a positive Na$^+$ balance would be appropriate for both volume and osmotic homeostasis in patients with Addison's disease, water intake poses a potential conflict, since a positive water balance would help to promote volume homeostasis but at the expense of worsening hyponatremia. It appears that volume regulatory mechanisms prevail in most cases, and such patients generally manifest both thirst and stimulated AVP secretion.

Adrenal insufficiency should be considered in any patients with the classical triad of hyponatremia, hyperkalemia and hypoglycemia – the first two as a result of mineralocorticoid deficiency and the last from glucocorticoid deficiency. Other useful diagnostic clues are the presence of clinical manifestations such as hyperpigmentation, vitiligo and salt craving. Because the salt-wasting and hypovolemia are the results of mineralocorticoid rather than glucocorticoid deficiency, only patients with primary adrenal insufficiency, i.e. Addison's disease, rather than secondary adrenal insufficiency, e.g. pituitary deficiency of adrenocorticotropic hormone (ACTH), will manifest these symptoms. In this regard, it is important to remember that withdrawal from pharmacologic steroid therapy causes secondary rather than primary adrenal insufficiency, since mineralocorticoid secretion remains intact in such patients. Consequently, the hypovolemia characteristic of patients with Addison's disease does not usually occur (although there may be hypotension due to the absence of permissive effects of glucocorticoids on vascular tone). Whenever the diagnosis is entertained it is essential to perform a rapid ACTH stimulation test. The criteria for normal adrenal function are straightforward: a plasma cortisol of >18 mg/dl at 30–60 min following 250 μg of intravenous cosyntropin (synthetic ACTH). Lower values require additional testing (plasma ACTH level and/or prolonged ACTH stimulation testing) to differentiate primary from secondary adrenal insufficiency.

Diuretics, osmotic diuresis

As discussed in Chapter 8, therapy with diuretic drugs is one of the most common causes of hyponatremia. Although the resulting Na$^+$ losses often induce some degree of hypovolemia as well, the magnitude of ECF volume reduction is generally mild and often subclinical. In contrast, obligatory solute diureses, particularly those associated with glucosuria, can cause substantially greater urinary Na$^+$ losses and severe hypovolemia relatively quickly, primarily because of the continuing natriuresis

and diuresis. A manifestation of this is the circulatory collapse which represents a major cause of early mortality in patients with diabetic ketoacidosis.

Salt-wasting nephropathy

Analogous to primary adrenal insufficiency, disorders of renal salt wasting also predispose to clinical hypovolemia. These include chronic interstitial nephropathy, polycystic kidney disease, medullary cystic disease, obstructive uropathy, Bartter's syndrome, and drugs such as cisplatinum. Most cases will manifest some degree of renal insufficiency. The sodium losses in these diseases are usually relatively mild and only rarely cause clinically significant hypovolemia, since dietary Na$^+$ intakes in the developed world are generally more than sufficient to replace daily urinary Na$^+$ losses even when these are fairly large.

Clinical manifestations

The hallmarks of hypovolemia are clinical signs of inadequate ECF and plasma volume, most of which reflect increased activity of the sympathetic nervous system to maintain mean arterial pressure via release of norepinephrine from nerve terminals and epinephrine from the adrenal medulla (Table 24.2). Associated symptoms are those of orthostatic dizziness, dry mucus membranes and thirst. The last symptom is a crucial part of compensatory mechanisms that maintain ECF volume. However, as noted in Chapter 8, the absence of increased sodium

Table 24.2 Correlation of clinical signs and symptoms with the magnitude of extracellular fluid volume contraction

Sign/symptom	Degree of dehydration		
	<5%	5–10%	>10%
Skin			
Turgor	↓	↓↓	↓↓↓
Color	Pale	Dusky	Mottled
Mucosae	Dry	Very dry	Parchment-like
Temperature of extremities	Cool	Cooler	Cold
Hemodynamics			
Pulse[a]	↑	↑↑	↑↑↑
Blood pressure[a]	→	↓	↓↓
Thirst	Mild	Moderate	Extreme

[a] Pulse and blood pressure changes augmented by upright posture.
Modified from Rudnick and Narins (1983).

appetite in response to hypovolemia limits the effectiveness of thirst to restore ECF volume, and contributes to the production of hypo-osmolality as a result of ingestion of hypotonic fluids. In addition, age-related changes appear to impair some of the compensatory homeostatic responses to hypovolemia. Elderly patients are known to be particularly prone to hypovolemia regardless of the cause. This suggests the presence of defects in the various mechanisms subserving osmotic and volume homeostasis. Studies in humans have consistently demonstrated intact or enhanced AVP secretion in response to osmotic stimuli. Although elderly patients generally have a decreased renal response to AVP, given the nature of the urine volume–urine osmolality relationship (Chapter 7; Figure 7.3), a small decrease in urinary concentrating ability will not cause markedly increased urine volume losses under most conditions. The most significant defect in the elderly appears to be a decreased sensation of thirst. After 24 h of fluid deprivation, elderly subjects have been found to report lesser degrees of subjective thirst and a less dry mouth than younger subjects, and this is accompanied by less spontaneous drinking after periods of water deprivation.

Therapy

The therapy of all hypovolemic disorders is ECF volume repletion and, if possible, correction of ongoing Na$^+$ losses. In most cases the preferred treatment is intravenous infusion with isotonic saline (0.9% NaCl) at a rate commensurate with the severity of the ECF volume depletion. Because estimation of ECF losses is relatively crude, it is generally wiser to choose an initial infusion rate based on the severity of clinical signs and then adjust the rate depending on the patient's clinical response, rather than to attempt to use formulae for calculating the volumes required to repair the volume deficit. The importance of adequate fluid replacement in hypovolemic patients cannot be stressed too strongly; one striking example of this is the historical observation that patients presenting with Addisonian crisis could often be stabilized with isotonic saline infusions well before the advent of synthetic corticosteroid replacement therapy. Today, such patients should be treated promptly with corticosteroid therapy in addition to isotonic saline, which completely reverses all the abnormalities of this disorder. Initial therapy of acutely ill adrenally insufficient patients should consist of stress doses of hydrocortisone (100 mg i.v. every 8 h). At these doses glucocorticoids crossreact sufficiently with renal mineralocorticoid receptors so that specific mineralocorticoid therapy is not required; however, once patients are tapered to physiologic replacement doses of hydrocortisone (i.e. 25–30 mg/day) they should also receive synthetic mineralocorticoids such as fludrocortisone acetate (0.1–0.2 mg/day). When clinically hypovolemic patients present with either hypo- or hypernatremia, ECF deficits should be treated with isotonic saline first and therapies to correct the osmolality second.

This will have the effect of achieving hemodynamic stability most rapidly, and because the infusate is isotonic it will also begin the correction of plasma osmolality regardless of the direction of the osmotic derangement.

Hypervolemia

Pathogenesis

Hypervolemia results from excess ECF and plasma volume. Because water distributes across all body fluid compartments, excess sodium is much more effective at producing ECF and plasma volume expansion because of its more restricted extracellular distribution. It should be remembered, however, that hyperosmolality from excess of other solutes does not invariably lead to volume expansion. Patients with renal failure have high levels of blood urea that often increase total plasma osmolality by as much as 20–30 mosmol/kg H$_2$O, yet this causes neither intracellular dehydration nor ECF and plasma volume expansion. This is because urea is an ineffective solute that freely permeates cell membranes. Only increases in concentrations of impermeable solutes are accompanied by ECF volume expansion; such clinical disorders are caused almost exclusively by sodium retention.

Most clinical disorders characterized by increased total body Na$^+$ and fluid are the result of a perceived deficit in the effective ECF volume (Chapter 8). Thus, in diseases such as congestive heart failure (CHF) and cirrhosis the kidney avidly retains Na$^+$ and water despite a body surfeit of both of these substances. Numerous experimental and clinical studies have attempted to understand the pathophysiological processes underlying such edema-forming states. This has been hampered by the existence of multiple mechanisms for sensing changes in ECF volume (Chapter 8). It is physiologically beneficial to have redundancies in important regulatory systems, but they make interpretation of experiments (including clinical experiments with drugs that block various components of renal Na$^+$ retention) exceedingly difficult. Although many questions about specific disease processes remain to be answered, evidence over the last decade has supported the concept that the critical component of the 'effective' ECF volume that represents the primary determinant of renal Na$^+$ retention is the effective arterial blood volume (EABV), which represents only approximately 15% of the blood volume, or about 0.5–0.71 of the total body water of a 70-kg man. Although this term is certainly more precise, the ambiguity of the qualifier 'effective' is still unavoidable, because the information that the arterial baroreceptors convey to the brain stem regarding the adequacy of the arterial circulation is exceedingly complex and a function of multiple components.

Since all baroreceptors are basically mechanoreceptors, they alter their electrical output according to the degree of stretch of the arterial wall, which is a function of the arterial pressure (both mean arterial pressure as well as dynamic changes in pulse pressure) and of the intrinsic tensile properties of the arterial wall. Although the latter can change with age and disease processes, under normal conditions the major determinant of arterial baroreceptor activity is the pressure in the large vessels of the arterial circulation, primarily the aorta and carotid arteries. The arterial pressure is in turn primarily determined by two factors: cardiac output and peripheral arterial resistance. Similarly, renal perfusion pressure determines the activity of the baroreceptors of the renal afferent arterioles which control renin secretion from the juxtaglomerular apparatus. Acute decreases in either variable are interpreted as a decreased EABV: in CHF this occurs as a result of the fall in cardiac output (and possibly pulse pressure) as myocardial function is compromised, and in cirrhosis as a result of the decrease in peripheral arterial resistance due to arteriovenous shunting and circulating vasodilators. In response to either of these factors, the activity of arterial and renal afferent arteriolar baroreceptors is increased and a cascade of neural and humoral responses is activated to increase arterial pressure back to normal ranges (Figures 24.1 and 24.2). These responses include activation of the sympathetic nervous system (both norepinephrine release from sympathetic nerve terminals and epinephrine release from the adrenal medulla), which increases peripheral arteriolar resistance and stimulates renin production by the kidney, suppression of brain-stem vagal efferent output to the heart, which causes a reflex tachycardia, activation of the renin–angiotensin system, which promotes renal Na^+ conservation via angiotensin-stimulated aldosterone secretion, and stimulation of AVP secretion, which promotes renal water retention. If these compensatory responses are sufficient to allow the EABV to return to normal, then cardiac output and mean arterial pressure will also return to normal, but this is only because they are now being supported by the secondary effects set in motion as a result of the initial perceived decrease in EABV. Thus, a new steady state is achieved in which an increase in total body Na^+ and water supports the maintenance of EABV at acceptable levels. Nonetheless, just as for the phenomenon of aldosterone escape (see Chapter 8), one should not construe the normalization of some physiological end-points as indicating the absence of ongoing pathological stimuli; in the case of early CHF, blood pressure and cardiac output remain relatively normal because of the compensatory mechanisms that are sustained by the baroreceptor-mediated responses to the initial decreases in cardiac output. A similar situation occurs when the cause of the decreased EABV is peripheral arterial vasodilation, as occurs in cirrhosis and a variety of other physiological and pathophysiological conditions (Figure 24.2). Although Figures 24.1 and 24.2 represent oversimplifications of complex pathophysiological processes, they provide a logical and relatively simple framework for understanding the basic processes underlying the pathogenesis of edema-forming states.

Differential diagnosis

The clinical evaluation of patients with edema entails assessing the same parameters evaluated in hypovolemic patients. Because the disease states are more varied, however, additional attention must be paid to careful

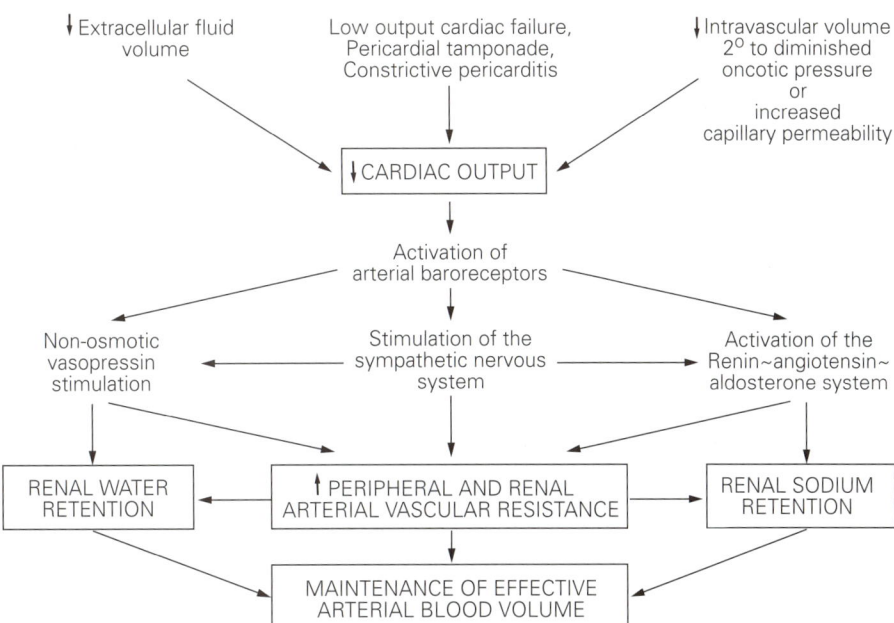

Figure 24.1 Summary of the secondary effects of decreased cardiac output on neural and humoral systems that act to maintain effective arterial blood volume by promoting renal Na^+ and water retention and stimulating arterial vasoconstriction. (Reproduced with permission from Schrier, 1990.)

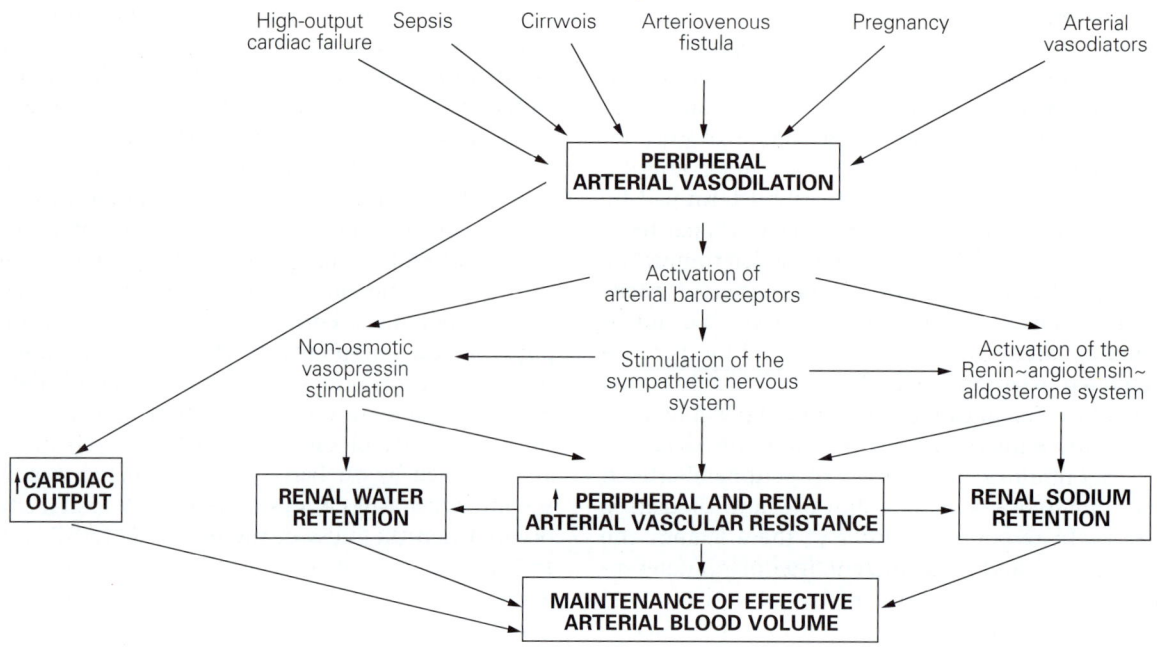

Figure 24.2 Summary of the secondary effects of arterial vasodilation on neural and humoral systems that act to maintain effective arterial blood volume by promoting renal Na⁺ and water retention and stimulating arterial vaso-constriction. (Reproduced with permission from Schrier, 1990.)

Table 24.3 Pathogenesis of hypervolemic disorders

Primary renal sodium retention
1. Renal failure
2. Primary hyperaldosteronism
   Adrenal adenoma
   Adrenal hyperplasia
   Exogenous mineralocorticoid therapy

Secondary renal sodium retention
1. Congestive heart failure
2. Cirrhosis
3. Nephrotic syndrome

evaluation of possible dysfunction of other organ systems such as the heart, liver, and kidneys. Hypervolemic states can be broadly divided into those in which pathological Na⁺ and water retention occurs as a result of primary renal or adrenal disease and independently of the ECF volume status, and those in which renal Na⁺ and water retention occurs secondarily to stimuli that signal an insufficiency of EABV (Table 24.3).

Primary renal sodium retention (baroreceptor suppression)

Diseases of primary renal Na⁺ retention produce an expansion of all components of the ECF, including the circulating arterial volume. As a result, these disorders are characterized by suppression of most of the neural and humoral mechanisms that act to maintain EABV.

Renal failure

Acute and chronic renal failure represent the quintessential example of primary renal Na⁺ retention. For the purpose of this discussion it is sufficient to state that as GFR decreases the kidney eventually becomes unable to excrete sufficient Na⁺ and water to balance fluid and salt intake and the water generated by tissue metabolism. At what stage of renal failure clinically significant fluid retention and edema occur, depends on the patient's salt and water intake as well as the degree of renal impairment. Because all ECF compartments are expanded, the renin–angiotensin–aldosterone system and the sympathetic nervous system are suppressed via the effects of baroreceptor activity, both arterial and venous. Although baroreceptor mechanisms would also be expected to suppress plasma AVP levels, the degree to which this occurs depends on the plasma osmolality (Chapter 7; Figure 7.4), the presence of other stimuli such as nausea, and effects of decreased renal clearance of AVP. Regardless of whether plasma AVP levels are elevated, the markedly reduced distal delivery of water to the distal collecting duct is the primary explanation for the water retention. Hypertension is also a common manifestation of overfilling of the arterial circulation, and the increases in blood pressure in this situation illustrate the importance of pressure-induced natriuresis as a regulator of ECF volume and EABV under normal conditions.

Primary hyperaldosteronism

Hyperaldosteronism is a classic example of primary sodium retention with subsequent ECF volume expansion. Although the kidneys are normal and the disease is secondary to elevated mineralocorticoid activity, because this process occurs independently of the ECF volume status it falls into the category of primary renal Na⁺ retention. High plasma mineralocorticoid activity can result from an adrenal tumor or hyperplasia (primary hyperaldosteronism) or from pharmacological therapy with synthetic mineralocorticoids. Regardless of the etiology, the net effect is sodium retention and potassium excretion. Thus, as in patients with the syndrome of inappropriate antidiuretic hormone secretion (SIADH), hyperactivity of a normal regulatory system leads to an abnormality of body fluid homeostasis.

As shown in Figure 8.4 (Chapter 8) (category IV), primary Na⁺ expansion should activate mechanisms to produce a negative Na⁺ balance to return body Na⁺ towards normal, and these consist almost exclusively of mechanisms to enhance Na⁺ excretion. But because aldosterone-induced sodium retention occurs in the distal nephron, the ability of other more proximal mechanisms to induce sufficient sodium excretion to produce a negative sodium balance and correct the sodium overload is limited. However, as discussed previously with regard to the water retention of SIADH, there are limits to the degree of volume expansion that can be tolerated. Just as a pressure–mediated renal escape from antidiuresis occurs when water loading becomes excessive in some patients with SIADH, a similar 'escape' from the antinatriuretic effects of aldosterone occurs in response to the chronic volume expansion in this disorder (Chapter 8).

A potential conflict arises with regard to water balance because of opposite needs for maintenance of osmotic versus volume homeostasis in this case. The increased osmolality should stimulate thirst and AVP secretion to produce a positive water balance and thereby blunt further increases in osmolality, whereas volume expansion should inhibit thirst and enhance water excretion. The net result depends on the chronicity as well as the severity of the sodium excess. With an acute sodium excess, as would be the case with hypertonic saline infusions in normal subjects, increases in thirst and AVP secretion clearly occur and lead to a positive water balance. However, with the more chronic and severe volume expansion that occurs with hyperaldosteronism, both pituitary and renal responses have the effect of facilitating increased excretion of water. Although AVP is secreted in response to increases in osmolality in patients with hyperaldosteronism, the chronic volume expansion shifts the threshold and sensitivity of the response so that less AVP is secreted per unit increase in osmolality. Modulation of the AVP response is likely mediated by baroreceptor inhibition of AVP secretion, and allows an increased urine flow in volume-expanded states despite plasma hyperosmolality. In addition to this pituitary

effect, the renal mechanisms producing aldosterone escape (Chapter 8) also result in increased urine flow even in the presence of AVP activity at the collecting tubules, analogous to renal escape in SIADH. In addition, hypokalemia, when present, reduces the sensitivity of the collecting tubular epithelium to AVP contributing to the diuresis. Corresponding effects are not apparent with regard to thirst, however, and patients with primary hyperaldosteronism are persistently polydipsic. This indicates that, similar to the lack of prominent thirst inhibition as a result of hyponatremia in SIADH, hypervolemia is not a very potent inhibitor of thirst. One might expect that another homeostatic mechanism in chronic hyperaldosteronism would be inhibition of sodium intake. However, this does not occur, and patients with hyperaldosteronism require sodium restriction since they do not spontaneously decrease their salt ingestion. These observations provide further evidence against regulation of sodium intake in man under most physiological and pathological circumstances, other than the occurrence of a stimulated salt appetite in some cases of Addison's disease.

Whenever primary hyperaldosteronism is suspected, particularly if hypokalemia is present, the initial evaluation should include simultaneous measurement of plasma renin activity (PRA) and plasma aldosterone levels. High aldosterone and suppressed PRA suggests primary hyperaldosteronism. Elevated levels of both aldosterone and PRA are more consistent with secondary hyperaldosteronism, although in most cases this diagnosis will be apparent from the underlying disease process and will not require these measurements.

Secondary renal sodium retention (baroreceptor activation)

In diseases of secondary renal Na⁺ retention, high plasma aldosterone levels are produced by activation of the renin–angiotensin system and angiotensin II stimulation of adrenal aldosterone secretion (Figure 24.3). Normally this occurs under physiological conditions of hypovolemia to promote renal Na⁺ conservation; however, when this cascade is activated in response to a perceived selective decrease in EABV, as discussed earlier, then pathological Na⁺ and fluid retention often results. Many different pathophysiological states can cause such sodium retention and its sequelae. For the most part, by the time significant hypervolemia occurs as a result of these disorders, the underlying diagnosis should be readily apparent.

Congestive heart failure

Congestive heart failure is the best-known cause of secondary sodium and fluid retention. Although the pathophysiology seems straightforward (Figure 24.1), because the disease evolves slowly over long periods of time, many of the clinical manifestations with regard

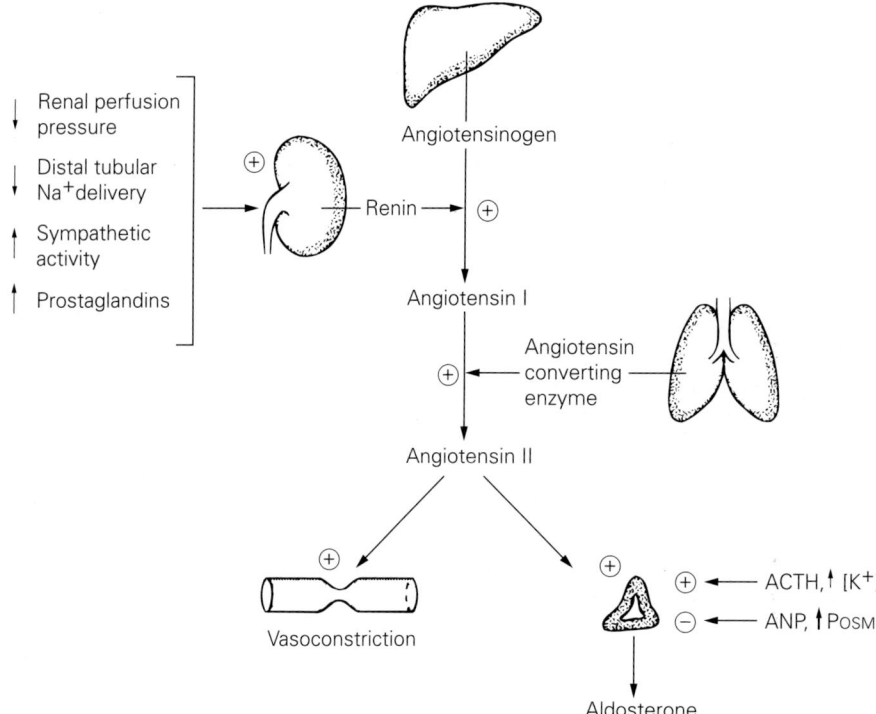

Figure 24.3 Cascade of biosynthetic steps involved with activation of the renin–angiotensin system. Renin is an enzyme secreted by the kidneys in response to hypovolemia, sensed by baroreceptors in the carotid sinus and renal afferent arterioles, as well as several other stimuli. Renin cleaves four amino acid fragments from liver-synthesized angiotensinogen to produce angiotensin I, which itself has little biological activity. Further cleavage of an additional two amino acids, primarily by angiotensin converting enzyme activity in the lungs, produces the bioactive octapeptide angiotensin II (AII). AII is a potent vasoconstrictor and is one of several stimulators of adrenal aldosterone secretion. The latter effect, along with possible direct intrarenal effects of AII, promotes renal Na^+ conservation which complements the pressor effects of AII to stabilize arterial pressure and volume.

to sodium and fluid balance depend on the point in the disease process at which the patient is evaluated. As cardiac output continues to fall, more defense mechanisms will be called into play to support EABV. Recruitment of different systems, all of which have similar vasoconstrictor effects, accounts for the failure of any one pharmacological intervention to work in all patients with CHF. For example, angiotensin converting enzyme (ACE) inhibitors will eliminate the effects of angiotensin II on vasoconstriction and aldosterone secretion, but not the effects of the sympathetic nervous system. Because sympathetic overactivity becomes more marked as the severity of the CHF increases, single agents such as this will be less effective in later stages of the disease.

One confusing aspect of CHF is the high output failure in patients with hyperthyroidism, anemia, beri-beri and arteriovenous fistulae. Such patients exhibit activation of the renin–angiotensin, sympathetic and vasopressin systems similar to those with low-output cardiac failure, yet obviously have an increased rather than decreased cardiac output. To some extent these findings can be explained by taking into consideration the second major determinant of EABV, peripheral vascular resistance, since many of these disorders are accompanied by vasodilation and/or arteriovenous shunting. In either case, the net effect on secondary activation of neurohumoral mechanisms to support EABV is similar (Figure 24.2). As these disorders progress, the myocardium eventually is unable to maintain the high level of cardiac output necessary to support blood pressure and tissue perfusion, and full-blown congestive failure then ensues.

Cirrhosis

The pathophysiology underlying the fluid and electrolyte abnormalities of cirrhosis remains debatable. It seems clear that the sodium and fluid retention is not a primary renal defect, but rather is secondary to a perceived decreased EABV, since all the defense systems for maintenance of EABV are activated as they are in CHF. However, the cause of the decreased EABV is uncertain. It has been proposed that a key factor in the pathophysiology is decreased peripheral vascular resistance, as a result of both the arteriovenous shunting in the splanchnic and other vascular beds in this disease, as well as from the decreased metabolism and clearance of a variety of vasoactive agents that accumulate during hepatic insufficiency.

Although this hypothesis could help to explain the Na^+ retention that is characteristic of this disorder even at early stages, other factors must clearly be operative as well. In this regard, it is helpful to contrast cirrhosis with a physiological state of chronic vasodilation, pregnancy. Pregnant females have a decreased peripheral resistance as a result of early hormonal changes and later arteriovenous shunting through the placenta. Presumably in response to perceived decreases in EABV, there is activation of the renin–angiotensin system, reflex increases in heart rate and cardiac output, and secretion of AVP at lower than normal plasma osmolatities. As a result, sufficient Na^+ and water is retained to expand blood and ECF volume by as much as 30–50%. Unlike in CHF and cirrhosis, however, pregnant women rarely manifest significant edema or ascites, unless fetal size becomes large enough to impede venous return to the heart. The greater edema of CHF patients may be explained by their lower arterial pressure, which prevents them from escaping from the Na^+-retaining effects of elevated aldosterone levels via increases in renal perfusion pressure. This is unlikely to be the case in most cirrhotic patients, however, many of whom have increased cardiac output and blood pressure similar to that observed in pregnant women. Cirrhotic patients must also have abnormal capillary function that predisposes them to increased exudation of fluid and solutes. Although it has been proposed that this effect is a function of arterial vasodilation, in this case these effects should also occur during pregnancy. It therefore seems more likely that defects specific to the cirrhotic process, such as the increased portal pressure known to occur in more advanced disease, act together with vasodilation-induced Na^+ retention to produce the characteristic clinical manifestations of this disorder. This would also explain the clinical observation that ascites formation generally precedes the development of subcutaneous edema in most cirrhotic patients.

Nephrotic syndrome

The hypervolemia of nephronic syndrome is not easily explained by a single mechanism. Evidence suggests that a subset of nephrotic patients indeed act as though a decreased EABV is the stimulus to activation of Na^+-retaining neural and humoral systems. Presumably this is primarily attributable to the decreased plasma oncotic pressure as a consequence of the hypoalbuminemia and hypoproteinemia produced by the ongoing proteinuria in this disease (Chapter 8; Figure 8.1). This effect would not only decrease intravascular volume, but would also directly increase the amount of interstitial fluid, since the

plasma oncotic pressure (π_C) at the venous end of the capillaries would be insufficient to counterbalance the hydrostatic forces favoring fluid exudation. Unlike in most cases of CHF and cirrhosis, however, in nephrotic syndrome the kidney itself is impaired as part of the disease process. Consequently, as the glomerulopathy progresses, patients will eventually manifest the increased plasma and ECF volumes characteristic of renal failure, with subsequent suppression of the neural and humoral systems that initially mediated Na^+ retention. This represents another example of differing presentations and different pathophysiological processes that occur during progression of diseases from milder to more severe degrees of organ function impairments.

Clinical manifestations

The clinical manifestations of hypervolemia depend on the underlying disease process. Patients with primary aldosteronism will generally have mild hypernatremia and hypokalemia and show varying degrees of hypertension but less frequently subcutaneous edema. When plasma $[K^+]$ is <3 mEq/l, symptoms of hypokalemia, such as muscle weakness, often predominate. Patients with hyperaldosteronism secondary to perceived reduced EABV generally do not have hypertension but tend to have greater degrees of edema, reflecting more sodium and water retention. As primary and secondary hyperaldosteronism often produce equivalent increases in plasma aldosterone levels, why does secondary hyperaldosteronism produce more pronounced degrees of edema? This can be understood by referring to the intrarenal mechanisms responsible for escape from the Na^+-retaining effects of aldosterone (Chapter 8). Because renal artery perfusion pressure is one of the major determinants of mineralocorticoid escape, this phenomenon would be expected to occur primarily in patients with primary hyperaldosteronism or mineralocorticoid therapy in whom sodium and fluid retention elevate arterial pressure. Patients with secondary hyperaldosteronism mostly have renal hypoperfusion from decreased EABV, and consequently cannot as easily 'escape' the continued mineralocorticoid effects on Na^+ retention. Despite considerable edema from sodium retention, these patients continue to retain more sodium and fluid because of persistent aldosterone effects in addition to intrarenal hemodynamic mechanisms causing sodium retention. It is noteworthy that plasma atrial natriuretic peptide (ANP) concentrations are quite high in patients with secondary hyperaldosteronism – substantially higher than those following physiological volume expansion in normal subjects. This suggests that, although ANP may contribute to the natriuresis occurring during escape from hyperaldosteronism, its effects are not sufficiently strong to override the intrinsic intrarenal hemodynamic mechanisms causing sodium conservation. It is also possible that a putative oubain-like natriuretic hormone, the release of which is thought to be controlled by arterial baroreceptors, may be stimulated in primary more than secondary hyperaldosteronism.

Therapy

Hypervolemic/edema-forming diseases are pathologically diverse, and therapy must be individualized to each disease. Nonetheless, some common guidelines are possible with regard to the fluid and electrolyte abnormalities common to these processes. For each, the most beneficial treatment is to arrest the underlying disease process, for example by corticosteroid treatment of patients with the nephrotic syndrome, or by improving the function of the chronically diseased organ, such as by inotropic therapy of the heart in CHF. However, these diseases eventually progress to the point where the hypervolemia itself becomes an impairment, by causing further organ dysfunction and by limiting the patient's activities.

Initial therapy in all these disorders should involve dietary sodium restriction. As discussed earlier, typical dietary Na$^+$ intakes in Western societies (6–8 g/day) are far in excess of body needs. Consequently, when pathological Na$^+$ retention is present, marked decreases are necessary. Although standard 'low sodium' diets often contain 1–4 g/day, in the presence of significant edema or ascites limitation of sodium intake to 250–500 mg/day may be required, but is difficult to achieve. For patients in whom this is not sufficiently restrictive, or who are unable to maintain this degree of sodium restriction, diuretic therapy is required. The initial therapy of CHF patients typically involves use of a thiazide diuretic. Although such therapy is generally sufficient during early stages of CHF to prevent sodium retention, as cardiac function worsens patients become refractory to simple diuretic therapy. At this point, in addition to increasing the dose of the diuretic agents, it is also helpful to combine agents that act in different parts of the nephron, such as

furosemide, a loop-acting diuretic, metolazone, a thiazide diuretic which acts at the distal tubule and spironolactone, an aldosterone receptor antagonist which acts at the cortical-collecting tubule. Given the prominent activation of aldosterone secretion in cirrhotic patients, spironolactone is often the diuretic of first choice in these patients, with thiazides and furosemide reserved for later use as the patients become refractory to this single agent.

An important caveat in the treatment of all edematous disorders is that all treatments act to antagonize the defense mechanisms activated to maintain EABV in these patients. Even though these defenses in many cases have become deleterious, rapid and/or excessive treatment will always entail the risk of compromising EABV too much, with subsequent hypotension, tissue hypoperfusion and further organ injury. Thus, diuresis should proceed only at rates commensurate with the rate at which edema fluid can be mobilized into the intravascular space: for CHF this should generally not exceed 1–2 pounds (0.45–0.9 kg) of weight loss per day, and in cirrhotic patients with ascites diuresis should be even slower (0.5–0.75 pounds (0.23–0.34 kg)/day) because of the slower fluid resorption rate from the peritoneal cavity. Similarly, a major limitation on the use of ACE inhibitors as vasodilator therapy in CHF is the hypotension due to blockade of the vasoconstrictor effects of angiotensin II. Such therapies only work to the extent that cardiac afterload can be reduced sufficiently to improve myocardial function short of reducing mean arterial pressure to levels which will negate these beneficial effects by impairing tissue perfusion. Thus, all therapies in hypervolemic patients must be cautiously titrated, with particular care taken when several different components of the body's normal defense mechanisms are being blocked or otherwise compromised (e.g. combined diuretic therapy and ACE inhibition).

Further reading

Bichet, D.G. and Schrier, R.W. (1993) Cardiac failure, liver disease and nephrotic syndrome, in *Diseases of the Kidney* (eds R.W. Schrier and C.W. Gottschalk), Little, Brown, Boston, pp. 2453–91.

Chonko, A.M. and Grantham, J.J. (1994) Treatment of edema states, in *Clinical Disorders of Fluid and Electrolyte Metabolism* (ed. R.G. Narins), McGraw-Hill, New York, pp. 545–82.

Cohn, J.N. (1988) Current therapy of the failing heart. *Circulation*, **78**, 1099–107.

Conrad, K.P. (1988) Possible mechanisms for changes in renal hemodynamics during pregnancy: studies from animal models. *Am. J. Kidney Dis.*, **9**, 253–9.

Epstein, M. and Perez, G.O. (1994) Pathophysiology of the edema-forming states, in *Clinical Disorders of Fluid and Electrolyte Metabolism* (ed. R.G. Narins), McGraw-Hill, New York, pp. 523–44.

Gonzalez–Compoy, J.M., Romero, J.C. and Knox, F.G. (1989) Escape from the sodium-retaining effects of mineralocorticoids: role of ANF and intrarenal hormone systems. *Kidney Int.*, **35**, 767–77.

Hall, J.E., Granger, J.P., Smith, M.J. Jr and Premen, A.J. (1984) Role of renal hemodynamics and arterial pressure in aldosterone 'escape'. *Hypertension*, **6**, 183–92.

Kirchner, K.A. and Stein, J.H. (1994) Sodium metabolism, in *Clinical Disorders of Fluid and Electrolyte Metabolism* (ed. R.G. Narins), McGraw-Hill, New York, pp. 45–80.

Leaf, A. (1976) Significance of the serum sodium concentration, in *Renal Pathophysiology* (eds A. Leaf and R.S. Cotran), Oxford University Press, New York, pp. 235–41.

Levine, T.B., Francis, G.S., Goldsmith, S.R. *et al.* (1982) Activity of the sympathetic nervous system and renin–angiotensin system assessed by plasma hormone levels and their relation to hemodynamic abnormalities in congestive heart failure. *Am. J. Cardiol.*, **49**, 1659–66.

Lindheimer, M.D., Barron, W.M. and Davison, J.M. (1991) Osmotic and volume control of vasopressin release in pregnancy. *Am. J. Kidney Dis.*, **17**, 105–11.

Philips, P.A., Rolls, B.G., Ledingham, J.J.G. *et al.* (1984) Reduced thirst after water deprivation in healthy elderly man. *N. Engl. J. Med.*, **311**, 753–9.

Rascher, W., Tulassay, T., Seyberth, H.W. *et al.* (1986) Diuretic and hormonal responses to head-out water immersion in nephrotic syndrome. *J. Pediatr.*, **109**, 609–14.

Riegger, G.A.J., Liebau, G. and Kochsiek, K. (1982) Antidiuretic hormone in congestive heart failure. *Am. J. Med.*, **72**, 49–57.

Robertson, G.L., Aycinena, P. and Zerbe, R.L. (1982) Neurogenic disorders of osmoregulation. *Am. J. Med.*, **72**, 339–53.

Rudnick, M.R., Bastl, C.P., Elfinbein, I.B. and Narins, R.G. (1983) The differential diagnosis of acute renal failure, in *Acute Renal Failure* (eds B.M. Brenner and J.M. Lazarus), W.B. Saunders, Philadelphia, pp. 176–222.

Schrier, R.W. (1988) Pathogenesis of sodium and water retention in high-output and low-output cardiac failure, nephrotic syndrome, cirrhosis and pregnancy. *N. Engl. J. Med.*, **319**, 1065–72 and 1127–34.

Schrier, R.W. (1990) Body fluid volume regulation in health and disease: a unifying hypothesis. *Ann. Inern. Med.*, **113**, 155–9.

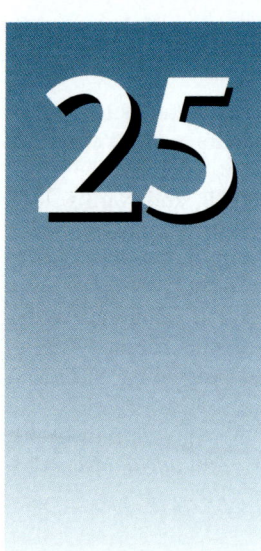

25

Potassium disorders

Rex L. Jamison

Introduction

To understand disorders of potassium (K⁺) regulation, it is essential to understand the normal regulation of K⁺ balance. Please see Chapter 9. The focus of this chapter will be on disorders of K⁺ in patients with pre-existing renal disease, but the same principles and approach to diagnosis and treatment apply to those with normal renal function. Disorders of K⁺ regulation can be conveniently divided into hyperkalemia and hypokalemia [1]. The frequency of hyperkalemia in patients with kidney disease depends on the pre-existing glomerular filtration rate, the extent to which potassium intake is increased and the suddenness with which deterioration of renal function occurs [2]. If the loss of kidney function is sudden and substantial, hyperkalemia often occurs, sometimes with fatal consequences. On the other hand, hyperkalemia (serum $K^+ \geq 5.5$ meq/l) rarely develops in a patient with progressive renal insufficiency until the glomerular filtration rate (as measured by the creatinine clearance) drops below 10–15 ml/min, unless another disturbance of potassium balance is superimposed. When K⁺ is ingested or administered parenterally, K⁺ is transferred temporarily into cells by the membrane enzyme, Na⁺,K⁺-ATPase, the activity of which is increased by insulin and β_2-adrenergic agonists. The excess K⁺ is eventually excreted by a mechanism that depends on the secretory capacity of the collecting tubule rather than the filtered load of K⁺. As described in Chapter 9, the source of K⁺ excreted in the urine is almost entirely K⁺ secreted into the collecting tubule. In fact it was an observation that the total urinary K⁺ excretion by a patient with severe chronic renal failure exceeded the filtered load of K⁺ which led to the suggestion that K⁺ undergoes secretion by the renal tubule [3]. Potassium secretion is enhanced by several factors: an increase in the plasma K⁺ concentration, a decrease in the luminal K⁺ concentration in the collecting tubule, a rise in aldosterone secretion and an increase in the flow of sodium and water to the K⁺ secretory site [4]. In patients with reduced renal mass, these factors operate more frequently and intensely. The remaining nephrons and cortical collecting ducts hypertrophy accompanied by an increase in the Na⁺,K⁺-ATPase activity in the basolateral membrane, which increases K⁺ secretory capacity.

Hypokalemia may also occur in patients with kidney disease, notably those with renal tubular acidosis. Gastrointestinal disturbances which accompany azotemia and the side effects of the drug and dietary treatment of patients with renal insufficiency are the most frequent contributors to K⁺ deficiency.

This chapter reviews the disturbances in K⁺ balance that occur in the patient with renal disease and their treatment and prevention.

Hypokalemia

Causes

The major causes of hypokalemia (serum $K^+ < 3.5$ meq/l) are listed in Table 25.1.

Nephrology, Edited by Rex L. Jamison and Robert Wilkinson.
Published in 1997 by Chapman & Hall, London. ISBN 0 412 60930 4

Pseudohypokalemia

Blood samples drawn from patients with very high numbers of white cells, e.g. acute myelogenous leukemia, may become low in potassium upon standing, as the cells take up potassium.

Table 25.1 Causes of hypokalemia

Pseudohypokalemia

Redistribution of potassium from extracellular fluid to cell
1. Metabolic alkalosis
2. β_2-Adrenergic agonists or increased β_2-adrenergic activity
3. Exogenous insulin or intravenous glucose
4. Hypokalemia periodic paralysis
5. Poisoning or overdose (barium, chloroquin, toluene, theophylline)

Potassium depletion
1. Decreased intake
   Alcoholism
   Anorexia nervosa
   Bulimia
   Starvation
2. Excessive perspiration
3. Gastrointestinal losses
   Vomiting (loss of sodium and acid)
   Diarrhea
   Laxatives
   Villous adenoma of the colon
4. Urinary losses
   Acid–base disorders
      renal tubular acidosis, types I and II
      chloride depletion/metabolic acidosis
      diabetic ketoacidosis
   Diuretics
      thiazide class
      inhibitors of thick ascending limb transport
         class ('loop' diuretics)
   Diuresis following renal injury
      postobstructive diuresis
      recovery phase of acute renal failure
   Bartter's syndrome
   Mineralocorticoidism
      primary hyperaldosteronism
      excess exogenous steroid therapy
      renal vascular disease
      licorice
   Pseudomineralocorticoidism (Liddle's syndrome)
   Magnesium depletion
   Drugs
      penicillins
      aminoglycosides
      amphotericin and other polyene antibiotics

Redistribution of potassium

The first step in evaluation of true hypokalemia is to distinguish between K^+ redistribution, in which there is a normal body K^+ content, and K^+ depletion. The factors causing K^+ redistribution (shift of K^+ into cells) are reviewed in Chapter 9. See Table 9.1. They include metabolic alkalosis, increased β_2-adrenergic activity or administration of β_2-adrenergic agonists, insulin treatment and poisoning with theophylline, barium, toluene or chloroquin [5–7]. β_2-Adrenergic agonists may be administered by the oral or parenteral route, or inhaled from a nebulizer.

There is a rare hereditary disorder, hypokalemic periodic paralysis, in which the victim has periodic attacks of paralysis associated with hypokalemia [8]. The pattern of inheritance indicates an autosomal dominant gene. The paralysis may be provoked by eating a heavy carbohydrate or a high sodium-containing meal, unusual physical exertion, or the administration of catecholamines. Attacks can be diminished by avoiding the foregoing inducers and by treatment with β_2-adrenergic blockers. For reasons that are not apparent, use of acetazolamide reduces the number of attacks.

Potassium depletion

The following disorders cause K^+ depletion [1].

Decreased food intake

This may reflect poor appetite, anorexia nervosa, bulimia or alcoholism. Diminished eating causes K^+ depletion, because the K^+ content of the urine and stool, although low, is not zero, so that the patient enters a net negative K^+ balance. By itself, low K^+ intake is infrequently a cause, but in combination with other factors, such as a diuretic, it may be important.

Excessive perspiration

If perspiration is prolonged and heavy, such as occurs with prolonged physical exertion under a hot sun, it can lead to a K^+ deficit. The associated volume reduction may sustain a normal plasma K^+ concentration; but there is a paradoxical high urinary K^+ excretion secondary to stimulation of aldosterone by sodium loss.

Gastrointestinal loss

The most common cause of hypokalemia is gastrointestinal loss. Vomiting induces K^+ depletion primarily from a combination of Na^+ depletion, which stimulates the renin–angiotensin–aldosterone axis, and loss of HCl, which leads to Cl^- depletion and metabolic alkalosis. As explained in Chapter 9, the low tubule fluid Cl^- obligates the secretion of K^+ in exchange for Na^+ reabsorption (see below). Diarrhea from any condition can cause K^+ depletion directly and indirectly due to the associated NaCl depletion. Laxative abuse should be suspected in the case of an abnormally dark colon ('black colon' or melanosis coli) and confirmed by detecting phenolphthalein, an ingredient of most laxatives, which with alkalization causes the urine to turn pink. A rare tumor of the colon, villous adenoma, secretes fluid containing K^+.

Urinary loss

Potassium depletion from urinary loss of K^+ usually requires two conditions: elevated mineralocorticoid concentration and increased delivery of Na^+ to the collecting tubule.

Acid–base disorders

Renal tubular acidosis (RTA)

RTA is a group of disorders of the kidney in which there is impairment of either collecting tubule secretion of H^+ (type I RTA) or proximal tubule reabsorption of HCO_3^- (type II RTA) and consequent systemic acidosis (Chapter 26). Type IV RTA occurs most often in patients with renal insufficiency due to diabetic nephropathy and is caused by hyporeninemic hypoaldosteronism. (Another form of RTA was proposed and named type III, but was later shown not to be a distinct entity.) Hypokalemia is associated with both types I and II [9]. In type II RTA, reabsorption of HCO_3^- is primarily impaired and delivery of $NaHCO_3$ to the thick ascending limb (TAL) is increased. There is a low capacity for HCO_3^- reabsorption in the TAL, so that $NaHCO_3^-$ flow to the distal and collecting tubule rises, where the reabsorptive capacity for HCO_3^- is also limited. As a consequence bicarbonaturia occurs, accompanied by Na^+ or K^+ and causing hypovolemia. Renin and aldosterone secretion are increased, which stimulate K^+ secretion. The serum HCO_3^- and K^+ fall and Cl^- rises, until a steady state is reached with a much lower serum HCO_3^-, at which point the urine becomes acid again and the loss of Na^+ and K^+ with HCO_3^- in the urine stops.

In type I RTA there are three possible defects in H^+ secretion. Each leads to a disturbance in K^+ balance. The most common is a reduction in H^+-Na^+ATPase (the proton pump) in the intercalated cell. The urine pH cannot be lowered below about 5.5. The fall in H^+ secretion obligates a reciprocal increase in K^+ to provide the essential electrical neutrality if Na^+ reabsorption by the principal cell is to occur. Consequently K^+ depletion and hypokalemia are quite common in type I RTA. Treatment with HCO_3 corrects the defect because it facilitates H^+ secretion without reaching the limiting pH gradient. A second defect is caused by nephrotoxic agents of which amphotericin is the prototype. The low collecting duct H^+ membrane permeability is essential for a low urine pH to be sustained. Amphotericin injures the membrane such that it becomes permeable to H^+ and the pH gradient

cannot be sustained. The effect and the treatment with HCO_3 are the same as with the defective proton pump. A third cause of H^+ impaired secretion is a defect in Na^+ reabsorption by the neighboring principal cell, such as occurs in tubulointerstitial disease (e.g. urinary tract obstruction, lupus nephritis, sickle cell disease). In this instance, however, the impaired luminal electronegativity will impair both H^+ and K^+ secretion leading to hyperkalemia (see below).

Diabetic ketoacidosis

This causes increased urinary losses of K^+ from the osmotic diuretic effect of glucosuria and ketonuria.

Chloride depletion–metabolic alkalosis

Depletion of Cl^-, for example from vomiting and diuretics, results in metabolic alkalosis and K^+ deficiency. As the HCO_3^- concentration rises in the proximal tubule, some of it escapes reabsorption and is delivered to the distal nephron and collecting tubule. The presence of a non-reabsorbable anion in the collecting tubule promotes K^+ secretion.

Inherited hypokalemic alkalosis

Two autosomal recessive genetic disorders with distinctive phenotypes produce hypokalemia with alkalosis. They have recently been shown to be due to mutations in genes encoding a thiazide-sensitive NaCl cotransporter in the distal tubule or the bumetanide (a 'loop' diuretic)-sensitive $Na^+K^+2Cl^-$ cotransporter in the loop of Henle [10]. Mutations in the latter gene are the underlying defect in some patients with Bartter's syndrome. The disorder manifests as Na^+ wasting and enormous urinary K^+ losses, high plasma renin and aldosterone levels, juxtaglomerular hyperplasia and metabolic alkalosis. Prostaglandin production is strikingly increased, presumably from the K^+ depletion. These cases occur in infants and are accompanied by hypercalciuria. Quite often the syndrome is mimicked in adults by surreptitious diuretic ingestion [11]. Mutations in the thiazide-sensitive NaCl cotransporter result in Gitelman's syndrome, which closely mimics Bartter's syndrome except that these patients are older with predominantly musculoskeletal abnormalities, and exhibit hypocalciuria and hypomagnesemia. A third, rarer type, the so-called antenatal hypercalciuric variant or hyperprostaglandin E syndrome, has been identified in which mutations in the gene encoding a specific potassium channel cause hypokalemia and metabolic alkalosis [12]. Therapy requires massive exogenous K^+, which is disagreeable, causing gastric distress. Other measures, such as prostaglandin synthetase inhibitors, K^+ sparing diuretics, or angiotensin-converting enzyme inhibitors are usually not sufficient, and have their own complications.

Diuretics

Except for the K$^+$-sparing diuretics, diuretics produce K$^+$ depletion by causing Na$^+$ and Cl$^-$ depletion, by inducing secondary hyperaldosteronism and by increasing the delivery of Na$^+$ to the K$^+$ secretory site [1]. Two classes of diuretics in particular, used in the treatment of patients with renal disease, create these conditions – the 'loop' diuretics, which inhibit Na$^+$K$^+$2Cl$^-$ apical transport in the TAL, and the thiazide-type diuretics, which inhibit Na$^+$ reabsorption in the distal tubule. In each case there is an increase of delivery of Na$^+$ to the collecting duct and enhanced K$^+$ secretion.

Elevated mineralocorticoid concentration

This occurs in primary hyperaldosteronism from an adrenal adenoma or bilateral hyperplasia of the zona glomerulosa [13]. It can reflect an underlying congenital disorder of steroidogenesis, adrenal carcinoma, pituitary adenoma (Cushing's disease) or chronic corticosteroid treatment [14, 15]. (Even though a primary glucocorticoid is prescribed, the doses are usually so high that there is 'spillover' occupancy of the mineralocorticoid receptors.) It may also be secondary to renovascular disease or very rarely to a renin-producing tumor in which increased renin secretion stimulates aldosterone secretion [16]. Patients often retain Na$^+$ and develop hypertension. A rare form of hyperadrenalism develops from licorice excess [17]. Licorice contains glycyrrhetinic acid, which inhibits the enzyme 11β-hydroxysteroid dehydrogenase, that converts cortisol to cortisone. Cortisol binds avidly to the aldosterone receptor.

Liddle's syndrome

Liddle's syndrome, or pseudoaldosteronism, is an autosomal dominant form of hypertension characterized by hypokalemia, metabolic alkalosis, urinary loss of K$^+$ and low renin and aldosterone levels. Warnock and his collaborators have demonstrated that it is caused by mutations in the β subunit of the epithelial sodium channel in the epithelium of the distal and collecting tubule [18]. These abnormal channels avidly reabsorb sodium, causing hypertension and K$^+$ wasting.

Magnesium depletion

This causes depletion of K$^+$ [19]. Although the link is not understood, speculation includes the fact that Mg^{2+} depletion may lower Na$^+$,K$^+$-ATPase, impairing the cellular accumulation of K$^+$, and it somehow induces an increase in urinary K$^+$ excretion.

Drugs

Drugs other than diuretics are associated with K$^+$ wasting [1]. These include members of the penicillin family, when administered in high doses. Penicillin is secreted in the proximal tubule and acts as a poorly reabsorbable non-Cl$^-$ ion. Aminoglycosides increase the permeability of the renal tubule to both K$^+$ and Mg^{2+} – side effects which may precede acute tubular necrosis. Amphotericin and other polyene antibiotics increase the tubule permeability to K$^+$ and Na$^+$.

Clinical manifestations of hypokalemia

Often patients have no symptoms; the diagnosis is first made from a routine serum K$^+$. Approximately 2% of the body K$^+$ is in the extracellular fluid; potassium depletion may be severe despite a modest hypokalemia. In general the fall in plasma K$^+$ is disproportionately greater than the fall in cell K$^+$, with the results that the transmembrane K$^+$ gradient is enhanced, and the cell interior becomes hyperpolarized.

Cardiovascular manifestations

Controversy surrounds the effect of hypokalemia on blood pressure; authorities state that the pressure falls or rises [20]. The weight of evidence in humans seems to favor hypertension. Administration of K$^+$ to normotensive persons lowers their blood pressure. It is well to keep this in mind in the treatment of hypertension, since diuretics are commonly prescribed and may lead to K$^+$ depletion. If the plasma K$^+$ is below 3.0 mEq/l, typical changes in the EKG may occur: flattening of the T wave, ST segment depression and the development of a U wave. With more severe falls in the plasma K$^+$, ventricular arrhythmias erupt. Hypokalemia predisposes to digitalis toxicity, presumably because it interferes with the renal excretion of digitalis and enhances binding of digitalis to the myocardium.

Neuromuscular manifestations

The hyperpolarization makes nerve and muscle cells less excitable. The patient may present with weakness or even paralysis of the skeletal muscle. A particularly dangerous complication is paralysis of the respiratory muscle. Severe hypokalemia impairs the microcirculation of the muscle and increases the risk of rhabdomyolysis. There may be constipation or ileus.

Renal fluid and electrolyte manifestations

Depletion of K$^+$ impairs the response to vasopressin, producing a mild nephrogenic diabetes syndrome which is compounded by the stimulation of the thirst center. Nevertheless it is rare to see extreme polyuria. A more important effect is on ammonia metabolism. Potassium depletion stimulates renal NH$_3$ production [1]. This may increase urinary pH and simulate an impaired distal acidification capacity, mimicking renal tubular acidosis. It may increase blood ammonia and precipitate coma in a patient with liver disease. If severe (plasma $K^+ < 2.0\,mEq/l$), a chloride depletion metabolic alkalosis may be generated leading to a vicious circle (see above). Various structural abnormalities have been described in the collecting ducts in experimental animals subjected to K^+ depletion, but have not been seen in humans. Instead vacuoles have been described.

Diagnostic approach to hypokalemia

Kamel *et al.* [20] have outlined a useful approach to determining the cause of hypokalemia (Table 25.1). It begins by ruling out pseudohypokalemia and redistribution of K^+ from the extracellular fluid (ECF) to the cell. This leaves true K^+ depletion. The differential depends on a few measurements made in a patient eating a normal sodium diet, established by demonstrating that the 24 h urine sodium excretion exceeds 100 mEq/day. These measurements are the blood pressure, the serum electrolytes, the plasma renin, the urinary excretion of K^+, Cl^- and specific tests that establish the diagnosis.

If the 24 h K^+ excretion is less than 20 mEq, then the K^+ depletion is due to extrarenal losses. A metabolic acidosis suggests lower gastrointestinal (GI) losses; a metabolic alkalosis implies gastric losses or previous use of diuretics. A normal acid–base balance suggests losses from sweating or use of laxatives.

If urinary K^+ excretion exceeds 20 mEq and the blood pressure is high, then the plasma renin will be decisive. If it is high, then renovascular hypertension or a renin-secreting tumor (very rare) should be ruled out. Malignant hypertension should also be included, but it is much less common than it was a decade ago. If the plasma renin is low, then plasma aldosterone should be measured. A high value indicates primary hyperaldosteronism; a low value indicates other abnormal steroid secretion, Cushing's syndrome or licorice ingestion. A normal plasma renin requires a review of the serum bicarbonate level. A metabolic acidosis indicates renal tubular acidosis. A metabolic

alkalosis requires measurement of urinary Cl^- excretion. A low value (<10 mEq) points to gastric losses; higher values can be found with diuretic use, Bartter's syndrome, Mg^{2+} depletion and severe K^+ depletion.

Treatment of hypokalemia

The first goal is to treat the underlying cause. To replenish K^+ losses via the lower GI tract K^+ is given as the alkaline salt (citrate, bicarbonate); if losses are due to vomiting and loss of Cl^-, then KCl is given. Patients with RTA require potassium citrate or $KHCO_3$. Urgent circumstances, such as cardiac arrhythmias and infarction, hepatic encephalopathy and neuromuscular paralysis, or the threat of any of these conditions, require intravenous replacement.

The prevention of hypokalemia is clearly preferable and is germane to a large population at risk, namely the patients prescribed diuretics. Determination of serum K^+ two weeks after initiation of diuretics is a safeguard against K^+ depletion. The use of K^+-supplements or so-called K^+-sparing diuretics may then be considered.

Hyperkalemia

Potassium tolerance

The rise in plasma K^+ after an acute K^+ load is less if the daily K^+ intake is gradually increased beforehand [1, 21] (Figure 25.1). Eventually an acute K^+ load, which if given before the conditioning by the increased K^+ intake would be fatal, is tolerated without event. This phenomenon is called potassium adaptation or potassium tolerance. It is primarily accounted for by an increase in the rate of urinary K^+ excretion. Figure 25.1 shows the changes which follow an increase in K^+ intake from 100 mEq to 400 mEq/day. The underlying adaptation that occurs is a striking increase in Na^+,K^+-ATPase activity in the cortical and medullary segments of the collecting tubule

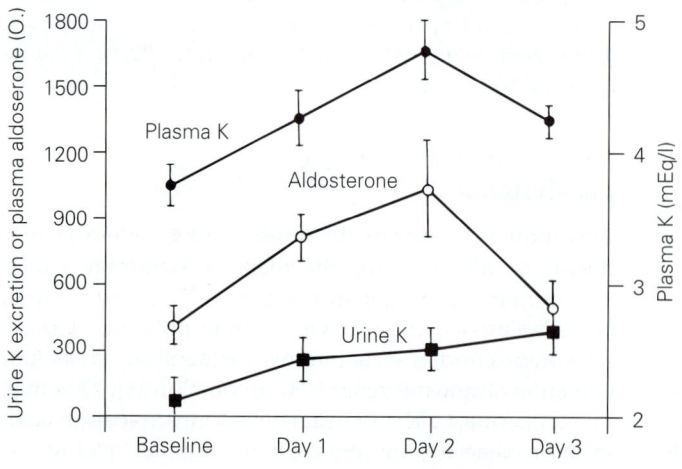

Figure 25.1 Effect of increasing potassium intake from 100 to 400 mEq/day on plasma K^+ (●), plasma aldosterone (○, pmol/l) and urinary potassium excretion (■, mEq/24 h). By day 2, urinary K^+ excretion equals intake. The modest rise in plasma K^+ and increase in plasma aldosterone are the stimuli to the kidneys. (Reproduced, with permission, from Rose, B.D. and Rennke, H.G. (1994) *Renal Pathophysiology*, p. 176, Williams & Wilkins, Baltimore). The figure is an adaptation of data from Rabelink *et al.* [21].

Table 25.2   Causes of hyperkalemia

Pseudohyperkalemia

Redistribution of potassium from cell to extracellular fluid
1. Metabolic acidosis (inorganic anions)
2. β_2- or non-selective β-adrenergic blocking agent
3. Insulin deficiency
4. Rhabdomyolysis
5. Hyperkalemic periodic paralysis
6. Poisoning or overdose
    Digitalis intoxication
    Arginine hydrochloride
    Succinylcholine
    Fluoride intoxication

Impaired urinary excretion of potassium
1. Reduction in effective extracellular fluid volume or circuating blood volume
2. Hypoaldosteronism
    Primary adrenal insufficiency
    Secondary adrenal insufficiency
    Hyporeninemic hypoaldosteronism
    Medications
        angiotensin converting enzyme inhibitors
        abrupt withdrawal of steroids
        heparin
        cyclosporin
3. Renal tubule disorders in which hyperkalemia is not explained simply by reduced GFR
    Gordon's syndrome
    Sickle cell nephropathy
    Diabetic nephropathy with hyporeninemic
        hypoaldosteronism
    Systemic lupus erthematosus
    Interstitial nephritis
        sulfonamides
        penicillin
        non-steroid anti-inflammatory drugs
        many other drugs
    Amyloidosis
    Renal tubular acidosis, type IV
    Urinary tract obstruction
    Transplant kidney
4. Drugs which directly interfere with potassium secretion, or block aldosterone
    Spironolactone
    Triamterene
    Trimethoprim
    Cyclosporin

[22]. A similar adaptation presumably occurs in the surviving collecting tubules in renal insufficiency and explains why hyperkalemia is uncommon in a patient with chronic renal failure until the glomerular filtration rate (GFR) is reduced to a very low level, less than 10 ml/min.

Causes of hyperkalemia

The major causes of hyperkalemia (serum $K^+ > 5.3$ mEq/l) are listed in Table 25.2 [1, 2, 20]. Hyperkalemia is due either to a redistribution of K^+ from cell to ECF (impaired cell uptake or increased cell loss of K^+) or decreased urinary excretion. It is rarely caused by an increased intake of K^+ unless the load is large or administered intravenously, or the K^+ excretory capacity is greatly reduced.

Pseudohyperkalemia

This is a term which refers to a high plasma K^+ concentration that occurs after the specimen of blood has been collected although the true plasma K^+ concentration is not increased. The most common reason is an improper collection in which red cell hemolysis releases K^+. Pseudohyperkalemia also occurs in thrombocytosis and leukemia. Potassium is normally released from platelets and white blood cells after the blood clots. If there is a high platelet count ($500\,000/mm^3$) or very high white cell count ($>100\,000/mm^3$) this phenomenon is more apt to happen. If there is no reason to suspect hyperkalemia, another blood specimen should be obtained carefully. If there is an outside possibility that the hyperkalemia could be real, an EKG will help to settle the matter.

Redistribution

Hyperkalemia due to redistribution is usually temporary, because eventually the kidney will excrete the excess K^+. See Table 9.1 in Chapter 9.

Decreased cell K^+ uptake or increased cell K^+ release

In metabolic acidosis, the acidemia is buffered in part by H^+ uptake by the cell. This is usually described as exchange for K^+ release. A more accurate description is that if the excess ECF anion is inorganic (Cl^-, SO_4^{2-}), the anion is unable to accompany the H^+, the resting membrane potential is reduced, allowing K^+ to diffuse out of the cell. If the anion is organic (ketones, lactate), the anion can permeate the cell, the potential is sustained and no K^+ diffuses out [20]. Potassium loss from cells is more common and more severe in inorganic metabolic acidosis than in organic acidosis or respiratory acidosis. A low plasma HCO_3^- will be the indicator. Insulin deficiency makes the diabetic patient more likely to have hyperkalemia, because insulin facilitates K^+ uptake by cells. The accompanying hyperglycemia also induces loss of water from the cells because glucose in this setting is osmotically effective, creating serum hypertonicity; loss of K^+ accompanies the loss of cell water.

Non-selective β_2 adrenergic blocking agents

When used to treat hypertension these agents lead to hyperkalemia because they block cell uptake of K^+ facilitated by the β_2 adrenergic receptor [6]. These agents rarely cause severe hyperkalemia unless combined with an impaired ability to excrete K^+.

Insulin deficiency

In a patient with uncontrolled diabetes mellitus, the lack of insulin makes the glucose an osmotically effective solute. Hyperglycemia draws water and K^+ from cells into the extracellular fluid [23].

Exercise

A mild rise in plasma K^+ concentration occurs in exercise, reflecting the K^+ loss that occurs in depolarization, temporarily exceeding the capacity of Na^+,K^+-ATPase to restore cell K^+. The more severe the exercise, the greater the rise in plasma K^+ [24]. In marathon runners, plasma K^+ may exceed 6 or 7 mEq/l. The rise in K^+ concentration in the ECF within the muscle causes vasodilatation and increased blood flow to the muscle.

Tissue necrosis

Rhabdomyolysis, necrosis of muscle caused by ischemia, metabolic, toxic, infectious or traumatic muscle damage, results in the loss of large amounts of K^+ and myoglobin from muscle. Hyperkalemia is frequent and may be exacerbated if acute tubular necrosis also occurs due to myoglobin-mediated renal tubule injury. Two other conditions of widespread cell necrosis are, on rare occasions, associated with hyperkalemia – hemolysis if acute and overwhelming, and the tumor lysis syndrome that accompanies the treatment of cancer patients with chemotherapy. In these latter cases, acute tubular necrosis may also occur, increasing the severity of the rise in K^+.

Drug overdose and toxins

Digitalis overdose, which causes cardiac toxicity, may also be accompanied by hyperkalemia. It is thought that this reflects digitalis inhibition of Na^+,K^+-ATPase. Among the treatments is the use of the digoxin-specific fab antibody, which promotes the excretion of digitalis drugs and, along with it, K^+. In the recovery phase, hypokalemia may occur [25]. Two drugs may induce hyperkalemia. As reported by Mazze et al. [26], succinylcholine used in the operating rooms to facilitate the endotracheal intubation of soldiers with massive traumatic tissue injury caused hyperkalemia that often led to ventricular fibrillation (Figure 25.2). The paralysis induced by the post-tetanic potentiation action of succinylcholine releases additional K^+ from the dying cells. Arginine hydrochloride, used in the treatment of severe metabolic alkalosis, causes hyperkalemia secondary to the exchange of arginine with cell

K^+ [27]. Cocaine intoxication leads to hyperkalemia from muscle damage, acidosis and acute renal failure.

Hyperkalemic periodic paralysis

As previously mentioned, there are two forms of periodic paralysis. One of them is associated with hyperkalemia [8]. This is a rare inherited autosomal dominant disease. The victim has a sudden onset of severe generalized weakness or paralysis, usually following ingestion of K^+, or exposure to cold temperature or after exercise. Mutations that impair inactivation of the sodium channel in skeletal muscle have been proposed to explain the pathogenesis of this disorder. Normally with the activation of muscle contraction, when the cell is depolarized, the Na channels close, allowing the restoration of the low Na^+, high K^+ state in the cell. A small fraction of the Na^+ channels fail to close, but these cells are sufficient so that the muscle is paralyzed [28]. The resting membrane potential of these cells is closer to the activation potential, such that a rise in serum K^+ may suffice to trigger the mechanism. The frequency of attacks may be reduced by taking steps to prevent hyperkalemia. Acetazolamide is effective.

Decreased urinary excretion of K^+

The primary abnormality in patients with severe renal insufficiency is a reduction in delivery of sodium and water to the collecting tubule, reflecting the loss of functioning nephrons [2]. The critical reduction may be precipitated by sodium deficiency induced by a diuretic or diarrhea. An abnormality in distribution of K^+ may also be a factor, since there is evidence for reduced activity of Na^+,K^+-ATPase in cells in uremia. The so-called K^+-sparing diuretics, amiloride, triamterene and spironolactone, used to reduce the urinary loss of K^+ that usually accompanies thiazide or loop diuretic treatment, may precipitate hyperkalemia in the patient with renal insufficiency.

Depletion of 'effective' extracellular fluid volume or circulating plasma volume, as in congestive heart failure, hepatic insufficiency, or sodium depletion, is sufficient to cause hyperkalemia by reducing sodium delivery to the collecting tubule. A patient with chronic renal insufficiency is especially vulnerable.

Hypoaldosteronism

Hypoaldosteronism has many causes [1,2]. There are several steps in the pathway between kidney and adrenal cortex, interruption of which can cause hypoaldosteronism. These steps include diminished renal renin production, deficiency of angiotensinogen, inhibition of converting enzyme, blockade of the angiotensin II receptor, impaired production of aldosterone in the adrenal cortex, blockade of the aldosterone receptor or inhibition of the Na^+ reabsorptive mechanism and associated secretion of K^+ and H^+ in the collecting duct.

Primary adrenal insufficiency, for example, from Addison's disease, results in failure of synthesis of both

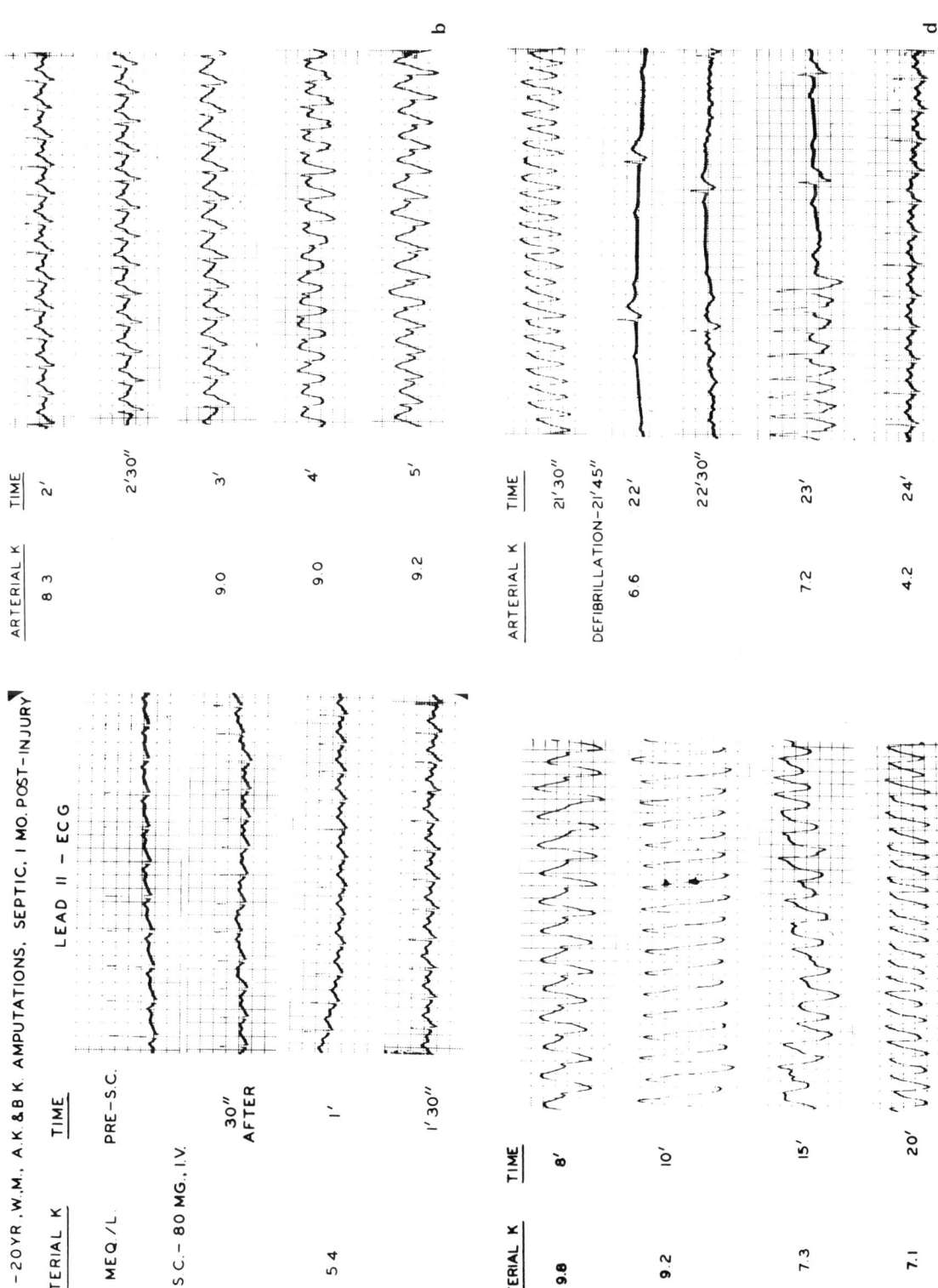

Figure 25.2 Arterial plasma K+ and electrocardiographic changes following the administration of succinylcholine to a traumatized patient. The patient was premedicated with pentobarbital and atropine. Anesthesia was induced with thiopental. Succinylcholine was administered to facilitate tracheal intubation. Arterial blood samples were obtained at the times indicated. The patient was monitored continuously with an electrocardiography. The EKG changes following succinylcholine are: (a) increasing height of the T wave; (b) widening of the QRS complex, decreasing QRS voltage and disappearance of the P wave; (c) ventricular tachycardia and fibrillation; (d) defibrillation and resumption of normal cardial rhythm. Resuscitation measures, begun at 2 min (b), included discontinuing anesthesia, ventilation, closed-chest cardiac compression and electrical defibrillation. Treatment of hyperkalemia included intravenous calcium chloride, lidocaine, and sodium bicarbonate. (Adapted from Mazze et al. [26], with permission.)

glucocorticoids and aldosterone. In addition there are congenital forms [1, 20]. Secondary adrenal insufficiency has a variety of etiologies. Hyporeninemic hypoaldosteronism is a disorder in patients with chronic renal insufficiency most commonly form diabetic nephropathy. The GFR is reduced but not to a level sufficient by itself to account for the elevated plasma K^+. The prevailing hypothesis is that renin synthesis by the juxtaglomerular apparatus is impaired, causing reduced angiotensin II formation and decreased aldosterone release, but this remains to be proven. The associated metabolic acidosis is thought to be due to the hypoaldosteronism and impaired ammonia metabolism secondary to the hyperkalemia. Treatment with mineralocorticoid (fludrocortisone) or sodium bicarbonate corrects both the hyperkalemia and the acidosis, but risks hypertension. Alternatively, a K^+-restricted diet plus a thiazide or loop diuretic is normally effective.

Medications whose complications may mimic secondary adrenal insufficiency include angiotensin converting enzyme (ACE) inhibitors and non-steroid anti-inflammatory drugs. Steroids (e.g. prednisone), if abruptly discontinued after chronic high-dose administration, may expose an inactive adrenal cortex. Treatment with losartan, an angiotensin II receptor blocker, has not yet been reported to cause hyperkalemia, to our knowledge, but it seems likely that it will. K^+-sparing diuretics, which interfere with the action of aldosterone (spironolactone, amiloride or triamterene) lead to hyperkalemia, especially in patients with renal insufficiency.

Renal disease associated with hyperkalemia

Besides hyporeninemic hypoaldosteronsim, there are other renal disorders in which the frequency of hyperkalemia is disproportionate to the reduction in GFR. These include urinary tract obstruction, distal RTA and some forms of interstitial nephritis.

Urinary tract obstruction is associated with hyperkalemia when the GFR is reduced even after the obstruction is relieved. It is probable that this reflects the fact that the initial and most severe injury is to the collecting tubules.

In systemic lupus erythematosus interstitial nephritis, secretion of both K^+ and H^+ is impaired. Patients with sickle cell nephropathy have been shown to exhibit hyperkalemia despite a normal GFR. As discussed in Chapter 40, the primary injury in sickle cell disease is to the renal medulla, eventuating in papillary necrosis. This is likely to result in a particularly widespread injury to the collecting duct system. Renal transplant recipients often have hyperkalemia following transplantation. It is now known that many cadaveric transplant kidneys undergo some degree of acute tubular necrosis secondary to the time between removal and transplantation [29].

Renal tubular acidosis has been described above, because of the association of the syndrome with hypokalemia. But type 1 RTA may also frequently be accompanied by hyperkalemia. In this case the problem is defective sodium reabsorption which in turn reduces K^+ and H^+ secretion. This form of type 1 RTA is observed in patients with urinary tract obstruction and sickle cell nephropathy (above). Type IV RTA has an associated hyperchloremic metabolic acidosis due to decreased excretion of NH_4^+. There is a hypoaldosteronemic state, either because of low circulating aldosterone, or because of a postulated defect in the mineralocorticoid receptor.

Gordon's syndrome is a rare familial disorder, presumably autosomal dominant, characterized by hyperkalemia despite a normal GFR, and hypertension [30]. The proposed defect is an abnormal increase in the reabsorption of Cl^- by the distal tubule or Cl^- shunting. This enables the accompanying cation, Na^+, to be reabsorbed as well, resulting in diminished Na^+ delivery to the K^+ secretory site. The hyperkalemia can be corrected by the administration of poorly reabsorbable anions, such as SO_4^{2-}, which is what established the pathophysiology of the mechanisms but this is impracticable as a treatment. The high serum K^+ can be prevented by the use of a diuretic such as hydochlorothiazide.

Drugs

Drugs that cause hypoaldosteronism have been summarized above. Trimethoprim and pentamidine have been shown to interfere directly with K^+ secretion in the collecting tubule [31]. Cyclosporin probably induces hyperkalemia by several pathways – renal ischemia, reduced plasma renin and aldosterone and Cl^- shunting in the distal tubule [32].

Clinical manifestations of hyperkalemia

Cardiovascular manifestations

Often there are no symptoms until a cardiac arrhythmia occurs. This may be an emergency. Figure 25.2 characterizes the electrocardiographic changes associated with a rising plasma K^+ concentration. The T waves rise and assume the characteristic 'peaked' configuration, the PR interval increases; the QRS complex widens until it becomes a sine wave and then ventricular fibrillation occur. Even before an arrhythmia impairs the cardiac output, the blood pressure may decline.

Neuromuscular manifestations

The patient may complain of numbness or tingling of the extremities; weakness and even paralysis may develop, as K^+ depletion in the respiratory muscle may be affected.

Treatment of hyperkalemia

The principal methods of treatment of hyperkalemia are summarized in Table 25.3. In nearly every case, K^+ must be removed from the body. The exception is the hyper-

Table 25.3 Treatment of hyperkalemia

Treatment	Rapidity	Duration	Comments
Reduce membrane excitability (intravenous)			
Calcium gluconate	min	1/2 to 1 h	Done with EKG attached
Calcium chloride			
Shift K^+ into cells			
$NaHCO_3$ (intravenous)	min	1–2 h	Observe for excess Na^+ loading
Insulin with glucose (intravenous)	30 min	4–6 h	Check blood glucose regularly
β_2-Adrenergic agonists	30 min	2–4 h	
(intravenous or nebulizer)			
Remove K^+			
Furosemide (intravenous)	1 h	4–6 h	
Cation exchange resin (oral or rectal)	1–2 h	4–6 h	Administer with an osmotic agent (sorbitol)
Dialysis	Immediate	Duration of dialysis	

kalemia observed in diabetic patients with insulin deficiency and hyperglycemia. The hyperkalemia is corrected by insulin and often reveals an underlying K^+ deficiency, owing to the glucose-induced osmotic diuresis and urinary excretion of K^+. The treatment is guided by the urgency of the clinical picture, which is established by the clinical manifestations, and the EKG.

Antagonism of membrane effects of hyperkalemia

More severe hyperkalemia requires antagonism of the membrane potential effects of hyperkalemia by calcium and measures to drive K^+ into the cells (redistribution). The former is achieved by inducing hyperpolarization of the electrically excitable cell, that is, raising the threshold of activation. Calcium, either as gluconate or chloride, administered intravenously, is the most effective treatment. Treatment is guided by the EKG. Beware of the patient taking digitalis; calcium may increase the risk of digitalis toxicity.

Increase cellular uptake of K^+ (redistribution)

The combination of insulin and glucose is a tried and true measure to induce K^+ entrance into cells and is often the first treatment to be instituted. β-Adrenergic agonists such as albuterol may be given intravenously or intranasally. This latter therapy, although effective in patients with some renal function, is often ineffective in patients with ESRD, perhaps because it has been shown that the circulating level of catecholamines in these patients is already above normal. If the serum HCO_3^- level is low from metabolic acidosis, the administration of $NaHCO_3$ may be effective.

Increase K^+ removal

Cation exchange resins work by exchanging Na^+ for K^+ in the GI tract. The resin may be administered orally or per rectum. Its effectiveness is proportional to the surface area of intestine exposed to it. Often an osmotic agent, like sorbitol, is given to encourage evacuation. Since hyperkalemia usually occurs in the setting of renal insufficiency, the physician should always consider hemodialysis therapy, the most effective and the fastest way to remove K^+.

References

1. Tannen, R.L. (1991) Disorders of potassium balance, in *The Kidney*, 4th edn (eds B.M. Brenner and F.C. Rector Jr), Saunders, Philadelphia, pp. 805–40.
2. Allon, M. (1995) Hyperkalemia in end-stage renal disease: mechanisms and management. *J. Am. Soc. Nephrol.*, **6**, 1134–42.
3. McCance, R.A. and Widdowson, E.G. (1937) Alkalosis with disordered kidney function. *Lancet*, **ii**, 247–9.
4. Giebisch, G., Malnic, G. and Berliner, R.W. (1991) Renal transport and control of potassium excretion, in *The Kidney*, (eds B.M. Brenner and F.C. Rector Jr), Saunders, Philadelphia, pp. 283–317.
5. DeFronzo, R.A., Sherwin, R.T., Dillingham, M. *et al.* (1978) Influence of basal insulin and glucagon secretion

on potassium and sodium metabolism. *J. Clin. Invest.*, **61**, 472–9.

6. Rosa, R.M., Silva, P., Young, J.B. *et al.* (1980) Adrenergic modulation of extrarenal potassium disposal. *N. Engl. J. Med.*, **302**, 431–4.

7. Howes, L.G. (1995) Which drugs affect potassium? *Drug Safety*, **12**, 240–4.

8. Griggs, R.C. and Ptacek, L.J. (1992) The periodic paralyses. *Hosp. Pract. (Off Ed)* **27**, 123–6, 129–30, 136–7.

9. Sebastian, A., McSherry, E. and Morris, R.C., Jr (1971) Renal potassium wasting in renal tubular acidosis (RTA). Its occurrence in types 1 and 2 RTA despite sustained correction of systemic acidosis. *J. Clin. Invest.*, **50**, 667–78.

10. Simon, D.B. and Lifton, R.P. (1996) The molecular basis of inherited hypokalemic alkalosis: Bartter's and Gitelman's syndromes. *Am. J. Physiol.*, **271**, F961–6.

11. Jamison, R.L., Ross, J., Kempson, R. *et al.* (1982) Surreptitious diuretic ingestion and pseudo-Bartter's syndrome. *Am. J. Med.*, **73**, 142–7.

12. International Collaborative Study Group for Bartter-like Syndromes (1997) Mutations in the gene encoding the inwardly-rectifying renal potassium channel, ROMK, cause the antenatal variant of Bartter's syndrome: evidence for genetic heterogeneity. *Hum. Mol. Genet.*, **6**, 17–26.

13. Funder, J.W. (1995) Apparent mineralocorticoid excess. *Endocrinol. Metab. Clin. North Am.*, **24**, 613–21.

14. Corry, D.G. and Tuck, M.L. (1995) Secondary aldosteronism. *Endocrinol. Metab. Clin. North Am.*, **24**, 511–29.

15. Kater, C.E. and Biglieri, E.G. (1995) Disorders of steroid 17-alpha-hydroxylase deficiency. *Endocrinol. Metab. Clin. North Am.*, **24**, 341–57.

16. Corvol, P., Pinet, F., Plouin, R.F. *et al.* (1995) Renin-secreting tumors. *Endocrinol. Metab. Clin. North Am.*, **24**, 255–70.

17. Walker, B.R. and Edwards, C.R. (1995) Licorice-induced hypertension and syndromes of apparent mineralocorticoid excess. *Endocrinol. Metab. Clin. North Am.*, **24**, 359–77.

18. Shinkets, R.A., Warnock, D.G., Bositisi, C.M. *et al.* (1994) Liddle's syndrome: Heritable human hypertension caused by mutations in the beta subunit of the epithelial sodium channel. *Cell*, **79**, 407–14.

19. al-Ghamdi, S.M., Cameron, E.G. and Sutton, R.A. (1994) Magnesium deficiency: pathophysiologic and clinical overview. *Am. J. Kidney Dis.*, **24**, 737–52.

20. Kamel, K.S., Halperin, M.L., Faber, M.D. *et al.* (1995) Disorders of potassium balance, in *The Kidney* 4th edn (eds B.M. Brenner and F.C. Rector Jr), Saunders, Philadelphia, pp. 999–1037.

21. Rabelink, T.J., Koomans, H.A., Hené, R.J. *et al.* (1990) Early and late adjustments to potassium loading in humans. *Kidney Int.*, **38**, 942–7.

22. Doucet, A. and Katz, A.I. (1980) Renal potassium adaptation: Na-K-ATPase activity along the nephron after chronic potassium loading. *Am. J. Physiol.*, **238**, F380–6.

23. Adrogué, H.J., Lederer, E.D., Suki, W.N. *et al.* (1986) Determinants of potassium levels in diabetic ketoacidosis. *Medicine (Baltimore)*, **65**, 163–72.

24. Thomson, A. and Kelly, D.T. (1989) Exercise stress-induced changes in systemic arterial potassium in angina pectoris. *Am. J. Cardiol.*, **63**, 1435–40.

25. Kelly, R.A. and Smith, T.W. (1992) Recognition and management of digitalis toxicity. *Am. J. Cardiol.*, **69**, 108G–18G.

26. Mazze, R.I., Escue, H.M. and Houston, J.B. (1969) Hyperkalemia and cardiovascular collapse following administration of succinylcholine to the traumatized patient. *Anesthesiology*, **31**, 540–7.

27. Bushinsky, D.A. and Gennari, F.J. (1978) Life-threatening hyperkalemia induced by arginine. *Ann. Intern. Med.*, **89**, 632–4.

28. Cannon, S.C. and Corey, D.P. (1993) Loss of Na$^+$ channel inactivation by anemone toxin (ATX II) mimics the myotonic state in hyperkalemia periodic paralysis. *J. Physiol.*, **466**, 501–20.

29. Veludina, S.J.A., Nelson, W.J., Huie, P. *et al.* (1995) Postischemic injury, delayed function and Na$^+$/K$^+$-ATPase distribution in the transplanted kidney. *Kidney Int.*, **48**, 1301–15.

30. Take, C., Ikeda, K., Kurasawa, *et al.* (1991) Increased chloride reabsorption as an inherited renal tubular defect in familial type II pseudohypoaldosteronism. *N. Engl. J. Med.*, **324**, 472–6.

31. Velazquez, H., Perzaella, M.A., Wright, F.S. *et al.* (1993) Renal mechanism of trimethoprim-induced hyperkalemia. *Ann. Intern. Med.*, **119**, 296–301.

32. Oster, J.G., Singer, I. and Fishman, L.M. (1995) Heparin-induced aldosterone suppression and hyperkalemia. *Am. J. Med.*, **98**, 575–86.

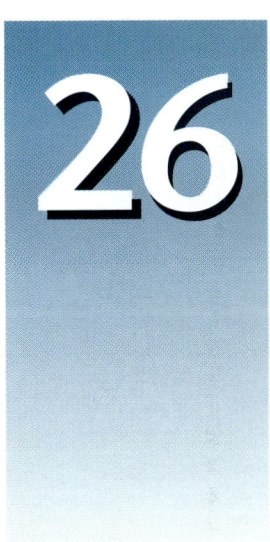

26

Acid–base disorders and their management

Kevin D. Burns and David Z. Levine

Introduction

This chapter, building on the groundwork laid in Chapter 11, will offer an approach to the care of the renal patient with acid–base disorders by providing typical case presentations, and by highlighting certain topics. Insights from abnormal tubular and cellular function will direct a pathophysiological approach to the assessment of the cases. For example, for each case presentation, it is appropriate to ask: what are the renal and extracellular components of the acid–base disturbance (what accounts for a given fall in the plasma [HCO_3^-] in the patient with renal disease, as well as the rate of fall), which nephron segments are likely to be involved, and what cell function is affected by the disease process?

First is the most common acid–base presentation in the renal patient: the ubiquitous fall in plasma [HCO_3^-] and metabolic acidosis that accompanies progressive loss of nephron mass, encountered in the vast majority of patients destined for dialysis or transplantation. Attention will be given to the susceptibility of these patients to other life-threatening acid–base disturbances. Second is an urgent acid–base presentation in renal patients: the metabolic acidosis associated with sepsis, cardiovascular catastrophes, or trauma, accompanied by acute renal failure. Finally, we will study the syndromes of renal tubular acidosis (RTA), with emphasis on the pathogenesis of proximal and distal acidification disorders, and discussion of specific abnormalities in renal transplant patients.

The reader will note that this approach differs in two respects from the usual presentation of acid–base disturbances. First, we will concentrate on problems afflicting renal patients primarily. Accordingly, for the patient with diabetic ketoacidosis or respiratory acidosis without accompanying renal disease, the information provided in other monographs will suffice [1–3]. The second difference is that a clinical setting, e.g. urinary tract obstruction, is provided here and therein acid–base disorders are discussed. We believe this approach will suit the busy clinician who will turn to this book with a patient in mind, rather than with a more general acid–base query.

Chronic renal failure

Adaptation of surviving nephrons to augment acid secretion

It has been recognized, both clinically and experimentally, that loss of nephron mass is associated with morphologic processes and adaptations in transport that protect acid–base balance. In patients with chronically diseased kidneys, there is a reduction in ammoniagenesis and a decreased generation of new HCO_3^- as the quantity of normal functioning proximal tubule tissue falls. Similarly, the overall capacity to secrete normal and increased rates of protons into the tubular lumen is impaired. However, at the level of the single surviving nephron, ammoniagenesis and HCO_3^- retrieval may be increased so that 5% of surviving nephrons may perform the work of many more normal nephrons.

Nephrology, Edited by Rex L. Jamison and Robert Wilkinson.
Published in 1997 by Chapman & Hall, London. ISBN 0 412 60930 4

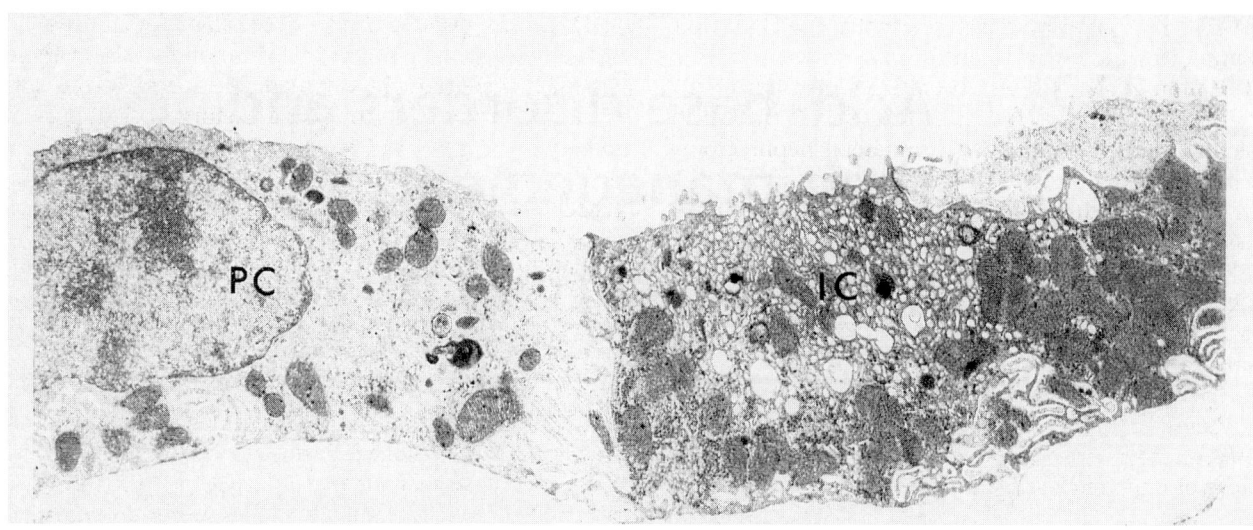

a

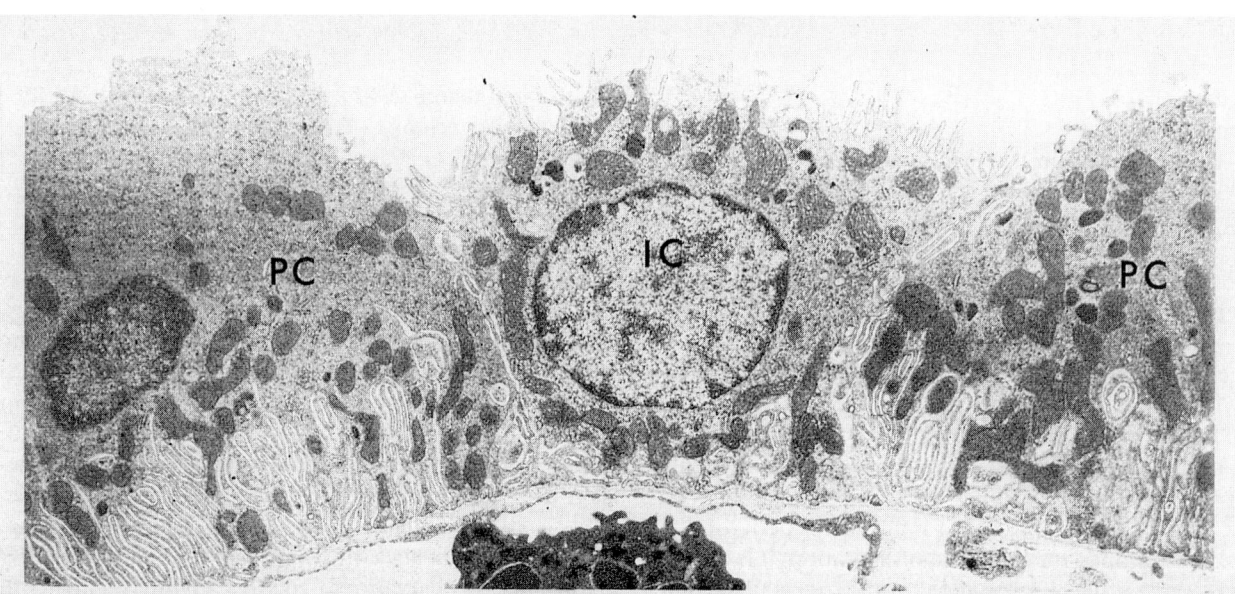

b

Figure 26.1   Principal (PC) and intercalated (IC) cells from cortical collecting tubule of a normal (a) or a 75% nephrectomized rat (b). The basolateral membrane of the principal cell is considerably greater following partial renal ablation, and cell size is increased. The luminal membrane of the intercalated cell is increased following partial renal ablation, but the number of apical cytoplasmic vesicles is reduced. (Reproduced, with permission, from ref. 7.)

What accounts for this adaptation? In the proximal tubule, there is hypertrophy of surviving nephrons in remnant kidney models, which creates a larger surface area for H⁺ transport. In proximal tubular brush border vesicles derived from remnant kidneys of rats [4] and dogs [5], there is an increase in Na⁺–H⁺ exchanger activity. Despite this increased ability to reabsorb filtered HCO_3^-, the net effect for the whole kidney is still a decrease in absolute H⁺ secretion, because the increased capacity does not offset the reduction in nephron mass. Similarly, although there is enhanced ammoniagenesis by individual proximal tubular cells in remnant kidneys, whole kidney ammonium (NH_4^+) excretion is impaired. Indeed,

Buerkert *et al.* [6] have shown that there is impaired re-entrapment of ammonia (NH_3) along the collecting ducts in a rat remnant kidney model, despite enhanced proximal tubule ammoniagenesis.

In the distal tubule, remnant kidney studies [7] have shown that cells of the initial collecting tubule increase their surface area in a manner consistent with an increased ability for α-intercalated cells to secrete H⁺ (Figure 26.1). Comprehensive functional data on distal tubule acidification in chronic renal failure are provided by Kunau and Walker [8]. After a three-quarter nephrectomy in rats, HCO_3^- reabsorption in the superficial distal tubule was enhanced, even when the increased HCO_3^-

load and more negative transepithelial voltage were accounted for in separate control experiments. In contrast, Hamm *et al.* [9] found no alteration in net HCO_3^- reabsorption in cortical collecting tubules and medullary collecting ducts in rabbits with unilateral nephrectomy and partial infarction of the remaining kidney.

In summary, currently available studies from renal ablation models indicate that hypertrophied proximal tubules have enhanced transporter activities and increased levels of ammoniagenesis, which serve to retrieve the higher than normal HCO_3^- load in surviving nephrons. The distal tubule also participates in this process of adaptation, whereas the collecting ducts may not. Increased proximal tubule ammoniagenesis has a limited salutary effect on overall generation of HCO_3^-, because of impaired re-entrapment of NH_3 along the collecting ducts.

The effect of this impaired renal capacity to excrete H^+ in chronic renal failure is now examined in the following two clinical cases.

Case 26.1: A 63-year-old man, a recluse who rarely saw his physician, was known to have chronic renal failure for many years. He presented to the emergency room hyperventilating and confused. On physical examination, there was no evidence of extracellular fluid (ECF) volume contraction. Laboratory studies revealed a serum creatinine of 950 μM (10.7 mg/dl). Arterial blood gas pH = 7.02, $[HCO_3^-]$ = 4 mM, arterial PCO_2 ($PaCO_2$) = 16 mmHg. Electrolytes were: Na^+ 140 mM, Cl^- 110 mM, K^+ 6.0 mM, with an anion gap (Na^+ − $[HCO_3^-$ + $Cl^-]$) of 26 mM. An ultrasound of his abdomen revealed bilateral shrunken kidneys, with no evidence of obstruction. On further enquiry, this patient was known not to have taken any medications, and not to have any factors known to precipitate acute renal failure.

Case 26.2: A patient well known to the nephrology service is a 55-year-old woman with lupus nephritis of 15 years duration. A renal biopsy at initial presentation with lupus revealed membranoproliferative glomerulonephritis. She presented on a routine clinic visit with arterial blood pH = 7.33, plasma $[HCO_3^-]$ = 21 mM, and $PaCO_2$ = 38 mmHg. The serum $[K^+]$ was normal, but her serum creatinine was 820 μM (9.2 mg/dl). An ultrasound of her abdomen revealed a reduction in renal size with increased echogenicity of the cortices.

What accounts for the difference in presentations of these patients, both with severe reduction in renal function? Patient no. 1 has small kidneys, severe metabolic acidosis and, quite possibly, no reversible component to his renal failure. The acidemia and azotemia are based on the irretrievable loss of renal mass. Patient no. 2, in contrast, has only a mild degree of metabolic acidosis, despite an equally severe depression of the glomerular filtration rate (GFR). In fact, this latter patient, who appeared relatively well, with a mild metabolic acidosis, is typical of a large number of patients approaching end-stage renal disease who are carefully managed in outpatient clinics. Indeed, they may remain asymptomatic, with no clini-

cally relevant disorder of acid–base balance demonstrable, virtually up to the point of initiation of dialysis. In these patients, there must be a remarkable adaptation of surviving nephrons to do the acid excretory work of normal kidneys.

As discussed in Chapter 11, the reduction in plasma $[HCO_3^-]$ in the patient with renal insufficiency will reflect, as in the patient without renal failure, the balance between net addition of H^+ to the ECF and its removal. Assuming that in the patients described above there is no diarrhea, sepsis, circulatory failure, ketoacidosis or exogenous poisons, the source of acid addition is presumed to be the metabolism of ≈1 mEq/kg/day of dietary acid. In both patients, to a greater or lesser degree, there is an inability of the damaged kidneys to excrete dietary-derived acid, so that the plasma $[HCO_3^-]$ is progressively titrated downwards. Patient no. 1 has seemingly exceeded the limits of adaptation, however, and over a period of days to weeks, has titrated his plasma $[HCO_3^-]$ down to very low levels. From a clinical standpoint, the patient with chronic renal failure may present with either mild or severe depression of the plasma $[HCO_3^-]$.

The anion gap

In the case studies above, the anion gap was increased. In chronic renal failure, metabolic acidosis progresses slowly. Generally, the increase in the anion gap correlates, but only to a limited degree, with the fall in plasma $[HCO_3^-]$ [10]. The increase in the anion gap is thought to be the result of accumulation of filtered anions (e.g. HPO_4^{2-}). The clinician should not be surprised, however, to find the elevations in the anion gap in patients with chronic renal failure are minor, despite very severe reductions in GFR. When the anion gap is greatly elevated (>30 mM) in a patient with chronic renal failure, one should be alerted to the presence of another process causing high anion gap metabolic acidosis. For example, the diabetic patient with renal disease may be prone to diabetic ketoacidosis or cardiovascular catastrophes leading to hypoperfusion and sepsis, causing lactic acidosis. In each case, the marked elevation in the anion gap, associated with a rapid fall in the plasma $[HCO_3^-]$, provides a valuable clue to a serious non-renal process contributing to life-threatening metabolic acidosis.

Thus, in the patient with chronic renal failure and an anion gap exceeding 30 mM, a second cause of high anion gap metabolic acidosis should be sought.

Rate of fall of plasma [HCO₃⁻]

The rate of fall of the plasma $[HCO_3^-]$ also provides a clue to the etiology of metabolic acidosis in patients with chronic renal failure. Consider patient no. 2 with lupus nephritis. Let us assume this patient came to the emergency room one day after her uneventful clinic visit in a state of severe metabolic acidosis, with a plasma $[HCO_3^-]$ of 5 mM. Could this be explained by a further deterioration of renal function? The answer is clearly no. Assuming the patient weighted 70 kg, she would accumulate approximately 70 mmol of H^+/day (1 mmol/kg/day on a typical Western diet). Since HCO_3^- distributes into a volume equal to 50% of total body weight, the 70 mmol H^+ would be buffered in approximately 35 l. Thus, the plasma $[HCO_3^-]$ would fall by 70 mmol/35 l/day = 2 mM/day. Since the plasma $[HCO_3^-]$ has fallen more rapidly than can be explained by the ability of the kidneys to handle the daily dietary acid load (from 21 mM to 5 mM), another process must be considered. If the anion gap has been increased further, the clinician must rule out sepsis or other causes of lactic acidosis, diabetic ketoacidosis or exogenous poisons.

Plasma osmolal gap

In the renal patient with unexpectedly severe metabolic acidosis and a markedly elevated anion gap, a clue suggesting ingestion of toxic alcohols or methanol is the presence of unaccounted for osmoles in the plasma. When the sum of: $(2 \times serum [Na^+]) + [urea] + [glucose]$ (in mM) exceeds the measured osmolality, the presence of methanol, ethylene glycol or isopropyl alcohols should be suspected. Thus, for example, the unconscious patient with absent blood ethanol, serum $[Na^+]$ = 140 mM, [urea] = 22 mM (61 mg/dl) and glucose = 8 mM (143 mg/dl), should have a serum osmolality of 310 mosmol/kg H_2O. A measured value of 350 mosmol/kg H_2O should alert the physician to the presence of one of these toxins.

Mixed acid–base disorders in chronic renal failure

It is not unusual for patients with chronic renal failure to develop superimposed acid–base disorders as renal function deteriorates. Perhaps the most common uremic symptoms are anorexia and nausea, which may progress to vomiting. Indeed, we have cared for a patient who presented with a serum [creatinine] of 3900 μM (44 mg/dl), associated with normal plasma $[HCO_3^-]$ and $[K^+]$. In this patient, metabolic alkalosis was superimposed on uremic acidosis, to render the patient in normal acid–base balance. The mechanism for the alkalosis was loss of gastric HCl, which alkalinized the ECF to offset the acidifying effect of retained dietary acid. Similarly, patients with diabetic gastroparesis may have protracted vomiting, and thus may present with metabolic alkalosis, despite the presence of renal failure. As discussed in Chapter 11, it is the impaired glomerular filtration of HCO_3^- that contributes to maintenance of the alkalosis in these patients, by virtue of impaired ability to excrete HCO_3^-.

Mixed acid–base disturbances are also likely to occur in patients with chronic renal failure who have coexistent respiratory disease. In the patient with chronic respiratory acidosis, the Pa_{CO_2} will not be appropriately decreased for the amount of the depression of the plasma $[HCO_3^-]$ associated with uremia. Thus, the rule of the ≈ 1 mmHg fall in Pa_{CO_2} for every 1 mM fall in $[HCO_3^-]$ (see Chapter 11) will be violated. In contrast, if the Pa_{CO_2} is abnormally low for the degree of metabolic acidosis in a patient with chronic renal failure, the clinician should search for a cause of superimposed respiratory alkalosis. This is not uncommon in renal patients, who may have congestive heart failure and interstitial pulmonary edema, pneumonia, or chronic anxiety.

The renal patient with chronic respiratory acidosis is in a precarious state. A diarrheal illness may lead to superimposition of a normal anion gap metabolic acidosis, due to gastrointestinal HCO_3^- loss, along with the high anion gap acidosis of renal insufficiency. Normally, such an acidosis would be accompanied by increased urinary NH_4^+ excretion. However, in the presence of chronic renal disease this cannot occur. Clearly, therefore, these combinations may result in severe acidemia with life-threatening consequences.

Table 26.1 summarizes four important clues to the presence of mixed acid–base disorders in patients with chronic renal failure.

Patients with chronic renal failure may develop superimposed severe normal anion gap metabolic acidosis from certain medications, as illustrated in the following case, and discussed in more detail in the section on RTA.

Case 26.3: A 75-year-old woman presented to the emergency room (ER) with a chief complaint of general malaise for several days. She had a history of diabetes mellitus, and for 20 years regularly visited her ophthalmologist for treatment of diabetic eye disease. The patient had recently begun therapy with acetazolamide, for glaucoma. Physical examination in the ER was unremarkable. Laboratory results: Na^+ 140 mM, K^+ 3.3 mM, HCO_3^- 19 mM, Cl^- 109 mM, anion gap 12 mM, serum creatinine 350 μM (3.9 mg/dl), arterial pH 7.36, Pa_{CO_2} 33 mmHg. The serum creatinine was unchanged over the previous year. The mild hypokalemia and metabolic acidosis with normal anion gap were thought to be consistent with acetazolamide ingestion. She was advised to stop taking the drug and to return to her ophthalmologist.

Unfortunately, there was some confusion about these instructions, and the patient continued to take the acetazolamide. One week later, she returned to the hospital with increasing malaise. Laboratory studies revealed: Na^+ 140 mM, K^+ 4.0 mM, HCO_3^- 9 mM, Cl^- 115 mM, anion gap 16 mM, serum creatinine 650 μM (7.3 mg/dl). The patient had developed

---

Table 26.1 Clues to the presence of superimposed acid–base disorders in the renal patient

1. Rapid fall in plasma $[HCO_3^-]$
2. Very high plasma anion gap (>30 mM).
3. Elevated plasma osmolal gap
4. Pa_{CO_2} inappropriate for the degree of reduction in plasma $[HCO_3^-]$

severe metabolic acidosis: since the plasma [HCO₃⁻] fell more than the increase in the anion gap, a high anion gap acidosis had developed superimposed on the normal anion gap acidosis. The increase in anion gap is consistent with her degree of renal dysfunction.

This case demonstrates that patients with reduced renal capacity to excrete the daily dietary acid load are at risk of developing severe metabolic acidosis when H^+ excretion is impaired further by the addition of an inhibitor of carbonic anhydrase, acetazolamide. Elderly patients with chronic renal failure are particularly prone to develop severe metabolic acidosis following use of this agent, and further deterioration of renal function may ensue [11]. Thus, in the patient with chronic renal failure who presents with a metabolic acidosis in which the decrease in plasma [HCO₃⁻] exceeds the increase in the anion gap, the clinician should be alerted to the possibility of ingestion of drugs impairing renal HCO₃⁻ reabsorption, or to other sources of HCO₃⁻ loss, such as diarrhea.

Therapy of metabolic acidosis in chronic renal failure

Should the patient with chronic renal failure and a persistent reduction in plasma [HCO₃⁻] receive alkali therapy? Recent studies suggest that the metabolic acidosis of uremia may contribute to development and maintenance of renal osteodystrophy. Bone is the largest reservoir of base in the body, and acts as a source of buffer in states of chronic metabolic acidosis. In most patients with chronic renal failure the plasma [HCO₃⁻] remains stable at a reduced level despite the state of chronic positive acid balance induced by the inability to excrete the daily dietary acid load. Investigators have suggested that significant losses of calcium and carbonate from the bones of uremic patients are proportional to the duration of disease and to duration of acidosis [12].

In children with RTA, alkali therapy reduces urinary calcium and phosphate excretion [13] and causes a sharp increase in bone growth [14]. Alkali therapy in chronic renal failure, however, does not appear to have the same benefit as it does in RTA. This may relate to the differences between uremic acidosis and other forms of chronic metabolic acidosis. Uremic acidosis is associated with major alterations in calcium, phosphate, parathyroid hormone, and vitamin D metabolism not found in other forms of metabolic acidosis. For example, negative calcium balance in chronic renal failure is due to decreased gastrointestinal reabsorption of calcium, rather than increased urinary loss, as is the case with chronic metabolic acidosis of other etiologies. Alkali therapy has only a modest effect on gut calcium reabsorption. Nevertheless, alkali therapy may be beneficial in certain uremic patients: a recent study in humans with chronic renal failure revealed that continuous HCO₃⁻ infusions to rapidly correct metabolic acidosis reduced serum parathy-roid hormone and alkaline phosphatase levels, and increased both plasma calcium and 1,25(OH)₂ vitamin D concentrations [15].

An additional reason to consider alkali therapy in uremic patients is suggested [16]. Metabolic acidosis stimulates muscle protein breakdown and catabolism of branched-chain amino acids, via increased activity of branched-chain amino acid decarboxylase. In humans with chronic renal failure, correction of metabolic acidosis with $NaHCO_3$ over a four-week period significantly reduced protein catabolism [17].

The mechanism for the proteolytic effect of acidosis is unclear, but an intact adrenal–glucocorticoid axis is required, and ATP-dependent proteolytic pathways are likely involved [16]. Uremic inhibition of transporters involved in maintenance of intracellular pH has also been implicated.

To return to the original question posed above, based on existing evidence, it seems reasonable to try to maintain plasma [HCO₃⁻] above 20 mM. This can be achieved with $NaHCO_3$ tablets, 600 mg q.i.d. (28.8 mEq HCO₃⁻ per day), although up to 1200 mg q.i.d. may be necessary to correct acidemia. The clinician must be alert to the complications of $NaHCO_3$ therapy: exacerbation of edema and hypertension from the Na^+ load, hypokalemia (especially in patients on continuous ambulatory peritoneal dialysis (CAPD)), and tetany induced by a decrease in ionized calcium concentration.

Acid–base disorders in the dialysis patient

Patients on CAPD and hemodialysis often have multiple disease processes and are more susceptible to acid–base disorders than other patients. Indeed, since the patient with no residual renal function cannot excrete the daily acid load, maintenance of a normal plasma [HCO₃⁻] depends on the addition of alkali to the ECF by the dialysis procedure. In hemodialysis patients, acetate or HCO₃⁻ added to the blood during dialysis raises predialysis plasma [HCO₃⁻] from approximately 19–23 mM to 28 mM, during the typical 4 h dialysis session. CAPD patients, exposed during the day to lactate-containing dwell solutions, obtain their base from the metabolism of lactate to HCO₃⁻ (note that acetate is converted into HCO₃⁻ in hemodialysis patients). CAPD patients tend to have nearly normal plasma [HCO₃⁻], however, in contrast to the mild metabolic acidosis in hemodialysis patients caused by progressive titration of the plasma [HCO₃⁻] between dialysis sessions.

It is generally true that hemodialysis patients tend to have their own acid–base and electrolyte 'signatures', as revealed by predialysis blood tests. A patient with a normal anion gap, and a plasma [HCO₃⁻] of 22 mM, for example, will not often vary from this predialysis presentation. This is not surprising insofar as dialysis parameters and hence alkali loading are predetermined, and dietary acid intake may vary little over time in the stable patient without intercurrent disease.

With these preliminary remarks, let us examine what may underlie the disturbances in the following patients.

Case 26.4: A chronic hemodialysis patient who has had an unvarying course is six days late for treatment, having been stranded in a remote rural area. He seems quite well, but for some breathlessness. Plasma [HCO$_3^-$] = 11.2 mM; arterial pH = 7.27; PaCO$_2$ = 25.2 mmHg; anion gap = 23 mM.

The metabolic acidosis in this patient cannot be attributed to the usual peridialysis fluctuations. As noted above, patients generally have plasma [HCO$_3^-$] above 19 mM and some patients even present with normal acid–base values before dialysis. Can the value of 11.2 mM [HCO$_3^-$] be attributed to missing the dialysis treatments? This is quite plausible, particularly since the patient is noted to be well. If plasma [HCO$_3^-$] falls by 1.5–2 mM/day postdialysis, this presentation is consistent with the effects of dietary acid addition to the ECF, unrelieved by intermittent alkali addition provided by regular dialysis. The corollary must be that if the patient has a severe metabolic acidosis despite regular dialysis, a cause of metabolic acidosis other than renal failure must be sought.

Case 26.5: A patient in the cardiac intensive care unit has postoperative oliguria, and pulmonary edema, associated with a 6 kg weight gain. BP is 160/93. A first hemodialysis is performed with acetate dialysate, and the patient becomes hypotensive during ultrafiltration of 6 kg. Plasma [HCO$_3^-$] falls to 8 mM from a predialysis value of 20 mM.

This patient became acidotic and hypotensive during dialysis, suggesting that the procedure, rather than cardiac disease, was the cause. With rapid fluid removal, especially in the elderly, acetate dialysis is known to induce hypotension, associated with failure of the normal conversion of acetate to HCO$_3^-$ and accumulation of acetate in the blood. In this clinical setting, HCO$_3^-$ dialysis with gentle ultrafiltration or continuous arteriovenous hemofiltration (CAVH) or continuous venovenous hemodialysis (CVVH-D) may be preferable. CAVH and CVVH-D induce less hemodynamic instability than conventional hemodialysis, since they are continuous processes and hourly fluid removal requirements are lower. In general, with hemodialysis, although HCO$_3^-$ baths are more difficult to maintain than acetate, very ill patients tolerate HCO$_3^-$ better. The important diagnostic point in this case is that hemodialysis should rapidly correct metabolic acidosis, rather than induce it. If the same events described above occurred with the patient undergoing dialysis in which the dialysate contained HCO$_3^-$, the most likely cause of the circulatory collapse might be sepsis, or some other cause of a fall in cardiac output. Finally, it is worth noting that after removal of a substantial volume of fluid, if this is replaced by the infusion or ingestion of non-HCO$_3^-$-containing solutions, 'expansion acidosis' would ensue, due to dilution of the plasma [HCO$_3^-$] by chloride-containing fluid. This acidosis might require correction at the subsequent dialysis treatment.

Case 26.6: A chronic hemodialysis patient, 71 years old, comes to the ER complaining of dizziness and anorexia. BP is 105/72. Plasma [HCO$_3^-$] is 14 mM, serum [K$^+$] = 3.9 mM. He was last dialyzed two days earlier, and states he drinks a lot of fluids. The anion gap is 16 mM.

This puzzling patient actually knew his diagnosis, enjoying the confusion of the ER physician. Could there have been simply too much weight removed during the last dialysis? This is unlikely, as it would not explain the superimposed metabolic acidosis, in a patient with good cardiac output. What about the normal serum [K$^+$], two days after the last dialysis? When asked about his urinary output, the patient replied that he was anuric. What kind of metabolic acidosis is associated with a loss of HCO$_3^-$, fluid, and presumably, K$^+$? This patient had longstanding Crohn's disease with ileal diarrhea, and had neglected to take his NaHCO$_3$ supplements.

Case 26.7: A 27-year-old female on chronic hemodialysis is asymptomatic, but for occasional hand cramps. Predialysis plasma [HCO$_3^-$] is 38 mM, with arterial pH 7.60, and PaCO$_2$ = 37 mmHg.

This young woman was in no distress when assessed. She had undergone regular, uneventful hemodialysis with a 38 mM HCO$_3^-$ dialysate concentration. Review of her laboratory results revealed variable elevation of the plasma [HCO$_3^-$], although the metabolic alkalosis was never so severe. Metabolic alkalosis in the dialysis patient is invariably due to loss of HCl, either by nasogastric suction, or vomiting. This patient was a surreptitious vomiter, leaving the clinician with the lingering alkalemia as a diagnostic clue: unlike other such patients, she is unable to intermittently excrete the excess HCO$_3^-$. Treatment involved counselling, and dialysis against a 28 mM HCO$_3^-$ bath.

Acute renal failure

Acute renal failure is often accompanied by severe metabolic acidosis, as the following case illustrates.

Case 26.8: A 54-year-old male underwent right femoral–popliteal bypass surgery. Preoperative renal function and acid–base status were normal. At 24 h postoperatively, he was noted to be oliguric, cold and clammy and poorly responsive. Physical examination revealed a blood pressure of 90/60, pulse 126/min, and absent pulses in the right foot. Laboratory studies revealed arterial pH 7.00, [HCO$_3^-$] 8 mM, PaCO$_2$ 32 mmHg, serum creatinine 220 μM (2.5 mg/dl), serum K$^+$ 6.4 mM and anion gap 31 mM.

This patient developed a severe metabolic acidosis, complicated by a superimposed respiratory acidosis (the PaCO$_2$, assuming normal compensation, should have been

24–26 mmHg). In this postoperative patient, respiratory acidosis was probably secondary to oversedation. The cause of the metabolic acidosis was multifactorial and could not be attributed solely to renal failure. Elevation of the anion gap suggests increased organic acid production. Indeed, this patient had lactic acidosis from impaired perfusion of his right leg, and acute renal failure was due to rhabdomyolysis in combination with impaired renal perfusion.

Since acute renal failure is often accompanied by lactic acidosis due to sepsis, hypovolemic shock or severe congestive heart failure, the clinician can expect profound high anion gap metabolic acidosis in these patients. In addition, acute renal failure occurs often in the setting of hypercatabolic states (e.g. burns, rhabdomyolysis) in which increased production of sulfuric and phosphoric acids contributes to the high anion gap. The finding of an unusually high anion gap (>30 mM), elevation of the osmolal gap (see earlier), and the presence of oxalate crystals in the urine, should alert the clinician to ethylene glycol poisoning as a cause of acute renal failure.

Therapy

In acute renal failure, treatment of metabolic acidosis is indicated when the plasma [HCO_3^-] is low (less than 10–12 mM), or when a patient is fatigued or dyspneic from the effort of respiratory compensation. Why should this acidosis be treated aggressively? As illustrated in Table 26.2, small changes in plasma [HCO_3^-] or Pa_{CO_2} can have dramatic effects on the pH in patients with serious acidosis.

Initial therapy must remove patients from immediate danger by raising the plasma [HCO_3^-] to 10 mM. The amount of $NaHCO_3$ required is determined by assuming that the volume of distribution of HCO_3^- is at least 50%

Table 26.2 Impact of small changes in [HCO_3^-] or Pa_{CO_2} on the acid–base status of a patient with plasma [HCO_3^-] of 7 mM

Condition	[HCO_3^-] (mM)	Pa_{CO_2} (mmHg)	pH
A. Stable metabolic acidosis	7	22	7.12
B. Patient develops respiratory fatigue	7	30[a]	6.99
C. Patient has small decrease in plasma [HCO_3^-]	5	20	7.02[a]

[a] Note that the slight increase in Pa_{CO_2} in example B, or the small decrease in plasma [HCO_3^-] in example C, converts a serious acidemia into a dangerous one. (Adapted from ref. [26], with permission.)

of the body weight. With increasing acidemia, the volume of distribution of HCO_3^- progressively increases and, accordingly, more $NaHCO_3$ is required for correction. Each ampoule of $NaHCO_3$ contains 50 mEq of HCO_3^- (44 mEq in the US). Therefore, an 80 kg patient (volume of distribution of HCO_3^- = 40 l) with a plasma [HCO_3^-] of 5 mM requires at least four ampoules of $NaHCO_3$ to raise the [HCO_3^-] to 10 mM, assuming no ongoing H^+ generation.

Of course, it is critical to arrest ongoing H^+ production in conditions where there is a rapid rate of H^+ addition to the ECF. For example, improving tissue oxygenation in lactic acidosis may be life saving, as can other measures to improve the cardiac output.

In patients with renal failure and diabetic ketoacidosis, the organic acids which are overproduced are not excreted in the urine as they are in patients with normally functioning kidneys. Thus, these patients can regenerate HCO_3^- consumed in buffering excess acid production if production can be halted and metabolism of the organic anions to CO_2 and H_2O proceeds in a normal fashion. If acidemia is not severe in these situations, insulin therapy alone is often sufficient to restore acid–base status.

The use of $NaHCO_3$ therapy in type A lactic acidosis (characterized by impaired tissue oxygen delivery) is controversial, with some investigators advocating administration [18] and others providing evidence for detrimental effects of HCO_3^- [19, 20]. In experimental animals, use of HCO_3^- for treatment of hypoxia-induced lactic acidosis is associated with development of venous hypercapnea and decreased intracellular pH, tissue hypoxia and accelerated lactate production [20]. Alkali therapy may increase lactate production at least in part by blocking the inhibitory effect of H^+ on anaerobic glycolysis [2]. Although further lactate production may lead to H^+ accumulation, it is also accompanied by ATP generation, which might improve cardiac contractility and tissue oxygenation. However, in humans with type A lactic acidosis, HCO_3^- therapy has not been shown to improve prognosis, and is probably of minimal value. In addition to the risks of HCO_3^- therapy noted in experimental studies, the high rate of lactic acid production with tissue hypoxia mandates large amounts of HCO_3^- infusion, associated with dangerous ECF volume expansion and hypernatremia. The stimulator of pyruvate dehydrogenase, dichloroacetate, reduces arterial lactate concentration and raises blood pH in patients with type A lactic acidosis, but has not been shown significantly to affect mortality rate.

How can $NaHCO_3$ be administered to the patient with acute renal failure? Since the majority of these patients have a limited capacity to excrete Na^+, alkali therapy is usually accompanied by a procedure to simultaneously remove fluid, i.e. dialysis. Dialysis against HCO_3^- bath is extremely effective at increasing plasma [HCO_3^-] especially when predialysis plasma [HCO_3^-] is low. Hemodialysis is also particularly useful in patients with acute renal failure and severe metabolic acidosis from toxic ingestions. Hemodialysis against an acetate bath should not be utilized in critically ill patients, since they may have impaired capacity to metabolize acetate to HCO_3^-.

In some hypercatabolic patients acid generation may exceed the removal rate by daily hemodialysis. In these patients institution of peritoneal dialysis, CAVH or CVVH-D will elevate plasma $[HCO_3^-]$. In both instances lactated Ringer's solution is used to replace the filtrate. In situations where there is diminished ability to metabolize lactate the clinician can substitute HCO_3^--containing solutions.

Challenging situations

Dialysis therapy is not readily available in all institutions. In such instances the clinician must correct metabolic acidosis associated with acute renal failure without causing excessive ECF volume expansion. There are a number of ways in which this can be achieved prior to transferring the patient to a dialysis facility. First, in the patient with pulmonary edema, severe metabolic acidosis, and acute renal failure, phlebotomy can be performed to permit administration of $NaHCO_3$. Second, mechanical ventilation should be considered to lower the $PaCO_2$. Indeed, this treatment can raise low blood pH much faster than intravenous administration of $NaHCO_3$, and can also improve the well-being of patients with pulmonary edema. This is a particularly attractive option in patients with chronic lung disease in whom $NaHCO_3$ loading is not possible. Third, significant amounts of HCl and fluid can be removed from the stomach by nasogastric suction. Gastric HCl secretion can be stimulated by pentagastrin. This may permit the intravenous administration of $NaHCO_3$ while the patient is being prepared for eventual dialysis. Fourth, diarrhea can be induced by sucrose enemas followed by $NaHCO_3$ administration.

Severe metabolic alkalosis in acute renal failure

As noted above, severe metabolic alkalosis can develop rapidly in the patient with marked reduction in GFR. This is especially true in acute renal failure.

Case 26.9: A 40-year-old male was transferred to our hospital from a chronic care mental health institution. He had been vomiting for several days and was unable to keep food or fluids down. His physical examination revealed profound ECF volume contraction. Abdominal radiographs revealed massive gastric dilatation consistent with pyloric stenosis. Laboratory values: arterial pH 7.61, PaCO2 49 mmHg, plasma [HCO3−] 49 mM, Na+ 140 mM, Cl− 80 mM, K+ 2.8 mM, serum creatinine 512 μM (5.8 mg/dl), urine Cl− 3 mM.

The patient had a Cl⁻ depletion metabolic alkalosis, secondary to gastric losses from vomiting. There was an associated profound K⁺ loss. In addition the patient had a severe reduction in GFR from volume contraction.

Failure to filter plasma HCO_3^- contributed to the maintenance of the metabolic alkalosis. The patient responded to intravenous infusion of KCl and NaCl to augment GFR.

Clearly this therapy will not benefit patients who have acute irreversible renal failure and metabolic alkalosis. In these patients, body HCO_3^- stores can be titrated down by the addition of acid as intravenous infusion of HCl. Alternatively, a simple way to reduce plasma $[HCO_3^-]$ in a patient receiving hemodialysis is to change the bath alkali source from HCO_3^- to acetate or to reduce the HCO_3^- concentration in the dialysate. In patients on peritoneal dialysis, intravenous fluids lacking lactate may be used as HCO_3^--free dialysate. However, it must be noted that peritoneal infusion of fluids with low pH is poorly tolerated by most patients [21].

Renal tubular acidosis (RTA)

The RTAs are a heterogeneous group of disorders characterized by the presence of hyperchloremic metabolic acidosis (normal anion gap) due to impaired renal net acid excretion, in association with a normal or nearly normal GFR. Chapter 11 presented a molecular approach to these disorders, based on existing knowledge about nephron segment transporters responsible for acid–base regulation. This section gives a clinical approach to these conditions and speculates about the specific etiologies.

The basic defect leading to renal acidosis in these conditions is present in the proximal or distal nephron, hence the separation into proximal and distal RTA.

Proximal RTA

Pathogenesis

In Chapter 11, it was noted that the proximal tubule is the major site of renal HCO_3^- reabsorption. In proximal RTA, a defect in this reabsorptive process occurs, resulting in the delivery of large amounts of HCO_3^- from the proximal tubule. Acidemia ensues due to bicarbonaturia, because of the limited ability of the distal tubule for HCO_3^- reabsorption.

What is the defect responsible for proximal RTA? Figure 11.2 (Chapter 11) shows a limited number of possibilities to account for defective HCO_3^- reabsorption in the proximal tubule. These include: (1) defect in apical Na^+-H^+ exchange; (2) impaired H^+-ATPase activity; (3) defective basolateral Na^+-$3HCO_3^-$ co-transport; (4) impaired carbonic anhydrase activity (either luminal or intracellular); or (5) impaired ability to maintain low intracellular Na^+ concentration [22]. Any of the first four conditions may result in impaired proximal HCO_3^- reabsorption. A defect in generation of low intracellular Na^+ concentration would impair Na^+-coupled transport, and could account for the clinical features of the Fanconi syndrome, a generalized defect in proximal tubule reabsorption leading to HCO_3^- wasting, glycosuria, amino aciduria and increased excretion of phosphate and uric acid. Such a widespread defect could include several possible mechanisms: increased membrane Na^+ permeability, decreased basolateral Na^+,K^+-ATPase activity, or impaired generation of ATP. These would result in an impaired electrochemical Na^+ gradient for Na^+ entry from the tubule lumen [22]. An attractive unifying hypothesis to explain the Fanconi syndrome is that it is due to a primary defect in the Na^+-$3HCO_3^-$ co-transporter, since this might raise the intracellular Na^+ concentration as well as impair HCO_3^- reabsorption. The elevated cell Na^+ concentration would impede all apical Na^+-coupled transport processes.

Chapter 11 discussed the important role of proximal tubule ammoniagenesis in acid–base balance. In proximal RTA it is intriguing that the urinary excretion of NH_4^+ is low despite the presence of chronic metabolic acidosis. Halperin et al. [23] have postulated that features of proximal RTA are explained by a primary elevation of the intracellular pH of proximal cells. This would account for the low HCO_3^- reabsorption and the impaired ammoniagenesis, as well as the normal to high rate of citrate excretion in this condition. We speculate that a primary defect in the basolateral Na^+-$3HCO_3^-$ co-transporter is responsible for the syndrome. With modern molecular methods testing of this hypothesis may soon be possible.

Clinical features

Proximal RTA is rare in adults. Most forms are accompanied by multiple defects in proximal tubule function (Fanconi syndrome). The genetic and acquired diseases and drugs that are associated with either selective HCO_3^- wasting or the Fanconi syndrome are shown in Table 26.3.

Most patients with proximal RTA maintain plasma $[HCO_3^-]$ greater than 15 mM. Severe metabolic acidosis is unusual, and it is possible for these patients to excrete an acid urine (pH < 5.5), as long as plasma $[HCO_3^-]$ is maintained below the low renal threshold for HCO_3^- reabsorption. A consistent finding in proximal RTA is hypokalemia due to increased distal delivery of $NaHCO_3$ and to secondary hyperaldosteronism from ECF volume contraction.

Osteomalacia is common in proximal RTA. Urinary calcium excretion is high. Interestingly, nephrolithiasis and nephrocalcinosis are rare. This may be due to the normal to high urinary citrate excretion in proximal RTA, in contrast to other forms of chronic metabolic acidosis, in which citrate excretion is low.

Diagnosis

The diagnosis of proximal RTA is straightforward. The fractional excretion of HCO_3^- is greater than 15% in patients with proximal RTA, when the plasma $[HCO_3^-]$ exceeds 20 mM.

Table 26.3   Causes of proximal RTA

Isolated HCO_3^- wasting
Idiopathic or genetic
Carbonic anhydrase deficiency, or inhibition
   acetazolamide
   carbonic anhydrase II deficiency

Generalized proximal tubule defect (Fanconi syndrome)
Primary genetic
Hereditary diseases
   Cystinosis
   Tyrosinemia
   Wilson's disease
   Hereditary fructose intolerance
   Galactosemia
Acquired diseases
   Dysproteinemias: multiple myeloma, monoclonal gammopathy
   Associated with secondary hyperparathyroidism
   Drugs and toxins: outdated tetracycline, gentamicin, lead, mercury, glue
   Interstitial nephritis: Sjögren's syndrome
   Renal transplantation
   Amyloidosis
   Nephrotic syndrome

$$FE_{HCO_3^-} = \left[U_{HCO_3^-}\right]/\left[P_{HCO_3^-}\right]/\left[U_{creatinine}\right]/\left[P_{creatinine}\right] \times 100\%.$$

Thus, administration of $NaHCO_3$ to the acidemic patient can be used as a diagnostic measure.

Specific disorders may be recognized in other ways. For example in cystinosis cystine crystals are present in the urine, and tyrosinemia is associated with urinary tyrosine crystals. In hereditary fructose intolerance, bicarbonaturia ensues after ingestion of fructose.

Treatment

In infants and children with proximal RTA alkali therapy improves bone growth. Urinary HCO_3^- losses can be compensated for by 10–15 mEq/kg/day of $NaHCO_3$. This increases K^+ losses and K^+ supplements are often necessary. K^+-sparing diuretics (amiloride, triamterene) may be used to prevent excessive K^+ losses. However, the clinician should be alert to the possibility of inducing an additional defect in distal acidification with these agents. Patients with hypophosphatemia and severe bone disease may require vitamin D and phosphate supplements.

In adults with proximal RTA, alkali therapy should be given to maintain plasma $[HCO_3^-]$ above 20 mM. Although there is no firm evidence for improvement of bone abnormalities with this treatment, the stimulatory effects of acidosis on protein catabolism, as discussed above, and the development of severe acidosis during intercurrent illness, can be prevented with maintenance of plasma [HCO_3^-] at the higher level.

Distal RTA

Distal RTA represents a heterogeneous group of conditions characterized by defective distal nephron acidification mechanisms. As discussed in Chapter 11, the distal convoluted tubule and collecting duct reclaim 10–15% of the filtered HCO_3^-, lower the urine pH to its final value and titrate non-bicarbonate urinary buffers. The collecting duct is able to maintain steep pH gradients of 10–100-fold compared to the limited capacity of the proximal tubule. In the cortical collecting duct, acidification is partly dependent on Na^+ transport and is therefore influenced by the transepithelial voltage. Na^+ reabsorption in this segment generates a lumen-negative electrical potential, which facilitates active secretion of H^+. Aldosterone increases H^+ secretion and Na^+ reabsorption and hence cortical collecting duct acidification.

Let us briefly review the transporters mediating urinary acidification in the distal nephron. The α-intercalated cell has apical membrane H^+-ATPase and H^+,K^+-ATPase, along with basolateral Cl^-/HCO_3^- exchange. Intercalated cells

also contain carbonic anhydrase. Thus, a number of defects could result in the syndrome of distal RTA: (1) diminished or defective H^+-ATPase or H^+,K^+-ATPase activity; (2) impaired generation of the lumen-negative electrical potential via diminished Na^+ delivery, Na^+ reabsorption or increased Cl^- reabsorption; (3) deficiency of aldosterone or resistance to aldosterone; (4) abnormal permeability of α-intercalated cells and/or principal cells, resulting in back-diffusion of H^+; (5) defective basolateral Cl^-/HCO_3^- exchange; or (6) carbonic anhydrase deficiency resulting in impaired removal of OH^-.

It is important to note that in distal RTA such defects alone cannot account for the impaired urinary net acid excretion. It is now widely recognized that these conditions are accompanied by defects in renal ammoniagenesis or decreased secretion of NH_3 in the collecting duct. In either situation, the net effect is a decrease in renal NH_4^+ excretion.

What accounts for impaired NH_4^+ excretion in distal RTA? Distal RTA encompasses numerous diseases affecting the kidneys (Table 26.4). In many of these diseases, hyperkalemia and diminished GFR both contribute to reduced renal ammoniagenesis. The inhibitory effect of hyperkalemia on ammoniagenesis may be secondary to elevation of pH within proximal tubule cells. In other conditions, characterized by medullary dysfunction from interstitial disease, there is impaired secretion of NH_3^+ into the collecting duct. Primary defects in the H^+ secretory mechanisms will also diminish the intraluminal trapping of NH_3 as NH_4^+.

Classical distal RTA

Classical distal RTA is characterized by hyperchloremic metabolic acidosis, hypokalemia, nephrocalcinosis and nephrolithiasis, osteomalacia and rickets. Because of inability to lower the urine pH below 5.5, these patients are prone to develop severe acidemia. Several comprehensive reviews on mechanisms and evaluation of classical distal RTA have been published [2, 22, 24–26]. Three cases of distal RTA are discussed here.

Case 26.10: This 37-year-old woman is the subject of a case report by Cohen et al. [27]. The patient has a long-standing history of neurological symptoms, in association with dry mouth, a positive Schirmer's test, and a lip biopsy revealing interstitial lymphocytic infiltrates, consistent with a diagnosis of Sjögren's syndrome. She presented in 1988 because of profound weakness and hypokalemia. At that time, her laboratory values were: serum Na^+ 145 mM, K^+ 1.6 mM, Cl^- 115 mM, HCO_3^- 15 mM, anion gap 15 mM, urea 8.5 mM, creatinine 141 μM. She had a urine pH of 7.0, with no glycosuria or amino aciduria. After administration of 6 g of NH_4Cl daily for 3 days, her lowest urine pH was 6.5, when the venous blood pH was 7.18. The urine anion gap (see below) was +16 mM. The fractional excretion of HCO_3^- after intravenous HCO_3^- loading ranged from 0.7 to 1.5%. The patient underwent renal biopsy, with fluorescent immunocytochemistry with an anti-

---

Table 26.4 Clinical classification of distal RTA

Associated with normal or low serum [K^+]
Nephrocalcinosis
Medullary sponge kidney
Sjögren's syndrome
Multiple myeloma
Hypercalcemia
Lupus erythematosus
Lithium
Primary
Amphotericin D (back-leak of H^+)

Associated with hyperkalemia
Hypoaldosteronism
Aldosterone resistance
Diabetic renal disease
Chronic pyelonephritis
Obstructive uropathy
Sickle cell hemoglobinopathies
Analgesic nephropathy
Mixed cryoglobulinemia
Amyloidosis
Drugs:
    Angiotensin converting enzyme inhibitors
    K^+-sparing diuretics
    NSAIDs
    Trimethoprim (in AIDS)
    Heparin

body against the 31 kDa subunit of the mammalian kidney H+-ATPase. Staining with the H+-ATPase antibody was absent in intercalated cells and in proximal tubular brush border microvilli, compared to abundance of staining in normal kidney (Figure 26.2). No evidence for anti-intercalated cell antibodies was demonstrated in the patient's serum.

Case 26.11: A 65-year-old woman presented to our hospital after she was found by a relative lying on her kitchen floor unable to move. She had been complaining of progressive weakness and had experienced sudden collapse and paralysis. Physical examination revealed severe generalized muscle weakness but no focal neurological defects. Past medical history was unremarkable, and she was taking no medications. Laboratory studies on admission revealed serum Na^+ 138 mM, K^+ 2.1 mM, Cl^- 112 mM, HCO_3^- 12 mM, anion gap 14 mM, urea 6.4 mM (17.8 mg/dl) and creatinine 100 μM (1.1 mg/dl). Arterial pH was 7.20, and Pa_{CO_2} was 31 mmHg. Urine pH was 6.8. With intravenous HCO_3^- loading, fractional excretion of HCO_3^- was never higher than 3.5%. Immunological screening was negative. The 24-h urine showed 1.1 g protein, however, and immunofixation revealed the presence of lambda light chains in the urine.

Case 26.12: A 52-year-old man presented to our hospital with a long-standing history of bilateral flank pain and dysuria. The patient, a particularly stoic individual, had a 10-year history of nephrolithiasis, passing 2–3 small stones per day. On admission, an intravenous pyelogram revealed multiple discrete calcifications in both kidneys, and abnormal renal papillae, consistent with medullary sponge kidney disease. Serum creatinine was normal. Random past urinalyses were reviewed: urinary pH values were 8.5, 7.5, 8.0, 6.5 and 7.0. However, plasma [HCO_3^-] was always within normal limits, as were serum [K^+] and calcium. Furthermore, there was no history of urine infection, and urine was sterile on admission. Urinary stones were analysed and shown to contain calcium, magnesium and phosphate. The patient was loaded with NH_4Cl to determine if distal acidification was impaired (Table 26.5).

Recent work has dramatically altered thinking about the pathogenesis of distal RTA. Whereas this disorder was long thought to represent an inability to maintain steep H+ concentration gradients across the distal nephron rather than a defect in H+ secretion, the pathogenesis is probably more complicated and varies depending on the etiology of the RTA syndrome.

The patient in case 26.10 establishes, for the first time, the specific cause of a form of distal RTA, as an H+ secretory defect secondary to absence of H+-ATPase [27]. By immunofluorescence studies, this patient with Sjögren's syndrome had no H+-ATPase in any nephron segments.

Could this same mechanism explain the distal RTA in cases 26.11 and 26.12 above? This answer remains unclear, and, indeed, one would also have to consider other pathogenetic mechanisms, including a primary decrease in the number of intercalated cells, an abnormally slow rate of activity of the H+-ATPase, or reduced apical insertion of H+-ATPase pumps from their cytoplasmic position. In the patient with renal stones (case 26.12), nephrocalcinosis might induce interstitial renal scarring, which could impair NH_3 diffusion into the tubular lumen.

The potential role of renal H+,K+-ATPase should also be considered in mediating distal acidification defects. In the patient with Sjögren's syndrome (case 26.10), staining for this enzyme was not performed on the renal biopsy. Impaired function of the H+,K+-ATPase would be expected to result in an acidification defect, accompanied by excessive urinary K+ loss. This could explain the hypokalemia which commonly accompanies hyperchloremic metabolic acidosis in distal RTA. To date, kaliuresis in distal RTA has been ascribed to secondary hyperaldosteronism induced by Na+ wasting.

Vanadate inhibits H+,K+-ATPase activity in experimental animals, associated with development of distal RTA [27a]. Distal RTA is common in northeastern Thailand, where it has been suggested that an environmental inhibitor of the H+,K+-ATPase may be responsible for the syndrome, since these patients also have gastric achlorhydria, and cattle apparently also suffer from the disorder [28].

In the case of the 65-year-old woman with distal RTA (case 26.11) and urinary light chains, it could be speculated that the paraprotein deposition in the renal interstitium directly or indirectly impairs H+-ATPase activity.

These three cases illustrate important clinical features of distal RTA. Because of severe K+ depletion, patients may

Table 26.5 NH_4Cl loading of patient with medullary sponge kidney disease and recurrent nephrolithiasis

	Time (h)							
	0	*1*	*2*	*3*	*4*	*5*	*6*	*7*
Plasma [HCO_3^-] (mM)	26	22	19	23	24	22	22	22
Blood pH	7.34	7.25	7.22	7.23	7.22	7.25	7.27	7.26
Urine pH	6.98	6.93	6.52	6.52	6.30	6.33	6.35	6.54

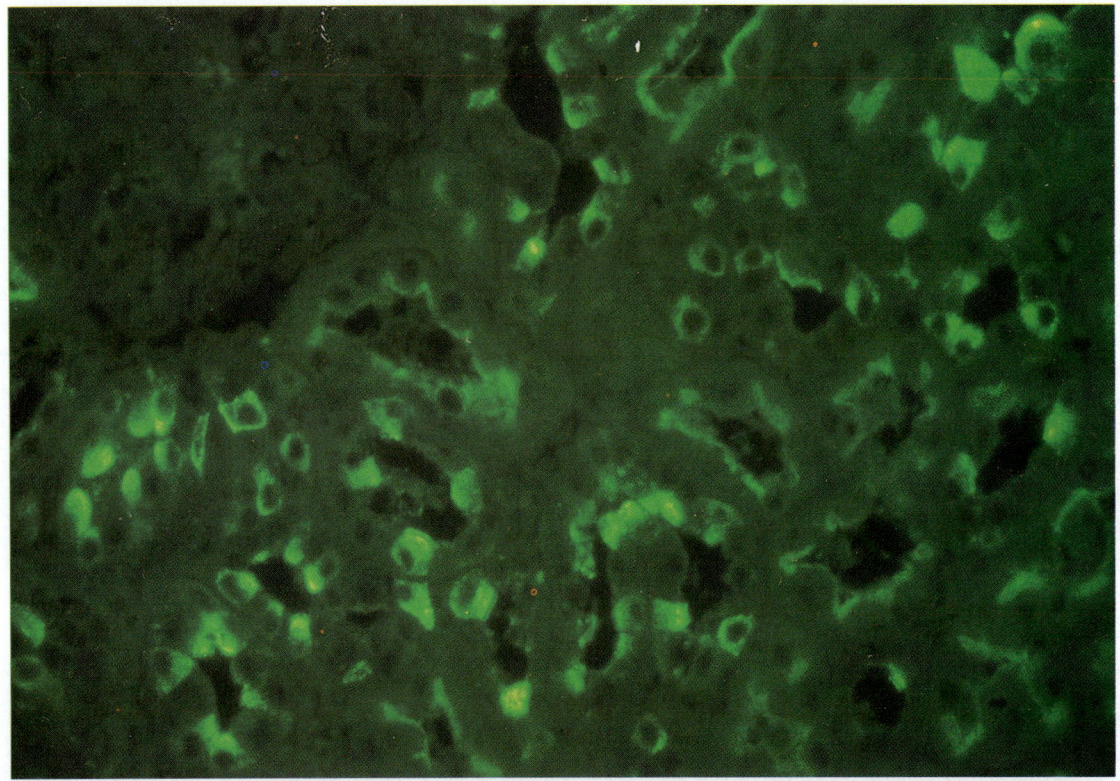

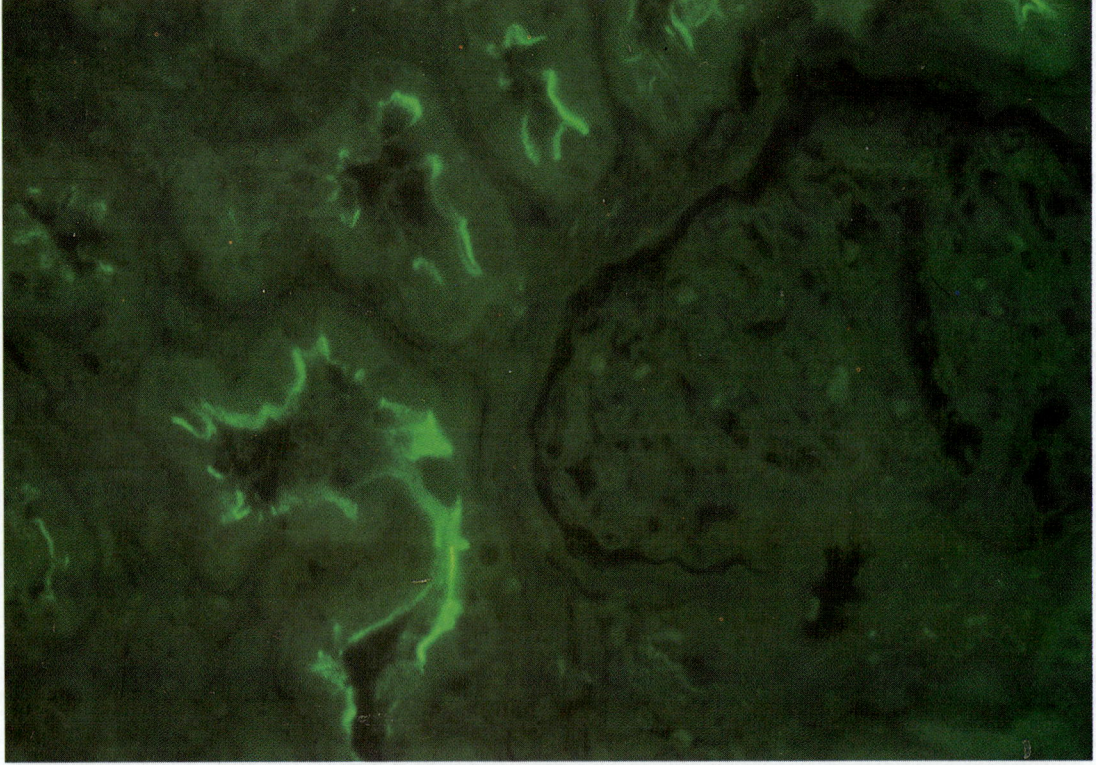

Figure 26.2   Anti-H⁺-ATPase immunofluorescence staining in normal human kidney (a), and in the renal biopsy of a patient with Sjögren's syndrome (case 26.10) (b). Note the lack of immunofluorescence in the intercalated cells of (b). Photographs were kindly provided by Dr B. Bastani.

present with paralysis, associated with severe metabolic acidosis. In case 26.11, the patient had undergone extensive neurological investigations for muscle weakness, prior to being transferred to our hospital following sudden collapse. With K$^+$ replacement therapy, she improved rapidly and has remained symptom-free. In contrast to these dramatic presentations, the patient with nephrolithiasis (case 26.12) was neither acidotic nor hypokalemic and, indeed, the diagnosis of distal RTA was not evident until a formal NH$_4$Cl challenge test was performed. In this case, the urine pH did not fall below 6.3 while the plasma [HCO$_3^-$] and blood pH decreased as a result of acid loading. There was failure of urine acidification (urine pH should fall below 5.5) with the induced metabolic acidosis. These cases highlight the spectrum of clinical presentations accompanying patients with distal RTA: patients with recurrent nephrolithiasis may have an underlying distal acidification defect that is not evident on first inspection.

Hyperkalemic distal RTA

In 1958 Lathem [29] described four patients with chronic pyelonephritis who presented with hyperchloremic metabolic acidosis, associated with hyperkalemia and acidic urine pH. The severity of acidosis and hyperkalemia was out of proportion to the degree of renal insufficiency in these patients. Subsequently, the presence of hyperkalemia in various forms of distal RTA has been well documented (Table 26.4). Hyperkalemia implies that mineralocorticoid is deficient or unable to act or that some process is interfering with the ability of the distal nephron to generate and maintain a lumen-negative electrical potential difference.

Aldosterone deficiency is the most frequent etiology of hyperkalemic metabolic acidosis in adults. This is usually in the form of hyporeninemic hypoaldosteronism and is associated with diabetic nephropathy and tubulointerstitial nephritis. Mild to moderate renal insufficiency is usually present. These patients are able to lower urine pH below 5.5. At least part of the problem is an inability of the adrenal cortex to respond appropriately to hyperkalemia by increasing aldosterone secretion. Aldosterone deficiency leads to impaired distal nephron H$^+$-ATPase activity. In addition, hyperkalemia inhibits ammoniagenesis, making it easier to lower urine pH, if some ability to secrete H$^+$ is retained. Both aldosterone deficiency and resistance have been described in patients with sickle cell disease and sickle cell trait presenting as hyperkalemic distal RTA [30].

Several disorders have been referred to as 'voltage-dependent' causes of hyperkalemic distal RTA, due to presumed primary inability to generate lumen-negative potential difference in the cortical collecting duct. In Gordon's syndrome, there is increased distal nephron permeability to Cl$^-$, which causes dissipation of the lumen-negative potential difference, and inhibits both H$^+$ and K$^+$ secretion. The patients are volume expanded and hypertensive and have suppressed renin–aldosterone systems. The syndrome may be familial and is associated with abnormal facies, short stature and intellectual impairment [24].

Obstructive uropathy, amiloride and lithium are considered classic causes of voltage-dependent distal RTA. With obstruction or amiloride, there is an inability to lower urine pH below 5.5, whereas in the nephropathy from lithium administration, urine can be rendered acidic with infusion. Recent information suggests that the pathogenesis of these disorders is more complex than previously thought.

In unilateral ureteral obstruction in rats, H$^+$-ATPase activity is decreased in both the cortical (CCT) and medullary (MCT) collecting tubules, whereas H$^+$,K$^+$-ATPase activity is increased in CCT and decreased in MCT [31]. Immunocytochemistry reveals an abnormal distribution of H$^+$-ATPase within the intercalated cells in kidneys of postobstructed rats [32]. Since the MCT is not a site of Na$^+$-dependent urine acidification, the defect in H$^+$-ATPase cannot be ascribed to a voltage-dependent mechanism. In the CCT, however, obstruction may lead to impaired reabsorption of Na$^+$ since Na$^+$,K$^+$-ATPase activity is suppressed, and this would further impair luminal acidification [31].

Amiloride administration in rats decreases H$^+$-ATPase activity, but only in the CCT. It inhibits Na$^+$ channels in the CCT and Na$^+$,K$^+$-ATPase in cortex and medulla, yet has no effect on H$^+$,K$^+$-ATPase activity.

In contrast to urinary tract obstruction and amiloride, the distal RTA of lithium administration is not usually accompanied by hyperkalemia. Lithium inhibits renal H$^+$-ATPase and H$^+$,K$^+$-ATPase. Decreased H$^+$,K$^+$-ATPase activity may prevent development of hyperkalemia with this agent.

Drugs as causes of hyperkalemic distal RTA

In addition to amiloride, other drugs cause hyperkalemic distal RTA, most commonly in patients who are elderly or have underlying renal insufficiency. Angiotensin converting enzyme inhibitors decrease plasma aldosterone levels, whereas K$^+$-sparing diuretics directly inhibit the action of aldosterone at the level of the principal cell. In patients with cirrhosis and ascites, the use of spironolactone must be carefully monitored: the combination of impaired distal nephron Na$^+$ delivery and blockade of aldosterone action by this drug renders these patients particularly susceptible to develop hyperkalemic distal RTA.

The use of non-steroidal antiinflammatory drugs (NSAIDs) in patients with renal insufficiency may also induce hyperkalemic distal RTA. These agents inhibit prostaglandin synthesis, and lead to hyporeninemic hypoaldosteronism. NSAIDS also increase Na$^+$ reabsorption in the thick ascending limb of the loop of Henle, by blocking the inhibitory effect of prostaglandins, resulting in decreased distal delivery of Na$^+$, further impairing urinary acidification. Recently, development of acute renal failure and hyperkalemia was described in three patients following administration of the NSAID, ketorolac, for management of postoperative pain [33].

The use of high-dose trimethoprim in patients with AIDS is associated with development of hyperkalemic distal RTA. Velasquez *et al.* [34] examined this phenomenon in human subjects and experimental animals. Intratubular trimethoprim blocked distal nephron apical Na^+ channels, reducing the lumen-negative voltage, resembling the action of amiloride. Thus, the coexistence of hypoadrenalism and renal insufficiency in many patients with AIDS renders them particularly sensitive to developing hyperkalemia and metabolic acidosis from use of trimethoprim.

Diagnosis of distal RTA

Laboratory evaluation of a patient with distal RTA involves the following steps.

1 In any patient with normal anion gap metabolic acidosis, first determine if urinary NH_4^+ excretion is adequate. When metabolic acidosis is the result of an extrarenal process, the urine $[NH_4^+]$ will be high. Since measurements of urinary $[NH_4^+]$ are not readily available, an indirect method of measurement is a useful determination of the urinary anion gap [35, 36]. The urine anion gap (in mM) is defined as urine $[Na^+] + [K^+] - [Cl^-]$. In metabolic acidosis from diarrhea, for example, the urine anion gap has a negative value, signifying that an unmeasured cation (i.e. NH_4^+) is present. Patients with distal RTA syndromes typically have reduced NH_4^+ excretion, and the sum of urine $[Na^+] + [K^+]$ usually exceeds urine $[Cl^-]$. Thus, in metabolic acidosis, when the urine anion gap has a positive value, urine excretion of NH_4^+ is insufficient.

Occasionally, the urine anion gap does not reflect the $[NH_4^+]$. This occurs when large quantities of unmeasured anions are excreted in the urine (ketoacidosis, toluene ingestion, negatively charged drugs). In these instances, one can calculate the urine osmolality, and subtract this from the measured osmolality. Calculated osmolality = $[urea] + [glucose] + 2 \times ([Na^+] + [K^+])$ (in mM). The difference is the urine osmolal gap.

$$\text{Urine osmolal gap} = \text{measured urine osmolality} - \text{calculated urine osmolality}$$

Because the urine osmolal gap consists of NH_4^+ and an equal number of anions, the quantity of NH_4^+, if accompanied by a monovalent anion, is half the difference of the measured and calculated osmolalities.

$$NH_4^+ \text{ excretion} = 0.5 \times (\text{measured osmolality} - \text{calculated osmolality})$$

2 Rule out proximal RTA. An alkaline urinary pH (>7.0) is diagnostic of proximal RTA. If urine is not alkaline, administer HCO_3^- until the urine pH exceeds 7.4. If the plasma $[HCO_3^-]$ is below normal at this point and the frac-

tional excretion of HCO_3^- exceeds 15%, the patient has proximal RTA. If the plasma HCO_3^- returns to normal before the urine pH becomes alkaline, proximal RTA is not present.

3 Patients with classical distal RTA (problem with H^+ secretion) typically have urine pH exceeding 5.5 and hypokalemia. A low urine pH with hyperkalemia signifies that the major defect is impaired ammoniagenesis or NH_3 secretion in the collecting duct. Measurement of aldosterone and renin levels is helpful in these instances.

4 When the patient is not acidotic (plasma $[HCO_3^-] > 24$ mM), as in the patient with nephrolithiasis and medullary sponge kidney disease (case 26.12), the diagnosis of a distal acidification defect requires oral acid loading with NH_4Cl (0.1 g/kg). Urine pH is measured sequentially between 2 and 8 h after acid loading. With a distal acidification defect, the urine pH will not decrease below 5.5 despite induction of systemic acidosis.

Treatment of distal RTA

Alkalinizing agents are the mainstays of treatment for distal RTA. Alkali may be administered as $NaHCO_3$ (1–2 mEq/kg/day), or as sodium citrate solution, if there is gastric intolerance to $NaHCO_3$. Correction of acidosis improves hypokalemia and increases urinary citrate excretion, thus preventing further nephrocalcinosis. Profound K^+ depletion requires K^+ supplementation. In hyperkalemic distal RTA, correction of the acidosis promotes K^+ movement into cells and K^+ excretion. Furosemide may be required in cases of ECF volume expansion or hypertension. Some patients respond to treatment with mineralocorticoid (fludrocortisone 0.5–2 mg/day). This is best achieved in combination with furosemide to prevent fluid overload and severe hypertension. Patients with Gordon's syndrome respond well to thiazide diuretics, which control blood pressure and hyperkalemia. Alkalinizing agents are occasionally required as well.

RTA in renal transplant patients

Hyperchloremic metabolic acidosis is the most common acid–base disturbance in renal transplant patients. Several disorders can be classified into those occurring early post-transplant, and those in longstanding renal allografts (Table 26.6). In the first few weeks after transplantation, proximal RTA can occur, with urinary HCO_3^- wasting due to resolving secondary hyperparathyroidism. This defect typically resolves within a few months. The Fanconi syndrome has been described after transplant surgery [37, 38], and also appears to be transient.

Acute tubular necrosis (delayed graft function) is not uncommon in the early post-transplant period. In these cases, the capacity of the distal nephron to acidify the urine may lag behind recovery of GFR, causing a temporary hyperchloremic metabolic acidosis. In long-standing renal transplants, chronic allograft rejection may be

Table 26.6 RTA syndromes in renal transplantation

Early
Associated with recovery from acute tubular necrosis
Selective proximal HCO_3^- wasting
Fanconi syndrome
Associated with resolving secondary
   hyperparathyroidism
Acute rejection (distal RTA)

Late (>6 months)
Acute and chronic allograft rejection (H^+ secretory
   defect)
Cyclosporin A toxicity (hyperkalemic distal RTA)

accompanied by distal RTA [39]. Distal RTA is also associated with acute allograft rejection in the early post-transplant period. In patients with chronic rejection and distal RTA, distal H^+ secretion is defective. Renal biopsy reveals interstitial mononuclear cell infiltrates, resembling those of patients with Sjögren's syndrome or hypergammablobulinemia. It is interesting to speculate that, as in Sjögren's syndrome, there may be deficient H^+-ATPase activity in chronic rejection. Aldosterone deficiency and hyperkalemia have been reported, however.

Cyclosporin A induces distal RTA in up to 20% of renal transplant recipients. These patients typically have hyporeninemic hypoaldosteronism and present with hyperkalemic distal RTA [40]. Distal tubular response to aldosterone may be impaired and data suggest augmented distal Cl^- reabsorption is a pathogenetic mechanism in some patients [41]. Adjustment of the cyclosporin A dose and administration of thiazides or loop diuretics are the mainstays of therapy.

In the authors' renal transplant population, development of RTA has been unusual. In a retrospective study of 38 renal transplant patients, all treated with cyclosporin A, at the time of discharge from hospital post-transplant, 8/38 patients (21%) had mild hyperchloremic metabolic acidosis, with plasma $[HCO_3^-] < 20$ mM, out of proportion to any degree of renal dysfunction. By six months post-transplant, no patient in this group had metabolic acidosis. *De novo* normal anion gap metabolic acidosis developed in 5/38 patients (13%), at 1–6 months post-transplant. Two of these patients continued to have plasma $[HCO_3^-] < 20$ mM at 12 months, associated with mild hyperkalemia. Base supplements were not required in any other patients.

In our center, serious acid–base disturbances in renal transplant patients are infrequent. In patients with persistent proven distal RTA, however, one should suspect chronic rejection or cyclosporin A toxicity.

References

1. Kraut, J.A. and Madias, N.E. (1995) Approach to the diagnosis of acid–base disrrders, in *Textbook of Nephrology*, 3rd edn (eds S.G. Massry and R.J. Glassock), Williams & Wilkins, Baltimore, pp. 487–93.

2. Halperin, M.L. and Goldstein, M.B. (1994) *Fluid, Electrolyte and Acid Base Physiology: A Problem-based Approach*. W.B. Saunders, Philadelphia.

3. Salem, M.M. and Batlle, D.C. (1995) Metabolic acidosis, in *Textbook of Nephrology*, 3rd edn (eds S.G. Massry and R.J. Glassock), Williams & Wilkins, Baltimore.

4. Harris, R.C., Seifter, J.L. and Brenner, B.M. (1984) Adaptation of Na^+-H^+ exchange in renal microvillus vesicles: role of dietary protein and uninephrectomy. *J. Clin. Invest.*, **74**, 1979–87.

5. Cohn, D.E., Klahr, S. and Hammerman, M.R. (1982) Increased Na^+–H^+ exchange in brush border vesicles from dogs with renal failure. *Am. J. Physiol.*, **243**, F293–9.

6. Buerkert, J., Martin, D., Trigg, D. *et al.* (1983) Effect of reduced renal mass on ammonium handling and net acid formation by the superficial and juxtamedullary nephron of the rat. Evidence for impaired reentrapment rather than decreased production of ammonium in the acidosis of uremia. *J. Clin. Invest.*, **71**, 1661–75.

7. Zalups, R.K., Stanton, B.A., Wade, J.B. *et al.* (1985) Structural adaptation in initial collecting tubule following reduction in renal mass. *Kidney Int.*, **27**, 636–42.

8. Kunau, R.T. and Walker, K.A. (1990) Distal tubule acidification in the remnant kidney. *Am. J. Physiol.*, **258**, F69–74.

9. Hamm, L.L., Hering-Smith, K.S. and Vehaskari, V.M. (1989) Control of bicarbonate transport in collecting tubules from normal and remnant kidneys. *Am. J. Physiol.*, **256**, F680–7.

10. Widmer, B., Gerhardt, R.E., Harrington, J.T. *et al.* (1979) Serum electrolyte and acid base composition: the influence of graded degrees of chronic renal failure. *Arch. Intern. Med.*, **139**, 1099–102.

11. Levine, D.Z. (1990) Acid–base complications induced by diuretics, in *Diuretics III: Chemistry, Pharmacology, and Clinical Applications* (eds J.B. Puschett and A. Greenberg), Elsevier, Amsterdam, pp. 228–34.

12. Eiam-ong, S. and Kurtzman, N.A. (1994) Metabolic acidosis and bone disease. *Miner. Electrolyte Metab.*, **20**, 72–80.

13. Mautalen, C., Montoreano, R. and Laberre, C. (1976) Early skeletal effect of alkali therapy upon the osteomalacia of renal tubule acidosis. *J. Clin. Endocrinol. Metab.*, **42**, 875–81.

14. McSherry, E. and Morris, R.C., Jr (1978) Attainment and maintenance of normal stature with alkali therapy in infants and children with classic renal tubular acidosis. *J. Clin. Invest.*, **61**, 509–27.

15. Lu, K.C., Shieh, S.D., Li, B.L. *et al.* (1994) Rapid correction of metabolic acidosis in chronic renal failure: effect on parathyroid hormone activity. *Nephron*, **67**, 419–24.

16. Price, S.R. and Mitch, W.E. (1994) Metabolic acidosis and uremic toxicity: protein and amino acid metabolism. *Semin. Nephrol.*, **14**, 232–7.

17. Reaich, D., Channon, S.M., Scrimgeour, C.M. *et al.* (1993) Correction of acidosis in humans with chronic renal failure decreases protein degradation and amino acid oxidation. *Am. J. Physiol.*, **265**, E230–5.

18. Narins, R.G. and Cohen, J.J. (1987) Bicarbonate therapy for organic acidoses: the case for its continued use. *Ann. Intern. Med.*, **106**, 615–18.

19. Graf, H., Leach, W. and Arieff, A.I. (1985) Evidence for detrimental effect of bicarbonate therapy in hypoxic lactic acidosis. *Science*, **227**, 754–6.

20. Arieff, A.I. (1991) Indications for use of bicarbonate in patients with metabolic acidosis. *Br. J. Anaesth.*, **67**, 165–77.

21. Gennari, F.J. and Rimmer, J.M. (1991) Acid–base disorders in renal failure. *Cont. Management Crit. Care*, **1**, 117–35.

22. Eiam-ong, S. and Kurtzman, N.A. (1995) Renal tubular acidosis, in *Texbook of Nephrology*, 3rd edn (eds S.G. Massry and R.J. Glassock), Williams & Wilkins, Baltimore, pp. 457–69.

23. Halperin, M.L., Kamel, K.S., Ethier, J.H. *et al.* (1989) What is the underlying defect in patients with isolated, proximal renal tubular acidosis? *Am. J. Nephrol.*, **9**, 265–8.

24. Arruda, J.A.L. and Cowell, G. (1994) Distal renal tubular acidosis: molecular and clinical aspects. *Hosp. Pract.*, **15**, 75–88.

25. Lash, J.P. and Arruda, J.A.L. (1993) Laboratory evaluation of renal tubular acidosis. *Clin. Lab. Med.*, **13**, 117–29.

26. Levine, D.Z. and Burns, K.D. (1997) Acid–base disorders in azotemic patients, in *Caring for the Renal Patient* (ed. D.Z. Levine), W.B. Saunders, Philadelphia, pp. 50–60.

27. Cohen, E.P., Bastani, B., Cohen, M.R. *et al.* (1992) Absence of H^+-ATPase in cortical collecting tubules of a patient with Sjogren's syndrome and distal renal tubular acidosis. *J. Am. Soc. Nephrol.*, **3**, 264–71.

27a.Dafnis, E., Spohn, M., Lonis, B. *et al.* (1992) Vanadate causes hypokalemic distal renal tubular acidosis. *Am. J. Physiol.*, **262**, F449–53.

28. Nilwarangkur, S., Nimmannit, S., Chaovakul, V. *et al.* (1990) Endemic primary distal renal tubular acidosis in Thailand. *Q. J. Med.*, **74**, 289–301.

29. Lathem, W. (1958) Hyperchloremic acidosis in chronic pyelonephritis. *N. Engl. J. Med.*, **258**, 1031–6.

30. Batlle, D., Itsarayoungyuen, K., Arruda, J.A.L. *et al.* (1982) Hyperkalemic hyperchloremic metabolic acidosis in sickle cell hemoglobinopathies. *Am. J. Med.*, **72**, 188–92.

31. Eiam-ong, S., Dafnis, E., Spohn, M. *et al.* (1993) H^+-K^+-ATPase in distal renal tubular acidosis: urinary tract obstruction, lithium, and amiloride. *Am. J. Physiol.*, **265**, F875–80.

32. Purcell, H., Bastani, B., Harris, K.P.G. *et al.* (1991) The cellular distribution of H^+-ATPase following acute unilateral ureteral obstruction in rats. *Am. J. Physiol.*, **261**, F365–7.

33. Haragism, L., Dalal, R., Bagga, H. *et al.* (1994) Ketorolac-induced acute renal failure and hyperkalemia: report of three cases. *Am. J. Kidney Dis.*, **24**, 578–80.

34. Velazquez, H., Perazella, M.A., Wright, F.S. *et al.* (1993) Renal mechanisms of trimethoprim-induced hyperkalemia. *Ann. Intern. Med.*, **119**, 296–301.

35. Batlle, D.C., Hizon, M., Cohen, E. *et al.* (1988) The use of the urinary anion gap in the diagnosis of hyperchloremic metabolic acidosis. *N. Engl. J. Med.*, **318**, 594–9.

36. Goldstein, M.B., Bear, R., Richardson, R.M.A. *et al.* (1986) The urine anion gap: a clinically useful index of ammonium excretion. *Am. J. Med. Sci.*, **292**, 198–202.

37. Massry, S.G., Preuss, H.G., Maher, J.F. *et al.* (1967) Renal tubular acidosis after cadaver kidney homotransplantation. *Am. J. Med.*, **42**, 284–92.

38. Vertuno, L.L., Preuss, H.G., Argy, W.P. *et al.* (1974) Fanconi syndrome following homotransplantation. *Arch. Intern. Med.*, **133**, 302–5.

39. Batlle, D.C., Mozes, M.F., Manaligod, J. *et al.* (1981) The pathogenesis of hyperchloremic metabolic acidosis associated with kidney transplantation. *Am. J. Med.*, **70**, 786–96.

40. Adu, D., Turney, J., Michael, J. *et al.* (1983) Hyperkalemia in cyclosporine-treated renal allograft recipients. *Lancet*, **ii**, 370–2.

41. Stahl, R.A.K., Kanz, L., Maier, B. *et al.* (1986) Hyperchloremic metabolic acidosis with high serum potassium in renal transplant recipients: a cyclosporine A-associated side effect. *Clin. Nephrol.*, **25**, 245–8.

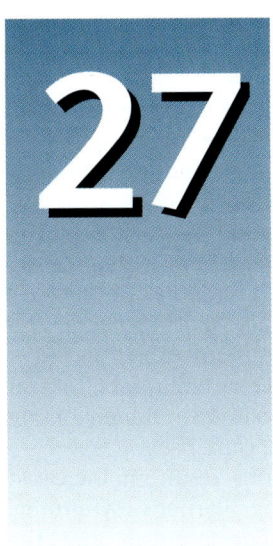

27

Magnesium disorders

Christopher J. Lote

Introduction

Magnesium is the second most abundant intracellular cation. A 70 kg adult contains about 25 g of magnesium. Only a small proportion of this (about 2.5%) is in the extracellular fluid; over 60% of the total body magnesium is in bone, and most of the rest is in muscle. The normal plasma concentration of magnesium is 0.9 mmol/l, of which about 20% is protein-bound. The clinical symptoms associated with magnesium disorders correlate well with the plasma magnesium concentration.

On a diet containing the normal magnesium content (300 mg/day), about 40% of the magnesium intake is absorbed, although absorption is higher (70%) in children. Urinary magnesium is typically 100–150 mg/day. With a high-magnesium diet (e.g. containing magnesium-based antacids), urinary excretion may be 600 mg/day or more, with no change in the plasma magnesium concentration. In both adults and children, the fraction of magnesium absorbed by the gastrointestinal tract increases when dietary magnesium is restricted, i.e. fractional magnesium absorption varies inversely with intake.

Gastrointestinal magnesium absorption occurs primarily in the distal small intestine (i.e. jejunum and ileum), so magnesium deficiency is common after surgical resection of the ileum.

Hypomagnesemia

Clinical manifestation of the disorder

Experimental magnesium depletion was first described in rats, in 1932 [1]. Within 5–7 days of the initiation of a magnesium-deficient diet, the rats had peripheral vasodilatation which was followed by seizures many of which were fatal. In 1960, a clearly defined group of hypomagnesemic patients was investigated [2]; they had tetany, and three (of five) had convulsions. A later study [3] showed that hypomagnesemic human subjects also have generalized weakness, anorexia, nausea and apathy, and are hypokalemic and hypocalcemic. There may be generalized tetany and the central nervous system symptoms can include delirium and psychoses.

Pathophysiology

The various causes of hypomagnesemia are listed in Table 27.1. The kidneys can be the cause of hypomagnesemia, or may be involved homeostatically in attempting to correct hypomagnesemia of other causes. When renal function is normal, renal homeostatic adjustments to maintain magnesium balance are rapid. If the dietary intake of magnesium is reduced to less than 50 mg/day, urinary magnesium excretion decreases within hours, and within a week is less than 12 mg/day. This rapid renal response represents magnesium reabsorption in the cells of the thick ascending limb of the loop of Henle (TALH) [4].

Nephrology, Edited by Rex L. Jamison and Robert Wilkinson.
Published in 1997 by Chapman & Hall, London. ISBN 0 412 60930 4

Table 27.1 Causes of magnesium disturbances

Hypomagnesemia	Hypermagnesemia
Gastrointestinal tract	
Decreased dietary Mg	Excessive dietary Mg (usually only possible in renal failure)
Severe diarrhea	Magnesium infusion (e.g. in treatment of eclampsia)
Steatorrhea	
Selective Mg malabsorption	
High dietary phosphate	
Intrinsic renal	
Acute tubular necrosis (diuretic phase)	Renal failure (with anuria or oliguria)
Familial Mg loss	
Bartter's syndrome	
Extrinsic renal	
Drugs	Drugs
Alcohol	
Diuretics	
Aminoglycosides	Mg-containing antacids
Cisplatin	Mg-containing cathartics
Cyclosporin	
Hypernatremia	
Hypercalciuria	
Hyperaldosteronism	Adrenal insufficiency
Ketoacidosis	
Inappropriate ADH secretion	
Severe burns	
Volume expansion	

When the kidney is the cause of hypomagnesemia, this may be due to a defect in renal function *per se*, or to drugs or other conditions altering renal function. Primary renal magnesium wasting can be a congenital condition, or may be acquired. A number of genetic disorders can influence magnesium excretion. Gitelman's syndrome, caused by a defect in the gene coding for the thiazide-sensitive sodium-chloride cotransporter [4a], is characterised by hypermagnesuric hypomagnesemia. About 20% of Bartter's syndrome patients also have hypermagnesuria, although there is considerable genetic heterogeneity in this syndrome [4b]. Acquired magnesium wasting is generally due to drugs. Aminoglycosides and cisplatinum (cisdichloradiamine platinum) induce renal magnesium loss as a consequence of tubule damage, and the defect can persist for months. Cyclosporin can also cause impaired renal magnesium absorption and hypomagnesemia [5, 5a].

Diuretics, with the exception of acetazolamide, all increase magnesium excretion. Since the majority of diuretics are short acting, they rarely induce hypomagnesemia, but thiazides can do so [5].

Because the tubular reabsorption of magnesium is associated with absorption of other cations (Chapter 10), disorders or abnormalities in the excretion of other ions can influence magnesium balance. Both sodium and calcium infusions increase magnesium excretion. So if saline infusions are given, together with diuretics, to treat hypercalcemia, then three magnesuric stimuli are acting in concert, and hypomagnesemia can ensue.

Several other disease conditions result in increased magnesium excretion, including Bartter's syndrome, primary and secondary hyperaldosteronism and the syndrome of inappropriate ADH secretion [6]. Insulin increases renal magnesium excretion, and this could explain the magnesium depletion sometimes observed in a number of hyperinsulinemic conditions [5b].

Hypomagnesemia also occurs as a consequence of starvation. This is generally not directly due to low magnesium intake, but occurs as a result of a large urinary loss of magnesium (typically 100–150 mg/day). It is likely that this is a consequence of a combination of two factors, ketoacidosis, and phosphate depletion. High urinary magnesium excretion also occurs in patients with diabetic ketoacidosis. It is not clear exactly how ketoacidosis leads to hypermagnesuria. Factors which could be involved are the complexing of magnesium with acetoacetate and, in diabetic ketosis, the osmotic diuretic effect of glycosuria [7].

One of the commonest causes of hypomagnesemia is excessive alcohol intake. As in the case of starvation, the problem is not primarily that of reduced magnesium intake, but excessive urinary magnesium loss. Ethanol acutely increases urinary magnesium excretion, but only if the plasma ethanol concentration is increasing. The chronic urinary loss of magnesium in alcoholic subjects is likely to be due to ketoacidsosis and to phosphate depletion [8].

Severe magnesium depletion is almost invariably associated with hypokalemia as a result of a large urinary potassium loss. This interaction between magnesium balance and potassium balance is poorly understood, since a major site of potassium excretion regulation in the nephron is the distal tubule and collecting tubule, which play no significant part in magnesium reabsorption.

Consequences of hypomagnesemia

There is a complex relationship between calcium homeostasis and magnesium homeostasis, such that hypomagnesemia is one of the commonest causes of hypocalcemia [7]. If either the plasma magnesium or calcium concentration is increased, there is inhibition of magnesium transport in the TALH [9, 10]. These effects are demonstrable in isolated perfused tubules, and are not due to hormonal changes, but are also not due to calcium and magnesium sharing a common transport process [10, 11]. They may be attributable to the effects of calcium on epithelial tight junctions [12], whereby Ca^{2+} binds to fixed negative charges in the paracellular pathways, and hence decreases the ability of Mg^{2+} to traverse the pathway [13].

Both magnesium and calcium have direct effects on parathyroid hormone (PTH) secretion, with PTH secretion being stimulated by decreased plasma concentrations of either ion. Indeed, it is the combined concentrations of calcium and magnesium which appears to determine PTH secretion. If there is an experimentally induced decrease in the plasma concentration of one of the ions, with a corresponding increase in concentration of the other, PTH secretion does not change [7, 14].

In contrast to the above acute studies, there is evidence that chronic magnesium depletion reduces PTH secretion, and leads to a diminished PTH response to hypocalcemia [15]. However, not all hypomagnesemic patients have decreased PTH but they do all tend to have hypocalcemia.

There is a similarly confusing picture with regard to vitamin D. Hypomagnesemia-induced hypocalcemia leads to decreased plasma levels of 1,25 $(OH)_2$ vitamin D_3 [16]. However, the hypocalcemia responds rapidly to replacement of magnesium, whereas the low 1,25 $(OH)_2$ D_3 level does not [7]. The low level of 1,25 $(OH)_2$ D_3 is not due to failure of conversion of 25 (OH) D_3 to 1,25 $(OH)_2$ D_3, and its cause is at present not clear.

As mentioned earlier, another consequence of hypomagnesemia is potassium depletion. When potassium-losing diuretics are administered, it is often not possible to restore normokalemia simply by administering potassium. Magnesium must also be given. Alfrey [7] has pointed out that under a variety of conditions it is only possible to replete intracellular deficits of magnesium and potassium by giving the ions together, whether the deficiency resulted from either primary potassium or magnesium depletion.

Diagnosis and treatment of hypomagnesemia

The plasma magnesium concentration is normally 0.9 mmol/l (1.8 mEq/l). Symptoms of hypomagnesemia become apparent at plasma magnesium concentrations of less than 0.5 mmol/l. Generally, a normal diet will restore magnesium to normal when plasma magnesium is above 0.5 mmol/l. However, patients with magnesium wasting (e.g. of gastrointestinal or renal origin) may require oral supplementary magnesium, usually up to 500 mg (20 mmol) Mg, four times daily, as magnesium oxide.

Hypomagnesemia with plasma magnesium below 0.5 mmol/l should be treated by intravenous or intramuscular magnesium, but close monitoring of the plasma magnesium is necessary, particularly in patients with reduced renal function. A typical intramuscular dosage would be 2 ml of 50% $MgSO_4$ (delivering 4 mmol Mg), administered 4 hourly for 4–6 doses. For small children (below 6 kg), the dose would be 0.5 ml of 50% $MgSO_4$ (1 mmol Mg), administered as a single dose with subsequent monitoring of plasma magnesium.

Intravenous magnesium (which should not be used in children) can be administered in a variety of ways; e.g. 12 ml of 50% $MgSO_4$ (containing 24 mmol Mg) can be added to 1 l of dextrose infusion and administered over 3–5 h [17].

Hypermagnesemia

Clinical manifestations of the disorder

In general, no symptoms of hypermagnesemia appear until the plasma magnesium concentration is over 4 mmol/l (i.e. more than four times the normal value), when neuromuscular symptoms become apparent (i.e. deep-tendon reflexes are depressed). At plasma concentrations of magnesium in excess of 5 mmol/l a flaccid quadriplegia develops, with deep-tendon reflexes absent. There is also lethargy, nausea, papillary dilatation and respiratory depression. Hypotension and bradycardia occur and complete cardiac arrest is possible [18].

Pathophysiology

Hypermagnesemia often occurs as a consequence of adrenal insufficiency [19], and in advanced renal failure [20]. In the latter, impaired magnesium excretion with maintained dietary intake, and in some cases the use of magnesium-containing antacids or cathartics [5], leads to rapid accumulation of magnesium. Most dialysis fluids contain magnesium in a concentration of 1–2.5 mmol/l, which generally maintains a normal plasma magnesium concentration, but may lead to increased intracellular levels.

Chronic hypermagnesemia as a consequence exclusively of renal failure is rare. It usually occurs when a renally compromised patient is given an exogenous load of magnesium.

Diagnosis and treatment of hypermagnesemia

There are generally no symptoms of hypermagnesemia until the plasma magnesium is about 4 mmol/l. The main risk factor for the development of hypermagnesemia is magnesium administration, either parenterally (e.g. for the treatment of eclampsia) or orally (e.g. in patients with reduced renal function receiving magnesium-containing laxatives or antacids. Treatment in such circumstances consists of discontinuing any magnesium administration.

If there is respiratory depression or cardiac arrhythmia, calcium administration (2–2.5 mmol i.v.) alleviates the symptoms. Renal magnesium excretion can be enhanced by giving furosemide (with saline to maintain diuresis). In patients with severe renal impairment, dialysis using a magnesium-free dialysate is the best treatment.

References

1. Kruse, H.D., Orent, E.R. and McCollum, E.V. (1932) Studies on magnesium deficiency in animals: symptomatology resulting from magnesium deprivation. *J. Biol. Chem.*, **96**, 519–39.
2. Vallee, B., Wacker, W.E. and Ulmer, D.D. (1960) The magnesium deficiency tetany syndrome in man. *N. Engl. J. Med.*, **262**, 155–61.
3. Shils, M.E. (1964) Experimental human magnesium depletion. I. Clinical observations and blood chemistry alterations. *Am. J. Clin. Nutr.*, **15**, 133–43.
4. Gitelman, H.J. and Welt, L.G. (1969) Magnesium deficiency. *Am. Rev. Med.*, **20**, 233–42.
4a. Simon, D.B. and Lifton, R.P. (1996) The molecular basis of inherited hypokalemic alkalosis: Bartter's and Gitelman's syndromes. *Am. J. Physiol.*, **271**, F961–6.
4b. Simon, D.B., Koret, F.E., Rodriguez-Soriano, J. *et al.* (1996) Genetic heterogeneity of Bartter's syndrome revealed by mutations in the K$^+$-channel, ROMK. *Nature Genet.*, **14**, 152–6.
5. Dirks, J.H. and Alfrey, A.C. (1986) Normal and abnormal magnesium metabolism, in *Renal and Electrolyte Disorders*, 3rd edn (ed. R.W. Shrier), Little, Brown, New York, pp. 331–59.
5a. Rob, P.M., Lebeau, A., Nobiling, R. *et al.* (1996) Magnesium metabolism: Basic aspects and implications of ciclosporine toxicity in rats. *Nephron*, **72**, 59–66.
5b. Djurhuus, M.S., Skott, P., Hothernielsen, O. *et al.* (1995) Insulin increases renal magnesium excretion – a possible cause of magnesium depletion in hyperinsulinaemic states. *Diabetic Medicine*, **12**, 664–9.
6. Alfrey, A.C., Terman, D.S., Brettschneider, L. *et al.* (1970) Hypermagnesemia after renal homotransplantation. *Ann. Intern. Med.*, **73**, 367–71.
7. Alfrey, A.C. (1992) Disorders of magnesium metabolism, in *The Kidney: Physiology and Pathophysiology*, 2nd edn (eds D.W. Seldin and G. Giebisch), Raven Press, New York, pp. 2357–73.
8. Wong, N.L.M., Quamme, G.A., Sutton, R.A.L. *et al.* (1980) Renal and tubular transport in phosphate depletion: a micropuncture study. *Can. J. Physiol. Pharmacol.*, **58**, 1063–71.
9. Le Grimellec, C., Roinel, N. and Morel, F. (1974) Simultaneous Mg, Ca, P, K, Na and Cl analysis in rat tubular fluid. III During acute Ca plasma loading. *Pflugers Arch.*, **346**, 171–89.
10. Quamme, G.A. (1982) Effect of hypercalcemia on renal tubular handling of calcium and magnesium. *Can. J. Physiol. Pharmacol.*, **60**, 1275–80.
11. Quamme, G.A. and Dirks, H.J. (1980) Effect of intraluminal and contraluminal magnesium on magnesium and calcium transfer in the rat nephron. *Am. J. Physiol.*, **238**, 187–98.
12. Quamme, G.A. (1992) Magnesium: cellular and renal exchanges, in *The Kidney: Physiology and Pathophysiology*, 2nd edn (eds D.W. Seldin and G. Giebisch), Raven Press, New York, pp. 2339–55.
13. Wright, E.M. and Diamond, J.M. (1968) Effects of pH and polyvalent cations on the selective permeability of gall-bladder epithelium to monovalent ions. *Biochim. Biophys. Acta.*, **163**, 57–74.
14. Targounik, L.H., Rodman, J.S. and Sherwood, L.M. (1971) Regulation of parathyroid hormone secretion *in vitro*. Quantitative aspects of calcium and magnesium ion control. *Endocrinology*, **88**, 1477–82.
15. Anast, C.S., Winnacker, J.L., Forte, L.R. *et al.* (1976) Impaired release of parathyroid hormone in magnesium deficiency. *J. Clin. Endocrinol. Metab.*, **42**, 707–17.
16. Fuss, M., Cogan, E., Gillet, G. *et al.* (1985) Magnesium administration reverses the hypocalcaemia secondary to hypomagnesemia despite low circulating levels of 25-hydroxyvitamin D and 1.25 dihydroxy vitamin D. *Clin. Endocrinol.*, **22**, 807–15.
17. Flink, E.B. (1969) Therapy of magnesium deficiency. *Ann. NY Acad. Sci.*, **162**, 901–5.
18. Randall, R.E., Chen, M.D., Spray, C.C. and Rossmeisl, E.C. (1964) Hypermagnesemia in renal failure. *Ann. Intern. Med.*, **61**, 73–88.
19. Wacker, W.E. and Vallee, B.L. (1958) Magnesium metabolism. *N. Engl. J. Med.*, **259**, 431–8, 475–82.
20. Spencer, H., Lesniak, M., Gatzo, C.A. *et al.* (1980) Magnesium absorption and metabolism in patients with chronic renal failure and in patients with normal renal function. *Gastroenterology*, **79**, 26–34.

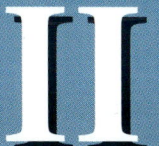

Impaired Renal Function

Section 3
Other Disorders
Secondary to Kidney
Disease

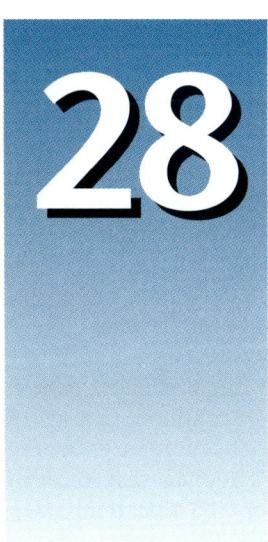

28

Proteinuria and the nephrotic syndrome

Bryan D. Myers

Introduction

A small amount of protein (usually less than 100 mg) is normally excreted in the urine of healthy subjects each day. Up to one-half is composed of plasma-derived proteins that have been filtered at the glomerulus and escaped reabsorption in the proximal tubule. Reflecting the fact that it is the most abundant protein in plasma, albumin is also the most abundant of the plasma-derived proteins in normal urine. The remainder of the protein excreted in normal urine is added beyond Bowman's space by the epithelial cells that line the tubules and the urinary tract. The most prominent of 'postglomerular' proteins is Tamm–Horsfall protein, a secretory product of distal tubule cells.

Clinical proteinuria is defined as a protein excretion rate in excess of 150 mg per 24 h. It represents the single most useful indicator of the presence of an injury to glomeruli. Such injury impairs the barrier to protein passage imposed by the walls of glomerular capillaries. A consequent enhancement of permeability to large plasma proteins elevates proteinuria into a pathological range and alters its composition such that albumin and other plasma-derived proteins account for >90% of the excreted protein.

Although proteinuria is usually a manifestation of glomerular injury, it should be borne in mind that it can also result from pathological processes not involving the glomerulus. For example, high circulating levels of pro-

teins that are produced by malignant clones of B cells or polymorphonuclear leukocytes can lead to substantial 'overflow' proteinuria. The secreted protein products of such cells (light chains and lysozyme, respectively) are readily filtered into Bowman's space by virtue of their small molecular size, notwithstanding a normal glomerular capillary wall. Another example is the presence of a defect in proximal tubule cells that prevents interiorization of the normal load of filtered protein, thereby permitting its escape into final urine, so-called 'tubular' proteinuria. A final example, and probably the commonest cause of 'non-glomerular' proteinuria, is that which results from infection of the urinary tract. Under these circumstances, proteinuria can result from either enhanced protein release from inflamed uroepithelial cells, or from local extravasation of serum proteins when the inflammation is hemorrhagic. Once these 'spurious' or non-glomerular causes of proteinuria have been excluded, however, the detection of an elevated urinary protein excretion rate should be regarded as signifying an alteration in the intrinsic barrier properties of glomerular capillary walls. Sometimes, such alterations are functional and lead only to transient proteinuria of modest proportions. More commonly, however, they result from structural disruption of the glomerular capillary wall by a disease process. Under these circumstances the proteinuria is likely to be sustained and can be substantial. It is the latter combination of findings that will be emphasized in the remainder of this chapter.

Nephrology, Edited by Rex L. Jamison and Robert Wilkinson.
Published in 1997 by Chapman & Hall, London. ISBN 0 412 60930 4

Detection and quantitation of proteinuria

Proteinuria is usually first detected by examining urine with a dipstick that has been impregnated with buffered tetrabromophenolphthalein. This indicator dye produces a graded color change (trace – 4+), which is proportional to the albumin concentration over a 20–2000 mg/l range. An older screening test that has withstood the test of time is the precipitation of protein by addition of 3% sulfonylsalicylic acid to urine. The turbidity that results is also graded on a scale of trace to 4+, and spans a similar concentration range to that detected by the dipstick. Once proteinuria has been detected by either of these screening methods, it should be quantified by more precise methods. This is best done by assay of total protein in a 24-h urine collection with the Biuret reagent. Knowledge of the level of proteinuria permits it to be classified into two broad categories, which are a useful guide to the subsequent evaluation of the proteinuric patient. Urinary protein losses in excess of 3.5 g/24 h are often associated with features of the nephrotic syndrome and hence known as nephrotic-range proteinuria. To avoid performing a 24 h urine collection, the urine protein : creatinine ratio (g/g) in a spot urine can be used as a surrogate. However, differential effects of diet, exercise, gender, posture and circadian rhythm on protein and creatinine excretion make this a less satisfactory measure than a timed excretion rate. In adults, creatinine excretion approximates 1 g per 24 h. Thus, a protein : creatinine ratio above 3.5 signifies nephrotic-range proteinuria. Lower levels of proteinuria are referred to as subnephrotic-range proteinuria. In most cases the latter does not result in symptoms or signs. Rather, it is typically detected either incidently during routine urinalysis of an otherwise asymptomatic patient, or coincidently during investigation of a patient who presents with other manifestations of renal disease, such as azotemia, hematuria or hypertension.

Clinical and laboratory manifestations of the nephrotic syndrome

Nephrotic-range proteinuria is attended by a constellation of abnormalities that are known collectively as the nephrotic syndrome. This includes a state of sodium retention, abnormalities that result from a profound alteration in the composition of the body protein pool, and a variable degree of renal insufficiency.

Features of nephrotic-range proteinuria

Schreiner [1] observed that manifestations of the nephrotic syndrome only became evident in patients with daily levels of proteinuria in excess of 3.5 g/24 h. Pro-teinuria in the overtly nephrotic subject is most likely to exceed this lower bound by a factor of 2 or 3, however. Immunochemical analysis of its composition shows that albumin accounts for >80% of the excreted protein. The second most copious of the excreted proteins is immunoglobulin G (IgG), which after albumin is the next most abundant protein in plasma.

Gross examination of nephrotic urine reveals it to be unusually frothy, and this early manifestation of the nephrotic syndrome may prompt an observant patient to seek medical advice. Another common feature of nephrotic-range proteinuria is an abundance in the urinary sediment of lipid-laden macrophages, or so-called 'oval fat bodies'. It has been proposed that lipid-laden macrophages represent a response to the uptake and processing of an enhanced load of filtered albumin by proximal tubule cells [2]. After processing, the free fatty acids normally transported by albumin are released and form complex lipids, which then permeate the basolateral cell membrane and enter the interstitium. They serve as chemoattractants for infiltrating macrophages. Once the macrophages have ingested the newly formed lipid, they find their way from the interstitum to the final urine via a pathway that remains to be determined.

It is the cumulative magnitude of urinary albumin losses that accounts for and best correlates with the severity of most features of the nephrotic syndrome. In contrast, the prevailing level of albuminuria is not always closely related to the extent of intrinsic injury to the glomerular capillary wall, and the reasons for the variability of this relationship are worthy of further consideration. Equation (28.1) shows that the albumin excretion rate (UV_{alb}) represents the difference between the load of albumin that is filtered (FL_{alb}) and the amount of that load which is reabsorbed in the proximal tubule (TR_{alb})

$$UV_{alb} = FL_{alb} - TR_{alb} \tag{28.1}$$

The most direct measure of the extent of injury to the glomerular barrier is provided by the glomerular sieving coefficient for albumin (θ_{alb}), which is the Bowman's space fluid-to-plasma albumin concentration ratio. The more permeable the glomerular barrier to albumin, the higher the value for θ_{alb}. Equation (28.2) shows that θ_{alb} is directly related to the filtered albumin load.

$$FL_{alb} = [S_{alb}] \times (GFR \cdot \theta_{alb}) \tag{28.2}$$

The two remaining determinants of the filtered albumin load are the serum albumin concentration (S_{alb}) and the glomerular filtration rate of water (GFR). These latter two quantities can vary independently of θ_{alb}, with the result that changes in the direction of FL_{alb}, and hence UV_{alb}, can become dissociated from those in the direction of θ_{alb}.

Consider, for example, a nephrotic glomerular injury which goes into partial remission. GFR (and perhaps S_{alb}) will increase toward the normal range, while θ_{alb} will decline. The offsetting effects of the former changes on FL_{alb} can leave UV_{alb} unchanged. In this example persisting and constant albuminuria can obscure the fact that glomerular capillary wall function is, in fact, improving. Alternatively, consider a worsening nephrotic glomerular injury in which GFR declines progressively and persistent, constant albuminuria leads to worsening hypoalbuminemia. Constancy of albuminuria under these circumstances requires that θ_{alb} increased in the interim (equation 28.2), but is often misinterpreted to indicate that the glomerular injury is 'stable'. An even more striking disparity between the level of albuminuria and the extent of glomerular injury is seen in sclerosing glomerulopathies. Here obliteration of glomeruli leads to a reduction in nephron number. Although FL_{alb} per nephron remains high, the progressive glomerulopenia results in the delivery of a smaller amount of albumin into the final urine. Declining albuminuria under these circumstances can be misinterpreted to reflect improving glomerular capillary wall function, when precisely the opposite is likely to be true. These examples illustrate the need to take the prevailing S_{alb}, the GFR and the number of functional glomeruli into account when attempting to infer the extent of glomerular barrier dysfunction from serial measurement of the level of albuminuria.

Sodium retention and edema

The clinical manifestation that most frequently brings the nephrotic patient to medical attention is the formation of edema. This represents an increase in the size of the interstitial fluid compartment. The interstitial fluid accumulates most readily in dependent areas where tissue pressure is low. It thus manifests as periorbital edema upon awakening in the morning, and pedal edema at the end of the day. Even when edema is generalized and massive, a condition referred to as anasarca, it remains most marked in the lower extremities. Not infrequently anasarca is also accompanied by serous effusion into the peritoneal, pleural and pericardial spaces.

Examination of the edema-forming, nephrotic patient during consumption of a known amount of sodium reveals a state of positive sodium balance. This can be partly explained by a lowered filtered sodium load, a consequence of the GFR depression that frequently accompanies nephrotic range proteinuria. Judged by the finding of low fractional sodium excretion, however, enhanced tubular sodium reabsorption appears to be the predominant cause of sodium retention in the nephrotic patient. Analysis of segmental sodium transport along the nephron of the nephrotic rat has identified the collecting duct as the major site of enhanced sodium reabsorption [3]. Refractoriness to the natriuretic action of the atrial natriuretic peptide (ANP) also indicates the distal tubule segment as the likely site of sodium retention in nephrotic humans. Both enhanced release of endogenous ANP during water immersion and infusion of exogenous ANP fail to promote an appropriate natriuretic response in nephrotic patients [4, 5]. It is the inner medullary segment of the collecting duct that is the tubule segment

most richly endowed with biological receptors for ANP [6, 7]. Thus, the blunted natriuretic response to ANP in nephrotic humans can be inferred to point to some alteration in the intrinsic transport properties of this tubule segment that renders it unresponsive to the natriuretic action of ANP.

An invariable finding in the sodium-retaining nephrotic subject is depression of S_{alb} to below 3 g/dl, and a corresponding fall in plasma colloid osmotic (or oncotic) pressure to below 20 mmHg (Figure 28.1). This has led to the hypothesis that a fall in plasma oncotic pressure permits extracellular fluid to be translocated from the vascular to the interstitial compartment [8]. An ensuing reduction of 'effective' plasma volume is then postulated to result in a series of neurohormonal adaptations which stimulate distal tubular reabsorption of sodium. In the absence of diuretic therapy, however, evidence of plasma hypovolemia is rarely forthcoming. In the majority of cases, the plasma and blood volumes, the central venous pressure and circulating levels of renin, angiotensin II and aldosterone are within the normal range [8]. That enhanced distal tubular sodium reabsorption is, in fact, independent of events in the systemic circulation is suggested by a model of unilateral proteinuric injury in the rat. This injury can be induced by infusion of aminonucleoside into a single renal artery while

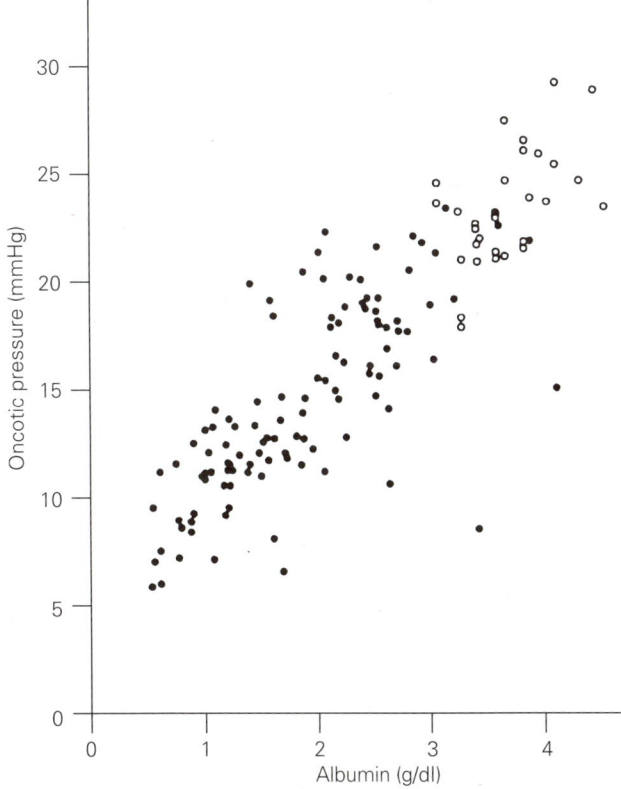

Figure 28.1 Serum albumin concentration plotted as a function of plasma oncotic pressure for 102 nephrotic patients (●) and 27 healthy controls (○).

clamping the opposite renal artery to prevent access to the contralateral kidney. Although the latter is exposed to the same systemic and hormonal influences, only the aminonucleoside-injected kidney exhibits proteinuria and avid sodium retention [9]. When all of the available evidence is weighed, it seems likely that enhanced tubular sodium reabsorption is the primary cause of sodium retention and edema in the nephrotic syndrome, and that systemic hormonal and hemodynamic alterations exert only a secondary influence on the extent and distribution of the retained extracellular fluid.

Altered plasma protein composition

An alteration in the composition of the plasma proteins is a consistent feature of the nephrotic syndrome, and likely contributes to many of its manifestations. The impact of massive proteinuria on plasma protein composition is shown by Table 28.1. These data allow a comparison of findings in 102 patients who presented consecutively with a nephrotic syndrome to those of 27 healthy controls [10]. Given a median urinary albumin excretion rate of 7.3 g/24 h (5053 µg/min), it is not surprising that serum albumin in the nephrotic subjects was reduced by 50% on average (Table 28.1). Because of its high concentration in plasma and its a relatively low molecular weight, albumin exerts most of the colloid osmotic (or oncotic) pressure that prevails within the plasma compartment. Thus, hypoalbuminemia in the nephrotic population was accompanied by a profound depression by 9 mmHg on average, in the oncotic pressure of plasma (Table 28.1).

Current evidence suggests that the oncotic pressure of the plasma perfusing the liver is the major regulator of protein synthesis and that the low oncotic pressure that characterizes the nephrotic syndrome stimulates hepatic protein synthesis, including that of albumin [11, 12]. Assuming a plasma volume of 41 in the nephrotic population, the plasma albumin pool can be estimated from

the mean plasma albumin concentration of 2 g/dl to approximate 80 g. The albumin lost in urine each day likely represents ~75% of the filtered albumin load. The remaining ~25% is catabolized in proximal tubule cells, such that about 10 g of albumin or 13% of the plasma albumin pool is lost following glomerular permeation each day. Apparently, enhanced hepatic synthesis of albumin cannot compensate for losses of this magnitude [12]. As stated previously, however, increased hepatic protein production is a generalized phenomenon, with the result that other hepatic-derived proteins are synthesized at a sufficiently rapid rate to elevate the concentration of non-albumin plasma protein in nephrotic subjects compared to healthy controls. (Non-albumin protein concentration in nephrotics can be estimated at 3.07 vs 2.59 g/dl in controls by subtracting albumin from total protein concentration in Table 28.1.) This results in a proportionately smaller reduction in nephrotic subjects of total plasma protein than albumin concentration, 33 vs 50%, respectively (Table 28.1). Of note, IgG, the second most abundant of the plasma proteins, does not contribute to the elevated non-albumin protein concentration in nephrotic plasma. IgG is a product of B cells and not hepatocytes, and in light of considerable urinary losses amounting to 0.5 g/24 h, serum IgG concentration, like that of albumin is significantly depressed in the nephrotic group (Table 28.1). The identity of the hepatic-derived proteins that elevate non-albumin plasma protein concentration has not been fully established. It seems likely, however, that an excess of the hepatic protein synthesis rate over corresponding urinary and tubular losses results in modest elevation in the plasma concentration of numerous protein species, and that the cumulative effect of this phenomenon is to defend against a precipitous fall in total plasma protein concentration and oncotic pressure [13].

An example of how the integrity of the circulation is defended by this adaptive response is the finding that the decline in plasma oncotic pressure in nephrotic subjects is proportionately smaller than that of serum albumin (Table 28.1). Figure 28.1 shows that the prevailing oncotic

	Controls (n = 27)	Nephrotics (n = 102)
Urinary albumin excretion (µg/min)	6.00 (2–51)	5053 (2003–26 300)
Urinary IgG excretion (µg/min)	1.10 (0.2–3.9)	350 (22–2719)
Serum albumin (g/dl)	4.02 ± 0.07	2.01 ± 0.08
Serum IgG (g/dl)	0.91 ± 0.04	0.60 ± 0.05
Serum total protein (g/dl)	6.61 ± 0.08	5.08 ± 0.09
Serum oncotic pressure (mmHg)	23.1 ± 0.5	14.3 ± 0.4

Table 28.1 Protein excretion and composition[a]

[a] Values are means ± SE, except for urinary protein excretion rates which are expressed as the median and (range). All values in nephrotics are significantly different from control values.

pressure in both nephrotic and normal subjects is related to albumin concentration in plasma. With the use of principal component analysis it can be shown that the relationship between oncotic pressure and albumin concentration is stronger in healthy controls than in nephrotic subjects [10]. In contrast, although there is no significant relationship between oncotic pressure and non-albumin protein concentration in healthy controls, there is a strong positive relationship between the two quantities in nephrotic subjects [10]. This suggests that a higher concentration of non-albumin protein may play an important role in maintaining oncotic pressure in the hypoalbuminemic nephrotic subject.

The altered levels and composition of circulating protein can be implicated in four common and important clinical manifestations of the nephrotic syndrome.

Maldistribution of extracellular fluid

As alluded to above, renal sodium retention results in an expansion of the extracellular fluid volume that manifests as a selective increase in the volume of the interstitial compartment [8], until a new steady state is reached. The rate of water flux from the plasma to the interstitial compartment (J_v) is a function of the prevailing Starling forces and the hydraulic permeability (k) and reflection coefficient for protein (σ) of systemic capillary walls. (The reflection coefficient is a measure of the extent to which protein is excluded, and thus is inversely related to the sieving coefficient.)

$$J_v = k(P_c - P_i) - \sigma(\pi_c - \pi_i) \qquad (28.3)$$

P_c and P_i are the hydraulic pressures in systemic capillaries and the interstitial compartments, respectively, and π_c and π_i, the corresponding oncotic pressures. The negative sign in front of the oncotic pressure difference indicates that it opposes water flux out of the plasma compartment. Under steady state conditions, the interstitial oncotic pressure in nephrotic subjects has been shown to decline in exact proportion to that in plasma, thereby maintaining a normal transvascular oncotic pressure difference and constancy of the relative volumes of the plasma and interstitial compartments [8]. Nephrotic patients are likely intermittently to experience unsteady state conditions, however. One example is during the rapid decline in plasma protein concentration that follows an abrupt onset of massive proteinuria. Another example is the patient with established nephrosis in whom plasma protein concentration declines suddenly as a result of hemodilution when the kidney fails to excrete a large fluid load. It is under these unstable circumstances before a new equilibrium can be reached that a diminished transvascular oncotic pressure difference could promote a net outward flux of fluid from the plasma to the interstitial compartment. A simultaneous increase in ($P_c - P_i$) during such acute episodes of plasma volume expansion would facilitate the outward movement of fluid (equation 28.3). Net flux of fluid into the interstitium will eventually dilute the interstitial fluid, restoring the ($\pi_c - \pi_i$) difference to normal. Simultaneously, enhanced lymphatic flow will return some of the interstitial fluid to the plasma compartment. Thus, an intermittent but incremental expansion of the interstitial compartment during periods of rapid hemodilution likely accounts for the extent of edema. Eventually, a new steady state will be reached and the absence of net fluid flux in either direction will maintain the disparate enlargement of the interstitial over the plasma compartment (and the attendant edema) that typifies the nephrotic syndrome.

Protein malnutrition

As stated previously the loss of a high filtered albumin load through both tubular catabolism and urinary excretion results in negative albumin balance [12]. This can be readily visualized in the integument. The skin overlying areas of edema exhibits white stretch marks, which result in a 'crazy paving' appearance. The nails exhibit parallel horizontal bands of dense and white opacity, a phenomenon known as Muehrcke's bands. Studies of nitrogen balance are difficult to perform because the level of proteinuria varies directly with the dietary protein intake [12]. Nevertheless, many nephrotic patients appear to be in a state of negative nitrogen balance, as judged by muscle wasting. In cases of prolonged and truly massive proteinuria, the loss of lean body mass can more than offset the accumulation of total body water, such that the patient may manifest progressive weight loss, despite the persistence of edema. Perhaps the most serious complication of protein malnutrition is impairment of cell-mediated immunity. This defect can combine with concurrent IgG deficiency secondary to massive immunoglobulinuria, and renders the nephrotic patient highly susceptible to infection. Although such susceptibility to infection is generalized, there seems to be a particular vulnerability to local infection at the sites of edema formation. Examples include cellulitis in swollen lower limbs and 'spontaneous' peritonitis in patients who have ascites. Because supplementation of dietary protein intake leads to enhancement of proteinuria, it is often difficult to achieve neutral or positive nitrogen balance, and the manifestations of protein malnutrition are likely to persist for the duration of the nephrotic syndrome.

Hypercoagulability

Urinary losses of some of the proteins in the coagulation cascade (e.g. antithrombin III) and adaptive hypersynthesis of others (e.g. fibrinogen) can tip the nephrotic patient into a hypercoagulable state [14]. Although thromboses have been reported within the arterial circulation, it is venous thrombosis that occurs with a particularly high incidence in nephrotic subjects [15]. The two major sites of phlebothrombosis are the deep veins of the calf and the renal veins [15, 16]. Whereas the former are not specific to any underlying disease, renal vein thrombosis is found dysproportionately in nephrotic subjects with membranous nephropathy. The incidence of phlebothrombosis in nephrotic subjects has been the subject of a controversy. Where imaging procedures have been used as a matter of routine, deep calf vein thrombosis has been reported with an incidence of 8–44%. A similarly variable incidence, 2–60%, has been reported for renal vein thrombosis. Because either form of venous thrombosis is likely to be associated with pulmonary thromboembolism, hypercoagulability represents the most lethal complication of the nephrotic syndrome. A high index of suspicion when the nephrotic subject manifests respiratory symptoms, such as pleuritic pain, hemoptysis, recurrent breathlessness and cough, should prompt the immediate initiation of diagnostic and imaging tests that are appropriate to the detection of phlebothrombosis and pulmonary embolism.

Hyperlipidemia

Either the low albumin concentration or, more likely, the low oncotic pressure of plasma perfusing the liver leads to an increase in hepatic lipid and apolipoprotein synthesis in the nephrotic syndrome [17]. In addition the catabolism of chylomicrons and very low density lipoproteins is reduced. Urinary losses of liporegulatory substances may contribute to the defective lipolysis, but multiple separate defects in the catabolism of triglyceride-rich lipoproteins have been implicated in their diminished peripheral clearance. The abnormalities of lipoprotein metabolism that attend the nephrotic syndrome are discussed in detail in Chapter 38. Their net effect is to increase the plasma total cholesterol substantially, notably that found in low density, intermediate density and very low density lipoprotein fractions [18, 19]. Although the incidence of atherosclerotic disease should be increased in light of the increase in total plasma cholesterol, this has been difficult to establish. The presence of co-existent risk factors for atherosclerosis, notably hypertension and chronic renal failure, makes the potency of hyperlipoproteinemia as a risk factor difficult to isolate in nephrotic patients. Given the natural history of atherosclerosis, one would predict that it is the patient with protracted nephrosis of many years duration who is most at risk of dying of premature cardiovascular disease [20].

Renal insufficiency

Impairment of kidney function is the rule in patients with the nephrotic syndrome and usually manifests in two ways. One is the inability of the kidney to maintain sodium and fluid homeostasis. The other is a loss by glomerular capillary walls of their intrinsic ultrafiltration capacity, a phenomenon that leads, in turn, to depression of the GFR. When viewed in physiological terms the GFR can be defined as the net rate of water flux across the walls of all capillaries in the two million glomerular tufts of the two human kidneys. It is determined by the product of the net pressure for ultrafiltration and the ultrafiltration coefficient, K_f, a measure of intrinsic ultrafiltration capacity.

$$\text{GFR} = (\Delta P - \pi_{GC}) \times K_f \qquad (28.4)$$

The net ultrafiltration pressure represents the imbalance between the transcapillary hydraulic pressure gradient (ΔP) and the intraluminal oncotic pressure that prevails along the glomerular capillaries (π_{GC}). K_f is the product of the available filtering surface area (S) and the hydraulic permeability of the glomerular capillary walls (k). With the exception of ΔP, each of the terms in equation (28.4) can be estimated to reasonable approximation. GFR can be equated with the clearance of inulin; π_{GC} can be calculated from a determination by membrane osmometry of systemic or afferent arteriolar oncotic pressure and knowledge of the filtration fraction; and K_f can be calculated by performing a morphometric analysis of pertinent glomerular structures in a renal biopsy [21]. When GFR, π_{GC} and K_f are known, equation (28.4) can be used to infer ΔP.

Using this approach it has been shown that GFR depression in some forms of the nephrotic syndrome (minimal change and membranous nephropathy) is exclusively a consequence of a profoundly lowered hydraulic permeability, k [21–23]. In other forms of nephrotic injury, associated glomerulosclerosis curtails the surface area for filtration; examples include proliferative lupus nephritis, idiopathic focal and segmental glomerulosclerosis, and diabetic nephropathy [23–25]. In each of the latter injuries an impairment of hydraulic permeability also contributes to K_f depression. The principal cause of impaired hydraulic permeability in nephrotic disorders is broadening and effacement of epithelial foot processes [21]. This lowers the frequency of interpodocytic slit diaphragms through which water must pass to gain access to Bowman's space, thereby increasing the resistance to water flow. The low K_f is partially offset by an increase in net ultrafiltration pressure, which is due in large part to a substantial lowering of π_{GC}. As a result the GFR falls less than in proportion to the K_f.

The disparity between GFR and K_f is illustrated in Figure 28.2 by a comparison of these two quantities in 80 nephrotic subjects with membranous nephropathy with corresponding values in 100 healthy volunteers. Membranous nephropathy has been chosen for this comparison because it is a generalized glomerular injury that produces morphologically similar changes in all glomerular tufts. Further, the incidence of global glomerulosclerosis is not different from normal, so that estimated K_f depression can be attributed exclusively to impairment of hydraulic permeability [21, 22]. As shown K_f depression is substantial; the median value in membranous nephropathy is 82% below normal, 3.0 vs 16.2 ml/min mmHg, respectively. Although the corresponding GFR depression is blunted by elevation of ultra-

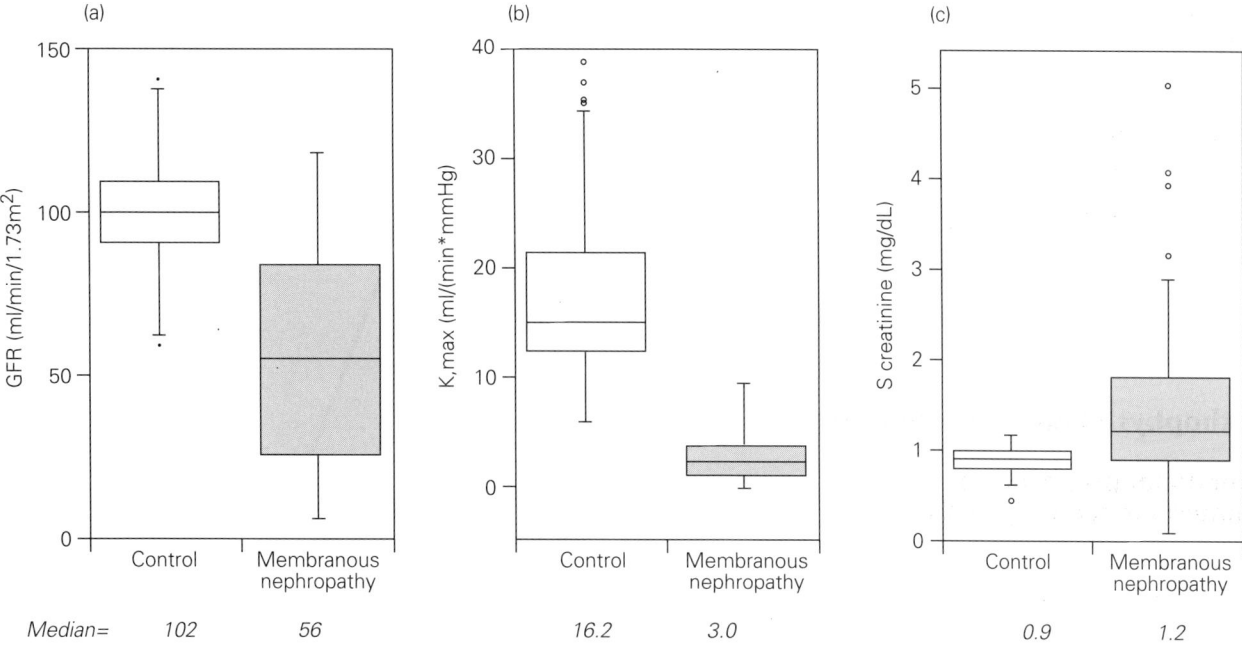

(a)

(b)

(c)

| Median= | 102 | 56 | 16.2 | 3.0 | 0.9 | 1.2 |

Figure 28.2 Quartile box plots of GFR (a), estimated K_f (b) and serum creatinine concentration (c) in 80 nephrotic patients with membranous nephropathy (hatched) vs 100 healthy volunteers (controls, open). The 25th, 50th and 75th percentiles (in ascending order) are the horizontal lines of the box; the rest of the range is indicated by vertical lines. Outliers are indicated by open circles.

filtration pressure, it too is substantial, the median GFR is only half that in normal controls, 56 vs 102 ml/min, respectively, and in most instances the GFR is below the normal 25th percentile (Figure 28.2).

Whereas median values for GFR and K_f in membranous nephropathy were depressed by 50 and 82%, respectively, the serum creatinine level was reciprocally elevated by only 33% (Figure 28.2). Further, whereas there was little or no overlap in the range for GFR and K_f between patients with membranous nephropathy and normal controls, there was considerable overlap between the corresponding range of serum creatinine levels. Because serum creatinine is the usual measure by which GFR is estimated in clinical practice, the treating physician will experience difficulty in appreciating the extent to which K_f (and the GFR) have decreased in nephrotic patients, irrespective of whether they are suffering from membranous nephropathy or other underlying gomerular disease. This is because a non-specific effect of nephrotic glomerular injury is to stimulate a creatinine transporter on the basolateral membrane of proximal tubule cells. The ensuing tubular hypersecretion of creatinine results in a creatinine clearance which overestimates the true GFR (inulin clearance) by 70% on average [26]. The relative enhancement of creatinine clearance in the nephrotic subject serves to maintain serum creatinine levels within or close to the normal range, despite substantial depression of the GFR and profound depression of the K_f (Figure 28.2). The failure of the serum creatinine to rise in inverse proportion to the reduction of GFR is often compounded

by a reduced production rate of creatinine, a consequence of the reduced muscle mass that accompanies protein malnutrition and corticosteroid therapy. These limitations of creatinine as a filtration marker in the setting of the nephrotic syndrome can mislead the treating physician to seriously underestimate the extent of glomerular injury, and to make inadvertent errors of judgement regarding the need for and optimal dosing of appropriate treatment.

The extent to which K_f, and hence GFR, is depressed in the nephrotic subject is, for the most part, a function of the underlying glomerular disease. Elements of the nephrotic syndrome *per se*, or its treatment, can also adversely influence the prevailing level of GFR, however. Both protein malnutrition and hypoalbuminemia have been separately shown to lower K_f in the non-glomerulopathic rat [27, 28]. A recent study of renal biopsies from children with kwashiorkor suggests that the low K_f results from broadening and effacement of foot processes with an ensuing impairment of hydraulic permeability [29]. The low ultrafiltration capacity induced by glomerular disease and protein depletion makes the nephrotic subject particularly vulnerable to acute exacerbations of hypofiltration and renal insufficiency. This is because the prevailing level of GFR is in large part maintained by an offsetting elevation of ultrafiltration pressure. Any maneuver that lowers the glomerular capillary perfusion pressure can, therefore, cause precipitous falls in the GFR. A common example is the overzealous use of diuretic agents to the point of causing plasma hypovolemia and glomerular underperfusion. Another example is the use of treatment modalities that are designed to lower the level of proteinuria, but which also lower glomerular capillary perfusion pressure. Widely used 'antiproteinuric' therapies which have this potentially adverse action include cyclosporin, angiotensin converting enzyme inhibitors and cyclo-oxygenase inhibitors. The susceptibility of the nephrotic patient to episodes of acute renal insufficiency should thus be constantly borne in mind when initiating treatments that can compromise the ultrafiltration pressure in such individuals.

Pathophysiology of proteinuria

Functional properties of glomerular capillary walls

The walls of glomerular capillaries (GC) behave as high-capacity ultrafiltration membranes. In humans, for example, a very high rate of ultrafiltration, approximating 150 l/day, is achieved, despite a pressure for ultrafiltration that is estimated to approximate only 10 mmHg. Despite their remarkably low resistance to water flow, GC walls impose an extremely efficient barrier to the passage of proteins the size of albumin and larger. Fluid sampled by the micropuncture technique from the first part of the proximal tubule conforms closely to that of an ideal ultra-filtrate of plasma. The concentrations of uncharged substances with a molecular radius (r_s) the size of inulin or smaller (±16 Å) in Bowman's space fluid are essentially identical to those in plasma. In contrast, the corresponding Bowman's space concentration of albumin is <1 mg/dl, a value 3–4 orders of magnitude lower than plasma albumin concentration, which is typically 4 g/dl [30, 31].

The Bowman's space-to-plasma concentration ratio of a given macromolecule is known as its sieving coefficient (θ) and provides the most precise measure of the permeability of the GC well to that macromolecule. Attempts have been made to determine θ for various proteins in the rat by sampling the earliest accessible part of the proximal tubule, and correcting for water reabsorption up to the site of sampling [31, 32]. An alternative approach has been to determine the urinary clearance of a protein and correct for proximal tubular reabsorption of that protein by measuring its accumulation in renal tissue [33–35]. Together these two methods for estimating θ of a protein have yielded the relation between the molecular properties of several proteins and glomerular barrier selectivity illustrated in Figure 28.3. Each θ is plotted as a function of the effective molecular radius of the protein. Transmural transport of the largest proteins (albumin and γ-globulin) is considerably more restricted than that of the smallest proteins (monomeric immunogloblin light chains). A clear trend toward progressive restriction of transmural transport with increasing size of the test protein only becomes obvious, however, when the mole-

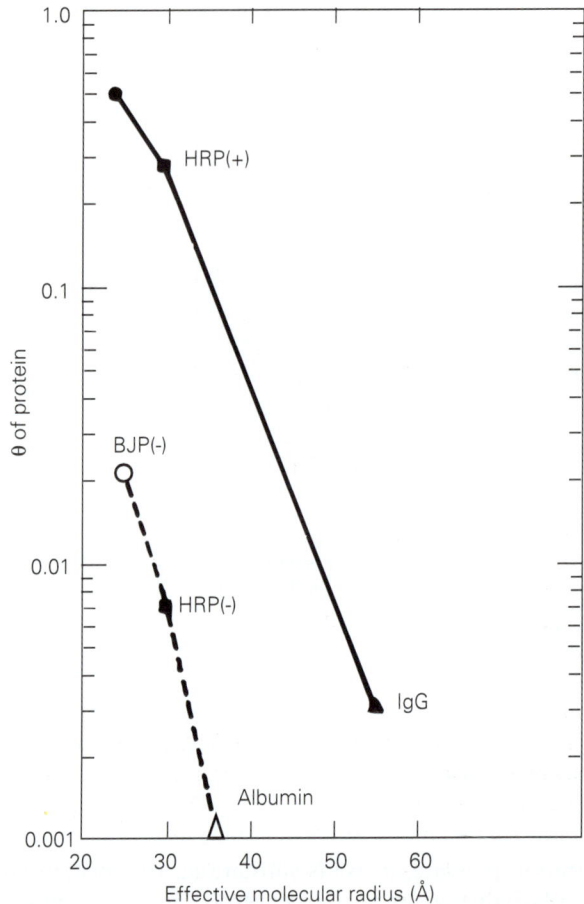

Figure 28.3 Sieving coefficients (θ) of proteins that are either cationic (+) or anionic (−) plotted as a function of molecular radius. BJP, Bence Jones protein (Ig light chains); HRP, horseradish peroxidase.

cular charge of each protein is taken into account. Thus, the inverse relation between the θ and molecular radius of either anionic or cationic proteins indicates that the glomerular capillary wall (GCW) has the properties of a size-selective filter. On the other hand, the greater restriction of anionic than cationic proteins of equivalent or similar radius points to the existence within the GCW of an electrostatic barrier, and indicates that it also functions as a charge-selective filter (Figure 28.3).

Tubular reabsorption of filtered protein

Few observations of the type shown in Figure 28.3 have been made because of technical complexities associated with such determinations. In the case of the micropuncture approach, these include the inaccessibility of Bowman's space fluid and limitations to the accurate measurement of protein concentration in the nanoliter quantities of the fluid that can be sampled. To circumvent these difficulties attempts have been made in experimental animals to calculate θ for a given protein from its urinary clearance and an estimate of the fractional reabsorption of the filtered load of that protein in the proximal tubule. Using either micropuncture techniques or the accumulation in renal tissue of a radiolabeled protein that has been infused, it has been estimated that >90% of the load of protein that is normally filtered by the healthy glomerular capillary wall undergoes reabsorption by proximal tubule cells [30–35] (Figure 28.4). After interiorization, the protein is catabolized to amino acids, and the latter then enter the peritubular circulation, whence they are transported to the liver. However, the proximal tubule transport system, although possessed of a high capacity, becomes rapidly saturated. Thus, increments in the filtered protein load as a result of glomerular injury result in a monotonic decline in the fraction that is reabsorbed (Figure 28.4). Studies in nephrotic rats suggest that fractional reabsorption can decline to as little as 20% of the filtered load [31–33]. Cationic proteins are more readily bound by the anionic glycocalyx of proximal tubule apical cell membranes with the result that they are interiorized and reabsorbed preferentially when compared to anionic proteins (Figure 28.4) [35]. Since the tissue accumulation technique of estimating tubular protein reabsorption requires removal of the kidney it can obviously only be used in experimental animals. In the human (or intact animal) with proteinuria, attempts have been made to infer glomerular sieving behavior from the clearance of discrete proteins into urine. Given the large and unknown level of fractional reabsorption and its charge-dependency, however, such extrapolations are too imprecise to be meaningful.

Exogenous probes of the glomerular filtration barrier

Because of the limitations in determining θ for a given protein, glomerular permeability has been most extensively studied by determining the fractional clearance of exogenous and non-reabsorbable macromolecules. The

fractional clearance of a probe macromolecule (M) is defined as the clearance of M divided by the GFR of water. With the clearance of inulin used to measure the latter, the fractional clearance (FC) is calculated from the urine (U) and plasma concentrations (P) of M and inulin (in) as follows:

$$FC_M = (U/P)_M / (U/P)_{in} \qquad (28.5)$$

If the probe macromolecule is neither reabsorbed nor secreted by the tubule, then dividing its U/P ratio by that of inulin corrects for water reabsorption along the tubule, and the fractional clearance of M will be exactly equal to the Bowman's space-to-plasma concentration ratio of M (θ).

Three non-protein polymers, namely, polyvinylpyrrolidone, dextran (a polymer of glucopyranose) and Ficoll (a polymer of sucrose) all of which are neither reabsorbed nor secreted by the tubule, have been used for this purpose [36–38]. The size-selective properties of the GCW have been elucidated by using uncharged, polydisperse preparations of these polymers. The absence of charge eliminates the consequences of electrical interaction between the permeating macromolecule and charged sites within the GCW; the use of preparations of broad size distribution permits θ to be determined over a wide range of molecular radii.

Of the foregoing exogenous polymers, uncharged dextran has been the most extensively used to examine the alterations in glomerular barrier size-selectivity that accompany the development of massive proteinuria. Such studies suggest that all nephrotic glomerular injuries are associated with an impairment of barrier size-selectivity [37]. An example of this approach is illustrated in Figure 28.5. Uncharged dextran 40 has been infused into 20 healthy volunteers and 27 patients with a nephrotic syndrome due to membranous nephropathy. Once again, this glomerular disease has been selected for purposes of illustration because of the homogeneity of the injury among glomeruli. A semilog scale has been used to plot θ for dextrans as a function of the effective molecular radius, r_S, with the latter determined by elution of the dextrans in urine and plasma from calibrated gel columns. A value below 1.0 indicates that there is measurable restriction to the transmural passage of dextran, a phenomenon which first becomes evident for the 28 Å r_S dextran eluate in the healthy control population. With increasing r_S, the θ for dextran in the control subjects declines in a monotonic fashion, approaching zero for dextran molecules of $r_S = 60$ Å (Figure 28.5). As shown in Figure 28.5, barrier size-selectivity has become altered in the nephrotic subjects. The sieving coefficients for relatively permeant dextrans of $r_S < 46$ Å are severely depressed. In contrast, the sieving coefficients for large, nearly impermeant dextrans of $r_S > 50$ Å are elevated above normal. Furthermore, the extent of the latter elevation becomes magnified with increasing r_S, indicating a glomerular membrane with a less sharp cut-off than normal.

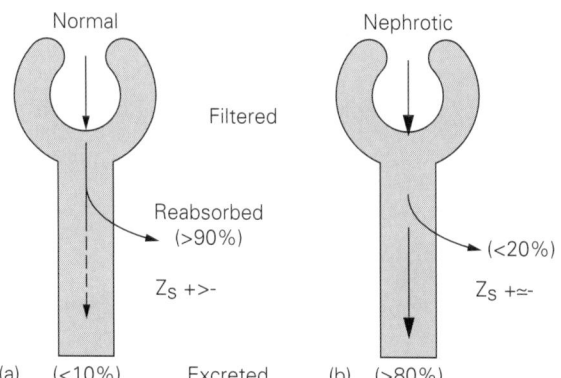

Figure 28.4 Schematic diagram of the amount of protein filtered, reabsorbed and excreted by the normal (a) or nephrotic (b) rat nephron. Z_s is the charge density of the filtered protein.

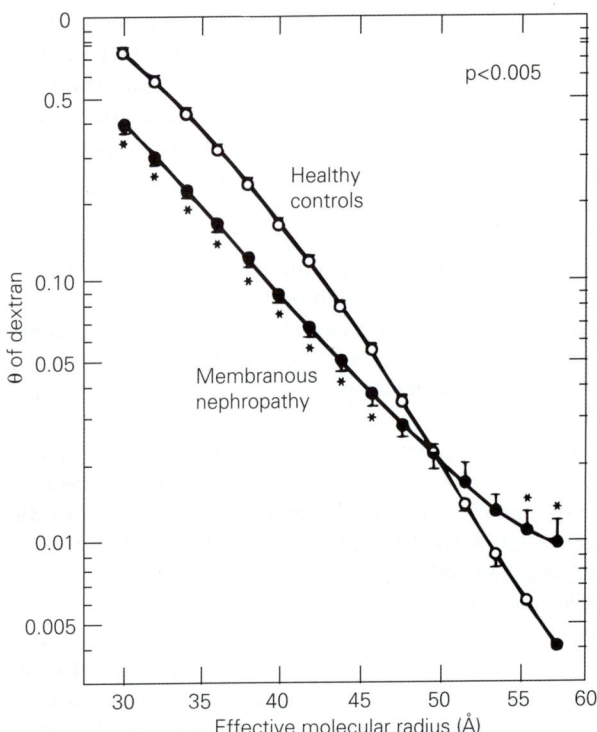

Figure 28.5 Dextran sieving coefficients (θ) plotted as a function of molecular radius for nephrotic patients with membranous nephropathy (●) vs controls (○). *$P < 0.005$.

Pore theory and size-selectivity

The most widely used descriptions of macromolecule transport across the glomerular capillary wall are based on a hydrodynamic theory of hindered solute transport through water-filled pores. Deen *et al.* [39] give a detailed description of how pore theory can be used to interpret the alterations in dextran sieving found in proteinuric disorders. In brief, a variety of distributions that are commonly used in probability analysis has been examined by a curve-fitting technique to select those pore-size distributions which successfully replicate the observed values of θ. According to the foregoing analysis, several hetero-porous membrane models can satisfactorily represent the glomerular capillary wall [39]. One adequate representation that has the virtue of simplicity is the isoporous + shunt model, in which the major portion of the GCW is assumed to be perforated by cylindrical restrictive pores of uniform radius. A second population of large pores, which are non-discriminatory for dextrans of up to $r_S = 60$Å, serves as a parallel shunt pathway.

The isoporous + shunt model has two pore parameters. These are: r_0, the mean restrictive pore radius, and ω_0, a parameter which represents the fraction of filtrate permeating the parallel shunt pathway. In addition to r_0 and ω_0, the membrane barrier to filtration of water and uncharged macromolecules is characterized by an ultrafiltration coefficient (K_f) and a ratio of effective pore area-to-pore length (S'/l). Assuming that variations in pore length (l) are minor in the presence of glomerular disease, changes in S'/l should primarily reflect the total number of pores in all GCWs of the two kidneys. The approach used for calculating these intrinsic membrane parameters separates their effects on fractional dextran clearances from those of purely hemodynamic changes [39].

The computed pore-parameters are summarized in Table 28.2. Compared to normal controls the nephrotic syndrome in membranous nephropathy is associated with a substantial reduction in K_f, pore density and restrictive pore radius (Table 28.2). Judged by ω_0, the shunt-pathway has become more prominent, such that the fraction of filtrate volume by which it is permeated increases by approximately 16-fold. Thus, according to this analysis, depression of θ for the low radius dextrans in nephrotic patients with membranous nephropathy is a consequence of a diminution in pore density together with a shift to smaller size of the restrictive pores that dominate the membrane. The increased resistance to water flow that results from these alterations explains the depression of GFR in membranous nephropathy that has been described above. On the other hand, the increased fraction of filtrate volume that is shunted serves to explain the massive increases in the filtered load and urinary excretion rate of protein that typify this glomerular disease.

Table 28.2 Membrane parameters

	Controls	Membranous nephropathy
Restrictive pore radius (r_0, Å)	57.5	54.2
	(55.9–60.6)	(49.5–57.5)
Pore density (S'/l, Km)	306	76
	(156–818)	(16–176)
Fraction of filtrate shunted	0.4	6.3
($\omega_0 \times 10^{-3}$)	(0.1–1.6)	(2.6–31.2)

All results are expressed as the median and (range): all values in membranous nephropathy are significantly different from control values.

Charge- and shape-selectivity

There is a large disparity between θ for albumin and that for an uncharged dextran of equivalent gel chromatographic radius, <0.0001 vs 0.25, respectively. This points to an influence of biophysical properties other than size on the transglomerular transport of circulating macromolecules. One such property is molecular shape. Whereas proteins behave as rigid spheres, dextran molecules display asphericity under shear, and thus do not behave as the ideal neutral spheres assumed in the pore-size calculations. In diffusion experiments using synthetic membranes of uniform and independently measured pore size, dextran and polyvinylpyrrolidone have been shown to diffuse more rapidly than a neutral sphere of equivalent r_S, whereas Ficoll closely follows the predictions for solid spheres [40, 41]. Quantitatively similar findings have been reported for the rat, where the fractional clearance of dextran exceeds that of Ficoll [38] or a neutral horseradish peroxidase [34] of equivalent radius. Thus, the application of the conventional solid-sphere model to dextran data will tend to overestimate GCW permeability to proteins.

Numerous studies using experimental animals have

shown that the normal GCW is also a charge-selective barrier. In rats and dogs, values of θ for various anionic macromolecules have been shown to be lower than θ for neutral macromolecules of similar size and chemical structure, which in turn are lower than values of θ for otherwise similar cationic macromolecules [42]. In other words, transport of negatively charged macromolecules is hindered, and that of positively charged macromolecules is enhanced, relative to uncharged macromolecules. Depletion of negatively charged components of the GCW has been shown to lead to the loss of such charge-selectivity in a variety of experimental glomerular diseases in the rat [42]. That this is also likely true of the nephrotic patients with membranous nephropathy is suggested by the renal handling of albumin and IgG in this disorder [43].

Figure 28.6 compares the fractional clearances of albumin and IgG in nephrotic patients with membranous nephropathy to the corresponding fractional clearance attributable to the shunt pathway (θ_∞), where the value for θ_∞ has been calculated from each individual's dextran-sieving curve using the isoporous + shunt model. Because luminal concentration of a retained macromolecule will increase with distance, as water is removed by ultrafiltration during axial plasma flow along the GCs, θ_∞ slightly exceeds ω_0, the fraction of filtrate volume passing through the shunt pathway. θ_∞ exceeds the fractional IgG clearance in almost all instances (Figure 28.6). Although molecular charge varies among its subclasses, IgG is a large protein of $r_S = 55\,\text{Å}$. As discussed above, the radius of the restrictive pores in membranous nephropathy has been calculated using dextran molecules and thus overestimates the effective radius presented by the restrictive pores to rigid protein spheres. This makes it unlikely that IgG can permeate the restrictive pores and suggests that IgG passes into Bowman's space exclusively via the shunt-like pores. The almost invariable finding of a fractional IgG clearance-to-θ_∞ ratio <1.0 is consistent with this possibility. In contrast, the fractional albumin clearance-to-θ_∞ ratio often exceeds 1.0 in membranous nephropathy (Figure 28.6). Because albumin r_S is only $36\,\text{Å}$, it is entirely possible that this protein could traverse restrictive pores, which according to the isoporous + shunt model present an effective mean radius towards dextrans in membranous nephropathy that varies between 49 and $58\,\text{Å}$. Studies in the rat reveal that passage through the restrictive pores of albumin, a polyanion, is normally prevented by electrostatic retardation [33]. Should the negatively charged sites of the GCW become depleted in membranous nephropathy, albumin could traverse both the restrictive pores as well as those of the shunt pathway, thereby explaining a fractional albumin clearance/θ_∞ ratio of >1.0, and accounting for the observed magnitude of albuminuria in this disorder.

Evidence in support of this has been provided by infusing a narrowly dispersed preparation of anionic dextran sulfate into 11 nephrotic patients with membranous nephropathy and eight healthy controls [43]. The θ for

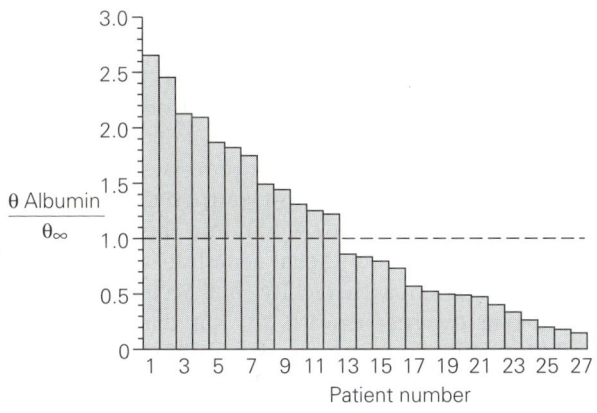

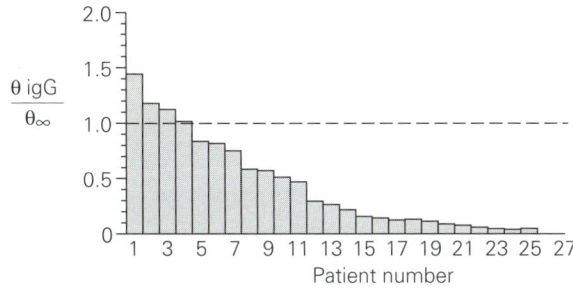

Figure 28.6 The ratio of the fractional clearance of albumin (upper) of IgG (lower) to θ_∞; the fractional clearance of a hypothetical molecule through the shunt pathway. The ratios are shown for each of the 27 nephrotic patients with membranous nephropathy in Figure 28.5. Ratios in excess of unity (the dashed horizontal line) indicate more protein filtration than can be attributed to the shunt pathway.

dextran sulfate of $r_S = 16\,\text{Å}$ was determined by separating this fraction of the preparation by size-exclusion chromatography of urine and an ultrafiltrate of plasma in each instance, and found in the healthy controls to be 0.63 ± 0.03 (Figure 28.7). In comparison uncharged dextrans of similar r_S were unrestricted, $\theta = 1.0 \pm 0.04$. We were thus able to demonstrate for the first time that the GCW in healthy humans normally exhibits charge-selectivity similar to that reported for experimental animals. In the nephrotic subjects, by contrast, charge discrimination was lost. The θ for the $16\,\text{Å}$ r_S dextran sulfate fraction was 0.91 ± 0.5 ($P < 0.001$ vs controls). The latter value was not significantly different from unity, or from the corresponding θ for uncharged dextran molecules of similar radius (Figure 28.7). From these findings, it was inferred that the albuminuria observed in membranous nephropathy reflects a combination of size- and charge-selective

defects. A schematic representation of the barrier defect in the nephrotic subjects with membranous nephropathy is depicted in Figure 28.8. Because dextran overestimates the effective pore size of the GCW, however, it is not yet possible to calculate the relative importance of the two types of defect. This must await similar studies with a more ideal species of macromolecular probe that behaves as a sphere during transglomerular permeation.

Pathogenesis and pathology of proteinuria

It should be emphasized that the computation of effective pore radii from the θ for probe macromolecules is mainly useful for making comparisons within the context of a particular model. The definition of structural counterparts to these 'functional' pores has proven elusive. A large body of literature has implied that the extracellular matrix that comprises the glomerular basement membrane (GBM) provides the barrier to the passage of proteins. The bulk of available evidence points away from a prominent role for the GBM in filtration barrier function, however. Daniels et al. [44] have shown that glomerular sieving coefficients for albumin and large dextran molecules are orders of magnitude lower in vivo in the rat with an intact GCW than are corresponding values in vitro for the isolated rat GBM.

In accord with the latter observation, morphological studies which use particulate and electron-dense macromolecules as tracers suggest that the slit diaphragm which separates adjacent epithelial foot processes is most likely to be the ultimate and most restrictive size-selective barrier. Despite an r_S of $61\,\text{Å}$, cationic species of ferritin can penetrate the endothelial fenestrae and the dense layer of the GBM with facility, but accumulate in the lamina rara externa beneath the slit diaphragms [45]. Similarly, neutral or cationic IgG antibodies have little difficulty in penetrating the GBM and attaching to antigens on the soles of epithelial foot process to initiate the glomerular injury in membranous nephropathy. In contrast, anionic species of ferritin or albumin are restricted to the level of the endothelial fenestrae, suggesting that

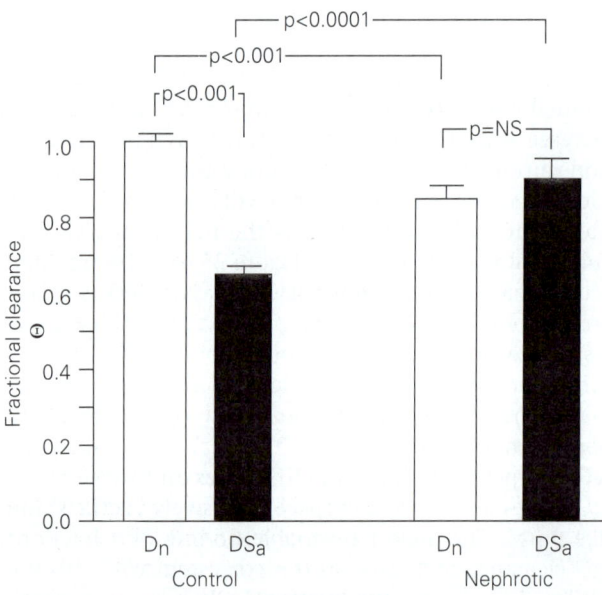

Figure 28.7 Sieving coefficients for a neutral dextran (D_n) or anionic dextran sulfate (DS_a) molecule of 16–18 Å radius in humans. Healthy control values are the left hand bars, nephrotic values in membranous nephropathy are the right hand bars.

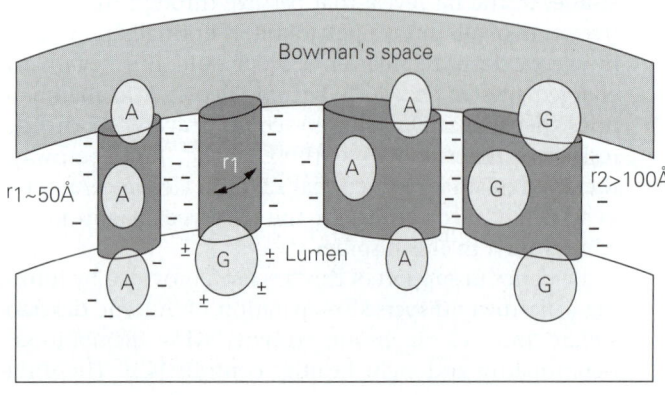

Figure 28.8 Schematic representation of functional glomerular pores in nephrotic subjects with membranous nephropathy. Restrictive pores of radius r_1 (~50 Å) dominate the barrier, shunt-like pores of radius r_2 (>100 Å) are permeated by only 1–2% of filtrate volume, and are freely permeable to albumin (A) and IgG (G). Restrictive pores are relatively depleted of associated negatively charged sites, permitting anionic albumin to permeate into Bowman's space. IgG is excluded by restrictive pores on the basis of its large size.

they are electrostatically hindered by the anionic glycocalyx that occupies much of the endothelial fenestral space. Thus, the GCW may be thought of as containing three barriers in series. A proximal endothelial electrostatic barrier and a distal epithelial size-selective barrier appear to be the most important. An intermediate barrier of less quantitative importance but with both size- and charge-selective properties is provided by the GBM.

That the slit diaphragm constitutes a distal size-selective barrier is consistent with the finding that it contains rectangular apertures, the dimensions of which would prevent the passage into Bowman's space of proteins the size of albumin or larger [46]. The ubiquitous deformation (or so-called 'effacement') of adjacent foot processes that accompanies all nephrotic disorders could alter the shape and size of the apertures, such that a few become enlarged and permeable to proteins. Yet another potential size defect is a complete detachment of some foot processes and their associated slit diaphragms from the lamina rara externa of the basement membrane. It is precisely at such sites of basement membrane denudation that ferritin particles have been demonstrated to penetrate into Bowman's space in various rat models of proteinuric glomerular injury [47]. The latter are usually associated with focal and segmental glomerulosclerosis, however, and comparable defects are rarely apparent in nephrotic humans with non-sclerosing glomerular injuries such as membranous or minimal change nephropathy. Because our ability to detect an alteration in the dimensions of slit diaphragmatic apertures is beyond the resolution of conventional electron microscopy, the precise structural basis of impaired barrier size-selectivity in membranous nephropathy and other nephrotic disorders of humans must remain a matter for conjecture.

Foot process detachment or other severe structural alterations that permanently disrupt the anatomical integrity of the GCW cannot provide an exclusive explanation for impaired size-selectivity and massive proteinuria, however. Both the prominence of shunt-like pores and the magnitude of proteinuria can be enhanced within a matter of minutes by maneuvers which either elevate glomerular capillary pressure [48, 49] or neutralize negatively charged sites within the GCW [50, 51]. This adverse effect on barrier function can be reversed equally promptly upon either restoring capillary pressure to normal levels or repleting the net negative charge of the GCW. Similarly, the administration to nephrotic patients of drugs that block the intrarenal production of prostaglandins or angiotensin II can reduce the size of the shunt pathway and the level of proteinuria within a matter of days [52–55]. Upon withdrawal of these agents too, barrier size-selectivity and proteinuria are restored promptly to pretreatment levels [54]. Morphological studies suggest that the aforementioned perturbations of barrier function and the filtered protein load are accompanied by alterations in the conformation of epithelial foot processes [50, 51, 56]. Thus at least some of the changes in GCW structure that attend the phenomenon of massive proteinuria are temporary in nature. It seems likely that they represent a reversible and non-specific response by glomerular epithelial cells to a variety of glomerular injuries.

Differential diagnosis

Nephrotic range proteinuria

Numerous glomerular injuries result in nephrotic range proteinuria. The discrete disease entities or categories of injury which together encompass most of the known causes of the nephrotic syndrome are shown in Table 28.3. The classification is based on the morphological appearance of glomeruli, and thus implies that a renal biopsy is required to make a precise diagnosis. This requirement applies particularly to causes 1 through 4 (Table 28.3). All represent immune injuries and a precise diagnosis is an important guide to the selection of the most appropriate form of immunosuppressive therapy. An exception is often made in the case of a nephrotic child or adolescent. Because minimal change nephropathy is the most prevalent underlying cause of the nephrotic syndrome in this age group, an argument can be made for initiating a four-week trial of corticosteroid or cyclosporin therapy without renal biopsy. A complete remission of proteinuria during such therapy, particularly if observed within two weeks of initiating therapy, can reasonably be inferred to be diagnostic of minimal change nephropathy.

The category of glomerular injury encompassed by the term proliferative glomerulonephritis refers to a group of injuries that are characterized by glomerular hypercellularity. The basis for the latter can be an infiltration by non-resident leukocytes or, more commonly, a proliferation of one or more of the three glomerular cell types. In some entities the proliferation tends to be endocapillary; that is, mesangial or endothelial cells are those that proliferate. Common examples are IgA nephropathy and post-infectious glomerulonephritis. In other entities the proliferation is extracapillary; that is, the proliferating cell type is the epithelial cell, producing the morphological

Table 28.3 Common causes of the nephrotic syndrome

1. Minimal change nephropathy
2. Idiopathic focal, segmental glomerulosclerosis
3. Membranous nephropathy
4. Proliferative glomerulonephritides
5. Diabetic nephropathy
6. Intraglomerular deposition of monoclonal immunoglobulin fragments, amyloid and non-amyloid fibrils
7. Secondary focal, segmental glomerulosclerosis

phenomenon of a 'cellular crescent'. Notable examples are systemic vasculitides such as Wegener's granulomatosis and polyarteritis nodosa. Whereas proliferation of either endo- or extracapillary cells may be predominant, at least some proliferation of all three cell types is often encountered in many forms of glomerulonephritis, and generalized involvement of all glomerular cell types is often a feature of proliferative lupus nephritis. The diagnoses of some of the glomerulonephritides that cause the nephrotic syndrome can be further refined by identifying pathognomonic serological markers, notably the presence of antibodies to DNA in lupus nephritis, or anti-neutrophil cytoplasmic antibodies in Wegener's granulomatosis, or anti-GBM antibodies in Goodpasture's syndrome. As a category, moreover, the presence of proliferative glomerulonephritis can be strongly suspected by a greater propensity than in the remaining categories of Table 28.3 to cause glomerular bleeding. The presence of an excess of dysmorphic erythrocytes in the urinary sediment is suggestive of glomerulonephritis, particularly when accompanied by erythrocyte or hemoglobin-pigmented casts. Unfortunately, the urine sediment is not diagnostic of glomerulonephritis. Although a less common feature of the remaining glomerular diseases, each entity listed in Table 28.3 can result in some glomerular bleeding, albeit of only modest proportions in most cases.

The case for always making a biopsy diagnosis in categories 5 through 7 is less compelling. On the one hand, there is no specific therapy for these disorders. On the other hand, the natural history and co-existent features of the underlying disease often permit a clinical diagnosis to be made with a relatively high degree of confidence.

Diabetic nephropathy is a case in point [57]. It typically manifests after more than a decade of diabetes mellitus and when first detected the proteinuria is of subnephrotic proportions. With the passage of time the proteinuria usually increases, often into a nephrotic range. By this time, however, the GFR is likely to be severely depressed and hypertension prevalent. Also, the almost invariable presence of other microvascular complications, such as retinopathy and neuropathy, allows the diagnosis to be made on clinical grounds with a high degree of precision. A reasonable compromise therefore is to limit the performance of a diagnostic renal biopsy to diabetic patients in whom nephrotic-range proteinuria is not fully consistent with the diagnosis of diabetic nephropathy. A common example is the sudden onset of nephrosis in a patient with diabetes of short duration, a well-preserved GFR and a lack of coexistent retinopathy and neuropathy. Under these circumstances a coincident glomerular injury unrelated to diabetic nephropathy may be found in the biopsy. Sometimes a normal appearance of glomeruli on light microscopy with foot process effacement on electron microscopy is interpreted to indicate coexistent minimal change nephropathy in a patient who happens to be diabetic. In our experience, however, this combination of findings is unresponsive to corticosteroid therapy. We infer therefore that it represents a disproportionate diabetic injury to epithelial cells, and thus merely a variant of diabetic nephropathy. It accounts for the small subset of diabetic patients whose diabetic nephropathy presents with a nephrotic syndrome and runs an unusually rapid downhill course [25].

Nephrotic-range proteinuria occurs in a number of glomerular diseases which are characterized by the deposition of monoclonal light chains, light chain-related amyloid or monoclonal immunoglobulin. In most cases the deposition of these substances is associated with a malignant proliferation of lymphoplasmacytic cells. Another association of the nephrotic syndrome that is being recognized with increasing frequency in biopsy material is the intraglomerular deposition of non-amyloid fibrils [59]. Depending on the size and ultrastructural characteristics of the fibrils these entities have been labeled 'fibrillary glomerulonephritis' or 'immunotactoid glomerulopathy'. Like light chain, amyloid and monoclonal immunoglobulin deposition disease, non-amyloid fibril deposition has been associated on occasion with lymphoplasmacyte cell malignancy, but this association is considerably weaker. The diagnosis of one of the foregoing entities can be suspected by demonstrating the presence of a monoclonal 'paraprotein' in serum or a proliferating clone of lymphocytes or plasma cells in a bone marrow or lymph node biopsy. The precise diagnosis and characterization of the substance being deposited in the glomeruli can only be made by morphological analysis, however. Thus, the accurate identification of this class of glomerular injuries also depends on the performance of a renal biopsy.

Finally, a host of diseases which are primarily tubulo-interstitial can in their terminal stages produce glomerular damage sufficient to result in nephrotic-range proteinuria. Common examples include obstructive nephropathy, analgesic-abuse nephropathy, and adult polycystic kidney disease. Focal and segmental glomerulosclerosis is the morphological hallmark of this secondary form of glomerular injury, albeit a non-specific one. The taking of a careful history and appropriate imaging of the kidneys and urinary collecting systems should identify the specific underlying diseases of these structures that can sometimes lead to nephrotic-range proteinuria.

Subnephrotic proteinuria

Diagnosing the precise cause of subnephrotic proteinuria presents a much more formidable challenge than in the case of nephrotic-range proteinuria. It has been estimated that the dipstick test is positive within a subnephrotic range (trace–2+) in up to 3% of apparently healthy individuals undergoing routine urinalysis. Several categories of disorders that encompass most of the causes of mod-

Table 28.4 Causes of subnephrotic-range proteinuria

Non-glomerular:	(a) Tubular
	(b) Overflow
	(c) Uroepithelial
Glomerular:	(a) Functional
	(b) Structural

erate proteinuria are shown in Table 28.4. A false positive dipstick test can occasionally reflect a detectable albumin concentration in a highly concentrated but essentially normal urine; a measurement of the protein excretion rate reveals it to be within normal limits.

As stated previously the finding of modest proteinuria can also occur in the absence of glomerular disease. Tubular proteinuria should be suspected when glycosuria, phosphaturia and amino-aciduria point to a generalized impairment of proximal reabsorption (Fanconi's syndrome). A demonstration of increased excretion of proteins of low molecular weight that are normally filtered in measurable quantities confirms the diagnosis. β_2-Microglobulin and lysozyme are the low molecular weight protein markers that are most widely used for this purpose. However, there is increasing evidence that tubular reabsorption of these proteins can be impaired in a non-specific fashion in the presence of a large filtered albumin load. From a practical point of view therefore, it is useful to estimate the albumin excretion rate when tubular proteinuria is suspected. The widespread and growing use of sensitive immunochemical techniques to detect minor increases in albuminuria (so-called 'microalbuminuria') has shown that the upper limit of the normal albumin excretion rate is 30 mg/24 h. Assuming a normal fractional albumin reabsorption rate of ±90% [31–35], it can be estimated that the upper limit for a normal filtered albumin load should approximate 270 mg/24 h. The finding of an albumin excretion rate in excess of this amount is inconsistent with purely tubular proteinuria, and points strongly to a coexistent glomerular injury.

The diagnosis of overflow proteinuria depends on the identification of an excess in urine of a single filtered protein species, one that is not normally present in significant amounts in the urine. Examples include myoglobin, hemoglobin, lysozyme and, most commonly, monoclonal light chains or Bence Jones proteins. Each can be identified and quantitated by specific immunochemical techniques. It is worth emphasizing that either the transcapillary passage *per se* of high filtered loads of monoclonal light chains or their intraglomerular deposition can damage the glomerular filter. That the patient has a combination of Bence Jones and glomerular proteinuria can once again be diagnosed by demonstrating an albumin excretion rate in excess of 270 mg/24 h.

Functional glomerular proteinuria can be defined as an elevated albumin excretion rate that is hemodynamically mediated, rather than attributable to a discrete disease process of the structures that comprise the filtration barrier. Examples of underlying conditions that are associated with functional glomerular proteinuria are congestive cardiac failure, constrictive pericarditis, the unaffected contralateral kidney of a patient with renovascular hypertension, fever and recent intensive exercise. All are associated with elevation of the filtration fraction and activation of the renin–angiotensin system, findings which in turn, suggest the presence of glomerular capillary hypertension. Although glomerular structure is not known to be altered, the use of the dextran sieving technique has revealed impairment of barrier size-selectivity under these circumstances [60]. The level of albuminuria is almost always subnephrotic, but anecdotal examples of functional proteinuria that have reached nephrotic proportions have been reported. Confirmation of the functional nature of the proteinuria requires the demonstration that it resolves rapidly when glomerular hypertension is reversed by effective treatment of the underlying condition.

The phenomenon of 'orthostatic proteinuria' refers to proteinuria that is within the pathological range only in the upright posture. Renal biopsy has revealed that some subjects who exhibit this phenomenon have abnormal glomerular morphology, but in others no glomerular pathology has been observed. It is likely that orthostatic proteinuria in the latter represents a functional proteinuria, one that is associated with an exaggerated circadian rhythm of glomerular filtration dynamics, such that daytime capillary pressure and flows enter a range that is elevated [61].

Subnephrotic proteinuria that cannot be attributed to non-glomerular or functional causes is likely to reflect a significant glomerular injury. The same glomerular diseases that cause nephrotic-range proteinuria can manifest as subnephrotic proteinuria (Table 28.3). Either a milder form of the injury or a stage of partial remission could account for a relatively low level of proteinuria in these disorders. Paradoxically, proteinuria can also fall from a nephrotic to a subnephrotic level in the terminal stages of these diseases. This is because the extreme depression of GFR that eventuates will substantially lower the prevailing filtered protein load (equation 28.2). Among patients who persistently demonstrate only subnephrotic-range proteinuria, glomerular damage secondary to vascular or tubule-interstitial disease is likely to be a far more prevalent cause than is the case in those with nephrotic range proteinuria. The same diagnostic approach described for the nephrotic syndrome, including urine microscopy, serology, renal imaging and renal biopsy, can be used to distinguish the underlying cause of persistent glomerular proteinuria of subnephrotic proportions. Because of a less urgent need for therapy, diagnostic renal biopsy is usually not resorted to under these circumstances, however, and the precise cause of sub-nephrotic proteinuria often remains unknown.

Principles of treatment

Treatment of the nephrotic syndrome is in the first place symptomatic and directed towards ameliorating the clinical manifestations. Dietary sodium restriction and administration of diuretic agents are the mainstays of treating edema. Venous thrombosis and pulmonary thromboembolism should be treated with heparin therapy initially, followed by prolonged anticoagulant therapy with coumadin. When the nephrotic syndrome is protracted, it is also reasonable to initiate dietary and appropriate drug therapy to lower the level of total plasma cholesterol. Symptomatic treatment aside, the main focus of managing the nephrotic patient should be on reducing the level of proteinuria into the subnephrotic range. If successful, such treatment will have tangible short-term benefits and potential long-term advantages.

In the short term reducing the level of proteinuria into a subnephrotic range will, by itself, reverse or ameliorate many of the clinical and laboratory manifestations of the nephrotic syndrome. Either reduced trafficking or lower intraluminal concentrations of protein along the nephron are associated with the restoration of normal renal tubular handling of sodium. Simultaneously, diminished tubular catabolism and urinary losses of albumin will gradually lead to elevation of the serum albumin concentration towards or into the normal range. Thresholds that appear to herald the end of the sodium retaining state are the attainment of levels of proteinuria below 3.5 g/24 h and a serum albumin concentration above 3 g/dl. Once these thresholds have been crossed, it is almost always possible to ease dietary sodium restriction and withdraw diuretic therapy. The increased serum albumin concentration is accompanied by a parallel increase in oncotic pressure, thereby removing the signal for enhanced hepatic synthesis of albumin, non-albumin protein species and lipoproteins. The ensuing normalization of plasma protein composition and tissue protein content is accompanied by reversal of protein malnutrition and the hypercoagulable state, and an improvement in hyperlipidemia.

Minimal change nephropathy is usually and some forms of proliferative glomerulonephritis are often self-limited injuries, and likely to resolve completely. However, the other causes of the nephrotic syndrome (Table 28.3) are chronic injuries and exhibit a high incidence of progression to end-stage renal failure. A growing body of evidence implicates a cumulative filtered protein load of large magnitude in the genesis of such progression [62]. Thus, a sustained therapeutic effort to minimize the filtered protein load may have the long-term benefit of being renoprotective and staving off progressive renal failure.

Three findings at presentation that have been found most strongly to predict progression to end-stage renal failure, regardless of the underlying disease, are massive proteinuria, azotemia and the finding on renal biopsy of tubular atrophy and interstitial fibrosis [63]. Clearly, the first two of these predictors signify severe glomerular dysfunction. The finding that histological damage to the tubulointerstitial compartment rather than to glomeruli is most strongly predictive of progression is, at first sight, a paradox. However, recent evidence suggests that enhanced transglomerular trafficking of protein and damage to the tubulo-interstitial compartment are linked [2]. Diverse experimental injuries that induce high-grade proteinuria in the rat are followed within several weeks by morphological evidence of tubular protein overload and an infiltration of the interstitium by macrophages and T cells. With further passage of time increasing collagenization of the interstitium along with focal and segmental glomerulosclerosis become evident [62]. Thus in the rat, at least, the induction of persistently heavy proteinuria *per se* can initiate virtually all the changes that are associated with progression. Several mechanisms have been postulated to explain how a high filtered protein load with subsequent tubular protein overload might trigger a mononuclear interstitial infiltrate. These include backleak of Tam–Horsfall protein, escape from tubular cytosol of lysozymal enzymes, activation of a local tubular complement system, and the formation of lipid chemotaxins from free fatty acids that are released during the uptake and processing of filtered albumin by proximal tubule cells [2, 62].

Both disease-specific and non-specific modalities of therapy are available to effectively lower the filtered protein load in nephrotic subjects. Disease-specific therapy applies only to the immune gomerular injuries that comprise categories 1 through 4 (Table 28.3). The therapy is based on immunosuppression and its efficacy varies widely among the various listed categories. Thus, for example, corticosteroids alone or in combination with cytotoxic drugs are very effective in minimal change nephropathy, quite effective in proliferative glomerulonephritis and only marginally effective in idiopathic focal and segmental glomerulosclerosis and membranous nephropathy. The newer immunosuppressive agent cyclosporin A appears to be more efficacious than corticosteroid and cytotoxic therapy in lowering the level of proteinuria in the latter two disorders [64, 65]. It is also extremely effective in minimal change nephropathy and could eventually replace corticosteroid therapy as first line therapy in this disorder by virtue of causing fewer side effects.

Non-specific therapy involves the use of modalities that lower the filtered protein load irrespective of the underlying disease. They include dietary protein restriction and the administration of agents that inhibit local formation of either angiotensin II or prostaglandin in the vicinity of the injured glomerulus. Inhibition of angiotensin II formation is usually achieved by the administration of an angiotensin converting enzyme inhibitor (ACEi) [66]. However, preliminary studies suggest that direct antagonists of type I angiotensin II receptors will prove to be equally effective [67]. The class of cyclo-oxgenase inhibitors that are known collectively as non-steroidal anti-inflammatory drugs (NSAIDs) should all be effective in lowering proteinuria via inhibition of prostaglandin production, but indomethacin and meclofenimate have been the most widely used for this purpose [68]. Dietary protein restriction and ACEi therapy have been shown in rats with experimental glomerular disease to lower glomerular capillary perfusion pressure, and this common effect may underlie their antiproteinuric effect [69]. Each form of therapy has also been shown by the dextran sieving technique to improve barrier size-selectivity in nephrotic glomerular injuries in both rats and humans. In human nephrotics moreover, the antiproteinuric effect of ACEi therapy has been shown by the dextran sieving technique to be accompanied by significant reduction in the prominence of shunt-like pores in the absence of measurable hemodynamic alterations [54, 55]. This raises the possibility that the antiproteinuric effect of this class of agents, and perhaps also that of dietary protein restriction, is via a primary membrane-modulating action on the glomerular filtration barrier. Indomethacin has also been shown by the dextran-sieving technique to reduce the shunt pathway, but in this case a simultaneous fall in glomerular perfusion rate and pressure does not permit hemodynamic and membrane-modulating effects to be distinguished [52, 53]. Although dietary protein restriction and ACEi therapy appear to exert their actions through diverse pathways, each has been shown to be renoprotective in the glomerulopathic rat. Common to such renoprotection is substantial lowering of the cumulative filtered protein load, blunting of the extent to which the interstitial compartment becomes collagenized, and a reduced prevalence of glomerulosclerosis. It is this combination of findings that underpins the rationale for therapy aimed at minimizing proteinuria in glomerulopathic humans [62].

It should be emphasized that the renoprotective efficacy of non-specific antiproteinuric therapy as observed in the rat has not yet been convincingly demonstrated in humans with severe glomerular disease. It is, thus, important to bear in mind that all three modalities can have adverse effects in the nephrotic patient, and should thus be used with caution. As stated previously, nephrotic glomerular injury is invariably associated with K_f depression. When K_f depression is profound, the GFR may be critically dependent on an elevated ultrafiltration pressure. It follows that lowering glomerular capillary pressure by initiating the foregoing antiproteinuric therapies may precipitate acute renal insufficiency. Also, lowering the dietary protein intake could aggravate negative nitrogen balance in a nephrotic patient, and thereby worsen protein malnutrition. Thus, care must be taken when initiating such therapy. Serum creatinine and potassium levels should be monitored frequently until it becomes clear that the patient is tolerant of the therapeutic manipulation, and is maintaining a stable and adequate level of renal function. It is probably also prudent to introduce these maneuvers sequentially and not simultaneously. A suggested sequence would begin with ACEi therapy, followed after several weeks by dietary protein restriction to supplement the antiproteinuric effect of the former. If there is an inadequate response to ACEi therapy combined with dietary protein restriction, a trial of a NSAID could be attempted. In this event the NSAID should be substituted for rather than added to the ACEi. A final precaution when making this substitution is to allow an adequate period to elapse between the two therapeutic maneuvers. It can take up to three weeks before ACEi is washed out of the tissues. So as to avoid precipitating severe renal insufficiency, it is wise to wait for this interval to pass before introducing treatment with an NSAID. In the event that ACEi therapy does not control hypertension or is replaced by an NSAID, it is important to ensure that hypertension is adequately treated in all patients who have a severe glomerular disease. Simply restoring normotension, regardless of the antihypertensive agent(s) used for this purpose, has been shown to delay progression to end-stage renal failure [70]. That such therapy is also antiproteinuric provides yet one more piece of evidence to support the hypothesis that transglomerular protein trafficking contributes to the progressive nature of many glomerular diseases.

Acknowledgment

The studies in this chapter that were performed in the author's laboratory were supported by NIH grant DK 29985.

References

1. Schreiner, G.E. (1971) The nephrotic syndrome, in *Diseases of the Kidney* (eds M. Strauss and L. Welt), Little, Brown, Boston, pp. 503–636.
2. Kees-Folts, D., Sadow, J.L. and Schreiner, G.F. (1994) Tubular catabolism of albumin is associated with the release of an inflammatory lipid. *Kidney Int.*, **330**, 1129–35.
3. Bernard, D.B., Alexander, E.A., Couser, W.G. *et al.* (1978) Renal sodium retention during volume expansion in experimental nephrotic syndrome. *Kidney Int.*, **14**, 478–87.
4. Peterson, C., Madsen, B., Perlman, A. *et al.* (1988) Atrial natriuretic peptide and the renal response to hypervolemia in nephrotic humans. *Kidney Int.*, **34**, 825–31.

5. Koepke, J.P. and DiBona, G.F. (1987) Blunted natriuresis to atrial natriuretic peptide in chronic sodium-retaining disorders. *Am. J. Physiol.*, **252**, F865–71.

6. Nonoguchi, H., Knepper, M.A. and Manganielle, V.C. (1987) Effects of atrial natriuretic factor on cyclic guanosine monophosphate and cyclic adenosine monophosphate accumulation in microdissected nephron segments from rats. *J. Clin. Invest.*, **79**, 500–7.

7. Healy, D.P. and Fanestil, D.D. (1986) Localization of atrial natriuretic peptide binding sites within the rat kidney. *Am. J. Physiol.*, **250**, F573–8.

8. Dorhout–Mees, E.J., Geers, A.B. and Koomans, H.A. (1984) Blood volume and sodium retention in the nephrotic syndrome: A controversial pathophysiological concept. *Nephron*, **36**, 201–11.

9. Ichikawa, I., Rennke, H.G., Hoyer, J.R. *et al.* (1983) Role for intrarenal mechanisms in the impaired salt excretion of experimental nephrotic syndrome. *J. Clin. Invest.*, **71**, 91–3.

10. Canaan-Kühl, S., Venkatraman, E.S., Ernst, S.I.B. *et al.* (1993) Relationships among protein and albumin concentrations and oncotic pressure in nephrotic plasma. *Am. J. Physiol.*, **246**, F1052–9.

11. Pietrangelo, A., Panduro, A., Chowdhury, J.R. *et al.* (1992) Albumin gene expression is down-regulated by albumin or macromolecule infusion in the rat. *J. Clin. Invest.*, **89**, 1755–60.

12. Kaysen, G.A., Kirkpatrick, W.G. and Couser, W.G. (1984) Albumin homeostasis in the nephrotic rat: nutritional considerations. *Am. J. Physiol.*, **247**, F192–202.

13. Al–Bander, H.A., Martin, V.I. and Kaysen, G.A. (1992) Plasma IgG pool is not defended from urinary loss nephrotic syndrome. *Am. J. Physiol.*, **262**, F333–7.

14. Kanfer, A. (1990) Coagulation factors in nephrotic syndrome. *Am. J. Nephrol.*, **10**, 63–8.

15. Llach, F. (1985) Hypercoagulability, renal vein thrombosis, and other thrombotic complications of nephrotic syndrome. Editorial review. *Kidney Int.*, **28**, 429–39.

16. Zucchelli, P. (1992) Renal vein thrombosis. *Nephrol. Dial. Transplant.*, **1**, 105–8.

17. Davis, R.A., Engelhorn, S.C., Weinstein, D.B. *et al.* (1980) Very low density lipoprotein secretion by cultured rat hepatocytes: inhibition by albumin and other macromolecules. *J. Biol. Chem.*, **255**, 2039–45.

18. Kaysen, G.A., Don, B. and Schambelan, M. (1991) Proteinuria, albumin synthesis and hyperlipidemia in the nephrotic syndrome. *Nephrol. Dial. Transplant.*, **6**, 141–9.

19. Vega, G.L. and Grundy, S.M. (1988) Lovastatin therapy in nephrotic hyperlipidemia: effects on lipoprotein metabolism. *Kidney Int.*, **33**, 1160–8.

20. Ordonez, J.D., Hiatt, R.A., Killebrew, E.J. *et al.* (1993) The increased risk of coronary heart disease associated with nephrotic syndrome. *Kidney Int.*, **44**, 638–42.

21. Drumond, M.C., Kristal, B. and Myers, B.D. (1994) Structural basis for reduced glomerular filtration capacity in nephrotic humans. *J. Clin. Invest.*, **94**, 1187–95.

22. Ting, R.H., Kristal, B. and Myers, B.D. (1994) The biophysical basis of hypofiltration in nephrotic humans with membranous nephropathy. *Kidney Int.*, **45**, 390–7.

23. Guasch, A., Hashimoto, H., Sibley, R.K. *et al.* (1991) Glomerular dysfunction in nephrotic humans with minimal changes or focal glomerulosclerosis. *Am. J. Physiol.*, **29**, F728–37.

24. Chagnac, A., Kiberd, B.A., Fariñas, M.C. *et al.* (1989) Outcome of the acute glomerular injury in proliferative lupus nephritis. *J. Clin. Invest.*, **84**, 922–30.

25. Austin, S.M., Lieberman, J.S., Newton, L.D. *et al.* (1993) Slope of serial GFR and the progression of diabetic glomerular disease. *J. Am. Soc. Nephrol.*, **3**, 1358–70.

26. Shemesh, O., Golbetz, H., Kriss, J.P. *et al.* (1985) Limitations of creatinine as a filtration marker in glomerulopathic patients. *Kidney Int.*, **28**, 830–8.

27. Baylis, C., Ichikawa, I., Willis, W.T. *et al.* (1977) Dynamics of glomerular ultrafiltration IX. Effects of plasma protein concentration. *Am. J. Physiol.*, **232**, F58–64.

28. Ichikawa, I., Purkerson, M.L., Klahr, S. *et al.* (1980) Mechanism of reduced glomerular filtration rate in chronic malnutrition. *J. Clin. Invest.*, **65**, 982–8.

29. Golden, M.H.N., Brooks, S.E.H., Ramdath, D.O. *et al.* (1990) Effacement of glomerular foot processes in kwashiorkor. *Lancet*, **336**, 1472–4.

30. Tojo, A. and Endou, H. (1992) Intrarenal handling of proteins in rats using fractional micropuncture technique. *Am. J. Physiol.*, **263**, F601–6.

31. Oken, D.E., Kirschbaum, B.B. and Landwehr, D.M. (1981) Micropuncture studies of the mechanisms of normal and pathologic albuminuria. *Contrib. Nephrol.*, **24**, 1–7.

32. Baldamus, C.A., Galaske, R., Eisenbach, G.M. *et al.* (1975) Glomerular protein filtration in normal and nephritic rats. *Contrib. Nephrol.*, **1**, 37–49.

33. Bertolatus, J.A. and Hunsicker, L.G. (1985) Glomerular sieving of anionic and neutral bovine albumins in proteinuric rats. *Kidney Int.*, **28**, 467–76.

34. Rennke, H.G., Patel, Y. and Venkatachalam, M.A. (1978) Glomerular filtration of proteins: clearance of anionic, neutral, and cationic horseradish peroxidase in the rat. *Kidney Int.*, **13**, 324–8.

35. Christensen, E.L., Rennke, H.G. and Carone, F.A. (1983) Renal tubular uptake of protein: effect of molecular charge. *Am. J. Physiol.*, **244**, F436–41.

36. Robson, A.M., Giangiacomo, J., Kienstra, R.A. *et al.* (1974) Normal glomerular permeability and its modification by minimal change nephrotic syndrome. *J. Clin. Invest.*, **54**, 1190–9.

37. Scandling, J.D., Black, V.M., Deen, W.M. *et al.* (1992) Glomerular permselectivity in healthy and nephrotic humans. Necker's Seminar in Nephrology. *Adv. Nephrol.*, **21**, 159–76.

38. Oliver, J.D. III, Anderson, S., Troy, J.L. *et al.* (1992) Determination of glomerular size-selectivity in the normal rat with Ficoll. *J. Am. Soc. Nephrol.*, **3**, 214–28.

39. Deen, W.M., Bridges, C.R., Breener, B.M. *et al.* (1985) Heteroporous model of glomerular size-selectivity: application to normal and nephrotic humans. *Am. J. Physiol.*, **249**, F374–89.

40. Bohrer, M.P., Patterson, G. and Carroll, P.J. (1984) Hindered diffusion of dextran and ficoll in microporous membranes. *Macromolecules*, **17**, 1170–3.

41. Davidson, M.G. and Deen, W.M. (1988) Hindered diffusion of water-soluble macromolecules and membranes. *Macromolecules*, **21**, 3474–81.

42. Maddox, D.A., Deen, W.M. and Brenner, B.M. (1992) Glomerular filtration, in *Handbook of Physiology*, section 8: Renal Physiology, Vol. 1 (ed. E.E. Windhager), Oxford Univsity Press, New York, pp. 545–638.

43. Guasch, A., Deen, W.M. and Myers, B.D. (1993) Charge-selectivity of the glomerular filtration barrier in healthy and nephrotic humans. *J. Clin. Invest.*, **92**, 2274–82.

44. Daniels, B.S., Deen, W.M., Mayer, G. *et al.* (1993) Glomerular permeability barrier in the rat: functional assessment by *in vitro* methods. *J. Clin. Invest.*, **92**, 929–36.

45. Rennke, H.G. and Venkatachalam, M.A. (1977) Glomerular permeability: *in vivo* tracer studies with polyanionic and polycationic ferritins. *Kidney Int.*, **11**, 44–53.

46. Scheeberger, E.E., Levey, R.H., McCluskey, R.T. *et al.* (1975) The isoporous substructure of the human glomerular slip diaphragm. *Kidney Int.*, **8**, 48–52.

47. Kanwar, Y.S. and Rosenzweig, L.J. (1982) Altered glomerular permeability as a result of focal detachment of the visceral epithelium. *Kidney Int.*, **21**, 565–74.

48. Shemesh, O., Deen, W.M., Brenner, B.M. *et al.* (1986) Effect of colloid volume expansion on glomerular barrier size-selectivity in humans. *Kidney Int.*, **29**, 916–23.

49. Yoshioka, T., Rennke, H.G., Salant, D.J. *et al.* (1987) Role of abnormally high transmural pressure in the permselectivity of defect of glomerular capillary wall: a study in early passive Heymann nephritis. *Circ. Res.*, **61**, 531–8.

50. Bridges, C.R. Jr, Rennke, H.M., Deen, W.M. *et al.* (1991) Reversible hexadimethrine-induced alterations in glomerular structure and permeability. *J. Am. Soc. Nephrol.*, **1**, 1095–108.

51. Hunsicker, L.G., Shearer, T.P. and Shaffer, S.J. (1981) Acute reversible proteinuria induced by infusion of the polycation hexadimethrine, *Kidney Int.*, **20**, 7–17.

52. Tiggeler, R.G.W.L., Hulme, B. and Hijdeveld, P.G.A.G. (1979) Effect of indomethacin on glomerular permeability in the nephrotic syndrome. *Kidney Int.*, **16**, 312–21.

53. Golbetz, H., Black, V., Shemesh, O. *et al.* (1989) Mechanism of the antiproteinuric effect of indomethacin in nephrotic humans. *Am. J. Physiol.*, **25**, 44–51.

54. Morelli, E., Loon, N., Meyer, T. *et al.* (1990) Effects of converting enzyme inhibition on barrier function in diabetic glomerulopathy. *Diabetes*, **39**, 76–82.

55. Remuzzi, A., Ruggenenti, P., Mosconi, L. *et al.* (1993) Effect of low-dose enalapril on glomerular size-selectivity in human diabetic nephropathy. *J. Nephrol.*, **6**, 36–43.

56. Olivetti, G., Giacomelli, F. and Wiener, J. (1985) Morphometry of superficial glomeruli in acute hypertension in the rat. *Kidney Int.*, **27**, 31–8.

57. Mogensen, C.E., Christensen, C.K. and Vittinghus, E. (1983) The stages in diabetic renal disease with emphasis on the stage of incipient diabetic nephropathy. *Diabetes*, **32**, 64–78.

58. Myers, B.D., Nelson, R.G., Blouch, K. *et al.* (1995) Progression of overt nephropathy in non–insulin–dependent diabetes. *Kidney Int.*, **47**, 1781–9.

59. Alpers, C.E. (1994) Glomerulopathies of dysproteinemias, abnormal immunoglobulin deposition, and lymphoproliferative disorders. *Curr. Opin. Nephrol. Hypertens.*, **3**, 349–55.

60. Carrie, B.J., Hilberman, M., Schroeder, J.S. *et al.* (1980) Albuminuria and the permselective properties of the glomerulus in cardiac failure. *Kidney Int.*, **17**, 507–14.

61. van Acker, B.A.C. (1994) *Glomerular Filtration Rate – Accurate Measurement and Circadian Rhythm.* Drukkerij Elinkwijk BV, Utrecht, The Netherlands, pp. 113–14.

62. Remuzzi, G. and Bertani, T. (1990) Is glomerulosclerosis a conseqence of altered glomerular permeability to macromolecules? *Kidney Int.*, **38**, 384–94.

63. D'Amico, G. (1992) Influence of clinical and histological features on actuarial renal survival in adult patients with idiopathic IgA nephropathy, membranous nephropathy, and membranoprofilerative glomerulonephritis: survey of the recent literature. *Am. J. Kidney Dis.*, **20**, 325–33.

64. Ponticelli, C., Rizzoni, G., Edefonti, A. *et al.* (1993) A randomized trial of cyclosporine in steroid–resistant idiopathic nephrotic syndrome. *Kidney Int.*, **43**, 1377–84.

65. Guasch, A., Suranyi, M., Newton, L. *et al.* (1992) Short-term responsiveness of membranous glomerulopathy to cyclosporine. *Am. J. Kidney Dis.*, **5**, 472–81.

66. Kasiske, B.L., Kalil, R.S.N., Ma, J.Z. *et al.* (1993) Effect of antihypertensive therapy on the kidney in patients with diabetes: a meta-regression analysis. *Ann. Intern. Med.*, **118**, 129–38.

67. Gansevoort, R.T., de Zeeuw D. and de Jong, P.E. (1994) Is the antiproteinuria effect of ACE inhibition mediated by interference in the renin–angiotensin system. *Kidney Int.*, **45**, 861–7.

68. Michielson, P. and van Renterghen, Y. (1983) Proteinuria and non-steroidal anti-inflammatory drugs. *Adv. Nephrol.*, **12**, 139–50.

69. Anderson, S., Meyer, T.W., Rennke, H.G. *et al.* (1985) Control of glomerular hypertension limits glomerular injury in rats with reduced renal mass. *J. Clin. Invest.*, **76**, 612–19.

70. Parving, H.H., Andersen, A.R., Smidt, U.M. *et al.* (1987) Effect of antihypertensive treatment on kidney function in diabetic nephropathy. *Br. Med. J.*, **294**, 1443–7.

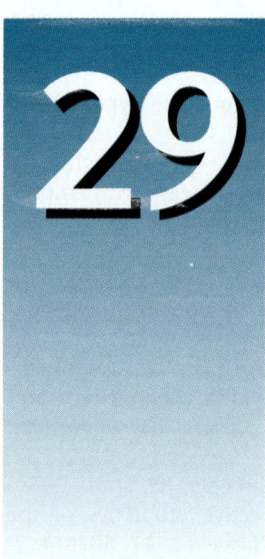

29

Calcium and phosphate metabolism

Michael Pazianas and John B. Eastwood

Normal homeostasis

Calcium and phosphorus are among the most abundant elements in the body. They are the dominant constituents of bone and present in the majority of body fluids. Both are an integral part of many of the body's fundamental enzyme and cellular pathways. Hence conservation of these elements is of considerable importance, especially calcium, as it is less readily available in food compared with phosphorus.

Physiological role of calcium

There are two major ways in which calcium exerts its influence in the body: structural and functional. The structural role is most clearly seen in the skeleton but it should be remembered that calcium (together with phosphorus) is an important element in the integrity of cell walls. The element is also essential in the ability of the cells to stick together.

Of more diverse importance is the involvement of calcium in elementary metabolic functions [1–3]. Calcium ions are central to the integrity of the clotting cascade and are of fundamental importance in muscle contraction. They are also important in cell division and motility, hormone secretion, the transfer of other inorganic anions across membranes and in intracellular signal transduction. They also modulate the activity of crucial enzymes involved in glycogen and cyclic nucleotide metabolism. Calcium ions are important because they can become complexed with organic compounds to form salts with a wide range of solubilities.

The normal range for total plasma calcium is 2.15–2.60 mM   (4.3–5.2 mEq/l,   8.6–10.4 mg/dl)   and 1.17–1.33 mM   (2.34–2.66 mEq/l,   4.68–5.32 mg/dl)   for ionized calcium. Approximately 40% of plasma calcium is protein bound, mostly to albumin (90%). About 50% is in ionic form and the remaining 10% is complexed with citrate, phosphate and other ions. Albumin concentration can alter total plasma calcium concentration and pH can change the ratio of ionized to bound calcium. At pH 7.4 it is estimated that 1 g/dl of albumin binds 0.8 mg/dl of calcium. In patients with hypoalbuminemia (liver disease, nephrotic syndrome) it is important to calculate the 'corrected' calcium to determine whether or not true hypocalcemia is present (measured total calcium + 0.025 (40 – serum albumin)). Binding of calcium to albumin is highly pH dependent. Acute acidosis decreases the binding and as a result more calcium ions will be available. Acute alkalosis has the opposite effect and is the explanation for the tetany inducible by hyperventilation (acute respiratory alkalosis). It is noteworthy that the calcium involved with the cellular and human mechanisms described above as well that in the plasma amounts to less than 1% of total body calcium.

The vast majority of the body's calcium is in the skeleton (males 1200 g, females 900 g) as hydroxyapatite $(Ca_{10}(PO_4)_6(OH)_2)$ but only about 1% of bone calcium is available for exchange with the extracellular fluid [4]. This exchangeable skeletal calcium plus that in the extracellular fluid are together known as the miscible pool of calcium (Figure 29.1).

The concentrations of calcium in plasma and extracellular fluid are maintained within a narrow physiolog-

Nephrology, Edited by Rex L. Jamison and Robert Wilkinson.
Published in 1997 by Chapman & Hall, London. ISBN 0 412 60930 4

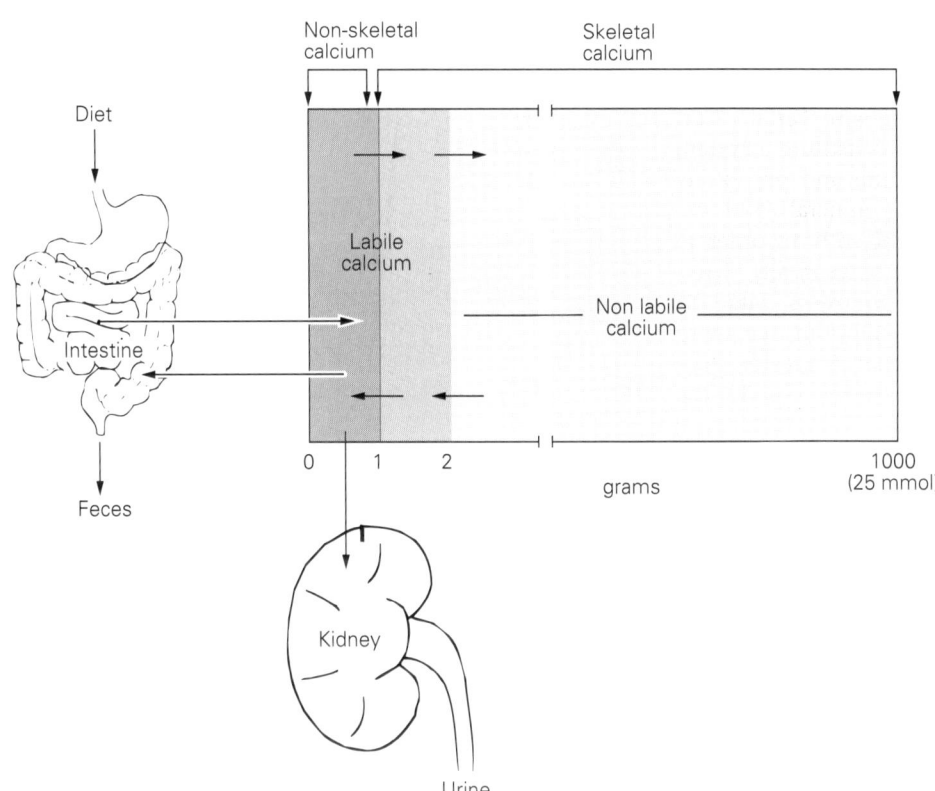

Non-skeletal calcium

Skeletal calcium

Diet

Labile calcium

Non labile calcium

Intestine

Feces

0   1   2   grams   1000 (25 mmol)

Kidney

Urine

Figure 29.1 Schematic representation of calcium distribution and flux. (Modified from Potts, J.T. Jr and Deftos, L.J. (1974) Parathyroid hormone, thyrocalcitonin, vitamin D, bone and mineral metabolism, in *Duncan's Diseases of Metabolism*, 7th edn (eds P.K. Bondy and L.E. Rosenbery), W.B. Saunders Company, Philadelphia, pp. 1225–430, with permission.)

ical range [5, 5a]. The concentration of calcium ions in the extracellular fluid is high (10^{-3} M) but intracellularly (in the cytoplasm) is usually $<10^{-7}$ M. This very steep gradient is maintained by mechanisms regulating the cellular entry and extrusion of calcium ions and by mechanisms that regulate uptake and release of calcium ions by intracellular stores [6, 7].

Physiological role of phosphorus

Phosphorus, like calcium, supports life in living species by contributing significantly to their structural and functional needs [1–3]. As mentioned above, phosphorus is a principal component of the skeleton. Phosphorus in combination with fatty acids (phospholipids) has a major structural role in the integrity of cell walls. Its functional contribution is equally important. Storage and decoding of genetic information requires phosphorus. Nucleotides contain one or more phosphate groups and in combination with a phosphate ester are known as nucleic acids, the most important of which are RNA and DNA. Nucleotides themselves carry chemical energy in the form of adenosine triphosphate (ATP). Phosphorus ions modulate enzyme activity through ATP which supplies the energy for the binding of coenzymes to the surface of enzymes. The intracellular signaling network is also dependent on phosphorus. Cyclic adenosine monophosphate (cAMP), a phosphate-containing adenine derivative, and calcium ions form intracellular pathways that

participate in a second messenger role. Phosphorus also has a central role in the systemic regulation of pH. At body pH it is a titrable acid ($HPO_4^{2-} + H^+ \rightleftharpoons H_2PO_4^-$). In adults, the normal range for serum phosphorus is 0.9–1.45 mM (2.8–4.5 mg/dl). There is considerable diurnal variation, lowest levels being found in the morning.

The skeleton accommodates about 85% of the body's phosphorus (i.e. 500–800 g). The remaining 15% is found either as inorganic phosphate (P_i) in extracellular fluid or as phosphate esters in unmineralized tissues. About 10% of serum phosphate is protein bound and approximately 35% is complexed with calcium, magnesium or sodium; 55% is in ionic form. In total, therefore, 90% (nonprotein bound) is ultrafiltrable and available for renal excretion. The difference between extracellular (1×10^{-4} M) and intracellular ($2–5 \times 10^{-4}$ M) phosphorus concentration is not as great as in the case of calcium.

Regulation of calcium and phosphorus homeostasis

The total fluxes of calcium involved in calcium homeostasis are quite large. The free calcium concentration in the cytosol of resting cells can rise more than 100-fold when the cells are activated. Nevertheless, calcium concentration in plasma and extracellular fluid is remarkably constant. Throughout the day, it is estimated that serum calcium fluctuates by only 0.25 mM in normal individuals. On the other hand, plasma phosphate concentration varies considerably throughout the day and is significantly affected by diet.

The minerals themselves together with certain hormones and other agents (see below) constitute a system linking the organs involved in calcium and phosphate homeostasis. The availability of the minerals and the capacity of the organs to operate efficiently in order to meet the changing demands of the body finally determine the balance. When mineral intake is equal to mineral losses the body is in equilibrium, i.e. zero balance. Children have an intake that is greater than output (positive balance) whereas in the elderly the reverse is often true (negative balance).

Hormones (Figure 29.2)

Parathyroid hormone (PTH)

PTH is an 84 amino acid polypeptide secreted by the chief cells of the parathyroid glands. The gene is localized on chromosome 11. The primary stimulus for PTH secretion is the ionized calcium concentration in the plasma [5], a fall of which increases PTH secretion (Figure 29.3). It is now known that calcium controls the synthesis and secre-

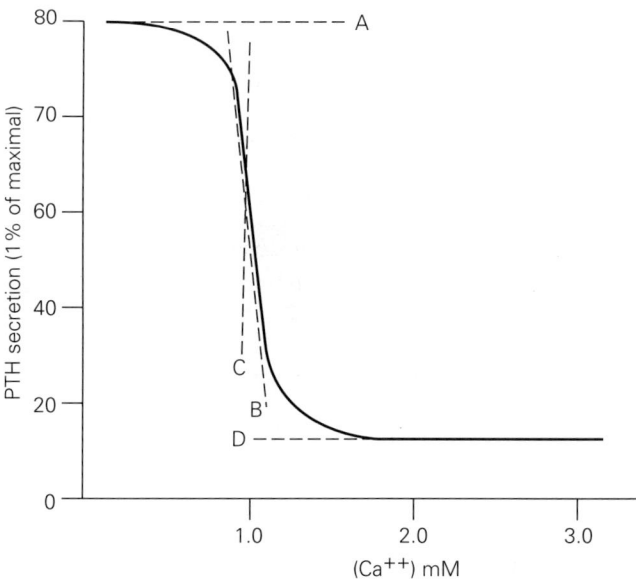

Figure 29.3 The inverse sigmoidal relationship between ionized plasma calcium concentration [Ca^{2+}] and PTH secretion rate. Small alterations in [Ca^{2+}] just below its physiological range can provoke large increases in PTH secretion rate. Below this level or if it exceeds 1.8 mM, the response to changes in [Ca^{2+}] is very small. A, maximal PTH secretory rate; B, slope of curve at its midpoint; C, Ca^{2+} concentration producing half-maximal change in PTH secretion (this is known as the 'set point'); D, minimal secretory rate (Adapted from Brown, E.M. (1983) Four parameter model of the sigmoidal relationship between PTH release and extracellular calcium concentration in normal and abnormal parathyroid tissue. *J. Clin. Endocrinol. Metab.*, **56**, 572–580, with permission.)

tion of PTH through a calcium sensing receptor [8–10]. There are also receptors to calcitriol (see below), the lack of which increases PTH [11].

In plasma PTH has a half-life of about 4 min. The liver and kidney are responsible for its clearance. The biological activity is contained within amino acids 1–34 of the N-terminal end of the molecule. The action of PTH is via receptors in bone and kidney. PTH stimulates osteoblasts and secondarily osteoclasts [12]. It is stimulation of the latter that leads to release of calcium and phosphate from the skeleton. In the kidney, PTH inhibits the reabsorption of phosphate causing phosphaturia and a fall in plasma phosphate. PTH also stimulates the reabsorption of calcium by the kidney. PTH also increases 1α-hydroxylase activity in proximal tubule cells to produce calcitriol which stimulates calcium and phosphate absorption in the gut.

1,25 (OH)₂ vitamin D₃ (calcitriol)

Cholecalciferol (vitamin D₃) is a steroid produced by the action of ultraviolet light on 7-dehydrocholesterol in the skin. Vitamin D is also obtained from the diet either as

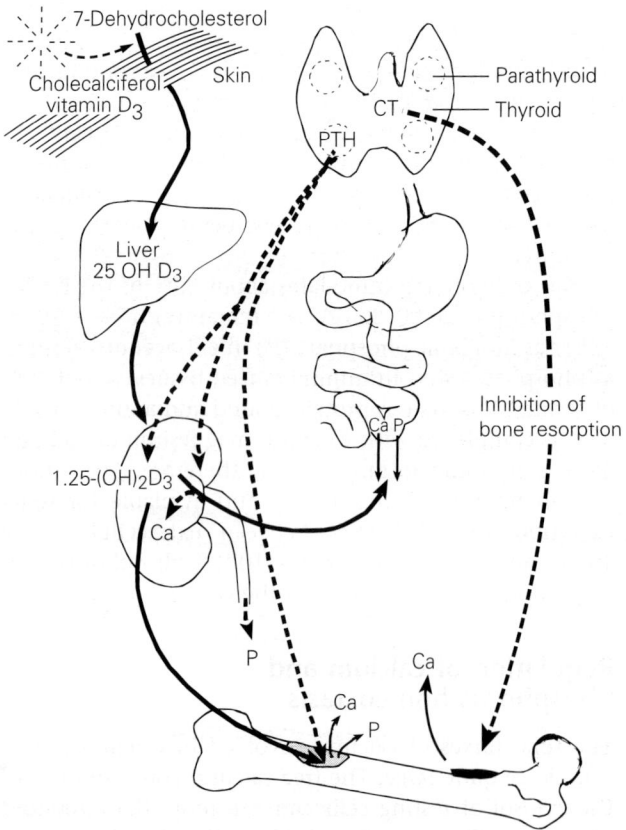

Figure 29.2 Hormonal influences on calcium and phosphate homeostasis. PTH, parathyroid hormone; CT, calcitonin; Ca, calcium; P, phosphate.

vitamin D_2 (ergocalciferol) or vitamin D_3. The dietary form is absorbed in the small intestine and, like the form synthesized in the skin, transported in the plasma bound to lipoproteins, albumin and a specific vitamin D-binding protein. When circulating vitamin D reaches the liver, it is hydroxylated to 25-OH vitamin D_3 (there is also a small amount of 25-OH vitamin D_2). A further metabolic step in the kidney converts 25-OH vitamin D_3 into 1,25-$(OH)_2$ vitamin D_3 [13].

There are receptors for 1,25-$(OH)_2$ vitamin D_3 in intestine, bone, parathyroid and kidney. In the intestine, 1,25-$(OH)_2$ vitamin D_3 increases absorption of calcium and phosphate. In the bone, it stimulates osteoblasts which in turn influence osteoclasts to proliferate and become active, which increases bone resorption and releases calcium and phosphate from bone. The effect of 1,25-$(OH)_2$ vitamin D_3 on the parathyroid gland is to reduce PTH synthesis and on the kidney to increase the excretion of calcium and phosphate.

Calcitonin

Calcitonin is a 32 amino acid peptide produced in the C cells of the thyroid gland. It inhibits bone resorption by direct action on the osteoclast. Indeed, calcitonin is the only known hormone that acts directly on osteoclasts (Figures 29.4 and 29.5). Acute changes in the concentration of calcium modulate its plasma level, i.e. a rise in plasma ionized calcium stimulates release of calcitonin. However, the physiological role of calcitonin in normal mineral homeostasis and skeletal metabolism has not yet been elucidated in humans [14].

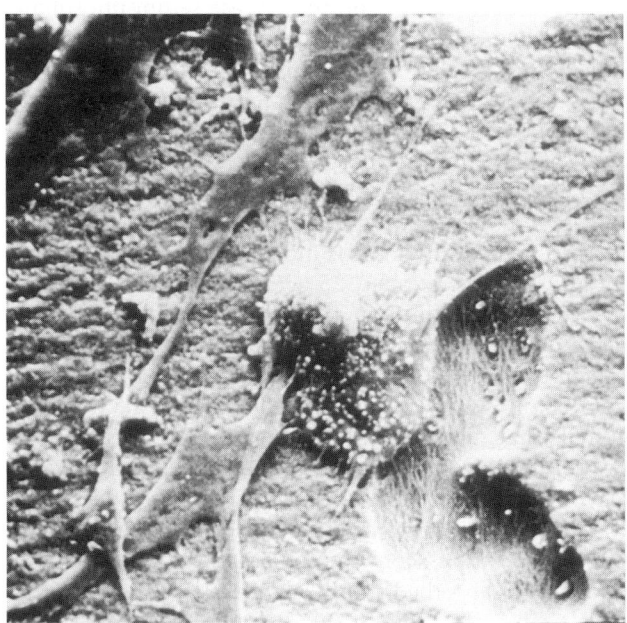

Figure 29.4 Scanning electromicrograph of an osteoclast which has moved to an adjacent site having created two resorption cavities (Courtesy of Professor A. Boyde, UCL, London, with permission.)

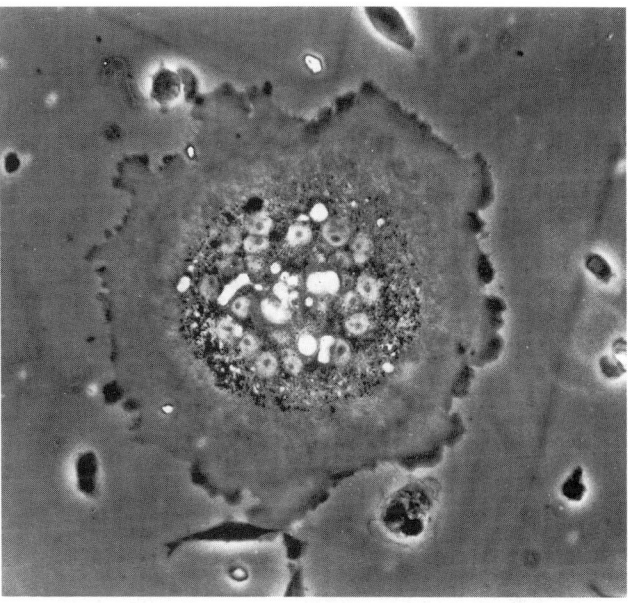

a

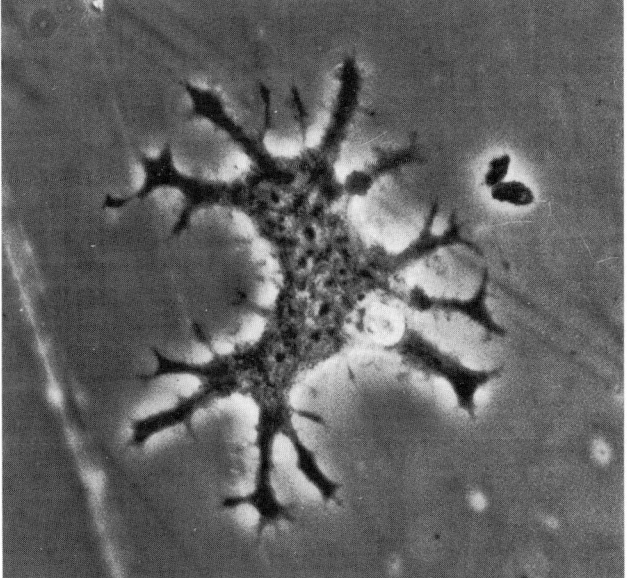

b

Figure 29.5 Effects of calcitonin on osteoclast membrane ruffling. The osteoclast plasma membrane adjacent to bone has complex folds, the 'ruffled border', which plays an important part in the bone resorbing system of the osteoclast. (a) An isolated rat osteoclast resorbing bone; (b) the same osteoclast after application of calcitonin; the ruffled border has been lost. (Courtesy of Professor T.J. Chambers, St George's Hospital Medical School, London, with permission.)

Parathyroid hormone-related protein (PTHrP)

PTHrP was discovered during the search for the cause of the hypercalcemia of malignancy [15]. The human PTHrP gene is located on chromosome 12 and expressed in the placenta, uterus, brain and smooth muscle. PTHrP is produced by many solid tumors. It shares the same receptor, the same mediator (cAMP) and many biological activities with PTH: it therefore causes hypercalcemia, hypophosphatemia, phosphaturia and an increase in $1,25\text{-}(OH)_2$ vitamin D_3 production in the kidney. However, homology with PTH is less than expected. Unlike PTH (84 amino acids) there are three PTHrP isoforms consisting of 139, 141 and 173 amino acids. Interestingly, the only homology with PTH is that eight of the first 13 amino acids in the molecule are the same.

The physiological role of PTHrP is yet to be established. Its presence in fetal tissues such as parathyroid has led to the suggestion that the hormone modulates placental calcium transport. This idea is supported by the observation that lack of the gene has lethal effects on the skeleton of the developing embryo.

Intestine

Calcium

In healthy adults, the net amount of calcium absorbed daily from the gut is 150–200 mg which in practice is only possible if the intake is more than 400 mg (10 mmol) [16] because there is an obligatory daily loss of calcium of around 200 mg from the intestine. Most of the calcium is absorbed in the jejunum and ileum where there is a large surface area and long exposure of minerals to the mucosa. Calcium absorption is a slow process which requires several hours to be completed. The absorptive efficacy of the duodenum is greater than that of jejunum and ileum, but its surface area is much smaller. Most normal individuals absorb 20–70% of the ingested calcium depending on intake; it is usually about 35%. There is a decline in calcium absorption with advancing age. The net calcium absorption in healthy individuals on the same diet varies widely; there is little relation between dietary intake of calcium and net absorption. A calcium intake in excess of 1000 mg daily will increase the amount of calcium absorbed but the increase in urinary calcium may offset any increase in calcium retention. Certain substances, including fatty acids, bile acids and lactose, can increase the rate of calcium absorption. On the other hand, calcium absorption is reduced with diets high in fiber, oxalate and phytate.

Transcellular calcium transport in the intestine is critically dependent on the presence of $1,25\text{-}(OH)_2$ vitamin D_3 and involves initial entry at the luminal brush border against a steep electrochemical gradient. This process is affected by variations in the lipid composition of the cell membrane, in particular its unsaturated fatty acid content, but the fundamental transport mechanism remains unknown. Recent evidence has shown the existence of a divalent cation sensing 'receptor' on the enterocyte and preliminary experiments suggest that this molecule is distinct from the cloned parathyroid calcium receptor [17].

Once inside the cell, calcium is transported to the opposite, basolateral membrane by means of calbindin,

an intracellular vitamin D-dependent calcium binding protein. At the basolateral membrane, calcium is pumped out of the cell again against a steep electrochemical gradient. There appear to be two mechanisms for this active transport. First, there is a calcium-ATPase that is sensitive to nanomolar concentrations of calcium. Second, there is a sodium–calcium exchange mechanism in which transport of calcium is driven by the inward electrochemical gradient for sodium ions, established by an Na,K-ATPase.

It is known that $1,25\text{-}(OH)_2$ vitamin D_3 increases the rate of calcium absorption. This may take place through either an increase in the permeability of the brush borders to calcium ions or alterations in the synthesis of the calbindin. $1,25\text{-}(OH)_2$ vitamin D_3 also increases calcium absorption by means of paracellular pathways.

In the colon there is an obligatory loss of calcium into the lumen which is why the expression 'net calcium absorption' is used in relation to the intestine, i.e. net absorption = intestinal absorption minus colonic loss.

Phosphorus

In healthy adults, the average daily phosphorus intake is 800–900 mg, though half of this would be sufficient to cover daily needs. In adults, the net absorption of phosphorus is estimated at 50–70% (80–90% in infants) and declines with advancing age. Jejunum (mainly) and duodenum are the most active sites for phosphorus absorption. Unlike calcium, absorption of phosphorus is directly proportional to dietary intake. Therefore, the quantity of dietary phosphorus determines its absorption in the gut. Serum phosphorus concentration reaches a peak about 1 h after a meal and returns to pre-meal values in 2–3 h. Carbohydrates tend to decrease serum phosphate, possibly by facilitating the movement of the mineral into cells.

As in the case of calcium, transcellular phosphorus transport in the gut takes place in three stages. At physiological pH, influx of phosphorus across the brush border is sodium dependent with both elements using the same transport system. In a more acidic environment (pH 6.0) the mechanism involved is independent of intraluminal sodium concentration. $1,25\text{-}(OH)_2$ vitamin D_3 facilitates the cellular transport in the duodenum by a calcium-dependent mechanism but its action on the jejunum is calcium independent. The other two stages in the transport of phosphorus are not well understood. It is suggested that a microtubular microfilament system is responsible for transport across the cell whereas calcium leaves the enterocyte by means of a passive process.

Like calcium, there is also a paracellular transport for phosphate but its contribution to the total amount of phosphorus absorbed is unlikely to be large.

Kidney

The kidney plays a crucial role in mineral homeostasis [18, 19]. It is responsible for the excretion of calcium and phosphate and is the major source of calcitriol. In practice, the maximum capacity of the kidney for calcium excretion is 600 mg/day, and the minimum is around 100 mg/day. This limited range of excretion has led to the suggestion that the kidney plays only a supportive role to the bone in mineral homeostasis.

Calcium (Figure 29.6)

Only the calcium not bound to protein (60%) is filtrable. Normal human kidneys filter about 10 g of calcium daily but only 1–5% reaches the urine. About 60% of the filtered calcium is reabsorbed in the proximal tubule. This process is probably predominantly unvarying since this segment of the nephron is not under the influence of calcitropic hormones. Despite the striking similarities in the handling of calcium and sodium, it is unlikely that both ions share the same transport mechanism.

A further 20–30% of the filtered calcium is reabsorbed in the thick ascending limb of the loop of Henle. In the cortical portion there is evidence of active transport. It is in this segment that PTH and calcitonin increase calcium reabsorption, and diuretics block directly (furosemide and ethacrynic acid) or promote indirectly (thiazides) calcium reabsorption. In the medullary portion calcium flux is voltage driven.

The distal convoluted tubule and early portion of the cortical collecting duct reabsorb about 10% of the filtered load of calcium. In this segment calcium transport takes

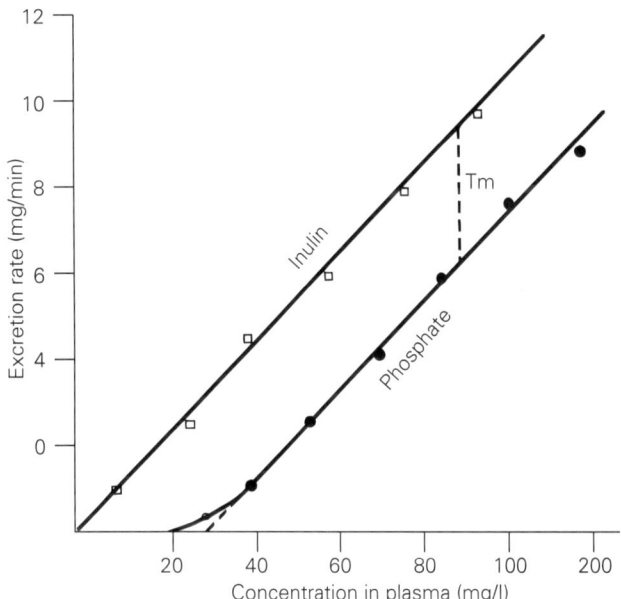

Figure 29.7 The relationship between plasma concentration and urinary excretion of phosphate in humans. The intercept of the projected phosphate slope (dotted line) with the x axis is known as the T_mP/GFR or the renal phosphate threshold. Mass units used for both inulin and phosphate. (From Bijvoet, O.L.M. (1969) Relation of plasma phosphate concentration to renal tubular reabsorption of phosphate. *Clin. Sci.*, **37**, 23–36, with permission.)

place against an electrochemical gradient. PTH is the primary regulator by stimulating the production of cAMP which increases transcellular transport. It is probable that calcitriol also plays a part since calbindin has been found in this region.

Phosphorus

In normal subjects, 7 g of phosphate passes into the glomerular filtrate each day. As has been mentioned above, intestinal absorption of phosphate is largely determined by intake; in other words, there is no mechanism for limiting absorption. For this reason the kidney is crucial in maintaining the plasma phosphate within acceptable limits [20, 20a]. Most phosphate reabsorption occurs in the proximal tubule. PTH blocks this process by a cAMP-dependent mechanism. The maximum rate of reabsorption of phosphate (Tm_{Pi}) in the kidney, normalized for the rate of glomerular filtration (GFR), represents the limit on the transport capacity or the 'renal threshold' for phosphate [21]. Above that level, all additional filtered phosphate is excreted (Figure 29.7). In a steady state the intake of phosphorus determines its excretion [22].

About 70–80% of the filtered phosphate is reabsorbed in the proximal tubule, 10% in the distal convoluted tubule and up to 3% in the collecting duct. Transport of

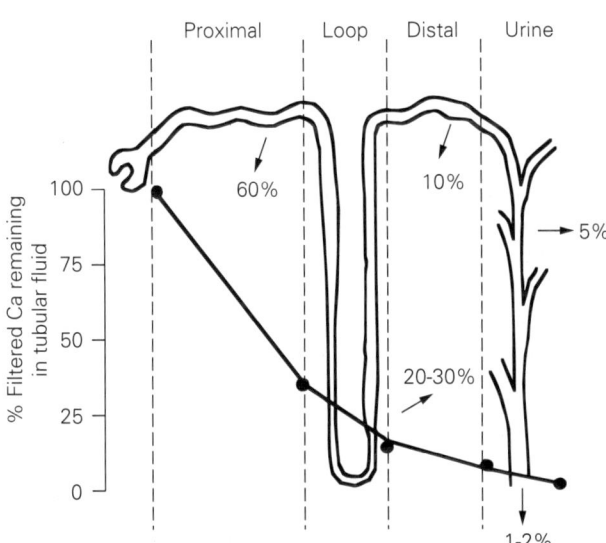

Figure 29.6 Diagram showing the proportion of filtered calcium remaining in the lumen (•) at different sites along the nephron. Arrows show the percentage of calcium reabsorbed in each segment of the nephron. (Modified with permission from Suki, W.N. and Rouse, D. (1991) Renal transport of calcium, magnesium and phosphate, in *The Kidney*, 4th edn (eds B.M. Brenner and F.C. Rector), W.B. Saunders, Philadelphia, with permission.)

phosphorus across the luminal brush border membrane of the proximal tubule is an active process and involves an Na^+-P_i co-transporter which is modulated by intracellular and luminal pH. PTH is the most significant hormonal regulator of phosphate excretion. It inhibits phosphate reabsorption in both proximal and distal convoluted segments of the renal tubule. The effect of vitamin D on phosphate excretion is less clear. Exogenous calcitonin causes phosphaturia but only at supraphysiological plasma concentrations. Growth hormone preserves phosphate probably through the action of insulin-like growth factor-I (IGF-I). Thyroxin and insulin are also hypophosphaturic. Phosphate reabsorption is inhibited by atrial natriuretic factor and glucocorticoids. The non-hormonal factors affecting the renal handling of phosphorus include dietary phosphate (the most significant modulator in the system), acid–base status, extracellular volume, serum calcium and diuretics.

Bone

Bone is the major store for calcium and phosphorus. Daily calcium turnover has been estimated to be 6400 mg. Interestingly, during remodeling the net accretion of calcium cannot exceed 400 mg/day.

Perturbations in chronic renal failure

Calcium

Plasma calcium tends to be low in patients with chronic renal failure for several reasons. It has long been recognized that the calcium intake of individuals with renal failure tends to fall as GFR falls, possibly as a consequence of increasing anorexia. In normal individuals, periods of calcium lack can be compensated for by an increase in calcitriol secretion with a consequent increase in the fractional absorption of calcium from the gut. This cannot happen in patients with chronic renal failure because their ability to manufacture calcitriol is impaired.

A second influence on the plasma calcium is the plasma concentration of phosphate. As renal failure progresses the plasma phosphate tends to rise and, as a physicochemical consequence, the plasma calcium tends to fall. A third factor is that the ability of PTH to produce a rise of calcium is blunted in patients with chronic renal failure.

Parathyroid hormone

The association between parathyroid enlargement and renal failure was first noted in the 1930s when it was found that children with renal rickets had hyperplastic parathyroid glands [23]. Albright *et al.* [24] pointed out that in adults with chronic nephritis there were sometimes radiological and histological appearances in the bone that resembled those of primary hyperparathyroidism. They considered the condition to be the 'adult counterpart of so-called renal rickets'.

It was not until the 1970s that assays for measuring circulating PTH became available. The earlier assays recognized fragments as well as the hormone itself and, in patients with renal failure, levels were found to be very high. Indeed, they were considerably higher than those found in patients with primary hyperparathyroidism. Modern assays, however, are sufficiently specific to recognize whole hormone and not fragments.

Hyperparathyroidism starts relatively early – when the GFR is in the region of 60–90 ml/min – as shown by increased circulating plasma levels of intact PTH [25] as well as by changes in bone histology.

Phosphate

As GFR falls an early effect is a fall in the absolute excretion of phosphate. Under these circumstances, one would expect the plasma phosphate to be high but it is generally normal or even decreased in early chronic renal failure [26, 27]. It is probable that the plasma phosphate is maintained at normal levels by a compensatory PTH-induced phosphaturia. Variations in intestinal phosphate absorption are not believed to play any part in these changes. As GFR continues to fall, however, the kidneys fail to excrete appropriate quantities of phosphate so the plasma phosphate rises [28].

The effects of hyperphosphatemia are threefold. First, there is a direct physicochemical effect on the level of ionized calcium, i.e. the plasma ionized calcium falls. If the calcium × phosphate product exceeds a certain value – 60 mg/dl (4.84 mM) – there is a risk of soft tissue calcification. In practice, the plasma phosphate has a much greater influence on the product than the plasma calcium since it is not unusual for the plasma phosphate to double (or even treble) whereas the plasma calcium is usually low, and only rarely high.

The second effect of hyperphosphatemia is to reduce calcitriol production [29]. The fall in circulating calcitriol means that intestinal calcium absorption is inadequate; indeed, there may be a net loss of calcium from the intestine, i.e. the obligatory 200 mg colonic loss of calcium may exceed that absorbed in the duodenum. The net result is a further reason why the plasma calcium may be low. The third effect of hyperphosphatemia is on the parathyroid gland. It has been known for many years that plasma PTH rises if plasma phosphate rises, the mechanisms being as described above. There is evidence from work with animals that phosphate itself may directly increase PTH secretion in uremia [30, 31], and more recently there is evidence in man [32].

To conclude, hyperphosphatemia has a number of effects on calcium–phosphate–vitamin D homeostasis, all of which are likely to increase the hyperparathyroid state.

Vitamin D (Figure 29.2)

Vitamin D₃ (cholecalciferol)

Cholecalciferol is formed in the skin from 7-dehydrocholesterol by the action of sunlight. There is evidence that skin synthesis in patients with renal failure is normal and unaffected by the pigmentation that may accompany chronic uremia.

25-OH vitamin D₃

The liver metabolite, 25-OH vitamin D_3, is the major circulating form of vitamin D. It has a half-life of 20–30 days. In many parts of the world there is sufficient sunlight to ensure sufficiency of vitamin D but in northern latitudes there is marked seasonal variation in plasma levels, with the lowest plasma concentrations being in April and the highest in October. In this state of marginal vitamin D deficiency there is greater reliance on diet. A good example of what can happen when individuals ingesting a very low vitamin D diet move from a tropical climate to a temperate one is that of the movement of Gujaratis from Uganda to Britain. Within around four years many of the women had developed clinical osteomalacia [33].

In patients with renal failure, 25-OH vitamin D levels can be low, especially in northern Europe. There is evidence that the individuals with renal failure who have the lowest 25-OH vitamin D levels are those who develop osteomalacia.

1,25-(OH)₂ vitamin D₃ (calcitriol)

The major kidney metabolite of vitamin D is calcitriol which is the most active of all the metabolites of vitamin D. The enzyme responsible for conversion of 25-OH vitamin D_3 to calcitriol is 1α-hydroxylase which is found in proximal tubular epithelial cells. Enzyme activity is inhibited by hyperphosphatemia and is one reason why circulating levels of calcitriol are usually low in patients with renal failure. The parathyroid glands escape from the inhibitory effect of calcitriol; mRNA of pre-pro-PTH and PTH production increase. PTH stimulates 1α-hydroxylase but usually not enough to prevent the fall in circulating calcitriol. On the other hand, calcitriol is sometimes maintained at the expense of an elevated PTH level [34]. Infusing PTH in patients with early renal failure does not produce an appropriate rise in calcitriol concentration, i.e. the 1α-hydroxylase system is failing. It has been shown in dogs that hyperparathyroidism can develop in renal failure even if the plasma calcium is deliberately kept high [35]. The rise of PTH, however, could be prevented by administration of calcitriol. Thus calcitriol lack

may be the primary event in the development of hyperparathyroidism in patients with renal failure.

Hyperparathyroidism in chronic renal failure: aetiology and mechanisms

There are three major factors in the genesis of the increased PTH secretion in patients with renal failure: low plasma calcium and calcitriol and high plasma phosphate [36].

Calcium

The direct rapid stimulatory effect of low plasma ionized calcium on the parathyroid gland has been known for many years. PTH is released from preformed secretory granules causing plasma PTH to rise within minutes. In the chronic hypocalcemic state, other mechanisms, including alterations in intracellular degradation of PTH, reutilization of degraded hormone and mobilization of a secondary storage pool come into play [37].

It is now known that hypocalcemia exerts its effect through the calcium-sensing receptor in the parathyroid gland [10]. Discovery of this mechanism should give new impetus to the search for medical means of treating hyperparathyroidism, i.e. by competitive inhibitors.

Vitamin D

Historically, the link between hypercalcemia and hyperparathyroidism is well established and, until the discovery of calcitriol, it was thought that the calcium–PTH relationship depended on simple chemical 'negative feedback'. The discovery of metabolites of vitamin D other than the liver metabolite (25-OH vitamin D_3) occurred in the late 1960s; Fraser and Kodicek [38] found the most active of them all, 1,25-(OH)₂ vitamin D_3, now known as calcitriol. They discovered that the metabolite seemed to be made only in the kidney, and this led to speculation that it might be deficient in patients with renal failure and, furthermore, that it might have a role in the genesis of renal bone disease.

It is now known that a relative or absolute deficiency of calcitriol develops early in the course of chronic renal failure. Calcitriol has a number of effects on PTH secretion, all via vitamin D receptors. First, it stimulates the intestinal absorption and skeletal mobilization of calcium leading to a rise in plasma calcium and inhibition of PTH. On the other hand, calcitriol also causes a rise in plasma phosphate which tends to lower the plasma calcium. Second, calcitriol causes a fall in transcription of mRNA for pre-pro-PTH production and a fall in PTH secretion.

In patients with uremia, there is not only less calcitriol but also possibly a decrease in the number of vitamin D receptors, though there is debate about the latter. Some authors believe that the effect of calcitriol is simply to modify the sensitivity of the parathyroid cell to calcium. This area remains controversial.

Phosphate

Any influence that phosphate has on the parathyroid was believed to be through its effects on plasma ionized calcium. For example, according to the 'trade-off' hypothesis [28], failure to excrete appropriate qualities of phosphate as renal failure progresses leads to elevation of plasma phosphate with, on a physicochemical basis, a consequent fall in plasma ionized calcium. Such falls in ionized calcium would cause incremental increases in PTH secretion and partial restoration of the status quo by means of increased urinary phosphate excretion. As renal failure progresses, the need to reduce the plasma phosphate and maintain plasma calcium requires higher and higher concentrations of PTH. The elevated plasma phosphate inhibits calcitriol production the consequence of which, as described above, is further stimulation of the parathyroid gland. Recent work suggests that phosphate has a direct effect on the parathyroid.

Aluminum

Plasma aluminum inhibits PTH secretion. Interest in this element has arisen because of the aluminum toxicity that can occur in hemodialysis patients as a result of contaminated water or malfunctioning machinery. In patients suffering from aluminum toxicity (dementia, osteomalacia, seizures, fractures) PTH levels are characteristically low.

Vitamin D and chronic renal failure: osteomalacia

As long ago as 1883 it was noted that children with late rickets could have albuminuria [39]. Further observations on the condition revealed that such individuals often had osteomalacia. In 1927, Parsons coined the term 'renal rickets' so creating a link with vitamin D deficiency rickets [40]. When it became clear in the 1920s that classical rickets could be cured by exposure to artificial ultraviolet light, sunlight or cod liver oil, such treatments were naturally used in individuals with 'renal rickets'. Unfortunately, the treatments were ineffective although it was found in 1928 that large amounts of viosterol (the first commercially available irradiated ergosterol (vitamin D_2)) could produce beneficial effects. However, many of the children died, probably of hypercalcemia in many cases [41, 42]. It was these experiences that gave rise to the notion of vitamin D-resistant rickets in patients with chronic uremia.

In the 1930s it became clear that (a) the dominant histological appearance in the bones of individuals with renal failure (whether adult or child) is osteitis fibrosa, i.e. hyperparathyroidism and (b) such individuals have large parathyroid glands. Thus, the link was made between the parathyroid gland and chronic renal failure [23, 24]. Since renal rickets was commonly osteitis fibrosa rather than osteomalacia, it was not surprising that the condition was resistant to vitamin D. What was new was that hyperparathyroidism could present clinically as 'rickets'.

In 1968 the first of a number of metabolites of 'parent' vitamin D (vitamin D_3, cholecalciferol) was identified. It was produced by hydroxylation of vitamin D_3 in the liver and was named 25-OH vitamin D_3 [43]. Two years later it was realized that an even more powerful metabolite, 1,25-$(OH)_2$ vitamin D_3, was present in plasma [38].

It is now clear that in individuals with chronic renal failure a proportion have histological evidence of osteomalacia. The notion of vitamin D resistance has remained but there is no convincing evidence that uremic osteoid is any less able to form bone than normal osteoid. On the other hand, there are disturbances in the plasma levels of certain vitamin D metabolites. 25-OH vitamin D_3 may be low [44] and there is some evidence that those with the lowest plasma levels have osteomalacia [45]. Calcitriol levels tend to fall as renal failure progresses to undetectable levels in end-stage renal disease. It is tempting to conclude that lack of calcitriol is causally related to osteomalacia but it should be remembered that individuals without kidneys (for example, dialysis patients rendered anephric) do not necessarily develop osteomalacia despite, presumably, the complete lack of calcitriol.

It is probable that vitamin D and osteomalacia are causally linked in patients with renal failure but the widespread emergence of aluminum as a cause of osteomalacia in dialysis patients in particular, and also in patients who have never been dialysed, has made interpretations of studies where the aluminum status has not been known, particularly difficult.

Soft tissue calcification in chronic renal failure

Deposition of mineral in soft tissues is an important complication of chronic uremia that has been recognized for almost 150 years [46]. Clinically, the deposition can be in skin and subcutaneous tissue, in the arterial wall, in cornea and conjunctiva, in peri-articular tissues, and in the viscera – particularly the heart and lungs. There is a close relationship between the presence and extent of soft tissue calcification and the level of the plasma calcium × phosphate product. Deposition occurs when the product is greater than 60 (using mg/100 ml) or 4.84 (using mM). In practice, it is the plasma level of phosphate that is the major determinant since its level can fluctuate to a greater extent than that of calcium. It is important to ensure in patients with renal failure that the plasma phosphate is kept below 2 mM (normal range 0.75–1.50 mM). Ensuring an optimal level of plasma phosphate is perhaps the most important therapeutic measure that one can take in individuals with chronic uremia whether or not they are on dialysis.

Contiguglia *et al.* [47] analysed material from individuals with soft tissue calcification and found that the material from around joints in subcutaneous tissues and in arterial walls ('non-visceral') was similar in composition to hydroxyapatite with a Ca:Mg:P ratio of 30:1:18, whereas the material found in heart and lungs ('visceral') had a much higher concentration of magnesium with a Ca:Mg:P ratio of 4.9:1:4.6 and resembled the composition of magnesium whitlockite. This study reminds us that attention should be paid not only to the intake and plasma levels of phosphate but also to those of magnesium, and that magnesium-containing compounds, e.g. antacids containing magnesium should not be given to patients with renal failure.

References

1. Bringhurst, F.R. (1995) Calcium and phosphate distribution, turnover and metabolic actions, in *Endocrinology*, vol. 2, 3rd edn (ed. L.J. DeGroot), W.B. Saunders, Philadelphia, pp. 1015–43.

2. Slatopolsky, E., Hruska, K. and Klahr, S. (1993) Disorders of phosphorus, calcium and magnesium metabolism, in *Diseases of the Kidney*, vol. III, 5th edn (eds R.W. Schrier and C.W. Gottschalk), Little, Brown, Boston, pp. 2599–644.

3. Broadus, A.E. (1993) Physiological functions of calcium, magnesium and phosphorus and mineral ion balance, in *Primer on the Metabolic Bone Disease and Disorders of Mineral Metabolism*, 2nd edn (ed. M.J. Favus), Raven Press, New York, pp. 41–6.

4. Phang, J.M., Berman, M., Finerman, G.A. *et al.* (1969) Dietary perturbation of calcium metabolism in normal man: compartmental analysis. *J. Clin. Invest.*, **48**, 67–77.

5. Brown, E.M. (1994) Homeostatic mechanisms regulating extracellular and intracellular calcium metabolism, in *The Parathyroids* (eds J.P. Bilezikian and M.A. Levine), Raven Press, New York, pp. 15–54.

5a. Kurokawa, K. (1996) How is the plasma calcium held constant? Milieu interieur of calcium. *Kidney Int.*, **49**, 1760–4.

6. Carafoli, E. (1992) The Ca^{2+} pump of the plasma membrane. *J. Biol. Chem.*, **267**, 2115–18.

7. Tsien, R.W. and Tsien, R.Y. (1990) Calcium channels, stores, and oscillations. *Annu. Rev. Cell. Biol.*, **6**, 715–60.

8. Brown, E.M. (1990) Extracellular Ca^{2+} sensing, regulation of parathyroid cell function, and role of Ca^{2+} and other ions as extracellular (first) messengers. *Physiol. Rev.*, **71**, 371–411.

9. Brown, E.M., Gamba, G., Riccardi, D. *et al.* (1993) Cloning and characterization of an extracellular Ca^{2+} sensing receptor from bovine parathyroid. *Nature*, **366**, 575–80.

10. Brown, E.M., Pollak, M., Seidman, C.E. *et al.* (1995) Calcium-ion-sensing cell surface receptors. *N. Engl. J. Med.*, **333**, 234–40.

11. Silver, J., Russell, J. and Sherwood, L.M. (1985) Regulation by vitamin D metabolites of messenger RNA for preproparathyroid hormone in isolated bovine parathyroid cells. *Proc. Natl. Acad. Sci. USA*, **82**, 4273–9.

12. Kronenberg, H.M. (1993) Parathyroid hormone: mechanism of action, in *Primer on the Metabolic Bone Disease and Disorders of Mineral Metabolism*, 2nd edn (ed. M.J. Favus), Raven Press, New York, pp. 58–60.

13. Reichel, H., Koeffler, H.P. and Norman, A.W. (1989) The role of the vitamin D endocrine system in health and disease. *N. Engl. J. Med.*, **320**, 980–91.

14. Zaidi, M., Shankar, V.S., Huang, C.L-H. *et al.* (1994) Molecular mechanisms of calcitonin action. *Endocr. J.*, **2**, 459–67.

15. Orloff, J.J., Wu, T.L. and Stewart, A.F. (1989) Parathyroid hormone-like proteins: biochemical responses and receptor interactions. *Endocr. Rev.*, **10**, 476–95.

16. Nordin, B.E.C. (ed.) (1988) *Calcium.* Springer–Verlag, New York.

17. Pazianas, M., Adebanjo, O., Shankar, V.S. *et al.* (1995) Extracellular cation sensing by the enterocytes: prediction of a novel divalent cation 'receptor'. *Biochem. Biophys. Res. Commun.*, **210**, 948–53.

18. Suki, W.N. and Rouze, R. (1996) Renal transport of calcium, magnesium and phosphate, in *The Kidney*, 5th edn (ed. B.M. Brenner), W.B. Saunders, Philadelphia, pp. 472–515.

19. Kurokawa, K. (1987) Calcium regulating hormones and the kidney. *Kidney Int.*, **32**, 760–71.

20. Dennis, V. (1992) Phosphorus homeostasis, in *Handbook of Physiology* (ed. E.E. Windhager), Chapter 37, Section: Renal Physiology, Oxford University Press, New York.

20a. Tenenhouse, H.S. (1997) Cellular and molecular mechanisms of renal phosphate transport. *J. Bone Miner. Res.*, **12**, 159–64.

21. Bijvoet, O.L. (1969) Relation of plasma phosphate concentration to renal tubular reabsorption of phosphate. *Clin. Sci.*, **37**, 23–36.

22. Trohler, U., Bonjour, J.P. and Fleisch, H. (1976) Renal tubular adaptation to dietary phosphorus. *Nature*, **261**, 145–6.

23. Langmead, F.S. and Orr, J.W. (1933) Renal rickets associated with parathyroid hyperplasia. *Arch. Dis. Child.*, **8**, 265–78.

24. Albright, F., Drake, T.G. and Sulkowitch, H.W. (1937) Renal osteitis fibrosa cystica. Report of a case with discussion of metabolic aspects. *Bull. Johns Hopkins Hosp.*, **60**, 377–99.

25. Reichel, H., Deibert, B., Schmidt-Gayk, H. and Ritz, E. (1991) Calcium metabolism in early chronic renal failure. Implications for the pathogenesis of hyperparathyroidism. *Nephrol. Dial. Transplant.*, **6**, 162–9.

26. Llach, F. and Massry, S.E. (1985) On the mechanism of secondary hyperparathyroidism in moderate renal insufficiency. *J. Clin. Endocrinol. Metab.*, **61**, 601–6.

27. Wilson, I., Felsenfeld, A., Drezner, M.K. and Llach, F. (1985) Altered divalent ion metabolism in early

renal failure: a role for 1,25(OH)$_2$D$_3$. *Kidney Int.*, **27**, 565–73.

28. Bricker N.S. (1972) On the pathogenesis of the uremic state – an exposition of the trade-off hypothesis. *N. Engl. J. Med.*, **286**, 1093–9.

29. Tanaka, Y. and DeLuca, H.F. (1973) The control of 1,25 dihydroxyvitamin D metabolism by inorganic phosphorus. *Arch. Biochem. Biophys.*, **159**, 566–70.

30. Kilav, R., Naveh-Many, T. and Silver, T. (1993) Phosphorus regulates parathyroid hormone gene expression. *J. Bone Miner. Res.*, **8**, S200.

31. Lopez-Hilker, S., Dusso, A., Rapp, N. *et al.* (1990) Phosphorus reduction reverses hyperparathyroidism in uremia independent of changes in calcium and calcitriol. *Am. J. Physiol.*, **259**, F432–7.

32. Combe, C. and Aparicio, M. (1994) Phosphorus and protein restriction and parathyroid function in chronic renal failure. *Kidney Int.*, **46**, 1381–6.

33. Finch, P.J., Ang, L., Eastwood, J.B. and Maxwell, J.D. (1992) Clinical and histological spectrum of osteomalacia among Asians in South London. *Q. J. Med.*, **83**, 439–48.

34. Ritz, E., Matthias, S. and Stefanski, A. (1995) Genesis of distubed vitamin D metabolism in renal failure. *Nephrol. Dial. Transplant*, **10**, 3–10.

35. Lopez-Hilker, S., Galceran, T., Chan, Y.L. *et al.* (1986) Hypocalcaemia may not be essential for the development of secondary hyperparathyroidism in chronic renal failure. *J. Clin. Invest.*, **78**, 1097–102.

36. Hruska, K.A. and Teitelbaum, S.L. (1995) Renal osteodystrophy. *N. Engl. J. Med.*, **333**, 166–73.

37. Felsenfeld, A, and Llach, F. (1993) Parathyroid gland function in renal failure. *Kidney Int.*, **43**, 771–89.

38. Fraser, D.R. and Kodicek, E. (1970) Unique biosynthesis by kidney of a biologically active vitamin D metabolite. *Nature*, **228**, 763–4.

39. Clement Lucas, R. (1883) On a form of late rickets associated with albuminuria, rickets of adolescence. *Lancet*, **i**, 993–4.

40. Parsons, L.G. (1927) The bone changes occurring in renal and coeliac infantilism and their relationship to rickets. *Arch. Dis. Child.*, **2**, 1–25.

41. Duken, J. (1928) Beitrag zur Kenntnis der malacischen Erkrankungen des kindlichen Skelettsystems. II Spatrachitis, tetanie und chronische schrumpfniere (Renale rachitis). *Z. Kinderheilk.*, **46**, 137–55.

42. Karelitz, S. and Kolomoyzeff, H. (1932) Renal dwarfism and rickets. *Am. J. Dis. Child.*, **44**, 542–55.

43. Blunt, J.W., DeLuca, H.F. and Schnoes, H.K. (1968) 25-Hydroxycalciferol. A biologically active metabolite of vitamin D$_3$. *Biochemistry*, **7**, 3317–22.

44. Bayard, F., Bec, P., Ton That, H. and Louvet, J-P. (1973) Plasma 25-hydroxy cholecalciferol in chronic renal failure. *Eur. J. Clin. Invest.*, **3**, 447–50.

45. Eastwood, J.B., Harris, E., Stamp, T.C.B. and de Wardener, H.E. (1976) Vitamin D deficiency in the osteomalacia of chronic renal failure. *Lancet*, **ii**, 1209–11.

46. Virchow, R. (1855) Kalk Metastasen. *Virchow's Arch. Path. Anat.*, **8**, 103–13.

47. Contiguglia, S.R., Alfrey, A.C., Miller, N.L. *et al.* (1973) Nature of soft-tissue calcification in uremia. *Kidney Int.*, **4**, 224–35.

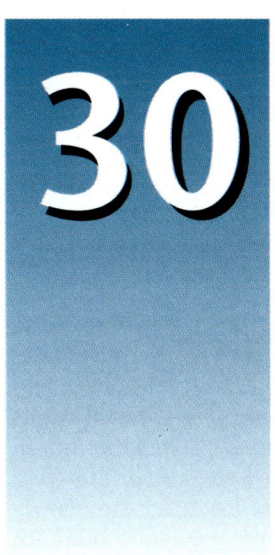

30 Renal osteodystrophy

David A. Bushinsky

Bone

The skeleton is a large, heterogeneous organ that has an important role in the structural integrity and ionic homeostasis of humans. The skeleton allows us to walk upright and contains, supports and protects virtually all of our other organs. The mineral phases of bone contain the largest store of calcium within the body and bone participates in buffering the additional hydrogen ions during acidosis. Renal insufficiency and renal failure alter the ionic and hormonal environment of bone leading to perturbations in its structure and function. To understand renal osteodystrophy we must first understand normal bone and its formation and resorption.

Mineral

In adults, bone consists of dense outer cortical bone found on the surface of the long and short bones of the extremities, the irregular bones such as the vertebrae and the flat bones of the skull and a softer interior of trabecular or cancellous bone [1]. Trabecular bone consists of a network of bony trabeculae which contains the hemopoietic marrow. The skeleton of normal infants and children also have woven bone, which is loosely organized, irregularly mineralized bone. Woven bone may reappear in the adult in pathologic conditions, such as hyperparathyroidism, Paget's disease or uremia [2].

Bone is made up of an inorganic, or mineral phase, and an organic phase. The inorganic phase, which makes up approximately two-thirds of the weight of mature bone, contains small crystals that have an X-ray diffraction pattern most consistent with hydroxyapatite [3]. However, it is widely recognized that bone apatite is also associated with other anions and cations [4]. There are other calcium phosphate complexes contained within the bone mineral, including brushite and octacalcium phosphate, in addition to non-phosphate compounds such as carbonate, associated with calcium, potassium, and/or sodium [5–8].

Organic phase

The organic phase of bone consists of collagen, non-collagen proteins and bone cells. Collagen makes up approximately 85–90% of all protein in bone [9]. It is a $1.5 \times 300\,nm$ rigid rod formed from three alpha chains that are linked both end-to-end and side-to-side to form fibrils that are several collagen molecules thick [1]. Fibrils are then arranged in bundles or fibers that can be seen on light microscopy. The collagen is predominantly type I collagen [9]. In addition, several non-collagen proteins including sialoproteins (such as osteopontin), proteoglycans, osteonectin and osteocalcin are found within bone [10].

Cells

The four principal differentiated cell types found in bone are osteoblasts, osteoclasts, osteocytes and lining cells. The osteoblasts are bone-forming cells which are cuboidal secretory cells that stain strongly for alkaline phosphatase

Nephrology, Edited by Rex L. Jamison and Robert Wilkinson.
Published in 1997 by Chapman & Hall, London. ISBN 0 412 60930 4

[11]. These cells originate from the marrow stromal fibroblastic system [12] and are responsible for secreting the organic bone matrix, or osteoid which is subsequently mineralized. Active osteoblasts are large in volume whereas inactive cells are thin. When an osteoblast becomes embedded in the matrix and stops secreting protein it is then termed an osteocyte. The actual function of the osteocyte is not clear though it may have a role in maintaining the integrity of the surrounding bone [13]. The lining cells line the majority of trabecular bone surfaces and may play a role in separating the bone from the marrow space [14].

Osteoclasts are the bone-resorbing cells of apparently mononuclear–phagocytic origin [15, 16]. They are large (50–100 µm), multinucleated (approximately 2–10 nuclei) cells involved in the vectorial transport of lysosomal enzymes and hydrogen ions toward the interface of the cell with the bone mineral [17–19]. At this narrow interface (0.2–0.5 nm), located at the apical pole of the cell, there is a ruffled border delineated by a clear zone that appears to seal the cell to the bone mineral, forming a microenvironment into which hydrogen ions and lysosomal enzymes are secreted [20]. The attachment of the osteoclast to the mineral appears to be directed by binding to osteopontin [21].

The lysosomal enzymes secreted by the osteoclast consist principally of tartrate-resistant acid phosphatase, arylsulfatase, β-glycerophosphatase, β-glucuronidase and cathepsins B and C and other cysteine proteases [22–25]. The cysteine proteases are primarily responsible for breakdown of the organic matrix [19, 22]. The cysteine proteases may operate co-operatively with collagenase, produced by the osteoblast, in removal of the organic matrix during bone resorption [26]. Osteoclasts also actively secrete hydrogen ions into the microenvironment of the attachment zone between the cell and the mineral [18, 19]. Hydrogen ion secretion appears to be secondary to a vacuolar, electrogenic H^+-transporting adenosine triphosphatase which is located at the apical pole of the cell, directly adjacent to the mineral [18]. The intracellular hydration of CO_2 is catalyzed by carbonic anhydrase isoenzyme II [27]. The HCO_3^- produced by the generation of H^+ appears to exit the cell via a Cl^-/HCO_3^- exchanger [28]. The increase in H^+ concentration in the microenvironment between the osteoclast and the mineral promotes solubilization of the mineral phase of bone leading to the release of calcium [22].

Bone mineral homeostasis

Regulation of bone formation

The process of mineralization of the organic matrix of bone requires proliferation and differentiation of osteogenic progenitor cells and stimulation of existing osteoblasts with subsequent deposition of mineral. Mineralization appears to be regulated by a variety of factors, both local and systemic, including hormones, ions and specific growth factors, in addition to physicochemical forces. The mechanisms involved in regulation of mineralization are less well understood compared with bone resorption.

Osteoinductive factors have been solubilized and extracted from devitalized bone matrix [12]. The best characterized of these factors is bone morphogenetic protein (BMP), a non-collagenous protein that stimulates morphologically unspecialized mesenchymal cells and induces cartilage and bone formation [29]. Prostaglandins may regulate multiple aspects of bone cell metabolism. In addition to their well-characterized effect in stimulating bone resorption, recent studies demonstrate a stimulatory effect on bone formation. Hormonal regulation does not appear to be as prominent a factor in homeostatic control of mineralization as in resorption, but there is evidence for some regulatory role of calciotropic hormones. Although the primary effect of calcitonin is to directly inhibit the activity of the osteoclast, some evidence suggests that this hormone may also have a direct anabolic effect on bone formation.

An anabolic effect of parathyroid hormone (PTH) has been demonstrated that appears separate from its better characterized effect of stimulating bone resorption [30]. Although necessary for normal bone formation, the steroid hormone $1,25(OH)_2D_3$ does not directly promote skeletal growth and mineralization, but rather has that effect by acting to normalize plasma calcium and phosphorus levels in the intact animal [31]. Loss of estrogen production in females is associated with decreased bone mass (osteoporosis) resulting from an increased rate of osteoclastic bone resorption and a reduced rate of bone formation [32].

Supplemental fluoride causes an increase in the rate of bone formation and in the number of osteoblasts [33]. Since the skeleton is composed of calcium and phosphate these ions are clearly needed for mineralization. Increasing the concentration of either increases bone deposition [7].

Acidosis has been found to decrease osteoblastic activity [34, 35]. There is a decrease in osteoblastic collagen synthesis and alkaline phosphatase activity in response to acidosis produced by a decrease in the medium bicarbonate concentration, metabolic acidosis, but not by acidosis produced by an increase in the partial pressure of carbon dioxide, respiratory acidosis [35]. In experimental situations acidosis decreases bone formation [36].

Regulation of bone resorption

Bone resorption is the process of osteoclast-mediated release of calcium from the mineralized matrix of bone, followed by degradation of the collagenous matrix [13]. There is histologic evidence demonstrating an increase in the activity and number of active osteoclasts on the bone surface in response to a variety of treatments which increase calcium release from bone mineral [22, 37].

The two major hormones that activate physiologic bone resorption are PTH and $1,25(OH)_2D_3$. PTH contributes to acute regulation of blood calcium levels by mobilizing calcium from skeletal reserves. PTH has been shown to increase the activity of existing osteoclasts and the development of new osteoclasts on the bone surface [37], leading to a release of calcium from the bone mineral. The osteoblast, and not the osteoclast, appears to be a direct target for PTH [22, 38–40]. The biologic responses to PTH in the osteoblast include decreased collagen synthesis [41] and inhibition of osteoblast maturation [42]. The action of PTH on the osteoblast mediates the subsequent activation of the osteoclast [43].

Specific proteolytic, lysosomal and acid-producing enzyme activities are increased in the osteoclast in response to PTH treatment of bone, including acid phosphatase [44], β-glucuronidase [45], cathepsins L and B [26] and carbonic anhydrase [45]. The activation of carbonic anhydrase is necessary to provide the hydrogen ions for secretion by the osteoclast to promote bone demineralization [22]. The acidity of the microenvironment delineated by the clear zones around the ruffled border area of the osteoclast has been shown to be increased by PTH and prostaglandin E_2 (PGE_2) [46]. PTH may also stimulate the production of other acids, including lactate and citrate, in parallel with resorption [22].

$1,25(OH)_2D_3$ stimulates bone turnover [47] and is a potent stimulator of osteoclastic bone resorption [48]. As with other steroid hormones, the receptors for $1,25(OH)_2D_3$ are intracellular [49]. Specific nuclear binding has demonstrated that the osteoblast is also the target cell for this hormone. The activity and number of osteoclasts in bone are increased after the injection of $1,25(OH)_2D_3$ into vitamin D-deficient rats [50].

Hydrogen ions have been shown to alter bone mineral metabolism directly [51, 52]. An acute fall in medium pH, well within the physiologic range, causes bone mineral dissolution. The mechanism by which hydrogen ions induce the release of bone calcium over an initial 24 h appears due to alterations in the physicochemical factors that govern the deposition and dissolution of the bone mineral and not to alterations in bone resorptive activity. The mechanism by which chronic metabolic acidosis induces the release of bone calcium appears to be a combination of a direct physicochemical effect of hydrogen ions on the bone mineral, as in acute metabolic acidosis, and enhanced cell-mediated bone resorption. Metabolic, but not respiratory, acidosis has been found to increase osteoclastic activity [34].

In addition to PTH, $1,25(OH)_2D_3$ and hydrogen ions, several other agents may have important regulatory effects on bone resorption. Thyroid hormone has been shown to increase bone resorption directly [53]. Prostaglandins, especially those of the E series (PGE_1 and PGE_2) directly stimulate bone resorption [54]. Exogenous agents can also have direct effects on bone resorption. An example of this is aluminum which can pathologically interfere with normal bone turnover and mineralization [55–57]. The predominant effect of aluminum is due to inhibition of osteoblast activity [55, 56, 58]. *In vitro* studies have shown that aluminum, in the concentrations observed in many dialysis patients, increases osteoclastic bone resorption [59] and decreases bone formation [60].

Remodeling

Bone remodeling encompasses the co-ordinated regulation of formation and resorption. Remodeling consists of activation of resting cells at a specific site in the bone, the slow resorption of the matrix by the osteoclasts, a reversal phase where mononuclear cells prepare the resorption lacunae for subsequent formation and finally deposition of mineralized bone by the osteoblasts [61]. About 10% of the adult skeleton is thought to be involved in remodeling on a yearly basis. This process is integral in mineral homeostasis by exchanging calcium and other ions as needed from the skeletal reservoir in the body; in addition it allows continual renewal and strengthening of old bone.

Bone cells synthesize several different growth factors and cytokines which have important effects on differentiated cell function and may act as local regulators of cell growth [62]. They may also play a critical role in remodeling, both by themselves and by mediating the effects of systemic hormones [29, 62]. In addition, systemic factors may be accumulated in the bone matrix and contribute to the local regulation of remodeling [63]. This could account for the coupling of resorption and formation during remodeling; factors previously deposited in matrix are released during resorption and then activate the formation process. Transforming growth factor β (TGF-β), $β_2$-microglobulin ($β_2$-M) insulin-like growth factor I (IGF-I) and platelet-derived growth factor (PDGF) are synthesized in cultured bone and isolated bone cells. Although their synthesis and effects are not limited to skeletal tissue, these agents have significant effects on bone remodeling *in vitro* and may be important regulators when acting in concert in skeletal tissue.

Calcium, phosphorus, PTH and vitamin D: actions and interactions

The synthesis of $1,25(OH)_2D_3$ is governed by the 1α-hydroxylase located in the mitochondria of the proximal tubule cells [52, 64]. $1,25(OH)_2D_3$ is the most potent stimulator of intestinal calcium and phosphorus absorption and suppresses the secretion of PTH. $1,25(OH)_2D_3$ can stimulate bone resorption and/or formation depending on the ionic environment and its secretion is controlled by PTH, calcium and phosphorus. PTH mobilizes bone calcium through increased osteoclastic bone resorption and by increasing the secretion of $1,25(OH)_2D_3$. PTH is phosphaturic and hypocalciuric and is regulated by calcium and $1,25(OH)_2D_3$ and perhaps by phosphorus.

Elevations in the concentration of calcium and phosphorus, and especially their product, can not only increase bone mineralization but induce soft tissue calcification as well. Hydrogen ions are primarily excreted by the kidney. An increase in the concentration of hydrogen ions can stimulate direct physicochemical bone dissolution as well as cell-mediated bone resorption. Renal failure directly disrupts this fine-tuned homeostasis on a number of fronts, including causing phosphate and proton retention and decreased $1,25(OH)_2D_3$ conversion with resultant hypocalcemia and elevated PTH. These ionic and hormonal perturbations alter bone accretion, physicochemical dissolution and cell-mediated resorption leading to disruption of the composition and structure of the bone.

Renal osteodystrophy

Clinical presentation

Patients with renal osteodystrophy present with a wide variety of non-specific signs and symptoms usually relating to the musculoskeletal system. A common complaint is one of bone pain; often there is a gradual onset of pain especially in the lower back, hips and legs. Another common complaint is that of the gradual onset of proximal muscle aching and weakness. Children with renal insufficiency usually have retarded linear growth and often exhibit skeletal deformities including frontal bossing, enlargement of the wrists and ankles, genu valgum and bowing of the long bones.

Although not strictly related to the skeleton, soft tissue and/or vascular calcification are not infrequently observed in patients with disorders of calcium and phosphorus metabolism. Soft tissue calcifications tend to occur in patients with a calcium phosphorus product (calcium × phosphorus, both in mg/dl) greater than 65–75. Many patients with renal failure, especially diabetics, have vascular calcification localized to the medial layer of small and medium sized arteries. In severe cases the impaired blood supply can lead to loss of digits. With 'calciphylaxis' there is necrosis of the skin, subcutaneous tissue and/or muscle. Calciphylaxis has been linked to marked elevations in PTH, calcium and phosphorus levels.

Types of renal osteodystrophy

There are two principal types of bone disorder observed in patients with end-stage renal disease; a high turnover disorder characterized by osteitis fibrosa and a low turnover state characterized initially by osteomalacia and more recently by adynamic or aplastic bone disease [65–67]. In osteitis fibrosa the number and size of the osteoclasts are increased, as are the number and depth of the osteoclastic resorption lacunae. The deposition of collagen is less ordered and the rate of bone formation is markedly increased. Osteomalacia results from defective bone mineralization. In osteomalacia the rate of mineralization is slower than that of collagen synthesis resulting in excessive accumulation of unmineralized osteoid and widened osteoid seams. In aplastic or adynamic renal osteodystrophy there is a similar marked reduction in the rates of mineralization and collagen synthesis resulting in osteoid seams of normal width. Although these disorders are discussed as distinct entities, there is enough of an overlap to suggest a continuous distribution between the extremes. Indeed many patients have bone biopsy evidence of both high and low turnover renal osteodystrophy, a so-called mixed lesion.

High turnover renal osteodystrophy

Pathogenesis

The approximately 25 mmol phosphate absorbed by the intestine each day must be quantitatively excreted by renal mechanisms for total body phosphate balance to be maintained (Figure 30.1). Any decrease in excretion that is not balanced by a decrease in absorption must lead to an increase in the concentration of extracellular fluid phosphate and/or an increase in bone or soft tissue phosphate deposition (Figure 30.2). With renal insufficiency there is a decrease in urine phosphorus excretion with resultant hyperphosphatemia [68, 69]. There is a strong inverse correlation between creatinine clearance and serum phosphate levels [68]. Recent evidence suggests that alterations in phosphate regulate PTH secretion through mechanisms that are not clear at this time [70].

$1,25(OH)_2D_3$ has been shown to fall with a decline in renal function especially when the creatinine clearance falls below 50 ml/min [65, 68, 71] (Figure 30.3). The fall is due in part to the increase in serum phosphate inhibiting the activity of 1α-hydroxylase [72] and in part to the decrease in the number of functional proximal tubule cells. The decrease in $1,25(OH)_2D_3$ causes a lowering of biologically active ionized calcium due, in most part, to a decrease in $1,25(OH)_2D_3$-stimulated intestinal calcium absorption [73]. There may also be a component of soft tissue calcium–phosphorus deposition due to an increase in the calcium phosphorus product [74]. The fall in ionized calcium will stimulate the synthesis and release of PTH [75].

Parathyroid cells have specific receptors for $1,25(OH)_2D_3$ [76] and $1,25(OH)_2D_3$ suppresses PTH gene expression and secretion [77, 78]. In addition, during renal failure there is decreased binding of $1,25(OH)_2D_3$ to the parathyroid cells [79]. Thus, during renal failure the combination of decreased levels of $1,25(OH)_2D_3$ and decreased binding of the available $1,25(OH)_2D_3$ to the parathyroid cells results in a marked increase in secretion of PTH at all levels of ionized calcium. This so called 'altered set point' for PTH secretion can be reversed by the administration of $1,25(OH)_2D_3$ [80], a non-calcemic analog of vitamin D [81] and perhaps by retinoic acid

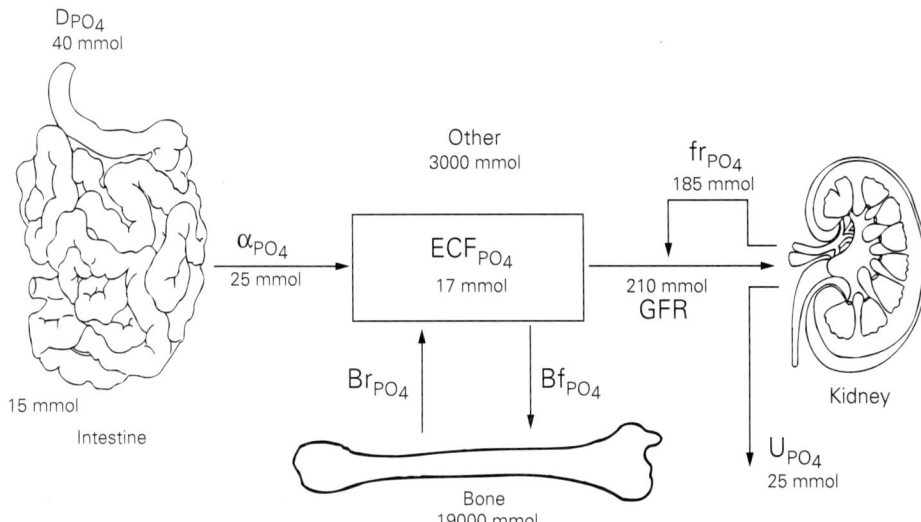

Figure 30.1 Distribution of phosphate between the gastrointestinal tract, bone, kidney and the extracellular fluid. Abbreviations: D_{PO_4}, dietary phosphorus supply; α_{PO_4}, fraction of intestinal phosphate absorbed; Br_{PO_4}, phosphate released during bone resorption; Bf_{PO_4}, phosphate being deposited in bone; GFR, glomerular filtration rate; fr_{PO_4}, renal fractional reabsorption of phosphate; U_{PO_4}, urinary phosphate excretion; ECF_{PO_4}, extracellular fluid phosphate.

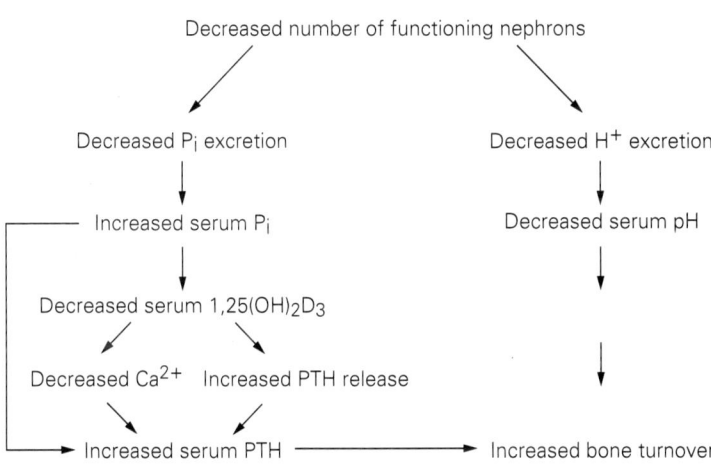

Figure 30.2 Diagram of the mechanisms leading to increased PTH release and bone turnover during renal failure. Abbreviations: Ca^{2+}, arterial blood ionized calcium concentration; P_i, concentration of blood phosphorus; PTH, parathyroid hormone; $1,25(OH)_2D_3$, concentration of 1,25-dihydroxyvitamin D_3. (Modified from ref. 52.)

[82]. PTH is degraded, principally in the liver and the kidney, into carboxyterminal fragments and these fragments are catabolized by the kidney [83]. With renal failure there is accumulation of PTH and carboxyterminal fragments in the serum, some of which are also biologically active [84].

Thus with declining renal function there is a progressive increase in the serum level of PTH (Figure 30.4) [68]. This increase in PTH leads to an increase in renal phosphate excretion, stabilizing the level of serum phosphate. However, a progressive decline in renal function leads to a continuing increase in serum phosphate and thus PTH. Although the elevated PTH level will stabilize the serum phosphate level, it will adversely affect the bone mineral by stimulating osteoblastic and then osteoclastic activity. A decline in renal function will also impair the ability to excrete endogenously produced hydrogen ions resulting in metabolic acidosis [51]. The metabolic acidosis will stimulate osteoclastic bone resorption and physicochemical bone dissolution [85]. In experimental conditions acidosis and PTH have an additive effect to stimulate

calcium release from bone, stimulate osteoclastic and inhibit osteoblastic function [86].

Bone biopsy and laboratory findings

With high turnover renal osteodystrophy, osteofibrosis, there is a marked increase in both bone formation and bone resorption with no defect in bone mineralization. The number and size of the osteoclasts are increased as is the number and depth of the osteoclastic resorption lacunae. Osteoblastic activity is increased and the osteoblasts lay down a disordered bone matrix which leads to abnormal woven bone formation. Fibrous tissue is found next to, and sometimes replacing, bone trabecula and in the marrow space. An increased bone formation rate, sometimes 3 to 4 times normal, is found when double tetracycline labeling is utilized before bone biopsy. The disorder can range from mild to severe. The absence of fibrosis and modest increases in osteoclastic activity indicate mild osteodystrophy.

The hallmark of this disorder is a marked elevation of

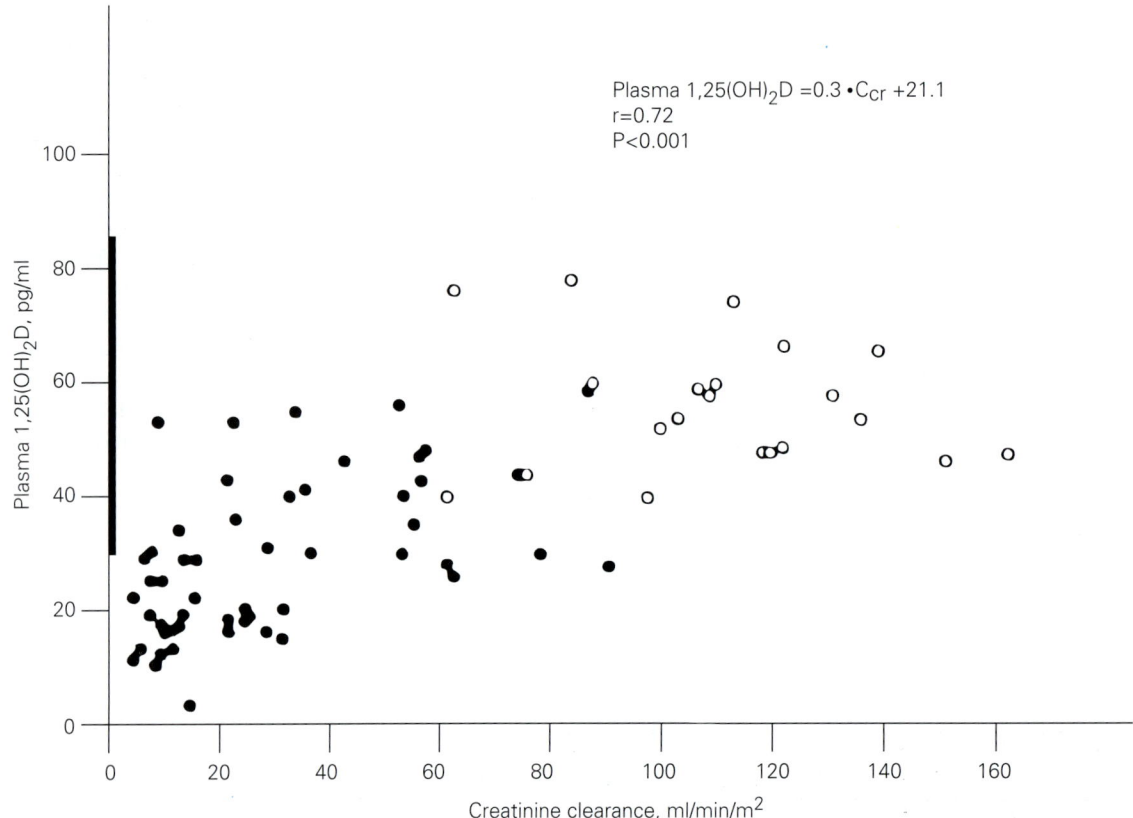

Figure 30.3 The correlation between plasma 1,25(OH)₂D₃ concentration and endogenous creatinine clearance in normal subjects (○) and patients with renal insufficiency (●). (From ref. 68.)

Table 30.1 Indications for parathyroidectomy

Calciphylaxis
Extraskeletal calcifications
Persistent serum calcium >11.5 mg/dl
Persistent hyperphosphatemia
Skeletal pain or fractures
Intractable pruritus

the serum PTH level (Table 30.1). In patients with renal insufficiency or failure it is important not to utilize a carboxyterminal assay to measure PTH [87, 88]. Normally biologically inactive carboxyterminal fragments are excreted by the kidney. With renal insufficiency these fragments accumulate and are detected as active PTH if a carboxyterminal assay is utilized. The newer immunoradiometric assays for PTH, in which binding to both amino and mid-terminal sites are necessary for hormone detection, appear to measure PTH levels more accurately in patients with renal insufficiency and failure. Elevated levels of PTH may be associated with hypocalcemia (secondary hyperparathyroidism) or hypercalcemia (tertiary hyperparathyroidism); phosphorus levels are usually ele-

vated. The magnitude of the PTH elevation correlates well with the severity of the osteitis fibrosa [65]. Increased PTH will stimulate osteoblastic alkaline phosphatase release causing an elevation in serum levels. Confirmation of a skeletal source for the alkaline phosphatase is necessary especially in patients with hepatic disease. Normally there will not be a marked elevation in basal serum aluminum levels and infusion of deferoxamine will not lead to a substantial increase in aluminum levels.

Radiographic examination will often reveal subperiosteal resorption in the phalanges and distal head of the clavicles and there may be erosion of the phalangeal tufts. The use of fine-grain radiographic film and a hand lens is helpful in detecting bone resorption. The extent of these changes often correlates with the magnitude of increase in PTH. Slipped epiphyses in children are indicative of severe osteitis fibrosa [65].

Low turnover renal osteodystrophy

Pathogenesis

Originally thought to result from vitamin D deficiency, osteomalacia has been closely associated with aluminum toxicity. Aluminum as a toxin in dialysis patients was first identified as a presumed cause of dialysis dementia [89,

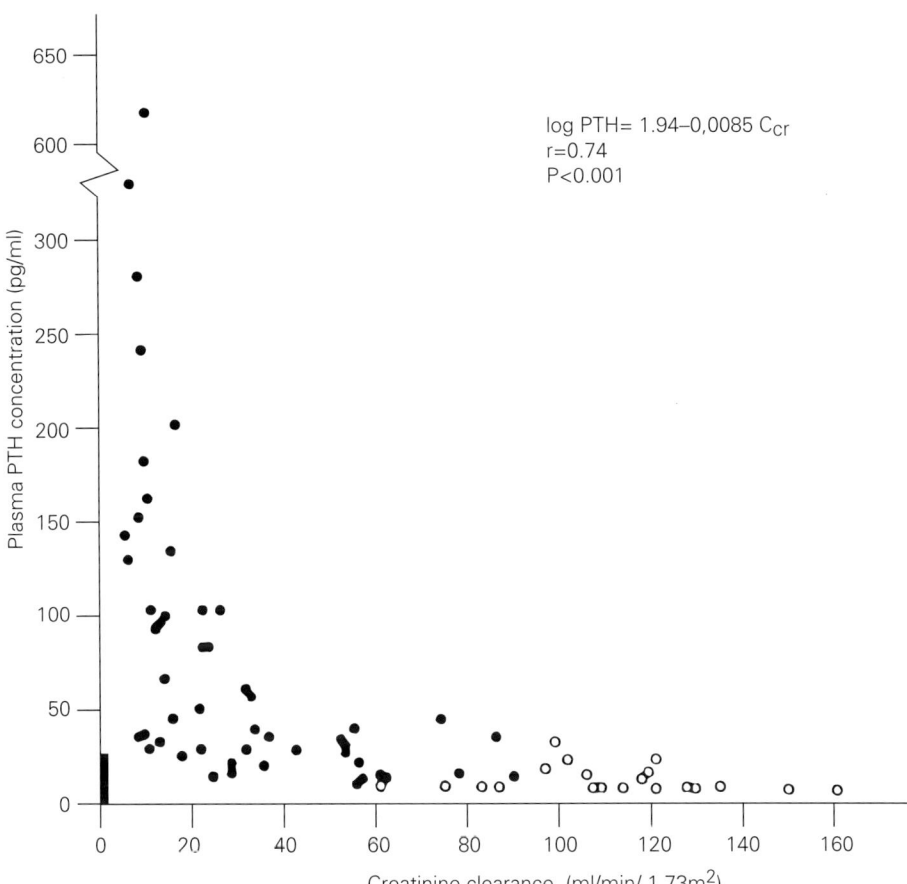

$$\log PTH = 1.94 - 0{,}0085\ C_{cr}$$
$$r = 0.74$$
$$P < 0.001$$

Figure 30.4 The correlation between plasma PTH concentration and endogenous creatinine clearance in normal subjects (○) and patients with renal insufficiency (●). (From ref. 68.)

90] and shortly thereafter aluminum deposition in bone was associated with osteomalacia [91, 92]. The source of aluminum was contamination of water used in making dialysate and ingestion of aluminum as a phosphate binder [93]. Although aluminum no longer contaminates dialysate it is still widely utilized as a phosphate binder. Most estimates are that approximately 30% of dialysis and predialysis patients are still ingesting at least some aluminum. Aluminum deposits within the mineralization front [94], the surface where the osteoid meets the mineralized bone, and is believed to adversely affect mineralization [95]. In addition, aluminum appears to reduce the number and activity of osteoblasts [96]. *In vitro* aluminum has been shown to decrease osteoblastic bone formation [60] and to increase osteoclastic bone resorption [59].

Recently aplastic renal osteodystrophy has been found in many patients who have no evidence for excess aluminum accumulation [97, 98]. Analysis of these patients suggests that they have extremely low levels of PTH. The disorder is associated with supraphysiological peritoneal dialysate calcium concentrations and use of oral calcium carbonate which together may lower serum PTH to levels which are inadequate to maintain normal bone turnover [97].

Bone biopsy and laboratory findings

With low turnover osteodystrophy there is an increase in osteoid width and volume and an increase in the bone surface covered with osteoid indicating impaired bone mineralization. There is also decreased osteoclastic activity. In patients with aluminum-induced osteomalacia deposits of aluminum are detected along the trabecular bone surfaces and on the cement lines. In adynamic osteodystrophy there is actually a decrease in osteoid volume with few osteoclasts or osteoblasts present. Many patients with adynamic osteodystrophy have no evidence of aluminum deposition. With double tetracycline labeling little or no bone formation is generally found.

Serum aluminum levels are often elevated in osteomalacia and administration of deferoxamine leads to a marked increase over the baseline (Table 30.1). After an initial serum aluminum level deferoxamine (40 mg/kg) is infused and aluminum is remeasured 24–48 h later. However, serum aluminum levels, even after deferoxamine infusion may not be accurate; if aluminum intoxication remains a diagnostic possibility then a bone biopsy is indicated. Aluminum is difficult to measure accurately: electrothermal atomic absorption spectrometry has proven reliable. PTH levels are often normal with osteomalacia and suppressed with adynamic osteodystrophy. Osteoblastic alkaline phosphatase levels are not elevated. Often patients with aluminum overload will develop hypercalcemia when calcium is utilized as a phosphate binder or with the introduction of $1,25(OH)_2D_3$ treatment. Anemia may be severe and poorly responsive to recombinant erythropoietin.

Radiographic examination will often demonstrate multiple fractures involving the ribs, hips and pelvis. There may be pseudofractures, radiolucent bands in the cortex perpendicular to the long axis of the bone, and diffuse osteopenia and compression fractures of the vertebrae. Children may exhibit rickets.

Changing spectrum of renal osteodystrophy

Initial descriptions of patients with biopsy-proven renal osteodystrophy indicated that almost 50% of patients had mild disease and the remaining patients were divided almost equally between those with osteitis fibrosa and those with osteomalacia (Figure 30.5) [99]. However, recent studies suggest that the disease spectrum has changed. Half of the patients now tend to present with adynamic (aplastic) disease and another quarter with osteitis fibrosa [100]. The reasons for this evolution are not clear but almost certainly reflect the attempts of physicians to decrease the use of aluminum containing phosphate binders and to better control serum phosphorus and calcium, and thus PTH, in dialysis patients.

Prevention and treatment of renal osteodystrophy

Phosphorus binding

As renal function declines phosphorus intake should be restricted to prevent phosphorus accumulation. However, most patients can not tolerate the degree of phosphorus restriction, 400–800 mg/day compared to the usual intake

of greater than 1 g per day, necessary to prevent hyperphosphatemia. As renal function declines below approximately 25% of normal most patients require binding of intestinal phosphorus to prevent its absorption and accumulation.

Dialysis will remove phosphorus from the body. Hemodialysis removes approximately 1 g per treatment and peritoneal dialysis approximately 0.3 g/day. In spite of these phosphorus losses it is a rare patient who will not require phosphorus binders in addition to dietary phosphorus restriction to control serum phosphorus.

Aluminum-containing compounds were utilized extensively as phosphorus binders until it was recognized that during renal insufficiency some of the absorbed aluminum was not excreted and accumulated in vital organs, such as the brain and bone, leading to severe toxicity. The extent of aluminum accumulation is related to the amount ingested, the degree of renal function, and the co-administration of compounds such as citrate that increase absorption. In view of the severe toxicity associated with aluminum current practice dictates restriction, as far as possible, of aluminum-containing compounds.

Calcium carbonate is an effective phosphate binder and has been shown to be effective in the control serum of phosphorus. The usual starting dose of calcium carbonate is 0.5 g with each meal and generally is rapidly increased until control of phosphorus is achieved; patients usually require between 5 and 15 g per day. Calcium carbonate must be taken with meals to increase phosphorus binding and the tablets should be chewed to increase the availability of calcium for binding. Hypercalcemia is a frequent side effect that can be lessened by lowering the dialysate calcium concentration to 2.5 mEq/l or less. Co-administration of $1,25(OH)_2D_3$ will increase calcium absorption and may lead to hypercalcemia. Calcium acetate is a very good phosphorus binder; however, calcium citrate should be avoided as the citrate enhances the absorption of aluminum. Magnesium-containing antacids also bind phosphorus but should be avoided as they may induced hypermagnesemia.

The goal of therapy is to keep the serum phosphorus below 5.5–6.0 mg/dl by a combination of phosphorus restriction and interstinal binding. To prevent precipitation of calcium phosphate complexes it is prudent to keep the calcium × phosphorus product below approximately 65. If the patient has a product greater than 65, aluminum-containing antacids can be utilized until the product falls below this number, at which time the calcium-containing antacids should be substituted for aluminum.

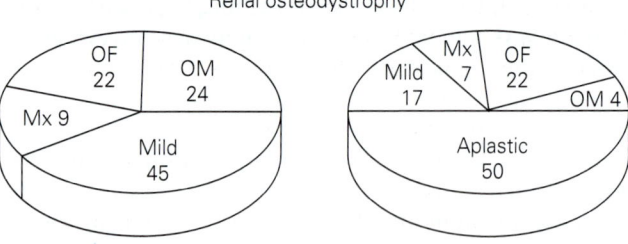

Figure 30.5 Changes in the distribution of renal osteodystrophy between (a) 1972 and (b) 1993. OF, osteitis fibrosa; OM, osteomalacia; Mx, mixed renal osteodystrophy; Mild, mild renal osteodystrophy; Aplastic, aplastic or adynamic renal osteodystrophy. (Reproduced from (a) ref. 99 and (b) ref. 100.)

Vitamin D

Various vitamin D sterols are effective in decreasing PTH secretion and bone turnover and increasing serum calcium. Calcitriol ($1,25(OH)_2D_3$), administered either through the oral or parenteral route, is effective and has a short half-life allowing discontinuation if hypercalcemia occurs.

In patients with renal insufficiency not yet on dialysis oral calcitriol may be utilized to help prevent secondary hyperparathyroidism. Initially there were scattered case reports that calcitriol may accelerate the progression toward renal failure by inducing hypercalcemia and nephrocalcinosis [101]. However, a careful double-blind controlled study failed to document an increase in the rate of progression toward renal failure [102]. Prior to initiating dialysis most patients require approximately 0.25 µg of oral calcitriol per day.

When patients are initiated on hemodialysis the usual practice is to administer $1,25(OH)_2D_3$ intravenously at the conclusion of the treatment; most patients on peritoneal dialysis continue on oral $1,25(OH)_2D_3$. Patients require up to 2 µg per treatment to effectively control the level of PTH. Calcitriol has been shown to decrease serum PTH levels in response to hypocalcemia and to improve the histologic appearance of osteitis fibrosa. Patients also report decreased bone pain and increased muscle strength.

The goal of therapy is to reduce serum PTH levels to 1.5–2 times normal to decrease the risk of osteitis fibrosa yet not induce adynamic renal osteodystrophy. The lowest dose of $1,25(OH)_2D_3$ that achieves the required reduction in PTH should be utilized. Often a fall in serum alkaline phosphatase will indicate an improvement in bone histology. The principal risks of calcitriol therapy are hypercalcemia, hyperphosphatemia and excessive suppression of serum PTH. Hypercalcemia can sometimes be controlled by decreasing the amount of oral calcium or decreasing the dialysate calcium concentration. Hypercalcemia is more frequent in patients with aluminum intoxication.

Acidosis

Acidosis has been shown to induce physicochemical bone mineral dissolution and to increase osteoclastic bone resorption and decrease osteoblastic bone formation [35, 85, 103]. Recent studies have indicated that acidosis and PTH have an additive effect on promoting calcium release from bone, and in stimulating osteoclastic function and inhibiting osteoblastic activity [86]. In a carefully controlled clinical study restoring predialysis bicarbonate concentration to the normal range decreased hyperparathyroid bone disease in patients with osteitis fibrosa and increased bone turnover in patients with osteomalacia [104]. Calcium carbonate is an effective buffer and has been shown to increase the extracellular fluid bicarbonate concentration [105, 106]. If calcium carbonate can not be used in sufficient quantities to increase the bicarbonate concentration without inducing hypercalcemia then sodium bicarbonate can be used. The goal of therapy is to raise the predialysis bicarbonate concentration to 22–24 mEq/l [85]. Alkalosis should be avoided as it will promote calcium phosphate deposition in soft tissues. However, there is no clinical evidence that increasing the predialysis bicarbonate to physiologic levels will promote metastatic calcification [107].

Parathyroidectomy

Patients with renal insufficiency often develop secondary hyperparathyroidism which is defined as an acquired disorder which develops in response to physiologic stimuli. For reasons that are not yet defined the parathyroid glands may become hypertrophied. Refractory secondary hyperparathyroidism develops when PTH secretion is no longer suppressible after correction of the underlying metabolic disorder. If hypercalcemia develops in patients with secondary hyperparathyroidism the disorder is termed tertiary hyperparathyroidism.

Often administration of $1,25(OH)_2D_3$ and correction of the underlying calcium and phosphorus abnormalities can lead to correction of secondary hyperparathyroidism; however, there are indications for parathyroidectomy in patients with refractory secondary or tertiary hyperparathyroidism (Table 30.1). As with all indications for surgery clinical judgement must weigh heavily on the decision to operate. Most commonly the choice of surgery is either subtotal parathyroidectomy in which three and a half glands are removed or total parathyroidectomy with reimplantation of some parathyroid tissue in the forearm. Either approach can be successful and success depends principally on the skill and experience of the surgeon. In the majority of cases surgery, correctly done, will be successful; however, second or subsequent surgery in the neck is far more complex than the initial operation.

Aluminum overload

Intravenous deferoxamine mobilizes aluminum from bone and soft tissues into the circulation and promotes more rapid aluminum removal from patients undergoing hemodialysis or peritoneal dialysis [108]. Deferoxamine treatment over many months leads to clinical and biopsy improvement of aluminum-induced osteomalacia [109]. On biopsy the amount of stainable aluminum decreases and there is increased bone formation. Prior parathyroidectomy not only appears to increase aluminum deposition but also inhibits the response to deferoxamine treatment [109, 110].

However, deferoxamine therapy is not without significant hazard. Serious, and at times lethal, infections with *Yersinia* and *Rhizopus* have been reported in patients given deferoxamine [111, 112]. Because of these complications deferoxamine should only be given to patients with severe symptomatic, biopsy-proven aluminum toxicity. Meticulous removal of all potential sources of aluminum, including aluminum-containing antacids, has been shown to improve bone histology in cases of aluminum overload without resorting to deferoxamine administration [113].

β₂-Microglobulin and amyloid

Dialysis-related amyloidosis is a serious and not uncommon complication of long-term dialysis treatment. In the early 1980s several groups found amyloid deposits in the carpal synovia and perineural tissue of long-term hemodialysis patients with carpal tunnel syndrome. In 1985 Gejyo *et al.* [114] demonstrated that the lesions contained amyloid with β₂-M as the constituent protein. This unique β₂-M amyloid stains with anti-β₂-M antibodies and has a characteristic electron-microscopic appearance with short, thick fibrils arranged in parallel bundles [115].

The major diseases associated with dialysis-related amyloidosis are carpal-tunnel syndrome and destructive arthropathy of large and medium-sized joints associated with cystic bone lesions. Both disorders are clearly related to the duration of time on dialysis and age at initiation of dialysis treatment. Charra *et al.* [116] have shown that no patients dialyzed for up to 8 years required surgery for carpal-tunnel syndrome whereas by 14 years 50% and by 20 years 100% required surgery. The cystic bone lesions are large (≥5 mm diameter in the wrists and ≥10 mm diameter in the shoulders and hips), have a normal adjacent joint space and are generally multiple [117]. In the report of the Working Party on Dialysis Amyloidosis [117] an increased age at onset of dialysis had a significant correlation with the development of carpal-tunnel syndrome and bone amyloidosis.

β₂-M is an 11 800 dalton protein composed of a single polypeptide chain which is expressed on the surface of all nucleated cells and is also released during degranulation of neutrophils [115]. Cytokines such as tumor necrosis factor, interleukin-2 and both alpha- and gamma-interferon increase β₂-M synthesis and release. Due to cell turnover and release approximately 200 mg of β₂-M per day is released into the extracellular space where it circulates freely in the plasma and is excreted by glomerular filtration, tubular reabsorption and subsequent degradation. Levels of β₂-M are correlated inversely with renal function. β₂-M, perhaps after limited proteolysis by the synovial cells, appears to deposit in collagen rich areas causing disease.

The type of membrane utilized during hemodialysis appears to significantly influence clearance and production of β₂-M. Hemodialysis utilizing a cuprophane membrane leads to an increase in the serum levels of β₂-M and tumor necrosis factor whereas utilization of a more biocompatable (less inflammatory response) polyacrylonitrile membrane reduced levels of both β₂-M and tumor necrosis factor. A marked decrease has been shown in the levels of β₂-M when patients were dialyzed with a biocompatable porous polysulfone membrane compared with cuprophane whether or not the dialyzers were reused [118]. The decrease in β₂-M with porous biocompatible membranes appears secondary to increased loss through the membrane, increased adherence of the protein to the membrane and decreased cytokine stimulation which increases β₂-M release. Importantly in a retrospective, large (221 patients), multicenter (12), long-term (up to 15 years) study the Working Party on Dialysis Amyloidosis has shown that patients dialyzed solely with a biocompatible porous membrane had significantly less radiological signs of bone amyloidosis than those treated with a cuprophane membrane [117].

Acknowledgment

This work was supported by National Institutes of Health Grants AM-33949 and AR-39906.

References

1. Aurbach, G.D., Marx, G.J. and Spiegel, A.M. (1985) in *Textbook of Endocrinology* (eds Wilson and Foster), W.B. Saunders, Philadelphia, pp. 1218–55.
2. Rasmussen, H. and Bordier, P. (1974) *The Physiological and Cellular Basis of Metabolic Bone Disease.* Williams & Wilkins, Baltimore.
3. Bonar, I.C., Roufosse, A.H., Sabine, W.K. *et al.* (1983) X-ray diffraction studies of the crystallinity of bone mineral in newly synthesized and density fractionated bone. *Calcif. Tissue Int.,* **35**, 202–9.
4. Bushinsky, D.A., Levi-Setti, R. and Coe, F.L. (1986) Ion microprobe determination of bone surface elements: effects of reduced medium pH. *Am. J. Physiol.,* **250**, F1090–7.
5. Nancollas, G.H., Lore, M., Perez, L. *et al.* (1989) Mineral phases of calcium phosphate. *Anat. Rec.,* **224**, 234–41.
6. Neuman, W.F. and Neuman, M.W. (1958) *The Chemical Dynamics of Bone Mineral.* University Chicago Press, Chicago.
7. Bushinsky, D.A. and Lechleider, R.J. (1987) Mechanism of proton-induced bone calcium release: calcium carbonate dissolution. *Am. J. Physiol.,* **253**, F998–1005.
8. Roufosse, A.H., Landis, W.J., Sabine, W.K. and Glimcher, M.J. (1979) Identification of brushite in newly deposited bone mineral from embryonic chicks. *J. Ultrastruct. Res.,* **68**, 235–55.
9. Miller, E.J. and Martin, G.R. (1968) The collagen of bone. *Clin. Orthop.,* **59**, 195–232.
10. Franzen, A. and Heinegard, D. (1985) Isolation and characterization of two sialoproteins present only in bone calcified matrix. *Biochem. J.,* **232**, 715–24.
11. Rodan, G.A. and Rodan, S.B. (1984) in *Bone and Mineral*

Research, Annual 2 (ed. W.A. Peck), Elsevier Science Publishers, Amsterdam, pp. 244–85.

12. Triffitt, J.T. (1987) Initiation and enhancement of bone formation. *Acta Orthop. Scand.*, **58**, 673–84.

13. Vaughan, J. (1981) *The Physiology of Bone.* Clarendon Press, Oxford.

14. Menton, D.N., Simmons, D.J., Orr, B.Y. and Plurad, S.B. (1982) A cellular investment of bone marrow. *Anat. Rec.*, **203**, 157–64.

15. Ko, J.S. and Bernard, G.W. (1981) Osteoclast formation in vitro from bone marrow mononuclear cells in osteoclast-free bone. *Am. J. Anat.*, **161**, 415–25.

16. Burger, E.H., Van der Meer, J.W.M., Van de Gevel, J.S. *et al.* (1982) *In vitro* formation of osteoclasts from long term cultures of bone marrow mononuclear phagocytes. *J. Exp. Med.*, **156**, 1604–14.

17. Baron, R. (1989) Molecular mechanisms of bone resorption by the osteoclast. *Anat. Rec.*, **224**, 317–24.

18. Blair, H.C, Teitelbaum, S.L., Ghiselli, R. and Gluck, S. (1989) Osteoclastic bone resorption by a polarized vacuolar proton pump. *Science*, **245**, 855–7.

19. Baron, R., Neff, L., Louvard, D. and Courtoy, P.J. (1985) Cell-mediated extracellular acidification and bone resorption: evidence for a low pH in resorbing lacunae and localization of a 100Kd lysosomal membrane protein at the osteoclast ruffled border. *J. Cell Biol.*, **101**, 2210–22.

20. Schenk, R.K., Spiro, D. and Wiener, J. (1967) Cartilage resorption in tibial epiphyseal plate of growing rats. *J. Cell Biol.*, **34**, 275–91.

21. Reinholt, F.P., Hultenby, K., Oldberg, A. and Heinegard, D. (1990) Osteopontin – a possible anchor of osteoclasts to bone. *Proc. Natl. Acad. Sci. USA*, **87**, 4473–75.

22. Vaes, G. (1988) Cellular biology and biochemical mechanism of bone resorption. A review of recent developments on the formation, activation, and mode of action of osteoclasts. *Clin. Orthop.*, **231**, 239–71.

23. Delaisse, J.M., Eeckhout, Y. and Vaes, G. (1984) *In vivo* and *in vitro* evidence for the involvement of cysteine proteinases in bone resorption. *Biochem. Biophys. Res. Commun.*, **125**, 441–7.

24. Krieger, N.S., Sukhatme, V.P. and Bushinsky, D.A. (1990) Conditioned medium from ras oncogene transformed NIH3T3 cells induces bone resorption *in vitro*. *J. Bone Miner. Res.*, **5**, 159–64.

25. Miller, S.C. (1985) The rapid appearance of acid phosphatase activity at the developing ruffled border of parathyroid hormone activated medullary bone osteoclasts. *Calcif. Tissue Int.*, **37**, 526–9.

26. Delaisse, J-M. and Vaes, G. (1992) in *Biology and Physiology of the Osteoclast* (eds B.R. Rifkin and C.V. Gay), CRC Press, Boca Raton, FL, pp. 289–314.

27. Sundquist, K.T., Leppilampi, M., Jarvelin, K. *et al.* (1987) Carbonic anhydrase isoenzymes in isolated rat peripheral monocytes, tissue macrophages and osteoclasts. *Bone*, **8**, 33–8.

28. Teti, A., Blair, H.C., Teitelbaum, S.L. *et al.* (1989) Cytoplasmic pH regulation and chloride/bicarbonate exchange in avian osteoclasts. *J. Clin. Invest.*, **83**, 227–33.

29. Urist, M.R., DeLange, R.J. and Finerman, G.A.M. (1983) Bone cell differentiation and growth factors. *Science*, **220**, 680–6.

30. Tam, C.S., Heersche, J.N.M., Murray, T.M. and Parsons, J.A. (1982) Parathyroid hormone stimulates the bone apposition rate independently of its resorptive action: differential effects of intermittent and continuous administration. *Endocrinology*, **110**, 506–12.

31. Brommage, R. and DeLuca, H.F. (1985) Evidence that 1,25-dihydroxyvitamin D$_3$ is the physiologically active metabolite of vitamin D$_3$. *Endocr. Rev.*, **6**, 491–511.

32. Hahn, T.J. (1989) in *Metabolic Bone Disease: Cellular and Tissue Mechanisms* (eds C.S. Tam, J.N.M. Heersche and T.M. Murray), CRC Press, Boca Raton, FL, pp. 223–37.

33. Briancon, D. and Meunier, P.J. (1981) Treatment of osteoporosis with fluoride, calcium and vitamin D. *Orthop. Clin. North Am.*, **12**, 629–48.

34. Krieger, N.S., Sessler, N.E. and Bushinsky, D.A. (1992) Acidosis inhibits osteoblastic and stimulates osteoclastic activity *in vitro*. *Am. J. Physiol.*, **262**, F442–8.

35. Bushinsky, D.A. (1995) Stimulated osteoclastic and suppressed osteoblastic activity in metabolic but not respiratory acidosis. *Am. J. Physiol.*, **268**, C80–8.

36. Sprague, S.M., Krieger, N.S. and Bushinsky, D.A. (1994) Greater inhibition of *in vitro* bone mineralization with metabolic than respiratory acidosis. *Kidney Int.*, **46**, 1199–206.

37. Holtrop, M.E., Raisz, L.G. and Simmons, H.A. (1974) The effects of parathyroid hormone, colchicine and calcitonin on the ultrastructure and the activity of osteoclasts in organ culture. *J. Cell Biol.*, **60**, 346–55.

38. Rao, L.G., Murray, T.M. and Heersche, J.N.M. (1983) Immunohistochemical demonstration of parathyroid hormone binding to specific cell types in fixed rat bone tissue. *Endocrinology*, **113**, 805–10.

39. Pliam, N.B., Nyiredy, K.O. and Arnaud, C.D. (1982) Parathyroid hormone receptors in avian bone cells. *Proc. Natl. Acad. Sci. USA*, **79**, 2061–3.

40. Rao, L.G. and Murray, T.M. (1985) Binding of intact parathyroid hormone to rat osteosarcoma cells: major contribution of binding sites for the carboxyl-terminal region of the hormone. *Endocrinology*, **117**, 1632–8.

41. Kream, B.E., Rowe, D.W., Gworek, S.E. and Raisz, L.G. (1980) Parathyroid hormone alters collagen synthesis and procollagen mRNA levels in fetal rat calvaria. *Proc. Natl. Acad. Sci. USA*, **77**, 5654–8.

42. Liskova-Kiar, M. (1979) Mode of action of cortisol on bone resorption in fetal rat fibulae cultured in vitro. *Am. J. Anat.*, **156**, 63–75.

43. Rodan, G.A. and Martin, T.J. (1981) Role of osteoblasts in hormonal control of bone resorption – a hypothesis. *Calcif. Tissue Int.*, **33**, 349–51.

44. Minkin, C. (1982) Bone acid phosphatase: tartrate resistant acid phosphatase as a marker of osteoclast function. *Calcif. Tissue Int.*, **34**, 285–90.

45. Vaes, G. (1968) On the mechanisms of bone resorption. The action of parathyroid hormone on the excretion and synthesis of lysosomal enzymes and on the extra-

cellular release of acid by bone cells. *J. Cell Biol.*, **39**, 676–97.

46. Anderson, R.E., Woodbury, D.M. and Jee, W.S.S. (1986) Humoral and ionic regulation of osteoclast acidity. *Calcif. Tissue Int.*, **39**, 252–8.

47. Marie, P.J. and Travers, R. (1983) Continuous infusion of 1,25-dihydroxyvitamin D₃ stimulates bone turnover in the normal young mouse. *Calcif. Tissue Int.*, **35**, 418–25.

48. Nijweide, P.J., Burger, E.H. and Feyen, J.H.M. (1986) Cells of bone: proliferation, differentiation, and hormonal regulation. *Physiol. Rev.*, **66**, 855–86.

49. Stern, P.H. (1980) The D vitamins and bone. *Pharmacol. Rev.*, **32**, 47–80.

50. Holtrop, M.E., Cox, K.A., Clark, M.B. *et al.* (1981) 1,25-dihydroxycholecalciferol stimulates osteoclasts in rat bones in the absence of parathyroid hormone. *Endocrinology*, **108**, 2293–301.

51. Bushinsky, D.A. (1995) in *The Principles and Practice of Nephrology* (eds H.R. Jacobson, G.E. Striker and S. Klahr), Mosby, St Louis, MO, pp. 924–32.

52. Bushinsky, D.A. and Krieger, N.S. (1992) in *The Kidney: Physiology and Pathophysiology* (eds D.W. Seldin and G. Giebisch), Raven Press, New York, pp. 2395–430.

53. Krieger, N.S., Stappenbeck, T.S. and Stern, P.H. (1988) Characterization of specific thyroid hormone receptors in bone. *J. Bone Miner. Res.*, **3**, 473–8.

54. Klein, D.C. and Raisz, L.G. (1970) Prostaglandins: stimulation of bone resorption in tissue culture. *Endocrinology*, **86**, 1436–40.

55. Dunstan, C.R., Evans, R.A., Hills, E. *et al.* (1984) Effect of aluminum and parathyroid hormone on osteoblasts and bone mineralization in chronic renal failure. *Calcif. Tissue Int.*, **36**, 133–8.

56. Plachot, J.J., Cournot-Witmer, G., Halpern, S. *et al.* (1984) Bone ultrastructure and x-ray microanalysis of aluminum–intoxicated hemodialyzed patients. *Kidney Int.*, **25**, 796–803.

57. Smith, A.J., Faugere, M.C., Abreo, K. *et al.* (1986) Aluminum-related bone disease in mild and advanced renal failure: evidence for high prevalence and morbidity and studies on etiology and diagnosis. *Am. J. Nephrol.*, **6**, 275–283.

58. Parisien, M., Charhon, S.A., Arlot, M. *et al.* (1988) Evidence for a toxic effect of aluminum on osteoblasts: a histomorphometric study in hemodialysis patients with aplastic bone disease. *J. Bone Miner. Res.*, **3**, 259–67.

59. Sprague, S.M. and Bushinsky, D.A. (1990) Mechanism of aluminum-induced calcium efflux from cultured neonatal mouse calvariae. *Am. J. Physiol.*, **258**, F583–8.

60. Sprague, S.M., Krieger, N.S. and Bushinsky, D.A. (1993) Aluminum inhibits bone nodule formation and calcification *in vitro*. *Am. J. Physiol.*, **264**, F882–90.

61. Vaananen, H.K. (1993) Mechanism of bone turnover. *Ann. Med.*, **25**, 353–9.

62. Canalis, E., McCarthy, T. and Centrella, M. (1988) Growth factors and the regulation of bone remodeling. *J. Clin. Invest.*, **81**, 277–81.

63. Hauschka, P.V., Mavrakos, A.E., Iafrati, M.D. *et al.* (1986) Growth factors in bone matrix. Isolation of multi-

ple types by affinity chromatography on heparin–sepharose. *J. Biol. Chem.*, **261**, 12665–74.

64. Bushinsky, D.A. (1994) in *Primer on Kidney Diseases* ed. A. Greenberg), National Kidney Foundation, pp. 406–13.

65. Goodman, W.G., Coburn, J.W., Ramirez, J.A. *et al.* (1993) in *Primer on the Metabolic Bone Diseases and Disorders of Mineral Metabolism*, 2nd edn (ed. M.J. Favus), Raven Press, New York, NY, pp. 304–23.

66. Llach, F. and Bover, J. (1996) in *The Kidney*, 5th edn (ed. B. Brenner), W.B. Saunders, Philadelphia, pp. 2187–273.

67. Malluche, H. and Faugere, M.-C. (1990) Renal bone disease 1990: an unmet challenge for the nephrologist. *Kidney Int.*, **38**, 193–211.

68. Pitts, T.O., Piraino, B.H., Mitro, R. *et al.* (1988) Hyperparathyroidism and 1,25-dihydroxyvitamin D deficiency in mild, moderate and severe renal failure. *J. Clin. Endocrinol. Metab.*, **67**, 876–81.

69. Delmez, J.A. and Slatopolsky, E. (1992) Hyperphosphatemia: its consequences and treatment in patients with chronic renal disease. *Am. J. Kidney Dis.*, **19**, 303–17.

70. Kilav, R., Silver, J. and Naveh-Many, T. (1995) Parathyroid hormone gene expression in hypophosphatemic rats. *J. Clin. Invest.*, **96**, 327–33.

71. Slatopolsky, E., Caglar, S., Pennell, J.P. *et al.* (1971) On the pathogenesis of hyperparathyroidism in chronic experimental renal insufficiency in the dog. *J. Clin. Invest.*, **50**, 492–9.

72. Kumar, R. (1984) Metabolism of 1,25-dihydroxyvitamin D₃. *Physiol. Rev.*, **64**, 478–504.

73. Theofan, G., Nguyen, A.P. and Norman, A.W. (1986) Regulation of calbindin-D28K gene expression by 1,25-dihydroxyvitamin D₃ is correlated to receptor occupancy. *J. Biol. Chem.*, **261**, 16943–7.

74. Reiss, E., Canterbury, J.M., Bercovitz, M.A. *et al.* (1970) The role of phosphate in the secretion of parathyroid hormone in man. *J. Clin. Invest.*, **49**, 2146–9.

75. Russell, J., Lettieri, D. and Sherwood, L.M. (1983) Direct regulation by calcium of cytoplasmic messenger RNA coding for pre-proparathyroid hormone in isolated bovine parathyroid cells. *J. Clin. Invest.*, **72**, 1851–5.

76. Brumbaugh, P.F., Hughes, M.R. and Haussler, M.R. (1975) Cytoplasmic and nuclear binding components for the 1α,25-dihydroxyvitamin D₃ in chick parathyroid glands. *Proc. Natl. Acad. Sci. USA*, **72**, 4871–5.

77. Silver, J., Russell, J. and Sherwood, L.M. (1985) Regulation by vitamin D metabolites of messenger ribonucleic acid for pre-proparathyroid hormone in isolated bovine parathyroid cells. *Proc. Natl. Acad. Sci. USA*, **82**, 4270–3.

78. Cantley, L.K., Russell, J., Lettieri, D. and Sherwood, L.M. (1985) 1,25-Dihydroxyvitamin D₃ suppresses parathyroid hormone secretion from bovine parathyroid cells in tissue culture. *Endocrinology*, **117**, 2114–19.

79. Korkor, A.B. (1987) Reduced binding of [³H]-1,25-dihydroxyvitamin D₃ parathyroid glands of patients with renal failure. *N. Engl. J. Med.*, **316**, 1573–7.

80. Andress, D.L., Norris, K.C., Coburn, J.W. *et al.* (1989) Intravenous calcitriol in the treatment of refractory

osteitis fibrosa of chronic renal failure. *N. Engl. J. Med.*, **321**, 274–9.

81. Brown, A.J., Ritter, C.R., Finch, J.L. *et al.* (1989) The noncalcemic analogue of vitamin D, 22-oxocalcitriol, suppresses parathyroid hormone synthesis and secretion. *J. Clin. Invest.*, **84**, 728–32.

82. MacDonald, P.N., Ritter, C., Brown, A.J. and Slatopolsky, E. (1994) Retinoic acid suppresses parathyroid hormone (PTH) secretion and preproPTH mRNA levels in bovine parathyroid cell culture. *J. Clin. Invest.*, **93**, 725–30.

83. Martin, K.J., Hruska, K.A., Freitag, J.J. *et al.* (1979) The peripheral metabolism of parathyroid hormone. *N. Engl. J. Med.*, **301**, 1092–8.

84. Goltzman, D., Henderson, B. and Loveridge, N. (1980) Cytochemical bioassay of parathyroid hormone: characteristics of the assay and analysis of circulating hormonal forms. *J. Clin. Invest.*, **65**, 1309–17.

85. Bushinsky, D.A. (1995) The contribution of acidosis to renal osteodystrophy. *Kidney Int.*, **47**, 1816–32.

86. Bushinsky, D.A. and Nilsson, E.L. (1995) Additive effects of acidosis and parathyroid hormone on mouse osteoblastic and osteoclastic function. *Am. J. Physiol.*, **269**, 1364–70.

87. Cohen Solal, M.E., Sebert, J.L., Boudailliez, B. *et al.* (1991) Comparison of intact, midregion, and carboxy terminal assays for parathyroid hormone for the diagnosis of bone disease in hemodialyzed patients. *J. Clin. Endocrinol. Metab.*, **73**, 516–24.

88. Quarles, D.L., Lobaugh, B. and Murphy, G. (1992) Intact parathyroid hormone overestimates the presence and severity of parathyroid-mediated osseous abnormalities in uremia. *J. Clin. Endocrinol. Metab.*, **75**, 145–50.

89. Alfrey, A.C., LeGendre, G.R. and Kaehny, W.D. (1976) The dialysis encephalopathy syndrome: possible aluminum intoxication. *N. Engl. J. Med.*, **294**, 184–8.

90. Platts, M.M., Goode, G.C. and Hislop, J.S. (1977) Composition of the domestic water supply and the incidence of fracture and encephalopathy in patients on home dialysis. *Br. Med. J.*, **2**, 657–60.

91. Ott, S.M., Maloney, N.A., Coburn, J.W. *et al.* (1982) The prevalence of bone aluminum deposition in renal osteodystrophy and its relation to the response to calcitriol therapy. *N. Engl. J. Med.*, **307**, 709–13.

92. Hodsman, A.B., Sherrard, D.J., Alfrey, A.C. *et al.* (1982) Bone aluminum and histomorphometric features of renal osteodystrophy. *J. Clin. Endocrinol. Metab.*, **54**, 539–46.

93. Pierides, A.M., Edwards, W.G., Jr, Cullu, U.S. *et al.* (1980) Hemodialysis encephalopathy with osteomalacic fractures and muscle weakness. *Kidney Int.*, **18**, 115–24.

94. Maloney, N.A., Ott, S.M., Alfrey, A.C. *et al.* (1982) Histological quantitation of aluminum in iliac bone from patients with renal failure. *J. Lab. Clin. Med.*, **99**, 206–16.

95. Goodman, W.G., Henry, D.A., Horst, R. *et al.* (1984) Parenteral aluminum administration in the dog: II. Induction of osteomalacia and effect of vitamin D metabolism. *Kidney Int.*, **25**, 370–5.

96. Goodman, W.G., Gilligan, J. and Horst, R. (1984) Short-term aluminum administration in the rat. Effects on

bone formation and relationship to renal osteomalacia. *J. Clin. Invest.*, **73**, 171–81.

97. Hercz, G., Pei, Y., Greenwood, A. *et al.* (1993) Aplastic osteodystrophy without aluminum: The role of 'suppressed' parathyroid function. *Kidney Int.*, **44**, 860–6.

98. Salusky, I.B., Coburn, J.W., Brill, J. *et al.* (1988) Bone disease in pediatric patients undergoing dialysis with CAPD or CCPD. *Kidney Int.*, **33**, 975–82.

99. Sherrard, D.J., Baylink, D. and Wergedal, J. (1972) Bone disease in uremia. *ASA/O Trans.*, **28**, 412–15.

100. Sherrard, D.J., Hercz, G., Pei, Y. *et al.* (1993) The spectrum of bone disease in end-stage renal failure – An evolving disorder. *Kidney Int.*, **43**, 436–42.

101. Christiansen, C.L., Rodbro, P., Christensen, M.S. *et al.* (1978) Deterioration of renal function during treatment of chronic renal failure with 1,25-dihydroxycholecalciferol. *Lancet*, **ii**, 700–3.

102. Baker, L.R.I., Abrams, S.M.L., Roe, C.J. *et al.* (1989) 1,25(OH)$_2$D$_3$ administration in moderate renal failure: a prospective double-blind trial. *Kidney Int.*, **35**, 661–9.

103. Bushinsky, D.A., Wolbach, W., Sessler, N.E. *et al.* (1993) Physicochemical effects of acidosis on bone calcium flux and surface ion composition. *J. Bone Miner. Res.*, **8**, 93–102.

104. Lefebvre, A., de Vernejoul, M.C., Gueris, J. *et al.* (1989) Optimal correction of acidosis changes progression of dialysis osteodystrophy. *Kidney Int.*, **36**, 1112–18.

105. Clarkson, E.M., McDonald, S.J. and DeWardener, H.E. (1966) The effect of high intake of calcium carbonate in normal subjects and patients with chronic renal failure. *Clin. Sci.*, **30**, 425–38.

106. Makoff, D.L., Gordon, A., Franklin, S.S. *et al.* (1969) Chronic calcium carbonate therapy in uremia. *Arch. Intern. Med.*, **123**, 15–21.

107. Harris, D.C.H., Yuill, E. and Chesher, D.W. (1995) Correcting acidosis in hemodialysis: effect on phosphate clearance and calcification risk. *J. Am. Soc. Nephrol.*, **6**, 1607–12.

108. Hercz, G., Salusky, I.B., Norris, K.C. *et al.* (1986) Aluminum removal by peritoneal dialysis: intravenous vs. intraperitoneal deferioxamine. *Kidney Int.*, **30**, 944–8.

109. Ott, S.M., Andress, D.L., Nebeker, H.G. *et al.* (1986) Changes in bone histology after treatment with desferrioxamine. *Kidney Int.*, **29**, S108–13.

110. McCarthy, J.T. and Kumar, R. (1995) in *The Principles and Practice of Nephrology*, 2nd edn (eds H.R. Jacobson, G.E. Striker and S. Klahr), Mosby, St Louis, pp. 1032–45.

111. Windus, D.W., Stokes, T.J., Julian, B.A. and Fenves, A.Z. (1987) Fatal rhizopus infections in hemodialysis patients receiving deferoxamine. *Ann. Intern. Med.*, **107**, 678–80.

112. Hoen, B., Renoult, E., Jonon, B. and Kessler, M. (1988) Septicemia due to *Yersinia enterocolitica* in a long-term hemodialysis patient after a single desferrioxamine administration. *Nephron*, **50**, 378–9.

113. Hercz, G., Andress, D.L., Nebeker, H.G. *et al.* (1988) Reversal of aluminum-related bone disease after substi-

tuting calcium carbonate for aluminum hydroxide. *Am. J. Kidney Dis.*, **11**, 70–5.

114. Gejyo, F., Yamada, T., Odani, S. *et al.* (1985) A new form of amyloid protein associated with chronic hemodialysis was identified as β_2-microglobulin. *Biochem. Biophys. Res. Commun.*, **129**, 701–6.

115. Koch, K.M. (1992) Dialysis-related amyloidosis. *Kidney Int.*, **41**, 1416–29.

116. Charra, B., Calemard, E. and Laurent, G. (1988) Chronic renal failure treatment duration and mode: their relevance to the late dialysis periarticular syndrome. *Blood Purif.*, **6**, 117–24.

117. van Ypersele de Strihou, C., Jadoul, J., Malghem, J. *et al.* (1991) Effect of dialysis membrane and patient's age on signs of dialysis–related amyloidosis. *Kidney Int.*, **39**, 1012–19.

118. Petersen, J., Moore, R.M., Jr, Kaczmarek, R.G. *et al.* (1991) The effects of reprocessing cuprophane and polysulfone dialyzers on β_2-microglobulin removal from hemodialysis. *Am. J. Kidney Dis.*, **2**, 174–8.

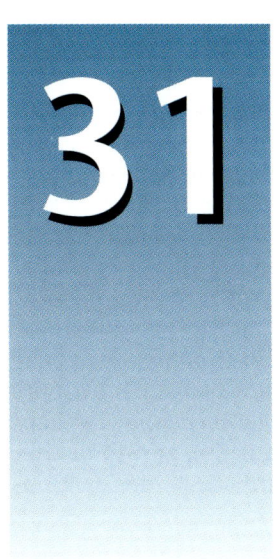

31

Hypertension and cardiovascular disorders

Robert Wilkinson

Introduction

Life expectancy for patients with end-stage renal disease (ESRD) is markedly reduced; vascular disease is the major cause of death. By the time patients with renal failure reach dialysis, coronary heart disease, congestive heart failure and cardiomegaly are each present in around 40% of patients and left ventricular hypertrophy in 30% [1]. Although other comorbid conditions such as diabetes, hyperlipidemia and smoking are important predisposing factors, hypertension is pre-eminent and observed at all stages of renal disease, affecting 80–90% of patients reaching ESRD, and is likely to be a major contributor to the development of vascular disease.

This chapter examines the pathogenesis of hypertension in renal failure and its clinical and pathological consequences, in particular vascular disease. In addition, left ventricular hypertrophy (LVH), a major risk factor for cardiac death, is discussed. Hypertension, anemia, high cardiac output due to arteriovenous fistulae, and the possible effects of growth factors such as angiotensin II, all contribute to increase the prevalence of LVH in patients with renal failure. Other factors which contribute to the development of vascular disease are also discussed.

Definition of hypertension in renal failure

Blood pressure in the general population has a Gaussian distribution with a tail at the higher values. Hypertension is operationally defined as the level of blood pressure above which treatment does more good than harm. The diagnostic criteria must, therefore, vary with the characteristics of the population treated, which determine the potential for doing good, and the treatments available which determine the hazards of intervention. In patients with renal failure, the risks of vascular disease are much higher than those in the general population so that the possibility for benefit from treatment is greater. Although it has not yet been demonstrated that control of blood pressure in patients with renal failure reduces the incidence of myocardial infarction and stroke, it seems likely from studies of control of pressure in those with essential hypertension that it will. In addition there is evidence to show that control of blood pressure in diabetic and non-diabetic patients delays progression of renal failure (Chapters 43 and 68). Based on the foregoing considerations, treatment of diastolic blood pressure (DBP) of 90 mmHg or more is recommended in patients with renal disease. By contrast, in the UK, Canada and New Zealand,

Nephrology, Edited by Rex L. Jamison and Robert Wilkinson.
Published in 1997 by Chapman & Hall, London. ISBN 0 412 60930 4

treatment of essential hypertension in patients aged less than 60 years is recommended only when DBP exceeds 100 mmHg. In the USA, however, treatment is recommended at levels of 90 mmHg.

Prevalence of hypertension in patients with various renal diseases

The prevalence of hypertension differs among patients with similar degrees of renal impairment depending on the underlying renal disease. Within a single disease category, however, blood pressure is inversely correlated with renal function [2].

Data from the UK Medical Research Council Glomerulonephritis Registry show that, in patients with normal renal function, hypertension was most frequent (40%) in mesangiocapillary glomerulonephritis (type I) and least common (16%) in minimal change nephropathy [2]. About 10% of the control population were hypertensive and 46% of patients with adult polycystic disease (APCKD) mean age 46 years, with normal renal function, were hypertensive [2]. Hypertension has been reported in young children who have inherited APCKD before there is evidence of cysts or of impaired renal function indicating that the hypertension cannot be solely due to impaired renal function.

Hypertension is present in approximately 30% of patients with chronic pyelonephritis (CPN) at presentation, increasing to around 50% after five years and 70% in patients reaching end-stage renal failure [2]. Both glomerular and tubulointerstitial renal diseases are commonly accompanied by hypertension. The suggestion that tubulointerstitial diseases often cause salt wasting and are, therefore, less likely to be accompanied by hypertension cannot be sustained.

Clinical manifestations

Hypertension in patients with impaired renal function may be of any degree of severity.

Malignant hypertension

Malignant hypertension is defined by the presence of bilateral fundal hemorrhages and exudates in a patient with hypertension. Its development is related to the severity of hypertension and in adults it is uncommon if diastolic pressure of less than 120 mmHg. It is also related to the rate of development of hypertension so that it is unusual in old people with long-standing hypertension, despite blood pressures as high as 260/150 mmHg, whereas it may occur at much lower pressures when the onset of hypertension is more rapid in patients with renal

or renovascular disease. The reduced susceptibility to retinopathy in long-standing hypertensives may be due to hypertrophy of resistance arterioles providing protection for the capillary beds.

It used to be thought that there was a specific 'uremic retinopathy' but it seems more likely that it is simply hypertensive retinopathy coming on at a lower pressure than in essential hypertension [3] probably because there has been less time for arteriolar hypertrophy. However, it is possible that higher levels of angiotensin II in some patients with renal disease may, by increasing capillary endothelial permeability and stimulating growth of arteriolar smooth muscle cells, contribute to the development of malignant hypertension.

Left ventricular hypertrophy

LVH is more common in hypertension associated with renal impairment than in essential hypertension probably because the former is often accompanied by anemia which leads to an increase in cardiac output. In addition, the blunting of the nocturnal fall in blood pressure in renal impairment may contribute to LVH. In normal subjects, and in most patients with essential hypertension, there is a diurnal variation in blood pressure, with a fall during sleep; in renal hypertension this is blunted or lost (Figure 31.1). The 24 h blood pressure load is therefore greater, increasing the risk of LVH. Hormones which may also act as growth factors, e.g. angiotensin II, may also contribute to the development of LVH. In patients who are treated by hemodialysis the construction of an arteriovenous fistula, by increasing cardiac output, also contributes to the development of LVH.

Fluid overload

Although sodium retention is probably the central pathogenetic factor in the hypertension of renal impairment, there is often no evidence of edema, because it does not appear until total body water is approximately 3 kg above normal. This amount of fluid retention is sufficient to trigger increased salt and water excretion to prevent further salt retention. The mechanisms involved include a rise in blood pressure which increases filtration pressure and reduces proximal tubular sodium reabsorption [4]. There is also release of atrial natriuretic peptide (ANP) and suppression of aldosterone secretion. There may also be release of a digitalis-like 'natriuretic hormone' which inhibits Na,K-ATPase in the renal tubule. The hypertension which accompanies renal failure may be regarded as a trade-off which allows preservation of salt balance despite the reduction in glomerular filtration rate (GFR) (Figure 31.2).

Salt overload may be difficult to detect unless there is a gallop or triple cardiac rhythm. Otherwise it may be assumed to be present and a loop diuretic is often an essential part of the drug regimen.

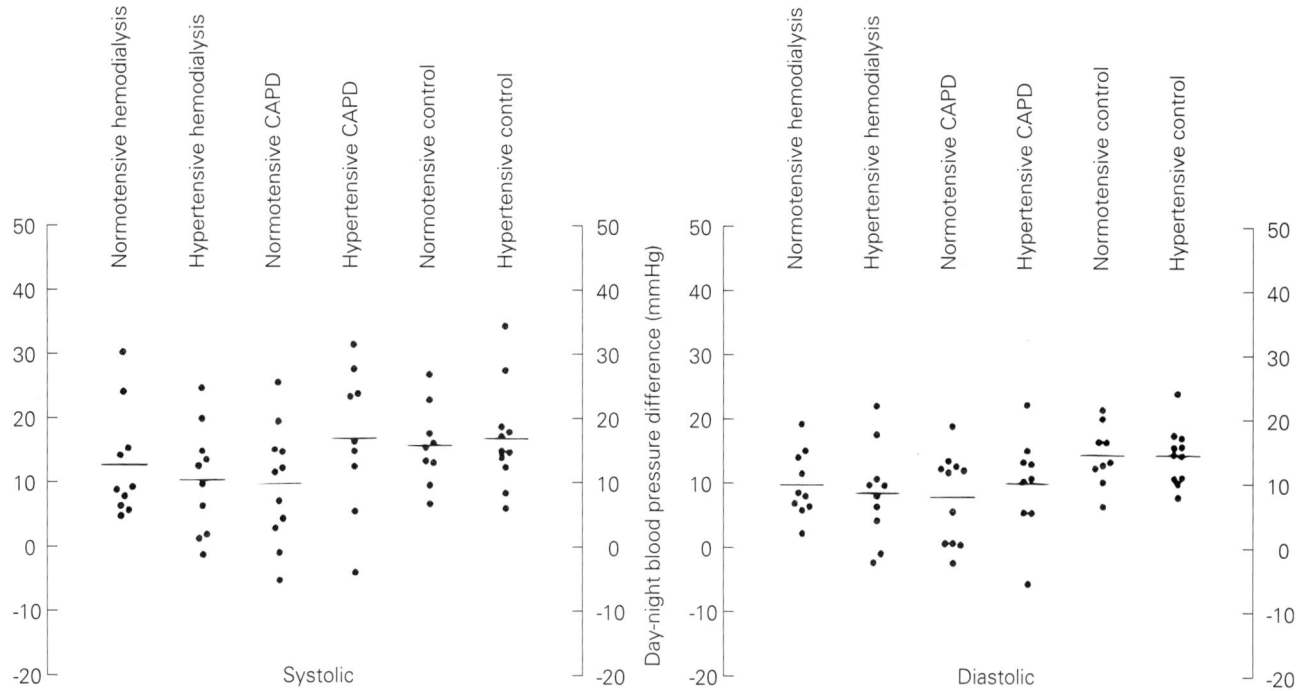

Figure 31.1 Attenuation or loss of nocturnal dip in blood pressure in dialysis patients. The day–night blood pressure differences in individual dialysis and control patients is shown. (Reproduced, with permission, from Luik, A.J., Struijk, D.G., Gladziwa, U. *et al.* (1994) *Nephrol. Dial. Transplant.*, **9**, 1616–21.)

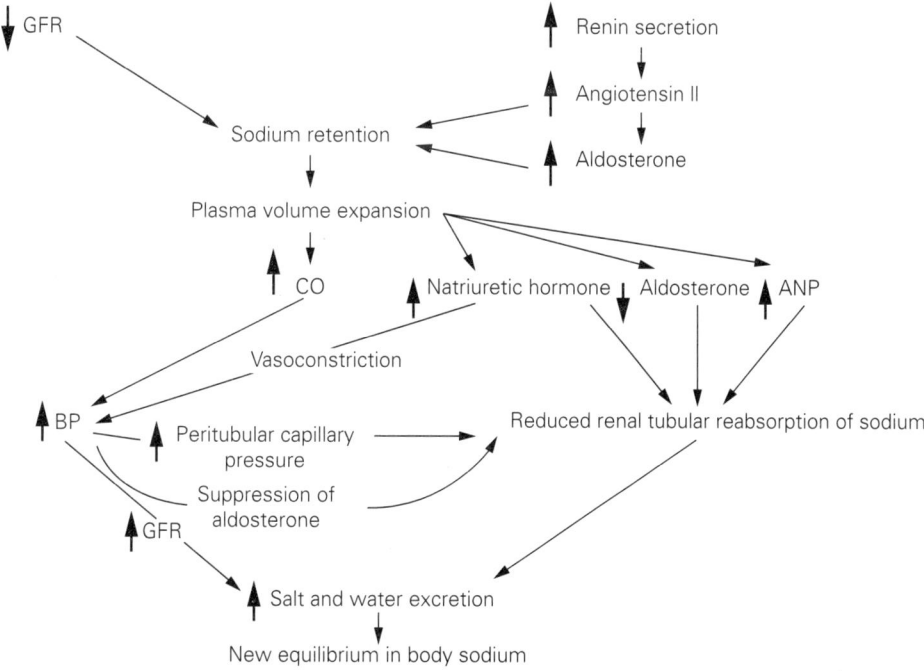

Figure 31.2 Diagram showing sodium homeostasis in chronic renal failure. The primary changes of reduced GFR and increased renin secretion lead to sodium retention, which is limited by a rise in BP and hormonal changes, which together increase sodium excretion. The new equilibrium may be reached before the point of clinically evident fluid retention.

GFR and treatment of hypertension

In the normal kidney GFR remains constant within a wide variation of arterial blood pressure as the result of autoregulatory mechanisms. In renal insufficiency, however, autoregulation is impaired and glomerular capillary pressure and GFR become much more dependent on the blood pressure. As a result GFR may fall when antihypertensive treatment is introduced. From animal work it seems likely that the loss of autoregulation is due to dependence on afferent arteriolar dilatation to maintain GFR in renal insufficiency [5]. When angiotensin converting enzyme inhibitors (ACE-I) or angiotensin II receptor blockers are administered the superimposition of efferent arteriolar dilatation on a reduction in systemic blood pressure and a reduced capacity to increase filtration pressure by further afferent dilatation may cause a more profound reduction in GFR than that accompanying an equivalent reduction in blood pressure with other antihypertensive agents (Figure 31.3). A marked reduction in GFR does not always occur because the fall in renal vascular resistance, brought about particularly by

ACE-I, leads to an increase in renal blood flow that diminishes the rise in colloid osmotic pressure opposing filtration along the glomerular capillary (Figure 31.4). This principle would still explain the maintenance of GFR even if, as may be the case, filtration equilibrium is not achieved.

GFR and fluid balance

In the normal kidney autoregulated GFR remains constant despite wide variations in fluid balance, but this capability is also disturbed in renal failure. The GFR falls with salt depletion and increases in parallel with a rise in blood pressure with salt loading [4]. This sensitivity of both blood pressure and GFR to salt balance is much less marked in essential hypertension. In renal failure it may be regarded as a 'trade-off' allowing the maintenance of sodium balance despite a reduction in functioning nephrons. The practical implication of this increased sensitivity to sodium balance is that in advanced renal failure a relatively minor illness causing salt depletion may be accompanied by a deterioration in renal function.

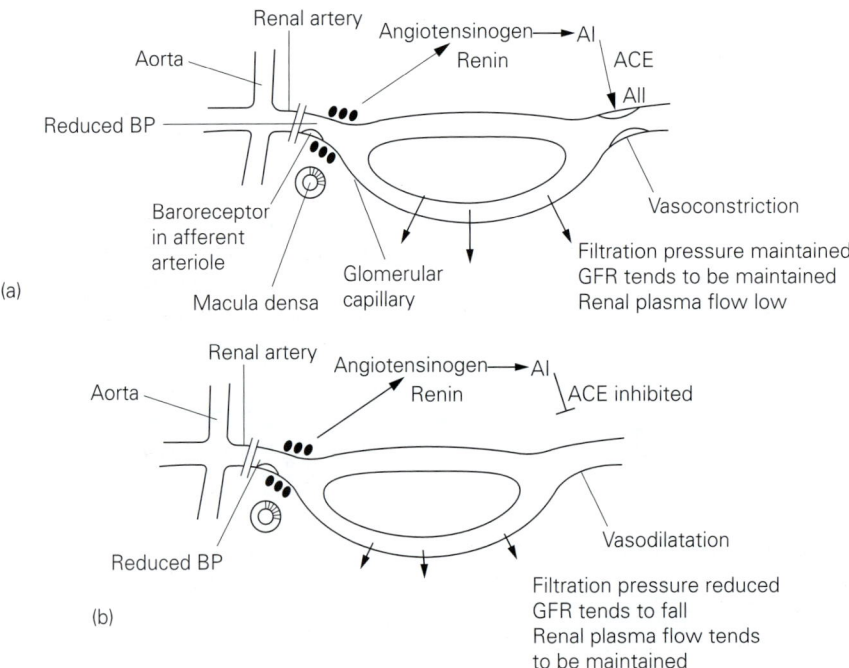

Figure 31.3 The role of angiotensin II (AII) in maintaining GFR in conditions of reduced renal perfusion pressure. Angiotensin II can be generated within the kidney because of the local availability of its substrate angiotensinogen together with renin and angiotensin converting enzyme. Reduced pressure at the afferent arteriolar baroreceptor stimulates renin release. (a) In the presence of AII efferent constriction maintains filtration pressure. (b) With ACE inhibition the efferent arteriole dilates and filtration pressure falls although renal plasma flow is maintained because of reduced renal vascular resistance (see Figure 31.4). (Reproduced in modified form from *Oxford Textbook of Clinical Nephrology*, Oxford Medical Publications, by permission of Oxford University Press.)

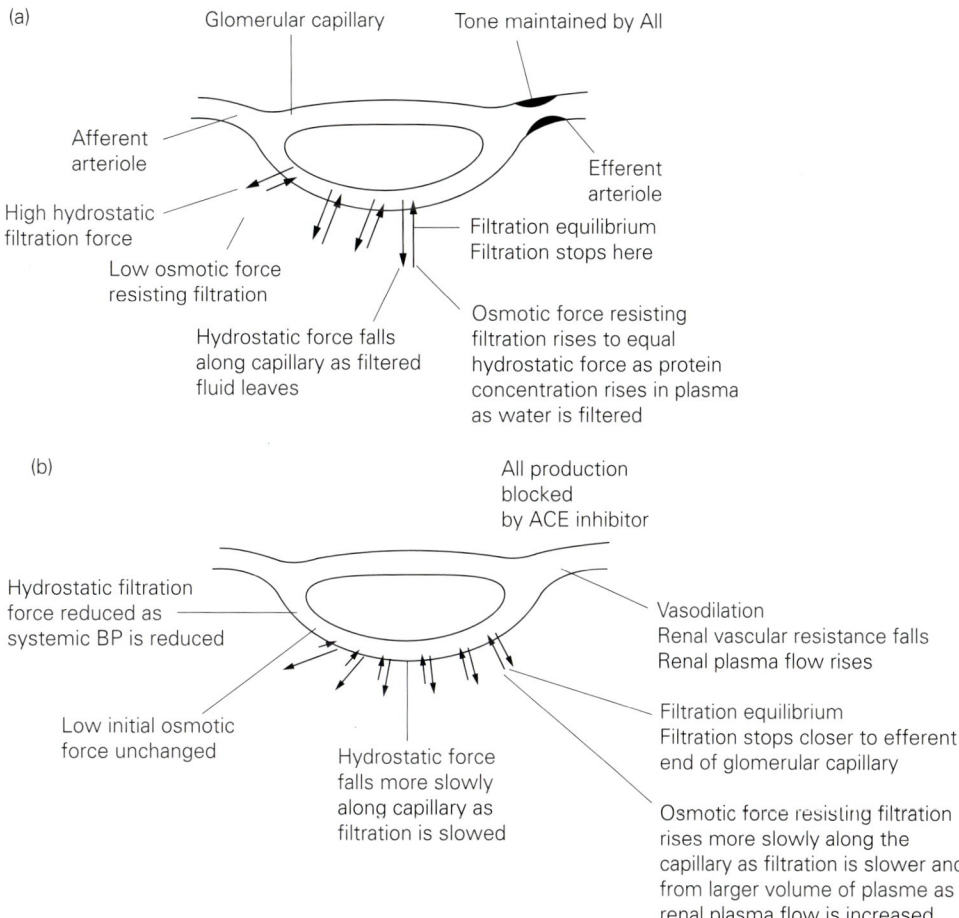

Figure 31.4 A possible mechanism for the maintenance of GFR in patients with impaired renal function despite the reduction in filtration pressure consequent on ACE inhibition (see Figure 31.3). (a) Filtration equilibrium is reached early in the glomerular capillary in the presence of angiotensin II and (b) slower filtration further along the capillary in the presence of an ACE inhibitor. (Reproduced from *Oxford Textbook of Clinical Nephrology*, Oxford Medical Publications, by permission of Oxford University Press.)

Pathogenesis of hypertension in renal disease

It would be naive to believe that the pathogenesis of hypertension in renal disease is completely understood. Guyton's computer model of blood pressure control in 1972 was based on animal studies and appeared to be almost complete and yet came before the discovery of ANP, nitric oxide (NO), endothelin and other vasoactive peptides. It is unlikely that there are no more vasoactive substances awaiting discovery and the precise role of currently known substances is not certain, so that any theory of the pathogenesis of renal hypertension must be provisional.

The role of the sympathetic nervous system and of vasoactive peptides in blood pressure control and the control of sodium balance and its disturbance in renal disease are discussed elsewhere in this book.

Hypertension in patients with parenchymatous renal disease without uremia

As mentioned there is an increased prevalence of hypertension in renal disease even before plasma creatinine rises above normal.

Renin

Plasma renin activity (PRA) is normal in hypertensive patients with glomerulonephritis [2] and in hypertensive and normotensive patients with APCKD [2] and those with CPN [2]. Nevertheless the renin–angiotensin system may be of importance since PRA was increased in 30% of normotensive patients with glomerulonephritis [2] and was higher in APCKD patients with hypertension than in matched patients with essential hypertension [2]. Furthermore an increase was found in PRA, plasma angiotensin II, plasma aldosterone (PA) and total body exchangeable sodium in patients with CPN (in whom the prevalence of hypertension is increased) even though these measurements did not vary according to blood pressure [2]. Hyperplasia of renin-containing cells in the kidney has been demonstrated in patients with CPN but again did not differ between those with normal and those with elevated pressure [2]. In patients with APCKD, the tubular epithelium lining the renal cysts can synthesize renin and contains increased amounts of immunoreactive renin. Cyst fluid contains renin, most of which is in the active form [2].

Further evidence supporting the role of a humoral factor, probably renin, rather than simply loss of nephrons in the pathogenesis of hypertension of non-uremic renal disease, comes from the observations of the effect of nephrectomy in predominantly unilateral CPN. Although not often performed now because of the availability of effective antihypertensive drugs and the appreciation of the value of conserving renal tissue, nephrectomy results in cure or improvement in hypertension in about half of those treated [2], although there have been no controlled trials of medical versus surgical treatment.

In patients with APCKD who have hypertension there is an increase in renal vascular resistance and the filtration fraction both of which are reversed by ACE-I indicating an active intrarenal role for renin possibly contributing to hypertension through sodium retention [2].

Sodium retention

The existence of sodium retention in non-uremic renal disease is difficult to establish because although total body exchangeable sodium can be measured reproducibly, it must be related to lean body mass, which is difficult to measure. However, we have found an increase in body sodium in patients with CPN [2] and an increase in ANP levels has been demonstrated in patients with APCKD [2].

'Natriuretic hormone'

The observations by Brod and co-workers give a possible explanation for the imperfect association of hypersecretion of renin and volume expansion with hypertension in renal disease. They found an initial hypervolemia and increased cardiac output in patients with renal disease but without hypertension. After two to eight years, 11 of the 12 patients with volume expansion had developed hypertension with an increase in peripheral resistance and a fall in cardiac output towards normal [2]. It seems possible that the sequence of events leading to hypertension in patients with renal disease but without impaired renal function is similar to that in patients with impaired renal function (Figure 31.2). Initial renal damage leads to

increased renin production and sodium retention, either directly from loss of nephrons or indirectly owing to angiotensin-stimulated hyperaldosteronism. Salt retention causes hypervolemia and increased cardiac output, initially without hypertension. Volume expansion stimulates the release of a digoxin-like (possibly ouabain) inhibitor of Na,K-ATPase, 'natriuretic hormone', which increases intracellular sodium and calcium and thereby causes a rise in peripheral resistance. Hypertension develops in some patients with time [2] perhaps influenced by the patient's genetic susceptibility to hypertension.

Other vasoactive substances

The role of other vasoactive substances including NO, endothelin, the kallikrein–kinin system, parathyroid hormone, parathyroid hypertensive factor, prostaglandins and renomedullary lipids in the hypertension of non-uremic renal disease is not known.

Neurogenic factors

In animal models of renal hypertension there is evidence that neurogenic factors are important in the development of hypertension. The hypertension is prevented or reversed by contralateral renal denervation following unilateral nephrectomy and the norepinephrine content in the remaining kidney is reduced [6]. In this model renal denervation also reduced peripheral sympathetic activity, suggesting that renal afferent nerves may be important in generating hypertension. In humans, although the findings have been inconsistent, patients with mild impairment of renal function appear to have an increased sensitivity to norepinephrine, suggesting a role for the autonomic nervous system in the development of hypertension.

Patients with parenchymatous renal disease with uremia

Sodium

In ESRF sodium retention is probably the dominant factor in causing hypertension since, in the majority of patients, treatment of fluid overload by removal of sodium by dialysis corrects hypertension. There is a loose correlation between total body exchangeable sodium and blood pressure [7]. As in the hypertension of non-uremic renal disease, the sodium retention may be translated into hypertension by stimulation of the release of the postulated digoxin-like 'natriuretic hormone' although the nature, the role, and even the existence of this hormone is not universally agreed.

Renin

Renin is probably a cofactor with sodium retention in causing hypertension in many ESRF patients. It may be the major factor in the hypertensive ESRF patients resistant to correction of salt and water overload. In these patients (10–20%) blood pressure is correlated with plasma renin, and hypertension is abolished by bilateral nephrectomy. Although taking into account that both plasma renin and body sodium improve the correlation with blood pressure, over sodium alone, the correlation remains weak [7].

Endothelin

There are three endothelins (-1, -2 and -3, Chapter 13). Endothelial cells probably produce exclusively endothelin-1 and this appears to be of greatest importance in hypertension. Endothelins (ET) act primarily as local hormones. Most of the ET released by endothelial and epithelial cells is directed into the interstitum; that which spills over into the bloodstream is rapidly removed in the lung, kidney and liver. Blood levels are not a reliable marker of ET activity. Understanding of the role of ET in the hypertension of renal failure awaits the development of specific antagonists [8]. However, in the absence of methods of studying tissue activity, plasma levels have been studied in the hope that they will give some clues to the importance of the endothelins.

In essential hypertension plasma ET concentration is normal [9] although vascular sensitivity to ET may be increased [10]. In uremia plasma ET is increased, probably due to reduced renal clearance of the hormone together with reduced inhibition of secretion by NO; the levels of which fall due to accumulation of dimethylarginine (see below). In addition there may be stimulation of ET secretion by uremic toxins and by the sympathetic nervous system during dialysis-induced hypovolemia. Raised plasma ET levels in patients with vascular tumors are associated with hypertension which resolves when the tumor is removed, suggesting a causal relationship and it is, therefore, conceivable that the raised ET levels in uremia also contribute to the development of hypertension even though endothelins are predominantly local hormones.

Arginine vasopressin

Arginine vasopressin (AVP) is metabolized in the kidney. Renal clearance is reduced in renal failure, raising plasma levels of AVP. The administration of an AVP antagonist to patients with ESRD and raised plasma AVP was accompanied by a fall in blood pressure [11]. It remains to be established, however, whether the increased AVP levels contribute to the development of hypertension.

Insulin resistance

Uremia is accompanied by insulin resistance and by raised plasma insulin levels due to reduced renal metabolism of insulin. This may contribute to the development of hypertension since insulin stimulates the sympathetic nervous system [12], increased activity of which has been demonstrated in uremia, and increases tubular reabsorption of sodium since the renal tubules are not affected by the resistance to insulin [13].

Renomedullary lipids

Renomedullary lipids are hypotensive substances but despite investigations over the past 30 years their role in hypertension remains uncertain.

Nitric oxide

Endothelium-derived relaxing factor, now known to be NO, is also a candidate for a role in hypertension associated with uremia. The enzyme NO synthase (NOS) acting on L-arginine forms NO when one of the terminal guanidino nitrogens is oxidized. In the endothelium NO maintains a basal state of vasodilatation. Inhibition of NO causes vasoconstriction whereas stimulation of NO, for example by acetylcholine, brings about further vasodilatation. In uremia the analog of L-arginine, asymmetrical dimethyl arginine, accumulates and inhibits NO production, which may contribute to the development of hypertension [14].

Bradykinin

Bradykinin, the vasoactive product of the kallikirein–kinin system, is a vasodilator but its role in the hypertension of ESRF is not known.

Atrial natriuretic peptide

ANP levels are elevated in patients with renal failure [15] in proportion to their degree of volume expansion. ANP appears to be responding to increased atrial filling pressure to modulate the rise in pressure. There is no evidence that a deficient ANP response contributes to the pathogenesis of hypertension in ESRF.

Prostaglandins

Prostaglandins (PG) may be vasodilators (PGI_2, prostacyclin, PGE_2 and PGD_2) or vasoconstrictors (thromboxane A_2 and PGF_2). There is no evidence of abnormal production of PG in ESRF. Like ANP, the vasodilator PG appear to be secreted appropriately in renal failure and act to modulate the rise in pressure caused by vasoconstrictor substances. Thus if cyclo-oxygenase is inhibited (by non-steroidal anti-inflammatory drugs) and PG production reduced, blood pressure rises due to unopposed action of vasoconstrictors. Thromboxane A_2 and PGF_2 are also inhibited, but any vasodilatory effect of this is outweighed by the loss of the vasodilatory prostaglandins.

Investigation of hypertension in renal disease

When the underlying cause of renal failure is known, further investigation of the cause of hypertension is not usually indicated. However, if the hypertension seems out of keeping with the severity of renal disease, or if there is an unexpected increase in the blood pressure or resistance to antihypertensive treatment, then further investigation may be worthwhile. As will be discussed the prevalence of atheromatous vascular disease is increased in uremia and renal artery stenosis may develop in previously healthy vessels and contribute to worsening hypertension. In rare situations, such as in renal failure due to renal vascular disease in neurofibromatosis, and in renal failure following nephrectomy for bilateral renal tumours in von Hippel–Lindau's syndrome, the possibility of co-existing pheochromocytoma should be borne in mind.

A reasonable approach to the search for correctable causes of hypertension in chronic renal disease is summarized in Table 31.1. In patients with poor renal function intravenous pyelography gives poor definition and is generally unhelpful; isotope renography is also of limited value but can be useful in deciding whether a small kidney is making a useful contribution to GFR prior to nephrectomy. Renal ultrasound is useful to determine kidney size – asymmetry suggests the possibility of renal vascular disease – and to exclude hydronephrosis. Renal artery stenosis can only be excluded with certainty by angiography.

Although, as discussed, there is evidence that in some patients hypertension is predominantly renin dependent and in others salt dependent, total body sodium is not usually determined and renin studies are not usually undertaken. This is because these measurements are difficult to undertake and difficult to interpret. They need to be taken under standard conditions, ideally after withdrawal of antihypertensive and diuretic therapy, and body sodium has to be related to lean body mass, which is difficult to measure accurately. Furthermore, from a practical point of view, this information is not necessary since sodium retention and hyperreninemia are assumed to be present in chronic renal disease and dealt with by inclusion of diuretics and beta-blockers or ACE-I in the treatment regimen.

Table 31.1 Investigation of disproportionate hypertension in a patient with known chronic renal disease

1. Renal ultrasound	Kidney size Hydronephrosis
2. Renal angiography	Renal vascular disease
3. Isotope renography	Contribution of small kidney to total GFR

Management of hypertension associated with impaired renal function

The drug treatment of hypertension is discussed in Chapter 67, and the importance of treatment in relation to progression of renal disease in Chapter 68. The control of blood pressure in hemodialysis and peritoneal dialysis is also covered elsewhere (Chapter 73 and Chapter 79). In this section the role of nephrectomy is discussed.

With the availability of a wide range of effective antihypertensive agents nephrectomy is very rarely considered. Since long-term compliance with complex antihypertensive regimes is often poor and control of blood pressure less than optimal, perhaps the role of nephrectomy in selected cases should be reconsidered.

Unilateral nephrectomy (Table 31.2)

In patients with predominantly unilateral CPN, nephrectomy cures or improves the blood pressure in about half of those operated upon. However, there have been no controlled trials of medical versus surgical treatment; in our experience, following the criteria for nephrectomy listed in Table 31.2, not only was blood pressure control facilitated but renal function at follow-up tended to be preserved [2] suggesting that any immediate loss of function arising from nephrectomy was outweighed in the long term by the protection conferred on the remaining kidney by improved blood pressure control. Renal vein renin studies are not of proven value to select patients for surgery [2].

Nephrectomy is only worthwhile if the disease is confined to one kidney and only justified if that kidney contributes less than 20% of total renal function as assessed by isotope renography. Medical control is preferred, but if the other criteria are met and blood pressure cannot be controlled with maximal drug therapy, or the patient

Table 31.2 Unilateral nephrectomy for patients with hypertension associated with chronic pyelonephritis

Necessary criteria
1. Unilateral disease
2. Diseased kidney contributes less than 20% of total function

Selection of patients
1. Difficult medical control of blood pressure
2. A woman planning pregnancy after severe hypertension in a previous pregnancy
3. Troublesome recurrent urinary tract infection not controlled by antibiotics

Surgery is in fact rarely necessary in chronic pyelonephritis (see text for details)

cannot tolerate the drugs which are necessary, then nephrectomy should be discussed. In a woman who fulfils the criteria of unilateral disease contributing less than 20% of function and who has suffered severe hypertension during her previous pregnancy, nephrectomy should be considered before embarking on a further pregnancy.

A further unusual indication for consideration of nephrectomy is in a patient fulfilling the same criteria of function and normality of the contralateral kidney in whom urinary tract infection cannot be controlled despite adequate antibiotic treatment over a prolonged period.

Unilateral nephrectomy is also a reasonable option in renovascular hypertension, if the affected kidney is badly damaged and isotope renography shows that it contributes less than 20% of total renal function, although again there have been no controlled trials.

Nephrectomy may also be considered in patients with unilateral disease due to renal calculi, hydronephrosis or renal tuberculosis. Its value in lowering blood pressure is not well established in these situations and nephrectomy would only be considered if medical treatment were ineffective or unacceptable to the patient, or if nephrectomy were indicated for other reasons.

Bilateral nephrectomy

In a very few instances of uncontrollable severe hypertension bilateral nephrectomy has been undertaken in patients not requiring dialysis. However, this is now exceptionally rare. Even in dialysis and transplant patients it is very rarely necessary to remove the native kidneys to control hypertension but the procedure can be very effective and the risk of surgery is low.

Vascular disease

Introduction

There is an increased prevalence of coronary, cerebral and peripheral vascular disease in patients with chronic renal disease [1, 16]. Vascular disease is present at the outset of renal replacement therapy and progresses in patients despite treatment by dialysis and transplantation [17]. Vascular disease is the commonest cause of death in patients with ESRD and is responsible for a markedly reduced life expectancy. At the age of 49 the life expectancy for the general population in the USA is 29.8 years but only 7.1 years in ESRD; at the age of 59 years the figures are 21.6 and 4.3 years, respectively [1].

Clinical manifestations

Vascular disease manifests in patients with chronic renal disease in the same way as it does in the general population, except that it occurs at a much earlier age and has a much greater prevalence. Coronary artery disease is present in 41% of US patients starting hemodialysis [1]; it is more difficult to diagnose the presence of underlying cerebrovascular disease at the start of dialysis but cerebrovascular disease accounts for 5% of deaths in dialysis patients. In patients with coronary artery disease, angina may develop at an earlier stage because of anemia but may resolve with erythropoietin therapy.

The same criteria for investigation and intervention should be applied for angina in dialysis patients as for non-renal failure patients. There has been a tendency in the past for cardiologists to regard dialysis patients as having a very poor prognosis and to be less worthy candidates for coronary artery by-pass grafting or angioplasty. In fact, since cardiac disease is the major cause of death in these patients, an active approach to the treatment of their disease is particularly important.

In the USA all patients with ESRD who are candidates for transplantation undergo cardiac evaluation but this is not universal practice in Europe. However, in all countries it is accepted that in patients with angina being considered for renal transplantation cardiac catheterization to assess the need for coronary artery by-pass or angioplasty should be undertaken prior to transplantation. It is much less commonly necessary to consider carotid surgery but duplex Doppler examination and digital vascular imaging should be considered in patients with a history of stroke or of transient cerebral ischemic attacks.

Peripheral vascular disease is common, affecting 8% of patients starting dialysis in one report [16]. It is much more common in diabetics of whom approximately 15% require some form of amputation following renal transplantation. In asymptomatic patients no formal assessment of the peripheral vascular system is necessary prior to transplantation. However, radiographs of the lower abdomen and pelvis should be obtained to detect vascular calcification and, if present, duplex Doppler and possibly angiography are necessary prior to consideration of renal transplantation.

Sometimes in uremic patients with chest pain at rest it is difficult to distinguish between unstable angina and pericarditis. It should be remembered that uremic pericarditis is not closely correlated with plasma creatinine levels and can develop in underdialysed patients when the plasma creatinine level seems satisfactory.

Pathogenesis

In the elderly patient with uremia the increased prevalence of vascular disease may reflect pre-existing vascular disease. In fact vascular disease of the renal vessels may have caused the renal failure. The cause of the increased prevalence of vascular disease is not fully understood. Several factors are likely to be involved.

Hypertension

There is an increased prevalence of hypertension at all stages of renal disease, reaching 80–90% in ESRD. Life insurance statistics first showed the association of even mild increases in blood pressure with ischemic heart disease and stroke in the general population. This was confirmed by the Framingham Study, which shows that hypertension is a major risk factor for myocardial infarction, stroke and heart failure. The effectiveness of anti-hypertensive treatment in reducing stroke and myocardial infarction confirms that the relationship between hypertension and these manifestations of vascular disease is causal. An analysis of 17 randomized trials of the treatment of essential hypertension has shown that a blood pressure reduction of 10–14 mmHg systolic and 5–6 mmHg diastolic was associated with a reduction of 38% in the incidence of stroke and 16% in that of coronary artery disease [18]. Such studies have not been done in renal hypertension but in the absence of evidence to the contrary it seems reasonable to conclude that hypertension is a risk factor for vascular disease that can be reduced by control of blood pressure. Since the reduction in the risk of vascular disease is proportional to the reduction in blood pressure in both high and low risk individuals [19], the reduction in vascular disease with control of blood pressure may therefore be great in patients with renal disease, who are in a high risk category.

In essential hypertension the risk of vascular events falls progressively as the level of achieved blood pressure, with treatment, falls. There is no J-shaped curve, i.e. increasing morbidity at levels of achieved pressure less than 80 mmHg [18], except in patients which pre-existing coronary artery disease. However, when the achieved blood pressure is 80 mmHg the risk of vascular disease attributable to blood pressure is low and there is little to gain by further reduction in pressure, whereas side effects from treatment may be increased.

Insulin resistance and glucose intolerance

The vascular complications of diabetes are covered elsewhere (Chapter 43). Insulin resistance, particularly in skeletal muscle, is a feature of non-diabetics with uremia and via hyperlipidemia may contribute to the development of vascular disease. Insulin resistance is partially corrected by dialysis [20] and is improved by low protein diet in the dialysis patient. It has been suggested that a dialysable factor may be responsible for insulin resistance; however, this has not been identified and it seems more likely that several factors are involved.

Insulin resistance does not lead to clinically manifest glucose intolerance in most uremic patients, except when the insulin secretory response to glucose is sufficiently impaired. Hyperparathyroidism may be responsible for the reduced insulin response since glucose intolerance has been reported to improve following correction of hyperparathyroidism by surgery or medical treatment with phosphate binders [21].

Hyperlipidemia

Lipid disorders in renal failure are covered elsewhere (Chapter 38). The role of lipid peroxidation in the pathogenesis of atheroma and the possible role of antioxidant treatment in prevention are briefly discussed.

Oxidative stress in chronic renal failure increases the susceptibility of low density lipoproteins (LDL) to oxidation. This may be accompanied by reduced antioxidant activity, particularly vitamin E, increasing the likelihood of lipid peroxidation. The triglyceride content of LDL is increased in renal failure which increases susceptibility to oxidation. The importance of lipid peroxides in the pathogenesis of atherosclerosis in renal disease has not been established, but evidence of increased levels in non-renal patients with atheroma has been reported.

Smoking

Many patients find it difficult to give up smoking because of the restrictions placed on other aspects of their lives by their renal disease. In one survey, 18% of patients were smokers [1] and smoking increased relative mortality by 26%.

Exercise

Regular exercise lowers blood pressure in patients with hypertension by 11 mmHg systolic and 6 mmHg diastolic [22]. It also increases insulin sensitivity [23], improves plasma high density lipoprotein levels and may contribute to regression of LVH. Patients with chronic renal disease are often unable to exercise regularly for a variety of reasons including general debility, anemia, renal bone disease and pre-existing vascular disease. This may contribute to the development of vascular disease.

Renin

Renin levels in tissue and plasma may be inappropriately high, in relation to sodium balance and blood pressure, in patients with renal disease (see above). Angiotensin II is a growth factor, as well as a powerful vasoconstrictor, and causes vascular smooth muscle hypertrophy and hyperplasia which may be the first stage in the development of atheroma. It has been shown in an animal model of high renin hypertension that treatment with an ACE inhibitor reversed aortic wall thickening. Laragh's group [24] has shown an association between the risk of myocardial infarction and pretreatment renin levels (related to urinary sodium) in a group of 1717 patients with mild to moderate essential hypertension.

Arterial stiffness and vascular calcification

Hypertension in end-stage renal failure is predominantly systolic, due largely to increased arterial stiffness, as in normal aging. The increase in stiffness may be due to arterial calcification, which is common in renal failure (Figure 31.5) (particularly in patients with hyperparathyroidism) or to lipid abnormalities, but it is not correlated closely with either.

Increased vascular stiffness may contribute to left ventricular hypertrophy by exaggerating the peak of systolic pressure [25].

Treatment and prevention

Treatment of vascular disease in uremic patients does not differ from that in non-uremics. Given the presence of multiple risk factors for the high overall risk, an active approach to correction of risk factors and to the treatment of the vascular disease itself is justified.

Hypertension

The consensus among those who treat patients with essential hypertension is that target blood pressure should be in the range 140–160 mmHg (systolic) and 80–85 mmHg (diastolic). Because of increased risk of vascular disease, as well as the effect of hypertension to accelerate progression of renal failure, the target blood pressures in renal disease should be even lower although the precise targets have not achieved a similar consensus.

Unfortunately the ideal blood pressure is difficult to achieve in practice because of side effects and imperfect compliance with drug and dietary regimes. Hypertension remains an important contributory factor to the development of atherosclerosis in renal disease.

Insulin resistance and glucose intolerance

Insulin resistance can be reduced by increased dialysis (see above); glucose intolerance, therefore, constitutes a clear indication for ensuring adequate dialysis time and efficiency.

Particular attention should also be paid to correction of hyperparathyroidism in patients with glucose intolerance. Since reversal of hyperparathyroidism is difficult without surgery, prevention by control of plasma phosphate and correction of vitamin D deficiency is essential. Physical exercise lowers insulin resistance (see below).

Lipid peroxidation

If lipid peroxidation is important in the pathogenesis of atherosclerosis in renal failure then antioxidants such as α-tocopherol (vitamin E) and ascorbic acid (vitamin C) may be of value in prevention. This has not been established and there is some risk in feeding large quantities of ascorbic acid to dialysis patients because of its conversion into oxalate which increases the risk of vascular calcification. Vitamin E is also not without risk and, until there is clear evidence of benefit, neither vitamin should be used as prophylaxis against vascular disease.

Smoking

Smoking should be strongly discouraged. Some patients may be helped by the use of nicotine chewing gum or transdermal patches.

Exercise

Patients should be encouraged to undertake moderate exercise. However, there is an increased risk of sudden death during exercise in patients with underlying heart disease and for this reason all patients should be advised on a cautious program, gradually increasing their level of exercise over several weeks under supervision. In view of the prevalence of heart disease in patients with uremia, it is probably wise to advise against intensive competitive exercise, unless patients have first undergone an exercise ECG stress test. It should be remembered that the incidence of renal bone disease remains high and that avas-

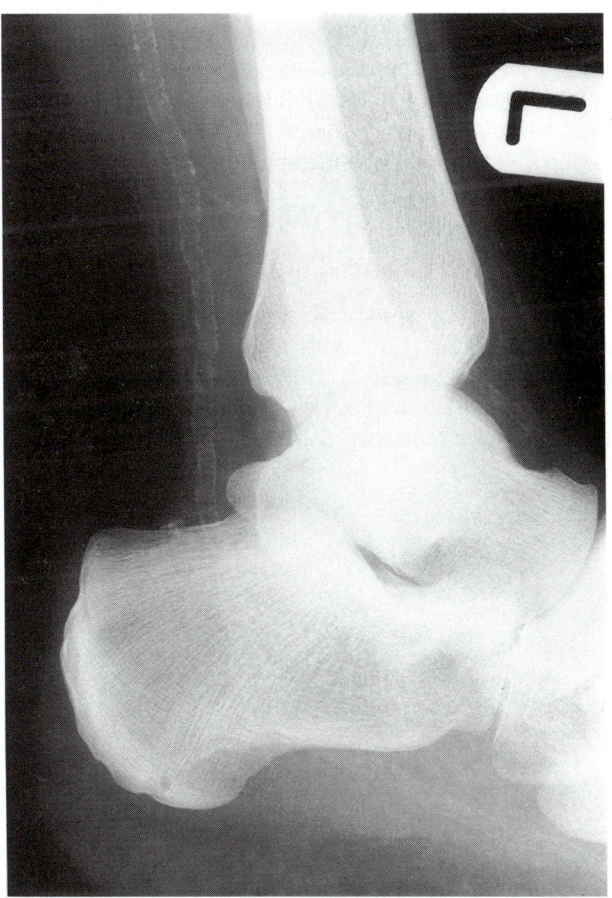

Figure 31.5 Calcification of the posterior tibial artery in a patient with long-standing chronic renal failure with secondary hyperparathyroidism requiring parathyroidectomy.

cular necrosis of bone due to steroid therapy may affect transplant recipients. Recurrent trauma to bones and joints incurred in jogging may accelerate joint damage and this type of exercise is best avoided. Swimming, cycling and walking are preferable.

Hyperreninism

If angiotensin II has a role in the pathogenesis of atherosclerosis in renal disease, then ACE-I or angiotensin II receptor blockers may be indicated for the prevention of vascular disease. There is some evidence that in the patient with chronic renal disease these drugs may delay progression of renal failure (Chapter 68). Here we consider extending their use to the patient with ESRD. These drugs are not without hazard, even when there is little renal function left to compromise, as they may cause hyperkalemia by reducing aldosterone secretion. At present, there is insufficient evidence to recommend ACE-I over other antihypertensive agents in patients undergoing dialysis for the specific purpose of reducing atheroma.

Vascular calcification and stiffening

Hyperparathyroidism is the major cause of vascular calcification in uremia. Approximately 70% of hyperparathyroid patients have radiological evidence of this malady. Unfortunately calcification does not usually regress after parathyroidectomy [26]. It is important to prevent hyperparathyroidism by preventing hyperphosphatemia and maintaining serum calcium in the high normal range by therapy with α-calcidol. It is often necessary to introduce these measures when plasma creatinine is still less than 2 mg/dl (170 μmol/l). The concept of vessel wall stiffness may be important in selecting the antihypertensive agent. Beta blockers tend to constrict small arteries and arterioles and therefore reduce aortic pressure less than calcium channel blockers and ACE-I. The latter two may, therefore, be more effective in pre-

venting left ventricular hypertrophy. It should be remembered that these differences have not been established in controlled trials and it would be premature to recommend a move away from beta blockers as initial therapy. Recent reports of increased cardiac events in patients with ischemic heart disease treated with short-acting calcium antagonists although flawed emphasize the need to base treatment strategies on prospective randomized controlled trials.

Outcome

Cardiac disease is the major cause of death in dialysis patients, accounting for 40% of deaths (see above). There is a pressing need for rigorous application of the preventative measures outlined above and for treatment of established vascular disease.

Left ventricular hypertrophy

Introduction

About 30% of patients starting renal replacement therapy in 1986 and 1987 had LVH in the United States [1]. In a prospective study of cardiovascular disease in Canadian centers, 74% of patients starting dialysis had echocardiographic evidence of LVH and 32% left ventricular dilatation. As in non-renal patients, the presence of LVH in renal patients is a major independent risk factor for death [16].

Clinical features and diagnosis

LVH is usually asymptomatic. It is more common in older patients, females, those with a wide pulse pressure (i.e. with more rigid vessels), and in those with malnutrition. Concentric LVH (without left ventricular dilatation) carries a lower mortality risk than eccentric LVH (with

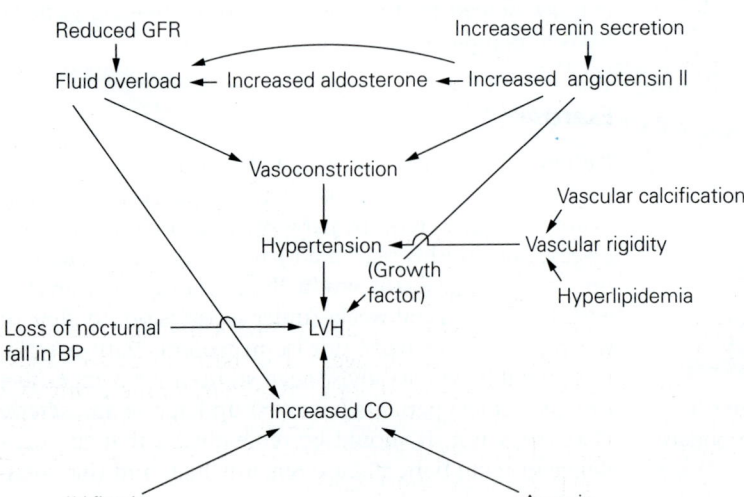

Figure 31.6 Factors contributing to the development of left ventricular hypertrophy in uremia.

dilatation) [16]. It may be possible to detect LVH by the presence of an apical heave but diagnosis is usually established by echocardiography. Electrocardiography is much less sensitive and identifies only about 10% of patients with LVH that are detected by echocardiography. The radiograph is usually normal in concentric LVH but may show left ventricular prominence.

Pathophysiology

Concentric LVH is thought to develop partly in response to pressure overload and eccentric LVH in response to volume overload. The development of concentric LVH is probably not simply dependent on pressure overload since the degree of hypertrophy varies from normal to severe LVH in patients with the same degree of hypertension. Angiotensin II stimulates proliferation of cardiac cells and is probably an important determinant of LVH. Increased cardiac expression of ACE messenger RNA and ACE activity has been demonstrated in experimental LVH. In a random sample of the population, LVH was associated with a double deletion (DD) polymorphism of the ACE gene, which is associated with increased tissue and plasma ACE activity [27].

In uremia there are two factors which may influence the development of LVH in response to pressure overload: increased renin secretion and vascular stiffness. As discussed above plasma renin, and possibly tissue renin, may be inappropriately high in relation to sodium status in uremia. Vascular stiffness results in systolic hypertension and a greater increase in aortic pressure than in brachial pressure (see above), thus increasing ventricular pressure overload.

Pathogenesis

Hypertension

Since blood pressure is an important determinant of left ventricular mass in patients with normal kidney function it is likely to have the same influence in patients with ESRD. Despite good control of blood pressure in patients with uremia, LVH may not regress, and in fact may progress. This reflects the importance of other factors in determining left ventricular mass in the ESRD patient. The changes in the ESRD patient which contribute to the development of LVH are summarized in Figure 31.6.

Loss of nocturnal 'dip' in blood pressure

As outlined above, there is a blunting or loss of the normal nocturnal fall ('dip') in blood pressure in patients with renal disease (Figure 31.1). This may put patients at greater risk of vascular disease, and in particular of LVH [28]. It is, of course, difficult to be certain whether non-dipping leads to LVH or the LVH is the cause of the loss of nocturnal dip.

Fluid overload

Fluid overload in uremia contributes to LVH predominantly through increased blood pressure rather than increased cardiac output. Although there is an initial increase in output with volume loading, in the steady state peripheral resistance rises and cardiac output returns towards normal.

Anemia

Patients with renal insufficiency are anemic because of deficiency in erythropoietin. Anemia often develops early in the course of renal disease and is, therefore, often present for several years before ESRD. Anemia results in an increased cardiac output which persists even when hypertension is corrected. LVH does not regress unless the anemia is corrected (Chapter 35).

Arteriovenous fistula

An arteriovenous fistula is the preferred form of vascular access for patients treated by hemodialysis. The exception is those patients with poor cardiac function who cannot tolerate the increased ventricular load imposed by the flow through the fistula. In patients with normal cardiac function, even a large fistula very rarely precipitates cardiac failure. However even a satisfactory fistula, which will often have a flow rate of around 500 ml per minute, may, over a prolonged period, contribute to the development of LVH. In a study in my own hospital fistula flow rate measured by Doppler ultrasound ranged from 575 to 2121 ml/min between dialyses and may be even higher during dialysis.

Arterial stiffness and vascular calcification

As has been discussed above, in relation to the development of vascular disease, increased arterial stiffness may contribute to the development of LVH by raising aortic systolic pressure.

Prevention and treatment

Hypertension

Hypertension in the earliest stages of renal disease should be treated vigorously. The level of blood pressure for treatment should be lower than that for essential hypertension. Although precise levels have not been agreed to, most nephrologists would treat patients with blood pressures persistently above 140/90 mmHg. The choice of antihypertensive agent has been discussed above. Although there are theoretical reasons for preferring ACE-I their superiority over calcium antagonists and beta-blockers in reducing or preventing LVH has not been established in clinical trials.

Anemia

Because of the cost of erythropoietin its use has usually been confined to those patients with more severe anemia, hemoglobin less than 8 g/dl, or who were symptomatic, certainly in the UK. Similarly the target hemoglobin with treatment has been limited to 10–11 g/dl partly on grounds of cost but also because this level has been considered adequate. The threshold for treatment and the target hemoglobin should be increased to prevent the development of LVH but the cost implications of a change in policy are considerable.

Arteriovenous fistula

If a fistula is very large and the patient has evidence of LVH, consideration should be given to reducing the size of the fistula. In extreme cases where there is left ventricular dilatation, the fistula should be closed and a central line used for access. Surgeons should be encouraged to construct radial rather than brachial fistulae, where possible, since they are less likely to have excessive blood flow.

The nephrologist is faced with the dilemma of whether to close a fistula following renal transplantation because of its possible contribution to LVH. In our unit we have adopted a formal policy of advising closure of the fistula at one year following transplantation. In practice, closure is rarely undertaken because of resistance by the patient and our own reluctance to lose an access site which may be vital in the event of graft failure. A reasonable compromise is to close the fistula following transplantation in those patients with echocardiographic evidence of LVH.

Arterial stiffness and vascular calcification

The prevention of arterial stiffness and vascular calcification has been covered in the section on vascular disease. The importance of prevention of hyperparathyroidism and the possible advantages of ACE-I and calcium channel blockers over other antihypertensive agents have been discussed.

Outcome

LVH progresses during dialysis treatment despite lowering blood pressure to normal [29]. It may be that treatment of anemia, of excessively large fistulae, hyperparathyroidism and the use of ACE-I or calcium channel blockers to achieve blood pressure control, will prevent or reverse LVH. Certainly LVH is at least partially reversible since wall thickness and mass have been reported to fall following successful renal transplantation [30].

Uremic cardiomyopathy

There has been controversy for years whether a specific uremic cardiomyopathy exists or whether the cardiomyopathy in uremic patients can be explained by the other derangements in renal failure. Intermyocardiocyte fibrosis in uremic patients was first described 50 years ago and has recently been confirmed [31]. It could not be attributed to hypertension or the duration or type of dialysis; indeed it occurs in patients who have not been dialysed. However, Dorhout Mees [32] has emphasized the danger in accepting uremic cardiomyopathy as a distinct entity since this may relax the vigilance over control of hypervolemia and hypertension. His group has shown that cardiac function in patients with uremic cardiomyopathy can be improved by careful ultrafiltration. The evidence, from measurements of ANP and vena cava diameter, shows that many dialysis patients do suffer chronic fluid overload and this may be misinterpreted as evidence of cardiomyopathy.

It seems wise, therefore, not to apply the label 'uremic cardiomyopathy' to dialysis patients with cardiac problems but rather to look for correctable causes of cardiac dysfunction.

Acknowledgments

I am grateful to Mrs Sheila Davidson, Mrs Pat Lawton and Mrs Rita Grieveson for their assistance in preparing the manuscript.

References

1. Port, F.K. (1994) Morbidity and mortality in dialysis patients. *Kidney Int.*, **46**, 1728–37.
2. Wilkinson, R. (1994) Renal and renovascular hypertension, in *Textbook of Hypertension* (ed. J.D. Swales), Blackwell, Oxford, pp. 831–57.
3. Heidland, A. and Heidbreder, E. (1987) Retinopathy in hypertension: increased incidence in renoparenchymal disease. *Contrib. Nephrol.*, **54**, 144–51.
4. Wilkinson, R., Luetscher, J.A., Dowdy, A.J. *et al.* (1972) Studies on the mechanism of sodium excretion in uremia. *Clin Sci.*, **42**, 711–23.
5. Dworken, L.D. and Feiner, H.D. (1986) Glomerular injury in uninephrectomized spontaneously hypertensive rats. A consequence of glomerular capillary hypertension. *J. Clin. Invest.*, **77**, 797–809.
6. Vari, R.C., Freeman, R.H., Davis, J.O. and Sweet, W.D. (1986) Role of renal nerves in rats with low sodium one-kidney hypertension. *Am. J. Physiol.*, **250**, H189–94.
7. Wilkinson, R., Scott, D.F., Uldall, P.R. *et al.* (1970) Plasma renin and exchangeable sodium in the hypertension of chronic renal failure. The effect of bilateral nephrectomy. *Q. J. Med.*, **39**, 377–94.

8. Luscher, T.F. and Wenzel, R. R. (1995) Endothelin in renal disease: role of endothelin antagonist. *Nephrol. Dial. Transplant.*, **10**, 162–6.
9. Davenport, A.P., Ashby, M.J., Easton, P. *et al.* (1990) A sensitive radioimmunoassay measuring endothelin–like immunoreactivity in human plasma: comparison of levels in patients with essential hypertension and normotensive control subjects. *Clin. Sci.*, **79**, 261–4.
10. Haynes, W.G. and Webb, D.J. (1994) Contribution of endogenous generation of endothelin-1 to basal vascular tone in man. *Lancet*, **344**, 852–4.
11. Gavras, H., Ribiero, A.B., Kohlmann, O. *et al.* (1984) Effects of a specific inhibitor of the vascular action of vasopressin in humans. *Hypertension*, **6**, I-156.
12. Reaven, G.M., Lithell, H. and Landsberg, L. (1996) Hypertension and associated metabolic abnormalities – the role of insulin resistance and the sympathoadrenal system. *N. Engl. J. Med.*, **334**, 374–81.
13. Skott, P., Vaag, A., Bruun, N.E. *et al.* (1991) Effect of insulin on renal sodium handling in hyperinsulinaemic type-2 diabetic patients with peripheral insulin resistance. *Diabetologia*, **34**, 275–81.
14. Calver, A., Collier, J., Moncada, S. and Vallance, P. (1992) Effect of local intra-arterial N^G-monomethyl-L-arginine in patients with hypertension: the nitric oxide dilator mechanism appears abnormal. *J. Hypertens.*, **10**, 1025–31.
15. Walker, R.G., Swainson, C.P., Yandle, T.G. *et al.* (1987) Exaggerated responsiveness of immunoreactive atrial natriuretic peptide to saline infusion in chronic renal failure. *Clin. Sci.*, **72**, 19 -24.
16. Foley, R.N., Parfrey, P.S., Harnett, J.D. *et al.* (1995) Clinical and echocardiographic disease in patients starting end-stage renal disease therapy. *Kidney Int.*, **47**, 186–92.
17. Sutherland, W.H.F., Walker, R.J., Ball, M.J. *et al.* (1995) Oxidation of low density lipoproteins from patients with renal failure or renal transplants. *Kidney Int.*, **48**, 227–36.
18. Collins, R., Peto, R., MacMahon, S. *et al.* (1990) Blood pressure, stroke and coronary heart disease, Part II. Effects of short-term reduction in blood pressure – an overview of the unconfounded randomised drug trials in an epidemiological context. *Lancet*, **335**, 827–38.
19. MacMahon, S., Peto, R., Cutler, J. *et al.* (1990) Blood pressure, stroke and coronary heart disease, part I: effects of prolonged differences in blood pressure – evidence from nine prospective observational studies corrected for the regression dilution bias. *Lancet*, **335**, 765–74.
20. DeFronzo, R.A., Tobin, J.D., Rowe, J.W. and Andres, R. (1978) Glucose intolerance in uremia. *J. Clin. Invest.*, **62**, 425–35.
21. Mak, R.H., Bettinelli, A., Turner, C. *et al.* (1985) The influence of hyperparathyroidism on glucose metabolism in uremia. *J. Clin. Endocrinol. Metab.*, **60**, 229–33.
22. Fagard, R., Bielen, P., Hespel, P. *et al.* (1990) Physical exercise in hypertension, in *Hypertension: Pathophysiology, Diagnosis and Management* (eds J.H. Laragh and B.M. Brenner), New York, Raven Press, pp. 1985–98.
23. Jennings, G., Nelson, L., Nestel, P. *et al.* (1986) The effects of changes in physical activity on major cardiovascular risk factors, hemodynamics, sympathetic function, and glucose utilization in man: a controlled study of four levels of activity. *Circulation*, **73**, 30–40.
24. Alderman, M.H., Madhavan, S., Ooi, W.L. *et al.* (1991) Association of the renin–sodium profile with the risk of myocardial infarction in patients with hypertension. *N. Engl. J. Med.*, **324**, 1098–104.
25. London, G.M. (1994) Increased arterial stiffness in end-stage renal failure: why is it of interest to the clinical nephrologist? *Nephrol. Dial. Transplant.*, **9**, 1709–12.
26. Nichols, P., Owen, J.P., Ellis, H.A. *et al.* (1990) Parathyroidectomy in chronic renal failure: a nine-year follow-up study. *Q. J. Med.*, **77**, **283**, 1175–93.
27. Schunkert, H., Hense, H-W., Holmer, S.R. *et al.* (1994) Association between a deletion polymorphism of the angiotensin-converting-enzyme gene and left ventricular hypertrophy. *N. Engl. J. Med.*, **330**, 1634–8.
28. Kawajima, I., Suzuki, Y., Shimosawa, T. *et al.* (1992) Diminished nocturnal decline in blood pressure in elderly hypertensive patients with left ventricular hypertrophy. *Am. Heart J.*, **67**, 1307–11.
29. Parfrey, P.S., Harnett, J.D., Griffiths, W. *et al.* (1990) The clinical course of left ventricular hypertrophy in dialysis patients. *Nephron*, **55**, 114–20.
30. Burt, R.K., Gupta-Burt, S., Suki, W.N. *et al.* (1989) Reversal of left ventricular dysfunction after renal transplantation. *Ann. Intern. Med.*, **111**, 653–40.
31. Mall, G., Huther, W., Schneider, J. *et al.* (1990) Diffuse intermyocardiocytic fibrosis in uremic patients. *Nephrol. Dial. Transplant.*, **5**, 39–44.
32. Dorhout Mees, E.J. (1995) Volemia and blood pressure in renal failure: have old truths been forgotten? *Nephrol. Dial. Transplant.*, **10**, 1297–8.

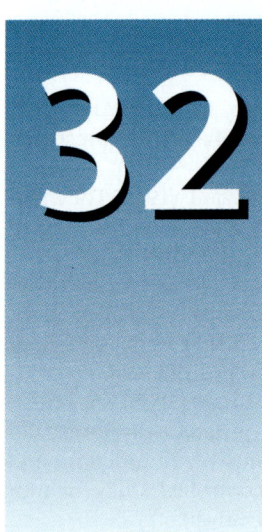

32

Gastrointestinal disorders

Kofi Oppong and Christopher Record

Gastrointestinal problems are an important cause of morbidity and mortality in dialysis-dependent patients and renal transplant recipients. There are also a number of gastrointestinal disorders that are attended by renal disease.

Gastrointestinal disorders in chronic renal failure

Upper gastrointestinal tract

Upper gastrointestinal tract symptoms are a common finding in individuals with chronic renal failure. Symptoms include nausea, vomiting, anorexia, heartburn, epigastric pain and hiccups. Most of these symptoms are relieved by dialysis and are not associated with endoscopically visible lesions.

Historically peptic ulceration and its complications were thought to have a higher frequency in dialysis patients but more recent endoscopic studies suggest no difference in the incidence of peptic ulcer disease from that of the general population [1]. Some disorders occur more frequently in uremia (Table 32.1) including erosive esophagitis, and angiodysplasia [2]. The pathogenesis of uremic lesions remains poorly understood. It has been suggested that there is an abnormal parietal cell response to gastrin, and impaired defensive mechanisms of the gastroduodenal mucosa in hemodialysis patients [3]. Serum gastrin is elevated in about half of patients with acute renal failure and most patients with chronic renal failure. However, basal and stimulated gastric acid secretion may be low, normal or high and does not correlate with symptoms or any lesions. The prevalence of *Helicobacter pylori* in patients with chronic renal failure and renal transplant recipients is no higher than that of age-matched healthy controls [4].

Angiodysplasia is now recognized as occurring more commonly in chronic renal failure and accounts for up to 20% of upper gastrointestinal bleeding in hemodialysis patients [5]. It is a more common cause of bleeding in patients with chronic renal failure than ulcers [2]. Lesions have been reported in the stomach, duodenum, jejunum and colon. The characteristic histological appearance is of tortuous thin-walled endothelium-lined venules and veins. Endoscopically the lesions of angiodysplasia appear as small, flat and bright red. Angiographically they appear as densely opacified tortuous intramural veins that empty contrast slowly. Since the main abnormality is submucosal, superficial endoscopic biopsies may fail to show the abnormality. The cause of the increased incidence in hemodialysis patients is unknown. Proposed explanations include aluminum hydroxide-induced constipation and chronic venous hypertension from fluid overload [6]. Spontaneous submucosal hemorrhage also occurs in uremia and may be mistaken for angiodysplasia at endoscopy. Treatments to reduce rebleeding and transfusion requirements include oral estrogen and neodymium: Yag laser photocoagulation.

Nephrology, Edited by Rex L. Jamison and Robert Wilkinson.
Published in 1997 by Chapman & Hall, London. ISBN 0 412 60930 4

Pancreatic disease

Abnormalities in the pancreas are common in end-stage renal disease (ESRD). In an autopsy study Vaziri *et al.* [7] found pancreatic abnormalities in 47 of 78 patients (60%) who had been treated with long-term hemodialysis. Although pancreatitis was the most common other abnormalities found included fibrosis, calcification, hemosiderin deposits, cystic changes, amyloidosis and abscess formation. Clinically apparent pancreatitis has been reported in 46 (6.4%) of 716 patients with ESRD [8], whereas Rutsky *et al.* [9] found that 2.3% of dialysis patients developed pancreatitis during a 10-year period. This compares with a yearly incidence of 0.1–1% in the general population. Chronic ambulatory peritoneal dialysis (CAPD) patients are at a greater risk than hemodialysis patients [9, 10]. In the study by Padilla *et al.* [8] pancreatitis was more common in patients with alcohol abuse, systemic lupus erythematosus, and polycystic kidney disease. It was not significantly associated with hyperlipidemia, biliary tract disease or hypercalcemia. Pancreatitis occurring for the first time after the onset of ESRD in patients is reported as having a generally benign course, with an uneventful recovery and few recurrent episodes [8].

Most patients have the typical presentation with abdominal pain and tenderness. The diagnosis of acute pancreatitis in chronic renal failure is complicated by the fact that serum amylase and lipase are frequently elevated in patients with chronic renal failure in the absence of pancreatitis, and symptoms of pancreatitis in a CAPD patient may be mistaken for peritonitis. However, a greater than threefold elevation of serum amylase activity or the presence of pancreatic enzymes in the peritoneal fluid suggests coexisting pancreatitis.

Miscellaneous gastrointestinal abnormalities

In HIV nephropathy-specific lesions contributing to gastrointestinal bleeding include Kaposi's sarcoma (found in the gut at autopsy in up to 70% of individuals dying of AIDS), cytomegalovirus colitis and non-Hodgkin's lymphoma.

Brunner's gland hyperplasia (manifesting as a nodular duodenum as revealed by barium meal examination) is associated with chronic renal failure. Dyspeptic symptoms are uncommon and there is no relationship between the nodules and peptic ulceration. In a renal transplant patient the differential diagnosis includes lymphoma, carcinoma and cytomegalovirus (CMV) infection.

Malabsorption may occur as a result of bacterial overgrowth, and also as a consequence of advanced β_2-microglobulin amyloidosis. The latter may also be associated with bleeding. Diarrhea can occur as a result of changes in concentration of normal bile acids or of the

Table 32.1 Gastrointestinal disorders found more commonly in chronic renal failure

Angiodysplasia
Brunner's gland hyperplasia
Esophagitis
Acute pancreatitis
Diverticular disease
Non-occlusive mesenteric ischemia
Colonic perforation
Diarrhea
Cecal and rectal ulceration
Malabsorption
Salmonella enteritidis septicemia

presence of unusual bile acids such as ursodeoxycholate in the gut lumen [11]. In diabetic patients diarrhea may be due to severe autonomic neuropathy.

Patients with chronic renal failure are more likely to develop rectal ulcers causing hemorrhage [12]. Dialysis patients have an increased risk of *Salmonella* enteritis and sepsis, and non-occlusive mesenteric ischemia [13] which is associated with a high mortality. The clinical signs are unreliable; a high index of clinical suspicion needs to be maintained. Non-occlusive mesenteric ischemia may occur as a complication of episodes of severe hypotension during dialysis.

Gastrointestinal disorders in renal transplantation

In a recent report of 416 transplant patients (399 cadaveric and 17 living related donor) [14] there were 31 major gastrointestinal complications with a 30% mortality rate. In another series of 614 transplant recipients 100 (16.2%) were found to have gastrointestinal and/or pancreatic complications [15] with a mortality of 35% in those with intestinal perforation and peritonitis or undergoing intestinal resection. Others have reported a gastrointestinal complication rate of 20% accounting for up to 50% of post-transplant deaths [16]. These complications occur primarily in the early post-transplant period.

Upper gastrointestinal complications of renal transplantation (Table 32.2) include peptic or infectious esophagitis (from candida, herpes simplex, and CMV) and gastroduodenal ulceration and erosion. Hepatobiliary complications (Table 32.3) arise due to immunosuppressive medication.

Routine endoscopy in the first two weeks post-transplant in a patient population not receiving prophylactic H_2 antagonists revealed 63% of patients had either a peptic ulcer, esophagitis, gastritis or duodenitis [17]. Less than half the patients with ulcers were symptomatic. Discrete ulcers of the esophagus and stomach are more likely to be viral (CMV or herpes simplex virus) in origin

Table 32.2   Gastrointestinal complications of renal transplantation

Pancreatitis
Peptic ulceration
Gastroduodenal erosions
Esophagitis
Colonic perforation
CMV infection
Colitis

Table 32.3   Hepatobiliary and pancreatic complications of immunosuppression

Peliosis hepatis[a]
Nodular transformation[a]
Venocclusive disease[a]
Cholestatic jaundice[a,b]
Symptomatic biliary calculi[b]
Pancreatitis[a]

[a] Associated with azathioprine.
[b] Associated with cyclosporin.

than peptic [16]. Peptic and viral causes of duodenal ulcers are approximately equal in incidence.

Gastrointestinal hemorrhage has been considered an important complication, reported to occur in over 20% of all patients following renal transplantation [18]. However, more recent series have a much lower incidence [14, 15], probably reflecting improved pretransplant assessment, prophylactic use of H_2 antagonists in the immediate post-transplant period and prompt investigation of symptoms. The period of highest risk of gastrointestinal bleeding is in the first few months after transplantation and coincident with high-dose steroid immunosuppression for acute rejection. Factors contributing to gastrointestinal bleeding in the post-transplant patient include immunosuppression-induced thrombocytopenia and the use of heparin for dialysis.

The small bowel and colon are the most common sites of serious gastrointestinal lesions in transplant recipients. Colonic perforation from ruptured diverticula was the most severe and frequent complication in one series [14]. The incidence of diverticular disease is known to be increased in uremia possibly due to chronic constipation and/or decreased tissue strength. Diverticular disease is also reported to be more common in polycystic kidney disease. Steroid treatment is associated with serious complications of diverticular disease and may mask the symptoms and signs of perforation. CMV infection may also cause colonic perforation [19].

Lower gastrointestinal hemorrhage [14, 20] has a high mortality rate. Causes include colitis from opportunistic infections, pseudomembranous colitis, ischemic or uremic colitis and idiopathic ulceration of the colon. Prompt diagnosis is facilitated by early colonoscopy. A small but definite increase in symptomatic biliary calculus disease has been reported in transplant patients taking cyclosporin A compared with those treated with prednisolone and azathioprine [21].

The incidence of post-transplantation pancreatitis is 1–7%, the mean incidence being 2.3% and the mortality 61% [22]. Pancreatitis may occur as a consequence of CMV infection and has also been related to azathioprine therapy. Azathioprine appears to cause injury via a hypersensitivity phenomenon and usually leads to pancreatitis within one month of exposure [23]. Other causes of pan-

creatitis include surgical injury, alcoholism, hyperlipidemia and hypercalcemia. Severe complications including hemorrhagic pancreatitis, abscess or pseudocyst formation contribute to the high mortality.

Cytomegalovirus infection

Symptomatic CMV infection of the gastrointestinal tract occurs in 6.4% of renal transplant recipients during the first year after transplantation [24]. Symptoms of gastrointestinal CMV disease include abdominal pain, malaise, anorexia, diarrhea and gastrointestinal bleeding [25], most symptoms arising as a result of mucosal ulceration. Endoscopic findings are non-specific and include erythema, erosions, ulceration, plaques, polyps and nodules [19]. It should be borne in mind at endoscopy that apparent peptic ulcers may be due to CMV infection. Biopsies should be taken from areas of abnormal looking mucosa. Any part of the gastrointestinal tract may be involved, although there is some evidence that a colonic location is predominant in renal transplant recipients.

Renal disease in patients with gastrointestinal disorders

Inflammatory bowel disease (IBD) is associated with a number of renal complications. The incidence of urinary calculi is 1.5–15%. Calcium oxalate stones are more common, although uric acid stones predominate after ileostomy. In Crohn's disease urinary tract infections and pneumaturia can occur as a result of enterovesical fistulae in 2–5% of patients. Crohn's disease is a cause of renal amyloidosis of the AA type.

Celiac disease can be associated with IgA nephropathy. Glomerular mesangial deposits of IgA may occur frequently in untreated celiac disease, but without complement deposition or overt glomerulonephritis [26]. However, in most patients with IgA nephropathy there is no evidence of latent celiac disease.

In diarrhea-associated hemolytic uremic syndrome (usually caused by verocytotoxin produced by *E. coli* or *Shigella dysenteriae*) rectal bleeding is an important presenting symptom. The condition may also mimic acute appendicitis or intussuception. Gastrointestinal complications include esophageal and colonic strictures, duodenal ulcers and colonic perforation [27].

Disorders of the liver and renal disease

Renal tubular acidosis (RTA) may be linked to chronic liver disease in up to one-third of cases. It is most strongly associated with primary biliary cirrhosis, although it has also been described in autoimmune chronic active hepatitis, alcoholic liver disease and cryptogenic cirrhosis. The defect is usually due to a distal RTA. There is no correlation between the severity of the liver disease and the presence of RTA.

Hepatic granuloma related to deposition of silicone (from silicone tubing) can occur in hemodialysis patients. The majority of these patients are asymptomatic although in some cases fever and malaise can occur. Liver involvement can occur in polycystic kidney disease. In the adult variant hepatic involvement is rare but hepatomegaly and portal hypertension can occur. Massive hepatomegaly may necessitate liver transplantation. Juvenile polycystic kidney disease is associated with congenital hepatic fibrosis. The extent of liver involvement varies from mild to severe. In patients with severe liver involvement, renal disease may be mild. Portal hypertension is the main clinical consequence of severe liver involvement.

The nephrogenic–hepatic dysfunction syndrome (Stauffer's syndrome) has been described in patients with hypernephroma without hepatic metastasis [28]. It is a rare condition the clinical features of which are hepatomegaly, splenomegaly, fever and weight loss. Laboratory findings include anemia, elevated alkaline phosphatase and prolonged prothrombin time. Liver biopsy characteristically shows minimal abnormality and liver function returns to normal after nephrectomy.

Renal transplantation is associated with hepatic vascular disease manifesting as either venocclusive disease (injury and occlusion of efferent hepatic venules) or peliosis hepatis (mottled blue liver) with or without nodular transformation. Venocclusive disease is rare.

Hepatitis B

Historically hepatitis B virus (HBV) infection has been a major problem for hemodialysis units. Between 1967 and 1971 the European Dialysis and Transplant Association reported annual incidence rates for HBV infection of 5–10% [30]. A survey in 1976 of 750 US dialysis centers found the prevalence of HBs antigenemia to be 7.8% with an annual incidence rate of HBV infection of 3% [31]. Blood transfusion and length of time on chronic hemodialysis were shown to be independent risk factors. The introduction of stringent infection control measures

such as the use of dedicated machines for HBsAg-positive patients and regular screening of patients for HBsAg and anti-HBs led to a fall in the prevalence and incidence of HBV infection. By 1989 the annual incidence of HBV infection among US dialysis patients had declined to 0.1% with a prevalence of 0.3% [32]. The risk of chronic infection and progression of liver disease following infection with HBV is increased in patients on hemodialysis probably due to an impairment of cell-mediated immunity [33]; also a significant proportion of HBsAg-positive ESRD patients remain HBeAg positive, indicating active viral replication.

The immune response to HBV vaccination tends to be sub-optimal in patients on chronic hemodialysis. Crosnier et al. [34] found only 26 of 43 (60%) hemodialysis patients developed anti-HBs titres >10 mIU/ml (the level required for protection). Even when an adequate anti-HBs response does occur it tends to be transient as Fleming et al. [35] reported that 13 of 23 (57%) vaccine responders had lost detectable anti-HBs within six months. Vaccination prior to the onset of end-stage disease, the use of a reinforced protocol (such as four vaccine injections and one booster one year later) and the co-administration of immune modulators may increase the effectiveness of vaccination.

HBV infection and transplantation

Immunosuppression following renal transplantation (RT) has been shown to lead to increased viral replication with an increase in HBV DNA levels [36] which could lead to an acceleration in the progression of the liver disease. However, the effect of HBV infection on graft and patient survival following RT remains controversial. Some authors report that HBV infection is associated with a bad prognosis in individuals with histological evidence of chronic liver disease [37], whereas other studies have not found chronic liver disease to be a common complication of RT in HBsAg-positive patients [38, 39] or HBeAg positivity to correlate with poor outcome [38]. A recent study of 151 HBsAg-positive renal transplant recipients [40] found a high rate of histological deterioration (85.3%) associated with cirrhosis in 28%. Liver disease was the leading cause of death in these HBsAg-positive individuals; however, there was not a significant difference in survival compared to HBsAg-negative transplant recipients.

Current knowledge would suggest that HBV-infected patients with mild disease on liver biopsy should not be precluded from RT, whilst RT should be avoided in individuals with severe chronic hepatitis or established cirrhosis as they appear to be at greatest risk of hepatic decompensation [37]. HDV infection is uncommon in haemodialysis or RT patients [41].

Hepatitis C

Hepatitis C (HCV) virus infection is the most common cause of liver dysfunction in chronic hemodialysis patients, anti-HCV antibody having been reported in between 10% to 40% of patients. The prevalence in CAPD patients is considerably lower. A multicenter study of 11 US hemodialysis centers found 52 of 499 patients (10%) and two of 142 staff (1%) to be anti-HCV positive [42] whilst a prospective study of 217 French dialysis patients over a period of 12 years found 39.6% to be anti-HCV positive and HCV accounted for 91% of dialysis-associated non-A non-B hepatitis [43]. The above figures compare with a prevalence in volunteer blood donors in the US of less than 1.4%. Even these figures may be underestimates however as the sensitivity of commercially available serological tests for HCV appears to be reduced in dialysis patients [44]. Duration of dialysis, history of IV drug abuse and blood transfusions are independent risk factors for hepatitis C seropositivity. The demonstration of length of time on dialysis as an independent risk factor for hepatitis C is strongly suggestive of nosocomial transmission of HCV in the dialysis setting, and the use of dedicated hemodialysis machines for HCV-infected patients is increasingly being advocated [45]. A high proportion of individuals infected with hepatitis C will go on to develop chronic liver disease although this may be asymptomatic for many years. Liver function tests are not an accurate guide to viral replication, or degree of liver damage in ESRD patients with hepatitis C, as Pol *et al.* [46] found only 16 of 52 (31%) patients with HCV RNA had abnormal liver function tests, and only 4 of 15 (26%) viremic patients with histological evidence of chronic hepatitis had elevated transaminases. Interferon alpha has recently been shown to be effective in the treatment of ESRD patients with chronic hepatitis C [47]. There is

now increasing evidence for a pathophysiological role for HCV infection in essential mixed cryoglobulinemia and cryoglobulinemic glomerulonephritis.

Renal transplantation and hepatitis C

Transmission of hepatitis C via solid organ transplantation has been well documented. In one study HCV RNA was detected in 7 of 26 (27%) recipients preoperatively and 23 of 24 (96%) following transplantation of an organ from an HCV carrier donor [48]. Anti-HCV positivity (prior to transplant) appears to be associated with a higher incidence of serious infection and episodes of acute rejection (49) post transplantation; however, in this study no difference was seen in patient or graft survival, and to date no other studies have reported an adverse effect of hepatitis C seropositivity on graft or patient survival. However, the presence of severe chronic hepatitis or cirrhosis on biopsy at the time of transplant assessment should probably be considered a contraindication to transplantation. All hepatitis C positive patients undergoing transplant assessment should therefore have a liver biopsy regardless of live function tests, to allow staging of the disease. HCV RNA should also be assayed. A recent study on the use of interferon alpha in renal transplant patients with chronic hepatitis C found a significant improvement in serum transaminase (during therapy) with no change in HCV viremia [50]. However, this was associated with irreversible deterioration in graft function in some patients. Interferon alpha should therefore not be used in the post-transplant setting.

References

1. Kang, J.Y., Wu, A.Y., Sutherland, I.H. and Vathsala, A. (1988) Prevalence of peptic ulcer in patients undergoing maintenance hemodialysis. *Dig. Dis. Sci.*, **33**, 774–8.
2. Zuckerman, G.R., Cornette, G.L., Clouse, R.E. and Harter, H.R. (1985) Upper gastrointestinal bleeding in patients with chronic renal failure. *Ann. Intern. Med.*, **102**, 588–92.
3. Muto, S., Asano, Y., Hosoda, S. and Miyata, M. (1988) Hypochlorhydria and hypergastrinemia and their association with gastrointestinal bleeding in undialyzed and hemodialyzed patients. *Nephron*, **50**, 10–13.
4. Davenport, A., Shallcross, T.M., Crabtree, J.E. *et al.* (1991) Prevalence of *Helicobacter pylori* in patients with end-stage renal failure and renal transplant recipients. *Nephron*, **59**, 597–601.
5. Dave, P.B., Romeu, J., Antonelli, A. and Eiser, A.R. (1984) Gastrointestinal telangiectasias. A source of bleeding in patients receiving hemodialysis. *Arch. Intern. Med.*, **144**, 1781–3.
6. Doherty, C.C. (1993) Gastrointestinal bleeding in dialysis patients (clinical conference). *Nephron*, **63**, 132–6.
7. Vaziri, N.D., Dure-Smith, B., Miller, R. and Mirahmadi, M. (1987) Pancreatic pathology in chronic dialysis

patients an autopsy study of 78 cases. *Nephron*, **46**, 347–9.
8. Padilla, B., Pollak, V.E., Pesce, A. *et al.* (1994) Pancreatitis in patients with end–stage renal disease. *Medicine*, **73**, 8–20.
9. Rutsky, E.A., Robards, M., Van Dyke, J.A. and Rostand, S.G. (1986) Acute pancreatitis in patients with end-stage renal disease without transplantation. *Arch. Intern. Med.*, **146**, 1741–5.
10. Caruana, R.J., Wolfman, N.T., Karstaedt, N. and Wilson, D.J. (1986) Pancreatitis: an important cause of abdominal symptoms in patients on peritoneal dialysis. *Am. J. Kidney Dis.*, **7**, 135–40.
11. Gordon, S.J., Miller, L.J., Haeffner, L.J. *et al.* (1976) Abnormal intestinal bile acid distribution of azotaemic man: a possible role in the pathogenesis of uraemic diarrhoea. *Gut*, **17**, 58.
12. Goldberg, M., Hoffman, G.C. and Wombolt, D.G. (1984) Massive hemorrhage from rectal ulcers in chronic renal failure. *Ann. Intern. Med.*, **100**, 397.
13. Valentine, R.J., Whelan, T.V. and Meyers, H.F. (1990) Nonocclusive mesenteric ischemia in renal patients:

recognition and prevention of intestinal gangrene. *Am. J. Kidney Dis.*, **15**, 598–600.

14. Bardaxoglou, E., Maddern, G., Ruso, L. *et al.* (1993) Gastrointestinal surgical emergencies following kidney transplantation. *Transplant Int.*, **6**, 148–52.

15. Benoit, G., Moukarzel, M., Verdelli, G. *et al.* (1993) Gastrointestinal complications in renal transplantation. *Transplant Int.*, **6**, 45–9.

16. Komorowski, R.A., Cohen, E.B., Kauffman, N. and Adams, M.B. (1986) Gastrointestinal complications in renal transplant recipients. *Am. J. Clin. Pathol.*, **86**, 161.

17. Steger, A.C., Timoney, A.S., Griffen, S. *et al.* (1990) The influence of immunosuppression on peptic ulceration following renal transplantation and the role of endoscopy. *Nephrol. Dial. Transplant.*, **5**, 289–92.

18. Lewicki, A.M., Saito, S. and Merrill, J.P. (1972) Gastrointestinal bleeding in the renal transplant patient. *Radiology*, **102**, 533–7.

19. Buckener, F.S. and Pomeroy, C. (1993) Cytomegalovirus disease of the gastrointestinal tract in patients without AIDS. (Review). *Clin. Infect. Dis.*, **17**, 644–56.

20. Stylianos, S., Forde, K.A., Benvenisty, A.I. and Hardy, M.A. (1988) Lower gastrointestinal hemorrhage in renal transplant recipients. (Review). *Arch. Surg.*, **123**, 739–44.

21. Lorber, M.I., Van Buren, C.T., Flechner, S.M. and Williams, C. (1987) Hepatobiliary and pancreatic complications of cyclosporine therapy on 466 renal transplant recipients. *Transplantation*, **43**, 35.

22. Fernandez–Cruz, L., Targarona, E.M., Cugat, E. *et al.* (1989) Acute pancreatitis after renal transplantation. *Br. J. Surg.*, **76**, 1132–5.

23. Steinberg, W. and Tenner, S. (1994) Acute pancreatitis. (Review). *N. Engl. J. Med.*, **330**, 1198–210.

24. Peterson, P.K., Balfour, H.H.,Jr, Marker, S.C. *et al.* (1980) Cytomegalovirus disease in renal allograft recipients: a prospective study of the clinical features, risk factors and impact on renal transplantation. *Medicine*, **59**, 283–300.

25. Mayoral, J.L., Loeffler, C.M., Fasola, C.G. *et al.* (1991) Diagnosis and treatment of cytomegalovirus disease in transplant patients based on gastrointestinal tract manifestations. *Arch. Surg.*, **126**, 202–6.

26. Pasternak, A., Collin, P., Mustonen, J. *et al.* (1990) Glomerular IgA deposits in patients with celiac disease. *Clin. Nephrol.*, **34**, 56–60.

27. de la Hunt, M.N., Morris, K.P., Coulthard, M.G. and Rangecroft, L. (1991) Oesophageal and severe gut involvement in the haemolytic uraemic syndrome. *Br. J. Surg.*, **78**, 1469–72.

28. Delpre, G., Ilie, B., Papo, J. *et al.* (1979) Hypernephroma with nonmetastatic liver dysfunction (Stauffer's syndrome) and hypercalcemia. Case report and review of the literature. *Am. J. Gastroenterol.*, **72**, 239–47.

29. Izumi, S., Nishiuchi, M., Kameda, Y. *et al.* (1994) Laparoscopic study of peliosis hepatis and nodular transformation of the liver before and after renal transplantation: natural history and aetiology in follow-up cases. *J. Hepatol.*, **20**, 129–37.

30. Marmion, B.P. and Tonkin, R.E. (1972) Control of hepatitis in dialysis units. *Br. Med. Bull.*, **28**, 169–79.

31. Alter, M.J., Favero, M.S., Petersen, N.J. *et al.* (1983) National surveillance of dialysis-associated hepatitis and other diseases, 1976 and 1980. *Dial. Transplant.*, **12**, 860–5.

32. Alter, M.J., Favero, M.S., Moyer, L.A. and Bland, I.A. (1989) National surveillance of dialysis-associated diseases in the United States, 1989. *ASAIO Trans.*, **37**, 97–104.

33. Lee, B.W., Yap, H.K., Tan, M. *et al.* (1991) Cell-mediated immunity in patients on haemodialysis: Relationship with hepatitis B carrier status. *Am. J. Nephrol.*, **11**, 98–101.

34. Crosnier, J., Jungers, P., Courouce, A.M. *et al.* (1981) Randomized placebo-controlled trial of hepatitis B surface antigen in French haemodialysis units. II Haemodialysis patients. *Lancet*, **i**, 797–800.

35. Fleming, S.J., Moran, D.M., Cooksley, W.G.E. and Faoagali, J.L. (1991) Poor response to a recombinant hepatitis B vaccine in hemodialysis patients. *J. Infect. Dis.*, **22**, 251–7.

36. Dusheiko, G., Song, E., Bowyer, S. *et al.* (1983) Natural history of hepatitis B virus infection in renal transplant recipients – A fifteen year follow–up. *Hepatology*, **3**, 330–6.

37. Rao, K.V., Kasiske, B.L. and Anderson, W.R. (1991) Variability in the morphological spectrum and clinical outcome of chronic liver disease in hepatitis B-positive and B-negative renal transplant recipients. *Transplantation*, **51**, 391–6.

38. Nelson, S.R., Snowden, S.A., Sutherland, S. *et al.* (1994) Outcome of renal transplantation in hepatitis BsAg-positive patients. *Nephrol. Dial. Transplant.*, **9**, 1320–3.

39. Agarwal, S.K., Dash, S.C., Tiwari, S.C. *et al.* (1994) Clinicopathologic course of hepatitis B infection in surface antigen carriers following living-related renal transplantation. *Am. J. Kidney Dis.*, **24**, 78–82.

40. Fornairon, S., Pol, S., Legendre, C. *et al.* (1996) The long-term virologic and pathologic impact of renal transplantation on chronic hepatitis B virus infection. *Transplantation*, **62**, 297–9.

41. Pol S., Dubois F., Mattlinger B. *et al.* (1992) Absence of hepatitis delta infection in chronic hemodialysis and kidney transplant patients in France. *Transplantation*, **54**, 1096–7.

42. Niu, M.T., Coleman, P.J. and Alter, M.J. (1993) Multicenter study of hepatitis C virus infection in chronic hemodialysis patients and hemodialysis center staff members. *Am. J. Kidney Dis.*, **22**, 568–73.

43. Simon, N., Courouce, A.M., Lemarrec, N. *et al.* (1994) A twelve year natural history of hepatitis C virus infection in hemodialyzed patients. *Kidney Int.*, **46**, 504–11.

44. Bukh, J., Wantzin, P., Krogsgaard, K. *et al.* (1993) High prevalence of hepatitis C virus (HCV) RNA in dialysis patients: failure of commercially available antibody tests to identify a significant number of patients with HCV infection. *J. Infect. Dis.*, **168**, 1343–8.

45. Blumberg, A., Zehnder, C. and Burckhardt, J.J. (1995) Prevention of hepatitis C infection in haemodialysis units. A prospective study. *Nephrol. Dial. Transplant.*, **10**, 230–3.

46. Pol, S., Romeo, R., Zins, B. *et al.* (1993) Hepatitis C virus RNA in anti-HCV positive hemodialysis patients: Significance and therapeutic implications. *Kidney Int.*, **44**, 1097–100.

47. Pol, S., Thiers, V., Carnot, F., Zins, B. *et al.* (1996) Effectiveness and tolerance of interferon-alpha-2b in the treatment of chronic hepatitis-C In hemodialysis-patients. *Nephrol. Dial. Transplant.*, **11**, 58–61.

48. Pereira, B.J. (1993) Hepatitis C in organ transplantation: its significance and influence on transplantation policies. (Review). *Curr. Opin. Nephrol. Hypertens.*, **2**, 912–22.

49. Roth, D., Zucker, K., Cirocco, R. *et al.* (1994) The impact of hepatitis C virus infection on renal allograft recipients. *Kidney Int.*, **45**, 238–44.

50. Rostaing, L., Izopet, J., Baron, E. *et al.* (1995) Preliminary results of treatment of chronic hepatits C with recombinant interferon alpha in renal transplant patients. *Nephrol. Dial. Transplant.*, **20**(suppl 6), 93–6.

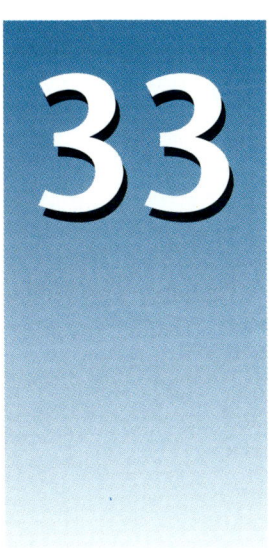

33

Endocrine disorders

R. Stuart C. Rodger

Introduction

Endocrine abnormalities are found in most patients with advanced renal failure and often contribute to the uremic syndrome. In renal failure circulating hormone levels are frequently abnormal and the hormone or target organ itself may be altered by uremia, changing its activity or responsiveness. These abnormalities are generally not ameliorated by dialysis therapy but are often reversed following successful renal transplantation. The pathogenetic mechanisms of endocrine abnormalities in uremia have been reviewed by Emmanouel *et al.* [1] and Handelsman [2] and are summarized in Table 33.1. The kidney itself has numerous endocrine functions but this chapter deals with the effects of loss of renal function and of uremia on extrarenal endocrine systems.

Hypothalamic–pituitary–gonadal function

Men

Clinical features

Sexual dysfunction has been known for many years to be prevalent in men with uremia. Reduced sexual activity is mainly due to erectile insufficiency coupled with some loss of libido. Noctural penile tumescence is significantly reduced in uremic men indicating that their impotence is organic rather than psychogenic in origin [3]. Studies

in the 1970s and 1980s indicated that up to 80% of men had diminished sexual function following the onset of uremia. The results of more recent surveys following the widespread use of erythropoietin, which may improve sexual function, have not yet been published. In patients whose primary renal disease is diabetes, impotence often occurs before severe renal failure ensues. Most men with end-stage renal disease will have testicular atrophy, histology from testicular biopsies showing decreased spermatogenic function [4].

Gynecomastia and galactorrhea may also be present less commonly. Semen analysis usually reveals a reduction in total volume, sperm count and motility.

Pathophysiology

Although the etiology of sexual dysfunction in men with chronic renal failure is usually multifactorial, endocrine abnormalities are thought to be of prime importance in most cases. When groups of patients have been studied the pattern of disturbance consistently found is of elevated gonadotropin and prolactin levels with low or low normal total and free testosterone levels. Adrenal androgens are normal whereas estrogen levels have been reported to be low, normal or high. Dynamic tests show an impaired testosterone response to human chorionic gonadotropin (HCG) stimulation and prolonged luteinizing hormone (LH) and follicle stimulating hormone (FSH) secretion following exogenous LH releasing hormone (LHRH). Prolactin release following a variety of stimuli such as thyrotropin releasing hormone (TRH)

Nephrology, Edited by Rex L. Jamison and Robert Wilkinson.
Published in 1997 by Chapman & Hall, London. ISBN 0 412 60930 4

Table 33.1 Pathogenic mechanisms of endocrine abnormalities in uremia

I. **Alterations of hormone levels**

A. Increased hormone levels
 1. Impaired hormone degradation
   (a) Impaired renal catabolism of hormones
   (b) Heterogeneity of hormone immunoreactivity
   (c) Impaired extrarenal hormone degradation
 2. Increased secretory rates
   (a) Augmented hormone secretion as an adaptive response to alterations in internal milieu
   (b) Augmented hormone secretion resulting from disorders of feedback control mechanisms

B. Decreased hormone levels
 1. Reduced secretory rates
   (a) Decreased hormone production by the diseased kidney
   (b) Dysfunction of other endocrine glands
 2. Impaired conversion of prohormones into the biologically active hormone

II. **Alterations of hormone effects on target tissue**

Reproduced from D.S. Emmanouel, M.D. Lindheimer and A.T. Katz, Pathogenesis of endocrine abnormalities in uremia. *Endocr. Rev.*, **1**, 28–44, 1980, © The Endocrine Society.

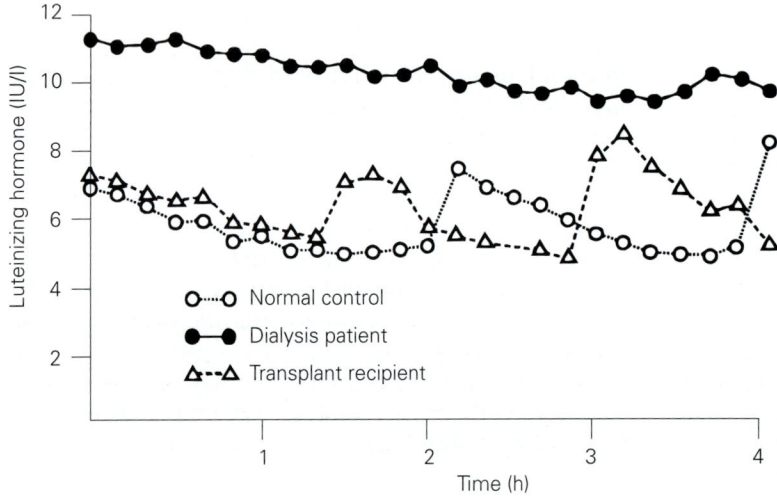

Figure 33.1 Luteinizing hormone secretory pattern in three subjects. (Reproduced from Rodger *et al.* [5], by permission of the BMJ Publishing Group.)

and insulin-induced hypoglycemia is blunted and serial venous sampling demonstrates absent or reduced pulsatile gonadotropin secretion (Figure 33.1) [5]. A reduction in the biopotency of LH resulting in reduced testosterone has been found in male dialysis patients and recently it has been shown that this is probably due to a preponderance of basic isoforms of LH compared with the more acidic forms found in normal men (Figure 33.2) [6].

Important non-endocrine factors which contribute to sexual dysfunction in uremic men include vascular disease, drugs and psychosocial stress. The role of hyperparathyroidism, autonomic neuropathy and trace element disturbance is more dubious.

Treatment and outcome

Sexual dysfunction tends to deteriorate after the initiation of dialysis therapy and the incidence of loss of libido and erectile insufficiency in patients treated by peritoneal dialysis is similar to that in age-matched hemodialysis patients although androgen levels may be higher. Successful renal transplantation offers the best prospect of recovery of sexual function for men with renal failure [7]. Fertility is also improved and there is a greater incidence of successful paternity. This is associated with a partial or complete correction of the endocrine abnormalities described above. The recovery of sexual function is by no means invariable or complete, however, and adverse

(a)

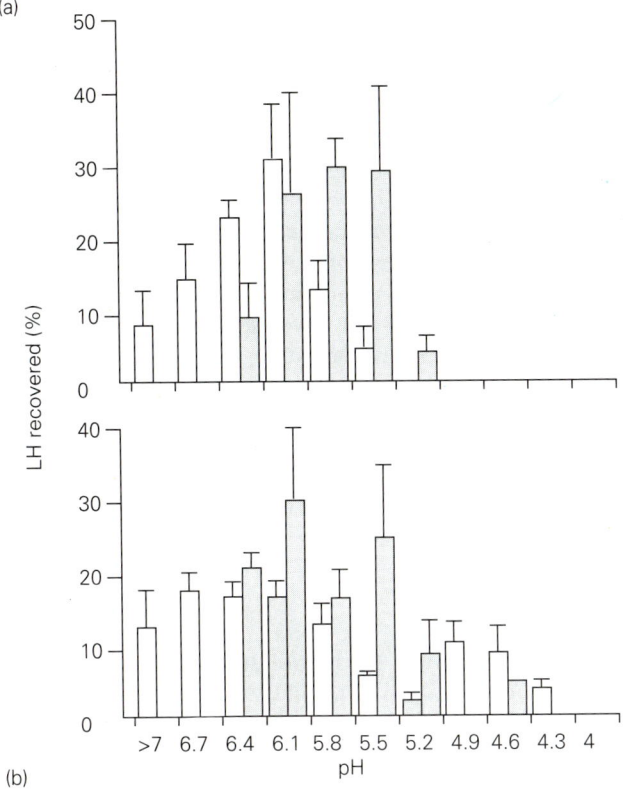

(b)

Figure 33.2 Combined LH distribution in subjects with CRF (open panels) and normal subjects (hatched panels) using (a) the immunoradiometric assay and (b) immunofluorimetric assay. (Reproduced from Mitchell *et al.* [12], with permission.)

prognostic indicators are increased age, prolonged duration of dialysis treatment, increased FSH levels prior to transplantation, poor graft function and division of the spermatic cord or the end-to-end anastomosis of the transplant renal artery to the internal iliac artery at the time of transplantation.

Several studies have suggested that the treatment of renal anemia with erythropoietin is associated with improved sexual function and a correction of some of the endocrine abnormalities of uremia. Controlled studies are needed to determine whether the reported beneficial effects of erythropoietin are merely due to an improved sense of well-being and fitness. Controlled studies have been conflicting with regard to the efficacy of zinc supplementation and dopamine agonist therapy; the use of either for treating uremic patients with sexual dysfunction remains controversial. Androgen therapy will correct some of the hormonal abnormalities in men with renal failure but this is usually not associated with an improved libido or potency.

If the patient with erectile insufficiency is a candidate for renal transplantation, penile autoinjection therapy with papaverine or prostaglandin can be offered until a functioning graft is obtained. If the patient is not a can-

didate for transplantation the choice is between autoinjection therapy and a penile implant.

Women

Clinical features

The literature concerning uremic women is less extensive than for men; however, it is clear that libido, sexual activity and orgasm are reduced in renal failure though possibly not to the same degree as in men [8]. Women with renal failure have irregular or absent menstruation and most women who menstruate have anovulatory cycles. Menometrorrhagia occurs in some patients and is exacerbated by anticoagulation during dialysis. Galactorrhea may be present. It has been suggested that there is a higher prevalence of ovarian cyst formation in women receiving hemodialysis. Older women may develop postmenopausal symptoms although flushing is said to be unusual.

Fertility is reduced and successful pregnancies are rare in women receiving dialysis treatment. Of 490 successful pregnancies in women on renal replacement therapy reported over a ten-year period to the European Registry, 11.6% occurred in patients undergoing dialysis [9]. The number of female hemodialysis patients of childbearing age who become pregnant has been estimated to be 1 in 200. The majority of pregnancies are thought to result in early spontaneous abortion.

Pathophysiology

In premenopausal uremic women, LH and prolactin levels are elevated whereas FSH levels are normal and estrogen and progesterone levels normal or low. Ovulatory surges and pulsatile secretion of LH are generally absent and there is loss of positive estrogen feedback on gonadotrophin secretion [10]. It is likely that these endocrine abnormalities account for sexual dysfunction in uremic women and that hypothalamic dysfunction plays a central role.

Treatment and outcome

Renal transplantation offers the best prospect of improvement in sexual function in women with severe renal failure. Correction of renal anemia with erythropoietin is also likely to be beneficial. In some patients peritoneal dialysis inhibits sexual activity because of the presence of the peritoneal dialysis catheter and the alteration of body image and in these circumstances a change to hemodialysis may be helpful.

If menometrorrhagia persists following endometrial curettage the menstrual bleeding can usually be controlled by medical treatment such as norethisterone, danazol or long-acting LHRH analogs. Resistant cases may require endometrial resection but hysterectomy is seldom necessary. Patients with galactorrhea are likely to be hyperprolactinemic. Treatment with a dopamine agonist such as bromocriptine should be effective, although this drug is poorly tolerated in patients with renal failure; correction of hyperprolactinemia may induce recovery of ovulation and fertility.

The prognosis for uremic pregnancy is poor, the main adverse features being anemia, hypertension and acidosis. Guidelines for management of pregnancies in patients with advanced renal failure are based on limited clinical experience. For patients receiving hemodialysis, frequent but short treatments using bicarbonate rather than acetate dialysate are generally advised to allow a liberal diet and prevent interdialytic hypertension. Correction of anemia with erythropoietin is probably advantageous provided hypertension does not develop, although this has not been demonstrated in a controlled study.

In postmenopausal women hormone replacement therapy reduces the incidence of osteoporosis and ischemic heart disease. In women with renal failure the same theoretical advantages apply although its use has not been carefully studied. Before embarking on hormone replacement therapy patients should be screened for cervical and breast malignancy and should continue to be monitored thereafter.

Children

Clinical features

The start of puberty is delayed by an average of two years in children with chronic renal failure; in addition the pubertal growth spurt is suppressed by 50%. In prepubertal children with chronic renal failure reproductive function may be permanently impaired.

Pathophysiology

The endocrine disturbance in uremic children is similar to that found in adults [11]. Gonadal steroids are reduced for pubertal stage and peripheral conversion of testosterone to dihydrotestosterone may be impaired. More recently immunoreactive inhibin levels have been shown to be elevated [12]. LH, FSH and prolactin levels are often elevated and LH pulsatility and bioativity are reduced, consistent with hypothalamic hypogonadism [13].

Treatment and outcome

At present treatment should be aimed at optimizing nutrition and renal replacement therapy. The use of low-dose testosterone or anabolic steroids is not advised because of their potential side effects and their disproportionate effect on skeletal maturity which will reduce overall capacity for growth. Successful renal transplantation is usually associated with recovery of normal endocrine function and pubertal development; however, growth may still be impaired at least in part due to the effect of corticosteroids.

Hypothalamic–pituitary–adrenal function

Clinical features

Many of the symptoms and signs of uremia such as muscle weakness, hyperpigmentation, hypotension, glucose intolerance and poor healing are also features of hypoadrenalism or hyperadrenalism. Although there are abnormalities of the hypothalamic–pituitary–adrenal axis in renal failure they are of uncertain clinical relevance and most patients do not have significant adrenocortical over- or underactivity. Patients with amyloidosis should be tested for adrenal insufficiency however, and uremic patients are more susceptible to hypothalamic–pituitary–adrenal suppression following steroid therapy. This is particularly relevant to patients with failed renal transplants returning to dialysis treatment in whom steroid withdrawal is contemplated.

Pathophysiology

The diurnal rhythm of cortisol secretion is retained in renal failure but diurnal profiles of serum cortisol levels may be elevated [14] and, in contrast to gonadotropin pulsatility, secretory episodes of cortisol are retained. The metabolites of cortisol accumulate in renal failure and care must be taken to use an assay which has low cross-reactivity with these metabolites. Similarly, adrenocorticotropic hormone (ACTH) precursors and bioinactive metabolic fragments may accumulate in renal failure and cross-react with radioimmunoassays for ACTH [15]. ACTH levels are probably normal or slightly elevated in most patients with renal failure and the adrenocortical response to ACTH stimulation is also normal.

The cortisol response to insulin-induced hypoglycemia is reduced in 10–50% of patients. However, the response to major stresses such as surgery is said to be preserved. Some studies have shown a reduced negative feedback suppression from oral and intravenous dexamethasone and also in the response to metyrapone [16]. Studies using corticotropin releasing factor in dialysis patients have shown a blunting of either ACTH or cortisol release.

In summary, the abnormalities of the hypothalamic–pituitary–adrenal axis in uremia occur at multiple levels. There is evidence of mild cortisol excess and loss of adrenal suppressibility. In addition to this the ability of the axis to increase cortisol secretion may be impaired in some circumstances. Further studies are needed to define the predominant defect and its clinical significance if any.

Treatment and outcome

Despite the endocrine abnormalities described above the diagnosis of coexisting pituitary adrenal disorders in patients with renal failure should not be difficult. Hypoadrenalism can be excluded by a normal short ACTH test and Cushing's syndrome diagnosed by the loss of diurnal rhythm of cortisol secretion and the failure to suppress cortisol levels following high dose dexamethasone. Renal transplantation inevitably causes some suppression of the hypothalamic–pituitary–adrenal axis unless corticosteroid therapy is completely avoided. Until the clinical significance of hypothalamic–pituitary–adrenal dysfunction is clarified no specific treatment is recommended.

Thyroid function

Clinical features

Kaptein *et al.* found a sixfold increase in the prevalence of goiter in dialysis patients compared to a group of hospital inpatients with normal renal function [17], and ultrasound studies have shown increased thyroid gland volume in 60% of dialysis patients. Patients with chronic renal failure frequently have symptoms such as cold intolerance and lethargy which might suggest hypothyroidism. Although most uremic patients are euthyroid the incidence of primary hypothyroidism but not hyperthyroidism is probably increased. In addition the hypothalamic–pituitary–thyroid axis is abnormal at multiple levels in the uremic patient, although the significance of this is uncertain as clinical indices of thyroid activity such as Achilles tendon relaxation time or myocardial contractility are usually normal and thyroid replacement therapy in these patients produces no clear clinical benefit.

Pathophysiology

Circulating total and free thyroxine (T4) concentrations are often low and both free and total tri-iodothyronine (T3) are usually decreased whereas those of reverse T3 are normal. The thyroidal response to thyrotropin stimulating hormone (TSH) and peripheral conversion of T4 into T3 are both reduced, although spuriously elevated free T4 levels may be occur in patients receiving hemodialysis due to interference in the assay by heparin.

The hypothalamic–pituitary control of thyroid hormone secretion is also deranged. Despite the low T4 and T3 concentrations, basal TSH levels are normal or only mildly elevated in patients with renal failure and there is a diminished TSH response to thyrotropin releasing hormone (TRH). The diurnal rhythm and pulsatile release of TSH secretion are both reduced with a loss of the normal nocturnal surge.

The pattern of thyroid function abnormalities in renal failure is similar to those described in 'sick euthyroid' patients apart from the normal reverse T3 concentrations and the blunted TSH response to TRH [18]. Thyroid function abnormalities found in patients treated by continuous ambulatory peritoneal dialysis (CAPD) are generally similar to those in patients on hemodialysis. Iodine-induced hypothyroidism has been described in two patients on CAPD caused by adding povidone iodine to the dialysis fluid to prevent peritonitis. Iodide concentrations are raised in patients with renal failure and excessive intake of iodine-rich foods has been shown to cause reversible hypothyroidism in three patients in Japan. Children and adolescents have a similar pattern of thyroid function test abnormalities to that in adults [19].

Treatment and outcome

At present there is no indication for treating the 'sick euthyroid' status of patients with chronic renal failure; indeed it may have a protective role in reducing protein catabolism [20]. The recognition of coexisting primary hypothyroidism is important, however, and depends on the presence of an elevated basal TSH level. Thyroid function tests revert to normal following successful renal transplantation, apart from the blunted TSH response to TRH which persists probably due to the effect of corticosteroids.

Growth hormone

Clinical features

In children with renal failure, abnormalities in the growth hormone (GH)–somatomedin axis are major factors causing growth retardation. In adults disturbances of this axis may be a factor in the loss of muscle mass but probably do not contribute to the glucose intolerance which occurs in chronic renal failure [21].

Pathophysiology

In adults, fasting levels of GH are elevated but mean GH concentrations over a 24-h period are decreased with a reduction in the normal sleep-associated increase in GH secretion [22]. In children, the pulsatility of GH secretion is retained with increased amplitude of pulses [23]. Both adults and children show hypersensitivity to many releasing stimuli; thus there is an exaggerated response to insulin-induced hypoglycemia and GH releasing hormone (GHRH) and a paradoxical rise in GH following TRH and glucose infusion. Although protein binding of GH is reduced there is peripheral resistance at the target tissue, probably due to a reduction in receptor binding.

Somatostatin levels are elevated and somatomedin (also known as insulin-like growth factor (IGF)) levels normal or reduced (IGF-I) or increased (IGF-II). Somatomedin bioactivity is reduced and this has been shown to be due to a greatly increased level of binding proteins [24].

Treatment and outcome

Abnormalities in GH secretion generally persist after the onset of dialysis therapy, although the exaggerated and paradoxical responses to hypoglycemia and glucose infusion may be less marked in patients on CAPD than hemodialysis. There is some evidence that growth in children may be better with CAPD than on hemodialysis although this is by no means conclusive. To maximize growth the aim should be to optimize the chosen mode of dialysis to ensure adequate nutrition and prevent renal osteodystrophy [25].

Renal transplantation results in a reduction in pulse amplitude of GH secretion, probably due to an effect of corticosteroids, but an increase in somatomedin bioactivity. Treatment of uremic prepubertal children with supraphysiological doses of recombinant human GH (rHGH) improves growth and increases somatomedin bioactivity probably by increasing IGF-I levels more than the binding protein levels [26]. rHGH also increasess growth in pubertal children with renal failure but is less effective. The use of GH therapy in renal allograft recipients could promote acute or chronic rejection although clinical studies have not demonstrated such effects.

Human GH has been shown to have an anabolic effect in normal aging men [28] and could have beneficial effects on muscle mass and bone density in adult and elderly dialysis patients. Its use in this setting, however, has only recently been investigated. Short-term studies show that GH may have an anabolic effect in patients treated by CAPD but the long-term effects are not yet known [29].

Conclusions

Over the last ten years our understanding of the endocrine abnormalities which occur in renal failure has improved greatly. The major therapeutic advance has been the use of rHGH to promote growth in uremic children. Priorities for future research should be to develop effective therapies for sexual dysfunction and delayed puberty in chronic renal failure and to investigate further the clinical implications of the disturbances of thyroid and adrenal function.

References

1. Emmanouel, D.S., Lindheimer, M.D. and Katz, A.T. (1980) Pathogenesis of endocrine abnormalities in uremia. *Endocr. Rev.*, **1**, 28–44.
2. Handelsman, D.J. (1985) Hypothalamic–pituitary gonadal dysfunction in renal failure, dialysis and renal transplantation. *Endocr. Rev.*, **6**, 151–82.
3. Procci, W.R., Goldstein, D.A., Adelstein, J. and Massry, S.G. (1981) Sexual dysfunction in the male patient with uremia – a reappraisal. *Kidney Int.*, **19**, 317–23.
4. Holdsworth, S., Atkins, R.C. and De Krester, D.M. (1977) The pituitary–testicular axis in men with chronic renal failure. *N. Engl. J. Med.*, **296**, 1245–9.
5. Rodger, R.S.C., Morrison, L., Dewar, J.H. *et al.* (1985) Loss of pulsatile luteinising hormone secretion in men with chronic renal failure. *Br. Med. J.*, **291**, 1598–600.
6. Mitchell, R., Banerfeld, C., Schaefer, F. *et al.* (1994) Less acidic forms of luteinising hormone are associated with lower testosterone secretion in men on hemodialysis treatment. *Clin. Endocrinol.*, **41**, 65–73.
7. Salvaterra, D., Fortima, J.L. and Belzer, F.O. (1975) Sexual function in males before and after renal transplantation. *Urology*, **5**, 64–6.
8. Mastrogiacomo, I., De Besi, L., Serafini, E. *et al.* (1984) Hyperprolacinemia and sexual disturbances among uremic women on hemodialysis. *Nephron*, **37**, 195–9.
9. Rizzoni, G., Ehrich, J.H.H., Broyer, M. *et al.* (1992) Successful pregnancies in women on renal replacement therapy Report from the EDTA Registry. *Nephrol. Dial. Transplant.*, **7**, 279–87.
10. Lim, V.S., Henriquez, C., Sieversten, G. and Frohman, L.A. (1980) Ovarian dysfunction in chronic renal failure: Evidence suggesting hypothalamic anovulation. *Ann. Intern. Med.*, **93**, 21–7.
11. Scharer, K., Schaefer, F., Trott, M. *et al.* (1989) Pubertal development in children with chronic renal failure, in *Growth and Endocrine Changes in Children and Adolescents with Chronic Renal Failure. Pediatric and Adolescent Endocrinology* (ed. K. Scharer), Karger, Basle, pp. 151–68.
12. Mitchell, R., Schaefer, F., Morris, I.D. *et al.* (1993) Elevated serum immunoreactive inhibin levels in peripubertal boys with chronic renal failure. *Clin. Endocrinol.*, **39**, 27–33.
13. Schaefer, F., Seidel, C., Mitchell, R. *et al.* (1991) Pulsatile immunoreactive and bioactive luteinising hormone secretion in pubertal patients with chronic renal failure. *Pediatr. Nephrol.*, **5**, 566–71.
14. Wallace, E.Z., Rosman, P., Toshav, N. *et al.* (1980) Pituitary–adrenocortical function in chronic renal failure: studies of episodic secretion and dexamethasone suppressibility. *J. Clin. Endocrinol. Metab.*, **50**, 46–51.
15. Grant, A.C., Rodger, R.S.C., Mitchell, R. *et al.* (1993) Hypothalamo–pituitary–adrenal axis in uremia: evidence for primary adrenal dysfunction? *Nephrol. Dial. Transplant.*, **8**, 307–10.
16. Rosman, P.M., Faraz, A., Peckman, R. *et al.* (1982) Pituitary adrenocortical function in chronic renal failure: blunted suppression and early escape of plasma cortisol levels after intravenous dexamethasone. *J. Clin. Endocrinol. Metab.*, **54**, 528–33.
17. Kaptein, E.M., Quion–Verde, H., Chooljian, C.J. *et al.* (1988) The thyroid in end–stage renal disease. *Medicine*, **67**, 187–97.
18. Wartosky, L. and Burman, K.D. (1982) Alterations in thyroid function in patients with cysteine illness: the euthyroid sick syndrome. *Endocr. Rev.*, **3**, 164–217.
19. Krogerush, L.J. and Sarna, L.S. (1996) Recombinant human growth hormone treatment. *Transplantation*, **61**, 898–903.
20. Verger, M., Verger, C., Hatt–Magnien, D. *et al.* (1987)

Relationships between thyroid hormones and nutrition in chronic renal failure. *Nephron*, **45**, 211–15.

21. Mak, R.H.K. and De Fronzo, R.A. (1992) Glucose and insulin metabolism in uremia. *Nephron*, **61**, 377–82.

22. Heaton, A., Johnston, D.G., Haigh, J.W. *et al.* (1985) 24 h hormonal and metabolic rhythm in uraemic patients before and during CAPD. *Clin. Sci.*, **69**, 449–57.

23. Schaefer, F., Hamill, G., Stanhope, R. *et al.* (1991) Pulsatile growth hormone secretion in peripubertal patients with chronic renal failure. *J. Pediatr.*, **119**, 568–77.

24. Blum, W.F., Ranke, M.B., Kietzmann, K. *et al.* (1991) GH resistance and inhibition of somatomedin activity by excess insulin like growth factor binding protein in uremia. *Pediatr. Nephrol.*, **5**, 539–44.

25. Shaefer, F. and Mehls, O. (1994) Endocrine, metabolic and growth disorders, in *Pediatric Nephrology* (eds M.A. Holliday, T.A. Barratt and E.D. Auner), Williams & Wilkins, Baltimore, pp. 1241–86.

26. Baumann, G., Shaw, M.A. and Amburn, K. (1989) Regulation of plasma growth hormone binding proteins in health and disease. *Metabolism*, **38**, 683–9.

27. Castellano, M., Turconi, A., Chaler E. *et al.* (1996) Thyroid fonction and serum thyroid binding proteins in pre-pubertal and pubertal children with chronic renal insufficiency receiving conservative treatment undergoing hemodialysis or receiving care after renal transplantation. *J. Pediatr.*, **128**, 784–90.

28. Rudmann, D., Feller, A.G., Nagraj, H.S. *et al.* (1990) Effects of human growth hormone in men over 60 years old. *N. Engl. J. Med.*, **323**, 1–6.

29. Ikizler, T.A., Wingard, R.L. and Breyer, J.A. (1994) Short–term effects of recombinant human growth hormone in CAPD patients. *Kidney Int.*, **46**, 1178–83.

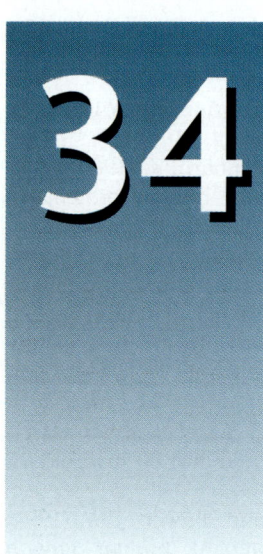

34

Neurological and psychiatric disorders

David J. Burn and David Bates

Introduction

Since the introduction of renal dialysis and transplantation 35 years ago, the neuropsychiatric disorders associated with renal impairment have changed from those produced by the untreated uremic state, to those which reflect the effects of the therapy, and the improved survival of the patients.

There are central and peripheral nervous system manifestations of acute and chronic renal failure. In addition, psychiatric disturbances may occur in the uremic state. Some conditions, such as diabetes mellitus and the systemic vasculitides, may produce both neuropsychiatric and renal disorders. The therapy of renal failure is associated with neuropsychiatric problems, some of which overlap with the untreated state, and some of which are unique to the treatment.

This chapter will concentrate upon the central and peripheral manifestations of the uremic state. Neurological disorders relating to the primary renal disease will then be considered, and in particular the neurological complications associated with diabetes. Finally, the neuropsychiatric complications of dialysis and renal transplantation will be discussed.

Central manifestations of the uremic state

Uremic encephalopathy

This term identifies the organic brain syndrome which occurs in patients with untreated renal failure and in association with dialysis. Uremic encephalopathy is usually more severe and progresses more rapidly in patients with an acute deterioration in renal function, whereas those with chronic renal impairment show a more gradual decline. The clinical course is characterized by variability from day to day, or even hour to hour. The early symptoms may be subtle, and comprise fatigue, apathy, clumsiness and impaired concentration. The patient may lose interest, so that repeated prompting may be required to elicit an answer; serial seven testing is useful to reveal loss of attention span. As the encephalopathy worsens, the patient may become emotionally labile, more obviously forgetful and sluggish, make perceptual errors, and develop sleep inversion (daytime sleepiness and nocturnal wakefulness). 'Frontal lobe' symptoms are manifest by impaired abstract thinking and behavioral change. In the late stages of uremic encephalopathy the patient may be delirious, with visual hallucinations, disorientation, and agitation, which evolves into torpor, preterminal coma and convulsions. Convulsions are invariable as a late feature of the uremic state and are usually generalized

Nephrology, Edited by Rex L. Jamison and Robert Wilkinson.
Published in 1997 by Chapman & Hall, London. ISBN 0 412 60930 4

tonic–clonic in type, although focal motor seizures are also common. Meningism, with nuchal rigidity and Kernig's sign, occurs in approximately one-third of patients.

Multifocal myoclonus and asterixis (a form of negative myoclonus, derived from the Greek *sterigma*, which means (*a*-, without) support), as well as a coarse postural and kinetic tremor characterize the later stages of the encephalopathy. Paratonia (gegenhalten, an involuntary and variable resistance to passive movement), grasp and palmomental reflexes (elicited by scratching the thenar eminence and observing contraction of the ipsilateral mentalis muscle) provide further evidence of frontal lobe dysfunction. Limb tone is usually increased in uremic coma, with hyperreflexia, ankle clonus and extensor plantar responses. The signs may be asymmetric, with frank hemiparesis occurring in up to 45% of patients. These signs may alternate sides during the course of the illness (so-called 'alternating hemiparesis').

In patients who have been treated with renal replacement therapy the severe manifestations of uremic encephalopathy are fortunately rare. Nevertheless, sluggishness, memory impairment and sleep disturbances are not uncommon and may lead to impaired quality of life. A number of studies have compared the effectiveness of chronic hemodialysis and continuous ambulatory peritoneal dialysis regimens on these symptoms, using both neuropsychological and neurophysiological parameters. The evidence appears to be that patients receiving either form of replacement therapy show significant deviations from normal controls in areas of attention/response speed, learning and memory and perceptual coding. Choice reaction time, which measures sustained attention, as well as speed of decision making, may be the most useful test to determine subtle cognitive impairment in uremia. The method of dialysis appears to make little or no difference to the neuropsychological parameters tested.

The investigation of uremic encephalopathy

The level of azotemia correlates poorly with the degree of neurological dysfunction, with widely varying blood urea values occurring in patients with similar symptoms. Laboratory blood tests confirm the patient has renal impairment, but do not exclude other causes for the encephalopathy, and provide little help in monitoring the neurological progress. Cerebrospinal fluid (CSF) analysis in the uremic patient with meningism may reveal an aseptic meningitis, with up to 250 lymphocytes and polymorphonuclear leukocytes per mm^3. The CSF protein may also be elevated up to 1.0 g/l (normal range up to 0.5 g/l).

Cerebral imaging with computed tomography (CT) or magnetic resonance imaging (MRI) of the patient with uremic encephalopathy is usually unhelpful, although it will exclude other causes of confusion, such as subdural

hematoma or hydrocephalus. Chronic renal impairment may be associated with cerebral atrophy. With MRI reversible signal changes (low signal intensity of T_1 weighted and high signal on T_2 weighted images) in the basal ganglia, periventricular white matter and internal capsule have been described in chronic uremic encephalopathy; the lesions disappear after dialysis. They are of uncertain significance and have not been widely reported.

The elecroencephalogram (EEG) is usually most abnormal in the acute encephalopathic state, within 48 h of the onset of renal failure. There is a generalized slowing of the EEG, most marked frontally, with an excess of delta and theta waves. In chronic renal failure the changes are less dramatic. As the uremic state progresses, the EEG becomes slower, with a reasonable correlation between the percentage of frequencies below 7 Hz and the increase in serum creatinine. Bilateral spike and wave complexes, in the absence of evident clinical seizure activity, have been reported in up to 14% of chronic renal failure patients.

The differential diagnosis of uremic encephalopathy

The diagnosis of uremic encephalopathy is usually straightforward, on the basis of history and examination, supported by appropriate laboratory findings. Hypertensive encephalopathy may, however, also produce seizures, focal neurological signs, delirium and stupor. Some helpful discriminating points are that uremic encephalopathy rarely causes papilledema, arterial spasm on fundoscopy, cortical blindness, or a substantial increase in CSF protein level. Hypertensive encephalopathy may cause all of these changes and produce more rapid fluctuations and fleeting neurological signs.

The hypercoagulable state associated with the nephrotic syndrome may lead to cerebral dural and venous thrombosis. The thrombosis may be extensive and become manifest with headache, vomiting, papilledema and focal neurological signs. If diagnostic doubt exists, MRI scanning is sensitive at detecting this problem, obviating the need for angiography.

A number of drugs, especially in the presence of renal impairment, may also produce an encephalopathy. Some of these drugs are listed in Table 34.1. A thorough review of the agents the patient is taking is essential.

Intercurrent infections and subdural hematomas are more common in the patient with renal impairment and should be excluded by appropriate neuroimaging and CSF analysis.

The pathophysiology of uremic encephalopathy

The pathophysiology of uremic encephalopathy is uncertain. Pathology studies have been unhelpful, since the changes found in the brain of patients dying with chronic

Category of drug	Examples
Cardiovascular drugs	Digitalis, amiodarone, β-blockers
Anticholinergic drugs	Benzhexol, tricyclic antidepressants
Tranquilizers and hypnotics	Benzodiazepines, phenothiazines
Antimicrobial drugs	Isoniazid, acyclovir, penicillin, cephalosporins, sulfonamides
Anticonvulsants	Phenytoin, sodium valproate
Anti-ulcer drugs	Cimetidine, ranitidine

Table 34.1 Drugs which may cause a toxic confusional state, with or without the presence of renal impairment

renal impairment are often mild, non-specific, and relate more to concomitant illnesses. There is no correlation between commonly measured indicators of renal failure and the severity of encephalopathy.

A number of findings have emerged from studies of uremic encephalopathy. The calcium content of the cerebral cortex is almost twice that of the normal value. This increase may be mediated by parathyroid hormone (PTH) activity, an effect probably independent of cyclic AMP. In dogs with experimentally induced acute or chronic renal failure, both EEG and brain calcium abnormalities may be prevented by parathyroidectomy. Also, in humans with renal failure, both EEG and psychological abnormalities may be improved following parathyroidectomy.

In renal impairment, the metabolic rate of the brain is reduced and this is, in turn, associated with a decrease in cerebral oxygen consumption. These changes occur despite normal levels of high-energy phosphates. One possibility which could explain these changes is a reduction in neurotransmission, leading to a reduction in metabolic activity. Synaptosomal preparations include vesicles derived from presynaptic terminals and allow the activities of the sodium/calcium exchanger and calcium ATPase pumps to be studied. These two pumps export calcium from excitable cells and are important in maintaining the calcium gradient of $10\,000:1$ (outside–inside cells) which normally exists. In the presence of uremia, there is a PTH-dependent enhancement of calcium transport by both transporter mechanisms. A number of studies have suggested that the ouabain-sensitive Na,K-ATPase pump activity is decreased in both acute and chronic uremic states. Since this pump is ultimately important in the release of neurotransmitters such as the biogenic amines, this could help to explain impaired synaptic function, and the reduction in the concentration of neurotransmitters which have been found in uremic rats.

Further evidence of impaired synaptic function in uremia comes from studies of the inhibitory effects of guanidino compounds, especially guanidinosuccinic acid, on the release of gamma-aminobutyric acid (GABA)

and glycine in animal models. These toxins, which are elevated in brain and CSF in renal failure, probably impair the release of neurotransmitters by blocking neuronal membrane chloride channels. In addition, methylguanidine has been shown to inhibit Na,K-ATPase pump activity.

Finally, the role of aluminum in chronic uremic encephalopathy is still uncertain; the balance of current evidence suggests that it is likely to be involved in producing a gradual deterioration in cerebral function over a prolonged period of time. The source of the metal is likely to be from diet and phosphate-binding drugs. Transport of aluminum into the brain almost certainly occurs via transferrin receptors on the lumen of brain capillaries. Once in the brain the aluminum may affect the expression or processing of the β/A4 precursor protein which, via a complex cascade of events, may lead to extracellular deposition of amyloidogenic β/A4 protein in senile plaques. It is unlikely, however, that the pathology so induced merely represents an Alzheimer-like change, since neurofibrillary tangles, which characterize Alzheimer's disease, are not commonly found in the cerebral cortex of renal dialysis patients.

The pathophysiology of uremic encephalopathy is therefore a complex and probably multifactorial process, with initial problems most likely to reflect a functional, primarily neurotransmission defect. Subsequent dysfunction may be due to increasingly evident histopathological change, and aluminum seems to be of key importance in this process.

Peripheral manifestations of the uremic state

Uremic neuropathy

This complication was probably first reported in 1863 by Kussmaul, who described a patient with weakness of the lower limbs in the presence of apparent kidney failure. Examination of the sciatic nerve at post-mortem revealed degeneration of peripheral nerve fibers.

Neuropathy occurs in up to 70% of patients who require therapy for chronic renal failure. Inexplicably, peripheral neuropathy in children with chronic renal failure is uncommon. The condition has an unexplained male predominance, and has a varied course, both in progression and severity. The classical uremic neuropathy is distal, sensorimotor and predominantly axonal. Clinically a typical 'glove and stocking' sensory loss is present, with distal muscle wasting and weakness, most pronounced in the lower limbs. Burning sensations in the feet or occasionally band-like sensations may be early sensory features, whereas weakness of foot dorsiflexion is usually the first motor complaint. Loss of the ankle jerk and impaired vibration sense in the feet are frequent early signs of uremic neuropathy. As the condition advances, wasting, weakness and ascending sensory disturbance become more pronounced. Although usually 'mixed' (i.e. sensorimotor in type), cases of either pure sensory or pure motor neuropathy have been reported.

In addition to the characteristic symmetrical distal sensorimotor polyneuropathy, isolated mononeuropathies, particularly carpal tunnel syndrome, are common in the uremic state. Although this may be due to vascular steal syndromes from forearm access shunts in some cases, such problems also occur in the non-hemodialyzed patient and presumably reflect an increased susceptibility to pressure palsies, due to a subclinical neuropathy.

The eighth cranial nerve (vestibulocochlear) is the most commonly affected cranial nerve in uremia. Variable hearing loss and occasionally complete deafness are reported, which may reverse with dialysis or renal transplantation. Primarily uremia-induced hearing deficits must be distinguished from the ototoxic effects of aminoglycoside antibiotics and other drugs, as well as conditions associated with hereditary hearing loss and nephropathy.

The investigation of uremic neuropathy

Serum creatinine and urea levels generally correlate poorly with the degree of clinical involvement. If, however, the degree of neuropathy is markedly out of proportion to the level of renal impairment, this should lead to a search for co-existing causes of neuropathy (such as drugs, e.g. nitrofurantoin).

Despite the pathology of uremic neuropathy (see below), a slowing of proximal nerve conduction (mainly reflecting the functional integrity of myelin in large axons) is the earliest neurophysiological finding, and may occur in the absence of a clinically evident neuropathy. Subsequently, as axonal loss and secondary demyelination occur, there is a decline in both conduction velocity and nerve action potential amplitude, which generally parallel the degree of clinical and pathological impairment. The CSF is rarely abnormal in uremic neuropathy, unless there is concomitant encephalopathy (see above).

The pathophysiology of uremic neuropathy

The condition has a predilection for large-diameter axons, with relative sparing of the unmyelinated and small myelinated afferent neurons. Post-mortem studies have confirmed the following changes: marked loss of axons and fiber breakdown in the distal nerve trunks of the legs with less severe changes proximally, normal spinal roots and degeneration in the cervical portion of the dorsal columns. Anterior horn cells are intact but may show chromatolytic changes. Paranodal demyelination and separation of the myelin sheath from the axolemma are also found, but are considered to be secondary to the primary axonal damage.

There is good evidence that uremic neuropathy is caused by retained, dialyzable toxins normally excreted by the kidneys. Uremic peripheral neuropathy does not develop if the glomerular filtration rate remains above approximately 12 ml/min. The neuropathy is reversed, at least partially, by dialysis and dramatically by renal transplantation. The so-called 'middle molecule hypothesis', with accumulation of one (or several) neurotoxic molecules of molecular weight 300–2000 which are slowly dialyzable, has been a popular explanation for the genesis of uremic neuropathy. There are so many potential candidates, however, that no one substance has yet been convincingly demonstrated to show a close correlation between plasma and tissue levels and the severity of the polyneuropathy. Compounds considered as candidates include guanidino compounds, polyamines, phenol derivatives, *myo*-inositol and parathyroid hormone. Enzyme inhibition by toxins has also been studied, particularly the enzymes transketolase, pyridoxal phosphate kinase and Na,K-ATPase. It may be that the etiopathogenesis of the neuropathy is multifactorial, explaining the apparent lack of correlation with any one parameter.

Treatment of uremic neuropathy

Following the institution of dialysis, mild neuropathies may clinically resolve completely, although impaired nerve conduction usually persists on neurophysiological testing. Severe cases slowly improve but do not fully recover, even after several years of dialysis. Paradoxically, a few patients have been reported to worsen on commencing dialysis. There is no good evidence that hemodialysis or continuous ambulatory peritoneal dialysis are superior to one another in treating uremic neuropathy.

Successful renal transplantation leads to a resolution of all but the most severe cases of neuropathy, with a dramatic improvement in neurophysiological parameters. Rapid recovery occurs in the first three months, followed by a slower phase over nine months to a year. Sensory symptoms and signs disappear within days to weeks in many cases. Wasting and weakness are next to improve, with deep tendon reflexes recovering last of all. It appears that uremia-related autonomic dysfunction and deafness are largely reversible within two years of transplantation.

Autonomic neuropathy

Autonomic dysfunction in uremia is usually mild and present only in severe cases. Parasympathetic involvement tends to be most pronounced: disturbance of sweating in the upper limbs has been reported. Further, occasionally troublesome, symptoms suggestive of autonomic failure are diarrhea, impotence and orthostatic light-headedness.

Postural hypotension, abnormalities in the Valsalva response and to induced hypotension, and abnormal heart-rate and blood-pressure responses to standing have also been documented in patients on chronic hemodialysis. However, autonomic neuropathy does not appear to be the only explanation for the sustained hypotension that may occur in some hemodialysis patients. The most likely sites of primary damage responsible for the autonomic dysfunction are the baroreceptors or their afferent fibers, or central nervous system (CNS) connections, since the efferent sympathetic system appears to be intact.

Myopathic disturbance in the uremic state

Myopathic disturbances may be associated with disorders of vitamin D metabolism, increased urinary calcium loss, phosphate depletion and PTH excess. Given the complex situation that exists in chronic renal failure, with reduced levels of 1,25-dihydroxycholecalciferol, hypocalcemia, hyperphosphatemia and hyperparathyroidism, myopathic dysfunction in the uremic state represents a combination of metabolic effects on skeletal muscle. The clinical picture, however, is similar to that produced by primary hyperparathyroidism and osteomalacia: proximal limb weakness and wasting occur, leading to a 'waddling' gait, with bone pain and tenderness adding to the functional incapacity. In the absence of a peripheral neuropathy, the knee jerks are preserved or even brisk.

Serum creatine kinase estimations are usually normal, whereas neurophysiological studies show a myopathic pattern without positive waves or fibrillations. Muscle biopsy yields non-specific findings, with type 2 ('fast-twitch') fiber atrophy.

The pathophysiology of the myopathy associated with chronic renal failure is poorly understood and probably multifactorial: PTH enhances muscle proteolysis and impairs energy production, transfer and utilization. Vitamin D has been shown to influence muscle contractility in rodents, possibly via the calcium-binding component of the troponin complex. The vitamin also accelerates protein synthesis and increases muscle ATP concentration. Some, but not all, patients with chronic renal impairment and myopathy respond to large doses of vitamin D.

Gangrenous calcification is a rare, but sometimes fatal complication of chronic renal failure. In this condition there is ischemia of skin and muscle due to a widespread deposition of calcium in the media and external elastic lamina of the arterial wall. A painful myopathy may ensue, with muscle necrosis and myoglobinuria.

Neurological disorders relating to the primary renal disease

This is a very extensive topic and attention is here briefly drawn to the variety of disorders which produce renal impairment and which are also associated with specific neurological dysfunction. Some of these conditions are shown in Table 34.2.

In diseases such as systemic lupus erythematosus the neuropsychiatric manifestations are protean, and the diagnosis is often arrived at through a process of exclusion: patients therefore require a battery of neurological investigations such as MRI scanning, CSF analysis, EEG and neuropsychometry.

As mentioned above, a careful check should always be made of the drugs a patient may be taking for the primary renal complaint, since these may lead to neurological complications in their own right.

Diabetes mellitus

Diabetes is the most common cause of end-stage renal failure and the neurological sequelae of this disorder are among the most frequent and severe that a nephrologist has to deal with. Some of the central and peripheral neurological disturbances caused by diabetes are therefore considered below. The neurological complications of insulin-dependent and non-insulin-dependent diabetes are similar and no further distinction between these two forms is made here. The incidence of neurological problems associated with diabetes is linked to the incidence of other complications, including nephropathy and retinopathy.

Peripheral disorders associated with diabetes

Diabetes is primarily associated with disorders of the peripheral nervous system, specifically peripheral and autonomic neuropathies. The prevalence of diabetic peripheral neuropathy varies from 10 to 50%, depending upon the series quoted. The precise figure is unknown, largely because of difficulties in defining the denominator in the prevalence data (for example, clinic-based studies exclude 'mild' cases looked after by their general practitioner) and because of the lack of agreed minimal criteria for the definition of diabetic peripheral neuropathy.

Table 34.2 Examples of conditions associated with renal impairment and specific neuropsychiatric involvement. The neuropsychiatric complications listed are not exhaustive, and only those most commonly associated with the condition are included

Condition	Renal lesion	Neuropsychiatric complications
Congenital disease		
Polycystic kidney disease	Polycystic kidneys	Intracranial aneurysm/subarachnoid hemorrhage
Metabolic disease		
e.g. Wilson's disease	Proximal and distal tubular dysfunction, nephrocalcinosis	Dystonia, dysarthria, dementia, Parkinsonism, psychosis
Fabry disease	Proteinuria, edema	'Young stroke', peripheral neuropathy
Inflammatory disease		
Sarcoidosis	Nephrocalcinosis, granulomatous interstitial nephritis	Cranial and peripheral neuropathies, basal meningitis, focal intracranial lesions, myopathy
Vasculitides, e.g.		
Wegener's granulomatosis	Focal and segmental necrotizing glomerulonephritis	Focal vasculitis, direct granulomatous extension, mononeuritis multiplex
Polyarteritis nodosa	Related to vasculitis and glomerulonephritis	Peripheral neuropathy, encephalopathy, stroke
Systemic lupus erythematosus	Lupus nephritis: varying patterns of involvement	Dementia, psychosis, seizures, coma, stroke and other focal neurological deficits

Table 34.3 A clinical classification of diabetic neuropathy

Symmetry of neuropathy	Neuropathies included
Symmetrical distal neuropathy	Small fiber predominant (painful or anesthetic)
	Large fiber predominant (ataxic or pseudotabetic)
	Autonomic neuropathy
Asymmetrical neuropathy	Cranial neuropathies
	Plexopathies (including amyotrophy)
	Mono- and polyradiculopathies
	Increased susceptibility to pressure palsies

Pathogenesis of diabetic peripheral neuropathy

The pathogenesis of diabetic peripheral neuropathy is unknown, with debate centering around metabolic and ischemic–hypoxic factors. Metabolic abnormalities include nerve cell hyperglycemia, which, via increased flux through the polyol pathway catalyzed by aldose reductase, raises neuronal levels of sorbitol and other alcohol sugars. *Myo*-inositol concentrations, on the other hand, are reduced. Vascular factors include reduced nerve blood flow, endoneurial capillary abnormalities, increased endoneurial vascular resistance and reduced endoneurial oxygen tension. Current evidence suggests that ischemic–hypoxic factors are of primary early importance in the causation of diabetic peripheral neuropathy.

Clinical features of diabetic-related peripheral neuropathies

A clinical classification of diabetic-related peripheral neuropathies is shown in Table 34.3. The clinical patterns of several of these neuropathies are considered briefly bleow.

Distal symmetrical neuropathy

This is the most common type of diabetic peripheral neuropathy. Initial symptoms are sensory and may be either positive (burning, pricking pains, supersensitivity, band-like sensations etc.) or negative (numbness 'like cotton wool' etc). If nociception is impaired, due to a relatively selective involvement of small myelinated and unmyelinated peripheral nerves, patients may present with painless metatarsal head ulcers or even Charcot joints of the ankle or foot (painless, but radiologically marked, disorganization of the joint). Predominant large fiber involvement leads to a loss of joint position sense, which symptomatically is worse with the eyes closed or in the dark (sensory ataxia or pseudotabetic presentation), and evolving distal weakness.

Autonomic neuropathy

Many patients with a distal symmetrical neuropathy will have symptoms attributable to autonomic dysfunction, if carefully questioned. These are usually minor, however. Although severe autonomic dysfunction due to diabetes is relatively uncommon, the frequency is probably higher in uremic diabetic patients, and is associated with reduced survivorship. Autonomic failure means that patients do not appreciate several of the somatic symptoms of hypoglycemia which are sympathetically mediated.

Pupillary abnormalities are usually asymptomatic; the pupil becomes small and fails to react to light and/or accommodation. Loss of sweating is common and may lead to impaired thermoregulation in hot climates. Elderly patients in particular may present with orthostatic hypotension, which is exacerbated by fluid depletion. A resting tachycardia is an early sign of cardiovascular involvement and is due to cardiac vagal autonomic dysfunction.

Gastroparesis and diarrhea are the two most commonly encountered gastrointestinal problems in diabetic autonomic neuropathy. The former problem may be asymptomatic, may present acutely with nausea and vomiting, or chronically, with vomiting of food eaten over 12 h previously. The diarrhea results from disordered small intestinal motility and may also be triggered by bacterial overgrowth. It is characteristically explosive, painless and watery, occurring mainly at night. Bouts of diarrhea may be interspersed with resistant constipation. It is, of course, important to exclude other gastrointestinal problems, such as colonic malignancies, before attributing the above problems to autonomic neuropathy.

Genitourinary problems may also occur. Impotence in men is particularly common and may be either due to erectile failure or failure of ejaculation.

Acute painful neuropathy with weight loss

This condition is associated with either poorly controlled diabetes or following the institution of tighter control. Weight loss may be up to 50% of original body weight. The pain is of rapid onset, burning or stinging in quality and primarily distal in site. Improvement occurs in 6–24 months when weight begins to increase.

Diabetic radiculopathy/ polyradiculopathy/plexopathy

These disorders often occur in relatively long-standing cases, and are uncommon in patients below the age of 40. A typical syndrome is the painful, unilateral truncal radiculopathy, with minimal accompanying sensory loss or weakness. A number of underlying visceral disturbances are often suspected if this condition is not recognized.

A characteristic polyradicular or plexopathic disorder is the so-called 'diabetic amyotrophy' which affects the upper lumbar plexus or roots. Patients present with severe anterior thigh pain, loss of muscle bulk in the quadriceps and buckling at the knee as the extensor mechanism weakens. There may also be significant weight loss which in the older patient may necessitate a search for underlying compressive lesions secondary to malignancy. The prognosis is excellent, with resolution of pain and weakness in a period of weeks to months.

Cranial neuropathy

Painless, pupil-sparing third nerve palsies and sixth nerve palsies are the characteristic diabetic-related cranial neuropathies.

Investigation of diabetic peripheral neuropathy

The investigation of a suspected diabetic peripheral neuropathy involves nerve conduction and electromyographic studies primarily. If the neuropathy is selectively small-fiber in type, conventional neurophysiological studies may be unhelpful. There are no pathognomonic findings to point to a diabetic cause for a peripheral neuropathy, so differentiation from uremic neuropathy may be difficult, particularly since both neuropathies are predominantly axonal. A full battery of autonomic function tests may also be required if significant autonomic symptoms are present.

Treatment of diabetic peripheral neuropathy

The symptomatic treatment of diabetic peripheral and autonomic neuropathy is currently all that can be offered. A number of treatments aimed at slowing down or reversing the underlying pathogenetic process, such as aldose reductase inhibitors, have proved largely disappointing. It is self-evident that meticulous attention to both diabetic control and the dialysis regimen is essential. Patients must be educated with regard to foot care. Physiotherapy may be very helpful in recovery following an acute plexopathy or radiculopathy. Pharmacologically, carbamazepine is useful if pain is lancinating or lightning in character, whereas amitriptyline is more suited to the treatment of persistent burning pain. Both drugs should be commenced in low doses initially.

Autonomic symptoms, especially orthostatic hypotension, may be difficult to treat. If orthostatism requires therapy, any potentially exacerbating factors should first be excluded, especially fluid depletion. Raising the bed head at night and avoiding late meals and alcohol may give some improvement. Pharmacological therapy in the renal patient is limited since several routinely used drugs rely on functioning nephrons, but the use of midodrine, an alpha receptor agonist, may be considered. Caution is required, however, in the treatment of postural hypotension because of the risks of severe supine hypertension. Gastroparesis may respond to domperidone (in reduced dosage) or metoclopramide. Erythromycin may also be helpful, probably as a result of its motilin-like activity. A percutaneous endoscopic gastrojejunostomy is advocated by some for intractable gastroparetic symptoms. Diarrhea may cease with broad-spectrum antibiotic treatment, but if this fails, loperamide or clonidine may be tried. Constipation is also treated with metoclopramide or domperidone.

Central disorders associated with diabetes

Diabetic ketoacidosis

Diabetic ketoacidosis (DKA) is a major cause of morbidity and mortality, especially in the younger patient. Despite therapeutic improvements, the mortality has remained largely unchanged at about 10% over the past 25 years, mainly due to neurological complications. DKA is characterized biochemically by hyperglycemia, dehydration and metabolic acidosis, and results from either accidental or intentional hypoinsulinism. Focal neurological signs such as hemiparesis and seizures are not uncommon, and 10% of cases progress to coma.

The underlying mechanisms behind the encephalopathy are not completely understood but serum hyperosmolality is certainly a significant contributing factor. Acidosis is unlikely to play a major role in most cases, since brain pH is well buffered. Infusion of β-hydroxybutyrate, the main ketone body present in DKA, into experimental animals does not induce coma. Toxic levels of lysolecithins and non-esterified fatty acids, or a primary defect in carbohydrate metabolism, are also possible contributing factors toward producing the encephalopathy.

The onset of cerebral edema after an initially good response to treatment is the most feared neurological complication in the management of DKA. Over 95% of cases occur in those aged under 20 years. At 2–24 h after treatment has started there is a sudden deterioration in the condition of the patient, with headache, confusion, incontinence and signs of transtentorial herniation with respiratory then cardiac arrest. The condition has a mortality in excess of 90%, with severe sequelae in those who survive. If given early, mannitol is the only conventional treatment that may help.

It is impossible to predict those who will develop cerebral edema, since the precise pathogenesis is unclear. 'Idiogenic osmoles', trapped within the CNS, and generated initially to counterbalance serum hyperosmolality, are thought to lead to fluid shifts into the brain as the serum osmolality is reduced. It is therefore advisable to use slow fluid replacement and low dose insulin (10 U/h) regimens as prophylactic measures.

Non-ketotic hyperosmolar coma

Non-ketotic hyperosmolar coma (NKC) is characterized by significant degrees of hyperglycemia, hyperosmolality and dehydration, usually in the elderly patient, without ketone body formation. The onset of NKC is insidious, and often provoked by intercurrent illness, combined with relative hypoinsulinism. In the renal patient, hypertonic peritoneal dialysis, infection and use of drugs known to interfere with insulin secretion or action (for example, β-blockers and diuretics) may be important triggers. In comparison with DKA, the frequency of seizures and coma is much higher in NKC. Stroke-like episodes may also occur. Level of consciousness is reasonably well correlated with serum osmolality, with values of less than 350 mosmol/l being associated with alertness in most cases. Adequate rehydration using normal or half-normal saline, a proper dosage of insulin, and treatment of intercurrent illness are the cornerstones for the management of NKC. The mortality of NKC is high, at around 40–50%, largely because of associated medical illness and delay in diagnosis.

Hypoglycemia

Hypoglycemia results from either accidental or intentional hyperinsulinism. Accidental insulin overdose may occur in the renal patient who adds insulin to their peritoneal dialysate, particularly if their vision is impaired secondary to retinopathy. Spontaneous, mild postprandial hypoglycemia may occur in patients with chronic renal failure. The warning 'sympathetic' phase of a hypoglycemic attack may be lost if there is an associated autonomic neuropathy.

Symptoms of neuroglycopenia include confusion and erratic behavior, seizures, focal signs, including reversible stroke-like events, choreoathetosis and coma. Rapid correction of blood glucose levels is the main priority in the treatment of hypoglycemia, and complete recovery is the rule, even after an hour or more of coma. Recurrent daily or nocturnal hypoglycemic attacks may lead to dementia, however. Prolonged and profound hypoglycemia leads to neuronal damage in the cerebral and cerebellar cortices as well as hippocampus, analagous to the areas that are damaged in ischemic–hypoxic brain injury. The mechanism for such neuronal loss is probably mediated via raised intracellular calcium and increased excitatory neurotransmitter levels.

Cerebrovascular disease

Stroke is 2 to 6 times more common in diabetics than in non-diabetics, and is involved in about 25% of diabetic deaths. Increased risk is largely mediated via a higher incidence of atherosclerosis and hypertension in diabetic patients. In the uremic patient hypertension is also common, thereby compounding the increased stroke risk in diabetic patients with renal failure. Hemorrhagic stroke frequency is not increased in the diabetic population, however.

Large post-mortem series have indicated 1.5–2.0 times the incidence of infarcts, particularly in deep hemispheric areas, suggesting small vessel disease. This increase in infarcts over non-diabetics was most apparent in cases below 60 years of age. Such infarcts are mediated by the interaction of hypertension and accelerated arteriolosclerosis.

Population-based prospective studies, such as the Framingham study, have confirmed that diabetes carries an increased relative risk for stroke of about 2 times normal, separate from other risk factors such as hypertension, obesity and hyperlipidemia. In addition, resulting neurological deficit tends to be greater, and survivorship poorer, in diabetic stroke.

Neurological disorders associated with dialysis

Dialysis dysequilibrium syndrome

Dialysis dysequilibrium syndrome (DDS) refers to a constellation of symptoms and signs that may occur during or after peritoneal dialysis or hemodialysis. The condition was first recognized in the 1960s when patients with severe uremia were often rapidly dialyzed over short periods of time. In its mildest form DDS may comprise only restlessness, muscle cramps, nausea and a severe throbbing headache. Patients with a prior diagnosis of migrainous-type headaches may find identical headaches occur during dialysis. Symptoms generally occur towards the end of dialysis and subside over several hours. A more advanced form of DDS is characterized by myoclonus, and delirium. These problems may persist for several days. In its most severe, and life-threatening form, DDS may produce generalized seizures, papilledema, raised intraocular pressure and cardiac arrthymias. Such features are now extremely uncommon, with most deaths from DDS being reported prior to 1970. Nowadays if a patient undergoing dialysis becomes obtunded or comatose, DDS is a diagnosis of exclusion and other disorders, such as intracranial bleeding and infection, should be sought first.

A number of early studies examined CT brain (parenchymal density) and EEG (increased slow waves burst) changes due to presumed DDS; these are of limited help and the diagnosis is primarily a clinical one. Although patients of all ages may develop DDS, children and the elderly have a higher risk.

The pathophysiology of DDS

A popular early theory was the 'reverse urea effect', which proposed that an osmotic gradient was set up between the plasma and brain during rapid dialysis because the shift of urea from brain to plasma lagged behind the removal of plasma urea by dialysis. Water would thus shift into the brain parenchyma as the osmotic gradient developed. Although urea is no longer thought to be responsible for such fluid shifts, Arieff et al. (1977) demonstrated in a uremic dog model that an intracellular acidosis occurs in the brain in association with an increase in unmeasured organic acids (idiogenic osmoles), so producing an osmotic gradient.

The treatment of DDS

Prevention of DDS is largely achieved by 'slow' dialysis, that is, low blood flow rates, at frequent intervals (every one to two days). A further preventative or, indeed, therapeutic measure includes adding osmotically active solute (e.g. urea, glycerol, mannitol, sodium) to the dialysate.

Wernicke's encephalopathy

Wernicke's encephalopathy is an acute syndrome comprising a combination of ophthalmoparesis (including combinations of nystagmus, lateral rectus palsy, conjugate gaze paresis), ataxia, mental changes and areflexia. In a minority of cases the patient may present with a Korsakoff psychosis (comprising defects in anterograde and retrograde memory and confabulation). The encephalopathy is due to deficiency of the water-soluble vitamin thiamine, and is characterized pathologically by petechial hemorrhages and capillary congestion in the hypothalamus and gray matter of the upper brain stem.

Although thiamine might therefore be expected to cross the dialysis membrane with ease, there have been few reports of Wernicke's encephalopathy in patients undergoing chronic dialysis. Studies have in fact indicated that thiamine is not removed by dialysis to any greater degree than that which is normally excreted in urine. This may be due to the tight plasma protein binding of the vitamin. The deficiency state probably only becomes manifest in special circumstances, such as a genetic predisposition, chronically malnourished patients with marked anorexia, and the use of glucose-containing intravenous fluids. A further, and cautionary, factor is that Wernicke's encephalopathy may not present in the classic way in chronic dialysis patients: for example, in one series of five pathologically proven cases ophthalmoplegia was recorded in only one. Other diagnoses were considered in all five cases prior to death, including dialysis dementia, brain-stem stroke and uremic encephalopathy. The disorder may therefore be underdiagnosed in dialysis patients.

Since Wernicke's encephalopathy is a preventable and potentially curable condition, it should be considered in all patients undergoing dialysis with an unexplained neurological picture and especially confusion. Parenteral thiamine should be given, particularly if the patient has developed anorexia or vomiting.

Subdural hematoma

A subdural hematoma is a collection of blood which forms when veins, often draining into the superior sagittal sinus, are torn. Blood oozes out into the space between the dura and arachnoid mater membranes and eventually coagulates with an outer wall of highly vascular granulation tissue which is prone to rebleeding.

Subdural hematomas have been reported in 1.0–3.3% of patients undergoing hemodialysis. All age ranges may be affected. Potentiating factors are coagulation problems associated with the uremic state, and the use of anticoagulants for dialysis. There is frequently no preceding history of trauma noted.

The clinical manifestations are protean and a high index of suspicion is necessary. The patient may be generally obtunded, cognitively impaired and ataxic, with marked day to day fluctuations, or may display focal signs such as hemiparesis. Gait ignition failure (inability to initiate walking) and locomotor failure (with short-stepped gait) may occur with bilateral subdural hematomas, which occur in up to 20% of cases.

The diagnosis is readily made by CT brain scanning, although care is necessary in interpretation if the subdural collections are bilateral and isodense with brain tissue. MRI scanning is an even more sensitive means of confirming the diagnosis, if available.

Treatment of all but the smallest hematomas (which should then be monitored by repeat neuroimaging studies to ensure they are not enlarging) is surgical. Unless irreversible damage has been caused by compressive effects, drainage of the clot is curative.

Dialysis dementia

Dialysis dementia (also known as dialysis encephalopathy, progressive myoclonic dialysis encephalopathy and hemodialysis encephalopathy) was first clearly documented by Alfrey *et al*. The disorder is progressive and is invariably fatal unless treated. Some authorities regard dialysis dementia as part of a multisystem disorder which also embraces vitamin D-resistant osteomalacia, proximal myopathy and non-iron-deficient, microcytic, hypochromic anemia.

In Europe, between 1976 and 1977, the prevalence for dialysis dementia was 600 per 100 000 dialysis patients, although there was a wide variation between different centers (see below). A slight male predominance has been reported. The mean age of those affected in a large series was 50 years, with an age range of 21–68 (Jack *et al.*, 1983–1984). Mean onset of symptoms after hemodialysis had commenced was 35 months in the same series (range 0.5–112 months), which is comparable with other reports. Death occurs at 6–9 months after the onset of symptoms in the majority of untreated cases.

One of the earliest signs of dialysis dementia is a disturbance of speech, with elements of both articulatory difficulties (dysarthria) as well as language problems (dysphasia). Such problems have been reported in up to 95% of dialysis dementia cases. The patient may initially have a stuttering, hesitant speech which only occurs during and immediately after dialysis. Dysgraphia (impaired writing ability) is also common. Other patients may present with either an expressive aphasia (low-output, effortful speech and word finding difficulties), or, less commonly, a receptive dysphasia (fluent speech, with altered words – paraphasias – or nonsense words – neologisms). In the early stages the patient may also be more apathetic and become depressed.

As the disorder progresses, the speech becomes more severely and persistently involved. Myoclonic jerks occur in up to 80% of cases and patients may become both ataxic, as well as developing inability to perform previously learned and familiar motor acts (apraxic).

In the later stages, convulsions develop in up to 60%, psychosis with hallucinations and paranoid delusions may be prominent, and frank dementia is obvious in over 95% of patients. Preterminally, the patient becomes immobile and mute, often succumbing to pneumonia.

The investigation of dialysis dementia

The EEG is of most help in supporting the clinical diagnosis. Abnormalities may actually precede clinically overt symptoms by up to six months. Intermittent bursts of high voltage slowing and spike-and-wave activity are noted, particularly in the frontal leads. Interestingly, the EEG may show an initial deterioration after treatment with deferoxamine has commenced (see below).

Neuroimaging studies and CSF analysis are of no positive help in making the diagnosis of dialysis dementia but are of use in excluding other diagnoses if the clinical picture is atypical. The roles of serum aluminum levels and deferoxamine infusion test are discussed briefly below.

The differential diagnosis of dialysis dementia

When epidemics of dialysis dementia occurred, the clinical diagnosis was invariably made without difficulty. Problems may arise however with continuing, albeit uncommon, cases of sporadic dialysis dementia. The prevalence of such cases has been estimated at around 0.6–1.0% of dialysis patients. Table 34.4 gives several

Table 34.4 Conditions which need to be considered in patients presenting with possible sporadic dialysis dementia

Condition	Investigations to confirm/refute diagnosis
Uremic encephalopathy	Review effectiveness of dialysis regimen
Drug intoxication	Reduce or withdraw suspected agent, EEG
Acute trace element intoxication	Blood levels
Hypercalcemia	Correction of serum calcium, EEG
Wernicke's encephalopathy	Red blood cell transketolase levels, 'Therapeutic trial' of thiamine
Subdural hematoma	CT or MRI brain scan
Normal pressure hydrocephalus	CT or MRI brain scan, lumbar puncture
Prion disease (Creutzfeldt–Jakob disease)	Peripheral blood DNA analysis for prion gene mutation, EEG
Alzheimer's disease	Neuropsychometry, EEG

other diagnoses which need to be considered in these cases, together with other investigations which may be useful if doubt exists.

The pathophysiology of dialysis dementia

Initial observations confirmed a marked disparity between gross clinical abnormalities, yet relatively minor pathological changes. More recently, neurofibrillary material has been found in cortical neurons of patients dying from dialysis dementia. There are considerable differences both in the composition of the tangle material and its distribution compared with Alzheimer's disease.

There is good evidence that aluminum is an essential toxin in the genesis of dialysis dementia, although the precise pathophysiological mechanism is still unclear. An early observation was the marked geographical variation in the incidence of the dementia, raising the possibility of an environmental toxin. Investigators first noted high concentrations of tin and decreased rubidium in the brains of dialysis dementia patients. Further work confirmed an 11-fold increased concentration of aluminum in the cerebral cortex of patients with dialysis dementia, compared with a three-fold increase in non-demented dialysed patients. These findings were rapidly linked to the aluminum concentration in the dialysate water supply. The European Dialysis and Transplant Association determined that 92% of dialysis dementia cases were linked with untreated or 'soft' water, compared with only 6% of cases who had received deionized water. It is now recognized that keeping the aluminum concentration in the water below 10 μg/l by reverse osmosis is not associated with the dementia in an epidemic form. Sporadic cases may relate to the use of aluminum phosphate binders (namely aluminum hydroxide), since even milligram absorption of aluminum binding agents can lead to considerable accumulation. However, since the use of these binders is so widespread, other, as yet unrecognized, factors must be involved, given the rarity of sporadic cases.

How aluminum interferes with neuronal function to cause the dementia, and why the transition between reversible and irreversible brain dysfunction occurs, is still unknown. Table 34.5 lists some of the potential neurotoxic effects of aluminum (several of which have only been demonstrated in *in vitro* models). These are probably not mutually exclusive and multiple mechanisms may operate to produce the clinical picture.

Serum and CSF aluminum levels have been studied for their predictive value in making the diagnosis of dialysis dementia. CSF levels are of absolutely no help, and should not be requested. Serum aluminum levels are of only limited assistance; dialysis dementia has been reported in patients with serum levels ranging from 15 to more than 1000 μg/l (normal range less than 15 μg/l). It may be stated that although the dementia is uncommon with serum levels below 50 μg/l, such levels by no means exclude the diagnosis.

Other workers have investigated the deferoxamine chelation test as a surrogate marker of dialysis dementia. Deferoxamine binds aluminum with greater avidity than plasma protein and tissue binding sites. The chelated complex has a molecular weight of 600 and so is removed by dialysis. The usual test protocol is to infuse deferoxamine (40 mg/kg) intravenously over the last 2 h of dialysis. The change in serum aluminum is measured between a baseline value and one taken 48 h after infusion. Although increments in excess of 200 μg/l have been reported to increase the sensitivity of predicting aluminum-associated osteomalacia, there is little additional predictive value to be gained from this test in the diagnosis of dialysis dementia over and above baseline serum aluminum levels.

Treatment of dialysis dementia

The use of aluminum-free dialysate is the most effective means of preventing dialysis dementia, although sporadic cases may still occur despite this measure (see above). The use of such dialysate may arrest, or even improve the established case, but since aluminum is so avidly plasma

Table 34.5 Potential neurotoxic effects of aluminum. Several have only been demonstrated in *in vitro* models. Multiple mechanisms may occur simultaneously

Possible mechanism	Example of effect
Complexing with high-energy phosphates	Binding with adenosine triphosphate
Impaired enzymatic function via interference with phosphate transfer	Reduced activity of dihydropteridine reductase (essential for dopamine synthesis)
Deoxyribonucleic acid binding	Reduced nuclear information transfer
Impaired hydrolysis of phosphoinositides	Deranged 'second messenger' function
Impaired microtubular function	Reduced axoplasmic transport
Reduced calmodulin activity via binding	Reduced calcium entry into neurons
Reduced neurotransmitter uptake	Impaired glutamic acid and GABA uptake in synaptosomal preparations

protein bound, very little is actually removed at subsequent dialyses.

Deferoxamine infusions are the mainstay of treatment of dialysis dementia, improving up to 70% of patients, sometimes to normal. Improvement is slow however, and therapy may need to be given once weekly for over a year. There is a similarity to chelation treatments used for other neurological illness (e.g. D-penicillamine therapy for Wilson's disease) in that there may be a period of paradoxical clinical and EEG worsening after treatment is commenced. The mechanism for this is uncertain but the deterioration may be profound, and occasionally fatal. In general, however, deferoxamine chelation is safe. Side effects reported include influenza-like symptoms, visual and auditory neurotoxicity, exacerbation of iron-deficiency anaemia, and increased occurrence of certain organisms which thrive in an iron-deficient environment (e.g. *Yersinia enterocolitica* and mucormycosis).

Psychiatric and sleep disorders associated with uremia and dialysis

Psychiatric disorders

The organic psychosis associated with uremic encephalopathy and the neuropsychological deficits reported in chronically dialyzed patients are discussed above. In patients undergoing hemodialysis, depression and anxiety are common and there is an increased risk of suicide. In males, impotence is common and often psychologically determined. In one nationwide series conducted in the United States 60% of patients were found not to manage any physical activity beyond self-care. With prolonged hemodialysis, many patients withdraw from their family responsibilities, leading other family members to respond with either overprotectiveness or resentment. Spouses of patients undergoing dialysis have been shown to have a high rate of psychiatric morbidity.

Psychosocial factors cause difficulties in the management of treatment, particularly if the dialysis is being conducted at the patient's home. Compliance with fluid restrictions and diet may be erratic, and such behavior occasionally has a suicidal motive. It is noteworthy that in one study of 285 patients on home dialysis for a minimum of 18 months it was concluded that psychosocial and demographic variables may be more important than physiological factors for survival.

If the patient undergoes renal transplantation, there is usually an initial sense of elation, accompanied by an increased feeling of well-being, both physical and mental. Sexual function also improves in many cases, unless there is an associated autonomic neuropathy. These feelings may be short-lived, however, particularly if there are episodes of graft rejection. Such episodes lead to anxiety, depression and anger. Organic psychoses and other mental disturbances associated with immunosuppressive agents are discussed below. For these, and a number of other reasons, including changes in familial psychodynamics, there is continued social and psychological morbidity in renal transplant recipients. It has been reported that such morbidity is greater in patients receiving a kidney from a living donor than in those patients who receive a cadaveric transplant.

Sleep disorders

A variety of sleep disorders have been described in uremic patients, which although not life-threatening can markedly interfere with quality of life. Daytime drowsiness is common in uremia. At night, sleep is affected by insomnia, which is multifactorial in nature. Polysomnographic recordings in uremic patients have indicated disorganized sleep staging and frequent wakening. Hypnotic drugs prescribed to promote sleep may have a paradoxical effect in uremic patients.

Restless legs syndrome is discussed specifically below. Other conditions which are associated with insomnia include 'burning feet', originally reported in 7% of uremic patients, although the incidence has fallen with the widespread prescription of B-vitamins. Despite this, other peripheral dysesthesias are common, affecting up to 40% of cases. Patients report 'swelling' or 'bursting' sensations in the limbs, especially the feet. Low-dose amitriptyline may be helpful in the treatment of such dysesthetic sensations. Muscle cramps in the legs are also troublesome at night, although are more frequent in acute uremia. Quinine sulphate is the drug of choice in treating these cramps.

Restless legs syndrome

Thomas Willis wrote in 1685: 'Wherefore to some, when being a Bed, they betake themselves to sleep, presently in the Arms and Leggs, Leapings and Contractions of their Tendons, and so great a Restlessness and Tossings of their Members ensue, that the diseased are no more able to sleep than if they were in a place of the greatest torture'. Although probably describing restless legs syndrome, Ekbom extended the description of this disorder in the 1940s to 1960s to such an extent that the syndrome now bears his name.

Restless legs syndrome is present in up to 40% of patients with varying degrees of renal impairment. It also occurs in association with other disorders, including diabetes, alcoholism, amyloidosis, Parkinsonism, pregnancy and may be idiopathic. In the uremic patient, there are often other symptoms present, such as cramps or burning feet, but restless legs syndrome may occur in isolation. Classically worse at night, the patients describe crawling, creeping, itchiness, pins and needles and other positive sensory disturbances which are located primarily between the knee and the ankle. Rubbing the skin, massage, stretching and often walking are required to alleviate the symptoms, leading to disturbed sleep. The condition is associated with periodic movements of sleep.

The pathogenesis of restless legs is uncertain, with contributions from both peripheral and central sources being postulated. Treatments used for the disorder are varied but currently preferred options are slow-release L-dopa preparations, opioids (such as codeine), or benzodiazepines, either singly or in combination.

Neurological complications of renal transplantation

More than 10 000 renal transplants are now carried out worldwide each year, with an 85–95% one-year graft survival. Approximately 30% of transplant recipients will develop neurological complications, although this figure may be higher if minor drug-related side effects are also included. Some of these are considered below.

Complications relating to the transplant procedure

Around 5% of patients acquire peripheral nerve injuries during the transplant procedure, usually because of intra-operative compression by retractors. The femoral and lateral femoral cutaneous nerves are most commonly affected. Unless the nerve has been severed (neurotmesis) the injury is usually neuropraxic in type and prognosis for recovery is generally good.

In some patients the caudal spinal cord is supplied by branches of the internal iliac arteries instead of the intercostal arteries. When the iliac artery is then used to supply blood to the allograft in these patients, spinal cord ischemia may then result. This comprises a combination of lower extremity pain and sensory abnormalities, sphincter disturbance and mixed upper and lower motor neuron signs.

Direct neurological side effects of immunosuppressive agents

Side effects relating to immunosuppressive therapy, especially cyclosporin, are some of the most common neurological problems encountered in the transplant recipient.

Table 34.6   Direct neurological side effects associated with immunosuppressive agents

Drug	Complications[a]
Cyclosporin[b]	Tremor (40%), encephalopathy (5%), seizures (2–6%), hemiparesis, paraparesis, quadriparesis, predominantly sensory neuropathy
Corticosteroids	Proximal myopathy, anxiety and dysthymia, psychosis (3%), 'steroid pseudorheumatism' and headache, fever, lethargy on withdrawal
OKT3 monoclonal antibody	Transient influenza-like symptoms <24 h[c] (>90%), aseptic meningitis 24–72 h[c] (2–14%), encephalopathy 1–4 days[c] (1–10%)

[a] Figures in parentheses are the approximate frequencies of the complications, if known.
[b] FK506 produces a similar spectrum of neurological complications to cyclosporin, but less commonly.
[c] Time after starting OKT3 treatment.

Many are relatively minor, but others are more serious and should be recognized because they are reversible on reduction or cessation of treatment. Table 34.6 summarizes the neurological complications caused by immunosuppressive agents.

Between 15 and 40% of patients receiving cyclosporin experience neurological side effects. Higher blood levels of cyclosporin are associated with an increased risk of complications, although the correlation is not a close one, and metabolites which are not assayed may also be important. Potentiating cofactors for cyclosporin neurotoxicity are previous cranial irradiation, hypocholesterolemia, hypomagnesemia, β-lactam antibiotic therapy, high-dose steroids, hypertension and uremia.

Rejection encephalopathy

This may occur in all age groups, and may be more common in young transplant recipients. Over 80% of cases occur within three months of transplantation but cases have been reported up to two years after surgery. The syndrome most commonly comprises convulsions, confusion and headache, combined with systemic features of graft rejection. The EEG, CT brain scan and CSF findings are non-specific. Although the cause is uncertain, the release of cytokines in the rejection process may be important. Symptomatic treatment of the seizures is usually necessary, but the prognosis overall is good for complete recovery.

Cerebrovascular disease

Cerebrovascular disease is second only to infection as the most common neurological complication after transplantation. Nearly one-quarter of transplant patients die because of vascular disease, with 50% of these deaths due to stroke. Predisposing pretransplant factors are diabetes mellitus, atherosclerosis and systemic lupus erythematosus. Post-transplant factors such as hypertension, hypercholesterolemia, and corticosteroid-mediated hyperglycemia also contribute to the high incidence of vascular disease. The use of aspirin (if no contraindication exists), as well as the stringent control of blood pressure, lipid status and blood glucose are essential prophylactic measures.

Central pontine myelinolysis

This devastating condition occurs in any age group and is associated with the excessively rapid correction of hyponatremia (greater than 12 mmol/l/day). The onset is subacute and often heralded by seizures and an acute confusional state. This metabolic encephalopathy may then mask the development of dysphagia, dysarthria, incontinence and a progressive flaccid then spastic quadriparesis. Reflex swallowing, coughing and respiration are preserved.

In the context of a rapid rise in serum sodium and initial hyponatremia, the investigation of choice is MRI brain scanning, which indicates an abnormal signal in the central pons, as well as extrapontine sites.

Central nervous system infections

Renal transplant recipients are predisposed towards developing CNS infection primarily because of drug-induced suppression of cell-mediated immunity. Contributing cofactors also include uremia, hyperglycemia and indwelling catheters. CNS infections, often fungal in type, have been reported in up to 45% of transplant patients coming to post-mortem. Table 34.7 lists the commonly encountered organisms in transplant recipients, and the neurological syndromes with which they are associated.

The timing of the infection after transplantation may give a clue to the nature of the likely pathogens. Broadly speaking, three phases exist. In the first of these, the first month post-transplantation, CNS infections are actually

Table 34.7 CNS infections in renal transplant patients (reproduced with permission from Conti, D.J. and Rubin, R.H. (1988) Infection of the central nervous system in organ transplant recipients. *Neurol. Clin.* **6**, 241–60)

Clinical syndrome	Microbial agent[a]
Acute meningitis[b]	*Listeria monocytogenes*
Subacute or chronic meningitis	*Cryptococcus neoformans, Mycobacterium tuberculosis* (*Listeria monocytogenes, Strongyloides stercoralis, Coccidioides immitis, Histoplasma capsulatum*)
Encephalitis or meningoencephalitis	*Listeria monocytogenes, Toxoplasma gondii* (varicella–zoster virus, JC papovavirus, *Strongyloides stercoralis, Cryptococcus neoformans*)
Localized mass lesion (brain abscess)	*Aspergillus* spp., *Nocardia asteroides, Toxoplasma gondii* (*Cryptococcus neoformans, Listeria monocytogenes, Mucorales*)

[a] Less common causes of each syndrome are shown in parentheses.
[b] Acute meningitis is defined as an illness of less than 24 h duration; subacute or chronic meningitis as an illness of longer duration, before the patient seeks medical attention.

very uncommon. When it does occur, infection is usually either acquired from the donor kidney, is related to the surgical procedure itself, or was present before transplantation. Pathogens are typically those found in the general, non-immunosuppressed population.

The second phase extends from one to six months post-transplantation. A combination of immunosuppressive drugs and the immunomodulating effect of common viruses means that immunosuppression is at its peak and the risk of CNS infection is greatest. Viruses (especially cytomegalovirus (CMV) and Epstein–Barr virus (EBV) and opportunistic organisms (especially *Aspergillus fumigatus*, *Nocardia asteroides* and *Listeria monocytogenes*) predominate.

The third phase of risk extends beyond six months after transplantation. Infections at this stage are either due to the lingering effects of previously acquired infections (such as CMV retinitis, for example), opportunistic infections in those patients who have often received higher than average immunosuppressive regimens because of chronic rejection (*Nocardia asteroides*, *Cryptococcus neoformans* and *Listeria monocytogenes* are the most common organisms involved), or due to the return of a pattern of infection seen in non-immunosuppressed individuals.

CNS infections in patients who have received a renal transplant may be difficult to diagnose. There are several reasons for this, but the main one is that in the presence of immune suppression the normal inflammatory response to infection is attenuated. Thus, for example, the usual signs of meningitis, including neck stiffness and fever, may be minimal. A high index of suspicion is needed therefore, particularly if there is infection present in extracranial sites, such as the lung. Neuroimaging, with either cranial CT or MRI, followed by lumbar puncture (assuming no intracranial mass effect), are obligatory. The CSF should be sent for white cell count and differential cytology, protein, glucose (always including a simultaneously taken blood glucose to allow meaningful interpretation), culture and sensitivity, viral titers, fungal studies and acid-fast stain, as well as culture for *Mycobacterium tuberculosis*. A number of recently developed tests, including polymerase chain reaction assays for JC virus (associated with progressive multifocal leukoencephalopathy) and fragments of mycobacterial DNA, also add to the diagnostic yield from lumbar puncture, but despite this, it is often not possible to make a definitive diagnosis in reasonable time, so empirical therapy must be commenced. Expert microbiological advice in these situations is vital, to ensure that the spectrum of likely pathogens is covered with drugs that penetrate adequately into the CNS.

Post-transplant lymphoproliferative disorder

Post-transplant lymphoproliferative disorder (PTLD) is a term used to define the range of abnormal proliferations of B lymphocytes which occur in renal transplant recipients. The spectrum of disease, from benign diffuse polyclonal lymphoid hyperplasia to highly malignant monoclonal B cell lymphoma, is thought to be closely connected with EBV infection of B lymphocytes, and subsequent EBV-driven lymphocyte proliferation.

Primary CNS lymphoma occurs 35 times more often in renal transplant recipients than normal, and may develop as early as three months postoperatively. Patients typically present with features of raised intracranial pressure and focal signs. Seizures are uncommon because of the deep-seated nature of the tumors. One-third of lymphomas are multicentric and 25% spread to the leptomeninges. CT brain scan appearance may show a surprisingly large lesion, in comparison with the clinical status of the patient. Lesions are isodense or hypodense and enhance strongly after contrast is administered. Brain biopsy is necessary to confirm the diagnosis. Malignant B cell lymphoma of the CNS in immunosuppressed patients carries a grave prognosis, and frequently responds poorly to chemotherapy and radiotherapy. Survival from time of diagnosis is usually only weeks to months.

Further reading

Alfrey, A.C., Le Gendre. G.R. and Kaelney, W.D. (1976) The dialysis encephalopathy syndrome: Possible aluminum intoxication. *N. Engl. J. Med.*, **294**, 184.

Arieff, A.I., Guisado, R., Massry, S.G. and Lazarowitz, V.C. (1977) Central nervous system pH in uremia and the effects of hemodialysis. *J. Clin. Invest.*, **58**, 306.

Bolton, C.F. and Young, G.B. (1990) *Neurological Complications of Renal Disease*. Butterworths, Boston.

Brown, T.M. and Brown, R.L. (1995) Neuropsychiatric consequences of renal failure. *Psychosomatics*, **36**, 244–53.

De Deyn, P.P., Saxena, V.K., Abts, H, Borggreve, F., D'Hooge, R., Marescau, B. and Crols, R. (1992) Clinical and pathophysiological aspects of neurological complications in renal failure. *Acta Neurol Belg.*, **92**, 191–206.

Fraser, C.L. (1992) Neurological manifestations of the uremic state, in *Metabolic Brain Dysfunction in Systemic Disorders* (eds A.I. Arieff and R.C. Griggs), Little, Brown, Boston, pp. 139–66.

Jack, R., Rabin, P.L. and McKinney, T.W. (1983–1984) Dialysis encephalopathy: a review. *Int. J. Psychiatr. Med.*, **13**, 309–26.

Jagadha, V., Deck, J.H., Halliday, W.C. and Smyth, H.S. (1987) Wernicke's encephalopathy in patients on peritoneal dialysis or hemodialysis. *Ann. Neurol.*, **21**, 78–84.

Jennekens, F.C.I. (1987) Peripheral neuropathy in renal and hepatic insufficiency, in *Handbook of Clinical Neurology*, Vol. 51, Neuropathies (ed. W.B. Matthews), Elsevier Science Publishers, Amsterdam, pp. 355–64.

Patchell, R. (1994) Neurological complications of organ transplantation. *Ann. Neurol.*, **36**, 688–703.

Raskin, N.H. and Fishman, R.A. (1976) Neurologic disorders in renal failure I. *N. Engl. J. Med.*, **294**, 143–8.

Raskin, N.H. and Fishman, R.A. (1976) Neurologic disorders in renal failure II. *N. Engl. J. Med.*, **294**, 204–10.

Schaumburg, H.H., Berger, A.R. and Thomas, P.K. (1992) Uremic neuropathy, in *Disorders of Peripheral Nerves*, 2nd edn. F.A. Davis, Philadelphia, pp. 156–63.

Windebank, A.J. and McEvoy, K.M. (1989) Diabetes and the nervous system, in *Neurology and General Medicine* (ed. M.J. Aminoff), Churchill Livingstone, New York, pp. 273–304.

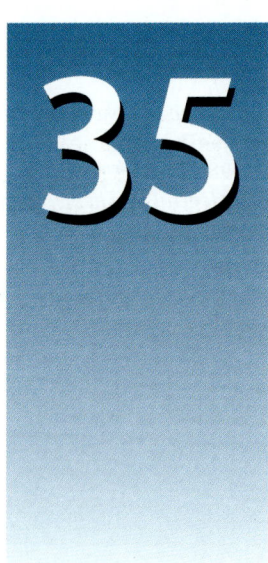

Hematological disorders

G.A. Coles and J.D. Williams

Introduction

Hematological disorders are common in both acute and chronic renal failure. In acute renal failure the hemoglobin concentration falls rapidly within a few days of onset of the condition and tends to plateau at 8–10 g/dl unless some other factor such as blood loss or infection occurs. Most patients with advanced chronic renal failure develop significant anemia but a few individuals, particularly those with autosomal dominant polycystic kidney disease, may maintain a normal hemoglobin level even up to the time when starting dialysis. In addition to anemia, bleeding disorders may also occur in uremia though their prevalence is considerably less. This chapter considers the causes and management of anemia and bleeding disorders particularly in chronic renal failure. Specific hematological problems such as the hemolytic uremic syndrome are discussed elsewhere in the book.

Clinical manifestations

In chronic renal failure anemia follows a gradual but progressive course. The first symptom is usually a reduced ability to undertake vigorous physical exertion. With time this worsens so that walking becomes restricted, particularly climbing stairs or hills. There is often increasing difficulty in sustaining a job or in carrying out household duties. Exertion makes the patient feel breathless, there is tiredness and lack of energy as well as a loss of libido. A common symptom is feeling cold. Palpitations may occur, particularly on exertion, and symptoms of angina pectoris may appear or worsen. Eventually the patient's activities are severely curtailed and self care becomes a problem [1].

The main physical sign is pallor of mucous membranes. Tachycardia may be present together with a systolic flow murmur. In severe cases there is evidence of cardiac enlargement and eventually cardiac failure may occur.

Physiological consequences of anemia

The physiological consequence of anemia is that there is a progressive decline in oxygen delivery to tissues since the falling red cell mass is unable to carry as much oxygen as normal. This is partly offset in chronic renal failure by a shift in the oxygen dissociation curve so that the hemoglobin more readily releases oxygen in the capillaries (Figure 35.1). This seems to be due at least in part to the renal retention of phosphate altering 2,3-diphosphoglycerate levels in the red cell which affect hemoglobin oxygen affinity. This compensatory mechanism only serves to slow the consequences of progressive anemia.

Nephrology, Edited by Rex L. Jamison and Robert Wilkinson.
Published in 1997 by Chapman & Hall, London. ISBN 0 412 60930 4

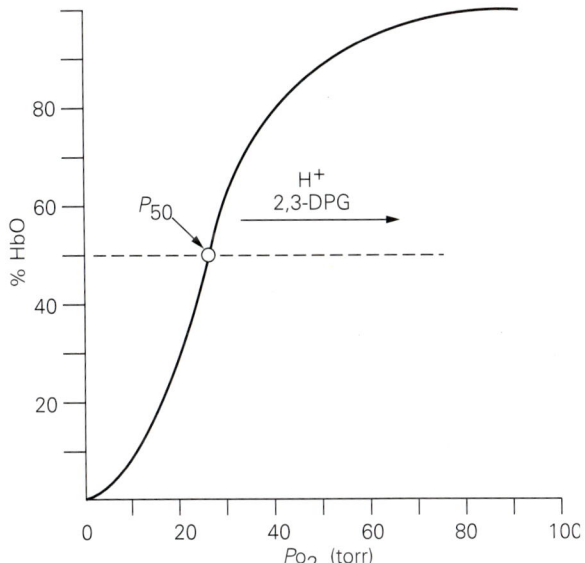

Figure 35.1 A typical oxygen dissociation curve of normal blood. The partial pressure of oxygen (Po_2) is plotted against percentage of oxygenated hemoglobin (HbO). P_{50} is the point at which 50% hemoglobin is oxygenated. Increase in acidity or in concentration of 2,3-DPG shifts the curve to the right, raising P_{50} and increasing the amount of O_2 released at a given Po_2. (Reproduced with permission from Massry, S. and Glassock, R.J. (eds) (1983) *Textbook of Nephrology.* Williams & Wilkins, Baltimore.)

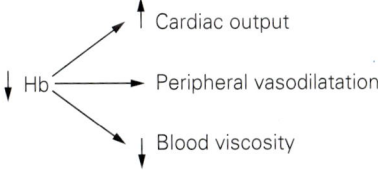

Figure 35.2 Cardiovascular effects of anemia.

There is, however, a fairly rapid increase in cardiac output. In addition the relative tissue hypoxia leads to peripheral vasodilatation which together with decreased whole blood viscosity causes decreased peripheral resistance (Figure 35.2) [2]. With time the increased cardiac output is accompanied by cardiac dilatation, particular of the left ventricle. This is usually evidenced as an increased end-diastolic diameter on echocardiography and clinically by signs of heart failure. Sometimes there is also hypertrophy of the interventricular septum or left ventricle particularly if there is an associated hypertension.

Pathophysiology of renal anemia

The characteristic blood picture in chronic uremia is a normochromic normocytic anemia with occasional fragmented or burr red cells (Figure 35.3). The absolute reticulocyte count is lower than normal. There is a reduced red cell mass but a normal whole blood volume unless fluid overload is present. The main cause of the anemia is a reduced red cell production by the marrow (Figure 35.4). There is also a mildly reduced red cell life span but this in itself is insufficient to explain the low blood count since non-uremic subjects with hemolysis due to a prosthetic heart valve are able to maintain a normal hemoglobin concentration despite a considerably shorter red cell half-life.

The reduction in erythropoiesis appears to be mainly due to a relative deficiency of erythropoietin. In most types of anemia, as hemoglobin concentration falls, there is a logarithmic rise in erythropoietin concentration in the serum. In chronic renal failure, however, erythropoietin levels remain within the normal range despite progressive anemia and are thus inappropriately low (Figure 35.5). This failure of erythropoietin production may in part be due to the destruction of the relevant cells in the kidneys but it is probably also due to down-regulation or resetting of the sensor mechanisms which normally respond to oxygen availability since in certain circum-

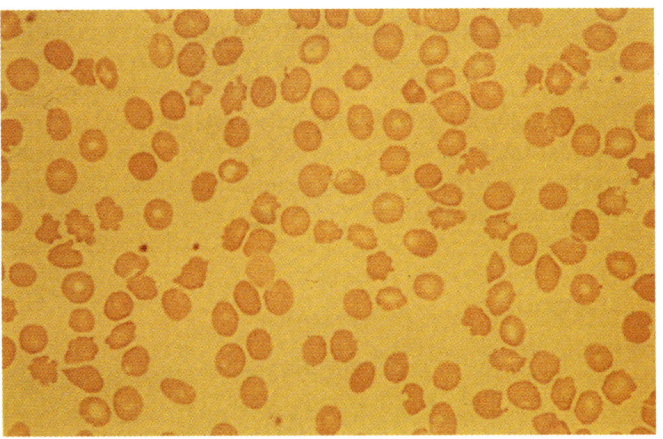

Figure 35.3 Renal failure: peripheral blood film showing coarse acanthocytes and 'burr' cells. (Reproduced with permission from Hoffbrand, A.V. and Pettit, J.E. (eds) *Clinical Hematology Illustrated.*)

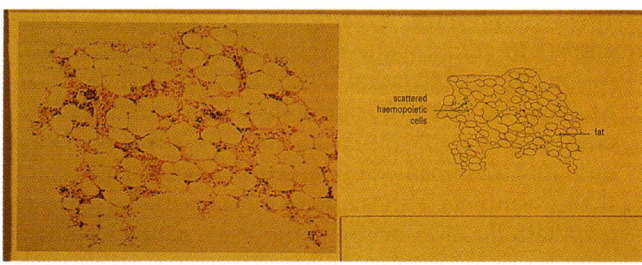

Figure 35.4 Histological section of marrow in chronic renal failure shows little evidence of hemopoiesis, the marrow having been replaced by fat. Hemotoxylin and eosin stain. (Courtesy of Dr C. Wardrop and reproduced with permission from Williams, J.D., Asscher, A.W., Moffat, D. and Sanders, E. (eds) (1991) *Clinical Atlas of the Kidney*, Gower Medical Publishing.)

Table 35.1   Factors contributing to renal anemia

Aluminum
PTH
'Uremic toxins'
Blood loss
Hematinic deficiency (nutritional)
Coincidental chronic disease – Rheumatoid arthritis
                                – Myeloma
                                – Malignancy

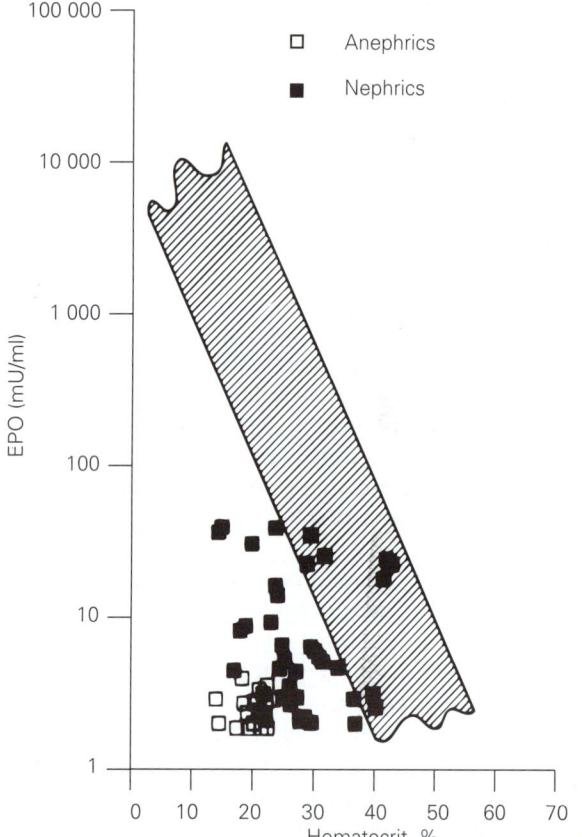

Figure 35.5 Erythropoietin titers in patients with anemia secondary to chronic renal disease. The hatched area represents the range in normal subjects. (Reproduced with permission from *Contrib. Nephrol.*, **66**, 1988.)

ence on the red cell count is iron deficiency due to poor intake and/or blood loss. Low protein diets can also be low in iron content. During hemodialysis there is an inevitable blood loss of up to 20 ml per session plus any taken for laboratory tests. Chronic gastrointestinal loss is not uncommon. Folate deficiency is relatively rare in chronic renal failure but may occur quickly in acute uremia unless care is taken to ensure an adequate intake, orally or intravenously. Vitamin B_{12} deficiency is not a feature of renal failure but may occur coincidentally.

Of particular importance is aluminum toxicity. The main sources are aluminum salts used as oral phosphate binders or aluminum contamination of water used to prepare dialysate. Toxicity may cause a microcytic anemia which initially can be misdiagnosed as iron deficiency.

Severe hyperparathyroidism may adversely influence uremic anemia. In particular it can blunt the response to exogenous erythropoietin in part because of the associated marrow fibrosis.

Both inflammation and malignancy may exacerbate the anemia. They can prevent an initial response to erythropoietin or may produce a drop in hemoglobin concentration during treatment. In the case of inflammation there may be a resistance to increased doses of erythropoietin for up to several weeks after the event has clinically resolved. It is thought that cytokines such as tumor necrosis factor-α (TNF-α) released by the disease process inhibit the action of erythropoietin on red cell precursors in the marrow [6].

Diagnosis

The diagnosis of renal anemia may be suggested by the symptoms and signs noted previously but is confirmed by

stances such as severe prolonged hypoxia, uremic patients may have increased serum erythropoietin levels [3, 4].

It has also been suggested that in uremia certain substances are retained which act as inhibitors of erythropoiesis. The data are conflicting and the initial response to exogenous erythropoietin appears similar in chronic renal failure patients as compared to normal subjects which would suggest that uremic inhibitors are not clinically relevant [5].

A number of other factors may also contribute to the anemia (Table 35.1). The second most important influ-

the finding of a normochromic normocytic anemia. The differential diagnoses with a low reticulocyte count include other causes of anemia. It is important to measure serum ferritin levels as a guide to iron deficiency and if these are low to exclude occult blood loss from the gastrointestinal tract. The need for other investigations will be determined by the specific clinico-laboratory findings of each affected individual [7].

Treatment

As already implied (Table 35.1, Figure 35.6) it is important to exclude other causes of anemia. In particular serum ferritin, folate and vitamin B_{12} concentration should be measured before commencing erythropoietin therapy. Transfusion can be given for temporary relief of symptoms or if the hemoglobin concentration is thought to be dangerously low, e.g. less than 6 g/dl. This therapy has its own dangers, however, and should not be used as a routine. Repeated transfusion runs the risk of producing iron overload. In addition, repeated exposure of the recipient to heterologous white cells/leukocytes could induce the formation of cytotoxic antibodies making it more difficult to find a compatible kidney for a subsequent transplant. In addition there is the risk of a blood-borne viral disease though this is low in those countries where blood products are carefully screened before release.

A fall in hemoglobin may well be an indication to start long-term dialysis. Sometimes there is a spontaneous

Hematinic deficiencies
Blood loss
Bone marrow suppression
myelofibrosis
myeloma
Hemolysis
Infection or inflammation
Aluminium toxicity

Figure 35.6 Causes of anemia in uremia other than erythropoietin deficiency.

improvement in the anemia during the first few months of replacement therapy particularly in patients receiving continuous ambulatory peritoneal dialysis (CAPD). In those individuals with persistent anemia, however, erythropoietin therapy should be offered. As a generalization any patient with a hemoglobin of 8 g/dl or less should receive the hormone as should those with symptoms such as angina with hemoglobin levels between 8 and 10 g/dl. Whether patients with a concentration of approximately 9 g/dl but who did not admit to significant symptoms should be treated is uncertain, not least because of the potential costs involved. At present the conventional target hemoglobin is 10–12 g/dl. The clinical benefits of values between 12 and 14 g/dl are currently the subject of study.

Erythropoietin can be given intravenously (i.v.) but the preferred route is subcutaneous (s.c.) as this will give a more sustained rise in serum erythropoietin concentrations as opposed to short sharp peaks (Figure 35.7) [8]. There is also some evidence that lower doses are required s.c. compared to i.v. (Figure 35.8). Treatment usually starts with a dose of 30 U/kg s.c. three times a week rounded to the nearest 1000 units to make dispensing easier. The hemoglobin concentration and blood pressure require monitoring at two-weekly intervals. If there is no response after four weeks then the dose should be increased to 50 U/kg and subsequently gradually to 200 U/kg three times weekly if necessary. Once the target hemoglobin has been reached then the dose is progressively reduced until the target hemoglobin is sustained. Usually dosing is first cut to twice a week and then reduced in amount per dose. It is of vital importance to ensure that adequate amounts of iron are available since functional iron deficiency can blunt the marrow activity (Figure 35.9) [9]. As a guide patients with a ferritin of 1000 µg/l or more are highly unlikely to develop this problem. Those with values between 100 and 1000 µg/l require oral iron supplements. Subjects with a level below 100 µg/l should have a therapeutic trial of iron therapy before starting erythropoietin since studies have shown that this group will almost invariably develop iron deficiency. After erythropoietin has been initiated then the serum ferritin concentration may not be a good guide to functional iron deficiency. Transferrin saturation is a better measure of functional iron availability. If this falls to less than 20% then iron therapy should be initiated or increased. An alternative guide to iron deficiency is the appearance of hypochromic cells in the blood film (Figure 35.10). This can be accurately measured by an automated hemocytometer and an appropriate alteration in iron supplementation made. Iron supplements can be given orally but not all patients can tolerate the large doses sometimes required. If iron deficiency occurs then a short course of i.v. iron dextran can be given.

The most prominent side effects of erythropoietin therapy are hypertension and an increased tendency to

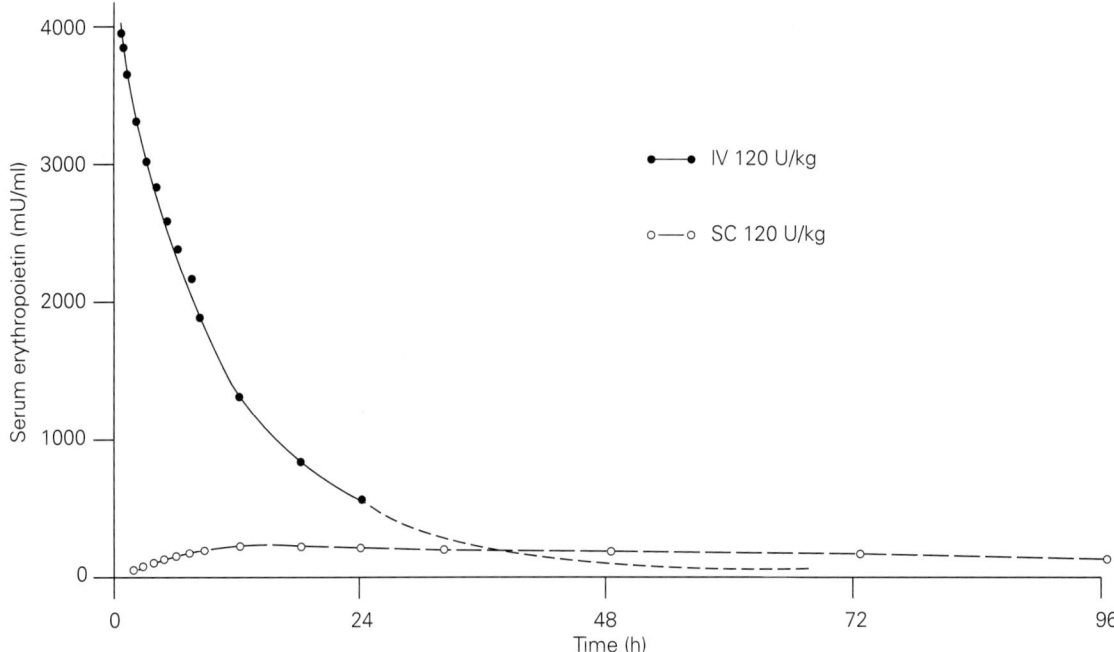

Figure 35.7 Bioavailability of erythropoietin following s.c. (0, 120 U/kg) administration in eight stable CAPD patients relative to an i.v. dose of 120 U/kg. Courtesy of Dr I.C. Macdougall.

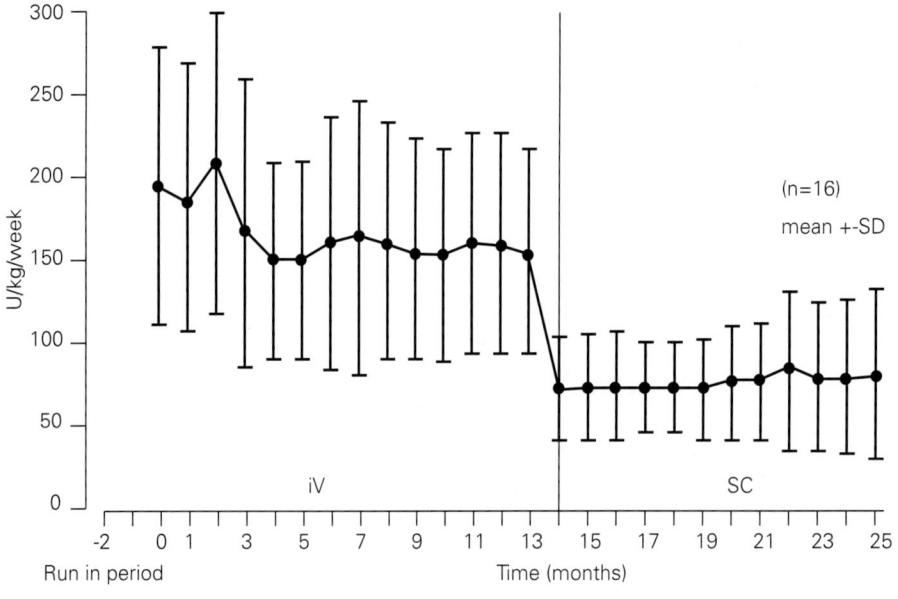

Figure 35.8 Weekly rhEPO dose (mean ± SD in hemodialysis patients treated 1–3 times/week with i.v. or s.c. rhEPO. (Reproduced with permission from *Contrib. Nephrol.*, **88**, 1991.)

fistula thrombosis in dialysis patients [10]. The rise in blood pressure can occur in previously normotensive individuals as well as those with treated hypertension (Figure 35.11). It usually occurs during the phase of a rising hematocrit and normally can be controlled by standard hypotensive drugs. It is essential to treat any hypertension before commencing erythropoietin. Subsequently, frequent monitoring of blood pressure is required until a new stable plateau concentration of hemoglobin is achieved. Clotting of fistulae seems to be confined to individuals who already have poor flow and/or a stenosis adjacent to their vascular access.

It has been suggested that the higher hematocrit may be associated with a tendency to hyperkalemia and reduced efficacy of dialysis during hemodialysis therapy. The data are conflicting and any effect is marginal. There is no good evidence that erythropoietin therapy significantly alters peritoneal membrane function during peritoneal dialysis. In experimental animals with renal failure human erythropoietin has been associated with a

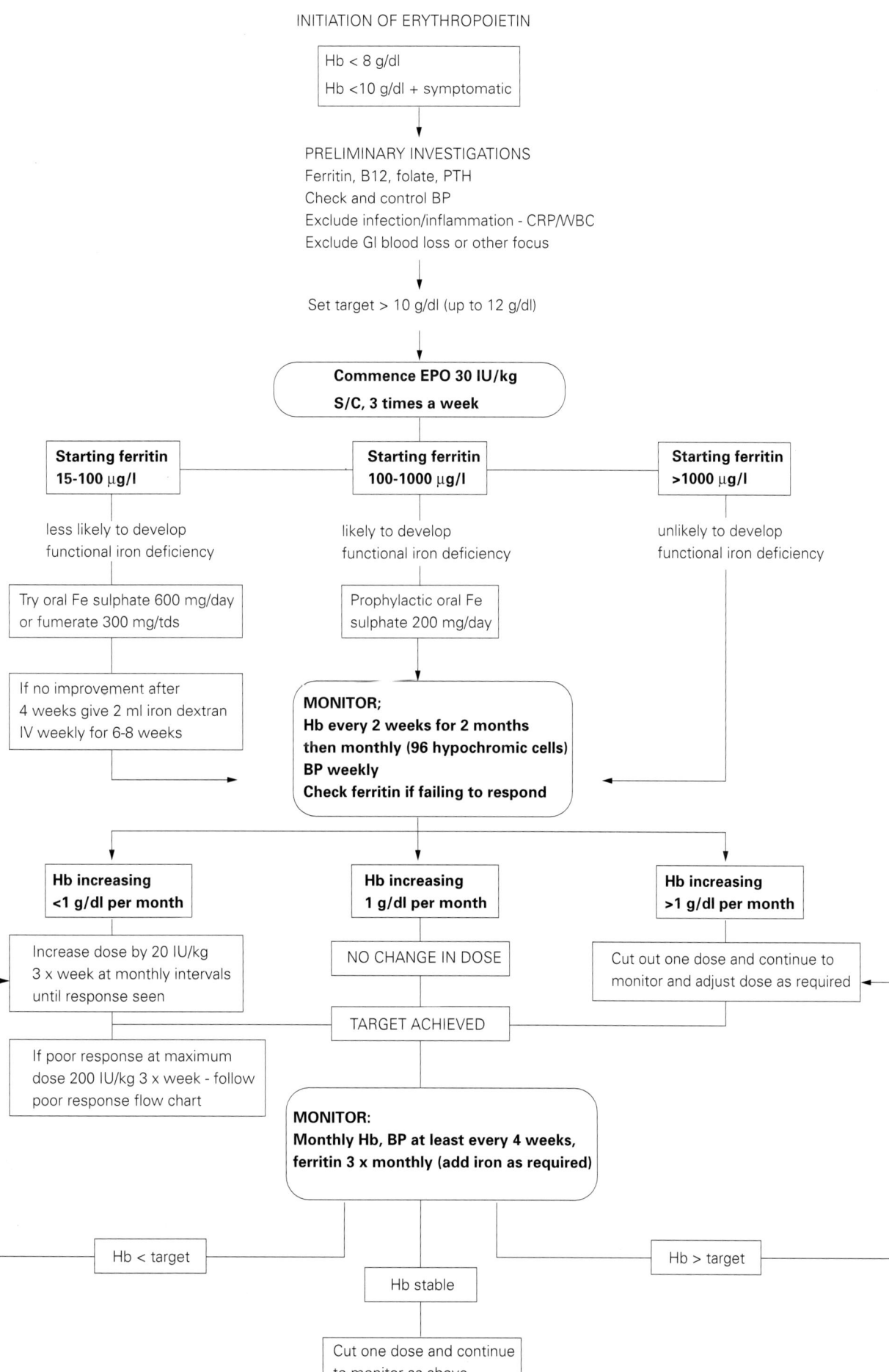

Figure 35.9 Algorithm for use of erythropoietin.

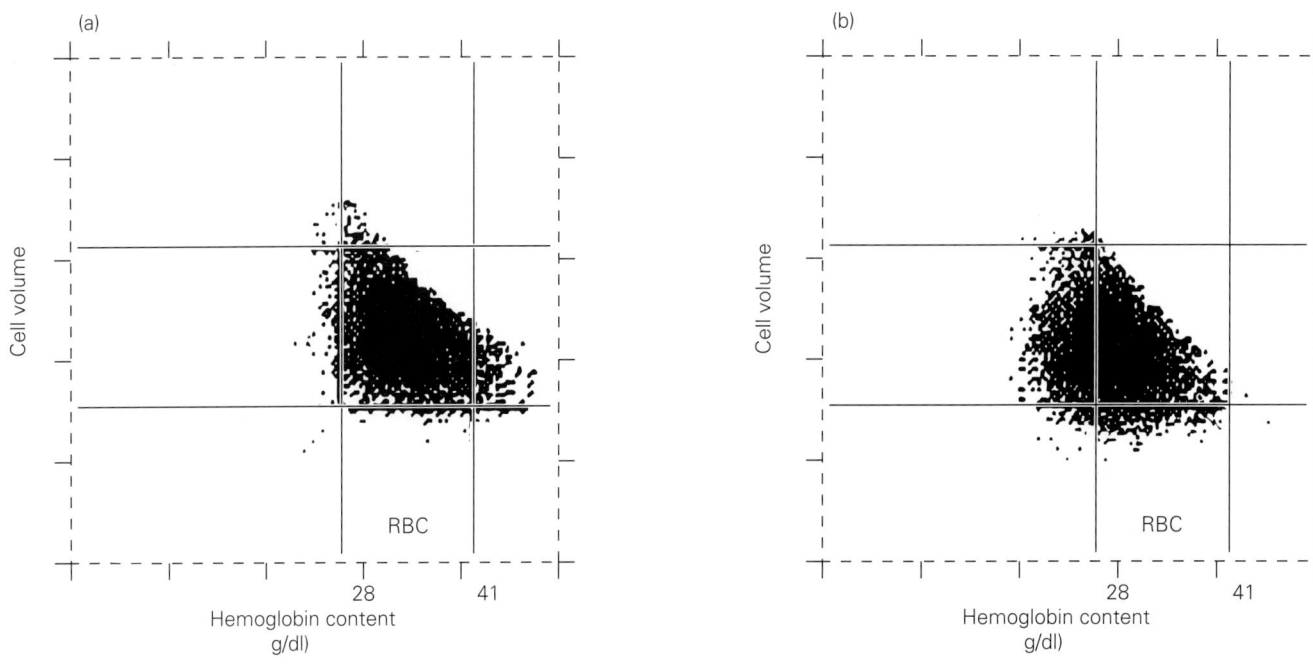

Figure 35.10 Calculated percentage of hypochromic cells in (a) a normal subject and (b) a patient with iron deficiency. Courtesy of Dr I. Cavill.

HYPERTENSION AND ERYTHROPOIETIN

CORRELATED WITH	INDEPENDENT OF
(I) Severity of anemia	(i) Erythropoietin dose
(ii) The time when hematocrit is increasing	(ii) Rate of rise of hematocrit
	(iii) Past history of hypertension

Figure 35.11 Hypertension and erythropoietin.

worsening of the uremia. Several studies in predialysis patients, however, have shown conclusively that the use of this hormone does not alter the rate of decline of renal function and thus it can be safely recommended in this group of subjects [11, 12].

Some patients may subsequently develop apparent resistance to erythropoietin. Should this occur then iron deficiency must be excluded. In its absence, other factors such as infection or malignancy should be considered. If any such factor is found then it should be corrected before increasing the dose of erythropoietin.

Treatment with erythropoietin leads to a reversal of hematological abnormalities (Figure 35.12) [13–15]. The first sign of a response is an increase in the absolute reticulocyte count which can occur one week after the start of treatment. Subsequently the blood count rises. The reticulocyte count may decrease after a few weeks but remains at a higher level than before as long as the hormone is administered. Marrow red cell production increases leading to an increase in red cell mass. Plasma volume tends to fall maintaining whole blood volume (Figure 35.13).

Red cell life span initially remains unchanged though there is some evidence that with prolonged therapy it increases. Whole blood viscosity rises exponentially but values are similar to those predicted from the blood count (Table 35.2) [16].

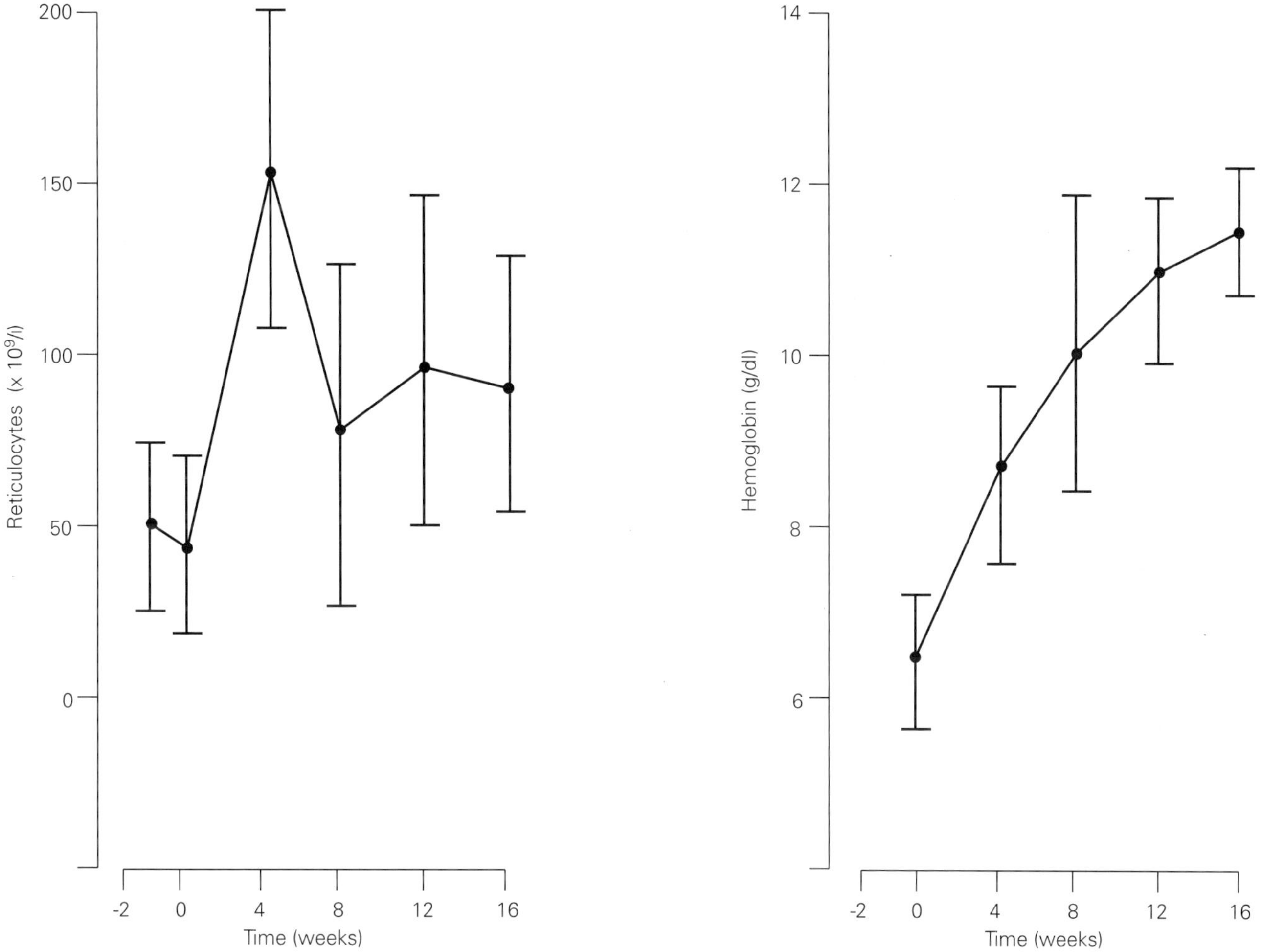

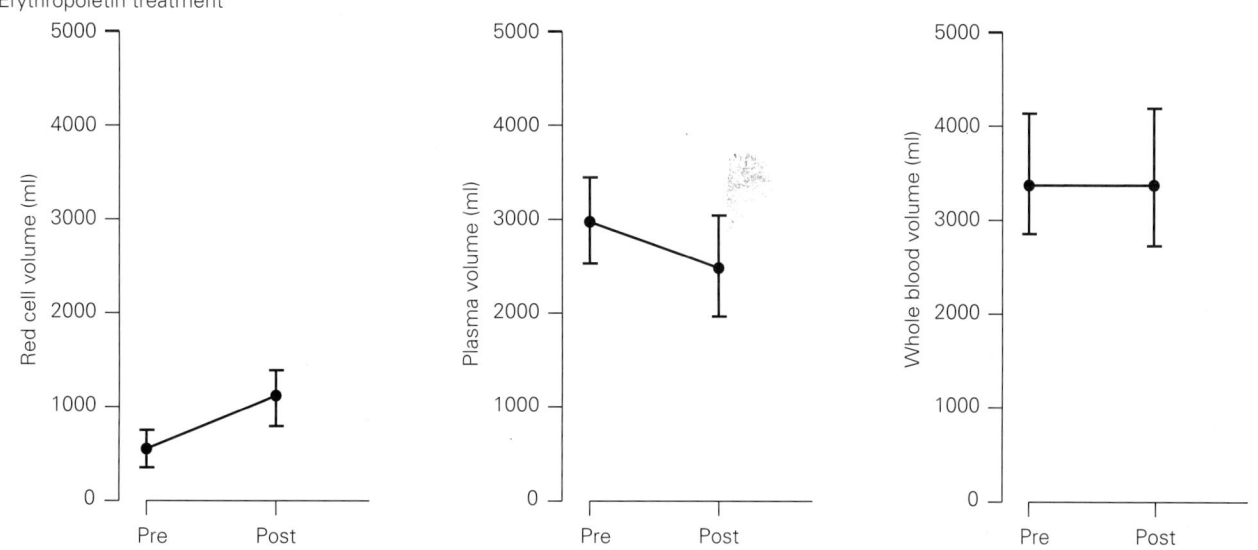

Figure 35.12 Serial changes in absolute reticulocyte count and hemoglobin concentration after initiation of erythropoietin therapy (Day 0). Courtesy of Dr I.C. Macdougall.

Erythropoietin treatment

Figure 35.13 Changes in red cell volume, plasma volume and whole blood volume before and after 16 weeks of erythropoietin therapy. Courtesy of Dr I.C. Macdougall.

Table 35.2 Rheological changes

	Normal volunteers	*Patients*	
		erythropoietin commenced	*52 weeks after erythropoietin*
Hb (g/dl)	14.6 (1.3)	6.4 (0.6)[a]	10.8 (0.7)[a]
WBV 3 s^{-1}	10.8 (1.92)	3.16 (0.62)[a]	7.37 (1.04)[a]
WBV 30 s^{-1}	4.92 (0.68)	2.12 (0.29)[a]	3.81 (0.03)[a]
WBC 300 s^{-1}	3.42 (0.44)	1.88 (0.29)[a]	2.81 (0.21)[a]
Plasma viscosity	1.26 (0.11)	1.21 (0.04)	1.19 (0.05)
Fibrinogen (mg/dl)	Not measured	276 (44)	Not measured
Cal vis Hb 10	2.60 (0.11)	2.61 (0.11)	2.76 (0.19)

[a] $P < 0.005$

WBV = whole blood viscosity measured at 3 s^{-1}, 30 s^{-1} and 300 s^{-1} shear rates.

Cal vis Hb 10 = calculated whole blood viscosity at 300 s^{-1} shear rate corrected to standard hemoglobin concentrations of 10 g/dl.

Results are expressed as means (SD).

Adapted from Macdougall *et al.* (1991) [8].

Outcome

With the amelioration of renal anemia, patients report an improved quality of life. There is a significant improvement in fatigue and physical symptoms. Interpersonal relationships are reported to improve and depression is less frequent [10]. Patients with angina may have a resolution of their symptoms and normalization of ischemic ECG changes on exercise testing have been reported (Figure 35.14) [17]. Specific testing has shown an increased exercise tolerance, improved oxygen uptake and an increase in the anerobic threshold – all signs of improved fitness (Figure 35.15). Echocardiographic data demonstrate a reduced left ventricular mass and decreased end diastolic volume (Table 35.3) [18]. These latter results are important since an increased left ventricular mass is an independent risk factor for death from a cardiac cause. Hopefully, the reduction will improve prognosis though this remains to be proven. There is also a reversal of the hemodynamic changes due to anemia with a fall in cardiac output and an increase in peripheral resistance (Figure 35.16). The latter is more than offset by the increased oxygen carrying capacity of the blood so that tissue oxygenation improves. Formal testing has also shown an improvement in brain function including cognition [19]. The long-term consequences of erythropoietin therapy are unknown though some patients have received this treatment for more than five years without obvious ill effects.

Polycythemia

Occasionally during renal replacement therapy polycythemia may develop as evidenced by a raised hemat-

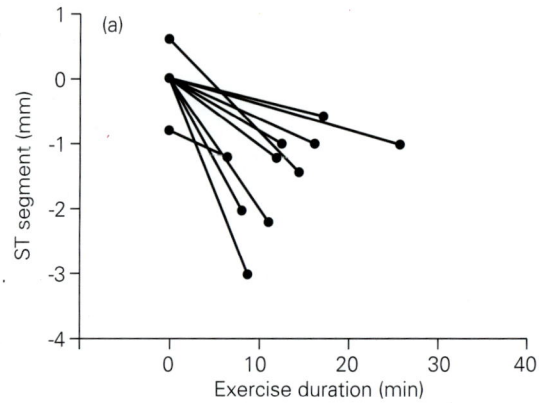

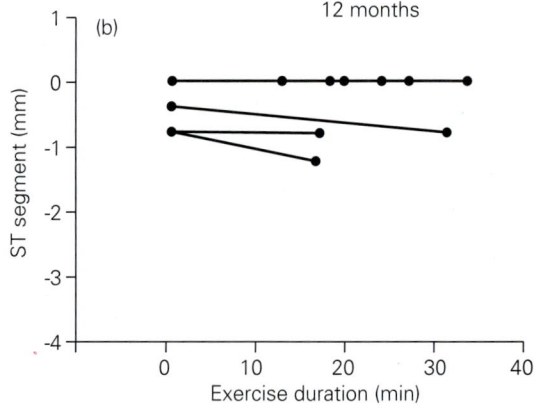

Figure 35.14 Maximal ST segment shift with exercise (a) before and (b) after 12 months of treatment with erythropoietin. Courtesy of Dr I.C. Macdougall, MD Thesis, University of Glasgow (1991).

Table 35.3   Echocardiographic parameters and the effects of erythropoietin (rHuEPO) treatment

	Control	*rHuEPO*	*P value*
Left atrial diameter (cm)	3.43 ± 0.33	3.22 ± 0.30	<0.03
Left ventricular mass index (g/m^2)	133.0 ± 30.8	109.8 ± 30.6	<0.05
Ejection volume (ml)	86.3 ± 24.0	75.2 ± 18.9	<0.03
Cardiac index (ml/min/m^2)	4175 ± 700	3635 ± 444	<0.01
Total peripheral resistance (dynes s cm^{-3} m^2)	1480 ± 162	1943 ± 250	<0.01

Values are mean ± SD.

Comparison of echocardiographic parameters in 11 HD patients before and after correction of anemia by recombinant EPO when Hb concentration was 6.8 ± 0.9 and 10.6 ± 0.66 g/dl (mean ± SD respectively).

Reproduced with permission from London *et al.* (1989) [18].

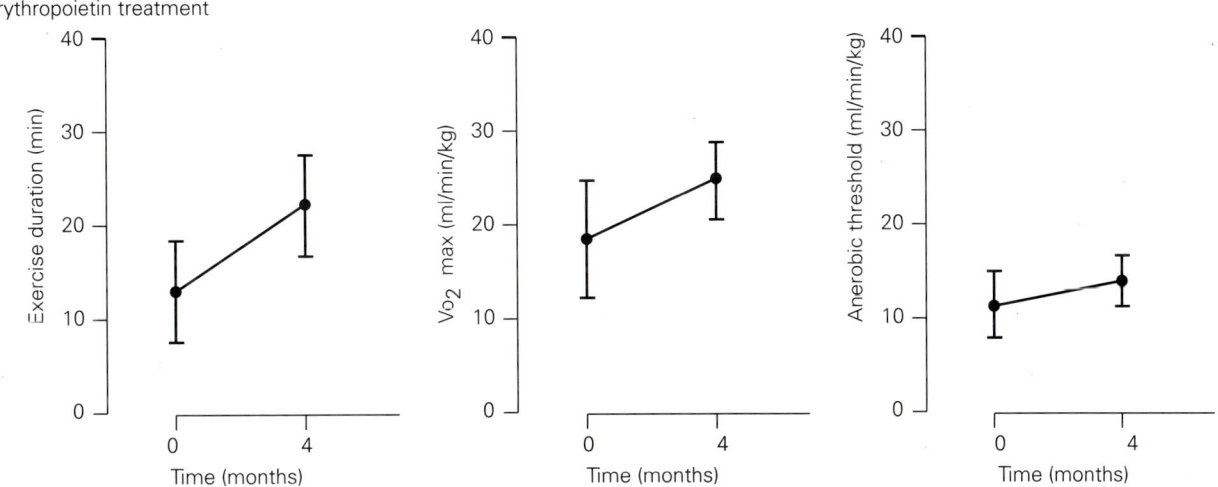

Figure 35.15   Changes in exercise duration, oxygen uptake (Vo_2) and anaerobic threshold before and after four months of treatment with erythropoietin. Courtesy of Dr I.C. Macdougall, MD Thesis, University of Glasgow 1991.

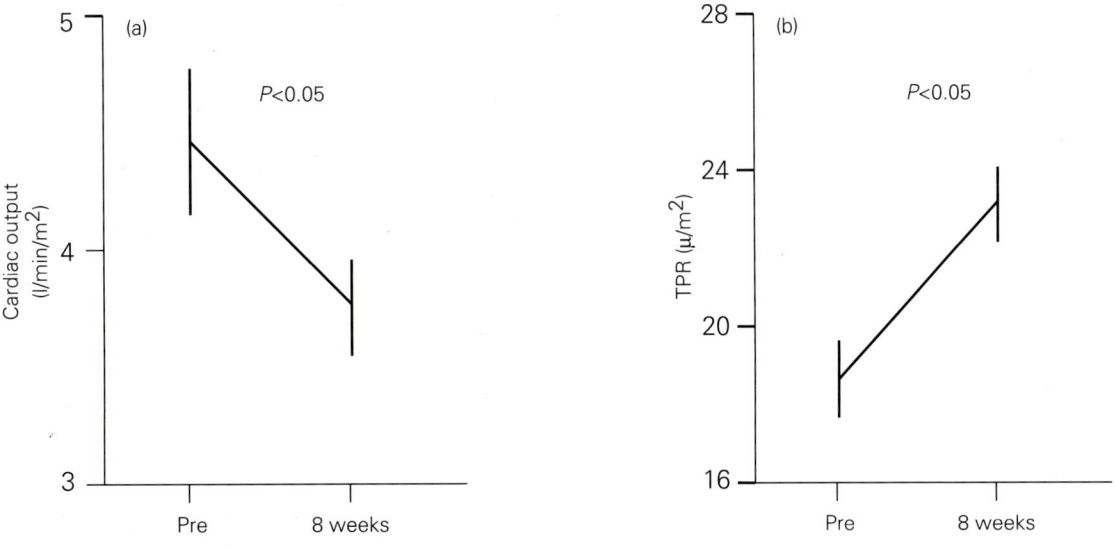

Figure 35.16   Changes of estimated hemodynamics with erythropoietin therapy. (a) Cardiac output; (b) peripheral resistance. (Reproduced with permission from Deschodt, G. *et al.* (1988) *Nephrol. Dial. Transplant.*, **13**, 494–5.)

ocrit. This may occur after many years dialysis therapy and is often associated with acquired cystic disease (Figure 35.17).

Following a renal transplant, polycythemia may also occur. This may be due to excess diuretic therapy similar to so-called stress polycythemia. In some patients there is a true increase in red cell mass, erythemia. This seems to be due to excess erythropoietin production. If necessary it can be treated by venesection but both theophylline and angiotensin converting enzyme inhibitors have been used with effect.

Acute renal failure

It has been reported that patients with acute renal failure may respond to erythropoietin. The use of this agent is not recommended at present since in this clinical situation other factors, such as gastrointestinal bleeding, shock, sepsis, etc., will make erythropoietin ineffective. Symptomatic treatment with red cell transfusion is suggested if necessary.

Bleeding disorders

Both acute and chronic uremia may be associated with disorders of bleeding. Clinically this may present with bruising or purpura. Some patients develop repeated epistaxes and less commonly there is overt bleeding from a wound which proves difficult to control.

The main abnormality is a prolonged bleeding time. The platelet count is usually normal but platelet function

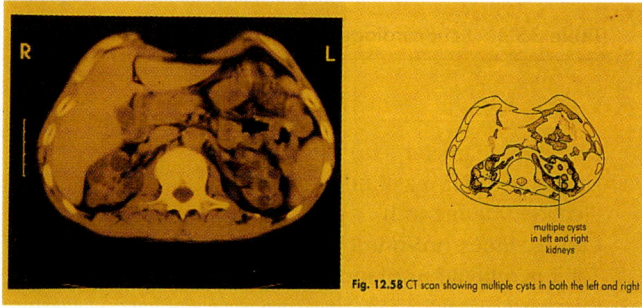

Figure 35.17   CT scan showing multiple cysts in both kidneys in a patient on long-term dialysis together with the change in hemoglobin concentration over the same time period. (Reproduced with permission from Williams, J.D., Asscher, A.W., Moffat, D. and Sanders, E. (eds) (1991) *Clinical Atlas of the Kidney*, Gower Medical Publishing)

tests can be disturbed with decreased aggregation in response to certain agonists. The intrinsic clotting mechanism is, however, normal. There are a number of possible lines of treatment. First, it is essential to check that the patient is not taking aspirin which can contribute to the bleeding problem. The effect of this drug takes a few days to wear off. Dialysis tends to improve bleeding time as does raising the hematocrit so that either transfusion (in the short term) or erythropoietin (in the long term) can benefit the patient [20]. The use of erythropoietin has also been reported to improve platelet aggregation *in vitro*. If invasive procedures such as biopsy are performed then it may be appropriate to correct the bleeding time with an agent such as Desmopressin.

References

1. Mayer, G., Thum, J. and Graf, H. (1989) Anemia and reduced exercise capacity in patients on chronic hemodialysis. *Clin. Sci.*, **76**, 265–8.
2. Creutzig, A., Capary, L., Nonnast–Daniel, B. *et al.* (1990) Skin microcirculation and regional peripheral resistance in patients with chronic renal anemia treated with recombinant human erythropoietin. *Eur. J. Invest.*, **20**, 219–23.
3. Eckardt, K.-U. (1994) Erythropoietin: oxygen dependent control of erythropoiesis and its failure in renal disease. *Nephron*, **67**, 7–23.
4. Erslev, A.J., Adamson, J.W., Eschbach, J.W. and Winearls, E.G. (eds) (1991) *Erythropoietin: Molecular, Cellular and Clinical Biology*. Johns Hopkins University Press, Baltimore.
5. Eschbach, J.W., Haley, N.R., Egrie, J.C. and Adamson, J.W. (1992) A comparison of the responses to recombinant human erythropoietin in normal and uremic subjects. *Kidney Int.*, **42**, 407–16.
6. Johnson, C.S., Cook, C.A. and Furmanski, P. (1990) *In vivo* suppression of erythropoiesis by tumor necrosis

factor α (TNFα): reversal with exogenous erythropoietin (EPO). *Exp. Hematol.*, **18**, 109–13.
7. Macdougall, I.C., Hutton, R.D., Cavill, I. *et al.* (1990) Treating renal anemia with recombinant human erythropoietin: practical guidelines and a clinical algorithm. *Br. Med. J.*, **300**, 655–9.
8. Macdougall, I.C., Roberts, D.E., Coles, G.A. and Williams, J.D. (1991) Clinical pharmacokinetics of epoietin (recombinant human erythropoietin). *Clin. Pharmacokinet.*, **20**, 99–113.
9. Van Wyck, D.B., Stivelman, J.C., Ruiz, J. *et al.* (1989) Iron status in patients receiving erythropoietin for dialysis-associated anemia. *Kidney Int.*, **35**, 712–16.
10. Canadian Erythropoietin Study Group (1989) The clinical effects and side effects of recombinant human erythropoietin in anemic patients on chronic hemodialysis. *Clin. Invest. Med.*, **12**(suppl.), B66.
11. Austrian Multicenter Study Group of rHuEPO in Predialysis Patients (1992) Effectiveness and safety of recombinant human erythropoietin in predialysis patients. *Nephron*, **61**, 399–403.

12. The US Recombinant Human Erythropoietin Predialysis Study Group (1991) Double-blind, placebo controlled study of the therapeutic use of recombinant human erythropoietin for anemia associated with chronic renal failure in predialysis patients. *Am. J. Kidney. Dis.*, **18**, 50–9.

13. Winearls, C.G., Oliver, D.O., Pippard, M.J. *et al.* (1986) Effect of human erythropoietin derived from recombinant DNA on the anemia of patients maintained by chronic hemodialysis. *Lancet*, **ii**, 1175–8.

14. Eschbach, J.W., Egrie, J.C., Downing, M.R. *et al.* (1987) Correction of the anemia of end-stage renal disease with recombinant human erythropoietin. *N. Engl. J. Med.*, **316**, 73–8.

15. Eschbach, J.W., Abdulhadi, M.H., Brown, J.K. *et al.* (1989) Recombinant human erythropoietin in anemic patients with end-stage renal disease. Results of a phase III multicentre trial. *Ann. Intern. Med.*, **111**, 992–1000.

16. Macdougall, I.C., Davies, M.E., Hutton, R.D. *et al.* (1991) Rheological studies during treatment of renal anemia with recombinant human erythropoietin. *Br. J. Haematol.*, **77**, 550–8.

17. Macdougall, I.C., Lewis, N.P., Saunders, M.J. *et al.* (1990) Long term cardio-respiratory effects of amelioration of renal anemia by erythropoietin. *Lancet*, **335**, 489–93.

18. London, G.M., Zins, B., Panier, B. *et al.* (1989) Vascular changes in hemodialysis patients in response to recombinant human erythropoietin. *Kidney Int.*, **36**, 878–82.

19. Marsh, J.T., Brown, W.S., Wolcott, D. *et al.* (1991) rHuEPO treatment improves brain and cognitive function of anemic dialysis patients. *Kidney Int.*, **39**, 155–63.

20. Moia, M., Mannucci, P.M., Vizzotto, L. *et al.* (1987) Improvement in the hemostatic defect of uremia after treatment with recombinant human erythropoietin. *Lancet*, **ii**, 1227–9.

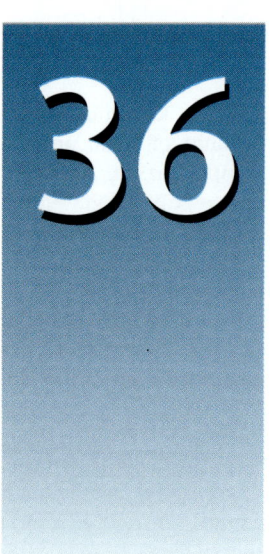

The immunological consequences of uremia

G.P. Spickett

Introduction

It has been appreciated for over 30 years that uremia has a significant effect on immunological function [1], leading predominantly to an increased incidence of infections but also possibly contributing to an increase in malignant disease through reduction of immunological surveillance and to a reduction in graft rejection. It has become clear that uremic immunosuppression is multifactorial, and affects many aspects of immunological function; however, there are two major contributing factors: the uremic state itself and hemodialysis. Disentangling these two has proved difficult. It seems that, although the problem of immune dysregulation is recognized, in practice it is underinvestigated and undermanaged.

The basis of the immune system

The immune system is divided into innate and specific arms (Table 36.1) but both arms are closely linked, through soluble factors (cytokines), which ensures that the immune response is co-ordinated. The innate system comprises a rapid response team of soluble factors with antibacterial activity and non-specific phagocytic or cytolytic cells. This system is active immediately but has no 'memory' of previous exposures. It provides the first line of defense against pathogens. In contrast the major feature of the specific immune response is the property of memory, so that subsequent re-exposure to a pathogen elicits a stronger and more rapid response. The antibody response is also capable through somatic mutation of hypervariable regions in the immunoglobulin genes of evolving on continued antigen exposure to provide antibodies of higher affinity against the pathogen. Immunological memory is persistent for long periods, tens of years, although it requires restimulation on a continuous basis, through antigen trapped on follicular dendritic cells within lymph nodes. Both T cells and B cells are required for a complete specific response and although some antigens, such as polysaccharides, are said to be 'T-independent', in reality these antigens also require T cells for optimal antibody responses by B cells.

Activation of either arm of the immune system tends to lead to activation of the other arm through the release of cytokines or the direct effects of activation products such as complement factors. The interrelations are depicted in Figure 36.1. The primary absence/failure of any major aspect of either system usually leads to problems with infection, the site and nature of the infections giving a clue as to the nature of the defect (Table 36.2). Acquired defects such as uremia may affect more than one component, leading to complex patterns of infection.

Nephrology, Edited by Rex L. Jamison and Robert Wilkinson.
Published in 1997 by Chapman & Hall, London. ISBN 0 412 60930 4

Table 36.1 Components of the innate and specific immune systems

Innate	Specific
Mucosal barriers	Cytotoxic T
Anti-bacterial secretions	lymphocytes (CD8+)
(lysozyme)	Helper T lymphocytes
Gastric acid	(CD4+)
Phagocytic cells	B lymphocytes
Natural killer cells	Antibody
Mast cells/eosinophils	
Complement cascade	
Kinin system	
Interferons	

Clinical consequences of immune dysfunction in uremia

It is recognized that sepsis is a major cause of death of uremic patients on dialysis, accounting for approximately 36% of deaths in a number of studies [2, 3]. It is the major cause of death in young dialysis patients, although cardiovascular deaths tend to be more common in older dialysis patients. The major bacterial pathogen appears to be *Staphylococcus aureus* [4], a marker pathogen for both humoral and phagocyte dysfunction. However, there is also an increased risk of tuberculosis in dialysis patients, indicating a significant T cell defect [5]. Viral infec-

tions are also problematic, particularly hepatitis B and cytomegalovirus. Furthermore, dialysis patients respond poorly to the hepatitis B vaccines, using conventional immunization schedules [6], which is a cause of significant concern. Responses to other vaccines such as pneumococcal polysaccharides are also reduced.

Mechanisms of immune dysfunction in uremia

Uremic patients are often lymphopenic, with a particular reduction in CD4+ T cells (T helper cells). Lymphoid organs mirror this depletion with thymic atrophy and loss of the follicular areas of lymph nodes with a reduction in plasma cells [7]. The T cells also show abnormalities of surface antigen expression, with reduced amounts of the CD3/Tcr complex, the T cells' antigen-specific receptor, and reductions of the level of expression of CD4 and CD8, molecules defining the T-helper and T-cytotoxic populations, respectively. These changes become less marked after long periods on dialysis [8].

In vitro tests of T cell function, such as proliferation to mitogens (phytohemagglutinin, PHA) and antigens (mycobacterial purified protein derivative, PPD) and alloantigens are reduced and *in vivo* tests (delayed-type hypersensitivity) are also poor or absent (anergy). It has been suggested that the poor T cell responses may be due to a reduction in interleukin-2 (IL-2) production, as the addition of IL-2 *in vitro* may restore the proliferative responses of uremic T cells. Paradoxically, the expression

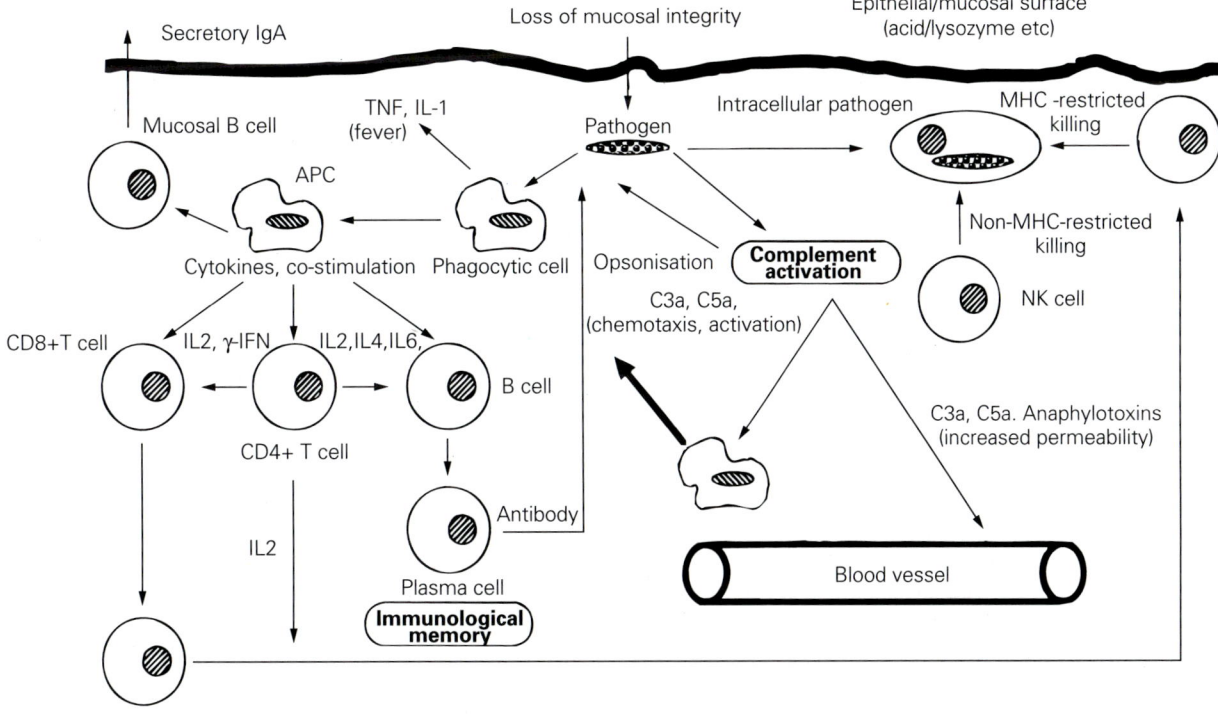

Figure 36.1 The immune response.

Table 36.2 Effects of deficiency of components of the immune system on susceptibility to infections

B lymphocyte deficiency	
Bacterial infections	*Streptococcus pneumoniae*
	Haemophilus influenzae
	Neisseria meningitidis
	Staphylococcus aureus
	Ureaplasma/Mycoplasma spp.
T lymphocyte deficiency	
Bacterial infections	Mycobacterial
Viral infections	Any type
	Papillomavirus
	Herpes viruses
Fungal/parasitic infections	*Candida* spp.
	Cryptococcus
	Cryptosporidium
	Toxoplasma gondi
	Pneumocystis carinii
Combined deficiency (T and B cell)	
Combination of all the above	
Phagocytic cell dysfunction	
Bacterial infections	Especially catalase-positive organisms; deep-seated abscesses
	Staphylococcus aureus
	Serratia marcescens
	Pseudomonas spp.
Fungal infections	*Aspergillus* spp.
Complement deficiency	
Bacterial infections	As for B cell deficiency (C3 deficiency)
	Recurrent Neisserial infection

of IL-2 receptors on T cells from uremic patients is increased. This is a feature usually seen in activated cells, although no studies have been carried out using other markers of T cell activation. Studies using flow cytometric assays during and after dialysis have shown that there is a significant increase in lymphocytes undergoing DNA replication (i.e. proliferating), strongly suggesting non-specific activation of T cells by the dialysis process [8], a process that the authors liken to 'lighting the stove under a pan of popcorn'.

Reports on B cell function are more conflicting. Total immunoglobulin levels may be normal, although *in vitro* production of immunoglobulin may give poor responses to T-dependent stimuli [9], although there may be high levels of spontaneous immunoglobulin M (IgM) and IgE production, suggesting polyclonal activation *in vivo*. Increased levels of membrane and soluble CD23, the Fc receptor for IgE which in its soluble form acts as a growth factor for B cells, have been recorded. Vaccine responses, as noted, are poor. It is not clear whether the humoral defects are due to an intrinsic B cell defect induced by uremia or are secondary to the impaired T cell function.

Most T cell proliferative responses are governed by interaction of the T cells with monocytes or other antigen presenting cells (APCs) such as dendritic cells. Not only are the antigens presented to the T cell in the context of the appropriate major histocompatibility complex (MHC) molecule, but the APCs provide additional cytokine stimuli to the T cells (IL-1) as well as co-stimulation through the interaction of other surface molecules with their cognate receptors on the T cells. If these co-stimulatory signals are missing then the T cell will become unresponsive. There is evidence that APC function in uremia is abnormal, with reduced expression of cognate molecules such as MHC class II (DR) and ICAM-1. If monocyte-independent T cell activation stimuli, such as triggering via the CD2 receptor (sheep erythrocyte receptor) are used, it has been shown that uremic T cells proliferate normally [10]. Monocytes also produce prostaglandins, which have an inhibitory effect on T cells and reduce IL-2 production. It has been suggested that uremia leads to increased monocyte prostaglandin production, which contributes to the T cell defect, although this is still controversial.

The key cytokines produced by monocytes are IL-1 and tumor necrosis factor-α (TNF-α), which both have T cell regulatory properties, in addition to their major role as endogenous pyrogens and contributors to the acute phase response through their effects on hepatic protein synthesis. Levels of both cytokines have been shown to be elevated in hemodialysis but not continuous ambulatory peritoneal dialysis (CAPD) patients or in undialyzed uremic patients. The production of these cytokines is a feature of activated monocytes, suggesting that hemodialysis is responsible for the activation. Although certain membranes, such as cuprophane, cause larger rises than other membranes, it has also been shown that trace quantities of endotoxin which may be found in dialysate fluids are more probably responsible for monocyte activation. Endotoxin (bacterial lipopolysaccharide) is also a potent polyclonal activator of B cells, leading to the high IgM production that has been recorded. An additional source of monocyte activation comes from the generation during dialysis of complement split products C3a and C5a (the anaphylotoxins) which are potent chemotactic and activation stimuli for monocytes, leading to release of IL-1 and TNF-α. Somewhat against the monocyte activation *in vivo* is the finding of reduced MHC class II and ICAM-1 on monocytes, as activation usually up-regulates these molecules.

The overall pattern of changes in the specific immune system seems to be a complex balance of direct suppressive effects of uremia, balanced by global activation by the dialysis process. Lymphocytes that are activated nonspecifically, particularly if they receive activating signals in the absence of proper co-stimulation, will proliferate and then die by apoptosis (programmed cell death). There will be two consequences of this process: first, the already activated cells will be unable to respond appropriately to infection and second, the pool of cells will be gradually depleted, leading to the lymphopenia noted in uremia. This process is analogous to one of the postulated mechanisms for the depletion of CD4+ T cells in HIV-1 infection.

In addition to the effects on the specific immune system, there are effects of uremia and dialysis on aspects of innate immunity. Mention has already been made of the effects on monocyte function and on the activation of complement by dialysis. Polymorphonuclear (PMN) cell function is also significantly deranged, with reduced chemotaxis, phagocytosis, bacterial killing and oxidative metabolism [11]. The degree of impairment may be related to the type of dialysis membrane, with cuprophane causing the largest effects on phagocytic activity, and newer membranes having lesser or no effects. Soluble factors have also been identified in uremic patients that inhibit granulocyte function (granulocyte inhibiting protein, GIP) or degranulation (degranulation inhibiting protein, DIP). In addition a molecule with significant homology to β2-microglobulin has also been identified which inhibits neutrophil function.

Natural killer cell (NK) activity is an essential part of the innate system for dealing with viral infections, before the specific immune system can generate specific, MHC-restricted cytotoxic T cells. NK activity is also likely to play a role in immune surveillance against tumor development. Uremia has been shown to reduce NK activity [12], although NK function was reported as normal in a group of patients on hemodialysis [13]. In the latter study, NK cell numbers were increased.

Many factors have been postulated to contribute to the immune defect in uremia, although which factors are most important remains a mystery. Urea itself alters the skin, reducing resistance to invasive infection, whereas uremic toxins such as methylguanidine are known to interfere with some immunological functions [12]. The role of other uremic toxins in the immune dysfunction is not known. Endorphins are known to accumulate in uremia and the met-enkephalins have been shown to reduce lymphocyte proliferation, IL-2 production and expression of CD71 (transferrin receptor) by T cells [14]; the effect was not reversible by naloxone. Parathyroid hormone (PTH) levels are elevated in uremia and it has been suggested that this hormone may also interfere with immune function through the elevation of intracellular calcium levels, as calcium flux is an essential part of the activation process for both lymphocytes and phagocytes [11, 15]. Reversal of the defects of phagocytic function and glucose uptake by uremic PMN can be achieved by treatment *in vivo* with verapamil, which is paralleled by normalization of intracellular Ca^{2+} concentration [11].

Iron overload has also been postulated to contribute to phagocytic cell dysfunction [16]. A correlation has been reported in uremic patients between infections and very high serum ferritin [17]. Iron overload is less likely to be a problem today as the anemia of chronic renal failure is more likely to be treated with erythropoietin rather than transfusion. Zinc deficiency may also occur in renal failure and may contribute to the immune deficiency. The effects of zinc deficiency on the immune system are widespread, with T and B cell dysfunction, thymic atrophy and lymphopenia [18, 19], all features which are found in uremia. Other vitamin and mineral deficiencies may also contribute to impaired immune function.

β2-Microglobulin levels are elevated in uremia, and it has been recognized that certain dialysis membranes fail to clear this protein adequately, leading to the development of β2-microglobulin amyloid. It has also been suggested that macrophage activation by dialysis leads to increased β2-microglobulin shedding, although it is more usually thought of as a marker of increased lymphocyte activation. Levels of IL-1, TNF-α and β2-microglobulin appear to rise in parallel, and are more likely to be increased by endotoxin rather than the intrinsic properties of the dialysis membranes [20]. High levels of β2-microglobulin have also been shown to further increase IgM production *in vitro* from uremic B cells [21].

Complement activation is a feature of dialysis and has important consequences in terms of activation of other

Table 36.3   Immunological abnormalities in uremia

Lymphocytes

Numbers	Lymphopenia (CD4+, CD8+)
In vivo activation	Increased CD25 (IL-2 receptor)
	Increased DNA synthesis
	Increased spontaneous IgM production
	Increased soluble and surface CD23 (B cells)
Reduced function	Reduced proliferation to mitogens and antigens
	Reduced monocyte-dependent IL-2 production
	Reduced/absent DTH[a] responses (anergy)
	Reduced antigen receptors (CD3/Tcr complex)
	Poor humoral responses to T dependent and T independent antigens
	Reduced NK cell function

Monocytes

In vivo activation	Increased IL-1/TNF-α production
	Increased prostaglandin synthesis?
Reduced function	Reduced expression MHC Class II/ICAM-1
	Poor support for T cell proliferation

Neutrophils

In vivo activation	Increased adhesion molecule expression (CD11b)
Reduced function	Reduced chemotaxis
	Reduced phagocytosis and bacterial killing
	Reduced oxidative metabolism

Complement

In vivo activation	Raised C3a, C5a anaphylotoxins during dialysis
Reduced function	Complement consumption

[a] DTH, delayed type hypersensitivity (Type IV hypersensitivity).

aspects of the immune cascade. It appears that certain dialysis membranes (cuprophane) have an increased tendency to activate complement. However, it appears that contaminating endotoxin may also be responsible for activation of the alternate (fluid phase) pathway of complement. As noted above, C3a and C5a will have profound effects on PMN function.

In considering the effects of uremia on immune function one should not lose sight of the disease causing the uremia in the first place. For example, systemic lupus erythematosus is strongly associated with deficiencies of complement components [22], and may also be associated with hypogammaglobulinemia rather than the more usual hypergammaglobulinemia [23]. Prior treatment with immunosuppressive drugs may also lead to long-term immunodeficiency, and other drugs that may be used in uremic patients such as anticonvulsants are well recognized to cause immunodeficiency [24].

Other facets to be considered in increasing the risk of infection include (1) the breach of cutaneous integrity through the need to develop access to either the vascular or peritoneal compartments for dialysis: this allows easy passage of bacteria from skin, bypassing the protection of the keratinized layers; (2) mechanical damage to cells

through extracorporeal circulation; (3) the development of amyloidosis. All these may contribute.

Table 36.3 summarizes the defects.

Investigation for immunodeficiency

The clinical investigation of suspected immunodeficiency in uremic patients is straightforward and should, as always, be driven by symptoms. It should follow the same lines as the investigation of primary immunodeficiency [25]. Patients with recurrent infections or unusual investigations merit further investigation (Table 36.2). There are no hard and fast guidelines as to when investigations should be carried out. However, two major infections (requiring i.v. antibiotics and hospital admission) in one year or one major and recurrent (>2) minor infections (documented bacterial infections, requiring antibiotics but not hospital admission) in one year should warrant further consideration of an underlying immunodeficiency. Similarly any patient with an unusual (opportunist) infection such as *Pneumocystis carinii* requires investigation.

Table 36.4 Investigation of immune deficiency in uremia

Suspected B cell defect

Total immunoglobulins (IgG, IgA, IgM)

IgG subclasses

Isohemagglutinins (natural IgM antibodies)

Antibacterial antibodies:	Pneumococcal
	Tetanus
	Diphtheria
	Haemophilus influenzae
Antiviral antibodies:	Polio
	Measles, mumps, rubella (MMR)
	Varicella zoster, HSV, EBV
	Hepatitis

(Full infection and immunization history is required to interpret results)

Dynamic tests:	*In vivo* immunization with testing for serological response (pneumovax, tetanus, hepatitis B)
	NB Avoid live vaccines in the immunocompromised

Suspected T cell defect

Total lymphocyte count (always look carefully at white cell differential)

Lymphocyte subpopulations	(CD4+ and CD8+ T cells, NK cells)
Dynamic tests:	*In vivo*: DTH[a] testing (multitest CMI)
	In vitro: T cell proliferation to antigens and mitogens (also tests monocyte function) cytokine production (research)

Phagocyte defect

Check for neutropenia on differential white count

Oxidative metabolism

Phagocytosis

Bacterial killing

(all these assays are difficult to standardize and are only available in specialist centers)

Complement defect

Hemolytic assays for alternate and classical pathways

(measurement of C3a and C5a is possible but requires tubes with futhan-EDTA)

[a] DTH, delayed type hypersensitivity.

The type of investigations should be driven by the type of infections present, as this identifies the likely deficiency (Tables 36.2 and 36.4). It is essential to undertake functional tests of immune function, as significant immunodeficiency may be present even with normal cell numbers and normal total immunoglobulins. Specialist immunological advice should always be sought in the investigation of recurrent or unusual infection.

Management

There is no therapy currently available that reverses the immunodeficiency of uremia, and although a successful renal transplant will relieve the uremia, this frequently substitutes an iatrogenic immunosuppression through the drug therapy required to prevent rejection. The patient therefore trades one type of immunodeficiency for another.

The most important aspects of management are firstly to appreciate the risks and to minimize those risks that are amenable to medical therapy. Attention should be paid to nutritional status, with correction of vitamin and mineral deficiency. The correction of zinc deficiency may not, however, restore lymphocyte responsiveness. Iron overload should be avoided or, if present, treated. Good uremic control through dialysis with biocompatible membranes is essential. This may be difficult to achieve due to the pressure on dialysis units. Efforts should be made to reduce or eliminate endotoxin from dialysates. Scrupulous aseptic technique, especially for those on home hemodialysis or CAPD, is essential.

Immunization, particularly against hepatitis B, is important but difficult. Regimens of multiple doses have been tried with some success, and it has been suggested that the recombinant vaccines are more immunogenic than the older plasma-derived vaccines [26]. The addition of IL-2 to the vaccination schedule has been advocated although whether this approach is helpful is still controversial [27].

For patients with recurrent infections, prophylactic antibiotics may be required and if there are documented bacterial infections with evidence of poor/absent humoral immune function on dynamic testing, then replacement therapy with i.v. immunoglobulin (200–600 mg/kg every three to four weeks), as for primary antibody deficiency, may be helpful [25]. This can be given during dialysis, so that the additional fluid load required to administer it can be removed.

Prompt antibiotic therapy for infections is required. A new cephalosporin, cefodizime, has been reported to enhance neutrophil phagocytosis in uremic patients and may have a specific role in the treatment of uremic sepsis. However, *in vitro* tests of neutrophil function are very often abnormal in untreated sepsis and improve with treatment of the underlying infection with any combination of antibiotics, so it is unclear whether this is a specific or generic antibiotic effect.

There have been reports that the use of recombinant erythropoietin (rh-EpO) to treat the anemia of chronic renal failure may be accompanied by improvements in immune function. Sennesael *et al.* [28] have reported that the response to hepatitis B vaccination is improved in patients on rh-Epo. At present financial constraints limit the use of rh-Epo in uremic patients, but if further studies confirm an additional effect of improving immune function and decreasing infections then the cost–benefit equation may be more favorable.

References

1. Lawrence, H.S. (1965) Uremia: Nature's immunosuppressive device. *Ann. Intern. Med.*, **62**, 409–14.
2. Lundin, A.P., Adler, A.J., Feinbrith, M.V. *et al.* (1980) Maintenance hemodialysis: survival beyond the first decade. *J. Am. Med. Assoc.*, **244**, 38–40.
3. Mailloux, L.U., Bellucci, A.G., Wilkes, B.M. *et al.* (1991) Mortality in dialysis patients: analysis of the causes of death. *Am. J. Kidney Dis.*, **18**, 326–35.
4. Bradley, J.R., Evans, D.B. and Calne, R.Y. (1987) Long-term survival in hemodialysis patients. *Lancet*, **i**, 295–6.
5. Garcia-Leoni, M.E., Martin-Scapa, C., Rodeño, P. *et al.* (1990) High incidence of tuberculosis in renal patients. *Eur. J. Clin. Microbiol. Infect. Dis.*, **9**, 283–5.
6. Mioli, V.A. and LaGreca, G. (1992) A special issue on viral hepatitis and the kidney. *Nephron*, **61**, 251–376.
7. Kirkpatrick, C.H., Wilson, W.E.C. and Talmage, D.W. (1964) Immunologic studies in human organ transplantation, I. Observation and characterisation of suppressed cutaneous reactivity in uremia. *J. Exp. Med.*, **119**, 727–42.
8. Stefoni, S., DeSanctis, L.B., Nanni-Costa, A. *et al.* (1995) Dialysis and the immune system. (Review). *Contrib. Nephrol.*, **113**, 80–91.
9. Kurz, P., Köhler, H., Meuer, S.C. *et al.* (1986) Impaired cellular immune responses in chronic renal failure: evidence for a T cell defect. *Kidney Int.*, **29**, 1209–14.
10. Meuer, S.C., Haver, M., Kurz, P. *et al.* (1987) Selective blockade of the antigen receptor mediated pathway of T cell activation in patients with impaired primary immune responses. *J. Clin. Invest.*, **80**, 743–9.
11. Haag-Weber, M. and Hörl, W.H. (1993) Uremia and infection: mechanisms of impaired cellular host defense. *Nephron*, **63**, 125–31.
12. Asaka, M., Iida, H., Izumino, K. *et al.* (1988) Depressed natural killer cell activity in uremia. *Nephron*, **49**, 291–5.
13. Baj, Z., Pokoca, L., Majewska, E. *et al.* (1992) T lymphocyte subsets and NK cell cytotoxicity in chronic hemodialysis patients. The effect of recombinant human erythropoietin (rHu-EPO) treatment. *Arch. Immunol. Ther. Exp.*, **40**, 201–6.
14. Zbrog, Z., Luciak, M., Tchorzewski, H. and Pokoca, L. (1991) Modification of some lymphocyte functions *in vitro* by opioid receptor agonists and antagonist in chronic uremic patients and healthy subjects. *Int. J. Immunopharmacol.*, **13**, 475–83.
15. Shasha, S.M., Kristal, B., Barzilai, M. *et al.* (1988) *In vitro* effect of PTH on normal T cells. *Nephron*, **50**, 212–16.
16. Flament, J., Goldman, M., Waterlot, Y. *et al.* (1986) Impairment of phagocyte oxidative metabolism in hemodialysed patients with iron overload. *Clin. Nephrol.*, **25**, 227–30.
17. Tielmans, C. and Lenclud, C. (1988) Respective role of hemodialysis and desferrioxamine therapy in the risk from infection of haemodialysed patients. *Q. J. Med.*, **68**, 573–4.
18. Bonomini, M., Manfrini, V., Cappelli, P. and Albertazzi, A. (1993) Zinc and cell-mediated immunity in chronic uremia. *Nephron*, **65**, 1–4.
19. Fraker, P.J., Gershwin, M.E., Good, R.A. and Prasad, A. (1986) Interrelationships between zinc and immune function. *Fed. Proc.*, **45**, 1474–9.
20. Gardinali, M., Calcagno, A., Conciato, L. *et al.* (1994) Complement activation in dialysis: effects on cytokines, lymphocyte activation and beta-2-microglobulin. *Int. J. Artif. Organs*, **17**, 337–44.
21. Paczek, L., Czarkowska, B., Schaefer, L. *et al.* (1992) Effect of beta-2-microglobulin on immunoglobulin production. *Immunol. Lett.*, **33**, 87–91.
22. Agnello, V. (1978) Lupus disease associated with inherited and acquired deficiencies of complement. *Springer Semin. Immunopathol.*, **9**, 161–78.
23. Baum, C.G., Chiorazzi, N., Frankel, S. and Shepherd,

G.M. (1989) Conversion of systemic lupus erythematosus to common variable immunodeficiency. *Am. J. Med.*, **87**, 149–56.

24. Aarli, J.A. (1985) Immunoglobulins in epilepsy. *Springer Semin. Immunopathol.*, **8**, 5–27.
25. Spickett, G.P., Misbah, S.A. and Chapel, H.M. (1991) Primary antibody deficiency in adults. *Lancet*, **337**, 281–4.
26. Jungers, P., Chauveau, P., Courouce, A.M. *et al.* (1994) Immunogenicity of the recombinant GenHevac B

Pasteur vaccine against hepatitis B in chronic uremic patients. *J. Infect. Dis.*, **169**, 399–402.
27. Jungers, P., Devillier, P., Salomon, H. *et al.* (1994) Randomised placebo-controlled trial of recombinant interleukin-2 in chronic uremic patients who are non-responders to hepatitis B vaccine. *Lancet*, **344**, 856–7.
28. Sennesael, J.J., Van der Niepen, P. and Verbeelen, D.L. (1991) Treatment with recombinant human erythropoietin increases antibody titers after hepatitis B vaccination in dialysis patients. *Kidney Int.*, **40**, 121–8.

Further reading

Descamps-Latscha, B., Herbelin, A., Nguyen, A.T. *et al.* (1994) Immune dysregulation in uremia. *Semin. Nephrol.*, **14**, 253–60.

Descamps-Latscha, B., Herbelin, A., Nguyen, A.T. *et al.* (1995) Dysrégulation du système immunitaire, chez l'urémique chronique et le dialysé. *Presse Med.*, **24**, 405–10.

Haag-Weber, M. and Hörl, W.H. (1993) Uremia and infection: mechanisms of impaired cellular host defense.

Nephron, **63**, 125–31.

Janeway, C.A. and Travers, P. (1996) Immunobiology. *The Immune System in Health and Disease*. 2nd edition. Blackwell Scientific, Oxford.

Stefoni, S., DeSanctis, L.B., Nanni-Costa A. *et al.* (1995) Dialysis and the immune system. (Review). *Contrib. Nephrol.*, **113**, 80–91.

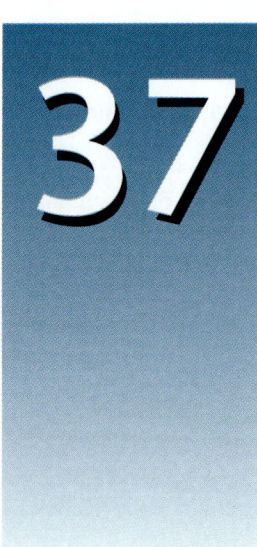

37

Skin–renal relationships

John A. Cotterill

Introduction

This subject is best approached under five headings:

1 Renal consequences of skin disease
2 Cutaneous consequences of renal disease
3 Diseases which commonly affect both skin and kidney simultaneously
4 Consequences of treatment of skin disease on the kidney
5 Consequences of treatment of renal disease on the skin.

Renal consequences of extensive skin disease

Some disturbances of renal function are an almost universal accompaniment of patients with extensive skin disease [1], such as exfoliative dermatitis, or erythroderma where there is an obligatory increase in skin blood flow, leading to a consequent decrease in blood flow to other organs, such as the kidneys. Plasma volume may be increased or decreased in patients with extensive skin disease. It is normally increased in patients with exfoliative dermatitis, but if capillary permeability is also increased, plasma volume may be reduced. Increased capillary permeability may be a feature of exfoliative dermatitis, and of extensive psoriasis, leading to edema,

particularly of dependent parts, such as the ankles and legs. This edema may be accentuated by the presence of hypoalbuminemia, which occurs because of excessive losses of protein through the skin and gut and also because of increased catabolism. Oliguria may occur in patients with exfoliative dermatitis and is associated with increased absorption of sodium by the kidney. Although renal blood flow is decreased, the glomerular filtration rate is preserved.

It is quite common for patients with extensive skin disease to feel thirsty, but this is not associated with significant changes in plasma osmolality. Significant proteinuria occurs in patients with extensive skin disease and the degree of proteinuria correlates with the activity and extent of the skin disease [2]. The D-xylose test performed to investigate for malabsorption may be abnormal in patients with extensive skin disease due to impaired renal function. Hyperuricemia is a feature of patients with extensive eczema and psoriasis and can be related in part to the extent of the eruption.

Cutaneous consequences of renal disease

There are several dermatological consequences of chronic renal failure [3]. The commonest and most troublesome is generalized pruritus. Other dermatological features of chronic renal failure include hyperpigmentation,

Nephrology, Edited by Rex L. Jamison and Robert Wilkinson.
Published in 1997 by Chapman & Hall, London. ISBN 0 412 60930 4

decreased sebum production, dryness of the skin and purpura.

Generalized pruritus

Generalized pruritus [4] is a feature in many patients with chronic renal failure. On the other hand, it is not usually a clinical feature of patients with acute renal failure.

The pathogenesis of generalized pruritus in chronic renal failure is poorly understood. The generally dry skin of patients with chronic renal failure may be one factor. Other factors may include secondary hyperparathyroidism and hyperuricemia. The presence of generalized pruritus may lead to excoriation of the skin and, occasionally, to thickening of the skin, sometimes with localized nodular changes. Fortunately, generalized, severe, troublesome pruritus occurs only in about a third of patients with chronic renal failure. It is noteworthy that hemodialysis, although improving the pruritus in some patients, may also initiate or exacerbate pruritus in up to 85% of patients so treated. Of this 85%, a third had pruritus before hemodialysis, whereas the others developed this symptom after dialysis [5]. It has been claimed that parathyroidectomy may relieve pruritus in some patients.

It has been postulated that unknown agents capable of inducing pruritus may be the cause of this symptom in patients with chronic renal failure. Possible pruritogens are calcium and/or magnesium and tissue levels of these ions may be more relevant to the development of pruritus than levels in the blood. Irradiation of the skin with ultraviolet light may be helpful in reducing pruritus and ultraviolet light B (UVB) 280–310 nm has been shown to reduce skin phosphorus to normal levels, suggesting that high phosphorus tissue levels may be important in mediating pruritus [6]. Therapy with cholestyramine or activated charcoal has been reported to be helpful.

Pigmentary changes in patients with chronic renal failure

Full-blown skin color changes seen in patients with chronic renal failure are now rarely seen, but patients with chronic renal failure develop a characteristic hyperpigmentation due to deposition of melanin in the skin. Other chromogens, such as urochromes, have also been blamed for the pigmentary changes, which are usually more marked on light-exposed skin. It has been claimed that beta-MSH (melanocyte-stimulating hormone) is increased in plasma in patients with chronic renal failure because of failure of the kidney to metabolize this hormone [7]. The anemia of chronic renal failure may also contribute to the overall perceived skin color.

Nail changes have also been described in patients with chronic renal failure. These changes have been described as 'half and half' nails (Figure 37.1). Individuals with this physical sign develop a distal hyperpigmentation of the nails, which contrasts with the normal, or white appearance of the proximal part of the nail. These changes have

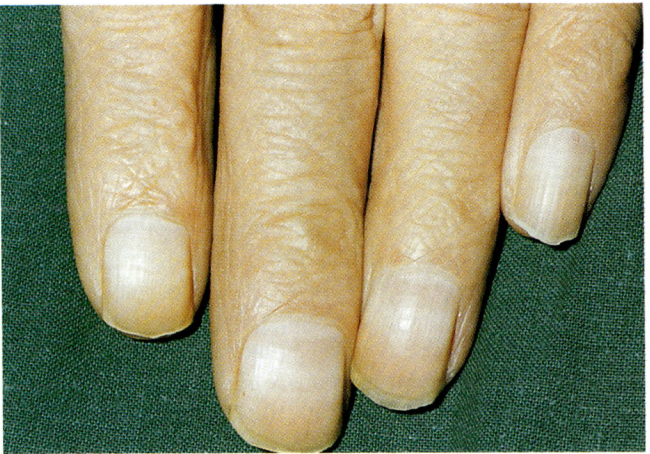

Figure 37.1 'Half and half' nails in chronic renal failure. The distal nail is hyperpigmented in contrast with the normal or white proximal nail.

been described in up to 10% of patients with chronic renal failure [8]. They are by no means specific to this condition, and may be seen also in patients with liver disease, and in some patients with malignant disease.

Hair changes

There may be a reduction of secondary sex hair of the face, suprapubic area and axillae, possibly due to changes in androgen metabolism [3]. For instance, up to 40% of patients with chronic renal failure may develop gynecomastia while receiving dialysis [9]. It has also been claimed that gynecomastia may be ameliorated by a phosphorus-restricted diet, coupled with oral phosphate-binding agents [10]. The scalp hair is often also affected and is said to resemble the appearances seen in patients with protein malnutrition.

Some rarer dermatological changes

Calcium deposition in skin

It is unusual for frank calcification to occur in the skin in uremic patients, but this change has been described, producing either papular or nodular changes, particularly around large joints or in the flexures. A calcifying panniculitis (inflammatory reaction of subcutaneous fat) has also been reported [4].

Perforating collagenosis

This is a rare clinical feature of patients with chronic renal failure [4]. It is possibly more common in patients with renal failure associated with diabetes mellitus and is seen in up to 10% or patients receiving hemodialysis. The condition is characterized by the presence of hypopigmented papules, up to 1 cm in diameter with a central perforating keratinous plug. It has been claimed that this is a feature more commonly seen in Afro-Caribbeans with chronic renal failure.

Porphyria cutanea tarda

This is a rare bullous condition which usually occurs on light-exposed areas, particularly over the knuckles. Following exposure to UV light, patients may develop painful blisters. Usual screening porphyrin tests are negative, although the clinical picture is clinically that of porphyria cutanea tarda. More sophisticated biochemical investigations usually confirm the diagnosis [11]. In the urine the main features include raised uroporphyrins and a moderate elevation of coproporphyrins and 7-, 6- and 5-carboxylate porphyrins.

The feces contain less soluble coproporphyrin, isocoprophyrin and protoporphyrin. Screening tests looking for a pink fluorescence using a Woods lamp as a source of UV light may be negative if the condition is in remission.

Urea frost

Urea frost, in which crystalline urea is deposited on the skin, has never been seen by this author. It was a cutaneous feature of chronic renal disease before effective treatment for this condition became available.

Purpura

Purpura is a fairly common accompaniment of patients with chronic renal failure and often will be accompanied by a mild thrombocytopenia.

Diseases that may affect both skin and kidneys

Some of the disorders that may present in this way are shown in Table 37.1.

Angiokeratoma corporis diffusum (Anderson–Fabry disease)

Clinical manifestations

Angiokeratoma corporis diffusum is an X-linked lysosomal disorder [12]. Most patients, therefore, are males and present with strange, but characteristic lancinating pain in the arms and limbs, and particularly the skin of the fingers and toes. The characteristic sphingolipid-containing angiokeratomas usually begin appearing shortly before puberty, particularly around the thighs, scrotum and umbilicus although they may occur on other parts of the body including the hands (Figure 37.2), and to the inexperienced non-dermatological eye, may be misdiagnosed as purpura.

The majority of patients develop renal disease as a result of sphingolipid deposition in glomerular vessels and death from renal failure in the third or fourth decade of life is usual without treatment, although a minority of patients survive beyond this age without apparent renal impairment. Proteinuria, together with hematuria and sphingolipid, may be found in the urine.

There are many other classical associated features of the disorder, including 'parrot-beaking' of the nails, increased tortuosity and dilation of conjunctival and retinal vessels and a specific superficial corneal dystrophy, which is of diagnostic importance. Other associated dermatological findings include dry, lax, hypohidrotic skin.

Genetic disorders	Anderson–Fabry disease (angiokeratoma corporis diffusum)
	Amyloidosis (Muckle Wells syndrome)
	Neurofibromatosis
	Tuberous sclerosis
	Sickle cell disease
	Von Hippel Landau disease
Acquired disorders	Amyloidosis
	Henoch Schönlein purpura and other vasculitides
	Collagen disease, including systemic lupus erythematosus
	Systemic sclerosis
	Polyarteritis nodosa
	Wegener's granulomatosis
	Erythema multiforme
	Toxic epidermal necrolysis
	Sarcoidosis

Table 37.1 Disorders which may affect both skin and kidneys

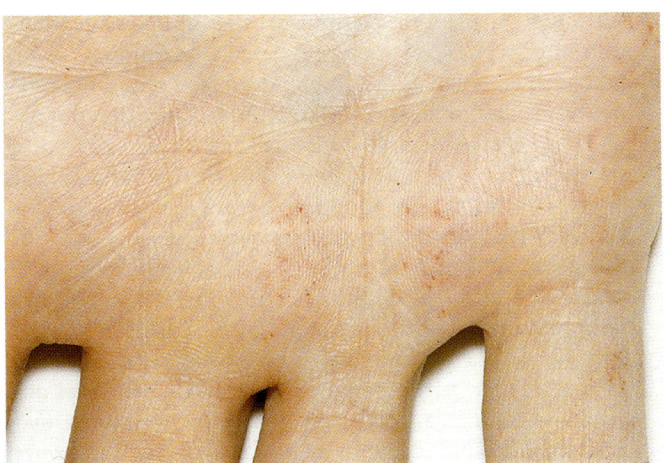

Figure 37.2 Typical angiokeratomas in an unusual site in a patient with Anderson–Jabry disease causing renal failure.

Pathogenesis

Patients with this condition are deficient in the enzyme lysosomal hydrolase α-galactosidase.

Treatment

It has been claimed that renal transplantation can supply a source of this deficient enzyme and lead to clinical improvement in patients with Anderson–Fabry disease [13]. However, abnormal lipid deposition has also been reported in a transplanted kidney.

Amyloidosis

Patients with myeloma-associated systemic amyloidosis may develop waxy, purpuric changes in their skin or mucosa in up to 40% of those affected [14]. The site of purpura, which often involves the eyelids (Figure 37.3), can be of diagnostic assistance. Other features present may include enlargement of the tongue and liver and the development of the carpal-tunnel syndrome. Much more rarely, excessively lax skin may be seen in association with amyloidosis [15].

Purpura involving the ear and eyelids may also be seen in patients following severe vomiting and retching, but this is usually a fairly transient phenomenon, whereas that seen in amyloidosis is usually quite persistent.

Muckle Wells Syndrome

This rare syndrome [16] is transmitted as an autosomal dominant and presents during childhood and adolescence with urticaria, often accompanied by fever. Subsequently patients develop sensory deafness, joint pain and effusions. These changes are associated with amyloidosis, and renal disease due to this condition may also occur and can result in premature death.

Neurofibromatosis (Von Recklinghausen's disease)

Several renal complications may occur in patients with neurofibromatosis. There are at least two distinct genetic types of neurofibromatosis (NF-1 and NF-2), but in both types neurofibromas form around nerves. NF-1 is characterized by café-au-lait spots. The presence of six or more such macular areas in the axillae is diagnostic (Crowe's sign) [17]. In addition, neurofibromas develop adjacent to peripheral nerves. In NF-2 acoustic neuromas, meningiomas and other central nervous system tumors develop. Inheritance is autosomal dominant.

Rarer clinical features include hypertension, due to pheochromocytoma of the adrenal gland, but hypertension may also occur because of renal artery stenosis. Renal artery thrombosis has been described, as has renal polycystic disease, and nephroblastoma. Problems with urinary outflow obstruction may occur secondary to pressure from a neurofibroma [18].

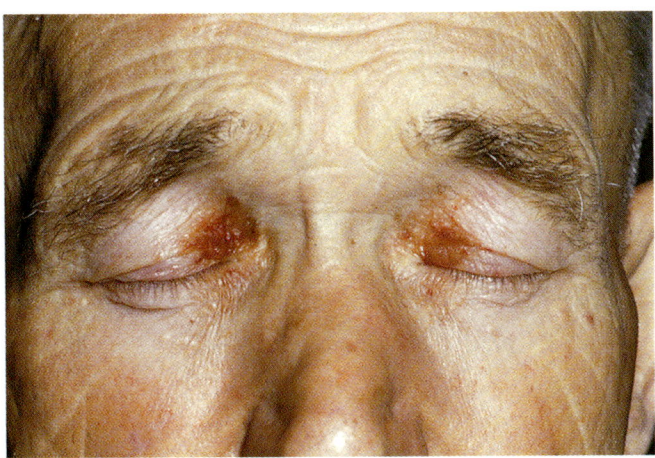

Figure 37.3 Purpura of the eyelids was the presenting feature in this patient with amyloidosis.

Tuberous sclerosis

Tuberous sclerosis [19] is characterized by the multiorgan formation of hamartomas in kidneys, skin, brain, eye and heart. Although the condition is thought to be transmitted by a single autosomal dominant gene on chromosome 9, the majority of patients appear to have no family history and are thought by geneticists to have developed the disease due to spontaneous genetic mutation.

Clinically, the skin lesions consist of facial angiofibromas (Figure 37.4), white macules, periungual fibromas and the characteristic shagreen patch. Other clinical features include mental retardation and epilepsy. Renal tumors of embryonic type, usually multiple, are reported to be present in up to 80% of patients at post mortem, but are mostly asymptomatic. Pathologically, the renal tumors are usually angiomyolipomas, but cystic renal disease may also be seen. Hematuria may be a rare presenting feature. It is easy to mistake the angiofibromas on the face for acne, particularly in children, but the lesions develop much earlier than classical acne. Diagnosis can be confirmed by the identification of the classical ash leaf-shaped white macules under Woods' light, in conjunction with other clinical features.

Von Hippel–Lindau disease

This rare, multiorgan disorder is transmitted as an autosomal dominant. Renal cell carcinoma, often bilateral, is reported to occur in about 25% of patients and is also reported to be the second commonest cause of death after cerebellar hemangioblastoma.

Dermatological features, such as café-au-lait macules and port wine stains, particularly of the face and neck, may also be seen [20].

Henoch Schönlein purpura

Henoch Schönlein purpura [21] is characterized by the deposition of immune complexes containing IgA.

Although the identification of the antigen in these immune complexes remains largely unknown, some autoantigens such as IgA rheumatoid factor, and IgA anti-neutrophil cytoplasmic antibody, have been described.

There is considerable doubt as to whether a preceding streptococcal infection is important in the pathogenesis of this condition. The condition occurs in both sexes, but the peak incidence is between four and seven years, and the peak incidence of nephritis is between six and 11 years. The classical clinical features include a purpuric rash, abdominal and joint pain. Purpura is seen particularly on the buttocks and legs, and is often palpable. Some of the lesions in the early stages may be urticarial and localized edema can occur on the scalp, around the eyes and distally on the hands and feet. Colicky abdominal pain may be accompanied by diarrhea and vomiting, or even by melena due to bowel involvement. Intussusception is a fairly rare clinical event.

Medium sized joints, such as the elbows, wrists, ankles and knees, are most frequently affected.

Up to 60% of patients may have hematuria or proteinuria. It has been claimed that up to 25% of affected children under the age of two years, and 50% of older children, show signs of renal involvement. Happily, in the majority of cases, the renal involvement is transient and only a small minority of children are left with permanent renal damage. Recurrent episodes are common, occurring in up to 50% of patients, and this may continue exceptionally for some years.

With regard to management, if streptococcal infection is present in either the patient or relatives, treatment with penicillin should be given. It is not thought that corticosteroids have any effect on renal disease or purpura. Regular urine analysis is important to identify any renal problems.

Other possible infective agents, such as cytomegalovirus, have been incriminated recently in the pathogenesis of this condition. More recently, an IgA anticardiolipin antibody has been detected in an adult patient with Henoch Schöenlein purpura [22].

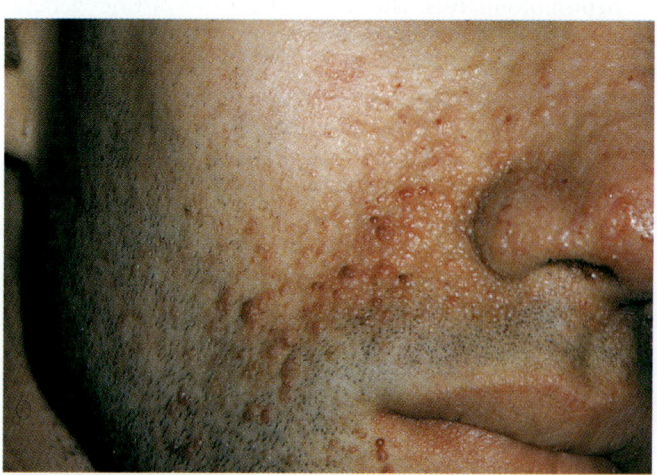

Figure 37.4 Facial angiofibromas in a patient with tuberous sclerosis.

Erythema multiforme (ectodermosis erosiva pleuriorificialis)

Although ectodermosis erosiva pleuriorificialis is quite a mouthful, it does describe in full the clinical features of erythema multiforme [23], which can involve all orifices, and which, when severe, is often referred to as the Stevens–Johnson syndrome, although Stevens and Johnson described the severe form of erythema multiforme many years after the original descriptions.

Pathogenesis

The cause of this relatively common condition is unknown, but it may be an immune complex disease. The commonest precipitating factor seems to be herpes simplex, but erythema multiforme can be associated with many other viral infections, including orf and glandular fever. It may be a feature of collagen disease and is a not uncommon complication of pregnancy. It may occur as a reaction to drugs, particularly long-acting sulfonamides, and possibly, the contraceptive pill. Erythema multiforme has been associated with primary atypical pneumonia (mycoplasma) infections.

Clinical manifestations

As the name erythema multiforme suggests, many different clinical forms exist, including the rarer, and often ill-diagnosed papular form, which may evolve to give the characteristic target lesions, particularly on the hands, arms and legs. Bullae are not uncommon and, characteristically, a central bullous lesion with a marginal ring of vesicles may be seen (herpes iris of Bateman). In this form, the mucous membranes, particularly of the mouth, may be involved. In the severe bullous form multiorgan involvement is usual. The mouth is almost always involved and the patient is unable to eat, and sometimes drink, and saliva runs constantly from the mouth. Eye involvement is also very common, and can be severe, leading to subsequent blindness, due to corneal opacities and synechiae. The urethra may be involved in up to half the patients with this severe bullous type of erythema multiforme. Lung involvement is not unusual, with a pneumonitis in up to a quarter of patients. Patients with the severe bullous from of this disease are ill, with high fever. Renal involvement, with hematuria, or even acute renal failure, can occur, and this may lead to progressive renal failure. Erythema multiforme, when severe, has many of the features of toxic epidermal necrolysis (see below), which has a significant mortality rate of 5–15%. It is usually easy to differentiate all clinical types of erythema multiforme from other more chronic bullous diseases, such as pemphigoid and pemphigus. A rare pustular type of erythema multiforme can also occur, and occasionally erythema multiforme and erythema nodosum can co-exist.

Treatment

In regard to treatment, the balance of the literature suggests that corticosteroids are not useful in this condition, but despite this they are often prescribed in a dose of 30–80 mg daily. Antibiotics are usually given. Perhaps erythromycin is the drug of choice to cover any possibility of mycoplasma infection.

Recurrent herpes simplex may be controlled quite well with long-term low-dose acyclovir therapy. The usual dose is 200 mg of acyclovir two or three times daily for six months.

Toxic epidermal necrolysis

Toxic epidermal necrolysis [24] is one of the most difficult conditions any dermatologist can be called upon to manage. It is also extremely distressing and very painful for the patient.

Pathogenesis

With regard to pathogenesis, toxic epidermal necrolysis can occur as a drug reaction, and a wide number of drugs have been incriminated, including the sulfonamides and allopurinol. Classically, allopurinol may give rise to toxic epidermal necrolysis if it is given to treat hyperuricemia in normal dosage in a patient with impaired renal function. In the classic scenario, such patients usually have a history of hypertension and are taking diuretics. Allopurinol can be given safely to patients with impaired renal function, but the dose must be adjusted downward as renal function falls, because allopurinol metabolites (oxypurinol) are cleared by the kidney. This author has seen several deaths from toxic epidermal necrolysis in elderly patients with impaired renal function following conventional dosage of allopurinol.

Other drugs which have been incriminated include ethambutol, phenolphthalein and the hydantoins and pentazocine. The condition may also arise as a complication of systemic disease, such as leukemia or lymphoma, following radiotherapy, and as a complication of viral infections or measles immunization. It has also been described following contact with the fumigant acrylonitrile.

Clinical manifestations

In this condition patients are constitutionally ill and marked skin redness and tenderness are initial physical signs. Subsequently, there is subepidermal blister formation due to basal cell damage and the Nikolsky sign (the ability to glide the involved epidermis over the underlying dermis due to damage at the epidermal–dermal border) becomes all too evidently positive (Figure 37.5). Even the slightest degree of oblique trauma to the skin results in stripping off of large sheets of necrotic epidermis. The mouth and other mucous membranes are also

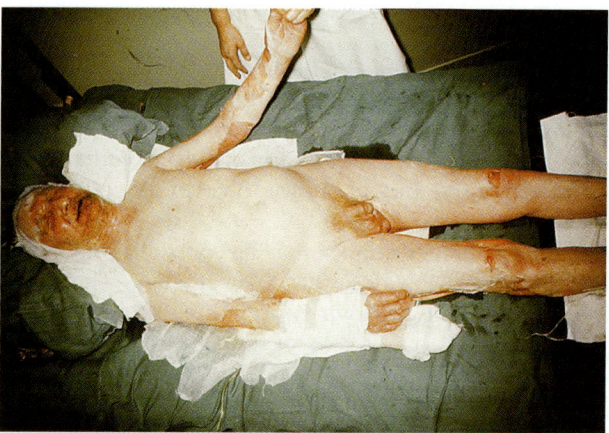

Figure 37.5   A patient with toxic epidermal necrolysis.

involved, which makes nutrition and fluid balance difficult.

The clinical appearance of toxic epidermal necrolysis can be simulated by the staphylococcal scalded skin syndrome (see below) which can occur in adults, but is much more common in children. However, it is important to exclude any staphylococcal infection by appropriate swabs, and, if necessary, a skin biopsy will demonstrate the level of the split. In toxic epidermal necrolysis there is always subepidermal blister formation, with basal cell damage, whereas in the scalded skin syndrome skin damage occurs just below the granular layer.

The mortality from toxic epidermal necrolysis can approach 50%, especially in the idiopathic group of patients, and permanent eye changes can result in corneal opacity and blindness. Clinically, it may be difficult initially to differentiate toxic epidermal necrolysis from erythema multiforme.

Treatment

The treatment of this condition is controversial. In the author's opinion, the patient should be managed in a burn unit. Steroids are not thought to be helpful. If there is any possibility of a staphylococcal cause for the skin problems, which is more likely in patients with impaired renal function, erythromycin or flucloxacillin should be prescribed. Nursing in a specialized burn unit on an air fluidized bed such as that manufactured by Clinitron is mandatory. Maintenance of fluid balance is vital and it may be necessary to debride wounds and apply either porcine xenografts or human cadaveric allografts.

Impaired renal function is common in elderly patients, and when the condition is associated with allopurinol therapy, excessive loss of water, electrolytes and protein through the skin exacerbates pre–existing renal problems.

The staphylococcal scalded skin syndrome (Lyell's disease)

Pathogenesis

This syndrome [25] is associated with staphylococcal infection and the changes in the skin are induced by an exotoxin elaborated by the staphylococcus, mainly of phage group II. The exotoxin, epidermolysin, is excreted by the kidney. Almost all adults who develop the staphylococcal scalded skin syndrome have a depressed immunity or impaired renal function or both, and diminished renal clearance of the exotoxin may be an important factor in pathogenesis.

Clinical manifestations

In contradistinction to toxic epidermal necrolysis, although the conditions can look very similar clinically, the split in the skin in the staphylococcal scalded skin syndrome is more superficial, occurring just below the granular layer. If there is any doubt about the diagnosis, a skin biopsy, processed as a frozen section, will establish the diagnosis rapidly.

Treatment

With regard to management, swabs should be taken to identify the staphylococcus involved and its sensitivity. If this condition occurs in a maternity hospital it is important to swab not only the parents, but also members of the medical and nursing staff to make sure there are no nasal carriers. Treatment of choice is either erythromycin or flucloxacillin. Topical treatment with antibacterial agents, such as silver sulfadiazine, may be helpful. Patients can die from this condition, usually when it has been diagnosed too late, or there has been failure of compliance with treatment by the parents. However, if treated properly and in time, recovery should be complete in children without impaired renal function. The prognosis of the older patient with the staphylococcal scalded skin syndrome, if recovery takes place, is usually the prognosis of the underlying disease. A good fluid intake seems a wise therapeutic measure to try to increase the renal clearance of the toxin.

Necrotizing fasciitis

Pathogenesis

Necrotizing fasciitis [26] is often associated with infection with group A β-hemolytic streptococci. Thirteen patients with this syndrome were recently reported from Norway. Of the 12 hospitalized alive, eight had clinical signs of shock, with a systolic blood pressure of 90 mmHg or less, and eight had impaired renal function. Seven patients had biochemical markers of disseminated intravascular coagulation and six patients fulfilled the criteria for streptococcal toxic shock syndrome. C reactive protein was elevated in ten patients.

Other organisms besides the streptococcus can be involved in pathogenesis, including anerobic bacteria, enterobacteria and streptococci other than serogroup Type A. *Staphylococcus aureus* and *Staphylococcus epidermidis* have also been incriminated.

Clinical features and treatment

Clinically, necrotizing fasciitis is characterized by the presence of soft tissue infection, which spreads rapidly, leading to subsequent necrosis of underlying fascia, subcutaneous fat and, at times, the overlying epidermis.

The condition is associated with a very high mortality rate, approaching 50%. It is important to diagnose the condition early and institute aggressive surgery to remove affected tissue. Aggressive appropriate antibiotic therapy is also necessary. Two of the patients in the Norwegian series required dialysis. The Norwegian authors stress the importance of early diagnosis, followed by aggressive treatment. Both the severity of infection and subsequent extent of surgical debridement increase with increasing time between onset and diagnosis.

Prompt surgery often reveals liquefaction necrosis of the fascia and subcutis confirming the diagnosis. Gram stains of tissue aspirate are useful in that Gram-positive cocci in chains are found in necrotizing fasciitis and such chains are rarely seen in patients with erysipelas.

Although all group A streptococci are always sensitive to benzyl penicillin, it is felt that this antibiotic may be inadequate for serious infections and large numbers of bacteria, so the addition of clindamycin is recommended. Treatment with clindamycin should cover possible infection with anerobes, but a third-generation cephalosporin or aminoglycoside should also be added to the antibiotic regimen to deal with any Gram-negative rods.

Partial lipodystrophy

This is a rare type of fat atrophy [27] which usually presents in childhood or in young adults and affects females up to five times more frequently than males. In some cases the condition seems to be familial whereas in others it seems to be precipitated by an acute febrile medical event such as measles.

Clinical features

The disease is characterized by complete loss of fatty tissue in the affected areas which are usually the face and upper half of the trunk. The facies (Figure 37.6) looks characteristically cadaverous.

The pattern of fat loss can vary. About 10% of patients have hemi-lipoatrophy involving just half the face or trunk. In a minority of cases there may be fat hypertrophy in the lower part of the body.

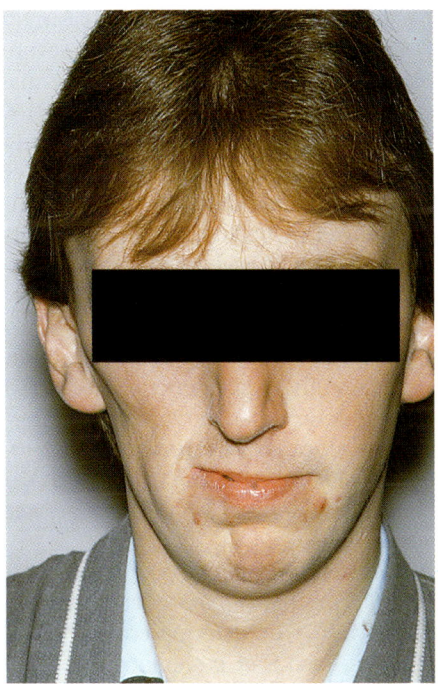

Figure 37.6 Typical facies of a patient with partial lipodystrophy.

Up to 90% of patients with partial lipodystrophy develop renal disease which can be precipitated by ergot derivatives, the contraceptive pill and pregnancy.

Pathologically there is a progressive mesangiocapillary (membranoproliferative) glomerulonephritis.

Immunologically there is a persistently low plasma concentration of the third component of complement (C3) accompanied by a serum factor capable of activating C3 termed nephritic factor (C3 NeF). Further associations with partial lipodystrophy include diabetes mellitus, which develops in a third of patients; more rarely retinitis pigmentosa and purpuric vasculitis have also been described.

Treatment

It is very important to follow female patients carefully during pregnancy and medication with an oral contraceptive is totally contraindicated. Renal transplantation in one patient has led to normalization of the immunological changes. The renal changes are usually progressive and lead to end-stage renal failure.

Consequences of treatment of skin disease on the kidney

Cyclosporin

Dermatologists prescribe relatively few drugs orally, but some of the drugs prescribed do have potential to cause renal damage [28]. Cyclosporin is being used increasingly for the long-term management of patients with severe psoriasis, severe eczema and rarer types of bullous diseases, such as pemphigus. Dermatologists usually use this drug in doses varying between 3 and 5 mg/kg/day. Only minimal nephrotoxicity is thought to develop with doses less than 2.5 mg/kg/day. At higher dose levels pathological change may be induced in both renal blood vessels and tubules. Once more, this damage may reverse if the drug is stopped, although some patients never fully recover renal function. In patients receiving cyclosporin therapy for dermatological problems, renal function should be monitored carefully. Renal function tests and blood pressure should be determined at two-weekly intervals during the first three months of treatment, and thereafter at monthly intervals in patients with psoriasis, eczema or pemphigus taking doses of cyclosporin greater than 2.5 mg/kg/day.

If patients with these conditions are maintained on lower daily doses than 2.5 mg/kg/day, renal function tests and blood pressure need only be determined every two months. It has been suggested that patients with atopic eczema should have blood pressure and renal function tests determined at two-weekly intervals, although in the author's experience this seems overzealous.

In patients receiving cyclosporin for a transplanted kidney, serum levels are measured periodically. Doses are adjusted to keep values within the therapeutic range.

If the serum creatinine rises 30% above the baseline reading on two consecutive occasions the dose of cyclosporin should be reduced, in patients with psoriasis, atopic eczema or pemphigus. Cyclosporin should be discontinued if this dose reduction is not successful in reducing creatinine levels within a month. It must be remembered that some patients with severe psoriasis can only be controlled with cyclosporin, having failed to respond to every other conceivable treatment. Discontinuing cyclosporin can have a devastating effect on the quality of their life. In these circumstances, it is important that the renal physician and dermatologist co-operate to optimize the patient's management.

Drug interactions

Decreased clearance of cyclosporin has been reported with concurrent use of erythromycin, ketoconazole or amphotericin B and therefore increases the risk of toxic effects of cyclosporin. Accelerated clearance of cyclosporin has been demonstrated in patients receiving phenytoin, carbamazepine, phenobarbitone, trimethoprim-sulfamethoxazole and rifampicin, presumably by inducing the P_{450} enzymes in the liver.

Topical medications which could affect renal function

Some dermatologists still use phenol topically on the skin [29]. Phenol is nephrotoxic and in the author's opinion

is best avoided. Severe systemic reactions, with abdominal pain, dizziness, hemoglobinurea, cyanosis and sometimes fatal coma, follow the application of phenol to extensive wounds. Even the accidental application of pure phenol to a small area of skin in a baby has been fatal.

Resorcinol can induce percutaneous toxic effects, with skin rash, hemolytic anemia and hemoglobinemia.

Fatal poisoning following carbon tetrachloride application to the skin to remove an adhesive plaster in an infant has been reported. Carbon tetrachloride is a recognized cause of hepatorenal failure.

It is known that repeated application of salicylic acid ointments to extensive skin disease, for instance, psoriasis, will produce salicylism. This effect is mostly seen in children and even fatal cases have been recorded as a result of acidosis. Salicylism can also occur in adults.

Consequences of renal replacement treatment on the skin

Venous hypertension of the hand associated with vascular access for hemodialysis

Venous hypertension of the hand is a rare complication following the creation of an arteriovenous access for patients receiving dialysis [30]. Venous hypertension leads to swelling, induration, hyperpigmentation, and even ulceration, most commonly in the thumb and index finger. These changes have been described in 0.1–0.5% of patients, mostly in those with a side-to-side arteriovenous fistula; end-to-side anastomoses carry less risk of vascular complications. These changes usually develop one to two years after creation of the anastomosis.

The histological findings with pericapillary fibrin cuffs are similar to those in patients with venous hypertension of the leg.

Skin cancer as a complication of renal transplantation

The incidence of non-melanoma skin cancer is much greater in patients who have undergone renal transplantation than in an age- and sex-matched control population [31–34]. This finding has been attributed to immunosuppressive therapy, ultraviolet light and the papilloma virus. A recent study from Holland of 764 patients treated by renal allograft between 1966 and 1988 showed a cumulative increase of skin cancer from 10% after 10 years to 40% after 20 years of graft survival. The sites of the squamous cell carcinoma were particularly frequent in light-exposed areas such as the backs of the hands, where solar damage was noted to be most pronounced [31].

Any squamous carcinoma is likely to behave more aggressively in immunosuppressed patients, than in non-immunosuppressed patients, so that radical excision may be followed by recurrence. It has been claimed that skin malignancy in these patients is more likely to metastasize than in the general population.

The Dutch authors proposed a new surgical technique to resurface the back of the hands of renal transplant patients with multiple skin cancers. The skin of the entire dorsum of the hand was excised and replaced with split skin grafts harvested from the thigh and buttocks. No recurrence of skin cancer was noted in the transplanted skin, with a mean follow-up time of 4.7 years, and the cosmetic appearances were acceptable. This technique looks very promising.

Malignant melanoma in renal transplant recipients

It has been claimed that an increased incidence of malignant melanoma occurs in patients who have undergone renal transplantation [32]. Besides immunosuppression, another important factor in pathogenesis is the pre-existence of clinically dysplastic nevi. Greene *et al.* [32] suggested that malignant melanoma in immunosuppressed patients evolves from precursor nevi. It is, therefore, important to examine pretransplant recipients for clinically atypical and potentially dysplastic nevi. A patient with clinically dysplastic nevi should be considered at an increased risk of developing malignant melanoma. Following transplantation the skin should be examined frequently to look for any sign of malignant change. Serial photography may be used. Any changes in a nevus warrants an excisional biopsy. It is important to counsel these patients to avoid excessive exposure to ultraviolet light, either by sunbathing or during a vacation in the tropics. Ultraviolet light-blocking agents and suitable clothing should be advised. If malignant melanoma is judged to be a risk, immunosuppression should be altered or consideration given to discontinuation if malignant melanoma is found.

Consequences of renal transplantation in a tropical environment

Of 157 renal allograft recipients that were followed for up to 23 months after transplantation cushingoid features were noted in 85%, striae in >40% and hypertrichosis in 22% [33]. Friable skin developed in about 20% of patients, and facial erythema in 27%. Fungal infections occurred in over 80% of patients and included candidiasis, cryptococcosis, tinea corporis and cruris and tinea versicolor. Viral infections included herpes zoster (11%), herpes simplex (3%) and the papilloma virus (warts 8%). Only one patient developed skin cancer, but the follow-up was rather short.

Acne associated with steroid therapy tended to occur during the first year of therapy and then disappear as the dose of steroids was reduced.

The authors comment that warts occur in 30% of patients receiving long-term immunosuppressive therapy and are frequently numerous and disfiguring. The high dermal melanin content of patients in the Indian subcontinent may protect them from development of malignant change.

Post-transplant cutaneous lymphoma

Four cases of primary cutaneous lymphoma were observed in a review of 673 transplant patients [34]. It appears to have a marked predilection for peripheral sites. Post-transplant lymphoma is closely associated with the Epstein–Barr virus. Primary cutaneous B-cell lymphoma is rare in normal individuals; in transplant recipients it usually presents as single or multiple nodules predominantly on the trunk and scalp.

Secondary cutaneous oxalosis

Oxalosis is characterized by the deposition of calcium oxalate in the tissues [35]. Secondary oxalosis from chronic renal failure or long-term hemodialysis rarely affects the skin and usually occurs in the lungs, spleen, pancreas, bones, joints and blood vessels. One patient was described with miliary calcified papules on the distal fingers, occurring after long-term hemodialysis. The crystals in the dermis were shown to be calcium oxalate in the form of the dihydrate crystal and a diagnosis, therefore, of secondary cutaneous oxalosis was made. In cutaneous oxalosis associated with hemodialysis miliary deposits occur in the fingers, but not the toes.

References

1. Shuster, S. (1978) The inter-relationship between systemic and skin disease, in *Dermatology and Internal Medicine*, Oxford University Press, Oxford, pp. 71–3.
2. Cotterill, J.A. and Cunliffe, W.J. (1971) Proteinuria associated with skin disease. *Lancet*, 403–405.
3. Schuster, S. (1978) Gastro-intestinal hepatic and renal disease, in *Dermatology and Internal Medicine*, Oxford University Press, Oxford, pp. 134–6.
4. Weismann, K. and Graham, R.M. (1992) Systemic disease and the skin, in *Textbook of Dermatology*, 5th edn (eds R.H. Champion, J.A. Burton and F.J.G. Ebling), Blackwell Scientific Publications, Oxford, pp. 2433–4.

5. Young, A.W., Sweeny, E.W., David, D.S. *et al.* (1973) Dermatological evaluation of pruritus in patients on hemodialysis. *N.Y. State J. Med.*, **73**, 2670–4.

6. Blachley, J.D., Blankenship, D.M., Munter, A. *et al.* (1985) Uraemic pruritus, skin divalent iron content and response to ultraviolet phototherapy. *Am. J. Kidney Dis.*, **i**, 752–93.

7. Gilkes, J.J., Eady, R.A., Rees, L.H. *et al.* (1975) Plasma-immuno-reactive melanatrophic hormones in patients on maintenance haemodialysis. *Br. Med. J.*, **i**, 656–7.

8. Knit, A., Bussels, F., El Fernandes, M. *et al.* (1975) Skin and nail disorders in relation to chronic renal failure. *Acta Dermatol. Venereol.*, **54**, 137–40.

9. Freeman, R.M., Lawton, R.L. and Fearing, M.O. (1968) Gynaecomastia: an endocrinologic complication of haemodialysis. *Ann. Intern. Med.*, **69**, 67–72.

10. Kolton, B. and Pederson, J. (1974) Calcinosis cutis in renal failure. *Arch. Dermatol.*, **110**, 256–7.

11. Poh-Fitzpatrick, M.B., Sosin, A.E. and Bemis, J. (1982) Porphyrin levels in plasma and erythrocytes in chronic haemodialysis patients. *J. Am. Acad. Dermatol.*, **7**, 100–4.

12. Wallace, H.J. (1973) Anderson–Fabry Disease. *Br. J. Dermatol.*, **88**, 1–21.

13. Maizel, S.E., Simmons, R.L., Kjellstrand, C.K. *et al.* (1981) Ten year experience in renal transplantation for Fabry's Disease. *Transplant Proc.*, **13**, 57–9.

14. Breathnach, S.M. (1988) Amyloid and amyloidosis. *J. Am. Acad. Dermatol.*, **18**, 1–16.

15. Newton, J.A., McKee, P.H. and Black, M.N. (1986) Cutis laxa associated with amyloidosis. *Clin. Exp. Dermatol.*, **11**, 87–91.

16. Muckle, T.J. (1979) The Muckle Wells syndrome. *Br. J. Dermatol.*, **100**, 87–92.

17. Crowe, F.W. (1964) Axillary freckling as a diagnostic aid in neurofibromatisis. *Ann. Intern. Med.*, **61**, 1142–3.

18. Harper, J. (1992) Genetics and genodermatosis, in *Textbook of Dermatology*, 5th edn (eds R.H. Champion, J.L. Burton and F.J.G. Ebling), Blackwell, Oxford, pp. 322–5.

19. Harper, J. (1992) Genetics and genodermatosis, in *Textbook of Dermatology*, 5th edn (eds R.H. Champion, J.L. Burton and F.J.G. Ebling), Blackwell, Oxford, pp. 327–31.

20. Harper, J. (1992) Naevi and developmental defects, in *Textbook of Dermatology*, 5th edn (eds R.H. Champion, J.L. Burton and F.J.G. Ebling), Blackwell, Oxford, p. 493.

21. Harper, J. (1992) Cutaneous vasculitis, in *Textbook of Dermatology*, 5th edn (eds R.H. Champion, J.L. Burton and F.J.G. Ebling), Blackwell, Oxford, pp. 1918–20.

22. Burden, D.A., Gibson, I.W., Rodger, R.S.C. and Toolman, D.M. (1994) IgA anticardiolipin antibodies associated with Henoch Schöenlein purpura. *J. Am. Acad. Dermatol.*, **31**, 857–60.

23. Champion, R.H. (1992) Disorders of Blood Vessels, in *Textbook of Dermatology*, 5th edn (eds R.H. Champion, J.L. Burton and F.J.G. Ebling), Blackwell, Oxford, pp. 1834–8.

24. Bastuji-Garin, S., Rzany, B., Stern, R.S. *et al.* (1993) Clinical classification of cases of toxic epidermal necrolysis, Stevens-Johnson Syndrome and Erythema Multiforme. *J. Am. Acad. Dermatol.*, **129**, 92–6.

25. Pye, R.J. (1992) Bullous Eruptions, in *Textbook of Dermatology*, 5th edn (eds R.H. Champion, J.L. Burton and F.J.G. Ebling), Blackwell, Oxford, pp. 1667–8.

26. Chelsom, J., Halstensen, A., Haga, T. *et al.* (1994) Necrotising fasciitis due to Group A streptococci in Western Norway: incidence and clinical features. *Lancet*, **ii**, **344**, 1111–15.

27. Burton, J.L. and Cunliffe, W.J. (1992) In *Text Book of Dermatology*, 5th edn (eds R.H. Champion, J.L. Burton and F.J.G. Ebling), Blackwell, Oxford, pp. 2158–60.

28. •• (1994) Immunosuppressive drugs and their complications. *Drugs Ther. Bull.*, **32**, 66–70.

29. Breathnach, S.M. (1992) In *Textbook of Dermatology*, 5th edn (eds R.H. Champion, J.L. Burton and F.J.G. Ebling), Blackwell, Oxford, pp. 3029–31.

30. Brakman, M., Faber, W.R., Zeegelaar, J.E. *et al.* (1994) Venous hypertension of the hand caused by hemodialysis shunt: immunofluorescence studies of pericapillary cuffs. *J. Am. Acad. Dermatol.*, **31**, 23–6.

31. van Zuuren, E.J., Posma, A.N., Scholtens, R.E.M. *et al.* (1994) Resurfacing the back of the hands as treatment and prevention of multiple skin cancers in kidney transplant patients. *J. Am. Acad. Dermatol.*, **31**, 760–4.

32. Greene, M.H., Young, T.I. and Clark, W.H. (1981) Malignant melanoma in renal transplant recipients. *Lancet*, **i**, 1196–8.

33. Chugh, K.S., Sharma, S.C., Singh, V. *et al.* (1994) Spectrum of dermatological lesions in renal allograft recipients in a tropical environment. *Dermatology*, **188**, 108–12.

34. McGregor, J.M., Yu, C.C.-W., Lu, Q.L. *et al.* (1993) Post-transplant cutaneous lymphoma. *J. Am. Acad. Dermatol.*, **29**, 549–54.

35. Ohtake, N., Uchiyama, H., Furue, M. and Tamaki, K. (1994) Secondary cutaneous oxalosis: cutaneous deposition of calcium oxalate dihydrate after long-term hemodialysis. *J. Am. Acad. Dermatol.*, **31**, 368–72.

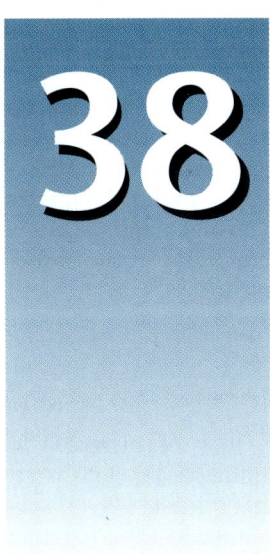

Disorders of lipids under conditions of impaired renal function

George A. Kaysen

Introduction

Both quantitative and qualitative changes occur in plasma lipoproteins when renal function is reduced (renal failure) and following the onset of proteinuria (the nephrotic syndrome). In each case disorders in lipid metabolism are in part a consequence of both increased synthesis and decreased catabolism of lipoproteins. In both cases composition of each lipoprotein class is also abnormal.

Lipid disorders of renal failure

Hyperlipidemia of chronic renal failure (CRF), although present in as many as 75% of dialysis patients, is usually of only moderate degree. Triglyceride concentration is increased whereas cholesterol is usually normal. The primary change in lipoproteins is qualitative rather than quantitative; however these qualitative changes have biological significance.

Triglycerides are increased predominantly in the very low density lipoprotein (VLDL) fraction, but intermediate density lipoprotein (IDL) reviewed in [1] and low density lipoprotein (LDL) triglyceride is also increased. High density lipoprotein (HDL) cholesterol is decreased whereas IDL and LDL cholesterol are increased. These changes in lipoprotein composition occur early in the course of renal failure, suggesting that they are a conse-

quence of renal failure *per se*, and not a consequence of treatment.

The lipid composition of each lipoprotein fraction is also abnormal. The triglyceride content of HDL and LDL is increased [1], whereas cholesterol concentration is increased in VLDL and chylomicron remnants. The protein content of each lipoprotein subfraction increases relative to lipid, in contrast to the nephrotic syndrome where the opposite situation pertains [2]. Thus CRF is associated with an increased quantity of apolipoprotein rich, lipid poor lipoproteins in plasma.

Lipoprotein(a) (Lp(a)) has been identified as a prominent and independent risk factor in atherogenesis in dialysis patients [3]. Generally the quantity of this lipoprotein in plasma is genetically determined [4]. Lp(a) consists of a molecule of LDL to which one molecule of the apolipoprotein apo(a) has been covalently attached to apo B 100. The size of the apo(a) molecule in Lp(a) is genetically determined and distributed in the population in a non-normal fashion [5]. A majority of individuals have the largest apo(a) and the lowest plasma Lp(a) concentration [5]. Lp(a) levels are increased in patients with a variety of renal diseases, including the nephrotic syndrome [6] and CRF [7]. Unlike inherited increases in plasma Lp(a) levels, acquired increases in Lp(a) are not associated with increased apo(a) size [6].

Apo A-I and apo A-II are apolipoproteins secreted by liver and intestine and are found predominantly in HDL. Apo A-I correlates inversely with atherosclerotic disease

Nephrology, Edited by Rex L. Jamison and Robert Wilkinson.
Published in 1997 by Chapman & Hall, London. ISBN 0 412 60930 4

in patients and is necessary for the action of lecithin cholesterol ester transferase (LCAT). Apo E is secreted by a variety of tissues and is recognized by both the remnant receptor in liver and the scavenger receptor in macrophages. Apo E is found on all lipoproteins.

Plasma apo A-I and apo A-II are decreased, and apo E is decreased in men with CRF. Decreased apo A-I is in part a consequence of reduced synthesis [8]. Since apo A-I is a necessary constituent of HDL, its reduced plasma concentration may cause the low HDL levels characteristic of CRF. Apo B, an apolipoprotein necessary for secretion of triglyceride rich lipoproteins (VLDL and chylomicrons (CM)), may be elevated. Apo B 48, an isoform only secreted by the intestine in humans, is increased in the VLDL fraction, suggesting the presence of CM remnant particles within the VLDL fraction. All apo C lipoproteins are increased [1] but the most noteworthy change is an increase in apo C-III relative to apo C-II leading to an increased apo C-III/apo C-II ratio. Apo Cs act to either catalyze (C-II) or inhibit (C-III) the action of lipoprotein lipase (LPL), the rate limiting enzyme hydrolyzing triglycerides within CM and VLDL, and also inhibit the uptake of remnants by the liver [9]. The changed apo C-III/C-II ratio should inhibit LPL and be important in the pathogenesis of hypertriglyceridemia in CRF.

Disordered lipoprotein metabolism in CRF

Although triglyceride production may be increased in CRF, decreased catabolism predominates [1]. LPL is reduced and serum from CRF patients inhibits LPL [1] suggesting the presence of a LPL inhibitor in CRF. Together these findings provide a basis for reduced lipolysis of triglyceride rich lipoproteins in CRF. VLDL is synthesized in the liver and catabolized on the vascular endothelium

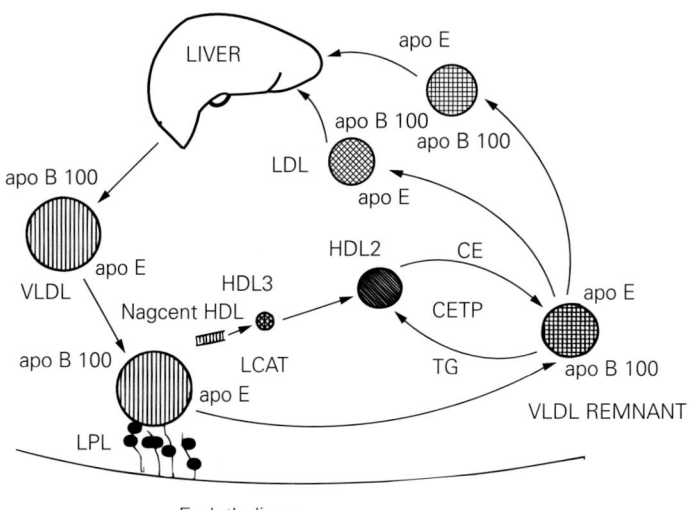

Figure 38.1 Metabolism of VLDL. Very low density lipoprotein (VLDL) is secreted by the liver and is hydrolyzed on the vascular endothelium by LPL. LPL, the small filled circles, is bound electrostatically to heparan sulfate and, in the presence of apo C-II, hydrolyzes triglycerides (TG) releasing free fatty acids, mono- and diglycerides for cellular uptake. Other surface constituents of VLDL, free cholesterol and phospholipids participate in the formation of nacent HDL. The free cholesterol on the surface of nacent HDL is esterified by the action of lecithin cholesterol ester transferase (LCAT) to produce cholesterol esters. These sink into the core as nascent HDL is metabolized to the small, dense HDL_3, and finally into the cholesterol ester (CE) rich HDL_2. The relatively TG-depleted VLDL remnant particle is released from the endothelial surface and then either taken up by the liver directly via the remnant receptor, which recognizes apo E, or interacts with CE-rich HDL_2. In that interaction, catalyzed by cholesterol ester transfer protein (CETP), the CE-rich core of HDL_2 is exchanged for the TG-rich core of the VLDL remnant, yielding a TG-rich HDL molecule (not shown) and LDL, which is then taken up by the LDL receptor in the liver, which recognizes apo B 100, the isoform secreted by the liver. HDL_2 is processed by lipases to HDL_3 to continue the cycle.

(Figure 38.1). Processed VLDL remnants are released and then may be either taken up directly by the liver by a receptor that recognizes apo E, or further metabolized to LDL, as discussed subsequently, and then taken up by the liver via the LDL receptor, which targets apo B 100. CM are synthesized in the intestine and are processed to remnants in much the same way as is VLDL, but are not processed to LDL and cannot be a target for the LDL receptor because they carry the apo B 48 isoform, one not recognized by the LDL receptor. Although CM themselves pose no significant risk for atherogenesis, CM remnants are atherogenic [10]. Remnant particles accumulate extensively in plasma of CRF patients [1].

HDL plays a pivotal role in the metabolism of both CM and VLDL. Mature HDL$_2$ is necessary for transport of the essential LPL cofactor, apo C-II to nascent VLDL and CM (Figure 38.2). Apo C-II is recycled by HDL$_2$ from both CM and VLDL remnants following their catabolism by LPL. Without recycling of apo C-II by HDL$_2$, the action of LPL on these large lipoproteins will be reduced.

Nascent (discoid) HDL arises in the plasma in part from phospholipids and cholesterol released during hydrolysis of CM and VLDL (Figure 38.1), with the addition of apo A-I and A-II [11]. Nascent HDL is a lipid bilayer and only becomes a spherical lipoprotein by the action of LCAT, an enzyme that esterifies free cholesterol. The cholesterol esters then sink into the core of the lipid bilayer transforming it into small spherical HDL$_3$ particles [12]. Further action of this same enzyme matures HDL to the larger HDL$_2$ species. It is this latter form that is most effective in shuttling apo C-II to nascent VLDL and CM and thus serves to facilitate their catabolism. Although all forms of HDL are reduced in CRF it is this latter form of the lipoprotein which is reduced the most, providing yet another mechanism for reduced lipolysis.

LCAT activity is reduced CRF [1]. Although some authors have found that dialysis normalizes LCAT activity [13]; this effect has not been universally observed and dialysis fails to correct disordered plasma lipoprotein composition [1]. The changes in HDL composition observed in CRF are precisely those anticipated to occur as a consequence of LCAT deficiency, suggesting that decreased activity of this enzyme may, in addition to reduced apo A-I synthesis, play an important role in causing reduced HDL in CRF.

Parathyroidectomy causes a prompt decrease both in cholesterol and triglycerides in patients with CRF [14], suggesting that the secondary hyperparathyroidism of CRF may also contribute to the lipid disorders of uremia. Primary hyperparathyroidism, however, causes increased synthesis of VLDL [1], not the decrease in catabolic rate that is characteristic of CRF. Furthermore, LPL activity is normal in patients with primary hyperparathyroidism, providing further evidence that secondary hyperparathyroidism is not the principal cause of the lipid disorders of CRF.

Effect of treatment modality on lipids in CRF

Treatment for end-stage renal disease has the potential to alter blood lipids. Lipid levels are higher in patients on continuous ambulatory peritoneal dialysis (CAPD) than in patients on hemodialysis [1], but the differences between patients treated with these different modalities are small. CAPD is accompanied by the transperitoneal loss of plasma proteins and by the absorption of large amounts of glucose. Both of these processes impact on lipoprotein metabolism. The latter induces increased synthesis of VLDL and the former process bears similarities to the nephrotic syndrome. A significant amount of HDL is lost across the peritoneal membrane [15]. The larger lipoproteins are cleared much less effectively by CAPD and thus are increased in plasma relative to HDL. HDL levels are, however, not uniformly lower in CAPD patients compared to hemodialysis patients [1]. Glucose absorption may also contribute to the greater plasma triglyceride concentration in CAPD patients, since reducing glucose

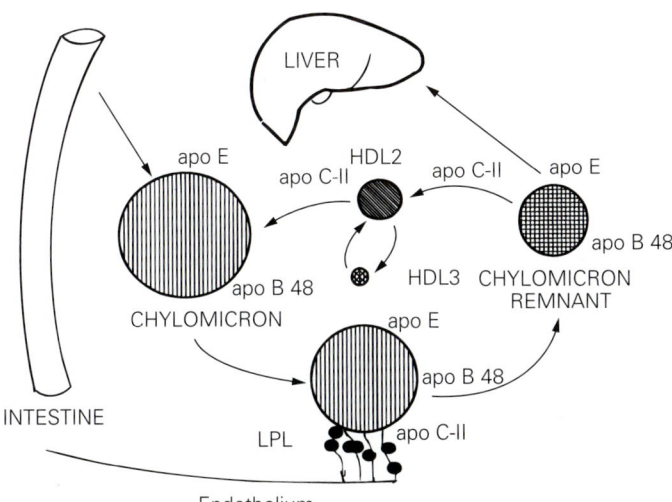

Figure 38.2 Metabolism of chylomicrons. CM are synthesized in the intestine. Apo B is required for their secretion. The isoform secreted by the liver is apo B 48 and is not recognized by the LDL receptor. HDL$_2$ transfers apo C-II to newly secreted CM. CM are then subjected to lipolysis by LPL. Once they have been depleted of much of their triglycerides, CM remnants are released, their apo C-II transferred back to HDL$_2$, and are then rapidly taken up by the remnant receptor on the liver. This receptor recognizes the apo E moiety, but not apo B 48.

absorption by using an amino acid based dialysate reduces plasma triglyceride, LDL, and apo B levels [1].

Transplantation

Once patients receive a transplant, plasma triglyceride levels promptly decrease [16] and cholesterol levels rise [17], usually to levels well in excess of 200 mg/dl. Although the increased cholesterol is predominantly in the HDL fraction [18], the incidence of cardiovascular disease remains elevated in patients following renal transplantation [1]. LDL cholesterol and apo B may also be elevated, and correlate with nephrotic range proteinuria, impaired renal function, diabetes and/or consumption of thiazides or beta blockers, and a steroid dose >12.5 mg/day [19]. Cholesterol may increase as a side effect of cyclosporin A [20] or glucocorticoids [21].

Lipid disorders of the nephrotic syndrome

There is general agreement that both hepatic lipid and apolipoprotein synthesis is increased [22], and that clearance of CM and VLDL [23] is reduced in the nephrotic syndrome. Marsh and Drabkin suggested that lipoprotein synthesis was increased in parallel with that of albumin in the nephrotic syndrome since all share a common secretory pathway [24]. This hypothesis was supported in part by the previous studies showing that infusion of albumin partially corrected nephrotic hyperlipidemia. Davis et al. [25] reported that apolipoprotein secretion (apo B) by hepatocytes in culture could be reduced by increasing oncotic pressure (π) in the culture medium, but albumin synthesis could not, supporting the hypothesis that extracellular π influences the rate of apo B synthesis by severing a link between albumin synthesis at that of apolipoproteins. Most evidence still supports the hypothesis that reduced extracellular albumin concentration and/or reduced extracellular π in some way regulates apolipoprotein synthesis and lipogenesis by the liver.

Although hepatic apolipoprotein synthesis is increased in the nephrotic syndrome, not all apolipoproteins are affected to the same degree, and mechanisms causing increased synthesis of the various apolipopproteins are also different. Secretion of apo A is increased approximately sixfold [24], whereas synthesis of apo B and E are only increased about twice. Synthesis of the C apolipoproteins is not increased. Apo A-I mRNA is increased transcriptionally in the livers of both nephrotic [2, 26] and analbuminemic rats [2], suggesting that reduced plasma π or albumin concentration, but not proteinuria, is responsible for the change in apo A-I gene expression. Although plasma apo B and E are both increased in nephrotic and analbuminemic rats, there is little or no change in the amount of these mRNAs in liver and no change in the rate of transcription of their cognate genes. Thus if increased synthesis of these apolipoproteins plays a role in estab-

lishing the increased levels of these apolipoproteins in plasma, the mechanisms involved are most likely post-transcriptional, at the level of translation or protein processing, in contrast to apo A-I.

Reduced lipoprotein catabolism in the nephrotic syndrome

Catabolism of CM and VLDL is greatly reduced in the nephrotic syndrome [23, 24, 27, 28]. Their clearance is reduced following the onset of proteinuria (the nephrotic syndrome), but is normal in rats with hereditary analbuminemia [23], suggesting that the urinary loss of a liporegulatory substance and not reduced albumin concentration or π may play a role in causing defective lipolysis in the nephrotic syndrome. LPL activity is reduced in nephrotic rats and provides a potential mechanism for delayed lipolysis [24]. It has been found that uptake of triglycerides was reduced to about 30% of normal in all organs [27], even in heart, reported to have normal levels of LPL activity. CM catabolism by hearts isolated from nephrotic rats was decreased in vitro and the LPL pool bound to the vascular endothelium was reduced by approximately 90%. LPL activity not bound to the vascular endothelium, and hence unable to interact with large lipoproteins, was normal [28]. Thus specific reduction of LPL attached to the vascular endothelium may play a role in the reduced catabolism of VLDL and CM in the nephrotic syndrome.

The relationship between reduced endothelial bound LPL activity and reduced catabolism of CM and VLDL is by no means clear. VLDL and CM catabolism by analbuminemic rats is normal despite a marked reduction in heparin releasable LPL activity [23]. Furukawa et al. [29] reported that HDL isolated from normal animals corrects defective lipolysis of VLDL isolated from nephrotic rats by LPL in vitro whereas HDL isolated from nephrotic rats does not, suggesting that HDL isolated from nephrotic animals may be dysfunctional; HDL isolated from nephrotic animals has been found to be structurally abnormal [29]. Thus multiple separate defects in the peripheral catabolism of triglyceride-rich lipoproteins may be responsible for delayed lipolysis.

Studies in patients with the nephrotic syndrome have not been as detailed as in the rat; however, when comparable studies are evaluated both species exhibit similar disturbances in lipid metabolism. The fractional turnover rate of triglycerides is reduced in nephrotic subjects compared to controls and the $t_{\frac{1}{2}}$ of triglyceride is prolonged from 4 to 11h in VLDL [30]. Not only is VLDL catabolism decreased, but the disappearance curve has an unusual shape presumed to result from a delay in the conversion of VLDL into IDL [31]. It is suggested that the delay in lipolysis in humans, as in rats, is due to a decrease in LPL activity. Evidence supporting this hypothesis is that LPL activity is reduced in children with the nephrotic syndrome and increases after remission. Furthermore, there is a strong inverse correlation between LPL and the concentration of triglycerides in the VLDL fraction [32], although not all investigators find a decrease in LPL activity in nephrotic patients [33].

Although total plasma apo C-II is raised in nephrotic patients, the amount of this LPL cofactor is reduced per unit of VLDL by more than 50%, since the total amount of VLDL is increased more than is total apo C-II [34].

Hepatic uptake of CM remnants is impaired in nephrotic rats [27] and plasma remnants are increased. LDL catabolism has been reported to be either normal or reduced [35] in patients with the nephrotic syndrome and only marginally reduced in nephrotic rats [34].

The effect of changes in the activities of liporegulatory enzymes

Cholesterol ester transfer protein (CETP) catalyzes the transfer of the cholesterol ester rich core of HDL_2 to VLDL remnant particles creating LDL (Figure 38.1) and increasing LDL cholesterol at the expense of HDL cholesterol. CETP is increased in the plasma of nephrotic patients and correlates positively with VLDL cholesterol and negatively with HDL cholesterol [36]. CETP levels decrease significantly following reduction of proteinuria after treatment with an angiotensin converting enzyme (ACE) inhibitor [48], in conjunction with a reduction in VLDL and LDL.

Plasma LCAT activity is increased in plasma of nephrotic patients when measured in assays using excess exogenous substrate [36]. HDL free cholesterol correlates inversely with LCAT activity. ACE inhibition results in a 40% reduction of proteinuria, a partial normalization of LCAT activity, and a decrease in VLDL and LDL cholesterol. LCAT activity is also increased in nephrotic rats when similar assay conditions are used [37]. These findings are opposite to those of Sestack et al. [38]. Differences may be explained by the different assay conditions used, but the physiologic consequences of these studies depend on the specific reaction catalyzed by LCAT in vivo. The protein LCAT catalyzes two separate reactions: the transfer of an acyl group, usually arachidonic acid, to free cholesterol, increasing the cholesterol ester content of HDL, and the lysoleithin acyltransferase (LAT) reaction, which takes place on LDL. Sestack et al. [38] found that whereas esterified cholesterol correlated positively with LCAT activity in normal rats it correlated negatively in nephrotic animals, suggesting that increases of the enzyme in vivo may increase the LAT rather than the LCAT reaction.

The observation that HDL_3 is preserved in plasma in nephrotic patients at the apparent expense of HDL_2 suggests that the LCAT reaction is reduced in nephrotic patients. However, increased activity of CETP could also explain this pattern of HDL distribution by rapidly cycling the core of HDL_2 to VLDL remnant particles, thus increasing the flux of cholesterol from the surface of nascent HDL into the core of LDL by increased activities

of both enzymes (Figure 38.1). This model would also clarify the HDL pattern in rats with the nephrotic syndrome characterized by increased HDL_2 and also of an even larger variety, HDL_1, found in humans to only a limited extent. Rats lack CETP and thus the cycle would be interrupted. Against this explanation is the observation that the transition of apo B from VLDL to LDL is impeded in nephrotic humans [39]. At this time it is unclear whether the LCAT reaction is indeed increased in the forward direction in the nephrotic syndrome.

Clinical implications of hyperlipidemia in renal disease

Cardiovascular disease is the leading cause of death in patients on dialysis [40]. The death rate from cardiovascular and cerebrovascular disease does not increase with time on dialysis [41]. Patients with CRF are frequently diabetic, hypertensive or both. Many smoke cigarettes. Many patients come to dialysis with advanced cardiovascular disease. Whether the specific lipid disorders of CRF contribute further to cardiovascular disease is unknown, despite the demographic data presented above.

The changes that occur in blood lipoprotein composition in the nephrotic syndrome [42], reduced HDL_2 cholesterol, a relative increase in HDL_3 cholesterol and the massive increase in total cholesterol, mostly found in the LDL, IDL and VLDL fractions, should be expected to cause increased risk of atherosclerotic disease. Indeed, accelerated atherosclerosis has been reported in patients with proteinuria and hyperlipidemia and in some studies has been associated with a sharply increased incidence of cardiovascular disease and stroke [43]. One study reported an 85-fold increase in the incidence of ischemic heart disease in such patients [44]. In another recent retrospective analysis of 142 patients with proteinuria greater than 3.5 g/day, the relative risk of myocardial infarction was found to be 5.5 and the risk of cardiac death 2.8 compared to age- and sex-matched controls [45]. It is not clear from this study, however, whether hyperlipidemia or some other manifestation of the nephrotic syndrome was responsible for the increased prevalence of coronary artery disease. The failure to identify the nephrotic syndrome as a risk factor for atherosclerotic disease in some studies may be due to the transient nature of proteinuria or to its short duration in some subjects [46]. It is generally difficult to find comparable groups of patients who have the same level of renal function, blood pressure and proteinuria with consistently different lipid levels for prolonged periods of time to independently analyze the effect of hyperlipidemia alone on the development of atherosclerotic vascular disease.

Hyperlipidemia of the nephrotic syndrome may be severe and is characterized by a high LDL/HDL cholesterol ratio. This pattern is associated with accelerated atherosclerosis in other clinical situations and there is no reason to believe that hyperlipidemia of the nephrotic syndrome would not have similar consequences, should this metabolic disorder persist. These abnormalities are further complicated by the increase in plasma Lp(a) levels, increased platelet aggregability, increased plasma viscosity, increased concentration of highly atherogenic remnants of VLDL and CM catabolism in plasma. It would be surprising indeed if hyperlipidemic patients with the nephrotic syndrome did not have considerable risk for development of serious atherosclerotic disease. For this reason, there is no rationale for leaving untreated pronounced hyperlipidemia for prolonged periods of time in a patient with the nephrotic syndrome.

Disordered lipid metabolism could also play a role in the cycle of progressive renal failure that occurs following the initiation of renal injury [47], although this link has not been established in humans or in animal models of renal disease that are not associated with substantial increases in cholesterol levels. Although the association between hyperlipidemia and progression of renal disease has not been as yet confirmed in humans, one disorder that causes hypercholesterolemia in humans, hereditary LCAT deficiency, may be linked to progressive mesangial and glomerular sclerosis [48].

Treatment of hyperlipidemia

Although there is no specific indication to treat the qualitative abnormalities that characterize the lipid disorders of both the nephrotic syndrome and CRF, if it is anticipated that the duration of hyperlipidemia will be prolonged, it is wise to initiate therapy.

Treatment of nephrotic patients with either ACE

inhibitors [49] or cyclooxygenase inhibitors [50] results in a decline in both proteinuria and blood lipid levels [24] even if plasma albumin concentration does not increase. The decline in blood lipid levels includes a decrease in total cholesterol, Lp(a) [6], a decrease in VLDL and LDL cholesterol and a decrease in the activities of CETP and LCAT [36]. The effect of ACE inhibitors is a class effect and appears to be shared by all drugs within this class.

It is probably prudent to restrict dietary cholesterol and saturated lipids in patients with the nephrotic syndrome. Omega 3 polyunsaturated fatty acids have been shown to be effective at reducing glomerular injury in a variety of experimental renal diseases in the rat; however, the long-term effects of dietary supplementation with fish oil in the nephrotic syndrome in patients are as yet unknown and it cannot be recommended for treatment of the nephrotic syndrome except within the context of a controlled investigative trial. If conservative therapy (reduction in proteinuria, dietary fat restriction) does not effectively reduce hyperlipidemia, a variety of lipid-lowering drugs, including the 3-hydroxy-3-methylglutaryl coenzyme A reductase (HMG CoA reductase) inhibitors, antioxidants and fibric acid derivatives, can be useful, but review of this subject is beyond the scope of this chapter.

Acknowledgment

This work was supported in part by a grant from the National Institutes of Health RO1 DK 42297 and in part by the research service of the United States Department of Veterans Affairs.

References

1. Kaysen, G.A. (1994) Hyperlipidemia of chronic renal failure. *Blood Purif.*, **12**, 60–7.
2. Sun, X., Jones, Jr., H., Joles, J.A. *et al.* (1992) Apolipoprotein gene expression in the analbuminemic rat and in the rat with Heymann nephritis. *Am. J. Physiol.*, **262**, F755–61.
3. Krolewski, A.S., Warram, J.H. and Christlieb, A.R. (1994) Hypercholesterolemia – a determinant of renal function loss and deaths in IDDM patients with nephropathy. *Kidney Int.*, **45**, S125–31.
4. Boerwinkle, E., Menzel, H.J., Kraft, H.G. and Utermann, G. (1989) Genetics of the quantitative Lp(a) lipoprotein trait. III. Contribution of Lp(a) glycoprotein phenotypes to normal lipid variation. *Hum. Genet.*, **82**, 73–8.
5. Gavish, D., Azrolan, N. and Breslow, J. (1989) Plasma Lp(a) concentration is inversely correlated with the ratio of kringle IV/kringle V encoding domains in the apo(a) gene. *J. Clin. Invest.*, **84**, 2021–7.
6. Wanner, C., Rader, D., Bartens, W. *et al.* (1993) Elevated plasma lipoprotein(a) in patients with the nephrotic syndrome. *Ann. Intern. Med.*, **119**, 263–9.
7. Guillausseau, P-J., Peynet, J., Chanson, P. *et al.* (1992) Lipoprotein (a) in diabetic patients with and without chronic renal failure. *Diabetes Care*, **15**, 976–9.
8. Fuh, M.M.T., Lee, C-M., Jeng, C-Y. *et al.* (1990) Effect of chronic renal failure on high-density lipoprotein kinetics. *Kidney Int.*, **37**, 1295–300.
9. Kowal, R.C., Herz, J., Weisgraber, K.H. *et al.* (1990) Opposing effects of apolipoproteins E and C on lipoprotein binding to low density lipoprotein receptor-related protein. *J. Biol. Chem.*, **265**, 10771–9.
10. Chung, B.H., Segrest, J.P., Smith, K. *et al.* (1989) Lipolytic surface remnants of triglyceride-rich lipoproteins are cytotoxic to macrophages but not in the presence of high density lipoprotein: A possible mechanism of atherogenesis? *J. Clin. Invest.*, **83**, 1363–74.
11. Tall, A.R. (1990) Plasma high density lipoproteins: metabolism and relationship to atherogenesis. *J. Clin. Invest.*, **86**, 379–84.
12. Eisenberg, S. (1984) High density lipoprotein metabolism. *J. Lipid Res.*, **25**, 1017–58.
13. Bories, P.C., Subbaiah, P.V. and Bagdade, J.D. (1982)

Lecithin:cholesterol acyltransferase activity in dialyzed and undialyzed chronic uremic patients. *Nephron*, **32**, 22–7.

14. Drüeke, T. and Lacour, B. (1985) Parathyroid hormone and hyperlipemia of uremia. *Contrib. Nephrol.*, **49**, 12–19.

15. Kagan, A., Bar-Khayim, Y., Schafer, Z. and Fainaru, M. (1990) Kinetics of peritoneal protein loss during CAPD: II. Lipoprotein leakage and its impact on plasma lipid levels. *Kidney Int.*, **37**, 980–90.

16. Kasiske, B. and Umen, A.J. (1987) Persistent hyperlipidemia in renal transplant patients. *Medicine*, **66**, 309–16.

17. Kobayashi, N., Okubo, M., Marumo, F. *et al.* (1983) De novo development of hypercholesterolemia and elevated high-density lipoprotein cholesterol: apoprotein A-I ratio in patients with chronic renal failure following kidney transplantation. *Nephron*, **35**, 237–40.

18. Rubiés-Prat, J., Romero, R., Chacón, P. *et al.* (1983) Apoprotein A and apoprotein B in patients with chronic renal failure undergoing hemodialysis and in renal graft recipients. *Nephron*, **35**, 171–4.

19. Lowry, R.P., Soltys, G., Peters, L. *et al.* (1987) Type II hyperlipoproteinemia, hyperapobetalipoproteinemia, and hyperalphalipoproteinemia following renal transplantation: Implications for atherogenic risk. *Transplant. Proc.*, **19**, 3426–30.

20. Jevnikar, A.M., Petric, R., Holub, B.J. *et al.* (1988) Effect of cyclosporine on plasma lipids and modification with dietary fish oil. *Transplantation*, **46**, 722–5.

21. Becker, D.M., Chamberlain, B., Swank, R. *et al.* (1988) Relationship between corticosteroid exposure and plasma lipid levels in heart transplant recipients. *Am. J. Med.*, **85**, 632–8.

22. Marsh, J.B. and Drabkin, D.L. (1960) Experimental reconstruction of metabolic pattern of lipid nephrosis: key role of hepatic protein synthesis in hyperlipemia. *Metabolism*, **9**, 946–55.

23. Davies, R.W., Staprans, I., Hutchison, F.N. and Kaysen, G.A. (1990) Proteinuria, not altered albumin metabolism, effects hyperlipidemia in the nephrotic rat. *J. Clin. Invest.*, **86**, 600–5.

24. Kaysen, G.A. (1991) Hyperlipidemia of the nephrotic syndrome. *Kidney Int.*, **39**, S8–15.

25. Davis, R.A., Engelhorn, S.C., Weinstein, D.B. and Steinberg, D. (1980) Very low density lipoprotein secretion by cultured rat hepatocytes: inhibition by albumin and other macromolecules. *J. Biol. Chem.*, **255**, 2039–45.

26. Marshall, J.F., Apostolopoulos, J.J., Brack, C.M. and Howlett, G.J. (1990) Regulation of apolipoprotein gene expression and plasma high-density lipoprotein composition in experimental nephrosis. *Biochim. Biophys. Acta*, **1042**, 271–9.

27. Kaysen, G.A., Mehendru, L., Pan, X.M. and Staprans, I. (1992) Both peripheral chylomicron catabolism and hepatic uptake of remnants are defective in nephrosis. *Am. J. Physiol.*, **263**, F335–41.

28. Kaysen, G.A., Pan, X.M., Couser, W.G. and Staprans, I. (1993) Defective lipolysis persists in hearts of rats with Heymann nephritis in the absence of nephrotic plasma. *Am. J. Kidney Dis.*, **22**, 128–34.

29. Furukawa, S., Hirano, T., Mamo, J.C.L. *et al.* (1990) Catabolic defect of triglyceride is associated with abnormal very-low-density lipoprotein in experimental nephrosis. *Metabolism*, **39**, 101–7.

30. Kekki, M. and Nikkilä, E.A. (1971) Plasma triglyceride metabolism in the adult nephrotic syndrome. *Eur. J. Clin. Invest.*, **1**, 345–51.

31. Vega, G.L. and Grundy, S.M. (1988) Lovastatin therapy in enphrotic hyperlipidemia: effects on lipoprotein metabolism. *Kidney Int.*, **33**, 1160–8.

32. Yamada, M. and Matsuda, I. (1970) Lipoprotein lipase in clinical and experimental nephrosis. *Clin. Chim. Acta*, **30**, 787–94.

33. Warwick, G.L., Packard, C.J., Stewart, J.P. *et al.* (1992) Post-prandial lipoprotein metabolism in nephrotic syndrome. *Eur. J. Clin. Invest.*, **22**, 813–20.

34. Joven, J., Masana, L., Villabona, C. *et al.* (1989) Low density lipoprotein metabolism in rats with puromycin aminonucleoside–induced nephrotic syndrome. *Metabolism*, **38**, 491–5.

35. McKenzie, I.F.C. and Nestel, P.J. (1968) Studies on the turnover of triglyceride and esterified cholesterol in subjects with the nephrotic syndrome. *J. Clin. Invest.*, **47**, 1685–95.

36. Dullaart, R.P., Gansevoort, R.T., Dikkeschei, B.D. *et al.* (1993) Role of elevated lecithin:cholesterol acyltransferase and cholesteryl ester transfer protein activities in abnormal lipoproteins from proteinuric patients. *Kidney Int.*, **44**, 91–7.

37. Agbedana, E.D., Yamamoto, T., Moriwaki, Y. *et al.* (1993) Studies on abnormal lipid metabolism in experimental nephrotic syndrome. *Nephron*, **64**, 256–61.

38. Sestak, T.L., Alavi, N. and Subbaiah, P.V. (1989) Plasma lipids and acyltransferase activities in experimental nephrotic syndrome. *Kidney Int.*, **36**, 240–8.

39. Warwick, G.L., Packard, C.J., Demant, T. *et al.* (1991) Metabolism of apolipoprotein B-containing lipoproteins in subjects with nephrotic-range proteinuria. *Kidney Int.*, **40**, 129–38.

40. Kooman, J.P. and Leunissen, K.M. (1993) Cardiovascular aspects in renal disease. *Curr. Opin. Nephrol. Hypertens.*, **2**, 791–7.

41. Kindler, J., Sieberth, H-G., Hahn, R. *et al.* (1982) Does atherosclerosis caused by dialysis limit this treatment? *Proc. EDTA*, **19**, 168–74.

42. Muls, E., Rosseneu, M., Daneels, R. *et al.* (1985) Lipoprotein distribution and composition in the human nephrotic syndrome. *Atherosclerosis*, **54**, 225–37.

43. Mallick, N.P. and Short, C.D. (1981) The nephrotic syndrome and ishcaemic heart disease. *Nephron*, **27**, 54–7.

44. Berlyne, G.M. and Mallick, N.P. (1969) Ischemic heart disease as a complication of nephrotic syndrome. *Lancet*, **ii**, 399–400.

45. Ordonez, J.D., Hiatt, R.A., Killebrew, E.J. and Fireman, B.H. (1993) The increased risk of coronary heart disease associated with nephrotic syndrome. *Kidney Int.*, **44**, 638–42.

46. Wass, V. and Cameron, J.S. (1981) Cardiovascular disease and the nephrotic syndrome: the other side of the coin. *Nephron*, **27**, 58–61.

47. Schmitz, P.G., Kasiske, B.L., O'Donnell, M.P. and Keane,

W.F. (1989) Lipids and progressive renal injury. *Sem. Nephrol.*, **9**, 354–69.

48. Larger, D.J., Rosenberg, B.F., Shapiro, H. and Bernstein, J. (1991) Lecithin cholesterol acyltransferase deficiency: ultrastructural examination of sequential renal biopsies. *Modern Pathol.*, **4**, 331–5.

49. Don, B.R., Kaysen, G.A., Hutchison, F.N. and Schambe-lan, M. (1991) The effect of angiotensin-converting enzyme inhibition and dietary protein restriction in the treatment of proteinuria. *Am. J. Kidney Dis.*, **17**, 10–17.

50. Gansevoort, R.T., Heeg, J.E., Vriesendorp, R. *et al.* (1992) Antiproteinuric drugs in patients with idiopathic membranous glomerulopathy. *Nephrol. Dial. Transplant.*, **7**, 91–6.

39

The uremic syndrome

Anders Alvestrand and Peter Stenvinkel

Introduction

A great number of different chronic renal diseases of inflammatory, infectious or metabolic etiologies may lead to renal insufficiency, and it is general experience that if renal insufficiency has advanced to a certain point, further deterioration to end-stage renal failure is almost inevitable. However, the disease process is often slow and may not become clinically evident until symptoms of uremia appear as a consequence of advanced renal impairment.

This chapter briefly describes the progressive course of renal insufficiency and its relation to the development of the uremic syndrome. The term uremia is defined and the clinical manifestations of uremia and its toxicological background are discussed. Finally, there is a discussion of the approach to the uremic patient and an outline of the different therapeutic alternatives available for the treatment of uremia.

The progressive nature of chronic renal disease

An important aspect of chronic renal disease is the great capacity for structural and functional adaptations of the diseased kidney. After an initial insult leading to loss of functioning nephrons, the development of chronic renal failure is generally characterized by a progressive decline in the capacity of the kidneys to eliminate water and solutes. During the course of the disease process, which is often slow, various compensatory or adaptive mechanisms become operative and contribute to maintaining homeostasis even when a substantial fraction of glomerular filtration rate (GFR) has been lost.

Glomerular and tubular adaptation to nephron loss

In animal models, the adaptive changes to nephron loss induced by subtotal renal ablation or experimental inflammatory disease have been extensively studied [1]. Reduction of functioning renal parenchyma leads to increases in single nephron GFR (SNGFR) which by some not yet well defined mechanisms are linked to and possibly cause glomerular and tubular hypertrophy. This adaptation occurs within several hours and increased filtration rate is maintained by an increase in glomerular plasma flow, variable rises in glomerular transcapillary pressure and an increased glomerular filtration coefficient, which probably depends on the increase in surface area in the hypertrophied glomeruli. Although it is not possible to study renal function at the single nephron level in the human, it is reasonable to believe that similar adaptive changes occur in the human kidney to those observed in animal studies. Thus, functional adaptation and renal hypertrophy are well documented in patients undergoing unilateral nephrectomy, in whom total GFR, after a short adaptation period, will generally remain at or near basal level, indicating that SNGFR in remnant

Nephrology, Edited by Rex L. Jamison and Robert Wilkinson.
Published in 1997 by Chapman & Hall, London. ISBN 0 412 60930 4

nephrons may double. However, the potential for functional adaptation depends on the character of the initial insult and appears to be less pronounced when the kidney is injured by a disease process involving primarily the glomeruli, e.g. glomerulonephritis.

The change in SNGFR is associated with adaptations in tubular transport, leading to an increased rate of rejection of the filtered load of solutes (i.e. an increase in fractional extraction). By these adaptive changes in glomerular and tubular functions the concentrations in the body fluids and whole body balance of a variety of substances that depend on the kidney for excretion can be maintained despite a marked reduction in the number of functioning nephrons. Clinically important accumulation of potentially toxic substances is, therefore, a late phenomenon in progressive renal failure.

The extent to which normal or only slightly increased serum concentration of a substance may be maintained in renal failure depends on whether its elimination is determined by filtration alone, filtration in combination with tubular reabsorption, or primarily by tubular secretion. With regard to substances that depend on tubular reabsorption or secretion for their elimination, it is important to note that each substance is regulated independently and that different modes of adaptation to nephron loss occur (Figure 39.1).

It is generally believed that mechanisms underlying the adaptive changes to nephron loss may contribute to further renal damage. These include the action of various growth factors and hormones, and the glomerular or tubular adaptations themselves, especially intraglomerular capillary hypertension, which may cause capillary damage and facilitate mesangial deposition of lipids and other macromolecules.

Clinical consequences of impaired renal function

From the clinical point of view the progression of renal disease can be considered to pass through four stages (Figure 39.2). The first stage is characterized by a diminution of the renal reserve capacity. At this stage, during which GFR is reduced to approximately 50% of normal, solute retention is minimal and electrolyte and acid–base balances are maintained. During the next stage of renal insufficiency GFR is further reduced (to 20–40% of normal) and retention of various solutes occurs and production of erythropoietin and $1,25(OH)_2$ vitamin D_3 becomes insufficient, but the patient is still asymptomatic. When GFR is reduced to less than 15–25% of normal, overt renal failure develops and the uremic syndrome becomes clinically evident. Lastly, end-stage renal failure is reached when life-sustaining renal excretory and homeostatic functions are lost (GFR less than 3–5% of normal).

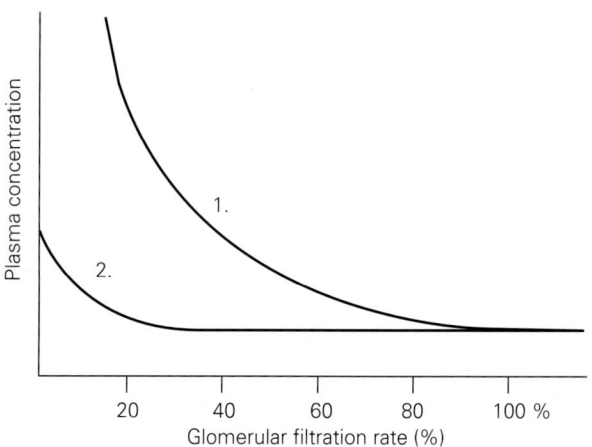

Figure 39.1 The accumulation of substances in plasma as glomerular filtration rate (GFR) decreases. (1) Substances mainly excreted by glomerular filtration (e.g. urea, creatinine). (2) Substances for which adaptation of tubular transport (secretion or reabsorption) takes place (e.g. urate, phosphate and potassium).

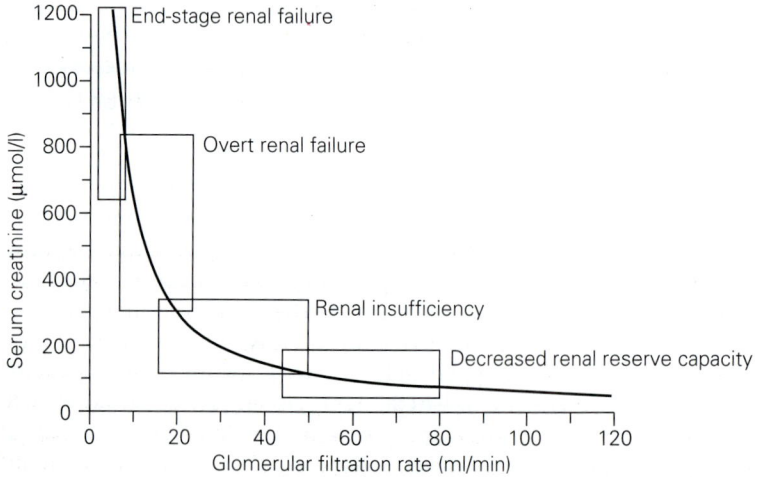

Figure 39.2 The relation between GFR and serum creatinine and the four clinical stages of renal insufficiency (see text).

Uremia

In the literature, the term uremia, which literally means urine in blood, is non-uniformly used to indicate the presence of abnormally elevated concentrations of small molecular nitrogenous substances in the blood, or to describe the pathophysiologic effects of one or more such substances ('uremic toxins') or the clinical manifestations of renal insufficiency or even a reduction in GFR *per se*. Such an arbitrary use of the term uremia is confusing and makes one think of the argument between Humpty Dumpty and Alice. '"When I use a word" Humpty Dumpty said in a rather scornful tone, "it means just what I choose it to mean – neither more nor less". "The question is" said Alice "whether you can make words mean so many different things". "The question is" said Humpty Dumpty "which is to be the master – that's all".'

A definition of uremia, which both emphasizes the toxic basis of the condition and is broad enough to cover all aspects of the uremic syndrome, was suggested by Bergstrom [2] and may well serve as the 'master definition':

> Uremia is a toxic syndrome caused by severe glomerular insufficiency associated with disturbances in tubular and endocrine functions of the kidneys. It is characterized by retention of toxic metabolites, derived mainly from protein metabolism, associated with changes in volume and electrolyte composition of the body fluids and excess or deficiency of various hormones.

According to this, and most other definitions, the term uremia clearly indicates a syndrome. To avoid confusion, more precise terms should preferably be used to describe specific aspects or components of the uremic syndrome.

Clinical presentation of uremia

The clinical picture of the uremic syndrome is characterized by its great variability with signs and symptoms from many organs. The most dramatic uremic picture is seen in patients with acute renal failure and anuria. In patients with chronic renal disease, on the other hand, clinically evident uremic symptoms often develop insidiously and late in the course of renal failure and multiorgan manifestations of severe uremia are seen only in untreated patients with terminal or near-terminal renal failure. However, patients in whom the presence of renal insufficiency is observed at a fairly early stage and who are regularly assessed and treated by a physician seldom develop signs or symptoms of severe uremia.

As discussed above, the kidneys have a substantial reserve capacity and clinical symptoms of renal failure and uremia do not develop until GFR is reduced to 25 ml/min or less (Figure 39.2). Early symptoms and signs include general fatigue, thirst and increased urinary volumes. At a more advanced stage (GFR ≤ 10–15 ml/min)

gastrointestinal symptoms occur. Anorexia is the earliest symptom followed by nausea and vomiting, which typically are most prominent in the morning. With decreasing renal function and increasing uremia a typical odor to the breath, uremic fetor, becomes evident and complications such as pericarditis and more severe disturbances of mentation and cognition and, finally, coma develop. The patient is also at risk of developing congestive heart failure and pulmonary edema due to fluid retention.

The spectrum of abnormalities is presented in Table 39.1 and the following section gives a brief overview of the clinical manifestations of uremia with emphasis on signs and symptoms of the untreated uremic patient.

Gastrointestinal manifestations

Among the most typical of symptoms of uremia are gastrointestinal manifestation such as anorexia, nausea and vomiting. Glossitis, stomatitis, esophagitis, gastritis, colitis and, more seldom, pancreatitis occur in advanced uremia and bleeding from the gastrointestinal tract is a fairly common problem in the uremic patient. Uremic fetor with an characteristic uriniferous odor to the breath often occurs even in mild uremia and tends to be associated with bitter or metallic taste sensations.

Neurologic manifestations

The development of renal failure is accompanied by alterations in central and peripheral nervous system functions. The constellation of symptoms ranges from slight changes in cognitive functions and memory deficits to the development of disorientation and coma. Cramps, tremor, fasciculations, twitching and myoclonia occur as manifestations of severe uremia. Less commonly severely uremic patients may present with behavioral abnormalities and psychotic symptoms.

Uremia is also associated with abnormalities of the peripheral nervous system. A symmetric mixed motor and sensory neuropathy that predominantly affects the lower extremities may develop, and the sensory symptoms, such as paresthesiae, burning sensations and pain, usually precede the motor symptoms, which reflect a more advanced disease stage. Loss of motor function can lead to muscle atrophy and, in later stages, paralysis.

Cardiovascular and pulmonary manifestations

The majority of patients with advanced renal failure retain sodium and water, which may result in peripheral edema, hypertension, congestive heart failure, pulmonary congestion, pleural effusion or ascites. Pulmonary edema is associated with a characteristic radiographic appearance, referred to as the 'uremic lung', in which opacities are limited to the central perihilar areas in a butterfly configuration.

Table 39.1   Manifestations of the uremic syndrome

Gastrointestinal system
  Anorexia
  Nausea, vomiting
  Stomatitis, gastritis, colitis
  Hiccoughing
  Hemorrhage

Cardiovascular system
  Hypertension
  Left ventricular hypertrophy
  Atherosclerosis
  Pericarditis
  Cardiomyopathy

Respiratory system
  Pulmonary edema
  'Uremic lung'
  Sleep apnea syndrome

Hematology
  Anemia
  Platelet dysfunction
  Bleeding

Musculoskeletal system
  Bone disease: osteitis fibrosa
  Osteomalacia
  β_2-Microglobulin amyloidosis
  Proximal myopathy
  Soft-tissue calcification

Immunology
  Susceptibility to infection

Endocrinology
  Hyperparathyroidism
  Insulin resistance
  Impaired renal breakdown of insulin
  Defective vitamin D metabolism
  Growth retardation
  Sexual dysfunction

Dermatology
  Pruritus
  Dry skin

Nervous system
  Fatigue
  Sleep disorders
  Memory dysfunction
  Behavior changes
  Peripheral neuropathy
  Coma
  Psychosis
  Restless legs

Fluid and electrolyte disorders
  Edema
  Metabolic acidosis
  Hyperkalemia
  Hyponatremia
  Hyperphosphatemia
  Hypo/hypercalcemia
  Hypermagnesemia

Miscellaneous
  Weight loss
  Uremic fetor
  Hypothermia

Uremic pericarditis may be clinically silent or present with chest pain and gives rise to a friction rub. In some patients a fibrinous pleuritis with pleural pain and a pleural friction rub coexists with pericarditis or occurs alone.

Hematological complications

Normochromic, normocytic anemia is a common feature and is caused by deficient renal production of erythropoietin. Other factors, such as gastrointestinal bleeding, multiple blood samplings and decreased red blood cell survival also contribute to the development of anemia in renal failure.

An increased tendency to bleeding is usually manifested by skin hemorrhage and bleeding at sites of surgery and trauma. Spontaneous, gross organ bleeding is unusual and a specific cause for bleeding should always be sought for when bleeding occurs.

Musculoskeletal manifestations

Unless prophylactic treatment is instituted fairly early, abnormalities in mineral metabolism invariably lead to renal osteodystrophy. Skeletal abnormalities develop slowly and do not generally give rise to clinical symptoms until the patient has been treated with dialysis for some time. In those in whom the rate of renal functional decline has been slow, proximal muscle weakness may manifest as a symptom of secondary hyperparathyroidism.

Cutaneous manifestations

Pruritus and excoriations at sites of itching are common problems in uremic patients. The skin, which tends to be dry and atrophic, is often characteristically discolored (café-au-lait). Precipitation of urea crystals on the skin, 'uremic frost', is a sign of very severe uremia.

Disturbances in fluid balance and electrolyte metabolism

Sodium homeostasis may be reasonably well preserved when GFR is substantially reduced. Owing to the loss of functioning nephron mass, the overall adaptability is reduced, however, which means that sodium loading and low sodium intake are less well tolerated than in normal individuals. Although the majority of patients tend to retain sodium and water, there is a very small subgroup of patients who tend to lose sodium and water while on a normal sodium intake and, therefore, are at risk of developing extracellular dehydration.

In patients with chronic renal failure metabolic acidosis generally does not occur until the GFR is reduced to about 25 ml/min. Bone carbonate participates as an extrarenal buffer, and acidosis is rarely severe until GFR is less than 10 ml/min. In patients with interstitial nephritis, acidosis tends to occur earlier than in those with glomerulonephritis. In acute renal failure which is often associated with markedly enhanced protein catabolism and negative nitrogen balance, more severe acidosis may develop.

Hyperkalemia may be especially marked in oliguric acute renal failure. Factors that enhance hyperkalemia are enhanced catabolism and severe metabolic acidosis. Severe hyperkalemia is less commonly a problem in chronic renal failure, because of increased secretion of potassium per nephron (a tubular adaptation). Enhanced fecal excretion of potassium also compensates for reduction in nephron mass to some extent.

Pathophysiology of the uremic syndrome

Uremic toxicity

The most frequently offered explanation for the clinical manifestations and symptoms of uremia (Table 39.1) is an autointoxication by metabolites normally excreted by the kidneys. This concept is supported by the relief of symptoms by dialysis, i.e. a combination of diffusive transport for removal of toxic substances and electrolytes and ultrafiltration for correction of overhydration. There is evidence that at least some 'uremic toxins' are products of protein metabolism, since increased protein intake promotes toxic symptoms, whereas protein restriction alleviates these symptoms. Uremic toxicity is the subject of several recent reviews [2–6].

Uremic sera and plasma ultrafiltrate from uremic patients have been shown to exert a variety of toxic effects in vitro. These include inhibition of cation transport, glucose utilization, mitochondrial metabolism, erythropoiesis, lymphocyte transformation, phagocytosis and various enzyme systems.

Abnormalities in intracellular and extracellular ion composition are well documented in chronic renal failure and depend on retention of water due to decreased renal excretory capacity and on abnormalities in ion transport. Impaired activity of Na^+,K^+-ATPase has been observed in erythrocytes, leukocytes and skeletal muscle of patients with uremia. Inhibition of active transport of sodium from the cell leads to impaired influx of potassium ions into cells and a decrease in the resting membrane potential. Measurements have shown that the electrical potential difference is reduced (i.e. less negative) in patients with near-terminal renal failure [7]. Abnormalities in ion transport and membrane potential might be an important factor for metabolic alterations in uremia. The defect in Na^+,K^+-ATPase activity is at least partially reversed following long-term dialysis treatment suggesting that a dialyzable factor in uremic serum might inhibit Na^+,K^+-ATPase activity or that dialysis removes the stimulus to the secretion of the inhibiting factor. Normalization of the resting membrane potential occurs following regular hemodialysis or treatment with low-protein diet supplemented with essential amino acids in combination with an infrequent hemodialysis schedule (which in itself did not correct the cell membrane depolarization) [8].

As a result of research using new methods for separation and identification of plasma compounds (e.g. high-performance liquid or gas chromatography and mass spectrometry), the list of substances with potentially toxic effects is growing. Comparatively little is known about the effects of uremic toxins in biological systems in vivo, however, and even less about the role of toxins in the development of clinical symptoms. Bergstrom and Fürst [3] proposed that a compound should meet four criteria to be considered a uremic toxin of clinical relevance. (1) It should be chemically identified and quantifiable in biological fluids. (2) Its concentration in tissue or plasma from uremic patients should exceed that present in nonuremic subjects. (3) Its concentration should correlate with uremic symptoms that disappear when the concentration is reduced to normal. (4) Toxic effects of the compound in a test system should be demonstrable at the concentration found in tissue or fluids from uremic patients. Very few substances have satisfied these criteria, and hence attempts to identify uremic toxins of clinical relevance have not been very successful. In a patient with advanced renal failure, metabolic disturbances are most likely caused by a combination of toxins, the concentrations of which do not change in parallel in response to a metabolic or therapeutic intervention. The effects of such substances may also be modified by adaptive processes, such that toxic effects take a long time to develop. Reliable methods for assessing various in vivo effects of substances under suspicion have often been lacking.

Potential uremic 'toxins' are often divided into three groups, according to their molecular weight: low-molecular substances (<350 Da, e.g. urea, creatinine) which are easily dialyzed through conventional cellulose membranes; middle molecules (350–5000 Da), which are poorly dialyzed; and large-molecular non-dialyzable substances (>5000 Da). These categories of substances are defined differently by different authors. Characteristics other than molecular weight (e.g. electrostatic charge, steric configuration, protein binding, multicompartmental behavior, etc.) may influence the ease by which a substance is removed by dialysis. The division of potentially toxic substances according to molecular weight is arbitrary and reflects the history of research on uremic toxins.

Small molecules

On the basis of the effectiveness of early hemodialysis (using cellophane membranes) to eliminate overt uremic symptoms, the likely toxic solutes were thought to be low-molecular-weight, non-protein bound substances. Retention of inorganic ions gives rise to various toxic effects and metabolic abnormalities; ions such as H^+, Na^+, K^+, Mg^{2+}, Al^{3+}, PO_4^{2-} belong, together with H_2O, to a small group of substances for which a toxic role of clinical importance in uremia is undisputed.

Urea

Urea is the principal end product of protein metabolism and accounts for at least 80–90% of urinary nitrogen excreted in the patient ingesting 40–60 g of protein per day. Its rate of excretion correlates with the protein catabolic rate, which in the metabolically stable patient is determined by protein intake. The serum urea concentration is proportional to the protein catabolic rate and inversely proportional to total urea excretion.

The role of urea as a uremic toxin is well established, although toxic symptoms and signs usually require concentrations above those that occur in patients. Some important features of the uremic syndrome are associated with retention of urea – changes in serum urea concentration presumably mirror the retention of other, toxic substances. Urea is recognized as a surrogate marker for uremic toxicity. As discussed further in Chapter 44, the clearance of urea in relation to body mass is widely used for quantifying the dose of dialysis.

Creatinine

Creatinine, a low-molecular weight (113 Da), water-soluble metabolite of creatine, is normally excreted by the kidney and is progressively accumulated in renal failure. There is no convincing evidence of the toxicity of either creatinine or creatine, however. In renal failure a substantial part (between 16 and 66%) of the creatinine produced each day is degraded, probably in the gut. The serum creatinine concentration is therefore useful as a marker of changes in renal function but therefore not a good index of either uremic toxicity or of absolute renal function.

Several other groups of small molecular compounds have been proposed as uremic toxins, for example, phenols, aliphatic and aromatic amines, polyamines, indoles and guanidines. Some of them are derived from naturally occurring amino acids by the action of bacteria in the gut. Although several compounds have been shown to interfere with biochemical and metabolic processes, toxic effects have, with few exceptions, only been observed at higher concentrations than those found in uremic sera.

It is well established that the L-arginine–nitric oxide signaling mediates the function of many different organ systems. On the basis of studies showing that inhibition of nitric oxide synthesis might account for various hemodynamic, gastrointestinal, neurologic and immunologic abnormalities that typically occur in renal failure, it has been proposed that retained endogenous inhibitors of nitric oxide synthesis might play a causative role in the multisystem toxicity of uremia [9]. On the other hand, inhibition of nitric oxide synthase may have some beneficial effects in reducing inflammatory damage in uremia, prevention of hypotension, improving myocardial function and possibly in reducing oxidative damage to lipids. The known endogenous and artificially synthesized compounds that inhibit nitric oxide synthase are structural analogs of its substrate, L-arginine, and contain guanidine nitrogens. In renal failure, accumulation of guanidine compounds, (e.g. asymmetrical dimethyl arginine, guanidinosuccinic acid and creatinine) is well documented and they could, conceivably, function as endogenous nitric oxide inhibitors.

Middle molecules

At the beginning of the 1970s many hemodialysis patients developed severe neuropathy, whereas this complication was not observed in patients undergoing long-term peritoneal dialysis despite lower clearance of small molecules in peritoneal dialysis as compared with hemodialysis. Neuropathy was considered as a manifestation of uremic toxicity and was proposed to be caused by some larger molecule(s) than urea, so called middle molecules (MM) which are more efficiently removed by peritoneal dialysis, probably because of the greater permeability of the peritoneal membrane than conventional hemodialysis membranes.

The MM hypothesis stimulated many researchers to try to identify toxic compounds in the middle molecular range. A large number of MM have been identified in uremic plasma of patients with creatinine clearances less than 10–15 ml/min but only a few of these compounds have been chemically characterized. Some MM have been shown to be glucuronide conjugates of amino acids and others to consist of fragments of known proteins. Although MM exert toxic effects in *in vitro* systems or bioassays, only a limited number of fully characterized MM have been tested for toxic effects *in vitro*. Recently, cross-linked advanced glycosylation end products (AGE) have been proposed to be uremic toxins [10]. AGE-peptides accumulate as a result of renal failure and might be of potential pathophysiological importance for the vasculopathy and macrophage dysfunction in uremia. No correlation has thus far been found between the concentration of different MM and specific uremic manifestations and it is not yet possible to evaluate their role as uremic toxins *in vivo*.

Large molecules

The normal kidney plays a role in removing molecules up to 40 000 Da. Several peptide hormones ≤40 000 Da pass the glomerular barrier and are reabsorbed and catabolized in the proximal tubules. Such substances may accumulate in the body fluids in patients with reduced GFR and are not efficiently removed by dialysis. High-molecular-weight fractions of uremic plasma ultrafiltrate inhibit metabolic processes *in vitro*, but few substances have been well characterized. Three peptides with clear inhibitory effects on specific polymorphonuclear cell functions have recently been characterized by amino acid sequence analysis [11]: (1) granulocyte inhibiting protein I (GPI I; MW 28 000 Da); (2) granulocyte inhibiting protein II (GPI II; MW 9500 Da) and (3) degranulation inhibitory protein (DPI; MW 14 000 Da) were found to be partly homologous with light chains, β2-microglobulin, and the angioplastic factor angiogenin, respectively. Although it is unclear whether high concentrations of these peptides are related to infectious complications in dialysis patients, the identification and characterization of these peptides suggest that other high-molecular-weight fragments or modifications of naturally occurring proteins may be retained in renal failure and interfere with cellular functions in various organs.

β2-Microglobulin

Deleterious effects of chronic accumulation of β2-microglobulin have been established. It is a 11 815 Da HLA class I light chain component of plasma membrane of all mammalian cells. When the HLA-complex is degraded, β2-microglobulin enters the extracellular fluid and is normally eliminated by the kidneys. Accumulation of β2-microglobulin in patients with renal failure causes deposition of amyloid, primarily in the carpal tunnel, the synovial membrane and bone. The elimination of β2-microglobulin by dialysis is inefficient. Clinical manifestations of β2-microglobulin amyloidosis develop in dialysis patients after 5–10 years. (Dialysis-related amyloidosis is further discussed in Chapter 76.)

Unfortunately, the results of the extensive research effort that has been made to elucidate the toxicological background of uremia have had little influence on the therapy of uremia. The identification of toxic substances or groups of substances with clinically significant effects would be of great importance and could have therapeutic implications. The production of substances with documented toxic effects might be blocked by metabolic manipulations or pharmacological therapy, and dialysis membranes and hemoperfusion systems or oral sorbents might be developed to eliminate specific substances.

The trade-off hypothesis

As discussed above, it is generally thought that uremic symptoms are caused by toxic compounds which accumulate in the body fluids as renal elimination decreases. Some components of the uremic syndrome are the consequences of adaptive responses to the loss of functioning renal mass which aim at maintaining homeostasis. For example, hypersecretion of certain hormones occurs to overcome end-organ resistance and may reach toxic concentrations. The classical example of such a 'trade-off' mechanism [12] is the rise in PTH secretion in response to hyperphosphatemia. Normal plasma concentrations of phosphate are restored but at the price of an elevated parathyroid hormone (PTH), which causes renal osteodystrophy, a common, in some cases disabling, complication in patients with advanced renal failure.

In addition to its effect on bone, PTH may have other toxic effects. Secondary hyperparathyroidism has been proposed as a factor in neuropathy, encephalopathy, pruritus, cardiomyopathy, sexual dysfunction, anemia and glucose intolerance. Experimental studies [13] show that chronic exposure of various cells to PTH is associated with a sustained rise in cytosolic calcium, which appears to lead to cellular dysfunction. The action of PTH is receptor mediated and utilizes different pathways in various cells. Experimental data [14] indicate that the increase in cytosolic calcium leads to down-regulation of the PTH–PTHrP receptor, and it has been suggested that an increase in intracellular [Ca2+] might lead to down-regulation of other receptors. Such a down-regulation could thus represent the trade-off for the maintenance of normal phosphate concentration in advanced renal failure, and could contribute to various hormonal abnormalities in uremia. However, it is important to emphasize that although a high PTH appears to exert adverse effects, the clinical significance of hyperparathyroidism for various organs (other than bone) is uncertain.

Other manifestations that occur in patients with advanced renal failure could represent 'adaptive injuries', too. Muscle wasting might be the 'trade-off' for the essential decrease in nitrogen, potassium and phosphate accumulation which results from a reduction in dietary protein intake. Clinical studies have demonstrated that an adaptive reduction in the intake of protein may start early during the course of renal insufficiency (GFR ≥ 25 ml/min) and continue in association with a reduction in energy intake as renal insufficiency progresses towards end-stage renal failure [15]. Such a reduction of nutrient intake before uremia might reflect the operation of a sensor–effector system that serves body homeostasis.

Potential role of uremic toxins in causing progression of chronic renal failure

Recent studies suggest that some compounds that accumulate as a consequence of reduction in the functioning nephron mass may promote glomerular sclerosis and contribute to further progression. In rats with sclerosis in remnant glomeruli seven weeks after subtotal nephrectomy, Motojima *et al.* [16] found that treatment for four weeks with either peritoneal dialysis or oral charcoal adsorbent markedly attenuated further progression of glomerular sclerosis as compared to that in untreated renal failure animals. These results suggest that some circulating substance(s) have the capacity to promote glomerular hypertrophy and sclerosis. Niwa *et al.* [17] showed that oral administration of indole or indoxyl sulfate to subtotally nephrectomized rats increased glomerular sclerosis and decreased inulin clearance compared to control uremic rats. Indoxyl sulfate is normally synthesized in the liver from indole, which is formed from tryptophan, by tryptophanase of intestinal bacteria. Indoxyl sulfate is normally excreted by glomerular filtration but accumulates in chronic renal failure. Stimulated by these findings Niwa and Ise [18] studied the effect of a low protein diet and oral adsorbent administration in subtotally nephrectomized animals on a high protein intake. They found that either treatment reduced plasma indoxyl sulfate levels and attenuated the glomerular sclerosis as compared to control animals on a high protein intake. The granulocyte inhibitory protein, GIP I, which, as discussed above, has been isolated from the plasma ultrafiltrate of patients with renal failure, amplifies the transcription and expression of important inflammatory

genes such as IL-6 and IL-8, both of which increase transcription and translation of collagen I, III and IV in cultured mesangial cells [19]. The results of these studies suggest that in renal insufficiency retention of toxic substances via disease-specific processes may promote progressive glomerular sclerosis and, thus, initiate a vicious cycle of progressive renal insufficiency (Figure 39.3).

The approach to the uremic patient

If renal failure is diagnosed before uremia develops, measures can be taken to forestall or delay the occurrence of uremia, as discussed below. Progressive renal failure may, however, pass unnoticed until advanced renal failure is reached. Sudden clinical worsening may also occur in chronic renal failure patients undergoing regular clinical check-ups. Thus, the clinical presentation differs from patient to patient. The approach to the care of the uremic patient includes several steps (Table 39.2).

Treatment of complications requiring immediate therapy

The first step is to look for complications that require immediate therapy. Severe sodium retention may lead to congestive heart failure and pulmonary edema and may

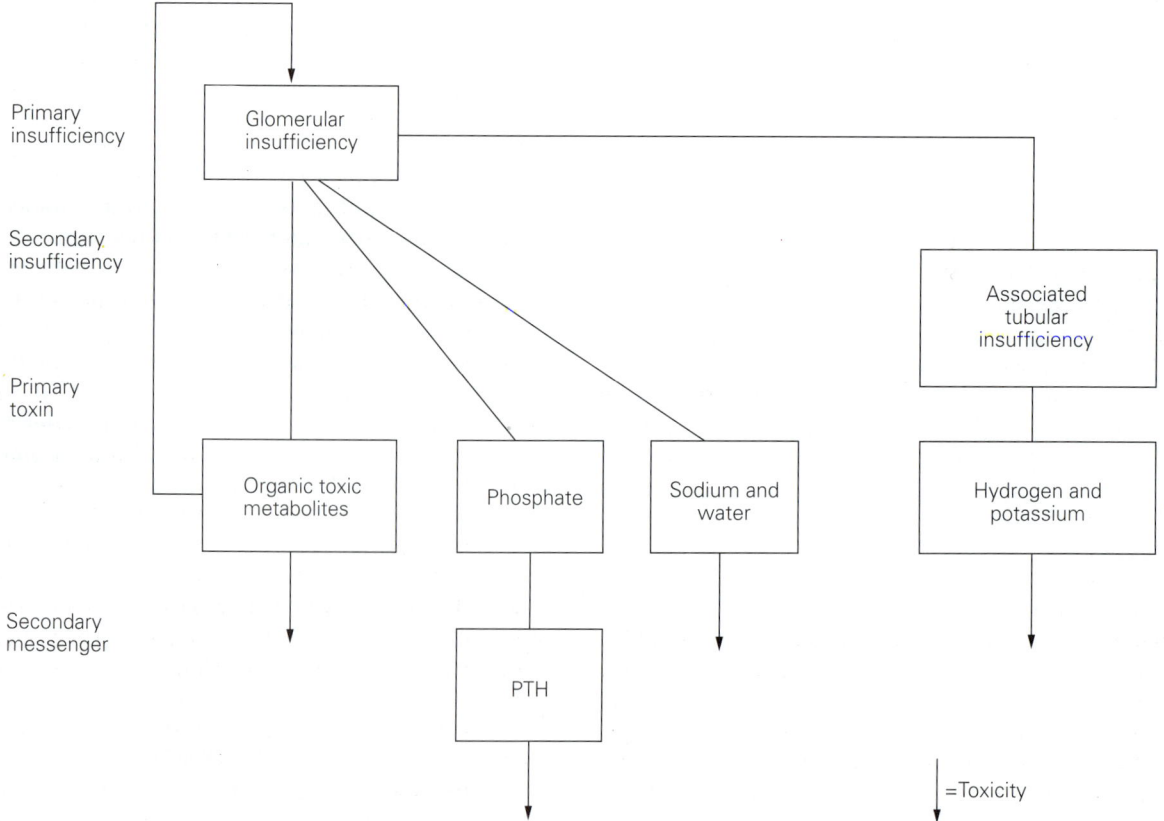

Figure 39.3 Simplified diagram of primary and secondary toxicity in uremia (Modified, with permission, from ref. [2]).

Table 39.2 The approach to the uremic patient

1. Treatment of life-threatening complications
2. Diagnosis of cause of renal failure
3. Correction of reversible factors exacerbating uremia
4. Prophylactic measures to slow progression of renal disease
5. Conservative management of uremia
6. Dialysis and transplant evaluation
7. Initiation of dialysis

require immediate treatment with loop-diuretics (e.g. furosemide). Hyperkalemia and metabolic acidosis should be diagnosed promptly and corrected. Potassium-containing foods should be reduced or totally excluded from the diet. Acidosis-induced hyperkalemia is treated by correcting acidosis with sodium bicarbonate. Potassium may also be lowered acutely by intravenous insulin and glucose or by the administration of a β-adrenergic agonist. An ion-exchange resin may then be given orally or rectally to eliminate potassium. Acute dialysis treatment may be indicated if fluid, acid–base and electrolyte balances cannot be adequately controlled by the above measures, and may also be indicated to relieve signs or symptoms of severe uremia such as pericarditis or encephalopathy.

Diagnosis

If the patient is known to have impaired renal function, it is usually not difficult to diagnose uremia. Few of the typical uremic symptoms are specific for uremia, however. Clinical symptoms or signs of uremia do not develop until GFR is reduced to about 15 ml/min or less. The likelihood that a sign or symptom is caused by uremia increases as GFR is reduced further. Differential explanations for potentially uremic symptoms should be considered in patients with less-advanced renal disease. Serum urea concentration may be used as a fairly reliable index of the severity of uremia, and uremic symptoms do not usually appear until serum urea concentration increases above 25–30 mmol/l. Such symptoms are usually alleviated or disappear if serum urea is reduced by conservative treatment or dialysis.

In the majority of patients the etiology of renal failure is known or may readily be diagnosed, but it is not unusual that it is not. It is important to distinguish between acute and chronic renal failure, as the approach to patients with acute and chronic renal impairment differs greatly. This is not always simple. The history is often of great help in distinguishing between acute and chronic renal failure, whereas physical examination and laboratory tests are often inconclusive. Most chronic renal diseases ultimately lead to reduction of kidney size;

renal sonography should be performed in all patients with renal failure to assess kidney size and exclude obstruction as a cause. Renal biopsy may be necessary for diagnosis in patients with normal kidney size, whereas renal biopsy is rarely informative in patients with small kidneys and may be associated with an increased risk of hemorrhagic complications. Once an advanced stage of renal insufficiency has been reached, therapeutic measures are directed towards complicating factors that exacerbate renal failure, correcting fluid, electrolyte and acid–base imbalances secondary to renal failure and alleviating uremic symptoms. In a patient with chronic renal failure of unknown etiology, the potential benefit of elucidating the underlying renal disease must be weighted against the risk of procedures, discomfort to the patient, and cost of further investigation.

Correction of reversible factors leading to exacerbation of renal failure or uremia

In patients with chronically impaired renal function small further reductions in GFR are associated with aggravation of the uremic syndrome. Conversely even slight improvements in renal function lead to alleviation of uremic symptoms in patients with severely impaired renal function (Figure 39.2).

Exacerbation of renal failure may be caused by cardiac insufficiency, antihypertensive medication and other drug treatment (e.g. non-steroidal anti–inflammatory drugs), urinary obstruction, pyelonephritis and hypercalcemia. Correction of these factors will lead to improvement of renal function and symptoms. Reversible exacerbation of chronic renal failure may be caused by decreased renal perfusion due to hypovolemia from various causes. Although the majority of patients with advanced renal failure tend to retain sodium and water, there is a very small subgroup of patients who tend to lose sodium and water while on a normal sodium intake and, therefore, are at risk of developing extracellular dehydration with low blood pressure and further lowering of GFR. The state of sodium balance should be carefully evaluated in all patients and salt-depleted patients should be prescribed sodium and fluid in amounts sufficient to stabilize blood pressure and optimize GFR. Metabolic acidosis accelerates the rate of muscle protein breakdown and enhances urea generation and may thus aggravate uremia. Sodium bicarbonate should be given to maintain serum bicarbonate above 22–22 mmol/l. In general, the amounts of sodium bicarbonate required will not result in sodium retention similar to that from quantitatively similar increases in sodium chloride intake [20]. Treatment with corticosteroids, intercurrent infections, and inadequate energy intake all increase protein breakdown and urea generation which may directly exacerbate uremia (without affecting GFR). Such causes of reversible aggravation of renal impairment and uremia should be corrected.

Prophylactic measures to prevent further damage to the kidneys

It is of the utmost importance to avoid factors that will further impair kidney function, such as the use of radio-contrast agents, intravascular volume depletion, hypertension, infection and nephrotoxic drugs (Table 39.3).

Conservative treatment of uremia

The primary goals of conservative treatment are to maintain fluid, electrolyte and acid–base homeostasis by adequate dietary regimens, and alleviate uremic symptoms while maintaining nitrogen balance. (The treatment of fluid, electrolyte and acid imbalances is discussed in Chapter 69.)

In renal failure, excessive dietary protein enhances production of nitrogenous, potentially toxic waste products and increases uremia. Restriction of dietary protein has an important role in management, provided that good nutrition can be maintained. The basic concept of treatment with a low-protein diet is to provide a restricted amount of protein together with generous amounts of energy.

To keep the patient free from uremia, the protein intake must be gradually reduced as renal function deteriorates. It is not certain when dietary protein should be restricted in patients with renal insufficiency. If a low-protein diet is prescribed primarily as a therapy to alleviate uremic toxicity, residual renal function is not the main guide for reducing protein intake. Protein restriction, on the other hand, may be used as a means to retard the rate of progression of renal insufficiency. The rationale, principles and results of such treatment are discussed in Chapters 68 and 71. As discussed above, uremic symptoms, in general, appear when serum urea concentration exceeds 25–30 mmol/l; this rarely occurs until GFR is below 15–20 ml/min. Dietary protein, therefore, should be gradually reduced to maintain serum urea below 25–30 mmol/l.

In patients with symptoms such as general fatigue, nausea and vomiting, restriction of dietary protein generally alleviates symptoms and decreases the serum urea concentration, whereas serum creatinine is not changed. Initially only a moderate restriction of dietary protein to about 0.9 g/kg/day is necessary. When renal function deteriorates further, and the urea concentration increases, toxic symptoms reappear and further restriction of protein intake to about 0.6 g/kg/day of protein is necessary. Provided that a large proportion of the dietary protein is of high biological value, neutral nitrogen balance is maintained. To reduce the risk of negative nitrogen balance and muscle wasting, it may be wise to supplement the diet with 5–8 g of essential amino acids (as tablets). It is also important to ensure a high energy intake ($\geq$35 kcal/kg/day). Patients who experience marked uremic symptom when on an unrestricted diet can, if the progression of the renal insufficiency is slow, manage for years on a diet of 0.6 g of protein/kg/day, and treatment with dialysis can be delayed. As the renal function deteriorates further urea accumulates and toxic symptoms develop in spite of dietary restriction to 0.6 g/kg/day. For certain patients, further dietary treatment with more severe protein restriction and amino acid or amino acid–keto acid supplementation may be a therapeutic alternative. (The dietary treatment of uremia is discussed in Chapter 68.)

Dialysis and transplant evaluation

Renal transplantation should be considered as a potential therapeutic alternative in all patients below 60–70 years of age with chronic progressive renal insufficiency. The question of transplantation should be discussed individually with all patients. A thorough medical and psychological evaluation of all potential transplant recipients to detect problems that may reduce the possibilities of a successful outcome of the surgical procedure and immunosuppressive treatment is useful. Contraindications for kidney transplantation include infection, such as tuberculosis and HIV, metastatic malignancy, extensive vascular disease, informed patient refusal, non-compliance and a high risk for perioperative mortality (see Chapter 69).

In all chronic renal insufficiency patients in whom progression to end-stage renal failure can be expected, dialysis treatment should be planned well ahead of time to allow time for careful explanation and discussion of the alternative treatments with the patients and family members and the creation of vascular or peritoneal access. The time at which to initiate dialysis treatment is a decision that requires consideration of laboratory parameters, and clinical signs and symptoms. Absolute indi-

Table 39.3 Potentially reversible causes leading to aggravation of renal failure or uremic symptoms

A. Exacerbation of chronic renal insufficiency
   Hypoperfusion
   Drug toxicity
   Urinary tract infection
   Obstruction

B. Exacerbation of systemic disease

C. Dietary
   Excessive protein
   Inadequate calories

D. Increased catabolism
   Intercurrent infection
   Corticosteroids

E. Metabolic
   Hypercalcemia
   Hypokalemia

cations to initiate dialysis treatment are signs of pericarditis, pulmonary edema not responsive to diuretics, therapy-resistant hyperkalemia and uremic encephalopathy. In most cases dialysis is started when symptoms such as anorexia and nausea progressing to vomiting occur and are not corrected by a weight-maintaining low protein diet that is readily accepted by the patient. Objective findings such as measurement of GFR with iohexol or creatinine clearance may be useful as guideposts for the decision to initiate dialysis and in general a GFR below 10 ml/min indicates that dialysis treatment may be needed in the near future.

References

1. Fine, L.G., Kurtz, I., Woolf, A.S. *et al.* (1993) Pathophysiology and nephron adaptation in chronic renal failure, in *Diseases of the Kidney* (eds R.W. Schrier and C.W. Gottschalk), Little, Brown and Co., Boston, pp. 2703–43.

2. Bergstrom, J. (1985) Uremia is an intoxication. *Kidney Int.*, **17**, S2–4.

3. Bergstrom, J. and Furst, P. (1983) Uremic toxins, in *Replacement of Renal Function by Dialysis* (eds W. Drukker, F.M. Parsons and J.F. Maher), Martinus Nijhoff, Boston, MA, p. 354.

4. Teschan, P.E. (1994) Uremia: an overview. *Semin. Nephrol.*, **14**, 199–204.

5. Vanholder, R., De Smet, R., Hsu, C. *et al.* (1994) Uremic toxicity: The middle molecule hypothesis revisited. *Semin. Nephrol.*, **14**, 205–18.

6. Bergstrom, J. and Wehle, B. (1995) Clinical implications of middle and larger molecules, in *Clinical Implications of Middle and Larger Molecules* (eds A.R. Nissenson, R.N. Fine and D.E. Gentile), Appleton & Lange, Norwalk, pp. 204–34.

7. Cottor, J.R., Woodward, T., Carter, N.W. and Knochel, J. (1979) Resting skeletal muscle membrane potential as an index of uremic toxicity. *J. Clin. Invest.*, **63**, 501–6.

8. Cotton, J.R. and Knochel, J. (1985) Correction of uremic cellular injury with protein-restricted amino acid-supplemented diet. *Am. J. Kidney Dis.*, **5**, 223–36.

9. Vallance, P., Leone, A., Claver, A. *et al.* (1992) Accumulation of an endogenous inhibitor of nitric oxide synthesis in chronic renal failure. *Lancet*, **339**, 572–5.

10. Ritz, E., Deppisch, R. and Nawroth, P. (1994) Toxicity of uremia – does it come of age? *Nephrol. Dial. Transplant.*, **9**, 1–2.

11. Haag–Weber, M., Mai, B., Cohen, C. and Horl W.H. (1994) GIP and DIP: A new view of uremic toxicity. *Nephrol. Dial. Transplant.*, **9**, 346–7.

12. Bricker, N.S. (1972) On the pathogenesis of the uremic state: An exposition of the 'trade–off' hypothesis. *N. Engl. J. Med.*, **286**, 1093–9.

13. Massry, S.G. and Smogorzewski, M. (1994) Mechanisms through which parathyroid hormone mediates its deleterious effect on organ function in uremia. *Semin. Nephrol.*, **14**, 219–31.

14. Tian, J., Smogorzewski, M., Kedes, L. and Massry, S.G. (1994) PTH–PTHrP receptor mRNA is downregulated in chronic renal failure. *Am. J. Nephrol.*, **14**, 41–6.

15. Kopple, J., Chumlea, W.C., Gassman, J.J. *et al.* (1994) Relationship between GFR and nutritional status. Results from the MDRD study. *J. Am. Soc. Nephrol.*, **5**, 335.

16. Motojima, M., Nishijima, F., Ikoma, M. *et al.* (1991) Role for 'uremic toxin' in the progressive loss of intact nephrons in chronic renal failure. *Kidney Int.*, **40**, 461–9.

17. Niwa, T., Ise, M. and Miyazaki, T. (1994) Progression of glomerular sclerosis in experimental uremic rats by administration of indole, a precursor of indoxyl sulfate. *Am. J. Nephrol.*, **14**, 207–12.

18. Niwa, T. and Ise, M. (1994) Indoxyl sulfate, a circulating uremic toxin, stimulates the progression of glomerular sclerosis. *J. Lab. Clin. Med.*, **124**, 96–104.

19. Kashgarian, M. and Block, L.G. (1995) GIP, a protein over-expressed in chronic renal disease. *Blood Purif.*, **13**, 77–8.

20. Husted, F.C., Nolph, K.D. and Maher, J.F. (1975) Na HCO$_3$ and NaCl tolerance in chronic renal failure. *J. Clin. Invest.*, **56**, 414–19.

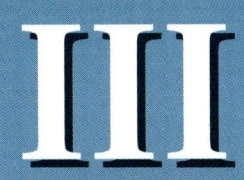

Diseases of the Kidney and their Treatment

Section 1
Inherited and Developmental Diseases

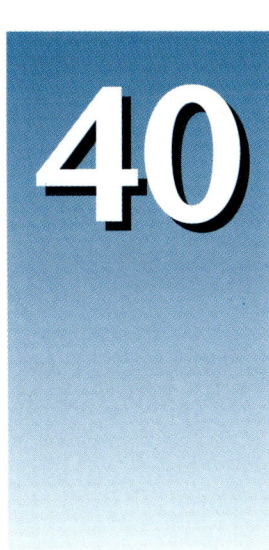

Hereditary and developmental diseases

Ashutosh S. Lohe and Rex L. Jamison

Introduction

Understanding of hereditary and developmental diseases of the kidney is constantly evolving as new information about their molecular and cellular mechanisms becomes available at an increasingly rapid rate. The clinical perspective alone is no longer sufficient. Genetic studies now play an increasingly important role in the diagnosis, classification and treatment of these diseases, because mutant genes cause the protein abnormalities that are responsible for the systemic manifestations of these illnesses. The first part of this chapter reviews the cystic diseases, hereditary and acquired, that have a predominantly renal presentation. The second part examines inherited disorders of the glomerular basement membrane and of metabolism that may affect the kidney. Elegant discoveries of the genetics of diabetes insipidus and Alport's syndrome, and experimental approaches to preventing cystogenesis in polycystic disease, are some of the advances that will be touched upon. Table 40.1 summarizes the inherited kidney diseases and their patterns of inheritance that are considered in this chapter.

Autosomal dominant polycystic disease of the kidney

Autosomal dominant polycystic kidney disease (ADPKD) is the most common cystic disease of the kidney, with an estimated prevalence of 1:400 to 1:1000. The disease is world-wide in its distribution and affects all races. It was responsible for about 10% of all end-stage renal disease (ESRD) in the United States and Europe, and 3% in Japan. In recent years it has fallen to 4–5% because of the increase in vascular and diabetic renal diseases in the more elderly patients accepted for dialysis. The prevalence of the disease in other populations is not well documented [1].

A monogeneic disease with complete penetrance (100% of gene carriers will show evidence of disease by the age of 80 years), ADPKD is genetically heterogeneous. Two and possibly three causative genes have been identified by linkage analysis. About 90% of all white European families have the gene located on the short arm of chromosome 16 (ADPKD1) [2]. A second gene locus has been identified on chromosome 4 (ADPKD2). Yet a third

Nephrology, Edited by Rex L. Jamison and Robert Wilkinson.
Published in 1997 by Chapman & Hall, London. ISBN 0 412 60930 4

	Chromosome
Autosomal dominant	
Autosomal dominant polycystic kidney disease	16 (ADPKD1), 4 (ADPKD2)
Medullary cystic disease	–
Nail–patella syndrome	9
Autosomal recessive	
Autosomal recessive polycystic kidney disease	6
Juvenile nephronophthisis	2
Cystinosis	17
Cystinuria	2 (type I)
Primary hyperoxaluria	2
Sickle cell anemia	11
Recessive nephrogenic diabetes insipidus	12
X-linked	
Fabry's disease	X
X-linked nephrogenic diabetes insipidus	X
Alport's syndrome	X
Unknown	
Fanconi's syndrome	–
Renal glucosuria	–

Table 40.1 Hereditary and developmental kidney disease: patterns of inheritance

ADPKD, autosomal dominant polycystic kidney disease.

locus has also been suggested. It is also possibly unique as it shows no linkage to chromosome 4 or 16. New mutations are rare. Absence of disease in parents, confirmation of paternity, typical clinical manifestations of ADPKD, and transmission to offspring, are all criteria which need to be satisfied in order to establish a new mutation.

Variable expression of the gene, even within families, and phenotypic differences between ADPKD1 and ADPKD2 may be responsible for the clinical heterogeneity of kidney disease in ADPKD. About 50–75% of all gene carriers will develop ESRD [3]. Extrarenal manifestations like hepatic cysts are unpredictable, although there is evidence to suggest that potentially lethal intracranial aneurysms cluster in members of a kindred. Unstable DNA or interaction of the ADPKD gene with modifying genes or the environment are the reasons proposed for the clinical spectrum observed.

Clinical manifestations

Autosomal dominant polycystic kidney disease is a systemic disease with both renal and extrarenal manifestations. An increasing number of patients without symptoms of kidney disease are now diagnosed when being investigated for hypertension, or incidentally during radiologic studies of the abdomen. Screening individuals in affected families is another reason for increased rate of detection.

Renal manifestations

The most common symptom of cystic enlargement of the kidney is chronic flank or back pain. Distension of the kidney and its capsule is the probable cause of this pain because it correlates well with renal and cyst size, and is relieved when cysts are decompressed.

Acute pain in contrast may be caused by hemorrhage, infection or obstruction of the kidney. Spontaneous intracystic hemorrhage is the usual cause. It may be accompanied by gross hematuria. Perirenal hematoma is an uncommon cause of pain and usually follows trauma. Infection within a cyst, often difficult to differentiate from pyelonephritis, is the second most common cause of pain. Nephrolithiasis secondary to stasis and metabolic factors like hyperuricemia and hyperoxaluria also causes pain. It can occur in 25–35% of all patients with ADPKD. Uric acid stones predominate [4].

Microscopic and gross hematuria and fever from infection are other common manifestations of kidney disease. Hematuria accompanies cyst hemorrhage, infection and stones. Occurrence of hematuria for the first time after age 50 should raise the suspicion of renal malignancy although there is no firm evidence for an increased incidence. Mild proteinuria may be found in a small percentage of patients but nephrotic-range proteinuria is rare and obligates a search for an additional etiology.

Hypertension

Arterial hypertension develops early and is present in approximately 50% of all pre-azotemic patients with ADPKD. The incidence of hypertension increases with age and with declining renal function and may affect 75–80% of patients with severe renal failure. Hypertension increases left ventricular mass. It contributes to cardiac and cerebrovascular morbidity and is thought to accelerate progression of renal disease.

Members of an ADPKD kindred unaffected by polycystic disease have lower levels of plasma renin when compared to their affected kin with normal renal function. Distortion of the renal vasculature by the cysts is believed to give rise to intrarenal ischemia. This leads to activation of the renin–angiotensin system, and subsequent hypertension [5]. It is noteworthy that decompression of painful cysts improves control over elevated blood pressure as well. Angiotensin converting enzyme inhibitors may be the agents of choice to control hypertension.

Liver and other gastrointestinal involvement

Cystic involvement of liver is the commonest extrarenal manifestation in ADPKD [6]. Rare in children, hepatic cysts develop later than renal cysts and show a striking female preponderance. These cysts are lined by biliary epithelium. Polycystic liver disease increases in severity with multiparity, suggesting a role of female hormones in modulating hepatic cystogenesis. The number and size of hepatic cysts also correlate independently with increasing age, and increasing renal insufficiency. Hepatic parenchymal volume is not reduced by cyst growth; hence liver function tests remain normal.

Any increase in liver enzymes suggests an intracystic complication like infection or carcinoma. The most common complication is infection, which may be life threatening. Patients with cyst infection present with fever, pain over the liver, leukocytosis and abnormal liver enzymes. Imaging procedures are more useful here than in the diagnosis of renal cyst infections. Enterobacteriaceae infections predominate [7] and antibiotic therapy may be required for as long as six weeks. Antibiotics useful for kidney infections, like ciprofloxacin and cotrimoxazole, are probably as effective as those which concentrate in the biliary tract like cefoperazone. Percutaneous and surgical drainage and partial hepatectomy may be needed if conservative therapy fails.

Unusual causes for abnormal liver function include: congenital hepatic fibrosis (although this is more common with autosomal recessive polycystic kidney disease), cholangiocarcinoma, and obstructive jaundice from compression of major bile ducts from extensive cystic involvement. Massive hepatic cystic disease may also cause portal hypertension with variceal hemorrhage, and cachexia from digestive discomfort. Octreotide, a somatostatin analog, has reportedly been used with some success in treatment of hepatic cystic disease. Surgical decompression of cysts, and hepatic resection, are other treatments which have been used with some success.

Other common gastrointestinal manifestations include colonic diverticulosis, hiatal hernia, pancreatic and splenic cysts.

Intracranial aneurysms

Intracranial aneurysm (ICA) is a rare but major vascular abnormality reported in ADPKD. This association is more frequent than by chance alone. The estimated prevalence of asymptomatic intracranial aneurysms by computed tomography (CT) scanning or magnetic resonance (MRI) angiography in ADPKD patients ranges from 5 to 11%. The corresponding figure in the general population is 1%. Aneurysm rupture may be the initial manifestation of ADPKD.

Other than family history of ruptured ICA, no clinical feature reliably predicts the presence of an aneurysm or its impending rupture. Headache is not a reliable symptom, although a change in its character may have prognostic implications in patients with demonstrable aneurysm. Rupture is not restricted to patients with chronic renal failure. The relative risk of rupture is four times higher in patients with a family history of ruptured ICA than in those without such history.

Most aneurysms rupture in the fourth to fifth decade of life (Figure 40.1) and carry a risk (40–60%) of morbidity

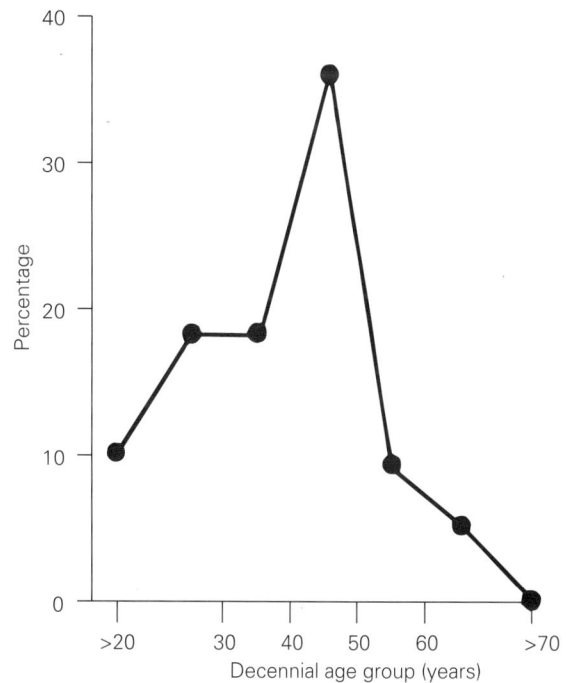

Figure 40.1 Age at intracranial aneurysm rupture in 71 patients with autosomal dominant polycystic kidney disease. (Reproduced from ref. [8] by permission of Blackwell Science, Inc.)

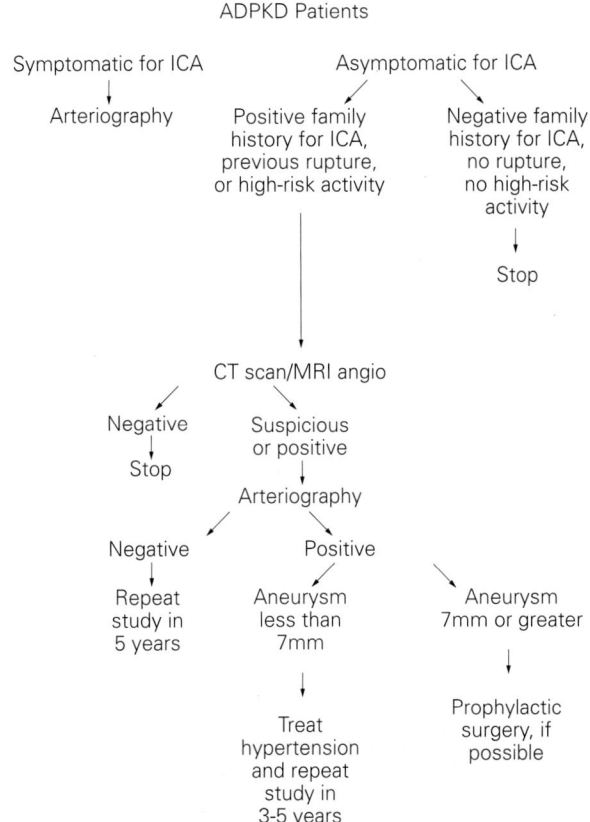

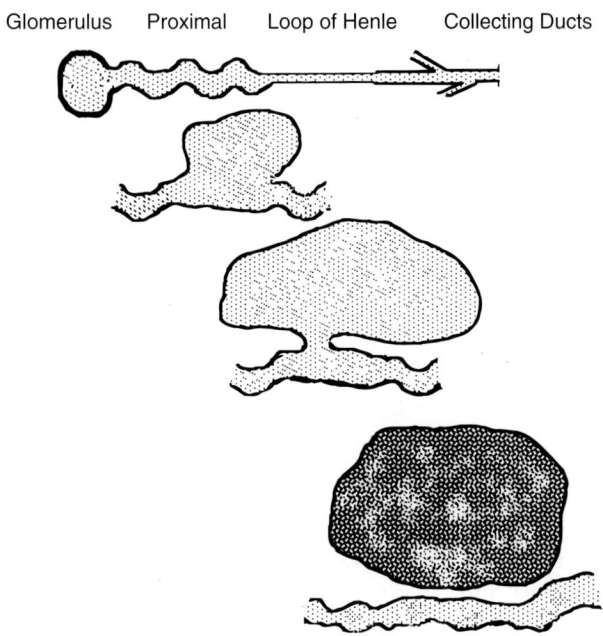

ADPKD Patients

Symptomatic for ICA   Asymptomatic for ICA

Arteriography   Positive family   Negative family
                   history for ICA,   history for ICA,
                   previous rupture,   no rupture,
                   or high-risk activity   no high-risk
                                            activity

                                            Stop

                   CT scan/MRI angio

Negative   Suspicious
              or positive
Stop
              Arteriography

Negative   Positive

Repeat   Aneurysm   Aneurysm
study in   less than   7mm or greater
5 years   7mm

                                 Prophylactic
              Treat   surgery, if
              hypertension   possible
              and repeat
              study in
              3-5 years

Figure 40.2 Current recommendations for screening for intracranial aneurysms in autosomal dominant polycystic kidney disease patients. (Modified, with permission, from Fick, G.M. and Gabow, P.A. (1992) The urgent complications of autosomal dominant polycystic kidney disease. *J. Crit. Illness*, **7**, 1905–20.)

Glomerulus   Proximal   Loop of Henle   Collecting Ducts

Figure 40.3 The isolation of a cyst. This schematic diagram depicts the process by which cysts disengage from the tubule of origin. Cysts originate as diverticula within the walls of the renal tubule. These diverticula enlarge and ultimately separate from the initial tubule. Fluid may enter this cyst from the tubule when the cyst is still in communication with the lumen. It will then resemble glomerular filtrate. Once the cyst disengages, further accumulation probably occurs by transepithelial secretion of fluid into the cyst lumen. (Adapted, with permission, from Martinez, J.R. and Grantham, J.J. (1995), Polycystic kidney disease: etiology, pathogenesis and treatment. *Disease-a-Month*, **41**, 695–766.)

and mortality at three months [8]. Ruptured aneurysms are saccular and are all present on the circle of Willis, mostly on the middle cerebral artery. MRI angiography can now detect aneurysms as small as 3 mm. Abnormal MRI findings must be confirmed by arteriography, however. Elective surgery or endovascular obliteration is indicated for all aneurysms greater than 10 mm. The growth of aneurysms greater than 7 mm needs to be monitored closely. Smaller aneurysms are generally not clipped because of their low rate of rupture and the high risk of surgery.

Routine screening of all patients with ADPKD for ICA is not cost effective [9]. Patients with ADPKD with previously ruptured ICA, and those with a family history of ruptured ICA, probably constitute the two major populations that should be screened every 5–10 years (Figure 40.2). Recurrent hemorrhage in the former may be from another aneurysm. MRI angiography or spiral CT are probably the screening procedures of choice because of their sensitivity and because arteriography in ADPKD patients has a higher rate of complications than in the general population.

Cardiovascular abnormalities

Mitral valve prolapse is detected in about 30% of patients with ADPKD. Aortic aneurysms have also been reported in ADPKD. Cerebrovascular accident resulting from ischemic stroke and hypertensive hemorrhage is far more common than those from ICA rupture and is the other major cardiovascular complication of ADPKD.

Pathogenesis of cyst formation

Renal cysts are present in many disorders of the kidney. While simple renal cysts usually arise from the distal tubule, the cysts in autosomal recessive polycystic kidney disease originate from any segment of the renal tubule. Many heritable or acquired factors that lead to disordered cell proliferation, fluid secretion, and extracellular matrix (ECM) abnormalities contribute to cystogenesis [10].

The growth rate of immature cells is faster than that of normal mature cells. It is hypothesized that epithelial cell proliferation occurs because certain tubular cells are arrested in a state of relative immaturity during the maturation process or are unable to redifferentiate following injury. Cysts are formed when these proliferating cells form a diverticulum that ultimately separates from the tubule of origin (Figure 40.3). Proto-oncogenes like c-myc, c-fos and c-jun, may be driving this growth.

Fluid accumulation within the proliferating epithelial cells is necessary for cyst formation and probably takes place by one of two mechanisms: sequestration of glomerular filtrate while the diverticulum is still connected to the parent segment, or transepithelial secretion into isolated cysts. The secretory capabilities of cyst epithelia has been further confirmed by the observation of rapid reaccumulation of fluid in drained cysts.

The cellular basis of fluid secretion by cyst epithelia has been studied in MDCK cells – an immortalized epithelial cell line. Cells suspended in a collagen matrix proliferate to form dense, solid balls of cells on addition of epidermal growth factor (EGF). Addition of a cyclic AMP-agonist leads to fluid secretion within these 'balls' and cyst formation. Stimulation of a basolateral Na, K, Cl transporter by increased intracellular cyclic AMP leads to increased intracellular concentration of chloride, disturbs the electrochemical balance and drives the chloride ions out of the cell through apical channels into the cyst cavity. Passive movement of Na into the cyst follows, through paracellular pathways. An increase in the NaCl concentration of cyst fluid leads secondarily to water flow and accumulation of fluid.

Finally, alterations in the ECM have been observed. The composition of ECM may have a regulatory role in directing growth, differentiation and function of epithelial cells. The extrarenal manifestations further support the notion that defective interaction between cells and ECM may be the initiating event in what is essentially a matrix disorder.

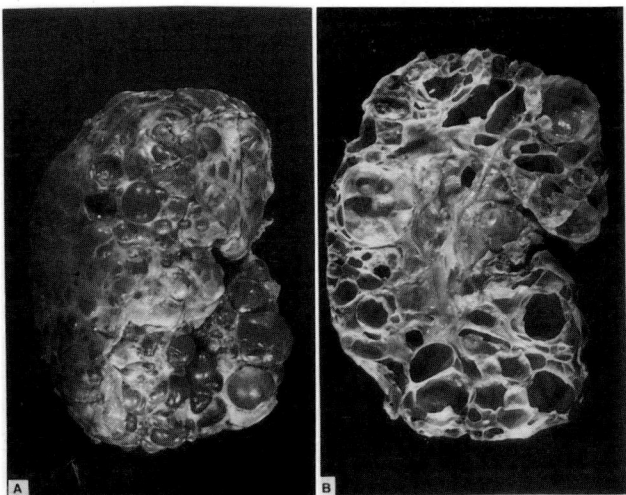

Figure 40.4 (a) Adult polycystic kidney disease (ADPKD) with cysts on the surface of the kidney. (b) Coronal section through the ADPKD kidney showing the cortical and medullary cysts of varying size. (Reproduced from ref. [3] by permission of Blackwell Science, Inc.)

Pathology

The renal cysts in ADPKD are distributed throughout the cortex and medulla of both kidneys (Figure 40.4). Areas of normal tissue must be demonstrable to differentiate it from cystic dysplastic kidney [11]. The walls of the cysts in ADPKD are usually lined by a single layer of mostly primitive epithelial cells.

Associated congenital anomalies are rare. Epithelial cysts occur in the thyroid, ovary, epididymis, seminal vesicles and endometrium. Cysts in the liver are lined by columnar cells resembling biliary epithelium. An increase in connective tissue is often observed in portal areas but hepatic fibrosis seldom results in liver dysfunction.

Diagnosis

Polycystic kidney disease is easily diagnosed in adults with enlarged kidneys. Difficulty may be encountered in younger subjects and in individuals lacking a family history especially when extrarenal manifestations like hepatic cysts are absent. There is no consensus on the criteria for diagnosing ADPKD in these situations. Criteria should be age-adjusted because cysts enlarge with time and may be too small to be detected in young patients; solitary cysts are common with increasing age (25% of all individuals over 50), and the reliability of ultrasound for ADPKD2 patients has not been defined. This is because the latter develop cysts, renal failure and hypertension at a later age than ADPKD1 patients.

CT is the most sensitive of radiologic modalities available to confirm the diagnosis. It can detect cysts with a diameter less than 10mm. Ultrasonography, though simpler and cheaper, can only resolve cysts if their diameter is greater than 10mm. The presence of three or more cysts with at least one cyst in either kidney is probably diagnostic beyond age 30 [12]. Two cysts may be sufficient in younger patients whereas five or more is necessary to establish the diagnosis in those over 50. Radioisotope scanning, intravenous urography or MRI are either too insensitive or too expensive to be useful as a routine screen.

Care must be exercised in distinguishing ADPKD from other hereditary cystic diseases like tuberous sclerosis, von Hippel–Lindau disease, juvenile nephronophthisis–medullary cystic disease complex and cystic dysplasia of kidney (Table 40.2). Problems with diagnosis are more likely when multiple renal cysts are detected in infancy and childhood.

Management of renal complications

Pain

Acute pain is often self limited and usually resolves with conservative management. Correction of the underlying cause like infection, obstruction or hemorrhage, along with bed rest, sedation and analgesia, is all that may be

Table 40.2 Differential diagnosis of cystic renal disease

	ADPKD	*ARPKD*	*JN-MCD*	*MSK*
Inheritance	Autosomal dominant	Autosomal recessive	JN–Autosomal recessive MCD–Autosomal dominant	None, developmental
Hypertension	Yes	Yes	Yes, late	No
Extrarenal features	Hepatic cysts, Intracranial aneurysms	Hepatic fibrosis	Retinal dysplasia, Hepatic fibrosis	?Hyperparathyroidism
Renal	Multiple large cysts	Medullary cysts	Sporadic medullary cyst	Medullary cysts
Kidney size	Increased	Increased	Normal or slightly reduced	Normal
Imaging choice	Ultrasound	Ultrasound	Not useful early in disease	Intravenous urography
Renal stones	Up to 35% of adults	No	No	Common

ADPKD, autosomal dominant polycystic kidney disease; ARPKD, autosomal recessive polycystic kidney disease; JN, juvenile nephronophthisis; MCD, medullary cystic disease; MSK, medullary sponge kidney.

necessary. Non-steroidal anti-inflammatory agents must be used with care as they may aggravate hemorrhage.

Chronic pain is a greater challenge because of the potential for narcotic abuse. Refractory pain has been managed successfully by reduction of cyst volume, either by percutaneous aspiration of cysts, or by surgical or laparoscopic decompression, with no deleterious effects on renal function. The probability of being pain-free at 18 months was 33% after needle aspiration and 81% after surgical decompression in one such study [13]. Nephrectomy is a treatment of last resort.

Hematuria

Most intracystic hemorrhages can be managed conservatively with analgesics and bed rest. Blood transfusions are seldom necessary. Rare cases of severe hemorrhage may require intra-arterial embolization or even nephrectomy. Secondary causes like stone and infection must be treated aggressively. Other measures that must be taken to prevent cyst hemorrhage in patients in whom this is a problem include avoiding physical activities that can cause bleeding, like contact sports.

Infection

Infection is common among females and elderly patients. Instrumentation of the urinary tract is a major predisposing factor and must be avoided unless absolutely necessary. Pyelonephritis and infected cysts present with fever and flank pain. Although the former can be diagnosed by the presence of white cell casts and positive urine culture, the latter is more likely when typical clinical features are present, urine findings are absent or ambiguous, and blood cultures are positive.

Pyelonephritis can be treated with standard antibiotics. Infections of the cyst are difficult to diagnose, treat and eradicate. They are difficult to identify by CT scanning or radionuclide scans, a problem which is compounded in patients on hemodialysis who may have had previous episodes of infection or intracystic bleeding. Treatment is difficult because of poor penetration by antibiotics into the cyst. Since most cysts do not communicate with the tubule lumen, diffusion of the antibiotic across the lipophilic cyst wall is critical for its action. Infected non-gradient cysts (those that do not develop an electrolyte concentration gradient between cyst fluid and plasma and which probably originate from the proximal tubule) are best treated by sulfamethoxazole, clindamycin, and ciprofloxacin whereas gradient cysts (distal tubular in origin) respond to clindamycin, trimethoprim and ciprofloxacin. Cotrimoxazole and ciprofloxacin are thus the agents of choice [14], since the type of cyst cannot be determined in routine clinical practice. Drainage of cysts is occasionally required in persistent infections. Nephrectomy may be necessary for cases with uncontrolled infection not responding to antibiotic treatment for more than four weeks.

Stones

The diagnosis of stone disease is best made by CT scanning. Anatomic distortion of the collecting system by enlarged cysts makes interpretation of intravenous urography difficult. Patients with stones are managed in the usual fashion. They should undergo metabolic evaluation and can be treated with lithotripsy as well as percutaneous and endourologic surgery.

Renal failure and its outcome

Type 2 ADPKD patients develop renal cysts, hypertension and ESRD at an older age than Type 1 ADPKD individuals (mean age at initiation of dialysis is 69.4 years versus 56.7 years). However, because of variable expression of the gene within families, prognosis is heterogenous and unpredictable. About 25–50% of all patients will not have ESRD at age 70. It is rare for ADPKD to cause renal failure in infancy. Renal failure occurs earlier in males. African–Americans develop renal ESRD earlier than whites and those with sickle cell trait even earlier [15]. Hypertension and infection should be treated aggressively as with any other renal disease. Protein restriction probably does not ameliorate the course of renal disease [16].

Renal replacement therapy (dialysis and kidney transplantation) is indicated when end stage renal failure ensues. Neither confer a survival advantage. Patient survival is 79% at five years after transplantation, similar to that of patients with chronic renal failure from other kidney diseases, compared to 73% on dialysis [17]. A special problem of ADPKD patients on hemodialysis is continued bleeding into cysts. Those on peritoneal dialysis have a higher incidence of abdominal and inguinal hernias. Pretransplant nephrectomy is advised only in patients with intractable or recurrent infections, bleeding, neoplasms, recurrent stones, intractable pain or massively enlarged kidneys encroaching on the transplant bed in the iliac fossa.

The mean age at death is about 59 years. The common causes of death are cardiac disease, infection and neurologic events (including ruptured cerebral arterial aneurysm, hypertensive intracranial hemorrhage and ischemic stroke) [18]. The incidence of death from cardiac disorder is similar in patients with or without ESRD. Increased left ventricular mass from hypertension and coronary artery disease probably play a significant role. The incidence of death from infections in ADPKD patients with ESRD is higher than in those without ESRD. It has not changed despite the introduction of modern renal replacement therapies (Figure 40.5). Access infections are responsible for less than 10% of all deaths from sepsis in ADPKD patients. In contrast, death from sepsis in the general ESRD population is usually related to dialysis access. Neurologic events are more likely to cause death in ADPKD patients without ESRD. Deaths from renal cancer are extremely rare.

Experimental approaches to therapy

In the future, pharmacologic therapy for hereditary renal cystic disease will probably focus on modifying the events that lead to cyst formation or growth. Many approaches are being tried in animal models of ADPKD.

Paclitaxel, by depolymerizing microtubules, blocks cell division and slows disease progression. Attempts are being made to modulate fluid accumulation with drugs that act selectively on cystic epithelia and interfere with the generation of cyclic AMP or with chloride transport. Finally, efforts are being made to prevent interstitial inflammation. This will reduce interstitial fibrosis and thereby retard the decline in renal function.

Genetic counseling

DNA linkage analysis can help identify affected individuals in ADPKD kindreds in whom radiologic studies are inconclusive. These tests can also help in prenatal diagnosis. At least two affected relatives must be included in the study to establish linkage to the ADPKD gene. Social, psychological, insurance and financial implications have generally limited the use of these tests.

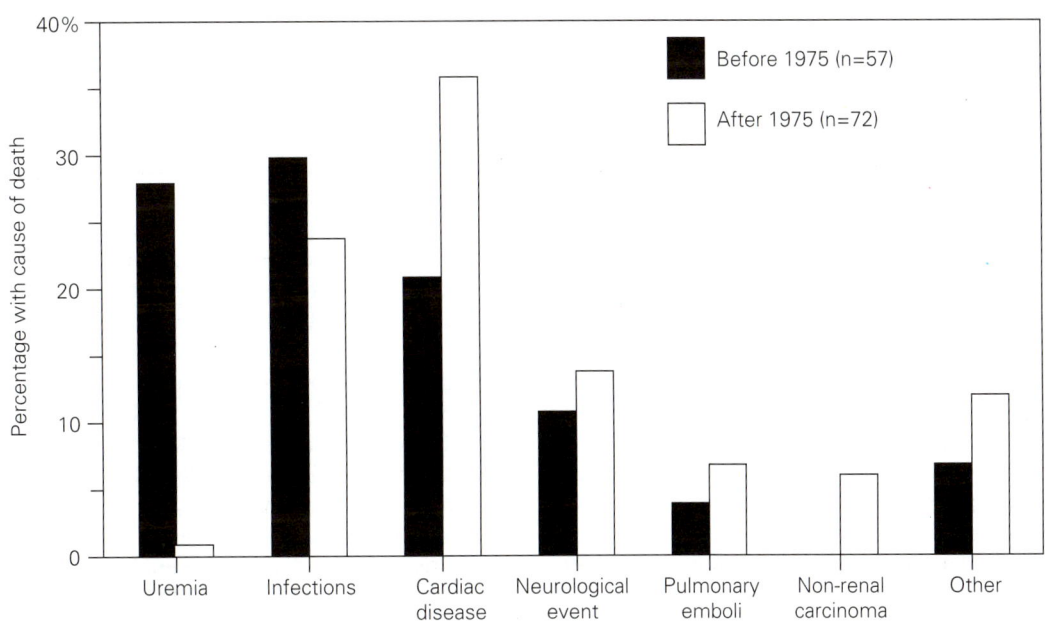

Figure 40.5 Primary causes of death in persons with autosomal dominant polycystic kidney disease with or without end-stage renal disease. (Reproduced, with permission, from ref. [18].)

Autosomal recessive polycystic kidney disease

Autosomal recessive polycystic kidney disease (ARPKD) is a rare disorder with an incidence of 1:6000 to 1:40 000 live births. The parents are almost never affected, and one of four siblings has a chance of developing disease by inheriting a defective gene from each carrier parent. The gene has been identified on chromosome 6 [19]. Perinatal, neonatal, infantile and juvenile variants have been described. Linkage analysis will provide further information about whether a single causative gene, with variable expression, is responsible for the different ages of presentation [20]. No genetic heterogeneity has been described.

Clinical manifestations

The most common variant is the perinatal form. It is rapidly fatal owing to pulmonary hypoplasia and respiratory failure. Early renal failure may be present. The kidneys in such patients are symmetrically and massively enlarged. Oligohydramnios from low urine output *in utero* results in poor development of lungs with or without associated Potter's facies. The liver is seldom affected.

Renal involvement is characterized by tubular dysfunction and a loss of ability to concentrate urine. Patients develop volume depletion and hypernatremia especially with illnesses that enhance extrarenal losses (diarrhea, vomiting) or impair fluid intake (altered sensorium). Hypertension appears in infancy and may be severe. Edema is a frequent complication and there is a high susceptibility of the cystic kidneys to infection.

Most deaths occur in the first month and another 10–20% of patients will die before the age of one year. Beyond the neonatal period, mortality and renal failure are less frequent. Renal involvement is less prominent after infancy and liver disease becomes more important. Patients in late childhood may manifest signs and symptoms related to congenital hepatic fibrosis like portal hypertension and ascending suppurative cholangitis rather than renal failure.

Pathology

The kidneys are enlarged (Figure 40.6). Their cut surface shows a radial arrangement of cysts extending from the subcapsular cortex to the medulla. Larger cysts are more common in the medulla. Glomeruli and tubules proximal to the collecting duct do not participate in cystogenesis. The pelvicocalyceal system is only slightly distorted. Kidneys are typically smaller in older children and have fewer cysts.

Hepatic lesions are limited to portal areas. The bile ducts are dilated and tortuous and the portal tracts fibrous (congenital hepatic fibrosis). This results from a develop-

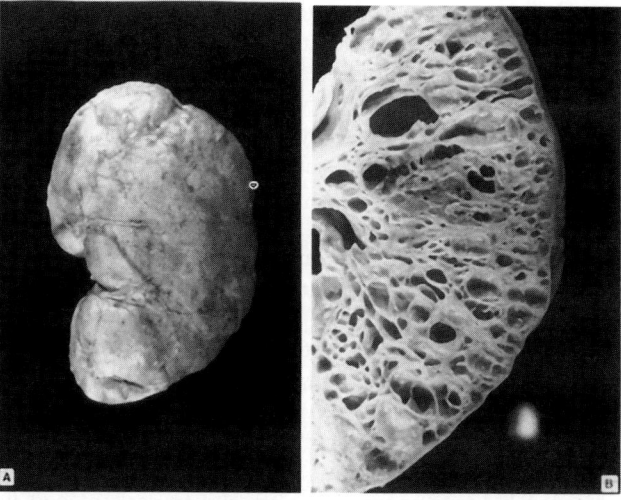

Figure 40.6 (a) Autosomal recessive polycystic kidney disease (ARPKD). The surface reveals little distortion compared to that of ADPKD. (cf. Figure 40.4). (b) Coronal section through the ARPKD kidney revealing the cysts. (Reproduced from ref. [3] by permission of Blackwell Science, Inc.)

mental arrest in the growth of intrahepatic bile ducts and is termed 'bile duct plate abnormality'. A similar histologic picture is also seen in Caroli's syndrome which is characterized by dilatation of intrahepatic ducts. It is either isolated or associated with congenital hepatic fibrosis.

Diagnosis

Ultrasonography is the preferred imaging technique especially for prenatal diagnosis. The typical picture is one of enlarged, echogenic kidneys with loss of corticomedullary junction. This picture may resemble that of ADPKD and other cystic diseases of childhood. Both parents have normal renal ultrasounds. A family history helps to differentiate between ARPKD and ADPKD. In the absence of a family history, biopsy of the liver is the only definitive means of diagnosis.

Intravenous urography is pathognomonic of the condition in younger children. It is seldom done because of the large dose of ionizing radiation. A delayed, mottled nephrogram is observed that may persist for several days. Opacification of the dilated collecting ducts produces linear contrast streaking in the cortex and a brush-like medullary opacification. Rare cases of neonatal ADPKD can still cause confusion.

The appearance of the kidneys in the older child depends on the degree of renal impairment and the extent of persisting cysts. A mottled nephrogram is uncommon. The medulla remains hyperechoic on ultrasound but the diffusely bright echo pattern is lost.

Treatment

Aggressive treatment of renal and hepatic complications has considerably reduced mortality. Survival is as high as 79% at 15 years in children who survive the first year of life. Treatment is directed at fluid replacement, correcting hypertension, managing infections, and offering dialysis and transplant when indicated. Older children also need to be treated for complications of portal hypertension and may on occasion need liver transplants.

Medullary sponge kidney

Medullary sponge kidney is believed to be a developmental abnormality (rarely inherited) of the medullary collecting tubules characterized by non-progressive cystic changes limited to the renal medulla. It is often asymptomatic. Usually found in adults in the fifth to seventh decades of life, the disease is present equally in both sexes and has an estimated prevalence in the general population of 1 in 5000–20 000 individuals.

Renal colic is the presenting complaint in a majority of patients although a subset will present with hematuria and urinary infection. Urolithiasis occurs more commonly in women than in men. Hypercalciuria should always be looked for and, if present, hyperparathyroidism ruled out. Distal renal tubular acidosis is associated with medullary sponge kidney and may aggravate the tendency to stone formation.

The tubular cysts arise in the medulla. They vary in size but almost never exceed 1 cm in diameter. Interstitial fibrosis occurs in patients with severe cystic disease. A mixture of calcium oxalate and calcium apatite intraluminal concretions are present in a majority of patients. High urinary pH and hypercalciuria promote their deposition and growth. Calculi are formed when these concretions erode the cyst wall and appear in the renal pelvis.

Excretory urography in early tubular ectasia characteristically shows a papillary blush that persists after clearance of contrast media from the pelvis in delayed films. As the disease progresses, linear radiations appear, giving a brush-like appearance to the renal papilla. Large cysts may produce large medullary opacification. Nephrocalcinosis is often present and supports the diagnosis. Papillary necrosis and bacterial and tuberculous abscesses may cause confusion but can be distinguished by their clinical features. Other causes of nephrocalcinosis like sarcoidosis, hypercalcemia and all causes of distal renal tubular acidosis must also be excluded.

Therapy is directed at correcting hypokalemia and acidosis, reducing hypercalciuria and treating complications like infection and urolithiasis. The long-term prognosis is very good; few patients progress to end-stage kidney disease.

Juvenile nephronophthisis–medullary cystic disease complex

Juvenile nephronophthisis (JN) and medullary cystic disease (MCD) are two diseases with similar renal morphology that are distinguishable by their patterns of inheritance, age of onset, and associated abnormalities. Whereas MCD has an autosomal dominant inheritance, JN is autosomal recessive. It is thus likely that different genes are responsible for producing these disorders that are pathologically identical. Recent linkage studies have also helped locate a gene for JN on chromosome 2. A homozygous deletion has been identified in affected subjects as well sporadic cases [21].

Children with JN usually become symptomatic at 9–10 years of age. Urinary concentration defects lead to polyuria and polydipsia in all patients. Salt wasting is prominent in most cases and moderate tubular proteinuria may be present. Slowly progressive renal insufficiency is accompanied by anemia, hypertension and growth retardation. ESRD occurs at the mean age of 13. Patients with MCD in contrast present late in life. They develop ESRD around age 35. Growth retardation and anemia are generally not present and some patients go undetected till the seventh decade of life. Flank pain, hematuria, and renal calculi seldom occur in the JN–MCD complex.

There is a strong association between JN (but not MCD) and retinal dysplasia. When present, this disease has been termed retinal–renal dysplasia. Changes in the retina include coarse clumping of pigment and diffuse mottling. Other ocular abnormalities described are tapetoretinal degeneration, coloboma, amblyopia and optic nerve atrophy. Hepatic fibrosis, skeletal abnormalities, cerebellar abnormalities and hypogonadism are additional extrarenal manifestations of JN.

The kidneys are normal or slightly reduced in size. Cut surface shows a thin fibrotic cortex and cysts in the outer medulla. Cysts are not essential for the diagnosis. Light microscopic findings include tubulointerstitial nephropathy with atrophic tubules surrounded by dense fibrosis. Tubular basement membranes are markedly thickened and multilayered. Imaging with ultrasonography or CT scanning shows medullary cysts, later in JN than in MCD.

Measures should be taken to avoid dehydration and salt depletion. Complications of renal insufficiency should be treated as they arise. Renal transplantation is the treatment of choice especially in children with ESRD. The disease does not recur in the allograft.

Acquired cystic kidney disease

The development of renal cysts in patients with chronic renal failure from non-cystic kidney disease is referred to as acquired cystic kidney disease (ACKD). Although neither inherited nor developmental, it is included for purposes of comparison to other cystic disorders of the kidney. It is generally accepted that more than three cysts should be present or more than 25% of the kidney involved for the diagnosis to be made [22]. This disease occurs in 7–22% of patients starting dialysis. The prevalence of cysts increases with the duration of dialysis, and 90% of all those on peritoneal or hemodialysis more than 10 years will have ACKD. Successful transplantation may cause regression of cysts in some patients, suggesting that a non-dialyzable renotropic factor is responsible for the cystic proliferation and neoplastic changes seen.

ACKD is usually silent but may occasionally present with hematuria, flank pain (from retroperitoneal or intracystic hemorrhage) or infection. Cysts are usually less than 5 mm but may grow to 3 cm. CT-scanning is more sensitive than ultrasound in detecting small cysts. A dreaded and infrequent complication is renal cell carcinoma – best identified by contrast-enhanced CT-scanning. It should be noted, however, that among ESRD patients with renal cell carcinoma, only 50–60% have acquired cystic disease at the time the cancer is diagnosed. Thus, the presence of renal cell cancer in ACKD may be incidental.

The annual incidence of renal cell carcinoma in dialysis patients is 3–6-fold that of an age-matched population and increases with the duration of dialysis, especially in male patients with cystic disease. It is difficult to distinguish a benign renal adenoma from a carcinoma although smaller tumors tend to show less indication of malignancy histologically and the majority of lesions smaller than 3 cm in diameter are histologically benign. Nevertheless, nephrectomy is recommended when a solid lesion – symptomatic or silent – is detected in the ESRD population, even if the lesion is less than 3 cm in diameter.

Since renal cell carcinoma is not a common cause of death in dialysis patients, screening is not cost effective. Neither is preventive nephrectomy because of surgical morbidity. It is important to note that only 0.2–0.5% of these cancers will be metastatic when detected. The five-year survival rate of those with renal cell cancer is 35% for dialysis patients, which compares favorably with a 42% survival for non-dialysis patients. Screening, if instituted, is probably most useful for young male dialysis patients with a good prognosis and multiple cysts in large kidneys.

Nail–patella syndrome

Nail–patella syndrome (NPS) is an autosomal dominant disorder characterized by dysplasia of the nails and bones. The kidney is affected in about half of cases. Linkage analysis has mapped the defect to chromosome 9, but the identity of the gene and its precise location remain to be determined.

Dysplastic changes in the nail are invariably present and are most marked in the thumb. Absent or hypoplastic patellae, deformed elbows and iliac horns are among the more frequent skeletal abnormalities. The kidney disorder usually manifests as asymptomatic hematuria and proteinuria. Nephrotic syndrome and chronic renal failure are uncommon.

Although light microscopy of a renal biopsy is unrevealing, electron microscopic studies reveal two characteristic lesions: irregularly thickened glomerular basement membranes with areas of rarefaction giving rise to a mottled and 'moth-eaten' appearance and the pathognomonic intramembranous fibrils with the periodicity of collagen, in the basement membrane (Figure 40.7).

There is no specific treatment. Renal transplantation is successful although the use of steroids may increase the risk of aseptic necrosis of the head of the femur.

Alport's syndrome

Alport's syndrome (AS) is an inherited disorder of type IV (basement membrane) collagen characterized by progressive nephritis and sensorineural hearing loss. Its estimated incidence is 1 in 5000, with males being predominantly affected. In view of the vast number of mutations reported, it is not surprising that there is marked interkindred variability in clinical manifestations. The predominant clinical types of AS, based on their rate of progression to ESRD, are juvenile-onset ESRD AS and adult-onset ESRD AS. Phenotypic variation is also determined by the presence or absence of extrarenal involvement.

Clinical features

Persistent microscopic hematuria is the key clinical feature of AS. Gross hematuria may be precipitated by upper respiratory infections. Proteinuria, initially absent, eventually appears with increasing age and may even reach nephrotic levels. Progression to renal failure, when it occurs, is fairly constant in affected males within a kindred. Prognosis in affected females is usually benign.

Hearing deficits are bilateral, sensorineural, cochlear in origin, and can be detected early by audiometry. Loss of hearing is usually moderate and does not worsen in affected males after the age 15; females have a more benign course. Sensorineural deafness is not an essential criterion for the diagnosis of AS.

About 15–30% of patients with AS have ocular abnormalities. Bilateral anterior lenticonus is pathognomonic of AS. It manifests as increasing myopia in the second to third decades of life. Cataracts have been reported. Other common abnormalities include pigmentary changes in the perimacular and macular region.

Other reported abnormalities in families with AS include thrombocytopenia with giant platelets, hearing

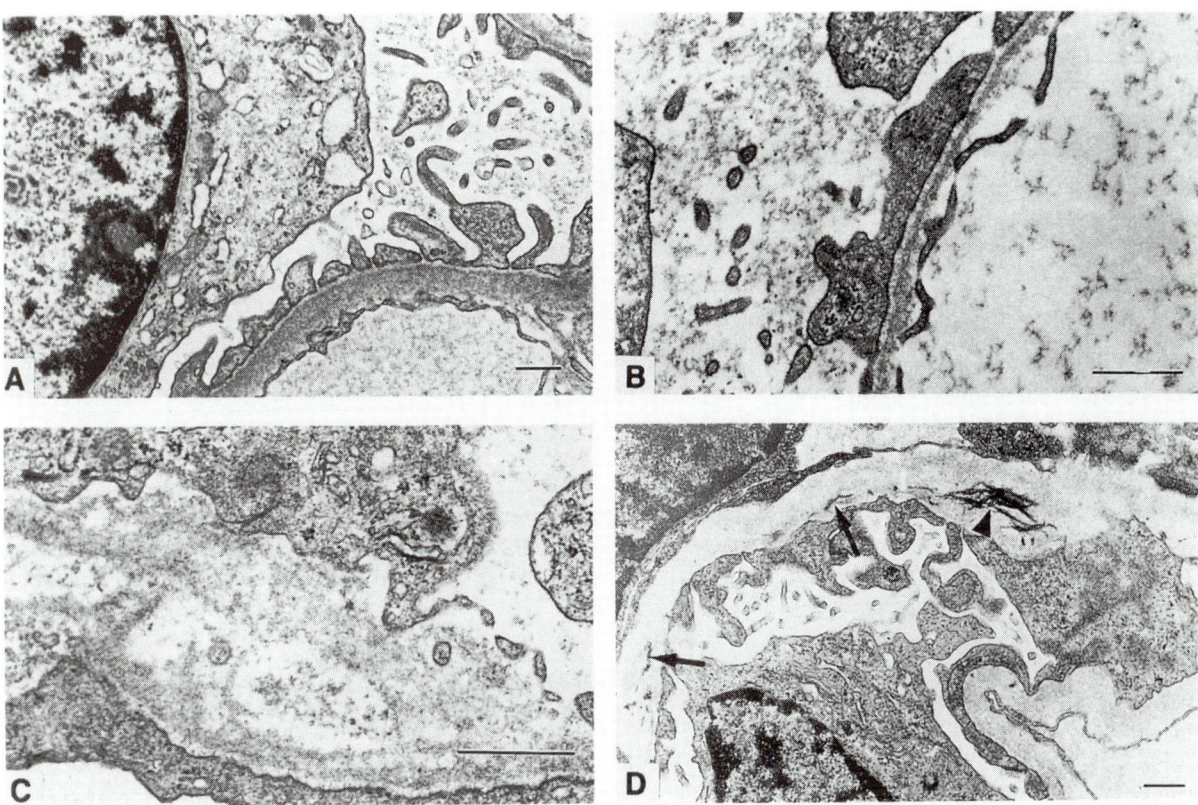

Figure 40.7 Electron micrographs of the glomerular basement membrane (GBM). (A) Normal kidney. (B) Thin basement disease; note the very thin GBM between the discontinuous thin endothelium of the glomerular capillary on the right and the podocytes of the epithelium on the left. (C) Alport's syndrome; note the fragmentation of the lamina densa into interlacing strands, simulating a 'basket-weave' appearance. (D) Nail–patella syndrome; the GBM is irregular and has areas of rarefaction resembling a 'moth-eaten' appearance. The arrows point to collagen fibrils within the GBM. Bar = 0.5 μm. (Reproduced, with permission, from Bodziak, K.A., Hammon, W.S. and Molitoris, B.A. (1994) Inherited disease of the glomerular basement membrane. *Am. J. Kidney Dis.*, **23**, 605–18.)

loss, cataracts, renal disease of variable severity and a bleeding diathesis. Another association that has been described is nephritis and hearing loss with diffuse leiomyomatosis. All patients with diffuse leiomyomatosis have dysphagia from esophageal involvement. Tracheobronchial leiomyomatosis is occasionally present and genital (clitoris and labia majora) involvement has been reported in affected females.

Pathology and pathogenesis

The glomerular basement membrane (GBM) shows characteristic ultrastructural changes (Figure 40.7). It is thickened with fragmentation of the lamina densa into multiple interlacing strands, giving the GBM a 'basket-weave' appearance. In more than 60% of patients with AS, immunofluorescence microscopy identifies a unique inability of the anti-α_3 anti-GBM antibody to bind to glomeruli. Affected males usually show no binding at all whereas affected females exhibit discontinuous and irregular binding. Normal kidneys show linear binding of these antibodies to the basement membrane.

Type IV collagen is made of three α chains organized in a triple helical structure. Each α chain has a 26–28 kDa carboxyl terminal non-collagenous domain and contains collagenous Gly-X-Y repeat sequences interrupted 21–23 times by non-collagenous sequences. Six α chains have been identified. The two major chains, α_1 and α_2, are found in all basement membranes and are coded by adjoining genes (COL4A1 and COL4A2) on chromosome 13. In contrast, the minor chains α_3, α_4, α_5 and possibly α_6, have more restricted distribution in specialized basement membranes of the kidney, eye and ear. The genes encoding α_3 and α_4 (COL4A3 and COL4A4) are on chromosome 2 whereas those encoding α_5 and α_6, COL4A5 and COL4A6 respectively, are on the long arm of the X chromosome (Figure 40.8). The triple helix of 'classical' type IV collagen consists of α_1 and α_2 chains in a 2:1 ratio. 'Novel' type IV collagen, on the other hand, contains the other α chains.

The anti-α_3 antibody is directed against the 'Goodpasture antigen' located in the non-collagenous domain (NC1) of the α_3 chain of a novel type IV collagen. It is collagen that is the primary defect in AS. Structural

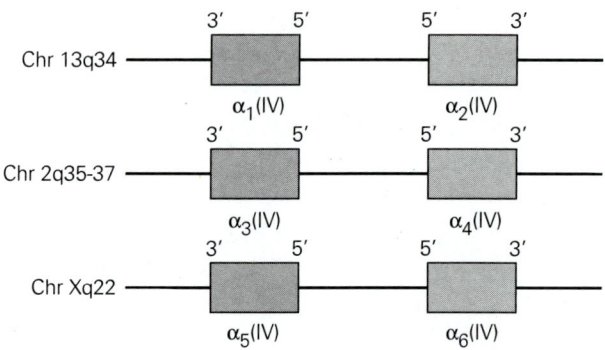

Figure 40.8 Schematic representation of the type IV collagen genes. The genes encoding for α_1(IV) and α_2(IV) are located head to head on chromosome 13q34. Similarly, the genes encoding for α_3(IV) and α_4(IV) are on chromosome 2q35–q37, and those encoding for α_5(IV) and α_6(IV) are on chromosome Xq22. (Adapted from Knebelmann, B., Antignac, C., Gubler, M.C. *et al.* (1993) A molecular approach to inherited kidney disorders. *Kidney Int.*, **44**, 1205–16 by permission of Blackwell Science, Inc.)

changes in the α_5 chain of AS patients impair the incorporation of α_3 and α_4 chains into the type IV collagen network [23]. This observation has been confirmed by immunohistochemical analysis of the collagen in the GBM of patients with mutations of COL4A5. α_3 and α_4 chain antigens were absent in these patients.

Genetics of Alport's syndrome

In the majority of cases (greater than 80%) the disease is linked to the X chromosome. Affected males transmit the mutant gene COL4A5 to daughters but not to sons. Autosomal recessive and dominant forms have also been described and should be suspected when affected members of the same generation born to unaffected parents have a similar progressive juvenile-onset ESRD (autosomal recessive) or there is father-to-son transmission (autosomal dominant), respectively. *De novo* mutations of the gene COL4A5 may account for 18% of all newborns with AS.

The Alport locus was mapped to the long arm of the X chromosome in the Xq22 region in 1988. Identification of the COL4A5 gene that encoded the α_5 (IV) chain at this site and the discovery of mutations in this gene in AS families helped to confirm this finding. Deletions of genetic material usually result in juvenile-type AS whereas base pair substitutions (point mutations) cause the adult-type AS. Mutations in COL4A3 and COL4A4 on chromosome 2 have been documented in autosomal recessive forms. Deletions in COL4A6 and COL4A5 are associated with AS with diffuse leiomyomatosis. The role of COL4A6 in AS needs to be better defined.

The discovery of the responsible gene in X-linked AS families has important clinical implications. In the future, DNA testing may identify the female carrier and

Table 40.3 Diagnostic criteria for Alport's syndrome

Positive family history of hematuria
Sensorineural deafness in proband or in affected member of family
Ocular changes (anterior lenticonus and/or macular changes)
Glomerular basement membrane ultrastructural changes
Absence by immunohistochemistry of α_3 and α_4 chains of type IV collagen in the glomerular basement membrane

permit prenatal diagnosis. The present criteria for the diagnosis of AS need to be revised to avoid underdiagnosing this disease in the general population (Table 40.3).

Therapy

Either dialysis or transplantation is appropriate for treating patients with AS with ESRD. Allograft rejection reaction in a transplanted AS patient may lead to severe crescentic glomerulonephritis and subsequent graft loss in 1–5% of those transplanted. Introduction of antigenic epitopes absent in the recipient probably triggers this process. Transplanted AS patients with allograft dysfunction must be evaluated for anti-GBM nephritis, not only because it is possible to treat such patients with plasmapheresis and cyclophosphamide, but also because it may have implications for future transplants in the patient and kindred members. It is not possible by current means of DNA testing to identify patients at risk for development of anti-GBM nephritis.

Thin basement membrane disease

Thin basement membrane disease is an inherited disorder of the peripheral capillary glomerular basement membrane with characteristic findings on electron microscopy.

Patients invariably present with asymptomatic microscopic hematuria without proteinuria. Males and females are affected equally. A small subset of patients may present with the loin pain–hematuria syndrome (LPH) [24]. There are no associated clinical features which allow diagnosis which can only be made on renal biopsy.

Glomeruli appear normal under light microscopy. Diffuse thinning of the basement membrane to 200 nm or less is observed under electron microscopy (Figure 40.7). Immunofluorescence studies are usually negative and distinguish the disorder from IgA nephropathy – another common cause for recurrent hematuria.

The prognosis is good and deterioration of renal function very rare. The incidence of hypertension is increased [25]. There is no therapy for this disorder. Angiotensin converting enzyme inhibitors may decrease the frequency of episodes of gross hematuria in the subset of patients presenting as LPH.

Fabry's disease

Fabry's disease (FD) also known by the descriptive name, 'angiokeratoma corporis diffusum universalis', is an X chromosome-linked inborn error of metabolism caused by a deficiency of α-galactosidase A, an enzyme necessary for the catabolism of ceramide trihexoside (a glycosphingolipid). This enzymatic defect interferes with intralysosomal degradation of glycosphingolipids and results in their accumulation in various tissues of the body outside the central nervous system, with protean manifestations.

The disease usually presents with a reddish purple macular skin rash on the trunk, legs, oral mucosa and upper limbs (Figure 40.9), but sparing the tongue. A majority of affected males experience dysesthetic pain in the extremities from autonomic involvement. Kidney involvement is usually evident in young adults and is characterized by lipiduria, proteinuria and hypertension. Cerebrovascular disease, polymyositis and arthropathy of the terminal interphalangeal joints, dilated venules in the conjunctive and retina, and corneal opacities are other manifestations.

Mutations in the gene or post-translational defects result in an inactive enzyme. Endothelial cells and vascular smooth muscle take up the undegraded circulating lipid. The consequences are widespread: aneurysmal dilatation of blood vessels in the eyes, skin and cerebral vasculature; hypertension; and premature coronary disease and strokes. Epithelial cells of the glomerulus and renal tubule also accumulate lipid. The cells have abundant cytoplasm which is finely vacuolated. Ultrastructural changes reveal that every renal cell type is affected despite a normal light microscopy appearance. The vacuoles are membrane-bound, electron-dense bodies with a lamellated appearance (zebra bodies) (Figure 40.9).

Characteristic physical and ultrastructural findings lead to the diagnosis which is confirmed by measurement of α-galactosidase A activity in peripheral leukocytes. The carrier state is more reliably identified by measuring urinary ceramide levels, since α-galactosidase A activity may be present in the low normal range. Prenatal diagnosis by amniocentesis is possible. Other skin lesions which may be confused with those of FD are present in hereditary telangiectasia and other angiokeratomoses. Glomerulonephritis associated with systemic diseases must be kept in mind.

The ESRD of FD can be treated by the usual means. Transplant is not contraindicated. Progressive vascular disease can complicate the course of the disease. Replacement enzyme therapy has not been found to be useful so far.

Cystinuria

Cystinuria is an autosomal recessive disorder with an overall prevalence of about 1 in 7000. The transport of cystine, ornithine, arginine and lysine is abnormal in the proximal renal tubule and in the jejunum in patients with cystinuria. Excessive renal excretion of cystine is responsible for the renal manifestations. No malnutrition occurs as enough dietary amino acids are absorbed as oligopeptides.

Three phenotypes have been described (I, II and III) in this basic aminoaciduria. Until recently, it was thought that they were due to multiple alleles of the same gene. Genetic heterogeneity has since been documented. Mutations of the amino acid transporter gene, SLC3A1, produce only homozygous type I cystinuria [26]. Another locus is probably responsible for homozygous types II and III.

The disease is usually detected in the second or third decade of life when the patient first passes a kidney stone. Cystine is highly insoluble (solubility limit, 250 mg/l from pH 4.5 to 7.5) and forms classic flat hexagonal crystals, easily detected by microscopic exam of the urine sediment (Figure 40.10). The definitive diagnosis of these radiopaque calculi requires measurement of urinary cystine excretion (more than 250 mg/g creatinine) and chromatographic analysis of the stone.

The medical approach to treatment is to reduce the urinary concentration of cystine below its solubility limit by increasing fluid intake, keeping pH of the urine above 7.5 by alkali therapy, and reducing cystine excretion by decreasing sodium intake. Patients who fail this therapy may respond to drugs containing a sulfhydryl group, like penicillamine and tiopronin, which form mixed disulfide complexes that are far more soluble than cystine itself [27]. Urinary cystine concentration monitoring is advisable to help individualize tiopronin therapy. The toxicity of penicillamine and tiopronin limits usage. Captopril, which also contains a sulfhydryl moiety, may be a useful and less toxic substitute.

Cystinosis

Cystinosis is an autosomal recessive disorder of excess lysosomal storage of cystine due to defective transport of cystine from lysosomes. The cystinosis gene has recently been linked to markers on the short arm of chromosome 17 [28]. Infantile nephropathic, intermediate, and benign cystinosis of adulthood are the three major forms of this disease. Unlike cystinuria, stones are not a feature of this illness.

Infantile disease is characterized by decreased growth, vomiting, polyuria and polydipsia and by Fanconi's syn-

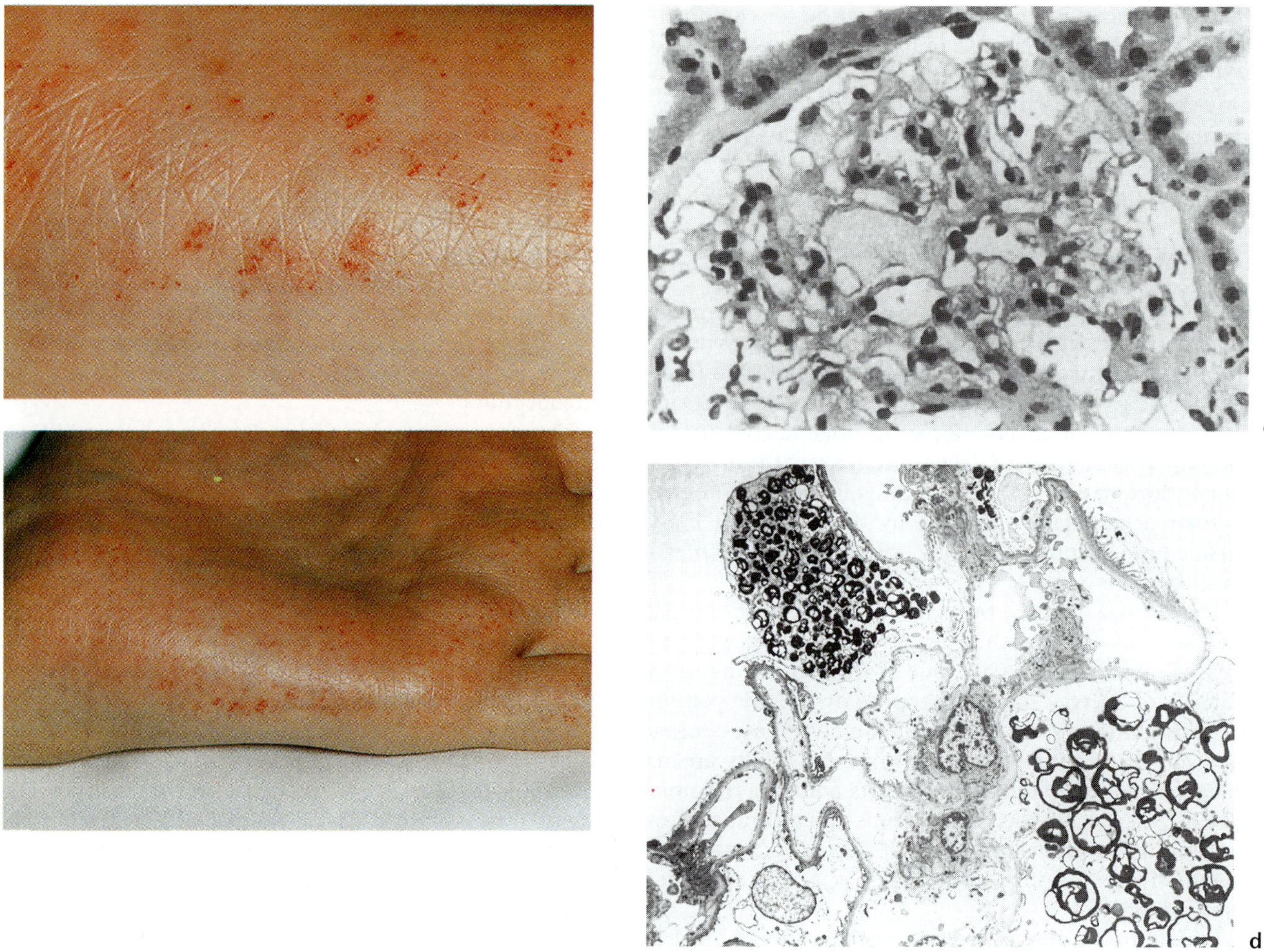

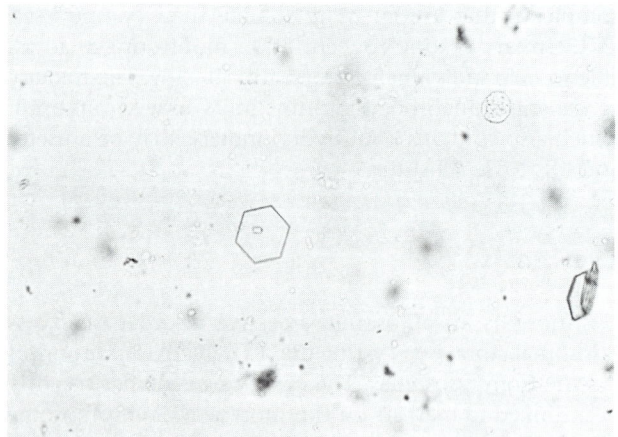

a

b

c

d

Figure 40.9 (a, b) The typical skin rash in Fabry's disease showing angiokeratoma, rather unusually, on the hands. (Photographs provided by Professor R. Wilkinson.) (c) The visceral epithelial cells are enlarged and have vacuolated foamy cytoplasm. (d) Electron micrograph of glomerular capillary loops. Lamellar and myelinoid inclusions are present in the visceral epithelial cell cytoplasm. (Reproduced, with permission, from Fukushima, M., Tsuchiyama, Y., Nakao, T. *et al.* (1995) *Am. J. Kidney Dis.*, **16**, 952–5.)

Figure 40.10 Cystine crystals in the urine. Typical hexagonal configuration. One leukocyte is also present. (Reproduced, with permission, from Birch, D.F., Fairley, K.F., Becker, G.J. and Kicaid-Smith, P. (1994) *A Color Atlas of Urine Microscopy*. Chapman & Hall Medical, London, p. 125.)

drome (see below) with proximal renal tubular acidosis, glucosuria and aminoaciduria. The onset is usually in the first year of life and ESRD occurs by age 10. As cystinosis progresses, other findings appear. These include hypothyroidism, corneal opacities and photophobia, insulin deficiency, signs of central nervous system involvement such as impaired motor skills and cerebral atrophy, and abnormalities of cardiac conduction. The intermediate form has similar manifestations, albeit with a slower progression. In contrast, the benign form is asymptomatic and has no abnormalities, by the light microscope, in the kidney.

Corneal or conjunctival crystals usually suggest the diagnosis which can be confirmed by measuring the cystine content of neutrophils. Histological examination reveals crystal deposition in various tissues. Prenatal diagnosis can be made by cell culture of amniotic fluid. The diagnosis should be considered in infants who present with vomiting, polyuria and dehydration. Diabetes insipidus and other disorders like galactosemia and urinary tract obstruction must be excluded. The young child will usually present with a failure to thrive and Fanconi's syndrome.

Specific therapy with cysteamine bitartrate, cysteamine hydrochloride or phosphocysteamine is effective in lowering the cystine content of leukocytes [29]. The bitartrate formulation is the least unpleasant. Patients treated early and aggressively have better glomerular function and may be able to avoid ESRD, as opposed to those who are untreated or non-compliant. Symptomatic therapy is necessary to prevent dehydration and to correct the consequences of Fanconi's syndrome like bicarbonaturia, phosphaturia and rickets. Hypothyroidism should be looked for periodically and treated promptly. Allograft survival at 10 years is not different from that in patients with non-inherited renal failure. Successful transplantation, however, does not affect cystine accumulation in non-renal tissues and has led to increased awareness of the multisystem manifestations of cystinosis.

Renal glucosuria

Primary renal glucosuria is a benign disorder of glucose reabsorption by the proximal tubule which is sometimes inherited. The condition should be diagnosed correctly to avoid confusion with diabetes mellitus.

Glucose is reabsorbed completely in the proximal tubule by glucose transporters that display saturation (first-order) kinetics. The rate of glucose transport increases linearly, as glucose concentration in the tubule increases, until the transporters are saturated. This point is called the saturation point and defines the maximum rate of glucose transport achieved – 'Tm' (tubular maximum). A further increase in tubular fluid glucose load has no effect on the Tm and glucosuria ensues. Different types of renal glucosuria can be defined by the Tm achieved. Type A has low maximal glucose reabsorption (low Tm). Type B has a normal Tm but some glucosuria may ensue before Tm is reached from one of two mechanisms: a gradual rather than sudden shift in the kinetics of absorption from first-order to zero-order (rate of absorption independent of glucose concentration) or heterogeneity in the nephron population with regard to glucose reabsorbing potential.

The glucosuria is asymptomatic, does not cause renal dysfunction, and does not require treatment. It is distinguished from other causes of glycosuria by the lack of hyperglycemia, a normal glucose tolerance test, and normal renal pathology.

Fanconi's syndrome

Fanconi's syndrome (FS) is a disorder characterized by excessive urinary losses of amino acids, glucose, phosphate, bicarbonate and other solutes. It is a congenital or

Table 40.4   Common causes of Fanconi's syndrome

Congenital or inherited disease
  Cystinosis
  Galactosemia
  Wilson's disease
  Idiopathic

Acquired disease
  Multiple myeloma
  Amyloidosis
  Medullary cystic disease
  Rejecting allograft
  Nephrotic syndrome
  Heavy metals
    lead, mercury, cadmium, bismuth
  Medications
    gentamycin, outdated tetracycline, salicylate
  Chemicals
    toluene, lysol, nitrobenzene

acquired syndrome that reflects a primary disorder of the proximal tubule. The glomerulus is unaffected.

The patient exhibits growth retardation, rickets, osteoporosis, polyuria and dehydration, muscle weakness and cardiac dysrhythmias. Biochemical abnormalities include hypokalemia, low carnitine levels, hypouricemia, generalized aminoaciduria, glycosuria, phosphate wasting with hypophophatemia, type 2 renal tubular acidosis and tubular proteinuria.

Most cases of Fanconi's syndrome are acquired. Table 40.4 lists the common causes of the syndrome. Therapy is directed towards the underlying cause and treatment of biochemical abnormalities. The treatment of acidosis requires large quantities of alkali (2–10 mEq/kg/day) as bicarbonate or citrate. Hypokalemia is corrected with 2–4 mEq/kg/day of potassium citrate, bicarbonate or phosphate. Neutral phosphates in a dose of 1–3 g, oral calcium and dihydroxycholecalciferol supplements (0.25–0.5 µg) are usually necessary. Adequate fluid intake must be assured to prevent dehydration. Patients with acquired FS who progress to renal failure can be dialyzed or even transplanted depending on the underlying disorder.

Hyperoxaluria

Hyperoxaluria may result from excessive absorption of oxalate from the gut or from metabolic overproduction of oxalate (oxalosis). Since the kidney is the only route of elimination of oxalate, ineffective renal clearance also results in accumulation and tissue deposition of oxalate, but not hyperoxaluria.

Enteric hyperoxaluria

The colon appears to be the major site of oxalate absorption. Dietary calcium interferes with oxalate absorption by forming insoluble complexes. Bile salts and fecal fat enhance it; the former probably by increasing permeability of the colonic mucosa to oxalate and the latter by binding calcium and so releasing oxalate for absorption. Short bowel syndromes and intestinal malabsorption states, e.g. Crohn's disease, lead to oxalate hyperabsorption in part by the above mechanisms. The treatment is to reduce the intake of oxalate and fat and to enhance the binding of enteric oxalate with oral calcium carbonate or cholestyramine.

Oxalosis

This term is used for two inherited inborn errors of metabolism that cause metabolic overproduction of oxalate. Both are autosomal recessive disorders. Excess endogenous synthesis also occurs in patients with pyridoxine deficiency, methoxyflurane excess or ethylene glycol poisoning.

Oxalosis is characterized as type I (from a deficiency of hepatic peroxisomal alanine:glyoxylate aminotransferase) or type II (from a lack of D-glyceric acid dehydrogenase). There is an infantile form with early renal failure from nephrocalcinosis, a juvenile form with recurrent stones and deposition of oxalate in the tissue and an adult form which has a more benign course. Oxalosis should be suspected when one finds hyperoxaluria, oxalate stones or nephrocalcinosis, if renal failure does not mask the diagnosis by lowering GFR or causing excess oxalate to be deposited in the tissues. The diagnosis is made by demonstrating the enzyme deficiency in liver biopsy specimens in type I oxalosis, and in peripheral blood leukocytes of type II.

Treatment consists of a high fluid intake, large doses of pyridoxine (250–1000 mg) to reduce oxaluria in type I patients, and phosphates to inhibit calcium oxalate crystal formation in the urine. Dialysis and renal transplantation are appropriate for ESRD, although oxalate deposition may cause recurrent disease in the allograft. Type I oxalosis is best treated by a liver transplant (with or without renal transplant) [30] to correct the primary enzymatic defect.

Congenital nephrogenic diabetes insipidus

Diabetes insipidus (DI) is a tubular disorder characterized by an inability of the kidney to concentrate urine. The ensuing polyuria is profound with excretion of large volumes (greater than 3 l/day) of dilute urine (<250 mosmol/kg H_2O). Vasopressin-sensitive neurogenic DI must be distinguished from the vasopressin-resistant variety. The former arises from a lack of endogenous argi-nine vasopressin (AVP) (central DI); the latter is due to renal insensitivity to the antidiuretic effect of AVP. The latter is also referred to as nephrogenic diabetes insipidus (NDI).

Physiology and genetics of diabetes insipidus

The release of AVP from the posterior pituitary is regulated by the tonicity information relayed by osmoreceptors in the anterior hypothalamus. A precursor of AVP preprovasopressin, and its carrier neurophysin II (NPII), are synthesized as a composite precursor in the supraoptic and paraventricular neurons of the hypothalamus, packaged into granules and axonally transported to the posterior pituitary. The composite precursor is cleaved and modified to form the active hormone during passage. AVP binds to arginine-vasopressin type 2 receptor (V2 receptor) present on the collecting tubule cells. Activation of this receptor promotes the incorporation of water channels (aquaporin-2, AQP2) into the luminal surface of these cells, thereby enhancing their water permeability.

There are three hereditary forms of DI: autosomal dominant central DI, X-linked NDI, and autosomal recessive NDI [31]. Mutations of different genes account for these disorders (Figure 40.11). The failure to manufacture AVP in central DI is due to mutations in the prepro-AVP-NPII gene. Renal resistance to the actions of AVP (nephrogenic DI) is due either to a mutation in the V2 receptor gene (X-linked NDI) or in the AQP2 gene (autosomal recessive NDI). X-linked NDI is fully penetrant in males. Heterozygous females exhibit varying degrees of penetrance (that is, variable polyuria and polydipsia) because of X inactivation. Autosomal recessive NDI can be distinguished clinically from X-linked NDI on the basis of gender, a history of parental consanguinity and normal urinary concentrating ability in the parents.

Clinical features, diagnosis and treatment of nephrogenic diabetes insipidus

Patients present shortly after birth with irritability, poor feeding, febrile episodes and failure to thrive. Untreated or undiagnosed disease invariably results in repeated episodes of dehydration, hypernatremia, hyperthermia and brain damage with mental retardation. Laboratory evaluation reveals hypernatremia, hyperchloremia, metabolic acidosis and prerenal azotemia.

The differential diagnosis is that of polyuria and polydipsia. Table 40.5 lists the common causes of polyuria in children. The diagnosis is established by performing the water deprivation test (Table 40.6). Failure of the urine osmolality to exceed 450 mosmol/kg H_2O, or the urine osmolality to exceed plasma osmolality by a factor of 1.5, after significant dehydration (defined as a loss of 2.5–5% of body weight) suggests the diagnosis. A failure of the

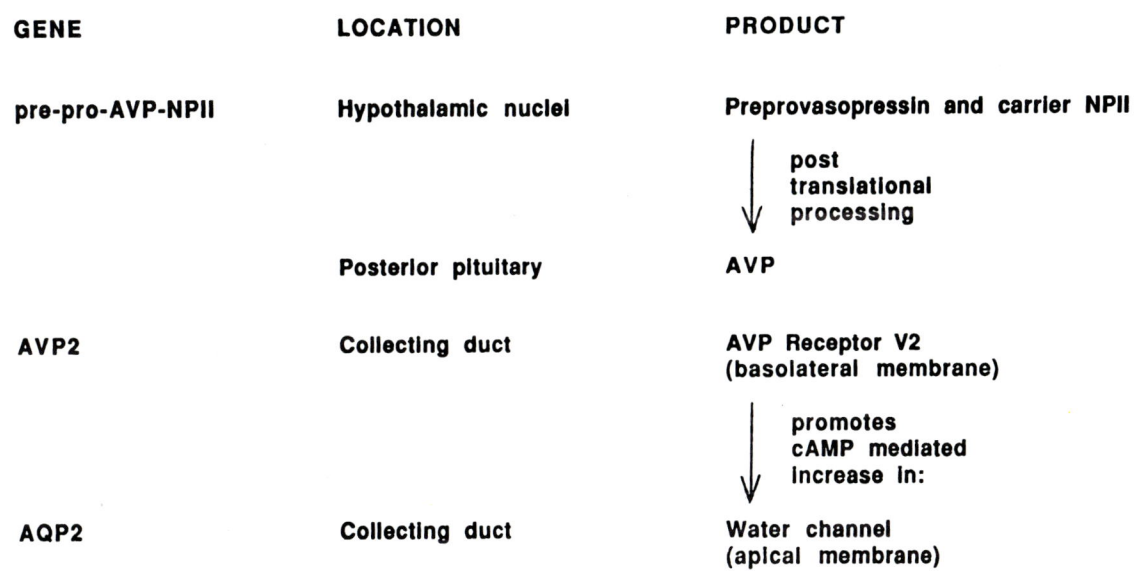

GENE	LOCATION	PRODUCT
pre-pro-AVP-NPII	Hypothalamic nuclei	Preprovasopressin and carrier NPII
		↓ post translational processing
	Posterior pituitary	AVP
AVP2	Collecting duct	AVP Receptor V2 (basolateral membrane)
		↓ promotes cAMP mediated increase in:
AQP2	Collecting duct	Water channel (apical membrane)

Figure 40.11 Genetics and physiology of nephrogenic diabetes insipidus. Central diabetes insipidus results from a failure to manufacture arginine–vasopressin (AVP) precursor due to mutations in the prepro-AVP-NPII gene or from destruction of the posterior hypophysis where AVP is stored. AVP binds to AVP type 2 receptor on the collecting tubule cells. Its activation promotes the incorporation of water channels (aquaporin-2, AQP2) into the luminal surface of these cells. Nephrogenic diabetes insipidus is due to either a mutation in the AVP type 2 receptor gene or in the AQP2 gene. cAMP, cyclic adenosine monophosphate; NPII, neurophysin II.

Table 40.5   Common causes of polyuria in children

Increased fluid intake
  Primary polydipsia
  Hypothalamic polydipsia

Increased osmotic load
  Glucose – diabetes mellitus, total parenteral
    nutrition
  Urea – hypercatabolic states, relief of obstructive
    uropathy
  Mannitol

Central diabetes insipidus – deficiency of AVP
  Idiopathic – congenital
  Neoplastic – leukemia, pituitary tumors,
    histiocytosis X
  Infections – encephalitis, tuberculous meningitis

Nephrogenic diabetes insipidus – tubular
unresponsiveness to AVP
  Inherited – Autosomal recessive, X-linked
  Acquired – obstructive uropathy, hypokalemia,
    hypercalcemia

AVP, arginine–vasopressin.
Adapted from Savage, J.M. and Postlethwaite, R.J. (1994) Symptoms and signs of childhood renal tract disease, in *Clinical Paediatric Nephrology* (ed. R.J. Postlethwaite), Butterworth-Heinemann, Oxford, pp. 75–88.

polyuria to respond to desmopressin (dDAVP) at this point, and of the urine osmolality to rise, confirms the diagnosis.

The treatment is directed to prevent dehydration and reduce urine output. Infants and young children should be given large volumes of fluid throughout day and night. Older children should be offered free access to fluids, since their thirst mechanism is usually adequate. Obligatory fluid losses should be minimized by giving a diet low in salt and with moderate restriction of protein (avoiding malnutrition). Thiazide diuretics and indomethacin, often in combination, are the most effective drugs, but their mechanism of action is not well understood. Hydrochlorthiazide (2–3 mg/kg) induces natriuresis and contraction of extracellular volume. This enhances the proximal tubule absorption of sodium and water and reduces the flow of urine to the vasopressin-resistant collecting tubules, resulting in a fall in urine output. Indomethacin (1–2 mg/kg) may limit water excretion by reducing the elevated levels of prostaglandins seen in NDI, that inhibit sodium and water reabsorption.

Sickle cell disease

Renal involvement in sickle cell anemia (homozygous SS haplotype, HbSS) was first described by Herrick in 1910. Sickle cell disease (SCD) includes patients with several combinations of abnormal hemoglobin (Hb) molecules, including hemoglobin SThal. In sickle cell trait, HbS is

Table 40.6 Water deprivation test for diagnosis of cause of polyuria

Performing the test

Free access to food and water for 3 days.

On the day before the test is to be performed determine the serum sodium concentration. The test should not be conducted if the serum sodium concentration is outside the normal range, which in most laboratories is usually 138–142 mEq/l.

There are two phases to the test:

Phase 1

Fluid and food are withheld after breakfast. The test is performed in a room where there is no source of water available to the patient or there is an observer present.

At the beginning of deprivation, the patient is weighed and the blood pressure and pulse recorded. A specimen of venous blood is obtained for serum AVP levels, osmolality, and sodium concentration; subsequent blood samples are subjected to the same measurements, except that after exogenous AVP is given, serum AVP levels are not measured. The patient is asked to void and urine obtained for specific gravity and osmolality.

Urine flow, osmolality and specific gravity, vital signs and body weight are measured every hour. Blood is obtained every 2 h.

Phase 1 ends when:

(a) The patient has lost ≥2.5% of body weight or serum sodium has risen by ≥4%, which represents a sufficient stimulus for endogenous AVP release.

or

(b) The urine osmolality reaches a plateau (change <30 mosmol/kg water in osmolality or ≤0.001 change in specific gravity). (The specific gravity is a less precise test than the osmolality.)

Phase 2

Administer 5 units AVP subcutaneously (s.c.) or 10 μg desmopressin (dDAVP) s.c. or by nasal insufflation.

Continue the test until urinary osmolality reaches a plateau, or until 14 h have elapsed since the test was began.

Interpretation of the Water Deprivation Test

There are five different patterns of response, each indicating a specific diagnosis.

1. In normal patients, the urine flow declines rapidly. Urine becomes maximally concentrated (≥800 mosmol/kg water) and urine osmolality does not rise after AVP administration, because endogenous AVP levels will rise sufficiently.

2. Patients with nephrogenic DI will lose weight, develop hypernatremia and high AVP levels and will show little or no change in urine flow or osmolality before or after exogenous AVP.

3. Patients with a complete lack of endogenous AVP (central DI) will lose weight and develop hypernatremia, but plasma AVP will be undetectable. Urinary flow may fall somewhat and urine osmolality may rise to ca. 200 mosmol/kg water. When exogenous AVP is given, urine flow will fall rapidly and urine osmolality will rise to ≥550 mosmol/kg water. The urine becomes concentrated because the patient lacks endogenous AVP, but it will not rise as high as normal because the renal medulla, having been subjected to chronic high volume flows, cannot become as concentrated as the normal medulla in a few hours.

4. Patients with a partial lack of endogenous AVP will partially respond to water deprivation (urine osmolality ca. 300–500 mosmol/kg water, detectable AVP in serum) but then respond further after exogenous AVP (urine osmolality ≥600 mosmol/kg water).

5. Patients with primary polydipsia will complain of thirst and make an attempt to obtain water (the test should be conducted with an observer). However, they will respond to water deprivation like normal patients, except that the urine osmolality will not reach normal levels, since the renal medulla has been subjected to chronic high volume flows, but should reach 600 mosmol/kg water. After exogenous AVP there will be no further rise in urine osmolality.

combined with normal Hb. The estimated incidence of renal disease, from mild chronic renal insufficiency to ESRD is 2.8–7%. Patients with HbSS, especially those with the Central African Republic haplotype, have an increased risk of developing renal failure. Well documented changes of medullary function and recent studies on cortical function have extended our understanding of the pathogenesis of nephropathy in sickle cell anemia.

Clinical presentation

Hematuria is a common presenting complaint in patients with SCD. It may be painless, microscopic or gross, and often unilateral and self-limited. When unilateral, the bleeding originates more often from the left kidney. A history of lumbar trauma, respiratory infection or unaccustomed exertion may be obtained. Obstruction of the collecting system may result from blood clots, after gross and protracted hematuria and its treatment with antifibrinolytic agents.

Renal papillary necrosis in patients with SCD may present as hematuria, acute renal failure, sepsis or urinary tract obstruction. The age at diagnosis is usually less than 40 and the prognosis is favorable. Papillary necrosis is not associated with an increased incidence of chronic renal failure [32].

Proteinuria occurs in less than 10% of patients with SCD. In a minority of patients with proteinuria, urinary protein excretion may be in the nephrotic range. Focal and segmental sclerosis in the setting of glomerular hypertrophy is the usual cause. Proteinuria is a strong predictor of ESRD in patients with SCD. Acute glomerulonephritis after human parvovirus B19-induced aplastic crisis is a rare cause of proteinuria in sickle cell patients.

Hypovolemia, sepsis, renal vein thrombosis, rhabdomyolysis, intravascular hemolysis, and ureteric obstruction from papillary necrosis or blood clot may all cause acute renal failure. Chronic renal failure is usually a consequence of glomerulosclerosis. HbSS, ineffective erythropoiesis with worsening anemia, proteinuria, nephrotic syndrome, and hypertension are important predictors of the development of chronic renal failure. Patients with chronic renal failure are at increased risk for cardiovascular complications including strokes. Table 40.7 summarizes the kidney pathology in SCD.

Pathophysiology

The primary abnormalities in renal function are confined to those with SCD, not trait. Effective renal blood flow (ERBF) and glomerular filtration rate (GFR) are increased in young adults with sickle cell anemia and decline thereafter with increasing age. The filtration fraction is reduced because the increase in GFR is less than that of ERBF. Correction of anemia with transfusions does not correct the

Table 40.7   Renal syndromes and diseases associated with sickle cell disease

Syndrome
   Hematuria (often unilateral)
   Hyposthenuria
   Nephrotic syndrome (most often from focal
      segmental sclerosis)
   Renal insufficiency (acute, chronic)

Disease
   Papillary necrosis
   Pyelonephritis
   Glomerulonephritis following parvovirus infection
   Renal infarction

increased ERBF and GFR. Indomethacin causes both to fall, however, suggesting that prostaglandins may mediate this phenomenon. A high urinary prostaglandin E_2/prostaglandin $F_{2\alpha}$ ratio may be responsible for some of these hemodynamic changes [33].

A combination of medullary ischemia and initial hyperfiltration by all nephrons probably leads to enlargement of superficial and juxtamedullary glomeruli. Secondary hemodynamic injury induced by glomerular hyperfiltration and hypertrophy may cause progressive nephron loss from glomerular sclerosis and ultimately chronic renal failure.

Sodium reabsorption is enhanced in the proximal tubule; phosphate reabsorption parallels the sodium reabsorption. Uric acid and creatinine secretion is enhanced. Creatinine clearance may thus overestimate GFR in SCD.

The decrease in the urinary concentrating capacity manifests as enuresis or vasopressin-resistant polyuria, and usually begins early in childhood. The maximal urine osmolality is usually less than 600 mosmol/kg H_2O. The likely cause is the severe anatomic derangement of the vasa recta, breakdown of the countercurrent blood flow and the failure to develop a maximal osmotic gradient in the renal medulla. Hematuria in this setting may be reversed by blood transfusion. The direct consequences of dehydration are sickle cell crises.

Distal urinary acidification is impaired and may manifest as incomplete renal tubular acidosis. A few patients may develop hyporeninemic hypoaldosteronism. Potassium excretion is impaired in patients with SCD. The pathogenesis of abnormalities in potassium excretion remain unclear. Hyperkalemia is rare. Table 40.8 lists the abnormalities in function seen in SCD.

Treatment

Infections, papillary necrosis, bleeding diathesis, vascular malformations, tumors and vasculitides must be first

Table 40.8 Functional renal abnormalities in sickle cell disease

Hemodynamic changes
    Increased glomerular filtration rate
    Increased renal plasma flow
    Decreased filtration fraction

Proximal tubule
    Reabsorption
        Increased sodium reabsorption
        Increased phosphate absorption
        Increased β_2-microglobulin reabsorption
    Secretion
        Increased uric acid secretion
        Increased creatinine secretion

Distal and collecting tubule
    Impaired urinary concentrating ability
    Impaired acidification
    Impaired potassium secretion

ruled out (as in the general population). The treatment of severe hematuria is hydration, alkalinization and blood transfusion. By reducing osmolality and increasing pH in the renal medulla and reducing the concentration of HbSS, one hopes to retard the sickling process in the vasa recta. Bleeding resistant to these measures may be treated with antifibrinolytic agents like ε-aminocaproic acid. This, however, carries the risk of urinary tract obstruction from blood clots. Other measures include high doses of oral urea – sufficient to raise the blood urea nitrogen concentration over 100 mg/dl to prevent irreversible sickling – and intravenous administration of triglycyl vasopressin or vasopressin to reduce renal blood flow. Uninephrectomy should be avoided if at all possible because of the risk of bleeding from the contralateral kidney.

Treatment of proteinuria with angiotensin converting enzyme inhibitors has not been shown to affect the progression of disease although it does reduce the proteinuria.

Outcome

Although the incidence of ESRD in SCD is less than 5%, the median survival of patients after the diagnosis of renal failure is only four years despite dialysis. Long-term survival is limited by an increase in the incidence of extrarenal complications like cerebrovascular accident and chronic restrictive lung disease. Since the number of kidney transplants is few, experience is limited. Graft survival is good although stroke, renal artery stenosis and recurrent painful crises are major post-transplant complications. Patients with HbSS have a much worse outcome, compared to those with HbSC or HbAS.

References

1. Chauveau, D., Knebelmann, B. and Grunfeld, J. (1995) Inherited kidney diseases: polycystic kidney disease and Alport's syndrome. *Adv. Intern. Med.*, **40**, 303–37.
2. The European Polycystic Kidney Disease Consortium (1994) The polycystic kidney disease 1 gene encodes a 14 kb transcript and lies within a duplicated region on chromosome 16. *Cell*, **77**, 881–94.
3. Fick, G.M. and Gabow, P.A. (1994) Hereditary and acquired cystic disease of the kidney. *Kidney Int.*, **46**, 951–64.
4. Torres, V.E., Wilson, D.M., Hattery, R.R. and Segura, J.W. (1993) Renal stone disease in autosomal dominant polycystic kidney disease. *Am. J. Kidney Dis.*, **22**, 513–19.
5. Chapman, A.B., Johnson, A., Gabow, P.A. and Schrier, R.W. (1990) The renin–angiotensin–aldosterone system and autosomal dominant polycystic kidney disease. *N. Engl. J. Med.*, **323**, 1091–6.
6. Everson, G.T. (1993) Hepatic cysts in autosomal dominant polycystic kidney disease. *Am. J. Kidney Dis.*, **22**, 520–5.
7. Telenti, A., Torres, V.E., Gross, J.B. *et al.* (1990) Hepatic cyst infection in autosomal dominant polycystic kidney disease. *Mayo Clin. Proc.*, **65**, 933–42.
8. Chauveau, D., Pirson, Y., Verellen-Dumoulin, C. *et al.* (1993) Intracranial aneurysm in autosomal dominant polycystic kidney disease. *Kidney Int.*, **45**, 1140–6.
9. Levey, A.S., Pauker, S.G. and Kassirer, J.P. (1983) Occult intracranial aneurysms in polycystic kidney disease. When is cerebral arteriography warranted? *N. Engl. J. Med.*, **308**, 986–94.
10. Grantham, J.J. (1994) Pathogenesis for renal cyst expansion: opportunities for therapy. *Am. J. Kidney Dis.*, **23**, 210–18.
11. Welling, L.W. and Grantham, J.J. (1991) Cystic and developmental diseases of the kidney, in *The Kidney* (eds B.M. Brenner and F.C. Rector), W.B. Saunders, Philadelphia, pp. 1657–94.
12. Bear, J.C., McManamon, P., Morgan, J. *et al.* (1984) Age at clinical onset and at ultrasonographic detection of adult polycystic kidney disease: Data for genetic counselling. *Am. J. Med. Genet.*, **18**, 45–53.
13. Bennett, W.M., Elzinga, L., Golper, T.A. and Barry, J. (1986) Reduction of cyst volume for symptomatic management of autosomal dominant polycystic kidney disease. *J. Urol.*, **137**, 620–2.
14. Martinez, J.R. and Grantham, J.J. (1995) Polycystic kidney disease: etiology, pathogenesis, and treatment. *Dis. Mon.*, **41**, 693–765.
15. Yium, J., Gabow, P.A., Johnson, A. *et al.* (1994) Autosomal polycystic kidney disease in blacks: clinical course and effect of sickle-cell hemoglobin. *J. Am. Soc. Nephrol.*, **4**, 1670–4.

16. Klahr, S., Levey, A.S., Beck, G.J. *et al.* (1994) The effects of dietary protein restriction and blood-pressure control on the progression of chronic renal disease. *N. Engl. J. Med.*, **330**, 877–84.

17. Pirson, Y. and Grunfeld, J.P. (1992) Autosomal dominant polycystic kidney disease, in *Oxford Textbook of Nephrology* (eds J.S. Cameron, A.M. Davision, J.P. Grufeld *et al.*), Oxford University Press, Oxford, pp. 2171–88.

18. Fick, G.M., Johnson, A.M., Hammond, W.S. and Gabow, P.A. (1995) Causes of death in autosomal dominant polycystic kidney disease. *J. Am. Soc. Nephrol.*, **5**, 2048–56.

19. Zerres, K., Mucher, G., Bachner, L. *et al.* (1994) Mapping of the gene for autosomal recessive polycystic kidney disease (ARPKD) to chromosome 6p21-cen. *Nature Genet.*, **7**, 429–62.

20. Lendon, M. and Postlethwaite, R.J. (1994) Cystic disorders of the kidney, in *Clinical Paediatric Nephrology* (ed. R.J. Postlethwaite), Butterworth–Heinemann, Oxford, pp. 305–18.

21. Konrad, M., Saunier, L., Heidet, L. *et al.* (1996) Large homozygous deletions of the 2q13 region are a major cause of juvenile nephronopthisis. *Human Mol. Gene.*, **5**, 367–71.

22. Chandhoke, P.S., Torrence, R.J., Clayman, R.V. and Rothstein, M. (1992) Acquired cystic disease: a management dilemma. *J. Urol.*, **147**, 969–74.

23. Antignac, C., Knebelmann, B., Druot, L. *et al.* (1994) Deletions in COL4A5 collagen gene in X-linked Alport's syndrome. *J. Clin. Invest.*, **93**, 1195–207.

24. Hebert, L.A., Betts, J.A., Sedmak, D.D. *et al.* (1996) Loin-pain hematuria syndrome associated with thin glomerular basement membrane disease and hemorrhage into renal tubules. *Kidney Int.*, **49**, 168–73.

25. Nieuwhof, C., Doorenbos, C., Grave, W. *et al.* (1996) A prospective study of the natural history of idiopathic non–proteinuric hematuria. *Kidney Int.*, **49**, 222–5.

26. Calonge, M.J., Volpini, V., Bisceglia, L. *et al.* (1995) Genetic heterogeneity in cystinuria: the SLC3A1 gene is linked to type I but not to type III cystinuria. *Proc. Nat. Acad. Sci. USA*, **92**, 9667–71.

27. Lindell, A., Denneberg, T. and Jeppsson, J.O. (1995) Urinary excretion of free cystine and tiopronin–cysteine–mixed disulfide during long term tiopronin treatment of cystinuria. *Nephron*, **71**, 328–42.

28. The Cystinosis Collaborative Research Group. (1995) Linkage of the gene for cystinosis to markers on the short arm of chromosome 17. *Nature Genet.*, **10**, 246–8.

29. Schneider, J.A., Clark, K.F., Greene, A.A. *et al.* (1995) Recent advances in the treatment of cystinosis. *J. Inher. Metab. Dis.*, **18**, 387–97.

30. Watts, R.W., Morgan, S.H., Danpure, C.J. *et al.* (1991) Combined hepatic and renal transplantation in primary hyperoxaluria type I: clinical report of nine cases. *Am. J. Med.*, **90**, 179–88.

31. Fujiwara, T.M., Morgan, K. and Bichet, D.G. (1995) Molecular biology of diabetes insipidus. *Annu. Rev. Med.*, **46**, 331–43.

32. Powars, D.R., Elliot-Mills, D.D., Chan, L. *et al.* (1991) Chronic renal failure in sickle cell disease: risk factors, clinical course, and mortality. *Ann. Intern. Med.*, **115**, 614–20.

33. de Jong, P.E. and Statius van Eps, L.W. (1985) Sickle cell nephropathy: new insights into pathophysiology. *Kidney Int.*, **27**, 711–17.

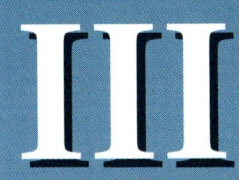

Diseases of the Kidney and their Treatment

Section 2
Diseases of the Kidney in Pregnancy

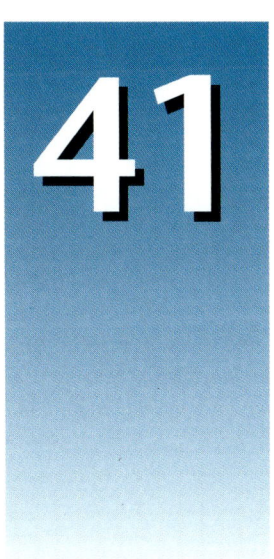

Diseases of the kidney in pregnancy

Mark Roberts, Chris Baylis and John M. Davison

Introduction

Renal tract disorders are one of the most frequent non-obstetric problems in pregnancy. Some relate to pre-existing renal disease, others arise *de novo* but may occur more commonly in pregnancy because of alterations in the renal tract and others are specific to pregnancy, often associated with pre-eclampsia (PE) (pregnancy-induced hypertension). The number of women with pre-existing renal disease that achieve a pregnancy has increased and relates to advances in medical care with improvements in their health, fertility and life expectancy. Familiarity with the renal tract alterations of pregnancy, in particular changes in physiology and pregnancy 'norms' for use in renal assessment, is essential for the diagnosis and appropriate management of renal disorders in pregnancy.

Renal tract alterations in normal pregnancy

The changes in structure and function in the renal tract are predominant among many other adaptations during pregnancy and seem to be non-reproducible by any other means.

Anatomical changes

Kidney length and volume increase by 15 and 70%, respectively, in normal pregnancy. There is no increment in the number of functioning nephrons. Ureteric dilatation, with or without pelvicalyceal dilatation, is usually apparent in the first trimester and both are present in 90% of women by term, persisting well into the puerperium (Figure 41.1). Non-pregnant standards for radiographic and ultrasound examinations cannot, therefore, be applied and postnatal assessments should be postponed until at least four months after delivery.

The cause of ureteric dilatation in pregnancy has not been resolved but it is not merely ureteric atony since ureteric tone actually increases with preservation of contraction frequency and amplitude. Local obstruction due to compression by the pregnant uterus or hypertrophied ovarian vessels could explain why dilatation stops at the pelvic brim and is often unilateral, usually right-sided. This would not explain why dilatation sometimes occurs in the first trimester when the uterus and ovarian vessels are small [1].

Alterations in renal hemodynamics and clinical implications

The gestational alterations in systemic hemodynamics are reviewed in Table 41.1. Cardiac output increases by 33% by the end of the first trimester and is maintained until term, facilitated by decreased cardiac afterload due to decreased peripheral resistance. Awareness of the normal mid-pregnancy reduction in diastolic blood pressure, which corresponds to changes in vascular tone, is neces-

Nephrology, Edited by Rex L. Jamison and Robert Wilkinson.
Published in 1997 by Chapman & Hall, London. ISBN 0 412 60930 4

sary for the diagnosis and management of hypertension in pregnancy. There is enhanced blood flow to many organs, including the kidneys, uterus and mammary glands; however, these changes are selective and blood flows to organs such as the brain and liver are unchanged [2].

Renal hemodynamics in human pregnancy

By the end of the first trimester renal plasma flow (RPF) has increased by 70–80% and is maintained until the end of the second trimester (28 weeks), thereafter decreasing slightly towards term. Glomerular filtration rate (GFR) also increases, reaching a plateau 50% greater than non-pregnant values by the end of the first trimester but, unlike RPF, is maintained until at least 36 weeks' gesta-

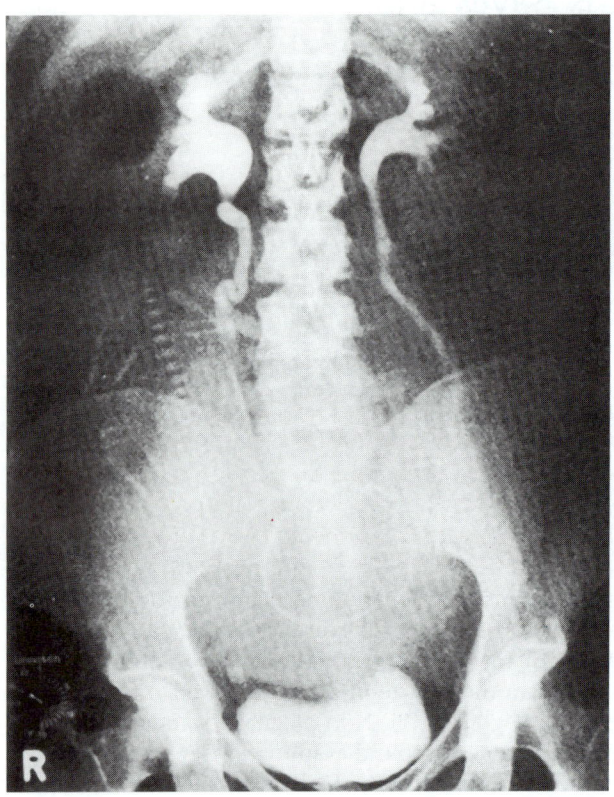

Figure 41.1   An intravenous urogram taken during pregnancy in a woman with spontaneous ureteric dilation, greatest on the right.

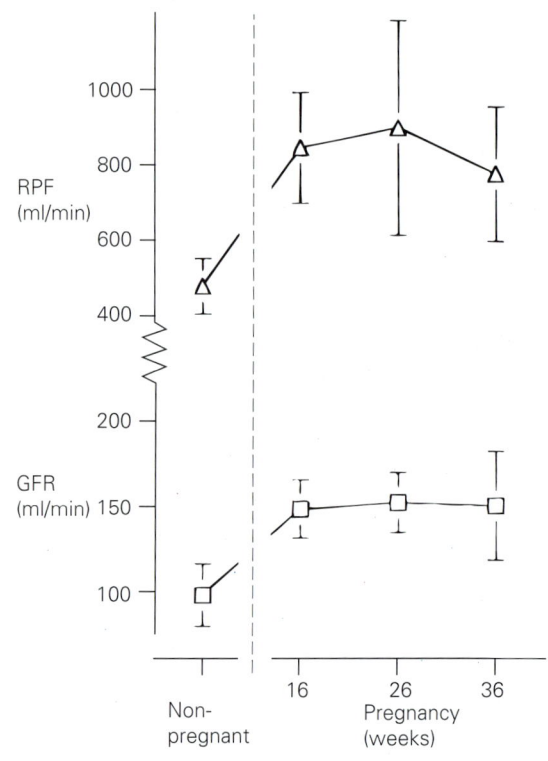

Figure 41.2   Relative changes in RPF and GFR in normal pregnancy (mean ± 1 SD). (Modified from ref. [3].)

Table 41.1   Systemic changes in pregnancy (modified from ref. [2])

		Non-pregnant	1st trimester	2nd trimester	3rd trimester
Cardiac output	(l/min)	4.5	6.0	6.0	6.0
Heart rate	(beats/min)	70	85	85	85
Stroke volume	(ml)	64	71	71	71
Total peripheral resistance	(dyn/s cm⁵)	1700	980	1010	1250
Blood pressure					
Systolic	(mmHg)	115	115	115	115
Diastolic	(mmHg)	70	55	60	70
Plasma volume	(l)	2.6	2.7	3.6	3.8

tion (Figure 41.2). During the last few weeks of pregnancy the 24 h creatinine clearance (see below) decreases towards non-pregnant values. These gestational changes are evident before the fetoplacental unit is fully developed and can be demonstrated in pseudopregnant rats, indicating that some maternal (humoral) factor is involved. Similar changes are evident in pregnant renal transplant recipients where the kidney, although partially renervated, is ectopic, receives an anomalous blood supply, is already hyperfiltering and may have come from a male donor [1]. In non-pregnant subjects comparable, physiologically mediated sustained increments in GFR do not occur.

Measurement of renal hemodynamics in animal models

Renal micropuncture measurements in rats have shown that both pre- and postglomerular arteriolar resistance vessels dilate in normal pregnancy which, as discussed in Chapter 2, increase GFR due to a selective rise in RPF without a change in glomerular blood pressure. Micropuncture studies also indicate that the glomerular ultrafiltration coefficient (K_f; the product of glomerular water

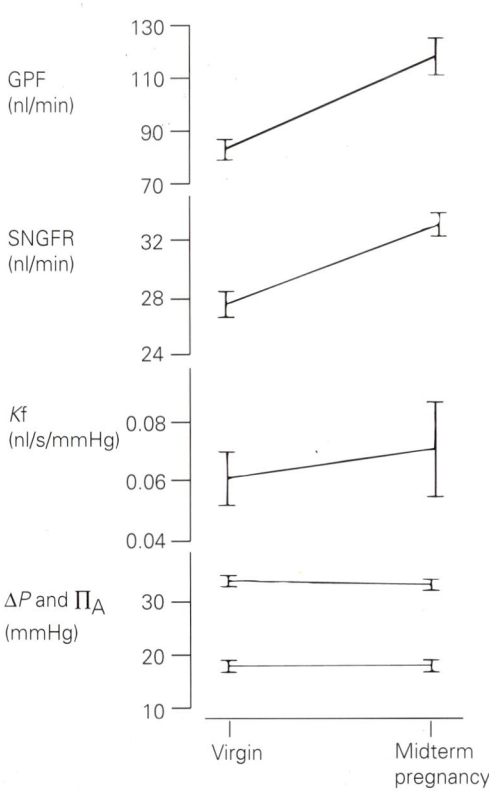

Figure 41.3 Changes in renal hemodynamics in rat pregnancy. GPF, glomerular plasma flow; SNGFR, single nephron GFR; K_f, ultrafiltration coefficient; ΔP, transglomerular hydrostatic pressure difference; Π_A, afferent glomerular oncotic pressure. (Adapted from ref. [4].)

permeability and filtration surface area) is not altered by pregnancy. Thus, the gestational rise in GFR is exclusively due to an increased RPF (Figure 41.3). The mechanism of the renal vasodilatation of pregnancy is still unknown although in recent years a possible role for the potent vasodilator nitric oxide has been suggested [5, 26]. Chronic renal vasodilatation has been associated with progressive glomerular injury in both animal models and humans; however, this is primarily due to selective preglomerular arteriolar dilatation which causes intraglomerular hypertension leading to glomerular sclerosis [5]. Gestational renal vasodilatation associated with recurrent pregnancies in both animals and women who have normal renal function is not associated with damage, probably because there is no change in glomerular blood pressure [1].

Assessment of renal function in pregnancy

Endogenous creatinine clearance, often used as an estimate of GFR, increases in pregnancy. The reliability of this measurement in non-pregnant subjects is hampered by collection errors and tubular secretion of creatinine, which may alter with renal impairment. In pregnancy the endogenous creatinine clearance may be additionally affected by the effects of ureteric dilatation and further increases in tubular secretion of creatinine. Inulin clearance is a safe and reliable alternative in pregnancy but its measurement is time consuming and errors due to supine hypotension and ureteric dilatation may still occur. Serum levels of creatinine, urea and urate decrease progressively throughout pregnancy (Table 41.2) and partly relate to changes in GFR. Despite limitations, creatinine clearance and serum creatinine values provide a useful measurement of the GFR response to pregnancy. Familiarity with the normal changes in serum chemistry due to changes in renal function is essential, if renal problems in pregnancy are to be properly diagnosed and managed [1].

Alterations in tubular function

Even allowing for small decrements of many plasma constituents in pregnancy, their tubular load still increases due to the large increase in GFR. In many instances this leads to parallel increases in tubular reabsorption to prevent excessive solute losses and, in the case of sodium, pregnancy actually results in net sodium retention.

Renal handling of glucose

In pregnancy glycosuria is normal and only rarely is it associated with abnormal carbohydrate metabolism. Both increases in the filtered load of glucose and a reduced tubular reabsorptive capacity contribute to the glycosuria. Studies in the rat suggest that the pregnancy-related reduction in tubular reabsorption occurs downstream

	Urea (mmol/l (BUN mg%))	Urate (mmol/l (mg%))	Creatinine (μmol/l (mg%))	Creatinine clearance (ml/min)
Non-pregnant	4.3 (12.0)	0.22 (3.7)	73 (0.82)	98
12 weeks	3.5 (9.8)	0.17 (2.9)	65 (0.73)	149
24 weeks	3.3 (9.2)	0.18 (3.0)	51 (0.58)	155
36 weeks	3.1 (8.7)	0.20 (3.4)	47 (0.53)	135
Term	3.6 (10.1)		58 (0.66)	122

Table 41.2 Mean values for serum creatinine, urea and creatine clearance in normal pregnancy

from the proximal tubule [1, 6]. Gestational glycosuria is often intermittent, unrelated to changes in plasma levels, pointing to the involvement of multiple factors.

Renal handling of urate

In non-pregnant women only a small proportion of filtered urate (~10%) is excreted and the final urinary excretion rate is a balance between tubular reabsorption and active secretion. Urate reabsorption decreases in early pregnancy, hence increasing excretion and lowering plasma levels. Urate levels increase again towards non-pregnant values near term (Table 41.2). Serum urate levels are higher in pregnancies complicated by PE or fetal growth retardation and serial measurements can be a useful predictive marker (see Hypertension in pregnancy).

Renal handling of protein

Total urinary protein excretion (TPE) increases progressively throughout pregnancy, attaining an upper limit at term of 300 mg/24 h (Figure 41.4). Many factors are involved, including increased filtration, altered glomerular permselectivity and changes in tubular function. Proteins which arise from the distal nephron (Tamm–Horsfall protein) are also present in significant quantities along with immunoglobulins and immunoglobulin light chains. A small proportion of TPE is due to albumin (Figure 41.4). Enhanced albumin excretion has been proposed as an early predictor of PE but specificity is lacking and pregnancy norms are not agreed upon, especially near term where changes may be related to the onset of labor and/or a subclinical phase of PE.

Regulation of acid–base ratio

The increased food intake and metabolism of pregnancy probably lead to an increased acid production. Pregnant women normally hyperventilate, however, the effect of which is to cause a relative arterial alkalosis (mean pH ~ 7.44 versus 7.40 in non-pregnant women). Plasma bicarbonate levels also decrease so that values of 18–22 mmol/l are normal. These changes need to be taken into account when assessing acid–base status.

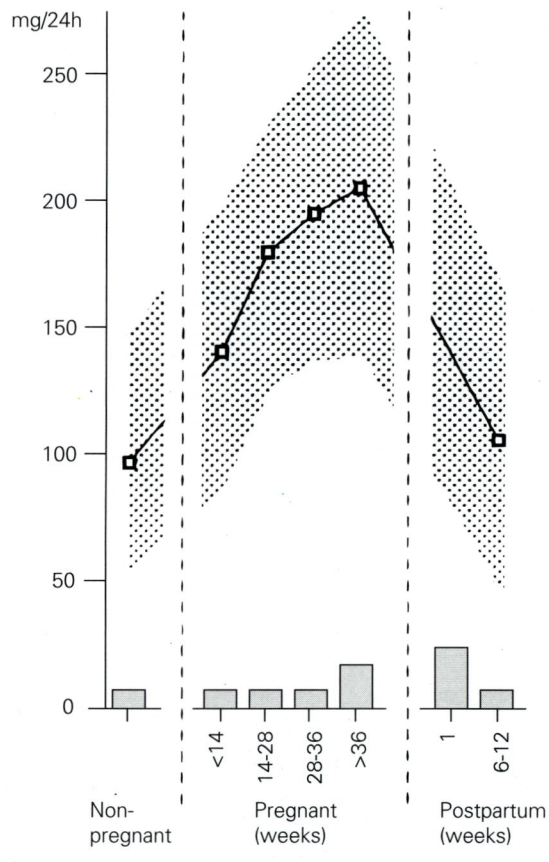

Figure 41.4 Changes in total urinary protein excretion (mean ± 1 SD, ⊡, shaded area) and urinary albumin excretion (median, □) in normal pregnancy. (Data extracted from refs. [7–10] and unpublished personal data.)

Renal handling of potassium

Serum potassium levels are reduced in pregnancy. Despite the relatively alkaline urine and increased mineralocorticoid activity (particularly aldosterone), expected to enhance potassium excretion, there is, in fact, a gradual increase in total body potassium taken up into fetal tissues and increased maternal mass. The antikaliuretic effect of progesterone is likely to cause the potassium conservation of pregnancy [1].

Osmoregulation

In pregnancy there is a decrease in plasma osmolality, reaching a baseline 8–10 mosmol/kg H_2O lower than non-pregnant values by the end of the first trimester (Figure 41.5) and remaining at this level until term. This decrement is due to water retention resulting in decreased plasma sodium and its attendant anions, with small contributions from other solutes (e.g. urea). Basal arginine vasopressin (AVP) levels are unaltered. The mechanisms underlying this resetting of osmotic thresholds for both thirst and AVP release (Figure 41.6) are unknown, although it is notable that exogenous human chorionic gonadotrophin (HCG) causes a reduction in plasma osmolality in non-pregnant subjects. Metabolic clearance of AVP is also increased. The latter may explain why some women with diabetes insipidus require more AVP in pregnancy.

Renal handling of sodium

There is retention of approximately 950 mEq of sodium by term in the products of conception and the expanded maternal extracellular space. Micropuncture studies in rats (who also show a marked renal sodium retention in the second part of pregnancy) suggest that increases in sodium reabsorption occur in the proximal tubule, loop of Henle and distal nephron [6]. The mechanism of this renal sodium retention is not known and is likely to be complex. As summarized in Table 41.3, sodium retention is due to the net effect of many natriuretic and antinatriuretic pregnancy adaptations. Recent interest has focused on the role of atrial natriuretic peptide (ANP), plasma levels of which are reported by some authors to increase in pregnancy, whereas others suggest a decrease; these disagreements may relate to methodological difficulties when measuring ANP in pregnancy [13]. Interestingly, recent studies have shown that pregnant rats become ·refractory to the tubular, natriuretic actions of ANP [14], but this is not the case for pregnant women [13].

Volume homeostasis

On average a healthy woman gains 12 kg in weight, most of it in the second half of pregnancy, including 6-71 of extracellular fluid taken up in interstitial fluid, plasma volume and products of conception. Red cell mass increases more gradually and to a lesser extent than plasma volume; thus hematocrit and hemoglobin con-

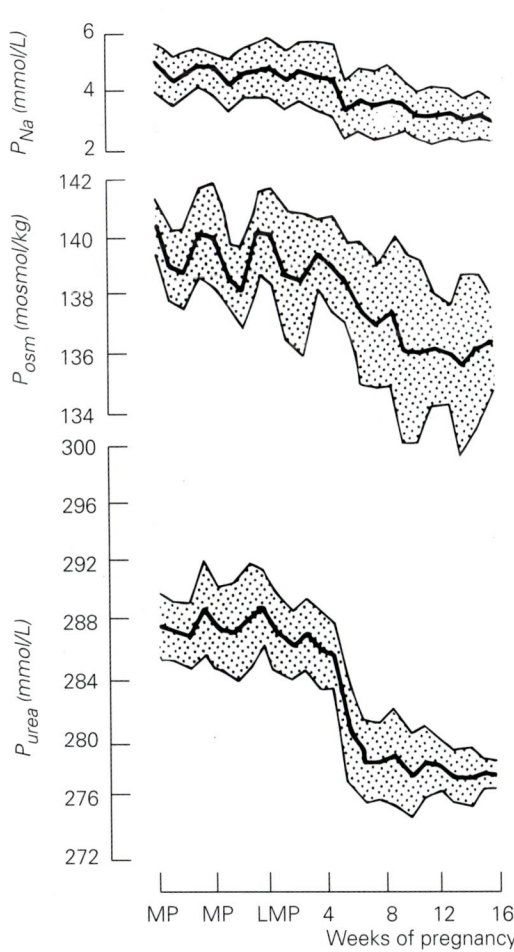

Figure 41.5 Mean values (±SD) for plasma urea (P_{urea}), sodium (P_{Na}) and osmolality (P_{osm}) measured at weekly intervals from before conception to the first trimester in nine women with successful obstetric outcome. MP, menstrual period; LMP, last menstrual period. (Reproduced, with permission, from ref. [11].)

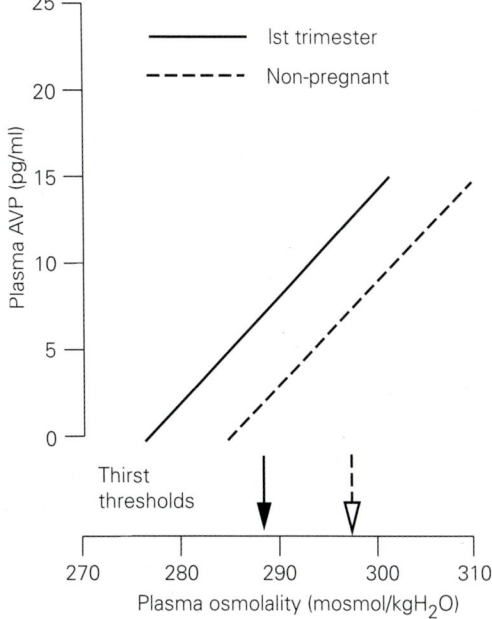

Figure 41.6 Relationship between plasma osmolality and AVP levels in pregnant and non-pregnant women. (Extracted from data supplied in ref. [12].)

Table 41.3   Sodium (Na) metabolism in pregnancy

	Natriuretic adaptations	Antinatriuretic adaptations
• Physical		Placental 'shunting' Exaggerated response to changes in posture
• Hemodynamic	Increased GFR (increased tubular load of Na)	Peripheral vasodilation (decreased 'effective' plasma volume)
• Hormonal	Increased progesterone (antagonism of mineralocorticoids)	Increased aldosterone (increased distal nephron reabsorption of Na) Increased renal deoxycorticosterone (mineralocorticoid effect) Increased plasma renin activity (stimulation of renin–angiotensin system) Increased estrogens (increased hepatic derived renin substrate)
	[a]Increased circulating and renal prostaglandins (vasodilation) *Increased neurophysins and melanocyte stimulating hormone*	*Increased circulating and renal prostaglandins (stimulation of renin release)* *Increased prolactin, corticotropic hormone, cortisol, growth hormone and placental lactogen*
• *Miscellaneous*	*Increased Na pump inhibition* *Decreased peritubular oncotic pressure*	*Increased net Na pump activity*

[a] Entries in italics refer to adaptations which have an uncertain role in Na metabolism.

centrations decrease (Figure 41.7). Plasma albumin concentration also decreases, making it difficult to interpret the activity of protein-bound drugs such as anticonvulsants or the levels of electrolytes such as calcium. Plasma levels of some carrier proteins actually increase (e.g. thyroid-binding globulin).

The mechanisms underlying these changes remain obscure. It appears that volume sensing and control systems recognize the expanded volume as normal or even contracted. This may be partly due to peripheral vasodilatation and blood pooling, giving the impression that despite increased intravascular volume, the 'effective' blood volume stays the same or even decreases. It is unlikely, however, that this is the primary event in volume adaptation as central volume expansion by water immersion has no effect on plasma osmolality or osmotic thresholds in pregnancy. The development of the physiological arteriovenous fistula, i.e. the placental circulation, may play a role in volume expansion as an arteriovenous fistula in non-pregnant subjects is associated with sodium and water retention. It is also of interest that increments in plasma volume are reduced in pregnancies complicated by PE or fetal growth retardation and may reflect diminished pregnancy adaptation(s) due to compromised placentation.

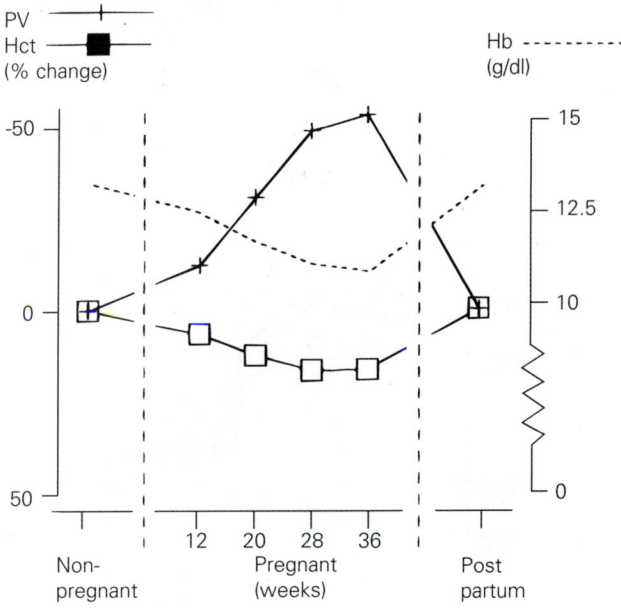

Figure 41.7   Serial measurement of mean hemoglobin (Hb) (g/dl), mean plasma volume and mean hematocrit (PV, Hct, % change) during normal pregnancy (*n* = 70). (Unpublished data, personal communication from Dr P.G. Whittaker, Newcastle upon Tyne, UK.)

Renal problems arising in pregnancy

Of the many renal problems that could arise *de novo* in pregnancy there are several which commonly occur. Some relate to anatomical changes in the urinary tract, particularly ureteric dilatation, and others are due to factors related to specific pregnancy disorders. Cystitis and upper tract infections, both acute and chronic, represent the commonest renal tract problems, occurring in up to 4% of pregnancies. Renal colic secondary to acute passage of a stone is the most frequent non-obstetric reason for an acute hospital admission in pregnancy. In developed countries the incidence of acute renal failure (ARF) associated with pregnancy complications has been dramatically reduced but it remains a relatively common problem in the Third World.

Urinary tract infections

Urinary tract infections are common in both pregnant and non-pregnant women. Susceptibility relates to basic immunological differences, structural/functional abnormalities and socioeconomic factors and may be further increased in pregnancy due to ureteropelvic dilatation, increased urinary nutrient content (glucose and amino acids) and altered immunity [15].

Since diagnosis is difficult because normal pregnancy symptoms include urinary frequency, dysuria, nocturia

and urgency, it must be based on laboratory evidence. A standard definition of infection is a colony count greater than 100 000 bacteria per ml of urine, although counts as low as 20 000 may represent active infection in pregnancy. Urinary white cell count tends to increase in pregnancy such that moderate pyuria may be normal. *Escherichia coli* is the predominant infecting organism (75–90% of cases); *Klebsiella*, *Proteus* and *Enterobacter* account for most of the remainder.

Asymptomatic bacteriuria

In pregnancy, 5% of women will have a covert urinary infection, 30% of whom will develop a symptomatic infection if untreated. Urinary infection confers an increased risk of pregnancy complications, including premature labor, fetal growth retardation and PE [16]. Most obstetricians advocate routine screening at antenatal booking, with additional screening (monthly) in women with a past history of urinary infections and/or renal disorders, a policy that would predict 70% of those destined to have symptomatic infections. Treatment should be governed by organism sensitivity and continued for at least 7–10 days for initial infections and 21 days for recurrences (some of the factors influencing choice of antibiotics are listed in Table 41.4). Regardless of the antimicrobial used or duration of treatment, 30% of women will relapse. Some authorities advocate prophylactic therapy following reinfections.

There is no evidence that asymptomatic infections cause permanent renal damage in adults with normal urinary tracts. Radiological abnormalities of the urinary tract are present in 20% of pregnant women with asymptomatic bacteriuria, although the association in some is incidental. A postpartum intravenous urogram (IVU) should be undertaken in women who fulfil certain criteria (Table 41.5), the aim being to identify abnormalities that require further management (e.g. chronic urinary tract obstruction).

Cystitis

Acute cystitis occurs in 2% of pregnancies, often in women who initially had negative screening in early

Table 41.4 Use of antibiotics in pregnancy

Antibiotic	Comments
Cephalosporins and penicillins	Safety and efficacy well established. Dose may need to be increased due to increased clearance.
Trimethoprim	Theoretical teratogenic risk in first trimester.
Nitrofurantoin	Once daily treatment makes it useful for prophylactic treatment. Risk of neonatal hemolysis if used within 2 weeks of delivery.
Aminoglycosides	Risk of auditory or vestibular nerve damage in fetus. Risk is small with gentamycin and tobramycin if plasma levels are monitored.
Quinolones (nalidixic acid, ciprofloxacin)	Associated with arthropathy in animal studies.

Table 41.5 Criteria indicating the need for an intravenous urogram 4 months postpartum

1. Asymptomatic bacteriuria in pregnancy
   and
2. Difficulty in eradicating the infection
   or episode(s) of symptomatic infection
   or symptomatic infections prior to pregnancy
   or recurrent infection(s) postpartum

pregnancy. It probably has a different pathogenesis than asymptomatic bacteriuria or acute pyelonephritis. Infection may be introduced by bladder catheterization, a procedure commonly employed on labor wards and following caesarean section. Treatment reduces the risk of ascending infections.

Acute pyelonephritis

Ureteric dilatation may increase susceptibility to pyelonephritis in pregnancy; despite routine screening it still complicates 1% of pregnancies (3% in unscreened populations). High fever (often fluctuating), vomiting, rigors and severe loin pain are common findings, but may be absent in the early stages. Diagnosis should be supported by urine microscopy and culture. Severe infections can have serious sequelae, including septic shock, adult respiratory distress syndrome and perinephric abscess formation.

The differential diagnosis in pregnancy is similar to that in non-pregnant subjects but, in addition, loin pain may be due to an acute hydroureter/hydronephrosis or it may be referred from the lumbosacral vertebra or sacroiliac joints (due to increased lumbar lordosis and softening of pelvic ligaments). Abdominal pain may be due to abruptio placentae, degenerating fibroids, chorioamnionitis or appendicitis, the latter presenting atypically in late pregnancy when the uterus is maximally enlarged.

Treatment should be aggressive and undertaken in hospital. Fluid and electrolyte balance should be monitored and intravenous fluids given to correct hypovolemia. Fetal tachycardia is common, making fetal heart monitoring difficult to interpret. There is a risk of premature labor, although prevention by treatment with beta sympathomimetics may exacerbate endotoxin-induced cardiovascular effects and increase the risk of respiratory complications. A penicillin or cephalosporin should be administered intravenously pending confirmation of organism sensitivity and oral therapy continued for two weeks. Failure to respond to treatment may indicate an underlying pelvi-ureteric or ureteric obstruction or the presence of calculi and warrants further investigation.

If Gram-negative sepsis is suspected, blood cultures should be taken and an aminoglycoside (gentamycin or tobramycin) added to the regime, although the new penicillins (e.g. piperacillin) appear to be equally effective with reduced risk to the fetus. Blood levels of an aminoglycoside should be monitored, since its clearance is altered in pregnancy.

Hydroureter/hydronephrosis

Ureteropelvic dilatation is common in pregnancy and may cause loin pain. Urine microscopy demonstrates few or no red cells, repeat urine cultures are negative and the diagnosis is confirmed by ultrasound. Positioning the patient in the knee–chest position may relieve discomfort and promote spontaneous drainage. Rarely is ureteric catheterization (stenting) or nephrostomy necessary to preserve renal function, unless there is a solitary kidney.

Table 41.6 Investigation of renal calculi in pregnancy

Laboratory investigation	Urine culture
	Urinalysis (protein, red and white cells and casts)
	Plasma urea and creatinine
	24 h creatinine clearance and protein excretion
	Analysis of any stones passed
Ultrasound (US)	Diagnosis and progress
Radiography (with uterine shielding)	Plain abdominal film (if warranted following US)
	IVU (limited exposure) only indicated if:
	Unresponsive to conservative therapy
	Declining renal function (especially in a solitary kidney)
	Severe pyelonephritis refractory to antibiotics
Future development	Magnetic resonance imaging

Hematuria

Spontaneous rupture of renal parenchyma, renal pelves or even a renal artery aneurysm are rare but may be more common in pregnancy, secondary to vascular or anatomical alterations.

Urolithiasis (renal tract calculi)

Although factors associated with renal stone formation are known to increase in pregnancy, namely, urinary stasis, ascending infections and excretion of stone-forming salts (e.g. calcium, urate and cystine), the incidence of renal calculi is low (1 in 2000 pregnancies). Furthermore, pregnancy does not appear to increase symptomatic calculi in known 'stone formers'. Enhanced excretion of inhibitors of calcium stone formation such as magnesium, citrate and nephrocalcin as well as increased alkalinity of the urine may afford some protection.

The presentation of renal calculi is similar to that in non-pregnant subjects. Most ureteric colic occurs in the second or third trimester when ureteric dilatation is greatest and perhaps previously asymptomatic stones pass into the ureter, only to become stuck at the pelvic brim. The mainstay of diagnosis of calculi is ultrasound. Interpretation of findings and visualization of the ureter can be difficult but may be enhanced with color flow Doppler scanning [17]. Radiological examination is undesirable because of potential effects on the fetus, although limited exposure may be warranted. Renal function should be assessed and infection excluded but any in-depth analysis of urine and plasma biochemistry to determine the cause of stone formation should be delayed until four months post-delivery when non-pregnant 'norms' can be applied (Table 41.6). Conservative management is usually successful or delivery can be effected before undertaking surgical or minimally invasive intervention (Table 41.7). Any definitive surgery should be delayed until at least four months post-delivery. The safety of lithotripsy has not been validated in pregnancy. Drugs used to treat 'stone formers' (thiazides, xanthine oxidase inhibitors, D-penicillamine) are best avoided.

Acute obstetric renal failure

Complications of pregnancy used to be a common cause of ARF but are now rate, except in Third World countries. Improved obstetric management, particularly of PE and acute hemorrhage, as well as liberalization of abortion laws, preventing the need for illegal procedures which may lead to sepsis, have dramatically reduced the incidence of ARF. Most cases are now related to PE and its complications, although any cause of ARF may arise in pregnancy (Table 41.8).

Management

In most cases, ARF is due to acute tubular necrosis but a higher proportion are due to renal cortical necrosis than

Table 41.7 Management of renal calculi in pregnancy

Conservative management	Hydration (ensuring a diuresis of >2 l/day)
	Analgesia (paracetamol, opiates)
	Diet (avoiding excess calcium)
	Treatment of infections (with follow-up prophylaxis if indicated)
Interventive management	Considered when obstruction is associated with:
	Worsening renal function
	A solitary kidney
	Persistent pyelonephritis
	Threatened premature labor
	Intractable pain
	Cystoscopy (ureteric stent or removal of stone)
	Nephrostomy
	Epidural analgesia
	Removal of stone(s) by open surgery
Follow–up at 4 months post-delivery	Routine investigation dictated by clinical findings

Table 41.8 Causes of acute renal failure (ARF) in pregnancy

Volume contraction/hypotension (± coagulopathy)	Antepartum hemorrhage (placenta previa, abruptio placentae, abortion)
	Postpartum hemorrhage
	Pre-eclampsia/eclampsia
	Amniotic fluid embolism
	Prolonged intrauterine death
	Acute fatty liver of pregnancy
	Idiopathic postpartum failure (hemolytic uremic syndrome)
	Hyperemesis gravidarum
	Adrenocortical failure (Sheehan's syndrome, failure to augment or prescribe maintenance steroids in labour)
Iatrogenic	Treatment for obstetric complications (transfusion and drug reactions)
Urinary tract obstruction	Damage to ureters (caesarean section or repair of genital tract injuries)
	Pelvic/broad ligament hematomas
	Pregnancy related hydroureter (rare cause unless in a solitary kidney)
Infection	Septic abortion
	Chorioamnionitis
	Pyelonephritis
	Puerperal sepsis
Acute-on-chronic renal disease	Exacerbation underlying renal disease
Incidental causes	Almost any cause of ARF may also occur in pregnancy

in non-pregnant subjects. Nevertheless, when ARF is associated with pregnancy-specific conditions such as PE and the hemolysis, elevated liver enzymes and low platelet (HELLP) syndrome (see below), spontaneous recovery can be surprisingly rapid following delivery.

Invariably pregnancy has advanced far enough for the fetus to be viable and co-ordination with the neonatal team allows optimal timing of delivery. In the obstetric setting, however, the current pregnancy may represent the best chance of perinatal success so, with the exclusion of PE, many would advocate early and frequent dialysis to prolong the pregnancy [18] (see below).

Pre-eclampsia (see hypertension in pregnancy)

This is a common condition, characterized by generalized vasoconstriction and often associated with minor renal dysfunction. ARF is rare unless PE is associated with other complications such as HELLP syndrome or abruptio placentae.

Uterine sepsis and pyelonephritis

Serious postpartum and postabortion sepsis is now rare. Improved supportive therapy and evacuation of retained products of conception usually prevent serious sequelae. Clostridial infection can rapidly supervene, resulting in ARF, hemolysis, coagulopathy and hypocalcemia,

although death is usually due to overwhelming sepsis rather than renal failure. Surgical removal of the uterus is often recommended but some prefer conservative management, stating that complications make surgery too risky.

Acute primary pyelonephritis is rarely associated with renal dysfunction or ARF in non-pregnant women. In pregnancy, however, decrements in creatinine clearance are common and the risk of ARF appears to be greater, perhaps due to increased sensitivity of renal vasculature to bacterial endotoxins.

Acute fatty liver of pregnancy

This condition occurs in late pregnancy or early puerperium and is associated with severe hepatic dysfunction and coagulopathy. Renal dysfunction may be mild, although ARF is not uncommon. Despite its rarity, awareness of acute fatty liver of pregnancy is essential as its initial presentation may be subtle (nausea, vomiting, mild jaundice) or complicated by other conditions such as PE, in which case there may be rapid progress to severe maternal and fetal compromise. Mortality rates for both mother and baby have been quoted at greater than 70%, although nowadays earlier recognition has led to earlier intervention that has reduced mortality rates to less than 20%. Other causes of hepatic dysfunction must be excluded and delivery effected immediately, followed by maximal supportive care.

Idiopathic postpartum renal failure

Idiopathic postpartum renal failure is rare but it is a recognized cause of ARF in the first few weeks after delivery. Its etiology is obscure but there are histological similarities with hemolytic uremic syndrome and malignant nephrosclerosis. The outcome of this condition is poor: few women make a complete recovery.

Hypertension in pregnancy

Hypertension complicates about 20% of pregnancies, has considerable impact on perinatal outcome and remains a major cause of maternal morbidity and mortality [19].

Classification

There are two main categories of hypertension in pregnancy – pre-eclampsia and chronic hypertension.

Pre-eclampsia (pregnancy-induced hypertension)

In this category women are usually normotensive before pregnancy and until 20 weeks' gestation, developing hypertension in late pregnancy (+/–proteinuria) which remits shortly after delivery. Different names have been proposed, the commonest being 'pre-eclampsia' (PE) and 'pregnancy-induced hypertension' (PIH). Some prefer to reserve PE for women with severe proteinuric hypertension in whom the term pre-eclampsia more accurately describes and highlights the adverse prognostic significance of proteinuria.

A further term, 'transient hypertension', has been proposed for non-proteinuric hypertension without features of PE [20]. The outcome of pregnancy is normally good but there is an increased risk of maternal hypertension in the years following pregnancy. Transient hypertension may actually represent covert chronic hypertension that is simply 'unmasked' by pregnancy. It is a diagnosis that can only be made reliably in retrospect of the pregnancy as severe complications, including eclampsia, still occur in non-proteinuric hypertensive pregnancy [21].

To avoid confusion the term PE will be used to describe all pregnancy-specific hypertensive disorders, although the reader should be aware that these terms mean different things to different people.

Chronic hypertension

This category includes women, often multiparous, with conditions that predate pregnancy. Hypertension is usually present in early pregnancy and if not previously noted should raise the suspicion of a chronic disorder. In most cases the diagnosis will be essential hypertension, although a few are secondary to disorders such as renal disease (see below).

Diagnostic difficulties are common as chronic hypertension predisposes to PE and the two conditions often co-exist. Furthermore, small increases in blood pressure (BP) and urinary protein excretion near term in women with chronic renal disease are normal, whereas larger increments may indicate progression of renal disease, rather than superimposed PE. The exact diagnosis may not be possible until several months after delivery when non-pregnant 'norms' can be applied. Finally, secondary hypertension may present *de novo* and although such instances are rare their consequences can be serious. Conditions such as pheochromocytoma should be considered, especially if the onset of hypertension is atypical.

Diagnosis and clinical features

Hypertension

Considering its importance, it is surprising that there is no universally agreed definition of hypertension in pregnancy. The main controversies concerning any definition focus on the use of Korotkoff phase IV or V sounds, the use of absolute BP values or changes from a baseline, the use of diastolic, systolic or mean arterial BP and the introduction of automated BP recorders. These controversies are outlined as follows.

1 The hyperdynamic circulation in pregnancy means that Korotkoff phase V (disappearance of sounds) may be very low or even unrecordable and has resulted in phase IV (muffling of sounds) being used to estimate diastolic BP. This approach has recently been questioned because Korotkoff V can, in fact, be measured reliably in most pregnant women and is more representative of intra-arterial pressure [22].

2 Complications of hypertension, such as cerebral hemorrhage, correlate with an absolute 'value' for BP. A 'cut-off' of 140/90 mmHg is commonly used for both pregnant and non-pregnant subjects. In pregnancy the major contributor to hypertensive complications is PE and increased BP is traditionally used in its diagnosis. If a change in BP from a baseline was included in the definition of hypertension in pregnancy it might highlight changes predictive of PE in women who commence pregnancy with very low BP (<90/60 mmHg) before an absolute level of 140/90 mmHg is reached [23]. There is, however, a risk of overdiagnosis if changes in diastolic BP are exaggerated or if baseline BP is not recorded in early pregnancy (see Renal tract alterations in normal pregnancy).

3 Although the diagnostic value of a raised diastolic BP is agreed, the value of systolic BP is debated. Routine use of the mean arterial pressure (MAP) has not simplified diagnosis or management of PE.

4 Automated BP recorders have been widely introduced into general medicine with great success but their accuracy in pregnancy has been questioned [24] and mercury sphygmomanometry remains the 'gold standard'.

Table 41.9 Definitions of high blood pressure (BP) in pregnancy

National High Blood Pressure Education Working Party [20]	*International Society for the Study of Hypertension in Pregnancy [21]*
Either: Systolic BP ≥ 140 mmHg *and/or* Diastolic BP ≥ 90 mmHg **or** Rise in systolic BP ≥ 30 mmHg from early pregnancy *and/or* Rise in diastolic BP ≥ 15 mmHg from early pregnancy	**Either:** Diastolic BP of ≥110 mmHg on one occasion **or** Diastolic BP of ≥90 mmHg on two consecutive occasions ≥ 4 h apart

In view of these controversies it is more important that each maternity unit adheres to a workable definition with which its staff are familiar and for which treatment protocols have been developed (see examples in Table 41.9). Furthermore, BP should be measured using the correct cuff size and avoiding supine hypotension due to vena caval compression by the pregnant uterus.

Proteinuria

Proteinuria is recognized as an adverse prognostic feature of PE but may be absent, or delayed in appearance in some women. Its definition (>0.3 g protein per 24 h) takes into account normal gestational increases in protein excretion (Figure 41.4). It is noteworthy that some normotensive women with proteinuria may still have PE, although the diagnosis can only be made in retrospect by exclusion of other renal diseases.

Edema

Edema is invariably emphasized in PE and can be rapid in onset in severe PE. Since it is also present in most normal pregnancies, edema is no longer considered diagnostic of PE.

Urate

Inappropriately high serum urate levels, often with normal creatinine levels, are commonly present in women with PE and may help differentiate PE from chronic hypertension. Specificity of hyperuricemia, however, is inadequate to be a reliable early marker of PE. Its use in assessing established PE can be confused by normal pregnancy changes (Table 41.2).

Pre-eclampsia

PE is usually a disease of first pregnancies (excluding abortion) but may occur in multigravidae, especially if certain

Table 41.10 Predisposing factors for pre-eclampsia

Maternal factors
- Primigravid (incidence = 6.1%)
- Chronic hypertension (renal disease, SLE)
- Family history (associated with HLA DR4 gene)
- Diabetes mellitus (including gestational diabetes)
- Advancing maternal age
- New partner

Fetal factors
- Multiple pregnancy
- Trisomy 13 and triploidy
- Hydrops fetalis (immune and non-immune)
- Hydatidiform mole

predisposing factors are present (Table 41.10). It is important to note that hypertension is only a sign of an underlying multisystem disorder, affecting hepatic, renal, hematological and vascular systems, and not a diagnosis. PE is closely associated with the HELLP syndrome and acute fatty liver of pregnancy and all may even be variants of a similar disease process. The fetus is at risk from placental insufficiency, abruptio placentae, and intervention on the behalf of the mother resulting in premature delivery.

The presentation of severe PE is variable as it may affect one or many systems (Table 41.11). In the developed world, grand mal convulsions (eclampsia) complicate 1 in 2000 pregnancies; 1 in 50 affected women die of the condition as do 1 in 14 of their offspring [21]. The commonest cause of maternal death is a cerebrovascular accident. Surprisingly, many women who have eclampsia do not have prior features of severe PE [25]. This is probably because cases with obvious features of PE are detected early and treatment instigated before eclampsia occurs so that a greater proportion of cases of eclampsia are now women with little or no warning signs.

Table 41.11 Features of severe pre-eclampsia

- Cerebral disturbances (headaches, visual disturbances)
- Epigastric pain (subcapsular liver hemorrhages?)
- Severe hypertension, often labile (≥160/110 mmHg)
- Hyperreflexia, especially clonus
- Retinopathy (usually a sign of chronic disease)
- Pulmonary edema
- Proteinuria (≥2.0 g/24 h)
- Hyperuricemia
- Hemoconcentration (increased hematocrit)
- High serum creatinine and urea (often only marginal)
- Elevated liver enzymes[a]
- Thrombocytopenia
- Microangiopathic hemolytic anemia

[a] Alkaline phosphatase is normally high in pregnancy due to placental contribution.

Pathogenesis

The exact etiology of PE remains obscure. The placenta is almost certainly involved as PE resolves after delivery and women with a hydatidiform mole, a condition with a large placental mass and no fetus, are predisposed to PE. Endotrophoblastic invasion of placental bed spiral arteries in early pregnancy, which normally increases their diameter by 4–6 times, is incomplete in women who subsequently develop PE (Figure 41.8). This results in constricted placental bed vasculature which remains responsive to circulating pressor agents; thus nutrient and oxygen supplies to the fetus are compromised, perhaps explaining why fetal growth retardation is common. Systemic changes, such as coagulopathy or vascular hyperreactivity, may be due to factors released by the placenta in response to 'relative ischemia'.

Dysfunction of vascular endothelium plays a role. It is notable that the renal lesion of PE is almost entirely limited to endothelium (see below). Endothelial cells are normally involved in maintaining vascular integrity, preventing intravascular coagulation and modifying vascular tone, functions which may be disrupted in PE [26]. Increased thromboxane concentration and decreased endothelial prostacyclin production may have a secondary effect on platelet function and coagulation. Circulating markers of endothelial function (endothelin, fibronectin) and of endothelial damage (endothelial antibodies) are increased and sera from women with PE can alter endothelial function *in vitro*.

Alterations in volume homeostasis also occur in PE, along with increased vascular tone, increased responsiveness to infused pressor agents (angiotensin II, catecholamines), increased plasma ANP and reduced plasma renin. Plasma volume is reduced and hematocrit often increased due to hemoconcentration.

Despite the advances in knowledge outlined above, a reliable and clinically applicable early marker of PE has not been identified. New areas of research include endothelium-derived relaxing factor (nitric oxide), which may be important in maintaining reduced vascular tone in pregnancy [5].

The renal lesion

PE is characterized by specific intraglomerular abnormalities often referred to as 'glomerular endotheliosis' (Figure 41.9). Extraglomerular alterations tend to be absent or non-specific. Unlike the situation in most other nephropathies, glomerular swelling is diffuse and extreme to the extent that herniation of glomerular contents into the proximal tubule is common (referred to as 'pouting'). Swelling is due to hypertrophy of endothelial cells (less commonly mesangial cells), resulting in large and bloodless glomeruli. There is little or no change in cell number or matrix, features which distinguish it from the proliferative nephropathies. Endothelial cells often contain heterogeneous vacuoles composed mainly of lipids. Foam cells, fibrin-like deposits and, less commonly, epithelial crescents or thromboses may be present. By light microscopy the basement membrane can appear artifactually thickened due to deposits, but this is not observed by electron microscopy. Immunochemistry has been disappointing; controversy surrounds the presence

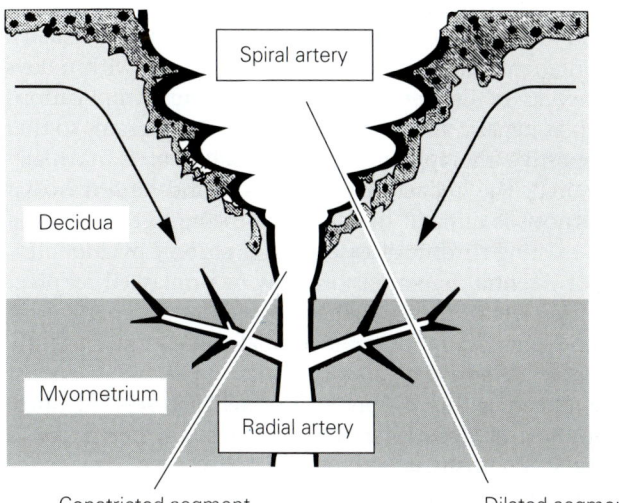

Figure 41.8 Drawing depicting invasion of spiral arteries by trophoblastic cells between 10 and 20 weeks gestation. In pre-eclampsia trophoblastic invasion does not extend beyond the deciduomyometrial junction and results in constricted segments of spiral artery.

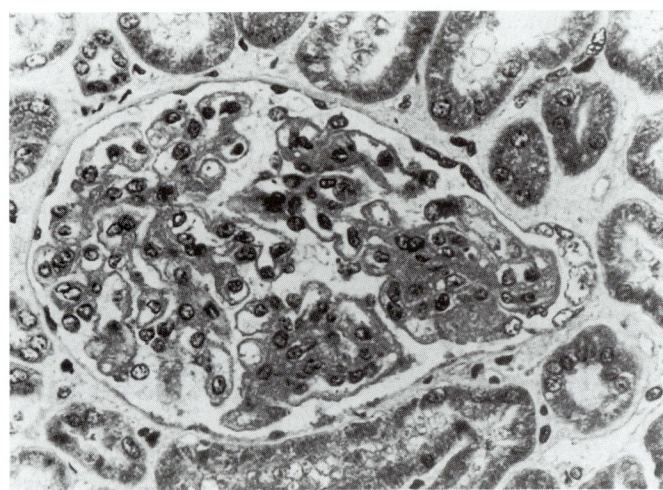

Figure 41.9 Glomerular capillary endotheliosis, the typical enlarged bloodlen glomerulus of pre-eclampsia with the capillary lumina obstructed by hypertrophised intracapillary and merangial cells and herniation of the glomerular tuft into the proximal tubule (H and E × 300).

and significance of IgM and IgG and fibrin. Lesions similar to focal segmental glomerulosclerosis have been reported but the benign long-term renal prognosis of PE suggests that they are not permanent.

The impact on the kidney and prognosis

Despite marked glomerular swelling, GFR and RPF undergo only small decrements. PE is rarely associated with acute renal failure unless treatment is neglected or complications such as abruptio placentae occur. Usually, spontaneous and complete resolution occurs within days or weeks of delivery, even when severe complications such as hepatic and renal dysfunction are present, so that supportive therapy postpartum is all that is normally required. The impact on remote renal and cardiovascular prognosis is difficult to determine owing to the fact that pre-existing chronic disease, such as chronic pyelonephritis or essential hypertension, may be unmasked by pregnancy. Overall the incidence of long-term hypertension is no higher than that in the normal population. In nearly all cases, glomerular abnormalities appear to disappear completely within 1–2 months of delivery, although proteinuria and glomerular abnormalities may persist for as long as 6 months.

Management of hypertension in pregnancy

Control of hypertension (Table 41.12)

The use of antihypertensives in mild/moderate hypertension (140/90–160/110 mm Hg) is controversial.

Reports of the use of antihypertensives causing reduced progression of PE together with improved neonatal outcome conflict with fears of reduced placental perfusion and the view that hypertension is but one sign of a more significant underlying disease. Generally there is agreement that overaggressive antihypertensive treatment can be detrimental; a target not lower than 120–140/80–90 mm Hg is, therefore, recommended. In severe hypertension (>160/110 mm Hg), treatment reduces the risk of hypertensive complications (intracranial hemorrhage) but probably does not prevent eclampsia.

With improved neonatal care treatment should not necessarily delay delivery, especially if pregnancy is near term, if BP control is difficult or if hypertension is accompanied by features of severe PE (Table 41.11) or fetal compromise (abnormalities of growth, cardiotocography or umbilical vessel Doppler velocimetry). After delivery, hypertension normally resolves within days or weeks.

Chronic hypertension

The outcome of pregnancy in women with mild/moderate essential hypertension (without superimposed PE) is similar to that of normotensive women but may be less favorable in those with secondary hypertension (e.g. renal disease). Prepregnancy counselling should be recommended and antihypertensive therapies reviewed before pregnancy is considered. Management depends on surveillance to detect superimposed PE or evidence of fetal compromise. The BP fluctuates, as in normotensive women, falling in mid-pregnancy and increasing in late pregnancy; thus antihypertensive treatment may need to be altered or temporarily stopped.

Pre-eclampsia

To date, no effective prophylaxis of PE has been identified and attempts to decrease its incidence by the use of diuretics, antiplatelet therapy (low-dose aspirin), dietary supplements (fish oil) or aggressive treatment of early hypertension ('hospitalized rest' and/or antihypertensive drugs) have not worked. A recent trial of low-dose aspirin in 10 000 'at risk' pregnancies suggested that it may only be of value in women especially likely to develop PE that is severe enough to warrant premature delivery [28]. The finding that women with PE have relative hypocalciuria prompted calcium supplementation for 'at risk' women. Although initial studies suggest a decreased risk of PE, large trials with long-term follow-up are essential before routine calcium supplementation can be recommended [29].

Once the disease process of PE commences it is progressive and only reverses following delivery. The timing of delivery is based on relative risks to the mother and fetus. Delays on fetal grounds are only warranted if maternal risks are small. Current management depends on early diagnosis, monitoring of progress and assessment of

Table 41.12 Use of antihypertensives in pregnancy

Antihypertensive	Comments
Alpha$_2$ adrenoreceptor agonists (methyldopa, clonidine)	Extensively used in pregnancy. Minor side effects such as lethargy and depression may limit use.
Beta adrenoreceptor antagonists (atenolol, metoprolol)	Reports of adverse neonatal outcome (depressed respiration, small size for dates, hypoglcemia and increased perinatal mortality) have not been borne out by most large controlled trials.
Combined alpha and beta adrenoreceptor antagonist (labetolol)	An IV bolus for hypertensive crises has fewer minor side effects than hydralazine.
Arterial vasodilators (hydralazine)	Reflex tachycardia, headaches and nausea are common but may be reduced if used as an adjunct to methyldopa or beta adrenoreceptor antagonists. Onset of action (20–30 min) and duration of control (6–8 h) following an IV bolus make it suitable for intermittent therapy on the labour ward.
Calcium channel blockers (nifedipine)	Effective in maintenance and acute control of hypertension but experience is less than with other drugs. Combination with magnesium sulphate (often used for seizure control) can cause severe hypotension.
Diazoxide	A third line therapy reserved for refractory hypertension. May result in profound vascular collapse.
Sodium nitroprusside	Use is limited because of fetal cyanide and thiocyanate toxicity but it may be required in exceptional circumstances when minute-to-minute control is necessary.
Diuretics (loop diuretics and thiazides)	Pre-eclampsia is associated with reduced intravascular volume and organ perfusion; therefore, diuretics are not recommended unless accompanied by invasive monitoring or as continued maintenance therapy for a chronic disease.
Angiotensin converting enzyme (ACE) inhibitors (Captopril)	ACE inhibitors have been associated with fetal death in animals as well as neonatal renal failure in humans and should be avoided in pregnancy.

Table 41.13 Anti-eclamptic therapy

Anti-convulsant	Complications
Magnesium sulfate	Respiratory or cardiac arrest at toxic levels.
Benzodiazepines (diazepam, clonazepam)	Effective for acute seizure control. Less effective for maintenance. Maternal respiratory and neurological depression. Respiratory depression in neonate.
Phenytoin	Hypotension and cardiac arrhythmias. IV bolus may be irritant. Troublesome minor side effects (dizziness, nystagmus, tinnitus, nausea, vomiting).
Chlormethiazole	Respiratory depression and obstruction. Sedation (neurological assessment difficult). Fluid overload with large doses.

fetal well-being. Up to 44% of eclamptic convulsions occur after delivery [21] so that close observation should be continued for at least the first 48 h.

Fluid management in severe PE

Although oliguria is common in PE, acute renal failure is rare. Inappropriate use of loop diuretics to treat oliguria may further reduce intravascular volume and organ perfusion. 'Blind' intravenous loading with crystalloids can be detrimental because, coupled with increased vascular permeability and decreased colloid osmotic pressure, it may lead to left ventricular dysfunction (due to increased afterload) and precipitate pulmonary edema. Therefore, if oliguria/anuria persists or if pulmonary edema is present, treatment should be guided by invasive surveillance (central venous pressure, pulmonary wedge pressure). Plasma volume expansion with colloids (e.g. 500–1000 ml of albumin) has been shown to help stabilize blood pressure in severe hypertension and is proposed as initial therapy for oliguria. Its effect is probably transient, however, since vascular permeability to colloids is increased.

Management of eclampsia and seizure prophylaxis (Table 41.13)

Eclampsia can occur without warning and be either self-limiting or associated with profound systemic and/or intracerebral disturbances [21]. Convulsions should be terminated with diazepam or clonazepam and maintenance therapy instituted while delivery is effected. Debate over the merits of magnesium sulfate, phenytoin, chlormethiazole and diazepam for seizure prophylaxis continues but the therapy with which each unit has the most experience is the safest. Many obstetricians commence anticonvulsant prophylaxis in the presence of severe hypertension or features of severe PE, continuing therapy for 24–48 h postdelivery.

Pregnancy in women with pre-existing renal disease

Over the last few decades advances in medical science have greatly improved the health, fertility and life expectancy of women with chronic renal disease. This has resulted in more women with chronic renal disease achieving a pregnancy. At least 1 in 200 pregnant women have a pre-existing renal disorder, the commonest being chronic pyelonephritis, but most only have mild renal impairment. Appropriate management of pregnant women with renal problems requires an understanding of the physiology of pregnancy and its interaction with renal pathology. This section discusses obstetric considerations for women with pre-existing renal disease and is intended as an adjunct to management issues discussed elsewhere in this textbook.

The interaction of renal disease and pregnancy

Pathophysiology

Women with mild or moderate renal impairment still undergo gestational increments in GFR and RPF, albeit to a lesser degree than healthy women. Although there have been concerns that gestational renal vasodilatation may accelerate long-term renal decline, this has not been supported by longitudinal studies comparing women who have conceived with those who have not. Data in humans are, admittedly, limited, especially in those with severe renal dysfunction. Studies of animal models with renal impairment have provided some reassurance as decline in renal function has not been accelerated by recurrent pregnancies. In rats, gestational hyperfiltration occurs without increased intraglomerular pressure [5], and might explain why the interaction of pregnancy and renal pathology is apparently benign.

Clinical implications

With most renal disorders fetal outcome and impact on renal prognosis appear to depend on the severity of renal disease prior to pregnancy rather than on the underlying disease. Increments in maternal BP, proteinuria and serum creatinine are common, especially in late pregnancy when they may be due to superimposed PE (see above). These changes are usually transient and reverse after delivery. Permanent renal decline can usually be attributed to the natural history of the disease but in some women, particularly those with severe disease or with specific disorders (see below), pregnancy may worsen long-term prognosis. The major contributors to adverse fetal outcome are placental insufficiency and premature delivery.

Specific renal disorders in pregnancy

The interaction of pregnancy and specific renal disorders is difficult to evaluate as randomized controlled trials will always be lacking and many conditions have a fluctuating course, making it difficult to differentiate between natural progression and gestationally mediated renal deterioration. Fetal prognosis is easier to define but can still be unpredictable. The comments listed below highlight the main areas of controversy and consensus.

Glomerulonephritis and focal segmental glomerulosclerosis

Transient renal decline and hypertension are common near term in pregnancies complicated by glomerulonephritis. If renal function is preserved and if hypertension is absent or well controlled prior to pregnancy, fetal and renal prognoses are good. This statement should be tempered for IgA nephritis, membranoproliferative (mesangiocapillary) glomerulonephritis and focal segmental glomerulosterosis, which have been associated with increased PE and fetal loss during pregnancy, followed by accelerated renal dysfunction and worsening hypertension after delivery. This view, however, is not universal [30, 31].

Tubulointerstitial disorders

Chronic pyelonephritis and/or reflux nephropathy are the commonest chronic renal disorders encountered in pregnant women. Providing renal impairment is minimal, obstetric outcome is favorable. Urinary tract dilatation may further increase ascending infections, the impact of which may be more important in pregnancy (see above). Women with urinary diversions and reconstructive surgery are also prone to ureteric dilatation and reflux. This is because the pregnant uterus may cause ureteric obstruction, but intervention is rarely required. As with all chronic renal diseases in pregnancy, urine should be screened regularly and infections treated promptly.

Women with adult polycystic kidney disease (PCKD) have a propensity to develop PE in pregnancy. In some cases where PE occurs, PCKD may not even be diagnosed at the time, becoming evident in later life. A family history is informative since adult PCKD is an autosomal dominant disease with 50% of offspring being affected. Prenatal diagnosis of PCKD is difficult as different gene loci have been identified necessitating studies identifying gene mutations within affected familial members [32].

Collagen disorders

The fluctuating course of systemic lupus erythematosus (SLE) makes evaluation difficult. In general, renal and fetal prognoses appear to be good when renal function is well preserved and prepregnancy remission of SLE exceeds six months. If a relapse occurs in pregnancy it can have severe consequences. The fetus is often severely compromised and maternal deaths have been reported. Differentiation between a renal 'flare up' and PE may be difficult, especially if extrarenal signs are absent. In pregnancy, the sedimentation rate is normally raised but a reduction of C3 complement, a positive fluorescent antinuclear antibody and an active urinary sediment may be indices of disease activity. Relapses following delivery are commonly reported and augmented steroid therapy to cover the puerperium is often advocated. However, one study suggested that the total number of relapses is not increased and that increasing the dose of steroids is not warranted [33].

There are a number of autoantibodies that are related to SLE but these can also occur in the absence of clinical disease. In pregnancy they are indicative of a poor prognosis, including spontaneous abortion, fetal death and/or

growth retardation and neonatal lupus syndrome. Aspirin (75–300 mg/day) together with corticosteroid therapy may improve outcome but the latter is normally reserved for patients with poor obstetric histories. If steroids are given in high doses there may be additional risks due to glucose intolerance. The potential benefit of plasma exchange or immunosuppressive regimes is uncertain.

Anticardiolipin antibodies may cause a false positive Wasserman reaction which is of note since pregnant women are usually screened by VDRL testing. Since there is an increased risk of thromboembolism with the 'lupus' anticoagulant in pregnancy, low-dose heparin is often prescribed, particularly if there is a history of thrombosis. Finally, anti-Ro antibody in SLE is linked with congenital heart block and is often associated with fibrosis or calcification of the conducting system, cardiomyopathy or structural abnormalities of the heart.

Pregnant patients with polyarteritis nodosa and systemic sclerosis with renal involvement have a poor prognosis and may develop malignant hypertension. Successful neonatal outcome is rare; even maternal deaths have been reported. In these diseases pregnancy is discouraged and early termination of accidental pregnancies is often recommended.

Diabetic nephropathy

Diabetes mellitus has considerable impact on fetal wellbeing (developmental anomalies, growth retardation and sudden death) and neonatal outcome (birth trauma, prematurity, respiratory distress and hypoglycemia). Diabetics are prone to urinary infections and PE. Management is aimed at achieving as near to 'normoglycemia' as possible and in nearly all cases results in a favorable perinatal outcome.

Microalbuminuria has been associated with increased complications in late pregnancy. When frank nephropathy is present the fetal prognosis is worse. Hypertension and increasing proteinuria (+/–PE) are common but usually reverse following delivery. Although previously disputed, it now appears that pregnancy in diabetics, in

Table 41.14 Example criteria for renal biopsy in pregnancy

- Experienced operator
- Less than 32 weeks' gestation
- Rapid deterioration in renal function
- Massive nephrotic syndrome of unknown origin
- Treatable condition suspected (e.g. rapidly progressive glomerulonephritis or minimal change nephropathy which may respond to steroids)
- Condition perhaps endorsing termination of pregnancy suspected (e.g. scleroderma or polyarteritis nodosa)

particular gestational renal vasodilatation, probably has no adverse effect on remote renal prognosis [34].

Solitary kidney

After surgical removal of a kidney there has been the concern that the compensatory renal vasodilatation in the remaining kidney may cause progressive glomerular damage, further exacerbated by pregnancy. This concern, however, is not supported by the limited data available [35].

Nephrotic syndrome

The commonest cause of the nephrotic syndrome in late pregnancy is PE. Other causes of the nephrotic syndrome also occur, but if renal function is preserved and hypertension minimal or absent, pregnancy is relatively uncomplicated. Fluid retention may be exacerbated by reductions in serum albumin concentration. Diuretics should be used with caution as uteroplacental blood flow may be compromised. Renal biopsy may rarely be required during the pregnancy and the criteria for this are outlined in Table 41.14.

Management of pregnant women with chronic renal disease

Prepregnancy counselling

Ideally management commences before pregnancy. Counselling should be available so that all implications of pregnancy in a woman with kidney disease are fully considered, timing is optimum and medications are reviewed to ensure compatibility with pregnancy. Life expectancy and long-term health may be adversely affected and the harsh reality(ies) of parenting may need to be carefully discussed. Not all women who are contemplating pregnancy will fit ideal preconception guidelines and each case requires individual consideration.

When contemplating pregnancy three questions are often asked:

'Will pregnancy make my kidney disease worse?'
'Will the kidney disease be harmful to my pregnancy?'
'Can I expect a healthy baby?'

Answers are based on retrospective studies of women categorized by prepregnancy renal function and whether hypertension is present (Tables 41.15 and 41.16). In general it appears that mild disease usually results in a successful obstetric outcome and is unlikely to cause further long-term renal impairment.

In moderate and severe renal disease many women experience accelerated renal decline, some of which can be attributed to natural progression, and certainly prognosis is worse if severe hypertension intervenes. A recent analysis [31] of 67 women in these categories in 82 pregnancies is important; maternal complications occurred in 70% and pregnancy-related loss of kidney function in almost 50% (of whom 10% quickly progressed to end stage failure), but the infant survival rate exceeded 90%, reflecting the specialist obstetric and neonatal care of those to tertiary centers.

Antenatal strategy

Patients must be monitored as high-risk cases with frequent antenatal review (every one to two weeks) with a team consisting of an obstetrician, nephrologist and neonatologist. A suggested plan for surveillance is outlined in Table 41.17.

The value of antiviral antibody screening in normal pregnancy is controversial but may be appropriate for women receiving immune suppression treatment. Urinary protein excretion may double and renal function normally declines by approximately 15% near term. If the changes are greater, then reversible causes of renal injury should be identified (urine infection, hypovolemia, diuretic therapy) and corrected, otherwise delivery should be considered. The recommended diet should simply be

Table 41.15 Assessment of renal impairment for prepregnancy counseling of women with chronic renal disease

Renal status	Plasma creatinine (μmol/l (mg%))	Hypertension
Mild	≤125 (1.4)	Absent/minimal
Moderate	125–250 (1.4–2.8)	Present/often requiring treatment
Severe	≥250 (2.8)	Severe/often difficult to control

Table 41.16 Prospects for and outcome of pregnancy in women with renal disease (%); based on 2813 pregnancies in 1902 women (1973–93). (Figures in parentheses refer to outcome when complications arise before 28 weeks)

Renal status	Problems in pregnancy	Successful obstetric outcome	Problems in long term
Mild	26	96 (85)	<3 (9)
Moderate	47	89 (59)	25 (71)
Severe	86	46 (8)	53 (92)

From Baylis and Davison, unpublished data.

Table 41.17 Surveillance of maternal and fetal well-being in pregnant women with chronic renal disease

1–2 weekly
Blood pressure
Plasma creatinine and electrolytes
Full blood count (including platelets)
Urinalysis

4–6 weekly
Plasma urate
24h creatinine clearance and protein excretion
Midstream urine specimen for microscopy and culture
Liver function tests and serum proteins
Calcium and phosphate levels

Assessment of fetal growth and liquor volume
   (ultrasound)
Fetal cardiotocography and Doppler velocimetry
Biophysical profiling

Table 41.18 Prepregnancy guidelines for renal transplant recipients

- Good general health 2 years post transplant
- Normal stature
- No (or minimal) proteinuria
- No hypertension
- No evidence of graft rejection
- No pelvicalyceal dilation
- Serum creatinine $\leq 125\,\mu$mol/l (1.4 mg%)
- Drug therapies at maintenance levels

normal diet as the impact of salt and protein restriction in pregnancy is uncertain. If necessary iron supplementation should be considered. Experience of recombinant human erythropoeitin (rHuEpo) use in pregnancy is limited.

Superimposed PE

Chronic renal disease increases the risk of PE by 3–7 times. If worsening renal function, hypertension or proteinuria occurs in pregnancy, it can be difficult to differentiate between PE and progression of renal disease [29]. Renal biopsy is rarely undertaken as delivery is usually indicated regardless of the cause (Table 41.14). Diagnosis may be easier if associated features of PE are present (see above) but often the final diagnosis can only be made following delivery when further investigations are performed or, as in the case of PE, the patient's condition resolves.

Delivery

The timing of delivery depends on both maternal and fetal well-being, although delays on fetal grounds are only warranted if maternal risks are small, especially as advances in neonatal care have dramatically improved the outcome for preterm infants. Although there are no specific contraindications to vaginal delivery, caesarean section is common and is usually performed because of fetal compromise or prematurity.

Renal transplant recipients

Approximately 1 in 50 women of childbearing age with functioning renal allografts become pregnant. Often it is unplanned; the increased libido and fertility relate to improved renal function. If at all possible prepregnancy counselling should be undertaken (Table 41.18).

Neonatal outcome and renal prognosis

Gestational increments in GFR and RPF still occur despite the ectopic location, anomalous blood supply and hyperfiltration of the transplanted kidney. The neonatal and renal prognoses relate to the degree of functional impairment. The frequency of spontaneous abortion is probably not increased but therapeutic termination is common. There is also the potential for ectopic pregnancies because of previous pelvic surgery. Approximately half the pregnancies that continue beyond the first trimester are complicated by hypertension (+/–PE), decline in renal function or graft rejection [36]. In 20% there is fetal growth retardation and in 50% there is either spontaneous or elective preterm delivery. If problems arise prior to 28 weeks gestation, successful obstetric outcome decreases from 93 to 70%. Complications are even greater in women transplanted for diabetic nephropathy, as most of them have generalized vasculopathy.

Remote complications (persistent hypertension, renal function deterioration, graft rejection) occur in 12% of pregnancies and double if complications had arisen prior to 28 weeks [36]. Pregnancy does not appear to alter the rate of graft rejection, although it might even be expected to decrease considering the immunological privileges afforded to the fetus.

Immunosuppressants (Table 41.19)

The risks of immunosuppressants, particularly long-term effects on the offspring, are still to be fully evaluated. Cyclosporin-A (CsA) appears to confer better graft survival than azathioprine but data concerning its use in pregnancy are limited. The theoretically deleterious effects of CsA nephrotoxicity (hypertension and renal dysfunction) as well as any contribution towards increased fetal growth retardation and PE are under review [36, 37].

Table 41.19 Immunosuppression and pregnancy

Drugs	Comments
General	Opportunistic infections (*Listeria monocytogenes*, hepatitis B, herpes simplex and cytomegalovirus are associated with an adverse fetal outcome)
	Glucose intolerance
	Neonatal immune suppression (B cell depletion)
	Neoplastic change (risk of hydatidiform mole?)
	Uncertain teratogenicity
Steroids (prednisolone)	Severe pregnancy dyspepsia
	Weakening of connective tissues (premature labor, uterine rupture)
Azathioprine	Neonatal leukopenia
	Decreased fertility in female rat offspring
	Hepatic toxicity
Cyclosporin A	Fetal growth retardation
	Nephrotoxicity
	Hypertension
	Hepatic toxicity
	Thromboembolism

The prepregnancy dose of azathioprine is usually continued. Bioavailability may be monitored by measuring metabolites of azathioprine (6-thioguanine nucleotides) and the dose adjusted accordingly. A simpler approach is to adjust the dose to maintain leukocyte counts normal for pregnancy, thus ensuring that the neonate has a normal blood count. The dose of CsA may need to be increased slightly to maintain blood levels in the therapeutic range but should be reduced again in late pregnancy or directly following delivery when CsA levels, and therefore nephrotoxicity, increase. It is unlikely that enhanced doses to cover 'rebound immunoresponsiveness' postpartum is of value but additional steroids are necessary to cover the stress of delivery. Neonatal adrenal suppression is not usually a problem as maintenance steroid doses are normally low by the time pregnancy is embarked on.

Obstetric management

Parathyroid dysfunction is common following renal transplantation and can have secondary effects on fetal parathyroid function. Maternal calcium and phosphate levels should be monitored and if parathyroidectomy has been performed calcium and vitamin D supplementation may be necessary.

Caesarean section is only indicated for obstetric reasons but is more common, mainly because of prematurity, pregnancy complications, pelvic osteodystrophy and fears of the unknown rather than dystocia caused by the transplanted kidney or risk of it being injured.

Dialysis patients

Despite decreased libido and relative infertility, women receiving hemo- and peritoneal dialysis still conceive, albeit rarely. Spontaneous abortion is common and exacerbated hypertension and altered volume homeostasis pose unnecessary risks considering that a successful outcome is unlikely. Pregnancy is strongly discouraged, at least until after a successful transplant. The use of contraceptives should be stressed and therapeutic termination should be considered for accidental conception.

Many patients present late as a *fait accompli*, as pregnancy is often unsuspected until the second trimester. If the pregnancy is to continue, control of hypertension must be a main priority. Rapid changes of plasma volume with the risk of hypotension should be avoided, particularly as pregnant women are prone to supine hypotension because of compression of the inferior vena cava by the pregnant uterus, decreasing venous return. Correction of uremia should be adequate and consequently frequency and duration of dialysis may need to increase. Maternal anemia is associated with fetal compromise. Iron supplementation should be considered and the dose of rHuEpo has been used in pregnancy without ill-effects and indeed requirements may double or triple [38]. Fetal/neonatal loss may still occur due to hypertension, abruptio placentae, growth retardation and calcium and electrolyte imbalance. Prematurity is common due to elective and spontaneous delivery and premature labor is sometimes directly associated with a dialysis session. Continuous ambulatory peritoneal dialysis would reduce the rapid changes in intravascular volume that occur in hemodialysis but may increase the risk of complications due to peritonitis (premature labor, ectopic pregnancy) [39].

Contraception in women with chronic renal problems

The prevailing message in this section is that pregnancy should not be discouraged in all women with chronic renal disease but should be timed such that the chance of a healthy infant is optimum with little detriment to the mother. No form of contraception is absolutely contraindicated but many would advise against oral contraceptives in women with hypertension and the intrauterine contraceptive device in women receiving immunosuppressants, due to potential risks of pelvic infection.

References

1. Baylis, C. and Davison, J. (1990) The urinary system, in *Clinical Physiology in Obstetrics* (eds F. Hytten and G. Chamberlain), Blackwell Scientific, Oxford, pp. 245–302.

2. Sturgiss, S.N., Dunlop, W. and Davison, J.M. (1994) Renal haemodynamics and tubular function in human pregnancy. *Ballière's Clin. Obstet. Gynaecol.*, **8**, 209–34.

3. Dunlop, W. (1981) Serial changes in renal haemodynamics during normal human pregnancy. *Br. J. Obstet. Gynaecol.*, **88**, 1–9.

4. Baylis, C. and Reckelhoff, J.F. (1991) Renal hemodynamics in normal and hypertensive pregnancy: lessons from micropuncture. *Am. J. Kidney Dis.*, **17**, 98–104.

5. Baylis, C. (1994) Glomerular filtration and volume regulation in gravid animal models. *Ballière's Clin. Obstet. Gynaecol.*, **8**, 235–64.

6. Atherton, J.C. and Green, R. (1994) Renal tubular function in the gravid rat. *Ballière's Clin. Obstet. Gynaecol.*, **8**, 265–85.

7. Brown, M.A., Wang, M., Buddle, M.L. *et al.* (1994) Albumin excretion rate in normal and hypertensive pregnancy. *Clin. Sci.*, **86**, 251–5.

8. Lopez-Espinoza, I., Dhar, H., Humphreys, S. and Redman, C.W.G. (1986) Urinary albumin excretion in pregnancy. *Br. J. Obstet. Gynaecol.*, **93**, 176–81.

9. Misiani, R., Marchesi, D., Tiraboschi, G. *et al.* (1991) Urinary albumin excretion in normal pregnancy and pregnancy-induced hypertension. *Nephron*, **59**, 416–22.

10. Wright, A., Steele, P., Bennett, J.R. *et al.* (1987) The urinary excretion of albumin in normal pregnancy. *Br. J. Obstet. Gynaecol.*, **94**, 408–12.

11. Davison, J.M., Vallotton, M.B. and Lindheimer, M.D. (1981) Plasma osmolality and urine concentration and dilution during and after pregnancy: evidence that lateral recumbency inhibits maximal urinary concentrating ability. *Br. J. Obstet. Gynaecol.*, **88**, 472–9.

12. Davison, J.M., Gilmore, E.A., Dürr, J. *et al.* (1984) Altered osmotic thresholds for vasopressin secretion and thirst in human pregnancy. *Am. J. Physiol.*, **246**, F105–9.

13. Irons, D.W., Baylis, P.H., Davison, J.M. (1996) Effects of atrial natriuretic peptide on renal hemodynamics and sodium excretion during human pregnancy. *Am. J. Physiol.*, **271**, 239–42.

14. Masilamani, S. and Baylis, C. (1994) Pregnant rats are refractory to the natriuretic actions of ANP. *Am. J. Physiol.*, **267**, 1611–16.

15. Peterson, C., Hedges, S., Stenqvist, K. *et al.* (1994) Suppressed antibody and interleukin-6 responses to acute pyelonephritis in pregnancy. *Kidney Int.*, **45**, 571–7.

16. Shieve, L.A., Handler, A., Hershow, R. *et al.* (1994) Urinary tract infections during pregnancy: its association with maternal morbidity and perinatal outcome. *Obstet. Gynecol. Surv.*, **49**, 596–7.

17. MacNeily, A.E., Goldenberg, S.L., Allen, G.J. *et al.* (1991) Sonographic visualization of the ureter in pregnancy. *J. Urol.*, **146**, 298–301.

18. Alcalay, M., Blau, A., Barkai, G. *et al.* (1992) Successful pregnancy in a patient with polycystic kidney disease and advanced renal failure: the use of prophylactic dialysis. *Am. J. Kidney Dis.*, **19**, 382–4.

19. Department of Health (1994) Trends in maternal mortality. *Report on Confidential Enquiries into Maternal Deaths in the United Kingdom 1988–1990.* HMSO, London.

20. National High Blood Pressure Education Program Working Group (1990) Report on high blood pressure in pregnancy. *Am. J. Obstet. Gynecol.*, **163**, 1689–712.

21. Douglas, K.A. and Redman, C.W.G. (1994) Eclampsia in the United Kingdom. *Br. Med. J.*, **309**, 1395–400.

22. Johenning, A.R. and Barron, W.M. (1992) Indirect blood pressure measurement in pregnancy: Korotkoff phase 4 versus phase 5. *Am. J. Obstet. Gynecol.*, **167**, 577–81.

23. Redman, C.W.G. and Jeffries, M. (1988) Revised definition of pre-eclampsia. *Lancet*, **i**, 809–12.

24. Franx, A., van der Post, J.A., Elfering, I.M. *et al.* (1994) Validation of automated blood pressure recording in pregnancy. *Br. J. Obstet. Gynaecol.*, **101**, 66–9.

25. Davey, D.A. and MacGillivary, I. (1988) The classification and definition of hypertensive disorders of pregnancy. *Am. J. Obstet. Gynecol.*, **158**, 892–8.

26. Baylis, C., Suto, T. and Conrad, K. (1996) Importance of nitric oxide in control of systemic and renal hemodynamics during normal pregnancy: studies in the rat and implications for pre-eclampsia. *Hypertension in Pregnancy*, **15**, 147–69.

27. Morris, N.H., Eaton, B.M., Dekker, G. (1996) Nitric oxide, the endothelium pregnancy and pre-eclampsia. *Br. J. Obstet. Gynaecol.*, **103**, 4–15.

28. CLASP (Collaborative Low-dose Aspirin Study in Pregnancy) Collaborative Group. (1994) CLASP: a randomised trial of low-dose aspirin for the prevention and treatment of pre-eclampsia among 9364 pregnant women. *Lancet*, **343**, 619–28.

29. Lindheimer, M.D. (1996) Pre-eclampia–eclampsia, 1996 Preventable? Have the disputes or its treatment been resolved? *Curr. Opinion Hypertension Nephrol.*, **5**, 452–8.

30. Abe, S. (1996) Pregnancy in glomerulonephritic patients with decreased renal function. *Hypertension in Pregnancy*, **15**, 305–12.

31. Jones, D.C. and Hayslett, J.P. (1996) Outcome of pregnancy in women with moderate or severe renal insufficiency. *N. Engl. J. Med.*, **335**, 226–32.

32. Anver, E.D. (1994) Gene time for polycystic kidney disease. *Lancet*, **344**, 833–4.

33. Lockshin, M.D., Reinitz, E. and Druzin, M.L. (1984) Lupus pregnancy: case–control prospective study, demonstrating absence of lupus exacerbation during or after pregnancy. *Am. J. Med.*, **77**, 893–8.

34. Gordon, M., Laudon, M.B., Samuels, P., Hissrich, S. and Gabbe, S.G. (1996) Peritoneal outcome and long term follow up associated with modern management of diabetic nephropathy. *Obstet. Gynecol.*, **87**, 401–9.

35. Foster, M.H., Sant, G.R., Donohoe, J.F. and Harrington, J.T. (1991) Prolonged survival with a remnant kidney. *Am. J. Kidney Dis.*, **17**, 261–5.

36. Davison, J.M. (1994) Pregnancy in renal allograft recipi-

ents: problems, prognosis and practicalities. *Ballière's Clin. Obstet. Gynaecol.*, **8**, 501–25.

37. Gowghan, W.J., Moritz, M.J., Redomski, J.S., Burke, J.F. and Armenti, V.T. (1996) National Transplantation Registry: Report on outcomes in treated recipients with an interval from transplant to pregnancy of greater than 5 years. *Am. J. Kidney Dis.*, **28**, 266–9.

38. Hou, S.H. (1994) Frequency and outcome of pregnancy in women on dialysis. *Am. J. Kidney Dis.*, **23**, 60–3.

39. Gadallah, M.F., Ahmad, B., Karubian, F. and Campese, V.M. (1992) Pregnancy in patients on chronic ambulatory peritoneal dialysis. *Am. J. Kidney Dis.*, **20**, 407–10.

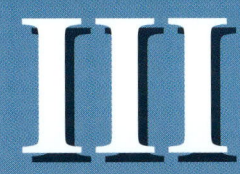

Diseases of the Kidney and Their Treatment

Section 3
Systemic Disease and Renal Involvement

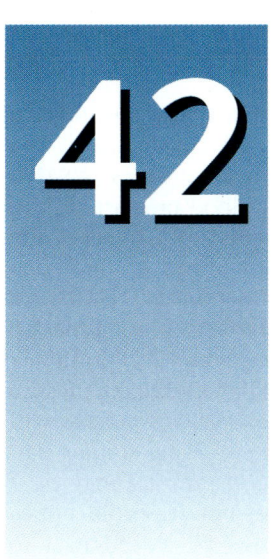

42

Diseases of the renal blood vessels and hypertension

Peter Rutherford and Robert Wilkinson

The detection of renal hypertension

Introduction

In the populations of developed countries blood pressure is a continuous variable which follows a normal distribution with a positive skew. Therefore, it is not possible to define hypertension with precision. The generally accepted level of >140/90 mmHg is based on epidemiological studies examining levels of blood pressure which are associated with greater morbidity and mortality and at which intervention influences these outcomes. Furthermore, this definition may be inappropriate in hypertension associated with renal disease since treatment of lower levels of blood pressure may retard the progression of renal disease.

In the UK, hypertension, defined as above, affects approximately 30% of adults aged between 35 and 64 years of age. However, only a small proportion, approximately 4%, of hypertensive patients have a primary renal disease. In contrast, although renal disease is uncommon among the hypertensive population, hypertension is common in all types of renal disease. Approximately 60% of patients with glomerular disease, in particular mesangiocapillary and sclerosing glomerulopathies, are hypertensive. Hypertension is very common in diabetic nephropathy and less so in tubulointerstitial disease, in patients with chronic pyelonephritis; 33% are hypertensive at presentation rising to 45% after five years of follow-up and 75% when end-stage renal failure is reached [1].

There is no simple way to distinguish those patients with renal disease from the much larger numbers referred with essential hypertension. Simple enrichment criteria may be useful; for example, in patients presenting with malignant hypertension the prevalence of renovascular hypertension (RVH) is higher than in patients presenting with uncomplicated hypertension, and may be as high as 30% [2]. However, the identification of patients presenting with hypertension in association with renal disease requires thorough clinical assessment followed by appropriate investigation in selected patients.

Clinical aspects of renal hypertension

It is useful to identify those few patients with underlying renal or renal vascular disease from within the large number of patients presenting with hypertension. Their response to antihypertensive treatment may be different and the choice of antihypertensive drugs may be different; for instance, angiotensin converting enzyme (ACE) inhibitors may be contraindicated in the patient with renovascular disease but the best choice in patients with diabetic nephropathy. Furthermore, the renal disease itself may require specific treatment whether or not this lowers blood pressure and correction of renal artery stenosis may be indicated not only to improve blood pres-

Nephrology, Edited by Rex L. Jamison and Robert Wilkinson.
Published in 1997 by Chapman & Hall, London. ISBN 0 412 60930 4

sure control but also to preserve renal function. It is important to recognize that the coexistence of renal disease and hypertension does not prove causation of the hypertension by the renal disease, indeed the reverse may be the case. For example, an inherited predisposition to hypertension may determine the development of nephropathy in diabetes mellitus [3]. In addition, there is evidence that the renal response to an immunological injury may be influenced by the blood pressure to which the kidney is exposed.

Clinical history

It is necessary to take a full medical history, including details of family, diet, exercise, smoking habits, alcohol intake and drug treatment. Reliable clues to underlying renal disease do not often arise in the history but certain features may be useful in selecting patients for further investigation (Table 42.1). The two most useful indicators are an early age of onset, with chronic pyelonephritis being the most common cause of hypertension in patients under the age of 20 years, and a history of a deterioration in renal function with an ACE inhibitor, suggesting bilateral renal artery stenosis or stenosis of the artery supplying a single functioning kidney. When the clinical characteristics of patients with RVH and essential hypertension were directly compared in the Cooperative Study of Renovascular Hypertension [2], however, although differences were observed, the overlap between the two groups was large.

Direct questioning regarding regular medications is also very important. The oral contraceptive pill is responsible for the development of hypertension in some women. The precise mechanism is unknown, but the estrogen component seems to be primarily responsible since the incidence of hypertension has decreased since the estrogen content was lowered [4]. Hypertension induced by the oral contraceptive pill may take as long as three months to disappear following withdrawal of the pill and in some patients may persist. The possibility of underlying renal disease should be considered at that point. Non-steroidal anti-inflammatory drugs (NSAIDs) may also produce an increase in blood pressure in both normotensive subjects and patients with hypertension and rarely may cause interstitial nephritis or glomerular abnormalities with proteinuria. In addition, NSAIDs can attenuate the antihypertensive effects of diuretics, β-adrenoreceptor blockers, vasodilators and ACE inhibitors [5]. This action is probably mediated by the suppression of renal and possibly extrarenal cyclooxygenase with inhibition of prostacyclin synthesis. Some studies have suggested that this effect on blood pressure may be of only minor clinical significance, but it would appear prudent to assess the response to withdrawal of NSAIDs, if possible, before embarking on extensive investigation.

Physical examination

A physical examination is of course necessary. Particular attention should be paid to the fundi, cardiovascular system and peripheral pulses to assess the extent of cardiovascular damage from the hypertension. Clinical clues to the presence of a renal cause can be found in some patients (Table 42.2). Most of these clinical features pertain to uncommon disorders and are self-explanatory. In patients with neurofibromatosis and hypertension, renal artery stenosis should be considered, as well as the more classically associated pheochromocytoma. The predictive value of an epigastric bruit is limited. A bruit is heard in 10% of essential hypertensives and only 50–60% of patients with RVH; therefore, the presence of a bruit only increases the likelihood of finding renal artery stenosis in a given patient from 1 to 10%, approximately.

Table 42.1 Features which make the diagnosis of renal hypertension more likely

1. Onset of hypertension before age 30 or after age 50 years
2. Short duration or recent worsening of hypertension
3. Symptoms of renal dysfunction, e.g. polyuria
4. Personal or family history of renal disease
5. Absence of family history of hypertension
6. Resistance to antihypertensive therapy
7. Extrarenal vascular disease
8. Severe hypertension
9. Retinopathy
10. Elevation in plasma creatinine with ACE inhibitors

Table 42.2 Features on physical examination suggesting renal hypertension

1. Bilateral enlarged kidneys
   (i)   Polycystic kidney disease
   (ii) Tuberous sclerosis
   (iii) Von Hippel–Lindau disease
2. Absence of peripheral pulses
3. Bruit in costovertebral angle or epigastrium – Renal artery stenosis
4. Facial rash, arthropathy – Systemic lupus erythematosus
5. Sensorineural deafness – Alport's syndrome
6. Partial lipodystrophy – Mesangiocapillary glomerulonephritis
7. Adenoma sebaceum – Tuberous sclerosis
8. Neurofibromatosis – Renal artery stenosis

Laboratory investigation

Clinical history and physical examination are useful in selecting patients for further investigation but fail to identify the majority of patients with renal disease in a population of hypertensives. Laboratory and radiological investigations are required in most cases. A suggested scheme for investigation is outlined in Table 42.3.

It is essential to perform a urinalysis and to measure plasma creatinine and electrolytes in all patients to assess end organ damage as well as to detect primary renal disease. These tests are not sensitive or specific, however. For instance only 40% of patients with chronic pyelonephritis have proteinuria and in RVH proteinuria, especially at nephrotic syndrome levels, rarely occurs, whereas proteinuria is common in essential hypertension.

The majority of patients with glomerulonephritis have either proteinuria or hematuria, although in some conditions, for instance IgA nephropathy, it may be episodic. Proteinuria may be absent despite quite advanced glomerular morphologic changes in lupus nephritis.

It is uneconomical to investigate fully all hypertensive patients for the presence of renal disease since the yield from investigation is low. Some guidelines concerning the indications for full investigation are given in Table 42.4.

Radiological investigations

Intravenous pyelography (IVP)

The traditional first step in the investigation of renal disease in hypertension has been the IVP. Conditions such as chronic pyelonephritis, obstructive uropathy and renal calculi can be reliably diagnosed. However, the IVP carries appreciable false-positive and false-negative rates, approximately 15 and 25%, respectively, in unilateral renal vascular disease, and is of little value in bilateral renal vascular disease. IVP is not feasible in patients with serum creatinine above about 300 μmol/l. Very rarely (about 1 in 100 000 injections) death due to anaphylactic shock may occur.

Renal ultrasound

This is a cheap and non-invasive investigation to measure renal size and detect polycystic kidney disease and

In all patients
1. Urinalysis
   Glomerulonephritis – blood and/or protein usually present
   Chronic pyelonephritis ⎫
   Polycystic kidney disease ⎬ blood and protein often absent
   Renovascular disease ⎭
2. Urine sediment
   Glomerulonephritis – red blood cells or casts
   Chronic pyelonephritis – possibly white blood cells
3. Plasma creatinine
4. Plasma electrolytes – hypokalemia suggesting primary or secondary aldosteronism
   – hypercalcemia suggesting hyperparathyroidism

In selected patients
1. Renal ultrasound
   Renal size
   Obstruction
   Polycystic kidneys
2. Intravenous pyelogram – particularly in young women
   Chronic pyelonephritis/reflux nephropathy
   Renovascular hypertension
   Polycystic kidneys
3. ^{99m}Tc-DTPA renogram with captopril and furosemide particularly in older patients
   Renovascular hypertension
4. ^{99m}Tc-DMSA scan
   Renal parenchymal scars
   Preferable to IVU in children
5. Renal arteriogram
   Renovascular hypertension

Table 42.3 Laboratory and radiological investigations to detect renal disease among hypertensive patients

hydronephrosis, although it may miss acute obstruction. The diagnosis of renal scarring in chronic pyelonephritis is operator-dependent, time-consuming and less reliable than IVP. Ultrasound is the first-line screening test for renal disease in hypertension.

Isotope renogram

This investigation is of undoubted value in the diagnosis and assessment of obstructive uropathy, particularly when combined with measurement of the drainage of the isotope from the kidney following administration of diuretic. In the context of the investigation of hypertension its main application is in the diagnosis of renal artery stenosis (see below).

Static renal isotope scan

^{99m}Tc dimercaptosuccinic acid is taken up by the proximal tubules and retained to give a static image of the renal parenchyma. It is the best technique for detecting and monitoring renal scars in the investigation of children with urinary tract infection or hypertension. It is more sensitive than the intravenous urogram and necessitates a much lower radiation dose. It is of much less value in adults. Since renal scarring is the common-

est cause of hypertension in children, this test should follow renal ultrasound in the investigation of children with hypertension.

Renal angiography

Renal angiography is necessary finally to exclude or confirm renal artery stenosis in the presence of suggestive clinical and radiological or renographic features.

The investigations outlined are arduous, expensive and carry some element of risk to the patient. In addition, they produce a low yield of patients with renal hypertension and an even lower yield of patients with correctable hypertension. The major decision to be taken is therefore whether to investigate rather than which tests should be applied.

Renovascular hypertension

Introduction

RVH is defined as hypertension caused by renal artery stenosis (RAS). RAS is not always functionally significant and is often found in normotensive patients being investigated for peripheral vascular disease. It may also be an 'incidental finding' without functional significance in patients with hypertension. There is no completely reliable means of determining the functional significance of RAS other than observing the effect on blood pressure of correcting the stenosis. This has led to RVH being defined as hypertension which is cured or improved by correction of RAS.

In the US approximately 17% of the population aged 18–74 years are hypertensive but only 1% have RVH. As long as blood pressure can be controlled and renal function remains stable, it is not vital to undertake tests to detect RVH but there are several advantages in making the diagnosis (Table 42.5). Against these advantages must be weighed the hazards and expense of investigation and interventional treatment involved. A conservative approach is often best, particularly in the elderly.

Table 42.4   Guidelines for the full investigation of hypertensive patients to exclude renal disease

1. Onset of hypertension before age 35 years
2. Severe or rapidly worsening hypertension
3. Clinical history or physical examination suggesting the presence of renal disease
4. Poor response to antihypertensive therapy
5. Intolerance of antihypertensive drugs
6. Prospect of pregnancy
7. Social indications, e.g. prejudice to employment if taking antihypertensive medication

---

Table 42.5   Advantages arising from the detection and correction of RAS in renovascular hypertension compared with medical treatment

1. In young patients hypertension may be cured
2. Even in older patients blood pressure control often improved
3. Number and dose of antihypertensive drugs can often be reduced with improved quality of life
4. Employment prospects and insurability improved
5. Prospects for pregnancy improved
6. In older patients atheromatous RAS is a major cause of renal failure, which in some patients may be preventable
7. ACE inhibitors and AII receptor blockers should be avoided before but may be given, if necessary, after correction of RAS

Clinical features of hypertension

Clinical history

There are no patient characteristics which reliably distinguish those with RVH. The clinical features which make renovascular disease more likely are listed in Table 42.1. Perhaps the commonest clinical clue is the development of impaired renal function following the administration of an ACE inhibitor.

Although it has been suggested that RVH is rare among Africans, in a study of patients selected for investigation on clinical grounds, the incidence in Africans and Caucasians did not differ [6].

Physical examination

There are some findings on physical examination which should raise the clinical suspicion of RVH. These are shown in Table 42.6. None is specific and in the majority of patients with RVH there is no clinical clue to its presence.

Simple screening tests

Most patients with RVH have normal plasma urea and creatinine levels and do not have proteinuria. Hypokalemia from secondary hyperaldosteronism is observed in approximately 15% of patients with RVH. Any asymmetry in renal size on ultrasonography is suggestive of RVH. A 1.5 cm difference in size is usually the upper limit of normal.

Selection by the clinical and simple laboratory screening tests outlined will increase the prevalence of RVH in a group of hypertensive patients from 1% to approximately 15% although some patients with RVH will be missed. The diagnostic yield from further investigation is relatively small and the therapeutic yield is even smaller. A prior decision should be made that intervention would be indicated if a suitable lesion were found before commencing any further tests. As discussed below, it is not proven that surgical intervention is superior to medical treatment in the patient with atheromatous renal artery stenosis.

Table 42.6 Features on physical examination suggestive of renovascular hypertension

1. Epigastric or costovertebral angle bruit
2. Lost or reduced peripheral pulses
3. Carotid bruit
4. Malignant hypertension
5. Neurofibromatosis

Pathophysiology of renal artery stenosis

In this section the pathophysiological consequences of RAS are discussed and in the next section the disease processes leading to it are described. The commonest consequence of RAS is hypertension. Bilateral RAS or stenosis of an artery to a single functioning kidney can result in renal failure or salt retention with pulmonary edema despite relatively good renal function. In 15–20% of patients, a hypokalemic metabolic alkalosis develops as a result of renin-stimulated hyperaldosteronism.

Hypertension

Hypersecretion of renin is the major pathogenetic factor in the development of hypertension in patients with unilateral RAS. Peripheral plasma renin levels are raised in only 50% of patients with RVH, but in the chronic stage of RVH there is an increased sensitivity to angiotensin II (AII). A significant positive correlation between plasma AII levels and arterial pressure has been reported in RVH, although the absolute levels of AII were lower than those required to achieve a similar level of hypertension with exogenous AII in normal subjects [7].

Renal failure

In unilateral renovascular disease plasma creatinine may not be increased, despite complete occlusion of the renal artery, because of compensatory hyperfiltration by the contralateral kidney. Renal function may also be preserved in bilateral renovascular disease because of an intrarenal compensatory mechanism. The reduction in renal plasma flow is detected by baroreceptors in the afferent arteriole (Figure 42.1), and local production of AII is stimulated which increases the glomerular filtration rate (GFR) and filtration fraction by efferent arteriolar constriction.

The effect of ACE inhibition uncovers the functional role of AII in RAS (Figure 42.2). The local physiological response is blocked, filtration pressure is reduced and GFR falls.

Many patients show no improvement in renal function following correction of RAS and often no moderation in the rate of decline of renal function. Reduced perfusion is therefore probably not the only factor in causing the renal impairment. Microembolization from the atheromatous plaque may be important. Perhaps more relevant is the fact that ischemic changes affect the proximal tubule as well as the glomerulus so progressive renal damage may be due to tubular ischemia, possibly related to AII-induced constriction of the efferent arteriole [8], and may be irreversible.

Pulmonary edema

Salt and water balance remain normal in unilateral RAS. The hemodynamic consequences of functionally significant RAS and the direct effect of AII on the tubule increase proximal tubular sodium reabsorption on the affected side (Figure 42.3). Secondary hyperaldosteronism increases distal tubular sodium reabsorption in both kidneys but contralateral pressure natriuresis maintains sodium balance. If both renal arteries are narrowed the balancing natriuresis is lost and salt retention develops. Diuretic resistant pulmonary edema may result despite normal left ventricular function. Intervention to correct the RAS can be very effective in preventing volume overload and improving renal function.

Hypokalemia

Secondary hyperaldosteronism and hypokalemia are present in many patients with RVH. Approximately 15% of patients have a serum potassium of less than 3.4 mmol/l [1].

Proteinuria

Mild proteinuria is frequent in RVH, occasionally being heavy in the absence of other glomerular pathology.

Treatment with an ACE inhibitor reduces proteinuria. Glomerular pore size (measured by dextran sieving analysis) is reduced by approximately 1 nm, suggesting that high AII levels are responsible for increased glomerular

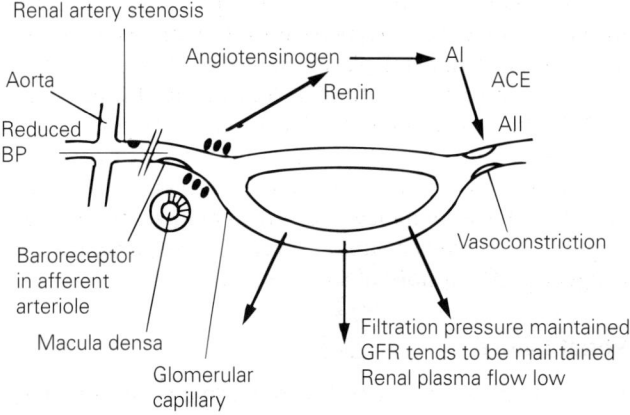

Figure 42.1 Intrarenal hemodynamic changes maintaining GFR in renal artery stenosis. ACE, angiotensin converting enzyme; AI, angiotensin I; AII, angiotensin II. (Redrawn, with permission, from ref. [1].)

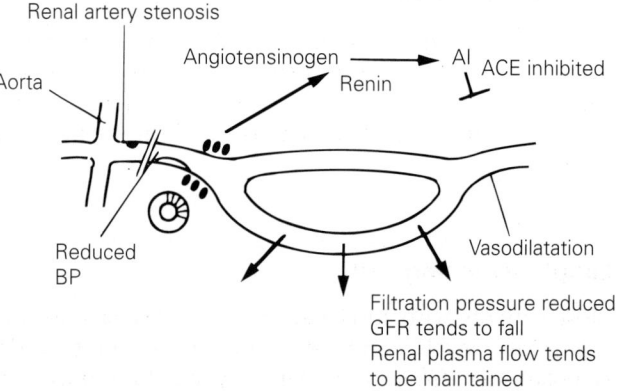

Figure 42.2 Following inhibition of ACE, glomerular pressure falls; despite the fall in renal vascular resistance there can be no increase in RPF.

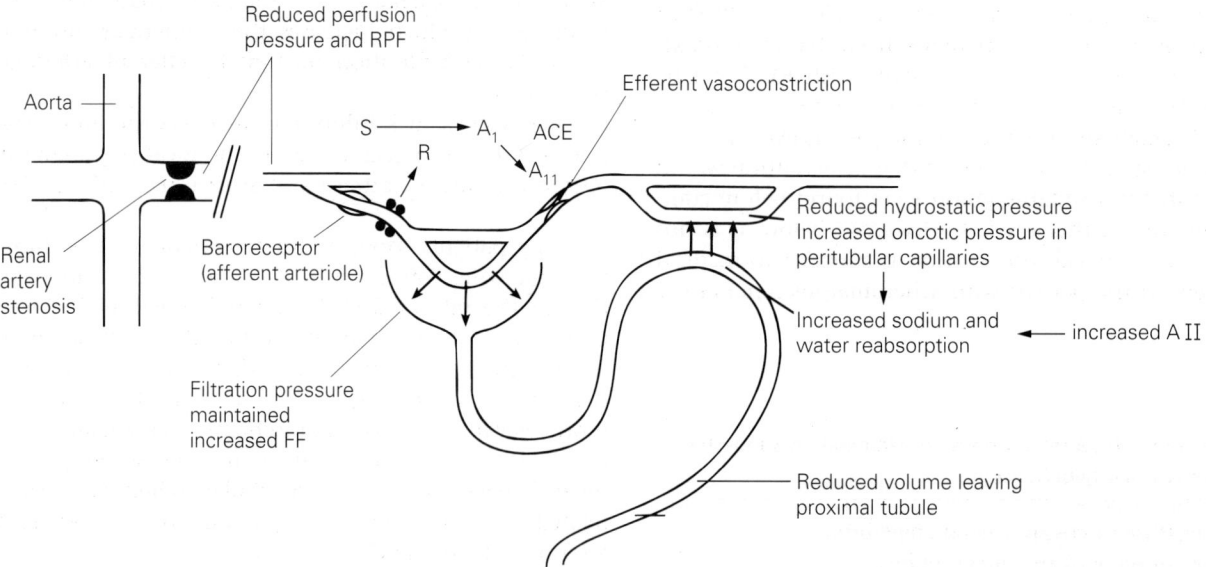

Figure 42.3 Intrarenal hemodynamic and hormonal changes in renal artery stenosis leading to sodium retention. In addition to hydrostatic and osmotic gradients facilitating proximal tubular sodium reabsorption, AII directly stimulates sodium reabsorption from the proximal tubule. FF, Filtration fraction; RPF, renal plasma flow; S, substrates (angiotensinogen); R, renin. (Redrawn, with permission, from Wilkinson, R. (1990) *Current Practice in Surgery*, Vol 2, Longman, London, pp. 38–46.)

permeability leading to proteinuria [9]. Indeed both plasma AII levels and proteinuria tend to be higher in patients with more severe RAS or occlusion of the renal artery. The effect of ACE inhibition is not simply due to its effect on blood pressure since other antihypertensive agents are less effective in reducing proteinuria.

Pathogenesis and natural history of renal vascular disease

General features

Several pathological processes may give rise to RAS. The relative incidence of the different conditions varies with the age and racial mix of the population (Table 42.7). In Western populations, atherosclerosis accounts for two-thirds of cases, predominantly in the elderly. The major cause in young people is fibromuscular dysplasia. Takayasu's arteritis is rare in the Caucasian population of Europe and US and more common in Asians. Rarely, RAS has been reported in association with pheochromocytoma and, very rarely, primary hyper-aldosteronism.

Histological examination of the renal vessels is generally not available unless the patient undergoes surgery. The diagnosis is based on radiological and clinical features.

Atheromatous RAS

This usually develops in patients with evidence of generalized atheromatous disease. The stenosis commonly affects the proximal portion of the renal artery (Figure 42.4). Atheromatous RAS is found in as many as half of patients undergoing angiography for peripheral vascular disease, many of whom are normotensive. Its presence in a hypertensive patient may not be of functional significance. Progression of RAS in this group occurs frequently, particularly in those with renal impairment at presentation or with severe stenosis.

Fibromuscular dysplasia (FMD)

In Western populations FMD is the commonest cause of RAS in young people, especially in females. Five different histological types are recognized: medial (65–75%), perimedal (10–25%) and intimal (10–15%) fibroplasia, medial hyperplasia (5–10%) and periarterial fibroplasia (<1%).

Medial fibroplasia (Figure 42.5) results in bands of renal artery fibrosis separated by dilated segments giving rise to the classical string of beads appearance. Occlusion of the renal artery is very rare. The process may involve other vessels including the abdominal aorta and the

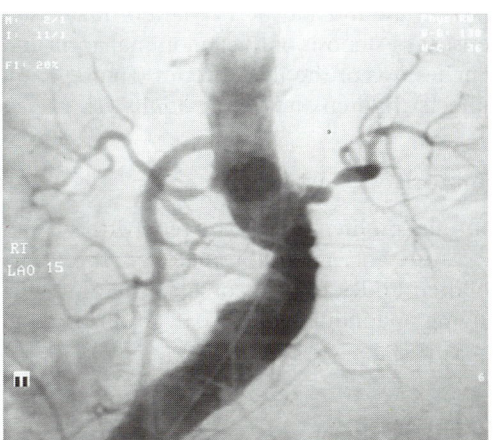

Figure 42.4 Atheroma of the renal arteries causing bilateral stenosis which is predominantly proximal. There is marked tortuosity and atheroma of the aorta. The patient, aged 70 years, presented with hypertension and mildly impaired renal function, plasma creatinine 190 μmol/l.

Table 42.7 Causes of renovascular hypertension

	Comments
1. Atherosclerosis	Male > female, elderly
2. Fibromuscular dysplasia	Female > male, young
3. Takayasu's arteritis	Young Asian females
4. Middle aortic syndrome	Young females
5. Neurofibromatosis	Children
6. Dissecting aortic aneurysm	
7. Dissection of renal artery	
8. Renal artery aneurysm	Usually part of (2)
9. Renal arteriovenous fistula	Usually following biopsy
10. Radiation arteritis	
11. Renal artery embolus	
12. Renal transplantation	
13. Extrinsic compression	Rare

carotid, coronary, femoral, iliac, popliteal, axillary, brachial and retinal arteries.

The etiology of fibromuscular disease is not understood; some consider it to be a low-grade arteritis.

Takayasu's arteritis

Takayasu's arteritis is a chronic inflammatory disease characterized by mononuclear cell infiltration and fibrous proliferation in the wall of the aorta and its major branches. This leads to stenosis or occlusion of the large vessels and coronary artery aneurysm. Although rare in Western populations, Takayasu's arteritis is a common cause of RAS in Asia, with a female:male ratio of 2.8:1 [10].

Middle aortic syndrome

This is a rare syndrome and may be a variant of Takayasu's arteritis. It consists of stenosis of the abdominal aorta and its major branches except the iliac arteries (Figure 42.6). It generally affects children and young adults [1].

Neurofibromatosis

RAS, due to intimal proliferation of the renal artery, is an uncommon feature of neurofibromatosis. It occurs usually in children under 16 years of age. There may be an accompanying abdominal aortic coarctation or renal artery aneurysm [11].

Renal artery aneurysm

Fusiform renal artery aneurysms although rare are quite common in patients with FMP. Saccular aneurysms (Figure 42.7), often at the bifurcation of the renal artery, however, most frequently occur in patients without FMP.

Hypertension can result from saccular aneurysms by several mechanisms, including renal ischemia due to turbulent flow, compression of the renal artery and emboli from thrombus within the aneurysm. Rupture of the renal artery aneurysm can occur during pregnancy but is rare.

Dissecting aneurysm of the aorta

In about one-fifth of hypertensive patients who develop dissection of the aorta, RAS predates the dissection [12]. In other patients the dissection may itself cause the RAS.

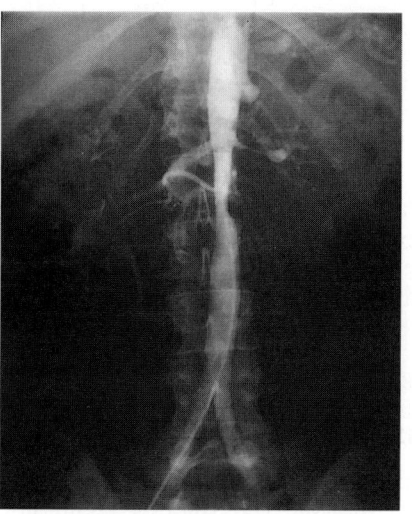

Figure 42.6 Aortogram in a woman aged 21 years with severe hypertension. There is aortic narrowing distal to the renal arteries with a very narrow left renal artery. This is an example of the 'middle aortic syndrome', a possible variant of Takayasu's arteritis. (Reproduced, with permission, from ref. [1].)

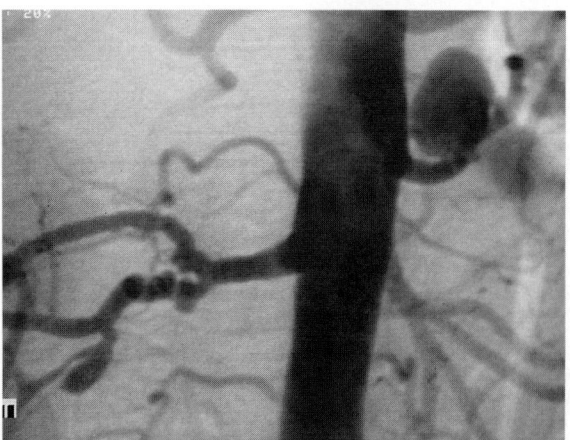

Figure 42.5 Medial fibroplasia in a hypertensive woman aged 43 years affecting predominantly the right renal artery. There is also, however, a saccular aneurysm of the left renal artery without evidence of stenosis of that artery.

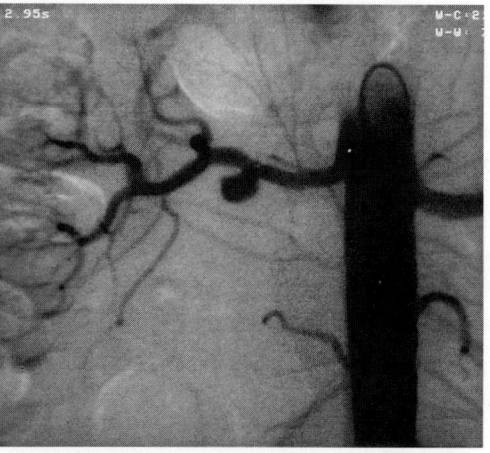

Figure 42.7 A saccular aneurysm of the right renal artery in a woman aged 38 years presenting with hypertension. (Reproduced, with permission, from ref. [1].)

Renal arteriovenous fistula

An arteriovenous fistula within the kidney usually announces itself with persisting hematuria following renal biopsy or trauma, although one quarter of fistulae are congenital. A systolic and diastolic bruit is often heard, raising the suspicion of RAS especially in the presence of hypertension. Ischemia of renal tissue distal to the fistula is thought to be responsible for the hypertension. Diagnosis is made by angiography which demonstrates early venous filling, as well as the fistula itself, and ischemia beyond the fistula (Figure 42.8).

Radiation arteritis

RAS may develop as a late complication of upper abdominal radiation, for example of para-aortic lymph glands in the treatment of conditions such as seminoma or lymphoma. Unlike postradiation nephritis this complication can be treated by angioplasty and the hypertension may be improved [13].

Extrinsic compression of the renal artery

This is a very uncommon cause of RAS. Fibrous bands are an extremely rare cause of external compression. Any tumor, including pheochromocytoma, can compress the renal artery. In the rare situation when RAS and pheochromocytoma co-exist, neurofibromatosis is the likely link. In this case RAS may be due to intimal proliferation rather than external compression.

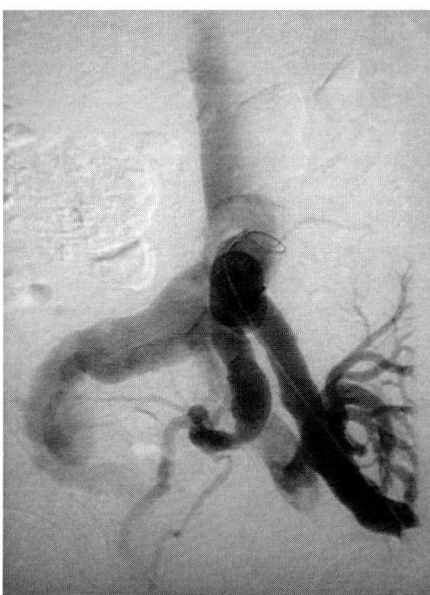

Figure 42.8 Renal arteriovenous fistula complicating renal biopsy in a renal transplant recipient. Contrast can be seen in the renal artery but also simultaneously in the renal vein due to early venous filling through the fistula.

Diagnosis of renovascular hypertension

General principles

In addition to the clinical history (Table 42.1) and physical examination (Table 42.6) which may give clues to the presence of RAS, certain features on simple screening make the diagnosis of RVH more likely. An increased plasma urea or creatinine not explained by known kidney disease, hypokalemia (usually without hypernatremia), and asymmetry of renal size on ultrasonography should raise the suspicion of RVH.

Specific tests for RVH are of three types. First, it may be necessary to apply additional specific screening tests. It may then be necessary to perform more invasive tests in selected patients to establish the diagnosis of anatomical RAS. Finally tests to assess the functional significance of RAS are widely used although they are of doubtful value.

Specific screening tests

Peripheral plasma renin activity (PRA)

PRA is increased in approximately 50% of patients with RVH and in up to 30% of those with essential hypertension. PRA is of no value in screening for RVH.

Captopril-stimulated PRA

Measurement of the PRA response to an ACE inhibitor has been used to increase the sensitivity and specificity of PRA measurement. Captopril-stimulated PRA is higher in renovascular disease than in essential hypertension. An upper limit of normal for this test has not been established, however, and almost all the commonly used antihypertensive drugs affect PRA levels; it is not feasible to withdraw these drugs in the majority of patients.

Tests to detect structural RAS

Rapid sequence IVP

The radiographic appearance of RAS is listed in Table 42.8 and Figure 42.9 demonstrates some features. In a meta-analysis of 20 studies, the sensitivity of the test was 75% and the specificity was 86% [14, 15]. The pathophysiology of the IVP changes in RAS are well understood. The reduction in renal size is due to reduced perfusion pressure although in long-standing cases it becomes irreversible as fibrosis develops. The delayed nephrogram is due to reduced renal blood flow. Hyperconcentration of the dye in the urine in the pelvis and calyces together with reduction in their volume is due to reduced tubule fluid flow from increased proximal tubular reabsorption of sodium and water upstream (Figure 42.3). This also accounts for the delayed washout of contrast. The patient

Table 42.8 Intravenous pyelography in renal artery stenosis

1. Reduced renal size
2. Delayed nephrogram
3. Hyperconcentration of contrast in later films
4. Reduced volume – 'spasticity' of renal pelvis
5. Delayed washout of contrast

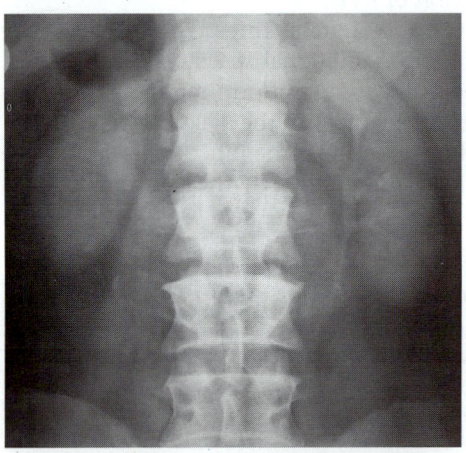

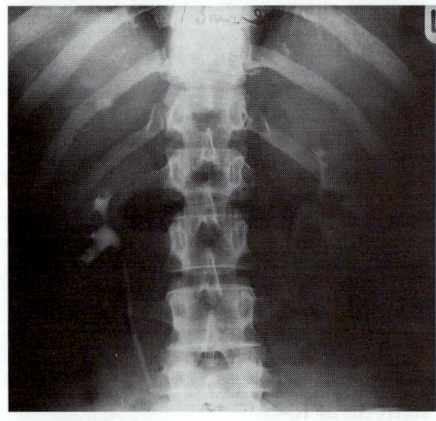

Figure 42.9 The IVP changes in a patient with right renal artery stenosis and hypertension. (a) Reduced renal length and delayed appearance of the pyelogram on the right in the 3 min film; (b) hyperconcentration on the right in the 15 min film. (Reproduced, with permission, from ref. [1].)

should not be dehydrated in preparation for the IVP because this delays washout of contrast from the renal pelvis on the non-affected side and may obscure differences between the two kidneys.

Magnetic resonance angiography

This technique avoids the need for X-ray and contrast media. It is useful in identifying stenoses within the

proximal 3 cm of the renal artery but may miss stenoses of branches [16]. At present it is not established for routine use.

Spiral computed tomography

This technique gives good visualization of the major renal vessels and correlates well with standard angiography. However, interpretation is more observer dependent than standard angiography [17] and is not yet recommended for routine use.

Renal angiography

Although this test provides no information regarding the functional significance of RAS, it is the 'gold standard' of structural information. Angiography defines the degree and site of stenosis and distinguishes atheroma from fibromuscular hyperplasia.

Femoral artery catheterization using the Seldinger technique is usually used, in patients with severe disease of the femoral or iliac vessels an approach via the axillary artery may be used to reach the renal vessels.

Intravenous digital subtraction angiography (IVDSA)

Femoral arterial puncture carries the risk of dissection, cholesterol embolus, arteriovenous fistula, false aneurysm and bleeding, particularly in older patients with atheroma. IVDSA has virtually replaced arterial puncture for visualization of the carotid arteries but has been less applicable in renal angiography. The contrast medium reaching the renal artery following the intravenous injection of a bolus of contrast medium, usually into a central vein, is in low concentration but can be visualized by computer subtraction of the preinjection image. Movement of the kidney with respiration may prevent the pre- and postinjection films from being superimposed and the subtracted image may be blurred. Bowel gas, obesity and overlying arteries can also interfere with the image. Central venous cannulation is not without risk and the larger volume of contrast required may be toxic. IVDSA has not gained widespread use in the investigation of hypertension.

Intra-arterial digital subtraction angiography (IADSA)

IADSA uses the same equipment as for IVDSA but the contrast is given by intra-aortic injection cephalad to the renal arteries. This enables much smaller volumes of contrast medium to be used than in conventional angiography. The findings by this technique correlate well with those of conventional angiography in the diagnosis of RAS [18].

Tests to detect the functional significance of renal artery stenosis

Isotope renography

A radiopharmaceutical which is filtered at the glomerulus and not significantly secreted or reabsorbed by the tubule, usually ^{99m}TcDTPA, is used for renography. With background subtraction to remove counts due to blood flow through the kidney, the curve generated by a normal kidney consists of a rapidly rising initial phase, representing glomerular filtration, reaching a peak as excretion of the isotope equals its accumulation by filtration. This is followed by a second phase as washout of the isotope exceeds filtration. In RAS the GFR is reduced and the upward slope of the curve is flattened. Because of increased proximal tubular sodium and water reabsorption (Figure 42.3) washout of ^{99m}TcDTPA is also reduced and as a result the peak is delayed and the downward slope of the excretory phase is also flattened (Figure 42.10a). Since the delayed washout can also be due to other conditions which increase distal reabsorption of sodium and water, the specificity of the renogram in the diagnosis of RAS can be improved by administering a loop diuretic which will reduce distal reabsorption without affecting proximal tubular reabsorption.

Captopril renography

The GFR may not fall detectably despite functionally significant RAS because of AII-mediated efferent arteriolar constriction, i.e. the isotope renogram is falsely negative. ACE inhibitors block this compensatory mechanism and improve the sensitivity of the renogram (Figure 42.10b). The use of captopril increased the sensitivity of the renogram from 71 to 91% without reducing specificity which remained at 95% [19]. Standard procedures and criteria have now been established which should enable a more reliable assessment of the value of the test in patients suspected of having RAS [20].

(a)

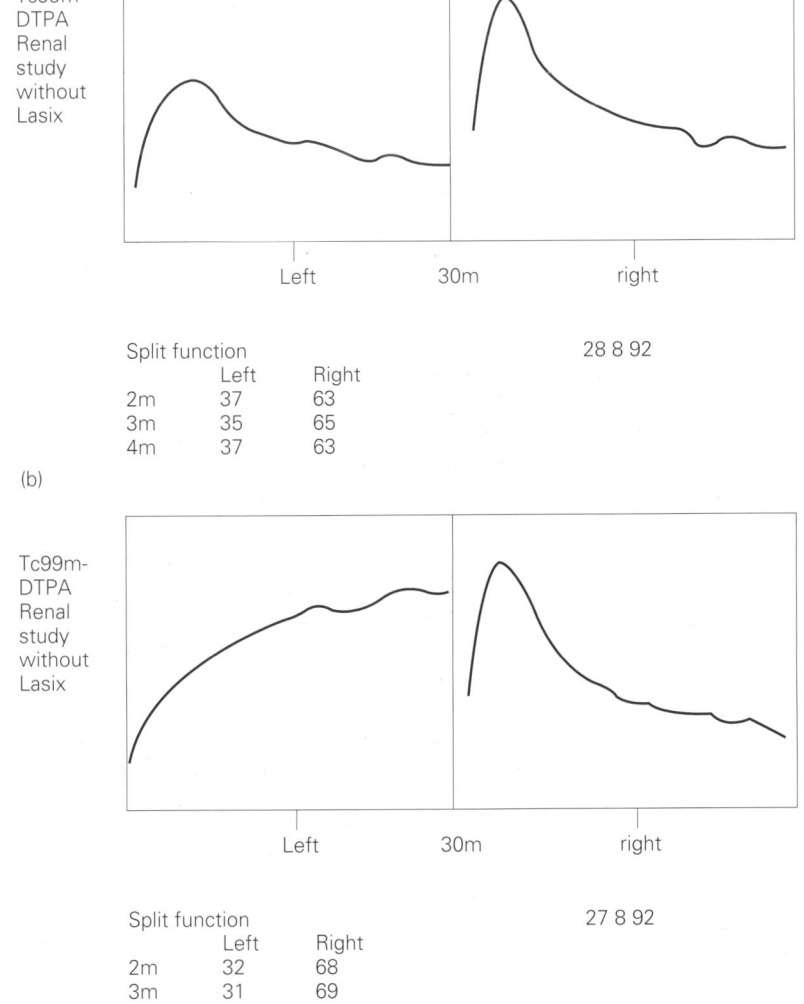

Figure 42.10 The isotope renogram in a man with left renal artery stenosis. (a) Without pretreatment with captopril, on the right there is an initial steep rise reflecting normal GFR, a sharp peak and a sharp fall indicating a brisk washout. On the left side the initial rise is slower, due to reduced GFR, and the peak is later and the washout slower due to reduced tubular flow. (b) Following captopril the right side remains normal but on the left the initial slope is flattened, indicating reduced GFR, and the washout phase is delayed beyond 30 min. (Reproduced, with permission, from ref. [1].)

Renal vein plasma renin ratio

It has been argued that an increase in the renal vein renin concentration on the affected side compared to the normal side (renal vein renin ratio) is the ultimate test of the functional significance of RAS. The plasma half-life of renin is long (30–45 min), however, so that renin in one renal vein may have originated in the other kidney. Thus, renal vein sampling must be done under active stimulation of renin to avoid the confounding effect of recirculation. Even with these techniques most studies have shown this test to have low specificity (around 70% [21, 22]) and sensitivity (around 65%) and it no longer has a place in the routine investigation of the patient with RAS.

Duplex Doppler ultrasonography

Blood flow velocity in the renal arteries can be measured by Doppler ultrasonography. However, the technique requires a high degree of operator skill and visualization of the renal arteries in some subjects may be difficult. Further assessment is required before it can be recommended for general use.

Proposed approach for the detection of RVH

A suggested approach to the investigation of hypertension is outlined in Table 42.9.

The IVP should follow clinical screening and abdominal ultrasound in a young female with hypertension in whom further investigation is indicated. Although 25% of patients with renal vascular disease will be missed, it remains the best test for the diagnosis of chronic pyelonephritis, which is the commonest cause of secondary hypertension in young women. In older patients and in young men, in whom chronic pyelonephritis is

Table 42.9 Approach for the diagnosis of renovascular hypertension[a]

In all patients
1. Clinical history
2. Physical examination
3. Urine analysis
4. Plasma creatinine and electrolytes

In selected patients
5. Abdominal ultrasound
6. a. Young females – rapid sequence IVP
   b. Males and older patients of both sexes – captopril renogram
7. Selective renal angiography

[a] The yield from investigation is low and only selected patients should undergo imaging investigation [5–7].

less likely, the captopril renogram with furosemide is preferred over the IVP.

Neither negative IVP nor renogram should preclude further investigation if clinically indicated. The next test is selective renal angiography with arterial puncture. If spiral CT scanning, magnetic resonance angiography or duplex Doppler examination are available they may be useful.

There are no reliable tests which predict the functional significance of RAS. The decision whether to intervene with either percutaneous angioplasty or surgery to correct stenosis is based on the clinical features.

Treatment of RVH

Medical treatment

Medical treatment does not differ from that of essential hypertension, except that AII converting enzyme inhibitors should be avoided if possible because of the risk of precipitating renal failure [23]. Multiple drug therapy is more commonly required in RVH than in essential hypertension.

The usual sequence of antihypertensive agents is diuretics followed by β-adrenergic blockers, long-acting preparations of calcium channel blockers, α-adrenergic blockers, methyldopa and, in resistant cases, minoxidil. In difficult cases, an ACE inhibitor may be used but only with careful monitoring of renal function. However, in unilateral RAS the loss of filtration on the affected side with ACE inhibitors may not be detected by monitoring plasma creatinine.

Percutaneous transluminal balloon angioplasty

This technique was first described in 1978 and is now the first-line treatment for the correction of RAS. Benefit following angioplasty occurs within a few days and is accompanied by a reduction in plasma renin. Correction of the stenosis is achieved in 50–90% of cases, and results are best in those patients with FMH. The success rate in dilating ostial lesions is relatively poor. Unfortunately, approximately 80% of atheromatous plaques are at the ostia or in the proximal one-third of the vessel. Success is also uncommon when the artery is occluded [1]. Preliminary results using a balloon-expandable stent for ostial lesions have been encouraging, although stenosis recurs in 30%. Stenting is now recommended in preference to angioplasty for ostial lesions [24].

Blood pressure response to angioplasty

Angioplasty is technically successful in 90% of patients with FMD and the blood pressure response in these patients is excellent, with cure of hypertension in 50% and improved blood pressure in another 40% [25]. In patients with atheromatous disease, however, the technical success rate is lower (56–100%, average 88%) and the blood pressure response is disappointing, even when the stenosis is fully corrected. In a single center study, 30% of patients were cured, 40% improved and 30% unchanged despite technically successful angioplasty [26]. There are no published prospective controlled trials comparing medical and interventional treatment to our knowledge. The preliminary results of a study in Scotland and the north of England suggest a slight advantage with intervention in controlling systolic blood pressure.

The assessment of the response to angioplasty is made difficult by the lack of an agreed definition of 'improvement' in blood pressure control. In the Cooperative Study of Renovascular Hypertension, improvement was defined as a decrease in diastolic blood pressure of 15% or more and a diastolic pressure of 91–109 mmHg without antihypertensive treatment. However, other studies have used a reduction in the number of antihypertensive agents without change in blood pressure as a definition of improvement.

Recurrence of renal artery stenosis

The reported recurrence rate of stenosis in the first year is around 15–20% for atheromatous disease and 5% for FMH.

Complications of percutaneous transluminal angioplasty

Serious complications are uncommon. They include renal artery occlusion or rupture and cholesterol emboli to the kidney, bowel or legs, myocardial infarction and stroke. The two latter conditions probably result from a profound fall in blood pressure. Overall mortality rate is approximately 1–2%, renal failure occurs in around 8%. Risks can be reduced by careful patient preparation for the procedure, reducing antihypertensive treatment beforehand and continuous monitoring during and following angioplasty to avoid hypotension. In the US, coronary and carotid atheromatous disease is often sought and corrected before renal artery surgery [27]; it may be that screening for these diseases and correcting them should also precede renal angioplasty.

Surgical correction of RAS

The results of surgery are very good in young patients with fibromuscular disease, Takayasu's arteritis or renal artery aneurysms. Hypertension is cured in 50–60% and improved in a further 30–35% of patients.

In atheromatous disease the results are generally much poorer. Hypertension is cured in only 20% and improvement in 60% of those with technically successful correction of stenosis. The long-term re-stenosis rate following successful surgery is approximately 20% at seven years [1].

Medical treatment or active intervention

Patients with FMD should be offered a corrective procedure since the risks are small and the results are good.

Overall, few hypertensives with atheromatous RAS are cured by intervention. The risks of correction are high and the renal vascular disease is usually not life-threatening. In fact patients often die of non-renal causes related to vascular disease elsewhere. On the other hand, progression of RAS to complete occlusion is common and generally silent. It remains to be determined whether intervention is worthwhile in atheromatous RAS. This will require large prospective trials. At present, a reasonable approach is to consider angioplasty or surgery in those cases in whom blood pressure control is unsatisfactory or renal function deteriorates. Even if renal function does not deteriorate, if the degree of stenosis exceeds 75% progression to total occlusion is probable and correction should be considered.

Survival of patients with renovascular disease

Patients with renovascular disease generally have vascular disease elsewhere. In a study from the Glasgow and Newcastle Hypertension Clinics, the 5- and 10-year survival of hypertensive patients with RAS was 83 and 67% compared to 90 and 79%, respectively, in those with essential hypertension. The excess deaths were mainly from coronary or cerebrovascular disease [28]. These results emphasize the need for careful studies of intervention; renal function is often not the limiting factor for survival and intervention may, in fact, increase the risk of death from other causes such as myocardial infarction and stroke.

Hypertension associated with chronic renal disease

Several aspects of hypertension in patients with chronic renal disease are covered elsewhere. The pathogenesis of hypertension is discussed in Chapter 31, and treatment of hypertension in Chapter 30. Hypertension in specific renal diseases is dealt with in chapters covering those diseases. In this section we will discuss the outcome of treatment of hypertension in chronic renal failure.

Outcome of antihypertensive treatment in chronic renal failure

Treatment of hypertension and cardiovascular risk

Cardiovascular disease accounts for 30–50% of deaths in patients with end-stage renal failure. Sustained hypertension and abnormalities of lipid metabolism, notably an increase in plasma triglycerides and reduction in high density lipoprotein (HDL) cholesterol, contribute to development of atherosclerosis.

Management of hypertension in patients with end-stage renal failure includes control of other risk factors, particularly plasma lipid abnormalities. Diuretics and β-blockers have adverse effects on plasma lipid metabolism whereas calcium channel antagonists and ACE inhibitors either have no effect or improve the lipid profile. These agents may have additional benefits when treating hypertension in patients with renal disease. However, diuretics used in low dose and highly cardioselective β-blockers have little adverse effects on lipids and may be used.

Interaction between hypertension, hyperlipidemia and renal damage

There is increasing evidence that the hyperlipidemia which frequently accompanies progressive renal disease contributes to glomerular injury. Animal studies have revealed that nephron injury can be aggravated by a high cholesterol intake [29]. Pharmacological treatment to reduce plasma lipids is associated with reduced glomerular injury and improved renal function [30]. Hyperlipidemia may alter vascular reactivity which could contribute to the development of hypertension and altered glomerular hemodynamic function. These observations reinforce the need to avoid the use of antihypertensive agents which have an adverse effect on plasma lipids.

Systemic hypertension and the kidney

The kidney plays a central role in the control of blood pressure and, conversely, is itself sensitive to a rise in blood pressure. This section will consider briefly these two issues.

No underlying cause for hypertension can be detected in 95% of patients with raised blood pressure and it must therefore be labeled as 'essential' or 'primary' hypertension. Although a strong genetic influence on human blood pressure has been recognized for many years, blood pressure does not segregate in families as a monogenic trait. Most studies of humans and experimental animals suggest that variation in blood pressure is secondary to the combined effects of many genes.

The role of the kidney in the pathogenesis of essential hypertension

Introduction

A few general statements should be made. Although three-quarters of current research is performed in experimental models, the relevance of the work to human essential hypertension is necessarily uncertain. There is a lack of data examining longitudinal changes in hemodynamic factors and renal function during the course of essential hypertension. Studies of adolescents with hypertension or adults with borderline hypertension may miss the initiating factors which become clouded by adaptive mechanisms. Within the population of patients with essential hypertension there may be variation in the importance of pathophysiological mechanisms at different stages.

This section will focus on the possible mechanisms of essential hypertension in which the kidney plays a major part.

Transplantation experiments

In the spontaneously hypertensive rat (SHR), cross-transplantation experiments have demonstrated that hypertension follows the kidney. If a kidney from a young rat of the normotensive strain is transplanted into a young rat of the hypertensive strain, before hypertension has developed, the blood pressure does not increase. Conversely, transplantation of a kidney from a hypertensive rat will result in a rise in blood pressure in a normotensive strain. A defect in renal sodium excretion is thought to be a major mechanism of hypertension in this rat strain [31].

Similar data are difficult to obtain in humans. In patients receiving renal transplants, the incidence of hypertension in the recipient is highest if the kidney originates from a donor with a familial predisposition to hypertension. Transplantation of kidneys from normotensive donors to patients with renal failure from malignant essential hypertension resulted in normotension in the recipients when the native kidneys were also removed [32].

Renal sodium retention – pressure natriuresis

In Western populations there is generally an excess of dietary sodium intake. It has been suggested that patients with essential hypertension are continuously correcting a slightly expanded extracellular fluid volume. The excessive dietary sodium intake is coupled with a defect in renal sodium excretion which leads to a disturbance of sodium handling in vascular smooth muscle, according to this theory.

Normal response to sodium loading

In normal subjects, as sodium intake increases, renal excretion of sodium rises to maintain an almost constant body sodium with very little change in blood pressure. The initial event is an increase in body sodium which results in a slight rise in blood pressure. Renin secretion is suppressed with a resultant fall in angiotensin formation and aldosterone secretion as well as release of atrial natriuretic peptide and possibly 'natriuretic hormone' an inhibitor of Na^+,K^+-ATPase. The fall in angiotensin production, in addition to reducing aldosterone secretion, leads to mesangial expansion and efferent arteriolar dilatation which result in an increased filtration coefficient and reduced filtration fraction, respectively. There is also a reduction in renal vascular resistance and an increase in renal blood flow. Efferent dilatation allows the transmission of increased pressure to peritubular capillaries. The reduced oncotic pressure of plasma in the efferent arteriole (due to the fall in filtration fraction) and the loss of the stimulating effect of AII on sodium reabsorption in the proximal tubule, combine to reduce proximal tubular sodium reabsorption. The increased filtration coefficient together with the increase in systemic blood pressure and afferent arteriolar dilatation result in an increase in filtered sodium and sodium excretion – a so-called pressure natriuresis. This sequence of events is illustrated in Figure 42.11a. In normal subjects ingesting the usual 'Western' diet of about 150 mEq of sodium per day, sodium balance is maintained with mean arterial pressure around 100 mmHg. Changes in dietary sodium intake have little effect on blood pressure.

Response to sodium loading in hypertensive subjects

The majority of patients with essential hypertension respond to sodium loading in the same way as normal subjects. Renal vascular resistance falls with afferent arteriolar dilatation, renal plasma flow rises and renin is suppressed resulting in efferent arteriolar dilatation and reduced proximal tubular sodium reabsorption (Figure 42.11b). In a subgroup of patients with hypertension (referred to as 'non-modulators'), renal vascular resistance does not fall and renin is not suppressed in response to sodium loading. In these patients sodium retention occurs until a rise in systemic pressure overcomes afferent resistance and is transmitted to the glomerular capillaries to cause a pressure natriuresis (Figure 42.11c). These patients have salt-sensitive hypertension ('non-modulators'). Those who are not salt sensitive ('modulators') do not require a substantial rise in blood pressure to maintain sodium balance in the face of increased sodium intake. In both groups increased renal venous tone in response to volume expansion may be important in reducing tubular sodium reabsorption. This increased tone may be mediated by the digoxin-like inhibitor of Na^+,K^+-ATPase (natriuretic hormone) released in response to volume expansion.

Treatment with ACE inhibitors can restore the response to sodium loading to normal in 'non-modulators', suggesting that the failure to suppress renin is of major importance in salt sensitivity.

Reduction in filtration surface area

It has been proposed [33] that hypertension may develop as a consequence of a primary reduction in the total number of nephrons or the filtration surface area per glomerulus. At any given glomerular pressure this would lead to reduced filtration of sodium resulting in salt retention and hypertension with restoration of sodium balance.

There is some evidence to suggest that Africans have a reduced number of nephrons and this may explain their increased susceptibility to hypertension and, because of glomerular hypertension, to hypertensive nephrosclerosis [34]. This remains an unproven hypothesis, however.

Nephron heterogeneity

Goldblatt's hypothesis was that essential hypertension was secondary to sclerosis of small intrarenal arterioles. He performed, now classical, experiments in dogs by clamping the main renal arteries. His work unraveled the pathophysiology of RAS but not that of essential hypertension. His hypothesis, however, formed the foundation for the work of Sealey and colleagues [35].

Sealey suggested that individuals with essential hypertension have nephron heterogeneity. A proportion of nephrons are ischemic and exhibit impaired sodium excretion. Other nephrons adapt with hyperfiltration and increased sodium excretion. The ischemic nephrons secrete renin which explains the normal renin levels in essential hypertension rather than the expected renin suppression by the raised blood pressure. The inappropriately high renin levels, through angiotensin and aldosterone, reduce sodium excretion in adjacent adapting nephrons by increasing tubular sodium reabsorption and enhancing tubuloglomerular feedback-mediated afferent arteriolar vasoconstriction. This hypothesis could explain the relative hyperreninemia of 'non-modulators'.

The renin–angiotensin system in essential hypertension

Plasma renin levels vary as a continuous variable in normal and hypertensive populations. Stimulation of renin release leads to sodium and water reabsorption in the kidney, vasopressin release, sympathetic nervous system stimulation and vasoconstriction. In addition to its role as a pressor hormone in hypertension, AII is an important growth factor.

Suppression of renin release and low levels of plasma renin activity would be expected in essential hypertension because of the effects of higher perfusion pressure in the afferent arteriole and the carotid sinus. In fact, approximately 20% of patients with essential hypertension have low plasma renin levels but most have normal or elevated plasma renin levels which could be secondary

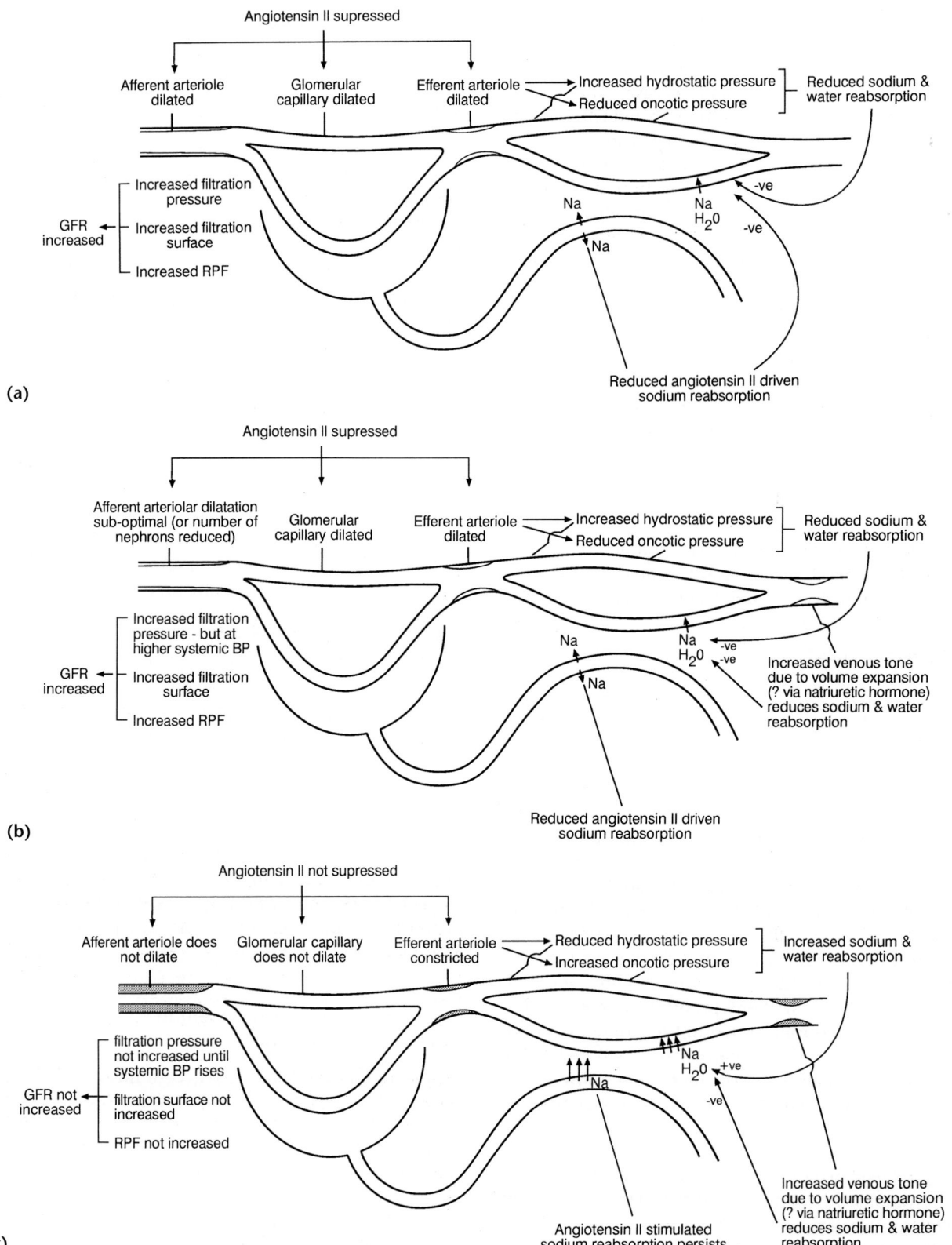

Figure 42.11   A simplified schema for the renal response to sodium loading in (a) normal subjects, (b) 'modulator' hypertensives, (c) 'non-modulator' hypertensives (see text).

to nephron heterogeneity (outlined above) or to enhanced sympathetic drive. An alternative explanation for the lack of suppression of renin in essential hypertension is a possible defective feedback mechanism. As discussed above inappropriate secretion of renin may be responsible for the sodium retention of non-modulators.

The essential hypertensive patients with low plasma renin are an interesting group. Possible mechanisms including volume expansion and mineralocorticoid excess have been excluded and plasma aldosterone levels are normal, not low. A possible explanation is that these subjects have increased adrenal cortical sensitivity to AII. To maintain normal aldosterone levels and volume control, less renin–angiotensin is required.

New techniques have allowed the molecular dissection of these peptide cascades. Conversion of circulating AI into AII is performed by ACE in the circulation and particularly in the lung. Tissue ACE is present in many organs including kidney, heart and blood vessels. There is evidence that a deletion polymorphism of the ACE gene, resulting in higher ACE levels, is associated with increased risk of myocardial infarction. Subsequent studies have not confirmed this finding and most studies show no association between high blood pressure and ACE polymorphisms.

Natriuretic peptide

The physiology of natriuretic peptides was described in a previous section. The role of natriuretic peptides in essential hypertension has been reviewed by Richards [36]. Plasma levels of atrial natriuretic peptide (ANP) and brain natriuretic peptide (BNP) are elevated in proportion to increasing blood pressure. There is an association of high natriuretic peptide levels with left ventricular hypertrophy. There is doubt, however, whether ANP is increased in mild uncomplicated essential hypertension. In the prehypertensive phase and in non-modulating hypertension (see above) there is an impairment in ANP secretion in response to increased AII or a rise in sodium intake.

The role of ANP in the pathogenesis of essential hypertension is uncertain. Modulation of the natriuretic peptide system using clearance receptor ligands or neutral endopeptidase inhibitors may offer a new therapeutic option in the management of established hypertension, however.

Conclusions

Although changes in renal physiology are linked to the pathogenesis of essential hypertension, the difficulties in studying them in a heterogeneous condition such as essential hypertension are clear. It is important to consider non-renal factors in essential hypertension including sympathetic nervous system activity, calcium metabolism, cell membrane abnormalities and resistance to insulin action.

The effect of essential hypertension on the kidney

Hypertensive nephropathy was the primary diagnosis in approximately 28% (9300 cases) of all patients beginning dialysis in 1988 in the US [37]. Between the ages of 20 and 59 years the rate in blacks was tenfold that in whites. The incidence of hypertension-related end-stage renal failure is increasing at an annual rate of 8.3%. This increase is largely due to the increasing acceptance of older patients for dialysis and to a greater readiness to attribute renal failure to hypertension rather than to 'cause unknown'. Nevertheless it is surprising when compared to the decline in cardiovascular deaths associated with better blood pressure control. This paradox can be partly explained by complications such as RVH, occlusive arterial disease, cholesterol emboli and interstitial nephropathy which are not directly related to blood pressure control. The adverse effects of accelerated or malignant hypertension on renal function are well established and are outlined briefly. This section then concentrates on the evidence suggesting that mild to moderate hypertension is associated with progressive renal disease.

Renal changes in malignant hypertension

The pathogenesis of malignant hypertension (MHT) has been discussed in Chapter 31 in relation to the changes in the optic fundus in patients with impaired renal function.

Clinical features

The definition of MHT has evolved over the years. The World Health Organization criteria, that the patient should have severe hypertension with bilateral fundal hemorrhages and exudates [38], are now generally accepted. The patient often presents with headache and in severe cases hypertensive encephalopathy, visual disturbance or breathlessness and is found to have retinal hemorrhages and exudates, with or without papilledema. Diastolic blood pressure is usually greater than 120 mmHg but in young people and those with rapid onset of hypertension MHT may occur at lower levels. Microscopic hematuria and/or proteinuria are usually present and renal function is often impaired and in severe cases acute oliguric renal failure may be the presenting feature.

Patients may present with microangiopathic hemolytic anemia (see below).

Pathology

Although the classical renal pathological change in MHT is of fibrinoid necrosis of the arteriolar wall (Figure 42.12), this may not be present. The fundamental change which

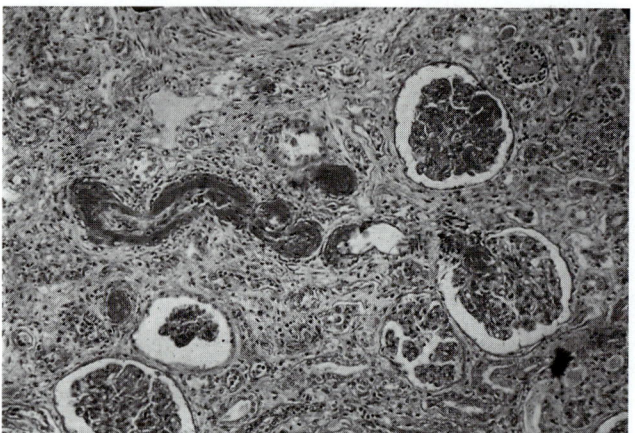

Figure 42.12 Malignant hypertension. Renal biopsy, haematoxylin and eosin × 250 mgn. An afferent arteriole showing necrosis of the wall and fibrinous exudation. The associated glomeruli contain fibrin thrombi.   (Courtesy Dr A R Morley.)

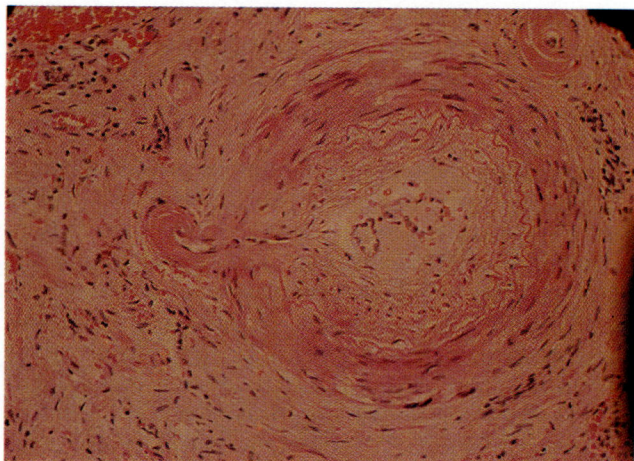

Figure 42.13 A hypertensive artery, hematoxylin and eosin × 250 mgn, narrowing due to subintimal proliferation and reduplication of the elastic laminae. Nearby small arteries and arterioles show marked hyalinization.   (Courtesy of Dr A R Morley.)

marks the transition from the benign to the malignant phase of hypertension is the transmission of the raised arterial pressure to the capillaries. This occurs when the intraluminal pressure is sufficient to overcome the capacity of the resistance vessels and can occur without histological evidence of disruption of the arteriolar wall. The increased pressure within glomerular capillaries, together with a possible direct effect of AII, increases capillary endothelial permeability so that fibrinogen can pass through the intima and even into Bowman's space. The presence of fibrin and possibly the direct effect of AII, leads to subintimal cellular proliferation in capillaries and interlobular arteries (Figure 42.13). These proliferative changes are similar to those seen in systemic sclerosis and may lead to occlusion of the small arteries and capillaries leading to permanent ischemic damage to the kidney.

When fibrinoid necrosis does occur it is thought to be due to disruption of the endothelium of the arteriole, from stretching, with passage of fibrin into the tissues of the vessel wall. In addition to the direct pressure effect and that of AII, it is thought that growth factors derived from platelets, which adhere to the damaged endothelium, may also contribute to the subintimal cellular proliferation. The adherent platelets may also trigger intravascular coagulation in patients with MHT.

Outcome

The treatment of malignant hypertension is often accompanied by an initial worsening of renal function due to reduced renal perfusion pressure. Renal function then usually stabilizes and thereafter may improve or very slowly deteriorate. In MHT due to essential hypertension progression of renal failure is usual if the plasma creatinine at presentation exceeds 300 μmol/l (mg/dl), but at levels below this renal function usually either stabilizes

or may improve with treatment [39]. An exception to this general rule is the syndrome of acute renal failure associated with malignant hypertension when there may be a gradual recovery of renal function, despite initial plasma creatinine levels far in excess of 300 μmol/l.

Before the advent of effective pharmacological therapy the survival of patients developing malignant hypertension was only 10% at one year, falling to almost zero by five years. With careful control of blood pressure and the availability of dialysis and renal transplantation five-year survival is now around 75% [40]. The predominant cause of death in patients with MHT is myocardial infarction [41].

Treatment

The major advance in the management of MHT over the past 30 years has been the realization that blood pressure should not be lowered too abruptly or too far. In the 1960s intravenous therapy was routinely used to lower blood pressure in MHT with often precipitous falls in blood pressure being achieved. Although this was usually surprisingly well tolerated it occasionally led to cerebral thrombosis or myocardial infarction. Even overvigorous oral antihypertensive therapy was not infrequently complicated by acute stroke.

Intravenous therapy for hypertension should be limited to those hemorrhage patients with hypertensive encephalopathy, dissecting aneurysm of the aorta, acute intracerebral hemorrhage, with pulmonary edema due to left ventricular failure (LVF) and to those patients unable to take drugs orally. LVF usually requires intravenous furosemide or bumetanide to treat the pulmonary edema and thereafter may be treated with orally administered drugs. Encephalopathy, if mild, may also be treated with bed rest and oral drugs but more severe cases require intravenous therapy, ideally with sodium nitroprusside (SNP). SNP has a rapid onset and short duration of action, each of only a few minutes; its administration requires constant supervision to achieve the required rate of reduction in pressure. SNP is difficult to use, since it requires the full-time attention of a nurse, it must be made up freshly before use, it is inactivated by light and has a toxic metabolite, thiocyanate, which should be measured daily if treatment extends beyond 48 h. Thiocyanate is excreted by the kidney and this limits the use of SNP in patients with renal impairment. When SNP is used it is usual to introduce a low dose of an orally acting antihypertensive agent at the outset so that prolonged treatment with SNP is not necessary.

Other antihypertensive drugs can be given intravenously in hypertensive emergencies but their more prolonged action increases the risk of inducing excessive hypotension. Hydrallazine is used in severe preeclampsia and eclampsia but rarely in other situations. Labetalol and diazoxide have both been used as repeated mini-boluses intravenously but may cause profound hypotension despite individual boluses being small. Nitrates must be given by continuous infusion and like nitroprusside require intensive monitoring. Nicardipine, a calcium channel blocker, can be given intravenously and appears less likely than the other drugs to cause excessive hypotension.

Oral therapy is appropriate for most patients with MHT. However, even oral therapy may induce excessive falls in blood pressure and be complicated by stroke. Target blood pressure for the first week should usually be around 180/110 mmHg and thereafter slowly reduced to 140–160 mmHg systolic and 80–90 mmHg diastolic over three months. This allows time for autoregulation of cerebral blood flow to reset and reduces the risk of stroke.

There has been a vogue for the use of sublingual nifedipine in the treatment of severe hypertension but this does occasionally cause severe hypotension and it is no longer recommended.

The majority of patients with malignant hypertension are best treated with bed rest and low initial doses of standard antihypertensive drugs. These drugs include β-adrenoreceptor blockers, calcium antagonists, labetalol and methyldopa; the combination of these drugs with a diuretic improves their effectiveness. ACE inhibitors may also be used but are usually avoided as initial therapy since up to 30% of patients with MHT will have underlying renal artery stenosis. The exception is scleroderma crisis when ACE inhibitor therapy is first choice.

Renal changes in benign essential hypertension

Clinical data

It is always difficult to be certain in a patient with hypertension and deteriorating renal function that there was no primary renal disease. In the absence of other conditions, increased serum creatinine with time is more pronounced in mild hypertensive than normotensive subjects [42]. The data from the Multiple Risk Factor Intervention Trial (MRFIT) have been examined for an association between baseline blood pressure and renal function [43]. A decline in renal function was greatest among those with elevated systolic or diastolic blood pressure, older individuals and blacks. Effective blood pressure control improved or stabilized renal function in all races except blacks.

Nephrosclerosis is the histological consequence of hypertension (see below). Using the UK MRC Glomerulonephritis Registry, 2.5% of all renal biopsies were classified solely as benign hypertensive nephrosclerosis [44]. Severe uremia and significant proteinuria can also be a consequence of nephrosclerosis. In the study by Rostand et al. [45], loss of renal function was noted in 15% of patients with essential hypertension. Elevated blood pressure causes a slow deterioration in renal function, usually becoming clinically evident in old age. The incidence of hypertensive nephrosclerosis is four to five times higher among blacks.

Pathology of renal disease associated with essential hypertension

The typical renal changes in essential hypertension at the time of biopsy or autopsy are the vascular changes of nephrosclerosis. Chronic hypertension is associated with structural changes affecting the endothelium, intima and the vascular smooth muscle cell layer. The afferent arterioles, interlobular and arcuate small arteries are particularly affected. The major pathological changes are shown in Figure 42.14.

Renal hemodynamic changes in essential hypertension

It is difficult to determine whether the renal hemodynamic changes observed in essential hypertension are a cause or the consequence of hypertension. In a comparison of the normotensive offspring of two hypertensives with those of two normotensive parents, those with hypertensive parents, and therefore themselves possibly 'prehypertensive', had lower RPF, increased renal vascular resistance and increased filtration fraction [46]. This suggests a primary increase in efferent arteriolar resistance in essential hypertension.

In established essential hypertension the increased renal vascular resistance persists but RPF and GFR are further reduced in parallel [47], suggesting an increase in afferent as well as efferent arteriolar resistance. This increase in afferent constriction may be a consequence of raised systemic pressure. However, fractional sodium excretion is increased in established essential hypertension which cannot be explained by either afferent or efferent arteriolar constriction [48]. It has been suggested that constriction of the renal venules may be responsible for the observed increase in fractional sodium excretion.

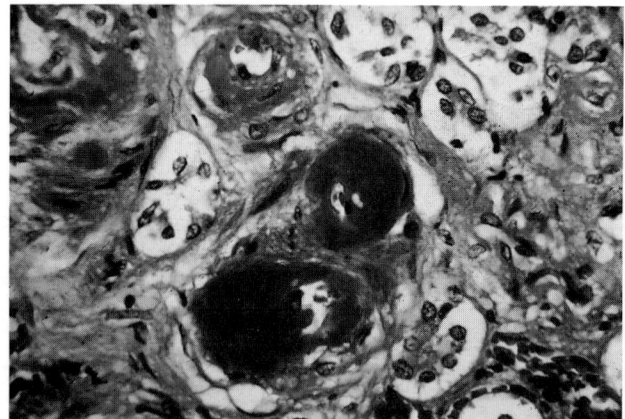

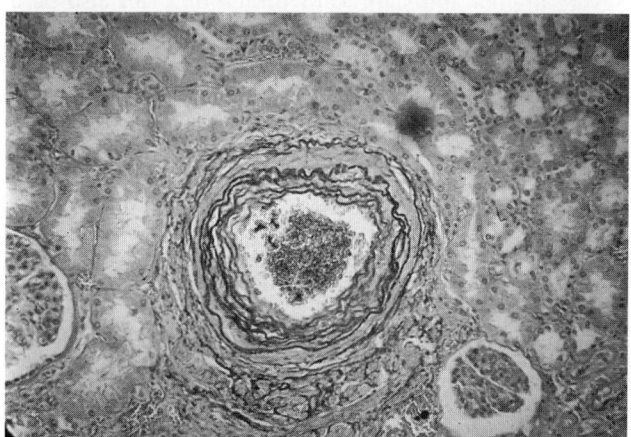

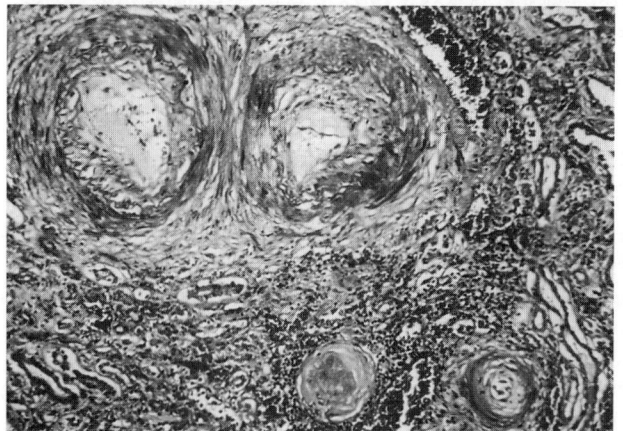

Figure 42.14   The renal histological changes in essential hypertension. (a) Arteriolar hyalinosis with irregular deposition of homogeneous eosinophilic material in the subendothelial space; (b) fibroblastic intimal thickening and wastage of the media with acquisition of an inner layer of fibroblastic tissue and additional elastic laminae; (c) metaplastic replacement of the muscular tissue with sclerotic tissue. (Photographs kindly supplied by Dr A.R. Morley.)

The heterogenity of 'essential hypertension' is illustrated by the observation that some young hypertensives have increased RPF [49]. Whatever the initial value RPF falls with the duration and severity of hypertension as

well as with age. The rate of fall with age is steeper in hypertensives than in those with normal pressure [47]. In established hypertension the pattern is of reduced RPF, a lesser reduction in GFR and increased filtration fraction. At this stage in the disease it seems likely that the intrarenal hemodynamic changes include angiotensin-induced efferent constriction, certainly in the 'non-modulators' (see above), since ACE inhibitors restore the ability of these patients to excrete a sodium load.

The implications of these observations are that the ideal drug treatment of essential hypertension may depend on the subgroup to which the patient initially belongs, modulator or non-modulator, and on the duration of the hypertension.

Albuminuria in essential hypertension

Around 40% of patients with essential hypertension have microalbuminuria, defined as an albumin excretion rate of $\geq 30\,mg/24\,h$. This abnormality was first described in patients with type I (insulin-dependent) diabetes mellitus where it is a predictor of the development of progressive renal failure. In patients with essential hypertension, microalbuminuria is an independent predictor of cardiovascular morbidity and mortality. It is not known whether microalbuminuria represents an early sign of renal damage or simply predicts progressive renal disease.

The effect of treatment on renal function

Progression of renal damage may occur in essential hypertension despite what is considered good control of blood pressure, suggesting that the generally accepted target blood pressure of 140/90 mmHg may not be sufficiently low to protect the kidney. In patients with primary renal disease there is some evidence to suggest that lower levels of blood pressure may be renoprotective. In one study mean arterial pressure (MAP) <100 mmHg was associated with slower progression of renal disease; in another, patients with renal disease with MAP 92 mmHg progressed more slowly than those with MAP 97 mmHg [50]. These lower levels of blood pressure may be necessary to protect the kidney in essential hypertension.

If glomerular hypertension is a major determinant of renal damage then ACE inhibitors, which, in addition to lowering systemic blood pressure, reduce glomerular pressure by reducing efferent arteriolar resistance, may be particularly effective in protecting the kidney. This presumes that there is AII-induced efferent constriction, which as discussed above is not certain. To our knowledge, no prospective controlled studies have been reported, confirming a specific beneficial effect of ACE inhibitors on renal function in essential hypertension. Other drugs such as calcium antagonists may be equally effective, if the site of postglomerular increased resistance proves to be not in the efferent arterioles but in the venules and if the constriction in the latter is not dependent on angiotensin.

It may be the degree of renal impairment at initiation of therapy, rather than the nature of the antihypertensive agent, that determines outcome. In the hypertension, detection and follow-up programme, progression was found in 27% of patients with initial plasma creatinine >200 μmol/l (1.7 mg/dl) compared to only 2% of those whose plasma creatinine was lower [51].

Conclusions

Hypertension causes renal damage and a progressive increase in renal vascular resistance. Sufficient damage to cause end-stage renal failure has become a major clinical problem despite aggressive antihypertensive therapy which lowers cardiovascular risk. Further studies are necessary to define the pathogenesis of renal disease in essential hypertension and to understand why blacks, the elderly and the obese are more likely to develop end-stage renal failure. The increased understanding may point the way to therapy which will prevent renal damage or retard its progression.

References

1. Wilkinson, R. (1994) Renal and renovascular hypertension, in *Textbook of Hypertension* (ed. J.D. Swales), Blackwell, Oxford.
2. Brown, A.L. and Wilkinson, R. (1996) Clinical approach to hypertension, in *The Oxford Textbook of Nephrology* (eds J.S. Cameron, A.M. Davison, J.P. Grunfeld, D.N.S. Kerr and E. Ritz), Oxford University Press, Oxford.
3. Viberti, C.G. (1987) Raised arterial pressure in parents of proteinuric insulin-dependent diabetics. *Br. Med. J.*, **295**, 515–17.
4. Khaw, K.T. (1982) Blood pressure and contraceptive use. *Br. Med. J.*, **285**, 403–7.
5. Puddey, I.B., Beilin, L.J., Vandongen, R. *et al.* (1985) Differential effects of sulindac and indomethacin on blood pressure in treated hypertension subjects. *Clin. Sci.*, **69**, 327–36.
6. Svetkey, L.P., Kadir, S., Dunnick, N.R. *et al.* (1991) Similar prevalence of renovascular hypertension in selected blacks and whites. *Hypertension*, **17**, 678–83.
7. Brown, J.J., Casals-Stenzel, J., Cumming, A.M.M. *et al.* (1979) Angiotensin II, aldosterone and arterial pressure: a quantitative approach. *Hypertension*, **1**, 159–79.
8. Marcussen, N. (1991) Atubular glomeruli in renal artery stenosis. *Lab. Invest.*, **65**, 558–65.
9. Remuzzi, A., Schieppati, A., Battaglia, C. and Remuzzi, G. (1989) Angiotensin converting enzyme inhibition ameliorates the defect in glomerular size selectivity in hyponatremic hypertensive syndrome. *Am. J. Kidney Dis.*, **14**, 170–7.
10. Liu, L.S. and Zheng, D.Y. (1990) Aortoarteritis: a report of 480 cases. *J. Hum. Hypertens.*, **4**, 135–7.
11. Kuo, J.Y., Okada, Y., Takeuchi, H. *et al.* (1989) Neurofibromatosis associated with renovascular hypertension due to stenosis and aneurysm of the left renal segmental artery: report of a case. *Urol. Int.*, **44**, 177–80.
12. Rackson, M.E., Lossef, S.V. and Sos, T.A. (1990) Renal artery stenosis in patients with aortic dissection: increased prevalence. *Radiology*, **177**, 555–8.
13. Milutinovic, J., Darcy, M. and Thompson, K.A. (1990) Radiation-induced renovascular hypertension successfully treated with transluminal angioplasty: case report. *Cardiovasc. Intervent. Radiol.*, **13**, 29–31.
14. Havey, R.J., Krumlovksy, F., delGreco, F. and Martin, H.G. (1985) Screening for renovascular hypertension: is renal digital-subtraction angiography the preferred noninvasive test? *JAMA*, **254**, 388–92.
15. Thornby, J.R., Stanley, J.C. and Fryback, D.G. (1982) Hypertensive urogram: a non-discriminating test for renovascular hypertension. *Am. J. Roentgenol.*, **138**, 43–9.
16. Loubeyre, P., Revel, D., Garcia, P. *et al.* (1994) Screening patients for renal artery stenosis: value of three-dimensional time-of-flight MR angiography. *Am. J. Roentgenol.*, **162**, 847–52.
17. Rubin, G.D., Dake, M.D., Napel, S. *et al.* (1994) Spiral CT of renal artery stenosis: comparison of three-dimensional rendering techniques. *Radiology*, **190**, 181–9.
18. Kim, D., Porter, D.H., Brown, R. *et al.* (1991) Renal artery imaging: a prospective comparison of intra-arterial digital subtraction angiography with conventional angiography. *Angiology*, **42**, 345–57.
19. Mann, S.J., Pickering, T.G., Sos, T.A. *et al.* (1991) Captopril renography in the diagnosis of renal artery stenosis: accuracy and limitations. *Am. J. Med.*, **909**, 30–40.
20. Oei, H.Y. (1991) Captopril renography, early observations and diagnostic criteria. *Am. J. Hypertens.*, **4**(suppl 12, part 2), 678S–84S.
21. Sellars, L., Shore, A.C. and Wilkinson, R. (1985) Renal vein renin studies in renovascular hypertension: do they really help? *J. Hypertens.*, **3**, 177–81.
22. Geyskes, G.G., Oei, H.Y., Klinge, J. *et al.* (1988) Renovascular hypertension: the small kidney update. *Q. J. Med.*, **66**, 203–17.
23. Farrow, P.R. and Wilkinson, R. (1979) Reversible renal failure during treatment with captopril. *Br. Med. J.*, **1**, 1680.
24. Dorros, G., Prince, C. and Mathiak, L. (1993) Stenting of a renal artery stenosis achieves better relief of the obstructive lesion than balloon angioplasty. *Cathet. Cardiovasc. Diagn.*, **29**, 191–8.
25. Wise, K.L., McCann, R.L., Dunnick, R.N. and Paulson,

D.F. (1988) Renovascular hypertension. *J. Urol.*, **140**, 911–24.

26. Ramsay, L.E. and Waller, P.C. (1990) Blood pressure response to percutaneous transluminal renal angioplasty for renovascular hypertension: an overview of published series. *Br. Med. J.*, **300**, 569–72.

27. Novick, A.C., Straffon, R.A., Steward, B.H. *et al.* (1981) Diminished operative morbidity and mortality in renal vascularization. *JAMA*, **246**, 749.

28. Isles, C., Main, J., O'Connell, J. *et al.* (1990) Survival associated with renovascular disease in Glasgow and Newcastle: a collaborative study. *Scott. Med. J.*, **35**, 170–3.

29. Kasizke, B.C., Kim, Y., O'Donnell, M.P. *et al.* (1991) Cholesterol mediated glomerular injury: influence of age, glomerular macrophages, growth and mesangial matrix. *J. Am. Soc. Nephrol.*, **2**, 682–6.

30. Keane, W.F., Kasizke, B.C. and O'Donnell, M.P. (1988) Hyperlipidemia and the progression of chronic renal disease. *Am. J. Clin. Nutr.*, **47**, 157–60.

31. Bianchi, A., Fox, V., Difrancesco, G.F. *et al.* (1974) Blood pressure changes by kidney cross transplantation between spontaneously hypertensive rats and normotensive rats. *Clin. Sci. Mol. Med.*, **47**, 435–48.

32. Curtis, T.T., Luke, R.G. and Duston, H.P. (1983) Remission of essential hypertension after renal transplantation. *N. Engl. J. Med.*, **309**, 1009–15.

33. Brenner, B.M., Gavicra, D.C. and Anderson, S. (1988) The renal abnormalities in hypertension: a proposed defect in glomerular filtration surface area. *Am. J. Hypertens.*, **6**, 335–47.

34. McCellon, W., Tuttle, E. and Issa, A. (1989) Racial differences in the incidence of hypertensive end-stage renal disease (ESRD) are not entirely explained by differences in the prevalence of hypertension. *Am. J. Kidney Dis.*, **13**, 484–93.

35. Sealey, J.E., Blumenfield, T.D., Bell, G.M. *et al.* (1988) On the renal basis for essential hypertension: nephron heterogeneity with discordant renin secretion and sodium excretion causing a hypertensive vasoconstriction volume relationship. *J. Hypertens.*, **6**, 763–77.

36. Richards, A.M. (1994) The natriuretic peptides and hypertension. *J. Intern. Med.*, **235**, 543–60.

37. US Renal Data System Report (1990) Annual Report III. Causes of end-stage renal disease. *Am. J. Kidney Dis.*, **16**(suppl 2), 22–8.

38. World Health Organization (1978) Arterial hypertension. *WHO Tech. Rep. Ser.*, **628**, 57.

39. Isles, C.G. (1988) Malignant hypertension, in *New Clinial Applications – Nephrology: Management of Renal Hypertension* (ed. G.R.D. Catto), MTP Press, Lancaster, pp. 41–78.

40. Isles, C.G., Lim, K.G., Bouton-Jones, M. *et al.* (1985) Factors influencing outcome in malignant hypertension. *J. Hypertens.*, **3**(suppl 3), S405–7.

41. Webster, J., Petrie, J.C., Jeffers, T.A. and Lovell, H.G. (1993) Accelerated hypertension – patterns of mortality and clinical factors affecting outcome in treated patients. *Q. J. Med.*, **86**, 485–93.

42. Rossansky, S.J., Hoover, D.R., King, L. and Gibson, T. (1990) The association of blood pressure levels and changes in renal function in hypertensive and non-hypertensive subjects. *Arch. Intern. Med.*, **150**, 2073–6.

43. Walker, W.G., Neaton, J.D., Culler, J.A. *et al.* (1992) Changes in serum creatinine in hypertensive patients in the Multiple Risk Intervention Trial (MRFIT). Evidence that lowering blood pressure protects renal function in mild to moderate hypertension. *JAMA*, **268**, 3085–91.

44. Innes, A., Johnston, P.A., Morgan, A.G. *et al.* (1993) Clinical features of benign hypertensive nephrosclerosis at time of renal biopsy. *Q. J. Med.*, **86**, 271–5.

45. Rostand, S.G., Brown, G., Kirk, K.A. *et al.* (1989) Renal insufficiency in treated essential hypertension. *N. Engl. J. Med.*, **320**, 684–8.

46. van Hooft, I.M.S., Grobbee, D.E., Dertex, F.H.M. *et al.* (1991) Renal hemodynamics and the renin–angiotensin–aldosterone system in normotensive subjects with hypertension and normotensive parents. *N. Engl. J. Med.*, **324**, 1305–11.

47. London, G.M., Safar, M.E., Sassard, J.E. *et al.* (1984) Renal and systemic hemodynamics in sustained essential hypertension. *Hypertension*, **6**, 743–54.

48. London, G.M., Levenson, J.A., London, A.M. *et al.* (1984) Systemic compliance, renal hemodynamics and sodium excretion in hypertension. *Kidney Int.*, **26**, 342–50.

49. Hollenberg, N.K., Bonicki, L.J. and Adams, D.F. (1978) The renal vasculature in early essential hypertension: evidence for a pathogenetic role. *Medicine*, **57**, 167–78.

50. Klahr, S. (1989) The kidney in hypertension. Villain and victim. *N. Engl. J. Med.*, **320**, 731–3.

51. Shulman, N.B., Ford, C.E., Hall, W.D. *et al.* (1989) Prognostic value of serum creatinine and effect of treatment of hypertension on renal function. *Hypertension*, **132**(suppl 1), 180–93.

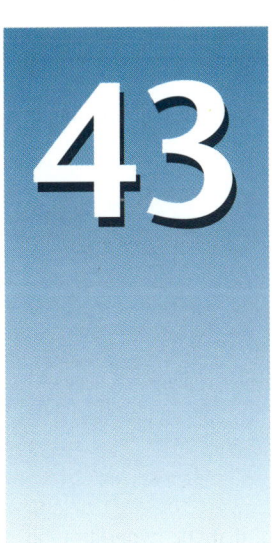

Diabetic nephropathy

Roberto Trevisan, James D. Walker and
GianCarlo Viberti

Introduction

Clinical diabetic nephropathy is defined by the presence of persistent proteinuria (urinary albumin excretion rate greater than 300 mg/day) in sterile urine of diabetic patients with concomitant retinopathy and elevated blood pressure, but without other renal disease or heart failure. Once manifest, diabetic nephropathy is characterized by a progressive decline in renal function, resulting in end-stage renal disease (ESRD). Histological changes of diabetic glomerulopathy are present in over 96% of insulin-dependent diabetic (IDDM) patients with clinical proteinuria and in approximately 85% of non-insulin-dependent diabetic (NIDDM) patients who develop proteinuria with concomitant retinopathy. In the absence of retinopathy 30% of proteinuric NIDDM patients have a non-diabetic renal lesion.

Between 25 and 50% of diabetic patients develop kidney disease although a smaller percentage require dialysis or kidney transplantation. The mortality from all causes in diabetic patients with nephropathy is 20–40 times higher than that of patients without nephropathy. Diabetic nephropathy is now the single most common cause of renal failure in the Western World and in some countries diabetic patients represent up to one-third of all patients entering renal replacement treatment programs.

In the United States the health-care cost for diabetic patients in renal failure exceeded $2 billion in 1993.

Natural history and clinical course of diabetic nephropathy in insulin-dependent diabetic patients

The evolution of diabetic nephropathy proceeds through several distinct but interconnected phases: an early phase of physiologic abnormalities of renal function, a 'microalbuminuria phase', and a clinical phase with persistent clinical proteinuria progressing to end-stage renal failure (Table 43.1).

Early renal abnormalities

After diagnosis of diabetes a clinically silent phase of variable duration occurs and during this period many renal abnormalities have been described.

Supranormal values of glomerular filtration rate (GFR greater than $135 \, ml/min/1.73 \, m^2$), often coupled with raised renal plasma flow, are found in approximately 20–40% of diabetic patients. Hyperfiltration is partially related to the degree of metabolic regulation; intensified

Nephrology, Edited by Rex L. Jamison and Robert Wilkinson.
Published in 1997 by Chapman & Hall, London. ISBN 0 412 60930 4

Table 43.1 Phases of diabetic nephropathy

Phase of disease progression	Urinary albumin excretion rate (µg/min)	Glomerular filtration rate	Blood pressure
Normoalbuminuria	<20	Normal or elevated	Increasing
Microalbuminuria	20–200	Normal or elevated	Rising further
Overt proteinuria	≥200	Decreasing	Elevated
Renal failure	≥200	Reduced	Elevated

insulin therapy with improvement of blood glucose control reduces GFR toward normal values [1]. These hemodynamic abnormalities are associated with an increase in kidney size which appears to be a prerequisite for the occurrence of glomerular hyperfiltration. Although normal GFR can be found in patients with large kidneys, supranormal GFR is exceptional in patients with normal kidney size. The prognostic significance of nephromegaly remains unclear.

Elevated GFR has been implicated in the initiation and progression of renal disease. There is convincing evidence in animal models of diabetes that hemodynamic factors, in particular intraglomerular pressure, play an important role in the development of glomerulopathy. In this regard, it is of note that in the presence of unilateral renal artery stenosis and systemic hypertension, diabetic glomerulopathic lesions seem confined to the non-stenosed kidney [2]. However, the prognostic significance of glomerular hyperfiltration remains controversial in humans. In small groups of selected 'hyperfiltering' patients two retrospective studies have shown a correlation between the initial high GFR and the subsequent increase in urinary albumin excretion. These findings were not confirmed in other reports. Two prospective studies of different designs, a case control and a cohort study, have failed to resolve the controversy after eight years of observation. No relationship between hyperfiltration and development of persistent proteinuria or hypertension was found in one study, whereas a positive association was claimed in the other. Both studies reported a faster rate of decline of GFR in diabetic patients with hyperfiltration, but the significance of the phenomenon remains presently unclear [3, 4].

Various metabolic and hormonal abnormalities of the diabetic state have been proposed as mediators of glomerular hyperfiltration (Table 43.2). Hyperglycemia *per se* has been demonstrated to increase GFR by approximately 6–10%. Ketone body infusion results in a dramatic rise in GFR of about 30%. Glucagon and growth hormone, two counterregulatory hormones often elevated in diabetic subjects, are also capable of inducing a modest increase in GFR either acutely or in the long term. Recent studies suggest that disturbances in prostaglandin production could play a role in the renal hemodynamic changes of diabetes. For example, an enhanced activity

Table 43.2 Potential mediators of diabetic hyperfiltration

- Hyperglycemia
- Increased plasma concentrations of ketone body and other organic acids
- Increased plasma levels of glucagon and growth hormone
- Disturbances in renal prostaglandin production
- Decreased renin activity
- Increased atrial natriuretic peptide
- Abnormalities of tubuloglomerular feedback mechanisms

of vasodilatory prostaglandins with an imbalance between vasoconstrictive and vasodilatory eicosanoids has been proposed as a mechanism of hyperfiltration. Findings that inhibition of prostaglandin production by aspirin reduces GFR in hyperfiltering diabetic patients would support this contention, but other studies have failed to confirm these results.

Several other mechanisms have been suggested as possible contributors to hyperfiltration, such as a decreased renin activity or reduced numbers of glomerular angiotensin II (AII) receptors, increased production of kinins, hyporesponsiveness to vasoactive substances, and abnormalities of tubuloglomerular feedback mechanisms [1]. Raised plasma level of atrial natriuretic peptide, in response to the increased exchangeable sodium and raised volume expansion of diabetes, has also been implicated as one important determinant. Some, but not all of these perturbations, increase GFR by elevating intraglomerular pressure, a factor strongly implicated in the pathogenesis of glomerular injury in diabetic animal models.

Microalbuminuria

A proportion of diabetic patients exhibit elevated rates of urinary albumin excretion well before clinically persistent proteinuria develops. An increase in albumin excretion rate in the range 20–200 µg/min is defined as microalbuminuria. Four longitudinal studies of cohorts of insulin-dependent diabetic patients have demonstrated that microalbuminuria is a predictor for the development of clinical diabetic nephropathy [5–8], and is associated with a 20-fold higher risk of progression to overt renal disease compared to normoalbuminuric patients (Table 43.3). Albumin excretion rates (AER) in healthy individuals range between 1.5 and 20 µg/min with a median around 6.5 µg/min. The average day-to-day variation of AER is about 40% and is similar both in normal and diabetic subjects. For this reason, an accurate classification of AER requires multiple measurements (usually three urine collections) over a period of a few weeks.

Persistent microalbuminuria is found after one year of insulin-dependent diabetes and can be present at diagnosis in non-insulin-dependent diabetic patients. The significance of microalbuminuria in patients with short-term diabetes is still unclear, but in individuals with five or more years duration of diabetes microalbuminuria is the consequence of definitive, albeit early, renal damage. Once microalbuminuria is established the albumin excretion rate tends to rise with time at an average rate of about 14% per year.

The excess albumin excretion rate in diabetic patients with persistent microalbuminuria is most likely the result of an increased transglomerular flux, as suggested by normal tubular function in these subjects. The increased fractional clearance of albumin at these early stages is likely to be a consequence of alterations in glomerular hemodynamics and, in particular, of an increase in transglomerular pressure gradient. As microalbuminuria becomes persistent and increases in degree, the selectivity index (i.e. the ratio between the clearance of albumin and that of immunoglobulin G (IgG)) starts to rise, reaching its higher value when albumin excretion is around 90 µg/min. The decrease is probably due to a disproportionate increase in the filtration of albumin compared to that of IgG. A probable reason for this phenomenon is a loss of the fixed negative electrical charge on the glomerular membrane. Experiments measuring the clearance of neutral dextrans have shown that pore size is unchanged at this stage. The transition to high selectivity proteinuria signals the advent of heavier proteinuria, suggesting an important role for the loss of the charge barrier in the evolution of diabetic nephropathy [1].

Microalbuminuria is consistently associated with higher levels of blood pressure. Several studies have confirmed a positive linear correlation between blood pressure and albumin excretion rate that is independent of age, sex, duration of diabetes, body mass index, and blood glucose control [9]. The magnitude of this rise in blood pressure is approximately 10–15% compared to the blood pressure of diabetic patients with normal albumin excretion. This phenomenon has been documented in a number of recent studies which have used 24 h blood pressure monitoring. The blood pressure increase which most often occurs within the so-called normal blood pressure range documents clearly that patients with microalbuminuria are not 'normotensive' relative to their counterpart with normoalbuminuria. At this stage of microalbuminuria, there is no hint of renal failure and GFR can even be supranormal. It is, therefore, difficult to ascribe hypertension to reduced renal function. Studies of transition from normo- to microalbuminuria have documented that the diabetic patients who progress show increases in blood pressure as the albumin excretion rate rises within the normal range. In non-Caucasian groups of non-insulin-dependent diabetic patients, similar observations have been made and in some cases there was evidence that the level of blood pressure which preceded the onset of diabetes was positively related to the development of proteinuria after the onset of diabetes. This raises the possibility that elevated blood pressure levels may be one factor contributing to the initiation of renal damage or, alternatively, that high blood pressure and an increase in urinary albumin excretion may represent concomitant manifestations of a common process responsible for the development of diabetic nephropathy.

Morphological studies have shown that structural lesions, such as increased mesangial fractional volume and decreased filtration surface density, are, on average, more advanced when albumin excretion rate exceeded 45 mg/24 h [10], confirming that microalbuminuria is a sign of renal disease. These findings underlie the importance of searching for earlier markers to identify those patients at risk of diabetic nephropathy.

Other associations of microalbuminuria are of note in relation to the enhanced risk of renal and cardiovascular complications of these patients (Table 43.4). Multiple lipoprotein and coagulation factor abnormalities,

Table 43.3 Predictive value of albumin excretion rate (AER) for overt nephropathy in IDDM patients

Study	No. of subjects	Baseline AER (µg/min)	Follow–up (years)	Type of collection	Predictive value (%)
Viberti *et al.* [5]	63	>30	14	Overnight	88
Parving *et al.* [6]	23	>28	6	24 h	63
Mathiensen *et al.* [7]	71	>70	6	24 h	70
Mogensen *et al.* [8]	43	>15	10	Short term	86

endothelial dysfunction, echocardiographic evidence of left ventricular hypertrophy, enhanced sodium retention and increased transcapillary escape rate of albumin have all been reported in patients with microalbuminuria and may have potentially important prognostic implications [1].

Using the euglycemic insulin clamp technique, diabetic patients with microalbuminuria have been found to be more insulin-resistant than normoalbuminuric patients (Figure 43.1) [11]. This altered insulin sensitivity which, by some authors, has been claimed to precede a rise in AER, may explain the reason why microalbuminuric patients have poorer metabolic control and other hemodynamic and lipid metabolism alterations in comparison with normoalbuminuric patients. Insulin resistance has been proposed as an independent risk factor for coronary artery disease in the non-diabetic population.

Thus, risk factors for both renal and cardiovascular complications cluster in diabetic patients with microalbuminuria. In a 23-year follow-up study of 63 IDDM patients, cardiovascular mortality was found to be more than twice as high in microalbuminuric IDDM patients than in normoalbuminuric subjects independent of attained age and duration of diabetes [12]. The importance of identifying and detecting these diabetic patients at an early stage is twofold. At the microalbuminuria stage patients may still respond to therapeutic interventions, and their study may provide insights into the pathogenesis of diabetic nephropathy before the clinical phase of the disease is overtly manifest.

Overt nephropathy

In diabetic patients who progress to overt, persistent albuminuria (albumin excretion rate >300 mg/24 h), GFR gradually declines in a linear fashion at a rate of 0.1–2.4 ml/min/month. The reason for differences in the rates of progression are not known but blood pressure control could be important. Before the introduction of early, intensive treatment for hypertension end-stage renal failure occurred on average seven years after the onset of proteinuria in patients with diabetes [1]. Comparison of life expectancy between cohorts, which received intensive antihypertensive therapy and older cohorts, not adequately treated, of insulin-dependent diabetic patients with proteinuria suggests that survival has been significantly extended by about two-fold.

Elevation of blood pressure is a feature of about 85% of patients with proteinuria and blood pressure increases about 7% per year in association with progressive renal failure. The excess of arterial hypertension in IDDM seems to be largely accounted for by patients with overt clinical nephropathy, whereas long-term uncomplicated diabetic patients tend to have lower blood pressure levels than those of age-matched normal controls.

Diabetic retinopathy and hyperlipidemia (characterized by raised cholesterol, low-density lipoprotein (LDL) cholesterol and triglycerides, and lower high-density lipoprotein (HDL) cholesterol) are present in most patients with nephropathy. At this stage, the course of

---

Table 43.4 Concomitants of microalbuminuria. 'The microalbuminuria syndrome'

1. Elevated blood pressure
2. Altherogenic lipid profile (increased VLDL-triglycerides, decreased HDL cholesterol, increased Lpa)
3. Elevated plasma fibrinogen levels
4. Decreased insulin sensitivity
5. Increased total body exchangeable sodium
6. Increased transcapillary escape of albumin
7. Impaired endothelium-dependent vasorelaxation
8. Increased left ventricular volume
9. High sodium–lithium countertransport activity
10. Diabetic retinopathy

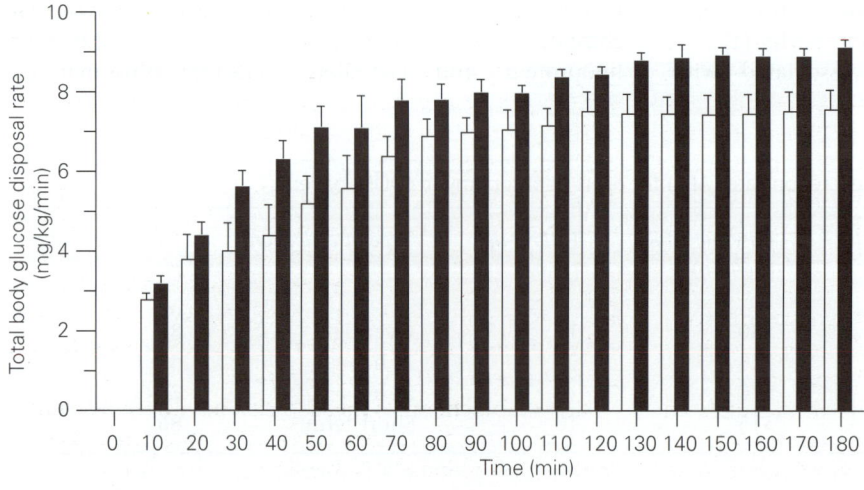

Figure 43.1 Total glucose disposal rate during euglycemic clamp in IDDM patients with (open bars) and without (filled bars) microalbuminuria. (Reproduced, with permission, from ref. [11].)

renal failure does not seem to be reversible, but available treatment modalities slow the rate of decline in renal function and delay the need for renal replacement therapy (see below). The degree of proteinuria is related to the extent of renal damage and the appearance of the nephrotic syndrome foretells a poor renal outcome.

Nephropathy in non-insulin-dependent diabetes

Renal failure in NIDDM develops in a smaller percentage of patients of European origin, but because the incidence of NIDDM is much greater, about one-half of the patients in end-stage renal failure belong to this group.

The prevalence of clinical proteinuria ranges between 10 and 40% in NIDDM patients, with large ethnic variations [1]. Diabetes duration and hypertension are related to the presence of proteinuria. Incidence data show that the cumulative risk of persistent proteinuria varies between 25 and 50% after a diabetes duration of 20 years or more. The clinical course of renal disease is less precisely defined in NIDDM patients, but progression to end-stage renal failure has been reported to be slower compared to that in IDDM patients. Recent observational studies of NIDDM patients with nephropathy have demonstrated that the rate of fall in GFR varies considerably from one patient to another but the increase in blood pressure to a hypertensive level is an early feature of diabetic nephropathy as in IDDM patients. Elevated systolic blood pressure accelerates the progression of diabetic nephropathy in NIDDM patients; however, end-stage renal failure is about 20 times less frequent in European subjects with NIDDM compared to those with IDDM. The reason for this discrepancy is not entirely understood, but it is possible that other competing causes of death, especially cardiovascular disease, in the older NIDDM group prevent progression to ESRF. In ethnic groups where ischemic heart disease is less common and NIDDM develops at a younger age (such as in the Japanese), the frequency of end-stage renal failure is similar to, if not higher than, that in IDDM patients.

Microalbuminuria in NIDDM patients appears to be not only a predictor of renal disease but also a powerful marker of cardiovascular mortality. Increased albuminuria is associated with coronary heart disease, cardiac failure and peripheral vascular disease. Several cardiovascular risk factors have been linked with microalbuminuria in NIDDM patients, such as lipoprotein abnormalities, hyperinsulinemia, insulin resistance and markers of endothelial dysfunction. None of these factors, however, can entirely explain the increased cardiovascular mortality in patients with abnormal AER. In a retrospective study of 503 NIDDM subjects, the 10-year survival rate was significantly poorer: around 30% in patients with microalbuminuria compared to 55% in patients with a normal AER. The majority of deaths were due to cardiovascular disease [13]. These findings were confirmed by a prospective study by Mattock et al. [14] who in a follow-up period of 7.5 years of a group of 145 patients with NIDDM found a highly significant excess mortality among those with microalbuminuria (49%) compared to those without (16%). In the whole cohort microalbuminuria conferred a relative risk for cardiovascular mortality of 5.5 which increased to 7.7 when patients with baseline evidence of cardiovascular disease were excluded and cardiovascular morbidity and mortality combined.

In conclusion, microalbuminuria in NIDDM patients indicates widespread vascular damage.

Pathogenesis of diabetic kidney disease

An understanding of the pathogenesis and pathophysiology of diabetic kidney disease is crucial to identifying intervention strategies to prevent or arrest the development of such a devastating long-term complication of diabetes. A number of recent studies, both in humans and in animal models of diabetes, have contributed to the understanding of some important pathogenetic mechanisms leading to the development of diabetic kidney disease.

There is no doubt that the diabetic milieu is necessary for diabetic glomerular lesions to develop. Microangiopathic lesions can be observed in chemically induced diabetes in the animal model and these can be prevented or greatly reduced by near-normalization of blood glucose levels, depending on the time of the start of intensified insulin treatment after the induction of diabetes. Moreover in the kidney, the morphological lesions typical of the diabetic state, such as mesangial expansion, are reversed by the transplantation of the diabetic kidney into a normal animal.

Renal lesions can also be seen in humans with chronic hyperglycemia secondary to pancreatitis and without any evidence of a genetic predisposition to diabetes. Both retrospective and prospective studies have suggested a relationship between blood glucose control and risk of diabetic nephropathy. The recently reported Diabetes Control and Complication Trial (DCCT) has now precisely documented that the rate of development and progression of diabetic proteinuria is closely associated with glycemic control [15]. Nevertheless, many patients, despite several years of poor diabetes control, develop no renal disease, as assessed by levels of urinary AER. It thus appears that in humans hyperglycemia is necessary, but not sufficient, to cause the renal damage that leads to kidney failure, and that other factors are needed for the manifestation of the clinical syndrome.

Several biochemical mechanisms have been advocated to explain the deleterious effects of high glucose concentrations in the kidney (Table 43.5).

Table 43.5 Biochemical basis for the effect of hyperglycemia on the pathogenesis of diabetic nephropathy

- Glucose toxicity
- Non-enzymatic glycation of protein
- Abnormal polyol metabolism
- Glucose-induced growth factor gene expression
- Increased sodium reabsorption
- Increased protein kinase C activity
- Increased cytokine production
- Alteration of extracellular matrix
- Disturbances in cell cycle and proliferation rate
- Decreased anionic charge of cell membranes
- Abnormal lipid metabolism
- Abnormal cation transport

Non-enzymatic glycation

A possible link between elevated glucose level and diabetic nephropathy resides in non-enzymatic glycosylation of cellular proteins [16]. The exposure of lysine amino terminal groups of circulating or structural protein to increasing amount of glucose would lead, by basic chemical stoichiometry, to increasing covalent binding of glucose to protein. These covalent products can then participate in cross-linking between or within proteins, producing advanced glycosylation end products (AGEs). The new combination may impair the original function of either protein and may affect normal processes of turnover and clearance, so that AGEs accumulate in tissues. The extent of glycation is dependent on protein half-life and the mean glucose level. Direct proof that these AGEs cause tissue injury in human diabetes is still lacking, although correlative studies have been performed and the amount of glycosylated products is related to the extent and severity of advanced complications of diabetes. Recent studies have shown that the AGEs lead to synthesis and secretion of cytokines when bound to a specific AGE receptor identified in macrophages. AGEs can induce an excess cross-linking of collagen molecules in the glomerular plasma membrane affecting the assembly and architecture of glomerular basement membrane (GBM) and mesangial matrix, and potentially act on mesangial cells via platelet-derived growth factor causing cells to synthesize more extracellular matrix. All these processes may lead to enhanced deposition of extracellular matrix proteins in the mesangium, interfere with the mesangial clearance of macromolecules and alter macrophage function, therefore contributing to mesangial expansion and glomerular occlusion.

Aminoguanidine, a hydrazine derivative which binds irreversibly to early glycation products, prevents AGE formation and AGE-induced protein crosslinking. The efficacy of this new drug in preventing some of the complications of diabetes in animal models speaks in support of the role of AGEs in the pathogenesis of diabetic complications.

The polyol pathway

Another possible mechanism of tissue injury involves excessive intracellular production of sorbitol from glucose, a reaction catalyzed by aldose reductase. Chronic hyperglycemia may lead to sorbitol accumulation in a variety of tissues, including renal tubuli and glomeruli. Sorbitol accumulation would cause tissue damage, via a disruption of cellular osmoregulation along with a depletion of myo-inositol [17]. Some beneficial effect of aldose reductase inhibition has been reported in diabetic animals. The increased GFR and proteinuria in rats with streptozotocin-induced diabetes were reduced by inhibitors of aldose-reductase or by supplementation of myo-inositol. Recent studies showed that cells may counterregulate inositol depletion and that the histological lesions of glomerular disease were unaffected by the administration of an aldose reductase inhibitor in the rat made diabetic with streptozotocin. Renal damage in the diabetic kidney is, therefore, unlikely to occur through a mechanism involving the polyol pathway.

Glucotoxicity

A further possibility is that glucose itself has a direct toxic effect on the cells. Lorenzi [18] demonstrated that cultured human endothelial cells chronically exposed to high glucose concentrations show important abnormalities in cell function, which could not be ascribed to alteration of the polyol pathway. High glucose levels determine alterations in cell cycle and proliferation and lead to increased gene expression and synthesis of collagen, fibrinonectin and laminin which may explain the increase in extracellular matrix production observed in the diabetic kidney. Mesangial cells exposed to elevated glucose concentrations synthesize less heparan sulfate and this could theoretically contribute to reduction of the electronegative charge which physiologically restricts the transcapillary flux of circulating albumin, thus giving rise to proteinuria. Moreover in mesangial cells high glucose levels induce the transcription and secretion of transforming growth factor-β (TGF-β), unique among the cytokines in stimulating matrix synthesis and inhibiting matrix degradation.

Hemodynamic and hypertrophic pathways

Glomerular hemodynamic disturbances with elevations of blood flow and filtration rate occur early in the course of diabetes. It has been suggested that these alterations are directly responsible for the development of glomerulosclerosis and its attendant proteinuria [19]. Several observations give support to the notion that renal hyperfusion and hyperfiltration contribute to renal damage (Figure 43.2). In several animal models with spontaneous or induced diabetes, both single nephron GFR and plasma flow are increased while intrarenal vascular resistance is reduced. Despite normal systemic blood pressure levels, transmission of systemic pressures to the glomerular capillaries is facilitated by proportionally greater reduction in afferent compared to efferent arteriolar resistances. Consequently, the glomerular capillary hydraulic pressure rises. Elevated intraglomerular pressure via increased mechanical stress and shear forces may damage the endothelial surface and disrupt the normal structure of the glomerular barrier, and eventually lead to mesangial proliferation, increase in extracellular matrix production and thickening of the glomerular basement membrane. Evidence that these glomerular hemodynamic abnormalities contribute to the development and progression of diabetic nephropathy has been provided by studies involving manoeuvres which aggravate or ameliorate glomerular hyperperfusion and hyperfiltration, without affecting metabolic control. For example both low protein diet or inhibition of angiotensin converting enzyme have been shown to prevent not only the disturbed hemodynamics but also the glomerular histologic lesions that occur in the untreated diabetic control animal. In other studies a dissociation between the hemodynamic perturbations and subsequent sclerosis has been reported. In different strains of diabetic rats, no relationship was found between level of glomerular hyperfiltration and pressure and subsequent degree of glomerular sclerosis.

The hemodynamic abnormalities so far described are usually associated with hypertrophic changes in the glomerulus. Marked renal hypertrophy is a very early event in diabetes and it has been argued that hyperplastic and hypertrophic changes in the diabetic kidney may precede the hemodynamic abnormalities. Although the exact role of growth factors in the development of diabetic kidney disease is not yet fully understood, growth hormone, insulin-like growth factors, transforming growth factor-β, platelet-derived growth factor and other growth promoters may be of importance for the long-term renal changes of diabetes. They may activate mesangial cell proliferation and increase mesangial matrix synthesis or decrease matrix degradation, giving rise to the histologic alterations that are pathognomonic of diabetic glomerulopathy.

Familial and genetic aspects

The annual incidence of diabetic nephropathy rises rapidly over the first 15–20 years of diabetes, but declines sharply afterward for longer diabetes duration. This leads to a cumulative incidence that, after approximately 20 years of diabetes, plateaus around 30–35%. This pattern of risk is compatible with an individual susceptibility to renal damage partly independent of the environmental perturbations caused by diabetes, and has stimulated the search for factors, other than glycemic control, which contribute to it.

That there is an individual predisposition to diabetic nephropathy is supported by the observation that this complication clusters in families. Seaquist et al. [20] reported that 83% of insulin-dependent diabetic siblings of probands with diabetic nephropathy have evidence of renal disease compared with only 17% of siblings of probands without nephropathy. This striking familial aggregation of diabetic kidney disease was also confirmed in a Danish population. A similar familial influence on development of nephropathy has been described in Pima Indians with NIDDM. Overt proteinuria occurred in 14% of the diabetic offspring of diabetic parents without pro-

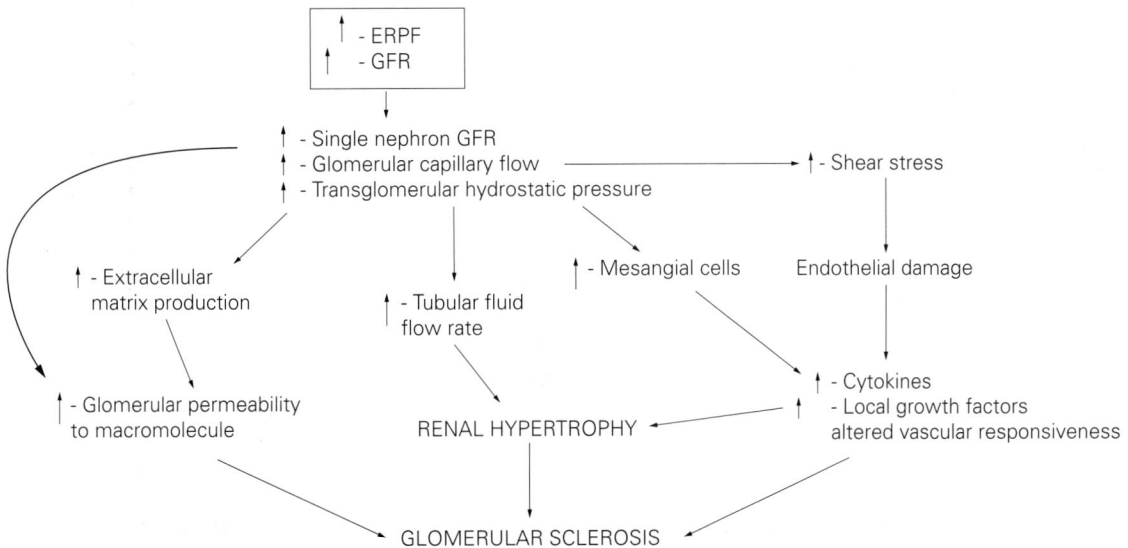

Figure 43.2 Possible sequence of events from intrarenal hemodynamic abnormalities to initiation of diabetic nephropathy.

teinuria, 23% if one parent had proteinuria, and 46% if both parents had proteinuria. Although these studies are consistent with the possibility that genetic factors play an important role in the susceptibility to diabetic nephropathy, they cannot entirely exclude shared environmental influences and do not provide insight into the nature of these factors.

Further information has come from other family studies of risk factors for nephropathy. Earle *et al.* [21] (Figure 43.3) demonstrated that a family history of cardiovascular disease greatly increases the risk of nephropathy in diabetic patients (odds ratio 3.2 compared to that of patients without a family history for cardiovascular disease) and enhances the likelihood of cardiovascular disease in diabetic patients who have nephropathy (odds ratio 6.2). This observation has been confirmed by recent studies which have also revealed that first degree non-diabetic relatives of IDDM patients with albuminuria have reduced insulin sensitivity and abnormal lipid profiles. This familial aggregation of renal and cardiovascular disease and their risk factors has led to the suggestion that these disorders may share a common pathogenetic basis.

Family studies of blood pressure have provided further insights. Higher arterial pressure was measured in parents of diabetic patients with proteinuria than in parents of patients without proteinuria. A higher prevalence of arterial hypertension among the parents of IDDM patients with nephropathy was also found by a subsequent study. The relative risk of developing overt nephropathy was found to be approximately 3.3 if at least one of the parents was hypertensive. These findings could not be confirmed in a Danish study of IDDM patients with nephropathy. However, in this study only parents of diabetic patients who had developed nephropathy before the age of 31 were analyzed and the presence of hypertension in deceased parents was not assessed.

That the hypertension associated with diabetic nephropathy is not merely a consequence of the renal disease is confirmed by several epidemiologial studies, the more recent using 24 h blood pressure monitoring, at different stages of renal involvement. A significant increase in arterial blood pressure has been reported in IDDM and NIDDM patients with microalbuminuria and a still well-preserved renal function. It is unlikely that this increase in blood pressure is a consequence of advanced renal impairment. A recent prospective study in normoalbuminuric normotensive IDDM patients has shown that those patients who progressed to microalbuminuria over a four-year period had significantly higher mean blood pressure values as well as glycated hemoglobin than those patients who did not progress. That higher arterial pressures precede and are related to the development of microalbuminuria has also been demonstrated in NIDDM patients of different ethnic origins. All these studies suggest that hypertension or a predisposition to it may be important components in determining the susceptibility to renal disease in diabetes.

The suggestion that hereditary causes are involved in the liability to diabetic nephropathy has stimulated the search for cell and genetic markers that would allow early diagnosis and identification of patients at risk as well as help clarify the molecular mechanisms of this complication.

Sodium–lithium countertransport

An increase in red blood cell sodium–lithium countertransport, a cell membrane cation transport system, is consistently associated with essential hypertension and its vascular complications. Up to 80% of the interindividual variability of the activity of this transport system is explained by genetic influence representing the sum of a major gene with polygene effects.

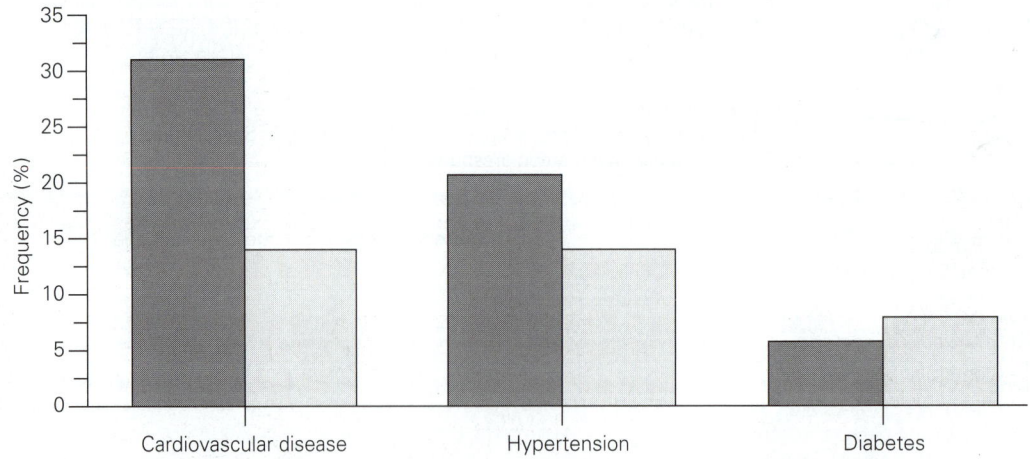

Figure 43.3 Frequency of cardiovascular disease, arterial hypertension and diabetes mellitus among the parents of diabetic patients with nephropathy (solid columns) and without nephropathy (light columns). The difference in the prevalence of cardiovascular disease was significant ($P < 0.03$). (Reproduced, with permission, from [21].)

Increased rates of sodium–lithium countertransport activity have been reported by several, though not all, authors both in IDDM and NIDDM patients with micro- or macro-albuminuria [22] (Figure 43.4). A significant correlation between the activity of this transport system in diabetic probands with nephropathy and their parents strongly suggested heritability of elevated activities in diabetic nephropathy. The importance of genetic factors was confirmed by the close association of sodium–lithium countertransport activities found in diabetic identical twins. That an increased sodium–lithium countertransport activity may confer an increased risk for nephropathy and its vascular complications is supported by a clustering of metabolic, hemodynamic and morphological abnormalities (such as poorer metabolic control, reduced insulin sensitivity, a more atherogenic lipid profile, greater proximal tubular reabsorption of sodium, higher GFRs, increased left ventricular thickness and larger kidneys size) in those patients with a high sodium–lithium countertransport activity, but without overt proteinuria [23].

Sodium–hydrogen antiporter

Sodium–lithium countertransport activity is determined by measuring sodium-driven lithium efflux from red blood cells loaded with lithium in an *in vitro* artifactual system. As this system does not operate *in vivo*, the relevance of this abnormality to the pathogenesis of diabetic renal disease remains uncertain. The close similarities between sodium–lithium countertransport and a physiological cell membrane exchanger, the sodium–hydrogen antiporter, has activated the search for abnormalities in this latter system in diabetic nephropathy.

Sodium–hydrogen antiport is an integral plasma membrane protein which catalyzes the electroneutral exchange of extracellular sodium for intracellular hydrogen with a stoichiometry of $1:1$. Molecular cloning studies have so far revealed the presence of five subtypes of sodium–hydrogen exchangers. These isoforms share a similar structure, but exhibit differences with respect to amiloride sensitivity, cellular localization, kinetic parameters, regulation by various stimuli and different plasma membrane targeting. They define a new gene family of vertebrate transporters [24]. The most widely studied sodium–hydrogen isoform, referred to as NHE 1, is ubiquitously expressed and is involved in a variety of cellular functions by virtue of its ability to control intracellular pH. It is inhibited by amiloride and its 5-amino-substituted derivatives. The gene for NHE 1 is located on the short arm of chromosome 1. It encodes a protein of 815 amino acids with two distinct domains. The N-terminal domain contains 10–12 transmembrane segments, whereas the C-terminal domain is cytoplasmic. Sodium–hydrogen antiport is involved in three important cellular functions: (1) intracellular pH regulation; (2) cell volume control and (3) stimulus–response coupling and cell proliferation. In the kidney, the isoform NHE 2 expressed on the apical membrane of polarized epithelia is directly involved in sodium reabsorption.

An essential feature of this transport system is its allosteric activation by intracellular protons which are presumed to interact at a 'modifier' site that is separate from the sites involved in sodium and hydrogen transport. The activity and expression level of this antiporter can be modulated by a large variety of chemical factors, including growth factors, tumor promoters, hormones as well as physical factors such as changes in cell volume, extracellular acidification and degree of cell spreading

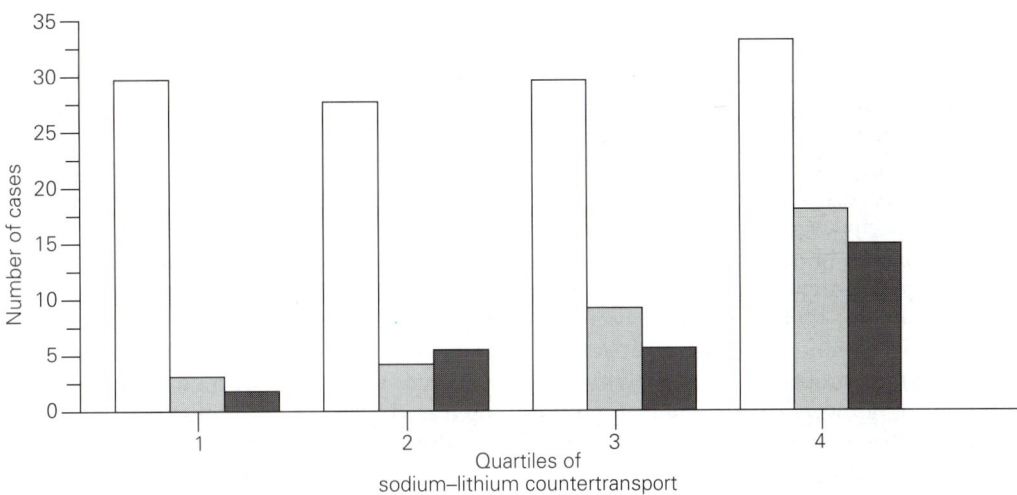

Figure 43.4   Sodium–lithium countertransport activity was measured in 185 IDDM patients. The figure shows the number of IDDM patients in each quartile of the distribution of sodium–lithium countertransport activity. Open, light and solid bars represent the number of patients with normo-, micro- and macroalbuminuria, respectively.

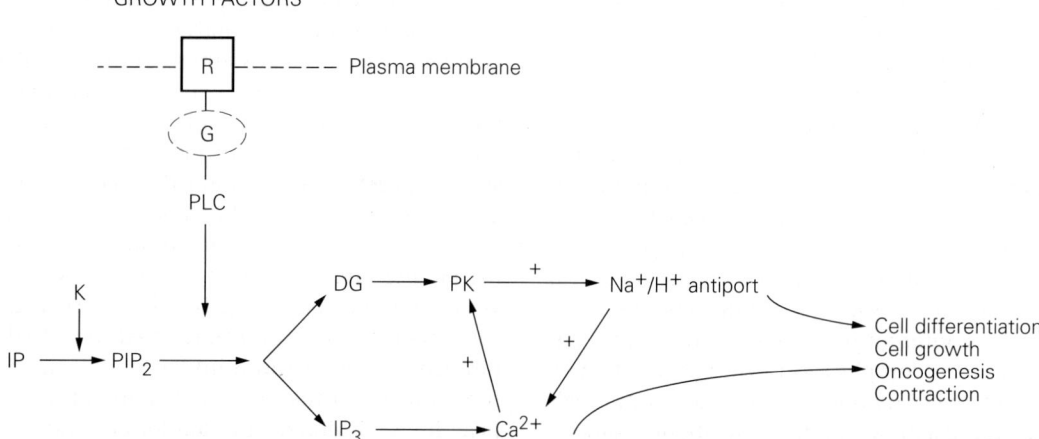

Figure 43.5 Schematic representation of interaction between growth factors and the sodium–hydrogen antiport and calcium-dependent activities. R, receptor; G, regulatory protein; PLC, phospholipase C; K, kinases; IP, inositol phosphate; PIP_2, phosphatidylinositol-4,5-biphosphate; DG, 1,2-diacylglycerol; IP_3, inositol-1,4,5-triphosphate; PK, protein kinase C.

(Figure 43.5). Protein kinases appear to play an important role in the regulation of the antiport, but the molecular mechanisms of activation are not yet fully elucidated. It has been reported that growth factors activate the antiporter by shifting the pH dependence of the 'modifier' site, adjusting the set point upward by 0.15–0.30 pH units. The alteration in the set point is probably mediated by phosphorylation of the antiporter itself or of an ancillary protein.

An increased sodium–hydrogen antiport activity has been reported in leukocytes of IDDM patients with nephropathy as well as in patients with essential hypertension. A higher activity was also found in red blood cells from IDDM patients with microalbuminuria. In these studies, however, measurements were performed soon after blood sampling and potential confounding effects of the disturbed diabetic environment on circulating cells could not be excluded. Skin fibroblasts, which can be cultured for several passages in well-defined conditions, were used by Trevisan *et al.* [25] to measure sodium–hydrogen antiport activity from IDDM patients with and without nephropathy. The kinetic parameters of sodium–hydrogen antiporter were determined by measuring the initial velocity of amiloride-sensitive net sodium uptake under pH gradient conditions. There was a significantly greater sodium–hydrogen antiport activity in the cells from patients with nephropathy compared to that of patients without nephropathy, whose activity was comparable to that of a non-diabetic control group (Figure 43.6). The raised activity was found to be caused by an increased maximal velocity for extracellular sodium, whereas the K_m for extracellular sodium was similar in all patients. The intracellular pH, measured using the distribution of [7-^{14}C]benzoic acid, was also higher in fibroblasts exposed to serum from IDDM

patients with nephropathy than in patients without. These findings in long-term cultured cells are consitent with an intrinsic overactivty of sodium–hydrogen exchange in patients with nephroapthy.

These results were confirmed by other studies in which sodium–hydrogen antiport activity was determined by a different technique, using a pH-sensitive dye. Resting intracellular pH was more alkaline in growing fibroblasts from IDDM patients with nephropathy than in those without. This was associated with a raised sodium–hydrogen antiport activity when intracellular pH was clamped at pH 6.5, but not when pH was clamped at 6.2. It was suggested that the abnormal activity of the exchanger in patients with nephropathy was accounted for by an increased apparent affinity of the antiporter for hydrogen ions at the internal hydrogen modifier site.

One study has established that this abnormal phenotype is conserved in Epstein–Barr-immortalized lymphoblasts. The maximal velocity was significantly elevated and the Hill coefficient for internal hydrogen binding was lower in lymphoblasts from IDDM patients with nephropathy compared with that of both normal controls and normoalbuminuric diabetic patients. By means of specific polyclonal antisera to the carboxyl terminus of NHE 1, it was shown that the elevated maximal velocity of sodium–hydrogen exchange was not due to an increased NHE 1 density, which was similar in IDDM patients with and without nephropathy, but to an increased turnover rate per site.

Although the enhanced sodium–hydrogen exchange activity could theoretically be caused by a reduced intracellular buffer capacity for hydrogen ions in nephropathic patients, this possibility has been excluded in all the above reported studies where intracellular buffer capacity was found to be similar in all subjects.

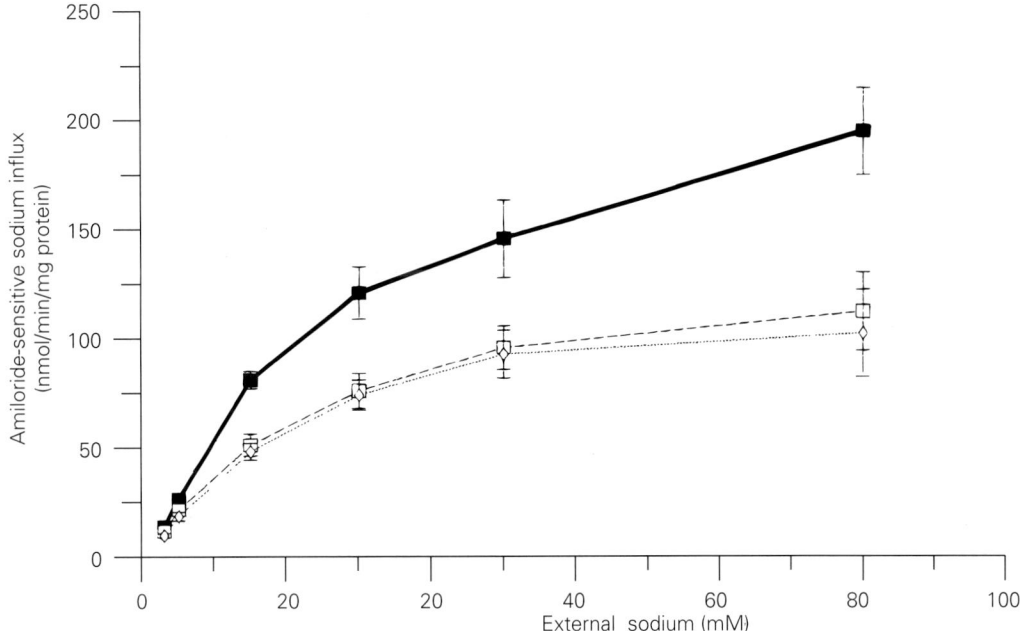

Figure 43.6 Amiloride-sensitive $^{22}Na^+$ influx as a function of external Na^+ concentration in acid-loaded fibroblasts from insulin-dependent diabetic patients with (filled squares) and without (open squares) nephropathy, and normal subjects (open circles). (Reproduced, with permission, from [25].)

Potential involvement of the sodium–hydrogen antiporter in the pathogenesis of diabetic nephropathy

The kinetic abnormalities of sodium–hydrogen antiport described in cells from IDDM patients with nephropathy are similar to those reported in cells from patients with essential hypertension and may be determined by genetic factors. This supports the contention that an inherited prediposition to essential hypertension increases the risk of diabetic nephropathy.

A critical question arises from these studies: is this altered cation transport system implicated in the pathogenesis of diabetic nephropathy and how? The abnormalities of sodium–hydrogen antiport seem unlikely to reflect modifications in sodium–hydrogen antiport gene(s). Genetic linkage analysis has yielded no evidence for NHE 1 as a candidate gene in hypertension. The possibility that the increased maximal velocity could be due to an increased gene expression of NHE 1 was excluded both in patients with essential hypertension and diabetic patients with nephropathy.

It seems more likely that some of the regulatory pathways of the sodium–hydrogen exchange may be important for its overactivity in diabetic nephropathy. Inhibition of protein kinase C in lymphocytes of IDDM patients with albuminuria normalizes the elevated activity of the antiporter. These preliminary findings suggest that a more extensive degree of phosphorylation may determine a more active antiport. Several other phenotypic abnormalities have been described in cultured cells from IDDM patients with nephropathy. Increased sodium–hydrogen antiport activity is closely associated with abnormal cell proliferation in several cell types, both in essential hypertension and in diabetic nephropathy. An enhanced DNA synthesis after stimulation of quiescent fibroblasts with serum has been described in skin fibroblasts from patients with diabetic nephropathy, suggesting a difference in the ability of these cells to enter the synthetic S phase after mitogen stimulation [25]. These preliminary data have been confirmed by the finding of abnormalities in the cell cycle and in the cell life span of these fibroblasts. Extracellular matrix synthesis, in particular collagen production, has also been found to be significantly greater in fibroblasts from patients with nephropathy. Since sodium–hydrogen antiport may be activated by extracellular matrix protein, this coexistence of an altered matrix synthesis with an overactive cation transport system may help to understand the reason for the excessive matrix deposition which leads to glomerular sclerosis in diabetic nephropathy.

Whether the enhanced activity of sodium–hydrogen antiporter reflects the appropriate response to an abnormal growth tendency or constitutes a primary permissive factor leading to cell function disturbances remains to be clarified. It is in any case clear that in diabetic nephropathy the reason for an increased susceptibility is likely to reside in the host cell response to the dysregulation brought about by diabetes. Many growth factors and vasoactive compounds are elevated in diabetes both in the circulation and at the tissue level. In glomeruli from rats made diabetic with streptozotocin, an increased and sustained mRNA expression of a variety of growth factors has been found.

More insight into the relationship between the disturbed milieu of diabetes and the sodium–hydrogen antiport activity has come from a study by Williams and Howard [26] which demonstrated that elevated glucose concentrations significantly increased sodium–hydrogen antiport activity in cultured vascular smooth muscle cells via a glucose-induced protein kinase C-dependent mechanism, thereby providing a biochemical basis for a further increase in the activity of the antiport in the vascular tissues of patients with diabetes mellitus. It is possible to speculate that increased concentrations of growth factors and plasma glucose may exert a more profound effect in that subset of patients characterized by an intrinsic overactivity of sodium–hydrogen antiport or predisposed to overreact to any hypertrophic or hyperplastic stimulus.

A possible sequence of the events leading to diabetic nephropathy is represented in Figure 43.7. Diabetic subjects exhibiting an overactivity of this membrane ion transporter could have increased tubular sodium reab-

sorption, which would raise renal plasma flow and lead to glomerular hyperfiltration in order to maintain sodium balance. The hypertrophic/hyperplastic processes of smooth muscle cells in arteries and arterioles associated with raised sodium–hydrogen antiport activity could lead to increased vascular tone and a rise in systemic and intraglomerular pressure. The same process could cause mesangial expansion. An altered extracellular matrix synthesis associated with sodium–hydrogen antiport overactivity may contribute to excessive matrix deposition in the mesangium and in the interstitium. These abnormalities would trigger a cycle of events producing systemic and glomerular hypertension, more severe glomerulosclerosis, and finally, glomerular occlusion and renal failure.

Candidate genes for diabetic nephropathy

The search for polymorphism in genes potentially involved in the susceptibility to the development of diabetic nephropathy has recently intensified with mixed results. Significant associations between DNA sequence differences at the locus of angiotensin I-converting enzyme (ACE) and diabetic nephropathy have been

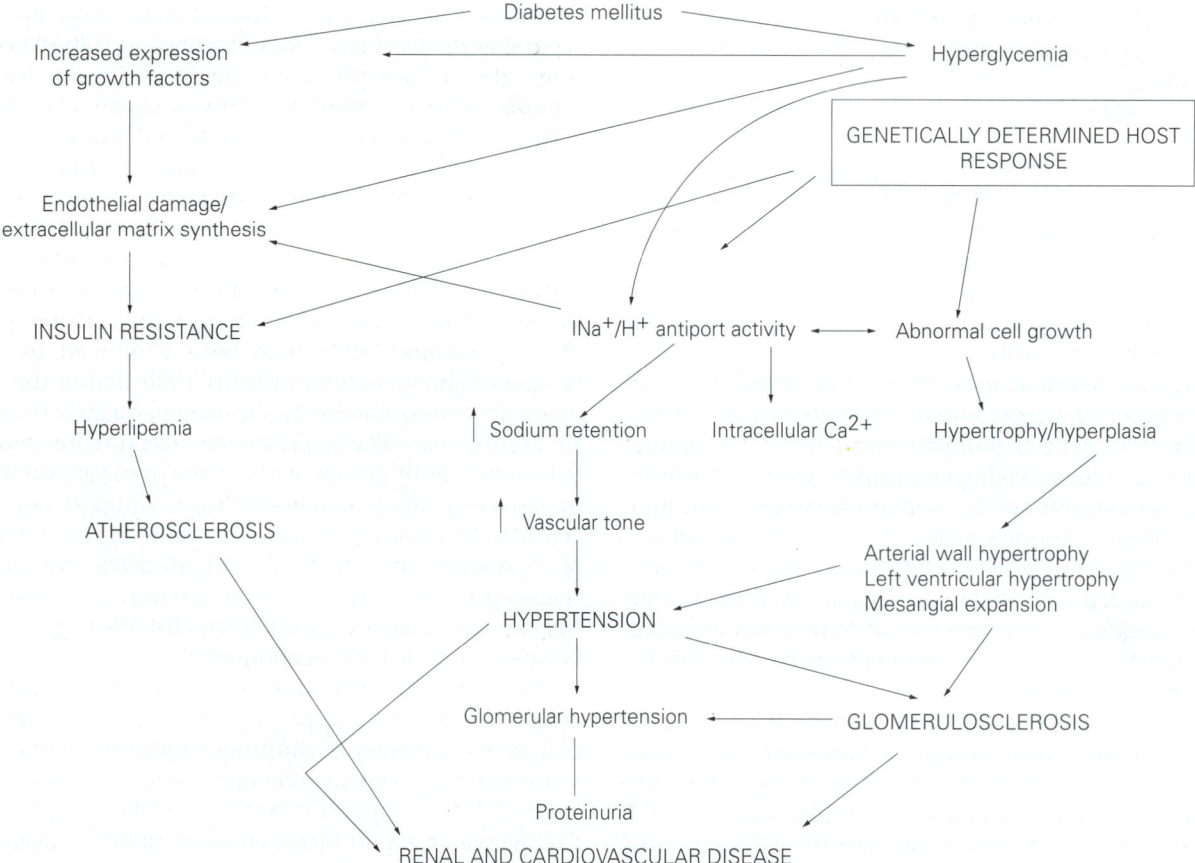

Figure 43.7 Hypothetical representation of a sequence of events leading to the development of renal and cardiovascular disease in a subset of susceptible IDDM patients.

reported by some groups. DNA from 151 insulin-dependent diabetic patients was genotyped at the ACE locus by a three-allele restriction fragment-melting polymorphism (Dde I) and a two-allele insertion/deletion recognized as an Xba I restriction fragment-length polymorphism. Carriers of Xba I/Dde I (+ =) haplotype had a fourfold risk of having diabetic nephropathy [27]. More recent data, however, in larger series have been unable to confirm an association between ACE polymorphism and nephropathy, but show a relationship with the cardiovascular complications of diabetic nephropathy.

The presence of the allele 2 of the anti-inflammatory interleukin-1 (IL-1) receptor antagonist gene has been reported to confer a fourfold increased risk for diabetic nephropathy in both IDDM and NIDDM patients. Moreover, a strong association has been described between allele frequency of the rarer allele of IL-1β gene and diabetic nephropathy in NIDDM patients. Whether these proinflammatory genes contribute to the pathogenesis or are a simple chromosomal marker remains to be established.

The candidate gene approach might not represent the best strategy to identify susceptibility genes for diabetic renal disease. Other techniques, including differential display of mRNA by polymerase chain reaction or genome search by microsatellite in multiplex diabetic nephropathy families, are being explored.

The pathology of diabetic nephropathy

Light microscopy

The light microscopic appearances of glomerular lesions in seven elderly patients with non-insulin-dependent diabetes described by Kimmelstiel and Wilson in 1936 [28] provided the impetus to the morphological and later morphometric study of diabetic renal disease. They reported nodular hyaline deposits, recognized the increase in 'intercapillary connective tissue', now known as mesangial expansion, suggested the term 'glomerulosclerosis' and linked the morphological changes to the clinical syndrome of proteinuria, edema, hypertension and a reduction in renal function. Subsequent light microscopic contributions were made by others, including Bell, who in 1942 described the more characteristic diffuse form of mesangial expansion [29]. The majority of light and electron microscopic studies have been undertaken in insulin-dependent diabetic patients although from the available data it appears that the pathological renal changes seen in non-insulin-dependent patients are similar [30].

The characteristic intraglomerular light microscopic changes of established diabetic nephropathy may be broadly divided into four categories.

1 The diffuse lesion. This common pattern represents an increase in the volume fraction of the mesangial region of the glomerulus in a relatively uniform distribution (Figure 43.8).

2 The nodular lesion. The nodules are well-demarcated hard masses, eosinophilic and PAS-positive, irregular in size and distribution, located in the central regions of peripheral glomerular lobules. Usually observed in more advanced glomerulosclerosis and after at least 14 years of diabetes. Several nodules may be present in each glomerulus and the remaining non-nodular mesangial regions frequently exhibit diffuse lesions (Figure 43.9).

3 The fibrinoid cap. These lesions are highly eosinophilic, rounded, homogeneous structures, situated within the peripheral capillary wall and are homogeneous in texture. These are not common.

4 The capsular drop. These exudative lesions, similar to the previous one, are also rarely observed, and may occur on the glomerular side of Bowman's capsule. They are appropriately named as they are frequently drop-shaped.

The tubules and interstitium may show a variety of non-specific changes as seen in other causes of chronic renal disease; however, arteriolar hyalinosis is character-

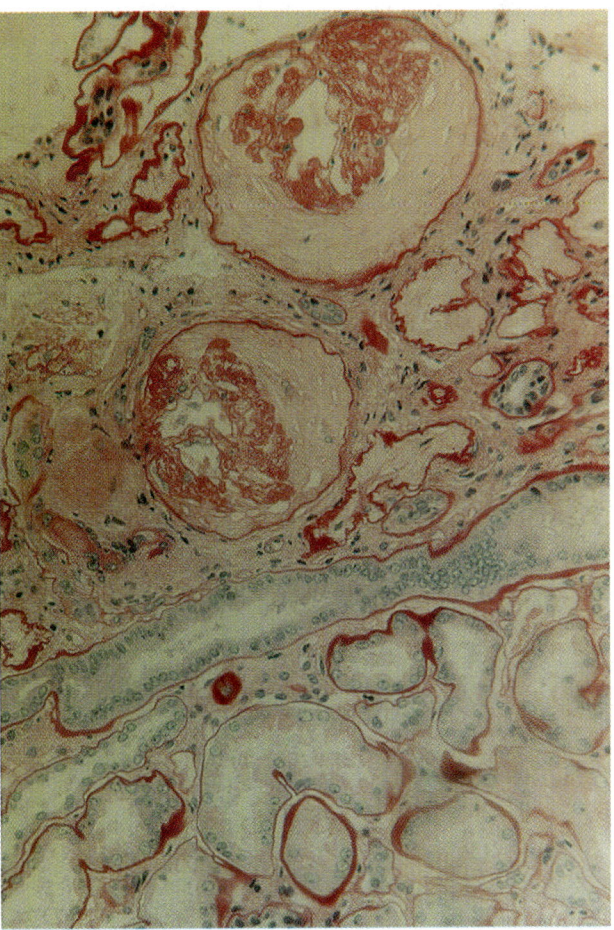

Figure 43.8 Diabetic glomerulosclerosis. Increase in periodic acid–Schiff-positive material in all mesangial regions with advancing sclerosis. A completely sclerosed glomerulus is visible next to the smaller glomerulus.

istic of diabetic renal disease (Figure 43.10). This is due to extraglomerular deposits of eosinophilic material which accumulate in the media or intima of afferent and efferent arterioles and is often the first pathological change of diabetic nephropathy detected using light microscopy and considered to be virtually pathognomonic. As glomerulopathy advances the expanded mesangium encroaches on the filtration surface ultimately leading to glomerular sclerosis (Figure 43.8).

Staining characteristics and immunopathology

A number of commonly used histological stains are employed for light microscopic examination. The most common is periodic acid–Schiff (PAS), which uniformly stains the diffuse, nodular and exudative lesions. The eosinophilic exudative lesions (fibrinoid cap, capsular drop and arteriolar hyalinosis) are particularly well stained red using hematoxylin–eosin, whereas a Masson–trichrome stain differentially stains the diffuse and nodular lesions blue and the exudative lesions red.

Thin linear staining of albumin and immunoglobulins along the capillary walls, Bowman's capsule and tubular basement membranes, is likely to represent a non-specific response to increased permeability rather than to represent specific binding due to the presence of specific binding sites. Using semiquantitative immunofluorescent techniques, increased levels of type IV and V collagen and fibronectin have been described in mesangial regions. Heparan sulfate proteoglycans are negatively charged components of the glomerular basement membrane which provide anionic sites believed to be important in regulating the permeability of the glomerular barrier. One study utilizing cytochemistry coupled with electron microscopy has demonstrated a reduction in these negatively charged sites in glomerular basement membrane from patients with established diabetic nephropathy [31]. Non-enzymatic glycosylation of fibronectin and collagen has been demonstrated *in vivo* and *in vitro* and this modification is associated with decreased binding of these proteins to heparan.

Electron microscopy

The majority of structural studies in patients with varying degrees of diabetic nephropathy have focused primarily

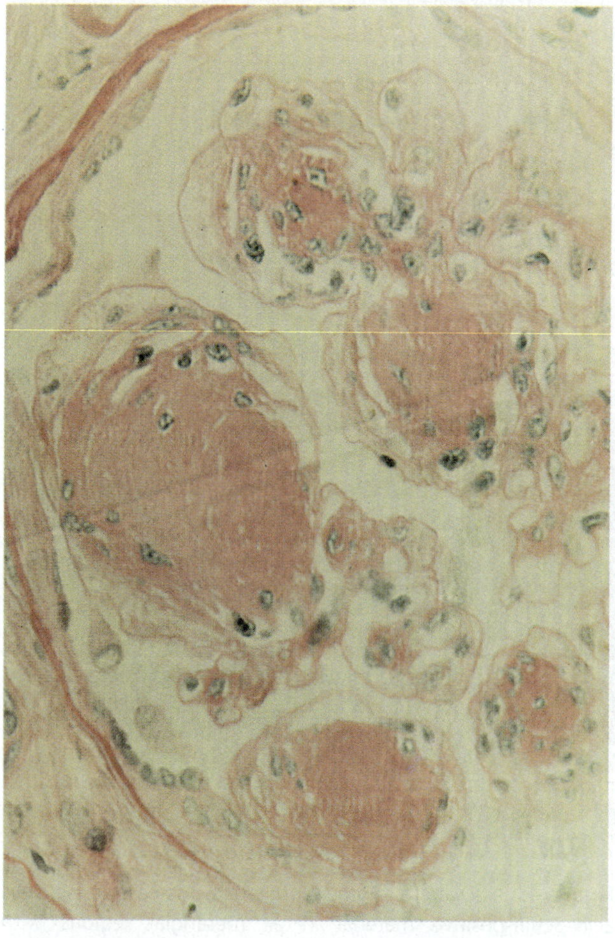

Figure 43.9 Gross nodular lesions in a single glomerulus (periodic acid–Schiff).

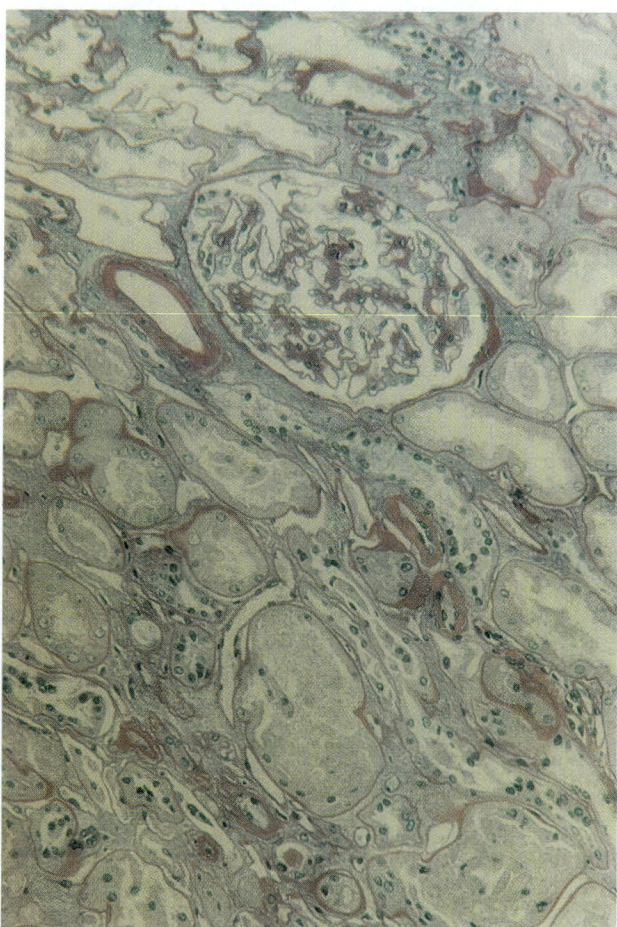

Figure 43.10 Arteriolar hyalinosis in diabetic nephropathy.

on glomerular pathology in type 1 subjects. However, structural and functional abnormalities of tubules, interstitium, interstitial renal vessels and the collecting system are likely to additionally determine overall function. Electron microscopic studies are performed on kidney biopsy samples which constitute a tiny fraction of the entire kidney. It is assumed, with some justification, that the sample taken is representative of the whole kidney. However, parameters may vary between and within individual glomeruli and small differences between groups may be masked if measurement techniques employed are not sufficiently sensitive. Glomerular and extraglomerular parameters seen on either light and electron microscopic sections can be quantitatively described using stereological methods. The peripheral glomerular basement membrane thickness and the volume of the glomerular mesangium expressed as a fraction of the glomerular volume are commonly quoted as estimates of filtration surface.

Peripheral basement membrane

In non-diabetic subjects glomerular capillary basement membrane thickness ranges widely from 250 to 450 nm. It increases by about 30% in the first five years of diabetes although appears to have no direct relationship with duration of diabetes in the absence of nephropathy. In a study of kidneys transplanted into diabetic recipients basement membrane thickness was increased by 55 nm from baseline two years post-transplantation compared to a 2 nm increase in non-diabetic kidney transplant controls. In native kidney the basement membrane thickness further increases with the transition from normoalbuminuria through microalbuminuria to proteinuria. From cross-sectional studies it is clear that there is overlap between cases with normalbuminuria and proteinuria. Thus the finding of a basement membrane thickness of 540 nm is consistent with either the functional finding of a urinary albumin excretion rate of <20 µg/min or >200 µg/min.

Mean values for basement membrane thickness fail to highlight local abnormal areas that may contribute to the increased leakage of albumin. Osterby et al. has described capillary loops with extremely thin and 'fluffy' basement membranes consisuting 1–5% of the total capillary length and surface in patients with advanced nephropathy and also at the stage of microalbuminuria [32]. It is conceptually difficult to envisage how a thickened basement membrane can be directly responsible for increased albumin leakage and this observation provides a possible structural expression of an area of 'large pores'. Areas of abnormally thin and 'fluffy' basement membrane and capillary formation within Bowman's capsule have been proposed as a expression of compensatory glomerular capillary growth analogous to the neovascularization of proliferative retinopathy.

Glomerular mesangium

Mesangial expansion, taken with increased thickness of the glomerular basement membrane, is the most characteristic electron microscopic change seen in patients with all forms of diabetic nephropathy. The mesangium is composed of mesangial cells and associated matrix and in a large study of 150 insulin-dependent patients with renal function ranging from normal to established proteinuria with reduced GFR, Steffes et al. [33] demonstrated that mesangial expansion is characterized by mesangial matrix expansion, rather than cellular expansion. Matrix expansion was, on average, three times that of cellular expansion.

In patients with microalbuminuria mean mesangial volume is clearly increased, but there is some overlap with non-diabetic controls and normoalbuminuric diabetic patients [32]. As albuminuria increases so the relative volume of mesangium increases and the available filtration surface necessarily decreases thereby reducing the GFR. Progressive mesangial expansion ultimately results in glomerular occlusion, sclerosis and resorption.

Glomerular epithelial cell

There have been few quantitative studies of epithelial foot processes and filtration slits and the data are not in complete agreement at the microalbuminuric stage. However, it appears that widening of filtration slits is not the long-awaited cause of the increased albumin leak in patients with diabetic nephropathy. Indeed, compared to the other intraglomerular pathology seen with the increasing severity of diabetic nephropathy the epithelial cell and its projections remain relatively unscared.

Glomerular volume and number

The accurate and precise measurement of glomerular volume is difficult. The glomerulus is a three-dimensional structure and application of the Cavalieri principle provides the best estimate of glomerular volume. The Cavalieri method requires complete sectioning of the glomerulus with repeated sections taken at a known distance apart and the area of each section measured: summing the area of each section and multiplying this by the distance between each section provides an estimate of volume. Other methods make assumptions regarding glomerular shape. Tissue procurement and preparation are likely to further confound the measurement. Diabetes is a cause of large kidneys and indeed large glomerular size has been reported particularly in non-insulin-dependent patients with no difference between those with or without nephropathy. In contrast Bilous et al. [34] described larger glomeruli in insulin-dependent patients who developed nephropathy after 24–26 years of diabetes compared to those who developed the complication after a duration of 14–16 years suggesting that the former group had either the capacity to enlarge their glomeruli and thereby protect filtration surface from the advancing mesangium or they were born with larger glomeruli [34].

Glomerular number is a further factor that may influence the functional effect of structural change and has recently received some attention. No significant differences have been found in glomerular number between non-diabetic patients and patients with uncomplicated insulin-dependent and non-insulin-dependent diabetes [35]. Patients with severe diabetic nephropathy have few glomeruli which is likely to be due in part to total sclerosis and resorption. A congenitally low number of glomeruli may also facilitate the loss of renal function.

Structure and function

After many careful light and electron microscopic studies the precise relationship between glomerular, tubular and interstitial structure and albuminuria is still not clear. Certainly the glomerular basement membrane is thickened and the mesangium expanded but these changes are unlikely to lead directly to an increased transglomerular passage of albumin. The most plausible structural component would be the epithelial filtration slits which remain remarkably normal despite heavy proteinuria. The loss of GFR is more easily explained from a structural viewpoint. Mesangial expansion with consequent loss of filtration surface and increased numbers of sclerosed glomeruli correlate well with GFR.

Interventions and glomerular structure

Two years of improved glycemic control in type 1 patients with microalbuminuria was associated with less basement membrane thickening and less mesangial matrix formation, suggesting a close relationship between blood glucose and the progression of morphological change in early diabetic nephropathy [36]. Other studies are presently investigating the structural effects of ACE inhibitor therapy in insulin-dependent patients with early renal disease.

Monitoring renal function in diabetic nephropathy

Though AER is a reliable indicator of the risk for overt renal disease and appears to be related to the severity of renal damage, its day-to-day variability makes it unsuitable for monitoring renal function over time. To evaluate the progression of renal disease and the impact of therapeutic intervention, a more precise method for the measurement of renal function is needed. Serum creatinine determination is the most commonly used method, but has several disadvantages. The relationship between serum creatinine and GFR is asymptotic in nature, and normal concentrations of serum creatinine are still found

even when as much as 50% of renal function is already lost. In addition, protein intake, lean body mass, metabolic disturbances and fluid losses can all influence serum creatinine levels. Endogenous creatinine clearance has similar shortcomings and, in renal insufficiency, overestimates renal function because of an increased tubular secretion of creatinine.

The renal clearance of inulin, using a primed continuous infusion technique, is the 'gold standard' for the determination of GFR, but is time consuming and relies on frequent urine sampling. These are some of the reasons that have led to the development of the plasma clearance of radioactive tracers. In Europe, the plasma disappearance of ^{51}Cr-labeled ethylene diaminetetraacetic acid (EDTA) after a single injection is one of the most widely used methods to evaluate GFR in diabetic patients and has proven reliable in several studies. Several blood samples over a period of at least 4 h should be collected for a precise estimation of renal function and an allowance should be made for an extrarenal clearance of about 4 ml/min, particularly in patients with advanced renal failure (GFR < 20 ml/min). As an alternative to tracer methods (e.g. ^{125}I-labeled iothalamate, ^{125}I-labeled diatrizoate, ^{99}Tc-labeled diethylenetriaminepenta-acetic acid (DTPA)), or to methods based on non-ionic, radiocontrast media (e.g. iohexol), the determination of serum β_2-microglobulin has been proposed. β_2-Microglobulin has the advantage of having a constant rate of synthesis, is also unaffected by factors that influence creatinine, is virtually freely filtered, not secreted by the renal tubules,

Table 43.6 Investigations routinely performed on all patients with abnormal albumin excretion rate

- General physical examination and dietary assessment (every 3–6 months)
- Blood pressure (every 3–6 months)
- Visual acuity (at least yearly)
- Fundoscopy (at least yearly)
- 12 lead ECG (yearly)
- Echocardiogram (when ECG is abnormal or symptoms are present)
- Exercise test (every 2–3 years or when symptoms are present)
- Serum urea and creatinine (yearly)
- Fasting lipid profile (yearly)
- Assessment of peripheral vascular disease (yearly)
- Glycated hemoglobin (every 3 months)
- Albumin excretion rates (every 6 months)
- Urinanalysis (every 6 months)
- ^{51}Cr-EDTA glomerular filtration rate (yearly if albumin excretion rate >300 mg/24 h)
- Renal ultrasound (initially)
- Serum complement levels (initially)
- Antinuclear factor (initially)

and once absorbed is not recycled. However, it is costly and the gains over serum creatinine, though significant, are of limited clinical use in the monitoring of changes in renal function in the normal and low-normal ranges. An abnormal rise in serum β_2-microglobulin is not detectable until GFR falls below 60 ml/min.

In diabetic patients with microalbuminuria, GFR should be determined yearly to assess progression and the effect of any therapeutic intervention. In patients with overt nephropathy, plotting GFR values over a period of months or years is a useful method for predicting the likely time for initiation of renal replacement therapy.

Table 43.6 summarizes the investigations that should be routinely performed on all diabetic patients with abnormal AER. All patients should be carefully followed up on a regular basis.

Treatment

Once diabetic nephropathy is established, its progression to end-stage renal failure cannot be reversed. However, treatment has been shown to slow the rate of decline in renal function and delay the need for renal replacement therapy.

Control of arterial hypertension

The positive relationship among levels of blood pressure, AERs and rate of progression of renal failure has led to changes in the treatment of hypertension in diabetic renal disease [1].

In an uncontrolled study of a small number of insulin-dependent diabetic patients, it was demonstrated that antihypertensive treatment slowed the rate of loss of GFR and decreased albuminuria. However, reducing the AER may not necessarily mirror an improvement in renal histologic lesions or in clinical outcome measures of end-stage renal failure or cardiovascular mortality. In a nine-year study in which a group of nine patients was used as its own control, it was shown that effective antihypertensive therapy could reduce the rate of decline in GFR from 0.94 to 0.22 ml/min/month. There was also a 50% reduction in AER. Such dramatic improvement in the rate of progression of renal disease could theoretically almost double the 'renal survival' of these patients. Recent retrospective studies have suggested a marked decrease in cumulative mortality rate 10 years after onset of nephropathy from approximately 60 to 18% in IDDM patients with clinical albuminuria receiving antihypertensive treatment.

In the early studies, blood pressure was lowered using multiple drugs, including beta-blockers, diuretics and vasodilators. More recently, ACE inhibitors have been used to obtain significant reduction of albuminuria and the rate of fall of GFR [37]. A prospective study of 409 IDDM patients with overt nephropathy provided clear evidence that captopril preserves renal function in patients with IDDM better than placebo and, more importantly, reduces both the need for dialysis or transplantation and the mortality rate (Table 43.7) [38]. The renoprotective effect of ACE inhibition appeared to be independent of its antihypertensive property.

In patients with microalbuminuria and normal blood pressure, Marre *et al.* showed that ACE inhibition could normalize AER in 50% of patients after one year of treatment. Blood pressure was slightly but significantly reduced while GFR remained unaltered. A four-year open study of normotensive IDDM patients with microalbuminuria demonstrated that captopril reduced AER without any effect on systemic blood pressure or GFR. In the control group, 30% of patients developed persistent proteinuria. In a double-blind randomized placebo-controlled trial of two years duration, ACE inhibition therapy significantly impeded progression to clinical proteinuria and prevented the increase in AER in non-hypertensive IDDM patients with persistent microalbuminuria (Figure 43.11) [39]. A stabilizing effect of ACE inhibition on proteinuria and serum creatinine has also been reported in a five-year controlled trial in normotensive NIDDM patients who had microalbuminuria. These results raise the possibility that at the stage of non-hypertensive microalbuminuria, the progression of renal damage in diabetic patients might be arrested. Recent reports indicate that treatment with ACE inhibitors reduce the fractional clearance of large-sized dextrans, suggesting a possible improvement in glomerular membrane size

	Captopril	Placebo
Mean blood pressure (mmHg)[a]	96 ± 8	100 ± 8
GFR decline (% per year)[a]	11 ± 21	17 ± 20
Doubling of serum creatinine (no. of patients)	25/207	43/202
No. of patients requiring dialysis, renal transplantation or died	23	42
Proteinuria	−30%	unchanged

[a] Data given as mean ± SD.

Table 43.7 Effects of ACE inhibition on diabetic nephropathy in 409 diabetic patients after a median follow-up time of three years [38]

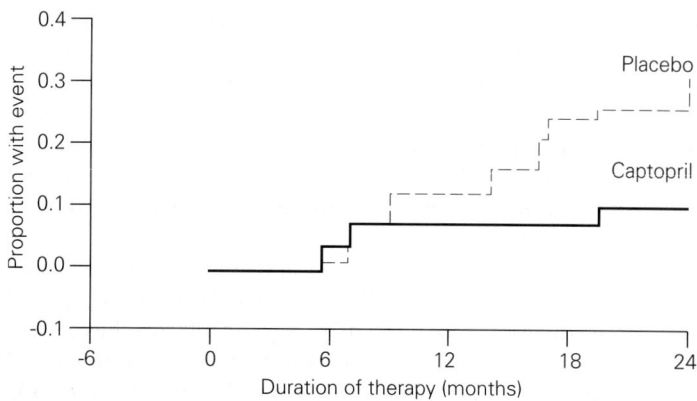

Figure 43.11 Probability of progression to clinical proteinuria after treatment with captopril (——) or placebo (– – –) in patients with insulin-dependent diabetes mellitus who had microalbuminuria. The difference between the two treatments was statistically significant (*P* = 0.03 by log-rank test). (Reproduced, with permission, from [39].)

selectivity independently of changes in systemic blood pressure. Direct modification of glomerular membrane permeability seems to be unique to this class of drugs.

No study has formally tested the optimal blood pressure necessary to prevent kidney damage. However, analysis of several small studies would suggest that the progressive fall of GFR might be halted by lowering mean blood pressure to below 105 mmHg; the progression of microalbuminuria should be stopped if mean blood pressure is kept below 93 mmHg.

Dietary treatment

Renal function and histology are influenced to a marked degree by dietary protein. GFR and renal plasma flow increase after a protein load in normal subjects. In experimental animals high protein intake is translated into sustained glomerular hyperfiltration and renal hypertrophy. Both phenomena are implicated in the pathogenesis of diabetic nephropathy. The precise effector mechanism of these hemodynamic alterations has only been partially elucidated, but changes in glucagon secretion, the production of renal vasodilatory prostaglandins, and other mediators may be involved. High protein intake accelerates the deterioration of most experimental renal diseases, including diabetes mellitus. Restriction of dietary protein limits further damage both in animal models of renal disease and in human renal failure. Evidence for a beneficial effect of protein restriction on progression of renal failure in patients with diabetic nephropathy has been provided. In a five-year self-controlled study of 19 diabetic patients with mean GFR at entry of 60 ml/min, Walker *et al.* [40] demonstrated a reduction of the rate of decline of renal function from 0.61 to 0.14 ml/min/month when the protein intake was decreased to 0.67 from an initial intake of 1.13 g/kg body weight/day. There was also a significant decrease in AER. This effect, which was comparable to that obtained with intensive antihypertensive treatment, was independent of systemic blood pressure changes. The individual response to a low protein diet was, however, heterogeneous, with some patients showing no reduction in the speed of progression of renal failure. The reason for this

variability is not known; it was independent of dietary compliance, blood glucose control, blood pressure and GFR at entry. The retarding effect of a low protein diet on the progression of diabetic renal disease was confirmed in another randomized prospective study. In these patients protein intake was reduced to 0.6 g/kg body weight/day and many of the patients on a low protein diet maintained stable renal function for an extended period of time. In both studies no untoward nutritional effects were seen with this degree of protein restriction.

The reduction in protein excretion rate and in the fractional clearance of albumin and IgG suggests that one of the beneficial effects of a low protein diet may be a decrease in intraglomerular pressure and improvement of glomerular membrane selectivity. Shorter-term studies have also shown that a low protein diet, independent of changes in plasma glucose and arterial pressure, reduces GFR and the fractional clearance of albumin in normoalbuminuric as well as microalbuminuric IDDM patients. All these data, taken together, provide evidence for an important role of reduced dietary protein in the management of patients with overt or incipient diabetic nephropathy. The best time to introduce protein restriction remains, however, to be determined. Because compliance with a low protein diet remains a critical aspect of therapy, attention has been drawn to the use of diets rich in vegetable proteins. In normal individuals, a diet rich in vegetable protein produces renal functional changes similar to those obtained by reducing animal protein. Whether vegetarian diets, with a protein content of about 1 g/kg body weight/day, would obtain the same effects as a lower amount of animal protein on the progression of diabetic renal disease remains an unresolved question. A vegetarian diet could theoretically be more acceptable to renal failure patients and compliance might improve.

Some caution should be applied in evaluating the findings of these studies, since a recent large trial in 1585 patients with various chronic renal diseases was unable to show any significant difference in a mean follow-up period of 2.2 years between the patients assigned to a usual protein diet or to a low-protein diet [41]. In this study there was a trend toward a slower decline in the

GFR only in the patients with more severe renal insufficiency on a very low-protein diet. In this study 3% of the patients had NIDDM. Therefore, although it seems reasonable to introduce a low-protein diet in the management of diabetic patients with advanced renal failure, the real value of this therapeutic maneuver in those patients with a renal function still in the normal range remains doubtful.

Control of hyperglycemia

Diabetic nephropathy is likely to be the result, to a considerable extent, of the disturbed metabolism of the diabetic state. Once established, however, the degree of glycemic control seems to have little impact on progression. A higher glycosylated hemoglobin has been related to a faster decline of GFR in patients with nephropathy by some authors, but this has not been confirmed by others. Strict metabolic control achieved by continuous subcutaneous insulin infusion has failed to halt the rate of decline of GFR or to decrease proteinuria [42]. Moderate hyperglycemia can increase GFR in proteinuric patients with subnormal levels of GFR, probably by changing the ultrafiltration coefficient. This effect may not be entirely negative in advanced renal disease. Though metabolic control does not play a crucial role in the progression of clinically overt diabetic kidney disease, an important impact of hyperglycemia in the pathogenesis of renal damage seems likely. Patients who develop

nephropathy have on average a record of poorer metabolic control than those who do not. Good metabolic control can postpone or possibly even halt progression to overt clinical nephropathy if applied at an early stage. Several studies have demonstrated that short periods of improved metabolic control not only reduce microalbuminuria, but also limit the exaggerated AER induced by physical exercise. Studies from Denmark have suggested that near-normal glycemia achieved using insulin infusion pumps can prevent the transition from microalbuminuria to clinical proteinuria. A recent meta-analysis found an association between metabolic control and urinary AER, and suggested that the rate of decline of GFR could be retarded by several years of improved glycemic control [43]. More recently the Diabetes Control and Complication Trial (DCCT) [15] has demonstrated that the rate of development of albuminuria may be significantly reduced by a good metabolic control. In this study 1441 IDDM patients were randomized to either conventional insulin treatment or to intensified treatment and followed for a mean period of 6.5 years. In the intensified treatment group (with a reduction of glycosylated hemoglobin around 1.5–2% in comparison with the other group), the risk of developing microalbuminuria (albumin excretion rate above 40 mg/24 h) was reduced by 39% and for developing clinical nephropathy (albumin excretion rate > 300 mg/24 h) by 54% (Figure 43.12). Most of the patients in the DCCT trial were normoalbuminuric at baseline. In the 73 patients with base-

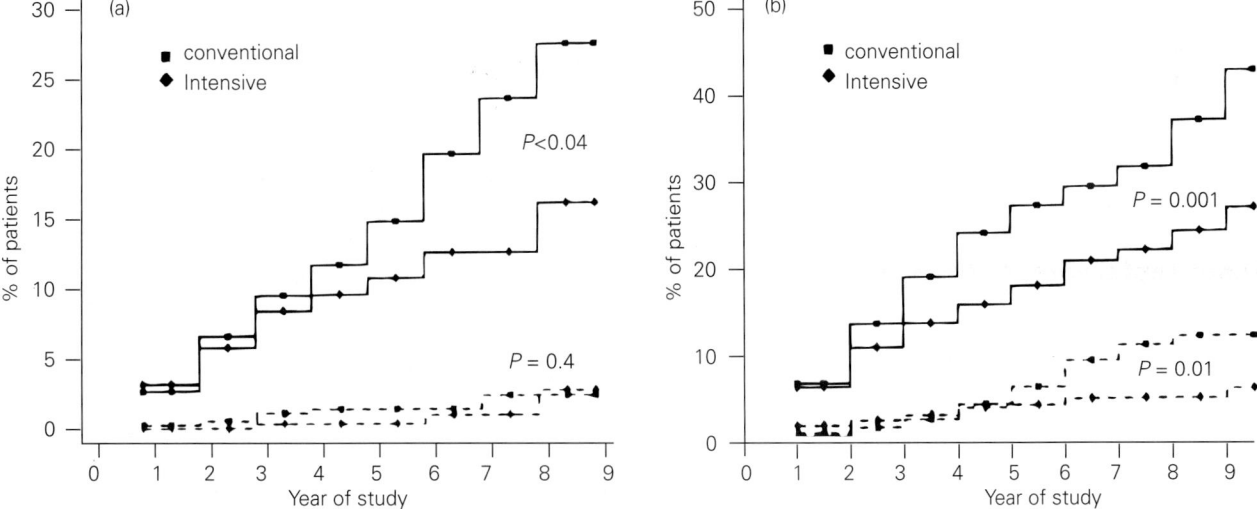

Figure 43.12 Cumulative incidence of urinary albumin excretion ≥300 mg/24 h (– – –) and ≥40 mg/24 h (——) in patients with IDDM receiving intensive or conventional insulin therapy. Patients included in the primary-prevention cohort were required to have had IDDM for 1–5 years, to have no retinopathy and urinary albumin excretion of less than 40 mg/24 h. Those included in the secondary-prevention cohort were required to have had IDDM for 1–15 years, to have very mild to moderate nonproliferative retinopathy and urinary albumin excretion of less than 200 mg/24 h. In the primary-prevention cohort (a), intensive therapy reduced the adjusted mean risk of microalbuminuria by 34% (P < 0.04). In the secondary-intervention cohort (b), patients with urinary albumin excretion of ≥40 mg/24 h at baseline were excluded from the analysis of the development of microalbuminuria. Intensive therapy reduced the adjusted mean risk of albuminura by 56% (P = 0.01) and the risk of microalbuminuria by 43% (P = 0.001), as compared to conventional insulin therapy. (Reproduced, with permission, from [15].)

line microalbuminuria no treatment effect was noted with 8 of 38 in the intensified treatment group and 8 out of 35 in the conventionally treated group progressing to persistent albuminuria. These negative findings have been supported by a recent report of the Microalbuminuria Collaborative Study Group which, in a five-year prospective study of 70 IDDM patients with microalbuminuria, was unable to show a reduction in the risk of progression to clinical albuminuria in the intensive diabetes therapy group. Six of 36 intensely treated patients and of 34 conventionally treated patients progressed. The sum of these results confirms blood glucose control as a key factor in the devolopment of diabetic albuminuria but, at the same time, raises the question of its limited efficacy once a degree of albuminuria has developed. This has to be viewed *vis-à-vis* the large risk reduction afforded by ACE inhibition in the treatment of diabetic patients with microalbuminuria.

These encouraging results do not prevent some patients from developing severe renal lesions despite meticulous glycemic control and little extra protection against complications seems to be obtained with glycosylated hemoglobin below 7.5%. Moreover, intensified metabolic control carries an increased risk of hypoglycemia, and ketoacidosis has been reported to be more frequent in users of subcutaneous insulin infusion pumps.

The DCCT achieved the goal for which it was designed and clearly demonstrated the importance of blood glucose control in the development of the microvascular complications in IDDM patients. However, there remains a major question regarding the extrapolation of these results to the much larger group of patients with NIDDM. The importance of this issue stems from the fact that the majority of patients with diabetes have NIDDM, and macrovascular morbidity and mortality is a greater burden in these patients than microvascular complications.

Renal replacement therapy

Renal failure due to diabetic nephropathy continues to provide an increasing number of patients on end-stage renal failure (ESRF) programs throughout the world. Incidence and prevalence figures vary between countries and reflect different rates of diabetic nephropathy, availability of renal replacement facilities and treatment policies. The number of new patients with diabetes taken onto ESRF programs varies from 7% in France to over 35% in some North American centers. Racial differences are clearly demonstrable in Europe and North America with Asian and black patients having a higher rate of ESRF than their white counterparts. Overall 16% of new renal replacement patients in Europe have diabetic nephropathy (1991 data) whereas the figure for the USA is double this at 34% [44].

Classifying patients on renal replacement therapy

(RRT) IDDM or NIDDM has been shown to be a major source of error, with misclassification of the type of diabetes seen in 31% of patients in a French study [45]. Many non-insulin-dependent patients are insulin treated, due to beta-cell failure, by the time they need RRT even though they are not strictly insulin-dependent and may be easily misclassified if a careful diabetes treatment history is not taken. Diabetic nephropathy is the primary cause of renal failure in over 90% of insulin-dependent patients but in only a third of non-insulin-dependent patients was this diagnosis given as the cause of the ESRF in France.

The method of renal replacement

Renal transplantation should be the aim for all patients with diabetes in ESRF. Patient and graft survival and rehabilitation are all superior after transplantation compared to dialysis. Clearly this ideal is limited by the availability of grafts and the local policies for organ harvesting. In Europe approximately 60–70% of diabetic patients are treated by hemodialysis, 15–20% by peritoneal dialysis and about 20% have a functioning graft (1991 data) [44]. However, major differences exist within Europe, with 63% of Swedish and 34% of British diabetic patients on RRT having a functioning renal graft at the end of 1985 compared to only 8 and 6% of German and French patients.

Particular problems for diabetic patients on renal replacement

Vascular access poses more of a problem in the diabetic patient. Arteriovenous fistulae tend to fail earlier whereas bovine or PTFE grafts appear to survive for longer. Blood pressure and blood glucose levels during hemodialysis tend to swing widely. Many units dialyze against a solution containing 10–12 mmol/l of glucose to minimize wide swings of blood glucose. Even though dialyzable inhibitors of insulin action exist, insulin requirements frequently fall as the GFR approaches single figures and hypoglycemia may be troublesome and dangerous, especially if the normal warning symptoms are diminished or lost. The expected half-life of insulin may increase in anephric patients and, coupled with anorexia, hypoglycemia is not infrequent and tight glycemic control difficult to achieve. The use of glycated hemoglobin as a measure of glycemic control in patients on hemodialysis or continuous ambulatory peritoneal dialysis (CAPD) is unreliable due to shortened red cell survival and the accompanying anemia [46]. The use of capillary blood glucose home monitoring is the preferred method for the assessment of glycemic control.

Up to 40% of patients starting on hemodialysis are blind, yet the incidence of new blindness on dialysis has declined over the last decade with no significant changes in anticoagulation regimens. This is likely to be due to better ophthalmological screening and treatment and improved blood pressure control. Loss of vision is the main reason for the low rate of employment in diabetics on hemodialysis: careful screening and appropriate therapy in the predialysis years should be associated with a reduction in the incidence of diabetic blindness. Although the majority of patients on hemodialysis consider themselves to be happy and leading active lives, 14% of patients in one series died due to termination of the dialysis. The patients in whom dialysis was terminated were not more likely to be blind or have had amputations compared to those who continued the RRT [1].

Peritonitis while on CAPD is often quoted as being more frequent in diabetic patients using intraperitoneal insulin. A survey by the National CAPD Registry, however, revealed similar peritonitis rates for patients using subcutaneous and intraperitoneal insulin [47]. Although no studies have directly assessed blood pressure levels in patients on hemodialysis and CAPD, it is the clinical impression that blood pressure control is better on the latter form of replacement.

Foot problems due to a combination of peripheral neuropathy with peripheral vascular disease are a constant source of morbidity especially in patients who have received a renal transplant. Approximately 30% of transplanted patients have had a major amputation at 10 years and it is particularly disappointing for patients with a successful renal graft to be incapacitated by foot ulcers, local surgery or a below-the-knee amputation. A careful watch must be kept on the feet in these patients with plentiful podiatry advice on foot care and footwear.

Survival on RRT

For all types of RRT, actuarial survival in patients with diabetes is worse than in matched non-diabetic patients and the differences appear to have been stable over recent years (Table 43.8). Cardiovascular disease and infection are the principal causes of death with relative mortality being 3–4-fold higher in diabetic patients under the age of 54 compared to non-diabetic patients on RRT. For the diabetic ESRF population aged 45–54, the death rate due to ischemic heart disease is 20–50 times that of the general population. Males are more affected than females [48]. Cardiac death is predictably associated with a preceding history of angina pectoris or myocardial infarction. Angioplasty or coronary bypass surgery was associated with less cardiovascular end points, including death, than with those medically treated in a small study of IDDM patients who had received a renal transplant (Figure 43.13) [49]. Despite these data many European centers do not routinely perform coronary angiography in asymptomatic diabetic patients prior to renal transplantation. The reasons for this policy include the observations that low-risk patients can be identified by algorithms, the restenosis rate after angioplasty is high, resources are limited and many non-diabetic symptomatic patients are considered to have a greater need.

Table 43.8 Diabetic patient survival on RRT

	1 Year (%)	5 Year (%)
Transplantation [49]		
Cadaver	84 (85)	63 (68)
Living-related donor	89 (94)	74 (85)
Hemodialysis [50]		
45–54-year-old IDDM	–	38 (70)
55–64-year-old NIDDM	–	31 (58)
CAPD [51]	78 (98)	–

Values in parentheses are for non–diabetic patients.

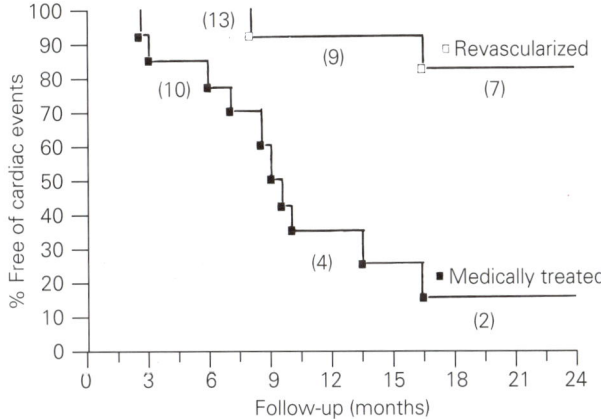

Figure 43.13 Cardiovascular events in medically treated and revascularized diabetic patients. Numbers in parentheses = patients available for follow-up. (Reproduced, with permission, from [49].)

Graft survival is longer with living-related rather than cadaver renal transplants. The University of Minnesota transplant group had more than 20 years experience with this technique and hare reported low perioperative mortality (0.03%) with no evidence of later progressive renal deterioration or other serious conditions [50].

Simultaneous pancreas and kidney transplantation

Isolated pancreatic transplantation is now rare and if a pancreatic transplant is performed it is common for both kidney and pancreas to be transplanted simultaneously. This procedure is more technically challenging than renal transplantation alone, requires higher levels of immunosupression, carries an increased rate of infection and cancer and has little or no proven benefits on the chronic complications of diabetes. However, combined kidney/pancreas transplantation has a higher one-year survival compared to pancreas transplant alone (75% vs

49%) [51]. Rates of rejection with combined procedures are up to three times higher compared to solo kidney transplants. The higher doses of immunosupressive agents used increase the risk of infection, especially cytomegalovirus and fungal infection, in the short term, and cancer, especially lymphoproliferative disorders, in the long term. The early mortality rate is appreciable with the combined transplant procedure even in the best centers; data from Minneapolis reveal a one-year survival of 85% compared to 96% for living-related kidney alone.

A successful kidney/pancreas transplant is likely to significantly improve the quality of life of a long-standing IDDM patient. A large contribution to this improvement will result from the alleviation of uremic symptoms. A fully functioning pancreas will enable the relaxation of dietary restrictions, allow the cessation of insulin injections and blood glucose monitoring and lift the fear of hypoglycemia. Against this must be balanced the data on survival and the progression of other diabetic complications. One indication for a combined procedure is patients with autonomic neuropathy and gastroparesis who frequently vomit after food having taken their preprandial insulin with resulting hypoglycemia. Although a successful pancreatic graft is unlikely to improve the autonomic neuropathy, the obviation of the need for insulin injections abolishes hypoglycemic episodes. There are only a few centers world-wide with a large experience of the combined procedure and patients who are contemplating this procedure should be referred to such a center.

Other renal conditions seen with diabetes

Renal papillary necrosis

Up to 50% of cases of renal papillary necrosis (RPN) occur in diabetic patients. It is associated with the duration of diabetes, is more common in older female patients (3:1 female to male ratio), is particularly common in those with frequent urinary tract infections (UTI) and is usually bilateral. Hematuria and a sterile pyuria are alerting signs as the condition may be asyptomatic. Alternatively a clinical picture resembling nephrolithiasis or pyelonephritis may present itself. Renal ultrasonography or an intravenous pyelogram will confirm or refute the diagnosis. Pathogenesis is multifactorial but ischemia is crucial and glomerulosclerosis is a frequent morphological concomitant. Superadded infection and analgesic abuse are probable precipitants and treatment involves eradication of infection and drainage of any obstruction.

Urinary tract infection

A distillation of the available data suggests that UTI is more common in female than male diabetic patients especially if pregnant (18% vs 4% in one series). Many infections are asymptomatic and it has been suggested that all pregnant diabetic women should be screened for bacteriuria. Chronic UTIs are often due to incomplete bladder emptying with large residual volumes. The prevalence of autonomic neuropathy affecting the bladder is unknown. Prophylaxis with continuous low-dose antibiotics has been shown in other groups of patients to prevent recurrent infection and the same is likely to hold true for patients with diabetes.

Diabetic nephropathy and pregnancy

Pregnancy should be planned in all women with IDDM. Advising women against pregnancy should only be done after a careful appraisal of all the factors in an individual case. There are few absolute contraindications to pregnancy in IDDM but the woman with established diabetic nephropathy, or even microalbuminuria, should be made aware of the current state of knowledge before making a decision. ACE inhibitors must be stopped before conception is planned as they are teratogenic and are associated with neonatal renal failure [52]. A suitable alternative is alpha-methyldopa.

A recent report has detailed the outcome of 26 women with proteinuria and a creatinine clearance of less than 80 ml/min [53]. The principal findings, which confirm the results of other small studies, were that heavier levels of proteinuria (>3 g/day) were more common as the pregnancy progressed and that 39% of the newborns were born before 34 weeks and 72% of these premature babies had the respiratory distress syndrome. More worrying was the finding that 20% of all children of diabetic mothers had evidence of psychomotor retardation at a mean follow-up of 4.5 years. Pregnancy did not appear to accelerate the decline of GFR in the mothers. Women with established nephropathy can thus expect to have an increase in urinary protein excretion as pregnancy advances and early delivery is likely. There is an increased rate of acute and chronic problems with the offspring.

Conclusions

Considerable progress has been made in our understanding of the pathogenesis of diabetic nephropathy and the therapeutic strategies to halt or delay the progression of this devastating complication. Arterial disease accompanies renal disease and its assessment and management is an important aspect of efforts to decrease the mortality and morbidity from ischemic heart disease and cerebral vascular accidents in proteinuric diabetic patients. Early detection of patients at risk of developing renal disease is critical. Microalbuminuria, a positive family history of essential hypertension, and elevated red cell sodium–lithium countertransport activity are useful markers of patients at risk of renal and cardiovascular disease. In these individuals, early antihypertensive treatment and strict control of blood glucose may arrest the progression of renal vascular damage. Diabetic patients make up an increasing proportion of patients on ESRF programs and survival on RRT is less than in non-diabetic patients. Renal transplantation is the preferred mode of renal replacement.

References

1. Viberti, G.C., Walker, J.D. and Pinto, J. (1992) Diabetic nephropathy, in *International Textbook of Diabetes Mellitus* (eds K.G.M.M. Alberti, R.A. De Fronzo, H. Keen and J. Pinto), John Wiley, Chichester, pp. 1267–328.
2. Berkman, J. and Rifkin, H. (1973) Unilateral nodular diabetic glomerulosclerosis (Kimmelstiel-Wilson). Report of a case. *Metabolism*, **22**, 715–22.
3. Rudberg, S., Persson, B. and Dalquist, G. (1992) Increased glomerular filtration rate as a predictor of diabetic nephropathy. An 8 year prospective study. *Kidney Int.*, **41**, 822–8.
4. Messent, J., Jones, S.L., Wiseman, M. and Viberti, C.C. (1991) Glomerular hyperfiltration and albuminuria – an 8 year prospective study. *Diabetologia* (suppl. 2 (abstract 3)), A1.
5. Viberti, G.C., Hill, R., Jarrett, R.J. *et al.* (1982) Microalbuminuria as a predictor of clinical nephropathy in insulin-dependent diabetes mellitus. *Lancet*, **i**, 430–2.
6. Parving, H-H., Oxenboll, B., Svendsen, P.A. *et al.* (1982) Early detection of patients at risk of developing diabetic nephropathy. A longitudinal study of urinary albumin excretion. *Acta Endoclinol.*, **100**, 550–5.
7. Mathiesen, E.R., Oxenboll, B., Johansen, K. *et al.* (1984) Incipient nephropathy in type 1 (insulin-dependent diabetes). *Diabetologia*, **26**, 406–10.
8. Mogensen, C.E. and Christensen, C.K. (1984) Predicting diabetic nephropathy in insulin-dependent diabetic patients. *N. Engl. J. Med.*, **311**, 89–93.
9. Wiseman, M.J., Viberti, G.C., Mackintosh, D. *et al.* (1984) Glycemia, arterial pressure and microalbuminuria in type 1 (insulin-dependent) diabetes mellitus. *Diabetologia*, **2**, 401–5.
10. Fioretto, P., Steffes, M.W. and Mauer, M. (1994) Glomerular structure in nonproteinuric IDDM patients with various levels of albuminuria. *Diabetes*, **43**, 345–9.
11. Yip, J., Mattock, M., Sethi, M. *et al.* (1993) Insulin resistance in insulin-dependent diabetic patients with microalbuminuria. *Lancet*, **342**, 883–7.
12. Messent, J., Elliott, T., Hill, R. *et al.* (1992) Prognostic significance of microalbuminuria in insulin-dependent diabetes mellitus: A twenty-three year follow-up study. *Kidney Int.*, **41**, 836–9.
13. Schmitz, A. and Vaeth, M. (1988) Microalbuminuria: a major risk factor in non-insulin-dependent diabetes. A 10 year follow-up study of 503 patients. *Diabetic Med.*, **5**, 126–34.
14. Mattock, M.B., Morrish, N.J., Viberti, G.C. *et al.* (1992) Prospective study of microalbuminuria as predictor of mortality in NIDDM. *Diabetes*, **41**, 736–41.
15. The Diabetes Control and Complications Trial Research Group (1993) The effect of intensive treatment of diabetes on the development and progression of long-term complications in insulin-dependent diabetes mellitus. *N. Engl. J. Med.*, **329**, 977–86.
16. Brownlee, M., Cerami, A. and Vlassara, H. (1988) Advanced glycosylation end products in tissue and the biochemical basis of diabetic complications. *N. Engl. J. Med.*, **318**, 1315–21.
17. Greene, D. (1988) The pathogenesis and its prevention of diabetic neuropathy and nephropathy. *Metabolism*, **37**(suppl 1), 25–9.
18. Lorenzi, M. (1992) Glucose toxicity in the vascular complications of diabetes: the cellular perspective. *Diabetes Metab. Rev.*, **8**, 85–103.
19. Vora, J.P., Anderson, S. and Brenner, B.M. (1994) Pathogenesis of diabetic glomerulopathy: the role of glomerular hemodynamic factors, in *The Kidney and Hypertension in Diabetes Mellitus*, 2nd edn (ed. C.E. Mogensen), Kluwer Academic Publishers, pp. 223–32.
20. Seaquist, E.R., Goetz, F.C., Rich, S. *et al.* (1989) Familial clustering of diabetic kidney disease. Evidence for genetic susceptibility to diabetic nephropathy. *N. Engl. J. Med.*, **320**, 1161–5.
21. Earle, K., Walker, J., Hill, C. and Viberti, G.C. (1992) Familial clustering of cardiovascular disease in patients with insulin-dependent diabetes and nephropathy. *N. Engl. J. Med.*, **326**, 673–7.
22. Mangili, R. (1994) Cation transport, hypertension and diabetic nephropathy, in *The Kidney and Hypertension in Diabetes Mellitus*, 2nd edn (ed. C.E. Mogensen), Kluwer Academic Publishers, pp. 273–84.
23. Trevisan, R., Nosadini, R., Fioretto, P. *et al.* (1992) Clustering of risk factors in hypertensive insulin-dependent diabetics with high sodium–lithium countertransport. *Kidney Int.*, **41**, 855–61.
24. Rosskopf, D., Dusing, R. and Siffert, W. (1993) Membrane sodium–proton exchange and primary hypertension. *Hypertension.*, **21**, 607–17.
25. Trevisan, R., Li, L.K., Messent, J. *et al.* (1992) Na/H antiport activity and cell growth in cultured skin fibroblasts of IDDM patients with nephropathy. *Diabetes*, **41**, 1239–46.
26. Williams, B. and Howard, R.L. (1994) Glucose-induced changes in Na/H antiport activity and gene expression in cultured vascular muscle cells. *J. Clin. Invest.*, **93**, 2623–31.
27. Doria, A., Warram, J.H. and Krowlewski, A.S. (1994) Genetic predisposition to diabetic nephropathy. Evidence for a role of the angiotensin I-converting enzyme gene. *Diabetes*, **43**, 690–5.
28. Kimmelsteil, P. and Wilson, C. (1936) Intracapillary lesions in glomeruli of kidney. *Am. J. Pathol.*, **12**, 83–97.
29. Bell, E.T. (1942) Renal lesions in diabetes mellitus. *Am. J. Pathol.*, **18**, 740–5.
30. Osterby, R., Gall, M-A., Schmitz, A. *et al.* (1993) Glomeru-

lar structure and function in proteinuric type 2 (non-insulin-dependent) diabetic patients. *Diabetologia*, **36**, 1064–70.

31. Vernier, R.L., Steffes, M.W., Sisson-Ross, S. and Mauer, S.M. (1992) Heparan sulphate proteoglycan in the glomerular basement membrane in type 1 diabetes mellitus. *Kidney Int.*, **41**, 1070–80.

32. Walker, J.D., Close, C.F., Jones, SL. *et al.* (1992) Glomerular structure in Type 1 (insulin-dependent) diabetic patients with microalbuminuria. *Kidney Int.*, **41**, 679–84.

33. Steffes, M.W., Bilous, R.W., Sutherland, D.E.R. and Mauer, S.M. (1992) Cell and matrix components of the glomerulus in type 1 diabetes. *Diabetes*, **41**, 679–84.

34. Bilous, R.W., Mauer, S.M., Sutherland, D.E.R. and Steffes, M.W. (1989) Mean glomerular volume and the rate of development of diabetic nephropathy. *Diabetes*, **38**, 1142–7.

35. Bendtsen, T.F. and Nyengaard, J.R. (1992) The number of glomeruli in type 1 (insulin-dependent) and type 2 (non-insulin-dependent) diabetic patients. *Diabetologia*, **35**, 844–50.

36. Bangstad, H-J., Osterby, R., Dahl-Jorgennsen, K. *et al.* (1994) Improvement of blood glucose control in IDDM patients retards the progression of morphological change in early diabetic nephropathy. *Diabetologia*, **37**, 483–90.

37. Bjorck, S. (1994) Clinical trials in overt diabetic nephropathy, in *The Kidney and Hypertension in Diabetes Mellitus*, 2nd edn (ed. C.E. Mogensen), Kluwer Academic Publishers, pp. 333–9.

38. Lewis, E.J., Hunsickler, L.G., Bain, R.P. and Rohde, R.D. (1993) The effect of angiotensin-converting-enzyme inhibition on diabetic nephropathy. *N. Engl. J. Med.*, **329**, 1456–62.

39. Viberti, G.C., Mogensen, C.E., Groop, L.C. and Pauls, J.F. (1994) Effect of captopril on progression to clinical proteinuria in patients with insulin-dependent diabetes mellitus and microalbuminuria. *JAMA*, **271**, 275–9.

40. Walker, J.D., Bending, J.J., Dodds, R.A. *et al.* (1989) Restriction of dietary protein and progression of renal failure in diabetic nephropathy. *Lancet*, **ii**, 1411–14.

41. Klahr, S.K., Levey, A.S., Beck, G.J. *et al.* (1994) The effects of dietary protein restriction and blood pressure control on the progression of chronic renal disease. *N. Engl. J. Med.*, **330**, 877–84.

42. Viberti, G.C., Bilous, R.W., Mackintosh, D. and Keen, H. (1983) Long term correction of hyperglycaemia and progression of renal failure in insulin-dependent diabetes. *Br. Med. J.*, **286**, 598–602.

43. Wang, P., Lau, J. and Chalmers, T.C. (1993) Meta-analysis of intensive blood-glucose control on late complications of type 1 diabetes. *Lancet*, **341**, 1306–9.

44. Raine, A.E.G. (1994) Evolution worldwide of the treatment of patients with advanced diabetic nephropathy by renal replacement therapy, in *The Kidney and Hypertension in Diabetes Mellitus*, 2nd edn (ed. C.E. Mogensen), Kluwer Academic Publishers, pp. 449–58.

45. Zmirou, D., Benhamou, P-Y., Cordonnier, D. *et al.* (1992) Diabetes mellitus prevalence among dialysed patients in France (UREMIDIAB study). *Nephrol. Dial. Transplant.*, **7**, 1092–7.

46. Paisley, R., Banks, R., Holton, R. *et al.* (1986) Glycosylated hemoglobin in uremia. *Diabetic Med.*, **3**, 445–8.

47. Balaskas, E.V. and Oreopoulos, D.G. (1994) Continuous ambulatory peritoneal dialysis in uremic diabetics, in *The Kidney and Hypertension in Diabetes Mellitus*, 2nd edn (ed. C.E. Mogensen), Kluwer Academic Publishers, pp. 469–85.

48. Brunner, F.P. and Selwood, N.H. (1992) Profile of patients on RRT in Europe and death rates due to major causes of death groups. *Kidney Int.*, **42**(suppl 38), S4–S15.

49. Manske, C.L., Wang, Y., Rector, T. *et al.* (1992) Coronary revascularisation in insulin-dependent diabetic patients with chronic renal failure. *Lancet*, **340**, 998–1002.

50. Basadonna, G., Matas, A.J. and Najarian, J.S. (1992) Kidney transplantation in diabetic patients: The University of Minnesota experience. *Kidney Int.*, **42**(Suppl 38), S193–6.

51. Remuzzi, G., Ruggenenti, P. and Mauer, S.W. (1994) Pancreas and kidney/pancreas transplants: experimental medicine or real improvement. *Lancet*, **343**, 27–31.

52. Hanssens, M., Keirse, M.J.N.C., Vankelecom, F. and Van Assche, F.A. (1991) Fetal and neonatal effects of treatment with angiotensin-converting enzyme inhibitors in pregnancy. *Obstet. Gynecol.*, **78**, 128–35.

53. Kimmerle, R., Zab, R-P., Cupisti, S. *et al.* (1995) Pregnancies in women with diabetic nephropathy: long-term outcome for mother and child. *Diabetologia*, **38**, 227–35.

44

IgA nephropathy and Henoch–Schönlein nephritis

John Feehally

Introduction

IgA nephropathy

IgA nephropathy (IgAN) is a glomerular disease defined by the mesangial deposition of IgA.

It was first recognized as a separate entity when immunofluorescence techniques were introduced for the study of renal biopsy and was described in 1968 by a Parisian pathologist, Jean Berger. Although its most common clinical presentation is hematuria, this is not universal nor necessary for the diagnosis. IgAN is unique among glomerular diseases in being defined by the presence of an immune reactant rather than any other morphological feature found on renal biopsy; the light microscopic changes are very variable.

Henoch–Schönlein nephritis

The nephritis associated with Henoch–Schönlein purpura (HSP) is also characterized by glomerular IgA deposition; indeed the renal histological features of HSP are indistinguishable from IgAN. It is the extrarenal disease which defines HSP – a systemic vasculitis most commonly involving the skin, joints and gut, in which tissue deposition of IgA is characteristic.

Relationship between IgAN and HSP

As well as the similarity of the glomerular disease, many immunological abnormalities have been identified in both IgAN and HSP. This suggests that IgAN may be a forme fruste of HSP, in other words that IgAN is 'HSP without the rash'. This idea remains speculative until the pathogenesis of these conditions is better understood.

IgA nephropathy

Renal histopathology (Figure 44.1)

Immune deposits

Diffuse mesangial IgA is the defining hallmark. IgG and C3, and less commonly IgM, may also be found in the same distribution. IgA also occurs sometimes along capillary loops.

Light microscopy

Light microscopic changes are, however, remarkably variable and do not correlate topographically with the IgA deposits. IgAN is usually an indolent lesion. The glomeruli may be virtually normal or there may be mesangial hypercellularity, either global or segmental. In long-standing disease there will be varying degrees of glomerular sclerosis in association with tubulointerstitial scarring.

Acute injury is much less common but focal segmental necrotizing glomerular lesions may occur with crescent formation. Another common finding in acute renal impairment in IgAN is tubular occlusion by red cells.

Nephrology, Edited by Rex L. Jamison and Robert Wilkinson.
Published in 1997 by Chapman & Hall, London. ISBN 0 412 60930 4

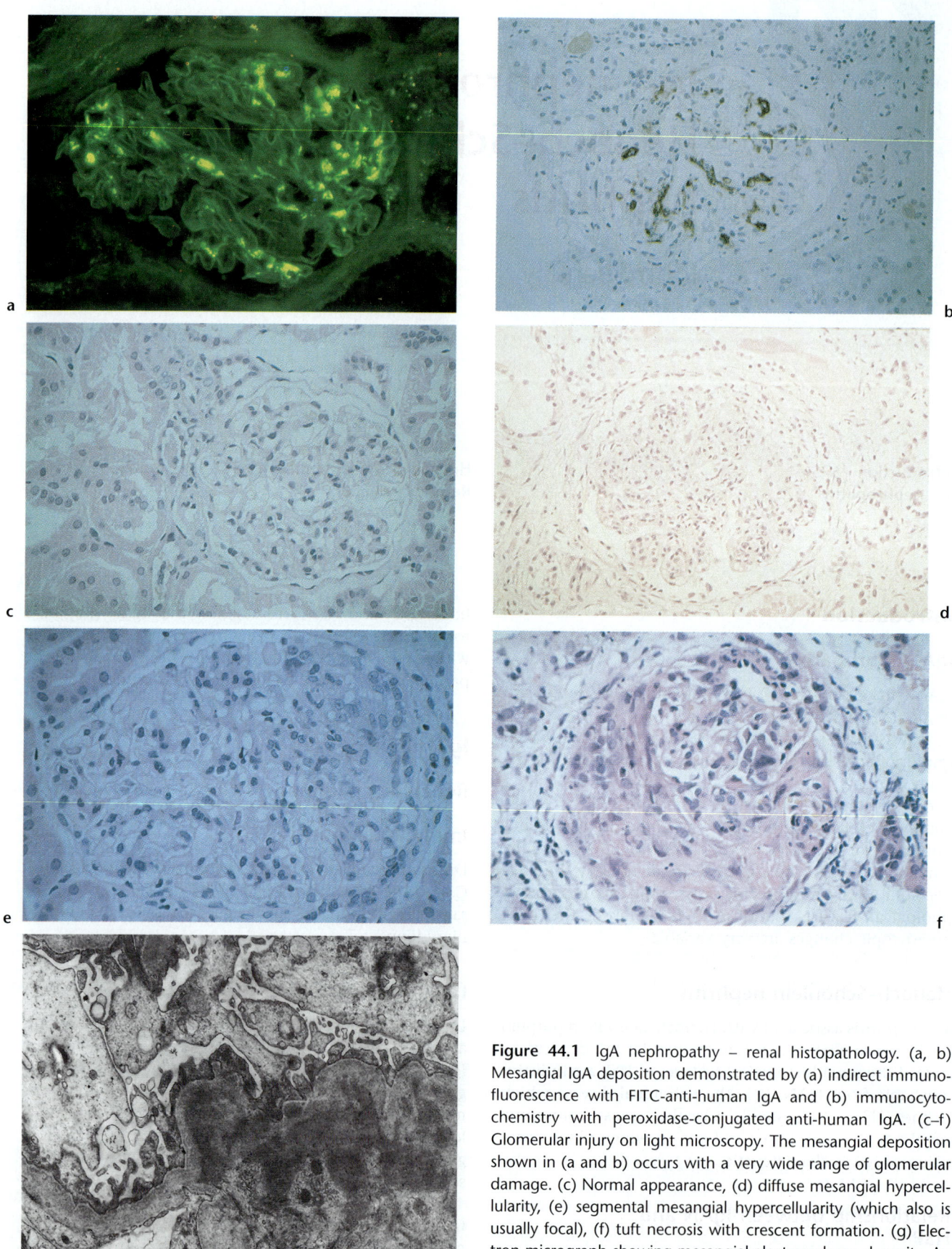

Figure 44.1 IgA nephropathy – renal histopathology. (a, b) Mesangial IgA deposition demonstrated by (a) indirect immunofluorescence with FITC-anti-human IgA and (b) immunocytochemistry with peroxidase-conjugated anti-human IgA. (c–f) Glomerular injury on light microscopy. The mesangial deposition shown in (a and b) occurs with a very wide range of glomerular damage. (c) Normal appearance, (d) diffuse mesangial hypercellularity, (e) segmental mesangial hypercellularity (which also is usually focal), (f) tuft necrosis with crescent formation. (g) Electron micrograph showing mesangial electron-dense deposits. An identical range of appearances can be seen in HSP nephritis (Micrographs kindly provided by Dr P.N. Furness.)

Electron microscopy

Electron-dense deposits correspond to the mesangial IgA.

Clinical

The range of presentations of IgAN are shown in Figure 44.2 and Table 44.1.

Hematuria

The most typical clinical presentation is episodic macroscopic hematuria. The urine is usually brown rather than red and clots are unusual. Occasionally there is loin pain. Hematuria usually follows intercurrent mucosal infection, upper respiratory tract or occasionally gastrointestinal. Hematuria is usually visible within 24h of the onset of the symptoms of infection, a clear distinction from the two- to three-week delay between the infection and subsequent hematuria in postinfections (for example, poststreptococcal) glomerulonephritis. Exercise alone will provoke hematuria in a few patients. There is persistent microscopic hematuria between attacks. This typical clinical pattern occurs most frequently in the second and third decades of life and is commoner in males by 3 to 1. The hematuria stops spontaneously over a few days at

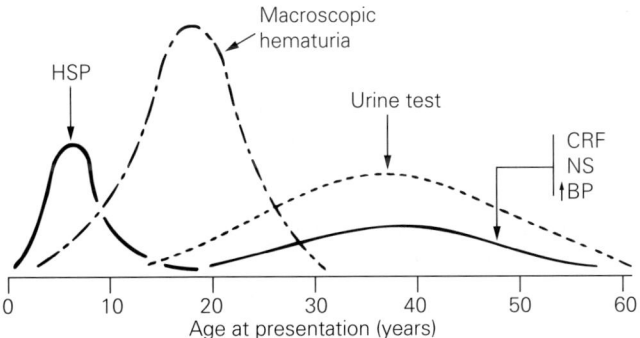

Figure 44.2 The pattern of clinical presentations in IgA nephropathy and Henoch–Schönlein purpura. The propensity of HSP for early childhood remains unexplained. The later presentation of IgAN with renal impairment, hypertension and nephrotic range proteinuria is presumed to indicate longstanding disease not previously identified through lack of macroscopic haematuria.

most. Most patients have only a few episodes of frank hematuria which become less frequent and stop over a few years at most.

Asymptomatic

Patients who do not report visible hematuria may be identified by asymptomatic urine testing when microscopic hematuria with or without proteinuria are identified. The number of patients thus identified will depend on local attitudes to routine screening of urine and also on the use of renal biopsy in patients with microscopic hematuria.

Proteinuria

There may also be proteinuria although nephrotic syndrome is uncommon (<10% of all cases). It is very unusual for proteinuria to occur without microscopic hematuria.

Renal function is usually preserved and blood pressure normal at this early stage.

Acute renal failure

Acute renal failure is very uncommon in IgAN and develops by two distinct mechanisms. There may be acute severe immune injury with necrotizing GN and crescent formation (Figure 44.1(f)). Alternatively it can occur with mild glomerular injury when heavy glomerular hematuria leads to tubular occlusion by red cells [1].

Chronic renal failure

Some patients already have renal impairment and hypertension when first identified; these patients tend to be older and it is usually assumed they have long-standing disease which went previously undiagnosed because there was never frank hematuria.

Geographical variation in the incidence of IgAN

Available epidemiological evidence suggests IgAN is common in Mediterranean countries and Japan and significantly less so in Northern Europe and North America [2]. Any cause for true variations in incidence is

Table 44.1 Clinical presentations of IgA nephropathy

Recurrent macroscopic hematuria (provoked by mucosal infection or exercise)
Asymptomatic microscopic hematuria ± proteinuria
Nephrotic syndrome
Acute renal failure – severe glomerular lesions
                  or – hematuria causing tubular occlusion
Chronic renal failure

unknown, although genetic factors may be important: for example in North America IgAN is less common in blacks than whites [3]. But it is also important to realize that attitudes to the identification and investigation of microscopic hematuria may bias the apparent differences. A country with an active program of routine urine testing will inevitably identify more individuals with microscopic hematuria; but only if renal biopsy is performed in such patients will those with IgAN be identified. A survey of nephrologists in the UK confirmed this view: those who offered renal biopsy to patients with isolated microscopic hematuria had the highest incidence of IgAN as a proportion of patients with glomerular disease in their practice [4].

Immunopathogenesis

Despite the accumulation of much information over the last 25 years about immune abnormalities in IgAN [5, 6], two crucial questions remain unanswered: why is IgA deposited in the mesangium? and what is the relationship between the IgA deposition and subsequent glomerular inflammation and sclerosis?

The IgA immune system

It is helpful to understand the design of the IgA immune system in man to appreciate the unanswered questions in IgAN [7].

The IgA system is compartmentalized. Circulating IgA is mostly derived from bone marrow; it is at least 90% monomeric (mIgA) and predominantly of the IgA1 subclass. The function of circulating IgA is uncertain.

Most IgA, however, is derived from mucosa and destined for mucosal fluids where it has a key role in defense against adherence and invasion of micro-organisms. This IgA is polymeric, IgA monomers covalently joined by J chain (pIgA), and may be IgA1 or IgA2. (Any functional differences in the two subclasses is unknown.) The IgA which reaches the mucosal fluids is secretory IgA, consisting of pIgA attached to secretory component, a protein which is part of the machinery of the endocytotic process by which pIgA reaches secretions.

The IgA system has significant differences in all experimental animals compared to man; a factor which limits the value of animal models of IgAN. Such models have therefore been used chiefly to examine events involved in glomerular IgA deposition and subsequent injury rather than the IgA immune environment which predisposes to IgA deposition.

The origin of mesangial IgA in IgAN

The mesangial IgA in IgAN is pIgA but is not secretory IgA (it has J chain but not secretory component). It is chiefly of the IgA1 subclass [6]. In view of the clinical association with mucosal infection, it has been proposed that the mesangial IgA is derived from the mucosa, rather than from the marrow. The tonsils in IgAN show up-regulation of IgA production compared to controls [8], but pIgA production is actually down-regulated in the lamina propria of duodenal mucosa (the main immunoglobulin production site in the mucosal system) [9] and up-regulated in the marrow [10]. This suggests that the mesangial IgA may be chiefly marrow derived but does not easily explain the clinical relationship between mucosal infection and episodes of hematuria, or the apparent role of the tonsil. The intriguing observation that manipulation of the tonsils during tonsillectomy may provoke immediate macroscopic hematuria remains unexplained.

Regulation of IgA production in IgAN

There is much evidence of abnormal regulation of IgA production in IgAN [5, 6]. Cultured peripheral blood lymphocytes produce excess IgA in a variety of experimental contexts without antigen. When antigen challenge is used, there may be evidence of increased and prolonged IgA production, particularly pIgA [11]. There is evidence for both B cell and T cell abnormalities in this control. These studies are all based on peripheral blood lymphocytes; it is not known to what extent such a population represents mucosa or marrow derived cells which are trafficking elsewhere.

Serum IgA

This altered control of IgA production may explain the increased serum total IgA found in IgAN, which is chiefly IgA1. The increase is in both pIgA and mIgA. However, this is not a sufficient explanation for the mesangial deposition of IgA. In other circumstances serum IgA may be much higher, due to monoclonal production in IgA myeloma or polyclonal IgA production in AIDS; yet IgA nephropathy is not a feature of myeloma, and the reports of IgAN in association with AIDS suggest an association little more than would be expected given the prevalence of these two common diseases.

Mechanism of IgA deposition in IgAN

Antigen-dependent mechanism

Mesangial immune deposits such as are seen in IgAN can be produced in experimental animals by infusion of antigen–antibody complexes, or by administering antibody directed against an intrinsic or extrinsic antigen already fixed in the mesangium. Search for relevant antigens within the mesangial deposits in IgAN has, however, been disappointing. At one time cytomegalovirus was reported in IgAN glomeruli but more sophisticated molecular studies did not sustain this proposition [12]. No viral or food antigens have been consistently identified. This may reflect a wide variety of antigens involved; or could mean that the initiating antigen may no longer be present by the time the diagnosis is made, deposits being perpetuated by the accretion of anti-idiotypic IgA directed against the original antibody.

Antigen-independent mechanism

Alternatively the IgA could be deposited in the mesangium by mechanisms other than classical antigen–antibody interactions. The glycosylation of the IgA molecule is a likely abnormality since changes in the carbohydrate structure of immunogobulins are known to modify interactions with cell surface receptors as well as other proteins. Recent observations of abnormal glycosylation of IgA1 in IgAN have therefore provoked much interest as a putative pathogenic abnormality [13, 13a]. However, little is known about the control of IgA glycosylation in normal B cells let alone in IgAN; and there is no direct evidence yet that altered IgA1 glycosylation promotes glomerular deposition.

Relationship of IgA deposition to glomerular injury

IgA is relatively non-inflammatory compared to IgG; it also activates complement poorly. Therefore, there is uncertainty as to whether IgA deposition alone is sufficient to provoke glomerular inflammation. This uncertainty is reinforced by the disparity between the diffuse IgA deposition and the injury on light microscopy which is often focal. In animal models IgG and C3 deposition as well as IgA are needed to provoke hematuria; but this is not reliably the case in humans where there may be clinical renal disease and structural glomerular injury even when IgA alone is found in the mesangium. Circulating IgG against a mesangial determinant (not fully defined) has been reported in IgAN [14]; this IgG correlated with clinical activity judged by hematuria but this finding has not been confirmed.

Immunogenetics and familial IgAN

A number of the abnormalities of IgA regulation seen in IgAN have also been described in first-degree relatives of patients.

Many studies have also sought associations between IgAN and major histocompatability complex (MHC) antigens as well as other candidate antigens relevant to control of IgA production, for example IgA switch region genes which control changes from IgM to IgA during an immune response. The most robust associations are with HLA DR4 and HLA DQw7 (which is in linkage disequilibrium with DR4) and with the rare complement component allele C4A. Overall these studies have been disappointing; genes apparently associated with IgAN or with the risk of IgAN progressing to renal failure have not consistently been identified in different populations.

The population variations in these studies suggest the reported genes may be close to, but cannot be identical

with, any disease susceptibility gene. Although these findings provoke ideas about the immunopathogenesis of IgAN, as yet they have no practical clinical value.

Despite this genetic and familial background, families with more than one affected member are uncommon, although one very large pedigree in the southern United States has been defined in great detail [15]. When they do occur, no single pattern of inheritance is consistently reported. Presumably additional environmental triggers are needed to provoke IgAN in the presence of a necessary, but not sufficient, genetic and immune background.

Diagnosis and differential diagnosis

Histopathology

By definition the diagnosis of IgAN requires identification of IgA in the glomeruli on renal histology. Mesangial IgA occurs in other conditions (Table 44.2), which can in general be differentiated without difficulty on clinical, serological and histological criteria.

Hematuria

In its most characteristic clinical setting (recurrent macroscopic hematuria coinciding with mucosal infection in a young male in the second or third decade of life) the diagnosis can be strongly suspected. However, the clinical suspicion can never be regarded as absolute proof without histological confirmation; frank hematuria occurs in a number of patterns of glomerular disease particularly in young people, where it often coincides with intercurrent infection (Table 44.3).

Nephrotic syndrome

Patients with IgAN occasionally develop a nephrotic syndrome, which is indistinguishable from minimal change nephrotic syndrome: there is a sudden onset of nephrosis with biopsy evidence of glomerular epithelial cell foot process effacement and a prompt absolute remission of proteinuria in response to corticosteroids. Only

---

Table 44.2 Causes of mesangial IgA deposition

IgA nephropathy
Henoch–Schönlein purpura nephritis
Systemic lupus
Alcoholic cirrhosis[a]

[a] Failure of normal liver clearance of IgA from the circulation leads to glomerular IgA deposits; hematuria or any other clinical manifestation of renal disease is very uncommon.

hematuria and IgA deposits persist after treatment. These patients are regarded as having two separate common glomerular diseases, IgAN and minimal change nephrotic syndrome. Other patients with IgAN develop nephrotic syndrome, lack the absolute response to corticosteroids and appear to have nephrosis as a manifestation of IgAN. The clinical differential diagnosis includes common causes of nephrotic syndrome appropriate for the age of the patient.

Chronic renal disease: hypertension, proteinuria, renal impairment

In this context IgAN will be clinically indistinguishable from many forms of chronic renal disease. Biopsy may be diagnostic, by identifying mesangial IgA, even when structural damage is so advanced on light microscopy that it can only be defined as 'end stage kidney'.

Clinical associations with IgAN

Although IgAN is clinically restricted to the kidney in most cases, associations with other conditions have been described. Since IgAN is common the importance of single case descriptions is uncertain. However, there are well-reported associations with IgAN, particularly with a range of immune diseases (Table 44.4). The relationship of these associated clinical diseases to the abnormalities of the IgA system is unclear.

Natural history

The overall prognosis of IgAN has now been defined in long-term natural history studies [16]. Large studies with follow-up in excess of 20 years indicate a slow attrition. By 20 years, a quarter of patients will have end-stage renal failure; a further 20% will have impaired renal function and will also progress eventually. The clinical impact of these outcomes must be appreciated in the context of a condition whose peak onset is in early adult life. These data also conceal a number of uncertainties. An active approach to investigation of microscopic hematuria is likely to increase the cohort of patients with IgAN but may include more with a good prognosis, thus altering the percentage risk of progression. Furthermore, the risk is not uniform. As in any glomerular disease the presence of hypertension, persistent heavy proteinuria and renal impairment at presentation, as well as histological evidence of glomerular and interstitial fibrosis, mark those with a poor prognosis from the point of diagnosis (Table 44.5). But onset of disease is extremely difficult to define when the early stages will be asymptomatic unless there is macroscopic hematuria. It is as yet unclear from available natural history data the extent to which the prognosis is better in those who have isolated hematuria. Perhaps unexpectedly, episodes of macroscopic hematuria do not confer a worse prognosis [17]; this may indicate that such episodes only occur early in the natural history, and that patients doing less well from the point

Table 44.3 Patterns of glomerular disease associated with episodic frank hematuria

Chronic	IgA nephropathy
	Mesangiocapillary GN
	Hereditary nephropathy (e.g. Alport's syndrome)
	Thin membrane nephropathy
Acute	Acute nephritic syndrome
	Rapidly progressive crescentic GN

Table 44.4 Clinical associations with IgA nephropathy

Rheumatoid arthritis
Seronegative spondylarthropathies
    ankylosing spondylitis
    Reiter's syndrome
Behçet's disease
Celiac disease
Scleritis
AIDS

	Renal survival			
	5 year (%)	10 year (%)	15 year (%)	20 year (%)
From time of renal biopsy	91	83	79	75
From time of first symptom	96	90	82	77

Adapted from [16].

Table 44.5 Natural history of IgA nephropathy; acturarial renal survival in 11 large series of patients with IgA nephropathy (total number of patients analyzed = 2653)

of diagnosis in fact were only identified well on in their disease. This is also suggested by the adverse influence age at diagnosis has on outcome.

Recurrence of IgAN in transplants

Mesangial IgA deposits recur in some 60% of patients with IgAN [18]. They may occur within days or weeks of transplantation, but the risk increases with the duration of the transplant. They seem benign in the short term and are not often associated initially with light microscopic changes. However, graft failure, associated with proteinuria and hypertension, will occur in up to half those with recurrent IgA deposits. It has been proposed that the risk of recurrence is increased in live related transplants (due to the likelihood of closer HLA matching) but this has not been confirmed. The choice of immunosuppressive regimen to prevent graft rejection does not influence the frequency of recurrent IgA deposits.

In occasional unwitting experiments cadaver kidneys with IgA deposits have been transplanted into recipients without IgAN. In all cases the IgA rapidly disappeared, supporting the concept that abnormalities in IgAN are in the IgA immune system and not in the kidney.

Treatment

There is no specific treatment available to prevent mesangial IgA deposition – a situation which will not change until the immunopathogenesis of IgAN is better understood. However, a number of immune and non-immune interventions have been tried over the last decade with, in general, disappointing results [19]. Unfortunately much of the available information is anecdotal with few well-designed randomized studies. Furthermore, follow-up has not always been as long as necessary to confirm or refute real benefit in a disease as indolent as IgAN.

Reduction of mucosal antigen challenge

The unproven presumption that IgAN is provoked by mucosal antigen challenge led to a number of studies designed to minimize mucosal antigen challenge. There are anecdotal reports of the benefit of oligoantigenic diets which remain unconfirmed. Short studies of sodium cromoglycate (known to reduce IgA antibody responses by reducing food antigen penetration) and 5-aminosalicylic acid (which reduces mucosal inflammation and might therefore reduce antigen entry) showed no benefit.

Tonsillectomy

The precise role of the tonsil in the immunopathogenesis of IgAN remains debatable. However, hematuria is reduced following tonsillectomy; although it is not known if this is followed by delay or prevention of chronic renal failure [20].

The observation that patients will occasionally have immediate frank hematuria following operative manipulation of the tonsil may perhaps provide an important pathogenic clue.

Reduction of circulating IgA levels

Phenytoin is known to reduce total serum IgA, but it proved of no benefit in a randomized controlled study.

Immunosuppressive drug treatment

Interventions have largely been restricted to patients with persistent proteinuria as well as hematuria, who are identified as having a poorer prognosis.

Corticosteroids

There have only between two short randomized studies of corticosteroids which showed no overall benefit. In one study the analysis focused on a subset of patients with heavy proteinuria and very minor histological changes in whom steroids induced a fall in protein excretion adequate to restore serum albumin. Three patients had complete abolition of proteinuria so may represent the coincidence of MCNS and IgAN described above. Information from uncontrolled studies also suggests benefit in those with heavy proteinuria but preserved renal function (GFR > 70 ml/min). Unfortunately many of these patients received non-steroidal anti-inflammatory drugs (NSAIDs) or dipyridamole as well.

Cyclosporin

One randomized trial shows significant reduction in proteinuria which reverts when cyclosporin is withdrawn and appears to parallel a fall in GFR. Cyclosporin is therefore of no benefit.

Cyclophosphamide

One controlled study suggests that cyclophosphamide may be of benefit in combination with dipyridamole and warfarin, in reducing the risk of progression to renal failure. The possibility that the anticoagulant alone produces the benefit has not yet been excluded.

A meta-analysis of the small number of randomized trials of immunosuppressive drugs in IgAN does suggest benefit confined to the small minority with nephrotic syndrome [21]. Nevertheless many nephrologists would regard the long-term effects of immunosuppression as unacceptable in typical young adult patients with IgAN.

Crescentic IgA nephropathy

Small numbers of cases are reported with short-term responses to various combinations of prednisolone and cyclophosphamide with plasma exchange, although the majority go on to end-stage renal failure within 12 months. Exactly which elements of the treatment are needed is not clear and will be hard to evaluate given the infrequency of such patients.

Non-immune treatments

Hypertension

Raised blood pressure is common in IgAN; indeed it may occur more frequently and earlier in IgAN than in other chronic glomerular disease, and may be associated with defects in red cell sodium–lithium countertransport. The benefit of different blood pressure-lowering agents has not been investigated in controlled studies although one retrospective study suggested benefit of an angiotensin converting enzyme (ACE) inhibitor over a regime based on beta blockers [22]. In a controlled study ACE inhibitor also significantly lowered proteinuria in normotensive patients with IgAN.

Fish oil

Although a two-year prospective randomized trial of fish oil supplementation showed benefit in delaying progression of renal impairment in IgAN with proteinuria [23], other controlled studies showed no benefit [24]. The reason for this discrepancy is unclear.

Summary of treatment options

With the possible exception of nephrotic patients in whom corticosteroids may be justified, there is no convincing evidence for specific therapeutic interventions in IgAN. Control of blood pressure, whatever class of agents is used, is the one available strategy to retard progression to renal failure.

Henoch–Schönlein purpura

Henoch–Schönlein purpura (HSP) is a systemic vasculitis defined by tissue deposition of IgA. It may occur at any age but is most common in the first decade of life. Organ involvement typically includes the skin (with recurrent vasculitic eruptions in a characteristic extensor distribution), the kidney and the gut. In practice, the diagnosis is made on clinical criteria in the great majority of children in whom it is a self-limiting illness. In adults, biopsy is used more freely to distinguish between HSP and other forms of systemic vasculitis; the diagnostic hallmark is the presence of IgA in affected tissues. The reasons for the predilection for the gut and the specific distribution of the rash are unclear. Many infective and environmental triggers have been associated with episodes of HSP in some patients; but no consistent pattern has emerged.

Henoch–Schönlein nephritis

The renal lesion in HSP is histologically indistinguishable from IgAN. Light microscopic appearances vary from near normal through diffuse mesangial hypercellularity to focal segmental GN. Mesangial IgA is diagnostic; IgA may also be seen on capillary loops. HSP is relatively uncommon in adults so much of the available information is derived from careful studies of children with HSP nephritis [25].

It is difficult to estimate the prevalence of renal involvement in HSP. In many patients it is only identified as transient hematuria with or without proteinuria during a self-limiting episode of HSP. Only a minority will therefore be seen by nephrologists and these are selected by the persistence of asymptomatic urine abnormalities, or because they become frankly nephrotic, or much less commonly because they develop rapidly progressive renal failure.

Of those who do reach nephrological care, predictors of poor prognosis are those common to IgAN and most other glomerular disease (Table 44.6).

Treatment

No specific treatment has ever been shown in controlled trials to influence the outcome of the nephritis or any other aspect of HSP.

The great majority of patients have transient urine abnormalities, which resolve as the rash and other clinical features recede. No treatment is required but they must be observed until after the urine has cleared.

Of those with persistent renal involvement who reach a nephrologist and undergo renal biopsy, the majority still have a good prognosis. If there is only mild histological change and preserved renal function, they should be observed without treatment, for as long as hematuria and proteinuria persist.

Irreversible chronic changes may be seen in the

Table 44.6 Markers of poor prognosis in IgA nephropathy and Henoch–Schönlein nephritis

Clinical	Older age
	Proteinuria – especially nephrotic range
	Hypertension
	Renal impairment
Histological	Glomerular sclerosis
	Interstitial fibrosis and tubular atrophy

These features are not specific for IgA nephropathy but are common to most chronic glomerular diseases.

absence of active glomerular inflammation. No immune treatment will influence this situation. As in other glomerular disease, control of blood pressure is the single most important factor in preserving renal function.

There are two circumstances where immune therapy is appropriate.

Rapidly progressive renal failure

The most aggressive pattern of HSP nephritis is focal segmental necrotizing glomerulonephritis (GN) (usually with crescent formation) which is histologically indistinguishable from the GN associated with other forms of systemic vasculitis, apart from deposits of IgA (Figure 44.1).

This is a very uncommon clinical circumstance and seems to occur less frequently than in antineutrophil cytoplasm antibodies (ANCA)-positive vasculitis. There is no specific evidence to guide treatment. A range of aggressive immunosuppressive regimes have been reported including oral corticosteroids in combination with azathioprine or cyclophosphamide, 'pulse' intravenous corticosteroids and plasma exchange. Most reports describe small numbers of patients with HSP nephritis in larger groups of patients with other forms of crescentic nephritis. Those with HSP appear to have as much chance of responding as other groups, but lack of numbers and absence of controlled data mean that no specific regimen has been identified.

Persisting nephrotic syndrome and deteriorating renal function

A small minority of patients have continuing nephrosis and will develop deteriorating renal function over months. Histology most commonly shows focal segmental proliferative GN without necrosis or crescents; with very variable degrees of chronic change. The renal prognosis is poor in the middle term, but there is no controlled evidence to guide treatment. Some anecdotal data in children favor 'pulse' methylprednisolone but the maintenance treatment thereafter is not defined.

IgA ANCA

IgA ANCA has been found in the serum of patients with active HSP but not in IgAN [26], although this is not confirmed in another study [27]. No direct pathogenic role has yet been identified for this circulating IgA, the antigen against which it is directed remains uncharacterized, and there are not enough longtitudinal data to confirm the clinical value in predicting relapse which has emerged for IgG ANCA in other types of systemic vasculitis.

Transplant recurrence

Recurrence of IgA deposits is common in HSP as in IgAN, though graft loss to recurrent nephritis is unusual. Delay-ing transplantation does not reduce the risk. Evidence from a single Japanese series of 15 children suggests that the risk of recurrence and graft loss is significantly higher in living related transplantation [28]; but this is yet to be confirmed.

Relationship between IgAN and HSP

These two distinct clinical entities are now seen as more and more closely related.

Clinical

Although IgAN is clinically confined to the kidney, IgA is also found in clinically and histologically normal skin in IgAN. HSP on the other hand is by definition a systemic illness, although nephritis with glomerular IgA deposition may persist years after the last clinical evidence of extrarenal disease. A patient whose primary renal disease was HSP has developed IgAN (with no systemic features) in a subsequent transplant. Identical twins who developed IgAN and HSP within days of each other have also been described.

Renal histopathology

The renal involvement of IgAN and HSP are effectively indistinguishable. IgA deposition is definitive; mesangial deposits are characteristic, but capillary wall deposits may occur in both. The wide gamut of light microscopic changes is seen in both (Figure 44.1).

IgA immune phenomena

Many abnormalities of the IgA immune system have been measured in HSP, and parallel those in IgAN [6]. Recent observations on the origin of the pIgA in IgAN, including studies based on bone marrow and gut lamina propria, have not been performed yet in HSP. Likewise, it is not yet known if abnormalities of IgA1 glycosylation also apply to HSP.

Graft recurrence

Both IgAN and HSP frequently produce recurrence of IgA deposits in transplants, with frank nephritis being much less common.

Differences between IgAN and HSP

Clinical

HSP nephritis appears to be a more active disease with shorter progression to end-stage renal failure in those with a poor prognosis.

IgAN is a more indolent disease but eventual prognosis may be poor even when initial histology appears very favorable. Any pathogenic events which underlie this difference are poorly understood.

The different age of onset – HSP most commonly in the first decade, IgAN in the second and third decades – remains unexplained.

Immunogenetics

Some of the immunogenetic associations are described in HSP, but none of the immunogenetic studies in HSP are of adequate size to draw firm conclusions.

The fundamental relationships between IgAN and its systemic counterpart, HSP, are of great interest in helping to unravel the pathogenesis of the two conditions; however this debate has no practical impact as yet on the clinical management of these patients.

References

1. Bennett, W.M. and Kincaid-Smith, P. (1983) Macroscopic hematuria in mesangial IgA nephropathy. *Kidney Int.*, **23**, 393–400.
2. Schena, F.P. (1990) A retrospective analysis of the natural history of primary IgA nephropathy worldwide. *Am. J. Med.*, **89**, 209–15.
3. Jennette, J.C., Wall, S.D. and Wilkman, A.S. (1985) Low incidence of IgA nephropathy in Blacks. *Kidney Int.*, **28**, 944–50.
4. Feehally, J., O'Donoghue, D.J. and Ballardie, F.W. (1989) Current nephrological practice in the investigation of microscopic haematuria in relationship to the incidence of IgA nephropathy. *J. R. Coll. Phys. Lond.*, **23**, 228–31.
5. Emancipator, S.N. (1990) Immunoregulatory factors in the pathogenesis of IgA nephropathy. *Kidney Int.*, **38**, 1216–29.
6. Feehally, J. (1988) Immune mechanisms in glomerular IgA deposition. *Nephrol. Dial. Transplant.*, **3**, 361–78.
7. Conley, M.E. and Delacroix, D.L. (1987) Intravascular and mucosal immunoglobulin A: two separate but related systems of immune defense? *Ann. Intern. Med.*, **106**, 892–9.
8. Bene, M.C., De Ligny, B.H., Kessler, M. and Faure, G. (1991) Confirmation of tonsillar anomalies in IgA nephropathy: a multicenter study. *Nephron*, **58**, 425–8.
9. Harper, S.J., Pringle, J.H., Wicks, A.C.B. *et al.* (1994) Expression of J chain mRNA in duodenal plasma cells in IgA nephropathy. *Kidney Int.*, **45**, 836–44.
10. Harper, S.J., Allen, A.C., Layward, L. *et al.* (1994) Increased IgA1 and IgA1 cells in bone marrow trephine biopsy specimens in IgA nephropathy. *Am. J. Kidney Dis.*, **24**, 888–92.
11. Layward, L., Allen, A.C., Hattersley, J. *et al.* (1992) Increased and prolonged production of specific polymeric IgA following systemic immunisation with tetanus toxoid in IgA nephropathy. *Clin. Exp. Immunol.*, **8**, 394–498.
12. Kanahara, K., Taniguchi, Y., Yorioka, N. and Yamakido, M. (1992) *In situ* hybridisation analysis of cytomegalovirus and adenovirus DNA in immunoglobulin A nephropathy. *Nephron*, **62**, 166–8.
13. Mestecky, J., Tomana, M., Crowley–Nowick, P.A. *et al.* (1994) Defective galactosylation and clearance of IgA1 molecules as a possible etiopathogenic factor in IgA nephropathy. *Contrib. Nephrol.*, **104**, 172–82.
13a. Allen, A.C., Harper, S.J. and Feehally, J. (1995) Galactosylation of N- and O-linked carbohydrate moieties of IgA1 and IgG in IgA nephropathy. *Clin. Exp. Immunol.*, **100**, 470–4.
14. Ballardie, F.W., Brenchley, P.E.C., Williams, S. and O'Donoghue, D.J. (1988) Autoimmunity in IgA nephropathy. *Lancet*, **ii**, 588–92.
15. Julian, B.A., Quiggins, P.A., Thompson, J.S. *et al.* (1985) Familial IgA nephropathy. Evidence of an inherited mechanism of disease. *N. Engl. J. Med.*, **312**, 202–8.
16. Ibels, L.S. and Gyory, A.Z. (1994) IgA Nephropathy: analysis of the natural history, important factors in the progression of renal disease, and a review of the literature. *Medicine*, **73**, 79–102.
17. Beukhof, J.R., Ockhuizen, T., Halie, L.M. *et al.* (1984) Subentities within adult primary IgA nephropathy. *Clin. Nephrol.*, **22**, 195–9.
18. Odum, J., Peh, C.A., Clarkson, A.R. *et al.* (1994) Recurrent mesangial IgA nephritis following renal transplantation. *Nephrol. Dial. Transplant.*, **9**, 309–12.
19. Feehally, J. (1996) Immunogobulin A nephropathy: fishoils and beyond. *Current Opinion in Nephrology and Hypertension*, **5**, 422–46.
20. Bene, M.C., Hurault de Lingny, B., Kessler, M. *et al.* (1993) Tonsils in IgA nephropathy. *Contrib. Nephrol.*, **104**, 153–61.
21. Schena, F.P., Montenegro, M. and Scivittaro, V. (1990) Meta-analysis of randomised controlled trials in patients with primary IgA nephropathy (Berger's disease). *Nephrol. Dial. Transplant.*, **1**, 47–52.
22. Cattran, D.C., Greenwood, C. and Ritchie, S. (1994) Long term benefits of angiotensin-converting enzyme inhibitor therapy in patients with severe IgA nephropathy. *Am. J. Kidney Dis.*, **23**, 247–54.
23. Donadio, J.V., Bergstralh, E.J., Offord, K.P. *et al.* (1994) A controlled trial of fish oil in IgA nephropathy. *N. Engl. J. Med.*, **331**, 1194–9.
24. Pettersson, E.E., Rekola, S., Berglund, L. *et al.* (1994) Treatment of IgA nephropathy with omega-3-polyunsaturated fatty acids: a prospective, double-blind, randomized study. *Clin. Nephrol.*, **41**, 183–90.
25. Haycock, G.B. (1992) The nephritis of Henoch–Schön-

lein purpura, in *Oxford Textbook of Clinical Nephrology* (eds J.S. Cameron, A.M. Davison, J.P. Grunfeld, D.N.S. Kerr and E. Ritz), Oxford University Press, Oxford, pp. 595–612.

26. Ronda, N., Esnault, V.L.M., Layward, L. *et al.* (1994) Antineutrophil cytoplasmic antibodies (ANCA) of IgA isotype in adult Henoch–Schönlein purpura. *Clin. Exp. Immunol.*, **95**, 49–56.

27. O'Donoghue, D.J., Nusbaum, P., Noel, L.-H. *et al.* (1992) Antineutrophil cytoplasmic antibodies in IgA nephropathy and Henoch–Schönlein purpura. *Nephrol. Dial. Transplant.*, **7**, 534–8.

28. Hasegawa, A. (1989) Fate of renal grafts with recurrent Henoch–Schönlein purpura nephritis in children. *Transplant. Proc.*, **21**, 2130.

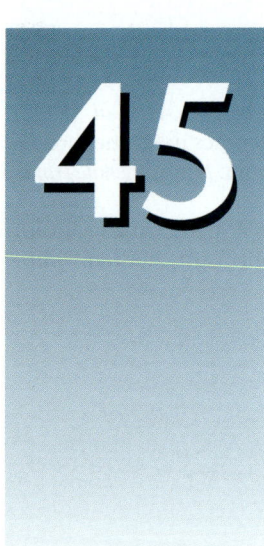

Rapidly progressive glomerulonephritis

A. Meguid El Nahas and Martin Wilkie

Introduction

Rapidly progressive glomerulonephritis (RPGN) refers to a form of glomerulonephritis (GN) characterized clinically by a rapid deterioration in renal function taking place over a short period of time ranging from a few days to a few weeks. If untreated, RPGN leads to end-stage renal insufficiency. Histologically, RPGN is characterized by severe inflammation and necrosis involving the glomeruli. The GN is often associated with glomerular crescent formation (crescentic GN).

Over recent years, it has become increasingly apparent that patients with RPGN have a spectrum of diseases. These could be divided and classified according to histological, serological and clinical findings (Table 45.1) [1–6].

This chapter focuses on RPGN in the context of anti-glomerular basement membrane (GBM) disease and anti-neutrophil cytoplasmic autoantibody (ANCA)-positive vasculitis. The diagnosis and management of patients with RPGN due to ANCA-negative vasculitis or an accelerated, crescentic, phase of a primary GN are discussed elsewhere.

Incidence

RPGN predominantly affects adults although the disease has been described in children as young as two to four years of age [2]. Patients with ANCA-positive microscopic renal vasculitis tend to be older than those with anti-GBM disease. In those with anti-GBM disease, the male:female ratio varies between 1.5 and 2 [1–5]. By contrast, there appears to be a female predominance in patients with RPGN associated with a systemic vasculitis [6–9]. This is particularly true of patients with ANCA-negative vasculitis (such as systemic lupus erythematosus (SLE)) and those with perinuclear (p)-ANCA (anti-myeloperoxidase (MPO))-positive renal microscopic vasculitis. Rapidly progressive glomerulonephritis is more common in Caucasians than in Afro-Caribbeans and Asians [1–7], in whom it is rare.

The incidence of RPGN in unselected series of renal biopsies varies between 2 and 5% [1, 2, 5, 10]. This overall incidence has been consistent in series reported from Europe, the United States, the Far East and Australasia. Anti-GBM disease is rare with an estimated annual incidence of 0.5 cases per million population [3–5]. The incidence of ANCA-associated vasculitis ranges from 4.6 to 7 cases per million population [7, 10]. There appears to be an increase in the incidence of renal vasculitis over recent years, in particular in elderly patients [10]. It is, however, difficult to ascertain whether this reflects a genuine increase in the number of cases or merely an increased awareness and improved diagnostic tests. Seasonal variations in the incidence of RPGN, with a predominance of cases in winter, have been described in patients with anti-GBM disease [3, 10a] as well as those presenting with ANCA-positive renal vasculitis [8, 11]. Clustering of cases

Nephrology, Edited by Rex L. Jamison and Robert Wilkinson.
Published in 1997 by Chapman & Hall, London. ISBN 0 412 60930 4

Table 45.1 Histological, serological and clinical classifications of RPGN

Glomerular immunofluorescence pattern	Serological markers	Clinical entities
1. Linear deposition of anti-GBM autoantibody	Circulating anti-GBM autoantibody	(a) Goodpasture's syndrome in the presence of lung hemorrhage (b) Anti-GBM disease in the absence of lung hemorrhage
2. No or scanty (pauci) immune deposits	Circulating antineutrophil cytoplasmic autoantibodies (ANCA)	(a) Systemic vasculitis (Wegener's granulomatosis (WG) or microscopic polyarteritis (mPA)). (b) Renal limited vasculitis (renal microscopic vasculitis)
3. Granular, immune complex, deposits	ANCA negative Other autoantibodies such as antinuclear antibodies may be positive	(a) ANCA-negative systemic vasculitis; systemic lupus erythematosus (SLE), Henoch–Schönlein purpura (HSP), cryoglobulinemia and other vasculitides. (b) RPGN associated with an underlying primary or secondary GN; primary GN such as IgA, membranous or membranoproliferative GN Secondary GN; postinfectious, drug-induced or neoplasia associated (c) Idiopathic RPGN

of anti-GBM disease has been reported from England, the United States and New Zealand.

Immunogenetics

Goodpasture's syndrome has been reported to occur in siblings and identical twins. Associations have been described between Goodpasture's syndrome and specific class I and II HLA antigens. An association with the class II HLA antigen DR2 (DRw 15) was identified in 50–88% of patients with Goodpasture's syndrome [12]. Additional associations have been identified between Goodpasture's syndrome and HLA-DR4 and the HLA-DQβ chain genes DQwlb and DQw3 [12]. This may be explained by the close linkage dysequilibrium between the DR and DQ genes. Further associations have been described with the class I antigen HLA-B7 which is also in linkage dysequilibrium with DR2 [12]. Patients who carry the HLA-DR2 and B7 antigens appear to have a worse renal prognosis, suggesting that B7 is a marker of severity of the disease whereas DR2 indicates susceptibility [12]. By contrast, it has been suggested that the DR1 and DR7 alleles may confer protection against Goodpasture's syndrome [12]. A higher risk (risk ratio = 5.75) for Goodpasture's syndrome has been described in carriers of the heavy chain constant region Gm haplotype 1,2,21 (axg) of IgG [12].

In patients with Wegener's granulomatosis (WG) and microscopic polyarteritis (mPA), a strong association has been reported with the DR4 DQw7 haplotype [12]. An increased incidence of HLA-DR2 has also been associated with WG [12]. Over-representation of HLA-B8 and under-representation of HLA DR3 have also been reported in this disease.

More recently, associations with α-1-antitrypsin [14] and the type IIa receptor for IgG (FcγRIIa) [15] gene polymorphisms have been described [16]. An increased frequency of the α-1-antitrypsin Z allele was noted in patients with c-ANCA positive vasculitis [14]. On the other hand, patients with p-ANCA had an increase in the S allele [14]. The demonstration of an association between the deficiency phentoypes of α-1-antitrypsin and ANCA-positive vasculitis is of interest in view of the fact that α-1-antitrypsin is the major physiological inhibitor of proteinase 3. However, these associations await confirmation in a larger number of patients with ANCA-positive vasculitis.

Environmental factors

Links have been suggested between Goodpasture's syndrome and viral infections since the original description of the disease linked it to the influenza virus [13]. Research has not substantiated the association between the disease and a virus. Associations between arboviruses and renal microscopic vasculitis have also been put forward [14]. This impression is reinforced by the flu-like prodromal symptomatology that often precedes the onset of RPGN. However, it remains doubtful whether these agents are pathogenic or merely activate the underlying immune-mediated disease. Systemic viral and bacterial infections are known to exacerbate immune-mediated diseases including Goodpasture's syndrome and renal vasculitis. The mechanism of such infection-induced flare-up is discussed below.

Numerous case reports have linked the onset or exacerbation of Goodpasture's syndrome with exposure to organic solvents and hydrocarbons [15]. A causal association remains to be confirmed. Cigarette smoking has also been implicated in the pathogenesis of lung hemorrhage in patients with Goodpasture's syndrome [16]. In an epidemiological study, 100% of smokers had lung hemorrhage compared to only 20% of the non-smokers [16]. Clinical recurrence of lung hemorrhage has been reported in patients who have resumed cigarette smoking. Experimental data support the notion that a toxic pulmonary insult, including cigarette smoke, increases the susceptibility to autoantibody-mediated alveolar injury. An association between smoking and lung hemorrhage has not been observed, however, in patients with WG or mPA.

Clinical manifestations

The spectrum of clinical presentation depends on the underlying disease. In patients with anti-GBM disease, a prodromal flu-like illness is common followed by symptoms related to anemia and lung hemorrhage [3–5, 10a]. Patients with pulmonary hemorrhage may be asymptomatic or have hemoptysis with or without dyspnea. In patients with ANCA-positive vasculitis, symptoms will depend on whether the patient is suffering from systemic vasculitis (WG or mPA) or renal microscopic vasculitis. In the latter disease, the symptoms may be non-specific symptoms of flu-like illness, pyrexia, lethargy, malaise, weight loss, arthralgias and myalgias [8, 9]. Patients with an ANCA-positive systemic vasculitis may also present with symptoms related to the systems involved: skin, joints, eyes, sinuses, ears, lungs or the nervous system [8, 9, 17]. It is important to have a high index of suspicion of ANCA-positive vasculitis in elderly patients with rapidly declining renal function since they often have little extrarenal involvement [8]. Many of those classified in the past as having idiopathic RPGN have recently been found to be ANCA positive [18, 19].

Renal manifestations

Renal involvement in anti-GBM disease tends to be severe with oliguria, macroscopic hematuria and some proteinuria (<5 g/24 h) [3–5, 10a]. By contrast, patients with renal vasculitis may exhibit the full range of renal abnormalities from isolated microscopic hematuria to a full blown nephritic syndrome although the latter is rare [7–9, 11, 20]. Hypertension is a late complication and is related to renal insufficiency and fluid overload in patients with

anti-GBM disease and those with ANCA-positive renal vasculitis. In severe cases, a rapid deterioration of renal function is observed. Oliguria or the requirement for dialysis carry a poor prognosis. Such clinical signs justify early diagnosis and intervention as the success of therapy in these patients depends to a large extent on the early institution of immunosuppression (see below).

Extrarenal manifestations

The extrarenal manifestations of anti-GBM disease are usually confined to the organs affected by circulating antibasement membrane autoantibodies. Pulmonary hemorrhage occurs in approximately two-thirds of patients [3–5, 10a]. Iron-deficiency anemia or radiological lung shadowing are suggestive of lung hemorrhage. Hemoptysis is common [3–5]. The time interval between the onset of hemoptysis and the development of renal disease varies considerably but is usually about three months. Ocular symptoms, including retinal detachment, related to the binding of the autoantibodies to the Bruch's membrane and the membranes of the choroidal vessels have been described [3].

In ANCA-positive vasculitis, a wide range of extrarenal involvement is often observed. Although the respiratory tract is most commonly affected, almost any organ can be affected [8, 9, 11, 17]. In a large series of ANCA-positive GN, 37 of 70 patients had pulmonary disease manifested by hemoptysis, radiological lung infiltrate and pulmonary hemorrhage [11]. Other upper respiratory tract disease, including sinusitis, epistaxis, rhinorrhea and disfiguring granulomatous nasal disease, occurs commonly [8, 9, 17]. Otitis media causing conductive hearing loss has been described. Laryngeal involvement may contribute to hemoptysis and can cause hoarseness. Rash is common and may be erythematous, macular or papular and associated with splinter hemorrhages. Skin biopsy usually reveals a leukocytoclastic vasculitis. Patients often complain of arthralgias or musculoskeletal symptoms. Many patients have established rheumatological diagnoses other than ANCA-positive vasculitis before renal disease becomes apparent [8]. Ocular involvement includes conjunctivitis and uveitis, orbital and retro-orbital masses as well as retinal vasculitis and optical neuropathy [8, 9, 17]. Patients may have mononeuritis multiplex, convulsions, dysphoria or a stroke. Oral and bowel ulcerations or perforations have been described. Gastrointestinal hemorrhage is a frequent complication. The vasculitis may involve the heart valves, myocardium or pericardium.

Physiology and pathophysiology

Regardless of the etiology of the RPGN glomerular crescent formation is the hallmark of the disease. These are observed in patients with anti-GBM disease, those with ANCA-associated renal vasculitis as well as those with ANCA-negative vasculitis and granular immune deposits. Glomerular crescents consist of an aggregation of cells within the Bowman's space, whose configuration accounts for its name. Cells, derived from blood, migrate into the space through holes in the capillary and from parietal epithelial cells lining the space. The latter predominate initially when the capsule is intact; monocytes, macrophages and lymphocytes (T cells) predominate later when the capsule is disrupted. Fibrinogen escapes into the Bowman's space through capillary holes [21, 26]. Activated monocytes may express a procoagulant that promotes fibrin polymerization. Fibrin, in turn, is chemoattractant to inflammatory cells such as monocytes, which constitute an important cellular element of crescent formation. Defibrination of experimental animals with ancrod, derived from snake venom, prevents crescent formation in experimental GN, which suggests a major role for fibrin in the initiation of glomerular crescent formation. Experimental evidence also suggests a role for delayed-type hypersensitivity in the pathogenesis of glomerular crescents through recruitment of macrophages [21]. Interventions aimed at depleting experimental animals of monocytes/macrophages have proved effective in attenuating the severity of experimental crescentic GN. Macrophages may, in turn, through the release of cytokines and growth factors, contribute to glomerular injury. Cytokines such as interleukin-1 (IL-1), tumor necrosis factor-α (TNF-α), platelet-derived growth factor (PDGF) and transforming growth factor-β (TGF-β) have been identified in the glomeruli of rodents with crescentic GN [22a, 22c]. Cytokines such as IL-1 and TNF-α have been shown to exacerbate the acute injury in experimental GN [22b] whereas growth factors such as PDGF and TGF-β have been implicated in mesangial proliferation and glomerulosclerosis respectively [22a, 22c]. Therapeutic interventions based on the inhibition of these cytokines and growth factors have proved effective in minimizing experimental glomerular injury and sclerosis [22a, 22c].

With the progression of glomerular scarring and in the presence of capsular adhesions or holes, interstitial myofibroblasts infiltrate crescents and contribute to their progression to fibrous scars. Crescents usually progress with the compression and subsequent collapse of the underlying glomerular tuft. They evolve within a few weeks into fibrous scars consisting of myofibroblasts and collagenous matrix. There is also some evidence that crescents can resolve without scarring. In general, the severity of RPGN is proportional to the degree of involvement of the glomeruli by crescents [4]. However, caution has to be exerted in the interpretation of renal biopsies in view of the limitations due to the selection bias in needle biopsy material [3].

Pathology and pathogenesis

Pathology

Light microscopy

Renal pathology in RPGN is characterized by glomeruli that are partially or completely surrounded by crescents (Figure 45.1a). The architecture of the glomerular tuft varies from normal to segmental and ultimately total necrosis. Extensive glomerular necrosis is often observed in anti-GBM disease. Focal and segmental glomerular necrosis is a feature of ANCA-associated GN (Figure 45.1b). Segmental glomerular necrosis also occurs in lupus nephropathy. These glomerular changes can also be observed in the absence of crescentic transformation. By contrast, the glomerular architecture is better preserved in patients with a crescentic GN superimposed on a primary GN such as IgA, membranous or membranoproliferative GN. In these patients, histological features of the underlying GN are often discernible.

In RPGN, an element of tubulointerstitial

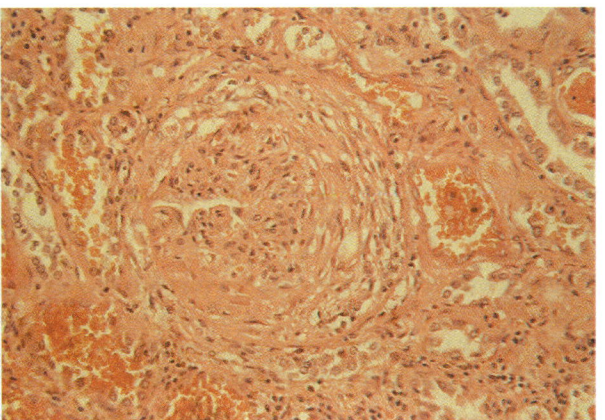

a

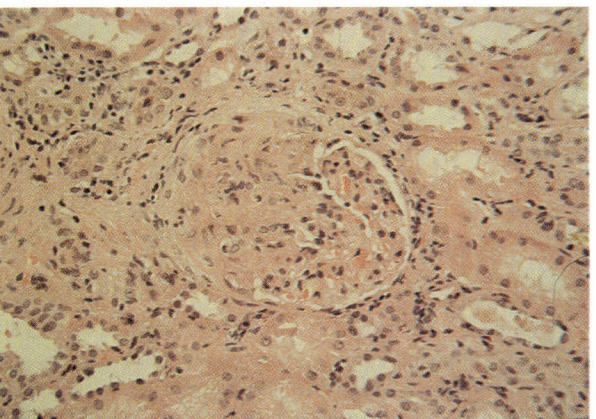

b

Figure 45.1 (a) Glomerular crescent surrounding the glomerular tuft in a patient with rapidly progressive glomerulonephritis. (b) Segmental glomerular necrosis in a patient with microscopic polyarteritis. (Courtesy of Dr J. Shortland, Mr B. Wagner, Department of Histopathology, Northern General Hospital Trust, Sheffield, UK.)

inflammation is also present [2, 3, 23]. It is characterized by inflammatory interstitial infiltrate consistent of macrophages and lymphocytes (helper and suppressor T cells) [2, 3]. Occasionally, an interstitial eosinophilic infiltrate is noted, in particular in patients with allergic angiitis. In anti-GBM disease, it has been suggested that the severity of the tubulointerstitial infiltrates may correlate with the extent of anti-TBM antibody deposition. Interstitial granulomas are very occasionally detected in patients with WG. However, these are not necessary to establish the diagnosis in the presence of a suggestive clinical and serological picture. In GN in general, the severity of the tubulointerstitial changes is a reliable marker of outcome [24].

Vasculitic changes are also observed in extraglomerular vessels in patients with anti-GBM disease as well as those with ANCA-positive renal vasculitis.

Immunohistology

Direct immunofluorescence-tagged antibody studies of tissue obtained by renal biopsy from patients with RPGN reveals three distincts patterns. The first, observed in patients with anti-GBM disease, is characterized by the linear deposition of the anti-GBM autoantibody along the GBM (Figure 45.2a). The deposited anti-GBM antibodies are usually of the IgG1 and IgG4 subclasses. However IgA anti-GBM antibodies have also been reported. Glomerular fibrin and complement deposition are also detectable by immunofluorescence. There is also a linear deposition fo anti-TBM antibodies along the basement membrane of distal tubules.

The second immunofluorescence pattern is observed in patients with ANCA-positive vasculitis; it consists of scanty (pauci) deposition of immunoglobulins within glomeruli (Figure 45.2b). Fibrin and complement can also be detected.

The third immunofluorescence pattern is observed in ANCA-negative vasculitis where granular deposition of immunoglobulin and complement (C3) occurs along the GBM (Figure 45.2c). Immune deposits are also detected on occasion along the tubular basement membrane (TBM). In patients with a primary GN complicated by crescent formation, the immunofluorescence pattern is that of the underlying GN.

Electron microscopy

A characteristic feature of crescentic glomeruli by electron microscopy consists of the presence of breaks (holes) within the GBM and Bowman's capsule [25]. As discussed above, fibrin is present within Bowman's space and is thought to attract inflammatory monocytic cells to initiate the formation of crescents. In anti-GBM disease, wrinkling of the GBM takes place. In RPGN, areas of dissolution of the mesangial matrix (mesangiolysis) are also observed. Electron-dense deposits are observed in a similar distribution to that described above; these are

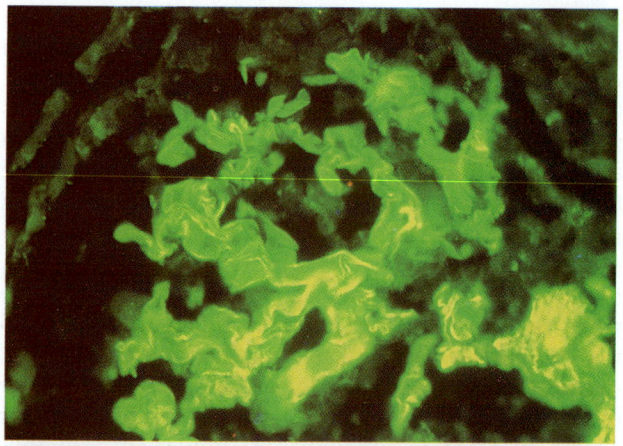

a

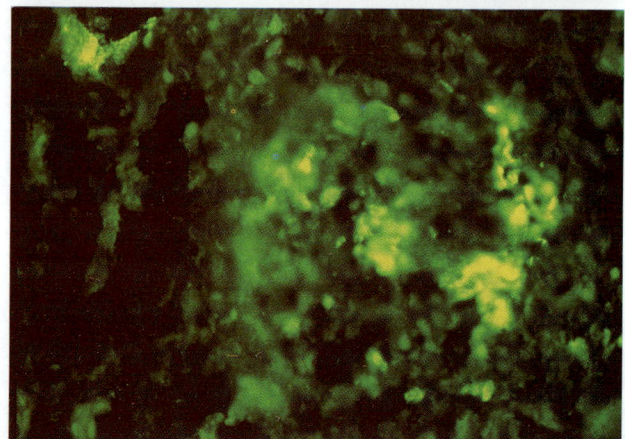

b

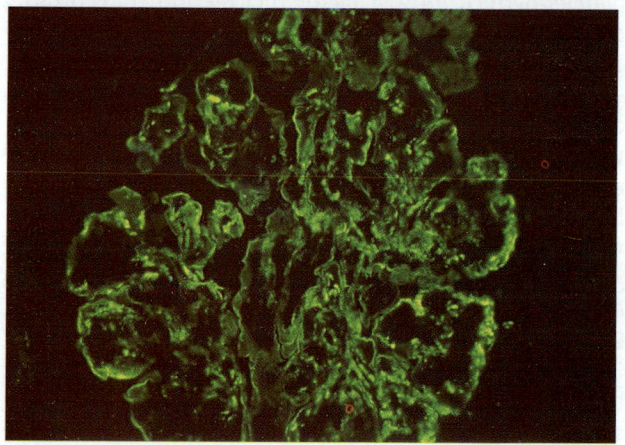

c

Figure 45.2 (a) Linear deposition of IgG (anti-GBM antibody) detected by direct immunofluorescence along the glomerular basement membrane of a patient with Goodpasture's syndrome (courtesy of Dr A Milford-Ward, Department of Immunology, Northern General Hospital NHS Trust, Sheffield, UK). (b) Scanty (pauci) glomerular immune deposits in a patient with an ANCA-positive vasculitis. (c) Granular glomerular deposition of immune deposits, detected by direct immunofluorescence, in a patient with an ANCA-negative vasculitis (SLE).

linear or granular depending on the type of RPGN. In SLE, mesangial and paramesangial immune deposits may be present.

Pathogenesis

The pathogenesis of RPGN depends on the entity studied (see above). It can be divided into an autoimmune phenomenon in patients with circulating anti-GBM autoantibodies and an immune-mediated vasculitis in patients with systemic or renal vasculitis. The latter can be subdivided into ANCA-positive and ANCA-negative conditions. A third group of patients with RPGN have an underlying primary or secondary GN. The pathogenesis of crescent formation will be discussed below.

Antiglomerular basement membrane disease (Goodpasture's syndrome)

Linear deposition of the autoantibody along the GBM is a feature of anti-GBM disease. In Goodpasture's syndrome, the titer of circulating anti-GBM antibodies correlates directly with the severity of the disease [3–5, 10a]. Remission is associated with a fall or disappearance of the circulating autoantibodies. Experimental models of anti-GBM disease support a close association between circulating as well as renal anti-GBM antibody levels and the severity of the GN.

The anti-GBM antibody is now known to be directed to the C-terminal, non-collagenous globular domain (NC1), of type IV collagen [26], specifically, against a 28 kDa monomeric component of the NC1 domain. Native hexameric $\alpha 3$(IV)NC1 is not immunogenic. Circulating antibodies isolated from patients with Goodpasture's syndrome react mainly with the $\alpha 3$ chain of type IV collagen ($\alpha 3$(IV)NC1) [26]. The spectrum of anti-GBM disease may be related to the distribution of the Goodpasture's antigen. The network of collagen containing the $\alpha 3$ and $\alpha 4$ type IV collagen chains appears to be restricted to a few basement membranes including the GBM, the TBM, the alveolar basement membrane (ABM), and those of the choroid plexus and the ciliary body. These basement membranes are characterized by their origination during embryogenesis from the fusion of endothelial and epithelial basement membranes. The involvement of these membranes in Goodpasture's syndrome is restricted by their inaccessibility to the circulating autoantibodies. In the glomeruli, the $\alpha 3$ and $\alpha 4$ chains of collagen IV appear to be localized in the lamina densa of the GBM confirming early findings based on indirect immunofluorescence. Antibodies reacting with other α chains have also been described although they seem to have a lower reactivity and may be less pathogenic [27]. Patients have also been described who have circulating anti-GBM antibodies that react with an antigen hidden in the NC1 epitope of the $\alpha 1$ chain of type IV collagen [27]. These antibodies are associated with a mild GN and no significant lung disease [27].

It has been suggested that exposure of the 28 kDa monomeric epitope of the $\alpha 3$(IV)NC1 or its dissociation from the native hexamer is necessary to trigger autoimmunity [26]. Such exposure of the pathogenic epitope by infection, hydrocarbons or cigarette smoke may initiate the disease. This would explain the role of these environmental factors in the pathogenesis of Goodpasture's syndrome.

Experimental models of anti-GBM disease, in particular nephrotoxic serum nephritis, suggest roles for cell-mediated immunity, the complement system as well as the coagulation system in the pathogenesis of the GN [28].

ANCA-positive vasculitis associated with pauci-immune deposits

The second group of patients with RPGN are those with an ANCA-associated vasculitis. The vasculitis, as in WG or mPA, can be systemic affecting a wide range of organs. It can also be confined to the kidney as in renal microscopic vasculitis. Many of these patients, previously thought to have idiopathic crescentic GN, were found to have circulating ANCAs [19, 29]. Renal biopsies in these patients show a characteristic scanty (pauci) amount of immune deposits within the glomeruli.

The association between ANCA and renal disease was first described in 1982 [14]. In 1985, the association between these autoantibodies and WG was established [29]. ANCA was also found in a high percentage of patients with mPA [6, 7, 30]. ANCA are highly specific (>80%) and sensitive (>90%) for the diagnosis of these systemic vasculitides [6, 7, 13c]. They are also detected in over 80% of patients with idiopathic crescentic GN [18, 19]. This has led to the identification of these patients as suffering from a form of microscopic vasculitis localized to the kidney with positive ANCA and the absence of extrarenal involvement [6, 7].

Two different indirect immunofluorescence patterns are observed when the patient's serum containing ANCA is incubated with normal human neutrophils. The first pattern consists of a diffuse cytoplasmic stain (c-ANCA) and is observed in patients with WG (Figure 45.3a). The second pattern is characterized by an artifactual perinuclear distribution of the antibody (p-ANCA) in ethanol-fixed neutrophils and is seen predominantly in patients with mPA [6, 7, 13c] (Figure 45.3b). Patients with renal microscopic vasculitis tend to have circulating p-ANCAs [6, 7, 13c].

The antigens for ANCA are enzymes of the neutrophil primary azurophilic granules; a 29 kDa serine proteinase-3 (PR3) for c-ANCA and myeloperoxidase (MPO) for p-ANCA [2, 27]. The perinuclear staining pattern observed for MPO is due to its release from intracellular stores during ethanol fixation and its binding to DNA. A perinuclear staining pattern (p-ANCA) is occasionally observed in patients with antibodies against other neutrophil cytoplasmic enzymes such as elastase, lactoferrin

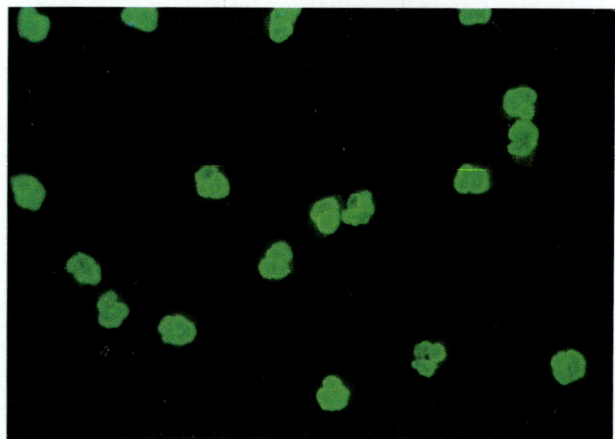

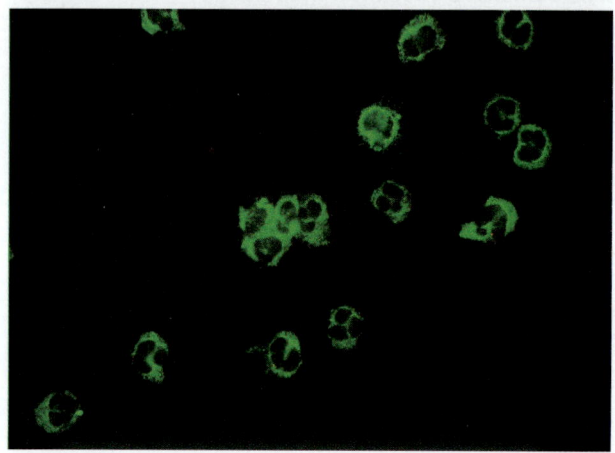

Figure 45.3 (a) c-ANCA indirect immunofluorescence staining pattern in a patient with Wegener's granulomatosis. (b) p-ANCA indirect immunofluorescence staining pattern in a patient with microscopic polyarteritis. (Courtesy of Dr A. Milford-Ward, Department of Immunology, Northern General Hospital Trust, Sheffield, UK.)

or eosinophilic peroxidase [6, 7, 13c] or bacterial/permeability-increasing (BPI) protein. Few patients display both ANCA staining patterns [6, 7, 19, 30] whereas others have been described with circulating anti-GBM and ANCA antibodies, in particular anti-MPO antibodies [19]. The latter tend to have low titers of circulating anti-GBM antibodies [19]. The clinical characteristics of these patients remain ill-defined, although there is some evidence to suggest that those with pauci-immune deposits have a better prognosis than those with linear GBM staining [19]. This is consistent with the better prognosis of patients with ANCA-associated renal disease when compared to those with anti-GBM disease [6, 10a] (see below).

In most studies, circulating levels of ANCA correlate with the activity of the associated vasculitis [6, 7, 19, 30]. Treatment leads to a fall in ANCA levels whereas recrudescence of the vasculitis is associated with a rise in the circulating titers [6, 7, 19, 29, 30]. The disappearance of circulating ANCA is associated with remission in the majority of patients [6, 7, 19, 29, 13c]. However, patients have been described with persistently raised ANCA levels despite quiescence of the underlying vasculitis and others have been described with a rise in the ANCA levels without reactivation of their vasculitis [6, 7, 31]. The role of ANCA in the pathogenesis of necrotizing vasculitis remains speculative. It is, however, known that the incubation of neutrophils with ANCA *in vitro* leads to their activation, degranulation and release of oxygen free radicals and proteolytic enzymes [7, 30]. There is evidence to suggest that cytokines, such as TNF-α, can stimulate neutrophils to express ANCA antigens on their cell surface, making them susceptible to antibody attack [30]. Cytokines can also stimulate the expression of cell adhesion molecules on the surface of neutrophils, facilitating their adhesion to vascular endothelium [30]. In susceptible individuals, these events would lead to a flare-up of the vasculitis. It is believed that such a process may underly the activation of vasculitis by intercurrent infections.

ANCA-negative crescentic glomerulonephritis associated with granular, immune complex, deposits

This group incorporates patients with ANCA-negative systemic vasculitis as well as those with primary and secondary GN. The former includes patients with systemic vasculitis such as SLE, Henoch–Schönlein purpura (HSP) and cryoglobulinemia. The latter includes patients with primary GN such as IgA, membranous or membranoproliferative GN. Secondary GN is associated with infections (poststreptococcal, endocarditis or visceral abscess), drugs (rifampicin, hydralazine, streptokinase, enalapril, penicillamine and phenylbutazone) and neoplasia (solid tumors and lymphomas).

Most patients with ANCA-negative GN display granular immune deposits within their glomeruli. This has led to the assumption that most of these conditions are due to the deposition of circulating immune complexes on the glomerular capillaries. *In situ* formation of immune complexes cannot be excluded. However, recent evidence suggests that the granular distribution of immunoglobulin is also compatible with autoimmunity to glomerular antigens.

Most of the RPGNs previously classified as idiopathic now appear to be ANCA-associated vasculitides confined to the kidneys [18]. However, a small percentage of patients with RPGN remain ANCA-negative and have scanty glomerular immune deposits, which justifies their classification as idiopathic [18].

Diagnosis and differential diagnosis

Faced with a patient with isolated rapidly declining renal function it is imperative to have a high index of suspicion for a crescentic GN. The history may clarify whether the patient is known to suffer from an underlying primary GN (undergoing a crescentic exacerbation), had a preceding pharyngeal, cutaneous or systemic infection or has consumed drugs known to cause an RPGN. The history and physical examination may suggest an underlying malignancy. Similarly, physical examination may indicate an infective endocarditis.

In the presence of respiratory symptoms and radiological lung shadowing, the differential diagnosis is widened. Infectious diseases associated with pneumonitis and renal failure have to be considered including atypical pneumoniae such as Legionnaire's disease. Other causes of pulmonary–renal syndrome include systemic vasculitides and occasionally poisoning (for instance by paraquat).

When patients present with rapidly declining renal function, it is imperative to search, through the history and physical examination, for systemic manifestations (listed above). Their presence points towards a systemic vasculitis. Appropriate serological tests will confirm the diagnosis (see below).

When faced with a patient with rapidly declining renal function and normal size kidneys a renal biopsy should be performed and treatment instituted promptly. It is often advisable to initiate treatment even before the result of the renal biopsy is available in order to avoid delay and maximize the chances of a good response (see below).

Investigations

In patients with active Goodpasture's syndrome microcytic anemia is a prominent feature. A normocytic anemia is also observed in patients with ANCA-positive vasculitis. In both groups of patients, there may be a leukocytosis. Eosinophilia has been described in some patients with ANCA-positive vasculitis [8]. ANCA-positive patients often have thrombocytosis, but thrombocytopenia has also been described [8, 17]. Raised erythrocyte sedimentation rate and, more specifically, a high C-reactive protein indicate disease activity in patients with vasculitis. Hypergammaglobulinemia is not uncommon.

Serum biochemistry reflects the degree of renal impairment. In patients with ANCA-positive vasculitis, an elevated alkaline phosphatase reflects hepatic involvement [17].

Serological investigations reveal high circulating titers of anti-GBM antibodies in patients with Goodpasture's syndrome. Those with WG will have high titers of c-ANCA whereas p-ANCA will be elevated in patients with mPA or renal-limited vasculitis. As mentioned above, some patients will have both autoantibodies, p- and c-ANCAs [19], and a few have a combination of ANCA (anti-MPO) and low titer anti-GBM antibodies [19]. As far as the ANCA serology is concerned, ANCA seropositivity by indirect immunofluorescence should be confirmed by ELISA as the combination of positivity by the two

methods increases the diagnostic specificity to 99% (European Union BCR project for ANCA assay standardization) [16]. Other tests may help to identify an underlying primary vasculitis such as SLE (raised antinuclear antibodies levels), cryoglobulinemia or a GN such as IgA nephropathy (raised circulating IgA levels).

In active GN, the urinalysis reveals an increased number of red cells, some of which are dysmorphic, as well as red cell casts. Leukocyturia is also observed. Proteinuria is below the nephrotic range [3, 5].

Radiological investigations show lung infiltrates in Goodpasture's syndrome and ANCA-positive systemic vasculitis. In the former, the infiltrate tends to be diffuse and symmetrical reflecting intra-alveolar hemorrhage. Typically, it involves the central lung fields, sparing the periphery. Vasculitic infiltrates are often asymmetrical and nodular in nature. Lung infiltrates due to vasculitic changes or hemorrhage may also be observed in ANCA-negative vasculitides. It is possible to confirm alveolar hemorrhage by measuring the total lung carbon monoxide (CO) uptake (TLCO) [3]. The transfer factor for CO [K_{CO}] (TLCO divided by lung volume) is increased with pulmonary hemorrhage because CO is trapped in the alveoli by free hemoglobin.

Radiological investigations usually reveal normal size kidneys, but occasionally large kidneys due to edema. Sinus X-rays may show abnormalities in patients with WG.

Ultimately, the diagnosis is confirmed by a renal biopsy (discussed above). In patients with WG, biopsies of the nasal septum or of the upper respiratory airways have variable yields and do not always show granulomatous lesions. Renal granulomas are not often detected in patients with WG.

Treatment

Conventional treatment

As described above, RPGN is a heterogeneous group of immunopathological conditions and the response to treatment varies accordingly. This heterogeneity often hampers interpretation of published clinical trials. Although the initial response to treatment if often good, for instance in ANCA-associated renal diseases, relapse is common necessitating long-term follow-up and careful determination of treatment end points.

The cornerstone of the treatment of RPGN, regardless of the underlying pathology or classification, is early and intense immunosuppression. In general, the response to treatment is good when it is initiated before end-stage renal insufficiency is reached and the patient is oliguric and requires dialysis [3, 5, 11, 20, 32]. This also applies to patients with anti-GBM disease [3, 5, 20, 32] and ANCA-positive systemic or renal vasculitis [11, 33]. Besides immunosuppressive treatment, management of these extremely ill patients often requires dialysis, nutritional supplements and the ability to distinguish between the complications of the disease and the side effects of treatment. The last point is extremely important as the morbidity and mortality of these patients are often related to complications of treatment [11, 17, 20, 32–34].

Immunosupressive therapy consists of steroids and an alkylating agent such as cyclophosphamide or an antimetabolite such as azathioprine [10, 33]. A consensus is emerging that the initial administration of intravenous methylprednisolone provides a therapeutic advantage over oral steroid therapy [10]. Debate continues as to the relative benefits of pulsed intravenous cyclophosphamide [10, 33].

In patients with anti-GBM disease, a combination of steroids and cyclophosphamide has been shown to be effective in improving renal function when instituted early in the course of the disease before a significant loss in renal function has taken place [3]. Delay in the institution of therapy leads to a poor response [3, 20, 34]. Initial therapy with a combination of prednisolone 1 mg/kg of body weight/day, cyclophosphamide 3 mg/kg/day and azathioprine 1–2 mg/kg/day and plasma exchange 3–4 l/day has been recommended [3, 34]. The value of plasma exchange in patients with anti-GBM disease has been evaluated in a controlled study and shown to lead to a more rapid disappearance of circulating anti-GBM autoantibodies when compared to treatment with immunosuppression alone [20]. This would justify plasma exchange in patients with high titers of circulating autoantibodies and in those with severe and life-threatening lung hemorrhage where prompt removal of the circulating autoantibodies may be life-saving [3, 10]. The effect of plasma exchange on renal functional outcome was difficult to interpret in this study as the patients were not well matched with regard to the percentage of crescents in the biopsy specimens. The main prognostic factors determining outcome were the percentage of crescents and the severity of renal impairment at the onset [20]. Patients with preserved renal function at the onset and less than 30% crescents had an excellent outcome regardless of treatment modality. By contrast, the response to either immunosuppression alone or with additional plasma exchange was poor in patients with greater than 70% crescents [20].

In patients with ANCA-associated renal disease, a combination of steroids and cyclophosphamide is effective in controlling the disease and preserving renal function when started early (serum creatinine <500–600 μmol/l) [11, 33, 35]. A large controlled trial of plasma exchange in these patients showed little additional advantage [36], although another study suggested that such therapy increases the likelihood of recovery of some renal function in dialysis-dependent patients [37]. In general, ANCA-positive patients respond better to therapy than those with anti-GBM disease [19]. The response to treatment in those with ANCA-positive systemic vasculitis and those with renal-limited disease is similar [11]. Patients

with c-ANCA and those with p-ANCA appear to have a similar response to treatment [11].

Evidence is accumulating to suggest that early and aggressive steroid therapy with intravenous methylprednisolone (ivMP) is an important factor in the success of the therapy of patients with RPGN [10]. In various series of patients with ANCA-positive vasculitis, ivMP appears to be more effective in restoring renal function when compared to oral, conventional, steroid therapy [10]. In a recent study of ANCA-positive patients, treatment with ivMP led to renal functional recovery in 41% of patients who were dialysis-dependent at the onset [8]. Others have suggested that ivMP is as effective as plasma exchange in patients with RPGN [38]. In Goodpasture's syndrome, ivMP is effective in reducing the severity of lung hemorrhage [20].

We recommend intravenous methylprednisolone 1 g/day (500 mg/day for patients over the age of 60) for three consecutive days. This is followed by oral prednisolone therapy 1 mg/kg of body weight/day for four weeks after which the dose is tapered. Steroid therapy is associated with oral cyclophosphamide (2 mg/kg/day, 1 mg/kg/day in the over sixties). Although anecdotal reports suggest a therapeutic advantage of cyclophosphamide over azathioprine in patients with ANCA-positive vasculitis [17], this has not been evaluated by a large-scale randomized trial. It is possible that initial treatment with azathioprine (2 mg/kg/day) is equally effective and possibly less toxic. We and others recommend a change at three months from cyclophosphamide to azathioprine (1 mg/kg/day) to prevent the long-term toxicity of cyclophosphamide. Plasma exchange is reserved for patients with Goodpasture's syndrome and severe lung hemorrhage.

Other therapies

An increasing number of therapies have been suggested for the treatment of patients with RPGN, in particular those who are ANCA-positive [13c, 39]. Many treatments consist of variations in the administration of immunosuppression including pulse intravenous methylprednisolone in association with monthly pulses of intravenous cyclophosphamide (0.5–1 g/m^2). As discussed above, the initiation of treatment with intravenous methylprednisolone appears to confer a therapeutic advantage over oral steroids [10]. Intravenous cyclophosphamide has been promoted as an effective and safe alternative to oral therapy in patients with SLE [32] and in those with RPGN [40] and WG [41]. However, when intravenous cyclophosphamide was compared to oral therapy in patients with ANCA-positive vasculitis, no difference in patients or renal survival was noted [11]. Others warned that intravenous cyclophosphamide had a high initial failure rate and did not sustain long-term remission [42]. It was concluded that at the present time low-dose oral cyclophosphamide in combination with steroids remain the treatment of choice in patients with WG [42].

Additional treatment modalities have been suggested for patients with RPGN [10, 33, 39]. The addition of monthly injections of high-dose intravenous immunoglobulins has been suggested. The use of protein A immunoadsorption columns to remove circulating autoantibodies has been advocated in patients with RPGN [43]. This form of therapy has been put forward as a safer alternative to plasma exchange. Treatment with other immunosuppressive agents such as methotrexate and cyclosporin A has also been reported [33, 39]. A combination of low-dose weekly methotrexate and corticosteroids has been found to be useful in some patients with mild to moderate Wegener's granulomatosis [50]. More recently, successful therapy has been achieved in the management of severe vasculitis with anti-CDw52 humanized antibodies (Campath 1H) [44]. This approach has also been applied with some success in patients with WG, in whom anecdotal reports have suggested that trimethoprim–sulfamethoxazole (Septrin) can induce remission in the initial phase of the disease [39].

Mose of these therapies are anecdotal and have not been formally tested in controlled clinical trials. They should not be a substitute for early and effective treatment with established regimens including high-dose methylprednisolone and cyclophosphamide or azathioprine. These therapies may also be associated with side effects, in particular a high incidence of infectious complications some of which may be fatal [37].

Complications of treatment

Complications of immunosuppressive therapy occur in a large number of the patients treated for an ANCA-positive crescentic GN. Toxicities are related to excessive glucocorticoids and cyclophosphamide. Infections, some of which are fatal, are not uncommon [8, 11, 35]. It is important to differentiate chest infections with lung shadowing from reactivation of the underlying vasculitis, for which an aggressive diagnostic approach is often warranted, including bronchoscopy, bronchial lavage and biopsy. Delay in therapy can be fatal. Judicious tapering of steroid therapy and the use of steroid-sparing drugs minimize steroid toxicity. Major toxicities associated with daily cyclophosphamide administration include infection, hemorrhagic cystitis, bladder fibrosis and ovarian failure [17]. Bone marrow suppression is common which justifies a close monitoring of peripheral blood count. Neoplastic complications include bladder cancer and leukemia. The long latency period for expression of malignancy, after discontinuation of treatment with alkylating agents, is of great concern [22]. Attempts to reduce these side effects include the use of pulsed monthly cyclophosphamide with concomitant mercaptoethanesulfonate to minimize bladder toxicity [41, 42]. A change at 3–4 months from cyclophosphamide to azathioprine

may also minimize the long-term side effects. Disease activity should be monitored with regular measurements of circulating autoantibodies (anti-GBM and ANCAs). In patients with long-term remissions and undetectable circulating autoantibodies the discontinuation of immunosuppression is justified [31]. In our unit, this is only considered after at least a year of sustained remission.

Outcome

If treatment is begun before irreversible loss of renal function, the initial response by patients with anti-GBM disease and those with ANCA-positive vasculitis is good. The survival of patients with anti-GBM disease has considerably improved over the last three decades [3]. The results of treatment of patients with anti-GBM disease show that the renal functional outcome at one year depends to a large extent on the severity of renal impairment at the onset of treatment; of those with initial serum creatinine in excess of 600 μmol/l, <18% had independent renal function at one year [3–5, 20]. Few dialysis-dependent anti-GBM patients recover independent renal function [3, 5, 20]. Caution against overzealous and potentially dangerous immunosuppression is warranted in this group especially when lung hemorrhage is absent or has subsided. The outcome for anti-GBM patients with an initial serum creatinine <600 μmol/l is more favorable with 36–90% showing a positive response to treatment [3–5, 20].

Factors that determine a poor outcome in patients with anti-GBM disease include oligoanuria and a serum creatinine >600 μmol/l [3–5, 20]. A poor prognostic value has also been assigned by some to the number of crescentic glomeruli [20], the percentage of glomeruli involved by circumferential crescents [5] and high titers of circulating anti-GBM autoantibodies [5].

As mentioned, the outcome of patients with ANCA-positive vasculitis is more favorable than that of patients with anti-GBM disease [19]. The outcome of p- and c-ANCA positive patients appears to be comparable [11, 32]. In a large series of patients with ANCA-positive vasculitis, survival was 75% at two years [11]. Recovery of renal function of 30–75% has been reported in dialysis-dependent ANCA-positive patients treated by immunosuppression [8, 11, 32, 36, 37]. Five-year patient survival varies between 38 and 56% [8, 11, 32, 36, 37]. This relatively high mortality has been attributed to extrarenal manifestations of the vasculitis and to the long-term infectious complications of immunosuppression [11, 27, 30].

Relapse is more common in patients with ANCA-positive vasculitis than in those with anti-GBM disease [19]. With that in mind, some have recommended continuing immunosuppression for at least two years after the induction of remission in ANCA-positive vasculitis

[35]. Long-term therapy should be guided by the levels of circulating ANCA antibodies [31]. Patients at risk of relapse are those with persistent or intermittent circulating ANCA levels [31]. When ANCA is undetectable for long periods of time the likelihood of relapses is minimal, justifying the discontinuation of immunosuppressive therapy [24]. Clearly, a more vigilant approach is recommended in the former group where clinical relapses have been described a short time after a rise in circulating ANCA levels [31].

Lung hemorrhage conveys a poor prognosis in ANCA-positive patients. Renal survival depends on renal function at the onset of treatment, with a more favorable response in patients with serum creatinine levels of <600 µmol/l [11, 32, 33, 35–37]. Other studies reported a good response to intensive immunosuppression regardless of the initial level of renal function in these patients [8]. In one study, a high histological activity index (glomerular neutrophil infiltration, crescent formation and necrosis) as well as a high chronicity index (fibrotic glomerular, tubulointerstitial and vascular sclerosis) indicated a poor prognosis [23]. In another, the degree of active glomerular lesions (crescents and necrosis) did not predict outcome whereas indices of chronicity did [32].

In some patients with RPGN, progressive renal scarring takes place long after the initial immune-mediated insult has subsided. It is important to differentiate between this type of progressive chronic renal failure (CRF) and reactivation of the underlying disease. Urinalysis as well as the measurement of serological markers of the disease (anti-GBM antibodies, ANCAs or other autoantibodies) and if necessary a renal biopsy will clarify the cause of progression. Such an approach is advisable to prevent unnecessary and potentially harmful prolonged immunosuppression. Recurrence of the immune-mediated disease should be treated in a similar fashion to the initial episode. Progressive renal scarring would justify the tapering of immunosuppression and increased emphasis on the control of other causes of progression of chronic renal failure such as systemic hypertension [45].

Conclusion

A better understanding of the spectrum of RPGN has emerged over the last decade. The discovery of the association between ANCA and RPGN has simplified their classification and helped to rationalize therapy. The classification of patients with RPGN into ANCA-positive and -negative vasculitis with renal involvement as well as anti-GBM disease allows early diagnosis and avoids confusion and delay. Very few patients with crescentic GN remain classified as idiopathic. Early diagnosis leads to prompt immunosuppression and good functional recovery. Delay in the initiation of therapy is associated with a poor response. The key to the success of the management of patients with RPGN is a high index of suspicion and the judicious use of immunosuppression.

Acknowledgment

The authors wish to thank Dr C.B. Brown for his review of the manuscript. They are also grateful to Drs J. Shortland and A. Milford-Ward for their assistance with the histological and immunological illustrations respectively.

References

1. Couser, W.G. (1988) Rapidly progressive glomerulonephritis: Classification, pathogenetic mechanisms, and therapy. *Am. J. Kidney Dis.*, **11**, 449–54.
2. Rees, A.J. and Cameron, J.S. (1992) Crescentic glomerulonephritis, in *Oxford Textbook of Clinical Nephrology* (eds S. Cameron, A.M. Davison, J.-P. Grunfeld, D. Kerr and E. Ritz), Oxford University Press, Oxford, pp. 418–38.
3. Turner, N. and Rees, A.J. (1992) Antiglomerular basement membrane disease, in *Oxford Textbook of Clinical Nephrology* (eds S. Cameron, A.M. Davison, J.-P. Grunfeld, D. Kerr and E. Ritz), Oxford University Press, Oxford, pp. 438–56.
4. Briggs, W.A., Johnson, J.P., Teichman, S. *et al.* (1979) Antiglomerular basement membrane antibody-mediated glomerulonephritis and Goodpasture's syndrome. *Medicine*, **58**, 348–61.
5. Herody, M., Bobrie, G., Gouarin, C. *et al.* (1993) Anti-GBM disease: predictive value of clinical, histological and serological data. *Clin. Nephrol.*, **40**, 249–55.
6. Falk, R.J. (1990) ANCA-associated renal disease. *Kidney Int.*, **38**, 998–1010.
7. Jennette, J.C. and Falk, R.J. (1990) Antineutrophil cytoplasmic autoantibodies and associated diseases: a review. *Am. J. Kidney Dis.*, **6**, 517–29.
8. Garrett, P.J., Dewhurst, A.G., Morgan, L.S. *et al.*, (1992) Renal disease associated with circulating antineutrophil cytoplasmic activity. *Q. J. Med.*, **85**, 731–49.
9. Bindi, P., Mougenot, B., Mentre, F. *et al.* (1993) Necrotizing crescentic glomerulonephritis without significant immune deposits: a clinical and serological study. *Q. J. Med.*, **86**, 55–68.
10. Levy, J.B. and Winearls, C.G. (1994) Rapidly progressive glomerulonephritis: what should be first-line therapy? *Nephron*, **67**, 402–7.
10a.Kline Bolton, W. (1996) Goodpasture Syndrome. *Kidney Int.*, **50**, 1753–66.
11. Falk, R.J., Hogan, S., Carey, T.S. *et al.* (1990) Clinical course of anti-neutrophil cytoplasmic autoantibody-associated glomerulonephritis and systemic vasculitis. *Ann. Intern. Med.*, **113**, 656–63.
12. Rees, A.J. (1994) The immunogenetics of glomerulonephritis. *Kidney Int.*, **45**, 377–83.
13. Goodpasture, E.W. (1919) The significance of certain pul-

monary lesions in relation to the etiology of influenza. *Am. J. Med.*, **158**, 863–70.

13a. Griffith, M.E., Lovegrove, J.U., Gaskin, G. *et al.* (1996) C-antineutrophil cytoplasmic antibody positivity in vasculitis patients is associated with the Z allele of alpha-1-antitrypsin, and P-antineutrophil cytoplasmic antibody positivity with the S allele. *Nephrol. Dial. Transpl.*, **11**, 438–3.

13b. Porges, A.J., Redecha, P.B., Kimberley, W.T. *et al.* (1994) Anti-neutrophil cytoplasmic antibodies engage and activate human neutrophils via Fc gamma RIIa. *J. Immunol.*, **153**, 1271–80.

13c. Savage, C.O.S. (1997) Primary systemic vasculitis. *Lancet*, **349**, 553–8.

14. Davies, D.J., Moran, J.E., Niall, J.F. and Ryan, G.B. (1982) Segmental necrotizing glomerulonephritis with anti-neutrophil antibody: possible arbovirus aetiology? *Br. Med. J.*, **285**, 606.

15. Daniell, W.E., Couser, W.G. and Rosenstock, L. (1988) Occupational solvent exposure and glomerulonephritis. A case report and review of the literature. *JAMA*, **259**, 2280–3.

16. Donaghy, M. and Rees, A.J. (1983) Cigarette smoking and lung hemorrhage in glomerulonephritis caused by autoantibodies to glomerular basement membrane. *Lancet*, **ii**, 1390–3.

17. Hoffman, G.S., Kerr, G.S., Leavitt, R.Y. *et al.* (1992) Wegener granulomatosis: an analysis of 158 patients. *Ann. Intern. Med.*, **116**, 488–98.

18. Angangco, R., Thiru, S., Esnault, V.L.M. *et al.* (1994) Does truly 'idiopathic' crescentic glomerulonephritis exist? *Nephrol. Dial. Transplant.*, **9**, 630–6.

19. Saxena, R., Bygren, P., Rasmussen, N. and Wieslander, J. (1991) Circulating autoantibodies in patients with extra-capillary glomerulonephritis. *Nephrol. Dial. Transplant.*, **6**, 389–97.

20. Johnson, J.P., Moore, Jr, J., Austin, H.A. *et al.* (1985) Therapy of antiglomerular basement membrane disease: analysis of prognostic significance of clinical, pathological and treatment factors. *Medicine*, **64**, 219–27.

21. Magil, A.B. (1985) Histogenesis of glomerular crescents. Immunohistochemical demonstration of cytokeratin in crescent cells. *Am. J. Pathol.*, **120**, 222–9.

22. El Nahas, A.M. (1992) Growth factors and the pathogenesis of glomerulosclerosis. *Kidney Int.*, **41**, S15–S20.

22a. Atkins, R.C. (1995) Interleukin-1 in crescentic glomerulonephritis. *Kidney Int.*, **48**, 576–86.

22b. Tomosugi, N.I., Cashman, S.J., Hay, H. *et al.* (1989) Modulation of antibody-mediated glomerular injury by bacterial lipopolysaccharide, tumor necrosis factor, and IL-l. *J. Immunol.*, **142**, 3083–90.

22c. Johnson, R.J. (1994) The glomerular response to injury: Progression or resolution? *Kidney Int.*, **45**, 1769–82.

23. Gans, R.O.B., Kuizinga, M.C., Glodschemeding, R. *et al.* (1993) Clinical features and outcome in patients with glomerulonephritis and antineutrophil cytoplasmic autoantibodies. *Nephron*, **64**, 182–8.

24. Risdon, R.A., Sloper, J.C. and de Wardener, H.E. (1968) Relationship between renal function and histological changes found in renal biopsy pecimens from patients with glomerular nephritis. *Lancet*, **i**, 363–6.

25. Burkholder, P.M. (1969) Ultrastructure demonstration of injury and perforation of the glomerular capillary basement membrane in acute proliferative glomerulonephritis. *Am. J. Pathol.*, **56**, 251–65.

26. Hudson, B., Kalluri, R., Gunwar, S. *et al.* (1993) Molecular characteristics of the Goodpasture autoantigen. *Kidney Int.*, **43**, 135–9.

27. Johansson, C., Butkowski, R., Swedenborg, P. *et al.* (1993) Characterization of a non-Goodpasture autoantibody to type IV collagen. *Nephrol. Dial. Transplant.*, **8**, 1205–10.

28. El Nahas, A.M. (1993) Masugi's nephritis: a model for all seasons, in *Experimental and Genetic Rat Models of Chronic Renal Failure* (eds N. Gretz and M. Strauch), Karger, Basle, pp. 49–67.

29. van der Woude, F.J., Rasmussen, N., Lobatto, S. *et al.* (1985) Autoantibodies against neutrophils and monocytes: tool for diagnosis and marker of disease activity in Wegener's granulomatosis. *Lancet*, **i**, 425–9.

30. Kallenberg, C.G.M., Brouwer, E., Weening, J.J. and Cohen Tervaert, J.W. (1994) Anti-neutrophil cytoplasmic antibodies: current diagnostic and pathophysiological potential. *Kidney Int.*, **46**, 1–15.

31. Gaskin, G., Savage, C.O.S., Ryan, J.J. *et al.* (1991) Anti-neutrophil cytoplasmic antibodies and disease activity during long-term follow-up of 70 patients with systemic vasculitis. *Nephrol. Dial. Transplant.*, **6**, 689–94.

32. Geffriaud-Ricouard, C., Noel, L.H., Chauveau, D. *et al.* (1993) Clinical spectrum associated with ANCA of defined antigen specificities in 98 selected patients. *Clin. Nephrol.*, **39**, 125–36.

33. Balow, J.E. (1993) Renal vasculitis. *Curr. Opin. Nephrol. Transplant.*, **2**, 231–7.

34. Lockwood, C.M., Pearson, T., Rees, A.J. *et al.* (1976) Immunosuppression and plasma exchange in the treatment of Goodpasture's syndrome. *Lancet*, **i**, 711–14.

35. Andrassy, K., Erb, A., Koderisch, J. *et al.* (1991) Wegener's granulomatosis with renal involvement: patient survival and correlation between initial renal function, renal histology, therapy and renal outcome. *Clin. Nephrol.*, **35**, 139–47.

36. Cole, E., Cattran, D., Magil, A. *et al.* (1992) A prospective randomized trial of plasma exchange as additive therapy in idiopathic crescentic glomerulonephritis. *Am. J. Kidney Dis.*, **20**, 261–9.

37. Pusey, C.D., Rees, A.J., Evans, D.J. *et al.* (1991) Plasma exchange in focal necrotizing glomerulonephritis without anti-GBM antibodies. *Kidney Int.*, **40**, 757–63.

38. Stevens, M.E., McConnell, M. and Bone, J.M. (1982) Aggressive treatment with pulse methylprednisolone or plasma exchange is justified in rapidly progressive glomerulonephritis. *Proc. Eur. Dial. Transplant. Assoc.*, **19**, 724–37.

39. Gross, W.L. and Rasmussen, N. (1994) Treatment of Wegener's granulomatosis: the view from two non-nephrologists. *Nephrol. Dial. Transplant.*, **9**, 1219–25.

40. Kunis, C.L., Kiss, B., Williams, G. *et al.* (1992) Intravenous 'pulse' cyclophosphamide therapy of crescentic glomerulonephritis. *Clin. Nephrol.*, **37**, 1–7.

41. Haubitz, M., Frei, U., Rother, U. *et al.* (1991) Cyclophosphamide pulse therapy in Wegener's granulomatosis. *Nephrol. Dial. Transplant.*, **6**, 531–5.

42. Hoffman, G.S., Leavitt, R.Y., Fleisher, T.A. *et al.* (1990) Treatment of Wegener's granulomatosis with intermittent high-dose intravenous cyclophosphamide. *Am. J. Med.*, **89**, 403–10.

43. Palmer, A., Cairns, T., Dische, F. *et al.* (1991) Treatment of rapidly progressive glomerulonephritis by extracorporeal immunoadsorption, prednisolone and cyclophosphamide. *Nephrol. Dial. Transplant.*, **6**, 536–42.

44. Mathieson, P.W., Cobbold, S.P., Hale, G. *et al.* (1990) Monoclonal antibody therapy in systemic vasculitis. *N. Engl. J. Med.*, **323**, 250–5.

45. El Nahas, A.M. and Wight, J.P. (1991) Management of chronic renal failure: Ten unanswered questions. *Q. J. Med.*, **81**, 799–809.

46

Antiglomerular basement membrane disease

J.B. Levy and C.D. Pusey

Introduction

Antiglomerular basement membrane (GBM) disease is a rare autoimmune disorder characterized by autoantibodies directed against a component of basement membranes restricted predominantly to the glomeruli and the lung. The classical presentation is a patient with rapidly progressive glomerulonephritis (RPGN), pulmonary hemorrhage and anti-GBM antibodies. This triad is referred to as Goodpasture's disease. Patients may also present with isolated pulmonary or renal involvement in the presence of the pathogenic autoantibodies. The terminology is confused because the clinical syndrome of pulmonary hemorrhage and RPGN is frequently referred to as Goodpasture's syndrome, but has many causes. Approximately one-third of patients will have Goodpasture's disease but the majority will have vasculitis of one sort or another (Table 46.1). The patient described by Ernest Goodpasture in 1919 [1] had fulminant pulmonary hemorrhage and a proliferative glomerulonephritis which was ascribed to influenza, the great pandemic raging at the time. It was 40 years later that Stanton and Tange described nine more patients with lung and renal disease and labeled the combination Goodpasture's syndrome [2]. Incidentally the patient described by Goodpasture himself probably had systemic vasculitis since the autopsy findings included splenic infarcts and hemorrhagic lesions in the small intestine as well as the kidney and lung pathology.

The pathogenic nature of anti-GBM autoantibodies in Goodpasture's disease was initially suggested in 1962 by Steblay's experiments in sheep, in which the injection of heterologous GBM resulted in fatal glomerulonephritis. This nephritis could be induced in normal animals by passive transfer of serum or by cross-circulation. In humans, Scheer and Grossman observed the binding of antibody to GBM in two patients with Goodpasture's syndrome, and subsequently Lerner *et al.* induced severe proliferative glomerulonephritis in squirrel monkeys by the passive transfer of human antibodies eluted from the kidney of a patient with Goodpasture's disease (reviewed in 3).

During the 30 years since these classic studies the Goodpasture antigen has been identified as the carboxy terminal, non-collagenous domain of the α3 chain of type IV collagen (α3(IV)NC1), recombinant human antigen has been produced, susceptibility genes in the major histocompatibility complex (MHC) have been identified and evidence for the involvement of autoreactive T cells has been produced and there has been development of highly successful treatment regimens.

Incidence

Goodpasture's disease is uncommon, with an estimated incidence of 0.5–1 new case per million population per year in Great Britain, and 0.9 in Sweden. In unselected series of renal biopsies from Europe and America 1–2% of

Nephrology, Edited by Rex L. Jamison and Robert Wilkinson.
Published in 1997 by Chapman & Hall, London. ISBN 0 412 60930 4

Table 46.1 Causes of Goodpasture's syndrome (RPGN with pulmonary hemorrhage)

Common	Microscopic polyarteritis
	Wegener's granulomatosis
	SLE
	Goodpastrue's disease
Less common	Churg–Strauss syndrome
	Henoch–Schonlein purpura
	HUS or TTP
	Behçet's
	Essential mixed cryoglobulinemia
	Rheumatoid vasculitis
	Penicillamine therapy

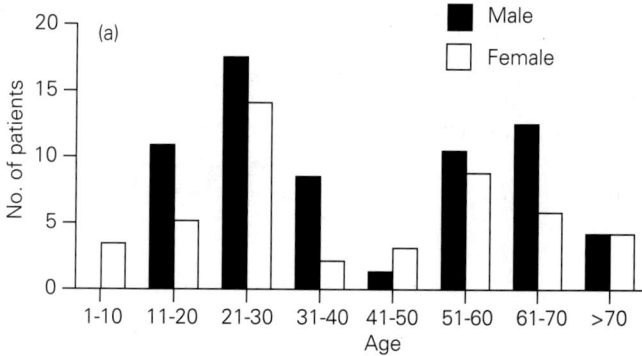

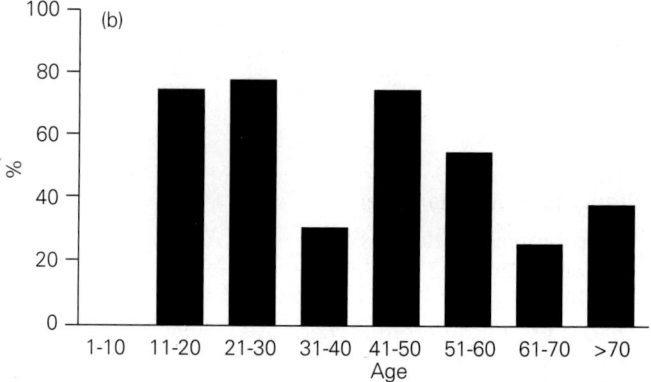

Figure 46.1 Age distribution (a) and incidence of pulmonary hemorrhage (b) in 112 patients with Goodpasture's disease. (Data combined from Hammersmith Hospital and all published series since 1990 containing patient details.)

patients have anti-GBM disease. It accounts for up to 7% of patients with end-stage renal failure. The majority of patients reported are Caucasian, with Asians and Afro-Caribbeans accounting for less than 10% of cases in the United States and 3% in the United Kingdom. In New Zealand the disease may be more common in Maoris. These racial differences may reflect the population immunogenetics, as Goodpasture's disease is known to be tightly associated with specific MHC molecules (see later).

The more widespread use of specific diagnostic tests (direct immunofluoresence, radioimmunassay and ELISA) has established a bimodal age distribution with peaks occurring in the third and sixth decades (Figure 46.1). The disease is only slightly more common in men despite earlier reports of a substantial male predominance, though the sex distribution is uneven with more men in the younger age groups. Pulmonary hemorrhage is much commoner in men, whereas glomerulonephritis alone is predominantly a feature of older patients and women (Figure 46.1).

Three clusters of cases have been reported, one each from New Zealand, America and the United Kingdom, and a seasonal variation was noted in the 1980–1984 British series with a peak in the spring and early summer [4]. The significance of these rare clusters is unclear and no pathogens (viral or other) were identified.

Clinical manifestations

Most patients present acutely with lung hemorrhage or RPGN, and occasionally with both. Lung hemorrhage tends to lead to early presentation as it is a particularly alarming symptom, whereas renal failure even in the context of RPGN may be insidious. However, the spectrum of disease is wide; some patients have chronic recurrent alveolar hemorrhage manifest only as iron deficiency, a few patients report recurrent minor episodes of

hemoptysis prior to a fulminant hemorrhage or symptoms of uremia, and some patients have no lung involvement at all and are simply investigated for hematuria or renal failure.

General features

Patients often give a history of several months of nonspecific symptoms with malaise, weight loss and headaches, but in contrast to patients with systemic vasculitis these are not prominent features. More commonly patients report minor hemoptysis over several weeks with symptoms of anemia. In some patients this has led to investigation for occult blood loss. The anemia is usually microcytic with occasional features of microangiopathy, in contrast to the anemia in systemic vasculitis which is usually normocytic. Many patients also report symptoms of upper respiratory tract infection but not of systemic inflammation.

Pulmonary features

Pulmonary hemorrhage occurs more commonly in young men. It is reported in about two-thirds of patients in more recent series (Figure 46.1 and Table 46.4) and almost always precedes or occurs synchronously with glomerulonephritis. Rarely pulmonary hemorrhage is the only manifestation of Goodpasture's disease. Patients often give a history of breathlessness over several weeks with or without episodes of minor hemoptysis. Pulmonary hemorrhage remits and relapses markedly but overt hemoptysis bears little relationship to the degree of alveolar bleeding. There is a strong association between pulmonary hemorrhage and cigarette smoking [5], and in some patients this can lead to dramatic recurrence of bleeding despite apparent resolution of underlying disease (see Figure 46.2). Smoking is likely to act as a local trigger rather than play a causative role. Pulmonary hemorrhage is rare in non-smokers, though several reports have noted associations with exposure to inhaled toxins (hydrocarbons, metal dusts, chlorine gas), fluid overload and intercurrent infections, both local and systemic. Isolated hemoptysis in Goodpasture's disease must be distinguished from truly local lung pathology, for example idiopathic pulmonary hemosiderosis, by careful examination of urine for red blood cells and casts, and serum for anti-GBM antibodies. In mild cases examination of the lung is often normal apart from tachypnea. More severe disease causes respiratory distress, cyanosis and frank hemoptysis, with inspiratory crackles audible over the mid and lower lung fields, and occasionally bronchial breathing. These signs can be difficult to distinguish from volume overload or even infection.

The chest radiograph is rarely normal, but neither are the features specific for pulmonary hemorrhage. Alveolar shadowing usually involves the central lung fields, sparing the apices and supradiaphragmatic regions. The opacities are often fleeting and rarely bounded by fissures, but may contain air bronchograms (Figure 46.3). These changes are very similar to those caused by pulmonary edema or infection; however in hemorrhage they usually clear within 48 h of an episode of bleeding. Minor abnormalities may persist for longer, but failure to clear may indicate recurrent bleeding.

Other signs of pulmonary hemorrhage include sudden falls in hemoglobin and an elevated K_{CO} – the diffusing capacity for carbon monoxide (see Figure 46.2). The K_{CO} is an extremely useful diagnostic aid both to confirm the existence of alveolar hemorrhage and to follow serially the clearance of blood. Repeated investigation will also facilitate the early recognition of new bleeding. Hemoglobin binds carbon monoxide avidly, and normally the measurement of carbon monoxide uptake by the lungs is a measure of the effectiveness of gas exchange across the alveolar membranes. The presence of blood within the alveoli, however, increases the amount of free hemoglobin available to bind inhaled carbon monoxide, and thus the measured K_{CO} rises. The K_{CO} is a much more sensi-

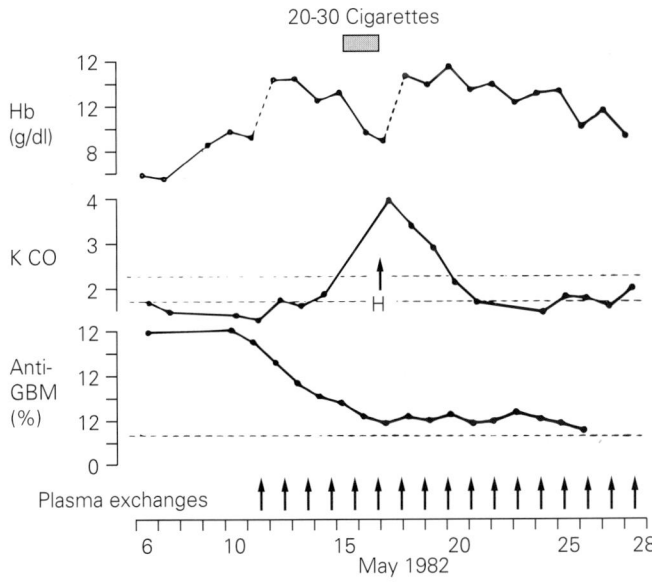

Figure 46.2 Smoking-induced relapse of pulmonary hemorrhage. This patient with nephritis and high titers of anti-GBM antibodies at presentation was improving with plasmapheresis and immunosuppression, when he resumed smoking. His K_{CO} rose substantially (middle), and hemoglobin fell by 20 g/l (top), coincident with symptomatic hemoptysis (H), and despite concurrent plasmapheresis. The anti-GBM antibody titer continued to fall during this episode of relapse. (Reproduced, with permission, from ref. [5].)

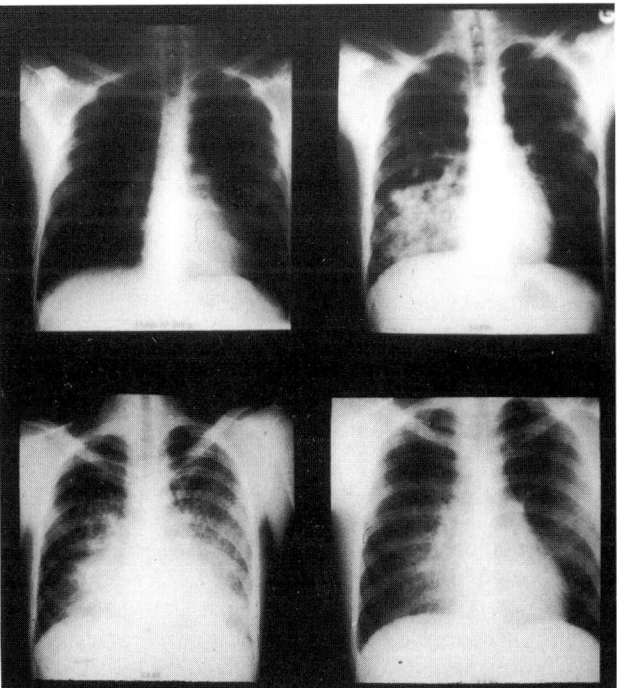

Figure 46.3 Chest radiographs of a patient with Goodpasture's disease taken over three days. (a) and (b) were taken 8 h apart, after the patient had an episode of hemoptysis. (c) and (d) were taken two days later and 12 h apart. Note the changing pattern of shadowing between the second (b) and third (c) radiographs, and the rapid resolution of the radiographic changes.

tive and specific marker of alveolar hemorrhage than a radiograph, and a rise in the KCO precedes radiographic evidence of bleeding. A rise of KCO of 30% above a stable baseline generally indicates fresh hemorrhage.

Bronchoscopy is sometimes performed in the investigation of a patient with purely pulmonary manifestations and is usually normal. During active hemorrhage blood may be visible oozing from the bronchi. Transbronchial biopsy is not a useful diagnostic tool as characteristic pathological immunofluoresence findings on the alveolar basement membrane are often absent. Hemosiderin-laden macrophages are characteristic, but not diagnostic. In difficult cases open lung biopsy is the preferred method for obtaining useful lung tissue.

Renal features

The range of renal presentation is similarly wide. At the severe end of the spectrum the progression of RPGN is inexorable with loss of renal function within days and little tendency to remit spontaneously. Very few untreated patients will retain useful renal function – only two of 52 patients in Benoit's 1964 review [6]. The manifestations of the nephritis *per se* are indistinguishable from those of RPGN of any other cause with sudden onset, hematuria (usually microscopic), cellular casts and moderate proteinuria (less than 5 g/24 h). Hypertension is uncommon early in the disease in the absence of volume overload. Oliguria is a late feature with a poor prognosis.

Many patients with recurrent pulmonary hemorrhage, however, have minor renal disease. Renal function may be normal, but microscopic hematuria is almost always detectable. Renal biopsy in these patients may show linear binding of immunoglobulin to GBM as the sole abnormality. This state can continue for months or years before some event triggers the onset of RPGN. Very rarely patients have chronic progressive renal disease. One patient has been described who presented with renal vein thrombosis. Renal imaging is not specifically useful and kidney size is normal.

Other organs

Despite the presence of the Goodpasture antigen in basement membranes of the eye, ear, choroid plexus, liver and some endocrine glands (Table 46.2), there is little evidence for injury in other organs apart from the eye. Jampol described two patients with retinal detachment and in one confirmed antibody binding to Bruch's membrane and choroidal basement membrane. Other patients have been described in whom retinal detachment appeared to be a specific complication of Goodpasture's disease. Retinal capillary leakage using fluoroscein angiography has been seen in some patients and a hemorraghic and exudative retinopathy has also been described. There is no good evidence for a specific encephalopathy of Goodpasture's disease despite occasional reports of

Table 46.2   Distribution of the Goodpasture antigen

Kidney	Glomerular basement membrane Bowman's capsule Distal tubular membrane
Lung	Alveolar basement membrane
Eye	Choroid Ciliary body Bruch's and Descemet's membrane Basement membranes of retinal capillaries, cornea and lens capsule
Ear	Cochlear basement membrane
Brain	Choroidal epithelial basement membrane
Liver	Hepatic artery in portal tracts
Other	Basement membranes of adrenal, pituitary, thyroid and breast

convulsions in patients with severe disease. This more likely reflects severe metabolic derangement in an acutely sick patient, rather than choroid plexus involvement, although antibody deposition on the choroid plexus basement membrane has been reported at post-mortem.

Pathogenesis

Anti-GBM disease has the best understood immuno-pathology of all autoimmune renal diseases, and yet the precise etiology remains largely unknown. The supposition is that the disease results from an unidentified environmental insult acting in a genetically predisposed individual. This predisposition is increasingly understood at a molecular level; however, the triggering factors remain elusive. We will first discuss the factors involved in susceptibility to Goodpasture's disease, the possible environmental triggers, and then the nature of the target antigen. Finally the autoimmune response leading to the observed pathology is described.

Immunogenetics

Goodpasture's disease has been reported in two sets of identical twins and four sibling pairs. In both twin pairs the disease onset was remarkably close in both individuals (five months and six weeks apart) supporting the role of an environmental trigger. However, several pairs of twins discordant for Goodpasture's disease are known. The rarity of the disease precludes any precise calculation of the concordance rate.

Anti-GBM disease is strongly associated with specific MHC antigens (HLA system in man). This was first noted in 1978 when Rees *et al.* [7] reported the presence of HLA DR2 serologically in 88% of patients compared with an incidence of 30% in controls. Subsequent studies from Australia and the United States have confirmed this association, with 87% and 50% of patients, respectively, bearing the DR2 antigen. More recently, molecular studies have confirmed and extended this association. Using restriction fragment length polymorphism (RFLP) analysis of genomic DNA, Burns *et al.* [8] demonstrated that 94% of patients with Goodpasture's disease carried either the haplotype HLA DRw15(DR2)/DQw6 or HLA DR4/DQw7. Furthermore, DR1 was negatively associated with Goodpasture's disease. This intriguing finding was confirmed in 82 patients by allele sequence specific oligonucleotide probing of specifically amplified DNA and subsequent nucleotide sequencing. In this study 79% of patients had DRB1*15 and 90% of patients had either DRB1*15 or DRB1*04 alleles (the genetic loci for DR2 and DR4, respectively), whereas the frequencies of DRB1*01 (DR1) and DRB1*07 (DR7) were significantly reduced and appeared to confer protection [8a]. Comparisons of derived amino acid sequences of expressed DRβ chains showed that the DRβ chains of DRB1*15 and DRB1*04 shared a five amino acid sequence motif which was not shared with DRB1*01 or *07. This motif, which lies on the floor of the antigen binding groove, has a stronger association with Goodpasture's disease than any individual allele, and was present in two patients who were neither DR2 or 4 (Figure 46.4). Intriguingly, American blacks rarely carry the DRB1*1501 or 1502 alleles but rather a rare allele DRB1*1503. The only difference between *1501 and *1503 is a point mutation within the motif associated with the disease. Thus specific charac-

teristics of the amino acid motif of DRB1*15 may determine susceptibility to Goodpasture's disease by influencing the binding of peptides and thus epitopes presented by class II molecules to T cells.

T cells are almost certainly pivotal in the development of Goodpasture's disease, with the central interaction being between the MHC, T cell receptor and the antigenic peptide. T cells are crucially important for the development of experimental anti-GBM disease and T cell help is required for the development of most antibody responses. Patients' T cells are known to respond to purified Goodpasture antigen and preliminary studies have demonstrated that T cell receptor Vβ gene expression is highly restricted in proliferating T cells to only a few families of genes, particularly Vβ2,8 and 18 (Fisher, unpublished observations).

Two other genetic influences have been described. First, HLA B7 is associated with Goodpasture's disease. This class I MHC antigen is in linkage disequilibrium with DR2 which may in part explain its increased incidence; however, patients carrying both antigens have more severe disease, with higher crescent scores and serum creatinines, than patients carrying DR2 alone. The mechanism involved remains unknown. Finally, patients with Goodpasture's disease are more likely to have inherited specific variants of immunoglobulin heavy chains – Gm allotypes. Inheritance of various combinations has been associated with different concentrations of IgG subclasses, susceptibility to autoimmune diseases and development of antibody responses by healthy individuals. The incidence of the Gm haplotype 1,2,21 is significantly increased in Goodpasture's disease (54% versus 17% controls; relative risk 5.75) and patients heterozygous at the

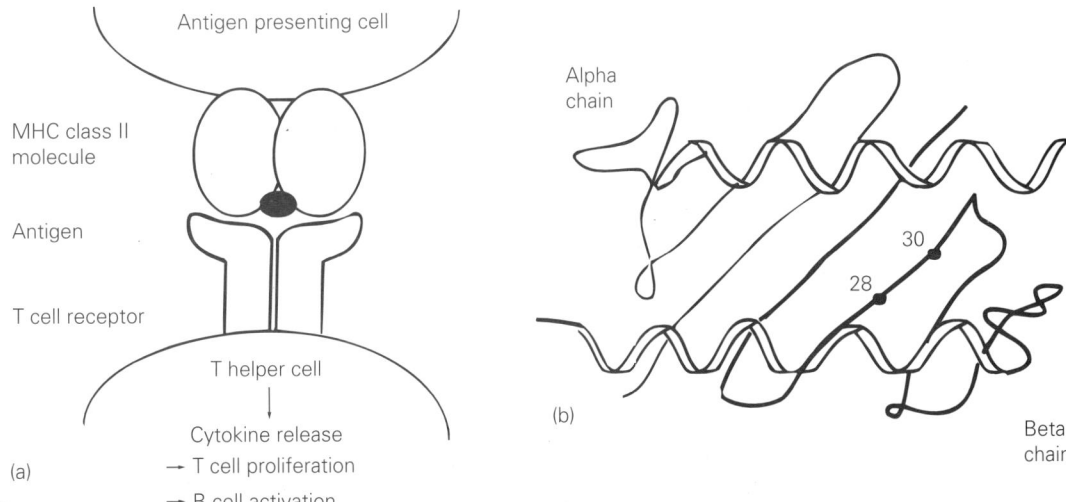

Figure 46.4 Diagrammatic representation of (a) the interaction between the MHC class II molecule on an antigen presenting cell, the antigen itself, and the T cell receptor. (b) The MHC class II peptide-binding cleft visualized from above. The conserved amino acids of the class II molecule most strongly associated with Goodpasture's disease lie on the floor of the peptide-binding cleft, between positions 26 and 30 of the β chain. (Modified from Dr Fisher.)

Gm complex have an increased titer of anti-GBM antibodies. The significance of this is also unknown.

Environmental factors

Investigation of environmental initiators is beset with difficulties, not least because many agents are known which will precipitate pulmonary hemorrhage or hematuria in patients with circulating anti-GBM antibodies. No specific pathogen or toxin has been positively identified which can initiate Goodpasture's disease *de novo* (but see hydrocarbon exposure below), and the temporal association of infection, especially of the upper respiratory tract, with the development of clinical symptoms is common and does not reflect causation.

Bearing these difficulties in mind, three clusters of cases of Goodpasture's disease have been reported. The seasonality of the disease has been alluded to earlier. Several workers have tried to establish an association with influenza infection, and early studies noted an apparent increase in the number of cases during 'flu epidemics. However, the ability of infections non-specifically to precipitate clinical evidence of the underlying presence of autoantibodies may well explain many of these cases, and systematic studies of the incidence of various infections in series of patients with Goodpasture's disease have been negative.

Exposure to hydrocarbons or solvent fumes has frequently been implicated in the development of glomerulonephritides and especially Goodpasture's disease. Many cases have been published in which exposure to a wide variety of hydrocarbons, including gasoline, oils, paints and organic solvents, preceded the onset of pulmonary hemorrhage and/or glomerulonephritis [9]. Again causation is difficult to establish particularly as awareness of the possible links tends to lead to an increased level of reporting, and exposure to hydrocarbons is widespread in developed countries. However, several case control studies have reported significantly greater exposure to hydrocarbons in patients with glomerulonephritis, and a number of reports include patients with nephritis in the absence of pulmonary hemorrhage, which suggests a mechanism other than pulmonary irritation in an individual with pathogenic autoantibodies. Finally, factory workers chronically exposed to petroleum-based oils (but not solvent-based paints) have increased circulating levels of anti-GBM autoantibodies, in excess of their non-exposed colleagues. All of this evidence does suggest that some hydrocarbons may cause disruption of basement membranes and subsequent initiation of an autoimmune response. Careful case control studies may further elucidate the link but have yet to be done.

The ability of environmental toxins, especially cigarette smoking, to precipitate lung hemorrhage in patients with Goodpasture's disease is well documented and some authors would suggest that lung hemorrhage only occurs in patients with an additional insult to the lung. In 51 patients with Goodpasture's disease in the United

Kingdom all of the 37 current smokers had pulmonary hemorrhage compared with two of ten non-smokers [5]. More recently Herody *et al.* [10] reported a series of 29 French patients with anti-GBM disease in which 13 of the 14 with pulmonary hemorrhage were smokers. Anecdotally several patients have been reported in whom pulmonary hemorrhage recurred on resumption of smoking during apparent recovery from the disease (Figure 46.2).

Disease associations

Intriguingly, Goodpasture's disease is only rarely associated with other autoimmune diseases aside from the vasculitides (Table 46.3). However, patients are increasingly recognized with both anti-GBM and antineutrophil cytoplasmic autoantibodies (ANCA). This is particularly interesting as many patients with Wegener's granulomatosis and microscopic polyarteritis, in whom ANCA are characteristic findings, present with RPGN and pulmonary hemorrhage. The precise incidence of these so-called 'double positive' patients is variable and partially dependent on the rigor with which the autoantibodies are char-

Table 46.3   Associations of Goodpasture's disease

Renal disorders	Membranous nephropathy[a]
	Post-transplant (Alport's)[a]
	Membranoproliferative nephritis
	Cortical necrosis
	Postlithotripsy
	Postobstruction
Autoimmune disorders	Microscopic polyarteritis[a]
	Wegener's granulomatosis[a]
	Celiac disease
	Hashimoto's thyroiditis
	Myasthenia gravis
	Partial lipodystrophy
	Ulcerative colitis
	Dermatomyositis
	Behcet's
	Penicillamine therapy
Malignant disorders	Lymphoma (especially Hodgkin's)[a]
	Thymoma
	Carcinoma of the bronchus
	Bronchial carcinoid
	Pancreatic islet cell tumor
Inherited disorders	Alport's post-transplant[a]
	Nail–patella syndrome

[a] Multiple cases reported.

acterized. In our laboratory we have found that 4% of patients with ANCA also have anti-GBM antibodies and that 25% of patients with anti-GBM antibodies also have ANCA (Coulthart and Pusey, unpublished). This is a strikingly high incidence of ANCA in those patients with undoubted Goodpasture's disease, but the significance of the observation is unclear. In our patients all of the ANCA were of a perinuclear pattern and their sera specifically recognized myeloperoxidase in an ELISA. Other centers have reported mixed ANCA specificities. Whether these double-positive patients have clinically distinct disease is not known, though most seem to have evidence of systemic vasculitis. In some of the reported patients the anti-GBM autoantibody was only fleetingly present. It is possible that damage to the GBM by systemic vasculitis allows the development of autoantibodies; however, the lack of any patients in our series with cytoplasmic ANCA or antiproteinase 3 antibodies, would seem to militate against this hypothesis. Such an explanation has also been proposed to account for the presence of anti-GBM antibodies in some patients with crescentic deterioration in membranous nephritis. Disruption of basement membrane could also have occurred in the patients reported to have developed anti-GBM disease postlithotripsy and posturinary tract obstruction. Both of these patients carried the HLA DR2 allele, further emphasizing the importance of genetic susceptibility.

The Goodpasture antigen

The autoantibody response in Goodpasture's disease is undoubtedly pathogenic. The target antigen to which this response is primarily directed is known as the Goodpasture antigen and has been identified as a minority component of GBM, namely the α3 chain of type IV collagen [11, 12]. All patients produce antibodies against this target, though some also develop low titers of antibodies against other alpha chains of type IV collagen (Figure 46.5). The immunohistochemical and immunoblotting patterns of patients' sera can be entirely replicated by a monoclonal antibody (P1), adding further evidence that the autoantigen is common in all patients [13].

Immunoelectronmicroscopic studies have located the Goodpasture antigen within the lamina densa of the glomerular and alveolar basement membranes, and immunohistochemical studies have demonstrated a restricted tissue distribution of the antigen to a few specialized basement membranes (Table 46.2). This distribution is markedly different from that of the more widespread α1 and α2 chains of type IV collagen. The last decade has seen the precise localisation of the autoantigen within the α3 chain of type IV collagen and the gene encoding the α3 chain has been cloned. Recombinant Goodpasture antigen has been produced and is recognized both by patients' sera and monoclonal antibodies raised against purified native material.

The structure of the GBM is highly complex, and involves networks of different collagen molecules

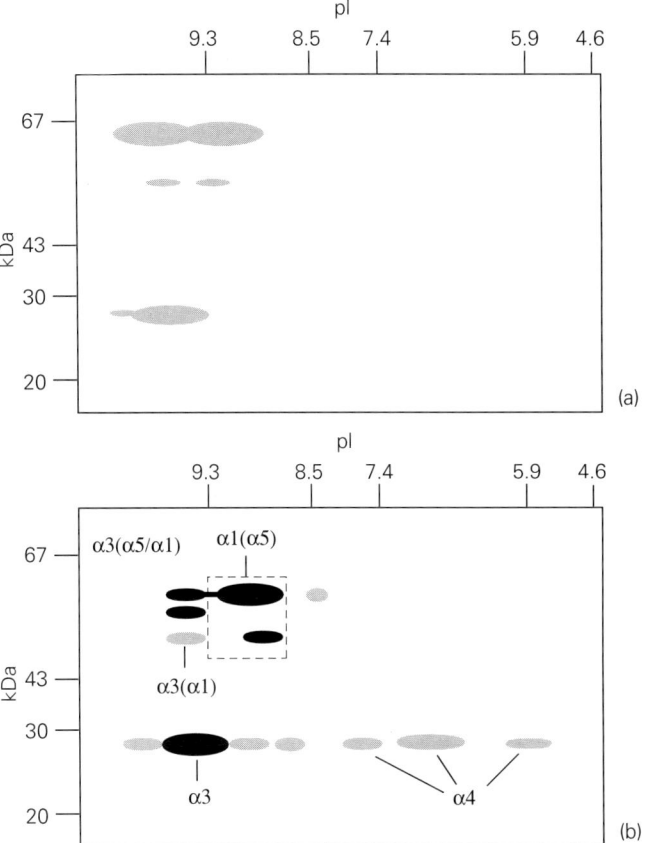

Figure 46.5 (a) Western blot of two-dimensional separated human GBM with anti-GBM antibodies from a patient with Goodpasture's disease. (b) Schematic diagram showing the identity of the separated human GBM components. The dominant components recognized by autoantibodies are the α3 monomers (28 kDa, pI > 9.3) and α3 containing dimers, though α4 monomers are also recognized by the patient's serum. Binding to α1/α5 containing dimers can in part be explained by their much higher concentration. (Reproduced, with permission, from Derry *et al.* (1994), *Experimental Nephrology*, S. Karger AG, Basel.)

together with several other distinct components (reviewed in [14]). Type IV collagen makes a chicken-wire-like structure with both N- and C-terminal ends cross-linked (Figure 46.6). Six different chains of type IV collagen have now been identified (α1–α6) and their genes cloned. α1 and α2 are ubiquitous whereas α3–α6 occur as minority components in specialized basement membranes. Triplets of these chains are formed within basement membranes with, for example, two α1 and one α2 chains entwined in a triple helix. Similarly α3 chains form helices with α4 chains. All of these molecules contain long collagenous regions capped with non-collagenous domains. The autoantigenic region of the α3 chain is contained within the C-terminal non-collagenous domain (NC1). Collagenase digestion releases hexamers of the NC1 domains and chaotropic

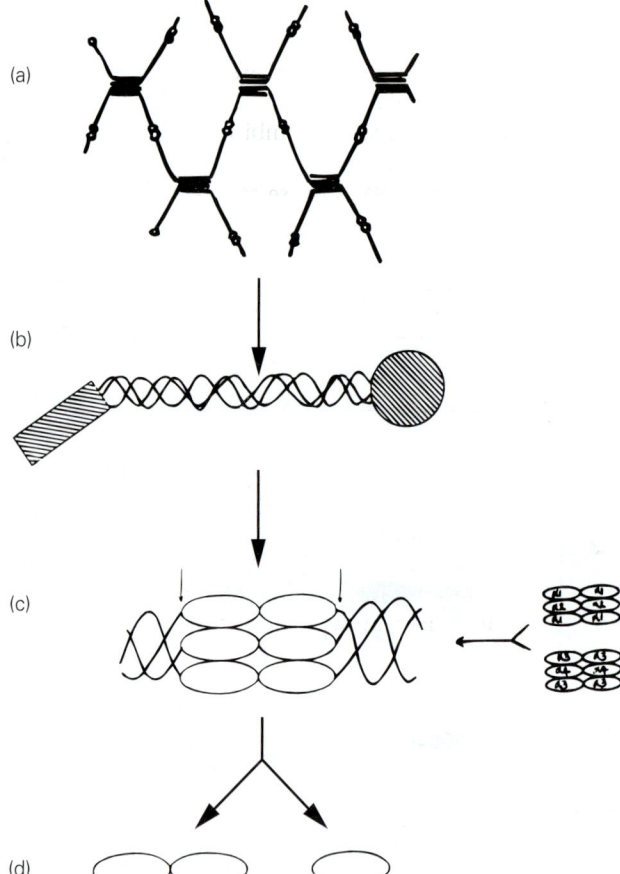

(a)

(b)

(c)

(d)

Figure 46.6 Schematic representation of the structure of type IV collagen. (a) The network of type IV collagen molecules. Triple helical protomers associate with each other at both their N and C termini. (b) An individual triple helical protomer composed of three α chains assembled from six genetically distinct isoforms (α1–α6). (c) The non-collagenous C-terminus of a protomer can be released by collagenase (arrows) and is made up of the three individual NC1 domains of one protomer closely associated with the three NC1 domains from the adjoined protomer (the hexameric subunit). This hexamer classically consists of $(\alpha1)_2\alpha2$ isoforms and probably $(\alpha3)_2\alpha4$ and $(\alpha5)_2\alpha6$ isoforms, and can be dissociated by chaotropic agents into the individual NC1 monomers or dimers. (d) The possible combinations of α chain monomers within the hexamer is not fully determined. The Goodpasture antigen is located within the NC1 monomer of α3 but is relatively concealed within the native hexamer.

agents can further release monomeric and dimeric components from these hexamers. Two-dimensional electrophoresis (SDS–PAGE and isoelectric focusing) can also separate collagenase-digested GBM into monomers and dimers of all six alpha chains. Immunoblotting of such separations confirms the restriction of antigenicity predominantly to the highly cationic, α3 chains (Figure

46.5). The epitope of the Goodpasture antigen recognized by autoantibodies is concealed within the three-dimensional structure of the hexamer and is only fully revealed on dissociation into the monomeric and dimeric components. More recently molecular biological techniques have localized the autoantibody binding site within the NC1 monomer [14a, 14b].

The Goodpasture antigen and Alport's syndrome

Alport's syndrome has provided important insights into glomerular basement membrane structure and the Goodpasture antigen in particular. Immunohistochemical studies using sera of patients with Goodpasture's disease or monoclonal antibodies against the α3 chain of type IV collagen show that the Goodpasture antigen, α3, is reduced or absent from the GBM of most patients with Alport's syndrome. The syndrome is usually X-linked or rarely autosomal recessive, and the gene for the X-linked variety has been mapped to Xq22. The gene for the α5 chain of type IV collagen maps to the same region, and recent sequencing studies have confirmed that most patients with Alport's have mutations within the α5 gene [15]. This is intriguing, not only because these patients have lost antigenic α3 reactivity within the GBM despite an apparently normal α3 gene, but also because a number of patients with Alport's develop Goodpasture's disease after receiving a kidney transplant. This phenomenon is not entirely understood, and there is controversy over the specificity of the antibody response. It seems likely that the failure of expression of normal α5 chains of type IV collagen somehow leads to a failure to incorporate the α3 chain correctly within the collagen network of basement membrane. This lack of expression of the α3 chain may lead to the failure to develop tolerance embryologically, and thus allow recognition of the α3 antigen as a foreign protein within an allograft. Mutations in both the α3 and α4 chains have been identified, particularly in patients with autosomal recessive disease.

The autoantibody response

The classic experiments of Lerner *et al.* [16] demonstrated the pathogenicity of the autoantibodies in Goodpasture's disease. In these experiments, purified immunoglobulin from patients with Goodpasture's disease was injected into uninephrectomized squirrel monkeys. Proteinuria developed rapidly with a proliferative, non-crescentic glomerulonephritis and linear binding of antibodies to the GBM. The animals did not develop hemoptysis or evidence of antibody deposition in the lungs. The human corollary is the recurrence of Goodpasture's disease in a transplant if performed while the autoantibody is still present. Furthermore, some studies show that the severity of nephritis correlates with antibody titer at presentation. Nevertheless, occasional patients have recurrence of autoantibody after treatment without evidence of target organ damage [17]. This may well relate to the effector mechanisms recruited by antibody deposition: the autoantibodies are usually IgG1 which can fix complement and bind macrophages, but occasionally an IgG4 response predominates. Patients with recurrence of antibody without nephritis usually possess the IgG4 subclass. Finally, in experimental models the threshold for injury can be markedly reduced by systemic infection, lipopolysaccharide, interleukin-1β and tumor necrosis factor. This probably explains the ability of infection to precipitate relapses of Goodpasture's disease (Figure 46.7).

Immunoregulation of autoantibodies

The strong association of Goodpasture's disease with HLA molecules suggests that T lymphocytes are critical in the pathogenesis of the disease. It is these cell surface molecules which present antigenic peptides to T cells responsible for the development and regulation of an immune response. Several studies have identified increased numbers of T lymphocytes and macrophages within the glomeruli of patients with Goodpasture's disease, and *in vitro* T cells from patients will proliferate specifically in response to both purified and recombinant Goodpasture antigen. In chickens the transfer of T cells from experimental birds with anti-GBM disease to irradiated recipients leads to glomerular disease without antibody production, whereas the transfer of B lymphocytes leads to production of anti-GBM antibodies but no nephritis [18]. In a rat model of anti-GBM disease (experimental allergic glomerulonephritis, EAG) transfer of T cells from affected animals to irradiated recipients fails to produce disease, but primes the response to subsequent antigen challenge [19]. Anti-T cell treatments such as anti-CD4 monoclonal antibody and cyclosporin can markedly reduce glomerular injury in EAG, though the antibody response is maintained in some animals.

Goodpasture's disease is unusual in that the autoimmune process tends not to recur after successful treatment despite the continued presence of the autoantigen. Explicit rechallenge in the form of an allograft after antibody levels have declined also rarely causes recurrence. It is unlikely that this is entirely due to the drug treatment as occasional cases of spontaneous remission have been reported, and in untreated patients the antibody levels decline naturally within one year. The mechanism of this immunoregulation is unknown.

Pathogenesis of lung hemorrhage

Lung hemorrhage is not a consistent feature of Goodpasture's disease and bears little correlation with antibody levels. This cannot be explained by a difference in the antigen itself, as immunofluoresence studies using patients' sera and monoclonal antibodies suggest the antigen in alveolar and GBMs is the same, and immunizing sheep with alveolar basement membrane induces glomerulonephritis and anti-GBM antibodies. Part of the explanation may be in a different presentation of the antigen within the collagen of the basement membrane. Alternatively the differential expression of lung and renal pathology may be due to the structural difference in the capillaries of the organs. The fenestrated endothelium of glomerular capillaries allows direct contact between antibodies and the basement membrane. This is not the case in the alveoli in which the endothelium forms a barrier between capillary lumen and basement membrane. Pulmonary hemorrhage may occur only when the barrier is disrupted, for example by cigarette smoking, inhalation of toxic agents such as solvents and chlorine gas, and infection. This can be demonstrated experimentally in rats and rabbits in which anti-GBM antibodies injected passively will only bind to alveolar basement membrane if a toxic pulmonary insult is co-administered. The epidemiological data on pulmonary hemorrhage in smokers supports this hypothesis.

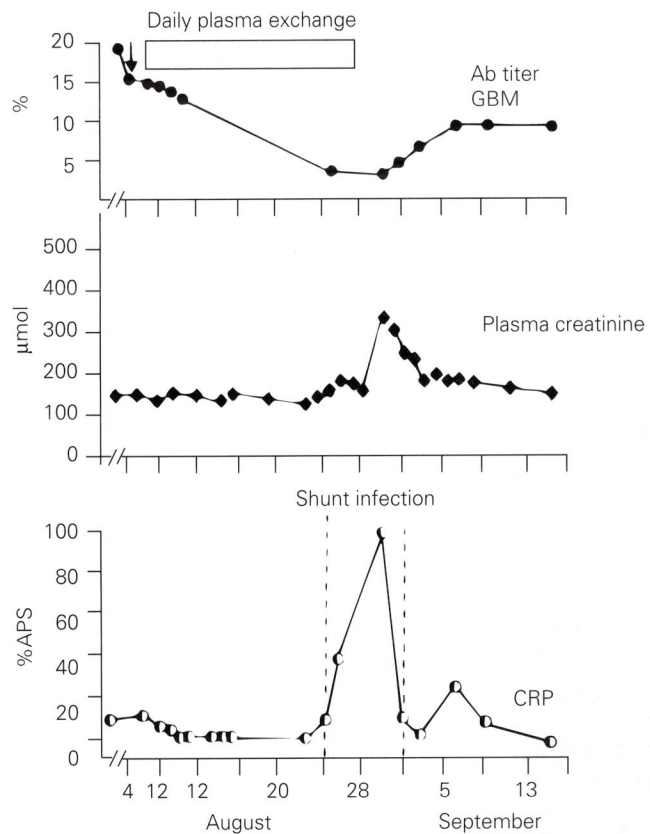

Figure 46.7 The effect of intercurrent infection in Goodpasture's disease. Note the rise in creatinine (middle) associated with a shunt infection and marked acute-phase response (bottom), despite the reduction in anti-GBM antibody level with immunosuppression and plasma exchange. (Reproduced, with permission, from Rees *et al.* (1977) *Br. Med. J.*, **2**, 723–6.)

Pathology

Renal

Light microscopic findings vary considerably from entirely normal to severe necrotizing crescentic nephritis despite the fact that all cases display fixed immunoglobulin along the glomerular capillary walls [20]. In milder cases the glomeruli show focal necrosis or proliferation interspersed with normal glomeruli (Figure 46.8). In more severe cases most glomeruli are involved with segmental or panglomerular necrosis and cellular crescent formation (Figure 46.9). Affected glomeruli contain T cells and occasional multinucleated giant cells in the periphery of the tuft. In some patients the glomeruli are sclerosed at presentation with fibrous crescents. An accompanying acute interstitial inflammatory cell infiltrate is common if not invariable. The blood vessels are usually normal though occasional patients show evidence of vasculitis. Whether these are patients who possess ANCA in addition to the anti-GBM antibodies remains to be clarified. Electron microscopy shows patchy foot process fusion with a minor degree of basement membrane thickening and frequently a rarified zone between the basement membrane and endothelium. Fractures of the basement membrane are also common.

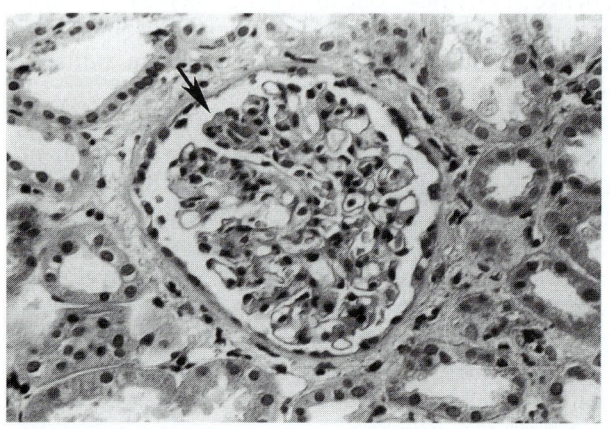

Figure 46.8 Glomerulus from a patient with Goodpasture's disease showing relatively minor changes only. The patient presented with pulmonary hemorrhage, hematuria and proteinuria, normal serum creatinine and high titers of anti-GBM antibodies. The biopsy showed small foci of segmental necrosis in some glomeruli only (*arrow*). (Histology courtesy of Dr M Thompson.)

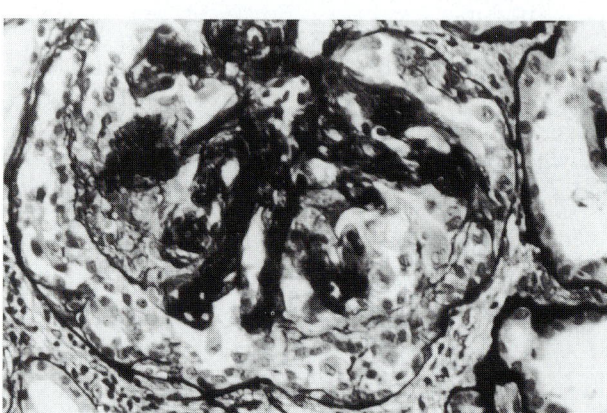

Figure 46.9 Biopsy from a patient presenting with RPGN, pulmonary hemorrhage, anti-GBM antibodies and a creatinine of 630 μmol/l. The biopsy shows a circumferential cellular crescent. (Courtesy of Dr M. Thompson.)

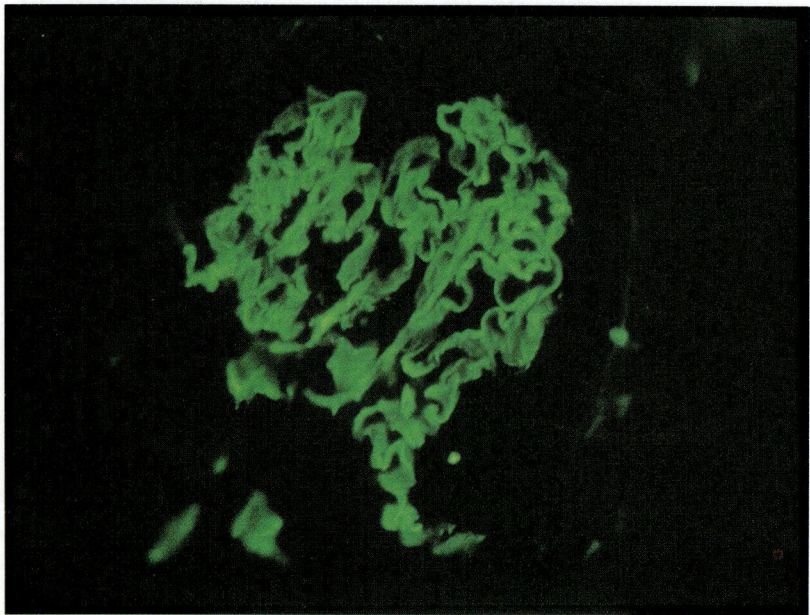

Figure 46.10 Direct immunofluorescence for IgG in the biopsy from a patient with Goodpasture's disease, showing linear binding of antibody to the GBM and faint staining of Bowman's capsule. (Courtesy Dr M. Thompson.)

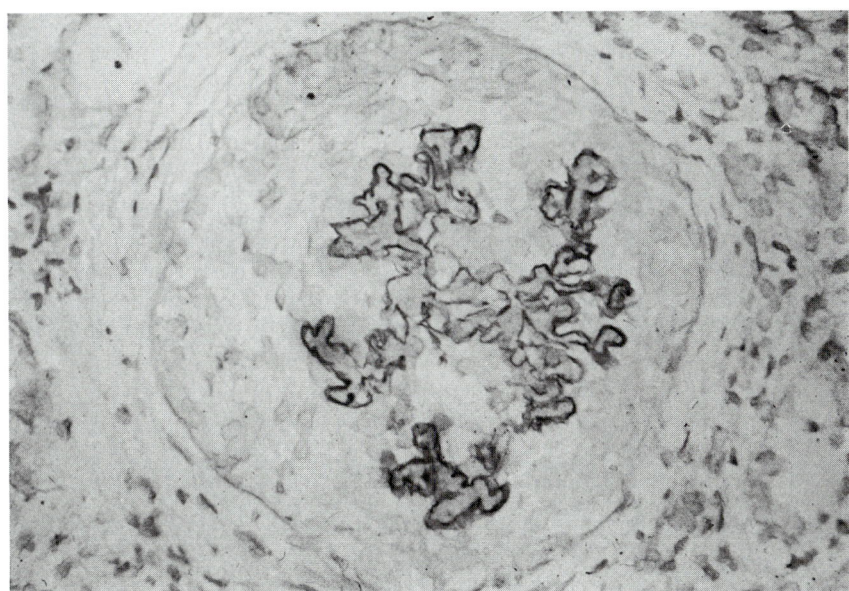

Figure 46.11 Immunoperoxidase staining for IgG in the biopsy from a patient with Goodpasture's disease, demonstrating how the glomerular tuft is compressed by a cellular crescent. (Courtesy of Dr M. Thompson.)

Neither the light nor the electron microscopic findings are diagnostic.

The characteristic linear staining of immunoglobulin along the GBM by direct immunofluoresence or imunohistochemistry is highly specific for Goodpasture's disease and occurs regardless of the antibody levels (Figures 46.10 and 46.11). However, linear staining may rarely be seen in systemic lupus erythematosus (SLE), diabetes, myeloma and fibrillary glomerulonephritis, usually because of high background with non-specific absorption of immunoglobulin along the glomerular capillary walls or fibrils. The deposited immunoglobulin is usually IgG, but can be accompanied by IgM or IgA in up to 20% of patients. A few patients have deposition of IgA alone. C3 is also deposited in a linear fashion along the glomerular capillary loops in about two thirds of patients. In many patients linear staining of distal tubular basement membrane is also seen, but this is usually focal and less intense than in the glomeruli. Bowman's capsule can also show deposition of antibody.

Lung

At autopsy, the lungs are enlarged and firm with obvious areas of underlying blood. The alveoli contain red cells, hemosiderin laden macrophages and fibrin and may be interspersed by relatively preserved alveoli. Interstitial hemorrhage and edema are common with relative preservation of the alveolar septa. Electron microscopy demonstrates thickened basement membrane with diffuse fragmentation and hyperplasia of pneumocytes [20].

The immunofluoresence findings are contradictory with reports of both absent binding and linear staining for IgG and C3. In most patients only patchy staining is detectable, hence the poor diagnostic yield of transbronchial biopsy.

Diagnosis and differential diagnosis

The diagnosis of Goodpasture's disease requires the demonstration of antibodies to the Goodpasture antigen either in the circulation, bound to the GBM or both. Detection of bound antibody by direct immunofluoresence requires renal or lung biopsy. A linear pattern of binding is both highly specific and sensitive for Goodpasture's disease. The major caveat is that bound antibody is retained for a long period and in no way reflects antibody titer, resolution of the disease or relapse. False negative results can occur in totally sclerosed glomeruli, whereas false positives have been reported post-transplantation and in diabetes, SLE and fibrillary glomerulanephritis. However, in the setting of a patient with crescentic nephritis and RPGN, a linear pattern of immunoglobulin is almost certainly diagnostic. The false negative rate from lung biopsy, particularly transbronchial, is high.

The measurement of circulating anti-GBM antibody by solid phase immunoassay has become invaluable in the diagnosis and management of patients with Goodpasture's disease. Our standard assay is now an ELISA based on highly purified antigen prepared from sheep kidney, with verification of equivocal results by western blotting using human GBM. Solid phase immunoassays allow the serial measurement of antibody titer to confirm the efficacy of treatment and also to demonstrate relapse or recurrence of antibody. Alternatively patient sera can be applied to sections of normal kidney and the characteristic linear pattern of binding visualized by a second antibody (indirect immunofluorescence). This technique has limited sensitivity and is difficult to quantitate.

A proportion of patients will also have circulating ANCA, the significance of which is as yet unclear. However ANCA should certainly be looked for as there is a suggestion that such double-positive patients behave more like they have vasculitis than pure anti-GBM disease. No other investigations are specifically useful. Serum immunoglobulins and complement are normal prior to plasmapheresis, and cryoglobulins, immune complexes, rheumatoid factors and antinuclear antibodies are not generally found. Patients are often anemic with a microcytic smear. The chest radiograph may be abnormal and the KCO will be raised if pulmonary hemorrhage has occurred.

The major differential diagnosis is from other causes of Goodpasture's syndrome (Table 46.1), pulmonary–renal syndromes (consider severe pneumonia, especially legionella, cardiac failure, pulmonary edema in acute renal failure of any cause and rare causes such as paraquat poisoning) and RPGN.

Treatment

The treatment of choice for most patients with Goodpasture's disease is plasmapheresis combined with corticosteroids and cyclophosphamide. This combination was introduced in the mid-1970s with dramatic impact on patient survival [21]. Previously most patients with anti-GBM disease died from either lung hemorrhage or renal failure. Benoit reported 96% mortality in 1964 [6], and in Wilson and Dixon's [22] series only 11% of patients who were not dialysis dependent at presentation survived with preserved renal function. At that time there was a suggestion that steroids may have been of some benefit, but no consensus as to the benefit of immunosuppressive agents. Bilateral nephrectomy was advocated in some patients with fulminant lung hemorrhage, with variable outcome. The introduction of combined immunosuppression, corticosteroids and intensive plasma exchange

Table 46.4 Outcome of patients with Goodpasture's disease. Data from all published series since 1964

Series	Number of patients	Pulmonary hemorrhage (%)	1-year patient survival (%)	1-year renal survival (%)	Notes
Benoit et al. 1964 [6]	52	100	4	4	Mortality at 3 years. Patients with Goodpasture's syndrome of all causes
Proskey et al. 1970 [25]	56	100	23	<23	Patients with Goodpasture's syndrome of all causes
Wilson and Dixon 1973 [22]	53	60	75	23	At analysis only 11.5% preserved renal function
Beirne et al. 1977 [26]	26	54	46	15	
Teague et al. 1978 [27]	29	100	62	31	Excluded patients without lung hemorrhage
Briggs et al. 1979 [28]	18	61	83	11	
Peters et al. 1982 [29]	41	56	76	39	Hammersmith Hospital single center
Simpson et al. 1982 [30]	20	100	90	59	Excluded patients without lung hemorrhage
Johnson et al. 1985 [24]	17	94	94	45	Randomized prospective study of treatment
Walker et al. 1985 [31]	22	62	59	45	Australian single center. All plasmapheresed
Savage et al. 1986 [4]	59	75	75	8.5	Data from multiple British centers
	49	52	84	35	Hammersmith Hospital single center
Williams et al. 1988 [32]	10	30	90	20	Single British unit. Patients presenting over 13 months
Bouget et al. 1990 [33]	14	21	79	29	French single center
Herody et al. 1993 [10]	29	52	93	41	French single center
Merkel et al. 1994 [34]	35	51	89	40	Survival at time of analysis

led to survival rates in excess of 70%, and this regimen has changed little in 20 years. The rationale was based on the known pathogenicity of the autoantibodies and the transient nature of the antibody response. Removal of circulating antibodies and suppression of further production, if accomplished early in the disease, should allow recovery. The results were dramatic with pulmonary hemorrhage often resolving within 48 h and renal function recovering in patients with even quite severe disease. Subsequent series of patients treated with similar regimes have demonstrated overall patient survival rates of 70–95% with particularly good results in patients treated before they require dialysis (Tables 46.4 and 46.5). Our current protocol is shown in Table 46.6.

Plasmapheresis regimens vary between units; however, given the aim of removing circulating antibodies as rapidly as possible, we propose an intensive protocol of daily 4 l plasma exchange initially for 14 days using 5% human albumin solution as replacement. This should be continued until antibody levels are suppressed. In patients with pulmonary hemorrhage or within 3 days of any invasive procedure (especially renal biopsy) 300–600 ml of fresh frozen plasma is given at the end of each exchange. Cyclophosphamide and prednisolone are given orally, with dose reduction in the elderly. There is no evidence for any additional benefit of azathioprine.

Recently several centers have addressed the use of intravenous methylprednisolone (0.5–1 g) and pulsed intravenous cyclophosphamide (0.5–1 g) in the treatment of RPGN. There is no evidence for any specific benefit in Goodpasture's disease, and the use of pulsed intravenous cyclophosphamide in particular may cause significant bone marrow suppression. Intravenous methylprednisolone is not an alternative to intensive plasma exchange either for lung hemorrhage or the nephritis, and there is a suggestion that it increases the risk of serious infection. In Bolton and Sturgill's [23] study of the use of pulsed intravenous methylprednisolone in RPGN, only two of 12 patients with anti-GBM disease maintained renal function (initial creatinines 130 and 430 μmol/l), and none of the patients with creatinine >600 μmol/l recovered.

Despite the widespread use of plasmapheresis there has only been one controlled trial of treatment in Goodpasture's disease in which just 17 patients were randomized to receive oral steroids and cyclophosphamide with or

Table 46.5 Renal recovery in patients with Goodpasture's disease. Series included if full treatment regimen available to patients, and data on renal function provided; untreated patients excluded from the analysis

Series (number of patients)	% of patients with independent renal function at 1 year with initial serum creatinine		Notes
	<600 μmol/l	>600 μmol/l	
Briggs et al. 1979 [28] (n = 15)	36 (11)[a]	0 (4)	Only four patients received plasmapheresis
Simpson et al. 1982 [30] (n = 12)	70 (10)	0 (2)	Eight patients received plasmapheresis
Johnson et al. 1985 [24] (n = 17)	69 (13)	0 (4)	Eight patients received plasmapheresis but with low intensity
Walker et al. 1985 [31] (n = 22)	82 (11)	18 (11)	Less intensive plasmapheresis Patients also received sulfinpyrazone and dipyridamole
Hammersmith Hospital 1976–88 (n = 56)	90 (21)	11 (35)	Some patients also received azathioprine
Bouget et al. 1990 [33] (n = 13)	50 (8)	0 (5)	Four patients with creatinine <600 μmol/l received <10 exchanges. Low overall intensity of plasmapheresis. Intravenous methylprednisolone used routinely. Mean delay of 5 days prior to treatment.
Herody et al. 1993 [10] (n = 29)	93 (14)	0 (15)	Four patients in first group and one in second did not receive plasmapheresis
Merkel et al. 1994 [34] (n = 32)	64 (14)	6 (18)	25 received plasmapheresis. Intravenous methylprednisolone used routinely. Some patients received i.v. pulsed cyclophosphamide

[a] Number in each group given in parentheses.

Table 46.6 Treatment protocol

Acute treatment
1. Plasma exchange, 4 l daily, for at least 14 days.
2. Cyclophosphamide 3 mg/kg/24 h orally (to nearest 50 mg). Reduced to 2 mg/kg in the elderly.
3. Prednisolone 1 mg/kg/24 h orally (maximum 60 mg)
4. Prophylactic amphotericin, nystatin suspension and ranitidine (consider low dose cotrimoxaole)

Subsequently
1. Stop cyclophosphamide at 12 weeks.
2. Prednisolone reduced weekly to 20 mg by 6 weeks, and then tailed off slowly over next 4 months

without plasmapheresis. Despite the limitations of the trial only two patients of eight receiving plasma exchange developed end-stage renal failure compared with six of nine receiving immunosuppressive drugs alone. The improved results with plasmapheresis occurred in spite of a low intensity of treatment-exchanges only every three days. This study confirmed the impression that patients with severe renal disease (>70% crescents and serum creatinine >600 μmol/l) have a uniformly poor prognosis, almost invariably progressing to ESRF (see later).

Should all patients therefore receive such intensive treatment? Since the disease can progress rapidly to death, all patients with progressive renal impairment and/or active lung hemorrhage should be aggressively managed with plasmapheresis and immunosuppressive drugs. Plasma exchange should be continued until antibody titers are suppressed. Patients with minor pulmonary hemorrhage alone, or with only trivial renal disease, could probably be treated with cyclophosphamide and prednisolone alone. The most difficult group are those patients with the most severe disease. If pulmonary hemorrhage is present then plasmapheresis will be useful in controlling this life-threatening feature, if not improving renal function. However, patients with severe renal disease in isolation are unlikely to recover, and in these patients the risks of treatment may well outweigh any benefit. Two caveats should be borne in mind: some patients with particularly fulminant disease and a short history, present with severe oliguric renal impairment and multiple crescents on biopsy, but occasionally recover renal function; and patients who also have ANCA may respond better despite apparently equally severe disease.

An alternative strategy to remove circulating antibodies is by immunoadsorption with staphylococcal protein A. The major advantage is the specific removal of immunoglobulin rather than depleting the patient of all circulating plasma proteins including clotting and complement factors, and avoiding the need for reinfusing large volumes of replacement blood products. The technique is difficult to administer, however, and not widely available. Specific immunoadsorption of anti-GBM autoantibodies remains for the future.

After the acute phase of treatment, if antibody levels are suppressed and the patient stable, cyclophosphamide can be completely withdrawn at three months. Prednisolone is reduced gradually from 60 to 20 mg over the first six weeks, and then more slowly, aiming for cessation of treatment by six months. Autoantibody has usually disappeared by eight weeks and rarely recurs.

Close monitoring of the patient is essential during this period for signs of recrudesence of disease activity, iatrogenic hematological toxicity or infections. Regular measurement of circulating anti-GBM autoantibody is important to confirm adequacy of treatment and identify relapse. Serum creatinine is the best guide to renal function and should begin to decline within one week, whereas the urea usually rises with steroid therapy. Lung hemorrhage can be identified by changes in Kco, chest radiograph or hemoptysis, or by sudden falls in hemoglobin. The Kco is the most sensitive and specific investigation. Blood counts are crucial to detect hemorrhage and drug induced leukopenia. The white cell count rarely declines before 10 days, and classically falls two to three weeks after oral cyclophosphamide is begun. The dose of cyclophosphamide should then be reduced to avoid severe leukopenia.

Finally, cyclosporin has been used with apparent success in at least one patient with disease unresponsive to plasma exchange, steroids and cyclophosphamide, though we have not found it to be useful as a sole agent. Anti-CD4 monoclonal antibody therapy will suppress nephritis in experimental models of the disease, and has been used successfully in a handful of patients with non-anti-GBM RPGN.

Outcome

Most patients with Goodpasture's disease now survive the acute illness, although lung hemorrhage remains an important cause of early death, especially in the setting of coincident infection. Over half the survivors still develop end-stage renal failure, however. One-year renal survival in the three series reported between 1990 and 1994 was still only 40% (Table 46.4). This is primarily due to the rapidity of progression of the disease and the severity of the renal damage. It is intriguing that unlike other diseases causing RPGN with histologically similar nephritis – in particular systemic vasculitis – the renal lesion of Goodpasture's disease seems to be relatively irreversible.

Many studies have now confirmed that patients presenting with a serum creatinine >600 μmol/l or dialysis dependent, oligoanuric and with crescents in >50% of glomeruli on biopsy have little chance of recovering renal function. Table 46.5 shows the response of patients from several centers to conventional treatments on the basis of the severity of their initial renal impairment. It should be noted that although most patients with creatinines >600 μmol/l do not recover renal function, there are exceptions. Before deciding not to treat patients with such severe renal disease with potentially toxic therapies, a biopsy is crucial. The appearance as well as the number of the crescents is important, as cellular rather than fibrotic crescents with patent glomerular capillary loops may indicate recent onset and potentially salvageable nephritis. Furthermore, many patients have superimposed acute tubular necrosis which may worsen the clinical presentation but allow response to treatment.

Despite this pessimism, patients with milder disease (creatinine <600 μmol/l) can recover with appropriate treatment. In the two studies reported in which adequate treatment was given, more than 90% of patients with creatinine <600 μmol/l had independent renal function at one year (Table 46.5). The published series also suggest that delay in institution of treatment, and too little (or no) plasmapheresis can lead to a reduced chance of recovery. Patients presenting with only minor renal impairment (creatinine <200 μmol/l) often recover fully. Given the uniform mortality prior to modern treatments these results are extremely impressive. However, in contrast to the renal lesion, lung damage resolves fully in almost all patients with no evidence of serious scarring or long-term functional deficits.

Relapse and recurrence

Relapse is the worsening of signs and symptoms of the disease while circulating autoantibodies are still present. Unlike recurrence (reactivation of disease and autoantibody production after resolution of the autoimmune response) relapse is relatively common and may be precipitated by a number of insults. Local infections, fluid overload and cigarette smoking can precipitate fresh lung hemorrhage, whereas systemic infection can exacerbate nephritis and pulmonary bleeding, presumably by alterations in the cytokine milieu (Figure 46.11). Intravascular catheters and chest infections are the most important source of sepsis. Early discontinuation of plasmapheresis or immunosuppression may also allow disease relapse.

Recurrence is very unusual. Most patients in whom antibody production has abated remain free of any further episodes of either nephritis or pulmonary hemorrhage. A few patients have recurrent mild pulmronay hemorrhage (usually precipitated by environmental toxins) with minimal nephritis, and rarely patients present with distinct episodes of renal disease. Although

such recurrences are almost always accompanied by a rise in antibody titer, detectable antibody production may also occur without apparent tissue injury. Renal transplantation can also precipitate recurrent autoantibody production if carried out before the autoimmune response has fully subsided. This can usually be avoided by delaying transplantation for at least six months, and preferably one year, after the disappearance of circulating antibody, and by confirming the absence of autoantibody over this period. Linear deposition of immunoglobulin along the GBM may occur in the graft without overt disease. One patient has been described who developed recurrence in an isograft from her identical twin sister two years after her initial Goodpasture's disease. She recovered fully on treatment with prednisolone and azathioprine. If transplantation is deemed necessary in the presence of antibody, the patient should be prepared using the acute treatment protocol described above. The immunosuppression for the transplant should then be sufficient to avoid disease recurrence. All patients receiving a transplant should have serial measurements of anti-GBM antibodies.

Anti-GBM disease in Alport's syndrome

The Goodpasture antigen is absent from the kidneys of many patients with Alport's syndrome (see above). Transplantation of a normal kidney may allow the development of anti-GBM antibodies as a result of the exposure of the immune system to a new antigen to which tolerance has not been established. The incidence of clinical anti-GBM antibody disease in transplanted Alport's patients is not known, but is probably only about 5%. These patients have circulating autoantibodies, nephritis and usually lose their grafts within the first year. Lung hemorrhage has not been reported in this context. Such a severe response is generally restricted to males developing end-stage renal failure before the age of 30, and all the patients reported have been deaf. Anti-GBM antibody formation as a lone phenomenon is commoner, and up to 50% of patients may demonstrate linear antibody binding along the GBM on immunofluoresence of the allograft biopsy, but without detectable circulating antibody or overt disease. These patients do well. The autoantibody response of Alport's patients developing Goodpasture's disease post-transplant is similar but not identical to that in typical Goodpastures. Antibodies are raised against α3(IV)NC1, the Goodpasture antigen itself, but probably also against the α4 and α5 chains.

Acknowledgment

JL is an MRC training fellow.

References

1. Goodpasture, E. (1919) The significance of certain pulmonary lesions in relation to the etiology of influenza. *Am. J. Med. Sci.*, **158**, 863–70.
2. Stanton, M.C. and Tange, J.D. (1958) Goodpasture's syndrome: pulmonary hemorrhage associated with glomerulonephritis. *Australas. Ann. Med.*, **7**, 132–44.
3. Turner, N., Lockwood, C.M. and Rees, A.J. (1993) Antiglomerular basement membrane antibody mediated nephritis, in *Diseases of the Kidney*, 5th edn (eds R.W. Schrier and C.W. Gottschalk), Little, Brown, Boston, pp. 1865–94.
4. Savage, C.O.S., Pusey, C.D., Bowman, C. and Rees, A.J. (1986) Anti-GBM antibody mediated disease in the British Isles 1980–1984. *Br. Med. J.*, **292**, 301–4.
5. Donaghy, M. and Rees, A.J. (1983) Cigarette smoking and lung haemorrhage in glomerulonephritis caused by autoantibodies to glomerular basement membrane. *Lancet*, **ii**, 1390–3.
6. Benoit, F.L., Rulon, D.B., Theirl, G.B. *et al.* (1964) Goodpasture's syndrome. A clinicopathological entity. *Am. J. Med.*, **37**, 424–44.
7. Rees, A.J., Peters, D.K., Compston, D.A. and Batchelor, J.R. (1978) Strong association between HLA DRw2 and antibody mediated Goodpasture's syndrome. *Lancet*, **i**, 966–8.
8. Burns, A., Fisher, M., Li, P. *et al.* (1995) Analysis of HLA class II genes in patients with Goodpasture's disease. *Q. J. Med.*, **88**, 93–100.
8a. Fisher M, Pusey, C.D., Vaughan, R.W., Rees, A.J. (1997) Susceptibility to anti-glomerular basement membrane disease is strongly associated with HLA-DRB1 genes. *Kidney Int.*, **51**, 222–9.
9. Bombassei, G.J. and Kaplan, A.A. (1993) The association between hydrocarbon exposure and anti-GBM antibody mediated disease (Goodpasture's syndrome). *Am. J. Ind. Med.*, **21**, 141–53.
10. Herody, M., Bobrie, G., Gouarin, C. *et al.* (1993) Anti-GBM disease: predictive value of clinical, histological and serological data. *Clin. Nephrol.*, **40**, 249–55.
11. Saus, J., Wieslander, J., Langeveld, J.P.M. *et al.* (1988) Identification of the Goodpasture antigen as the α3 (IV) chain of collagen IV. *J. Biol. Chem.*, **263**, 13374–80.
12. Butkowski, R.J., Shen, G.Q., Wieslander, J. *et al.* (1990) Characteristation of type IV collagen NC1 monomers and Goodpasture antigen in human renal basement membranes. *J. Lab Clin. Med.*, **115**, 365–73.
13. Pusey, C.D., Dash, A., Kershaw, M.J. *et al.* (1987) A single autoantigen in Goodpasture's syndrome identified by a monoclonal antibody to human glomerular basement membrane. *Lab. Invest.*, **56**, 23–31.
14. Hudson, B.G., Reeders, S.T. and Tryggvason, K. (1993) Type IV collagen: structure, gene organization, and role in human diseases. Molecular basis of Goodpasture and Alport syndromes and diffuse leiomyomatosis. *J. Biol. Chem.*, **268**, 26033–36.
14a. Levy, J.B., Turner, A.N., George, A.J.T. and Pusey, C.D. (1996) Epitope analysis of the good pasture antigen using a resonant mirror biosensor. *Clin. Exp. Immunol.*, **106**, 79–85.
14b. Kallursi, R., Sue, M.J., Hudson, B.G. and Neilson, E.G. (1996) The good pasture antigens structural delineation of two immunologically privileged epitopes on the α3 chain of type IV collagen. *J. Biol. Chem.*, **271**, 9062–8.
15. Tryggvason, K., Zhou, J., Hostikka, S.L. and Shows, T.B. (1993) The molecular genetics of Alport syndrome. *Kidney Int.*, **43**, 38–44.
16. Lerner, R.A., Glassock, R.J. and Dixon, F.J. (1967) The role of anti-glomerular basement membrane antibodies in the pathogenesis of human glomerulonephritis. *J. Exp. Med.*, **126**, 989–1004.
17. Hind, C.R., Bowman, C., Winearls, C.G. and Lockwood, C.M. (1984) Recurrence of circulating anti-glomerular basement membrane antibodies three years after immunosuppressive treatment and plasma exchange. *Clin. Nephrol.*, **21**, 244–6.
18. Bolton, W.K., Chandra, M., Tyson, T.M. *et al.* (1988) Transfer of experimental glomerulonephritis in chickens by mononuclear cells. *Kidney Int.*, **34**, 598–610.
19. Reynolds, J., Sallie, B.A., Syrganis, C. and Pusey, C.D. (1993) The role of T-helper lymphocytes in priming for experimental autoimmune glomerulonephritis in the BN rat. *J. Autoimmun.*, **6**, 571–85.
20. Heptinstall, R.H. (1994) Anti-glomerular basement membrane antibody disease, in *Pathology of the Kidney* (ed. R.H. Heptinstall), Little, Brown, Boston, pp. 677–712.
21. Lockwood, C.M., Rees, A.J., Pearson, T.A. *et al.* (1976) Immunosuppression and plasma exchange in the treatment of Goodpasture's syndrome. *Lancet*, **i**, 711–15.
22. Wilson, C.B. and Dixon, F.J. (1973) Anti-glomerular basement membrane antibody-induced glomerulonephritis. *Kidney Int.*, **3**, 74–89.
23. Bolton, W.K. and Sturgill, B.C. (1989) Methylprednisolone therapy for acute crescentic rapidly progressive glomerulonephritis. *Am. J. Nephrol.*, **9**, 368–75.
24. Johnson, J.P., Moore, J.J., Austin, H.J. *et al.* (1985) Therapy of anti-glomerular basement membrane antibody disease: analysis of prognostic significance of clinical, pathological and treatment factors. *Medicine*, **64**, 219–27.
25. Proskey, A.J., Weatherbee, L., Easterling, R.E. *et al.* (1970) Goodpasture's syndrome. A report of five cases and review of the literature. *Am. J. Med.*, **48**, 162–73.
26. Beirne, G.J., Wagnild, J.P., Zimmerman, S.W. *et al.* (1977) Idiopathic crescentic glomerulonephritis. *Medicine*, **56**, 349–81.
27. Teague, C.A., Doak, P.B., Simpson, I.J. *et al.* (1978) Goodpasture's syndrome: an analysis of 29 cases. *Kidney Int.*, **13**, 492–504.
28. Briggs, W.A., Johnson, J.P., Teichman, S. *et al.* (1979) Antiglomerular basement membrane antibody-mediated glomerulonephritis and Goodpasture's syndrome. *Medicine*, **58**, 348–61.
29. Peters, D.K., Rees, A.J., Lockwood, C.M. and Pusey, C.D.

(1982) Treatment and prognosis in antibasement membrane antibody-mediated nephritis. *Transplant Proc.*, **14**, 513–21.

30. Simpson, I.J., Doak, P.B., Williams, L.C. *et al.* (1982) Plasma exchange in Goodpasture's syndrome. *Am. J. Nephrol.*, **2**, 301–11.

31. Walker, R.G., Scheinkestel, C., Becker, G.J. *et al.* (1985) Clinical and morphological aspects of the management of crescentic anti-glomerular basement membrane antibody (anti–GBM) nephritis/Goodpasture's syndrome. Q. J. Med., **54**, 75–89.

32. Williams, P.S., Davenport, A., McDicken, I. *et al.* (1988)

Increased incidence of anti-glomerular basement membrane antibody (anti-GBM) nephritis in the Mersey region, September 1984–October 1985. *Q. J. Med.*, **68**, 727–33.

33. Bouget, J., Pogamp, P. Le, Perrier, G. *et al.* (1990) Glomérulonéphrites rapidement progressives a anticorps anti-membrane basale glomérulaire. *Ann. Med. Interne*, **141**, 408–15.

34. Merkel, F., Pullig, O., Marx, M. *et al.* (1994) Course and prognosis of anti-basement membrane antibody mediated disease: report of 35 cases. *Nephrol. Dial. Transpl.*, **19**, 372–6.

Further reading

Levy, J.B., Lachmann, R.H. and Pusey, C.D. (1996) Recurrent Goodpasture's disease. *Am. J. Kidney Dis.*, **27**, 573–8.

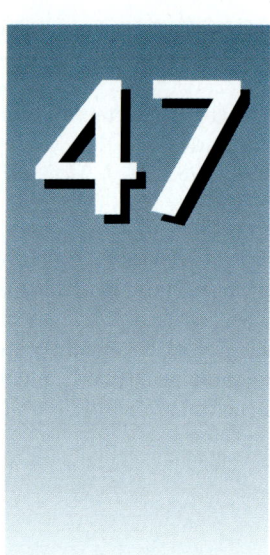

Acute postinfectious glomerulonephritis

Stephen H. Powis and Steven H. Sacks

Introduction

Postinfectious glomerulonephritis has traditionally been used to describe the acute nephritis which occurs following infection with group A β-hemolytic streptococcus. However, many other infections are associated with a wide variety of lesions within the kidney. For example, severe septicemia may result in acute tubular necrosis, HIV infection can lead to a form of focal segmental sclerosis, tuberculosis may lead to renal amyloid and *Escherichia coli* infection can be associated with the hemolytic–uremic syndrome. This chapter describes the features of classical poststreptococcal glomerulonephritis and discusses some of the renal abnormalities found in association with other bacterial infections. The renal complications of viral and parasitic infections are described in other chapters.

Poststreptococcal glomerulonephritis

Postreptococcal glomerulonephritis (PSGN) is usually an acute illness from which all but a few patients make a complete, spontaneous recovery [1–4]. The incidence of PSGN has declined in developed countries, although it is still relatively common in developing countries. The decline in westernized countries may be related to better public health and the use of antibiotics, but may also be due to intrinsic changes in the pathogenicity of the bac-

teria. PSGN can occur sporadically or as part of an epidemic. Children, typically in the age range 2–6 years, are affected more often than adults. Males develop nephritis more frequently than females, although the incidence of subclinical nephritis may be higher in females. During an epidemic of β-hemolytic streptococcal infection, around 5–10% of children with pharyngitis and 25% of children with skin lesions develop clinically detectable glomerulonephritis.

Pathophysiology

The demonstration of circulating immune complexes in the serum, the fall in serum C3 and the demonstration of IgG and complement components within glomerular deposits all suggest that PSGN is an immune complex-mediated disorder. However, the exact mechanisms responsible for immune complex formation and deposition in the glomeruli are unknown. Several different mechanisms have been suggested. Nephritogenic strains of β-hemolytic streptococci (group A, in contrast to group C which are very rarely nephritogenic) may posses unique antigens which have affinity for sites within the glomeruli. Subsequent reaction with circulating antibody results in *in situ* immune complex formation. Alternatively, the direct binding of antigenic protein to the glomeruli may stimulate the conversion of plasminogen into plasmin, that activates the complement cascade without requiring immune complex formation. It has also been proposed that streptococcal neuraminidase may

Nephrology, Edited by Rex L. Jamison and Robert Wilkinson.
Published in 1997 by Chapman & Hall, London. ISBN 0 412 60930 4

expose antigenic sites on circulating IgG molecules, resulting in an autoimmune reaction which drives immune complex formation and deposition. Finally, it has been suggested that cross-reacting antibodies directed against glomerular basement membrane (GBM) components are induced by nephritogenic streptococci which share antigenic epitopes with GBM epitopes (molecular mimicry).

Clinical manifestations and differential diagnosis

PSGN characteristically develops around ten days after an upper respiratory tract infection or three weeks after a skin infection, such as impetigo. The initial infection may be associated with a broad spectrum of symptoms, ranging from the severe (e.g. pharyngitis or impetigo) to patients who are asymptomatic. Although most patients present with features of an acute nephritis, the exact presentation may be variable, ranging from asymptomatic microscopic hematuria to a marked nephritic syndrome. Some individuals may present with acute renal failure. Hypertension is usually mild, but may be pronounced; hypertensive encephalopathy is rare, although encephalopathy has been reported in the absence of significant hypertension. Edema is also usually mild, but sometimes may be severe enough to produce pleural effusions and ascites. Some patients present with features of congestive cardiac failure. Other less specific symptoms include malaise, anorexia, nausea, vomiting and arthralgia.

Hematuria, often described as 'smoky', is an almost universal feature. Red cell casts are observed on urine microscopy. Proteinuria is frequent but moderate, rarely exceeding 2 g/24 h. About three-quarters of all patients have some degree of renal impairment on presentation, although in the majority this is mild. Acute renal failure requiring dialysis is unusual, occurring in less than 1% of children and slightly more frequently in adults.

Up to 4% of patients with non-streptococcal upper respiratory tract infection may also develop microscopic hematuria. These abnormalities are usually not detected unless urinalysis is performed and typically resolve within two to seven months. In the few patients in whom microscopic hematuria persists, renal biopsy may show a nonspecific mesangioproliferative glomerulonephritis. The outlook for such abnormalities is almost invariably benign.

In practice, PSGN most often needs to be distinguished from IgA nephropathy, which can have a poor long-term prognosis. Table 47.1 lists the differentiating features between PSGN and IgA nephropathy. A definitive diagnosis can be made following renal biopsy, although this is not required in most cases. Rarely, evidence of both IgA nephropathy and PSGN is found together in the same biopsy. Sometimes an acute infection is followed by tubulointerstitial nephritis (TIN), for example in pneumococcal pneumonia. The finding of abundant leukocytes in the urine deposit and of a tubulointerstitial monocytic infiltrate on tissue biopsy will usually confirm this diagnosis. Acute renal failure due to infection-associated ATN almost always occurs at the peak of the infection and is therefore relatively easy to distinguish, clinically, from a postinfectious nephritis. However, it may be more confusing when there is acute renal dysfunction during the course of chronic sepsis, when both ATN and postinfectious nephritis can occur. Lastly, postinfectious nephritis must be remembered in the differential diagnosis of a crescentic nephritis. The other causes, including systemic vasculitis and anti-GBM disease usually have distinct features on clinical and pathological evaluation.

Histological abnormalities

The most common lesion found on renal biopsy is a diffuse proliferative glomerulonephritis (Figure 47.1). The exact changes observed depend on when the biopsy is obtained. Within the first two weeks of the illness, an inflammatory infiltrate of neutrophils, eosinophils and monocytes appears within the capillary lumen and the

	PSGN	IgA nephropathy
Average time between infection and hematuria	10 days	Less than 5 days
History of recurrent gross hematuria	Rare	Common
Serum C3 and C4	Depressed	Normal
Antistreptolysin O and/or anti-DNAse B titers	Raised	Normal
Throat culture	Positive	Negative
Mesangial IgA deposition	Absent	Present
Persistent or progressive hematura, proteinuria and renal dysfunction following infection	Uncommon	Common

Table 47.1 Differentiating features between poststreptococcal glomerulonephritis and IgA nephropathy

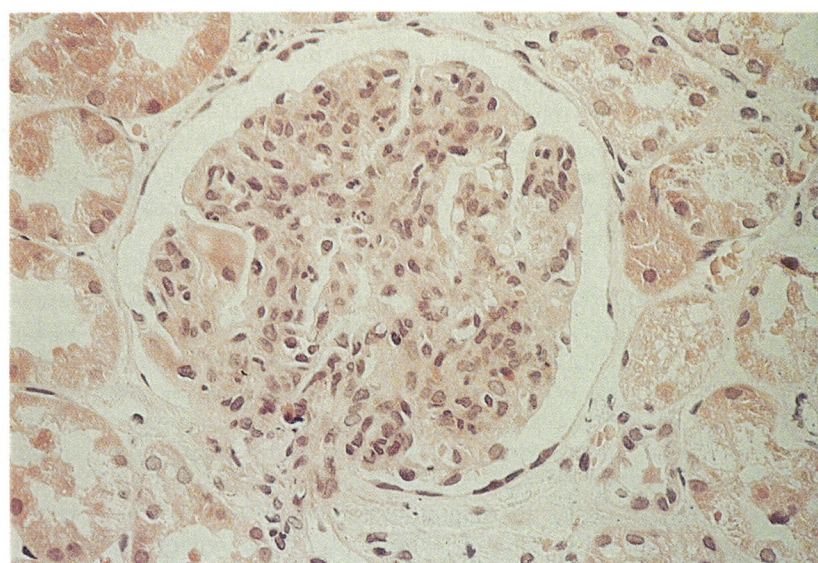

a

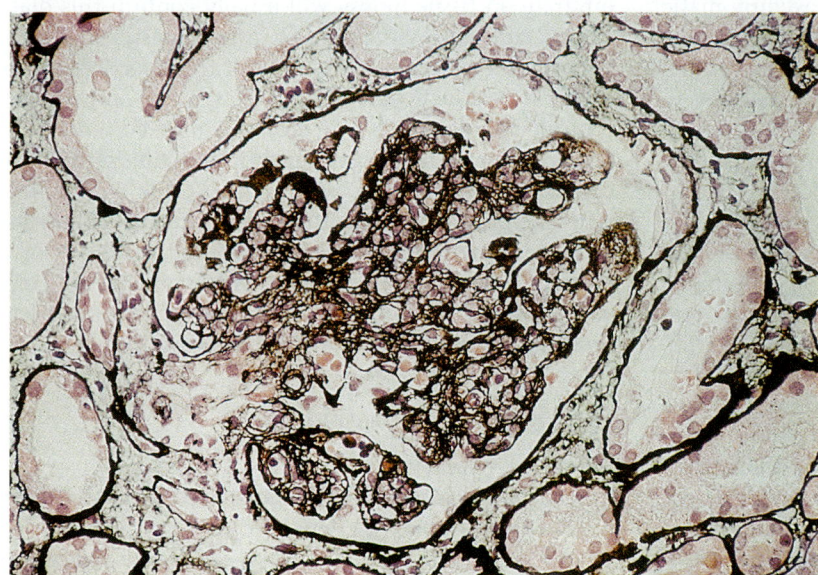

b

Figure 47.1 (a) H&E stain (×400) of a glomerulus with diffuse proliferative glomerulonephritis secondary to PSGN. Note the moderate numbers of polymorphonuclear leukocytes and the tuft occlusion by infiltrating cells. (b) A silver stain (×400) showing diffuse endocapillary proliferation. Some capillary walls show irregular thickening, although this is not a consistent feature of PSGN. The silver stain is also helpful in excluding crescent formation; this can be difficult on H&E stains because of the increased cellularity.

mesangium. Proliferation of endothelial and mesangial cells is also prominent. Focal capsular adhesions may be observed, but widespread crescent formation is uncommon. After two weeks, neutrophils begin to disappear and the infiltrate becomes predominantly mononuclear. Interstitial abnormalities, such as edema and infiltration by mononuclear cells, are generally mild.

Immunofluorescence or immunohistochemical microscopy usually demonstrates deposits of IgG and C3, or C3 alone and sometimes C1q in a diffuse, granular pattern (Figure 47.2). C3 deposition can be detected in the absence of IgG early in the disease or during resolution. IgM and IgA deposition is less frequent and C4 is usually not detected at all.

Electron microscopy shows characteristic subepithelial electron-dense deposits, often described as 'humps' (Figure 47.3). These are most frequent during the first month of the disease, after which they begin to resolve.

Often there is a rough correlation between the number of subepithelial deposits and the degree of proteinuria. Mesangial and subendothelial electron-dense deposits may also be observed, and these can persist after the resolution of subepithelial deposits.

Complete resolution of the histological abnormalities may take many years. Glomerulosclerosis may eventually develop in the rare patients with marked crescentic changes.

Treatment

Treatment of PSGN is predominantly symptomatic. Treatment of edema with diuretics such as furosemide generally results in a prompt diuresis. Hypertension can be controlled with diuretics and/or vasodilators. Uremia should be managed with control of serum potassium and dialysis if required. Immunosuppressive agents are gener-

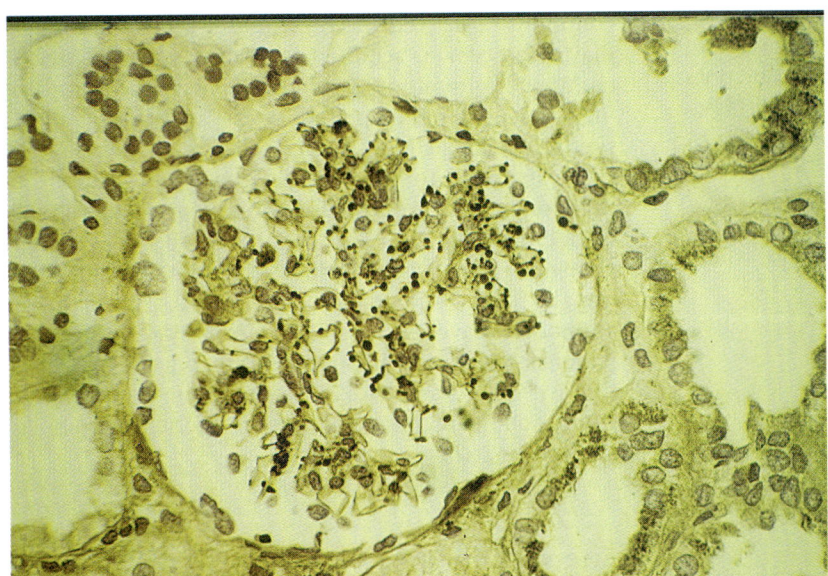

Figure 47.2 Indirect immunoperoxidase of a pronase-digested paraffin section (×400) stained with anti-human IgG. The predominant feature is the large number of humps around capillary walls.

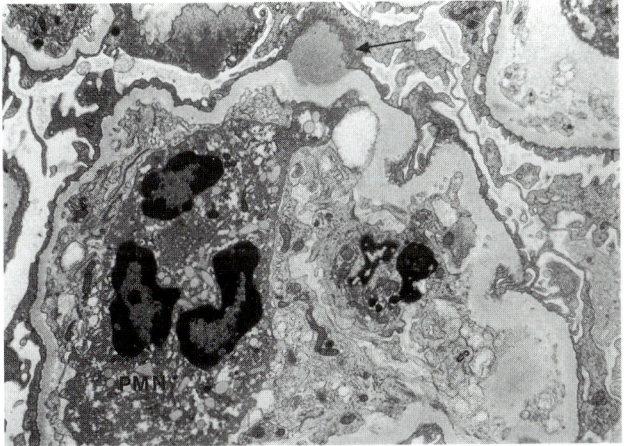

Figure 47.3 Electron microscopy showing a subepithelial hump (arrowed). Note the polymorphonuclear leukocyte (PMN) within the capillary.

ally not considered except in the case of rapidly progressive renal failure when a renal biopsy may be helpful. With severe crescentic nephritis, pulsed steroid therapy (such as methylprednisolone) has often been advocated. However, the benefit of such treatment is uncertain. A study of 10 children (with PSGN) in whom >50% of the glomeruli were occluded by crescents compared the effects of immunosuppression (prednisolone, azathioprine and cyclophosphamide; as well as dipyridamole and anticoagulants) with supportive therapy alone [5]. The authors concluded that although treatment may have hastened the recovery of renal function, there was no difference in outcome between those on immunosuppressive treatment and those on no treatment. Specific treatment for the streptococcal infection is only required if there is evidence of continuing active infection.

Outcome

The short-term outcome of PSGN is excellent. Most patients undergo a spontaneous diuresis after one week, the serum creatinine returning to normal within a month. Hypertension also resolves rapidly, but urinary abnormalities may take longer to resolve. Hematuria usually disappears within six months, but may persist for many years. The degree of proteinuria usually falls during the recovery phase but mild proteinuria may still persist several years later. C3 levels usually return to normal within two months.

The long-term prognosis of PSGN is generally very good and better in children than in adults. Less than 2% of patients can be expected to develop end-stage renal failure. However, these patients can develop hypertension, proteinuria and renal failure many years after the initial illness. These late complications have been associated with glomerulosclerosis on renal biopsy. One study found an increasing incidence of these three features after two years, but other studies have failed to produce similar findings [6–8]. It is not known why some patients deteriorate so long after PSGN, but one possibility is that sclerosis results from compensatory glomerular hyperfiltration following the loss of glomeruli in the acute illness.

Renal complications of other infections

A study by Montseny *et al.* [9] has underlined the changed spectrum of organisms, predisposing factors and outcomes associated with a proliferative glomerulonephritis in adults. Table 47.2 summarizes some of the many other viral, bacterial and parasitic infections that have been linked to proliferative glomerulonephritis. Many of these

Table 47.2 Infections associated with a proliferative glomerulonephritis; the list is not comprehensive and does not include many of the organisms found in infective endocarditis associated glomerular disease

Bacteria	Viridans streptococci
	Streptococcus pneumoniae
	Staphylococcus epidermidis
	Staphylococcus aureus
	Neisseria meningitidis
	Salmonella typhae
	Mycobacterium leprae
	Treponema pallidum
	Yersinia enterocolytica
Viruses	Hepatitis B
	Hepatitis C
	Cytomegalovirus
	Human immunodeficiency virus
	Epstein–Barr virus
Parasites	*Plasmodium malariae*
	Plasmodium falciparum
	Schistosoma haematobium
	Schistosoma mansoni
	Toxoplasma gondii

are discussed in detail in other chapters. Staphylococcal infection can occur at many different sites, but is most commonly associated with renal lesions in patients with infective endocarditis or shunt nephritis (see below). With antibiotic treatment, pneumococcal (*Streptococcus pneumoniae*) associated glomerulonephritis is rarely seen; renal biopsy usually shows a proliferative glomerulonephritis with subepithelial humps. Patients present with minimal proteinuria, hematuria and mild impairment of renal function.

Tuberculosis most commonly causes renal amyloid, but has also been associated with mesangiocapillary glomerulonephritis and focal proliferative glomerulonephritis. Severe leptospirosis (Weil's disease) is usually associated with an acute interstitial nephritis in the context of oliguric renal failure, but mesangial proliferation and immunoglobulin and complement deposition can occur. Typhoid fever (*Salmonella typhi* infection) results in glomerular involvement in 2–4% of patients. Renal abnormalities are most commonly microscopic hematuria (sometimes macroscopic), mild to moderate proteinuria and mild renal impairment. Renal biopsy usually shows mesangial proliferation, but IgA nephropathy has also been observed, possibly secondary to IgA stimulation within the gut. Although renal involvement is usually transient, patients with glomerulonephritis are reported to have a higher mortality.

The association between syphilis (*Treponema pallidum*) and nephrotic syndrome is well established. This is most commonly observed in congenital syphilis, although it may also occur in acquired secondary syphilis. Affected children commonly present in the first four months of life. A few patients present with an acute nephritic syndrome. Renal biopsy usually shows a membranous nephropathy with variable mesangial proliferation and occasional crescent formation. Complement and IgG can be identified in subendothelial deposits. More rarely, changes similar to poststreptococcal glomerulonephritis may be seen. Treponemal antigens and antitreponemal antibodies have been isolated from the glomeruli of patients with syphilitic glomerulonephritis, suggesting that the lesions are mediated by immune complex deposition. Following treatment with antibiotics, the glomerulonephritis resolves completely.

Site-specific infections

Bacterial endocarditis

A variety of different organisms can give rise to infective endocarditis. Following the introduction of antibiotics, the frequency of endocarditis-associated glomerulonephritis has fallen. Post-mortem studies show a frequency of around 20–25%. The symptoms and signs of endocarditis usually precede renal manifestations, although a few patients may initially present with renal failure. Hematuria, proteinuria and renal impairment are the most common abnormalities, but hypertension is not common. The presence of high titers of circulating immune complexes and hypocomplementemia are of little diagnostic value because they occur in endocarditis *per se* and are also found in other disorders such as systemic lupus erythematosus.

Renal biopsy in patients with acute endocarditis typically shows a diffuse membranoproliferative glomerulonephritis similar to that seen in PSGN. In chronic endocarditis, a more focal, segmental proliferative glomerulonephritis is observed, although these patients may also have a diffuse proliferative glomerulonephritis. Crescents may also be present. Immunological staining shows granular deposits of IgG, IgM and complement components. An interstitial nephritis may also be observed, although this may be a result of, or aggravated by, antibiotic treatment. A drug-induced interstitial nephritis may be suspected if the renal abnormalities worsen after the start of antibiotic therapy and by the presence of eosinophilia. Electron microscopy shows subepithelial, subendothelial and mesangial dense deposits. Bacterial antigens and antibacterial antibodies have been eluted from the kidneys of patients with glomerulonephritis-associated endocarditis.

Treatment is directed toward the organism responsible for the endocarditis. No specific therapy is required for the renal lesion. The severity, course and prognosis of the nephritis is primarily related to the severity of the underlying endocarditis. If the endocarditis is successfully treated with antibiotics, renal function can normalize within a few weeks. Hematuria and proteinuria take longer to resolve and may persist for months or years. If the endocarditis is severe or treatment delayed, renal function may not be fully regained even if the responsible organism is eradicated. If the patient responds poorly to antibiotic therapy, renal function may deteriorate to irreversible end-stage renal failure. In severe cases, the use of immunosuppressive agents or plasma exchange may be considered but their efficacy is unproven.

Shunt nephritis

Shunt nephritis is most often associated with infection of catheters inserted into the ventricle to treat hydrocephalus, although it can also occur following infection of other indwelling catheters. Ventriculoatrial shunts are associated with nephritis more frequently than ventriculoperitoneal shunts. Bacterial colonization of ventricular shunts probably occurs at the time of insertion. Although up to one-third of shunts may become colonized, nephritis occurs in less than 5% of infected patients. The most common infecting organism is *Staphylococcus epidermidis*, although a variety of other bacteria has been reported.

Patients present with evidence of infection. Fever is almost always present, although usually low grade, and may be accompanied by a rash, joint pains, anemia, hypertension and hepatosplenomegaly. There may also be signs of increased intracranial pressure. Hematuria is most often microscopic, but may be macroscopic. Proteinuria is great enough to cause a nephrotic syndrome in about one quarter of patients. Renal failure may be apparent. Serum C3 and C4 levels are depressed and a high titer of circulating rheumatoid factor, cryoglobulins and immune complexes may be observed.

Renal biopsy reveals a lesion similar to type I mesangiocapillary glomerulonephritis, with subendothelial dense deposits and deposition of IgG, IgM and C3. Mild mesangial proliferation and crescents are occasionally seen. Bacterial antigens have been identified in affected glomeruli.

Treatment consists of removal of the infected shunt and appropriate antibiotic therapy. Antibiotic therapy without shunt removal is not usually sufficient. Following treatment, urine abnormalities disappear and renal function improves over months, but abnormalities can persist long-term. A small number of patients may develop progressive renal dysfunction leading to end-stage renal failure.

Chronic suppurative infections

Chronic suppurative infections have been associated with a number of different renal lesions. These include lung abscess, subphrenic abscess, dental abscess and osteomyelitis. The commonest infecting organism is *Staphylococcus aureus*. Renal abnormalities develop after several months, in contrast to amyloid which develops over years. Renal histology has shown proliferative, mesangial proliferative, membranous and focal proliferative glomerulonephritis, sometimes with crescent formation.

Patients usually present with symptoms and signs of infection. Renal abnormalities range from mild urinary abnormalities to severe renal failure. Treatment is directed at the underlying infection. If successful, the renal abnormalities usually resolve. The renal prognosis is poorer if the patient has presented in acute renal failure or if the infection can not be controlled. A small number of successfully treated patients may develop progressive renal dysfunction.

Postinfectious glomerulonephritis in renal allografts

Postinfectious glomerulonephritis has only occasionally been described in renal transplant patients, in contrast to other forms of glomerulonephritis which are reported in about 6% of adult cases. This is perhaps surprising in view of the risk of infectious complications of transplantation. The scarcity of cases may in part reflect that the postinfectious complications are immunologically mediated and are suppressed by immunosuppressive treatment, or may reflect differences in the transplant population and the population at risk of postinfectious nephritis. Reports include cases of PSGN [10] and of postinfectious glomerulonephritis secondary to disseminated staphylococcal infection and to a mycotic aneurysm of the coronary artery [11]. The effect of treatment with higher doses of immunosuppression in such cases is unknown, though one child with PSGN received increased doses of prednisolone, and the transplant kidney began to improve within a few days.

References

1. Lewy, J.E., Salinas–Madrigal, L., Herdson, P.B. *et al.* (1971) Clinicopathologic correlations in acute poststreptococcal glomerulonephritis: a correlation between renal functions, morphologic damage, and clinical course of 46 children with acute poststreptococcal glomerulonephritis. *Medicine*, **50**, 453–501.

2. Potter, E.V., Lipscultz, S.A., Abidh, S. *et al.* (1982) Twelve to seventeen-year follow-up of patients with poststreptococcal acute glomerulonephritis in Trinidad. *N. Engl. J. Med.*, **307**, 725–9.

3. Rodriguez-Iturbe, B. (1984) Epidemic poststreptococcal glomerulonephritis. *Kidney Int.*, **21**, 109–20.

4. Tejani, A. and Ingulli, E. (1990) Poststreptococcal glomerulonephritis. Current clinical and pathologic concepts. *Nephron*, **55**, 1–5.

5. Roy, S., Murphy, W.M. and Arant, B.S. (1981) Poststreptococcal crescentic glomerulonephritis in children: comparison of quintuple therapy versus supportive care. *J. Pediatr.*, **98**, 403–10.

6. Baldwin, D.S. (1977) Post-streptococcal glomerulonephritis, a progressive disease? *Am. J. Med.*, **62**, 1–11.

7. Lien, J.W., Mathew, T.H. and Meadows, R. (1979) Acute poststreptococcal glomerulonephritis in adults: a long term study. *Q. J. Med.*, **48**, 99–111.

8. Perlman, L.V., Herdman, R.C., Kleinman, H. and Vernier, R.L. (1965) Poststreptococcal glomerulonephritis: a ten-year follow-up of an epidemic. *JAMA*, **307**, 725–8.

9. Montseny, J.J., Meyrier, A., Kleinknecht, D. and Callard, P. (1995) The current spectrum of infectious glomerulonephritis. Experience with 76 patients and review of the literature. *Medicine*, **74**, 63–73.

10. Sorof, J.M., Weidner, N., Potter, D. and Portale, A.A. (1995) Acute post-streptococcal glomerulonephritis in a renal allograft. *Pediatr. Nephrol.*, **9**, 317–9.

11. Sanfillipo, F. and Croker, B.P. (1983) The possible occurrence of staphylococcal postinfectious glomerulonephritis in a renal allograft. *Transplantation*, **35**, 25–9.

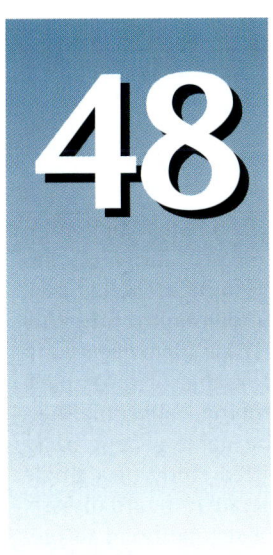

Nephropathy in systemic lupus erythematosus and other connective tissue disease

Francis W. Ballardie

Introduction

Clinical events in the progression of lupus nephritis to end-stage renal failure have a major impact on morbidity and mortality in patients with systemic lupus erythematosus (SLE). Renal diseases in other connective tissue diseases (CTD) are generally of lesser severity, rarer and have been studied in a less rigorous way. Management of the major problems of lupus nephritis has continued to perplex physicians in attempting to optimize therapeutic benefits versus risks of treatment regimens. A recent review [1] highlighted frustrations of nephrologists in defining these. Despite a new array of research data from application of developing technologies, analyzing the disturbances in cytokine networks, defining new autoantigens and delineating new mechanisms of renal injury, investigators have failed to define targets for interruption of the numerous abnormalities of the immune system in SLE. Why active organ disease in patients becomes quiescent with end-stage renal disease or after allograft transplantation remains unexplained. Although there are exceptions to this broadly held view, how can the suppression of disease activity by uremia be explained when our most powerful immunosuppressive agents may fail to do so? The heterogeneity of lupus nephritis and the inconclusive results of treatment by conventional therapies have confounded analyses to a much greater extent than those of treatment of other autoimmune multisystem diseases such as primary vasculitis. The

results of prospective multicenter trials with specific questions of therapy, exemplified by those of the Lupus Nephritis Collaborative Study Group [2] have provided little supporting evidence for intensive regimens, prompting reassessment of the benefits of immunosuppressive drugs [3], the value of serological parameters [4] and pathology indices [5], almost to the point of cynicism.

In the face of pessimism, however, 10-year life expectancy of patients with lupus nephritis during the past three decades has improved from less than 20% and there is more than 80% for kidney survival alone [6], even with severe grade IV (WHO classification [1]) forms of disease. The timing and choice of immunosuppression, better treatment of infection, hypertension, and the metabolic consequences of disease and dialysis, have contributed to this advance. The problem of appropriate treatment of indolent or inactive disease while attempting to prevent acute, possibly life-threatening flares of systemic lupus with nephritis remains, as does the need for vigilance in management of phases of the disease. The development of mild or severe nephropathy in autoimmune connective tissue disease that fail to fulfill the American Rheumatism Association (ARA) diagnostic criteria for SLE challenges the traditional view that the prognosis in affected patients is benign. This chapter focuses on the emergence of new concepts in the genesis of nephropathy in SLE, CTD, and on reappraisals of management of these diseases.

Nephrology, Edited by Rex L. Jamison and Robert Wilkinson.
Published in 1997 by Chapman & Hall, London. ISBN 0 412 60930 4

Detection of nephropathy

Nephritis is common in SLE, perhaps invariable. The local policy for renal biopsy in this disease influences its incidence. Clinical evidence of nephritis, as defined by significant proteinuria, abnormal urinary sediment or renal dysfunction, is present in 10% of adult patients with SLE at presentation, but will develop in about two of every three patients during the course of their disease. Renal biopsy performed on patients without clinical evidence of nephritis reveals that more patients have renal involvement – even severe diffuse proliferative glomerulonephritis in the absence of proteinuria – the 'silent nephritis' of SLE. The effects of subclinical nephritis on long-term renal function and glomerular scarring are not known. Radioimmunoassay of urine may reveal microalbuminuria in lupus patients. Steroid therapy suppresses this abnormality. The systemic lupus patient in the general medical or rheumatological clinic should therefore have, at least, urinalysis on each visit to detect clinical disease at an early stage. The variable association of nephritis with disease of other organs in some patients with SLE is perplexing; understanding may prove fundamental to understanding the link to organ injuries [1].

The modes of presentation of lupus with clinically evident nephritis are typical of SLE as a whole, often with more than one clinical feature being present. Arthritis is most frequently the main presentation with rash, pleurisy and thrombocytopenia less common. Proteinuria in the nephrotic range is present in more than half the cases, but rapidly progressive renal disease, progressing to renal failure is infrequent. Although SLE is very much less common in males, the clinical expression of disease in most has many similarities to that in females. Renal involvement is similar and pleurisy is common in males, but central nervous system disease dominates in females.

Episodic acute deteriorations in renal function associated with extrarenal manifestations are again common – averaging 1.6 features per episode. Central nervous system disorders dominate the clinical picture, however. It is also clear that severe nephritis may be unaccompanied by extrarenal manifestations, even though the patient has previously suffered symptomatic SLE with or without clinical evidence of nephritis. Such variations in the clinical expression of a patient's organ involvement in SLE merit constant vigilance.

In contrast to these typical patterns, of onset and episodic deterioration, of renal disease, it is clear that glomerulonephritis can herald the later diagnosis of SLE. Clinical evidence of renal disease, with glomerular lesions characteristic of those in unequivocal cases of SLE, may also precede by several years the clinical and serological expression of SLE.

Immunopathogenesis

Cytokines

The notion that peptide regulatory factors may be central in immunopathogenetic defects in SLE and CTD has developed from murine models, and fundamental knowledge of perturbations of immunoglobulin structure inducible by cytokines, in B cells. These have been compared with human disease. Three strains of mice have been used in delineating cytokine abnormalities: MRL/lpr-lpr, NZB/W and BXSB. The stable genetic background in these strains has permitted study of a single gene, or other alterations that accelerate or retard disease. Experimental evidence that cytokine regulation of autoreactivity is important – both quantitative and qualitative aspects – is derived from these models. First, splenic B cells from lupus-prone mice are polyclonally activated early in life, before autoantibody detection, suggesting mononuclear cell-derived factors are responsible. Second, maintenance of the normal, non-autoimmune state is achieved by 'functional silencing' of autoreactive B cell clones in transgenic mice, rather than by clonal deletion. Third, cytokines modify disease expression; interleukin-2 (IL-2) not only ameliorates murine nephritis, a phenomenon similar to the effects of IL-2 on other models of autoimmune nephritis, but also reduces immunoglobulin synthesis in MRL/lpr-lpr lupus-prone mice. There is evidence that genes which determine cytokine dysregulation are expressed in renal tissue. Cultured mesangial cells from MRL/lpr-lpr mice have a decrease in secreted, and surface macrophage-colony stimulating factor (M-CSF), a macrophage chemoattractant and differentiation factor. Progressive kidney disease is associated with mesangial cell proliferation and accumulation of macrophages in the glomerulus, with increased mRNA encoding for proinflammatory cytokines tumor necrosis factor (TNF-α) and IL-1β [7]. Mesangial cell membrane M-CSF was expressed at high intensity on cell membranes, further stimulated by coculture with TNF-α. Persistently high serum M-CSF was present at age one week, preceding clinical disease.

Comparison of these key findings with SLE and CTD in humans has revealed striking parallels. Patients with SLE and Sjörgen's syndrome have elevated expression of IL-3 in peripheral blood mononuclear cells and elevated serum levels of cytokine IL-3, a growth factor with multilineage effects. Proliferating marrow stem cells, and differentiating hemopoietic lineages similarly express these abnormalities. There are more specific maintenance and induction effects of IL-3 on differentiated T and B cells, and serum IL-3 is elevated in patients with SLE and Sjörgen's syndrome, excessively so in a patient who subsequently developed lymphoma [8]. Conversely IL-2 is reduced in these two conditions as it is in most auotimmune disease. Many regulatory, and mRNA transcription, factors govern *in vivo* cytokine synthesis, which may not show direct correlations with mRNA expression. These findings suggest similar pathogenetic mechanisms between humans and murine models of disease. Clearly, a complete analysis of all components of transcription – from mRNA to proteins – of the cytokine network, in SLE and CTD is an immense task, and other variables such as disease activity, or which human tissue – mononuclear cell or renal – is examined, may initially confuse conclusions in emerging studies. These concepts have been developed in Berger's disease, IgA nephropathy (more recently and correctly termed IgA-related nephropathy), the nephritis which now shows several broadly similar immunopathogenetic disturbances to SLE. In IgA-related nephropathy distinct and selective patterns of disturbance in the cytokine network have been found, and unexpected evidence for paracrine, not autocrine, roles for cytokine transforming growth factor (TGF-β) has been found [9]. Similar analyses in SLE, of this rapidly developing field are soon likely to provide more complete profiles of peptide regulatory factors.

Autoimmune profiles and nephropathy

Friou's pioneering discovery of antinuclear factor (ANF), now expanded to a panoply of autoantibody profiles, has not provided clear explanations of organ injury, although there are associations between ANF and injury. The cause and effect relationship between autoantibody deposition and organ injury, established beyond reasonable doubt in antiglomerular basement membrane disease, remains ill-defined in SLE/CTD patients. Further, at least three different assays are available for each of the common autoantibodies, each assay dependent on varying physicochemical properties, specificities and clonal restrictions, of the autoantibody types. These tests yield variable results. The sensitivity of current assays, and their association with disease of organs other than the kidney have been reviewed [10–12]. The value of assays has been best evaluated in anti-DNA systems, in which the polyethylene glycol (PEG)-precipitation assay reveals positivity in less than 50% of sera, which are positive in assay by *Crithidia lucilliae*, and in other assays, e.g. ELISA, counterimmunoelectrophoresis and Farr, which are of intermediate sensitivity. Table 48.1 summarizes current knowledge of nephropathy-associated autoantibody profiles for both SLE and CTD.

The long-standing observation that double-stranded DNA is not an immunogen in experimental animals has focused research on the properties of anti-DNA antibodies which are associated with pathogenicity. These properties include immunoglobulin isotype (predominantly IgG), complement fixation properties, the charge present on the antibodies – mainly cationic, and avidity, as well as the breadth and type of specificity: polyreactivity and idiotype. Abnormalities in the regulation of variable

region (Vr) genes encoding for anti-DNA antibody has also been proposed as a central defect in the pathogenesis of SLE [13]. These Vr genes are identical by Southern blot analysis in normal and autoimmune subjects. In lupus, polyclonal B cell activation could account for overexpression of Vr genes and spontaneous production of self-reactive autoantibodies. However, this hypothesis does not explain the cytokine abnormalities, so simultaneous inheritance of genes encoding for peptide regulatory factors, and autoreactive germline Vr genes has been proposed to explain the genetic predisposition to SLE. Cloned Vh (hypervariable) gene subgroups in murine models appear intrinsically autoreactive, consistent with this hypothesis. Analysis of the nucleotide sequence of human IgG anti-DNA hybridomas show intrinsic (somatic) mutations of Vh, suggesting that pathogenic anti-DNA is derived from the natural autoantibody repertoire. However, the presence of a gene in a germline does not necessarily mean it will be transcribed. Generally an additional stimulus is required, such as antigen exposure or induction by an abnormal cytokine network. Other stimuli have been proposed. One of them is molecular mimicry, in which SmD, a small ribonucleoprotein, shares peptide sequences with Epstein–Barr virus (EBV)-encoded nuclear antigen I, suggesting that autoimmunity is induced by cross reactivity mechanisms, in addition to the known potential for EBV to polyclonally activate B cells [14]. The polyclonal B cell activation characteristic of SLE patients, and in some clinically unaffected relatives, may be explained by invoking one or more of these mechanisms.

Advances in understanding these perturbations of the immunoglobulin network in SLE and CTD has prompted fresh interest in modulation of the network as a therapeutic tool. The expression of antibodies of anti-DNA idiotype in the resolving phase of experimental lupus-like disease [15], and the use of monoclonal antibody reagents with anti-idiotype activity have shown that nephritis is delayed in BW mice after injection of these antibodies. Only antibodies with restricted anti-idiotype activities were effective, and elution of kidneys of animals with terminal nephritis showed deposition of subsets of the polyclonal anti-DNA antibody only [16]. These findings argue that within the (polyclonal) group of antibodies with anti-DNA activity, certain subgroups of restricted specificity only, are capable of inducing renal injury, and that idiotype modulation in SLE is potentially of therapeutic benefit. However, much has to be learned about the details of anti-DNA specificities before this avenue can be safely explored in humans with lupus or CTD nephropathy.

In human lupus nephritis, several cross-sectional, and longitudinal studies of anti-DNA antibodies in sera, with assessment of clinical disease activity, have proved inconclusive about their value, prompting evaluation of the subset with nephritogenic potential. The finding that nephritis is heralded by steadily rising high avidity anti-

Table 48.1 Autoimmune profiles of SLE/connective tissue diseases with nephropathy

Autoantibody	Autoantigen	Disease	Autoantibody prevalence	Organs	WHO grade nephritis
ANF anti-DNA (high–low avidity)	nuclear dsDNA ssDNA	SLE SLE	90–95% diagnostic: 50–100%	All; Vasculitis	O to V (high avidity anti-DNA)
anti-Sm anti-RNP	ENA: snRNA–70 kDa protein complex	SLE specific: Sjögren's systemic sclerosis Rheumatoid arthritis polymyositis	30%	Nephritis Cerebritis Myositis Arthritis	I to III
anti-SSB/La	sRNA–46.7 kDa protein	SLE Sjögren's	5–30%	Low grade nephritis: Skin: photosensitivity	interstitial
anti-SSA/Ro	sRNA–60 and 52 kDa protein	Heartblock			
antiphospholipid	–ve charge phospholipids	Thromboses: arterial + venous; CNS High fetal loss		All	I to V, and glomerular thrombosis
antiheparan sulfate proteoglycan	shared DNA determinants, or indirect (histones)	Glomerular basement membrane targets		Active nephritis	
anti-dsDNAId	ssDNAId	Remitting SLE [15]		Cerebritis in remission	Inactive phase

Abbreviations: ds/ss, double/single strand; kDa, kilodaltons; ENA, extractable nuclear antigen; RNP and Sm, ribonucleoprotein antigen (components of ENA): ribonuclease sensitive, and insensitive, respectively; SSB/La, ribonucleoprotein antigen (distinct from ENA); SSA/Ro, cytoplasmic RNA antigens; s, small; sn, small nuclear; –ve, negative; IF, immunofluorescence; Id, idiotypes.

DNA antibody whereas lower avidity antibodies are associated with cerebritis [17], is now clear. Cross reactivity of certain anti-DNA antibodies with heparan sulfate proteoglycan, (HSPG), the major, highly negatively charged basement membrane component of basement membranes, initially suggested a direct autoimmune pathogenesis of lupus nephritis by the formation of glomerular *in situ* immune complexes between anti-DNA and HSPG [1, 17]. However, this analysis proved too simple for two reasons. First, initial and most subsequent studies used commercially available HSPG of bovine source, and second, rigorous purification of the HSPG used as ligand in ELISA, to remove highly charged, bound, histones from HSPG, was not undertaken. Dissociation of these histones abrogates anti-DNA binding to HSPG, restored by reconstitution with histones [18]. Formation of *in situ* glomerular complexes in lupus nephritis is thought to be mediated *in vivo* by these mechanisms (Figure 48.1). These concepts have been further evaluated and yet further rationalization has taken place. Purified, histone-free human HSPG from human source shows much higher avidity for purified IgG anti-DNA antibodies than either histone-free, or even crude bovine HSPG, suggest-

ing that direct anti-DNA-human HSPG binding, not requiring histones occurs *in vivo* [19].

The increased affinity of anti-DNA antibodies associated with active lupus nephritis has been shown to parallel serum reactivity to HSPG [20], in the crude ELISA system, suggesting at least that antibodies complexed to histones may be pathogenic. Further analysis with purified human HSPG is merited, since these data also suggest that human HSPG may have some epitope-related antigenic properties not shared by bovine HSPG or native DNA.

Genetics

Hereditary deficiences of complement components encoded for on non-linked loci, C1q (chromosome 1p), C1r-C1s (chromosome 12p), C4, C4A, C2 (chromosome 6q, MHC region), are all associated with lupus and lupus-like diseases. Class II MHC linkages to lupus have also been reported, with allele polymorphisms associated with specified autoimmune profiles and expression of clinical organ disease (Table 48.1). T cell receptor genes (chromosome 14), not linked to MHC, are associated, at least

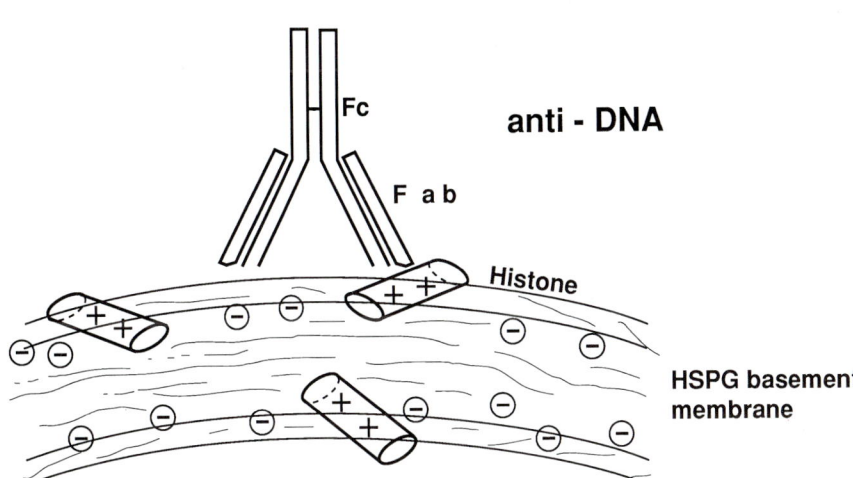

anti - DNA

Figure 48.1 Proposed *in situ* complex formation of glomerular immune deposits in lupus nephritis. Models using HSPG of bovine source require histones for binding [17] but pure human HSPG alone binds anti-DNA [19].

in some populations, with SLE. Immunoglobulin gene mapping studies have shown conflicting results. A major area of interest in humans is cytokine gene polymorphism, a concept supported by findings of variation in TNF-α genes in murine models of lupus.

Concordance rates for lupus-like disease in monozygotic twins is lower than expected, reported to be 24–60%, and for dizygotic twins 2%. These findings argue that environmental stimuli in genetically susceptible individuals contribute more than expected. For further information on concepts in genetics of SLE, the reader is referred to excellent reviews [21–23].

Pathology and serological indices in management

Evaluation of disease activity and hence the therapy for SLE and CTD nephritis are, perhaps, the most difficult in clinical nephrology. The capricious nature of the disease, the propensity for transformations in type and severity of nephropathy in 10–20% of patients and the uncertainty about the mechanism by which end-organ injury is mediated all contribute to the problems of defining reliable indices of disease activity.

Serological and cellular abnormalities detected in SLE and other CTD express the associated immunoregulatory abnormalities. A decade ago, available serological assays were evaluated longitudinally; no single test was found to be of value as a discriminant for alteration of the clinical features [24]. No single test was found that helped place SLE patients into those manifesting cerebritis, arthralgias, or cutaneous vasculitis. The tests differed in their ability to reflect disease activity when these subgroups were analysed. Circulating IgG anti-ds (double stranded) DNA antibodies of high avidity which fix complement are said to be markers of severity of nephritis. Others claim IgM, anti-dsDNA antibodies to be of significance. Severe nephritis, in general, is usually accompa-

nied by high dsDNA binding, often with low C3 and C4 levels. In the Mayo clinic trial of type IV lupus nephritis in 1978, addition of cyclophosphamide to prednisolone altered impaired CH_{50} levels, but not other serological parameters, and was of limited benefit to clinical disease. Cellular abnormalities, with subtle changes of lymphopenia and thrombocytopenia, should not be overlooked [24].

The lack of consistency among published studies evaluating clinicopathological correlants is, in part, explained by their experimental design. In a long-term prospective study of 143 patients with SLE, 33 developed active SLE nephritis. Of these, 21 had acute nephritis or deterioration in pre-existing renal disease [25]. A rising anti-dsDNA antibody preceded flares in each patient, with a usual doubling time of antibody titer of six weeks, but the actual flares were characterized by a rapidly decreasing antibody level. Decreasing levels of C4, then C1q and C3 accompany the early phase and flare. The novel data on HSPG/histone complex reactivity referred to may not affect these conclusions. Changes in the serological titers of indices of an individual patient may be of greater value than absolute levels and provides useful reassurance to the clinician that a new clinical feature is probably a consequence of SLE.

The renal pathology indices of lupus nephritis have been revisited. Glomerular morphology has been evaluated by a semiquantitative scoring system divided into 'Activity' and 'Chronicity' indices (AI and CI, respectively), Table 48.2 [26]. These indices signify potentially reversible and irreversible renal injury, respectively. In the prospective controlled multicenter trial of the Lupus Nephritis Collaborative Study Group, in which 86 patients were entered, the predictive value of AI and CI was assessed in severe lupus glomerulonephritis against two cut-off points: chronic renal failure (serum creatinine >600μmol/l or rise of >300μmol/l) or death (from renal and non-renal causes). Neither index by itself predicted an individual's outcome. The authors concluded that this form of renal biopsy assessment is not sufficient as a therapeutic guide and does not aid patient management. In contrast, the NIH study of grade IV nephritis [27] showed that a high CI, particularly the presence of fibrous crescents, glomerular sclerosis, tubular atrophy and interstitial fibrosis, strongly predicted a poor outcome.

It is important to note that neither study delineated AI as a poor prognostic index which most nephrologists and other specialists accept as meriting aggressive immunosuppressive treatments.

Treatments of nephritis in SLE and CTD

The controversies concerning renal disease in SLE highlight the problems of developing rational therapeutic regimens. The intensity of arguments have continued unchanged since Wagner's excellent review [28]. The natural history of untreated renal disease in SLE is now difficult to determine. Improvement in survival in recent decades has been associated initially with corticosteroid, and later with additional immunosuppressive regimens, and there is unlikely ever to be a formal trial comparing therapies with no treatment. Most physicians believe patients may improve, or at least stabilize temporarily, with judicious use of either steroid or immunosuppressive agents. Few studies have examined issues of remission–induction therapies, distinct from remission–maintenance, yet in practice these are central in decisions of patient management. Until these studies have been undertaken, scepticism based on outcome parameter trials [3] will remain, with some foundation.

Activity evaluation: acute phase

A suggested scheme for assessing disease activity of SLE with nephritis is depicted in Tables 48.3 and 48.4. Since progressive renal failure in SLE is not usually considered as a stepwise phenomenon [29], evaluation in this way may provide a more critical appraisal of requirements for immunosuppresion. Episodes of acute renal dysfunction are reported in 18% of lupus nephritis, most frequently in the first 12 months after presentation, but also at any time subsequently. The differential diagnosis of their cause is that of any potentially acute glomerulonephritis and each patient requires careful assessment before treat-

Table 48.2 Glomerular morphology evaluated by a semiquantitative scoring system

Activity	Chronicity
Glomerular cell proliferation	Glomerular sclerosis
Leukocyte exudation	Fibrous crescents
Fibrinoid necrosis[a]	Tubular atrophy
Cellular crescents[a]	Interstitial fibrosis
Hyaline deposits	
Interstitial mononuclear cell infiltrate	

Features marked [a] are weighted by a factor of two because of their ominous prognostic significance.

Table 48.3 Causes of acute renal dysfunction in lupus nephritis

1 Rapidly progressive glomerulonephritis
2 Hemodynamics – volume depletion
3 Thrombosis – renal vein
          – micro/macroarterial
4 Sepsis
5 Sepsis + rapidly progressive glomerulonephritis

Table 48.4 Scheme for assessing activity of SLE with nephritis

1. Eliminate possibility of infection; treat appropriately
2. Eliminate other causes of renal dysfunction, e.g. renal vein thrombosis
3. Evaluate clinical response:
    (a) Severity of extrarenal manifestations (ARA criteria)
    (b) Nephritis: urine deposit: red cell ⎫ excretion
                                         cast ⎭
             proteinuria
             glomerular morphology: repeat renal biopsy (in minority)
4. Consider relevant serological or immunological factors known to correlate with disease activity in the individual, e.g. rising DNA binding; falling C3, CH50; CRP[a]; leukopenia; thrombocytopenia

[a] SLE is associated with relatively low CRP values when active. CRP values above 60 mg/l generally indicate superadded infection.

ment. Since the precise time course of deterioration is often not known, the general approach is to define whether the SLE is active – suggesting more severe, or transformed, forms of glomerulonephritis which occur in 15% of SLE nephropathy – or whether a hemodynamic, septic, or thrombotic event has occurred. The decision to repeat a renal biopsy on such patients is usually made after adequate information on other factors has been obtained (Table 48.3).

Difficulties in excluding thrombotic events persist. In the presence of lupus anticoagulant or anticardiolipin (Table 48.1), the index of suspicion is higher. Doppler ultrasound, dynamic computer tomographic scanning with contrast or venography for large vessel renal vein thrombosis have been advocated, with varying sensitivity of detection, but small thromboses are unlikely to be detected. Arteriography with venous phase imaging of renal veins is likely to be the most sensitive and specific imaging, but is seldom undertaken in the setting of acute renal dysfunction.

Lupus vasculopathy

Vascular disease usually affects small vessels, and is of two types, present more often in SLE than CTD: thrombo-occlusive disease (Figure 48.2), or necrotizing vasculitis. Thrombotic disease which is more common, is associated with the most severe, type IV glomerular lesions, analyzed in the foregoing studies. No controlled study has evaluated the benefit or otherwise, of anticoagulation in addition to immunosuppression, in lupus nephritis. The presence of thrombi may denote a particularly poor prognosis [30] which many consider as an indication for anticoagulants.

Necrotizing vasculitis is characterized by the presence of cellular infiltrates of vessel wall media and is a rare occurrence. It is often associated with severe hyperten-sion. Anecdotal evidence suggests its presence is an indication for treatment with cyclophosphamide.

Lesions of lesser severity

Lupus membranous nephropathy is reported in 7–26% of SLE glomerulopathies, and does occur in CTD [1], encompassing the 'pure' morphological lupus membranous (WHO Class V(a) and (b)) and membranous nephropathy with associated glomerular cell proliferation (V(c) and (d)). Prognosis appears to be similar to that of idiopathic membranous nephropathy, 10–40% of affected patients reported as showing progressive impairment of renal function. Two studies have recently evaluated long-term outcome and the effect of treatment. A total of 42 affected patients with category V lesions had a 10 year kidney survival (93%) similar to that of patients with category IV, diffuse proliferative glomerulonephritis [31]. These class IV survivals are atypical, most studies suggesting that lupus membranous nephropathy has a more benign prognosis. Some authors consider that patients with types V(a) and V(b) do not require a high dose of immunosuppressive therapy [32]. However, repeated induction of remission of nephrotic syndrome, albeit with stable GFR, may be achieved in relapsing nephrotic syndrome in such patients [1].

For patients with low-grade proliferative lesions, types II and III, considerations for therapy have been reviewed [1]. There are outstanding problems, to optimize therapeutic risk : benefit ratios. Patients with low-grade disease, which can produce progressive renal scarring, are those least likely to benefit obviously from immunosuppressive drugs which have associated toxicity. Although progressive scarring may be reduced by use of cytotoxics in these patients, the most effective and least toxic regimens have not been evaluated in controlled studies.

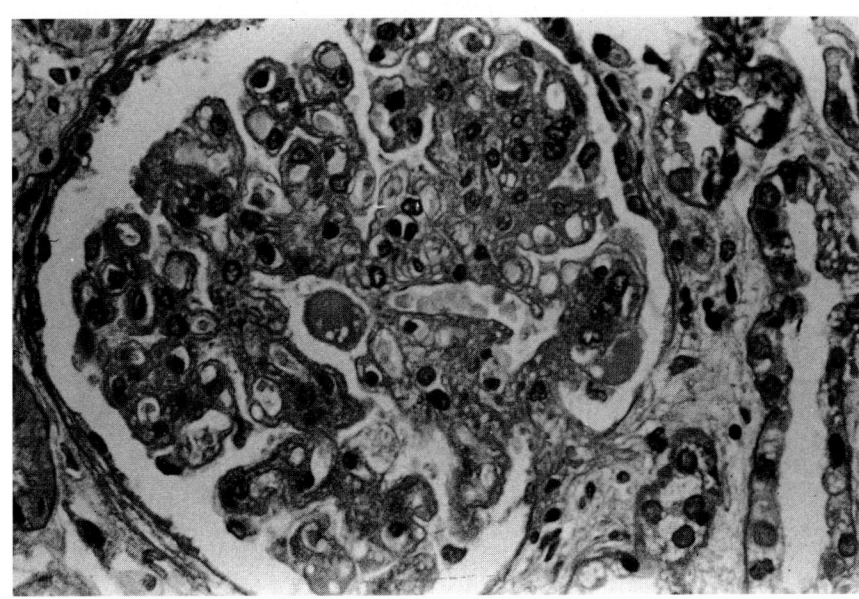

Figure 48.2 Intraglomerular hyaline thromboses in a patient with lupus nephritis and circulating anticardiolipin antibody. (Reproduced with permission and thanks: Dr I Roberts, Department of Pathology.)

Cyclophosphamide

Intravenous cyclophosphamide has been evaluated most extensively for nephritis in SLE with both acute and chronic disease phases (but generally not so defined). Studies have used regimens of $0.5-1.0\,g/m^2$, and from one to three monthly combination with corticosteroids. Since the analyses a decade ago [33, 34], which summarized benefits of prednisolone combined with cytotoxic therapy (azathioprine or cyclophosphamide) in reducing progression of renal scarring to irreversible lupus nephritis (in both functional and histological terms), and preventing nephropathy-related deaths (review, [1]), several new regimens have been proposed and evaluated.

In 1986, Austin *et al.* in the NIH trial [35] examined the outcomes of 107 patients with lupus nephritis. Most had type IV disease, a minority with III or V. Multiple treatment groups were entered: prednisolone only; prednisolone and azathioprine; prednisolone, azathioprine and oral cyclophosphamide; prednisolone and oral cyclophosphamide; prednisolone and intravenous cyclophosphamide. Life-table analyses suggested separation of renal survival curves, but this reached statistical significance only with prednisolone and intravenous cyclophosphamide when compared to prednisolone alone. This conclusion, of benefit of combined therapy, has been criticized [3].

Follow-up of the same cohort studied by Austin *et al.* has shown that renal survival in all cyclophosphamide-treated patients was improved beyond five years [36], but the numbers were small. It is noteworthy that patients survival did not differ among treatment groups. In the Mayo Clinic randomized trial [37], patients with type IV nephritis after four years had a higher incidence of clinically active nephritis after four years when treated with prednisolone alone (40 mg/day) compared to treatment with oral cyclophosphamide (100 mg/day) and prednisolone. However, the proportion of patients alive with stable or improve renal function was similar in both groups. Mortality did not differ between treatment groups, five years after trial entry [38].

Other therapeutic maneuvers: plasmapheresis/bolus steroids/cyclosporin A

In a randomized, controlled trial of 86 patients with type IV lupus nephritis, prednisolone and oral cyclophosphamide treatment was compared to this combination therapy plus 12 treatments with plasmapheresis over four weeks. No difference in clinical course was apparent, assessed by severity of exacerbations during reduction of prednisolone, or clinical outcomes – renal failure or death [2, 39]. These findings, like treatment in lupus of lesser severity [1], indicate that plasmapheresis is ineffective in SLE.

Bolus steroid treatment has received attention, with anecdotal favorable reports when compared to oral steroids [1]. Many physicians are convinced of its value in the treatment of acute, severe lupus with nephritis, and its popularity remains. Yet the only controlled trial of bolus steroids, was in patients with dominantly non-renal lupus, in 1988, and the number of patients studied was small. Several anecdotal reports of using cyclosporin A in lupus nephritis have been published. There is no convincing benefit, although considering the pathogenetic mechanisms of SLE, including the perturbations of cytokines, cyclosporin ought to be beneficial. Controlled studies of greater numbers of patients to evaluated outcome have not yet been undertaken. The significant vascular and other nephrotoxic side-effects of cyclosporin in an already injured kidney may offset any potential benefit in ameliorating the underlying inflammatory process. A review of alternative 'aggressive therapy' has been published [40]. Intravenous immunoglobulin may be primarily indicated for thrombocytopenia, after careful evaluation as to cause. Total lymphoid irradiation has been used experimentally, resulting in long-term CD4 lymphocyte depletion and there are anecdotes of improvement in renal function and proteinuria in lupus nephritis. Recombinant biological products have been studied: alpha interferon, and gamma interferon, which conceivably, could exacerbate disease; murine monoclonal antibody, against Fc receptors or CD5. These avenues and insights into the cytokine network, merit further study in the light of evolving concepts on immunopathogenesis.

Morbidity and mortality

Morbidity, considered a consequence of all corticosteroid or immunosuppressive regimens is common to all treatment groups in all studies [28–35]. Major infections, herpes zoster, avascular necrosis of bone, and malignancies occurred in all. In those receiving cyclophosphamide, hemorrhagic cystitis and transient leucopenia occurred. Gonadal toxicity is rare when the total cyclophosphamide dose is 8 g or less in adult males or premenopausal women. For further review, see [40]. Cumulative side effects were less common in those receiving intravenous compared to oral cyclophosphamide, although in the latter, those treated for less than 6 months, did not have hemorrhagic cystitis [35]. Although all studies in the last two decades show improvement in patient survival and renal function, Donadio and Glassock [3] believe these findings do not provide convincing support for use of cytotoxic agents. This view, with our present knowledge and therapies, will remain controversial until further studies with regimens more specifically aimed at disease activity are evaluated. In particular, use of the potentially more benign drug azathioprine, needs a more extensive evaluation.

The causes of mortality in patients with lupus nephritis are similar to those of all patients with SLE. Early deaths are the result of active lupus with intercurrent infection, with late deaths occurring from cardiovascular disease. This bimodal pattern has been observed in several studies. Mortality in the early phase reflects the difficulties in balancing suppression of lupus affecting the kidney and other organs while minimizing the risks of infection from therapy – especially in the patient with advancing uremia. Vascular disease is a result of accelerated atheroma in 50% of patients dying from SLE under the age of 40 and appears to be causally related to duration of disease, hypertension, hyperlipidemia and lupus carditis, rather than to the dose of steroid. Vasculitis of the coronary vessels is also reported, in children as well as adults [41]. It is likely that the presence of lupus anticoagulant exacerbates the tendency to occlusive arterial disease [1].

It is tempting to attribute reduced mortality in nephritis-related deaths in the pooled analysis [30], to a steroid-sparing effect although this is not reflected in controlled studies (Table 48.5). In an analysis of infection and immunosuppression in other immunologically-mediated diseases it was found that higher-dose steroids used in patients with impaired renal function proved to be a high-risk factor for serious infections [42]. Treatment with cyclophosphamide was associated with infection only in the presence of neutropenia. Frequency of infection was unrelated to the duration of plasma exchange. Bacteria accounted for the majority of infections. Serious opportunist pathogens, however, accounted for 14% of infections in patients with lupus nephritis. These findings support the conclusions of at least one analysis (Table 48.5), that appropriate and careful use of cytotoxic therapy, although minimizing steroid dose in lupus nephritis may reduce morbidity and mortality.

Patients who reach end-stage renal failure but who require therapy for control of SLE of organs other than the kidney may be particularly susceptible to steroid-induced mortality. Management of lupus patient in end-stage renal failure is as difficult as in other phases of the disease. Survival of patients undergoing long-term dialysis is comparable to that of the general dialysis population [1]. Patients with acute deterioration in renal function prior to dialysis are more likely to have continuing disease activity and higher mortality than those with slowly progressive renal failure. In survivors, clinical and serological evidence of lupus activity often abates [43], allowing immunosuppressive therapy to be reduced. A general approach to the lupus patient receiving maintenance dialysis is to adjust treatment meticulously to requirements, as in other, non-dialysis dependent states of disease. Recovery of renal function has been documented in a significant minority. The absence of active SLE as well as the rarity of recurrence of nephritis in those patients receiving allografts may have pathogenetic implications discussed previously, but, as yet, remains unexplained.

Major problems persist in the management of the nephropathies of systemic lupus erythematosis and other connective tissue disease. Our developing but incomplete understanding of its pathogenesis makes it difficult to identify any maneuver at present that will improve prognosis or reduce complications, other than excellence in management using current agents. Although important advances have been made, relevant immunotherapeutic strategies for the future are dependent on yet greater understanding.

Table 48.5 Summary of major analysis and trials in the last decade of therapy for lupus nephritis

Studies (Ref.)	Treatments[a]	Survival		Comment
		Renal	Patient	
Pooled analysis [34]	Pvs.	*	(*)	Not controlled
[33]	P + Cy; P + Az	*	–	Repeat renal biopsy
NIH (i) [35]	Pvs	*	NS	
(ii) [36]	P + o/i.v. cytotoxics	*	NS	>5 year follow-up
Mayo (i) [37]	Pvs P-oCy	NS	–	
(ii) [38]		NS**	NS	

*Statistically significant change (see text); ** $P = 0.06$; NS, not significant; –, not examined.
[a]P, prednisolone; Cy, oral (o) or i.v. cyclophosphamide; (++): q.v. text; Az = azathioprine.

References

1. Ballardie, F.W. (1989) Lupus nephritis, in *Multisystem Disease* (ed. G. Catto), Kluwer Academic, Dordrecht, pp. 42–63.
2. Lewis, E.J., Hunsicker, L.G., Lan, S.-P. *et al.* (1992) A controlled trial of plasmapheresis therapy in severe lupus nephritis. *N. Engl. J. Med.*, **326**, 1373–9.
3. Donadio, Jr, J.V. and Glassock, R.J. (1993) Immunosuppressive drug therapy in lupus nephritis. *Am. J. Kidney Dis.*, **21**, 239–50.
4. Smeenk, R., Brinkman, K., van den Brink, H. *et al.* (1990) Antibodies to DNA in patients with systemic lupus erythematosus. Their role in the diagnosis, the follow-up and the pathogenesis of the disease. *Clin. Rheumatol.*, **9**, 100–10.
5. Schwartz, M.M., Lan, S., Bernstein, J. *et al.* (1992) Role of pathology indices in the management of servere lupus glomerulonephritis. *Kidney Int.*, **42**, 743–8.
6. Moroni, G., Banfi, G. and Ponticelli, C. (1992) Clinical status of patients after 10 years of lupus nephritis. *Q. J. Med.*, **305**, 681–9.
7. Brennan, D.C., Jevnikar, A.M., Bloom, R.D. *et al.* (1992) Cultured mesangial cells from autoimmune MRL-*lpr* mice have decreased secreted and surface M-CSF. *Kidney Int.*, **42**, 279–84.
8. Fishman, P. and Shoenfeld, Y. (1993) Cytokines, interleukin–3 and autoimmunity. *Israel J. Med. Sci.*, **29**, 159–64.
9. Ballardie, F.W., Gordon, M., Sharpe, P. *et al.* (1994) Intrarenal cytokine mRNA expression and location in normal human and IgA nephropathy tissue: TGFα, TGFβ, IGF1, IL-4 and IL-6. *Nephrol. Dial. Transplant.*, **9**, 1545–52.
10. Ben–Chetrit, E. (1993) The molecular basis of the SSA/Ro antigens and the clinical significance of their autoantibodies. *Br. J. Rheumatol.*, **32**, 396–402.
11. Dhillon, V., Latchman, D. and Isenberg, D. (1991) Heat shock proteins and systemic lupus erythematosus. *Lupus*, **1**, 3–8.
12. Stratta, P., Canavese, C., Thea, A. *et al.* (1992) Clinical implication of antiphospholipid antibodies in systemic lupus erythematosus. *Contrib. Nephrol.*, **99**, 123–5.
13. Singh, A.K. (1993) Abnormalities in the regulation of variable region genes that encode for antibodies to DNA may be a central factor in the pathogenesis of systemic lupus erythematosus. *Ann. Rheum. Dis.*, **52**, 378–83.
14. Sabbatini, A., Bombardieri, S. and Migliorini, P. (1993) Autoantibodies from patients with systemic lupus erythematosus bind a shared sequence of SmD and Epstein–Barr virus-encoded nuclear antigen EBNA 1. *Eur. J. Immunol.*, **23**, 1146–52.
15. Suenaga, R. and Abdou, N.I. (1992) Expression of inactive stage anti–dsDNA idiotypes on anti–ssDNA antibodies in a lupus patient during active stage of lupus cerebritis. *J. Autoimmun.*, **5**, 379–92.
16. Mackworth–Young, C.G. and Madaio, M.P. (1992) Anti–DNA idiotype network: therapeutic considerations. *Lupus*, **1**, 339–40.
17. Faaber, P., Rijke, T.P.M. and van der Putte, L.B.A. (1986) Cross-reactivity of human and murine anti-DNA antibodies with heparan sulphate. *J. Clin. Invest.*, **77**, 1824–30.
18. Termaat, R.M., Brinkman, K., van Gompel, F. *et al.* (1990) Cross-reactivity of monoclonal anti-DNA antibodies with heparan sulphate is mediated via bound DNA/histone complexes. *J. Autoimmun.*, **3**, 531–5.
19. Yendle, J.E., Brenchley, P.E.C., Ballardie, F.W. and Anderson, J.C. (1992) Human, not bovine heparan sulphate preferentially binds autoantibodies, with comparable DNA affinities in lupus nephritis. *Lupus*, **1**, 9.
20. Kramers, C., Termaat, R.M., Ter Borg, E.J. *et al.* (1993) Higher anti–heparan sulphate reactivity during systemic lupus erythematosus (SLE) disease exacerbations with renal manifestations; a long term prospective analysis. *Clin. Exp. Immunol.*, **93**, 34–8.
21. Arnett, F.C. and Reveille, J.D. (1992) Genetics of systemic lupus erythematosus. *Rheum. Dis. Clin. North Am.*, **18**, 865–92.
22. Drake, C.G. and Kotzin, B.L. (1992) Genetic and immunological mechanisms in the pathogenesis of systemic lupus erythematosus. *Curr. Opin. Immunol.*, **4**, 733–40.
23. Batchelor, J.R. (1993) Systemic lupus erythematosus and genes within the HLA region. *Br. J. Rheumatol.*, **32**, 13–15.
24. Marrow, W.J.W., Isenberg, D.A. and Todd–Pokropek, A. (1982) Useful laboratory measurements in the management of systemic lupus erythematosus. *Q. J. Med.*, **51**, 125–38.
25. Swaak, A.J.G., Groenwold, J. and Bronsveld, W. (1986) Predictive value of complement profiles and anti-dsDNA in systemic lupus erythematosus. *Ann. Rheum. Dis.*, **45**, 359–66.
26. Gonzalez–Dettoni, H. and Tron, F. (1985) Membranous glomerulopathy in SLE. *Adv. Nephrol.*, **14**, 347–64.
27. Austin, H.A., Muenz, L.R., Joyce, K.M. *et al.* (1984) Diffuse proliferative lupus nephritis: Identification of specific pathologic features affecting renal outcome. *Kidney Int.*, **25**, 689–95.
28. Wagner, L. (1976) Immunosuppressive agents in lupus nephritis: a critical analysis. *Medicine*, **55**, 239–50.
29. Yeung, C.K., Ng, W.L. and Wong, W.S. (1985) Acute deteriorations in renal function in systemic lupus erythematosus. *Q. J. Med.*, **219**, 393–402.
30. Schwartz, M.M. (1992) Lupus vasculitis. *Contrib. Nephrol.*, **99**, 35–45.
31. Pasquali, S., Banfi, G., Zucchelli, A. *et al.* (1993) Lupus membranous nephropathy: long-term outcome. *Clin. Nephrol.*, **39**, 175–82.
32. Donadio, Jr, J.V. (1992) Treatment of membranous nephropathy in systemic lupus erythematosus. *Nephrol. Dial. Transplant.*, Suppl. 1, 97–104.
33. Felson, D.T. and Anderson, J. (1984) Evidence for superiority of immunosuppressive drugs and prednisolone over prednisolone alone in lupus nephritis. *N. Engl. J. Med.*, **311**, 1528–33.

34. Balow, J.E., Austin, H.A., Muenz, L.R. *et al.* (1984) Effect of treatment on the evolution of renal abnormalities in lupus nephritis. *N. Engl. J. Med.*, **311**, 491–5.

35. Austin, H.A., Klippel, J.H., Balow, J.E. *et al.* (1986) Therapy of lupus nephritis: controlled trial of prednisolone and cytotoxic drugs. *N. Engl. J. Med.*, **314**, 614–19.

36. Steinberg, A.D. and Steinberg, S.C. (1991) Long-term preservation of renal function in patients with lupus nephritis receiving treatment that includes cyclophosphamide versus those treated with prednisolone only. *Arthritis Rheum.*, **34**, 945–50.

37. Donadio, Jr, J.V., Holley, K.E., Ferguson, R.H. and Ilstrup, D.M. (1978) Treatment of diffuse proliferative nephritis with prednisolone and combined prednisolone and cyclophosphamide. *N. Engl. J. Med.*, **299**, 1151–5.

38. Donadio, Jr, J.V., Holley, K.E. and Ilstrup, D.M. (1982) Cytotoxic drug treatment of lupus nephritis. *Am. J. Kidney Dis.*, **2**, 178–81.

39. Lewis, E.J. and the Lupus Nephritis Collaborative Study Group. (1992) Plasmapheresis therapy is ineffective in SLE. *J. Clin. Apheresis*, **7**, 153.

40. Klippel, J.H. (1993) Is aggressive therapy effective for lupus? *Rheuma. Dis. Clin. North Am.*, **19**, 249–61.

41. Haider, Y.S. and Roberts, W.C. (1981) Coronary arterial disease in systemic lupus erythematosus. *Am. J. Med.*, **70**, 775–81.

42. Cohen, J., Pinching, A.J. and Rees, A.J. (1982) Infection and immunosuppression. *Q. J. Med.*, **201**, 1–15.

43. Cheigh, J.S., Stenzel, K.H. and Rubin, A.L. (1983) Systemic lupus erythematosus in patients with chronic renal failure. *Am. J. Med.*, **75**, 602–6.

49

Scleroderma: systemic sclerosis

Donal J. O'Donoghue

Introduction

Systemic sclerosis or scleroderma (literally meaning 'hardening of the skin') is characterized by vascular abnormalities, uncontrolled proliferation of connective tissue matrix and perivascular infiltration of monocytes. The classical clinical hallmarks are Raynaud's phenomenon, sclerodactyly and abnormal nail fold capillaries. The spectrum of disease is wide in both severity and extent, ranging from localized scleroderma, with only single patches of hard skin (morphea) of no clinical or functional importance, to diffuse cutaneous thickening, with rapidly advancing visceral involvement (Table 49.1) [1].

Systemic sclerosis is rare in children and men under the age of 30, but thereafter increases steadily with age, peaking in the 45–64 year age group. Overall, the female to male ratio is 3; the female excess is much more pronounced (15 : 1) in the 20–44 year age group. Scleroderma occurs throughout the world and in all races, but the reported incidence depends on definitions employed and case ascertainment. The community-based annual incidence of systemic sclerosis in the USA is approximately 10 new cases per million population, but there are differences within ethnic groups. Young black females seem to be at excess risk. Estimates of prevalence vary between 125 and 250 per million population [2].

Clinical manifestations

Systemic sclerosis usually begins insidiously, the first manifestation often being Raynaud's phenomenon or symmetrical swelling and stiffness of the fingers. The subsequent development of firm, taut, hidebound skin, proximal to the metacarpophalangeal joints permits a definitive diagnosis of systemic sclerosis in over 90% of patients. Changes confined to the fingers (and toes) – sclerodactyly – can occur in a number of conditions and are not specific for systemic sclerosis.

Localized scleroderma, in which by definition, visceral involvement does not occur, very rarely progresses into systemic sclerosis. It generally carries a benign prognosis and the lesions may soften spontaneously over time. Similarly, scleroderma-like syndromes, due to toxic, metabolic or inflammatory disorders, usually affect the skin predominantly. Vinyl chloride and bleomycin toxicity are associated with hepatic and pulmonary fibrosis but renal involvement is not a feature. Even in chronic graft-versus-host disease following bone marrow transplantation, in which there is widespread endothelial injury with internal organ involvement analogous to that of classical generalized scleroderma, renal involvement is rare and does not mimic the clinical or histological features of scleroderma renal crisis.

Early scleroderma can be difficult to distinguish from

Nephrology, Edited by Rex L. Jamison and Robert Wilkinson.
Published in 1997 by Chapman & Hall, London. ISBN 0 412 60930 4

Table 49.1 Classification of scleroderma and scleroderma-like syndromes

1. Localized (focal) forms of scleroderma
   (a) Morphea
   (b) Linear scleroderma
   (c) Scleroderma en coup de sabre[a] (with or without facial hemiatrophy)

2. Systemic sclerosis
   (a) Diffuse cutaneous systemic sclerosis
   (b) Limited cutaneous systemic sclerosis (CREST[b] syndrome)
   (c) Scleroderma *sine*[c] scleroderma (visceral disease without cutaneous involvement)
   (d) Overlap syndromes and early/undifferentiated connective tissue disease
      • systemic sclerosis/polymyositis overlap
      • mixed connective tissue disease
      • systemic lupus erythematosus/systemic sclerosis overlap
      • rheumatoid arthritis/systemic sclerosis overlap

3. Scleroderma-like syndromes
   (a) Drug induced
      • environmental e.g. vinyl chloride, toxic oil syndrome
      • pharmacological e.g. bleomycin, pentazocine, silicon implants
   (b) Metabolic and tumor associated
      • acromegaly
      • porphyrias
      • carcinoid syndrome
      • bronchoalveolar carcinoma
   (c) Inflammatory – immunological
      • amyloidosis
      • graft-versus-host disease
      • eosinophilic fasciitis

[a] en coup de sabre (French) – resembing the scar of a sabre wound.
[b] CREST – calcinosis, Raynaud's phenomenon, esophageal hypomotility, sclerodactyly and telangiectasia.
[c] *sine* (Latin) – without.

conditions such as primary Raynaud's phenomenon and other connective tissue diseases. Although scleroderma *sine* scleroderma (visceral disease without cutaneous involvement) occurs in 5% of patients, it is rare for renal scleroderma to be the first manifestation of disease: such cases may lead to diagnostic confusion, despite the majority of them having Raynaud's phenomenon and often abnormal nail fold capillaries.

The subsets of systemic sclerosis identified by the pattern of skin involvement, also distinguish prognostically different groups (Table 49.1). Diffuse cutaneous systemic sclerosis affecting the trunk, face and proximal as well distal portions of the extremities is associated with relatively early appearance of cardiopulmonary, renal and gastrointestinal involvement. Limited cutaneous systemic sclerosis is often preceded by 'isolated' Raynaud's phenomenon. Skin involvement is limited to sclerodactyly often with calcinosis (deposition of calcium in the skin, in the form of nodules or plaques) and facial tightening with telangiectasia.

Esophageal motility disorders occur early but other visceral features – pulmonary hypertension, biliary cirrhosis, trigeminal neuralgia and renal disease – may take years to develop. This subset of systemic sclerosis is often known by the acronym CREST – calcinosis, Raynaud's phenomenon, esophageal involvement, sclerodactyly and telangectasia.

Renal disease and hypertension are rare in the clearly established polymyositis/scleroderma overlap syndromes and scleroderma renal crisis has not been reported [3]. In the undifferentiated connective tissue syndromes, or mixed connective tissue disease, renal involvement is uncommon if the illness remains undifferentiated and after evolution follows the pattern of disease (either scleroderma or systemic lupus erythematosus) that has developed.

Visceral manifestations result from various combinations of inflammation, fibrosis and atrophy. Different organs may have different patterns of injury and the extent of involvement can vary. Detailed descriptions of the involvement of organs other than the kidney can be found in other texts and reviews.

The frequency of renal involvement in systemic sclerosis depends on the case mix of the study population, the timing of observation in relation to diagnosis and the criteria used to define renal involvement. Diffuse skin disease is a major risk factor for development of scleroderma renal crises but chronic renal disease and hypertension are both common in diffuse scleroderma and CREST syndrome (Table 49.2) [4]. Features of renal disease are usually apparent within two to three years of diagnosis and over 90% of patients who will develop renal failure do so within six years. Nevertheless, many patients have functional and structural renal vascular involvement without accelerated hypertension or chronic renal failure. Cold exposure leads to reduced renal blood flow analogous to cutaneous Raynaud's phenomenon. There is evidence of pathology in the renal vasculature in approximately 60% of cases, even in the absence of overt renal disease.

A direct relationship between scleroderma and acute renal failure was not recognized until Moore and Sheehan [5] described the clinical features of scleroderma renal crisis. Over the past 30 years, renal disease has been shown to be the most common cause of death in virtually every series. The introduction of angiotensin converting enzyme inhibitors has radically altered the outlook, but renal involvement remains a major cause of morbidity and mortality in scleroderma.

The spectrum of renal disease varies from asymptomatic urinary abnormalities or mild hypertension, to the distinctive medical emergency of scleroderma renal crisis [6]. Proteinuria, hypertension and renal impairment are frequent in patients with scleroderma. Cannon and colleagues [7], identified at least one of these abnormalities in 45% of 210 patients with systemic sclerosis. In another large series, proteinuria occurred in 109 of 271 patients, although severe renal failure was present in only 19. Proteinuria is often accompanied by microscopic hematuria correlating with the pathological changes of ischemic glomerular and tubulointerstitial disease; however macro-scopic hematuria and nephrotic range proteinuria are rare. These non-specific markers of renal disease should not be assumed to be secondary to scleroderma and should be fully investigated, as they may have other causes.

Scleroderma renal crisis is a life-threatening complication. The clinical features are those of severe, often accelerated hypertension, visual disturbances and left ventricular failure. Renal blood flow and glomerular filtration rate are decreased and renal failure rapidly progresses. The urinary sediment is active and, as a rule, there is microangiopathic hemolytic anemia, particularly in those in whom hypertension is not severe. In the absence of cutaneous disease, the diagnosis may be difficult to distinguish from other causes of accelerated hypertension or hemolytic uremic syndrome/thrombotic thrombocytopenic purpura.

Pathogenesis

The earliest pathological changes involve the microvascular endothelium and result in subendothelial edema, platelet aggregation and perivascular lymphocyte migration. Tissue fibrosis and atrophic changes are late events [8].

It is uncertain what initiates the uncontrolled proliferation of connective tissue in scleroderma and why the vascular injury progresses to fibrosis instead of repair. It is clear, however, that several mechanisms are involved, either simultaneously or sequentially. These include inflammatory and immune mechanisms, abnormal vascular responses and repair, fibroblast activation by cytokines and growth factors and interactions between different components of the extracellular matrix [9a].

Following injury and inflammation of the vascular endothelium, mononuclear inflammatory cells migrate through the vessel wall and bind to connective tissue matrix components where they stimulate a fibroblast fibrogenic response probably mediated by the interaction of transforming growth factor-beta (TGF-β), platelet

	Diffuse scleroderma (n = 351) (%)	CREST syndrome (n = 346) (%)	Poorly characterized syndromes (n = 49) (%)
Proteinuria	22	16	12
Hypertension	31	26	25
Chronic renal failure (creatinine >130 μmol/l)	25	13	10
Scleroderma renal crisis	19	1	6

(From Shapiro and Medsger (1988) [4] University of Pittsburg 1972–1984).

Table 49.2 Frequency of renal involvement in systemic sclerosis subsets

derived growth factor (PDGF) and basic fibroblast growth factor (BFGF). It has been suggested that fibroblast synthesis of interleukin-6 which appears to be up-regulated in systemic sclerosis, could lead to increased synthesis of tissue inhibitors of metaloproteinases. Metaloproteinases normally degrade matrix and their inhibition may therefore further contribute to uncontrolled fibrogenesis. The impaired T-cell synthesis of interferon gamma, recently reported in systemic sclerosis, may also contribute to fibrosis as this cytokine normally down-regulates the synthesis of collagen. Specific fibroblast abnormalities have also been described with increased spontaneous and stimulated collagen synthesis [9b], but the molecular basis of these abnormalities has not been elucidated.

The majority (90%) of patients with systemic sclerosis have positive antinucleolar or antinuclear antibodies showing a fine speckled nucleolar pattern on immunofluorescence. This family of antinucleolar autoantibodies is directed at a variety of antigens. Certain antibodies appear to define disease subsets with different genetic associations, patterns of organ involvement and prognosis [10] (Table 49.3). These antibody responses appear to be genetically determined [11] and are associated with specific HLA class II polymorphisms. Anticentromere antibodies are associated with HLA-DQ Beta I alleles with a polar tyrosine or glycine amino acid at position 26 of the outermost domain of the DQ Beta molecule as opposed to a hydrophobic leucine residue. Antitopoisomerase I antibodies are associated with specific motifs in the HLA-DQ Beta I molecule [12] and anti PM-SCL (antipolymyositis-scleroderma) are nearly 100% correlated with the presence of HLA-DR3 [13]. Antibodies to the RNA polymerase enzyme complex are thought to be predictive of renal crisis. Scleroderma renal crisis developed in 24% of patients with anti-RNA polymerase antibodies in contrast to 10% of patients with antitopoisomerase I antibodies. Although these scleroderma-associated antibodies are non-complement fixing, they may in some way interfere with gene transcription and thereby disrupt control of collagen formation. Therapies aimed at reducing these autoantibodies have not, however, led to clinical improvement/remission.

Renal pathology

The characteristic lesion of renal scleroderma is concentric intimal hyperplasia of the interlobular and arcuate arteries [14] (Figure 49.1). The larger arteries, including the main renal vessels and interlobar vessels may be normal or show only intimal sclerosis consistent with atherosclerosis or hypertension. In the interlobular arteries, the proliferating intimal cells are arranged concentrically in a mucoid matrix of ground substance composed of glycoproteins and mucopolysaccharides. This proliferation may damage the internal elastic lamina, allowing smooth muscle cells to migrate into the intima. The fibrous thickening of the adventitia and perivascular tissue that accompanies these changes is seldom found in

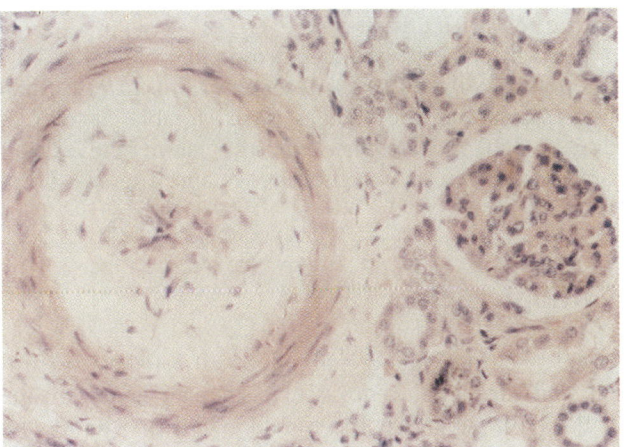

Figure 49.1 Photomicrograph of a renal biopsy specimen from a patient with scleroderma, concentric intimal hyperplasia with perivascular fibrosis resulting in gross vascular narrowing (right) and a resulting ischemic glomerulus (left).

Table 49.3 Autoantibodies and subsets of systemic sclerosis

Autoantibody specificity	HLA associations	Disease subset
1. Anticentromere antibodies (ACA)	HLA-DQβ1 tyr or gly 26	CREST[a] syndrome
2. Antitopoisomerase-I antibodies (Anti-Topo-1) (also known as Scl-70)	HLA-DQβ1 TRAELDT sequence 71–77, tyr 30 or 26	Diffuse cutaneous systemic sclerosis
3. Anti-RNA polymerase antibodies	Not yet determined	Diffuse cutaneous systemic sclerosis (high risk of scleroderma renal crisis)
4. Anti-PM-Scl antibodies	HLA-DR3	Polymyositis – scleroderma overlap

[a] Calariosis, Raynaud's phenomenon, esophageal hypomotility, sclerodactyly and telangiectasia.

other causes of hypertension [15]. The gross vascular narrowing results in distal ischemia and atrophy. Intravascular thrombosis may also occur which can result in necrosis and small wedge-shaped infarcts.

The fibrinoid necrosis of the smaller vessels is indistinguishable from the seen in malignant hypertension from other causes and can occur in scleroderma without severe hypertension.

Glomerular changes are secondary to ischemia (Figure 49.1) and include focal and diffuse basement membrane thickening with progressive glomerular sclerosis. There may also be non-specific hyperplasia of the juxta-glomerular apparatus. Superimposed microangiopathic changes can occur. Rarely there may be glomerular necrosis and crescent formation [16]. Immunofluorescent studies of affected glomeruli show non-specific changes consistent with ischemic injury and sclerosis – IgM, complement and fibrinogen deposition have all occasionally been reported. Immunohistochemical staining reveals a marked increase of type III collagen around the blood vessels and throughout the kidney, but particularly within the interstitium.

Even in patients without scleroderma renal crisis, the interlobular arteries frequently show concentric intimal hyperplasia and the tubules have variable degrees of diffuse ischemic atrophy, and the glomerulir exhibit ischemic changes with obsolescence and interstial fibrosis [15].

Pathophysiology

There is clear evidence for functional renal vasospasm [7] and structural renovascular changes [15a] in the majority of patients with systemic sclerosis. Scleroderma renal crisis and chronic renal impairment develop on the background of this established vasculopathy. The more frequent occurrence of crisis in winter implies that exposure to cold causes vasospasm and may precipitate acute renal failure, although this has not been confirmed in all series.

In crisis, plasma renin activity increases markedly, probably the result of renal ischemia consequent on renal vasoconstriction, rather than a primary causative event. However, the resulting activation of the angiotensin system is almost certainly the pivotal factor in amplifying the vicious cycle of vascular constriction and damage; the role of other pressor systems, such as endothelin, in the modulation of scleroderma renal crisis has not been adequately studied. A subgroup of patients who are at excess risk for accelerated hypertension can be identified on the basis of their clinical and serological features (Table 49.4).

Diagnosis

The diagnosis of early systemic sclerosis or prescleroderma is based on clinical criteria but can be difficult. It is aided by positive serology and abnormal capillaroscopy of the nail fold (Figure 49.2). This can be performed with an ophthalmoscope and reveals capillary dilatation, deformation and areas of capillary depletion in the nail folds. Renal involvement, however, nearly always occurs in the context of established disease and diagnostic dilemma is unusual because of the distinctive features of scleroderma renal crisis [17]. Rarely patients may develop antineutrophil cytoplasmic antibodies with an associated crescentic nephritis [16]. Drug-associated scleroderma-like syndromes infrequently cause a crisis or renal failure. When scleroderma renal crisis occurs in the classical clinical setting and responds to treatment, histological confirmation may not be necessary. In atypical cases, renal biopsy is required to confirm the interlobular changes, exclude coincidental renal disease, for prognostic purposes and to identify the extent and severity of vascular changes and resulting tubulointerstitial atrophy and fibrosis. Renal biopsy should be deferred until hypertension has been adequately controlled but even then it is associated with an increased risk of bleeding.

Table 49.4   Risk factors for scleroderma renal crisis

Major	Minor
Diffuse skin involvement	Recent onset of anemia
Rapidly progressive skin thickening	New cardiac events – pericardial effusion, congestive cardiac failure
Short duration of disease (<5 years)	
Anti-RNA polymerase III antibody	
	Drug therapy
	Corticosteroids
	Cyclosporin A
	NSAIDs
	Interferon gamma

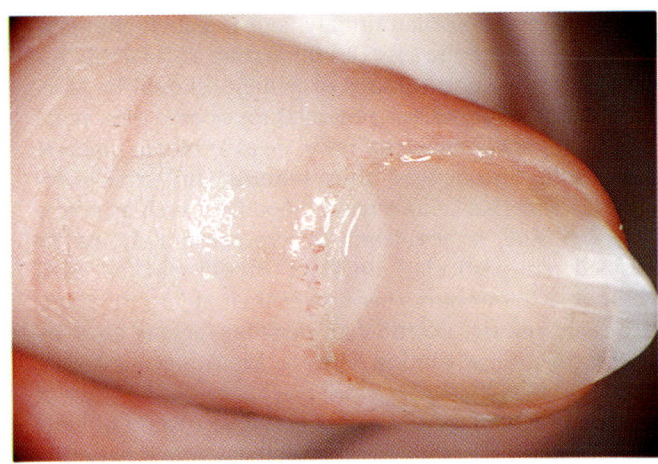

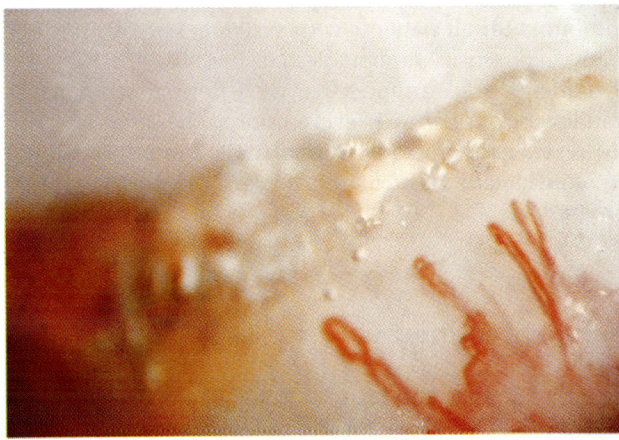

Figure 49.2 Abnormal nail fold capillaries in a patient with scleroderma. (a) Gross appearance. (b) Capillaroscopy, showing an area of capillary dilatation (right) and an avascular area of capillary depletion in the nail fold (left). (Photographs kindly given by Dr Gunter Holti, Newcastle.)

Treatment

A detailed review of the general treatment of systemic sclerosis is beyond the scope of this chapter [18]. The clinical heterogeneity, relatively low frequency and variable natural history have hampered controlled clinical trials. Even D-penicillamine, which is considered by many to be standard therapy, has not been shown to halt excessive fibrosis or vascular damage in the skin or internal organs [19, 20]. The management and outcome of scleroderma renal crisis has been transformed by the use of angiotensin converting enzyme (ACE) inhibitors [21]. Indeed, before their introduction, the average patient survival was rarely beyond three months [22]. Early bilateral nephrectomy was recommended for the control of hypertension [23].

Although no controlled trials have been performed, ACE inhibitors appear to have substantially reduced the mortality of scleroderma renal crisis. In a recent report of 108 patients from one center, the one-year survival increased from 18% to 76% after the introduction of ACE inhibitors [21]. Patients with systemic sclerosis who developed new severe hypertension (diastolic pressure >110 mm Hg) should be considered to have scleroderma renal crisis until proven otherwise. They should immediately be treated with a short-acting ACE inhibitor. Blood pressure should be lowered to the normal range within 72 h by increasing the ACE inhibitor dose every 6–8 h as necessary. If blood pressure control is not achieved with maximum ACE inhibition, other oral or parenteral antihypertensive agents should be added. It is not unusual for renal failure to progress over the next 7–10 days and some patients will still develop end-stage renal failure.

Steen *et al.* [21] observed progression to renal failure or death in 24 of 55 patients who were treated with ACE inhibitors. Of the 53 patients who did not receive this treatment, a poor outcome was observed in 49 (92%). The reasons why ACE inhibition does not rescue almost half of the treated patients are not clear. They may include the presence of advanced renal failure at the initiation of therapy, inadequate blood pressure control despite ACE inhibition and co-existing disease such as crescentic nephritis. In addition, the underlying pathophysiological mechanisms may persist and factors other than renin–angiotensin system activation may be important in promoting progression of the vasculopathy.

Several new agents have been used in the management of non-renal systemic sclerosis, including cyclosporin A and interferon gamma. Both appear to be associated with a high incidence of acute renal failure, despite concomitant use of ACE inhibitors in some of the patients [24].

Anticoagulants, antithrombotic drugs, corticosteroids, immunosuppressive therapy and plasma exchange (with or without fresh frozen plasma) have not established a place in the management of renal scleroderma. However, prostacyclin may be beneficial by further reducing blood pressure, and by direct endothelial effects. High-dose steroids have been reported as a risk factor for the development of scleroderma renal crisis but this association may be coincidental because rapidly progressive cutaneous disease is sometimes treated with steroids.

Outcome

Pulmonary hypertension has now replaced renal disease as the main cause of mortality in systemic sclerosis, but renal involvement remains a strong adverse prognostic factor for survival. In a prospective study of 237 patients, renal involvement at enrolment carried a relative risk of death of 7.5 [25]. In recent series, multiorgan involvement is frequently present at the time of death, emphasizing both the systemic nature of the disease and the absence of effective therapy.

The outcome for patients with scleroderma who receive renal replacement therapy is poor in comparison with other disease groups, perhaps reflecting the on-going systemic process. Hemodialysis may be complicated by the difficulty of creating and maintaining the vascular access and the hemodynamic instability of these patients. Similarly, continual ambulatory peritoneal dialysis (CAPD) can be complicated by peritoneal sclerosis, altered peritoneal permeability due to local vasospasm, poor wound healing and exacerbation of impaired pulmonary reserve. In one report of 311 patients with scleroderma-induced end-stage renal failure; overall survival was 33% at 3 years, compared to 71% for lupus nephritis [26]. The importance of continuing ACE inhibitors during dialysis was emphasized by a report of recovery of renal function in 11 of 20 patients with scleroderma renal crisis between 3 and 15 months after commencing regular dialysis; indeed, in the previous study just cited 6.8% of scleroderma patients recovered renal function, compared to only 3.3% of the lupus group [26].

Successful renal transplantation for scleroderma-induced renal failure was first reported by Richardson in 1973 [27] and although recurrence can occur in the allograft this is not frequent. Comorbidity often precludes transplantation, however, and large comparative studies have not been reported, but the progressive nature of systemic sclerosis suggests that the outcome will not be as good as with primary renal diseases.

Prevention

The patient at high risk of scleroderma renal crisis can be identified by the rapid development of diffuse cutaneous disease, anti-RNA polymerase III antibodies and disease duration of less than five years (Table 49.4). Pre-existing hypertension, abnormal urinalysis or impaired glomerular filtration rate are less discriminating risk factors for renal crisis but both groups of patients should be carefully educated about the potential for scleroderma renal crisis and encouraged to have regular blood pressure monitoring and at least three-monthly full clinical review. Factors that reduce renal blood flow such as severe cold exposure, hypovolemia or hypotension should be avoided. In particular, diuretics should not be used without ACE inhibitors because of their ability to stimulate renin release. Potential nephrotoxic agents must be used with utmost caution so as to avoid precipitating a renal crisis.

Prompt diagnosis and early aggressive treatment with ACE inhibitors is required when scleroderma renal crisis is considered. Prophylactic use of high-dose ACE inhibitors for all patients with systemic sclerosis has not gained consensus support perhaps because the majority of patients are normotensive with normal renin levels and low or normal ACE levels, prior to the onset of crisis. However, early introduction of ACE inhibitors should be considered, particularly if skin disease is rapidly progressive.

Acknowledgments

I would like to thank Miss Sarah J. Gilliard for secretarial assistance, Dr R. Reeve for the photomicrographs and Dr A. Herrick for the nail fold capillaroscopy illustration, and Drs P.A. Kalra, W.D. Plant and S. Waldek for kindly reviewing the manuscript.

References

1. Masi, A. (1980) Preliminary criteria for the classification of systemic sclerosis. *Arthritis Rheum.*, **23**, 581–90.
2. Steen, V. and Medsger, T. (1990) Epidemiology and natural history of systemic sclerosis. *Rheum. Dis. Clin. North Am.*, **16**, 1–10.
3. Marguerie, C., Bunn, C., Benyon, H. *et al.* (1990) Polymyositis, pulmonary fibrosis and autoantibodies to aminoacyl-tRNA synthetase enzymes. *Q. J. Med.*, **282**, 1–20.
4. Shapiro, A. and Medsger, T. (1988) Renal involvement in systemic sclerosis, in *Diseases of Kidney*, 4th edn (eds R. Schreiner and C. Gottschalk), Little, Brown, Boston, pp. 2272–83.
5. Moore, H. and Sheehan, H. (1952) The kidney of scleroderma. *Lancet*, **i**, 68–70.
6. Donohoe, J. (1992) Scleroderma and the kidney. *Kidney Int.*, **41**, 462–77.
7. Cannon, P., Hassar, M., Case, D. *et al.* (1974) The relationship of hypertension and renal failure in scleroderma to structural and functional abnormalities of the renal cortical circulation. *Medicine*, **54**, 1–46.
8. Prescott, R., Freemont, A., Jones, C. *et al.* (1992) Sequen-

tial dermal microvascular and perivascular changes in the development of scleroderma. *J. Pathol.*, **166**, 255–63.
9. Postlethwaite, A. (1993) Connective tissue metabolism including cytokines in scleroderma. *Curr. Opin. Rheumatol.*, **5**, 766–72.
9a. Hebbar, M., Gillot, J.-M., Hachulla, E. *et al.* (1996) Early expression of E-selecting, tumour necrosis factor α and mass cell infiltration in the salivary glands of patients with systemic sclerosis. *Arthritis and Rheumatism*, **39**, 1161–5.
9b. Jelaska, A., Arakawa, M., Broketa, G. *et al.* (1996) Heterogenecty of collagen synthesis in normal and systemic sclerosis skin fribroblasts. *Arthritis and Rheumatism*, **39**, 1338–46.
10. Kahaleh, B. (1993) Immunological aspects of scleroderma. *Curr. Opin. Rheumatol.*, **5**, 760–5.
11. Reveille, J. (1993) Molecular genetics of systemic sclerosis. *Curr. Opin. Rheumatol.*, **5**, 753–9.
12. Maul, G., Jimenez, A., Riggs, E. and Ziemnicka-Kotula, D. (1989) Determination of an epitope of the diffuse systemic sclerosis marker antigen DNA topoisomerase I: sequence similarity with retroviral p30gag protein sug-

gests a possible cause for autoimmunity in systemic sclerosis. *Proc. Natl. Acad. Sci. USA*, **86**, 8492–6.

13. Marguerie, C., Bunn, C., Copier, J. *et al.* (1992) The clinical and immunogenetic features of patient with autoantibodies to the nucleolar antigen PM-Scl. *Medicine*, **71**, 327–36.

14. D'Angelo, W., Fries, J., Masi, A. and Shulman, L. (1969) Pathological observations in systemic sclerosis. *Am. J. Med.*, **46**, 428–40.

15. Kovalchik, M., Guggenheim, S., Silverman, M. *et al.* (1978) The kidney in progressive systemic sclerosis. A prospective study. *Ann. Intern. Med.*, **89**, 881–7.

15a.Rivolta, R., Mascagni, B., Vittorio, B. *et al.* (1996) Renal vascular damage in systemic sclerosis patients without clinical evidence of nephropathy. *Arthritis and Rheumatism*, **39**, 1030–4.

16. Alvarez, V., Salazar, V., Ortega, A. *et al.* (1992) Pulmonary hemorrhage and focal necrotizing glomerlonephritis in a case of systemic sclerosis. *Clin. Rheumatol.*, **11**, 116–19.

17. Kahaleh, M. and Leroy, E. (1979) Progressive systemic sclerosis: kidney involvement. *Clin. Rheum. Dis.*, **5**, 167–84.

18. Jayson, M. (1988) Treatment of systemic sclerosis, in *systemic sclerosis – Scleroderma* (eds M. Jayson and C. Block), Wiley, Chichester, pp. 289–301.

19. Pope, J. (1993) Treatment of systemic sclerosis. *Curr. Opin. Rheumatol.*, **5**, 792–801.

20. Torres, M. and Furst, D. (1990) Treatment of generalized systemic sclerosis. *Rheum. Dis. Clin. North Am.*, **16**, 217–41.

21. Steen, V., Constanino, J., Shapiro, A. and Medsger, T. (1990) Outcome of renal crisis in systemic sclerosis: relation to availability of angiotensin converting enzyme (ACE) inhibitors. *Ann. Intern. Med.*, **113**, 352–7.

22. Traub, Y., Shapiro, A., Rodnan, G. *et al.* (1983) Hypertension and renal failure (scleroderma renal crisis) in progressive systemic sclerosis. Review of a 25 year experience with 68 cases. *Medicine*, **62**, 335–52.

23. Leroy, E. and Fleischmann, R. (1978) The management of renal scleroderma. Experience with dialysis, nephrectomy and transplantation. *Am. J. Med.*, **64**, 974–8.

24. Denton, C., Sweny, P., Abdulla, A. and Black, C. (1994) Acute renal failure in scleroderma treated with cyclosporin A: a report of three cases. *Brit. J. Rheum.*, **33**, 90–2.

25. Lee, P., Langevitz, P., Alderdice, C. *et al.* (1992) Mortality in systemic sclerosis. *Q. J. Med.*, **82**, 139–48.

26. Nissenson, A. and Port, F. (1990) Outcome of end stage renal disease in patients with rare causes of renal failure. III. Systemic/vascular disorders. *Q. J. Med.*, **273**, 63–74.

27. Richardson, J. (1973) Hemodialysis and kidney transplantation for renal failure from scleroderma. *Arthritis Rheum.*, **16**, 265–71.

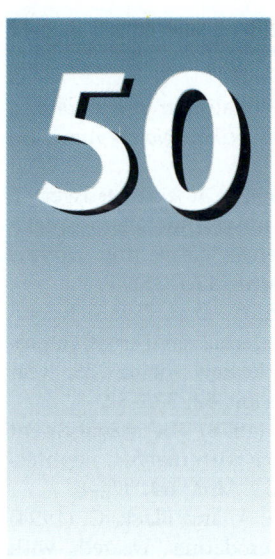

Pauci immune vasculitides: Wegener's granulomatosis, microscopic polyangiitis and polyarteritis nodosa

C.M. Lockwood and D.S. Peat

Introduction

Wegener's granulomatosis, microscopic polyangiitis and polyarteritis nodosa are the systemic vasculitides which are most frequently managed by nephrologists. They are members of a spectrum of clinical syndromes, most of which were defined eponymously. Hitherto they were classified morphologically, by the site and size of blood vessels involved, as well as the presence or absence of either accompanying granulomata or aneurysms, see Table 50.1.

There are two requisite features which characterize the pathology of the vasculitic lesion in the systemic vasculitides: first, there should be evidence of inflammation and necrosis of the vessel wall; second, this should be primary, exclusive to the vessel wall and not secondary to other pathology, such as adjacent to an abscess cavity or contiguous with ulcerated mucosa. Further detailed analysis has led to an appreciation that more subtle changes may herald the appearance of the early vasculitic lesion [1]. These include the development of endothelial cell swelling, as well as the display on the endothelial cell surface of adhesion molecules such as endothelial leukocyte adhesion molecule-1 (ELAM-1) (Figure 50.1). Recent studies suggest that the primary forms of small vessel vasculitis, including Wegener's and microscopic polyangiitis, are examples of classical autoimmune diseases in which both humoral and cellular mechanisms are operating, although, paradoxically, in neither of these two, nor polyarteritis nososa, are immune deposits a feature. This is called pauciimmune vasculitis. Most information has been obtained for Wegener's granulomatosis and microscopic polyangiitis which, in turn, has greatly helped development of strategies for their treatment. In this chapter the etiology, pathogenesis and treatment of Wegener's, microscopic polyangiitis and polyarteritis nodosa will be grouped for discussion, the clinical features of the syndromes, however, will be described individually as will their differential diagnoses.

Etiology

There are few clues to the etiology of the primary vasculitides: the rarity of the diseases and lack of suitable diagnostic markers have hampered efforts to understand how they arise. Genetic predisposition, infectious agents and abnormal responses to drugs have all received attention as responsible candidates. With respect to a genetic predisposition, one early study suggested a weak link between small vessel vasculitis and the DQw7 allele, another that DR1 was 3.8 times commmoner in patients with Wegener's granulomatosis; however, these findings remain controversial [2]. Alternatively, a series of reports have suggested a pivotal role for α_1-antitrypsin genetic polymorphism, at least in Wegener's granulomatosis, where it appears to be a useful predictor of progression of disease morbidity [3]. More recently the demonstration that in the small vessel vasculitides the polymorphonuclear leukocyte may be inappropriately activated through

Nephrology, Edited by Rex L. Jamison and Robert Wilkinson.
Published in 1997 by Chapman & Hall, London. ISBN 0 412 60930 4

Table 50.1 Morphological classification of systemic vasculitis

Vessel size	Granulomata helpful to diagnosis	Granulomata infrequent
Large	Takayasu's disease aneurysms	Temporal arteritis
Medium	Churg–Strauss disease	Polyarteritis nodosa aneurysms (nodes)
Small	Wegener's granulomatosis	Microscopic polyangiitis Henoch–Schonlein purpura Kawasaki disease aneurysms

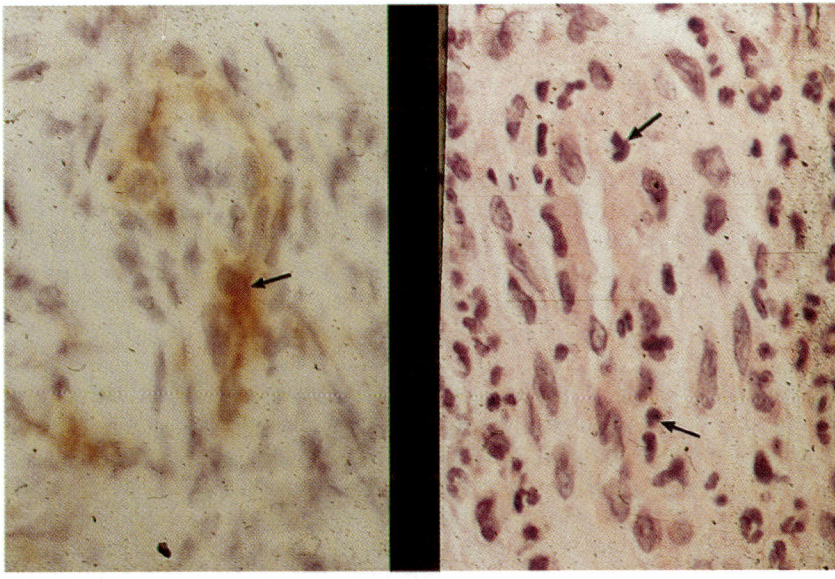

Figure 50.1 (a) Early vasculitis as shown by cloudy endothelial swelling, staining pink; note infiltrating leukocytes (arrow) in vessel wall. (b) Sequential sections from vessel in (a) showing endothelial cells stained for ELAM-1 expression (arrows).

its FcγRII receptor has led to the speculation that polymorphisms of this receptor may be relevant pathogenetically [4].

Infection with hepatitis B and hepatitis C has been implicated in the etiology of polyarteritis nodosa but only for a proportion of patients [5]. Hepatitis B virus has been isolated from circulating immune complexes and vasculitic lesions, although whether this merely reflects infection load has not yet been elucidated. Studies from dialysis centers which experience a high prevalence of hepatitis B infection have suggested that infected patients with vasculitis and associated aneurysmal dilation may experience regression of these features, as well as of the serological abnormalities, if they receive appropriate antiviral therapy. It should be remembered that generalized vasculitis may be a common complication, during the evolution of a variety of clinical infections. Such vasculitis has neither the serological associations nor the longevity of the pauci immune vasculitides.

That environmental factors may be important is sug-

gested by reports that vasculitis may have a seasonal incidence. However, whether these environmental factors such as epidemic infections are initiators or amplifiers of injury is uncertain, since, for example, it is well known that vasculitis may relapse in association with intercurrent infection.

Better evidence supports the role of drugs in producing vasculitis. Hydralazine is a frequently documented example. Rapidly progressive crescentic glomerulonephritis has been reported as a complication of hydralazine therapy in several studies with features which are clinically, histologically and serologically, indistinguishable from microscopic polyarteritis of the kidney [6]. Withdrawal of the drug alone was sometimes sufficient to achieve resolution of the nephritis, which otherwise usually responded to steroid treatment. Other small vessel vasculitic syndromes have been reported as adverse reactions to propyl thiouracil, again with appropriate histology and different serology [7].

Experimental models to study the etiology of vasculitis have been difficult to develop but, in both the Kinjoh mouse and the Brown Norway rat, a role for genetic factors in predisposing to vasculitic injury, which in the former incorporates a crescentic nephritis, is now emerging, as well as the identification of autoimmune phenomena, humoral and cellular, similar to those found in human vasculitis [8].

Pathogenesis

The demonstration by indirect immunofluorescence techniques that sera from patients with clinical syndromes typical of Wegener's granulomatosis or microscopic polyangiitis contained autoantibodies reactive with neutrophil cytoplasm antigens provided the first evidence that autoimmune mechanisms might underlie the development of the primary vasculitides (Figure 50.2). A variety of antigens have now been characterized, most of which are constituents of neutrophil granules. The two most important, proteinase 3 and myeloperoxidase, are linked to Wegener's granulomatosis and microscopic polyangiitis, respectively. Wegener's granulomatosis is closely associated with antibodies to proteinase 3; antibodies with such specificity have not consistently been reported in other clinical situations. The association is not absolute since autoantibodies with other specificities, particularly for myeloperoxidase, have been reported in patients with clinicopathological features compatible with classical Wegener's. Microscopic polyangiitis is associated with antibodies to myeloperoxidase, though the association is less close than is that for Wegener's with proteinase 3: diseases indistinguishable clinically from microscopic polyangiitis have been reported to be associated with antibodies with specificities for less common neutrophil antigens such as elastase, cathepsin

G and lactoferrin. Furthermore, antimyeloperoxidase antibodies have been reported in certain non-vasculitic disorders, thus raising questions as to whether variation in epitopic specificity may account for these discrepancies.

Nevertheless, clinical and laboratory studies have provided circumstantial evidence that antineutrophil cytoplasm antibodies are important in pathogenicity [9, 10]. Clinically a number of studies have shown that autoantibody levels correlate with disease activity. Relevant to this are findings that their subclass and affinity could be important variables explaining why certain patients with similar autoantibody levels had different degrees of disease activity. It must be remembered that there exists a small number of patients with biopsy-proven vasculitis, in whom such autoantibodies cannot be detected and for whom cellular mechanisms are perhaps of greater pathogenetic importance.

Laboratory studies have shown that *in vitro* antineutrophil cytoplasm antibodies may mediate the propagation of vasculitic injury by three main mechanisms. The first involves the binding of these antibodies to antigens such as proteinase 3 and myeloperoxidase expressed constitutively on the neutrophil membrane, thereby bringing about inappropriate neutrophil stimulation. There is concomitant cross linkage to the FcγR11 receptor, ostensibly by the Fc moiety of the autoantibody molecule. As a consequence, the neutrophil is activated, an effect enhanced if there is a degree of priming by cytokines such as tumor neurosis factor-α (TNF-α). Activation upregulates the expression of adhesion molecules of the β2 integrin family, particularly CD18, which facilitates binding of neutrophils to ligands such as ELAM-1, expressed on endothelium, and stimulates the neutrophil to release toxic oxygen species as part of the activation step. Co-culture experiments have shown that the com-

(a) (b)

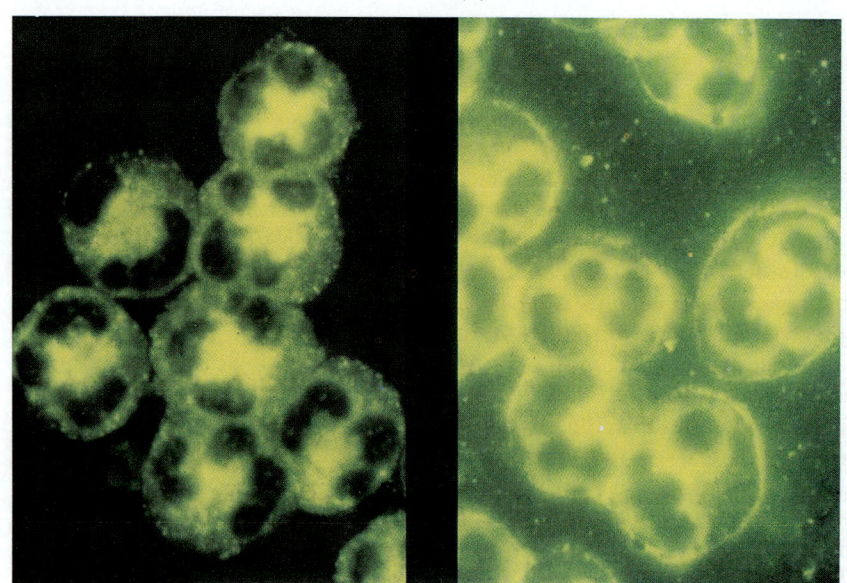

Figure 50.2 (a) c-ANCA staining of immobilized normal human polymorphonuclear leukocytes (PMN) from a patient with Wegener's granulomatosis; note granular staining with internuclear accentuation. (b) p-ANCA staining from a patient with microscopic polyangiitis; note perinuclear staining and the normal PMN cell membrane staining also.

bination of neutrophils and autoantibody on endothelial cell monolayers can produce endothelial injury. The second mechanism is dependent on the release of the relevant neutrophil autoantigens, together with the neutrophil constituents, as a consequence of autoantibody stimulation. The majority of these antigens are highly cationic and are attracted to the surface of the endothelium by the negative charge, an effect particularly important in the glomerulus which carries a particularly high anionic charge. Antineutrophil cytoplasm antibody binding to these previously planted antigens causes cytolysis, thereby initiating endothelial injury. Studies in the isolated experimental kidney, involving perfusion of myeloperoxidase followed by antimyeloperoxidase antibody, have shown that such injury may take place. A third mechanism postulates interference by autoantibodies with the complexing of the autoantigens, mostly enzymes, to their physiological inhibitors. This mechanism has been best elucidated in the context of proteinase 3, the physiological inactivators of which include α_1-antitrypsin. Patients with Wegener's granulomatosis, possessing a particular allelic polymorphism of the α_1-antitrypsin gene have been shown to have more extensive disease and to run a greater risk of mortality.

Clinical profiles

Wegener's granulomatosis

Wegener's granulomatosis [11] is a necrotizing granulomatous vasculitis which involves both the upper and lower respiratory tracts. Typically this is accompanied by a small vessel vasculitis of the kidney and to a variable extent other organs. Circulating autoantibodies to neutrophil cytoplasm antigens, usually to proteinase 3, can be found in most untreated patients at presentation.

Clinical presentation

Many patients develop clinical evidence of vasculitis against a background of non-specific symptoms such as malaise, weight loss, fever and night sweats, indicating a constitutional disturbance. There is also evidence of multisystem disease, reflecting the pattern of vasculitic involvement. The disease has an equal sex incidence and no ethnic group is exempt. The course is variable; some patients have indolent disease which takes months or years to declare itself, with long periods when the patient is relatively symptom-free; other patients develop fulminating life-threatening organ failure within weeks. Because any organ system may be involved the patient may be seen by a wide range of specialists, so that a varying spectrum of clinical involvement may be reported. With the predilection of the vasculitis to affect the airways, however, usually respiratory tract symptoms and signs predominate.

Upper respiratory tract

Bloody foul-smelling nasal discharge, paranasal sinus pain, nasal ulceration and septal perforation, and eventually a saddle nose deformity, may be present. Chronic suppurative otitis media due to a blocked eustachian tube, and occasionally painless deafness, due to eighth nerve involvement may develop. Hoarseness, due to granulomata on the vocal chords or stridor due to vasculitis in the trachea producing tracheal stenosis, may appear. Granulomatous space-occupying lesions in the sinuses may erode locally, leading to formation of fistula (Figure 50.3). Bacterial superinfection may be a significant clinical problem wherever the mucosal epithelium is breached.

Using whole-body scintiscanning techniques, to determine the distribution of autologous isotope-labeled neu-

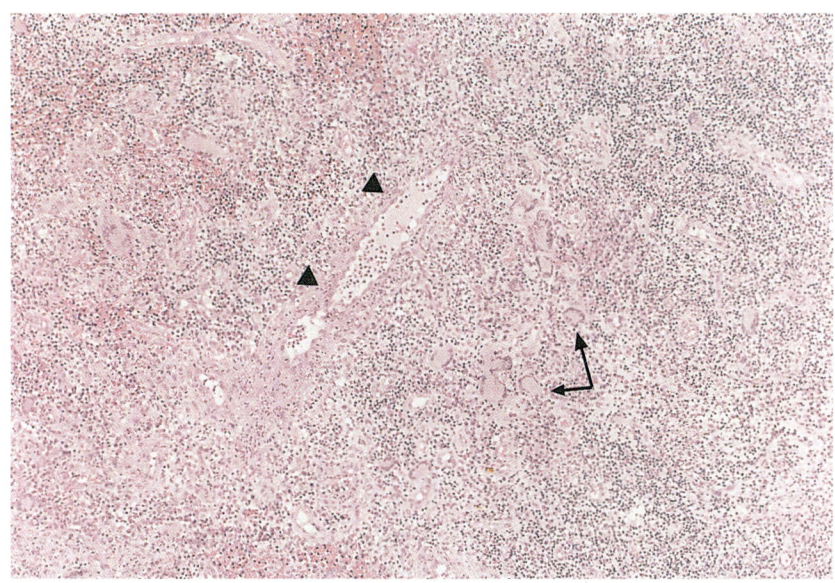

Figure 50.3 Granulomatous inflammation with many multinucleate cells (arrows) and vasculitis (arrowheads) in nasal soft tissue biopsy.

trophils, it has been possible to show that almost all patients with active Wegener's disease show abnormal focal uptake in or near the upper respiratory tract, particularly the paranasal airspaces [12]. This non-invasive assessment of the distribution of vasculitis has proved to be particularly helpful since it demonstrates involvement not ascertainable clinically even by ear, nose and throat specialists or computed tomography (CT) scanning. Sequential studies have proved invaluable in monitoring treatment.

Lower respiratory tract and lungs

Chronic non-productive cough, dyspnea, pleurisy and hemoptysis reflect vasculitis or granulomata in the airways or lung. Occasionally formation of exuberant endobronchial granulomatous tissue occludes the airway and leads to segmental collapse; more rarely an obliterative bronchiolitis may spread, sleeve-like along the bronchus or bronchiole. Extension into alveolar spaces either as a capillaritis (Figure 50.4) or necrotizing granulomatous pneumonic process may bring about a rapid deterioration in pulmonary function (Figures 50.5 and 50.6). It is an ominous development when accompanied by lung hemorrhage, this being particularly resistant to treatment. Although radiographs characteristically show there are pulmonary nodules which may cavitate, transient pulmonary infiltrates or more permanent changes of pulmonary fibrosis may also be found.

It has been shown the lung is almost always involved in Wegener's granulomatosis [13]. Bronchoscopy may reveal inflammatory endobronchial changes, even when CT is normal. Alveolar lavage in such circumstances reveals that the alveolitis is associated with pulmonary

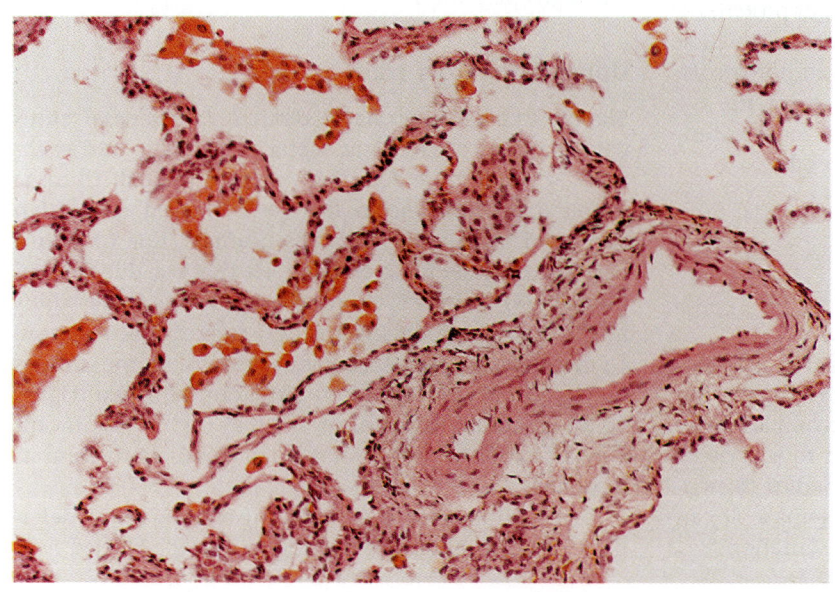

Figure 50.4 Capillaritis: capillary walls are expanded with inflammatory cells including neutrophils, and pigmented macrophages in the alveolar air spaces. Note the sparing of adjacent vessel.

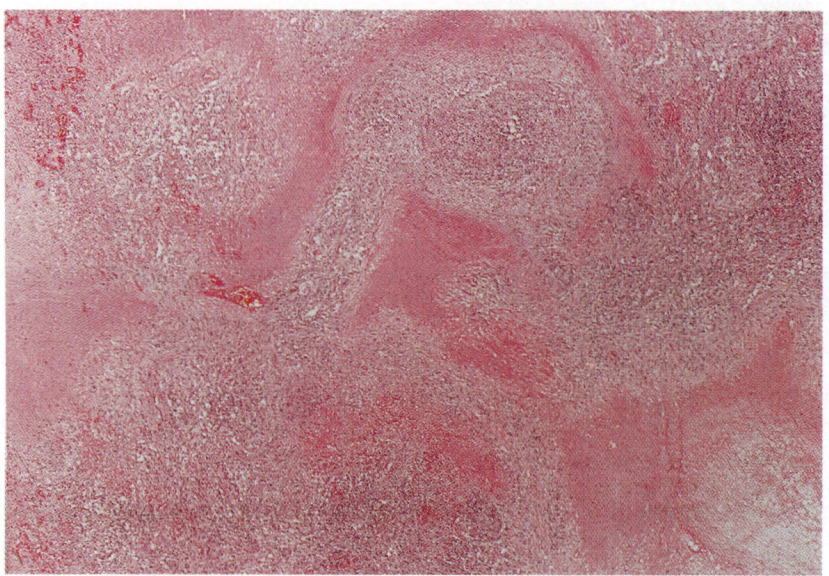

Figure 50.5 Palisading geographical necrosis of the lung with surrounding granulomatous inflammation.

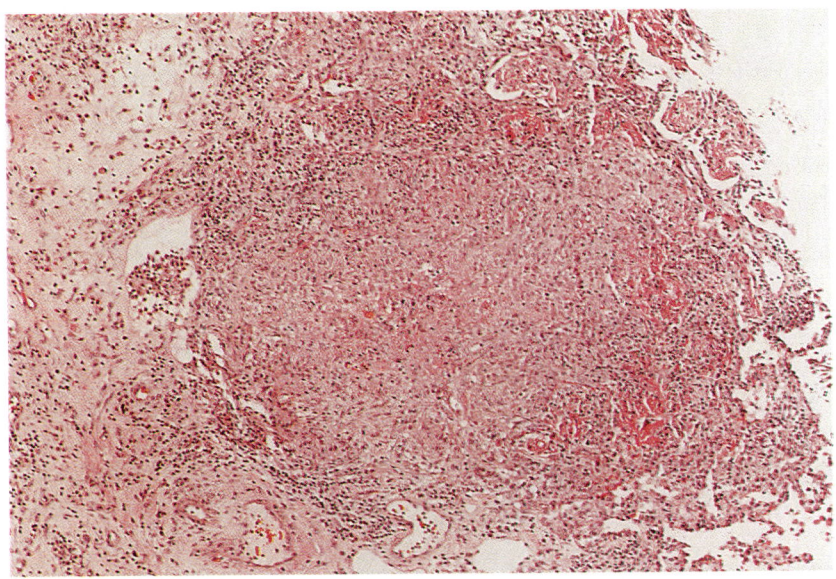

a

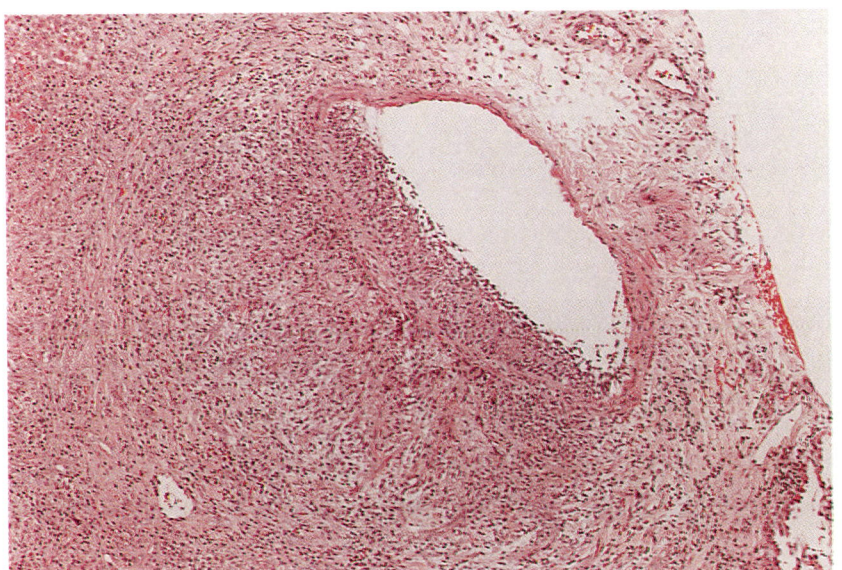

b

Figure 50.6 (a) Parenchymal granulomas and (b) granulomatous vasculitis seen in a florid case of pulmonary Wegener's granulomatosis.

production of antiproteinase 3 antibodies. This suggests that interaction between infection, the neutrophil response, autoantibodies and proteinase inhibitiors has a crucial bearing on pulmonary injury. Indeed, pulmonary injury can be generated experimentally by intratracheal instillation of proteinase 3 in hamsters.

Renal involvement

The renal injury has particular importance because until renal replacement therapy became widely available, the prognosis of the disease was determined by the nature of the renal injury and its response to treatment. Even in the presence of normal renal function, early renal involvement may be suspected if there is asymptomatic proteinuria or hematuria. At this stage renal biopsy may show only a minor focal proliferative glomerulonephritis (Figure 50.7). The tempo of the renal disease is unpre-

dictable and the sudden deterioration in renal function, in the presence of red cell casts in the urine, may indicate the development of an acute focal necrotizing glomerular capillaritis with crescent formation, the histological hallmark of rapidly progressive nephritis (Figure 50.8). Examination of the renal biopsy by immunofluorescence characteristically reveals few if any antibodies as immune deposits, i.e. pauci immune nephritis. Occasionally in a patient with impaired renal function, biopsy may show no evidence of actual vasculitis; segmental scarring and fibrosed crescents in glomeruli may indicate the previous involvement of the kidney in an episode of Wegener's granulomatosis which did not subsequently progress (Figure 50.9). Although the glomerulus usually bears the brunt of the disease, this is not always the case, so that occasionally the histological picture may be that of a granulomatous tubulointerstitial nephritis (Figure 50.10).

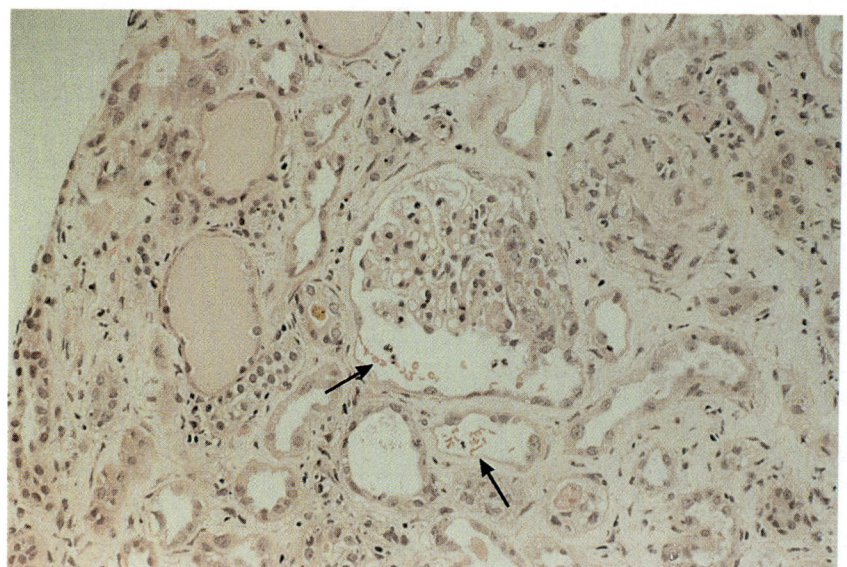

Figure 50.7 Red blood cells in Bowman's space and in proximal tubules (arrow), with mild proliferative changes in the glomerulus.

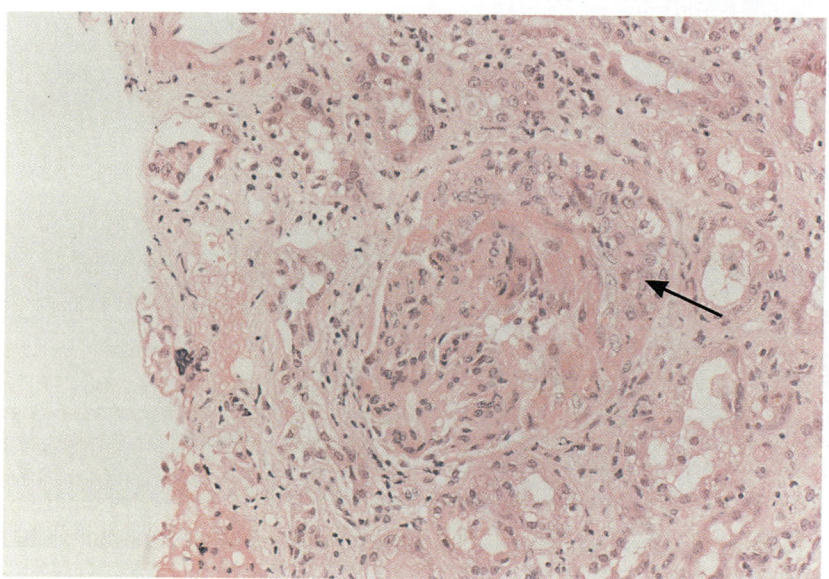

Figure 50.8 Necrotizing glomerulonephritis with destruction of capillary loops, fibrin, neutrophils and a cellular crescent (arrow).

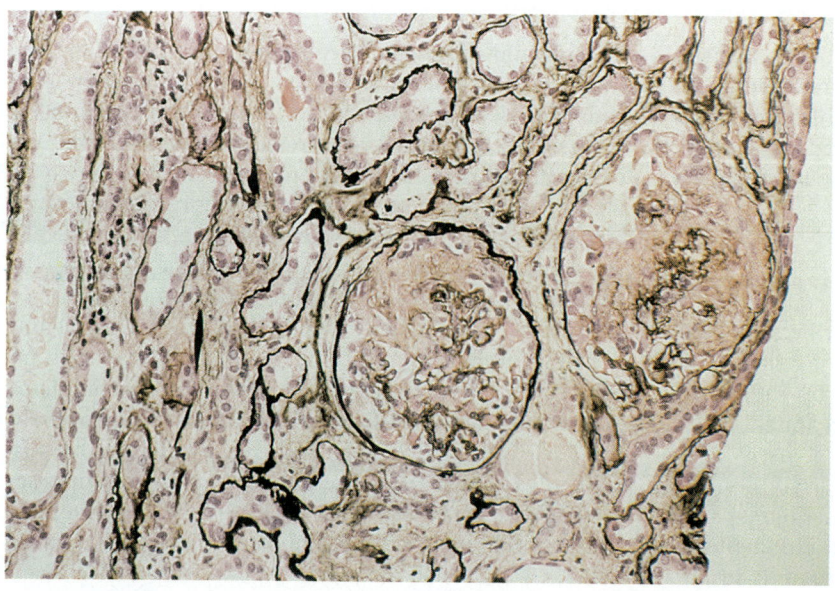

Figure 50.9 Segmental scarring with fibrous crescents indicative of previous active renal involvement.

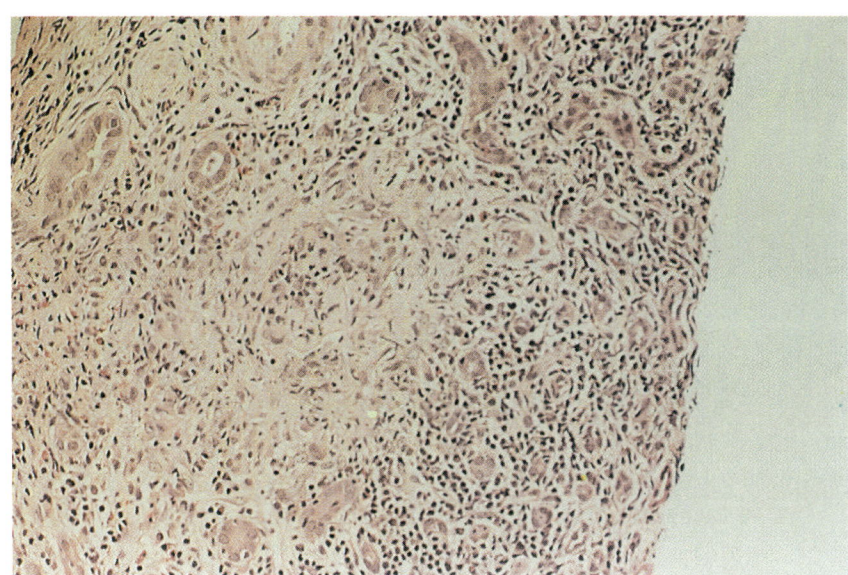

Figure 50.10 Granulomatous destruction of glomerulus with an accompanying tubulointerstitial nephritis.

Recurrent involvement of the transplanted kidney in a patient with known Wegener's disease is always a risk. Periodic measurements of GFR are an important component of postallograft management.

The eye

Conjunctivitis, uveitis and scleritis may all occur in Wegener's granulomatosis, but the finding of proptosis, due to retro-orbital development of granulomatous vasculitis forming a pseudotumor, is particularly important. First, in the context of respiratory tract disease or nephritis proptosis is strongly suggestive of Wegener's granulomatosis; second, in approximately 50% of patients it causes loss of vision because of optic nerve ischemia and third, due to involvement of the extraocular muscles, it may be responsible for the loss of conjugate gaze and diplopia.

Other manifestations

Most patients experience generalized myalgias and arthralgias at some stage in the disease, less frequently a symmetrical polyarthritis may develop. Occasionally the arthritis may be restricted to one or few joints. Joint deformity is not a feature of arthritis in Wegener's granulomatosis, however. A variety of lesions can be found in the skin. These vary from infarcts in nail folds and purpuric rashes to isolated ulcers, vesicles and papules. Biopsy occasionally discloses granulomata typical of Wegener's granulomatosis. Nervous system involvement is unusual but can be severely debilitating. Mononeuritis multiplex is the commonest neurological lesion; occasionally central nervous system abnormalities are found, including isolated lesions of the cranial nerves, meningeal involvement and stroke.

Wegener's granulomatosis of the heart is rare but pericarditis and coronary arteritis have been reported as well as arrhythmias attributed to granulomata in the conducting bundles of Hiss. Very rarely biopsy-proven disease has been described in the breast, ureter, vagina, cervix (Figure 50.11), spleen (Figure 50.12) and parotid gland.

'Limited' Wegener's granulomatosis is the term given to the condition in which there is only restricted involvement clinically and in most patients it means the disease is limited to the upper respiratory tract. Sometimes this situation persists for many years before progression to organs becomes manifest; occasionally subclinical disease is only discovered at autopsy. There was an impression that limited Wegener's granulomatosis ran a more benign course and was easier to treat, but with the advent of serological tests to diagnose the condition more readily it has become evident that milder, generalized forms of the disease also exist and so the prognostic and therapeutic distinction is no longer evident.

Diagnosis

The diagnosis may be suspected clinically from the combination of disease in the upper or lower airways and renal involvement. Usually there are constitutional symptoms; malaise, fever, night sweats and weight loss. Biopsy confirmation may prove to be frustrating, since histological evidence of granulomatous vasculitis is often hard to obtain.

Usually the kidney provides the most suitable tissue, although transbronchial biopsies are also useful. In the kidney the diagnostic requirement is the demonstration of focal necrosis of the glomerular capillary wall in the absence of other primary glomerular pathology. The differential diagnosis then lies between other small vessel vasculitides, such as microscopic polyangiitis and Henoch–Schönlein purpura, systemic lupus erythematosus or Goodpasture's syndrome associated with

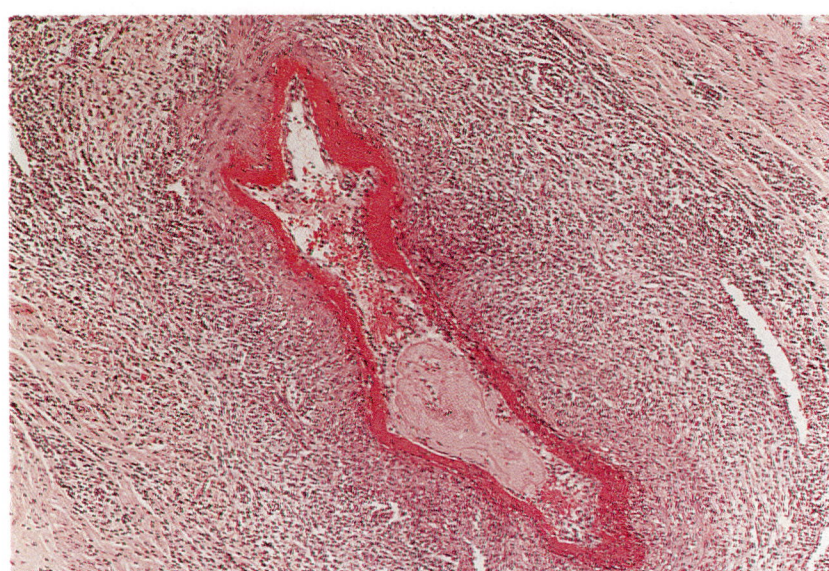

Figure 50.11 Incidental finding of a fibrinoid arteritis in serosal vessels of the cervix.

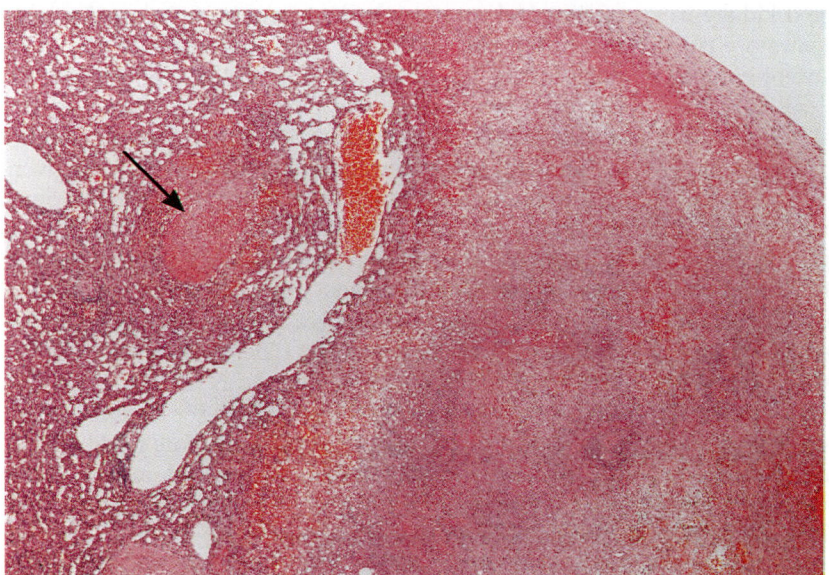

Figure 50.12 Characteristic geographical necrosis in the spleen with a fibrinoid arteritis (arrow).

antiglomerular basement membrane (GBM) antibodies. Immunofluorescence staining of the tissue may be helpful since: (1) mesangial deposits of IgA are characteristic of Henoch–Schönlein disease; (2) glomerular and extraglomerular capillary immunoglobulin deposits of any, and sometimes all isotypes, as well as complement, are found in lupus nephritis; and (3) linear deposits of IgG along the GBM are the hallmark of anti-GBM nephritis. Glomerular immunoglobulin deposits, if present, are typically scanty in Wegener's granulomatosis and microscopic polyangiitis, accounting for the term 'pauci immune nephritis' often used to describe the renal lesion in both diseases. Further distinction between these two disorders has to depend on the clinical context and autoantibody specificity, because granulomata are rarely found in the kidney.

Until recently there was no diagnostic laboratory test for Wegener's granulomatosis. However, growing evidence now suggests that antineutrophil cytoplasm antibodies with specificity for proteinase 3 are closely associated with the development of the disease; rarely have autoantibodies with this specificity validated by accepted criteria (immunoblotting, immunoprecipitation and competitive inhibition studies using pure molecular species) been reported in other conditions and in none consistently. Thus anti proteinase 3 antibodies are proving to be valuable for the diagnosis of Wegener's granulomatosis, frequently alerting the physician to the need for careful evaluation of multisystem symptomatology and close supervision of the patient during follow-up of a suspected case. As mentioned above, antibodies to proteinase 3 can be found in 85% of untreated patients with generalized Wegener's granulomatosis and in approximately 60% of those with limited disease. Other abnormal laboratory findings, characteristic of any small vessel vasculitis in the untreated acute phase, include, almost invariably, normochromic normocytic anemia, neutrophil leukocytosis, thrombocytosis and evidence of an acute phase response (raised erythrocyte sedimentation rate and C reactive protein), as well as in 80% of patients, a polyclonal increase in immunoglobulins and, in 50%, a positive rheumatoid factor.

Differential diagnosis

The clinical presentation with pulmonary renal involvement and distinctive serology has made the differential diagnosis of the patient with Wegener's granulomatosis relatively straightforward. Atypical forms with either limited disease or negative serology may still cause problems. In such circumstances lung tumors or other causes of granulomata, such as tuberculosis or sarcoid may be suspected. Differentiation from other vasculitides or connective tissue diseases may be difficult. Distinction from the pulmonary renal presentation of Goodpasture's syndrome may be difficult because the two can co-exist, but it is important because the implications for treatment are different. The presence of circulating anti-GBM antibodies in patients with Goodpasture's syndrome is usually helpful here.

Idiopathic 'lethal' midline granuloma may present with features suggestive of Wegener's granulomatosis limited to the head and neck. This condition is thought to be a variant of a T cell lymphoma that is locally invasive and not found elsewhere other than the head and neck. Unlike Wegener's disease it may produce destructive ulceration of facial tissues although both disease tissues can erode through upper airways. In idiopathic midline granuloma, laboratory tests reflect the absence of inflammatory vasculitis with near normal sedimentation rate or C reactive protein level, white blood cell count and platelet count.

Lymphomatoid granulomatosis is extremely rare but closely resembles Wegener's granulomatosis in multiorgan distribution including lungs, kidney, upper respiratory tract and central nervous system; it differs in the nature of the blood vessel involvement. There is no inflammatory infiltrate; instead the vessel destruction appears to be mediated by infiltrates of lymphocytes of either T or B cell lineage. Transformation to lymphoma eventually occurs in approximately half the patients. In keeping with absence of inflammation, elevated values of C reactive protein, sedimentation rate and white blood cell count are usually not present.

Microscopic polyangiitis

Microscopic polyangiitis [14] is a vasculitis of small blood vessels which may affect any organ in the body, either singly or in multisystem fashion. Disease limited to a single organ is not uncommon, and has been well described for the kidney, gut and skin. Evolution to a multisystem disease may occur later, up to several years after presentation. Circulating autoantibodies to a variety of neutrophil cytoplasm antigens, predominantly myeloperoxidase, can be found in many patients.

Clinical presentation

The disease has an equal sex incidence and is not restricted by age or race. Constitutional disturbance manifested by fever, night sweats, weight loss and profound malaise is common and it may be several weeks before organ-specific symptoms arise. In one-third of patients a 'flu'-like prodromal illness may occur prior to presentation.

Renal involvement

The kidney is almost always involved in microscopic polyangiitis and up to 100% of patients have proteinuria and hematuria during their illness. Although occasionally mild at first, there is usually a glomerulonephritis of moderate severity which may run a rapidly progressive course. However, it is not possible to predict the outcome, based on the level of serum creatinine at referral. Renal biopsy usually reflects the severity of the vasculitis. The presence of focal necrosis of glomerular capillary walls supports the diagnosis. For some time nephrologists have recognized idiopathic rapidly progressive nephritis as a form fruste of microscopic polyangiitis limited to the kidney, which should be treated in the same way as generalized polyangiitis (Figure 50.13).

Lung involvement

Angitis of the pulmonary circulation may manifest as cough, pleurisy, dyspnea or hemoptysis. Radiologically there may be opacification or segmental atelectasis. The most serious complication is lung hemorrhage which can be profuse and occasionally fatal.

Other manifestations

Purpuric rashes are common and splinter hemorrhages may be found. Arthralgias are a frequent complaint, the joint involvement usually being symmetrical; arthritis is less common and joint deformation is not a feature of this vasculitis. Mononeuritis multiplex is a particularly debilitating complication of polyangiitis. Gastrointestinal symptoms may include non-specific abdominal pain, diarrhea or gastrointestinal hemorrhage (Figure 50.14). Patients with microscopic polyangiitis do not frequently have upper respiratory tract or ocular symptoms, in contrast to patients with Wegener's granulomatosis, nor do they have asthma and flitting pulmonary infiltrates in contrast to the Churg–Strauss syndrome, neither do they present with severe hypertension and large viscus perfo-

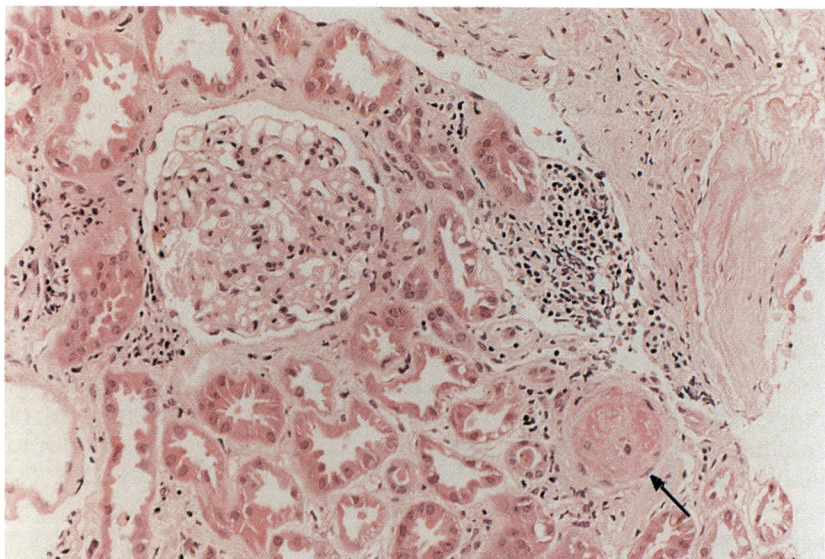

Figure 50.13 A fibrinoid arteriolitis (arrow) accompanies mild proliferative glomerular changes in microscopic polyangiitis.

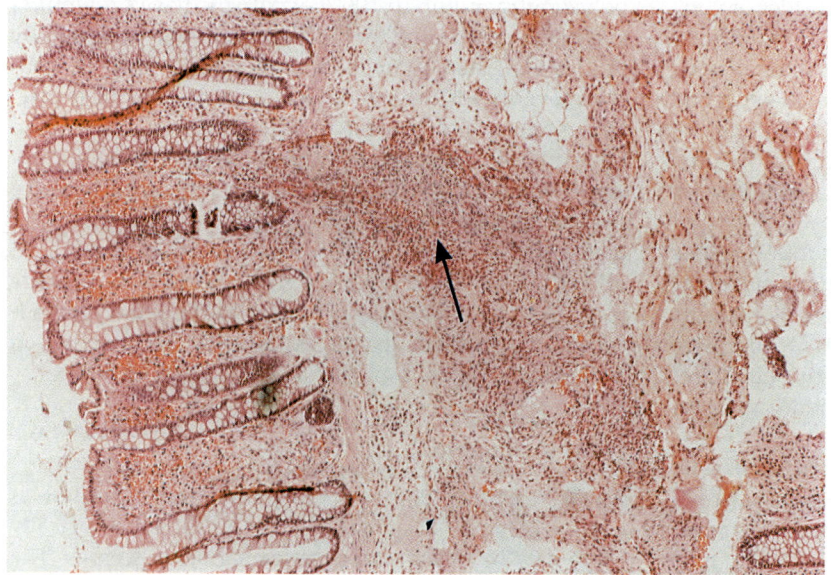

Figure 50.14 Mixed inflammatory cells infiltrate a submucosal vessel in the ileum (arrow).

ration or organ infarction as may occur in polyarteritis nodosa.

Diagnosis

The diagnosis of microscopic polyangiitis may be suspected in a patient with constitutional symptoms of malaise, fever, weight loss and night sweats not accounted for by infection and neoplasm, in whom there is evidence of multiple organ dysfunction. Confirmation of the diagnosis may come from biopsy of the affected organ, of which the organ with the highest postive yield is usually the kidney. Segmental vascular necrosis with an inflammatory cell infiltrate at any biopsy site may provide a useful clue to the diagnosis. It must be remembered that these pathological changes may be seen near epithelial surfaces that have been breached due to a variety of causes, such as infection, trauma or neoplasm, in association with other pathology such as tumor and abscess, or in other connective tissue diseases such as rheumatoid arthritis and systemic lupus erythematosus. The finding of focal segmental necrosis of glomerular capillary walls does, however, restrict the diagnosis to microscopic polyangiitis or to other small vessel vasculitides, such as found in Wegener's granulomatosis, systemic lupus erythematosis, Goodpasture's syndrome, cryoglobulinemia or Henoch–Schönlein purpura. The first four of these respectively have distinctive circulating immunoglobulins, detectable as autoantibodies to proteinase 3, DNA, GBM or isolatable as cryoglobulins. All have characteristic deposits of immunoglobulin in the renal biopsy except microscopic polyangiitis and

Wegener's granulomatosis, where such deposits are not found.

The detection of circulating antineutrophil cytoplasm antibodies has contributed greatly to the laboratory diagnosis of microscopic polyangiitis. Usually they have specificity for myeloperoxidase but occasionally clinical syndromes present with antibodies to lactoferrin, elastase or cathepsin G. In the correct clinical context, the detection of these antibodies is very helpful but it must be remembered that autoantibodies with similar specificities may be found in other conditions which are not primary vasculitides, for example, inflammatory gastrointestinal diseases, such as chronic active hepatitis, sclerosing cholangitis, Crohn's disease and ulcerative colitis. Other laboratory findings which are abnormal as in other vasculitides, include a normochromic normocytic anemia, raised sedimentation rate or C reactive protein, and a leukocytosis. Frequently there is thrombocythemia. Hyperglobulinemia and, occasionally, positive rheumatoid factors may be found.

Differential diagnosis

The differential diagnosis usually has to be considered among three categories of patients, those presenting with pyrexia of unknown origin, with malignancies and with covert infection. The differential diagnosis may be particularly difficult since vasculitis may be evident as rash in patients from any of those, for example, associated with sarcoid or SBE in those with pyrexia of unknown origin, with carcinoma or leukemia in those with malignancy or with tuberculosis or syphilis in those with infection. All of these disorders may also show additional multisystem involvement due to the underlying disease. These diagnostic problems, therefore, emphasize the importance of antineutrophil cytoplasm antibody detection, since in none of the preceding conditions have such autoantibodies consistently been found.

Polyarteritis nodosa

Polyarteritis nodosa [15] is a vasculitis of medium sized arteries in which aneurysm formation is frequent. The clinical manifestations reflect the size of vessel involved: major organ infarction may affect the intestinal, renal or cerebral vasculature. Moderate to severe hypertension is common. In many patients an overlap with microscopic polyangiitis is apparent clinically and at biopsy. Circulating antineutrophil cytoplasm antibodies are rarely found and when present may indicate the coincident development of the smaller vessel vasculitis. An association with hepatitis B antigenemia is evident in certain patient populations.

Clinical presentation

The disease may present at any age and is commoner in men (male to female ratio 2:1). Constitutional disturbance with tachycardia, fever and weight loss is frequent and may be accompanied by striking clinical signs such as an acute abdomen, myocardial infarction, cerebrovascular accident in young people, or severe hypertension.

Renal involvement

Extraglomerular arteritis rarely occurs alone; often a glomerular capillaritis similar to microscopic polyangiitis is found. Proteinuria, hematuria and casts are evidence of renal involvement. Additional clinical findings such as malignant hypertension or frank hematuria may reflect the contribution of ischemia or infarction due to larger vessel vasculitis (Figure 50.15). Progressive renal failure

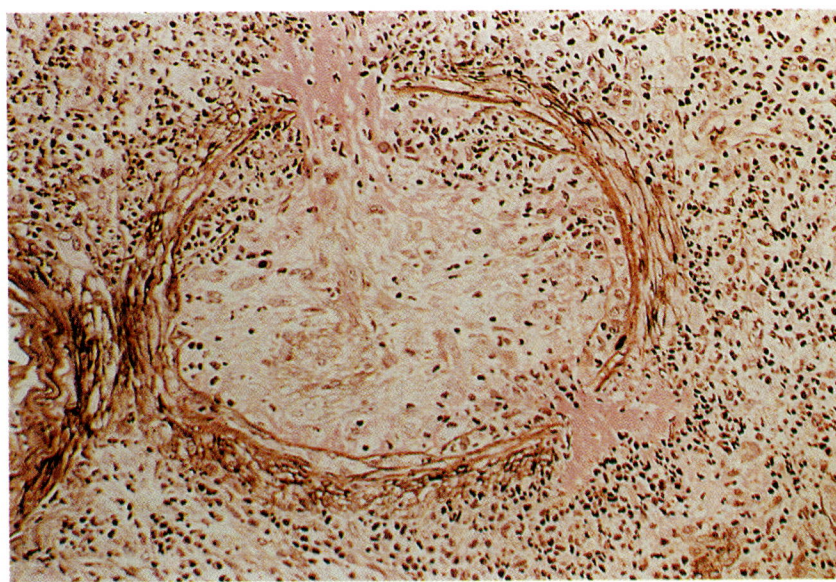

Figure 50.15 An active chronic arteritis in an arcuate renal artery. The lumen contains organizing thrombus with fibrin leaking through the disrupted vessel wall (methanamine silver).

was an important cause of death before renal replacement therapy became available.

Cardiac involvement

Coronary arteritis is an important cause of intractable heart failure or death due to myocardial infarction. The cardiac involvement may be compounded by other cardiac complications including acute vasculitic pericarditis and renovascular hypertension.

Gastrointestinal tract

Typically the patient presents with severe abdominal pain or gastrointestinal hemorrhage from mucosal ulceration or perforation. Polyarteritis may affect single organs mimicking acute cholecystitis, pancreatitis or appendicitis. Liver involvement may cause hepatitis or even necro-

sis. There is no distinctive clinical entity associated with hepatitis B polyarteritis, however.

Skin

Cutaneous involvement varies from vasculitic purpura or urticaria to subcutaneous hemorrhage with gangrene (Figure 50.16). The presence of palpable nodules near to the course of superficial arteries is a distinctive feature of polyarteritis nodosa. These may reach the size of a large pea, and can persist from days to months. Rarely these small 'nodose' aneurysms may cause ulceration in the surrounding skin.

Other manifestations

Arthralgias and myalgias are frequently present. Neurological manifestations are rare. A stroke from cerebral vas-

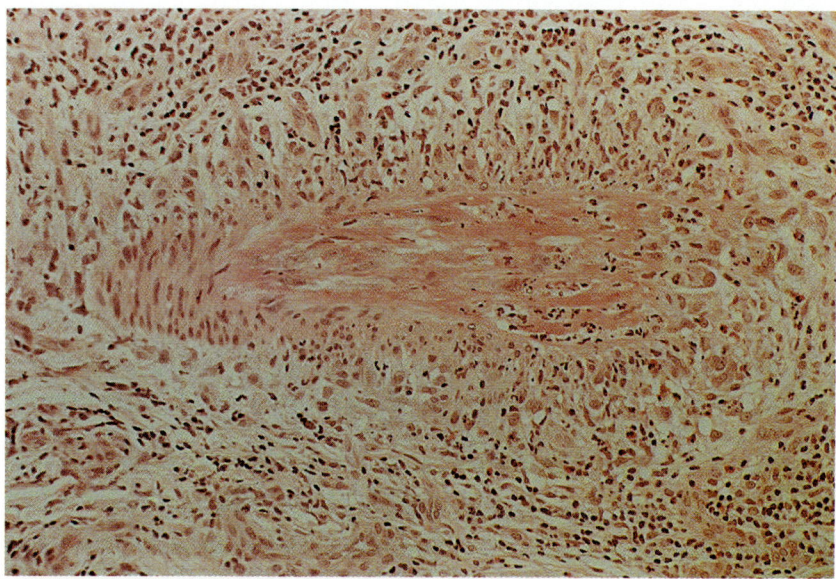

a

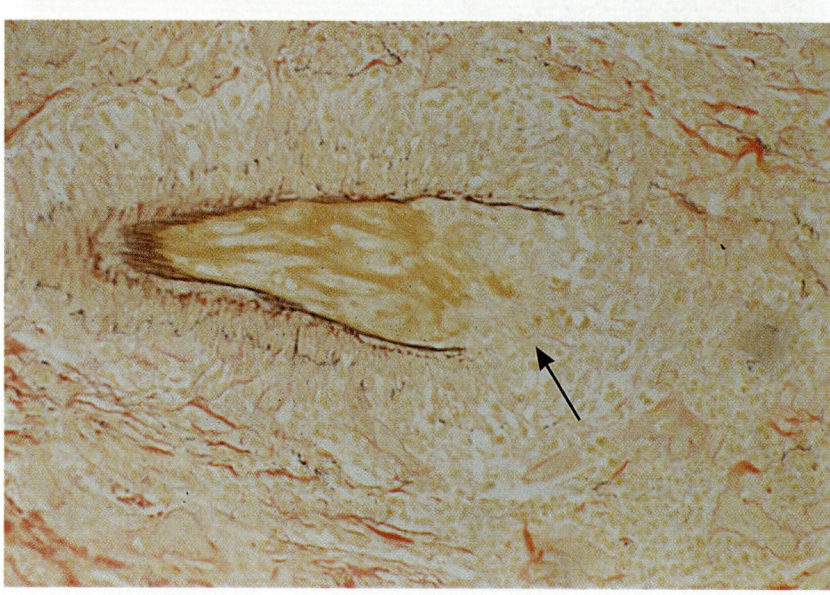

b

Figure 50.16 (a) Fibrinoid vasculitis in a subcutaneous vessel with transmural, almost granulomatous inflammation and (b) destruction of the elastic lamina (arrow).

culitis or visual disturbance due to retinal aneurysms and hemorrhage (visible fundoscopically) are the most striking. Mononeuritis multiplex secondary to arteritis of the vasa nervorum may produce peripheral neurological signs. Rarely, polyarteritis nodosa may affect the ovaries, testes (Figure 50.17), epididymi, salivary gland (Figure 50.18) or bladder.

Diagnosis

It is unusual for polyarteritis to present without clinical features of a microscopic polyarteritis but superimposition of dysfunction of any of the major organs, together with hypertension, are useful pointers to the diagnosis of polyarteritis nodosa. The diagnosis may be confirmed by angiography or by histology of affected tissue.

There are no specific laboratory tests for polyarteritis nodosa. However, almost all patients have a normochromic normocytic anemia, raised sedimentation rate or C reactive protein and leukocytosis.

Differential diagnosis

The differential diagnosis for the size of vessel involved in polyarteritis nodosa makes it worth excluding two other multisystem vascular occlusive diseases. First, thrombotic thrombocytopenic purpura is readily distinguished from thrombocytopenia and intravascular hemolysis; second, Degos disease, which is an occlusive arterial disease affecting skin, gastrointestinal tract and brain is distinguished by its skin lesions which are distributed centrifugally towards the extremities. They

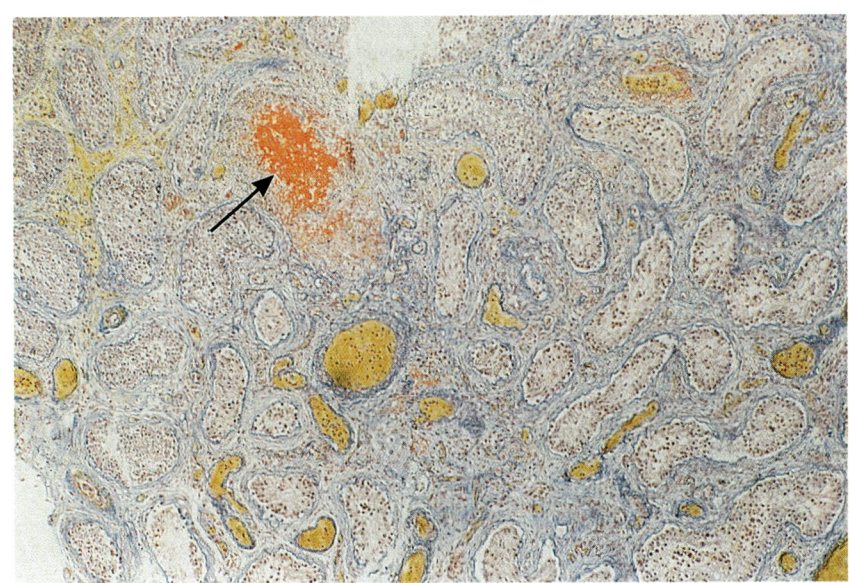

Figure 50.17 Testis with seminiferous tubules and dilated vessels (yellow). Fibrin (red arrow) marks destruction of an arterial wall (Trichrome).

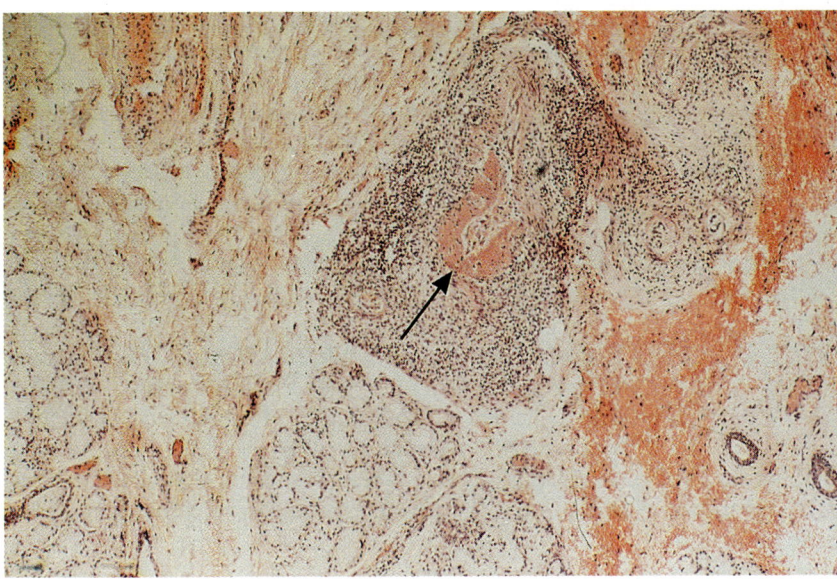

Figure 50.18 Minor salivary glands with a single small artery (arrow) showing fibrinoid inflammation.

undergo a typical course starting as pink–grey papules, which develop a depressed scaly center surrounded by an elevated red margin.

Management of the systemic vasculitides

Monitoring disease activity

Standard tests of organ function should be used to monitor the effect of treatment on disease activity. Serial measurements of the sedimentation rate and C reactive protein levels are a useful guide as to whether the vasculitis has been brought under control, but are relatively non-specific, being elevated by intercurrent infection, other causes of inflammation or vasculitic injury. Many centers use serial antineutrophil cytoplasm antibody measurements to monitor treatment [16, 17] with an aim to reduce these levels to background during induction therapy, withdrawing treatment at an earlier stage if control of the autoimmune response can be demonstrated in this manner. It must be noted, however, that certain patients have persistently raised autoantibody levels despite no evident disease activity. A very small number of patients exhibit the reverse discordancy, they have undetectable autoantibody but continuing vasculitis.

Autologous indium-labeled polymorph nuclear scanning has been used to detect covert vasculitis, unsuspected clinically and radiologically. Scans performed at 3 and 24 h after reinjection of labeled leukocytes have demonstrated that persistent foci of uptake, revealed by the gamma camera imaging, are commonly found in the upper airways in patients with Wegener's granulomatosis. Other foci can frequently be revealed in the lungs. Serial studies have enabled the effects of treatment to be monitored and, when performed prospectively have been valuable in predicting relapse.

Conventional treatment of systemic vasculitis

Cytotoxic drugs and steroids are conventionally the mainstays of treatment for the small vessel vasculitides [18]. Usually these are combined, at high dose, in an induction regimen to gain effective control of the disease activity at presentation which is followed after two months by a lower dose, maintenance regimen for the longer term, in which other immunosuppressive agents may substitute for cyclophosphamide.

Induction therapy

Empirically it has been determined that doses of cyclophosphamide at 3 mg/kg body weight (rounded down to the nearest 50 mg) are suitable for the induction

of remission. This dosage should be lowered or discontinued temporarily if the total white cell count falls to less than 4.0×10^9/l, or the neutrophil leukocyte count falls to less than 2.0×10^9/l. Cytotoxic therapy should also be modified if severe infection occurs. In the older patients, aged 55 years or over, a lower induction dose of 2 mg/kg is often given because of the greater susceptibility of the elderly to bone marrow immunosuppression and infection. Steroids are given at high dose, initially prednisolone 60 mg/day, tapering at weekly intervals until at two months the patient is receiving 10 mg/day.

Maintenance therapy

Usually cyclophosphamide can be substituted by the same dose of azathioprine at two months and at the same time steroid treatment may be converted into an alternate day regimen. Both drugs may then gradually be withdrawn at 12 months.

Other treatments

The use of pulse dose (0.75–1 g i.v.) cyclophosphamide or prednisolone has been advocated by some. Recent evidence suggests, however, that pulse cyclophosphamide is less effective at maintaining remission than oral cyclophosphamide. Furthermore, since the active metabolites of cyclophosphamide are in part excreted in the urine in patients with nephritis, lower dose oral therapy should allow more accurate titration of dose effect. It remains to be demonstrated whether pulse administration of prednisolone is superior for the management of systemic vasculitis.

For patients who are intolerant of cyclophosphamide perhaps the most useful drug is azathioprine. Where disease activity is not controllable by either drug, other immunomodulatory agents such as methotrexate or cyclosporin A have been tried. Although some patients benefit, as yet there is no substantial evidence to warrant their use as first-line agents in management.

The use of trimethoprim–sulphamethoxazole has enjoyed a vogue for the management of systemic vasculitis, particularly Wegener's granulomatosis. With the advent of better diagnostic criteria, however, careful exclusion of intercurrent infections (particularly a problem in Wegener's that affects the upper respiratory tract) and study of controls given trimethoprim–sulphamethoxazole alone, doubts have been cast over the efficacy of this agent.

In patients who have fulminating vasculitis, threatening vital organ function, then intensive plasma exchange may be beneficial. Evidence from several studies suggests that such an approach may benefit patients with severe renal vasculitis (requiring dialysis support), lung hemorrhage due to pulmonary vasculitis, or coma due to cerebral vasculitis.

Problems with conventional therapy

Conventional treatment for patients with multisystem vasculitis, such as Wegener's granulomatosis and microscopic polyangiitis, has usually combined steroids and cytotoxic agents, most frequently cyclophosphamide or azathioprine, in a high-dose induction regimen to achieve remission, followed by a lower dose maintenance regimen to safeguard the remission long term. This empirical approach was used for two main reasons: first, without a specific laboratory test, it was difficult to segregate the vasculitides into homogeneous syndromes and assign them to treatment protocols, since clinically they form a spectrum of closely related diseases; second, a limited understanding of the pathogenetic mechanisms underlying their evolution had hampered the development of more specific therapies. Experience with high dose induction regimens for patients with Wegener's granulomatosis has shown that, although marked improvement might eventually be achieved in 90% of patients, the median time to achieve remission on treatment was 12 months and relapses were frequent, occurring in up to 50% of patients during follow-up, necessitating further courses of therapy. Similar rates of relapse were found in other series. Substantial morbidity was encountered in these patients, not only due to the disease but directly due to the treatment itself. In Wegener's granulomatosis, glucocorticoid-induced cataract and osteopenic fractures complicated the course of patients receiving steroids in 21% and 11%, respectively, all of whom developed cushingoid features. Cytotoxic drug-induced female infertility or hemorrhagic cystitis were problems attendant on the use of cyclophosphamide in 57% and 43% respectively. Compared to an age and sex matched population, there was a 33-fold increased risk of the development of bladder cancer. There existed considerable scope for alternative treatments which might be safer and more specific.

New therapeutic strategies

High dose intravenous immunoglobulin therapy (IVIg)

The basis for the use of intravenous immunoglobulin (IVIg) [19, 20] in the management of patients with systemic vasculitis was formulated on laboratory and clinical observations. Laboratory experiments had shown that antineutrophil cytoplasm antibody reactivities could be neutralized by IVIg in a manner consistent with idiotypic reactivities predicted by the network theory. Anti-idiotypic activity could be identified in IVIg. Similar anti-idiotypic activity could be detected in normal sera from certain individuals and during remission in others who had been treated for systemic vasculitis. Sequential studies in these patients showed that circulating anti-idiotypic antibodies to antineutrophil cytoplasm antibody fluctuated with disease activity. Clinical observations were drawn most persuasively from experience of the use of IVIg for Kawasaki's disease, a childhood form of antineutrophil cytoplasm antibody-associated vasculitis. Treatment with IVIg reduced coronary artery aneurysms, a feature of this vasculitis. Other data from controlled trials all pointed to the efficacy of IVIg in the management of this disorder. Studies showed that for a range of autoimmune diseases a considerable potential existed for IVIg to bring about sustained remission.

Studies of IVIg in systemic vasculitis have been carried out in three stages. The first study used IVIg for the management of patients refractory to conventional high-dose steroids and cytotoxic agents [19, 20]. Encouraging results led to the establishment of a multicenter, placebo controlled, randomized prospective study of IVIg for patients with such refractory vasculitis, which is still in progress. A third study has tested the effect of IVIg alone in the management of previously untreated disease.

In the first study 26 patients have so far been treated [19]. Their diagnosis consisted of Wegener's granulomatosis (14), microscopic polyangiitis (11), and rheumatoid vasculitis (1). All patients had disease refractory to conventional therapy with steroids and cytotoxic drugs. Treatment consisted of IVIg (Sandoglobulin), given as a total dose of 2 g/kg. Effects of treatment were monitored by changes in sedimentation rate, C reactive protein, gamma camera imaging, and antineutrophil cytoplasm antibody titers. Results showed that by two months there was full remission in 50% of the patients and partial remission in the remainder: full remission was defined as the maximum improvement which could be achieved given the morbidity of the vasculitis judged on an individual patient basis. Clinical improvement was accompanied by falls in C reactive protein, sedimentation rate and autoantibody titers, and improvement in the paired white cell scans compared to pre-IVIg. After one year of follow-up 19 out of 26 patients were still in remission. Six patients were in partial remission and one patient died from overwhelming sepsis. As well as the clinical benefits the previous drug therapy could also be reduced. The mean dose of cyclophosphamide or azathioprine which was 55 mg daily, had fallen modestly to 50 mg daily by 12 months; the mean daily dose of prednisolone had fallen from 16 mg to 6 mg by the same time. Similar beneficial effects of the use of IVIg in refractory Wegener's have come from other groups in Europe and the United States. At the present stage the randomized placebo-controlled trial has now recruited some 28 of the 36 patients required for appropriate statistical analysis to be carried out.

The results of the open study have led us to try to determine whether IVIg has a place for the management of systemic vasculitis at first referral. Six patients with mild, seemingly stable and non-progressive disease were selected for such treatment. There were three patients with Wegener's and three with microscopic polyangiitis. Similar treatment and monitoring were carried out, as in the studies mentioned above. At one year four patients were still in remission. However, for two patients the response was only transient and conventional therapy was subsequently used for these two. Although the number of patients receiving IVIg alone for the treatment of vasculitis is small, the responses observed highlight the need to understand which component of the treatment interferes with the pathogenetic mechanisms underlying the development of the autoimmunity.

The complication of IVIg treatment for the groups of patients described above have been mild. Approximately one quarter of the patients experienced rashes and occasional arthralgias and headaches during infusion of the IVIg and for a few hours after that, were common problems as has been noted by others when IVIg was used for treatment of non-vasculitic conditions. The most worrisome observation was that the infusion was frequently accompanied by a transient and reversible deterioration in renal function in those patients who had a modest degree of renal impairment at the time of entry to the study. It appeared that those patients with a plasma creatinine of 200 µml/l or greater were the most likely to show such alteration. The mechanism underlying this nephrotoxicity is as yet unclear, but may be related to the osmotic agent used to stabilize the preparation of IVIg. Virus transmission as noted when IVIg was used for the treatment of other conditions has not so far been a problem in our experience with the management of patients with vasculitis.

Monoclonal antibody therapy [21]

There is less evidence for the active participation of T cells than for humoral mechanisms in the autoimmune processes in the systemic vasculitides; however, indirect involvement, by orchestrating B cell function, is considered likely. In certain groups of antineutrophil cytoplasm antibody-associated vasculitis patients, disease activity has been correlated with fluctuation in the levels of products of activated T cells. Attempts to establish antigen specific T cell lines or clones have not been successful, however. In addition to patients with autoantibody-associated disease, there are other patients with vasculitis in whom circulating autoantibodies are not found. Whether these patients have limited disease and are a form fruste of multisystem vasculitis or represent the consequence of a different pathogenetic mechanism is uncertain. Evidence suggesting the latter possibility comes from the identification of a small number of patients who have florid multisystem vasculitis, biopsy of which reveals lymphocytic infiltrates of T cells in and around vasculitic lesions, even though they do not have circulating autoantibodies nor do they respond to conventional immunosuppression.

The demonstration that cellular autoimmune mecha-

nisms might be operating in the development of systemic vasculitis encouraged the exploration of more specific forms of therapy. The opportunity arose with the availability for clinical use of humanized monoclonal antibodies with specificity for lymphocytes, particularly encompassing T lymphocytes. This coincided with the referral of certain patients with refractory, autoantibody negative, lymphocytic vasculitis. The success with monoclonal antibodies, such as anti-CD52 and anti-CD4, in the treatment of these rare patients with intractable vasculitis, led us to consider their use for other patients with the more usual autoantibody-associated vasculitis, either as a supplement for ineffective conventional immunosuppressive drug therapy or, as an alternative to it, since in the latter circumstance conventional treatment was contraindicated because of risks from cumulative toxicity or undesirable side effects.

The study group comprised 13 patients with Wegener's granulomatosis in whom the diagnosis was made on clinicopathological grounds. Clinically, there was evidence of multisystem disease in all 13, with paranasal involvement found in 11/11 by whole body scintiscanning after reinjection of isotopically labeled autologous leukocytes. Pathologically there was histological evidence of vasculitis in 12/13; radiotherapy and chemotherapy for an intractable lesion in the remaining patient before referral made subsequent histological interpretation difficult. The diagnosis was supported serologically by the presence of autoantibodies to proteinase 3 by antigen-specific ELISA in 12/13, including the patient without convincing findings by histology, and antineutrophil cytoplasm antibodies by indirect immunofluorescence in the remaining three. The patients were considered for monoclonal antibody therapy because conventional treatment had been ineffective or was contraindicated. All received humanized, monoclonal anti-CD52 with or without CD4 antibodies intravenously in doses up to 40 mg/day for up to 10 days.

Remission, defined by programmed withdrawal of drug therapy without return of active disease, was obtained in 12/13; the remaining patient died on treatment at day 7. Cytotoxic drugs were discontinued at the time of monoclonal antibody treatment in all patients; temporary reintroduction was required in 1/13 during follow-up at a time of minor relapse. Steroid therapy was tapered to zero during a nine-month reduction regimen. In three patients major relapse occurred at 1.5, 3 and 10 months and remission was achieved by further courses of monoclonal antibody therapy. At latest follow-up of the 12 patients who gained remission eight are well, five of these eight, the earliest treated are receiving neither cytotoxic drugs nor steroids; three patients died of causes other than vasculitis, and one has a recurrence in the ethmoid sinus for which she is undergoing local monoclonal antibody therapy to the lesion.

Humanized monoclonal antilymphocyte antibodies appear to provide an effective treatment for patients with systemic vasculitis, either refractory to or intolerant of steroids or cytotoxic agents. At this stage their use should be restricted to patients with severe disease, unresponsive to other therapies, including high dose intravenous immunoglobulin.

References

1. Granger, D.N. and Kabes, P. (1994) The microcirculation and inflammation: modulation of leucocyte–endothelial cell adhesion. *J. Leukocyte Biol.*, **55**, 662–275.

2. Zhang, L., Jayne, D.R.W., Zhao, M.H. *et al.* (1995) Distribution of MHC class II alleles in primary systemic vasculitis. *Kidney Int.*, **47**, 294–8.

3. Esnault, V.L.M., Testa, A., Audrain, M. *et al.* (1993) Alpha 1 antitrypsin genetic polymorphism in ANCA positive systemic vasculitis. *Kidney Int.*, **43**, 1329–32.

4. Porges, A.J., Redecha, P.B., Kimberlay, W.T. *et al.* (1994) Monoclonal ANCA (anti MPO and anti PR3) engage and activate neutrophils via the Fcα receptor IIa. *J. Immunol.*, **153**, 1271–80.

5. Guillevin, L., Visser, H. and Noel, L.H. (1993) Antineutrophil cytoplasm antibodies in systemic polyarteritis nodosa with and without hepatitis B virus infection and Churg–Strauss syndrome – 62 patients. *J. Rheumatol.*, **20**, 1345–9.

6. Short, A.K. and Lockwood, C.M. (1995) Antigen specificity in hydralazine associated ANCA positive systemic vasculitis. *Q. J. M ed.*, **88**, 775–83.

7. Dolman, K.M., Gans, R.O.B., Vervaart, Th.J. *et al.* (1993) Vasculitis and antineutrophilic cytoplasmic autoantibodies associated with propylthiouracil therapy. *Lancet*, **342**, 651–2.

8. Kettritz, R., Young, J.J., Kinjoh, K. *et al.* (1995) Animal models in ANCA vasculitis. *Clin. Exp. Immunol.*, **101 S1**, 12–15.

9. Kallenberg, C.G.M., Grouwere, E. and Weening, J.J. (1994) Antineutrophil cytoplasmic antibodies: current diagnostic and pathophysiological potential. *Kidney Int.*, **46**, 1–15.

10. Jennette, J.C. and Falk, R.J. (1994) Pathogenic potential of antineutrophil cytoplasmic autoantibodies. *Lab. Invest.*, **70**, 135–7.

11. Hoffman, G.S., Korr, G.S. and Leavitt, R.Y. (1992) Wegener's granulomatosis: an anlysis of 158 patients. *Ann. Intern. Med.*, **116**, 488–98.

12. Reuter, H., Wraight, E.P., Qasim, F.J. and Lockwood, C.M. (1995) Management of systemic vasculitis: contribution of scintigraphic imaging to evaluation of disease activity and classification. *Q. J. Med.*, **88**, 509–16.

13. Hoffman, G.S. (1993) Wegener's granulomatosis. *Curr. Opin. Rheumatol.*, **5**, 11–17.

14. Savage, C.O.S., Winearls, C.G., Evans, D.J. *et al.* (1985) Microscopic polyarteritis: presentation, pathology and prognosis. *Q. J. Med.*, **220**, 467–83.

15. Guillevin, L., Lê Thi Huong, D., Godeau, P. *et al.* (1988) Clinical findings and prognosis of polyarteritis nodosa and Churg–Strauss angiitis: a study in 165 patients. *Br. J. Rheumatol.*, **27**, 258–66.

16. De'Oliveira, J., Gaskin, G., Dash, A. *et al.* (1995) Relationship between disease activity and antineutrophil cytoplasmic antibody concentration in long term management of systemic vasculitis. *Am. J. Kidney Dis.*, **25**, 380–9.

17. Jayne, D.R.W., Gaskin, G., Pusey, C.D. and Lockwood, C.M. (1995) ANCA and predicting relapse in systemic vasculitis. *Q. J. Med.*, **88**, 127–33.

18. Savage, C.O.S. and Lockwood, C.M. (1993) The systemic vasculitides, in *Clinical Aspects of Immunology* (eds D.K. Peters and P.J. Lachmann), Blackwell, Oxford, pp. 1205–16.

19. Rossi, F., Jayne, D.R.W., Lockwood, C.M. and Kazatchkine, M.D. (1991) Antiidiotypes against antineutrophil cytoplasmic antigen antibodies in normal human polyspecific IgG for therapeutic use and in the remission sera of patients with systemic vasculitis. *Clin. Exp. Immunol.*, **83**, 298–303.

20. Jayne, D.R.W. and Lockwood, C.M. (1993) Pooled intravenous immunoglobulin in the management of systemic vasculitis. *Adv. Exp. Med. Biol.*, **336**, 469–72.

21. Lockwood, C.M., Thiru, S., Isaacs, J.D. *et al.* (1993) Long-term remission of intractable systemic vasculitis with monoclonal antibody therapy. *Lancet*, **341**, 1620–2.

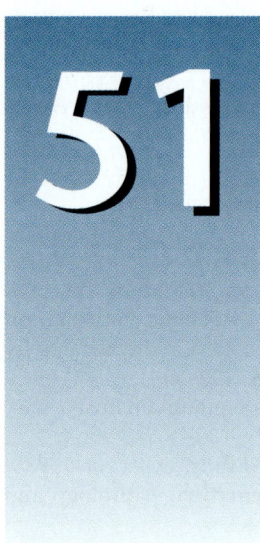

51 Dysproteinemias and renal disease

N.P. Mallick and G.S. Lucas

Introduction

The dysproteinemias are a fascinating group of disorders which have protean clinical features. Their detection is often a challenge to clinical acumen; their treatment can be very rewarding. This chapter concentrates on the renal aspects of these conditions and offers some guidance on the influence of renal manifestations on prognosis and management.

The dysproteinemias

Paraproteins are monoclonal immunoglobulins produced by a clone of B-lymphoid cells (Table 51.1). Most commonly, the paraprotein arises from a limited, apparently non-malignant, clonal expansion. Such 'monoclonal gammopathies of undetermined significance', or benign paraproteinemias, will either be asymptomatic or (less frequently) present with symptoms caused by the paraprotein. Monoclonal gammopathy of undetermined significance is increasingly recognized because of the sensitivity and more frequent use of modern screening techniques. It is commoner in the elderly: approximately 3% of patients over 70 years old will have a paraprotein [1].

Less frequently, paraproteins arise from an overtly malignant B cell clone; 4% of patients with lymphomas have paraproteins [2]. Such lymphomas are usually low-grade and diffuse. The paraprotein is most commonly IgM and may result in the clinical syndrome of Waldenstrom's macroglobulinemia. As a rule, such lymphomas produce paraproteins of normal structure, although there is frequently an imbalance in the rate of production of heavy and light chains, leading to the secretion of an excess of free light chains. In a minority of cases, the neoplastic clone does not produce heavy chains at all (the light chain diseases).

At the other end of the spectrum of dysproteinemias is myeloma (see below), an overt malignancy of plasma cells. In myeloma, immunoglobulin formation by the malignant monoclone is usually unbalanced; it may secrete fragments of immunoglobulin as well as free light chains in large amounts. These latter are responsible for much of the renal disease in myeloma but there is a striking variation in the frequency of renal disease associated with the different paraprotein disorders (Table 51.1). This is only partially explained on the basis of light chain production and other known predisposing factors and shows our imperfect understanding of the ways in which renal damage occurs.

Nephrology, Edited by Rex L. Jamison and Robert Wilkinson.
Published in 1997 by Chapman & Hall, London. ISBN 0 412 60930 4

Table 51.1 Paraprotein disorders and their renal complications

	Paraprotein/light chain	Renal complications
Myeloma	IgG, IgA, light chain (rarely IgD, IgE, non-secretory)	More than 50%
Monoclonal gammopathy of undetermined significance	IgG, IgA, IgM (rarely IgD, light chain)	Rare
Plasmacytoma (localized myeloma)	As myeloma	Rare
Amyloid (AL)	As myeloma (usually with lambda light chain)	75–90%
Waldenström's macroglobulinemia	IgM	Infrequent (mainly glomerular)

Cryoglobulins

Cryoglobulins are formed by the association of immunoglobulins either with each other or with an anti-IgG (IgM rheumatoid factor). They precipitate in the cold and dissolve on warming. Three types of cryoglobulins are described (I, II and III) depending on the composition. In types I and II there is a monoclonal immunoglobulin and so by inference a B cell monoclone to produce it.

In type I cryoglobulinemia, the monoclonal protein aggregates with itself; this phenomenon is usually associated with an overt lesion such as myeloma or macroglobulinemia. Occasionally the culprit monoclone is 'silent' and may be discovered only when, on appropriate staining, it is revealed in a bone marrow aspirate. In type II the rheumatoid factor is monoclonal but in the type III form both the IgM-RF and the IgG are polyclonal.

Cryoglobulin may be primary or secondary. The later are associated with infection and the rheumatoid factor (RF) is usually, but not always, polyclonal (type III cryoglobulinemia). The other immunoglobulin in the complex is primarily directed against an antigen derived from the infective agent.

Immunosuppressive therapy, which may have a place in the treatment of type I or II cryoglobulinemia, may aggravate any infection, especially if it is due to a virus, whereas treatment of the infection may produce a cure. An obvious difficulty arises if there is doubt as to whether there is an infective cause in a given case, especially since there is some evidence that an infection is sometimes associated with a type II cryoglobulinemia.

Renal involvement does not always occur in the cryoglobulinemias, being found in perhaps 20% of all cases. In general the cryoglobulinemias are characterized by relatively non-specific features including arthralgia, purpura, malaise, Raynaud's phenomenon and fever. There have been a number of authoritative reports, principally from European countries, of glomerulonephritis (usually of the mesangiocapillary form) associated with what has until recently been termed 'mixed essential cryoglobulinemia. Within the last few years, it has become clear that these lesions are associated with Hepatitis C virus infection and that the cryoglobulins are formed by monoclonal (type II) or polyclonal (type III) RF and IgG directed against viral antigenic determinants (epitopes). There are subtypes of the virus but the renal lesion does not appear to be associated with any subtype in particular, nor does a particular viral epitope appear always to be responsible.

The best treatment appears to be antiviral agents; controlled trials to assess the efficacy of alpha-interferon were in progress during 1996. Interestingly, as Pozzato *et al.* [3] point out, the type II abnormalities cannot occur without the presence of an appropriate B cell monoclone and this raises the question as to which came first. These authors showed that 39% of cases with the combination of type II or III cryoglobulin and hepatitis C infection had evidence of a low-grade non-Hodgkin's lymphoma. This finding points to the inadvisability of treating these patients, as has been done previously, with immunosuppressive agents which are likely to promote the replication of virus.

Myeloma

Myeloma, the best known dysproteinemia and commonest plasma cell malignancy, provides a challenge for both the nephrologist and the hematologist. It accounts for 1% of all malignant disease with an annual incidence of 3 per 10^5 in the European population. In 1958, before the introduction of melphalan, myeloma was viewed as a dismal disorder with a median survival of 3.5 months and frequent early death from renal failure [4]. Since then partially effective chemotherapy regimens have been introduced with median survival in most trials exceeding 24 months.

A better understanding of the biology of myeloma has revealed its heterogeneity and the variety of ways in which it can affect the kidney. Novel (and expensive) therapies continue to be introduced. The challenge for clinicians is to uncover the most effective use of such treatments at a time of increasing financial restraint.

The defining hallmarks of myeloma are: plasma cell infiltration within the bone marrow, osteolytic lesions on radiographs, and a serum paraprotein or urinary light chain. 55–60% of cases will produce an IgG paraprotein, 20–25% IgA, 20% light chain alone, and 1% IgD. Rarely, myeloma will be an IgE or IgM producing, biclonal or non-secretory clone. Of the common types of myeloma, IgG and IgA carry a better prognosis than light chain myeloma, principally because of the higher risk of renal failure associated with light chain production [5]. In two-thirds of myelomas, the associated light chain is kappa, mirroring the kappa : lambda ratio of 2 : 1 in normal, non-clonal immunoglobulins. In contrast, the uncommon IgD myelomas are virtually all lambda light chain. In IgG myeloma, about three-quarters of patients will have an excess of light chains small enough (molecular weight, monomer 22 kDa, dimer 44 kDa) to permit them to undergo glomerular filtration. Proximal tubular cells have a limited capacity to reabsorb and catabolize light chains which is readily exceeded in myeloma. Free light chains may damage these cells, or pass down the nephron to form casts in the tubular lumen. The remainder are excreted in the urine.

Renal manifestations of myeloma

The kidney is a major target of both the light chains and the paraproteins produced in myeloma. Histologists recognize three main types of renal lesions: tubular damage resulting in myeloma (or cast) nephropathy, light chain (AL) amyloid, and light chain deposition disease. Less commonly, in light and heavy chain deposition disease, intact immunoglobulin is found precipitated in glomerular and tubular basement membranes. In some patients, these different histological entities co-exist.

The commonest form of renal damage is myeloma nephropathy. It is principally found in patients who excrete free light chains, either alone or in association with an intact immunoglobulin. Light chains filter freely through the glomeruli and deposit in the tubular basement membranes. Lower down the nephron, casts containing light chain and Tamm–Horsfall protein are formed in the already damaged tubules. Rarely crystals may be found in the tubular cells; this may result in significant proximal tubular impairment ranging from the Fanconi syndrome to renal tubular acidosis. Most patients with myeloma kidney will have frank myeloma when their renal impairment is diagnosed. This is in sharp contrast to light chain amyloid and light chain deposition disease, in which the renal damage may occur without any other features of myeloma (Table 51.2 and Figure 51.1).

In AL amyloid, the form of amyloid in myeloma (Figure 51.2), fibrils derived from immunoglobulin light

Table 51.2 Presenting features of light chain amyloid and light chain deposition disease (LCDD)

	Amyloid (%)	LCDD (%)
Myeloma	20	31–60
Monoclonal immunoglobulin or light chain in serum or urine	87	80–82
Lambda light chain	73	15–20
Proteinuria	80–100	92
Nephrotic syndrome	48	23
Renal failure	58–70	85–93

Data principally taken from Gertz *et al.* [32] and Buxbaum et al. [33].

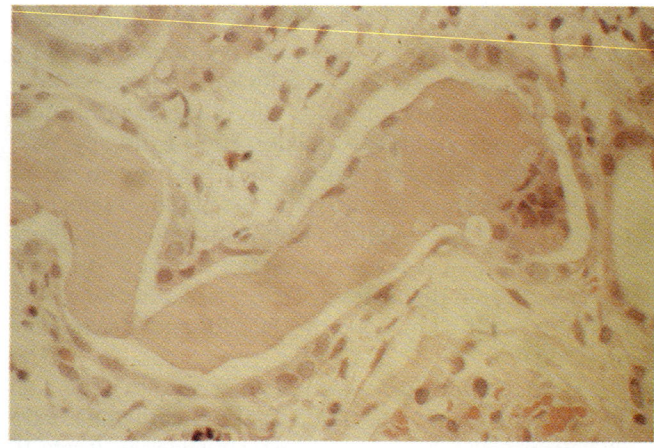

Figure 51.1 Myeloma kidney.

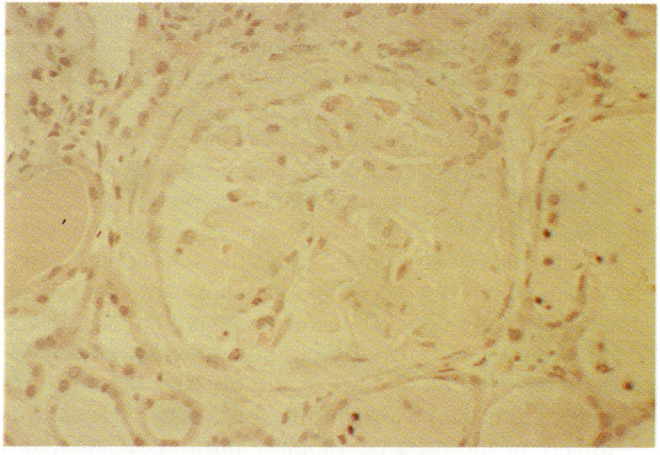

Figure 51.2 Amyloid deposition in myeloma.

chains deposit widely throughout the body. In early disease, the mesangium is involved, spreading to the glomerular basement membranes and arterial vessels. The tubular basement membranes and associated blood vessels are also involved. Approximately half the patients will present with the nephrotic syndrome, some with associated renal failure. Of the remainder, the majority will have less heavy but significant proteinuria (Table 51.2). Lambda light chains (especially lambda-6) are more likely to be responsible than kappa light chains. At present, there is no effective therapy for AL amyloidosis and it carries a very poor prognosis. The median time to end-stage renal disease (ESRD) for patients with renal amyloidosis is only 13.8 months, and median survival on dialysis is only 8.2 months [6].

Although light chain deposition disease (LCDD) is properly regarded as a systemic disease, the great majority of patients with LCDD present with renal disease (Table 51.2), principally renal failure. In 31–60%, there will be clear evidence of myeloma at presentation. Both glomeruli and tubules may be involved. The glomerular involvement is in the form of a nodular glomerulosclerosis or a mesangiocapillary glomerulonephritis, and the tubular basement membranes are thickened and often reduplicated. Ultrastructurally, microfibrils will be noted in the same distribution. In contrast to amyloid, the lesions do not stain with Congo Red, and kappa light chains are more frequently implicated in LCDD than lambda light chains. With treatment of the myeloma, 60–80% of patients with accompanying LCDD will have improvement or stabilization of their renal function. Left untreated, patients with LCDD progress to ESRD within 2–23 months [7, 8].

Why should some patients with very significant light chain excretion escape renal damage, whereas others present with renal disease at a very early stage, with little other evidence of myeloma, and a low tumor mass? Why should renal failure be very much commoner in myeloma than in Waldenström's macroglobulinemia in which patients may have pronounced light chain excretion for many years? The answers to these questions remain elusive.

Amyloid is clearly associated with lambda light chains, particularly lambda-6, and although there is a less clear-cut association between kappa light chains and LCDD, these observations suggest that the type of light chain may determine the risk and type of renal damage. There is conflicting evidence on the role of the isoelectric point of the light chain in determining whether or not nephrotoxicity develops. It may be that this is only one of the physicochemical properties of the light chain that is important and that its role cannot be assessed in isolation. At present we have no consistent evidence supporting a link between a given light chain type or property and myeloma nephropathy.

In a landmark paper, Soloman et al. [9] described the effect on mice of the intraperitoneal administration of purified monoclonal human light chains. The light chains were prepared from urine samples from patients with either myeloma or primary (AL) amyloid, and well-characterized renal lesions. There was a consistent association between the renal lesions induced in the mice, ranging from myeloma nephropathy (with and without tubular crystal formation) to LCDD and AL amyloid, and the renal lesions present in the corresponding human subject, suggesting that the (as yet ill-defined) physical properties of the light chain are a major determinant of the type of renal lesion. There is, however, some evidence (see below) that in myeloma cytokine overexpression (especially IL-6) may contribute to the renal lesions seen. This together with the commoner occurrence of (for example) hypercalcemia with IL-6 overexpression may help to explain the relative frequency of renal impairment in myeloma, by contrast with Waldenström's macroglobulinemia and other lymphoid malignancies associated with monoclonal light chains.

Presentation and management of renal complications in myeloma

Renal impairment is a common presenting feature of myeloma, and many other patients develop renal disease in the course of their disease. In most cases, the renal failure will be multifactorial in origin. Although light chain toxicity is the principal cause, hypercalcemia, hyperuricemia, or renal infection are other common contributing factors, and many patients are severely salt or water depleted because of intercurrent nausea and vomiting, poor water conservation because of hypercalcemia, and insensible loss because of fever (see Table 51.3). Renal impairment often occurs insidiously before the myeloma is discovered and may be exacerbated by clinical complications such that it becomes a major feature at presentation.

Although prompt management at presentation (principally by volume replacement or rehydration) will

Table 51.3 Factors contributing to renal failure in myeloma

Light chains
  tubular damage
  amyloid
  light chain deposition
Immunoglobulin – deposition
Hypercalcemia – dehydration
Infection
Nephrotoxic drugs
Hyperviscosity
Hyperuricemia
Plasma cell infiltration

improve renal function in many patients [10], some chronic renal impairment often remains. Of 1205 patients in the MRC fourth and fifth Myeloma trials, 42% had a serum creatinine greater than 130 µmol/l (1.48 mg/dl) after initial fluid depletion had been corrected, but before any chemotherapy. In 20% the creatinine was greater than 200 µmol/l (2.27 mg/dl) and in 12% greater than 300 µmol/l (3.4 mg/dl) [11]. These figures are broadly equivalent to a glomerular filtration rate already reduced to 60, 40 and 25 ml/min for a 50-year-old man of average size. Alexanian *et al.* [12], in a series of 424 previously untreated patients, identified Bence Jones proteinuria with or without hypercalcemia as the factors causing the presenting renal failure 97% of the time. After volume replacement, hydration and initial chemotherapy, 'normal' plasma creatinine or BUN values were achieved promptly in 51% of these patients. These findings are similar to the British experience [11]. Alexanian *et al.* [12] point out that patients who recovered normal renal function had only mild renal impairment at presentation and were not oliguric.

Early studies of outcome in myeloma emphasized the poor prognostic significance of renal impairment at presentation [13, 14]. Prompt volume restoration and rehydration of myeloma patients presenting with renal impairment has improved the outlook. Nephrologists and hematologists also recognize that even if renal function does not return promptly to normal on initial therapy, the condition may yet be reversible [15]. The serum β_2-microglobulin value on presentation has been recognized as the most important prognostic indicator in myeloma. β_2-microglobulin is the invariant polypeptide chain of HLA class I molecules, present on the surface of almost all nucleated cells. In disease, the serum β_2-microglobulin is a balance between the production rate (from cell turnover) and its clearance from the blood by glomerular filtration. Both factors may be abnormal in myeloma, contributing to the strong prognostic value of this parameter [16].

Features that predict a favorable (renal) outcome are normal size kidneys which show no evidence of advanced tubulointerstitial damage on biopsy; the prompt correction of reversible precipitating factors, such as urinary tract infection, dehydration, volume depletion or hypercalcemia; and withdrawal of nephrotoxic drugs or radioiodine contrast media. Nevertheless, recovery from acute renal failure due to myeloma may take months. During this time dialysis may be necessary. The place of plasma exchange as an additional therapy is debated. On first principles, there would appear to be a case for this treatment. In renal failure, the plasma level of the light chains is raised because their clearance by the kidney is impaired, so their rapid removal from the plasma might limit the damage that they inflict and hasten recovery. Some authors [17, 18] have reported evidence in favor of this approach, whereas others find the evidence inconclusive. Inevitably there are cases of myeloma that progress to end-stage renal failure. Usually this reflects the insidious damage caused by filtered light chains which cause toxic damage to proximal and more distal tubular cells and produce casts in association with Tamm–Horsfall protein in the tubular lumen.

The prognosis for patients who appear to require long-term renal replacement therapy is determined mainly by that of the underlying B cell lesion and its response to therapy. It should be remembered that even though over 50% of patients with myeloma develop renal impairment, perhaps less than 10% die from it [19]. The majority succumb to the progressive disease itself, to infection, or to other complications. In a number of recent studies, the one-year survival for myeloma patients on renal replacement therapy (RRT) is around 50% [17, 20–22]. Across Europe, the experience as reported to the EDTA Registry is that few patients survive more than a year (Figure 51.3).

If the lesion comes under control on therapy, then the patient may have several years of good quality life on dialysis. Some authors have pointed to the increased likelihood of infection in these inevitably immunosuppressed patients and have suggested that it is better to avoid peritoneal dialysis with its attendant risks of peritonitis. Nevertheless, peritoneal dialysis does provide adequate dialysis for one to two years and infection is not uncommon in the alternative RRT, hemodialysis, particularly if an indwelling venous catheter is used [23].

Renal transplantation has been performed in myeloma and up to four years of good renal function have been secured. At present, most physicians will see very few cases in which it seems appropriate to undertake renal transplantation. It may be appropriate in the rare case in which the myeloma has apparently been cured by bone marrow transplantation or chemotherapy, and the patient is in end-stage renal failure but otherwise in good health. As bone marrow transplantation is increasingly used, even for poor prognosis myeloma, such cases may be seen more often.

It must be recognized that there is a considerable cost to maintaining a patient with myeloma on RRT. Coward [24] has calculated that complications in the myeloma patient add up to a third to the costs of hemodialysis, mainly due to more frequent and longer hospital admissions for infection and other complications. The pain and suffering that some patients undergo is reflected in this increased requirement for hospital care. Although it is of paramount importance to give each patient the best chance of worthwhile survival, in some cases the march of the underlying disease and its other complications may make palliative therapy a better option. This is in keeping with the data of Alexanian *et al.* [12], who emphasized that it is in those cases in which the myeloma is already irreversible that terminal renal failure occurs, so that the opportunity for salvaging the patient are inherently limited.

The other form of presentation of myeloma to nephrologists is the onset of proteinuria. This is largely

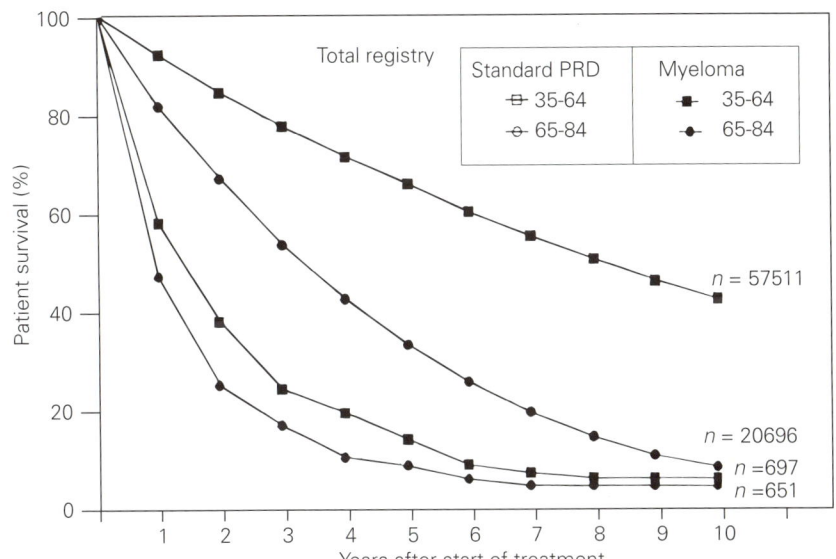

Figure 51.3 Patient survival in myeloma and standard PRD after start of treatment, 1982–92; males. (From the EDTA Registry.)

Table 51.4   Myeloma staging

Stage I Myeloma cell mass <0.6 × 10¹²/m² (low cell mass)	
All of the following:	Hemoglobin >10 g/dl
	Normal serum calcium
	Normal bone radiographs (or solitary plasmacytoma)
	Low serum paraprotein level/urinary light chain excretion
Stage II Intermediate cell mass	
	Fitting neither Stage I nor Stage III
Stage III Myeloma cell mass >1.2 × 10¹²/m² (high cell mass)	
One or more of the following:	Hemoglobin <8.5 g/dl
	Serum calcium >3.0 mmol/l
	Advanced lytic bone lesions
	High serum paraprotein level/urinary light chain excretion
Subclassification	A: Relatively normal renal function (<180 µmol/l)
	B: Abnormal renal function (>180 µmol/l)

Taken from Durie and Salmon [14].

due to the excretion of excess light chains (with or without an intact paraprotein), but there is frequently albuminuria also and this may sometimes be heavy enough for the patient to develop a full-blown nephrotic syndrome. In such cases there is a strong possibility of amyloid deposition in the glomeruli [25].

It is important to remember that light chains are not detected by the dipstick. In any patient suspected of dysproteinemia or with renal failure urine should be tested with sulfa salicylic acid (SSA). A positive SSA plus negative dipstick suggests light chains.

Erythropoietin therapy in patients with myeloma and ESRD

Anemia is a frequent complication of myeloma and may occur in the absence of massive bone marrow infiltration by myeloma, and in the presence of normal white cell and platelet counts. About 25% of patients with myeloma will have inappropriately low serum levels of erythropoietin (Epo), rising to 50% of those with stage III disease (Table 51.4 shows staging), and 60% of those with renal impairment and serum creatinine >170 µmol/l 1.9 mg/dl [26]. There is now extensive experience with the use of Epo to treat anemia in myeloma patients. The baseline serum Epo level has proved to be a good (inverse) predictor of response, and Epo has not, as feared, been shown to have any stimulatory effect on myeloma [27]. There is limited experience of the use of Epo in anemic patients with myeloma and ESRD, but early data suggest that Epo can be used to good effect in this group of patients, although the rise in hematocrit per unit of Epo is less than that seen in other forms of ESRD [28].

Cytokine-mediated renal damage in myeloma?

Interleukin-6 (IL-6) has been identified as a major cytokine involved in the emergence of the tumor clone and in tumor-associated toxicity in patients with myeloma [29]. It is not yet clear whether it acts as an autocrine or paracrine growth factor. About 42% of untreated patients with myeloma will have elevated serum IL-6 levels [30]. Patients with elevated IL-6 levels have a significantly worse prognosis with more advanced disease, more osteolytic lesions and lower hemoglobin and higher serum creatinine concentrations [30].

Overexpression of IL-6 has been implicated in a range of autoimmune disease, e.g. IgA nephropathy. Transgenic mice overexpressing IL-6 will develop myeloma and mesangial proliferative glomerulonephritis. Fattori *et al.* [31] constructed transgenic mice carrying the mouse metallothionein-I gene promoter fused to the human IL-6 gene. Such mice express IL-6 in the liver and secrete the cytokine in the blood. They have a polyclonal hyper-gammaglobulinemia, and an IgG plasmacytosis in the spleen, lymph nodes and thymus. Interestingly, most of mice die at 12–20 weeks of renal failure. Initially they develop membranous glomerulonephritis, which progresses to a focal glomerulosclerosis and extensive tubular damage with casts and tubular atrophy.

It is highly likely that other key cytokines will be identified over the next few years that have central roles in the development of myeloma and in the renal injury. IL-6 and other such cytokines may well go a long way to improve our understanding of the frequency of renal disease in myeloma, particularly advanced myeloma, and may offer new targets for therapeutic intervention.

References

1. Saleun, J.P., Vicariot, M., Deroff, P. *et al.* (1982) Monoclonal gammopathies in the adult population of Finisterre, France. *J. Clin. Pathol.*, **35**, 63–8.
2. Alexanian, R. (1975) Monoclonal gammopathy in lymphoma. *Arch. Intern. Med.*, **135**, 62–6.
3. Pozzato, G., Mazzaro, C., Crovatto, M. *et al.* (1994) Low-grade malignant lymphoma, hepatitis C virus infection, and mixed cryoglobulinemia. *Blood*, **84**, 3047–53.
4. Feinleib, M. and MacMahon, B. (1960) Duration and survival in multiple myeloma. *J. Natl. Cancer Inst.*, **24**, 1259–69.
5. Kelsey, P.R. and Delamore, I.W. (1986) Clinical features of multiple myeloma, in *Multiple Myeloma and Other Paraproteinemias* (ed. I.W. Delamore), Churchill Livingstone, Edinburgh, pp. 117–36.
6. Gertz, M.A., Kyle, R.A. and O'Fallon, W.M. (1992) Dialysis support of patients. with primary systemic amyloidosis. A study of 211 patients. *Arch. Intern. Med.*, **152**, 2245–50.
7. Ganeval, D., Noel, L.H., Preud'homme, J.L. *et al.* (1984) Light-chain deposition deposition disease: its relation with AL-type amyloidosis. *Kidney Int.*, **26**, 1–9.
8. Heilman, R.L., Velosa, J.A., Holley, K.E. *et al.* (1992) Long-term follow-up and response to chemotherapy in patients with light-chain deposition disease. *Am. J. Kidney Dis.*, **20**, 34–41.
9. Soloman, A., Weiss, D. and Kattine, A.A. (1991) Nephrotoxic potential of Bence Jones proteins. *N Engl. J. Med.*, **324**, 1845–51.
10. MRC Working Party (1984) Analysis and management of renal failure in fourth MRC myelomatosis trial. *Br. Med. J.*, **288**, 1411–16.
11. MacLennan, I.C.M., Cooper, E.C., Chapman, C.E. *et al.* (1989) Renal failure in myelomatosis. *Eur. J. Hematol.*, **43**, 60–5.
12. Alexanian, R., Barlogie, B. and Dixon, D. (1990) Renal failure in multiple myeloma. *Arch. Intern. Med.*, **150**, 1693–5.
13. MRC Working Party (1980) Prognostic features in the third MRC myelomatosis trial. *Br. J. Cancer*, **42**, 831–40.
14. Durie, B.G.M. and Salmon, S.E. (1975) A clinical staging system for multiple myeloma. Correlation of measured myeloma cell mass with presenting clinical features, response to treatment, and survival. *Cancer*, **36**, 842–54.
15. Mallick, N.P. (1994) Acute renal failure and myeloma. *Nephrol. Dial. Transplant.*, **9** (suppl 4), 108–10.
16. Cuzick, J., Cooper, E.H. and MacLennan, I.C.M. (1985) The prognostic significance of serum beta-2 microglobulin compared with other presentation features in myelomatosis. *Br. J. Cancer.*, **288**, 1411–16.
17. Pasquali, S., Casanova, S., Zuccheli, A. *et al.* (1990) Long–term survival of patients with acute and severe renal failure due to myeloma. *Clin. Nephrol.*, **34**, 247–54.
18. Johnson, W.J., Kyle, R.A., Pineda, A.A. *et al.* (1990) Treatment of renal failure associated with myeloma. Plasmapheresis, hemodialysis, and chemotherapy. *Arch. Intern. Med.*, **150**, 863–9.
19. Rayner, H.C., Haynes, A.P., Thompson, J.R. *et al.* (1991) Perspectives in multiple myeloma: survival, prognostic factors and disease complications in a single centre between 1975 and 1988. *Q. J. Med.*, **79**, 517–25.

20. Iggo, N., Palmer, A.B., Severn, A. *et al.* (1989) Chronic dialysis in patients with multiple myeloma and renal failure: a worthwhile treatment. *Q. J. Med.*, **73**, 871–2.

21. Brown, J.H., Maxwell, A.P., Bruce, I. *et al.* (1993) Renal replacement therapy in multiple myeloma and systemic amyloidosis. *Ir. Med. Sci.*, **162**, 213–17.

22. Molby, L., Hansen, H.H. and Jensen, E.L. (1994) Development and treatment of renal insufficiency in multiple myeloma. *Ugeskr–Laeger.*, **156**, 4343–7.

23. Korzets, A., Tam, F., Russell, G. *et al.* (1990) The role of continuous ambulatory peritoneal dialysis in end–stage renal failure due to multiple myeloma. *Am. J. Kidney Dis.*, **16**, 216–23.

24. Coward, R.A. (1989) The cost of chronic dialysis in multiple myeloma. *Postgrad. Med. J.*, **65**, 302–6.

25. Kyle, R.A. (1994) Monoclonal proteins and renal disease. *Annu. Rev. Med.*, **45**, 71–7.

26. Beguin, Y., Yerna, M., Loo, M. *et al.* (1992) Erythropoiesis in multiple myeloma: defective red cell production due to inappropriate erythropoietin production. *Br. J. Hematol.*, **82**, 648–53.

27. Barlogie, B. (1993) Treatment of the anemia of multiple myeloma: the role of recombinant erythropoietin. *Semin. Hematol.*, **30**, 25–7.

28. Powe, N.R., Griffiths, R.I., Gorer, J.W. *et al.* (1993) Early dosing practices and effectiveness of recombinant human erythropoietin. *Kidney Int.*, **43**, 1125–33.

29. Klein, B., Zhang, X.G., Lu, Z.Y. *et al.* (1995) Interleukin-6 in human multiple myeloma. *Blood*, **85**, 863–72.

30. Pelliniemi, T.T., Irjala, K., Mattila, K. *et al.* (1995) Immunoreactive interleukin-6 and acute phase proteins as prognostic factors in multiple myeloma. *Blood*, **85**, 765–71.

31. Fattori, E., Della Rocca, C., Costa, P. *et al.* (1994) Development of progressive kidney damage and myeloma kidney in Interleukin-6 transgenic mice. *Blood*, **83**, 2570–9.

32. Gertz, M.A., Kyle, R. and Greipp, P.R. (1991) Response rates and survival in primary systemic amyloidosis. *Blood*, **77**, 257–62.

33. Buxbaum, J.N., Chuba, J.V., Hellman, G.C. *et al.* (1990) Monoclonal immunoglobulin deposition disease: light chain and light and heavy chain deposition diseases and their relation to light chain amyloidosis. *Ann. Intern. Med.*, **112**, 455–64.

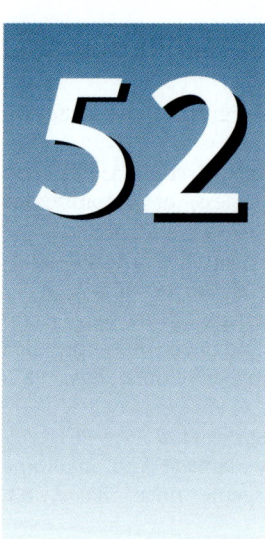

52

Sarcoidosis

Barry I. Hoffbrand

Introduction

Sarcoidosis is a disease of unknown etiology, characterized by non-caseating epithelioid granulomas involving many organs. The most frequent presentations are with hilar lymphadenopathy, pulmonary infiltration and eye and skin manifestations. The immunopathological hallmarks of active sarcoidosis are a high CD4/CD8 lymphocyte ratio at sites of active inflammation and depletion of circulating CD4 lymphocytes. A T cell subset, CD4+, HLA-DR+ is responsible for release of interleukin-2, a cytokine believed to be involved in the accumulation of CD4 cells at sites of granuloma formation. There is also B cell hyperactivity in tissues due to release of cytokines by helper T cells. The T cells express adhesion molecules that indicate that they are memory cells which recognize the unknown antigen(s) responsible for the disease [1] (Figure 52.1).

Sarcoidosis gives rise to renal disease by at least two manifestations of the granulomatous process. One is direct involvement of the kidneys leading to granulomatous interstitial nephritis. The other is granuloma-related abnormal calcium metabolism leading to hypercalcemic renal failure, nephrocalcinosis and/or urolithiasis. The two frequently coexist [2].

The evidence of a third renal manifestation of sarcoidosis, that of associated glomerular disease, is a good deal less compelling. Although there appears to be a relationship of sarcoidosis with membranous disease, this may, in fact, represent what appears to be a striking dearth of reports of minimal change disease in sarcoidosis [3]. Such a negative association, if real, would have

implications for the mechanisms involved in minimal change disease.

Granulomatous interstitial nephritis

Although the earliest reports of granulomatous changes in the kidney in sarcoidosis date from autopsy studies in the 1930s, it was only two decades later that percutaneous renal biopsy revealed the frequency of such involvement as a cause of renal failure, usually largely reversible [4]. The apparent prevalence of granulomatous changes in the kidneys in sarcoidosis varies dependent on the population studied and the methods used. Autopsy reports give figures of around 20% [5] whereas biopsy findings suggest a figure as high as 40% [2, 6, 7]. In the majority of such cases there is no detectable renal disease clinically. A large Italian multicentre study of renal biopsy has provided an incidence of sarcoidosis of 0.1 per million of population [7a]. The indications for biopsy and diagnostic criteria are not provided. The manifestations of renal sarcoidosis when of clinical importance are principally those reflecting renal failure.

Hannedouche *et al.* [8] reported six cases of granulomatous interstitial nephritis in sarcoidosis and reviewed 51 other published cases dating back to 1955 [4]. This condition, however, is by no means as rare as this figure would suggest. Ball *et al.* [9] found six cases of renal sarcoidosis among 408 native renal biopsies over a two-year period at a tertiary referral centre. This represented 1.5%

Nephrology, Edited by Rex L. Jamison and Robert Wilkinson.
Published in 1997 by Chapman & Hall, London. ISBN 0 412 60930 4

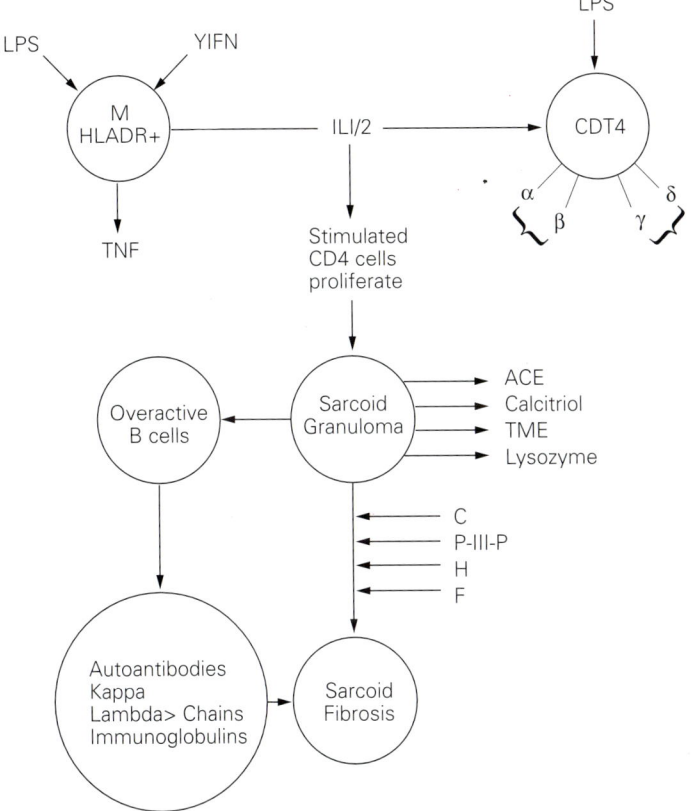

Figure 52.1 Sarcoid granuloma; interplay between macrophages, T and B cells, and cytokines. LPS, lipopolysaccharide; IFN-γ, interferon-γ; M, macrophage; CDH, thymus-mediated helper cell; IL1/2, interleukins 1 and 2; TNF, tumor necrosis factor; ACE, angiotensin converting enzyme; TME, metallopeptidase; P-III-P, type III procollagen N terminal peptide; C, collagenase; H, hyaluronic acid; F, fibronectin. (Courtesy Dr D.G. James and the editor of *Thorax*.)

of all the biopsies and 20% of all the cases of interstitial nephritis. Our own figures from three district general hospitals are similar [10]. Four cases of granulomatous interstitial nephritis due to sarcoidosis were found in 205 patients biopsied (1.9%) and constituted 31% of cases of interstitial nephritis. The indication for biopsy in both studies was renal failure. In our series renal sarcoidosis represented 7% of the patients biopsied for this indication. Two of our patients and all of Ball *et al*.'s [9] were not previously known to have sarcoidosis. Although there is an equal sex incidence in sarcoidosis in general, this does not hold for renal sarcoidosis, where 39 (68%) of 57 cases reviewed were male [8].

Pathology

By renal biospy, sarcoidosis affects primarily the interstitium and consists of variable numbers of sarcoid granulomas against a background of chronic inflammatory cells (Figure 52.2). The granulomatous inflammation has the cellular characteristics of granulomatous sarcoid in other tissues [11]. Interstitial fibrosis and tubular atrophy are of therapeutic significance as they indicate irreversibility as they do in other conditions. Granulomas may not be detected or may disappear with healing. Glomerular and vascular changes of uncertain significance are seen but immune complexes are absent [12]. Nephrocalcinosis and granulomatous interstitial nephritis frequently coexist [6, 8]. Calcific microspherules in glomerular structures

have been described [13] but are unlikely to be specific for sarcoidosis.

Clinical manifestations

The renal failure of renal sarcoidosis generally develops gradually over weeks or months. As with most other forms of interstitial nephritis, proteinuria is absent or mild and hypertension generally only complicates advanced uremia (Chapter 57). There may be leukocytes, red cells and granular casts in the urine. Tubular functional abnormalities occur, notably urinary concentration defects [14] or frank nephrogenic diabetes insipidus [15]; hyperglobulinemia may be involved as the mechanism in some cases [12]. Hypercalcemia or an inappropriately high plasma calcium and enlarged kidneys may be diagnostic clues to renal sarcoidosis in someone presenting with otherwise unexplained renal failure. Granulomatous interstitial nephritis may also rarely present with frank haematuria [8, 8a]. Serum angiotensin-converting enzyme levels and gallium-67 citrate scans are of little help in establishing the diagnosis or following the response to treatment [8, 16].

Treatment

The response to corticosteroid treatment, which will also suppress the associated hypercalcemia, is usually satisfactory with a substantial improvement in renal function.

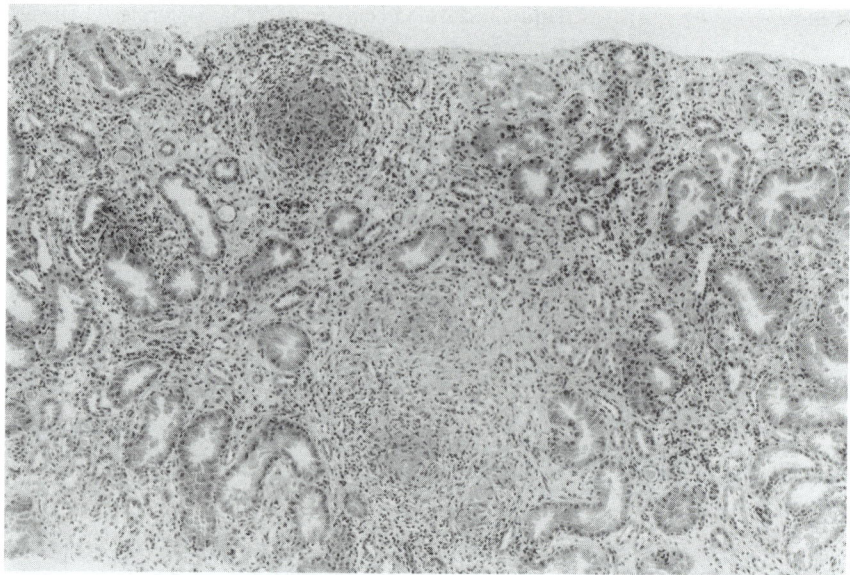

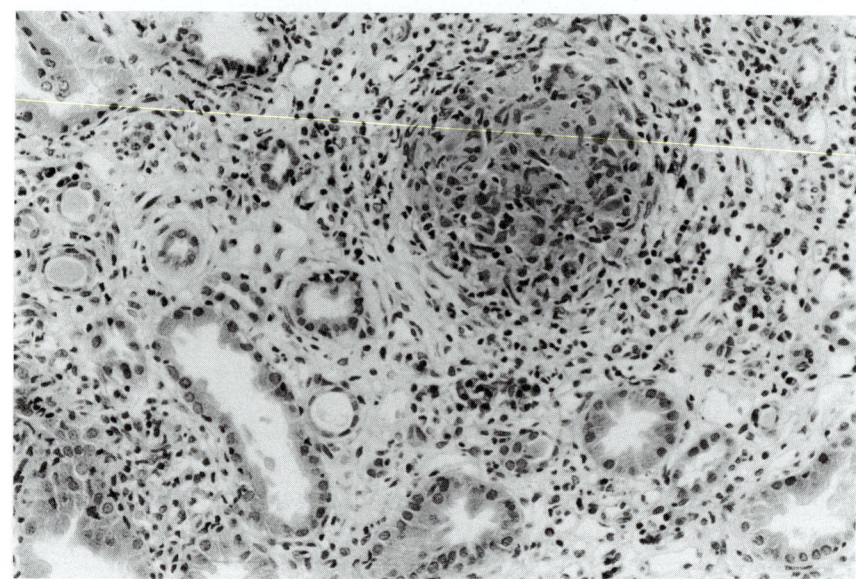

Figure 52.2 Granulomatous interstitial nephritis in sarcoidosis (a) ×100. (b) ×250. (H&E). (Courtesy of Dr Meryl Griffiths.)

Due to interstitial fibrosis and tubular atrophy, however, a majority of patients have residual irreversible renal impairment. Prolonged treatment with generally small maintenance doses is usually needed in view of the tendency for relapses to occur [8]. Tubular abnormalities with renal sarcoidosis also respond to corticosteroids [14].

Differential diagnosis

Granulomatous interstitial nephritis is by no means specific for sarcoidosis but also occurs in drug reactions, tuberculosis, glomerulonephritis and Wegener's granulomatosis as well as occasionally an idiopathic disorder [17, 18, 18a]. Renal involvement in sarcoidosis may, however, precede other manifestations of the disease by months or years [19].

A disorder with uveitis and interstitial nephritis was described by Dobrin *et al.* in 1975 [20]. Although there may be granulomatous changes in other tissues, the renal lesion is an acute interstitial nephritis with mononuclear cells and some eosinophils. Also in contrast to sarcoidosis, the condition is more or less confined to females. The immunopathology nonetheless resembles that found in sarcoidosis with cutaneous anergy, reduced lymphokine production from peripheral blood mononuclear cells and increased tissue T and B cell activity [21]. The interstitial nephritis responds well to corticosteroids but the uveitis tends to recur [21].

Abnormal calcium metabolism

Hypercalcemia was first recognized as a feature of active sarcoidosis in 1939 and has long been considered the major cause of renal impairment in this disease [2]. This is a view that might not now stand critical reappraisal. The frequency of hypercalcemia and of hypercalciuria is reported to be 2.5–17% and 7.5–65%, respectively in reported series [22], figures that will depend, among other variables, on whether or not corticosteroids have been given.

Pathogenesis

Following the demonstration that the abnormal calcium metabolism of sarcoidosis is due to increased serum calcitriol levels and that this does not depend on the presence of renal tissue, it was shown that alveolar macrophages and lymph gland homogenates from patients with sarcoidosis exhibit 1α-hydroxylase activity and can convert 25-hydroxycholecalciferol to calcitriol [23]. Macrophage 1α-hydroxylase differs from its renal counterpart in not being inhibited by the end product, calcitriol, and in being readily inhibited by corticosteroids [23]. These findings provide the basis for the clinical observations that sharp rises in plasma calcium occur with increased activity of the disease, falling renal function, light exposure and low-dose oral vitamin D, and that the hypercalcemia of sarcoidosis is steroid-responsive.

Calcitriol raises plasma calcium and phosphate concentrations primarily by increasing their transport from the lumen of the small intestine but also synergistically with parathyroid hormone by enhancing bone resorption [24].

Clinical manifestations

Hypercalcemia in sarcoidosis more commonly contributes to chronic rather than acute renal failure with interstitial calcium deposition, chronic inflammation and interstitial fibrosis, showing similarities to the interstitial nephritis discussed above. Impaired urine concentrating ability is an early and prominent feature of hypercalcemia leading to polyuria and polydipsia. However, the features of nephrogenic diabetes insipidus are accompanied by sodium depletion and impaired glomerular filtration rate and permeability attributed to direct effects of calcium on the kidney. Intravenous normal saline to correct the extracellular volume depletion and maintain a diuresis using furosemide is the major requirement in the treatment of hypercalcemic renal failure from all causes [25]. Corticosteroids are effective in relatively small doses in correcting the hypercalcemia of sarcoidosis thanks to their inhibitory effect on macrophage 1α-hydroxylase activity. The dosage regime will need to be adjusted for individual patients [12].

The reversibility of renal functional abnormalities with corticosteroids will depend on the degree of chronic changes present. Hypercalciuria may persist but other therapeutic options can be considered, namely chloroquine [26] and ketoconazole [27, 27a].

Hypercalciuria is responsible for a raised prevalence of renal stones in sarcoidosis – a figure of 10% is quoted [12, 28]. A recent retrospective study of 618 patients with sarcoidosis found that calculi were the presenting manifestation of the disease in six cases (1%) but occurred in a total of 14 patients (2.2%) before the diagnosis of sarcoidosis was made [29]. Radiological nephrocalcinosis is rare, is more frequent in patients with renal failure and is directly related to hypercalcemia [12]. Sarcoidosis has also been reported as a cause of hypercalcemia in an anephric patient on hemodialysis [30].

Sarcoidosis is much less frequently seen in children than adults and the incidence of renal involvement is unknown. However, the pattern of renal disease with granulomatous interstitial nephritis and calcium metabolism abnormalities appears to be similar [31].

The place of calcitriol in an immunomodulating role in sarcoidosis has not been established. It does, however, appear to contribute to the proliferation and differentiation of circulating monocytes into macrophages and epithelioid cells forming granulomas. There is also evidence that calcitriol is a down-regulator of T cell activity by inhibiting T helper cell proliferation and cytokine production [32].

Glomerular disease

There is no convincing evidence of an association of sarcoidosis with primary glomerular disease. Such evidence as there is consists of case reports with no clues such as time course or response to treatment that establishes an etiological relationship.

There is a widely held belief that membranous glomerulonephritis in particular is related to sarcoidosis. It has been suggested that the pattern of histological types of glomerulonephritis differs in sarcoidosis from that found in the general population and that membranous disease is overrepresented [3]. The dearth of reports of minimal change disease in sarcoidosis is believed to be a critical finding. A decade later, we are not aware of reports, a few atypical cases apart [12, 33, 33a] of minimal change disease and sarcoidosis co-existing. Membranous glomerulonephritis in a patient with granulomatous interstitial nephritis has been reported [34].

Although abnormalities of cellular and humoral immunity have been found in minimal change disease and are reviewed elsewhere in this volume (Chapter 15), there is no clear evidence to support Shalhoub's [35] hypothesis that it is secondary to a disorder of T-lymphocyte function. The immunological abnormalities of sarcoidosis could provide clues to the cause of minimal change disease or the expression of the changes in disordered glomerular basement membrane function [36].

Sarcoidosis and urological disease

Retroperitoneal lymph gland involvement in sarcoidosis may, rarely, lead to obstructive nephropathy or renovascular hypertension [12]. Renal sarcoidosis may mimic a renal tumor [37] and, conversely, sarcoid granulomas showing morphological and immunocytochemical features indistinguishable from those of sarcoidosis have been described in renal cell carcinoma [38].

Finally, it should be remembered that coincidental urinary tract disease and other causes of hypercalcemia may occur in patients with sarcoidosis [2, 16].

References

1. Semenzato, G., Agostini, C. and Chilosi, M. (1994) Immunology and immunopathology, in *Sarcoidosis and Other Granulomatous Diseases* (ed. D.C. James), Marcel Dekker, New York, pp. 153–79.
2. Romer, K. (1980) Renal manifestations and abnormal calcium metabolism in sarcoidosis. *Q. J. Med. NS*, **49**, 233–47.
3. Taylor, R.G., Fisher, C. and Hoffbrand, B.I. (1982) Sarcoidosis and membranous glomerulonephritis: a significant association. *Br. Med. J.*, **284**, 1297–8.
4. Berger, K.W. and Relman, A.S. (1955) Renal impairment due to sarcoid infiltration of the kidney. Report of a case proved by renal biopsies before and after treatment with cortisone. *N. Engl. J. Med.*, **252**, 44–9.
5. Longcope, W.T. and Freiman, D.C. (1952) A study of sarcoidosis based on combined investigation of 160 cases, including 30 autopsies, from the Johns Hopkins Hospital and Massachusetts General Hospital. *Medicine*, **31**, 1–132.
6. Lebacq, E., Verhaegen, H. and Desmet, V. (1970) Renal involvement in sarcoidosis. *Postgrad. Med. J.*, **46**, 526–9.
7. Casella, F.J. and Allon, M. (1993) The kidney in sarcoidosis. *J. Am. Soc. Nephrol.*, **3**, 1555–62.
7a. Schena, F.P. and the Italian Group of Renal Immunopathology (1997) Survey of the Italian Registry of Renal Biopsies. Frequency of the renal diseases for 7 consecutive years. *Nephrol. Dial. Transplant.*, **12**, 418–26.
8. Hannedouche, T., Grateau, G., Noël, L.H. *et al.* (1990) Renal granulomatous sarcoidosis. Report of six cases. *Nephrol. Dial. Transplant.*, **5**, 18–24.
8a. Mills, P.R., Burns, A.P., Dorman, A.M. *et al.* (1994) Granulomatous sarcoid nephritis presenting as frank haematuria. *Nephrol. Dial. Transplant.*, **9**, 1649–51.
9. Ball, S., Newman Saunders, A., Cattell, V. *et al.* (1993) Idiopathic interstitial nephritis in Indians. Paper presented at meeting of the Renal Association, London October 1993 and personal communication.
10. Restrick, L.J., Blomley, M.J.K., Drayson, R.A. *et al.* (1993) Percutaneous renal biopsy in the district general hospital. *J. R. Coll. Physicians*, **27**, 247–51.
11. Cheng, H.F., Nolasco, F., Cameron, J.S. *et al.* (1989) HLA-DR display by renal tubular epithelium and phenotype of infiltrate in interstitial nephritis. *Nephrol. Dial. Transplant.*, **4**, 205–15.
12. Kenouch, S. and Mery, J-P. (1992) Sarcoidosis, in *Oxford Textbook of Clinical Nephrology* (eds S. Cameron, A.M. Davison, J.P. Grunfeld *et al.*), Oxford University Press, Oxford, pp. 576–82.
13. Trillo, A., Orozco, R. and Jindal, K. (1992) Glomerular calcinosis in sarcoidosis. *Arch. Pathol. Lab. Med.*, **116**, 1221–5.
14. Muther, R.S., McCarron, D.A. and Bennett, W.M. (1980) Granulomatous sarcoid nephritis: a cause of multiple tubular abnormalities. *Clin. Nephrol.*, **14**, 190–7.
15. Panitz, F. and Shinaberger, J.H. (1965) Nephrogenic diabetes insipidus due to sarcoidosis without hypercalcemia. *Ann. Intern. Med.*, **62**, 113–20.
16. Pagniez, D.C. and Delvallez, L. (1989) Renal gallium scintigraphy and sarcoid nephritis. *Nephrol. Dial. Transplant.*, **4**, 76.
17. Mignon, F., Mery, J-P., Mourgnot, B. *et al.* (1984) Granulomatous interstitial nephritis. *Adv. Nephrol.*, **13**, 219–45.
18. Hoffbrand, B.I. (1994) The kidney in sarcoidosis, in *Sarcoidosis and Other Granulomatous Disorders* (ed. D.G. James), Marcel Dekker, New York, pp. 335–43.
18a. Viero, R.M., Caballo (1995) Granulomatous interstitial nephritis. *Hum-Pathol*, **26**, 1347–53.
19. Ford, M.J., Anderton, J.L. and MacLean, N. (1978) Granulomatous sarcoid nephropathy. *Postgrad. Med. J.*, **54**, 416–17.
20. Dobrin, R.S., Vernier, R.L. and Fish, A.J. (1975) Acute eosinophilic interstitial nephritis and renal failure with bone marrow–lymph node granulomas and anterior uveitis. A new syndrome. *Am. J. Med.*, **59**, 325–33.
21. Gafter, U., Kalechman, Y., Zevin, D. *et al.* (1993) Tubulo-interstitial nephritis and uveitis: association with suppressed cellular immunity. *Nephrol. Dial. Transplant.*, **8**, 821–6.
22. Coburn, J.W. and Barbour, G.L. (1984) Vitamin D intoxication and sarcoidosis, in *Hypercalciuric States. Pathogenesis, Consequences and Treatment* (ed. F.L. Coe), Grune & Stratton, Orlando, pp. 379–433.
23. Singer, F.R. and Adams, J.S. (1986) Abnormal calcium homeostasis in sarcoidosis. *N. Engl. J. Med.*, **315**, 755–7.
24. Holick, M.F., Krane, S.M. and Potts, J.T. (1994) Calcium, phosphorus and bone metabolism: calcium regulating hormones, in *Harrison's Principles of Internal Medicine* (eds K.J. Isselbacher, K.J. Braunwald, J.D. Wilson *et al.*), McGraw-Hill, New York, p. 2143.
25. Rainford, D.J. and Stevens, P.E. (1992) Acute renal failure from tubular injury, in *Oxford Textbook of Clinical Nephrology* (eds S. Cameron, A.M. Davison, J-P. Grunfeld *et al.*), Oxford University Press, Oxford, p. 1012.
26. Adams, J.S., Diz, M.M. and Sharma, O.P. (1989) Effective reduction in the 1,25-dihydroxyvitamin D and calcium concentration in sarcoidosis associated hypercalcemia

with short course chloroquine therapy. *Ann. Intern. Med.*, **111**, 437–8.

27. Bia, M.J. and Insogna, K. (1991) Treatment of sarcoidosis-associated hypercalcemia with ketoconazole. *Am. J. Kidney Dis.*, **18**, 702–5.

27a. Sharma, O.P. (1996) Vitamin D, calcium and sarcoidosis. *Chest*, **109**, 535–39.

28. Rizzato, G. (1992) Sarcoidosis in Italy. *Sarcoidosis*, **9**, 145–7.

29. Rizzato, G., Fraioli, P. and Montemurro, L. (1995) Nephrolithiasis as a presenting feature of chronic sarcoidosis. *Thorax*, **50**, 555–9.

30. Kalanter-Zadeh, K., Neumeyer, H-H., Wunsch, P.H. and Luft, F.C. (1994) Hypercalcemia and sarcoidosis in an anephric dialysis patient. *Nephrol. Dial. Transplant.*, **9**, 829–31.

31. Nocton, J.J., Stark, J.E., Jacobs, G. and Newman, A.J. (1992) Sarcoidosis associated with nephrocalcinosis in young children. *J. Pediatr.*, **121**, 937–40.

32. Costabel, U. (1994) Biochemistry, in *Sarcoidosis and Other Granulomatous Disorders* (ed. D.G. James), Marcel Dekker, New York, pp. 429–63.

33. Anwar, N. and Gokal, R. (1993) Simultaneous occurrence of IgA nephropathy and sarcoidosis in the context of pre-existent minimal change nephrotic syndrome. *Nephron*, **65**, 310–12.

33a. Taylor, J.E. and Ansell, I.D. (1996) Steroid sensitive nephrotic syndrome and renal impairment in a patient with sarcoidosis and IgA nephropathy. *Nephrol. Dial. Transplant.*, **11**, 355–6.

34. Khan, I.H., Simpson, J.G., Catto, G.R.D. and Macleod, A.M. (1994) Membranous nephropathy and granulomatous interstitial nephritis in sarcoidosis. *Nephron*, **66**, 459–61.

35. Shalhoub, R.J. (1974) Pathogenesis of lipoid nephrosis: a disorder of T cell function. *Lancet*, **ii**, 556–9.

36. Sewell, R.F. and Short, C.D. (1993) Minimal-change nephropathy: how does the immune system affect the glomerulus? *Nephrol. Dial. Transplant.*, **8**, 108–12.

37. Rohatgi, P.K., Liao, T.E. and Borts, F.T. (1990) Pseudotumor of left kidney due to sarcoidosis. *Urology*, **35**, 271–5.

38. Campbell, F. and Douglas-Jones, A.G. (1993) Sarcoid-like granulomas in primary renal cell carcinoma. *Sarcoidosis*, **10**, 128–31.

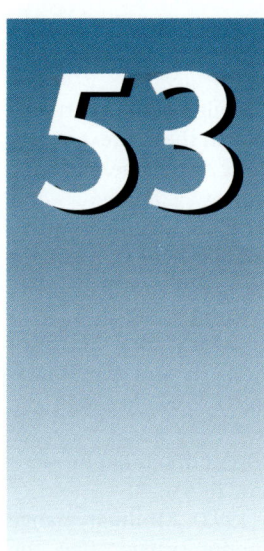

53

Diseases of the kidney secondary to malignant disease

Paul Mead and Adrian R. Morley

Introduction

Tumors are capable of affecting kidney structure and function through a number of mechanisms.

Prerenal causes of renal failure

Patients suffering from malignancy are at risk of renal hypoperfusion for a number of reasons. These include hypovolemia secondary to poor oral intake, vomiting and diarrhea, relative hypovolemia secondary to sepsis, and a severe capillary leak syndrome secondary to interleukin-2 therapy and poor cardiac output secondary to malignant pericardial effusion. Such hypoperfusion will lead to oliguria and varying degrees of renal insufficiency. Restoration of renal perfusion will reverse these abnormalities unless the hypotensive episode has been of sufficient severity and duration to induce acute tubular necrosis. Tumor present at the kidney hilum, either as metastases or lymphoma, may produce renal artery compression of sufficient degree to induce severe hypertension.

Intravascular coagulation

Diffuse intravascular coagulation (DIC), hemolytic uremic syndrome (HUS) and thrombotic thrombocy-topenic purpura (TTP) cause acute renal failure through renal ischemia secondary to microvascular damage. DIC, as well as being induced by sepsis, has also occurred in cases of carcinoma of the pancreas, lung and trophoblastic tumors. HUS and TTP, which present with the triad of acute renal failure, thrombocytopenia and a microangiopathic hemolytic anemia, have occurred in cases of mucin-secreting adenocarcinoma of stomach, pancreas and prostate. Additionally, HUS and TTP may occur with antitumor therapy, including mitomycin, the combination of bleomycin with cisplatin and of radiotherapy with high dose cyclophosphamide. Many tumors are capable of inducing a hypercoagulable state, predisposing to renal vein thrombosis. In addition, thrombosis or occlusion of one or both renal veins may arise from external compression or particularly with renal cell carcinoma, direct invasion of the renal veins and inferior vena cava by tumor. Such events may present acutely with loin pain, acute decline in glomerular filtration rate and hematuria or be clinically covert.

Direct infiltration of kidney substance

Probably the most obvious example of tumors affecting kidney structure is that of those arising directly from renal tissue, the most common of which is the renal cell carcinoma. This is the tumor type which had previously

Nephrology, Edited by Rex L. Jamison and Robert Wilkinson.
Published in 1997 by Chapman & Hall, London. ISBN 0 412 60930 4

been termed a hypernephroma under the mistaken belief that it arose from heterotopic adrenal nests within the kidney. It occurs with a worldwide incidence of 2–8 per 100 000 population. Presentation is classically with any combination of hematuria, pain and or the presence of a palpable mass. Treatment is largely surgical with a 5-year survival of approximately 40%. Metastatic spread of other tumors to the kidney does occur, although probably less commonly than one would expect, given that the kidney receives 20% of the cardiac output. In one series, postmortem examination of over 4000 cancer sufferers demonstrated the presence of renal metastases in approximately 18% of cases (hematological malignancies were excluded). Metastatic spread to the kidney tends to be a late event in patients with widely disseminated disease. Proteinuria and hematuria are common features, whereas pain and renal insufficiency rarely occur [1].

Interstitial disease

Disease primarily affecting the interstitial tissue of the kidney can occur in subjects with malignancy. Infiltration by tumor in cases of lymphoma or acute leukemia is not uncommon, although only rarely, when such a process is both extensive and rapid, does acute renal failure ensue. In this situation the renal prognosis depends on the responsiveness of the tumor to radiation or chemotherapy. In the treatment of malignancy many drugs, in addition to cytotoxics, are used including antibiotics, analgesics, antiemetics and, in the case of hematological malignancies, allopurinol. Such agents are capable of initiating an acute interstitial nephritis characterized by hematuria, proteinuria, acute renal failure, fever, rash, arthralgia, liver dysfunction and blood eosinophilia. Here the mechanism of damage is believed to be immunological with the drug acting as the initiating antigen. Cases of chronic interstitial nephritis have been described with certain cytotoxic agents of the nitrosourea class. Here the disease occurs over a period of months to years and is characterized by proteinuria and progressive renal impairment. The proposed mechanism of damage is thought to be through alkylation of tubular cell proteins. Radiotherapy involving the kidneys can produce similar effects.

Renal tubular disease

Renal tubular dysfunction may occur via a number of mechanisms in subjects suffering from malignancy. Once again, therapies directed at the malignancy may have adverse effects on function and lead to the tubular development of acute tubular necrosis. Aggressive treatment of hematological malignancies occasionally causes an acute nephropathy as part of the so-called tumor lysis syndrome. This is due to destruction of malignant cells with

the release of several substances, in particular urate, which exert a deleterious effect on the kidney. Chemotherapeutic strategies employing high dose methotrexate $(1–2\,g/m^2)$ carry an appreciable risk of nephrotoxicity associated with widespread intratubular deposition of methotrexate and its metabolites. Both non-oliguric and oliguric acute renal failure may occur. The risk of this can be reduced ny maintaining an alkaline diuresis throughout the treatment period. Ifosfamide has been associated with tubular dysfunction leading to hypokalemia, hypophosphatemia and acidosis and vincristine through its effect in augmenting the release of arginine vasopressin (AVP) is capable of causing hyponatremia.

The tumor itself is also capable of affecting renal tubules, the most obvious example being that of multiple myeloma where light chains, once filtered through the glomerulus, cause tubular dysfunction through both direct toxic effects on the tubular cells and also tubular obstruction. This is usually characterized by varying degrees of renal failure, but is also occasionally associated with other abnormalities of tubular function. Similarly, tubular cells may become dysfunctional because of the effects of filtered lysozyme released from leukemia cells in patients with acute monocytic or myelomonocytic leukemia. Tumors may cause hypercalcemia from dissolution of bone by metastases or production of a parathyroid hormone-like substance. Hypercalcemia exerts numerous adverse effects on the kidney, examples of which include, the development of renal calculi, nephrocalcinosis, decreased glomerular filtration rate secondary to renal vasoconstriction and nephrogenic diabetes insipidus from AVP antagonism at the level of adenylcyclase. Various tumors are capable of elaborating AVP, an excess of which leads to water retention and consequent hyponatremia [2]. Destruction of endocrine tissue by tumor may become clinically evident because of withdrawal of a hormone effect on the kidney, one example being malignant infiltration of the hypothalmus causing destruction of AVP-secreting tissue, leading to diabetes insipidus characterized by polyuria, hypernatremia and hypovolemia.

Urinary obstruction

When tumors involve the urinary tract, obstruction of urinary outflow may occur. Such tumors may be intrinsic, for example transitional cell carcinomas of the urinary tract and prostatic carcinoma, or extrinsic, in which tumors arising from local structures, e.g. the cervix uteri and rectum, either compress or infiltrate the ureters. Obstructive uropathy secondary to malignant disease is relatively uncommon, accounting for less than 10% of all cases of obstruction. The commonest cause being secondary to benign prostatic hyperplasia. Strictures of the ureter leading to obstructive uropathy can occur as a complication of radiotherapy. This has been most commonly described in cases of cervical carcinoma.

Glomerular disease

Introduction

The remainder of this chapter will discuss glomerular disease arising as a consequence of malignancy, under three headings: glomerular disease secondary to solid tumors; glomerular disease secondary to lymphoma and leukemia and glomerular disease secondary to plasma cell dyscrasias. With solid tumors, the most frequently observed glomerular lesion is membranous glomerulonephritis, probably resulting from deposition of tumor-derived antigen within the glomerular basement membrane (GBM) and its subsequent interaction with antibody to form immune complexes. In the second group, the most commonly described association is minimal change glomerulonephritis in subjects suffering from Hodgkin's lymphoma. It is proposed that the malignant cells elaborate and release lymphokines which alter the permeability characteristics of the GBM and cause proteinuria. In plasma cell dyscrasias, amyloidosis is the classic glomerular lesion encountered. It is due to light chain deposition and modification which ultimately leads to the formation of amyloid. Amyloid deposits in the GBM alter its structure and affect its function leading to proteinuria and later uremia by occluding glomerular capillary loops.

Glomerular disease secondary to solid tumors

Introduction

Urinary abnormalities such as mild proteinuria or hematuria occur commonly in patients suffering from malignancy. This is not necessarily associated with structural changes within the glomerulus [3, 4]. Histologically proven glomerulonephritis is rare in patients with malignant disease, the estimated prevalence is 1.6% [5]. Nephrotic syndrome is the most frequently described renal presentation associated with underlying malignancy. In an adult nephrotic population the reported prevalence of underlying malignancy ranges from <1% to 10.6% [6–8]. The most frequently reported glomerular lesion is membranous glomerulonephritis accounting for approximately 70% of cases [9]. In patients with membranous glomerulonephritis, the prevalence of an associated tumor lies between 6% and 11% [10, 11]. Most cases occur in subjects age 40 years or more.

Since the annual incidence of membranous glomerulonephritis in the UK is three per million adult population and only 10% of these are likely to be associated with malignancy, the association of a malignancy and membranous glomerulonephritis is uncommon.

The postmortem series mentioned earlier demonstrated glomerulonephritis in 1.6% of cancer sufferers [5]. Given the prevalence of malignancy in the general population one might expect the prevalence of malignancy-associated glomerulopathy to be higher. However, unless renal disease is life threatening, the investigations necessary to establish the nature of renal involvement in patients with advanced malignancy are usually considered inappropriate. Renal involvement is therefore probably underdiagnosed.

In 45% of cases, onset of the nephrotic syndrome predates discovery of an underlying tumor. In most of these cases, the underlying tumor becomes clinically evident within a year of the onset of the nephrotic state. In approximately 40% of cases the nephrotic state and underlying tumor are diagnosed simultaneously and in the remainder the nephrotic state develops after diagnosis of the malignancy. In 70% of the latter cases, the nephrotic syndrome develops within a year of the diagnosis of the malignancy [9].

In addition to membranous glomerulonephritis, many other types of glomerulopathy have been described in association with solid tumors (Table 53.1). Such associations, however, have usually been published as case reports or as very small series. The associated glomerulopathies described present similarly to their idiopathic counterparts. The underlying tumors vary, the most frequently described of which are tumors of the lung and gastrointestinal tract. These account for approximately 70% of cases [9].

Case report

This is a case of a patient presenting with nephrotic syndrome and subsequently developing symptoms of a malignancy. The rarity of the association is emphasized by the fact that this was one of only two cases in the last three years in a renal unit that serves a population of 1.5 million.

A 69-year-old female presented with nephrotic syndrome developing over four weeks and preceded by a two-day history of symptoms suggestive of an infection with associated diarrhea. She was receiving treatment with amlodipine for hypertension. Positive findings on physical examination included a raised jugular venous pressure, ascites and gross peripheral edema. Initial investigation revealed normal values for hematological indices, plasma urea, creatinine and electrolytes. Serum albumin was 12 g/l (normal range 38–48 g/l) and 24-h urinary protein excretion 5.33 g.

Autoantibodies were not present and electrophoresis of serum and urine failed to demonstrate evidence of a monoclonal gammopathy. Renal biopsy showed a mild immune complex nephritis (Figure 53.1).

She was treated with prednisolone, diuretics and an HMG-CoA reductase inhibitor. There was no reduction in urinary protein. After two months she developed left-sided weakness. A chest radiograph showed a lesion in the right mid zone and some widening of the mediastinum, suggestive of a primary lung neoplasm with paratracheal lymph node involvement (Figure 53.2). Brain scan revealed three rim-enhancing abnormalities: two in the right cerebral hemisphere and the third within the left

Table 53.1 Histological classification of glomerular lesions other than membranous glomerulonephritis associated with underlying solid tumors

Histological lesion	Associated tumor	Reference
Minimal change nephropathy	Renal cell carcinoma Bronchogenic carcinoma	Abouchacra *et al.* [12] Moorthy [13]
Crescentic glomerulonephritis	Gastric carcinoma Prostatic carcinoma	Irish *et al.* [14] Haskell *et al.* [15]
Amyloidosis	Renal cell carcinoma Ovarian carcinoma	Karsenty *et al.* [16] Fernandezmiranda *et al.* [17]
Congo red negative fibrillary glomerulonephritis	Metastatic adenocarcinoma of liver	Abraham *et al.* [18]
Mesangiocapillary glomerulonephritis	Carcinoma of esophagus	Walker *et al.* [19]
IgA nephropathy	Bronchial small cell carcinoma Squamous cell carcinoma of bronchus	Mustonen *et al.* [20] Cairns *et al.* [21]
Mesangial proliferative glomerulonephritis	Small cell anaplastic carcinoma of lung	Jermanovich *et al.* [22]
Focal segmental glomerulosclerosis	Adenocarcinoma of rectum	Kitano [23]

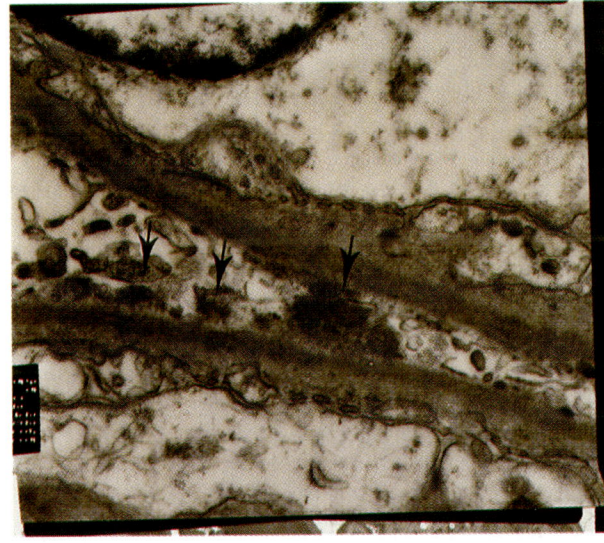

Figure 53.1 Electron microscopy of GBMs showing dense deposits on their epimembranous surfaces (×24 000). The patient presented with nephrotic syndrome and was subsequently found to have an underlying bronchial neoplasm.

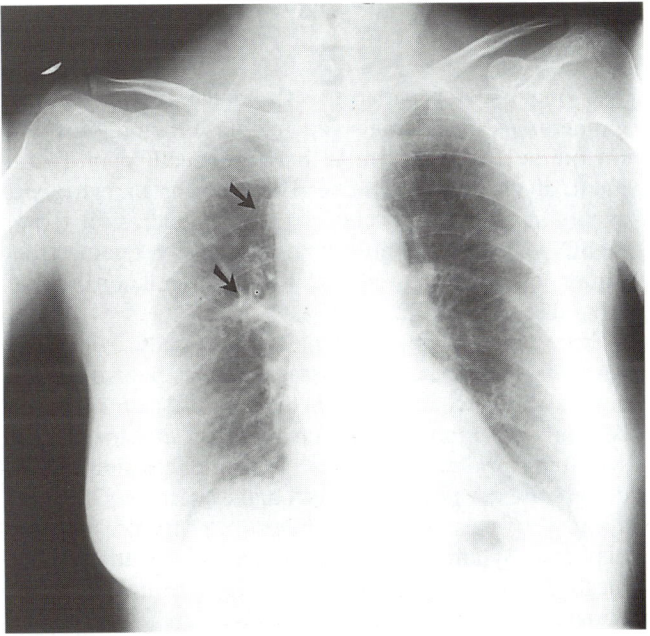

Figure 53.2 Chest radiograph showing abnormalities compatible with a diagnosis of malignancy (arrows) in the patient described in Figure 53.1.

cerebellar hemisphere, the appearances compatible with metastatic disease. Oral dexamethasone was instituted as palliative treatment. She deteriorated rapidly. A request for autopsy was refused.

Mechanisms of glomerular injury

Circulating immune complexes occur in a large proportion of patients suffering from solid tumors [9]. Evidence suggests, however, that preformed immune complexes do not have a role in the pathogenesis of glomerulonephritis [24]. It is now generally accepted that many forms of immune complex glomerulonephritis result from the initial interaction and deposition of circulating antigen within the GBM. Subsequent antibody attachment occurs and, through several effector mechanisms, leads to a local inflammatory response and ultimately glomerular dysfunction [24]. Studies of tumor-associated glomerulonephritis [9, 25, 26] have provided convincing evidence for the presence of tumor-derived antigen and appropriately directed antibody in the glomeruli. The antigens were tumor specific or the re-expressed fetal antigen, carcinoembryonic antigen (CEA). A slightly different sequence of events may occur in some cases of tumor-associated glomerulopathy. It is postulated that the tumor, through effects on the host immune system, causes development of autoantibodies which interact with host antigen deposited in the glomerulus or with antigenic determinants of the glomerular structure itself. Patients with malignancies have a high incidence of autoantibodies, a number of which have been implicated in the pathogenesis of glomerulonephritides [9]. The antigens have been either deoxyribonucleic acid (DNA) or renal tubular epithelial antigen (RTE).

This evidence, together with the histology of the glomerular lesions and the report of clinical and histological improvement after tumor resection [27], indicates that the most common glomerular lesions associated with solid malignancies are derived from *in situ* immune complex formation. Both tumor-derived antigens and autoimmune antibodies are implicated.

Outcome

The outcome for patients with malignancy-associated glomerulopathy, is largely dependent on the prognosis of the tumor [12, 14, 28] and is therefore usually poor. Treatment of glomerular disease with steroids or cytotoxic agents has been unsuccessful [12, 29]. Successful treatment, both medical and surgical, directed against the tumor has, however, generally led to remission of the renal disease [9, 22, 29, 30].

Recurrence of the malignancy is usually associated with a relapse of the renal disease [22, 31], but this is not always the case. Boon *et al.* described a case of small cell lung carcinoma, in which the associated nephrotic syndrome resolved with treatment and did not return despite the development of cerebral metastases [28]. The authors speculated that failure of recurrence of the nephrotic syndrome could be explained by the impermeability of the blood–brain barrier to tumor-derived antigens.

Conclusion

Solid tumor-associated glomerular disease is rare. The glomerulopathy commonly manifests as the nephrotic syndrome. Membranous glomerulonephritis is the most frequent lesion. Many different tumors have been implicated, with those of lung and gastrointestinal tract being the most frequent. In the vast majority, the tumor will either be clinically obvious at the onset of the nephrotic syndrome or become so within a year. Treatment of the nephrotic syndrome should be symptomatic. If the malignancy is successfully treated the nephrotic syndrome will resolve.

Re-emergence of the renal abnormalities may herald a tumor relapse. Overall, the prognosis of solid tumor-associated glomerular disease is poor and largely determined by the underlying malignancy. The need to screen for malignancy in patients with the nephrotic syndrome depends on the age of the patient, the renal lesion observed and the presence of other risk factors for tumor such as smoking, family history, occupation, etc. Screening in asymptomatic patients is usually limited to chest radiograph.

Glomerular disease secondary to lymphoma and leukemia

Introduction

Abnormalities of urinalysis are common in patients suffering from either lymphoma or leukemia [4]. They are rarely related to a specific glomerulopathy, but often reflect renal parenchymal infiltration with malignant cells [32]. The most frequently recognized specific association is that of nephrotic syndrome due to minimal change glomerulonephritis in Hodgkin's lymphoma. From 1930 to 1986 only 41 such cases had been described. In one series of 600 patients with Hodgkin's disease only four were found to have the nephrotic syndrome. In three of these histological examination of renal tissue showed minimal change glomerulonephritis [33]. Renal amyloidosis is also a complication of Hodgkin's disease. The amyloid deposit is usually the AA type and is a reflection of many years of active disease [34]. With the advent of more effective chemotherapeutic strategies for lymphoma only five cases of nephrotic syndrome due to amyloidosis in association with Hodgkin's disease have been described since 1962 [9]. Other glomerulopathies have been reported in patients with Hodgkin's lymphoma (Table 53.2), but they are rare. Even though non-Hodgkin's lymphoma is much more common than Hodgkin's lymphoma, the number of reported cases of associated glomerulopathy is less than that in Hodgkin's disease; up to 1986 only 35 cases had been described. The renal pathology varied widely.

Renal disease is also rare in patients with leukemias, only 36 cases with a glomerulopathy had been published up to 1986, most commonly in patients with chronic lymphocytic leukemia [33].

Taking lymphomas and leukemias together, the most frequent clinical manifestation of an underlying glomerulopathy is the nephrotic syndrome. Given the rarity of an associated glomerulopathy and the fact that these malignancies are themselves uncommon, the likelihood of an underlying lymphoma or leukemia in a patient with nephrotic syndrome is extremely small. In a series of 101 patients with nephrotic syndrome, none had a hematological malignancy whereas eleven had an associated solid tumor [8]. In contrast to patients with solid tumors,

Table 53.2 Glomerulopathies reported in association with Hodgkin's disease

Glomeropathy	Reference
Focal glomerulosclerosis	Watson *et al.* [35]
Membranous glomerulonephritis	Row *et al.* [11]
Mesangiocapillary glomerulonephritis	Pascal [5]
Mesangial proliferative glomerulonephritis	Hyman *et al.* [36]
Crescentic glomerulonephritis (anti GBM +ve)	Kleinknecht *et al.* [37] Mu *et al.* [38]

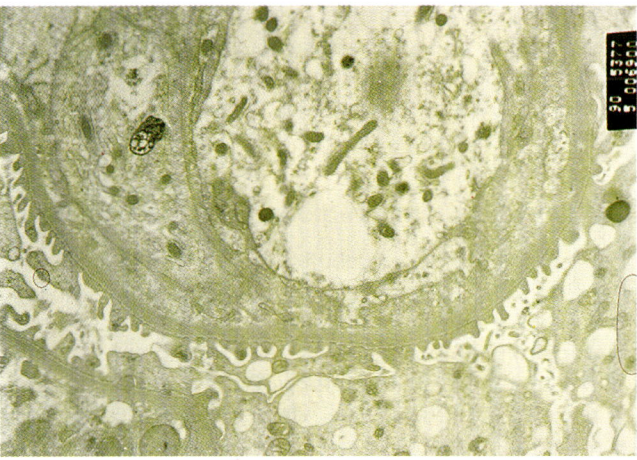

Figure 53.3 Electron microscopy showing a glomerular capillary loop with endothelial cell swelling and cytoplasm filling the capillary space (×6900). The patient had nephrotic syndrome associated with lymphoblastic lymphoma.

those with lymphoma or leukemia-associated glomerulopathies manifest the nephrotic syndrome simultaneously with the malignancy or with a recurrence or relapse [9].

The following case is a case of lymphoma-associated glomerulopathy.

Case report

A man aged 64 was found to have a high-grade lymphoblastic lymphoma, involving lymph nodes in his neck, left axilla, mediastinum and right groin but not the bone marrow. He responded to chemotherapy but developed recurrent disease after four years with cervical, axillary and para-aortic lymphadenopathy. Initially no treatment was given because he was well, however, he later developed marked bilateral leg edema, renal impairment and significant proteinuria. Renal biopsy revealed a glomerulopathy with endothelial swelling tending to obliterate the glomerular capillaries (Figure 53.3). Treatment consisted of high-dose diuretics, fluid restriction, intravenous human albumin infusion and high-dose steroids. His edema disappeared, renal function improved and proteinuria fell from 2.16 to 0.65 g/24 h. Subsequently he was given a further course of chemotherapy; he responded well and showed no evidence of recurrence of his renal disease. His long-term care was transferred to another center and no further details of this case have been sought. This case illustrates three aspects of glomerulopathy associated with lymphoma and leukemia. First, the association is very rare, since this was only one of two cases in five years in a region serving a population of 3 million. Second, the nephrotic syndrome responded to treatment specifically for glomerulopathy. Third, the renal disease may not be manifest at the initial presentation of the malignancy, but develop later when an apparently effectively treated disease shows evidence of recurrence.

Mechanisms of glomerular injury

The mechanism of glomerular injury associated with lymphoma and leukemia is unknown as is the case for the idiopathic glomerulopathies. Theories are many. Viral antigens may play a role in the immune complex-mediated glomerular injury linked to lymphoreticular disease [9, 36]. The virus may either be present because of the host's impaired immunity or as an oncogenic determinant initiating the malignancy. In minimal change disease (MCD) found in patients with Hodgkin's disease, abnormalities in the number or function of T cells may lead to the elaboration of lymphokines capable of increasing glomerular capillary permeability to macromolecules. (The same theory has been advanced to explain idiopathic MCD.) Proteases produced by tumor cells that cause vascular damage have also been proposed. Finally, cryoglobulinemia sometimes occurs in patients with lymphoma or leukemia and may play a pivotal role in the development of kidney dysfunction [39, 40]. This is discussed later.

Outcome

The prognosis of the glomerular disease is largely dependent on the underlying neoplastic process. Effective therapy directed towards the tumor generally leads to remission of the renal lesion [33, 41]. This does not exclude the possibility that the chemotherapeutic agents themselves have a beneficial effect on the renal lesion. In contrast with the situation with solid tumors, specific therapies directed against the glomerular lesion have shown a beneficial response in some cases with lymphoma or leukemia [33, 42]. Recurrence of a previously treated lymphoma or leukemia may lead to the reemergence of the renal disease [9]. Shapira *et al.* however, have reported minimal change glomerulonephritis in two patients who had previously undergone treatment for Hodgkin's disease and had no evidence of recurrence [43]. These patients were thought to have developed the glomerular lesion because of a persisting T-cell abnormality [44].

Waldenström's macroglobulinemia

Waldenström's macroglobulinemia is included here because it may be a variant of lymphocytic lymphoma. It is a condition in which the primary abnormality is of neoplastic proliferation of plasmacytoid lymphocytes. These activated abnormal B lymphocytes produce IgM which is released into the general circulation. This condition accounts for about 30% of monoclonal macroglobulinemias [45]. It is a rare condition, about one seventh as common as multiple myeloma. The median age at presentation is 63 years. Most of the morbidity is associated with the increased blood concentration of IgM. Patients commonly present with symptoms of fatigue, weakness, weight loss and bleeding. Examination may reveal hepatosplenomegaly, purpura, lymphadenopathy, neurological signs and retinopathy. It is incurable; with treatment, the median survival is 5 years [45]. Deranged renal function, although uncommon, can occur by a number of mechanisms. These include amyloidosis, cellular infiltration of the kidney, glomerular IgM deposition (Figure 53.4) glomerular immune complex deposition, minimal change glomerulonephritis and antiglomerular antibodies [45, 46]. The renal abnormalities tend to improve with the introduction of therapy directed towards the neoplasm.

Conclusion

The association of glomerular disease with lymphomas and leukemias is a rare phenomenon. The most frequent

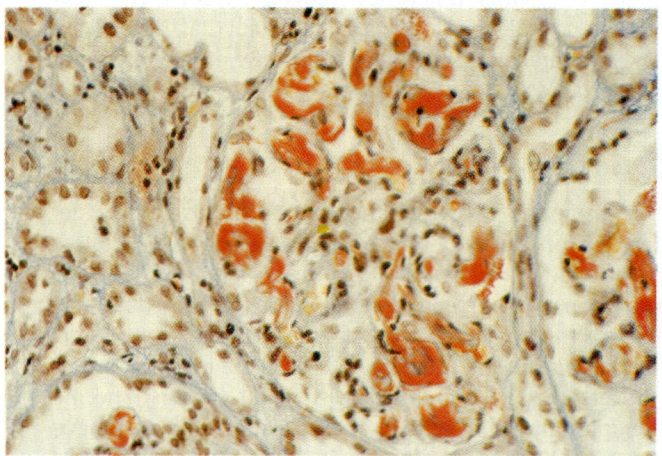

Figure 53.4 Renal histology from a case of Waldenström's macroglobulinemia showing glomerular change consistent with extensive intracapillary deposition of IgM (×200; hematoxylin and eosin).

neoplastic processes are Hodgkin's disease and chronic lymphocytic leukemia. Nephrotic syndrome is the commonest renal presentation and is usually manifest at the time of diagnosis of the neoplastic process or with a relapse. The most frequently observed renal lesion in association with Hodgkin's disease is minimal change glomerulonephritis. In chronic lymphocytic leukemia the renal pathology varies widely. Specific therapy directed against the neoplastic process is the most effective way of improving the renal abnormality. However, treatment directed specifically at the renal lesion, such as prednisolone, may also be effective, unlike the situation with solid tumors.

Glomerular disease secondary to plasma cell dyscrasias

Introduction

Plasma cell dyscrasias are a group of disorders characterized by an abnormal proliferation of a clone of plasma cells which have the potential to produce immunoglobulin. Such a process is responsible for a range of pathological conditions from an apparently harmless benign monoclonal gammopathy to an overt malignancy (multiple myeloma). This section briefly describes those glomerular lesions that occur in association with the malignant end of the spectrum. Multiple myeloma is a neoplastic disease of plasma cells, the diagnosis of which is based on three major criteria:

1   The presence of a monoclonal immunoglobulin in the blood and/or urine. This is not pathognomonic as other conditions can cause a paraproteinemia and also rarely no paraprotein may be detected despite the presence of obvious myeloma.
2   Bone marrow plasmacytosis. The monoclonality of such plasma cells can be inferred from appropriate immunocytochemistry.
3   Osteolytic bone lesions (Figure 53.5).

Multiple myeloma accounts for approximately 1% of all cancers with an incidence of approximately 3/100000 population per year. It occurs more frequently in older age groups. The disease carries a poor prognosis, cures are rare and the median duration of survival is two to three years with treatment.

Renal disease is common, it is found in 10% of patients at presentation and in half of all myeloma patients at some time during their illness. Renal involvement carries a poor prognosis with regard to survival. Since renal involvement common, patients frequently first appear in a nephrology clinic and the diagnosis of multiple myeloma made by renal biopsy. In the vast majority of cases, however, the renal disease is not due to glomerular pathology, but to tubular toxicity related to light chain excretion (Figure 53.6). Less commonly renal failure develops as a result of hypercalcemia. Glomerular involvement can occur by a number of mechanisms,

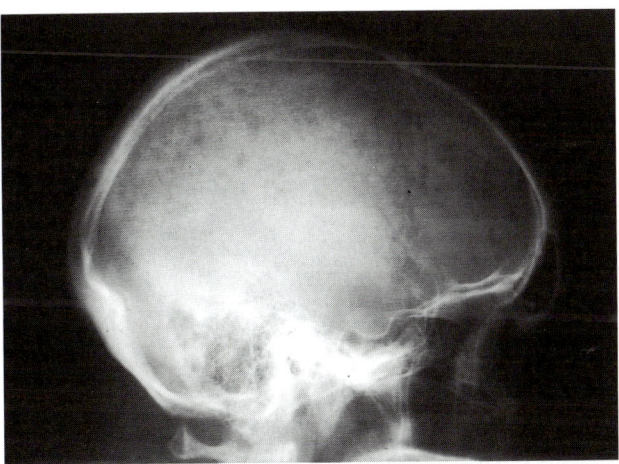

Figure 53.5 Skull radiograph showing the typical lytic lesions of multiple myeloma.

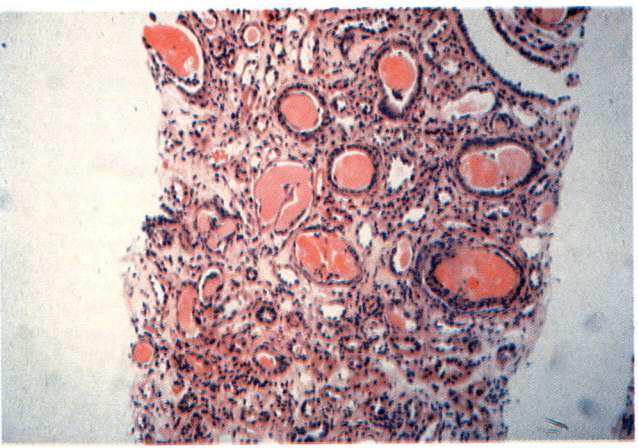

Figure 53.6 Myeloma kidney showing large irregular cracked and fissured casts with associated damage to tubular walls and the presence of multinucleated giant cells (×200; hematoxylin and eosin).

including amyloid deposition, light chain deposition disease and as a complication of cryoglobulinemia. Other glomerular lesions have been reported, but occur much less frequently. These include combined light and heavy chain deposition disease, heavy chain deposition disease and rapidly progressive glomerulonephritis. Amyloidosis is the most frequently encountered glomerular lesion, but it is relatively rare. In one series of over 2000 renal biopsies undertaken at a single center for all indications, a diagnosis of amyloidosis was made in only 25 cases and of these only two showed evidence of multiple myeloma [47]. The following case demonstrates that multiple myeloma can be present even in the absence of a demonstrable serum or urine paraprotein.

Case report

A 44-year-old fireman was referred because of hypertension, hematuria and proteinuria. General examination demonstrated borderline hypertension and mild peripheral edema. Investigations confirmed the hematuria, quantified the proteinuria at 7 g/24 h and demonstrated a low serum albumin of 34 g/l. Serum protein electrophoresis was normal. Renal biopsy showed features consistent with mesangiocapillary glomerulonephritis on light microscopy. Electron microscopy, however, raised the possibility of light chain deposition disease (Figure 53.7). Four further serum and two further urine samples over the course of the patient's illness failed to disclose a monoclonal gammopathy. Within a year he reached end-stage renal failure. Within a few months of commencing dialysis he developed hepatic encephalopathy. Liver biopsy also raised the possibility of light chain deposition disease (Figure 53.8). Skeletal survey, serum ionized calcium and serum and urine electrophoresis were all normal. Bone marrow examination showed 30% plasma cells, which appeared malignant. Immunocytochemical analysis of these cells was in keeping with their mono-

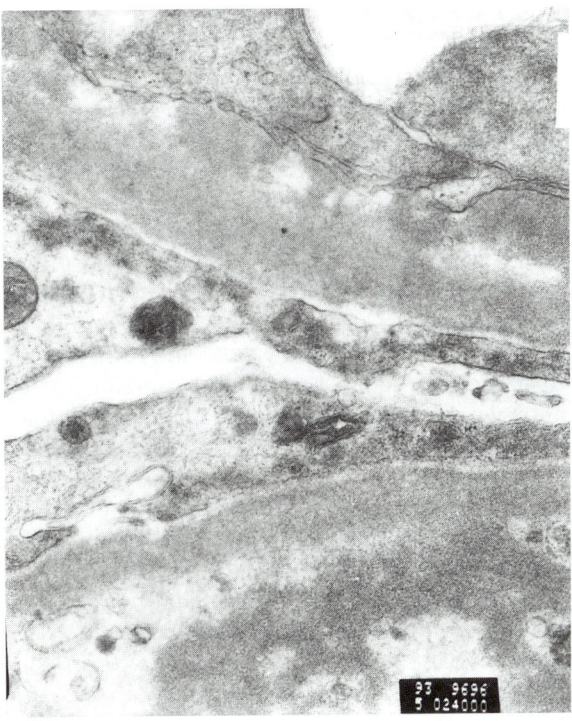

Figure 53.7 Electron microscopy of GBMs showing heavy infiltration with an electron-dense amorphous material (×24 000). The patient presented with nephrotic syndrome and was subsequently shown to have multiple myeloma although serum and urine electrophoresis failed to demonstrate a monoclonal gammopathy or light chains.

clonal nature and showed the presence of kappa light chains.

The patient deteriorated rapidly and died within a week of the diagnosis of multiple myeloma. Autopsy was not requested.

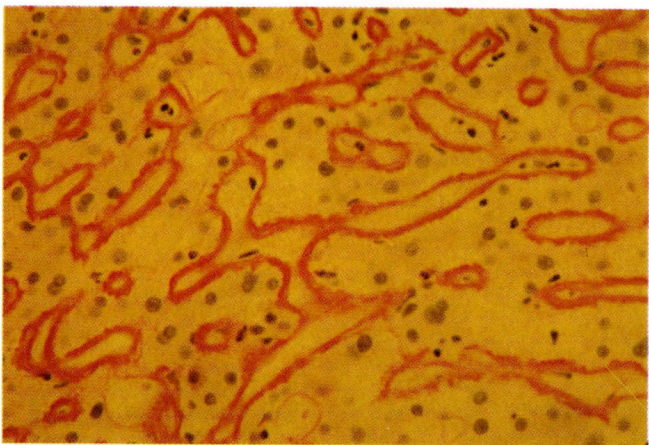

Figure 53.8 Liver histology showing the presence of an abnormal deposition of periodic acid–schiff-positive material (×400; PAS). This is the same patient as in Figure 53.7 after the development of hepatic encephalopathy.

Mechanisms of glomerular injury

Amyloidosis in the plasma cell dyscrasias is due to formation of amyloid protein from immunoglobulin light chain amino acid sequences. Observations suggest that certain light chains have structural peculiarities which predispose them to undergo amyloidogenesis [48]. The same is true for light chain deposition disease [49]. Amyloidosis and light chain deposition disease affect the kidney in the same way. Abnormal protein is deposited within the mesangium and near the GBM (Figure 53.9). This alters the permeability of the GBM and disrupts the glomerular capillary loops. The clinical consequence is proteinuria with or without renal insufficiency. Multiple myeloma is associated with type 1 and type 2 cryoglobulinemia [39]. In type 1 the pathogenic immunoglobulins are monoclonal, whereas in type 2 the cryoglobulins are mixed with a monoclonal component possessing antibody activity towards polyclonal IgG. Several different glomerular lesions have been described and two mechanisms have been proposed for their development. The first proposes that the cryoglobulin precipitates in the glomerular capillaries because of an increase in its concentration as a result of ultrafiltration. In this situation the cryoglobulin may precipitate at a higher temperature than normally required.

The second proposed mechanism suggests that there may be initial trapping of immunoglobulin in the glomeruli where it acts as an antigen for antibody deposition. In both types of cryoglobulinemia the antibodies have been shown to activate complement, thus providing an effector mechanism for inflammation.

Outcome

The prognosis in those individuals with multiple myeloma is poor. Light chain amyloidosis (AL) carries an

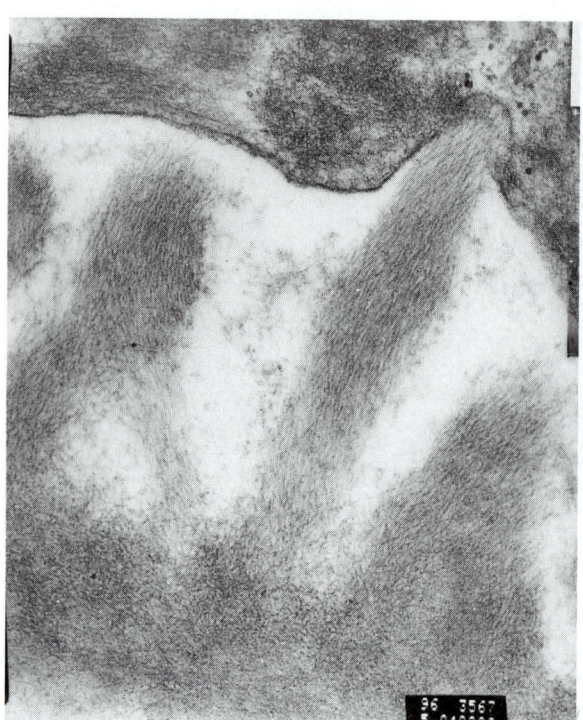

Figure 53.9 Electron microscopy of a GBM showing randomly distributed microfibrils characterstic of amyloidosis (×40 000). The patient had multiple myeloma with circulating and urinary light chains.

even worse prognosis with a median survival of between 7 and 12 months. In such individuals the presence of multiple myeloma has in some series been associated with a considerably worse prognosis, whereas in others it has not [49, 50]. Cardiac failure secondary to amyloid infiltration of cardiac muscle is the commonest cause of death. In patients with proven multiple myeloma cytotoxic therapy is indicated. Besides altering the course of the malignancy it may also improve amyloid glomerulopathy. Even in cases of AL amyloidosis not associated with overt malignancy, cytotoxic therapy may still be of benefit. The prognosis of light chain deposition disease is better than that of AL amyloidosis, with one series showing a survival for the former of 76% at three years. Cytotoxic therapy may benefit those without an overt malignancy [49]. The morbidity of patients with multiple myeloma can be severely adversely affected by an associated cryoglobulin. Severe cold sensitivity, cutaneous necrosis, vasculitic rashes, polyneuropathy and renal involvement can all occur. Here, as well as appropriate cytotoxic regimes, the use of plasmapheresis can be of benefit [51].

Conclusion

Renal dysfunction is common in myeloma and usually secondary to the toxicity of light chains or hypercalcemia.

Glomerular disease is rare. When it does occur, amyloidosis, light chain deposition disease or cryoglobulinemia are usually responsible. It manifests as proteinuria, sometimes to nephrotic levels and varying degrees of renal insufficiency. When renal biopsy suggests any of these conditions we recommend early bone marrow examination. Although the prognosis of multiple myeloma is poor, treatment is of benefit and has occasionally resulted in long-term survival. Such treatment may also have a beneficial effect on the associated glomerular diseases.

References

1. Wagle, D.G., Moore, R.H. and Murphy, G.P. (1975) Secondary carcinomas of the kidney. *J. Urol.*, **114**, 30.
2. Bartter, F.C. and Schwartz, W.B. (1967) The syndrome of inappropriate secretion of antidiuretic hormone. *Am. J. Med.*, **42**, 790–806.
3. Puoligoki, H., Mustonen, J., Petterson, E. *et al.* (1989) Proteinuria and hematuria are frequently present in patients with lung cancer. *Nephrol. Dial. Transplant.*, **4**, 947–50.
4. Sawyer, N., Wadsworth, J., Winnen, M. and Gabriel, R. (1988) Prevalence, concentration and prognostic importance of proteinuria in patients with malignancy. *Br. Med. J.*, **296**, 1295–8.
5. Pascal, R.R. (1980) Renal manifestations of extrarenal neoplasms. *Human Pathol.*, **11**, 7–17.
6. Kaplan, B.S., Klassen, J. and Gautt, M.H. (1976) Glomerular injury in patients with neoplasia. *Annu. Rev. Med.*, **27**, 117–25.
7. Heneghan, W., Rao, T.K.S., Nicastri, A.D. and Friedman, E.A. (1980) Low incidence of malignancy associated with nephrotic syndrome in the elderly (abstract). *Am. Soc. Nephrol. 13th Annual Meeting*, p. 20A.
8. Lee, J.C., Yamouchi, H. and Hopper, J. Jr (1966) The association of cancer and the nephrotic syndrome. *Ann. Intern. Med.*, **64**, 41–51.
9. Eagen and Lewis (1977) Glomerulopathies of neoplasia. *Kidney Int.*, **11**, 297–306.
10. Hopper, J. Jr (1974) Tumour related renal lesions. *Ann. Intern. Med.*, **81**, 550–1.
11. Row, P.G., Cameron, J.S., Turner, D.R. *et al.* (1975) Membranous nephropathy. Long-term follow-up and association with neoplasia. *Q. J. Med.*, **44**, 207–39.
12. Abouchacra, S., Duguid, W.P. and Somerville, P.J. (1993) Renal cell carcinoma presenting as nephrotic syndrome complicated by acute renal failure. *Clin. Nephrol.*, **39**, 340–2.
13. Moorthy, A.V. (1983) Minimal change glomerular disease: a paraneoplastic syndrome in two patients with brionchogenic carcinoma. *Am. J. Kidney Dis.*, **3**, 58.
14. Irish, A.B., Savdie, E. and Delprado, W. (1992) Simultaneous presentation of gastric carcinoma and crescentic glomerulonephritis. *Nephron*, **60**, 254.
15. Haskell, L.P., Fusco, M.J., Wadler, S. *et al.* (1990) Crescentic glomerulonephritis associated with prostatic carcinoma: evidence of immune mediated glomerular injury. *J. Med.*, **88**, 189–92.
16. Karsenty, G., Ulman, A., Droz, D. *et al.* (1985) Clinical and histological resolution of systemic amyloidosis after renal cell carcinoma removed. *Nephron*, **40**, 232–4.
17. Fernandezmiranda, C., Mateus, Gouzalezgomez, C. and Ballestin, C. (1994) Systemic amyloidosis and ovarian carcinoma. *Postgrad. Med. J.*, **70**, 505–6.
18. Abraham, G., Bargman, J.M., Blake, P.G. *et al.* (1990) Fibrillary glomerulonephritis in a patient with metastatic carcinoma of the liver. *Am. J. Nephrol.*, **10**, 251–3.
19. Walker, J.F., O'Neil, S. and Campbell, E. (1981) Carcinoma of the oesophagus associated with membrano-proliferative glomerulonephritis. *Postgrad. Med. J.*, **57**, 592–6.
20. Mustonen, J., Henn, H. and Pasternack, A. (1981) IgA nephropathy associated with bronchial small cell carcinoma. *Am. J. Clin. Pathol.*, **76**, 652–6.
21. Cairns, S.A., Mallick, N.P., Lawler, W. and Williams, G. (1978) Squamous cell carcinoma of bronchus presenting with Henoch–Schönlein purpura. *Br. Med. J.*, **12**, 174–5.
22. Jermanovich, N.B., Giammarco, R., Ginsberg, S.J. *et al.* (1982) Small cell anaplastic carcinoma of lung with mesangial proliferative glomerulonephritis. *Arch. Intern. Med.*, **142**, 397–9.
23. Kitano, S. (1984) Poorly differentiated adenocarcinoma of rectum in a nephrotic patient with focal segmental glomerulosclerosis. *Jpn. J. Surg.*, **14**, 155–8.
24. Cousser, W.G. (1985) Mechanisms of glomerular injury in immune complex disease. *Kidney Int.*, **28**, 569–83.
25. Borachovitz, D., Kam, W.K., Nolte, M. *et al.* (1982) Adenocarcinoma of the palate associated with nephrotic syndrome and epimembranous carcinoembryonic antigen deposition. *Cancer*, **49**, 2197–22-2.
26. Da Costa, C.R., Dupont, E., Hamers, R. *et al.* (1974) Nephrotic syndrome in bronchogenic carcinoma: report of two cases with immunochemical studies. *Clin. Nephrol.*, **2**, 245–51.
27. Walker, J.F., O'Neill, S. and Campbell, E. (1981) Carcinoma of the oesophagus associated with membrano–proliferative glomerulonephritis. *Postgrad. Med. J.*, **57**, 592–6.
28. Boon, E.S., Vrij, A.A., Nieuwhof, C. *et al.* (1994) Small lung cancer with paraneoplastic nephrotic syndrome. *Eur. Resp. J.*, **7**, 1192–3.
29. Wakashin, M., Wakashin, Y., Jesato, K. *et al.* (1980) Association of gastric cancer and nephrotic syndrome. An immunological study in three patients. *Gastroenterology*, **78**, 749–56.
30. Barton, C.H., Vaziri, N.D. and Spear, G.S. (1980) Nephrotic syndrome assoiated with adenocarcinoma of the breast. *Am. J. Med.*, **68**, 308–12.
31. Robinson, W.L., Mitas, J.A., Haerr, R.W. and Cohon, J.M. (1984) Remission and exacerbation of tumor related nephrotic syndrome with treatment of the neoplasm. *Cancer*, **54**, 1082–4.

32. Martinez-Maldonado, M. and Benabe, J.E. (1993) Non-renal neoplasms and the kidney, in *Diseases of the kidney*, 5th edn (ed. R.W. Schrier and C.W. Gottschalk), Little Brown and Company, pp 2265–85.

33. Dabbs, D.J., Striker, L.M., Mignon, F. and Striker, G. (1986) Glomerular lesions in lymphomas and leukemias. *Am. J. Med.*, **80**, 63–7.

34. Glenner, G.G. (1980) Amyloid deposits and amyloidosis. *N. Engl. J. Med.*, **302**, 1333–43.

35. Watson, A., Stachwa, I., Fragda, J. and Bourke, E. (1983) Focal segmental glomerulosclerosis in Hodgkin's disease. *Am. J. Nephrol.*, **3**, 228–32.

36. Hayman, L.R., Burkholder, P.M., Joo, P.A. and Segar, W.E. (1973) Malignant lymphoma and nephrotic syndrome. *J. Pediatr.*, **82**, 207–12.

37. Kleinknecht, D., Morel-Maroger, L., Callard, P. *et al.* (1980) Anti-glomerular basement membrane nephritis after solvent exposure. *Arch. Intern. Med.*, **140**, 230–2.

38. Mu, K.W., Golbus, S.M., Kunfanan, R. *et al.* (1978) Glomerulonephritis with Hodgkin's disease and Herpes zoster. *Arch. Pathol. Lab. Med.*, **102**, 527–9.

39. Brouet, J.C., Clauvel, J.P., Danon, F. *et al.* (1974) Biological and clinical significance of cryoglobulins. A report of 86 cases. *Am. J. Med.*, **57**, 775–88.

40. Lockwood, C.M. (1979) Lymphoma cryoglobulinemia and renal disease. *Kidney Int.*, **16**, 522–30.

41. Moulin, B., Ronco, P.M., Mongenot, B. *et al.* (1992) Glomerulonephritis in chronic lymphocytic leukemia and related B-cell lymphomas. *Kidney Int.*, **42**, 127–35.

42. Allon, M., Campbell, W.G., Nasr, S.A. *et al.* (1988) Minimal change glomerulopathy and interstitial infiltration with mycosis fungoides. *Am. J. Med.*, **84**, 756–9.

43. Shapiro, C.M., Vancer Laan, B.F., Jao, W. and Sloan, D.E. (1985) Nephrotic syndrome in two patients with cured Hodgkin's disease. *Cancer*, **55**, 1799–804.

44. Lauria, F., Foa, R., Gobbi, M. *et al.* (1983) Increased proportion of suppressor/cytoxic (OKT 8[+]) cells in patients with Hodgkin's Disease in long lasting remission. *Cancer*, **52**, 1385–8.

45. Kipps, T.J. (1995) Macroglobulinaemia, in *Williams Haematology*, 5th ed. (eds E. Beutler, M.A. Lichtman, B.S. Coller and T.J. Kipps), McGraw-Hill, pp 1127–32.

46. Kyle, R.A. (1989) Monoclonal gammopathies and the kidney. *Ann. Ren. Med.*, **40**, 53–60.

47. Zollinger, H.U. and Mihatsch, M.J. (1978) *Glomerulonephrosis and Glomerulosclerosis*, in *Renal Pathology in Biopsy: Light, Electron and Immunofluorescent Microscopy and Clinical Aspects.* (eds H.U. Zollinger and M.J. Mihatsch), Springer-Verlag, pp 380–406.

48. Auconturier, P., Khamlichi, A.A., Preud'Homme, J.L. *et al.* (1992) Complementary DNA sequences of human amyloidogenic immuniglubulin light chain precursors. *Biochem. J.*, **285**, 149–52.

49. Gallo, G., Picken, M., Buxbaum, J. and Frangione, B. (1989) The spectrum of monoclonal immunoglobulin deposition disease associated with immunocytic dyscrasias. *Semin. Haematol.*, **26**, 234–45.

50. Janssen, S., van Rijswizk, M.H., Meizer, S. *et al.* (1986) Systemic amyloidosis: a clinical survey of 144 cases. *Neth. J. Med.*, **29**, 376–85.

51. Kyle, R.A. (1991) Amyloidosis, in *Hematology: Basic principles and practise* (eds R. Hoffman, E.J. Benz Jr, S.J. Shattil, *et al.*), Churchill Livingstone, pp 1038–47.

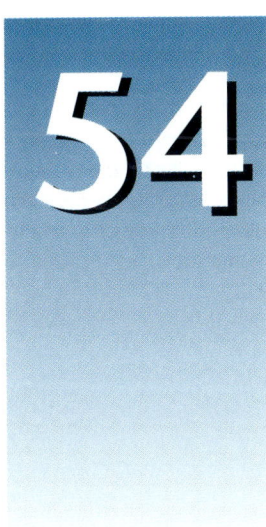

54

Glomerular disease in tropical countries

Clare M. Lloyd, R. Kasi Visweswaran and Steven H. Sacks

Introduction

Renal diseases in the tropics differ considerably from those in temperate climates in etiology, incidence and natural history. In part, these differences may be explained by differences in geography (temperature, climate and humidity), environment (toxins, chemical and pollutants), genetic considerations, society and economic conditions. Most developing countries have large populations in rural areas facing poverty, malnutrition, lack of education, lack of consciousness of personal hygiene, poor health care facilities and delays in hospitalization – conditions which are the epitome of underdevelopment. During the last century, industrially advanced countries have experienced a change in disease patterns due to substantial improvements in socioeconomic conditions and rapidly expanding medical facilities. Consequently, many diseases once prevalent do not now occur in Western countries although they remain relatively common in the tropics. In addition, tropical countries are not only exposed to diseases common to temperate and tropical climates but are also heavily burdened with diseases caused by etiologic agents specific to tropical regions.

An important point to consider is that data concerning the incidence of glomerular diseases in the tropics are not likely to be as accurate as those in more developed countries for a variety of reasons. Primarily, medical care is not universally available in many tropical countries; therefore early symptoms may be missed. For cultural reasons, patients may seek help at much later disease stages. In many cases, the true disease prevalence is unlikely to be known. Disease susceptibility is remarkably different in tropical regions. Altered immune responses to pathogens due to poor nutrition are recognized as important determinants of the pathogenesis and morbidity of glomerular disease in the tropics. Large-scale migration of people brought about by war and famine has resulted in the loss of natural immunity to particular strains of individual pathogens. A major consideration in determining pathogenesis of glomerular diseases in tropical regions is the probability that individuals are likely to be infected with several agents at any one time. Differences in disease severity and incidence may be explained by the interaction of particular pathogens during concomitant infections.

Of growing importance to clinicians in non-tropical areas is the risk of imported disease, via travelers returning from holidays in the tropics or immigrants who have lost their natural immunity returning to their native country to visit family. It is important for clinicians to be aware that a patient has traveled recently, as well as knowing the geographical spread of infectious agents in tropical areas. For the purposes of this chapter tropical areas are defined as geographical areas bounded by the tropics of Cancer and Capricorn, i.e. between latitudes 23.5° north and south of the equator, respectively. This chapter first considers the different patterns of primary disease in the tropics (compared with more developed countries) and then discusses specific renal diseases.

Nephrology, Edited by Rex L. Jamison and Robert Wilkinson.
Published in 1997 by Chapman & Hall, London. ISBN 0 412 60930 4

	Relative incidence in developed countries (%)	Areas of low incidence	Areas of high incidence
Minimal Change	15–20	Malawi S. Africa Zimbabwe Uganda Papua New Guinea	Kenya Jamaica Malaysia India
Focal glomerulosclerosis	10	Pakistan Uganda S. Africa	Brazil Mexico Malawi Thailand Guyana
Membranous GN	20–30	Indonesia Jamaica	S. Africa Sudan Pakistan
IgA GN	13	Tunisia S. Africa Mexico	Hong Kong Singapore Taiwan
Proliferative GN	10–15		Zimbabwe Tunisia Kenya Nigeria Uganda Jamaica India Malaysia

Table 54.1 Summary of the relative incidence of primary glomerular diseases in developing countries. Percentages represent the proportion of patients with each primary glomerular disease relative to the total number of cases of glomerulonephritis

GN, glomerulonephritis.

Primary glomerular diseases

Minimal change disease

Minimal change disease (MCD) is strikingly rare in tropical countries. Whereas the incidence of MCD is 15–20% of patients with glomerulonephritis (GN) in the adult population in Western countries it varies from 0 to 36% in tropical countries. The incidence is relatively low among blacks in South Africa (4%), in Malawi (0), Zimbabwe (1%), Uganda (4%) and Papua New Guinea (3%) but comparable to that in the West in other areas: Kenya (30%), Jamaica (25%), Malaysia (35%) and India (30%). The low incidence in certain areas may be explained by the relatively good prognosis of this disease coupled with poor access to health care facilities. Genetic resistance to MCD has been implicated in a study in South Africa which showed that the incidence of MCD among black children is significantly lower than in South African children of Indian descent (14% of GN cases versus 75%).

Focal segmental glomerulosclerosis

This disease comprises around 10% of cases of nephrotic syndrome in the West. The incidence in tropical areas varies from 0 in Pakistan, Uganda and S. Africa to a higher incidence in Brazil (20%), Mexico (24%), Malawi (33%), Thailand (20%) and Ghana (37%). No reasonable explanation is offered for this marked variability.

Membranous nephropathy

The incidence of primary membranous glomerulonephritis (MGN) is extremely variable in the tropics. Although MGN makes up 20–30% of cases of nephrotic syndrome in Western countries it is rare in Indonesia (4%) and Jamaica (4%), but more common in S. Africa (54%), Sudan (33%) and Pakistan (26%). MGN in Africa is frequently associated with hepatitis B infection.

Table 54.2   Summary of the association between infections and glomerular diseases and some of the countries in which this association is most prominent

Glomerular disease	Tropical disease association	Areas of high incidence
Immune complex GN	Typhoid	Developing countries
Interstitial nephritis	*P. falciparum* infection	Subsaharan Africa, SE Asia
Membranous GN	HCV HBV Typhoid	Developing countries Zimbabwe, Taiwan Developing countries
Mesangioproliferative GN	Leprosy Typhoid	India Developing countries
Mesangiocapillary GN	HCV HBVsAg carriers	Ethiopia S. Korea
FSGS	HIV Schistosomiasis	Worldwide – Africa, SE Asia in particular Brazil, Egypt
Cryoglobulinemia	HBV HCV (with IgA deposits)	S. Korea Developing countries
Renal amyloidosis	Leprosy Schistosomiasis	Papua New Guinea Brazil, Egypt
Eosinophillic GN	Filariasis	India, West and Central Africa
Acute tubular necrosis	*P. falciparum* infection	Africa, SE Asia
Nephrotic syndrome	*P. malariae* infection	Nigeria, Uganda, Yemen

GN, glomerulonephritis; HCV, hepatitis C virus; HBV, hepatitis B virus; FSGS, focal and segmental glomerulosclerosis; HIV, human immunodeficiency virus.

IgA nephropathy

IgA nephropathy is the commonest form of primary glomerular disease in Hong Kong, Singapore and Taiwan where it accounts for 25–39% of all patients compared to around 13% in the UK. Data for African countries are scarce. IgA disease seems to be rare in Tunisia (1% of biopsies), S. Africa (0.8%) and Mexico (1.4%), but more common in Brazil (10%), Chile (10%) and India (13%). This variability may reflect access to screening programs or diagnostic use of renal biopsy, as well as availability of immunofluorescent staining techniques.

Proliferative glomerulonephritis

This histological category is heterogeneous and includes pure mesangioproliferative, endocapillary proliferative, mesangiocapillary (MCGN) and crescentic GN. Proliferative GN constitutes 10–15% of all glomerular disease in Western countries and is relatively rare in children. It remains the most commonly reported lesion in many tropical countries, however. In several reports an associa-

tion with infectious agents is implicated (e.g. poststreptococcal infection in Zimbabwe, Tunisia, Kenya and Nigeria; and *Plasmodium malariae* infection in Uganda). In the majority of cases reported from Jamaica, India and Malaysia, an infectious etiology was ruled out, indicating pure mesangiocapillary GN.

The differences in pattern and distribution of primary glomerular diseases reported in the tropics compared to Western countries may be summarized as follows: (1) there is a high incidence of glomerular disease in tropical countries; (2) there is a low incidence of childhood MCD in children and adult Africans and a high incidence of MGN in African children; (3) there is a high incidence of proliferative lesions in most African countries; (4) there is a high incidence of MCGN in Mexico and Brazil; and (5) there is a low incidence of IgA nephropathy in tropical regions apart from South East Asia. Despite the evidence supporting an association between certain infectious agents and specific glomerular diseases, the variability in prevalence cannot be wholly explained. Further research into genetic, social, economic, geographic and environmental considerations is needed to provide answers for this conundrum.

Secondary glomerular diseases

Glomerular disease and bacterial infection

Typhoid

Hematuria and proteinuria are found in 60% of patients during the febrile phase of typhoid infections. Glomerular disease usually has a benign course with patients making a complete recovery after one to two weeks [1]. During a rarer form patients present with fever, generalized edema and hypertension mimicking poststreptococcal GN. Histology shows large glomeruli with mild to moderate mesangial proliferation. Immunofluorescent staining of biopsies demonstrates deposits of C3, IgG and IgM in variable amounts. In one study, *Salmonella* Vi antigen was observed in the glomerular capillary wall. Although the kidney disease is postulated to be an immune complex type GN, no circulating immune complexes (CIC) have been found in typhoid fever.

Leptospirosis

Leptospira is a common organism with a world-wide distribution, although it occurs more frequently in tropical areas where wild and domestic animals serve as reservoirs of infection, and water sources such as dams, wells and stagnant pools and ponds are frequently contaminated.

Renal changes occur early during infection, when interstitial nephritis is induced as leptospires migrate from peritubular capillaries through the renal interstitium before excretion in the urine. Glomerular changes occur but tend to be mild and are limited to mild hypercellularity [2].

Complement C3 is present in the mesangium but is not thought to be specific. Ultrastructural examination shows electron-dense deposits in mesangial, paramesangial and intramembranous areas. The organism itself is rarely seen in human biopsies but in hamster models leptospira can be seen initially in the glomeruli and then in the interstitium and renal tubules a few hours after inoculation.

The pathogenesis of renal failure during leptospirosis is unknown but is likely to be multifactorial. Circulating immune complexes have only been observed in one patient. In patients who recover from the acute illness, renal function returns to normal. The diagnosis should be suspected in patients presenting with sudden onset of fever, myalgia, jaundice and acute renal failure. The diagnosis is made by detecting antigen by immunofluorescent-labeled antibodies in the urine and tissue. The organism can be cultured only in the first week of infection, although specific antibody may be detected during the second week. Patients with leptospirosis are treated with penicillin. Clearance of infection is generally followed by resolution of the nephritis.

Leprosy

There are 12 million new cases of leprosy world-wide every year. Three million occur in India, the rest in Africa, Brazil, China, Southeast Asia and South America. There are several glomerular lesions associated with leprosy, namely, secondary amyloidosis and several types of GN.

The clinical course of GN associated with leprosy is characterized by a rapidly progressive renal disease manifesting as oliguric renal failure. Nephritis may occur years later, in conjunction with active leprosy, concomitant with amyloidosis, or alternatively, during treatment – as in the case of erythema nodosum leprosum reactions. Hypertension is rarely observed [3]. Progression to renal failure is well described in patients with renal amyloidosis or crescentic GN. The natural history of other glomerulopathies associated with leprosy is unclear. The incidence of amyloidosis in leprosy varies widely in different geographical areas. In India renal amyloidosis was only detectable in 2–8% of patients with leprosy, whereas in Papua New Guinea, 60% of all cases of amyloidosis were secondary to leprosy. Secondary amyloidosis is more frequent in patients with lepromatous and borderline leprosy than in those with tuberculoid leprosy [4]. There is no correlation between duration of disease and onset of amyloidosis which may occur as soon as two to three years after the initial diagnosis of leprosy. There is a positive association between erythema nodosum leprosum and development of amyloidosis, however (Figures 54.1 and 54.2). The amyloid fibril protein observed during leprosy is the AA type. During each episode of erythema nodosum leprosum, there is a rise in blood levels of serum amyloid A-related protein (SAA), the precursor of amyloid fibril, which persists for several months.

Glomerulonephritis associated with leprosy occurs more commonly than amyloidosis. The frequency varies from 6–50% according to biopsy studies, and 1.5% according to urinary abnormalities suggestive of GN. All

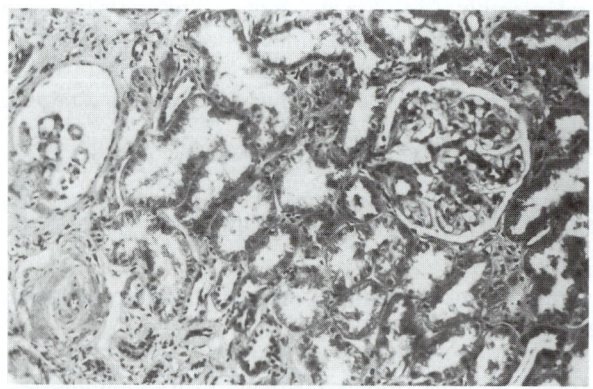

Figure 54.1 Amyloid deposits in glomeruli and blood vessels during an erythema nodosum leprosum reaction (hematoxylin and eosin). (Courtesy of Dr S. Lucas.)

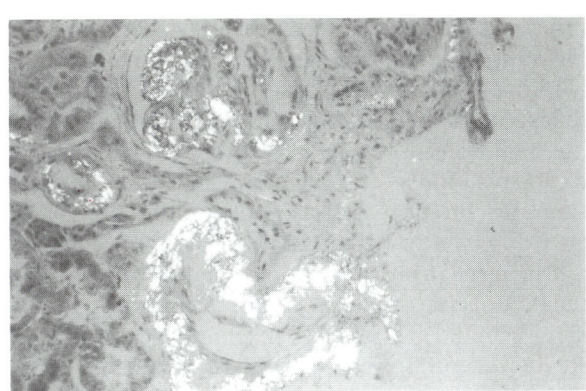

Figure 54.2 Extensive amyloid deposits in glomeruli and vessels during an erythema nodosum leprosum reaction (Congo red staining). (Courtesy of Dr S. Lucas.)

types of GN except focal glomerulosclerosis have been reported with each major form of leprosy. The two most common forms are diffuse endocapillary proliferative GN and mesangial proliferative GN. Immunofluorescence shows granular deposits of IgG, C3 and to a lesser extent, IgM, IgA and fibrin in the capillary walls and the mesangium. Electron microscopy shows electron-dense bodies in mesangial–subendothelial or subepithelial regions. Other changes include neutrophil infiltration, focal foot process fusion, basement membrane thickening, and mesangial proliferation, expansion and interposition.

Erythema nodosum leprosum is an immune complex disease which occurs when mycobacterial antigens are released by the breakdown of *Mycobacterium leprae* following drug treatment. During such an episode, GN and abnormalities of renal function have been observed. Hypocomplementemia has also been described in conjunction with immune complex formation. These observations, together with the demonstration of electron–dense deposits and the presence of immunoglobulins and complement within diseased glomeruli, suggest that the GN is immune-complex mediated. The exact nature of the immune complexes is undetermined, however. The antigen could either be specific to *Mycobacterium leprae* or non-mycobacterial and exogenous such as staphylococcal, streptococcal or hepatitis B virus antigen – all of which are common to patients with leprosy. It has also been postulated that the GN has an autoimmune component since autoantibody production in leprosy patents has been described. Antibodies observed include IgG-M cryoglobulins, as well as DNA-binding antibodies and antibodies directed against nuclear antigens. Glomerular lesions associated with leprosy are likely to have a multifactorial origin and this is probably reflected in the varied morphological expressions documented.

Leprosy should be suspected in those with skin or peripheral nerve lesions who have been in endemic areas, and is confirmed by skin biopsy. It is not known whether drugs given for treatment of leprosy affect the course of glomerular disease. Erythema nodosum leprosum reac-

tions predispose to renal complications, but episodes are less frequent when dapsone and clofazimine are used in combination (rather than alone). This combination is the treatment of choice for lepromatous leprosy.

Glomerulonephritides associated with viral infection

Hepatitis B virus

An association between persistent hepatitis B virus (HBV) surface antigenemia and glomerular disease was first reported in 1971. Hepatitis B infection remains a global problem but the prevalence varies. Areas of high endemicity (greater than 7%) include China, Taiwan, Southeast Asia, the Pacific islands, subsaharan Africa and southern India [5]. The association between HBV and GN is most evident in areas of high endemicity, for example in Zimbabwe, and in Taiwan HBV surface antigenemia (HBsAg) was recorded in 80–100% of children with membranous glomerular lesions.

Children (over 80% of whom are males) with membranous nephropathy present at 2–12 years of age with nephrotic or non-nephrotic proteinuria. Hypertension is present in fewer than 25%. Although the transaminases may be slightly elevated there is no clinical evidence of liver disease. In contrast, adults with HBV GN often have chronic active hepatitis. There is a striking association between the HBV carrier state and GN, however. For example, in South Korea 88% of adults with mesangio-capillary GN are HBVsAg carriers. Markers for identification of HBV-related GN include the presence of virus-associated antigens HBs, HB epsilon (HBe) or HB core (HBc) in the glomeruli or sera of patients. The reasons for the different predilection of glomerular lesions between children and adults are unknown, and within countries major differences in antigen prevalence occur between ethnic groups.

HBV-associated membranous nephropathy is indistinguishable from idiopathic membranous nephritis apart from the presence of small mesangial deposits in the former. Electron microscopic examination reveals subendothelial electron deposits and mesangial interposition. These are particularly prevalent in patients with HBeAg, implicating that antigen in the generation of capillary wall lesions. Microtubular virus-like structures are observed in glomerular endothelial cells in some patients with membranous or mesangioproliferative lesions. Immunohistological staining shows deposition of HBeAg, along with IgG and C3, in glomerular capillaries. Evidence suggests that HBV-MN is an immune complex-mediated disease due to subendothelial immune deposit formation from passive trapping of CICs rather than from *in situ* complex formation [6].

Spontaneous remission occurs in 30–60% of cases. Most patients remain symptomatic for 12 months or longer, however, and may progress to end-stage renal failure [7]. Steroid therapy may decrease proteinuria, but unfortunately there is an increase in serum HBeAg, HBV DNA and alanine transferase and the appearance of virus-like particles in glomeruli. These findings suggest that active viral replication occurs in the absence of overt clinical hepatitis and the use of steroids, although it may reduce the duration of nephrotic syndrome, may potentiate viral replication. Interferon treatment is accompanied by the eradication of markers of HBV in some, but not all, cases (reviewed in [1]). It may also resolve the proteinuria in isolated cases. This therapy is unlikely to be readily available in tropical areas.

Hepatitis C virus

Glomerular disease often accompanies chronic liver disease although the latter may be clinically silent. Cryoglobulinemic mesangiocapillary (MCGN), mesangio-proliferative, membranous, diffuse proliferative and sclerosing GN have all been described. Mesangial proliferative GN with IgA deposition is especially common. Hepatitis C virus (HCV) infection is an important cause of MCGN especially in areas where HCV is prevalent. Indeed the high incidence of MCGN in developing countries (e.g. Ethiopia) may be due to the high prevalence of HCV.

Patients present with nephrotic syndrome or non-nephrotic proteinuria in conjunction with mild to moderate renal insufficiency. As many as 60–70% have type II (or more rarely type III) cryoglobulinemia. Only 20% of patients show signs of liver disease, but the majority have elevated transaminases; the clinical presentation suggests primary renal disease. Other features of the disease include hypocomplementemia (decreased CH50, C4 and C3), rheumatoid factor and increased C1q binding.

Renal tissue from patients with HCV-associated nephropathy shows increased cellularity, accentuation of the lobular architecture and double contours of the basement membrane. Mesangial proliferation and sclerosis may also be present. IgM, IgG and C3 deposition occurs in the mesangium and capillary walls. Ultrastructural examination reveals subendothelial deposits characteristic of MCGN type I. Occasionally mesangial and subepithelial deposits are seen. In some cases the immune deposits have the ultrastructural features of cryglobulins, with a fibrillar or cylindrical substructure. The classic lesion is usually MPGN type I, with a relative lack of immune deposits as in some cases of acute exudative and proliferative GN. Areas of focal sclerosis may also be prominent.

Evidence that HCV is involved in the pathogenesis of the associated nephritis is based on the presence of HCV RNA and antibody in serum. Immune complexes and cryoglobulins have been located within the subendothelial space of glomerular capillary walls. Identification of HCV in the glomeruli is elusive, however, although there is one report which claims to detect virus-like particles in the mesangium [8]. HCV GN relates to glomerular deposits of CICs containing HCV ag, anti-HCV antibody and rheumatoid factor. Viremia usually persists despite a strong antibody response. The lack of neutralizing antibody response to HCV may reflect the ability of the virus to change its envelope antigens by mutation during the course of an infection resulting in spontaneous changes in antibody affinity and avidity. This fact potentially explains the chronic relapsing course of disease that is frequently observed in patients with mixed cryoglobulinemia. The mechanism responsible for the formation of rheumatoid factor is unclear. The histology supports the possibility that CICs localize in glomerular capillaries, where they deposit in subendothelial and mesangial areas and initiate local cell proliferation and leukocyte infiltration. A secondary hypothesis suggests that chronic HCV infection results in autoantibody formation, e.g. type 1 liver–kidney microsomal antibody, anti-smooth muscle antibody, antinuclear antibodies and occasionally perinuclear antineutrophil antibodies. In addition, antibodies directed towards intrinsic renal antigens may be formed, accounting for the renal pathology.

Infection with hepatitis C virus can be confirmed by an enzyme-linked immunosorbent assay (ELISA) for HCV antigen in patient serum, but due to the relatively high incidence of false positives infection is usually confirmed by polymerase chain reaction analysis, where available.

Pulse steroid therapy may improve renal function, but most patients continue to suffer significant proteinuria and low levels of circulating cryoglobulins [9]. Treatment with interferon-γ reduces proteinuria without any improvement in renal function in 45% of patients treated [10]. A good clinical response correlates with the disappearance of HCV RNA from the serum during treatment but relapse of viremia and renal disease are common after completion of therapy. Spontaneous remissions rarely occur.

Human immunodeficiency virus

As many as 10% of children and adults with human immunodeficiency virus (HIV) have chronic renal failure which manifests as HIV-associated nephropathy (HIVN) [11]. The risk is not uniform and although HIV remains a global problem, the impact of this virus on countries in tropical areas cannot be underestimated. Studies of HIV nephropathy are limited to the US and western Europe, but with the growing numbers of HIV-positive individuals in the tropics, especially Africa, this particular complication of HIV deserves further study.

HIV nephropathy does not only occur in terminal AIDS patients, indeed over 50% of patients are asymptomatic seropositive carriers or have AIDS related complex (ARC). By definition all patients are HIV positive, have a low CD4 count and a reversed CD4:CD8 ratio. The most common presentation is persistent proteinuria (>3.5 g/24 h) in conjunction with hypoalbuminemia and edema, although glomerular filtration rate (GFR) is usually normal. Serum complement is not usually depressed but there is usually non-specific elevation of IgG and IgM. Patients do not show hypertension during early or late disease. The GN has a malignant nature with a rapid deterioration in renal function in the absence of additional insult from anoxic injury or nephrotoxic agent. Most studies show that end-stage renal disease (ESRD) develops within four to six months. The development of ESRD in HIV nephropathy usually marks the beginning of a progressive clinical deterioration ending in death for most patients within a year, even if maintenance dialysis is available [12].

The most common histological manifestation is that of focal and segmental glomerulosclerosis (FSGS) which occurs in over 80% of patients (Figure 54.3). Mesangial changes include hyperplasia and matrix expansion. FSGS is associated with increased numbers of enlarged visceral epithelial cells containing large vacuoles and protein absorption droplets [13]. Affected glomeruli are shrunken with obliteration of capillary lumens (Figure 54.4) and may be filled with monocytes containing lipid (foam cells). Immunofluorescence shows deposition of IgM, C3, C1q in a granular formation in sclerotic areas, mesangium

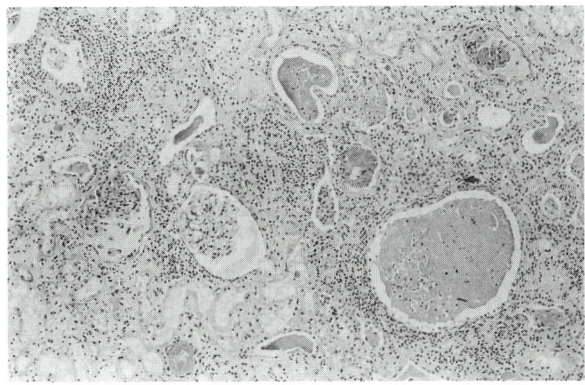

Figure 54.3 Focal segmental glomerulosclerosis during early HIV associated nephropathy showing interstitial infiltrates (hematoxylin and eosin). (Courtesy of Dr S. Lucas.)

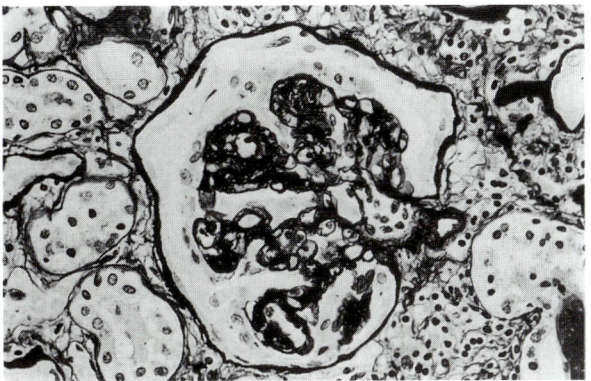

Figure 54.4 Focal segmental glomerulosclerosis during HIV associated nephropathy showing capillary collapse (silver methanamine). (Courtesy of Dr S. Lucas.)

and capillary walls. Some studies have reported linear staining for IgG and light chains along the glomerular basement membrane. IgM is the predominant immunoglobulin, but IgG and IgA are seen occasionally. Attempts to localize HIV antigen within the kidney have been uniformly unsuccessful. Electron microscopy is consistent with FSGS, with obvious effacement of foot processes, wrinkling and folding of the GBM and detachment of epithelial cells. Deposits are observed in the mesangium and (more rarely) in subepithelial or endothelial regions. In contrast to idiopathic FSGS various ultrastructural tubuloreticular inclusions are almost invariable and may involve glomerular endothelium, interstitial capillary endothelium and interstitial leukocytes. These intracytoplasmic collections of 24 nm interanastomosing tubules are generally large, often multiple in a given cell and average 0.92 inclusion per glomerular capillary studied [14].

The pathogenesis of HIV nephropathy has not been elucidated. There are no data to support immune complex involvement and the significance of localized immunoglobulin remains unclear. In one instance, proviral HIV DNA was demonstrated in renal tubular and glomerular epithelial cells, supporting a role for viral invasion in the pathogenesis of HIV nephropathy [15]. It is not known whether HIV alone can cause functional or structural changes in the kidney, however, or if other bacterial and/or viral agents are involved. It is unlikely that HIV nephropathy is solely due to opportunistic infection since it is seen in asymptomatic carriers, and glomerular lesions are not associated with various opportunistic infections in non-HIV patients. Whether HIV alone causes renal disease or other factors such as drug abuse, environmental or genetic factors, are necessary is unknown.

Corticosteroid treatment is unsuccessful and may precipitate infections in already immunosuppressed patients. Treatment for the renal disease is palliative.

Glomerular diseases associated with parasitic infections

Schistosomiasis

Schistosomiasis affects 300 million people, and is especially prevalent in Africa, Asia and South America. It is usually contracted in childhood or adolescence after ingesting water containing cercariae liberated from infected snails. The disease is characterized by granuloma formation resulting from eggs deposited by adult worms or traveling in the bloodstream to various organs. *Schistosoma haematobium* affects the bladder, ureters and genital tract. Bladder capacity is reduced and the ureters become stenosed resulting in hydronephrosis and insidious renal failure. Glomerular disease is rare. *S. mansoni* and *S. japonicum* cause glomerular disease in experimental studies, although clinical glomerular disease is reported only in *S. mansoni*, primarily in Brazil and Egypt.

The reasons for the differences in prevalence of renal disease among different strains is unclear. The incidence of renal disease is variable, although it is thought that 2.5% of patients in endemic areas have renal disease. However, 15% of patients with hepatosplenic disease also have overt renal disease.

Patients with a light worm load are asymptomatic. About 4–6% of patients with a heavy worm load develop hepatosplenic disease over several years and 12–15% of these patients develop glomerular disease. About 60% of patients with renal involvement have the nephrotic syndrome. The proteinuria tends be non-selective with the excretion of IgM, β_2-macroglobulins and lipoproteins. Levels of C3 are abnormally low and circulating immune complexes are observed.

Several patterns of glomerular pathology have been described. Transformation between types has been reported, although controlled longitudinal studies have not been conducted. These types are classified as follows: class I, mesangioproliferative GN; class II, exudative GN; class III, mesangiocapillary GN; class IV, focal and segmental sclerosis (FSGS); class V, amyloidosis [16]. In all types there is mesangial expansion (due to amorphous and fibrillar periodic acid–Schiff-positive material), and a mild to moderate increase in cellularity; mesangial cell proliferation is especially common in early disease. Immunofluorescence shows a heavy, granular pattern of deposition of IgM and to a lesser extent IgG, IgA and IgE in the glomerular wall, with C3 and C1q in the mesangium and along the capillary walls. Indirect immunofluorescent staining shows circulating cathodic antigen in the mesangium and capillary walls. This antigen is specific for schistosoma and is purported to be important in the pathogenesis of the disease [17]. Ultrastructural analysis reveals electron-dense deposits, which may be subepithelial, subendothelial or intramembranous, and laminar bodies in the mesangium. Schistosomal pigment, which is dark brown to black, may sometimes be found within the mesangial matrix.

There is convincing evidence that the initial glomerular injury in schistosomal glomerulopathy is a result of the immune response to specific parasitic antigens initiating an immune complex-mediated nephritis. Mesangial deposition of circulating gut antigens and (possibly) soluble egg antigens of different schistosomal species almost certainly causes the initial injury which usually manifests as mesangial hypercellularity (class I lesions) with few clinical sequelae. Progression into the second phase of overt renal disease is complex, involving many parasitic and host factors that ultimately determine the predominant transformation into another of the four classes of nephritis. Autoimmune mechanisms may be responsible for progression, as polyclonal B-cell activation has been recorded during schistosomiasis. In support of this, antinuclear antibodies, anti-DNA antibodies and anti-GBM antibodies have been detected in the serum of patients [18].

The diagnosis for schistosomiasis is confirmed by isolation of eggs in the urine or by biopsy of bladder tissue. The result of treatment with immunosuppressive drugs and antiparasitic agents is disappointing. Only 50% of patients respond to treatment with cyclophosphamide, with or without prednisolone. In addition, antischistosomal drugs and immunosuppressives cause complete remission in only 30% of patients. It seems that by the time that the lesion is expressed clinically, the course of disease is independent of the presence of the parasite.

Filariasis

Renal complications have been reported after *Onchoserca volvulus* (river blindness), *Wuchereria bancrofti* and Loa-Loa infections. Filarial GN is most prevalent in India and West and Central Africa. Renal involvement may manifest as an acute nephritic syndrome but more often as nephrotic syndrome with varying degrees of renal insufficiency [19]. During *W. bancrofti* infections, chyluria signals glomerular disease.

Patients with bancroftian filariasis generally develop mesangioproliferative, diffuse proliferative or acute eosinophillic GN, with microfilariae sometimes detectable in glomerular capillaries. Onchocercal infections are usually responsible for minimal change, mesangioproliferative mesangiocapillary and chronic sclerosing GN. In patients with Loa-Loa infection, membranous, mesangiocapillary and chronic sclerosing GN have been documented. Immunofluorescence staining shows IgM, IgG and C3 deposited within the glomerular mesangium and capillary walls. Onchocercal antigen is found in glomerular deposits in 50% of patients during one study, but specific antigens have not been looked at for other infections. Electron microscopy shows foot process fusion and electron-dense deposits in the mesangium.

The presence of immunoglobulin and complement together with filarial antigen in glomeruli implicates immune complex-mediated mechanisms in the pathogenesis of filarial GN. Patients may show marked eosinophilia and the diagnosis of filariasis can usually be confirmed by the presence of microfilaria in blood or lymph (Figure 54.5).

Patients with nephritis are treated with the antifilarial drug diethylcarbamazine, which generally leads to resolution of renal complications. Patients with nephrotic syndrome do not usually respond to any treatment.

Malaria

The World Health Organization estimates that there are 300 million cases of malaria per year. Total deaths from malaria in tropical Africa alone amount to one million per year. The relationship between glomerulonephritis and malaria has been suspected since the late nineteenth century but a cause and effect relationship was not described until 1930. Around 1% of patients infected with

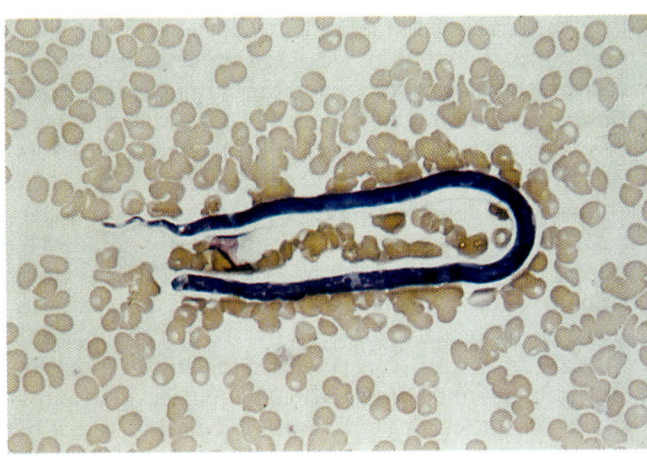

Figure 54.5 Microfilaria in the bloodfilm of a patient with Loa-Loa infection and membranous glomerulonephritis. (Courtesy Dr A. Morley.)

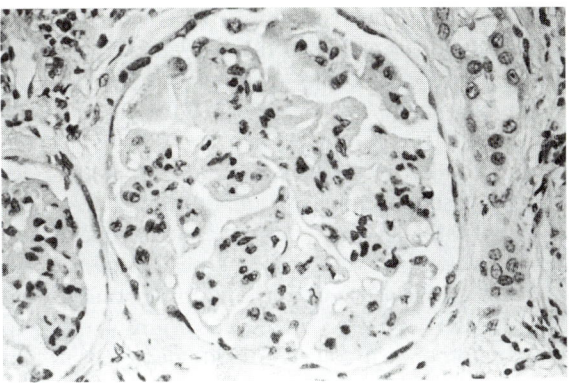

Figure 54.6 Increased mesangial matrix and an increase in cell numbers in a glomerulus during Quartan malaria nephrotic syndrome (hematoxylin and eosin). (Courtesy of Dr W. Akinsola.)

Plasmodium falciparum may develop acute tubular necrosis, from intravascular hemolysis and (more rarely) blackwater fever. In contrast, up to 58% of children infected with *P. malariae* develop the nephrotic syndrome.

The exact incidence of glomerular disease associated with malaria is unknown, although the incidence of nephrotic syndrome in malaria endemic areas is 20–60 times that in non-endemic areas. In northern Nigeria quartan malaria nephrotic syndrome accounts for 30% of children with nephrotic syndrome. In Nigeria, Uganda and Yemen nephrotic syndrome accounts for 2.5% of all hospital admissions, in contrast to 0.02–0.03% in the USA.

Falciparum associated GN

Infection with *P. falciparum* can induce an acute transient GN soon after the onset of fever, but this may remain undetected because of the absence of hypertension, edema or decline in renal function [20]. There are few cases of nephrotic syndrome or renal insufficiency. No correlation has been found between the degree of fever, proteinuria or urinary sediment. In the acute phase, serum C3 and C4 are reduced and *P. falciparum* soluble antigens, antiparasite antibodies and circulating immune complexes can be detected.

Renal biopsy shows mesangial expansion, mesangial and endothelial cell proliferation, irregular thickening of the glomerular basement membrane and monocyte infiltration. Eosinophilic granular material and pigment laden macrophages are present in the capillary lumens. Erythrocytes with parasites are observed in tubular but not glomerular capillaries [21]. Patients who develop disseminated intravascular coagulation show giant nuclear masses in the capillaries. Immunofluorescent staining shows IgM and C3 within the capillary walls; IgG and IgA staining occurs occasionally. Falciparum antigen may be detected in the mesangium and capillary walls in some circumstances. Electron microscopic examination reveals electron-dense deposits in the mesangium and subendothelial areas with widening of the foot processes.

Histological and experimental evidence indicates that GN is mediated by immune complexes. The pathology is similar to that observed during *P. berghei* infection in mice and *P. falciparum* infection in *Aotus* monkeys. Infection with *P. falciparum* is routinely confirmed by microscopic examination of thick and thin blood smears on several occasions. Nephritis is usually acute and transient and lesions resolve four to six weeks after initiation of antimalarial therapy.

Quartan malaria nephrotic syndrome

Quartan malaria nephrotic syndrome is associated with *P. malariae* infections and is characterized by chronic progressive lesions that lead to ESRF and are unresponsive to therapy. It is predominantly found in children and young adults, peaking at five years old [22]. A quartan fever is present only during the early stages of disease. A nephrotic state develops with generalized edema and ascites. In adolescents and young adults, renal failure tends to be combined with nephrotic syndrome. Blood pressure is normal but rises in those with advanced renal disease. Proteinuria is generally non-selective, but 20% of patients may show highly selective proteinuria. Quartan malaria nephrotic syndrome is particularly prevalent among malnourished individuals.

Mild changes in renal architecture can be seen in children whereas adolescents show more advanced mesangial sclerosis (Figure 54.6). There is focal and segmental thickening of capillary walls which may show double contours. This thickening is due to argyophilic fibrils arranged in a plexiform fashion in the subendothelium. As the disease progresses more capillaries become affected until the capillary lumen is completely obliterated. Cellular proliferation is absent, although small fibroepithelial crescents may be seen. On electron microscopy the basement membrane appears irregularly thickened and contains lacunae, many of which are full of electron-dense material. Basement membrane material also appears in the subendothelial zone. Immunofluorescence shows deposits of IgG, IgA, IgM and occasionally complement components within glomeruli (Figure 54.7). *P. malariae* antigen is also found in one-third of biopsies. A grading system has been devised according to the proportion of glomeruli involved and the degree of inflammation and sclerosis. Grade I describes biopsies in which up to 30% of glomeruli have lesions; in grade II 30–75% of glomeruli are affected; and in grade III biopsies more than 75% of glomeruli have lesions [23].

The quartan malaria nephrotic syndrome is an immune complex-mediated disease, with *P. malariae* antigen being demonstrable in one-third of cases in conjunction with *P. malariae* specific antibody. Several important issues remain unresolved however. It is unclear why only a small proportion of patients with *P. malaria* develop this nephrotic syndrome. Genetic factors are undoubtedly important in determining susceptibility to chronic disease. In particular, the HLA system may be important since it plays a role in the development of other complications of malaria infection [24]. Environmental factors also play a major role. Multiple infections may precipitate progression to chronic disease. For example, *P. falciparum* infection followed by infection with *P. malariae* has been associated with progressive glomerular lesions. Patients with *P. malariaie* also tend to be more malnourished compared to those with falciparum infections and the different immune responses to each strain may reflect these differences in nutritional status.

The most puzzling aspect of this disease is the fact that the lesion is persistent and progressive, even in the absence of discernible circulating antigen. Factors which might affect the persistence of infection include the affin-

ity of the antibodies produced, the efficiency of the reticuloendothelial system in clearing complexes, the site of localization of the antibody and the chronicity of antigen stimulation due to the presence of the exoerythrocytic stage. It may be that there is continuous release of antigens from the liver; however, this seems unlikely since antimalarial therapy is ineffective [25]. Autoantibodies directed towards a variety of antigens have been found in the sera of patients with malaria infection [26, 27]. These antibodies may be formed as a result of polyclonal activation of autoreactive B cells by the malaria parasite which is known to be a potent mitogen. Alternatively, autoantibodies may be stimulated by the release of autologous antigen released as a result of damage induced be the parasite. Cross reactivity of plasmodial antigens with autologous antigen is also suspected (reviewed in [28]). The high incidence of antinuclear factor in malaria endemic areas may represent cross-reacting antibodies induced by malaria nuclear material. Autoantibodies may be trapped as complexes within the kidney or react directly with kidney tissue as has been postulated in experimental malaria and for autoimmune renal diseases such as systemic lupus erythematosus.

Diagnosis of quartan malaria nephrotic syndrome is difficult since parasites are rarely observed, although they may be present during the early febrile stages. Treatment of quartan malaria nephrotic syndrome is also problematic, since antimalarial therapy has no effect on the course of renal disease even when parasites are eradicated from the bloodstream. Generally, patients are also unresponsive to the drugs usually used to treat renal disease, but histological grading has been found to have some value in predicting response to therapy. For example, those with grade I lesions respond to prednisolone or cytotoxic drugs whereas those with grade II or III lesions are unresponsive [23]. However, spontaneous remissions are rare in cases of quartan malaria nephrotic syndrome and the usual course is one of slowly progressive renal damage leading ultimately to renal failure in three to five years. Death is generally due to hypertension, renal failure or recurrent infection.

Other tropical infections

This chapter has described the main causes of glomerular disease secondary to infectious agents special to tropical areas. There exists a spectrum of diseases which are prevalent in the tropics which is beyond the scope of this chapter. If renal disease is observed during these diseases it will generally manifest as an immune complex nephritis due to a heavy antigenic load. As such, treatment with antibacterial, -viral or -parasitic agent will decrease the antigenic load and thus resolve the nephritis. In addition, postinfectious nephritis is very common in tropical areas due to increased prevalence of general infections because of poor social and economic conditions. Characteristics of this particular type of nephritis are covered in Chapter 47.

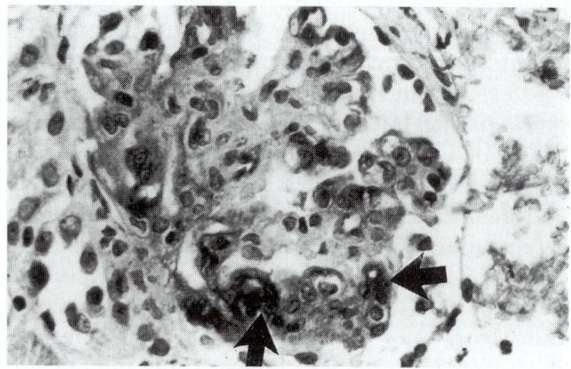

Figure 54.7 C1q binding in the glomerular mesangium (arrows) during quartan malaria nephrotic syndrome (immunoperoxidase). (Courtesy of Dr W. Akinsola.)

Acknowledgments

CML was supported by the National Kidney Research Fund and RKV was supported by an International Society for Nephrology Scholarship.

References

1. Sitpraja, V., Pipatanagul, V., Boonpucknavig, V. and Boonpucknavig, S. (1974) Glomerulonephritis in typhoid fever. *Ann. Intern. Med.*, **81**, 210–13.
2. Sitpraja, V., Pipatanagul, V., Mertowidjojo, K. *et al.* (1980) Pathogenesis of renal disease in leptospirosis. *Kidney Int.*, **17**, 827–36.
3. Cologlu, A.S. (1979) Immune complex glomerulonephritis in leprosy. *Lepr. Rev.*, **50**, 213–22.
4. McAdam, K.P.W.J., Anders, R.F., Smith, S.R. *et al.* (1975) Association of amyloidosis with erythema nodosum leprosum reactions and recurrent neutrophil leucocytosis in leprosy. *Lancet*, **ii**, 572–5.
5. Levy, M. and Chen, N. (1991) Worldwide perspective of hepatitis B-associated glomerulonephropathy in the 80s. *Kidney Int.*, **40**, S24–33.
6. Takekoshi, Y., Tochimaru, H., Nagata, Y. and Ikami, N. (1991) Immunopathogenetic mechanisms of hepatitis B virus-related glomerulopathy. *Kidney Int.*, **40**, S34–9.
7. Lai, K.N. and Lai, F.M.-M. (1991) Clinical features and the natural course of hepatitis B virus-related glomerulopathy in adults. *Kidney Int.*, **40**, S40–5.
8. Horikoshi, S., Okada, T., Shirato, I. *et al.* (1993) Diffuse proliferative glomerulonephritis with hepatitis C virus-like particles in paramesangial dense deposits in a patient with chronic hepatitis C virus. *Nephron*, **64**, 462–4.
9. DeVecchi, A., Montgnino, G., Pozzi, C. *et al.* (1983) Intravenous methylprednisolone pulse steroid therapy in essential mixed cryoglobulinemia nephropathy. *Clin. Nephrol.*, **19**, 221–7.
10. Johnson, R.J., Willson, R., Kamabe, H. *et al.* (1994) Renal manifestations in hepatitis C virus infection. *Kidney Int.*, **46**, 1255–63.
11. Rappaport, J., Kopp, J.B. and Kotman, P.E. (1994) Host virus interactions and molecular regulation of HIV-1: Role in the pathogenesis of HIV-associated nephropathy. *Kidney Int.*, **46**, 16–27.
12. Rao, T.K.S. (1991) Clinical features of human immunodeficiency virus associated nephropathy. *Kidney Int.*, **40**, 13–18.
13. Bougoignie, J.J. and Pardo, V. (1991) The nephropathology in human immunodeficiency virus (HIV-1) infection. *Kidney Int.*, **40**, S19–S23.
14. D'Agati, V., Suh, J-L., Carbone, L. *et al.* (1989) Pathology of HIV-associated nephropahy: A detailed morphologic and comparative study. *Kidney Int.*, **35**, 1358–70.
15. Cohen, A.H., Sun, N.C.J., Shapshak, P. and Imagawa, D.T. (1989) Demonstration of human immunodeficiency virus in renal epithelium in HIV-associated nepropathy. *Modern Pathol.*, **2**, 125–8.
16. Barsoum, R.S. (1993) Schistosomal glomerulopathies. *Kidney Int.*, **44**, 1–12.
17. Sobh, M.A., Moustafa, F.E., El-Housseini, F. *et al.* (1987) Schistosomal specific nephropathy leading to end-stage renal failure. *Kidney Int.*, **31**, 1006–1011.
18. Hillyer, G.V. (1971) Deoxyribonucleic acid and antibodies to DNA in the serum of hamsters and man infected with schistosomes. *Proc. Soc. Exp. Biol. Med.*, **136**, 880–3.
19. Chugh, K.S., Singhal, P.C., Tewari, S.C. *et al.* (1978) Acute glomerulonephritis associated with filariasis. *Am. J. Trop. Med. Hyg.*, **27**, 630–1.
20. Boonpucknavig, V. and Sitprija, V. (1979) Renal disease in acute *Plasmodium falciparum* infection in man. *Kidney Int.*, **16**, 44–52.
21. Bhamarapravati, N., Boonpucknavig, S., Boonpucknavig, V. and Yaemboonruang, C. (1973) Glomerular changes in acute *Plasmodium falciparum* infection: an immunologic study. *Arch. Pathol.*, **96**, 289–93.
22. Hendrickse, R.G. and Adeniyi, A. (1979) Quartan malaria nephrotic syndrome in children. *Kidney Int.*, **16**, 64–74.
23. Hendrickse, R.G., Adeniyi, A., Edington, G.M. *et al.* (1972) Quartan malaria nephrotic syndrome: a collaborative clinicopathological study in Nigerian children. *Lancet*, **i**, 1143–9.
24. Hill, A.V., Allsop, C.E., Kwiatkowski, D. *et al.* (1991) Common West African HLA antigens are associated with protection from severe malaria. *Nature*, **352**, 595–600.
25. Houba, V. (1979) Immunologic aspects of renal lesions associated with malaria. *Kidney Int.*, **16**, 3–8.
26. Adu, D., Williams, D.G., Quakyi, I.A. *et al.* (1982) Ant-ss DNA and anti-nuclear antibodies in human malaria. *Clin. Exp. Immunol.*, **49**, 310–16.
27. Zouali, M., Druilhe, P. and Equem, A. (1986) IgG-subclass expression of anti-DNA and anti-ribonuclearprotein antibodies in human malaria. *Clin. Exp. Immunol.*, **49**, 310–16.
28. Wozencraft, A.O. and Staines, N.A. (1990) DNA-binding antibodies and parasitic disease. *Parasitol. Today*, **6**, 254–9.

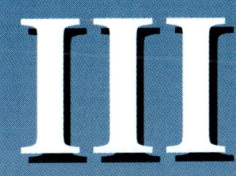

III

Diseases of the Kidney and Their Treatment

Section 4
Primary Diseases of the Glomerulus

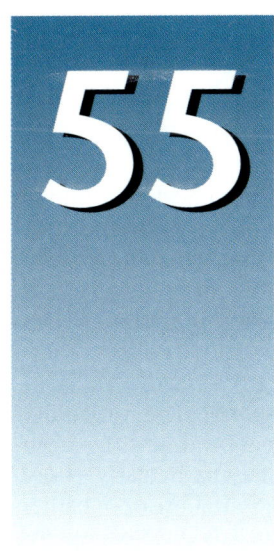

55

Primary diseases of the glomerulus

Michael Kashgarian

Introduction

The advances made in the study of the pathogenesis of renal disease in experimental animals has led to a more accurate description of the pathogenic events involved in many forms of glomerular disease. Although our knowledge is as yet incomplete, correlation of these experimental studies with clinical pathological studies in patients has led to a more detailed description of the morphological changes of specific disease categories and has given some insight into the role that these changes may play in progression of renal disease and in potential therapeutic modulation of the acute injury. It is therefore important to view the structural changes associated with specific disease entities, not only as pathologic correlations to a clinical syndrome but also as structural responses to specific pathogenic mechanisms which result in the observed alterations of both structure and function.

The glomerulus is a uniquely structured vessel designed for filtration. The combination of a fenestrated endothelium, a uniformly thin basement membrane and an epithelial cell broken up into small foot processes form the basis for the intrinsic porosity of the filter (Chapter 1). The relatively high density of negatively charged glycoproteins of the basement membrane and the surface coating of the cells provide an additional charge-related restriction barrier. Alteration of any individual or combination of components could result either in loss of the semi-permeability characteristics of the filtration membrane or in loss of its bulk filtration capacity. The former

leads to protein loss and the nephrotic syndrome and the latter to diminished filtration capacity and progression to renal failure. Another important component is the mesangium around which the glomerular capillaries are arranged. Filtration not only occurs across the capillary wall but also to a limited extent through the mesangium. Flow through the mesangium appears to act as a clearing mechanism for macromolecules which are not filtered and may accumulate in a relatively unstirred layer between the endothelium and the basement membrane. This clearing mechanism may remove immunocomplexes of intermediate size or macromolecules which may accumulate when the glomerular capillary permeability has been altered. It has a limited capacity which if exceeded could further aggravate the injury. In addition, the cells of the mesangium are capable of secreting a variety of inflammatory mediators and cytokines and may play a central role in orchestrating glomerular inflammation. Also of importance is the continuity of the mesangium with the juxtaglomerular apparatus. This indicates a potential role of the mesangial cell in regulating glomerular filtration directly, through contraction, and indirectly, by regulating cytokine release. Since the glomerular capillary bed receives some 20–25% of the cardiac output of which it filters one fifth, it is particularly vulnerable to a wide variety of injurious stimuli. As a result, the initiating factors in many forms of glomerular injury are unknown. This does not necessarily reflect a lack of understanding but does limit us to a more descriptive clinical pathological correlation. Hence the use of the term, primary glomerular diseases.

Nephrology, Edited by Rex L. Jamison and Robert Wilkinson.
Published in 1997 by Chapman & Hall, London. ISBN 0 412 60930 4

The primary diseases of the glomerulus most often present clinically as the nephrotic syndrome (Chapter 28) or, at least substantial proteinuria. Hematuria is less frequently associated with these diseases but may occur in individual circumstances, particularly when a degree of glomerular proliferation, inflammation or sclerosis accompanies the underlying lesion. Lesions which will be discussed under this heading include minimal change disease and its variants, focal segmental glomerulosclerosis, membranous glomerulopathy and mesangiocapillary glomerulonephritis all of which are classically associated with the clinical presentation of heavy proteinuria, hypoalbuminemia and a tendency to edema formation. The pathophysiology of the nephrotic syndrome is common to these disorders and has been discussed in an earlier chapter.

Minimal change glomerulopathy and its variants

Clinical manifestations and its natural history

Minimal change disease has been variously called lipoid nephrosis, nil disease, minimal change disease, foot process disease, visceral epithelial disease and primary nephrotic syndrome. The term lipoid nephrosis was used by pathologists before the advent of electron microscopic examination since the most prominent feature by light microscopy was vacuolization of the tubular epithelium.

Minimal change disease is 10–15 times more common in children than in adults. Over 80% of children with nephrosis have minimal change disease whereas only 20–30% of adults with nephrotic syndrome fall into this category [1–3]. In children, there is a male predominance. In the vast majority of pediatric cases, the lesion does not progress to renal insufficiency, although the patients frequently exhibit a relapsing or a cyclical course. Spontaneous remissions can occur and relapses diminish in frequency after puberty. The vast majority of pediatric patients are responsive to glucocorticoid therapy. Although the optimal regimen has not been fully standardized, four to six weeks of oral prednisone (60 mg/M²/day) is generally given as initial therapy, followed by alternate day steroid therapy for an additional four to six weeks. The response to therapy basically falls into three groups [4, 5]: Those who have a complete remission with no recurrences; those who have steroid-induced remissions but have relapses with recurrence of the nephrotic syndrome which is also steroid responsive; and those in whom the remission is steroid-dependent and who relapse either during or immediately upon steroid withdrawal. Patients who are either steroid dependent or steroid resistant have been noted to respond to more aggressive therapy which includes the addition of cytotoxic agents or immunosuppressive agents such as

cyclosporin [6–8]. Long term prognosis in children with uncomplicated minimal change disease is excellent with 25-year survivals in excess of 95% [9, 10].

The picture with adults is more complicated. Minimal change nephrotic syndrome often presents in adults in their 5th, 6th and 7th decades at a time when other unrelated underlying renal abnormalities, such as hypertension, nephrosclerosis, diabetes or chronic pyelonephritis may exist [1]. A greater percentage of adults appear resistant to steroid therapy and often longer periods of therapy are required to elicit a response. This variability makes it difficult to clearly separate steroid-sensitive from steroid-resistant patients. In adults, particularly those with cardiovascular complications, initial use of or earlier institution of alternate therapies, such as cytotoxic agents or immunosuppressive agents, is often considered [11]. Similarly, while the long term outcome in children is extremely favorable, it is less so in adults, especially when superimposed on a background of renal vascular disease. Progression to renal insufficiency appears to be more common in adults than in the pediatric population.

Pathology and pathogenesis

The term minimal change disease comes from the light microscopic histologic picture. Light microscopic examination generally reveals essentially normal (minimal change) appearing glomeruli (Figure 55.1). Subtle abnormalities can sometimes be identified, including swelling of visceral epithelial cells and a proteinaceous precipitate in Bowman's capsule. In some patients there may be mild mesangial prominence caused by increases in either mesangial cellularity and/or mesangial matrix. In some instances, the mesangial widening is enough to warrant the term mesangial proliferative glomerulonephritis (Figure 55.2). The proximal tubular epithelial cells may

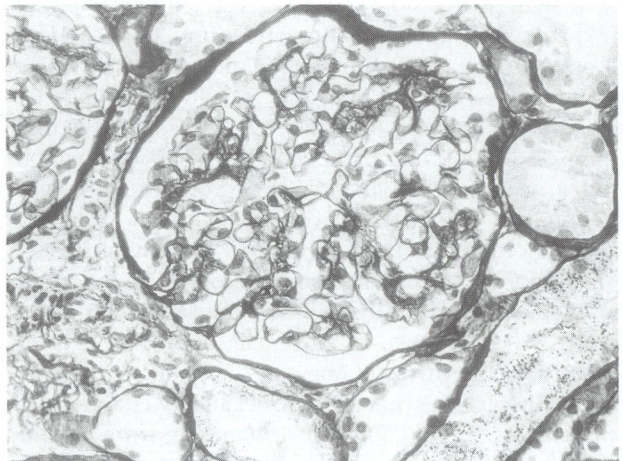

Figure 55.1 Minimal change glomerulopathy. The glomerulus is essentially normal by light microscopy. The capillary loops are thin and delicate and there is no significant increase in mesangial cells and matrix. (Hematoxylin and eosin, ×400.)

be vacuolated or show prominent hyaline droplets or lipid resorption droplets. Colloidal iron and Alcian blue stains reveal a loss of staining in the glomerulus reflecting the loss of negatively charged glomerular glycoproteins and therefore loss of the charge barrier of filtration. Glomerulosclerosis, focal areas of tubular atrophy and interstitial scarring are generally absent or inconspicuous in the pediatric population. In adults, the presence of glomerulosclerosis associated with aging or hyaline arteriolosclerosis may make the distinction between minimal change disease and focal segmental glomerulosclerosis more difficult. In children who have had multiple relapses, subsequent biopsies may show segmental or global sclerosing lesions. The presence of these lesions does not necessarily indicate a change to a more progressive lesion as it does in focal segmental glomerulosclerosis.

In the majority of cases, immunofluorescence examination is usually completely negative. Small amounts of complement and fibrinogen may be found in a comma-like pattern in the peripheral capillary walls or in the mesangium. In some patients with mesangial prominence, IgM and complement may be found in a typical mesangial pattern. On very rare occasions, mesangial IgE has been observed. The presence of these proteins does not seem to indicate any adverse clinical effects such as steroid resistance or potential for progression to renal insufficiency.

Electron microscopic examination of glomeruli is the gold standard for the diagnosis for this entity. The most prominent changes are found in the visceral epithelial cells. There is extensive loss of the normal epithelial cell foot processes on the external (urinary) side of the glomerular basement membrane, so-called 'foot process fusion' with basal condensation of the cytoplasmic microfilaments (Figure 55.3). The cell bodies of the visceral epithelial cells in Bowman's space show microvillus

formation and large intracellular pseudocysts. The glomerular basement membrane is of normal thickness and no evidence of immune complex deposition is identified although focal subendothelial fibrillar material may be found. It should be noted, however, that although the epithelial cell changes are characteristic of this entity, the diagnosis is essentially a diagnosis of exclusion.

One particular histologic variant of the primary nephrotic syndrome deserves some discussion. In 10–20% of patients within the spectrum of minimal change disease, there is a more pronounced degree of mesangial hypercellularity and increase in mesangial matrix [7, 12–14]. This is often associated with immunofluorescence staining for IgM and C3 and the presence of small mesangial electron dense deposits by electron microscopy. The presence of IgG or IgA argues against the diagnosis of primary nephrotic syndrome and other entities such as Berger's disease or post infectious glomerulonephritis must be considered. Generally these patients generally do not behave significantly differently from those with the very minimal changes although some may have hematuria and hypertension. It is likely that this group of patients represents only a variant in the spectrum of this disease process. Although some investigators believe that the mesangial deposits are involved in the pathogenesis of the lesion and may have a negative influence on the

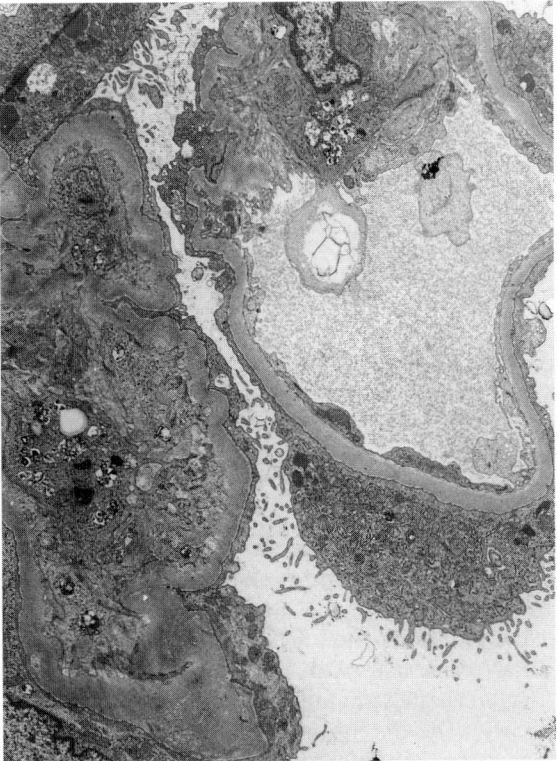

Figure 55.3 Electron micrograph of a glomerulus from a patient with minimal change glomerulopathy. There is obliteration of the foot processes of the epithelial cells with microvillous transformation in Bowman's space. No immune complex deposits are present. (×3975.)

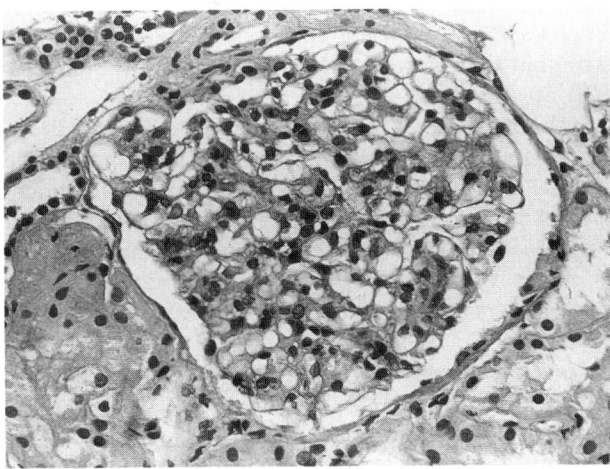

Figure 55.2 Mesangial proliferative variant of minimal change disease. There is a definite increase in mesangial prominence caused by an increase in mesangial cells and matrix. (Hematoxylin and eosin, ×400.)

Table 55.1 Conditions associated with minimal change disease

Primary

Secondary
- Drugs
  - Gold
  - Lithium
  - Non-steroidal anti-inflammatory drugs (often with acute interstitial nephritis)
  - Tiopronin
- Infections
  - Syphilis
- Neoplasia
  - Hodgkin's disease
  - Non-Hodgkin's lymphoma
  - Carcinoma (kidney, pancreas, colon, prostate)
  - Mesothelioma
- Microangiopathies
  - Bone marrow transplant nephropathy
  - Hemolytic uremic syndrome/thrombotic thrombocytopenia (healing phase)
  - Radiation nephritis
  - Sickle cell anemia
  - Syndrome of circulating antiphospholipid (anticardiolipin) antibodies
  - Transplant glomerulopathy
- Paraprotein deposition diseases
  - Cryoglobulinemia, type I
  - Fibrillary glomerulonephritis
  - Immunolactoid glomerulopathy
  - Light chain or heavy chain disease
  - Waldenström macroglobulinemia

clinical course, it is likely that the accumulation of IgM and C3 in the mesangium is merely the result of an overload of the capability of the glomerulus to clear unfiltered macromolecules [7, 14]. Although the presence of these mesangial abnormalities must be acknowledged, they do not alter the clinical approach to such patients in terms of therapy or prognosis.

The etiology and pathogenesis of minimal change disease is unknown, as is the mechanism of the glomerular permeability defect. The association in some cases with a viral prodrome and the occurrence of an identical lesion in a few patients with Hodgkin's disease suggests that a T-cell mediated immune response may be involved (Table 55.1). The recent identification of circulating factors suggests that cytokines may be involved in the permeability defect. The transfer of proteinuria from one animal to others using T cell transfers is consistent with this proposed mechanism [15]. Although many data strongly suggest the involvement of T cell mediated immunity, there are insufficient findings to draw any substantive conclusion as to the role of T cells or other immune mechanisms in the pathogenesis.

Focal segmental glomerulosclerosis

Clinical manifestations and natural history

The most important variant in the spectrum of lesions which comprise the primary nephrotic syndrome is the presence of focal and segmental glomerulosclerosis [16–20]. Although the lesion itself is relatively non-specific in that it can occur secondary to a variety of different types of glomerular injury, its presence in patients with the idiopathic nephrotic syndrome makes it a distinct clinical pathologic entity. Within this group of patients, there are at least two subgroups. First there are patients whose initial biopsies and clinical course are consistent with minimal change disease but who have multiple relapses responsive to therapy and develop focal sclerotic lesions late in the course of their disease. The presence of focal sclerosis late in the disease is not accompanied by any change in the pattern of responsiveness to steroids nor does it necessarily predict progression to chronic renal failure [19]. The second and more important group are patients who present with focal and segmental glomerulosclerosis early in the course of their disease shortly after the onset of the nephrotic syndrome. A rather distinctive clinical picture emerges with non-selective proteinuria, and hematuria, and often hypertension complicating the nephrotic syndrome. These patients frequently do not respond to steroid therapy or are, at best, steroid dependent. The prognosis is poor with a tendency to a rapidly progressive decline in renal function and a greater chance of recurrence of the disease in renal allografts. The lesion is more frequent in adults than in children and in African Americans [21]. Whether this is a characteristic of the lesion itself or due to genetic or co-morbid factors, such as hypertension or arteriosclerosis, is not clear.

Both subgroups of patients are initially clinically indistinguishable from individuals with uncomplicated minimal change disease. The possibility of focal segmental sclerosis as a diagnosis becomes considered only after atypical features are noted, such as hypertension, renal insufficiency, hematuria, non-selective proteinuria, or most commonly, poor or non-responsiveness to steroid therapy.

Since the prognosis of the subgroup of patients with early focal segmental glomerulosclerosis is generally poor, the effectiveness of different therapeutic approaches has been difficult to evaluate. Aggressive regimens such as the use of intravenous methylprednisilone combined with oral cyclophosphamide or treatment with cyclosporine may afford some protection from or at least retard progressive renal insufficiency [6, 22, 23]. The response to

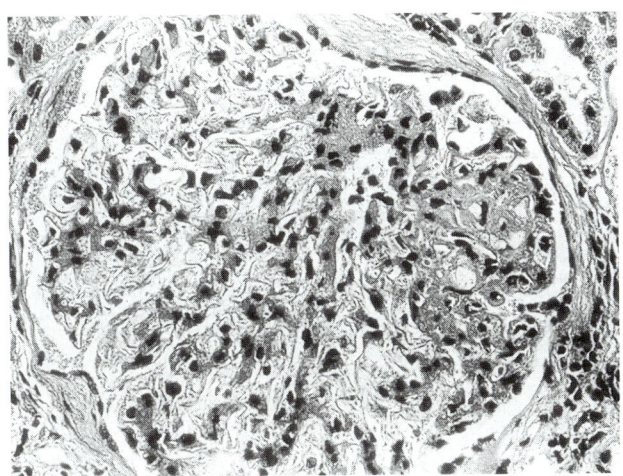

Figure 55.4 Focal and segmental glomerular sclerosis. The glomerulus is enlarged and there is a segmental area of sclerosis at the hilar region of the glomerulus. The remainder of the glomerulus has a more normal architecture. (Hematoxylin and eosin, ×400.)

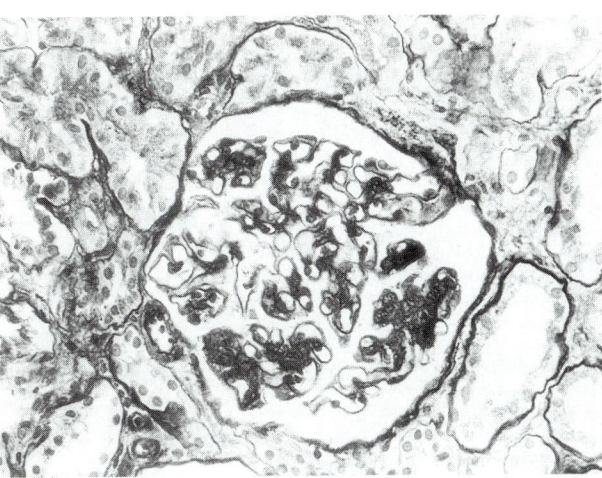

Figure 55.5 Glomerular tip lesion. There is a focus of glomerular sclerosis and adhesion to Bowman's capsule opposite to the vascular pole. The glomerulus is not enlarged and the capillary loops are patent. (Hematoxylin and eosin, ×400.)

various forms of therapy is extremely varied. Generally, when the lesion is present at the onset of the disease, it is associated with steroid unresponsiveness and relatively rapid progressive renal failure. Some patients, however, show a more typical relapsing course with some degree of steroid responsiveness or dependence and with a later slowly progressive onset of renal failure. Cyclosporin has also been suggested as an alternate therapy for all but as with minimal change disease, relapses are frequent following cessation of therapy [6].

Pathology and pathogenesis

By light microscopy, the glomerulosclerosis involves only portions of the glomerular tuft (segmental) (Figure 55.4) of a limited number of glomeruli (focal). Recently, there has been some discussion as to whether the location of the sclerotic lesions has any clinical significance. It has been suggested that the presence of tip lesions at the proximal tubule pole of the glomerulus indicates a good prognosis whereas multiple segmental lesions or hilar lesions are more likely to be steroid resistant and associated with renal insufficiency (Figure 55.5) [24]. Although there may be differences in the pathogenesis of the tip versus the 'hilar' lesion, at the present time, there is no convincing evidence that the distribution of lesions has any clinical pathological significance. The sclerotic lesions are generally more common in juxtamedullary glomeruli. Hyaline material is frequently seen in the vascular pole of the glomerulus and in the arterioles. Occasionally synechiae are present between the segmental sclerotic lesions and Bowman's capsule. Uninvolved portions of the glomerulus may be entirely normal or show mild mesangial hypercellularity and widening (mesangial proliferative glomerulonephritis with focal segmental glomerulosclerosis). Interstitial fibrosis and tubular atrophy are often prominent and may be the only finding present in some renal biopsies because of sampling error. Global glomerulosclerosis becomes more prominent as the lesion progresses. Immunofluorescence findings are variable and similar to those of minimal change glomerulonephropathy but more often reveal the presence of IgM and C3 in a mesangial pattern. By electron microscopy, the sclerotic lesions contain abundant matrix material associated with wrinkled and collapsed glomerular capillary loops (Figure 55.6). The hyaline deposits observed by light microscopy are electron dense material which does not have the typical characteristics of immune complexes. The epithelial cells show changes very similar to those of minimal change disease with obliteration of the epithelial cell foot processes, but occasionally show more severe alterations also including detachment from the basement membrane and denudation of the basement membrane.

Although the pathogenesis of the lesion is unclear, several possible mechanisms have been suggested. These include protein overload, hyperfiltration, disordered lipid metabolism and enhanced intraglomerular coagulation. One interesting anatomic explanation offered is that detachment of visceral epithelial cells from the basement membrane causing focal denudation leads to adhesion to the parietal epithelial cells of Bowman's capsule and forms a nidus for a region of sclerosis.

Collapsing glomerulopathy

A group of patients with nephrotic syndrome and rapidly progressive renal failure has been identified with biopsy findings of a form of glomerulosclerosis and has given rise to the concept of a distinct entity called collapsing glomerulopathy [25, 26]. The lesion appears to occur more frequently in African Americans and in males. One

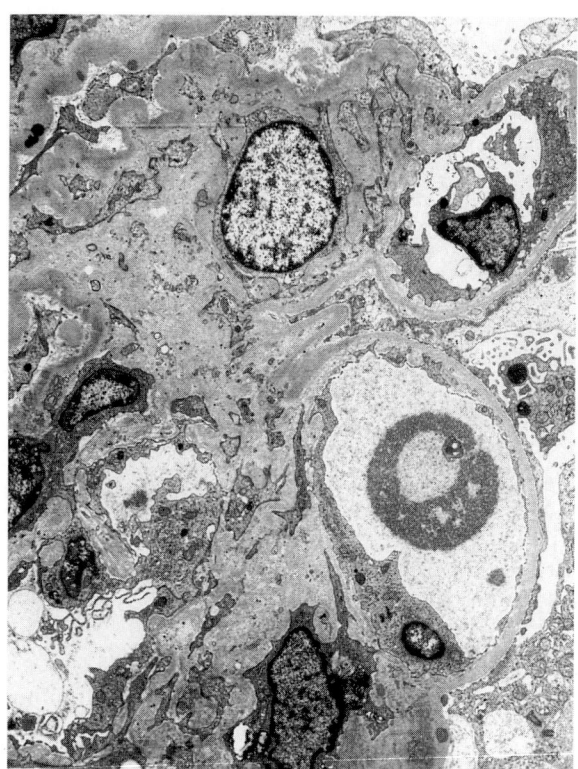

Figure 55.6 Electron micrograph of a glomerulus from a patient with focal segmental glomerular sclerosis. The findings are similar to minimal change glomerulopathy with effacement of the foot processes. In addition, there is evidence of mesangial sclerosis and irregular thickening of the basement membrane. (×3313.)

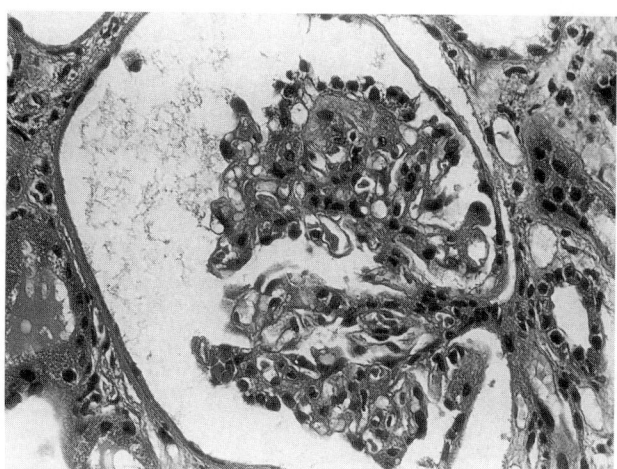

Figure 55.7 Collapsing glomerular sclerosis. The glomerulus has collapsed leaving a widely open Bowman's space. The epithelial cell nuclei are crowded together along the collapsed capillary loops. The mesangium is also prominent. (Hematoxylin and eosin, ×400.)

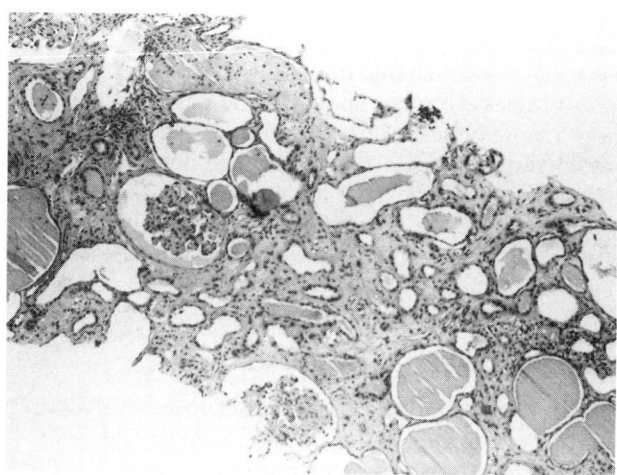

Figure 55.8 HIV nephropathy. There is evidence of collapsing glomerular sclerosis associated with an interstitial infiltrate and fibrosis. The tubules are dilated with flattened epithelium and are filled with proteinaceous casts. (Hematoxylin and eosin, ×100.)

probably should not apply the term focal segmental glomerulosclerosis to this entity since the lesion is not one of sclerosis per se but rather one of global glomerular capillary collapse (Figure 55.7). An associated feature is the presence of dilated tubules which contain proteinaceous casts. The picture is similar to that of HIV nephropathy except that it usually lacks an interstitial infiltrate and tubular reticular inclusions of the endothelial cells. Clinically these patients have hypertension, extremely heavy proteinuria, and elevated serum creatinine. Response to therapy is disappointing, progression is extremely rapid and renal survival is generally less than two years.

HIV nephropathy

A particular form of collapsing glomerulosclerosis is associated with patients with acquired immune deficiency disease (AIDS) [25, 27, 28]. The lesion has been implicated as a cause of chronic renal failure in some patients with HIV infection but not in others. There appears to be a predilection for focal and segmental glomerulosclerosis with a collapsing element among black intravenous drug users with AIDS, although this nephropathy is rare in white patients, with homosexuality as the only risk factor

for AIDS. The lesion has several distinct clinical and pathological characteristics. There is a relatively rapid clinical progression to renal failure. By light microscopy, focal and segmental sclerosis in all stages of evolution may be present in many glomeruli. The sclerotic process is characterized by global capillary collapse similar to collapsing glomerulopathy, and localized hyperplasia and vacuolization of the visceral epithelial cells overlying the sclerotic glomerular segments (Figure 55.8). In addition the tubules show striking alterations including the presence of large hyaline casts as well as degenerative changes and necrosis of epithelial cells. An active interstitial nephritis is frequently present. Immunofluorescent find-

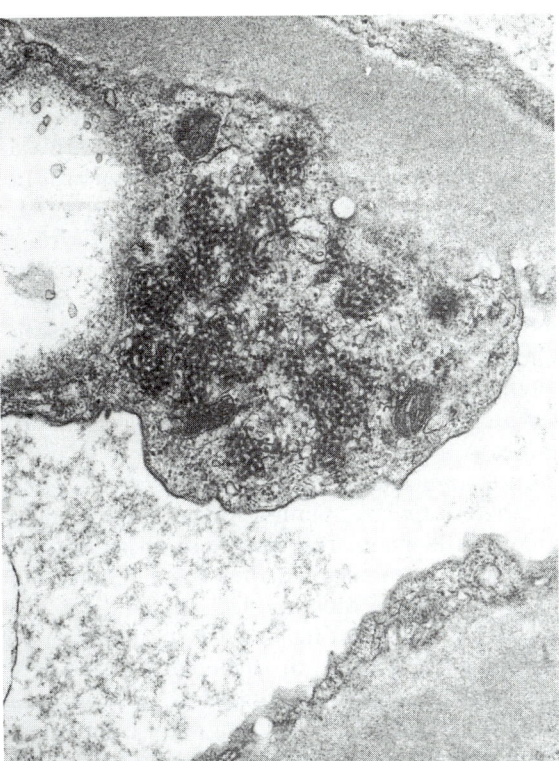

Figure 55.9 Electron micrograph of glomerular capillary wall of patient with HIV nephropathy. The endothelial cell contains tubular reticular inclusions thought to be induced by interferon-α. (×24 300.)

Table 55.2 Conditions associated with membranous glomerulonephropathy

Primary

Secondary
    Autoimmune disease
        Dermatomyositis
        Hashimoto's thyroiditis
        Primary biliary cirrhosis
        Rheumatoid arthritis
        Sjögren's syndrome
        Systemic lupus erthematosus
    Drugs
        Captopril
        Gold
        Formaldehyde
        Mercury
        Non-steroidal anti-inflammatory drugs
        Penicillamine
        Probenecid
        Tiopronin
        Trimethadione
    Infections
        Filiariasis
        Hepatitis B
        Hepatitis C
        Hydatid disease
        Leprosy
        Malaria
        Schistosomiasis
        Syphilis, secondary and congenital
    Microangiopathies
        Sickle cell disease
        Transplant glomerulopathy
    Neoplasia
        Carcinoma (lung, colon, stomach, breast)
        Lymphoma
    Other glomerular diseases
        Crescentic glomerulonephritis
        Diabetic glomerulonephropathy
        Focal glomerulosclerosis
        IgA nephropathy
    Other
        Sarcoidosis

ings are variable but frequently immunoglobulins and complement are found in an amorphous granular pattern and segmental distribution. By electron microscopy, the changes are like those of collapsing glomerulopathy or focal and segmental sclerosis in the absence of HIV infection. In some cases, mesangial dense deposits may be found. The endothelial cells are frequently filled with numerous and prominent tubular reticular structures (Figure 55.9). These structures have recently been thought to be associated with α interferon activity although a more direct relation to viral infection has also been suggested. Similar lesions have also been seen in patients with a history of intravenous drug abuse without concurrent AIDS.

Membranous glomerulonephropathy

Clinical manifestations and natural history

Membranous glomerulonephropathy (also termed membranous nephropathy, membranous glomerulonephritis, extramembranous glomerulonephritis and epimembranous nephropathy) is clinically similar to primary nephrotic syndrome with minimal change nephropathy in that it is characterized by massive proteinuria and the nephrotic syndrome. In contrast to minimal change nephropathy, however, there is an increased permeability of the glomerular capillaries to serum proteins of high as well as low molecular weight and, in the majority of instances, a gradual but progressive reduction in surface area for ultrafiltration leading to some renal insufficiency. In most series of adults with nephrotic syndrome, membranous nephropathy is the most common diagnosis, occurring in approximately 25%–30% of all adults with the nephrotic syndrome [29]. However, the percentage and incidence of membranous nephropathy in different populations vary. This is likely due to the fact that some cases of so-called idiopathic membranous glomerulonephropathy are associated with a specific identifiable antigen or are secondary to a malignancy, infection, or drug or toxin exposure (Table 55.2). Membranous nephropathy is unusual in children. The incidence increases with increasing age forming a continuum with young adults [4].

The disease usually has an insidious onset with increasing proteinuria eventually reaching the nephrotic range and, in most instances, manifesting as the nephrotic syndrome. Overall, the long term clinical course of such patients is one of gradually progressive renal failure with approximately 50% of patients developing significant renal failure after 10–15 years [29, 30]. On the other hand, a few patients exhibit an aggressive rapidly progressive course to renal failure. The long term prognosis may correlate with the degree of proteinuria. Patients who initially present with proteinuria but without the nephrotic syndrome appear to have a more favorable outcome than those who manifest the nephrotic syndrome at the outset. Although not typical, spontaneous remission of the nephrotic syndrome and decreases in protein excretion rate are not uncommon. The generally long clinical course and variability in protein excretion has made it difficult to assess critically the benefits of therapeutic approaches to modulation of this disease. Assessment is further complicated by the fact that idiopathic membranous nephropathy, a diagnosis by exclusion, made in the absence of association with known antigens as previously described. It is often difficult to exclude completely all of these possibilities. Since an older population group is affected, there is the possibility that an associated neoplasia goes undetected.

A variety of therapeutic approaches has been attempted [29, 31]. Although there have been reports that corticoid steroid therapy may improve the long-term prognosis, the results of various studies are often conflicting. Recently on the basis of a controlled study, it has been suggested that high dose intravenous methylprednisolone and oral chlorambucil improves renal function and increases the likelihood of remission [32]. Similar beneficial effects have been attributed to other cytotoxic drugs such as cyclophosphamide but the value of these therapeutic regimens is still open to debate [33, 34]. Regimens that address the symptoms have included angiotensin converting enzyme inhibitors, non-steroidal anti-inflammatory drugs and even omega 3 fatty acids.

Pathology and pathogenesis

By light microscopy, the glomeruli usually appear moderately enlarged and the mesangium has a mild to moderate degree of prominence. The thickness of the peripheral capillary walls varies from a minimal increase to a striking thickening, depending on the stage of dis-

order (Figure 55.10). Where the change is minimal, a stiffness of the glomerular capillary loops is sometimes apparent. Silver methenamine Masson stains are particularly useful in evaluating membranous nephropathy, because they reveal a classical spike-and-dome pattern with vacuolization of the thickened peripheral capillary walls. The interstitium may show varying degrees of scarring and tubular atrophy. Some studies suggest that the degree of tubulointerstitial alteration is the best predictor of progression to renal insufficiency. Glomerular capillary thrombosis may occasionally occur and suggests the possibility of large renal vein thrombosis. Margination of the polymorphonuclear leukocytes in the peripheral glomerular capillaries sometimes accompanies renal vein thrombosis.

Immunofluorescence staining generally reveals a granular peripheral capillary staining for immunoglobulins. The extent of the granularity may be so great as to give a pseudo-linear appearance. The immunoglobulins most commonly involved in order are IgG, IgM and IgA. It is of interest that in studies in which IgG subtypes have been identified, the IgG in membranous glomerulonephropathy is most commonly IgG 4. A granular deposition of C_3 is also common, but other complement components have not been demonstrated as consistently in a granular pattern. The membrane attack complex C_{5b}–C_9 has also been found. Mesangial deposits are present in a minority of cases. The finding of mesangial immunoglobulin deposits strongly suggests that an identifiable antigen such as hepatitis B may be involved.

Electron microscopic studies have described four stages of development of the membranous lesion [35]. While these stages may be useful for descriptive purposes, it is likely that there is a continuum of change from initial immune complex formation to incorporation into the basement membrane and to final dissolution. In stage 1,

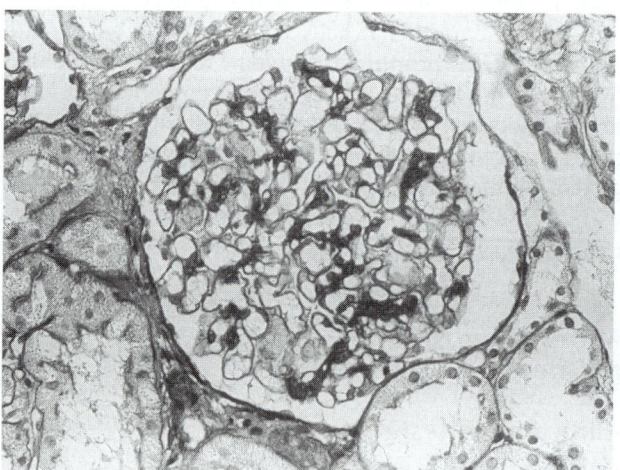

Figure 55.10   Membranous glomerulopathy. The glomerulus is enlarged and the capillary loops appear prominent with a rigid configuration and thickening of the capillary walls. The mesangium also shows an increase in matrix. (Hematoxylin and eosin, ×400.)

scattered electron dense deposits are noted in an epimembranous pattern with a relatively normal appearing glomerular basement membrane. Foot process effacement occurs in relationship to these deposits. The deposits are few and scattered along different portions of the capillary loops. In stage 2, subepithelial deposits are more abundant and are separated from each other by the deposition of basement membrane-like material, giving rise to the classical 'spike and dome' appearance by light microscopy (Figure 55.11). In stage 3, the apical portions of the spikes form an enclosed basement membrane-like structure so that the deposits are now completely surrounded by basement membrane material and are intramembranous rather than epimembranous. In stage 4, there is dissolution of the deposits with rarefaction and evidence of repair and irregular thickening of glomerular basement membrane repair.

Several possible pathogenic mechanisms have been proposed. All of them suggest that the immune complexes identified by immunofluoresence and electron microscopy are the result of *in situ* formation of immune complexes at specific sites [36, 37]. According to one idea, relatively low numbers of circulating immune complexes formed with antibodies of low affinity and avidity dissociate the antigens localized to the glomerular basement

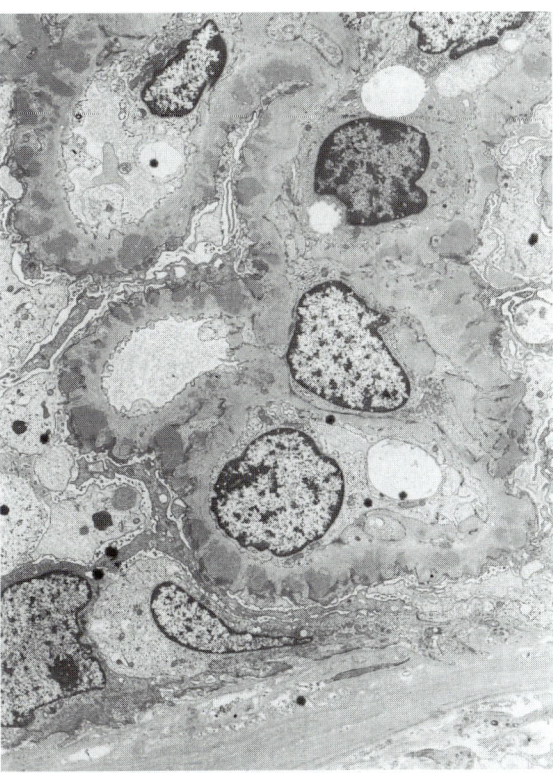

Figure 55.11 Electron micrograph of a glomerulus from a patient with membranous glomerulonephropathy. The basement membrane is thickened with numerous subepithelial deposits separated by 'spikes' of basement membrane material. There is effacement of the foot processes similar to that seen with minimal change disease. (×2650.)

membrane by filtration and form new complexes *in situ* that are stabilized in the basement membrane. A second theory is that intrinsic antigens such as specific basement membrane-associated glycoproteins or planted antigens such as bacterial components or lectins serve as the antigenic component of immune complexes formed *in situ*. Despite the anatomic evidence of an immune mediated lesion, described earlier, attempts to modulate this response have not been consistently clinically successful.

Mesangiocapillary glomerulonephritis

Clinical manifestations and natural history

Mesangiocapillary glomerulonephritis is known by a variety of synonyms. These include membranoproliferative glomerulonephritis, hypocomplementemic glomerulonephritis and lobular glomerulonephritis. This entity is defined more by its morphology than by its clinical presentation. As with membranous glomerulonephropathy, mesangiocapillary glomerulonephritis may be a primary disease or secondary to a variety of systemic, infectious, or hereditary diseases. The primary forms are heterogeneous and further subdivided based on immunofluorescent and electron microscopic findings. Type I has subendothelial deposits and type II has electron dense deposits within the basement membrane. Other types have been described. The clinical features are indistinguishable for all histologic types. Some cases are classified as primary with no known etiology, but the identical morphological lesion is secondary to a variety of infections and multi-system disorders such as lupus erythematosus or cryoglobulinemia [38] (Table 55.3). This certainly suggests that eventually an etiologic agent will be found in most cases we currently consider primary (or idiopathic). As a result of the heterogeneity of the morphologic findings and potential etiologic mechanisms, the clinical presentation is extremely varied.

Although all age groups are affected, primary forms of mesangiocapillary glomerulonephritis occur most common from late childhood to young adulthood [39]. The usual clinical presentation is the nephrotic syndrome complicated by acute nephritis, with hematuria and hypertension. Azotemia may be present and is a poor prognostic indicator. An important finding is hypocomplementemia, predominately C_3. Hypocomplementemia is very frequent in mesangiocapillary glomerulonephritis, but its etiology is related to histologic type. In type I, complement activation occurs by the classic pathway, while in type II, the alternative pathway is activated. The hypocomplementemia in type II is thought to be due to catabolism of C_3 by a circulating IgG, called nephritic factor (NeF). NeF is an autoantibody that binds C3bBb, a convertase enzyme, which prevents it from inactivation so that catabolism of C_3 continues [40]. The pathogenic role of NeF, however, is unclear. Although the clinical and pathological patterns vary depending on the subtype, the disease follows a generally relentless course to renal insufficiency ending in end stage renal disease after 5–10 years [39, 41–43]. Therapeutic approaches have included continuous and alternate day steroids, combined steroid and cytotoxic therapy and anticoagulants and platelet inhibitors [44]. No consistent beneficial effect of any modality has been demonstrated.

Pathology and pathogenesis

By light microscopy, the most prominent finding is glomerular enlargement with accentuation of the lobular architecture. Mesangial areas are expanded by increased numbers of mesangial cells and matrix (Figure 55.12). In some instances, nodular accumulation of matrix exists within lobules mimicking the lesion of Kimmelsteil–Wilson disease in diabetic nephropathy and giving rise to what has been termed lobular glomerular nephritis. The hypercellularity is predominantly mesangial but infiltration with leukocytes is common and may

be extensive. Another characteristic light microscopic feature is the marked thickening of the peripheral capillary wall. This is the result of extension of mesangial cells and matrix around the peripheral capillary resulting in a double contour or tram track appearance seen with special stains such as the Masson silver methenamine stain. This combination of proliferation and peripheral capillary wall thickening was formerly described as mixed membranous and proliferative glomerulonephritis. Necrosis is uncommon but crescents may be seen in approximately one fifth of cases. (A cresent is a lesion in a region in the glomerulus with a convex edge at the glomerular rim and a concave edge containing several types of cells which compress the glomerular capillary tufts.) Rarely, focal forms, in which only a portion of the glomeruli are involved, can be identified. Tubular and interstitial changes range from none to varying degrees of interstitial fibrosis and tubular atrophy often associated with a chronic inflammatory infiltrate. The overall light microscopic pattern is similar in all subtypes. The differences lie in the immunofluorescent and electron microscopic findings. The unique light microscopic pattern may reflect a direct attack on the integrity of the mesangial cells, since mesangiolysis is occasionally identified. Immunofluorescence and electron microscopic examination is necessary to separate subtypes.

In type I, immunofluorescence reveals deposition of immunoglobulins. These are most frequently IgG and IgM but also occasionally IgA. Prominent C_3 deposits are found in an irregular and granular distribution along the periphery of the lobule. Complement components early in the classic pathway are occasionally found as is properdin of the alternative pathway. In some cases, deposition of complement components is present in the absence of deposition of immunoglobulins. Electron

Table 55.3 Conditions associated with mesangiocapillary glomerulonephritis (Adapted from Rennke, H.G. (1995) *Kidney Int.*, **47**, 643–56)

Primary
    Type 1
    Type 2
    Type 3

Secondary
    Autoimmune diseases
        Rheumatoid arthritis
        Sjögren's syndrome
        Systemic lupus erythematosus
    Infections (chronic)
        Bacterial
            Endocarditis
            Infected ventriculoatrial shunt
            Leprosy
            Visceral abscesses (multiple)
        Myoplasma
        Protozoal
            Malaria
            Schistosomiasis
        Viral
            Cryoglobulinemia type II (mixed essential
                cryoglobulinemia)
            Hepatitis B
            Hepatitis C

    Liver disease
        α_1-antitrypsin deficiency
        Cirrhosis

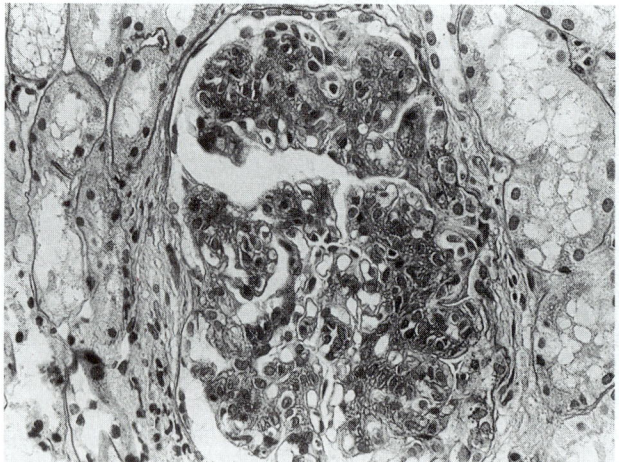

Figure 55.12 Mesangiocapillary glomerulonephritis. There is lobular accentuation of the glomerular architecture secondary to mesangial expansion by increased numbers of mesangial cells. The capillary walls appear thickened and the capillary loops are compromised. (Hematoxylin and eosin, ×400.)

microscopy correlates with the light microscopic picture. There is extensive mesangial cell proliferation with mesangialization of the peripheral capillary loops by extension of mesangial cells and mesangial matrix to the periphery of the capillary wall (Figure 55.13). The peripheral capillary basement membrane is usually identifiable as a distinct basement membrane but is separated from endothelial cells by mesangial cells and matrix continuous with the mesangial area thus giving rise to tram track or double contour appearance. In addition, there is a prominent increase in mesangial matrix. Electron dense deposits are found in the subendothelial and mesangial regions. Occasionally, subepithelial humps are present and when this is a prominent feature, a distinct subgroup has been suggested (type III of Burkholder). In areas of mesangialization of the peripheral capillary loop, the electron dense deposits may lie in the subendothelial mesangial matrix. The epithelial cells show foot process effacement and inflammatory cells including polymorphonuclear leukocytes; monocytes are often present within the capillary lumen and sometimes in a subendothelial site.

The immunofluorescence and electron microscopic findings strongly suggest that the pathogenesis of this subtype is an immune complex disease, perhaps related to an infectious agent [36]. The fact that the exact same histologic picture is seen in the glomerulonephritis associated with infected ventricular–atrial shunts, bacterial endocarditis and hepatitis B and C adds strength to this argument [38, 45].

Type II is also known as dense deposit disease [46, 47]. In addition to the other clinical features shared with type I patients, most patients with type II will have the presence of C_3 nephritic factor (NeF) in their serum. There is an apparent familial incidence of this type which is associated with the occurrence of partial peripheral lipodystrophy. By light microscopy in addition to the findings of type I mesangiocapillary glomerulonephritis, the basement membranes sometimes have a refractile appearance and more intensely take up histologic stains. The immunofluoresence findings in type II mesangiocapillary glomerulonephritis are very consistent. There is extensive deposition of C_3 along the peripheral capillary walls. Depending on the extent of deposition, it can be irregularly linear or discontinuous. Mesangial deposition of complement is also prominent. Immunoglobulins are usually absent although occasionally IgM may be noted.

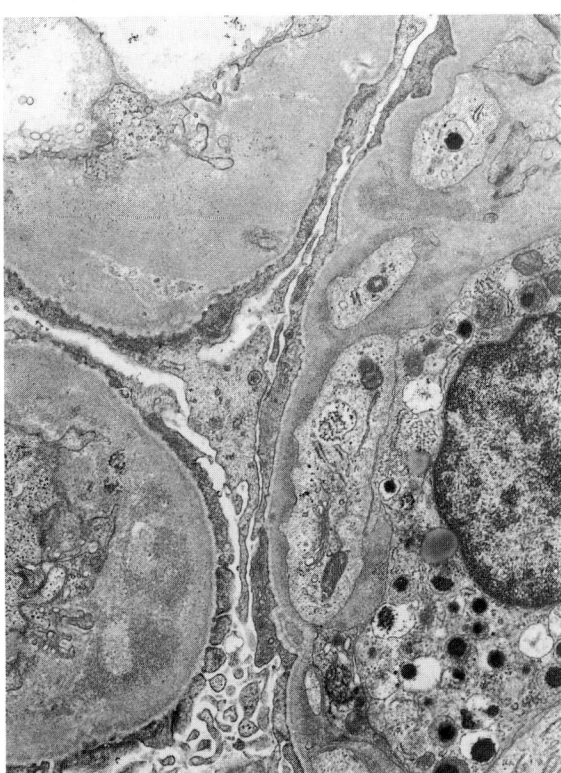

Figure 55.13 Electron micrograph of a glomerulus from a patient with type I mesangiocapillary glomerulonephritis. The capillary wall is thickened by peripheral extension of the mesangium with layering of epithelial cell basement membrane, mesangial cell, mesangial matrix duplicating the basement membrane and endothelial cell. The capillary lumen is occupied by a circulating leukocyte. Electron-dense deposits are present in the mesangium and beneath the basement membrane. (×10050.)

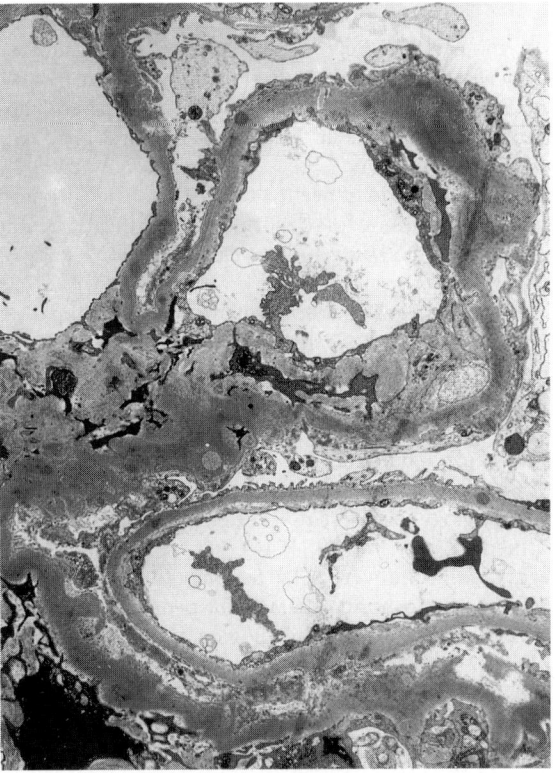

Figure 55.14 Electron micrograph of a glomerulus from a patient with dense deposit disease. The basement membrane is irregularly thickened and there are ill-defined dense deposits within the basement membrane. Focal reduplication by mesangialization of the peripheral capillary wall is also present. (×3313.)

Fibrin is also occasionally present. The most striking change is detected by electron microscopy. A very electron dense material is present within the lamina densa of the glomerular capillary basement membrane which is often widened by the presence of the deposit (Figure 55.14). The deposit forms a long ribbon of hazy electron dense material. In some instances, the ribbon is discontinuous and the electron dense material has a sausage like appearance. In some individual cases, subepithelial electron dense humps similar to deposits observed in poststreptococcal glomerulonephritis are identified. The epithelial foot processes are effaced. The dense deposits are sometimes also identified as being present in the tubular basement membrane as well.

The pathogenesis of this subtype is likely to be a combination of genetic and extrinsic factors. The anatomic characteristics of the deposits suggest that there may be a genetic alteration in the composition of the glycoproteins of the basement membrane. The association in some cases with a familial partial lipodystrophy helps support this concept. The deposition of complement following activation of the complement pathway with formation of $C_3bB\text{-}NeF$ is likely secondary to an external stimulus such as an antecedent infection but could also reflect an intrinsic defect in the complement cascade. Until further information is available the entity will continue to be considered as a primary subtype.

Burkholder described a third type (III) of mesangiocapillary glomerulonephritis that, like type I, is an immune complex mediated disease. Deposits are located in the subepithelial region, however, and there are gaps in the glomerular basement membrane.

References

1. Cameron, J.S., Turner, D.R., Ogg, C.S. *et al.* (1974) The nephrotic syndrome in adults with 'minimal change' glomerular lesions. *Q. J. Medicine.*, **43**, 461–88.
2. Churg, J., Habib, R. and White, R.H.R. (1970) Pathology of the nephrotic syndrome in children. A report for the International Study of Kidney Disease in Children. *Lancet*, **i**, 1299–302.
3. Anonymous (1978) Report of the International Study of Kidney Disease in Children: Nephrotic syndrome in children. Prediction of histopathology from clinical and laboratory characteristics at time of diagnosis. *Kidney Int.*, **13**, 159–65.
4. Habib, R. and Kleinknecht, C. (1971) The primary nephrotic syndrome of childhood. Classification and clinicopathologic study of 406 cases. *Pathol. Annu.*, **6**, 417–74.
5. Glassock, R.J. (1980) Management of the idiopathic nephrotic syndrome. *Contrib. Nephrol.*, **23**, 158–80.
6. Ponticelli, C. (1993) Cyclosporine in idiopathic nephrotic syndrome. *Immunopharmacol. Immunotoxicol.*, **15**, 479–89.
7. Siegel, N.J., Gaudio, K.M., Krassner, L.S. *et al.* (1981) Steroid–dependent nephrotic syndrome in children: histopathology and relapses after cyclophosphamide treatment. *Kidney Int.*, **19**, 454–9.
8. Gregory, M.J., Smoyer, W.E., Sedman, A. *et al.* (1996) Long–term cyclosporine therapy for pediatric nephrotic syndrome: a clinical and histologic analysis. *J. Am. Soc. Nephrol.*, **7**, 543–9.
9. Tejani, A., Nicastri, A.D., Sen, D. *et al.* (1983) Long term evaluation of children with nephrotic syndrome and focal segmental glomerular sclerosis. *Nephron*, **35**, 225–31.
10. Andenmatten, F., Bianchetti, M.G., Gerber, H.A., *et al.* (1995) Outcome of idiopathic childhood nephrotic syndrome. A 20 year experience. *Scand. J. Urol. Nephrol.*, **29**, 15–9.
11. Ittel, T.H., Clasen, W., Fuhs, M., *et al.* (1995) Long–term ciclosporine A treatment in adults with minimal change nephrotic syndrome or focal segmental glomerulosclerosis. *Clin. Nephrol.*, **44**, 156–62.
12. Anonymous (1983) Report of the Southwest Pediatric Nephrology Study Group: Chidhood nephrotic syndrome associated with diffuse mesangial hypercellularity. *Kidney Int.*, **23**, 87–94.
13. Anonymous (1981) Report of the International Study of Kidney Disease in Children: Primary nephrotic syndrome in children. Clinical significance of histopathologic variants of minimal change and of diffuse mesangial hypercellularity. *Kidney Int.*, **20**, 765–71.
14. Glassock, R.J. (1985) Natural history and treatment of primary proliferative glomerulonephritis: a review. *Kidney Int. Suppl.*, **17**, S136–42.
15. Ritz, E. (1994) Pathogenesis of 'idiopathic' nephrotic syndrome (editorial; comment). *N. Engl. J. Med.*, **330**, 61–2.
16. Anonymous (1985) Focal segmental glomerulosclerosis in children with idiopathic nephrotic syndrome. A report of the Southwest Pediatric Nephrology Study Group. *Kidney Int.*, **27**, 442–9.
17. Cameron, J.S., Turner, D.R., Ogg, C.S. *et al.* (1978) The long–term prognosis of patients with focal segmental glomerulosclerosis. *Clin. Nephrol.*, **10**, 213–8.
18. Siegel, N.J., Kashgarian, M., Spargo, B.H. and Hayslett, J.P. (1974) Minimal change and focal sclerotic lesions in lipoid nephrosis. *Nephron.*, **13**, 125–37.
19. Kashgarian, M. (1974) Lipoid nephrosis and focal sclerosis. Distinct entities on spectrum of disease. *Nephron*, **13**, 105–8.
20. Haas, M., Spargo, B.H. and Coventry, S. (1995) Increasing incidence of focal-segmental glomerulosclerosis among adult nephropathies: a 20-year renal biopsy study. *Am. J. Kidney Dis.*, **26**, 740–50.
21. Ingulli, E. and Tejani, A. (1991) Racial differences in the incidence and renal outcome of idiopathic focal segmental glomerulosclerosis in children. *Pediatr. Nephrol.*, **5**, 393–7.
22. Tune, B.M., Kirpekar, R., Sibley, R.K. *et al.* (1995) Intra-

venous methylprednisolone and oral alkylating agent therapy of prednisone-resistant pediatric focal segmental glomerulosclerosis: a long-term follow-up. *Clin. Nephrol.*, **43**, 84–8.

23. Mendoza, S.A., Reznik, V.M., Griswold, W.R. *et al.* (1990) Treatment of steroid-resistant focal segmental glomerulosclerosis with pulse methylprednisolone and alkylating agents. *Pediatr. Nephrol.*, **4**, 303–7.

24. Huppes, W., Hene, R.J. and Kooiker, C.J. (1988) The glomerular tip lesion: a distinct entity or not? *J. Pathol.*, **154**, 187–90.

25. Bourgoignie, J.J. and Pardo, V. (1991) The nephropathology in human immunodeficiency virus (HIV–1) infection. *Kidney Int. Suppl.*, **35**, S19–23.

26. Detwiler, R.K., Falk, R.J., Hogan, S.L. and Jennette, J.C. (1994) Collapsing glomerulopathy: a clinically and pathologically distinct variant of focal segmental glomerulosclerosis. *Kidney Int.*, **45**, 1416–24.

27. Friedman, E.A., Rao, T.K.S., and Nicastri, A.D. (1987) Heroin associated nephropathy. *Nephron.*, **13**, 421–6.

28. Rao, R.K.S., Friedman, E.A. and Nicastri, A.D. (1987) The types of renal disease in the acquired immunodeficiency syndrome. *N. Engl. J. Med.*, **316**, 1062–8.

29. Cameron, J.S. (1992) Membranous nephropathy and its treatment. *Nephrol. Dial. Transplant.*, **7**, 72–9.

30. Anonymous (1979) Collaborative study of the adult idiopathic nephrotic syndrome: A controlled study of short–term prednisone treatment in adults with membranous nephropathy. *N. Engl. J. Med.*, **301**, 1301–6.

31. Austin, H.A.D., Antonovych, T.T., MacKay, K. *et al.* (1992) NIH conference. Membranous nephropathy. *Ann. Intern. Med.*, **116**, 672–82.

32. Ponticelli, C., Zucchelli, P., Passerini, P. and Cesana, B. (1992) Methylprednisolone plus chlorambucil as compared with methylprednisolone alone for the treatment of idiopathic membranous nephropathy. The Italian Idiopathic Membranous Nephropathy Treatment Study Group [see comments]. *N. Engl. J. Med.*, **327**, 599–603.

33. Remuzzi, G., Schieppati, A. and Garattini, S. (1994) Treatment of idiopathic membranous glomerulopathy. *Curr. Opin. Nephrol. Hypertens.*, **3**, 155–63.

34. Hogan, S.L., Muller, K.E., Jennette, J.C. and Falk, R.J. (1995) A review of therapeutic studies of idiopathic membranous glomerulopathy. *Am. J. Kidney Dis.*, **25**, 862–75.

35. Ehrenreich, T. and Churg, J. (1968) Pathology of membranous nephropathy. *Pathol. Annu.*, **3**, 145–86.

36. Couser, W.G. and Salant, D.J. (1980) In situ immune complex formation and glomerular injury. *Kidney Int.*, **17**, 1–13.

37. Couser, W.G. (1993) Pathogenesis of glomerulonephritis. *Kidney Int. Suppl.*, **42**, S19–26.

38. Zamurovic, D. and Churg, J. (1984) Idiopathic and secondary mesangiocapillary glomerulonephritis. *Nephron*, **38**, 145–53.

39. Habib, R., Kleinknecht, C., Gubler, M.C. and Levy, M. (1974) Idiopathic membranoproliferative GN in children. Report of 105 cases. *Clin. Nephrol.*, **1**, 194–214.

40. Strife, C.F., Leahy, A.E. and West, C.D. (1989) Antibody to a Cryptic Solid Phase C1Q Antigen in Membranoproliferative Nephritis. *Kidney Int.*, **35**, 836–42.

41. Kin, Y. and Michael, A.F. (1980) Idiopathic membranoproliferative GN. *Annu. Rev. Med.*, **31**, 273–88.

42. Cameron, J.S., Turner, D.R., Heaton, J. *et al.* (1983) Idiopathic mesangiocapillary glomerulonephritis. Comparison of types I and II in children and adults and long term prognosis. *Am. J. Med.*, **74**, 175–92.

43. Pedersen, R.S. (1995) Long–term prognosis in idiopathic membranoproliferative glomerulonephritis. *Scand. J. Urol. Nephrol.*, **29**, 265–72.

44. Tarshish, P., Bernstein, J., Tobin, J.N. and Edelmann, CM, Jr. (1992) Treatment of mesangiocapillary glomerulonephritis with alternate-day prednisone – a report of the International Study of Kidney Disease in Children. *Pediatr. Nephrol.*, **6**, 123–30.

45. D'Amico, G. and Ferrario, F. (1992) Mesangiocapillary glomerulonephritis. *J. Am. Soc. Nephrol.*, **2**, S159–66.

46. Bennett, W.M., Fassett, R.G., Walker, R.G. *et al.* (1989) Mesangiocapillary glomerulonephritis type II (dense–deposit disease): clinical features of progressive disease. *Am. J. Kidney Dis.*, **13**, 469–76.

47. Habib, R., Gubler, M.C., Loirat, C. *et al.* (1975) Dense deposit disease. A variant of membranoproliferative GN. *Kidney Int.*, **7**, 204–15.

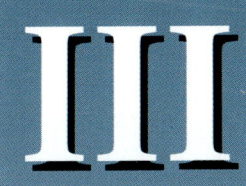

III

Diseases of the Kidney and Their Treatment

Section 5
Diseases of the Renal Interstitium

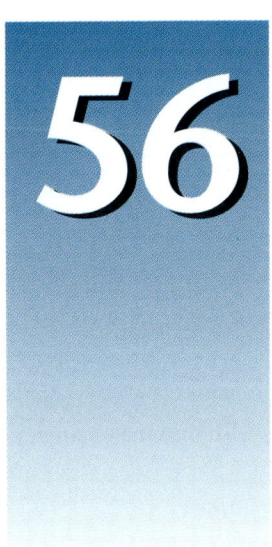

Tubulointerstitial nephritis

J.H. Stewart

Introduction

The hallmarks of interstitial nephritis are inflammatory cellular infiltrate and, in chronic disease, fibrosis in the interstitium, together with tubular damage or atrophy. The etiology is heterogeneous, with toxic, immunological or ischemic injury to the tubular epithelium, causing many cases whereas others result from disease within, or damage to, interstitial structures.

Although this chapter is principally concerned with those nephropathies which primarily involve the tubules or interstitium, tubulointerstitial nephritis is present to some extent in all chronic diseases of the kidney; it coexists in a pronounced fashion with arterial, arteriolar and glomerular sclerosis in end-stage renal failure, whatever the original disease. This non-specific secondary form of tubulointerstitial nephritis, which itself has a multifactorial pathogenesis, is an important element of the pathology of progressive renal failure.

This chapter is divided into three sections describing in turn acute tubulointerstitial nephritis, diseases which primarily cause chronic tubulointerstitial nephritis and tubulointerstitial nephritis occurring in chronic renal failure of glomerular or vascular etiology.

Acute tubulointerstitial nephritis

Of the diseases causing acute tubulointerstitial nephritis, the most common, acute pyelonephritis and renal tubular necrosis, and acute allograft rejection, are covered in other chapters (Table 56.1). This section describes the features common to acute tubulointerstitial injury, whatever its cause, and two forms of the disease which have an immune etiology – acute allergic nephritis and the particular form of acute interstitial disease associated with non-steroidal anti-inflammatory drugs (NSAIDs).

Clinical manifestations

The clinical presentation comprises local and systemic manifestations of acute diffuse inflammation of the kidneys. Often, perhaps usually, symptoms are mild and it is only a raised serum creatinine which draws attention to the condition.

Dull pain may be felt in the loins, or oliguria noted. Occasionally there is visible hematuria, especially in acute allergic interstitial nephritis. The kidneys are sometimes tender or enlarged, although the latter is frequently apparent only on ultrasonography. The urine contains evidence of inflammatory exudate – some protein, leukocytes, erythrocytes, epithelial cells and cellular casts, but not the combination of heavy albuminuria and numerous red cell and granular casts characteristic of acute glomerulonephritis. When the cause is an NSAID, there may be moderate or heavy albuminuria, even nephrotic syndrome, due to the associated minimal-change glomerulopathy – in a minority of such cases the interstitial disease or the glomerulopathy occurs alone.

Serum creatinine is raised even in the absence of oliguria; severe oliguria is uncommon except in renal tubular necrosis and acute allograft rejection. Blood pres-

Nephrology, Edited by Rex L. Jamison and Robert Wilkinson.
Published in 1997 by Chapman & Hall, London. ISBN 0 412 60930 4

Table 56.1 Diseases causing acute tubulointerstitial nephritis

	Etiological agent	Disease
Infective	Ascending bacterial	Acute pyelonephritis
	Hematogenous bacterial	Renal microabscesses
	Systemic – leptospiral, brucella, rickettsial, viral	Acute interstitial nephritis
Ischemic	Hemorrhagic, septic, or cardiogenic shock	Renal tubular necrosis
Toxic	Aminoglycosides, other tubular toxins	Renal tubular necrosis
	Non-steroidal anti-inflammatory drugs	Acute interstitial nephritis with minimal-change glomerulopathy
Immune	β-lactam antibiotics, other drugs	Acute allergic interstitial nephritis
	Allotransplantation	Acute (cellular) graft rejection
Idiopathic	–	Tubulointerstitial nephritis–uveitis syndrome
		Other acute interstitial nephritis

sure is usually not high except with oliguric renal failure. Specific tubular abnormalities are rarely evident.

Except in acute pyelonephritis which is frequently accompanied by bacteremia, systemic symptoms of the renal inflammation are usually not pronounced – mild fever and malaise may occur. The underlying conditions responsible for renal tubular necrosis, and the systemic bacterial, rickettsial and viral infections which involve the renal interstitium, nearly always declare themselves by their extrarenal manifestations.

Pathophysiology

In renal tubular necrosis, the (usually) mild interstitial inflammation is secondary to tubular disruption and leakage, and to cellular damage. The pathophysiology is dominated by impairment of proximal tubular sodium reabsorption, resulting in activation of tubuloglomerular feedback which switches off glomerular filtration – hence oliguria and often severe renal failure.

When the etiology is immune or infective, the disease is primarily interstitial, with only secondary involvement of tubular epithelial cells and, except in cases associated with NSAIDs and sometimes in acute allograft rejection, there is little or no glomerular or arterial pathology. However, in severe examples of acute interstitial nephritis there is sufficient tubular injury to cause significant renal impairment and sometimes oliguria.

Pathology and pathogenesis

Only the pathology and pathogenesis of acute allergic interstitial nephritis, and of the acute interstitial disease caused by NSAIDs, will be described here.

Acute allergic interstitial nephritis

This disease is most commonly seen in the third or subsequent weeks of treatment with a β-lactam penicillin or cephalosporin, the highest risk being with methicillin. A few cases have been described with each of a large number of other drugs, especially sulfonamides, thiazide diuretics and rifampicin.

The predominant pathology is interstitial, is cortical rather than medullary and comprises edema and inflammatory infiltrate which may be sparse, focal or intense. The most numerous cells are lymphocytes, with CD4+ T cells rather more frequent than CD8+ T cells, B lymphocytes and plasma cells, natural killer cells, or macrophages [1]. Polymorphonuclear granulocytes, usually eosinophils, are often present (Figure 56.1a). The inflammatory reaction may be concentrated around, or even be seen to be invading, tubular epithelium (so-called tubulitis) (Figure 56.1b). In more severe cases, tubulitis is associated with epithelial cell degeneration resembling patchy tubular necrosis, and some disruption of the tubular basement membrane. Granulomata may form in the interstitium, but vasculitis is uncommon. Increased extracellular matrix, followed by destructive fibrogenesis, may appear as early as the second week of acute inflammation [1].

Immunofluorescence microscopy or immunoperoxidase staining may show, with diminishing frequency: no complement or immunoglobulin; immune complexes sometimes with complement along the tubular basement membrane; or linear IgG and complement on the tubular basement membrane [1].

The pathology indicates a cell-mediated delayed-type hypersensitivity reaction directed against tubular cells or nearby interstitial structures. However,

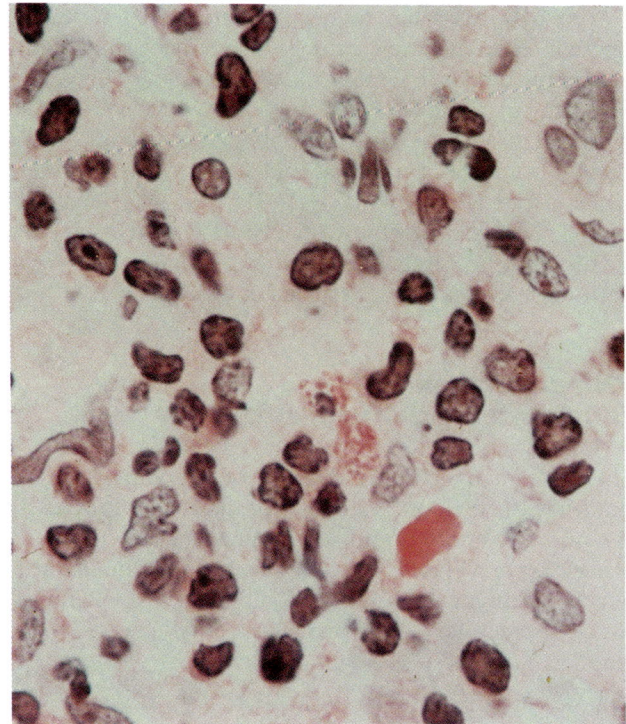

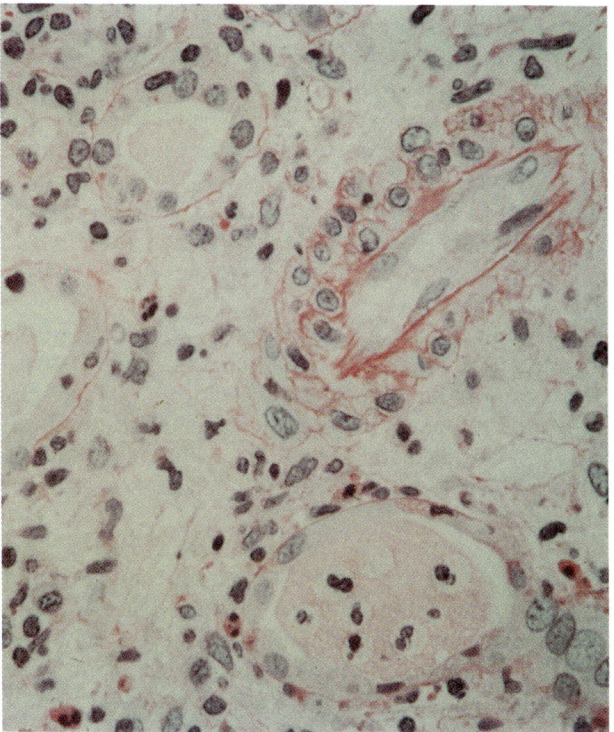

Figure 56.1 Acute allergic interstitial nephritis. (a) High power view of inflammatory infiltrate which is predominantly mononuclear but contains some eosinophils. (b) Lower power view showing that the infiltrate tends to surround, and may penetrate, the tubular basement membrane.

dimethoxyphenyl-penicilloyl radicals may attach to tubular basement membrane as hapten in β-lactam associated nephritis, and antibody to this combination is occasionally present. Coexisting fever, a maculopapular rash on trunk and upper extremities, blood eosinophilia and raised serum IgE levels in rather less than half the patients with acute allergic interstitial nephritis signifies that IgE-mediated hypersensitivity may be involved as well as delayed-type hypersensitivity.

Acute interstitial nephritis with minimal-change glomerulopathy

The combination of an acute interstitial nephritis with moderate or heavy albuminuria and otherwise nearly normal glomeruli showing extensive epithelial foot process spreading ('fusion') is characteristically seen in fewer than 0.2/1000 subjects who take an NSAID other than aspirin for several months [2]. Fenoprofen is the drug carrying the highest risk.

The interstitial inflammatory exudate in this disease resembles that of acute allergic interstitial nephritis except that cytotoxic T cells predominate, and eosinophils are uncommon [3]. There is no evidence of antibody-mediated injury in this form of interstitial nephritis, and extrarenal manifestations of hypersensitivity are rare.

This disease is believed to be a toxic effect of NSAIDs on the immune system, resulting from blockade of cyclo-oxygenase causing arachidonic acid metabolism to be directed towards the alternative lipoxygenase pathway within the kidney, thus increasing production of proinflammatory leukotrienes or expoxy- and hydroxy-eicosanoids [2]. However, that some cases of NSAID-related interstitial disease are in fact allergic is suggested by the presence in them of eosinophils in the infiltrate and other manifestations of IgE-mediated hypersensitivity.

A distinction must be made between this inflammatory disease and the functional renal failure which is sometimes associated with ischemic renal tubular necrosis and which is also an acute toxic effect of NSAIDs. The two conditions may coexist.

Diagnosis

Acute tubulointerstitial nephritis should be considered in any patient with a rising serum creatinine but little or no evidence of glomerular or arterial disease, no prerenal factors, and no dilatation of the urinary collecting system on ultrasonography.

The clinical history of exposure to a β-lactam or aminoglycoside antibiotic or an NSAID, susceptibility to ascending urinary infection, or a recent or coexisting condition causing shock, will indicate the diagnosis directly.

Most difficulty is experienced in those patients exposed to a nephritogenic or nephrotoxic agent at about the same time as a major operation, serious infection or other significant illness which may itself have caused tubular necrosis. The presence of other features of a hypersensitivity reaction or of significant eosinophiluria in the case of β-lactam antibiotics, or of moderate or heavy albuminuria when an NSAID is implicated, indicates a drug-related etiology.

Acute renal failure due to intrarenal obstruction, as in myeloma, uric acid nephropathy, or sulfonamide or other drug crystalluria, has a clinical presentation similar to that of acute tubulointerstitial nephritis, but oliguria is more prominent.

In the small proportion of cases where doubt remains, renal biopsy will nearly always provide the diagnosis. Tissue should be reserved for immunofluorescence microscopy (for immune complexes, linear tubular basement membrane staining or paraprotein), and electron microscopy (to demonstrate glomerular epithelial foot process spreading).

In the rare cases associated with leptospiral, brucella, rickettsial or viral infections, culture of the etiological agent from blood or urine may not be feasible, and serological confirmation of the infection may be delayed for a week or more. The responsible organism may be seen in the renal biopsy tissue, or a characteristic perivascular distribution of the infiltrate at the cortico-medullary junction may suggest an infective etiology.

Treatment and prognosis

When the etiology is toxic or allergic, the offending agent and all related drugs must be withdrawn; when infective, appropriate antibiotic therapy is given. By these means alone the majority of patients with acute interstitial nephritis recover satisfactory renal function, often slowly, and have no residual urinary abnormality. When caused by an NSAID, nephrotic range albuminuria usually resolves spontaneously within a month of ceasing the drug. However, except with tubular necrosis, precise measurement of glomerular filtration rate will often show some permanent reduction from the (presumed) pre-existing level, and in a substantial minority of patients with immune-mediated acute interstitial nephritis, serum creatinine remains elevated although severe renal failure is rare. For this reason, active treatment directed at the immune process must be considered.

In patients with acute allergic interstitial nephritis, there is some evidence that high-dosage corticosteroids (i.e. prednisolone ≈ 1 mg/kg body weight/day for 10 days to 6 weeks, or intravenous methylprednisolone 0.5–2 g for several days) may be advantageous [1], but these regimens provide no demonstrable benefit for patients with NSAID-associated acute interstitial nephritis. The presence of granulomata may indicate a worse prognosis and, by analogy with the response in renal sarcoidosis, corticosteroids are recommended.

Very few cases fail to regain useful renal function. These include the rare examples of tubular necrosis with extensive tubular basement membrane disruption, some instances of acute allograft rejection which cannot be reversed by potent anti-T-lymphocyte therapy, and a small percentage of drug-induced acute tubular or interstitial disease.

The relationship of the acute disease caused by NSAIDs to the chronic interstitial nephritis which is also seen with these agents [3] is discussed elsewhere.

Primary chronic tubulointerstitial nephritis

There are many chronic diseases of the kidney which primarily cause injury to tubules or interstitial structures; the more common and important are described in other chapters (Table 56.2). In this section, the features which distinguish chronic tubulointerstitial nephritis from glomerular and vascular renal disease are emphasized.

Clinical manifestations

Chronic tubulointerstitial nephritis is often covert until renal failure is sufficiently advanced to be symptomatic, although manifestations of tubular dysfunction, most often polyuria, may appear at an early stage. In the absence of coexisting arterial pathology, hypertension is not prominent, and urinalysis is negative or discloses only minor and non-specific abnormalities unless or until glomeruli are involved. Anemia may be more pronounced than in chronic renal failure of glomerular, arterial or cystic origin.

Many diseases causing chronic tubulointerstitial nephritis affect tissues elsewhere than in the kidney, with resultant non-renal clinical manifestations; or they may injure predominantly one segment of the nephron resulting in an identifiable renal tubular syndrome – proximal, distal, papillary, salt-wasting or nephrogenic diabetes insipidus.

With advancing renal damage, the clinical picture becomes less characteristic as tubulointerstitial injury extends throughout the kidney, and arteries and glomeruli become involved. Thus, end-stage renal failure due to chronic tubulointerstitial disease may prove to be indistinguishable from that due to other diseases.

Pathophysiology

Proximal tubular syndromes

Cystinosis and some cases of myeloma and heavy metal poisoning result in severe proximal tubular dysfunction (Fanconi syndrome) with clinically evident metabolic acidosis due to bicarbonate wasting, phosphaturia leading in time to hypophosphatemic rickets, aminoaciduria, and

Table 56.2 Diseases primarily causing chronic tubulointerstitial pathology

	% ESRF[a]
Cystic	
Polycystic kidney disease	7.7
Medullary cystic disease	0.3
Medullary sponge kidney	–
Transport	
Cystinosis	0.2
Immune	
Autoimmune (Sjögren's; systemic lupus erythematosus)	–
Dysproteinemia	0.1
Granulomata (sarcoid; drugs; Wegener's)	0.5
Allograft rejection	[b]
Metabolic	
Hypokalemia	–
Hypercalcemia	0.2
Toxic	
Analgesics; non-steroidal anti-inflammatory drugs	9.1
Heavy metals (lead; cadmium; germanium; platinum)	0.4
Endemic Balkan nephropathy	–
Drugs (lithium; aminoglycosides; cyclosporin)	0.2
Radiation	0.3
Infective	
Ascending (pyelonephritis; vesicoureteric reflux)	5.6
Hematogenous (tuberculous; other)	0.1
Obstructive	
Intrarenal (myeloma; gout; oxalosis)	1.8
Post-renal	3.9
Neoplastic	
Leukemia; lymphoma	–
Unknown etiology	1.7

[a] Percentage of all cases with primary end-stage renal failure attributed to this disease in Australia in 1992 (from the 16th Report of the Australian and New Zealand Dialysis and Transplant Registry).

[b] Chronic graft rejection was the cause of 29% of renal transplant failures in Australia in 1992.

renal glycosuria. More common is a lesser degree of proximal tubular injury which may be detectable only as tubular proteinuria, in which low-molecular-weight plasma proteins normally present in glomerular filtrate escape proximal reabsorption.

Distal nephron syndromes

When papillary damage is prominent, for example in analgesic nephropathy, or the distal nephron is the target of immune-mediated injury as sometimes in Sjögren's syndrome, impaired urinary concentration and distal renal tubular acidosis may dominate the clinical picture, but usually these functional abnormalities are too mild to cause symptoms.

Hyperkalemia more often is due to dysfunction of the juxtaglomerular apparatus – hyporeninemic hypoaldosteronism – than to distal nephron pathology.

Papillary necrosis, causes structural damage, manifest by hematuria, infection or obstruction, in addition to functional syndromes.

Salt-wasting nephropathy

Some impairment of sodium conservation may occur with proximal or distal tubular injury, but when the damage is proximal, activation of tubuloglomerular feedback is likely to limit the loss of salt and water. Severe salt-wasting is rare except when there is involvement of the thick ascending limb of Henle's loop, as may be the case in medullary cystic disease, or all segments of the nephron as in postobstructive uropathy [3].

Nephrogenic diabetes insipidus

Lithium and hypercalcemia both impair water conservation to a greater extent than other functions of the nephron, causing prominent polyuria and thirst.

Pathology and pathogenesis

Tubulointerstitial damage is commonly a consequence of one or more of: extra- or intrarenal urinary obstruction; toxic damage to tubular epithelium or interstitial structures; infection; an immune process; or diffuse infiltration of the kidneys by malignant cells or abnormal proteins.

As the most common and important diseases primarily causing chronic tubulointerstitial nephritis are covered elsewhere, the following sections illustrate the pathology and pathogenesis of some less common causes, or those which are informative.

Intrarenal obstruction

In two of the moderately common forms of interstitial nephritis, hyperuricemic nephropathy (Figure 56.2a) and myeloma kidney (Figure 56.2b), and in some rare conditions, such as oxalosis, precipitation of material which is relatively insoluble in the concentrated acidic urine of the collecting ducts causes tubular blockage and disruption followed by an inflammatory reaction around the damaged tubule. The pathogenesis of the interstitial lesion comprises elements of local inflammatory reaction to the foreign material, sometimes with giant cells, and more general sequelae of urinary obstruction, namely tubular dilatation and atrophy and interstitial fibrosis, with relative preservation of glomeruli and arteries [4].

Tubular epithelial injury

Most nephrotoxic drugs and chemicals have their primary effect on renal tubular epithelium. Important examples are described separately.

Hypercalcemia, lithium toxicity and hypokalemia share a common presentation (polyuria) but the underlying pathology differs. The microscopic lesion is predominantly distal tubular dilatation and microcyst formation in lithium nephrotoxicity [5], calcium deposition with cellular damage (Figure 56.3) and interstitial inflammation ultimately leading to medullary nephrocalcinosis in chronic hypercalcemic nephropathy and proximal tubular vacuolation in chronic hypokalemia. Only in the most severe and prolonged instances, such as in gross abuse of diuretics or purgatives, does hypokalemia cause significant permanent renal damage. In these cases, augmented ammoniagenesis (see below) may be responsible for the interstitial pathology.

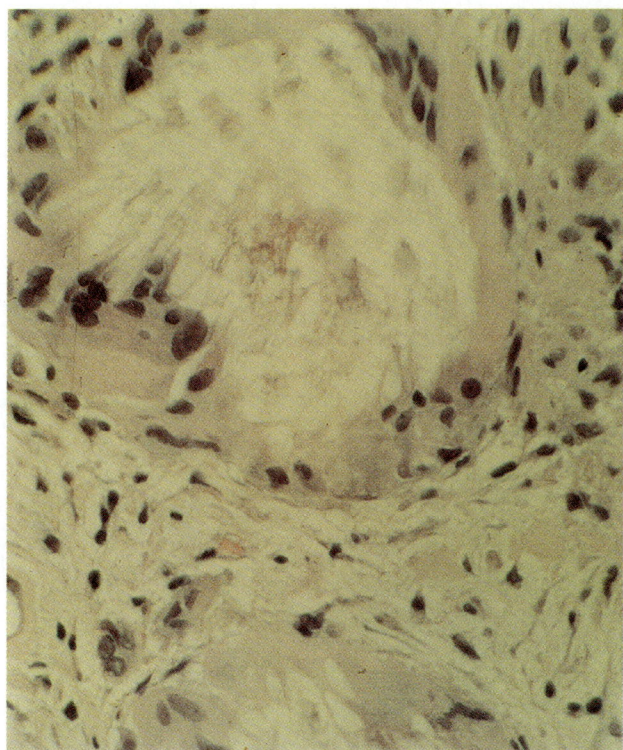

a

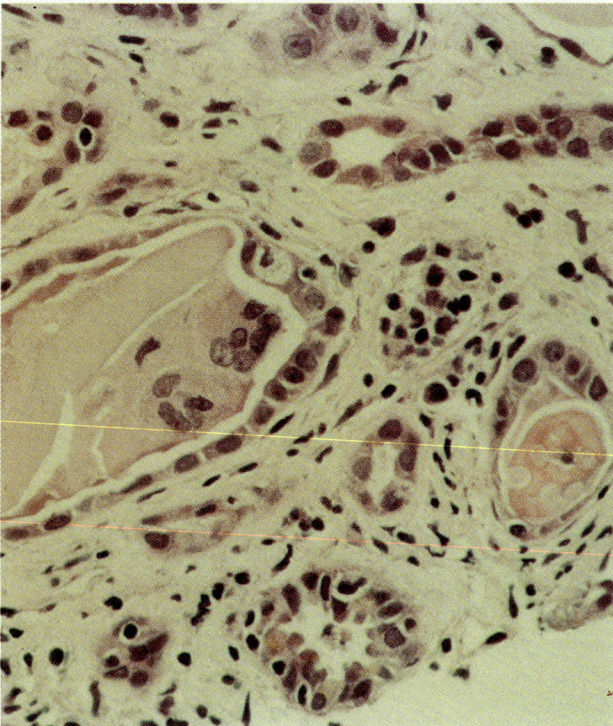

b

Figure 56.2 Tubulointerstitial nephritis secondary to intrarenal obstruction. (a) In hyperuricemic nephropathy, uric acid crystals precipitate in the collecting ducts causing a local inflammatory reaction which often includes giant cells as illustrated here. (b) Myeloma proteins may precipitate in the distal nephron resulting in obstruction, tubular damage and interstitial infiltration.

Immune chronic interstitial nephritis

Little is known about the immunopathogenesis of the interstitial renal disease that occurs in about one-tenth of patients with Sjögren's syndrome [6] and in a smaller proportion of those with other autoimmune diseases, especially systemic lupus erythematosus. Although autoantibodies are often present, neither humoral immunity against tubular antigens nor deposition of immune complexes seems responsible. The lymphocytic infiltrate comprises B cells which may have been subject to virally induced proliferation, and T cells whose role is uncertain. Most commonly the distal nephron is the main target.

Granulomas are prominent only in a minority of cases of sarcoidosis, allergic reactions to drugs such as NSAIDs, or Wegener's granulomatosis.

Vasculitis, most commonly Wegener's, may affect interstitial vessels as well as glomeruli.

Diagnosis

In the early stages of tubulointerstitial nephritis prior to a detectable fall in glomerular filtration rate, suspected proximal tubular damage may be verified by demonstrating one or more of the elements of the Fanconi syndrome – aminoaciduria, renal glycosuria, bicarbonate wasting – or tubular proteinuria in which β_2-microglobulin clearance is increased relative to creatinine clearance, or

lysozyme is present in the urine. Distal nephron injury may impair the ability to concentrate urine disproportionately, or to lower urinary pH below 5.3 in the presence of systemic metabolic acidosis.

A tubulointerstitial etiology will be suspected in patients with reduced kidney function when hypertension is mild, there is little or no albuminuria, or when tubular dysfunction is prominent. The clinical history, manifestations of extrarenal disease, or laboratory tests will identify the underlying disease in many cases, and imaging by ultrasonography or contrast pyelography in most of the remainder. When the diagnosis is not clear, renal biopsy is usually informative except in those cases due to a low-grade toxin such as a heavy metal or a NSAID [3], and in chronic radiation nephritis.

Treatment and outcome

Treatment is directed in the first place to the underlying cause, in particular ceasing exposure to nephrotoxins. In those cases with intrarenal obstruction, particularly by myeloma protein, uric acid or a relatively insoluble drug metabolite, reversal of renal failure depends on establishing an alkaline diuresis by rehydration and intravenously infusing sodium bicarbonate until the plasma bicarbonate is 30–33 mmol/l.

Acute infections must be treated, but in chronic pyelonephritis antibacterial therapy confers no benefit in the absence of demonstrable kidney infection. Moreover, unless given early, treatment of tuberculosis rarely restores kidney function which, in this disease, is compromised permanently by strictures of the urinary collecting system as much as by the infective process in the renal parenchyma.

When granulomata are present, as in sarcoidosis and some drug-induced interstitial nephritides, there is slow and often incomplete improvement with corticosteroids in medium dosage. For renal vasculitis, cyclophosphamide is the most effective agent. The tubulointerstitial component of Sjögren's syndrome, systemic lupus erythematosus, or the dysproteinemias does not resolve with corticosteroid, immunosuppressive or cytotoxic therapy.

Symptomatic therapy

Of the consequences of tubular dysfunction, only salt-wasting and acidosis frequently need treatment, but persistent hyperkalemia may require oral ion-exchange (polystyrene) resins or fludrocortisone.

Chronic renal failure due to tubulointerstitial disease is often not as troublesome as when glomerular or arterial pathology predominates – no nephrotic syndrome and less hypertension or symptomatic salt and water retention. However, acidosis, electrolyte abnormalities, bone disease, and anemia may appear earlier, be more severe, and require more active treatment when chronic nephritis is primarily tubulointerstitial.

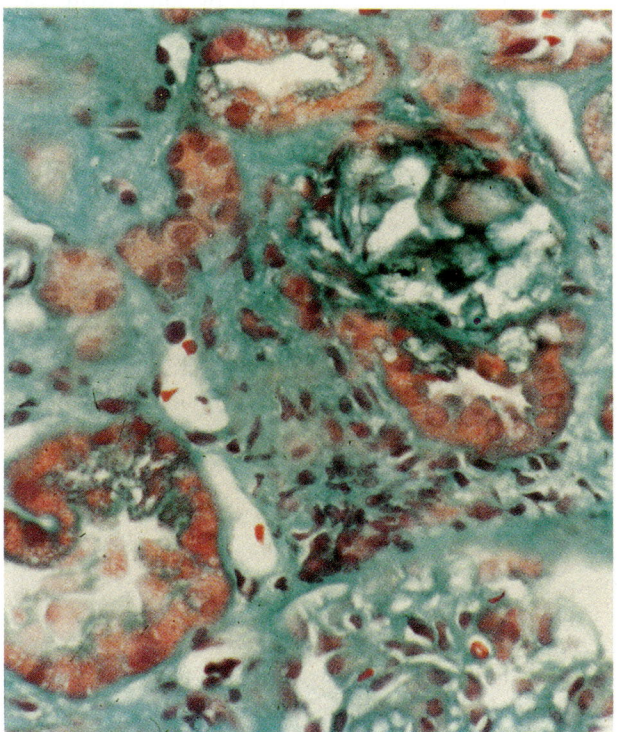

Figure 56.3 Precipitation of calcium salts in tubular epithelium is the initial lesion in hypercalcemic nephropathy.

Interstitial pathology in progressive renal failure

Fibrosis and mononuclear cell infiltration of the interstitial compartment together with tubular atrophy are pronounced features of end-stage renal disease, whatever the primary etiology (Figure 56.4). Indeed it has been observed that in glomerular disease the severity and extent of tubulointerstital damage is a more accurate indicator of prognosis than the glomerular pathology [7, 8]. Rather than being a passive and non-specific result of arterial or glomerular obliteration, chronic tubulointerstitial nephritis is increasingly recognized as being due to specific consequences of one or more of the following: glomerular or vascular dysfunction; extension of glomerular disease into the tubulointerstitial compartment; compensatory tubular hypertrophy; uremic toxicity.

Ischemia

Near-total renal artery occlusion is characterized by pronounced atrophy of tubular (especially proximal) epithelium and relatively well preserved glomeruli. The degree to which renal function is restored after revascularization is predicted by the severity of the tubular, not the glomerular, pathology. A similar phenomenon may occur to a lesser extent in advanced chronic renal failure as a consequence of hypertensive or atherosclerotic narrowing of intrarenal vessels.

Additionally, in human kidneys with glomerular disease, the peritubular capillary network shows a degree of obliteration and separation from epithelium by fibrosis sufficient to cause tubular ischemia [9]. This angiopathy is probably a consequence of hypertension and/or local production of vasoactive substances [8].

Extension of glomerular inflammation

In active glomerulonephritis, the inflammatory process may spill into the surrounding interstitial tissue through the hilum of the glomerulus or the damaged capsular basement membrane or into the glomerular filtrate, thereby delivering mediators of tissue injury to either surface of the tubular epithelium.

Uncommonly, an immune process involving the glomeruli may, because of shared antigens or the systemic nature of the disease, also involve other renal structures in the tubulointerstitial compartment [1, 10], examples being antitubular basement membrane specificity of antibodies in antiglomerular basement membrane nephritis, the involvement of interstitial capillaries in Wegener's granulomatosis, and interstitial immune complex deposition in systemic lupus erythematosus.

Proteinuric nephropathy

Most normally filtered serum proteins, and a significant amount of those that appear in the glomerular filtrate as a result of disease, are taken up by endocytosis and degraded by lysosomal enzymes in the proximal tubular epithelium. With the exception of minimal change nephrotic syndrome in which the filtered protein is virtually all albumin, the severity of proteinuria provides an index of the rate of progression in a variety of glomerular diseases and correlates with the degree of tubulointerstitial damage [11]. Various mechanisms have been suggested to account for this correlation.

There may simply be a non-specific effect of increased trafficking of protein across proximal tubular cells, perhaps mediated either by escape of lysosomal degradative enzymes into the interstitial compartment [12] or by increased metabolic activity [11]. In addition, it is at least theoretically possible that an interstitial autoimmune disease may be initiated when serum proteins are processed by proximal tubular cells, which are not only capable of presenting antigen but can also be induced to express on their surfaces those components of the major histocompatibility complex necessary for immune activation [1, 10].

Filtered proteins may themselves be toxic to proximal tubules, light chains being the best-known example. Complement can be activated by the brush border [13], and both minimally modified low-density lipoprotein [14] and glycated albumin may stimulate production of reactive oxygen species by tubular epithelium. Filtered

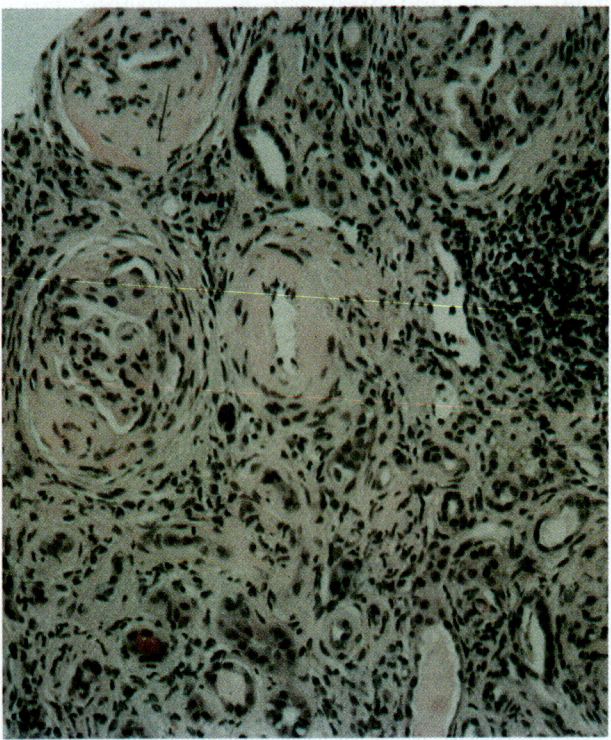

Figure 56.4 Extensive chronic interstitial inflammation and tubular damage in a patient with advanced crescentic glomerulonephritis due to antiglomerular basement membrane antibodies.

cytokines may induce excess tubular production of toxic metabolites such as nitric oxide [15].

Alternatively, the leaked serum protein may carry to the proximal tubular cells an injurious molecule, such as iron which catalyzes the formation of hydroxyl ions [16] or non-esterified fatty acid which results in the production of a lipid inflammatory factor [17].

Tubular hypermetabolism

The metabolic work of renal tubular epithelium, largely dedicated to sodium reabsorption, is usually increased in the surviving nephrons of chronically damaged kidneys quite apart from any effects of proteinuria. This is, among others, an inevitable consequence of elevated single nephron glomerular filtration rates. Measures which reduce tubular metabolism protect against that component of progressive parenchymal damage which has been attributed to increased mitochondrial production of reactive oxygen species and ammonia. These two metabolites respectively cause interstitial injury by lipid peroxidation and by generating amidated C′3, a C′3/C′5 convertase which activates the C′5–9 cascade [18]. Acidosis or hypokalemia also increases renal ammoniagenesis.

Uremic toxicity

Relatively insoluble uremic metabolites, such as inorganic phosphate [19] or oxalate [20], may be found as crystalline deposits in the tubules or interstitium in advanced

renal failure, contributing to autonomous progression by causing intrarenal obstruction or an interstitial inflammatory reaction. The accumulation of calcium phosphate in chronically damaged kidneys may be the single most important factor in the tubulointerstitial component of progressive renal failure.

Intrarenal obstruction

In chronically diseased kidneys, casts are frequently seen in distal nephrons which are often dilated and presumably obstructed (Figure 56.5). These casts may be formed by the interaction of filtered proteins or other macromolecules with Tamm–Horsfall mucoprotein [21], but as their occurrence is more characteristic of chronic pyelonephritis than glomerular disease, local tubular factors appear to be important in causation. Escape of Tamm–Horsfall protein into the interstitial compartment itself may cause inflammation [21]; however, the release of inflammatory mediators by the obstructed nephron is likely to be the main cause of the interstitial nephritis in this situation [22].

Pathogenesis of the interstitial component of progressive renal failure

The translation of tubular epithelial injury into interstitial fibrosis and reduced glomerular filtration rate involves a number of mechanisms, the contribution of each varying with nature of the tubular damage (Figure 56.6). The most severe lesions will result in disruption, even obliteration, of the tubule leaving atubular glomeruli which can have no excretory function [23]. Tubuloglomerular disconnection is most common in chronic pyelonephritis.

At the other end of the scale, functional tubular damage causing impairment of proximal sodium reabsorption activates tubuloglomerular feedback, thereby reducing glomerular filtration rate [7]. Although no further structural damage should result, a more-or-less permanent activation of tubuloglomerular feedback might account in part for the correlation of reduced glomerular filtration rate with tubulointerstitial, rather than glomerular, pathology [24].

A variety of immune events set in motion either by mediators released from tubular cells, or by loss of tolerance consequent upon renal tissue injury, may contribute significantly to disease progression [1, 10].

The chronic interstitial disease, comprising fibrosis, mononuclear cell infiltration and attenuation of the capillary network, which is chiefly responsible for the tubulointerstitial component of autonomous renal disease, however, is caused for the most part by release of paracrines from one or more of the following: partially damaged tubular epithelium or glomeruli; interstitial capillary endothelium; circulating or infiltrating leukocytes and platelets. Numerous mediators have been implicated,

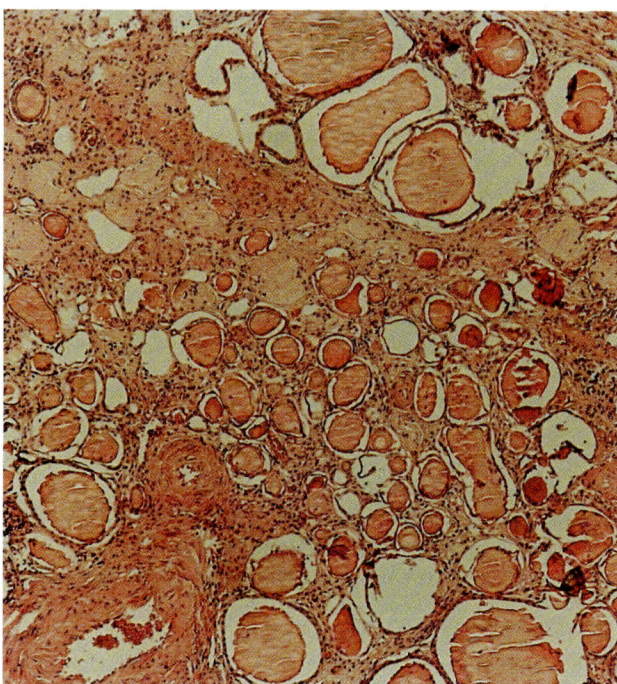

Figure 56.5 'Thyroidization' of the kidney characteristic of advanced chronic renal failure, especially in chronic pyelonephritis.

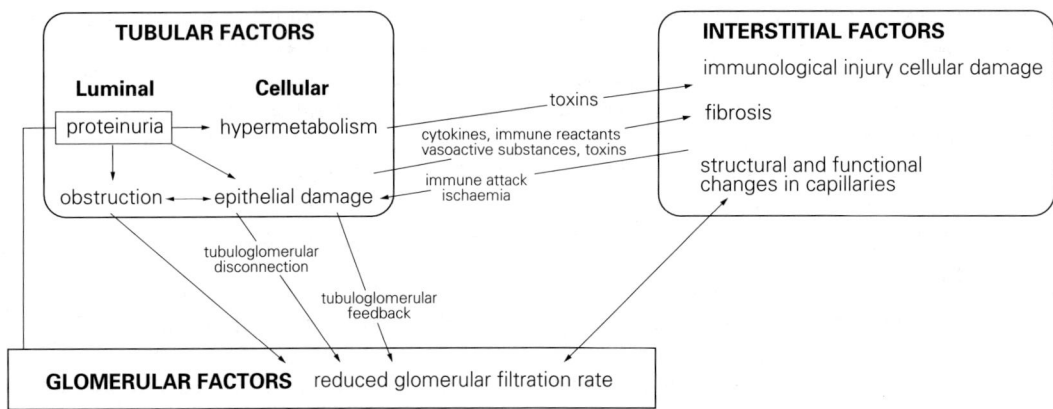

Figure 56.6 The interrelationship of tubular, interstitial and glomerular factors in the pathogenesis of chronic tubulointerstitial injury.

including: chemotactic cytokines which recruit inflammatory cells, particularly T lymphocytes [25] and macrophages [22, 26]; growth factors such as transforming growth factor-β [27] and platelet derived growth factor [8] which promote fibrosis; vasoactive substances which may have a structural or functional effect on peritubular capillaries [8], and local toxins such as proteolytic enzymes, reactive oxygen species, nitric oxide [15], and ammonia or other nucleophilic amines [11, 18] which may themselves be toxic to extracellular matrix or to interstitial or tubular cells, or activate other injurious processes.

The recruitment and activation of macrophages and T cells by tubular and inflammatory cell-derived attractant factors is the major cause of fibrosis and injury to interstitial structures [8, 25, 26]. The resultant ischemic and immunological damage to the tubular epithelium completes the cycle of events which comprises the tubulointerstitial component of autonomous progressive renal pathology.

References

1. Neilson, E.G. (1989) Pathogenesis and therapy of interstitial nephritis. *Kidney Int.*, **35**, 1257–70.
2. Murray, M.D. and Brater, D.C. (1993) Renal toxicity of the nonsteroidal anti-inflammatory drugs. *Annu. Rev. Pharmacol. Toxicol.*, **32**, 435–65.
3. Kleinknecht, D. (1995) Interstitial nephritis, the nephrotic syndrome and renal failure secondary to nonsteroidal anti-inflammatory drugs. *Semin. Nephrol.*, **15**, 228–235.
4. Iványi, B. (1993) Development of chronic renal failure in patients with multiple myeloma. *Arch. Pathol. Lab. Med.*, **117**, 837–40.
5. Kling, M.A., Fox, J.G., Johnston, S.M. *et al.* (1984) Effects of long-term lithium administration on renal structure and function in rats. A distinctive tubular lesion. *Lab. Invest.*, **50**, 526–35.
6. Kater, L. and de Wilde, P.C.M. (1992) New developments in Sjögren's syndrome. *Curr. Opin. Rheumatol.*, **4**, 657–65.
7. Mackensen-Haen, S., Bohle, A., Christensen, J. *et al.* (1992) The consequences for renal function of widening of the interstitium and changes in the tubular epithelium of the renal cortex and outer medulla in various renal diseases. *Clin. Nephrol.*, **37**, 70–7.
8. Fine, L.G., Ong, A.C.M. and Norman, J.T. (1993) Mechanisms of tubulo-interstitial injury in progressive renal diseases. *Eur. J. Clin. Invest.*, **23**, 259–65.
9. Bohle, A., Gise, H.V., Mackensen-Haen, S. and Stark Jakob, B. (1981) The obliteration of the post-glomerular capillaries and its influence upon the function of both glomeruli and tubuli. *Klin. Wochenschr.*, **59**, 1043–51.
10. Wilson, C.B. (1989) Study of the immunopathogenesis of tubulointerstitial nephritis using model systems. *Kidney Int.*, **35**, 938–53.
11. Rustom, R., Jackson, M.J., Critchley, M. and Bone, J.M. (1992) Tubular metabolism of aprotonin ^{99m}Tc and urinary ammonia: effects of proteinuria. *Miner. Electrolyte Metab.*, 18, 108–12.
12. Eddy, A.A. (1989) Interstitial nephritis induced by protein-overload proteinuria. *Am. J. Pathol.*, **135**, 719–33.
13. Camussi, G., Rotunno, M., Segoloni, G. *et al.* (1982) *In vitro* alternative pathway activation of complement by the brush border of proximal tubules of normal rat kidney. *J. Immunol.*, **128**, 1659–63.
14. Ong, A.C.M. and Moorhead, J.F. (1994) Tubular lipidosis: epiphenomenon or pathogenetic lesion in human renal disease? *Kidney Int.*, **45**, 753–62.
15. Markewitz, B.A., Michael, J.R. and Kohan, D.E. (1993) Cytokine-induced expression of a nitric oxide synthase in rat renal tubule cells. *J. Clin. Invest.*, **91**, 2138–43.
16. Harns, D.C.H., Tay, C. and Nankivell, B.J. (1994) Lysosomal iron accumulation and tubular damage in rat puromycin nephrosis and ageing. *Clin. Exp. Pharmacol. Physiol.*, **21**, 73–81.
17. Kees-Folts, D., Sadow, J.L. and Schreiner, G.F. (1994) Tubular catabolism of albumin is associated with the

release of an inflammatory lipid. *Kidney Int.*, **45**, 1697–709.

18. Nath, K.A., Hostetter, M.K. and Hostetter, T.H. (1985) Pathophysiology of chronic tubulo-interstitial disease in rats. Interactions of dietary acid load, ammonia, and complement component C3. *J. Clin. Invest.*, **76**, 667–75.

19. Lau, K. (1989) Phosphate excess and progressive renal failure: the precipitation-calcification hypothesis. *Kidney Int.*, **36**, 918–37.

20. Fayemi, A.O., Ali, M. and Braun, E.V. (1979) Oxalosis in hemodialysis patients. A pathologic study of 80 cases. *Arch. Pathol. Lab. Med.*, **103**, 58–62.

21. Kumar, S. and Muchmore, A. (1990) Tamm–Horsfall protein – uromodulin (1950–1990). *Kidney Int.*, **37**, 1395–401.

22. Rovin, B.H., Harris, K.P.G., Morrison, A. *et al.* (1990) Renal cortical release of a specific macrophage chemoat-tractant in response to ureteral obstruction. *Lab. Invest.*, **63**, 213–20.

23. Marcussen, N. (1992) Atubular glomeruli and the structural basis for chronic renal failure. *Lab. Invest.*, **66**, 265–84.

24. Persson, A.E.G., Boberg, U., Hahne, B. *et al.* (1982) Interstitial pressure as a modulator of tubuloglomerular feedback control. *Kidney Int.*, **22**, S 122–8.

25. Strutz, F. and Neilson, E.G. (1994) The role of lymphocytes in the progression of interstitial disease. *Kidney Int.*, **45**, S 106–10.

26. Pichler, R., Giachelli, C.M., Lombardi, D. *et al.* (1994) Tubulointerstitial disease in glomerulonephritis. Potential role of osteopontin (uropontin). *Am. J. Pathol.*, **144**, 915–26.

27. Border, W.A. and Noble, N.A. (1993) Cytokines in kidney disease: the role of transforming growth factor-β. *Am. J. Kidney Dis.*, **22**, 105–13.

Diseases of the kidney due to analgesics

J.H. Stewart

Classical analgesic nephropathy

Introduction

Analgesic nephropathy emerged only in the 1950s, becoming common probably because women drafted into manufacturing industry during the Second World War adopted the practice of taking analgesics to cope with the stress of working, and passed the habit to their teenaged daughters. Consumption for more than a year of several tablets or powders per day of analgesic preparations containing at least three ingredients unequivocally causes the classical form of this disease in which the primary lesion is papillary necrosis [1–3]. Renal pathology caused by single analgesics or nonsteroidal anti-inflammatory drugs (NSAIDs) will be described separately.

For two decades analgesic nephropathy caused some 20% of chronic renal failure in Switzerland, Scandinavia and Australia and also occurred in Great Britain, North America and South Africa. In addition it was an important cause of acute renal failure. By 1986, the prevalence of analgesic nephropathy in end-stage renal failure programs was 18% in Switzerland and Belgium, and 13% in West Germany, but had fallen to 12% in Australia and 2% in Sweden. Apart from four countries of North–Central Europe with prevalences of 4–5%, the recorded proportion of end-stage renal failure due to this disease was 2% or less in North America, the rest of Europe and Asia [1].

Clinical manifestations

The clinical picture comprises the manifestations of (1) the renal and urinary pathology: papillary necrosis, chronic interstitial nephritis, and urothelioma; (2) minor drug dependency; and (3) the non-renal toxicity of heavy analgesic consumption (Table 57.1).

Renal and urinary manifestations

Papillary necrosis of any etiology may be silent or may cause one or more florid clinical syndromes [1, 4]. Asymptomatic pyuria, indolent urinary infection or acute pyelonephritis are frequent. Hematuria may be microscopic or macroscopic. Necrotic papillae may separate and be retained in the collecting system as filling defects or as calculi which can become staghorn; more often they are passed and cause colic; occasionally they obstruct the ureter. When infection is present, pyonephrosis results in a serious acute illness due principally to Gram-negative septicemia and its complications, frequently including acute renal failure.

Chronic interstitial nephritis is insidious, manifest only as a decline in renal function, hypertension which is often difficult to control, and proteinuria in advanced disease. With renal impairment, salt-wasting, acidosis and uremic bone disease may appear early and be unduly severe.

Urothelial cancer nearly always presents with hema-

Nephrology, Edited by Rex L. Jamison and Robert Wilkinson.
Published in 1997 by Chapman & Hall, London. ISBN 0 412 60930 4

Table 57.1 The non-renal manifestations of analgesic abuse

Drug	Effect
Phenacetin	Methemoglobinemia, splenomegaly, pigmentation
Caffeine	Withdrawal headache, insomnia, psychomotor stimulation
Codeine	Constipation, laxative abuse, addiction
Aspirin, other NSAIDs	Peptic ulcer, milk-alkali syndrome, bleeding, iron deficiency, salicylism, perinatal morbidity, accelerated atherogenesis
Uncertain etiology	Premature aging, encephalopathy

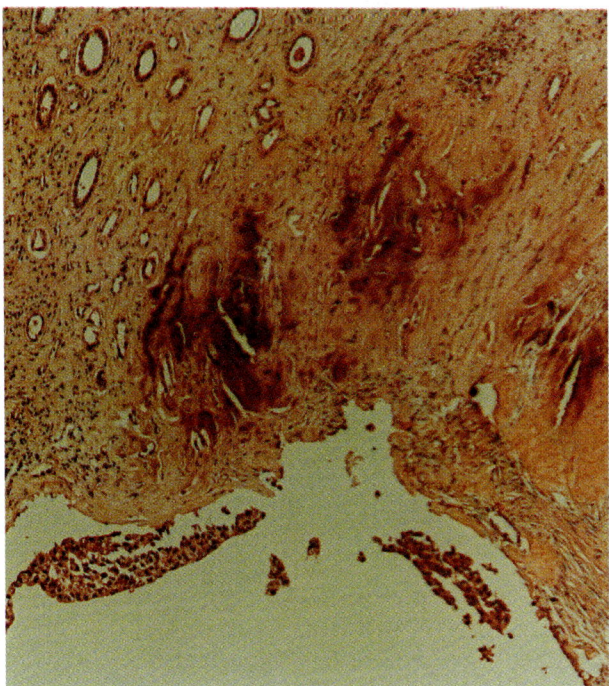

Figure 57.1 Papillary necrosis in the kidney of a patient who had consumed approximately 20 kg of aspirin, phenacetin and caffeine (APC) powders over a period of 30 years. The tip of the papilla has separated, the inner medulla shows necrosis and calcification centrally, and there is mononuclear infiltration of the adjacent tissue.

turia, but some cases are detected by contrast pyelography or urinary cytology, or because of late complications such as urinary obstruction or metastases.

Manifestations of minor analgesic dependency

Personality traits associated with non-medical use of analgesics include nervousness, depression and emotional lability; a lack of security in interpersonal relationships may manifest as a propensity to seek medical solutions for a variety of problems [5]. Frank neurosis or psychosis infrequently underlies the habit. A minority of patients take excessive amounts of analgesics for painful musculoskeletal conditions such as backache or arthritis.

Women are more than twice as likely as men to abuse analgesics, and the disease takes 20 years on average to appear; thus most persons with this diagnosis are middle-aged or elderly females.

Pathophysiology

The susceptibility to ascending infection of retained necrotic papillae accounts for the frequency and persistence of urinary infection. Hematuria is microscopic if aspirin or other NSAIDs are being taken, or macroscopic from papillary separation or cancer. Impaired urinary concentration, salt-wasting, and distal renal tubular acidosis are a corollary of the predominantly medullary site of the lesion, and reduced excretion of citrate, a result of acidosis, may account for the propensity to medullary nephrocalcinosis. Proteinuria appears only when focal glomerulosclerosis supervenes as a consequence of compensatory hypertrophy.

Hypertension may be renin-dependent due to salt-wasting, intrarenal arterial disease or atheromatous renal artery stenosis, or it may reflect the salt retention characteristic of advanced renal failure.

Pathology and pathogenesis

Papillary necrosis

To the naked eye the papillae initially appear nearly normal. At an early stage, necrosis of interstitial and capillary endothelial cells and of the epithelium of the thin segment of the ascending limb of Henle's loop, thickening of the subjacent basement membranes and increased medullary ground substance are seen on microscopy [3]. Advanced cases show necrosis of all elements of the medulla, often with partial or complete papillary separation; characteristically there is pigmentation and calcification in the inner medulla and mononuclear infiltration in the outer medulla (Figure 57.1), but unlike papillary necrosis of diabetic, infective or obstructive etiology, there is no acute inflammatory component (Table 57.2).

The pathogenesis generally involves heavy and prolonged exposure simultaneously to three ingredients of compound analgesic preparations [1, 2]. The role of one of the ingredients, usually caffeine, sometimes codeine or a barbiturate, is to promote habituation, in the case of caffeine by causing withdrawal headache or a perception of improved psychomotor performance [5]. The second

Table 57.2 Causes of renal papillary necrosis

Disease	Pathology
Compound analgesics	Toxic, non-inflammatory, calcification
NSAIDs	Ischemic, non-inflammatory
Sickle cell disease	Ischemic, non-inflammatory
Profound shock	Ischemic, non-inflammatory
Diabetes	Ischemic, acute inflammation
Urinary obstruction	Acute inflammation
Acute pyelonephritis	Acute inflammation

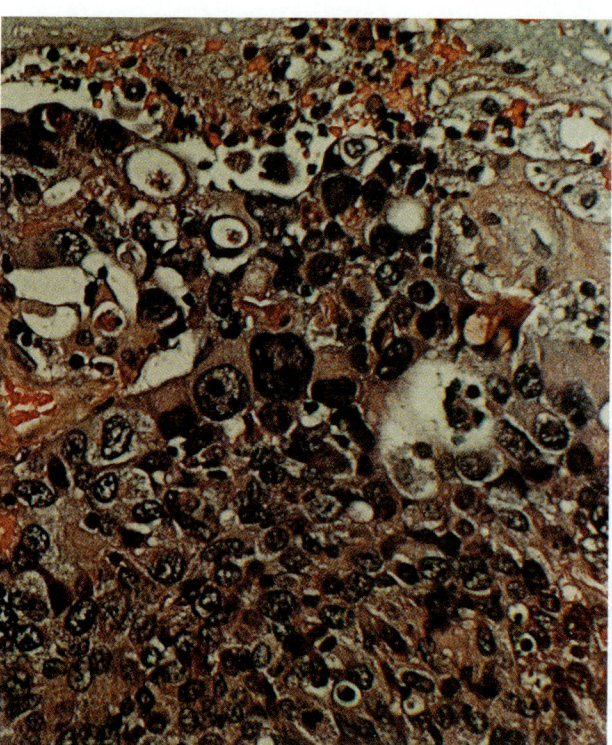

Figure 57.2 A pleomorphic transitional cell carcinoma of the renal pelvis arising adjacent to an area of analgesic-related papillary necrosis.

ingredient, if aspirin, depletes glutathione which protects the renal medulla from the toxic metabolites of the third ingredient, phenacetin (or possibly paracetamol – acetaminophen in America) [1, 6]. In continental Europe and Scandinavia, the second ingredient often was not aspirin, but a pyrazolone (e.g. phenazone or antipyrine) whose role in pathogenesis is not known.

Huge doses of single analgesics, particularly aspirin and other NSAIDs, may cause papillary necrosis in laboratory animals [7] – medullary ischemia may be responsible.

Chronic interstitial nephritis

Due to intrarenal urinary obstruction, cortical tissue atrophies over those necrotic papillae which are retained; there is tubular atrophy, fibrosis, mononuclear infiltration and in advanced disease glomerular obsolescence and arterial intimal thickening. As they empty into calyces more peripherally, nephrons situated in the columns of Bertin are relatively spared and may hypertrophy, ultimately showing focal glomerulosclerosis [1, 3].

Paracetamol (acetaminophen) causes nephrotoxic tubular necrosis [8], and there may also be a direct toxic effect of other analgesic metabolites or NSAIDs on renal tubular epithelium [7]. Thus the pathogenesis of the cortical tubulointerstitial component of analgesic nephropathy may be multifactorial.

Capillary sclerosis

This, the earliest lesion, appears as basement membrane thickening, revealed by electron microscopy to be concentric layers of thin lamellae entrapping cellular debris and lipid (which may be pigmented) in the capillaries underlying the urothelium, maximally at the pelvi-ureteric junction [9]. Diffusion through the urothelium of urinary metabolites of phenacetin causes repeated toxic lysis of the vascular endothelial cells, accounting for this pathology.

Transitional cell carcinoma

Precancerous lesions or urothelioma may be seen anywhere in the urinary tract, most commonly in the renal pelvis or bladder [10]. The tumors are transitional cell carcinomas, not commonly showing extensive squamous change, but on the whole they are more malignant than tobacco-related urothelial cancers (Figure 57.2). Although *N*-hydroxy metabolites of phenacetin (but not of paracetamol/acetaminophen) are carcinogenic, papillary necrosis is itself considered to be the risk factor accounting for the location, frequency and malignancy of analgesic-related tumors in the nearby urothelium [11].

Diagnosis

The diagnosis of analgesic-abuse nephropathy depends on demonstrating (1) excessive analgesic intake and (2) the characteristic lesion, usually by imaging, occasionally by histological examination of a passed papilla or a removed kidney.

Detection of analgesic abuse

If analgesic intake is denied or understated, as is likely if the habit is deemed to be reprehensible, the detection in the urine of salicylate (by Phenistix) or *N*-acetyl-*p*-aminophenol (by colorimetry) [12] indicates surreptitious consumption which usually is heavy.

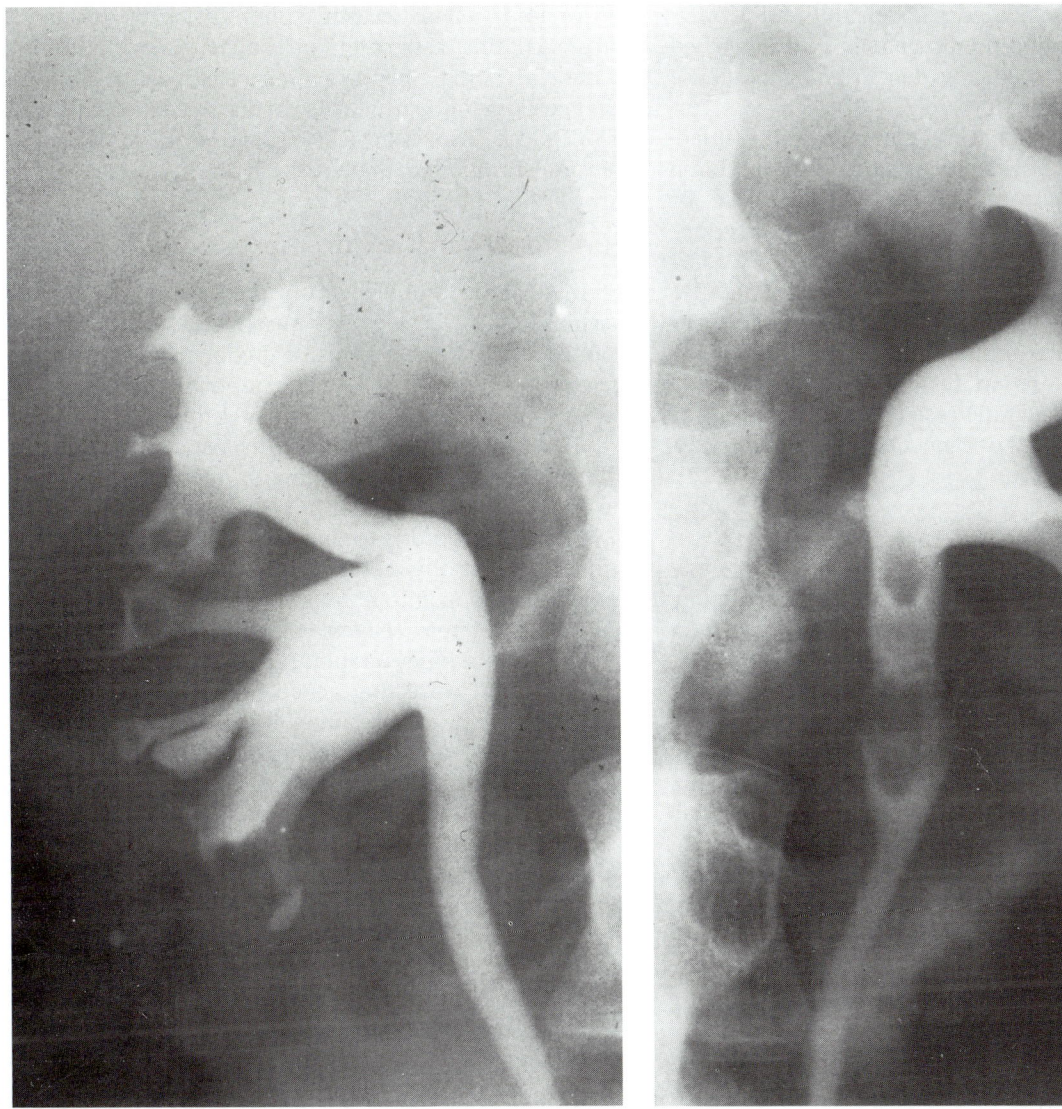

a   b

Figure 57.3 An excretion urogram of a patient with analgesic-associated renal papillary necrosis. (a) In the right kidney, several papillae are separated but retained in the calyces, whereas other calyces show clefts at their fornices as a result of partial separation, or are clubbed following passage of necrotic papillae. (b) In the region of the left pelviureteric junction, there are several filling defects which have the characteristic appearance of separated papillae, but could be blood clot or urothelioma.

Capillary sclerosis, if seen in nephrectomy or autopsy specimens, is pathognomonic of heavy phenacetin intake [9].

Imaging

Only contrast pyelography demonstrates papillary separation both sensitively and specifically. The diagnosis of analgesic nephropathy is based on a characteristic combination of calyceal irregularity, sometimes including manifest papillary pathology (Figure 57.3a), with overlying cortical atrophy, whereas cortical thickness is relatively preserved between the calyces [13]. The abnormality is usually distinguishable from papillary necrosis of different etiology, normal renal lobulation, reflux nephropathy, tuberculosis, medullary nephrocalcinosis from metabolic causes, and medullary sponge kidney. However, the pyelogram may be normal in the early stages of the disease, and when papillae remain *in situ* there may be no distortion of calyces. Plain radiography, ultrasonography or computed tomography may show cortical scarring or papillary calcification.

In suspected or proven analgesic nephropathy, a radiolucent filling defect in the collecting system may be a separated papilla, blood clot or tumor (Figure 57.3b).

Treatment

All analgesics must be stopped. Although single drugs rarely cause the disease there is evidence that, even when used in recommended dosage, paracetamol and NSAIDs other than aspirin may cause progression of established renal injury whether originally due to analgesic abuse [14] or to other causes [15].

Intervention is directed at the complications – infection, obstruction, tumor, hypertension, acidosis, bone disease, symptomatic renal failure. The presence of retained necrotic tissue impedes eradication of infection, mandating prolonged antibiotic therapy which may not be successful. Normal surgical principles apply to the treatment of obstruction and urothelial cancer, and there are no special considerations with regard to maintenance dialysis and transplantation for these patients except perhaps in respect of their increased propensity to occlusive arterial disease [4, 12] or cancer of the upper urinary tract.

Outcome

Since many patients present with infection or obstruction and may be critically ill with pyonephrosis, septicemia or acute renal failure, they often improve rapidly with treatment. In the stable patient, autonomous progression is less likely than in other chronic renal diseases [14], perhaps because of their older age and female sex. It is the propensity to renin-dependent hypertension and atheroma which represents the greatest risk of renal failure and of non-renal morbidity and mortality [4, 12].

Cancer of the renal pelvis is fatal in about 70% of cases, mainly from dissemination of this aggressive tumor, but sometimes from renal failure hastened by nephrectomy [1].

Prevention

It has only been in countries where phenacetin was removed and not replaced by another agent, as in Scandinavia in 1961–2, Canada in 1973 and Australia in 1979, that analgesic nephropathy has declined rapidly [1, 2]. However, there was evidence that public education and medical intervention was reducing the incidence of end-stage renal failure due to this disease in Australia in the 1970s before these measures were taken [1]. Because of the long latent interval, analgesic nephropathy is still being diagnosed in older Australian women 17 years after effective prevention was adopted.

The incidence of renal pelvic cancer has also declined, the effect being apparent some 10 years after banning phenacetin.

Kidney disease due to nonsteroidal anti-inflammatory drugs

About 1% of persons taking NSAIDs other than aspirin suffer functional syndromes attributable to suppression of cyclooxygenase causing diminution of intrarenal prostaglandins. Less common is a characteristic form of acute interstitial nephritis associated with minimal change glomerulopathy which is described in Chapter 56. NSAIDs are also believed to have significant role in causing chronic renal failure.

Functional renal syndromes

NSAIDs have little effect on the kidney in healthy persons. However, because vasodilator prostaglandins counterregulate the actions of angiotensin and norepinephrine when the renal circulation is under stress or when it is reduced as in old age or chronic renal disease, NSAID administration in these circumstances readily precipitates functional renal failure or, rarely, acute tubular necrosis [16–18]. High risk situations include shock, volume depletion due to diuretics or an alcoholic binge, surgical operations, cardiac or liver failure, hypoalbuminemia or concomitant usage of angiotensin converting enzyme inhibitors. Unless there is ischemic tubular damage, the kidneys rapidly recover on ceasing the NSAID and correcting the predisposing factor(s). However, as the renal failure is usually asymptomatic until advanced, and the patients are often frail or suffering from significant comorbidity, a critical illness may result.

The renal prostaglandin, PGE_2, has a mild natriuretic action in the loop of Henle and collecting duct, and PGI_2 stimulates renin release; thus inhibition of PGE_2 and PGI_2 during prolonged use of NSAIDs causes sodium retention with a consequent rise in blood pressure or, in about 3% of subjects, edema. A form of hyporeninemic hypoaldosteronism may occur, but hyperkalemia with (usually) mild acidosis is uncommon in the absence of other contributing factors.

Two NSAIDs, sulindac and salicylates, are said to have less renal toxicity, in the case of sulindac because its active metabolite, the sulfide, is converted enzymatically within the kidney into the inactive prodrug, the sulfoxide [16]. Salicylates bind to renal cyclooxygenase, but inhibit the enzyme less than do other NSAIDs. Paracetamol (acetaminophen) does not inhibit cyclooxygenase, other than perhaps in the central nervous system, and so causes only cytotoxic injury, not functional renal syndromes.

The contribution of NSAIDs to irreversible renal disease

NSAIDs cause irreversible kidney disease which resembles classical analgesic nephropathy except that chronic tubulointerstitial nephritis, not papillary necrosis, is the dominant lesion. The cause clearly differs from classical analgesic nephropathy as no metabolite of phenacetin or paracetamol (acetaminophen) is involved. When present, papillary necrosis is caused by ischemia from the action of NSAIDs on the renal circulation [7]. In the majority of patients who do not have papillary necrosis, there may be an insidious and chronic form of the acute interstitial nephritis described in Chapter 55, thought to be due to diversion of arachidonic acid metabolism towards synthesis of proinflammatory leukotrienes [16].

With NSAIDs increasingly available to the public directly, and being misused by sportsmen and others for musculoskeletal pain or to improve performance, nephrologists fear the reappearance of 'analgesic nephropathy' as a major cause of acute and chronic renal failure. That this is unlikely to happen is due to two factors – the absence of an habituating ingredient coformulated with the NSAIDs, and the relative insensitivity of the kidneys of young and healthy persons to the injurious effects of these drugs. Because of their toxicity in the elderly and the sick, kidney disease either primarily from this source, or made significantly worse by NSAID consumption, is likely to be as frequent, but not as severe, as classical analgesic nephropathy once was [4, 15, 19].

Other causes of papillary necrosis

The acute inflammatory form of papillary necrosis that occurs in diabetes, acute pyelonephritis and urinary obstruction, is now rare. The usual presentation was of pyonephrosis in which Gram-negative septicemia is superimposed on ureteric obstruction, although less florid manifestations occur.

Ischemic papillary necrosis is seen in a substantial minority of persons with sickle cell disease, and in some of those with the trait [20]. The condition is usually silent or manifest only as painless hematuria, but all the complications of papillary necrosis described above can happen. As there is little cortical atrophy, kidney functional deterioration in sickle cell disease is generally due to other manifestations of the disease, chiefly glomerulopathy. Other causes of ischemic papillary necrosis, such as severe dehydration from gastroenteritis in infants, are uncommon.

References

1. Stewart, J.H. (ed.) (1993) *Analgesic and NSAID-induced Kidney Disease*, Oxford University Press, Oxford.
2. Noels, L.M., Elseviers, M.M. and de Broe, M.E. (1995) Impact of legislative measures on the sales of analgesics and the subsequent prevalence of analgesic nephropathy: a comparative study in France, Sweden and Belgium. *Nephrol. Dial. Transpl.*, **10**, 167–74.
3. Burry, A.F. (1967) The evolution of analgesic nephropathy. *Nephron*, **5**, 185–201.
4. Nanra, R.S. (1993) Analgesic nephropathy in the 1990s – an Australian perspective. *Kidney Int.*, **44**(suppl 42), 86–92.
5. Murray, R.M. (1973) The origins of analgesic nephropathy. *Br. J. Psych.*, **123**, 99–106.
6. Engelhardt, G. and Homma, I. (1996) Effects of acetylsalicylic acid, paracetmol and caffeine and a combination of these substances on kidney glutathione levels. *Ardnermittel Forschung*, **46**, 513–8.
7. Prescott, L.F. (1982) Analgesic nephropathy: a reassessment of the role of phenacetin and other analgesics. *Drugs*, **23**, 75–149.
8. Björck, S., Svalander, C.T. and Aurell, M. (1988) Acute renal failure after analgesic drugs including paracetamol (acetaminophen). *Nephron*, **49**, 45–53.
9. Mihatsch, M.J., Hofer, H.O., Gudat, F. *et al.* (1983) Capillary sclerosis of the urinary tract and analgesic nephropathy. *Clin. Nephrol.*, **20**, 285–301.
10. Bengtsson, U., Johansson, S. and Angervall, L. (1978) Malignancies of the urinary tract and their relation to analgesic abuse. *Kidney Int.*, **13**, 107–13.
11. McCredie, M., Stewart, J.H., Carter, J.J. *et al.* (1986) Phenacetin and papillary necrosis: independent risk factors for renal pelvic cancer. *Kidney Int.*, **30**, 81–4.
12. Dubach, U.C., Rosner, B. and Stürmer, T. (1991) An epidemiologic study of abuse of analgesic drugs. Effects of phenacetin and salicylate on mortality and cardiovascular morbidity (1968 to 1987). *N. Engl. J. Med.*, **324**, 155–60.
13. Elseviers, M.M., Waller, I., Nenov, D. *et al.* (1995) Evaluation of diagnostic criteria of analgesic nephropathy in patients with end-stage renal failure: results of the Anne study. *Nephrol. Dial. Transpl.*, **10**, 808–14.
14. Schwarz, A., Kunzendorf, U., Keller, F. and Offermann, G. (1989) Progression of renal failure in analgesic-associated nephropathy. *Nephron*, **53**, 244–9.
15. Perneger, T.V., Whelton P.K. and Klag, M.J. (1994) Risk of kidney failure associated with the use of acetaminophen, aspirin, and nonsteroidal antiinflammatory drugs. *N. Engl. J. Med.*, **331**, 1675–9.
16. Murray, M.D. and Brater D.C. (1993) Renal toxicity of the nonsteroidal anti-inflammatory drugs. *Annu. Rev. Pharmacol. Toxicol.*, **32**, 435–65.
17. Simon, L.S. (1995) Actions and toxicity of nonsteroidal anti-inflammatory drugs. *Current opinion in Rheumatology*, **7**, 159–66.
18. Kleinknecht, D., Landais, P. and Goldfarb, B. (1986) Analgesic and non-steroidal anti-inflammatory drug-associated acute renal failure: a prospective collaborative study. *Clin. Nephrol.*, **25**, 275–81.
19. Sandler, D.P., Burr, F.R. and Weinberg, C.R. (1991) Nonsteroidal anti-inflammatory drugs and the risk for chronic renal disease. *Ann. Intern. Med.*, **115**, 165–72.
20. Allon, M. (1990) Renal abnormalities in sickle cell disease. *Arch. Intern. Med.*, **150**, 501–4.

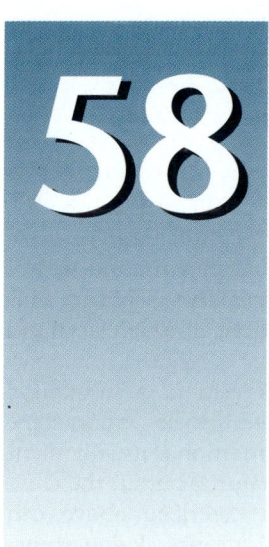

58

Injury to the kidneys from heavy metals and radiation

Richard P. Wedeen

Lead nephropathy

Clinical manifestations

Acute lead nephropathy

Acute lead poisoning is most frequently encountered in children three months to six years of age as a result of the ingestion of chips of paint (pica). When the blood lead concentration exceeds 150 µg/dl, encephalopathy is common and fatal seizures may occur. In this setting, the appearance of the Fanconi syndrome characterized by aminoaciduria, glycosuria, phosphaturia, and hypercalciuria is of relatively minor importance [1]. As with other forms of the Fanconi syndrome, vitamin D-resistant rickets may develop.

Removal of lead by chelation therapy reverses the proximal tubule reabsorptive defect and removes the intranuclear inclusion bodies of acute lead nephropathy [2]. If the child survives without chelation, chronic tubulointerstitial nephritis may develop several decades later. An epidemic of tubulointerstitial nephritis in young adults occurred in Queensland, Australia, at the turn of the century. Studies of 'Queensland nephritis' over seven decades suggest that the delayed development of chronic renal failure corresponded to the nephropathy in adults exposed to lead in their occupations [3].

Chronic lead nephropathy

The etiology of Queensland nephritis was identified because symptomatic lead poisoning had occurred in childhood. Symptomatic lead poisoning from occupational exposure, contaminated alcoholic beverages or other identifiable sources has similarly permitted the recognition of lead as the etiological agent in chronic interstitial nephritis [1]. Typically, renal failure is evident only after years of excessive lead absorption and is frequently associated with hypertension or gout [4–6]. About 50% of patients with lead nephropathy suffer from gout, and although hyperuricemia is universal in renal failure, gout is unusual in renal disease unrelated to lead exposure. In the absence of renal failure, gout cannot usually be attributed to lead exposure despite coexisting hypertension.

In contrast to cadmium nephropathy, in lead nephropathy the excretion of urinary 'marker' proteins such as human intestinal alkaline phosphatase, tissue non-specific alkaline phosphatase, retinol binding protein, Tamm–Horsfall glycoprotein, lysozyme, and β_2-microglobulin (β_2–M), [7] are not increased. The increase in urinary N-acetyl-β-D-glucosaminidase that occurs when blood lead levels are elevated may reflect the proximal tubule injury of acute lead poisoning rather than the chronic interstitial nephritis associated with occupational lead exposure [8, 9a].

Recent mortality data support the notion that hypertensive cardiovascular disease is a more frequent cause of death among lead workers than among the general population [9]. A role for lead in the induction of hypertension with renal failure was suggested by Batuman *et al.* [5] who studied patients using the EDTA lead-mobilization test. Patients with elevated levels of chelatable lead

Nephrology, Edited by Rex L. Jamison and Robert Wilkinson.
Published in 1997 by Chapman & Hall, London. ISBN 0 412 60930 4

in this study would have been designated 'essential' hypertensives had the chelation test not been performed. The value of the EDTA lead-mobilization test for identifying the contribution of previously unrecognized lead poisoning to renal disease in adults with hypertension or gout has recently been confirmed by Sanchez-Fructuoso et al. in Spain [11a].

A role for lead in hypertension gains further credence from epidemiological studies. The Second National Health and Nutrition Examination Survey (NHANES II), performed between 1976 and 1980, included blood lead and blood pressure measurements in almost 10 000 non-institutionalized Americans aged six months to 74 years. The correlation between blood lead and blood pressure (after confounding variables were accounted for) indicated that blood lead predicts blood pressure even when both measurements are within the 'normal' range [10, 11]. On the other hand, a number of epidemiological studies have failed to demonstrate a relationship between lead and blood pressure; possibly reflecting the reduced statistical power of small cohorts [12].

Pathophysiology

Acute elevations of blood lead concentrations result in selective accumulation of lead in the kidneys where it is sequestered in proximal tubules within characteristic acid-fast intranuclear inclusion bodies (Figure 58.1). With prolonged excessive absorption, the kidney becomes only a minor storage site and lead is retained primarily in bone. Since more than 95% of blood lead is bound to erythrocytes, clearance is difficult to measure, but like other cations, lead appears to undergo bidirectional transport across the tubular epithelium. Plasma clearance ranges from about 1 to 3 ml/min and is relatively independent of renal failure [6, 13].

In lead nephropathy, the kidney shows the characteristic morphology of relatively acellular tubulointerstitial nephritis (Figure 58.2). Intranuclear inclusion bodies are absent when there is no current exposure to lead. The appearance of arteriolar nephrosclerotic lesions before hypertension develops and the relatively short duration of hypertension suggest that the primary renal injury from lead may be to the renal microvascular endothelium. This view is consistent with the finding that creatinine clearance decreases with increasing blood lead in the general population independent of blood pressure [14].

Treatment

There is no evidence to suggest that advanced chronic lead nephropathy is reversed by removal of lead with chelating agents; indeed, it seems likely that no improvement in renal function can be anticipated after the steady-state serum creatinine has exceeded 3 mg/dl (265 µmol/l). Lead-induced focal interstitial nephritis, however, may have a reversible functional component that is at least in part prerenal in origin. Chronic volume depletion and hyporeninemic hypoaldosteronism may contribute to the reversible component of renal dysfunction [15, 16]. Prerenal azotemia is associated with the mesenteric vasospasm of acute lead poisoning which is believed to cause lead colic.

Diagnosis

The diagnosis of lead nephropathy can be substantiated by demonstrating excessive body lead stores in patients with tubulointerstitial renal disease when other identifiable causes of renal failure have been excluded. After cessation of exposure to lead, the blood lead concentration

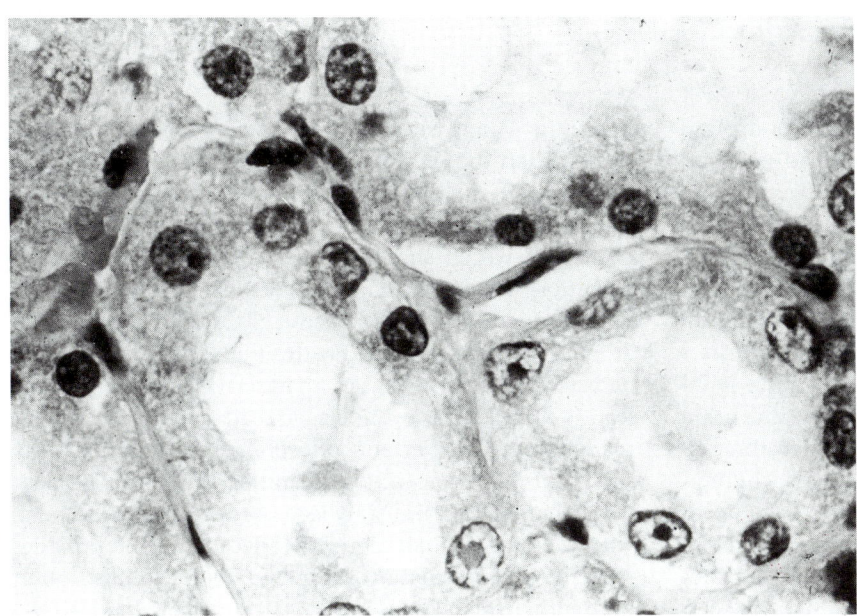

Figure 58.1 Post mortem renal tissue from a 56-year-old lead paint formulator who died from lead encephalopathy. At the time of death his blood lead was 65 µg/dl, and his hemoglobin was 6.5 g/dl. He had basophilic stippling of red blood cells, and his serum creatinine was 1.1 mg/dl (97 µmol/l). An acid-fast intranuclear inclusion body (light gray) is present in a proximal tubule cell. The brain contained 11.2 µg Pb/g and the kidney 16.6 µg Pb/g wet weight.

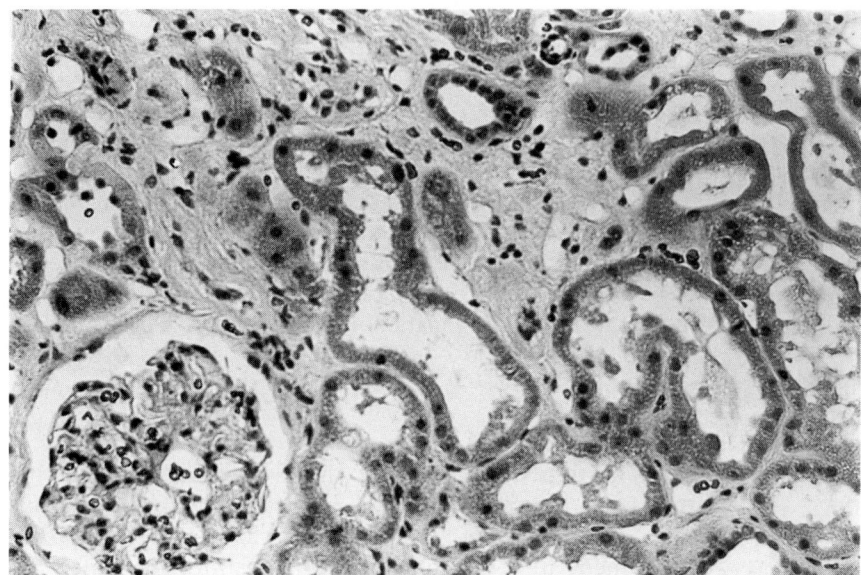

Figure 58.2 Light microscopy showing focal interstitial nephritis in a kidney biopsy from a 54-year-old man who had been a lead worker for 34 years. His blood lead was 46 μg/dl, glomerular filtration rate 80 ml/min/1.73 m² (¹²⁵I-iothalamate clearance) and EDTA chelation test 1,620 μgPb over three days. (Wedeen *et al.*, *Arch. Int. Med.*, 139:53–8, 1979).

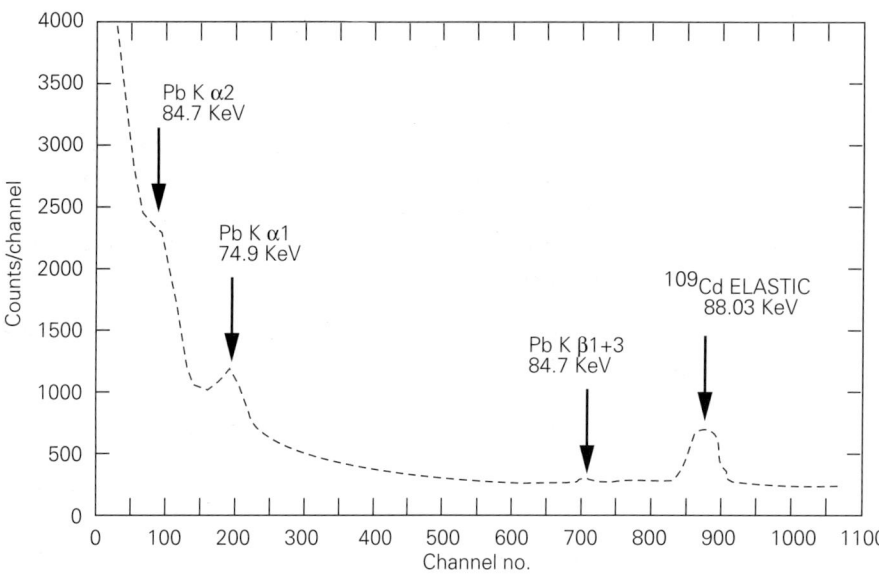

Figure 58.3 X-ray spectrum from the tibia of a 52-year-old woman with severe peripheral muscle weakness who was receiving chronic hemodialysis. She exhibited pica for leaded chips of paint while in the hospital. Her blood lead was 82 μg/dl and bone lead 120 ppm wet weight. *In vivo* tibial K XRF measures the ratio of the characteristic $K_{\alpha1} + K_{\alpha2}$ peaks emitted by lead to the elastic scatter. Using published values for the composition of bone, the concentration of lead in bone is calculated [19].

is inadequate for the detection of excessive body lead burden. Because the biological half-life of lead in blood is approximately 30 days, blood levels reflect recent, rather than cumulative, lead exposure. Cumulative lead absorption can be assessed by the $CaNa_2EDTA$ lead mobilization test. $CaNa_2EDTA$ binds to lead in soft tissues and bone and the lead–chelate complex is cleared in the urine at the glomerular filtration rate. Chelatable lead correlates well with bone lead concentration [11a, 17]. Since renal failure reduces the rate of excretion of lead–chelate, urine collections should be extended from one day to three to five days. When normalized to body surface area, children and adults without unusual lead exposure excrete up to about 650 μg/1.73 m²/day lead–chelate during the chelation test [12, 18]. The degree of renal failure that precludes reliance on the lead mobilization test has not been

determined, but the chelation test is probably inappropriate when the serum creatinine exceeds about 7 mg/dl (650 μmol/l). *In vivo* tibial K X-ray fluorescence (XRF) is a safe, non-invasive, and reliable technique for measuring bone lead which should replace the more cumbersome chelation test [19]. Characteristic K-shell fluorescent X-rays stimulated by a radioactive ¹⁰⁹Cd source from lead atoms in bone are recorded with a high purity germanium detector and multichannel analyzer (Figure 58.3). Bone lead is normalized to the elastic scatter which arises primarily from calcium and phosphorus so that the measurement is largely independent of geometry. Because more than 90% of the body lead burden is stored in bone with a biological half-life of two decades, bone provides more direct information on cumulative lead absorption than either the level of blood lead or chelatable lead.

Management

Lead can be removed from the body by chelation. However, the toxicity of chelating agents in the presence of renal failure has not been systematically examined. $CaNa_2EDTA$ is safe as a diagnostic test, but the cumulative effect of repeated administration of the compound when renal function is compromised is not known. The efficacy and adverse effects of the new oral chelating agent, succimer, has not been examined in renal failure.

Cadmium nephropathy

Introduction

Cadmium is widely used in the manufacture of plastics, pigments, glass, alloys and electrical equipment. The heaviest exposure occurs in smelting, electroplating and welding operations; absorption is primarily by inhalation but about 10% is retained following ingestion. Inhalation of as little as 10–15 mg causes severe gastrointestinal symptoms and may produce fatal acute pneumonitis or delayed chronic obstructive pulmonary disease [20]. After high parenteral doses, necrosis occurs in the testicles, sensory ganglia and the liver in experimental animals.

Proximal tubule dysfunction

An association between kidney disease and cadmium was first noted at the end of the nineteenth century, but the distinctive tubular proteinuria and osteomalacia were not recognized until the 1940s. Until recently, only a few cases of progressive renal failure due to occupational exposure to cadmium had been identified.

The kidney is considered the 'critical organ' for cadmium because the metal accumulates in the proximal tubule where it produces its most prominent toxic effect [21]. Individuals without excessive exposure accumulate cadmium in the kidney up to about 50 years of age, reaching a maximum level of 50–100 µg/g kidney. Hepatic accumulation, although less than renal accumulation, continues up to the eighth decade. When the intrarenal cadmium concentration reaches 200 µg/g tubular proteinuria, the Fanconi syndrome with glycosuria and hypercalciuria, and increased urinary excretion of cadmium begin.

Increased urinary excretion of low-molecular-weight proteins such as β_2-M or RBP is an early renal effect of cadmium. β_2-M has been the most extensively examined urinary protein in cadmium nephropathy, but because of its instability in acid urine, measurement of urinary RBP or NAG is probably more reliable [22, 23]. Slight increases in the excretion of albumin and transferrin in cadmium workers raise the possibility of glomerular injury but could also be explained by impaired tubular reabsorption/catabolism of these proteins that are normally filtered in small quantities. Proteinuria in cadmium workers rarely exceeds a few hundred milligrams per day and does not approach nephrotic levels (>3.5 g/day). The usual techniques for detecting albuminuria such as Albustix, heat and picric acid, or nitric acid are not sufficiently sensitive or specific to detect reliably tubular proteinuria. Although phosphotungstic, trichloroacetic, and sulfosalicylic acids are more sensitive tests for urinary protein, immunologic techniques are required for specific protein identification.

Calcium wasting

Hypercalciuria secondary to renal calcium wasting is responsible for kidney stones among cadmium workers, which may reach an incidence of 40% [23, 24]. Osteomalacia with pseudofractures and severe bone pain was the major clinical manifestation of environmental cadmium poisoning in Japan after the Second World War. This syndrome, known as 'Itai-itai byo' ('ouch-ouch disease'), arose from consumption of rice contaminated by cadmium, derived from rivers polluted by metal mining operations. The disease affected primarily postmenopausal multiparous women who had subsisted on diets deficient in calcium and vitamin D for decades. The victims developed a waddling gait, shortened stature, anemia, glucosuria and elevated serum alkaline phosphatase. Hypertension was absent. Excretion of β_2-M often exceeded the normal maximum (1 mg/g creatinine) 100-fold.

Chronic interstitial nephritis

The glomerular filtration rate was progressively reduced in the most severely affected individuals in Japan with Itai-itai byo [25]. Progressive interstitial nephritis has been observed among occupationally exposed workers in the United States [24] and in Belgium [26]. An increased relative mortality from kidney disease has been found among cadmium workers [20]. The effect of cadmium on blood pressure remains controversial in part because in experimental animals, a hypertensive effect has been found after low doses of cadmium which disappears after high doses.

Pathophysiology

Following absorption, cadmium is transported to the liver bound to albumin, where it induces the synthesis of a carrier protein, metallothionein, within 24 h. The cadmium–thionein complex is released from the liver into the blood and filtered in the glomerulus. It is reabsorbed by proximal tubules by pinocytosis and transferred to lysosomes. Catabolism of the cadmium–thionein complex with release of unbound cadmium into the cytoplasm is believed to contribute to the proximal tubule injury and to the continuous resynthesis of metallothionein and prolonged retention by the kidney. The biological half-life of cadmium–metallothionein is several days [20]. The complex is about 15 times more nephrotoxic than either cadmium alone or the zinc–thionein complex. Total body stores of cadmium in normal adults range from 10 to 30 mg, with roughly one-third present in the kidneys and another third in the liver. Under steady-state conditions, red cell cadmium concentration is 45–60 times that in the plasma.

Diagnosis

Although urinary cadmium excretion is normally less than 2 μg per day, after the critical concentration has been exceeded, urinary cadmium in excess of 10 μg per day is usual. Clinically important abnormalities of proximal tubular function are associated with urinary cadmium excretion in excess of 30 μg per day. The blood cadmium concentration is less reliable as an indicator of health effects. Nevertheless, blood levels greater than 1 μg/dl, as well as urine concentrations of over 10 μg/g of creatinine, are considered evidence of excessive exposure.

In vivo measurement of liver and kidney cadmium content by neutron capture gamma ray analysis has proved to be a safe, accurate, non-invasive and portable method for assessing cumulative cadmium retention in liver and kidney (Figure 58.4). Once renal failure is clinically apparent, the renal cortex begins to lose cadmium so that in renal failure neutron activation analysis shows falling, rather than increasing, cadmium content, even when exposure is continued. Concomitant with the reduction in renal cadmium, urinary cadmium excretion increases (generally exceeding 10 μg/l), but liver cadmium may continue to increase. Liver cadmium concentrations greater than about 60 μg/g may therefore indicate cadmium toxicity.

Differential diagnosis

Both lead and cadmium are associated with tubulointerstitial nephritis and hypertension, with chronic renal disease not becoming clinically apparent until years after the inception of exposure. The difference between lead and cadmium nephropathy is, nevertheless, striking. Both metals are retained in the body with biological half-lives of about 10 years, but, in contrast to lead, cadmium is stored in the liver and kidney cortex. Although both lead and cadmium accumulate in proximal tubule cells, lead is retained in intranuclear inclusion bodies, whereas

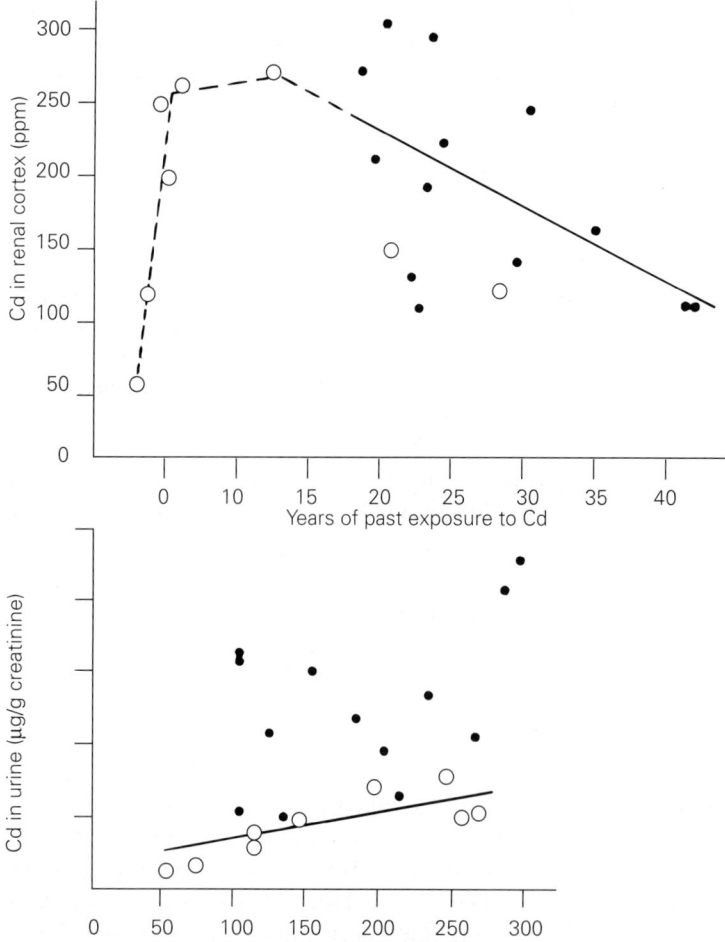

Figure 58.4 Renal cortical cadmium concentration determined by *in vivo* neutron activation analysis in cadmium workers without (open circles) and with (closed circles) increased urinary β_2-microglobulin excretion. Kidney cadmium increases with exposure up to the time at which urine cadmium concentration begins to rise and renal abnormalities appear following which renal cadmium content falls (from Roels *et al.*, 26:217–40, 1981, with permission).

cadmium is held in lysosomes. Cadmium nephropathy is characterized by tubular proteinuria. In cadmium nephropathy, proximal tubular dysfunction persists until renal failure supervenes whereas the Fanconi syndrome of acute lead poisoning is transient. The persistent hypercalciuria of cadmium nephropathy is responsible for the kidney stones and osteomalacia.

Management

Cadmium nephropathy cannot be reversed once tubulointerstitial disease has progressed sufficiently to produce clinical renal failure. There is evidence that even the early renal injury characterized by isolated tubular proteinuria may progress after termination of exposure [26, 27]. Chelation therapy with EDTA is ineffective after cadmium has accumulated in the kidney.

Mercury nephrotoxicity

Clinical manifestations

The principal symptoms following environmental or occupational exposure to mercury are neurological, although the disease of acrodynia is still occasionally encountered in infants following the application of mercurial ointments for skin rashes.

Diuretic effect

Certain organomercurials, including mercuhydrin and chlormerodrin, that are avidly accumulated in the proximal tubule and inhibit proximal tubular salt and water reabsorption were used as diuretics prior to the availability of furosemide and ethacrynic acid. Other organomercurials that accumulate within the proximal tubule, such as p-chloromercuribenzoate, have no diuretic effect themselves, but can block the action of mercurial diuretics [27].

Tubular proteinuria

Industrial effluents containing mercury undergo biotransformation in aquatic reservoirs and accumulate in freshwater and saltwater fish as methylmercury, which induces neurological disease and is teratogenic but does not cause renal failure [28]. Tubular proteinuria occurs after excessive methylmercury absorption, but total protein in the urine is trivial. Phenyl mercury is less neurotoxic than methylmercury but also induces tubular proteinuria [28]; long-term intake induces renal failure in experimental animals. Occupational exposure to elemental mercury for a decade with urine concentrations exceeding 50 µg/dl is associated with increased intestinal alkaline phosphatase excretion but little increase in other urinary proteins [29, 30]. There are no studies indicating that enzymuria from mercury exposure predicts the development of renal failure as it does for cadmium.

Acute tubular necrosis

Mercury bichloride ($HgCl_2$), given parenterally in doses of over 1 mg/kg regularly produces acute tubular necrosis in experimental animals. Incomplete recovery may leave calcified tubular remnants, persistent tubulointerstitial nephritis, and chronic renal insufficiency.

Immunologically mediated glomerulonephritis

The nephrotic syndrome

Case reports of the nephrotic syndrome (albuminuria >3.5 g/day) developing after occupational or therapeutic exposure to mercury suggest idiosyncratic allergic reactions in humans. Kidney biopsies frequently reveal immune complex deposits in glomerular basement membranes indicative of membranous glomerulonephritis. A specific antigen has not been identified within the immune complexes, and normal glomeruli or antiglomerular basement membrane antibody disease have also been reported.

The animal model

Multiple small subcutaneous doses of $HgCl_2$ have been shown to induce biphasic glomerulonephritis in rodents that is under precise genetic control [31]. Antiglomerular basement membrane antibodies are found after one week; these are replaced after two to three weeks by granular IgG deposits in the arteriolar walls and mesangium, as well as in the glomerular basement membrane simulating membranous glomerulonephritis. Immunoglobulin localization in the glomeruli is associated with heavy proteinuria, circulating immune complexes and polyclonal B-cell activation due to antiself Ia autoreactive T cells initiated by mercury inhibition of T-suppressor cell functions.

Pathophysiology

Inorganic mercury is selectively accumulated in the kidney, where it is retained with a half-life of about two months. The inorganic and organic mercurials bind avidly to sulfhydryl groups in circulating proteins, amino acids and intracellular glutathione, cysteine and metallothionein. Selective accumulation in the pars recta of proximal tubules is accomplished by absorptive endocytosis of mercury bound to amino acids or proteins in the tubular lumen. Mercury is released into the cytosol by intralysosomal enzymatic degradation [32]. It is less clear if mercury is transported in the secretory direction, entering proximal tubular cells from the peritubular surface. Excretion is primarily through bile in the feces. Neither elemental mercury (Hg^0) nor the mercurous salt (Hg_2Cl_2, calomel) produce sustained renal tubular injury despite induction of tubular proteinuria after more than 100 µg/l of mercury appears in the urine [33]. Biotransformation of inorganic mercury to mercuric ions is believed to account for renal accumulation.

Diagnosis

Blood mercury is a useful indicator of the body burden of methylmercury, but is inappropriate for biological monitoring of inorganic mercury. Although the presence of any mercury in urine is consistent with the diagnosis of mercury-induced nephrotic syndrome, variation in individual susceptibility appears to be critical in determining the renal response.

Management

The mercury-induced nephrotic syndrome disappears spontaneously after termination of exposure. British Antilewisite (BAL) is an effective chelating agent for mercury when administered at an initial dose of 5 mg/kg intramuscularly, followed by 2.5 mg/kg for 10 days.

Uranium, beryllium, arsenic and chromium

The injection of uranyl nitrate into experimental animals is a standard technique for the induction of acute tubular necrosis. Extensive experience during development of the atomic bomb made it clear that the kidney is the primary site of injury in acute uranium toxicity [34]. Hexavalent uranium readily enters the bloodstream after inhalation and is filtered at the glomerulus as a bicarbonate complex producing necrosis in the second and third parts of the proximal tubule. Catalase, alkaline phosphatase and β_2-M excretion are increased in uranium workers, but chronic renal failure induced by uranium has not been described in humans.

Beryllium induces the triad of pulmonary fibrosis, hypercalcemia, and hypercalciuria almost indistinguishable from sarcoidosis [35]. Although, the mechanism whereby beryllium increases blood calcium remains unclear, a reduction in circulating parathormone is believed to result from increased absorption and sensitivity to vitamin D. As with other types of hypercalcemia, interstitial nephritis may develop.

Chronic renal disease has not been reported to arise from industrial exposure to arsenic or chromium. Acute tubular necrosis, however, may result from arsine gas (AsH_3) in industrial accidents. Arsine, used as a poison gas in the First World War, is a colorless and odorless gas that is formed when arsenicals are mixed with acid. Inhalation produces massive hemolysis, hemoglobinuria, hematuria, jaundice and abdominal pain within a few hours and acute tubular necrosis within a few days. Hemodialysis is required, and exchange transfusion may be life saving by removing the arsenic–hemoglobin complex from the circulation. Incomplete recovery from acute tubular necrosis has resulted in persisting chronic tubulointerstitial nephritis in surviving victims [36]. Incomplete recovery from patchy cortical necrosis following consumption of 'moonshine' contaminated with arsenic has also been reported to result in persisting renal disease [37].

Acute oliguric renal failure and tubular necrosis occurs following massive absorption of hexavalent chromium as the chromate or dichromate. Renal failure is not produced by trivalent chromium. Minimal tubular proteinuria in the absence of reduced glomerular filtration has been reported in chromeplaters [38], but the implications of this finding for clinically important renal disease remain speculative. Like other heavy metals, chromium is selectively accumulated in the proximal tubule, but there is little evidence of chronic renal disease resulting from usual occupational exposure [39]. The finding of an odds ratio of 2.7 (confidence interval 1.2–6.3) for occupational exposure to chromium in a case control study of chronic renal failure warrants further evaluation of the association of environmental exposure to chromium with chronic renal disease [40].

Radiation injury to the kidneys

Clinical manifestations

Radiation injury to the kidneys has been recognized since the first decade of the twentieth century but did not become clinically important until the extensive use of radiotherapy for cancer in the 1950s. Radiation nephritis is characterized by the appearance of hypertension and progressive renal failure beginning more than six months after irradiation. Renal dysfunction follows administration of at least 2000 cGy (rad) over about five weeks to the kidneys or portion of a kidney. With appropriate shielding and field selection, radiation nephritis became uncommon following treatment of abdominal tumors but re-emerged as an important clinical entity with the widespread use of total body irradiation preparatory to bone marrow transplantation in the 1980s. About 25% of two-year survivors of bone marrow transplantation develop nephropathy [41]. The threshold of radiation dose to induce progressive renal failure is lower in children and those treated with nephrotoxic or radiomimetic drugs [42].

Luxton [43] described four phases of radiation nephritis: (1) 'Acute radiation nephritis' which is clinically evident at 6–12 months after radiation; (2) 'Chronic radiation nephritis'; (3) benign and (4) malignant hypertension which appear after 18 months. The apparent latent period may in part be attributable to the absence of clinical signs such as proteinuria in the early phases of interstitial nephritis. The most common presentation is hypertension with renal failure and disproportionate anemia. Hyperreninemic renovascular hypertension due

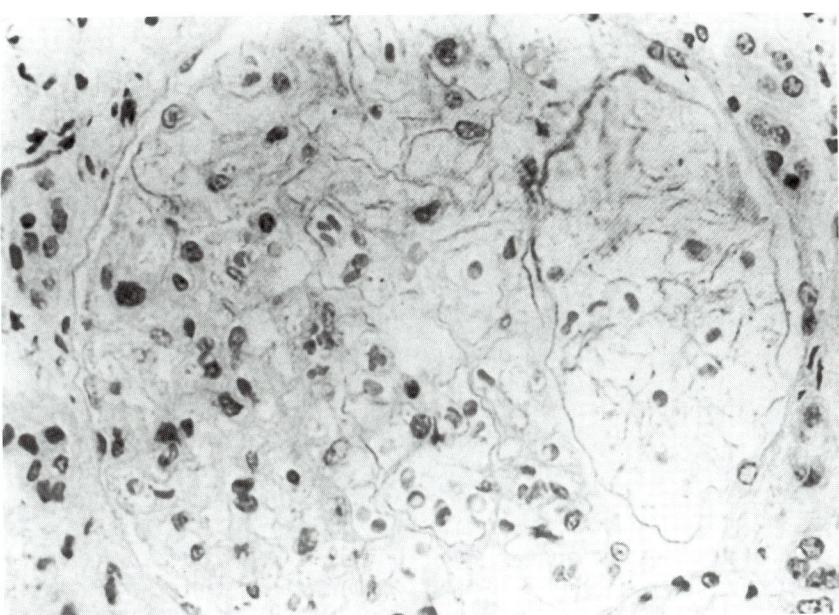

Figure 58.5 Renal biopsy from a bone marrow transplant recipient showing segmental mesangiolyisis and loss of endothelial cells (from ref. 40, with permission).

to unilateral radiation injury has been cured by nephrectomy [44]. In some patients, glomerular injury presenting as nephritis or nephrosis dominates the clinical picture [45]. Glomeruli tend to be enlarged and hypocellular. Microangiopathic hemolytic anemia has been described within six months of total body irradiation preparatory to bone marrow transplantation [46].

Pathology and pathogenesis

An understanding of the pathogenesis has been confounded by the presence of co-existing malignant disease, and the concurrent use of toxic pharmacologic agents. Nevertheless, there is considerable evidence that hypertension is associated with radiation nephritis and is renovascular in origin. The microvascular endothelium appears to be the target cell [47]. Thickening of the basement membrane, focal and segmental necrosis and microthrombi in glomerular capillaries are often observed in association with interstitial nephritis, microangiopathic hemolytic anemia and hypertension [48]. Mesangiolysis may be prominent (Figure 58.5).

Avioli *et al.* [49] observed a progressive fall in renal plasma flow and glomerular filtration rate within one month of radiotherapy and at renal doses of radiation below that generally believed to induce radiation nephritis. Micropuncture studies in rat have revealed reductions in glomerular filtration rate and renal plasma flow accompanied by an increase in total renal vascular resistance as early as 45 min after irradiation (1500 cGy) [50]. Reduction in renal function was not apparent two weeks later but reappeared after two months. Evidence of histologic

damage, increased proteinuria or overt renal failure was absent [50].

Differential diagnosis

Although the cause of radiation nephritis is obvious, differentiating among the potential mechanisms of renal injury in patients with abdominal tumors or marrow transplantation treated with nephrotoxic antibiotics and chemotherapeutic agents during the course of a complex illness is often impossible. When associated with renal failure, thrombocytopenia, and microangiopathic hemolytic anemia, the clinical picture resembles the hemolytic uremic syndrome.

Treatment

Studies in animals support the view that angiotensin converting enzyme inhibitors, particularly captopril, given early in the course of the disease can prevent the development of hypertension and slow the progression of renal failure [51].

Prevention

Radiation nephritis can usually be prevented in the treatment of abdominal tumors by shielding the kidneys.

Outcome

The clinical course of radiation nephritis is usually similar to that of slowly progressive interstitial nephritis.

References

1. Wedeen, R.P. (1984) *Poison in the Pot: The Legacy of Lead*. Southern Illinois University Press, Carbondale.

2. Goyer, R.A. and Wilson, M.H. (1975) Lead-induced inclusion bodies: results of ethylenediaminetetraacetic acid treatment. *Lab. Invest.*, **32**, 149–56.

3. Emmerson, B.T. (1973) Chronic lead nephropathy. *Kidney Int.*, **4**, 1.

4. Batuman, V., Maesaka, J.K., Haddad, B. *et al.* (1981) The role of lead in gout nephropathy. *N. Engl. J. Med.*, **304**, 520–3.

5. Batuman, V., Maesaka, J.K., Haddad, B. *et al.* (1983) Contribution of lead to hypertension with renal impairment. *N. Engl. J. Med.*, **309**, 17–21.

6. Behringer, D., Craswell, P., Mohl, C. *et al.* (1986) Urinary lead excretion in uremic patients. *Nephron*, **42**, 323–9.

7. Cardenas, A., Roels, H., Bernard, A.M. *et al.* (1993) Markers of early renal changes induced by industrial pollutants. I. Application to workers exposed to mercury vapour. *Br. J. Ind. Med.*, **50**, 17–27.

8. Endo, G., Horiguchi, S. and Kiyota, I. (1990) Urinary N-acetyl-β-D-glucosamindase activity in lead-exposed workers. *J. Appl. Toxicol.*, **10**, 235–8.

9. Nuyts, G., Roels, H.A., Verpooten, G.F. *et al.* (1991) Does lead play a role in the development of chronic renal disease? *Nephrol. Dial. Transplant.*, **6**, 307–15.

9a. Verberk, M.M., Willems, T.E.P., Verplanke, A.J.W., and De Wolff F.A., (1996) Environmental lead and renal effects in children. *Arch. of Environ. Health*, **51**, 83–7.

10. Pirkle, J.L., Schwartz, J., Landis, J.R. *et al.* (1985) The relationship between blood lead levels and blood pressure and its cardiovascular risk implications. *Am. J. Epidemiol.*, **121**, 246–58.

11. Schwartz, J. (1993) Beyond LOEL's p values, and vote counting: Methods for looking at the shapes and strengths of assciations. *Neurotoxicology*, **14**, 237–46.

11a. Sánchez-Fructuoso, I.A., Torralbo, A., Arroyo, M. *et al.* (1996) Occult lead intoxication as a cause of hypertension and renal failure. *Nephrol. Dial. Transplant.*, **11**, 1175–80.

12. Wedeen, R.P. (1988) Occupational and environmental renal diseases. *Curr . Nephrol.*, **11**, 65–106.

13. Campbell, B.C., Elliott, H.L., Meredith, P.A. *et al.* (1981) Lead exposure and renal failure: does renal insufficiency influence lead kinetics? *Toxicol. Lett.*, **9**, 121–4.

14. Staessen, J., Lauwerys, R.R., Ide, G. *et al.* (1994) Renal function is inversely correlated with lead exposure in the general population. *N. Engl. J. Med.*, **327**, 151–6.

15. Ashouri, O.S. (1985) Hyperkalemic distal tubular acidosis and selective aldosterone deficiency: combination in a patient with lead nephropathy. *Arch. Intern. Med.*, **145**, 1306–7.

16. Vander, A.J. (1988) Chronic effects of lead on the renin–angiotensin system. *Environ. Health Perspect.*, **78**, 77–84.

17. Van de Vyver, F.L., D'Haese, P.C., Visser, W.J. *et al.* (1988) Bone lead in dialysis patients. *Kidney Int.*, **33**, 601–7.

18. Rosen, J.F., Markovitz, M.E., Bijur, P.E. *et al.* (1989) L-line X-ray fluorescence of cortical bone lead compared with CaNa:2EDTA test in lead-toxic children: public health implications. *Proc. Natl. Acad. Sci. USA*, **86**, 685–9.

19. Wedeen, R.P., Ty, A., Favata, E.A. and Jones, K. (1995) Clinical application in *in vivo* tibial K–XRF for monitoring lead stores. *Arch. Environ. Health*, **50**, 355–61.

20. Friberg, L., Elinder, C.-G., Kjellstrom, T. and Nordberg, G.F. (eds) (1986) *Cadmium and Health: a Toxicological and Epidemiological Appraisal*. CRC Press, Boca Raton.

21. Jung, K., Pergande, M., Graubaum, H.J. *et al.* (1993) Urinary proteins and enzymes as early indicators of renal dysfunction in chronic exposure to cadmium. *Clin. Chem.*, **39**, 757–64.

22. Roels, H., Bernard, A.M., Cardenas, A. *et al.* (1993) Markers of early renal changes induced by industrial pollutants. III. Application to workers exposed to cadmium. *Br. J. Ind. Med.*, **50**, 37–48.

23. Jarup L. and Elinder C.G. (1993) Incidence of renal stones among cadmium exposed battery workers. *Br. J. Ind. Med.*, **50**, 598–602.

24. Thun, M.J., Osorio, A.M., Schober, S. *et al.* (1989) Nephropathy in cadmium workers – assessment of risk from airborne occupational cadmium exposure. *Br. J. Ind. Med.*, **46**, 689–97.

25. Kido, T., Nogawa, K., Ishizaki, M. *et al.* (1990) Long-term observation of serum creatinine and arterial blood pH in persons with cadmium-induced renal dysfunction. *Arch. Environ. Health*, **45**, 35–43.

26. Roels, H.A., Lauwerys, R.R., Buchet, J.P. *et al.* (1989) Health significance of cadmium-induced renal dysfunction: a five-year follow-up. *Br. J. Ind. Med.*, **46**, 755–64.

27. Wedeen, R.P. and Goldstein, M.H. (1963) Renal tubular localization of chlormerodrin labelled with mercury-203 by autoradiography. *Science*, **141**, 438–41.

28. Clarkson, T.W., Friberg, L., Norberg, G.F. and Sager, P.R. (eds) (1988) *Biological Monitoring of Heavy Metals*, Plenum Press, New York, pp. 199–247.

29. Cardenas, A., Roels, H., Bernard, A.M. *et al.* (1993) Markers of early renal changes induced by industrial pollutants. II. Application to workers exposed to lead. *Br. J. Ind. Med.*, **50**, 28–36.

30. Nuyts, G.D., Roels, H.A., Verpooten, G.F. *et al.* (1992) Intestinal-type alkaline phosphatase in urine as an indicator of mercury induced effects on the S3-segment of the proximal tubule. *Nephrol. Dial. Transpl.*, **7**, 225–9.

31. Goldman, M., Baran, D. and Druet, P. (1988) Polyclonal activation and experimental nephropathies. *Kidney Int.*, **34**, 141–50.

32. Zalups, R.K. and Lash, L.H. (1994) Advances in understanding the renal transport and toxicity of mercury. *J. Environ. Toxicol. Health*, **42**, 1–44.

33. Himeno, S., Pergande, M., Graubaum, H-J. *et al.* (1986) Urinary biochemical changes in workers exposed to mercury vapor. *Ind. Health*, **24**, 151–5.

34. Dounce, A.L. (1949) The mechanism of action of uranium compounds in the animal body, in *Pharmacology and Toxicology of Uranium Compounds* (eds C. Voegtlin and H.C. Hodge), McGraw-Hill, New York, pp. 951–91.

35. Stoeckle, J.D., Hardy, H.L., Weber, A.L. *et al.* (1969) Chronic beryllium disease. Long-term follow-up of sixty cases and selective review of the literature. *Am. J. Med.,* **46**, 545–61.

36. Muehrcke, R.C. and Pirani, C.L. (1968) Arsine-induced anuria. A correlative clinicopathological study with electron microscopic observations. *Ann. Intern. Med.,* **68**, 853–66.

37. Gerhardt, R.E., Crecelius, E.A. Hudson, J.B. (1990) Moonshine-related arsenic poisoning. *Arch. Intern. Med.,* **140**, 211.

38. Lindberg, E. and Vesterberg, O. (1983) Urinary excretion of proteins in chromeplaters, exchromeplaters and referents. *Scand. J. Work, Environ. Health,* **9**, 505–810.

39. Wedeen, R.P. and Qian, L. (1991) Chromium-induced kidney disease. *Environ. Health Perspect.,* **92**, 71–4.

40. Nutys, G.D., Van Viem, E., Thys, J. *et al.* (1995) New occupational risk factors for chronic renal failure. *Lancet,* **346**, 7–11.

41. Cohen, E.P., Lawton, C.A., Moulder, J.E. *et al.* (1993) Clinical course of late onset bone marrow transplant nephropathy. *Nephron,* **64**, 626–35.

42. Bergstein, J., Andreioli, S.P., Provisor, A.J. and Yum, M. (1986) Radiation nephritis following total-body irradiation and cyclophosphamide in preparation for bone marrow transplantation. *Transplantation,* **41**, 63–6.

43. Luxton, R.W. (1961) Radiation nephritis. A long term study of 54 patients. *Lancet,* **ii**, 1221–4.

44. Hulbert, W.C., Anderson, V.M., Ettinger, L.J. *et al.* (1988) Hyperreninemic hypertension secondary to radiation nephritis in a child. *Urology,* **26**, 153–6.

45. Jennette, J.C. and Ordonez, N.G. (1983) Radiation nephritis causing nephrotic syndrome. *Urology,* **22**, 631–4.

46. Guinan, E.C., Tarbell, N.J., Neimyer, C.M. *et al.* (1988) Intravascular hemolysis and renal insufficiency after bone marrow transplantation. *Blood,* **72**, 451–5.

47. Jaenke, R.S., Robbins, M.E.C., Bywaters, T. *et al.* (1993) Capillary endothelium. Target site for radiation injury. *Lab. Invest.,* **68**, 396–405.

48. Lawton, C.A., Cohen, E.P., Barber-Derus, S.W. *et al.* (1991) Later renal dysfunction in adult survivors of bone marrow transplantation. *Cancer,* **67**, 2795–800.

49. Avioli, L.V., Lazor, M.Z., Cotlove, E. *et al.* (1963) Early effects of radiation on renal function in man. *Am. J. Med.,* **34**, 329.

50. Teixeira, V. de P.C., Boim, M.A., Segreto, H.R. and Schor, N. (1994) Acute, subacute, and chronic x-ray effects on glomerular hemodynamics in rats. *Renal Failure,* **16**, 457–70.

51. Cohen, E.P., Moulder, J.E., Fish, B.L. and Hill, P. (1994) Prophylaxis of experimental bone marrow transplantation. *J. Lab. Clin. Med.,* **124**, 371–80.

59

Balkan nephropathy

K.C. Siamopoulos

Epidemiology

Balkan nephropathy (BN) is an endemic familial, chronic, tubulointerstitial disease which occurs in some restricted areas of Bulgaria, Yugoslavia and Romania along the tributaries of the Danube river. These areas are at an altitude of 150–500 m above sea level and generally have high humidity and rainfall. The disease has been described among the inhabitants of the endemic areas and after a latent period in emigrants from these affected areas. It is of note that within the endemic area not all villages are affected. The prevalence in the affected villages has been estimated to be 3% in Bulgaria, 0.5–4.0% in Yugoslavia, and from 0.5 to more than 10% in Romania. Despite the emphasis on the familial character of the disease in the older and more recent literature, there are many unaffected households living in close relationship to affected families [1, 2].

Clinical manifestations and laboratory characteristics

BN is a chronic, slowly progressive disease which usually appears in the third and fourth decade of life; affected individuals reach end-stage renal failure in the fifth to sixth decade. Overt or latent kidney disease has not been documented in children from endemic settlements.

Early symptoms or findings suggestive of the disease are not evident. The features of polyuria, polydipsia and nocturia are the result of the decreased concentrating capacity of the kidneys due to tubulointerstitial damage, BN could also be characterized as a salt-losing nephritis. Defects in urinary acidification as well as in ammonia and uric acid excretion have also been described. The findings from the urinary sediment examination are not helpful. A few red and white blood cells per high power field with some granular casts and uric acid crystals may be present. Although overt proteinuria is a feature of advanced disease, the presence of β_2-microglobulin, a marker of tubular dysfunction, has been well documented [3, 4]. α_1-microglobulin, which is another low-molecular-weight protein, has also been shown to be a reliable marker of disease onset [5]. Urinary cultures are usually sterile.

Hypertension is rare except in patients with advanced renal failure in whom a volume-dependent high blood pressure may be present. A normocytic, normochromic anemia may be detected in the early stages of the disease and becomes more severe with the progression of renal dysfunction. Apart from anemia, however, no other extrarenal manifestations, either systemic or organ specific are evident in the early stages.

Etiology and pathophysiology

Despite extensive work, the etiology of BN remains unknown. Since the first description of the disease in the

Nephrology, Edited by Rex L. Jamison and Robert Wilkinson.
Published in 1997 by Chapman & Hall, London. ISBN 0 412 60930 4

1950s, various etiologic factors have been implicated. Although lead has been found to be 10-fold higher in concentrations in the flour used in endemic settlements compared to that used in non-endemic areas, urinary excretion of lead after treatment with chelating agents was not increased or different from that of a control population. Similarly, a causal relationship between cadmium, silica or coal deposits and BN is lacking. The possibility that zinc or selenium deficiency could play a role in the etiology of the disease has not been confirmed. Attempts to isolate bacteria or viruses as etiological factors have been unsuccessful [5, 6].

It appears that there is a very close relationship between ochratoxin A, a mycotoxin occurring in plant products, and BN [7]. Ochratoxin A is nephrotoxic in all animal species tested and was detected in 9.8–13.5% of serum samples from inhabitants of an endemic area compared to 3.6% of serum samples from control areas. Lymphocytes of patients with BN have numerical and structural chromosomal aberrations and it was recently observed that ochratoxin A induced similar chromosomal aberrations in cultured human peripheral lymphocytes *in vitro* [8]. It has been suggested that these chromosomal aberrations may reflect the etiopathogenesis of urinary tract malignant tumors frequently seen in subjects with BN [9–13].

Aristolochic acid, a mutagenic and nephrotoxic alkaloid found in the plant *Aristolochia*, has been proposed as a cause of BN, but this hypothesis has not been confirmed. It has recently been hypothesized that aristolochic acid might be responsible for the nephropathy associated with Chinese herbs, which is similar to BN [12].

Studies from Bulgaria and Romania suggest that a genetic background with chromosomal anomalies is critical to the development of BN and as it has recently been published these chromosomal anomalies are found even in healthy relatives of BN patients, who were born in non-endemic areas [13, 14]. Other studies from Yugoslavia however, point to the presence of environmental rather than genetic factors [15]. Most investigators agree that, although predisposition to BN is inherited polygenetically, manifestations of the genotype are modified by environmental factors.

The role of immune mechanisms in the development of BN is not clear. However, the limited immunohistological findings in renal biopsies obtained in early stages of the disease suggest that immune mechanisms do not play an important pathogenetic role in BN. The role of β_2-microglobulin and other low-molecular-weight proteins in the progression of BN remains to be established.

Pathology and pathogenesis

The genesis of BN lesions remains a matter of speculation. Autopsies of patients with end-stage renal failure from BN showed shrunken, smooth surfaced kidneys with severe atrophy and sclerotic lesions primarily affecting the superficial cortex. Kidney biopsies performed on BN patients with either normal renal function or mild to moderate renal failure, revealed the predominant pathology is that of a chronic, non-destructive, multifocal interstitial nephropathy found more commonly in the superficial cortex [5] (Figure 59.1). The sclerotic and atrophic lesions involve all nephron components regardless of the disease stage. A recent study has shown an inverse correlation between the progression of histomorphologic involvement of the kidney and the EDTA clearance. Tubulointerstitial changes, such as interstitial sclerosis and tubular atrophy, were the most frequent findings with an incidence of 98% and 96% in the biopsies, respectively. Global glomerular sclerosis with microvascular hyalinosis/sclerosis was found in 80%. Renal vascular changes were present in 80% of the biopsies with hyalinosis being the most frequent alteration. By contrast, interstitial infiltration, mainly by mononuclear cells, was found in only 38%.

Immunostaining is negative or insignificant. Slight focal deposits of C_3, IgM and less often of IgG are found in the mesangium in about 30% of patients. In the extraglomerular vessels IgM deposits were found in 17% of cases and deposition of C_3 in 89%. The latter finding, however, was also frequent in control biopsies. Focal and segmental granular or linear C_3 deposition along the tubular basement membrane was noted in 15% of cases.

Electron-microscopic studies of renal tissue revealed abnormalities within cells and between cells (Figure 59.2). Thickening of the tubular basement membrane with splitting of the lamina densa and widening of the intercellular junction were frequent. Proximal tubules were more commonly affected than other tubule segments. Glomerular and vascular lesions were also detected by electron microscopy. Thickening and wrinkling of the glomerular basement membrane and fragmentation of the internal elastic lamina of the interlobular arteries with increased electron density, suggesting calcium deposition, were occasionally observed. The reported electron-microscopic findings, however, are not considered to be pathognomonic.

Diagnosis and differential diagnosis

The insidious onset and slow development of renal insufficiency with minor renal abnormalities and the absence of systemic manifestations make diagnosis and its differentiation from other chronic interstitial nephropathies difficult. Living in an endemic area is a prerequisite for the diagnosis of BN whereas the familial nature of the disease is also an indication. However, it has been suggested that there could be isolated cases of BN outside the endemic areas, but no such cases have been described in other Balkan countries or even in other areas of the countries in question. Nevertheless, BN should be suspected in

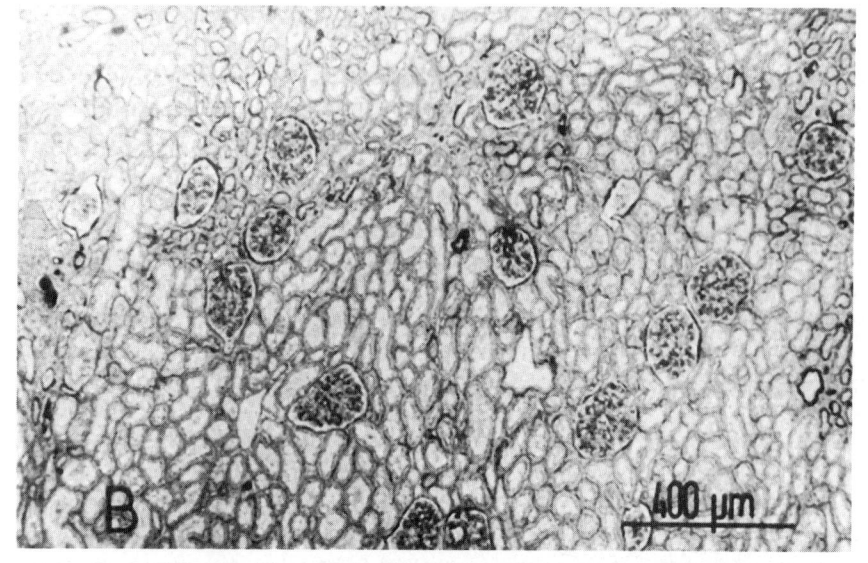

a

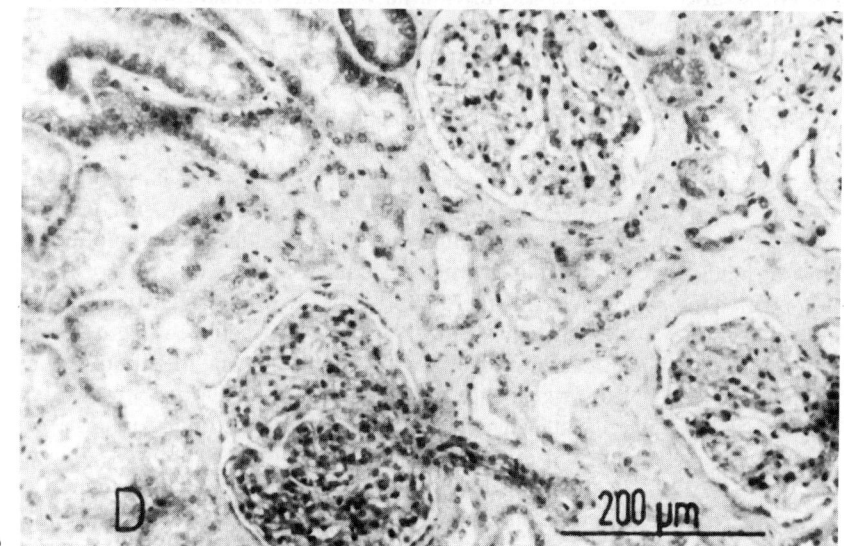

b

Figure 59.1 Renal biopsy appearances on light microscopy in patients with Balkan nephropathy. (a) Scattered areas of interstitial sclerosis with tubular atrophy and arteriolar and arterial hyalinosis mostly in the superficial cortex in a patient aged 40 years with glomerular filtration rate (GFR) 109 ml/min. (b) Interstitial sclerosis with little interstitial cellular infiltration, flattening of tubular cells of atrophic tubules. Hypertrophy of residual glomeruli and tubules in a patient aged 54 years with GFR 50 ml/min. (Reproduced, with permission, from Ferluga, D., Hvala, A., Vizjak, A. *et al.* (1991) *Kidney Int.*, **40**, S57–S67.)

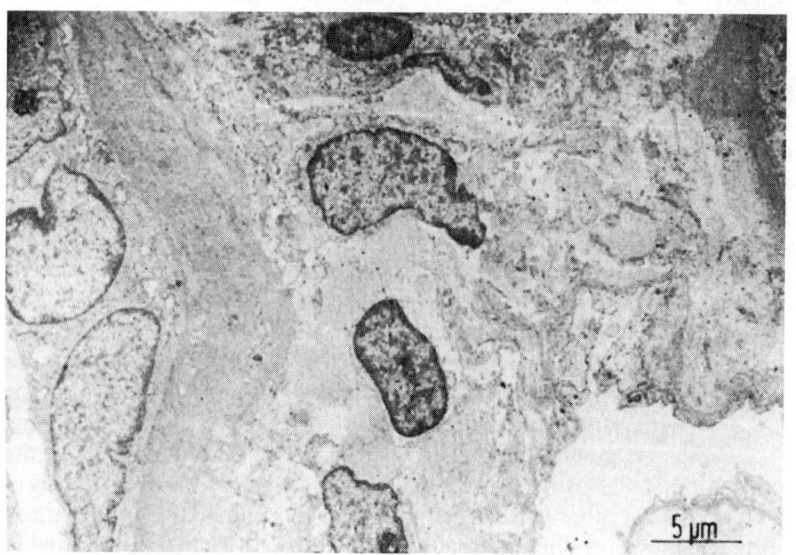

Figure 59.2 Electron miscroscopical appearance of renal biopsy in a patient age 47 years with Balkan nephropathy with glomerular filtration rate 30 ml/min. Flattening and absence of specific differentiation of the epithelial cells of atrophic tubules, irregular thickening and splitting of tubular basement membrane and mild thickening of the basement membrane of peritubular capillaries. (Reproduced, with permission, from Ferluga, D., Hvala, A., Vizjak, A. *et al.* (1991) *Kidney Int.*, **40**, S57–S67.)

any case with clinicolaboratory evidence of interstitial nephritis in the absence of other known etiologic factors [10]. 'It has recently been published that the serum activity of angiotensin-converting enzyme (ACE) was significantly increased in patients with BN even in those without arterial hypertension [16]. Accordingly the use of ACE inhibitors could slow down the progression of kidney damage.'

As in any case of acute or chronic nephropathy, ultrasonography and urinalysis should be the first examinations to evaluate the kidney and urinary tract. Kidney size varies from normal to severely reduced, depending on the stage of the disease. However, a preliminary observation in a recent study from Yugoslavia shows that kidney size is reduced even in BN patients with normal renal function. The renal outline is usually smooth and normal pelvicalyceal and ureteral morphology are common findings, except in cases of concomitant urothelial tumors. For purposes of differential diagnosis, a renal biopsy should be performed in selected cases. Urinary β_2-microglobulin excretion was increased not only in BN patients but also in some healthy members of nephropathic families, so it has been suggested that urinary β_2-microglobulin may serve as a marker of the early tubular damage in BN. However, this finding lacks the specificity required for screening purposes outside endemic areas.

Treatment

There is no specific treatment for BN patients. Conservative management including general measures that may slow the progression of renal failure and the detection and treatment of potentially reversible factors which could aggravate renal failure are important. Patients with end-stage kidney disease are treated by dialysis and kidney transplantation. Recurrence of endemic nephropathy in the grafted kidney has not been observed.

Outcome

BN is a very slowly progressive disease. It is clinically manifested during the fifth or sixth decade of life and the calculated incidence of deaths from or with BN in a susceptible population is 3.3/1000 persons/year. It has recently been reported that in endemic areas a positive test for urinary β_2-microglobulin is associated with ten times greater relative risk of developing BN when compared to the control population with no positive test after 15 years of follow-up. The finding that some individuals who had a repeatedly positive β_2-microglobulin test remained not only clinically unaffected but later had a negative test, after 14 years of follow-up, however, supports previous observations that non-progression and reversal of persistent azotemia occur in a few patients [5].

Prevention

Since the etiology of the disease and the pathogenetic mechanisms are unknown, prevention of BN is not yet possible. It has been suggested that migration of affected families outside the endemic regions could contribute to a lower incidence of the disease.

References

1. Polenakovic, M.H. and Stefanovic, V. (1991) Balkan nephropathy, in *Oxford Textbook of Clinical Nephrology* (eds Cameron, Davison, Grunfeld et al.), Oxford University Press, Oxford, pp. 857–66.
2. Wolstenholme, G.E.W. and Knight, J. (eds) (1967) *The Balkan Nephropathy* (Ciba Foundation Study Group no 33), Little, Brown, Boston.
3. Hall, P.W., Piscator M., Vasiljevic, M. and Popovic, N. (1972) Renal function studies in individuals with the tubular proteinuria of endemic Balkan nephropathy. Q. J. Med., **41**, 385–93.
4. Karlsson, F.A. and Lenkei, R. (1977) Urinary excretion of albumin and β_2-microglobulin in a population from an area where Balkan nephropathy is endemic. Scand. J. Clin. Lab. Invest., **37**, 169–73.
5. Hall, P.W. and Batuman, V. (eds) (1991) Balkan endemic nephropathy. Kidney Int., Suppl. 34.
6. Apostolov, K., Spasic, P. and Bojanic, N. (1975) Evidence of a viral etiology in endemic (Balkan) nephropathy. Lancet, **ii**, 1271–3.
7. Krogh, P., Hald, B., Plestina, R. et al. (1977) Balkan (endemic) nephropathy and foodborn ochratoxin A: preliminary results of a survey of foodstuffs. Acta Pathol. Microbiol. Scand., **85**, 238–40.
8. Manolova, Y., Manolov, G., Parvanova, L. et al. (1990) Induction of characteristic chromosomal aberrations, particularly X-trisomy, in cultured human lymphocytes treated by ochratoxin A, a mycotoxin implicated in Balkan endemic nephropathy. Mutat. Res., **231**, 143–9.
9. Puchlev, A., Popov, N., Astrug, A. et al. (eds) (1965) International Symposium on Endemic Nephropathy, Bulgarian Academy of Sciences Press, Sofia.
10. Stefanovic, V. and Polenakovic, M.H. (1991) Balkan nephropathy: kidney disease beyond the Balkans? Am. J. Nephrol., **11**, 1–11.
11. Strahinjic, S. and Stefanovic, V. (eds) (1979) Endemic (Balkan) nephropathy. Proc. 4th Symp. Endemic (Balkan) Nephropathy, University Press, Nis.
12. Cosyns, J.P., Jadoul, M., Squifflet, J.P. et al. (1994) Chinese herbs nephropathy: a clue to Balkan endemic nephropathy? Kidney Int., **45**, 1680–8.

13. Tonceva, D., Dimitrov, T. and Tzoneva, M. (1988) Cytogenetic studies in Balkan endemic nephropathy. *Nephron*, **48**, 18–21.

14. Toncheva, D. and Dimitrov, T. (1996) Genetic predisposition to Balkan endemic nephropathy. *Nephron*, **72**, 564–9.

15. Ceovic, S., Hrabar, A. and Radonic, M. (1985) An etiological approach to Balkan endemic nephropathy based on the investigation of two genetically different populations. *Nephron*, **40**, 175–9.

16. Huskic, J., Kulenovic, H. and Culo, F. (1996) Serum angiotensin converting enzyme activity in patients with endemic nephropathy. *Nephron*, **74**, 120–4.

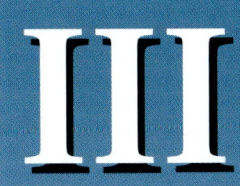

Diseases of the Kidney and Their Treatment

Section 6
Other Diseases

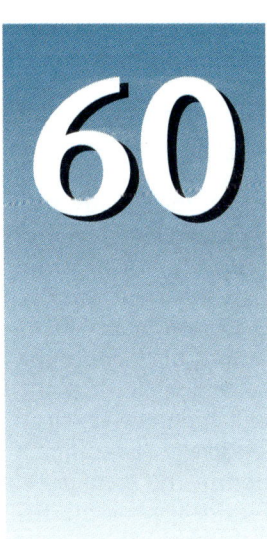

60

Urinary tract infection

M. Sussman and P.E. Gower

Introduction

Infections of the urinary tract are among the most common community-acquired infections, ranking in incidence with respiratory and gastrointestinal infections. In their life-time about 20% of women experience a urinary tract infection and 3% have more than one episode per year. The age-related incidence of community acquired urinary tract infection in the England and Wales is shown in Figure 60.1.

Though urinary tract infections cause a great deal of suffering and inconvenience, they do not usually represent a threat to life and in otherwise healthy adults they cause no permanent damage. In infancy and childhood, however, when urinary tract infection is frequently associated with vesicoureteric reflux, there is a serious risk of kidney damage. In up to 40% of pregnant women covert urinary tract infection may become acute, often in the form of acute pyelonephritis and this may be associated with an increased rate of prematurity, but this is still the subject of controversy. The increased incidence of urinary tract infection in elderly men and women is related to structural and functional changes associated with aging. The organisms responsible for urinary tract infection are also the commonest cause of septicemia in patients whose resistance is compromised by other conditions.

The urinary tract is normally sterile because direct access by bacteria is only by way of the urethra and the system is washed out by the continuous production of urine, which is regularly evacuated. Circumstantial evidence suggests that bacteria frequently find their way into the lower urinary tract and that the vast majority of urinary tract infections are ascending. The mechanisms are not entirely clear but epidemiological evidence from urinary tract infection in females suggests that entry may be passive, as during sexual intercourse. In uncircumcized males bacteria may accumulate under the prepuce and so find their way into the urinary tract.

The bacteria that have a predilection for the urinary tract posses virulence factors that allow them to colonize and damage the uroepithelium and the kidney. The combination of host susceptibility factors and bacterial virulence factors constitutes urinary tract infections classical examples of host–bacterial interactions.

Uncommonly, urinary tract infection may result from spread by way of the blood stream (hematogenous). This is sometimes termed descending urinary tract infection and the infecting organism settles in the kidney, where an abscess (renal carbuncle) may result, as in septicemia due to *Staphylococcus aureus*. Whether organisms localized in this way in the kidney appear in the urine will depend on the severity of the infection, but this is unusual. There is no reliable evidence that infection reaches the urinary tract by lymphatic spread.

Nephrology, Edited by Rex L. Jamison and Robert Wilkinson.
Published in 1997 by Chapman & Hall, London. ISBN 0 412 60930 4

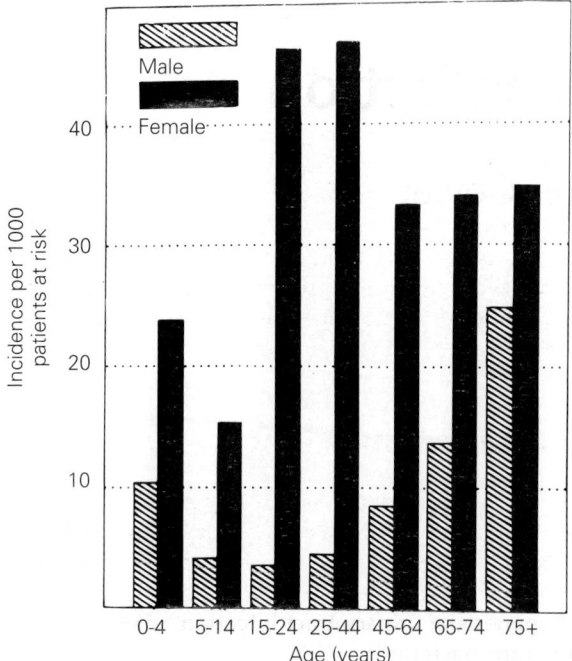

Figure 60.1 The incidence of cystitis and urinary tract infection in general practice. (After Morbidity Statistics in General Practice. Third National Study 1981–82. HMSO, 1986, By kind permission of Bayer Diagnostics.)

Susceptibility and defense

Host defenses

The defenses of the urinary tract against infection consist of general non-specific resistance mechanisms and immunity mechanisms that are specifically directed against individual pathogens. The main evidence for these two types of defense remains circumstantial but some important general conclusions of clinical significance can be drawn.

There is a reciprocal relationship between non-specific resistance and susceptibility. When resistance mechanisms are disturbed or fail, susceptibility ensues but the relationship is not direct. In many patients with urinary tract infection, the susceptibility factors cannot be identified and often, when known susceptibility factors prevail, infection does not occur. This strongly suggests that the mechanisms involved are not understood.

Structural and functional resistance mechanisms

The urethra is the first barrier to entry of infection into the urinary tract. This is consistent with the greater frequency of urinary tract infection in women, who have a short urethra, and the fact that urinary tract infection in

women is often related to sexual intercourse, during which it is thought that the infecting organisms may be 'massaged' into the bladder.

The constant flow of urine through the urinary tract and its regular and complete voiding are central mechanisms of resistance against infection [1, 2]. Any of a wide range of structural and functional abnormalities that interfere with urine flow or voiding are associated with an increased risk of infection. For example, bladder outflow obstruction may lead to incomplete voiding. If the resulting residual urine becomes infected, spontaneous clearance of infection by 'wash out' is less likely. The common occurrence of urinary tract infection in the presence of outflow obstruction is persuasive evidence for the frequent entry of bacteria into the urinary tract. Infection of residual urine is commonly asymptomatic but, as has long been recognized, represents a serious risk during diagnostic or other instrumentation, particularly if carried out against an obstruction. Passage of instruments may cause sufficient tissue damage to allow infected urine to enter the circulation to cause a bacteremia with resulting 'catheter fever' [3], and occasionally metastatic infection.

Urine may also be trapped by foreign bodies, such as calculi or indwelling catheters, which may then become infected. Conversely, if such conditions are relieved, the clearance of infection is often dramatic.

Ureteral peristalsis is part of the wash-out system and interference with it, as in vesicoureteric reflux can be expected to increase susceptibility to urinary tract infection. It is, therefore, significant that certain uropathogens produce substances that interfere with ureteral peristalsis [4, 5].

Vesicoureteric reflux is common in childhood and is significantly associated with a risk of infection. In this case small volumes of urine pass retrograde from the bladder into the ureter and even into the renal collecting duct system during voiding [6], later to return to the bladder at the end of voiding. Operationally this constitutes the equivalent of residual urine, which maintains the infection in the system. With maturation, vesicoureteric reflux often spontaneously resolves and with it the risk of infection.

Urine

Urine is an excellent bacterial growth medium [7] because it contains glucose and a full range of other bacterial nutrients. Other constituents, however, such as urea and hydrogen ions, may serve as relative growth inhibitors [8]. Thus, urine of high osmolarity and low pH is less supportive of bacterial growth than dilute urine. It should be emphasized, however, that the growth-promoting properties of urine probably always outweigh its inhibitory characteristics.

Throughout pregnancy, urine pH is such as to support the growth of Gram-negative urinary pathogens [7]. In diabetes, glycosuria supports the growth of larger bacterial populations than usual and this may affect the severity of such infections [9].

Urine also contains Tamm–Horsfall glycoprotein, the polysaccharide moiety of which includes mannose. Bacteria bearing type 1 fimbriae bind to the glycoprotein and tend to be washed out of the urinary tract (see below).

Mucosal resistance

After complete bladder emptying, the remaining film of contaminated urine would be expected to maintain infection even against the effect of wash-out [2]. That this is not so suggests that the bladder has effective antibacterial mechanisms. The bladder mucosa is covered by a layer of mucin, which tends to prevent bacterial attachment and experimental observations have shown that the bladder mucosa possesses antibacterial activity but the mechanism is not understood [10, 11].

The kidney

The renal medulla is far more susceptible to infection than the cortex. Thus, the dose of bacteria required to initiate infection by direct inoculation is some 10^4-fold higher in the cortex than in the medulla [12]. This may be related to the physiological state of the medulla with its low blood flow, high osmolality, low oxygen tension and high ammonia content, all of which tend to inhibit resistance and immunity [13].

Immunity

Urine contains IgG and secretory IgA (sIgA) [14]. A significant proportion of urinary sIgA originates in the urethra where it probably constitutes a partial barrier to the entry of infection. Urine also contains antibodies against bacterial O-antigens, K-antigens and adhesins and these may inhibit the adherence of bacteria to the uroepithelium.

The tissues of the urinary tract respond to infection with the expected local and systemic type-specific immune responses. However, the extent to which these play a protective role is probably small. Thus, in lower urinary tract infection the immune response is usually slight because of its superficial nature. In experimental renal infection, type-specific antibodies are, however, detectable in the urine before they appear in the circulation [15], which suggests that they are produced locally in the kidney. In acute pyelonephritis there is a systemic immune response in the course of which antibodies to bacterial surface components appear in the circulation; IgM antibodies appear first followed by IgG antibodies. In the urine sIgA appears first followed by IgG, which probably originates from the serum.

The cellular responses to infection in the urinary tract have been studied in experimental systems. In ascending infections, T-cell infiltration occurs in the kidney and appears to be related to the degree of chronicity [16] but bladder infiltration is transient. Later, suppressor T-cells appear in the kidney and this may lead to persistence of bacteria in the kidneys [17]. If cyclophosphamide is administered during such infections and an antibiotic is also given, the antibacterial effect is greater than if antibiotic is given alone. This effect may be due to modulation of suppressor T-cell activity and the resulting enhancement of helper T-cell activity. However, patients with T-cell deficiencies and increased susceptibility to opportunistic infections do not appear to have an increased susceptibility to renal infections.

Bacteria and the urinary tract

The introitus of adult women is colonized by a commensal flora that consists mainly of *Lactobacillus* spp., *Staphylococcus epidermidis*, corynebacteria and streptococci, but before the menarche and after the menopause, *Bacteroides* spp. predominate [18]. In women susceptible to urinary tract infection, enterobacteria are commonly present [19] and it is possible that *Escherichia coli* adheres better to the vaginal cells of girls and women with recurrent urinary tract infection [20].

In males the prepucial mucosa may become colonized with *Proteus* spp. [21].

Urinary pathogens

The origin of the vast majority of organisms involved in urinary tract infection is to be found in the fecal flora and the commonest organism responsible is *E. coli*. Thus, the serotypes of *E. coli* associated with urinary tract infection usually belong to a restricted range of O-serotypes identical to those present in the feces [22]. About 90% of covert urinary tract infection are due to *E. coli*, whereas in community- and hospital-acquired urinary tract infection the prevalence is about 64% and 47% respectively [23]. When septicemia results from community- and hospital-acquired urinary tract infection the prevalence of *E. coli* is 64% and 45%, respectively [24, 25], which supports the clinical observation that urinary tract infection is the commonest source of septicemia. As a general rule, the more 'complicated' the circumstances in which urinary tract infection arises, the lower the probability that *E. coli* is the cause.

Apart from *E. coli*, a variety of other Gram-negative organisms, that also originate from the fecal flora, may cause urinary tract infection. These include, *Klebsiella*, *Enterobacter* and *Pseudomonas aeruginosa* among others. Less frequently, urinary tract infection is due to Gram-positive organisms, including *Enterococcus faecalis* and *Streptococcus agalactiae* that also originate from the fecal flora. *Staphylococcus saprophyticus* is particularly associated with urinary tract infection in young sexually active women [26].

Fastidious organisms have been isolated on special culture media from the urine of women with the urethral syndrome [27] but their significance is uncertain. Similarly, anerobic bacteria are rarely of significance in urinary tract infection [28].

Urinary tract infection due to *E. coli* is less common in men than in women, because in males most urinary tract infection occurs in early life in the presence of congenital abnormalities, whereas in the elderly it is commonly associated with outflow obstruction. Particularly in young boys, infection may be due to *Proteus mirabilis*, and occasionally other species of *Proteus*, that originate from the prepucial sac [29]. These organisms have a powerful urease that releases ammonia, which raises the urine pH and leads to precipitation of phosphates with possible renal stone formation. Other uropathogens, including *Klebsiella*, *Pseudomonas* and *S. saprophyticus* are also urease-positive, but are not particularly associated with stone formation.

Catheterization and instrumentation of the urinary tract are associated with a high risk of sporadic infection. This is due to introduction of any of a wide range of exogenous organisms, not necessarily of fecal origin, including more unusual organisms such as *Gardnerella vaginalis*, *Serratia*, *Acinetobacter calcoaceticus* and *Candida albicans*. The same is true of indwelling devices, such as urinary drains. If such drains are open, epidemic infection with 'hospital' organisms, particularly *Ps. aeruginosa* is the rule. Infection with fungi such as *Aspergillus* spp. may also occur in patients with indwelling catheters.

Virulence mechanisms of uropathogens

In order to overcome the non-specific host resistance mechanisms, urinary pathogens possess a number of powerful and specific virulence factors. These are best understood in the case of *E. coli*, but similar mechanisms probably operate in the case of other Gram-negative organisms. Little is known of the virulence factors of Gram-positive organisms in the urinary tract.

Adherence

Colonization of the urinary tract by *E. coli* depends mainly on the presence of fimbriae. These are filamentous appendages, 5–7 nm in diameter and distinct from flagella (Figure 60.2), that adhere to a wide variety of cells, including erythrocytes [30] but adhesion may occasionally be due to non-fimbrial adhesins.

Fimbrial adhesins are classified on the basis of the cell receptors to which they attach. Adherence of type 1 fimbriae is due to binding to mannose present in cell surface macromolecules. Since this binding can be inhibited by D-mannose or mannosides, it and type 1 fimbriae are referred to as mannose-sensitive. Mannose-sensitive fimbriae also agglutinate erythrocytes and this hemagglutination is also mannose-sensitive [31]. The binding of mannose-sensitive fimbriae to the mannose-containing Tamm–Horsfall glycoprotein present in urine may be a defense against invasion at an early stage [32].

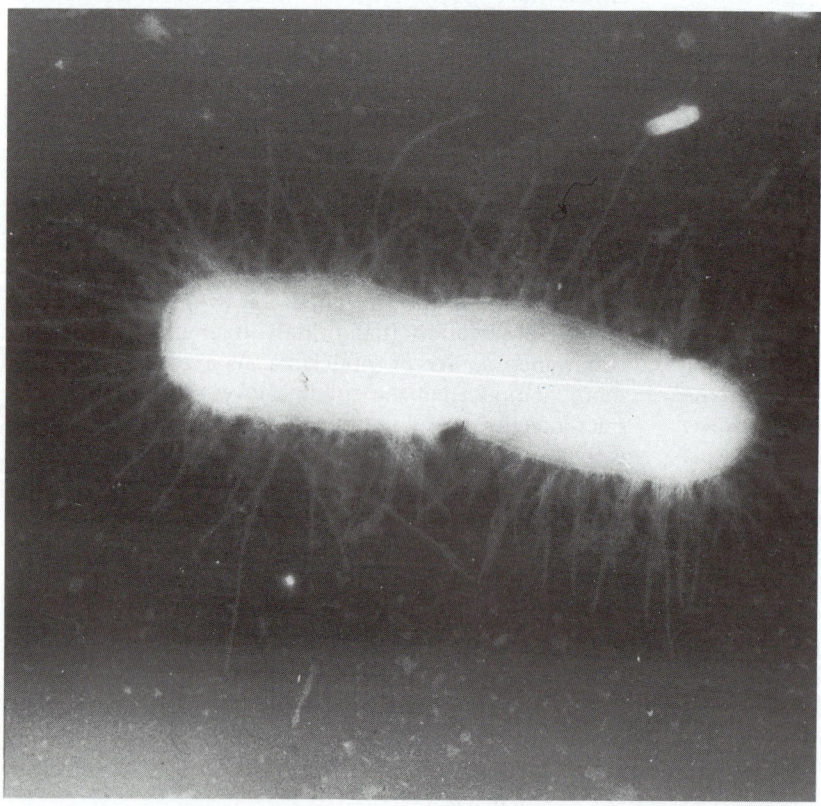

Figure 60.2 Electron micrograph of *Escherichia coli* negatively stained with phosphotungstate. Fimbriae are seen as a bristle-like fringe. (Negative print)

Adherence and hemagglutination by another large and heterogeneous group of fimbriae is not inhibited by mannose and such fimbriae are collectively referred to as mannose-resistant (MR). The best studied of this group of fimbriae (P fimbriae) bind to the receptor structure α-D-gal(–>)-β-D-gal that is present in P blood group glycolipid antigen [33]. P fimbriae are particularly associated with the urinary tract infection of childhood. MR fimbriae other than P fimbriae have occasionally collectively been referred to as X fimbriae. The receptors of some of these have been identified as glycophorin A and B of the M and S blood group antigens, the glycolipid Forssmann antigen and the glycoprotein Dr antigen [34].

The production of fimbriae is under the control of a complex genetic on–off switch that gives rise to phase variation. Current evidence points to the possibility that the controls that operate the switch may be common to MS and P fimbriae.

Though in parallel with other staphylococci *Staph. saprophyticus* does not possess fimbriae, it causes hemagglutination that is inhibited by *N*-acetylglucosamine-containing saccharides which are thought to represent the receptor in the urinary tract [34].

Lipopolysaccharide O-antigens

These are the classical endotoxins that are integral constituents of the Gram-negative cell envelope. Molecules of lipopolysaccharide (LPS) consist of polysaccharide side chains towards the surface of the organism that endow the organisms with their O-antigenic specificity, a polysaccharide core and lipid A, which is buried in the cell envelope.

Some evidence suggests that LPS is a virulence factor in acute urinary tract infection. Thus, rough strains of *E. coli* that have partially or completely lost their serotype-specific agglutinability are more common in covert bacteriuria than in symptomatic infection. As a result, in covert bacteriuria, which may be of long standing, the serotype concordance with fecal *E. coli* may be absent. In experimental models LPS induces shedding of bladder epithelial cells [35] and it plays a role in the induction of inflammation. LPS also interferes with ureteric peristalsis [4, 5] and causes renal damage by granulocyte activation [36].

Capsular K-antigens

Capsular K-antigens are acid polysaccharides with antiphagocytic activity present on the surface of *E. coli* and other organism [37]. As in the case of O-antigens, only a limited range of K-antigenic types of *E. coli* is associated with urinary tract infection. The presence of K-antigens is particularly associated with invasiveness and they appear to be of particular significance in urinary tract infection associated with renal invasion and this has been confirmed in experimental pyelonephritis.

Serum sensitivity

Depending on their surface components, strains of *E. coli* are more or less sensitive to the bactericidal action of serum that is due to the presence of antibody and complement. Thus, organisms with complete O-antigenic side chains, particularly if K-antigen is also present, are relatively resistant to serum and such strains are associated with acute urinary tract infection. In the absence of K-antigen, particularly if the polysaccharide side-chains are short or absent, *E. coli* is very serum-sensitive and such strains are common in covert infections [38]. Resistance to the effect of serum is probably not of great significance in lower urinary tract infection, but it may play a role in invasive infections.

Iron scavenging

Iron is an essential nutrient of bacteria and its acquisition is a central problem for all pathogens. Since free iron is extremely toxic for biological systems, it is retained and transported by powerful iron-binding proteins including transferrins and ferritins. Pathogens have highly specific and effective methods for obtaining iron from bound sources in their environment [39].

Urine contains sufficient free iron to support bacterial growth. It is, therefore, particularly during tissue invasion that organisms must exercise means of iron acquisition. For this purpose they produce low-molecular-weight substances called siderophores as part of a high-affinity iron transport system. *E. coli* and other Gram-negative uropathogens secrete enterochelin when iron is in short supply. The formation constant of the iron chelate of enterochelin is 10^{52}, so affording organisms the ability to acquire iron *in vivo* [40]. The chelate is taken up by the cells and the iron is released intracellularly. Some strains of *E. coli* responsible for urinary tract infection carry a plasmid (pColV) that codes for the production of aerobactin, another iron-binding compound, which forms a complex with transferrin and mobilizes bound iron. Aerobactin-producing strains of *E. coli* appear to be particularly associated with septicemia.

The long-suspected relationship between hemolysin production and pathogenicity [41] is now well-established. *E. coli* produces a secreted α-hemolysin and a cell-bound β-hemolysin [42]. A large proportion of *E. coli* strains isolated from patients with urinary tract infection produce α-hemolysin [43] and, in animal experimental infections, such strains are more virulent than non-hemolytic strains [44].

Pathogenesis of urinary tract infection

The pathogenesis of urinary tract infection can be conceived of taking place in several stages. These are colonization of the urinary tract, invasion and the production of tissue damage.

It is well-established that colonization of the urinary tract depends on the ability of uropathogens to adhere to epithelium by means of fimbrial adhesins. Though a number of other virulence factors have been identified, the precise mechanism by which they operate to give rise to various types and severity of urinary tract infection is not clear. There are, however, tantalizing clues that point to some general mechanisms.

Women with recurrent urinary tract infection tend to be periurethrally colonized with Gram-negative bacilli [45]. The presence of type 1 fimbriae on all strains of *E. coli* does not suggest that these play an important role in established urinary tract infection but they may play a part in the earliest stages of colonization, such as of the introitus and terminal urethra. Moreover, they tend not to be produced within the urinary tract [31]. However, persuasive evidence supports the view that MR fimbriae are involved in colonization of the bladder and kidney. Thus, P-fimbriae are produced in the urinary tract in acute urinary tract infection and by most strains of *E. coli* isolated from children with acute pyelonephritis [46]. The same is true of adults with pyelonephritis but less so of those with lower urinary tract infection.

Supporting evidence for the importance of MR fimbriae in acute urinary tract infection comes from pregnant women with acute urinary tract infections. They are six times more likely to be infected with a strain of *E. coli* bearing MR fimbriae than they are if the infection is covert. In addition, the presence of MR fimbriae on *E. coli* isolated from pregnant women with urinary tract infection correlates significantly with their past history of urinary tract infection [47].

A model for the colonization of the urinary tract in urinary tract infection suggests that colonization by *E. coli* is maintained in the colon by the binding of type 1 fimbriae to colonic mucus. If fecal organisms bearing only type 1 fimbriae enter the urinary tract, they will bind to urinary mucus and be removed during voiding. If, however, MR fimbriae are present, colonization of the urinary tract may take place [32].

Little is known of the mechanisms exploited by *E. coli* in invasive infections of the kidney and infections that lead to septicemia. Such invasive strains usually have K-antigens and O-antigens, are serum resistant and have active iron scavenging mechanisms, all of which would tend to favour survival in the face of host systemic resistance and immunity mechanisms.

Significant bacteriuria

The most significant advance in the laboratory diagnosis of urinary tract infection was the introduction of quantitative bacteriology. This was based on the observation by Kass [48] that, in the absence of symptoms, the presence of more than 10^5 colony forming units (cfu) per ml of urine indicated, with a probability of about 80%, that the

organisms were present in bladder urine rather than as mere contaminants. Repetition of the same observation in the same individual raises the probability to some 95%. The condition so identified became known as asymptomatic significant bacteriuria but is better termed covert bacteriuria because it is in reality part of a natural history of infection that includes symptomatic episodes [49].

The original definition of significant bacteriuria was derived from observations of asymptomatic women and specimens of total urine, rather than midstream urine. The organisms isolated were almost exclusively *E. coli*. It is hardly surprising, therefore, that it has been shown that in midstream urine collected from women with acute lower urinary tract infection the presence of as few as 10^2 cfu/ml correlates with bladder bacteriuria [50]. Because of the lower risk of contamination when urine is collected from males, a count of greater than 10^3 cfu/ml defines bacteriuria [51].

Laboratory diagnosis

The 'gold standard' for the bacteriological diagnosis of urinary tract infection depends on direct colony counting in which a measured volume of a suitable dilution of the urine is plated on a suitable medium. Texts on practical medical microbiology should be consulted for details of these techniques. The major disadvantage of these methods is that they are time-consuming and expensive. This has led to the development of a variety of semi-quantitative, chemical, enzymatic and automated methods for the diagnosis of bacteriuria, some of which have been applied for screening purposes.

Specimen collection

The single most important factor that can lead to the misinterpretation of urine bacteriology is contamination of the specimen during collection. The use of catheters for the collection of urine to avoid contamination is, however, to be frowned upon because of the high risk, up to about 6%, of initiating urinary tract infection in this way.

Collection presents few problems with men, from whom midstream urine can be collected with nothing more than retraction of the foreskin, but even this may be unnecessary [51]. In the case of women careful attention must paid to collection technique. The labia should be carefully separated and the area washed with plain water or a non-irritant soap that does not contain antibacterial agents. A midstream specimen should then be collected in a sterile or clean dish and transferred aseptically into a sterile universal container for transmission to the laboratory. Alternatively, the specimen can be collected directly into a suitably wide-necked screw-capped container. Collection of uncontaminated urine from infants and children presents problems. Specimens collected in urine bags are unsuitable because they are always contaminated. Suprapubic aspiration is, however, a safe and justifiable means for collecting urine from children.

Unless examination of specimens can be carried out without delay, they must be refrigerated at 4°C, but not frozen. If this is not possible specimens can be preserved with borate at a final concentration of 1.8%, but such specimens are not suitable for the detection of leukocytes with reagent strips.

Microscopy

For purposes of diagnosis of infection urine microscopy is mainly directed to detecting the presence of increased numbers of leukocytes (pyuria). For most purposes a wet film of urine is examined with the high power (×40) dry objective of the microscope. The volume of urine examined in one high-power field can be calculated from the volume of urine placed on the slide and the area of the cover slip. Significantly more than 10^4 leukocytes/ml is regarded as pyuria. Possible sources of confusion are tubular epithelial cells and leukocytes of vaginal origin.

Semiquantitative methods

Quantitative urine culture, as we have noted, is too time-consuming for routine use. It has, therefore, become conventional to use semiquantitative methods for the detection of bacteriuria. Many such methods are available [52] but only those that are widely used will be considered here. It is important that such methods give a reliable colony count, that the cultured organisms and contamination are easily recognized.

Small measured volumes of urine can be spread over the surface of suitable culture media with standard loops. These are available as disposable items and reliable viable counts can be obtained in this way.

A particularly useful method is the dipslide [53], which is attached to the lid of a standard universal container. The plastic slide carries a culture medium on each side, most commonly MacConkey and CLED (Cysteine Lactose Electrolyte-Deficient) media [54]. The former allows the multiplication of organisms capable of growth on bile salt media, whereas the latter supports the growth of all common urinary pathogens, allows their clear colonial differentiation and prevents the swarming of *Proteus*. Dipslides are particularly valuable for transport purposes, because the colony counts are 'frozen' when refrigeration is not available. After incubation, colony counts on dipslides can be determined by reference to standard regression plots.

In the filter paper strip method, a standardized strip of filter paper that absorbs a known volume of urine is dipped in the specimen and is then pressed on the surface of the culture medium. The density of growth after incubation is proportional to the colony count.

Rapid and screening methods

Chemical changes in urine due to bacterial growth can be exploited to provide a measure of the presence of bacteriuria. Thus, the growth of enterobacteria in urine leads to the reduction of urinary nitrate to nitrite, which can be identified by means of the diazo (Gries) reaction on reagent strips. Ideally, a first morning specimen of urine should be tested to ensure adequate nitrate reduction in the bladder overnight. A disadvantage of this method is that some uropathogens, such as *Pseudomonas* and *Enterococcus*, do not reduce nitrate.

Various urinalysis reagent strips ('dipsticks') with impregnated pads for the determination of a variety of urine constituents are commercially available. Such reagent strips can be used to screen for nitrite and the presence of leukocytes. When both tests are negative, the negative predictive value for bacteriuria is more than 90% and screening can be very reliable for the immediate discarding of urine specimens that do not require further examination. However, the low positive predictive value of these tests makes screening tests unsuitable for diagnostic purposes. They may, however, be useful for 'self follow-up' by patients with a long-term or recurrent problem of urinary tract infection.

Other methods

Many physical and biological methods have been proposed for the rapid automated detection of bacteriuria and some of these have come to the market. These include methods based on photometry, bioluminescence, electrical impedance, flow cytometry and fluorescence. None has, however, been widely accepted, mainly because of their expense and partly because of their unreliability.

Interpretation of urine bacteriology

When urine colony counts are carried out for screening purposes in asymptomatic individuals, for example in pregnancy, the standard 'Kass criteria' apply. If more than 10^5 cfu/ml are found, significant bacteriuria is present with a probability of about 80%. If greater precision is necessary, the test should be repeated. Strictly speaking, in the case of organisms that tend to grow in aggregates, such as *Staphylococcus* spp. and *Streptococcus* spp., significant bacteriuria is present at counts lower than 10^5 cfu/ml. Fortunately, this is not troublesome because under most circumstances uropathogens are present in numbers that far exceed the breakpoint of significance. This may, however, not be the case in the earliest stages of infection when counts have yet to reach their maximum.

Since the Kass criteria were defined in asymptomatic populations, it is hardly surprising that, in the presence

Table 60.1 Criteria for the diagnosis of significant bacteriuria in different types of patients [91]

	Colony forming units/ml[a]	
	Coliforms	Other organisms
Symptomatic		
female	$\geq 10^2$	$\geq 10^5$
male	$\geq 10^3$	$\geq 10^3$
Covert		
female[b]	$\geq 10^5$	$\geq 10^5$
male[b]	$\geq 10^5$	$\geq 10^5$
Catheterized patient	$\geq 10^2$	$\geq 10^2$
Suprapubic aspirate	any number	

[a] Specimens and midstream unless otherwise indicated.
[b] In two consecutive specimens.

particularly of acute symptoms, a diagnosis of bacteriuria does not require the presence of 10^5 cfu/ml [50]. The criteria, in terms of organism count, for the diagnosis of significant bacteriuria in different types of patient are presented in Table 60.1.

Urinary tract infections

Covert infections

Covert bacteriuria [55], which is also termed 'asymptomatic bacteriuria', is defined as the presence of microorganisms in urine in the absence of symptoms. It is defined as any number of organisms present in urine obtained by suprapubic bladder aspiration or more than 10^5 cfu/ml ($>10^9$ cfu/l) in a midstream urine, usually in pure culture.

Screening and treatment of populations with covert bacteriuria is the subject of considerable debate, but two groups deserve attention; children under the age of two and pregnant women.

Children

The prevalence of covert bacteriuria in neonates is less than 1% which rises to 3% in premature infants. Infections at this age may be difficult to diagnose and the incidence of urological abnormalities is high. In selected instances, neonates with covert infections should be investigated by ultrasound and cystography. Reflux nephropathy is an important cause of renal failure in children and to a lesser extent in adults, and although no screening test for reflux is available, urinary infection in neonates has been used as an indication to investigate for renal abnormalities including reflux.

Screening for covert bacteriuria in children over the age of five years is not cost-effective. There is no evidence

that treatment of children at this age with covert infections affects subsequent infection rates or the development of renal scars [56].

Pregnancy

The prevalence of covert bacteriuria in pregnancy is between 2.5 and 15%. In the absence of treatment, acute pyelonephritis may occur in 25–40% of such patients who develop a symptomatic infection. The evidence that bacteriuria is related to the development of premature labor and fetal malformations is conflicting, but screening for and treatment of covert bacteriuria in the first trimester of pregnancy is recommended. Approximately 15% of patients with covert bacteriuria during pregnancy have some underlying renal abnormality, particularly if it proves difficult to eliminate the bacteriuria with treatment [57].

Screening other population groups

There is no evidence that screening for bacteriuria in women who are not pregnant or men is cost-effective. However, the coincidental discovery of a covert infection in a man justifies further investigation, since such a finding is significantly associated with renal abnormalities, including stones and obstruction.

The prevalence of covert bacteriuria rises sharply in men and women after the age of 65, but there is very little evidence that the identification or treatment of elderly people with covert urinary tract infections affects subsequent symptoms, renal damage or mortality [55].

Covert bacteriuria in special categories

The following guidelines are suggested for the treatment of patients in special categories who have a covert urinary tract infection.

1   Patients who should be treated include those due for catheterization, instrumentation or operations on the urinary tract and who have known congenital or acquired renal abnormalities, for example, polycystic kidney disease, stones or obstruction.
2   Patients for whom treatment is reasonable but unsubstantiated include those with diabetes, valvular heart disease and immunosuppressed patients, including those after renal transplantation.
3   Patients for whom treatment is controversial include those with short-term indwelling catheters and ileal conduits.
4   Patients with long-term catheters should not be treated with antibiotics unless they are symptomatic.

Cystitis and acute pyelonephritis

The clinical differentiation between cystitis (acute bacterial infection confined to the bladder) and acute pyelonephritis (acute bacterial infection above the bladder involving one or both kidneys) is fairly straightforward [58], but tests used to define the site of infection have shown that symptoms are a rather poor guide to the site of infection. However, localization tests are not routinely used in clinical practice and at present there is merit in continuing to differentiate acute symptomatic urinary infections into cystitis and acute pyelonephritis on the basis of clinical findings and the result of urine culture.

Cystitis

This is defined as the presence of symptoms of a lower urinary tract infection, dysuria, frequency, backache and occasionally loin pain without tenderness, and an infected urine. Frequency of micturition often leads to bacterial counts lower than 10^5 cfu/ml, which are nevertheless considered to be significant [58]. Dysuria is almost always present and hematuria is found in up to 60% of patients. The commonest organisms found include *E. coli*, coliforms and staphylococci.

Cystitis tends to occur in women of child-bearing age, is often related to intercourse and is almost entirely treated in the community. Although single-dose treatment with ampicillin, trimethoprim, or cotrimoxazole has been recommended [59], relapses, especially after ampicillin treatment, are high and a three-day course of these antibiotics or a quinolone antimicrobial agent is now recommended [60]. Further investigations are rarely required and should be confined to patients with recurrent infections, macroscopic hematuria, or for patients with unusual organisms such as *Proteus* or *Pseudomonas* spp., where an underlying abnormality of the urinary tract, such as a stone or tumor of the bladder or kidney, are more likely.

Many women suffer recurrent bacterial cystitis and may be helped by simple methods such as postintercourse micturition, increased fluid intake and scrupulous perineal hygiene. Despite these measures some patients continue to complain of recurrent attacks and a dose of trimethoprim (100 mg) or nitrofurantoin (50 mg) nightly or postintercourse for three to six months has been shown to be very effective in preventing recurrences of lower tract infections.

Non-bacterial cystitis

About 50% of women with symptoms of cystitis do not have a conventional positive urinary bacterial culture and have been labeled as suffering from 'urethral syndrome'. Possible causes include anerobic or fastidious organisms [61], though this has been disputed [62], *Chlamydia trachomatis* [63], tuberculosis and other bladder pathologies such as stones or tumors. Careful physical examination and investigation should be undertaken in all women with persistent or recurrent symptoms of urinary infec-

tion before they are labeled as functional or hypochondriacal.

Acute pyelonephritis

Classically, patients with acute pyelonephritis present with loin pain, fever and an infected urine. There are undoubtedly atypical presentations, including absence of loin pain or fever, or pain referred to the chest or anterior abdomen that mimics, for example, acute appendicitis. Investigation should include blood cultures, renal function tests, ultrasound of the abdomen and, where appropriate, a pregnancy test. Treatment depends on the organisms present and the patient. Most patients with uncomplicated acute pyelonephritis respond to a two-week oral course of ampicillin, cotrimoxazole or a quinolone [58]. Short-term treatment is not recommended. Toxic patients or patients with complicated infections, especially if acquired in hospital, often require intravenous antibiotics, such as an aminoglycoside, a second or third generation cephalosporin or a quinolone. Treatment should be continued for 14 days.

The prognosis of patients with a normal urinary tract after an attack of acute pyelonephritis is considered to be excellent. Intravenous pyelography has demonstrated swelling of the affected kidney at the time of the attack of acute pyelonephritis [64] but the affected kidney usually returns to normal size. CT scans have shown that in a few patients minor scars develop in the kidney after an attack of acute pyelonephritis [65]. This has been confirmed in a study in which atrophy of kidneys was found in two of the 55 patients examined [66]. Prospective trials have, however, provided very little evidence to support the notion that such scars are associated with progressive glomerulosclerosis or hypertension [67].

Urinary tract infection in the elderly

Symptomatic and covert urinary infections are common in elderly people [68]. There is considerable controversy about the importance of infection in this age group and, in particular, the effect of bacteriuria on morbidity, hypertension, renal failure and mortality.

Urinary infections in the elderly are associated with underlying urinary tract problems, including prostatic obstruction, stones and malignancies in men, prolapse and malignancies in women, and indwelling catheters in both. These patients may present with lower or upper urinary tract symptoms, but incontinence, fever or general ill health may predominate. Symptomatic patients should be treated with short-term antibiotics, since long-term treatment is associated with a high risk of development and spread of resistant organisms. Patients with covert infections should be treated only to cover urological procedures.

Covert bacteriuria is common in elderly patients and ranges from 6 to 34% in men and 17 to 50% in women

have been reported [55]. It has been shown that there is no relation between bacteriuria and worsening renal function, hypertension, mortality and symptoms. Institutionalized or hospitalized patients seem at particular risk of developing resistant organisms if covert bacteriuria is treated. Data on the treatment of ambulatory elderly non-hospitalized patients with covert infections are controversial and further studies are needed to determine whether this group would benefit from treatment.

Urinary infections in men

Apart from the very young or very old, urinary infections are less common in men [51] as compared with women, but they are more likely to be associated with urological abnormalities at any age. The three groups that require special attention include neonates, men with acute symptomatic infections and the elderly.

Neonatal urinary infection

The incidence of urinary tract abnormalities is higher in males as compared with female infants. These abnormalities are associated with a higher incidence of both symptomatic and covert infections. All urinary infections in this age group should therefore be investigated by ultrasound of the urinary tract and, in selected cases, with urography and/or cystography. Treatment is determined by the causative organism, bearing in mind that there is a higher incidence of more unusual organisms such as *Proteus* spp. in uncircumcized boys [69].

Symptomatic infections in men aged 15–55 years

Covert bacteriuria is uncommon in this age group. Symptoms suggestive of a urinary infection should prompt a thorough search for the cause, including urethritis due to *Neisseria gonorrhoeae* or *Chlamydia trachomatis*. The usual Gram-negative or Gram-positive infections are uncommon and may be associated with urinary tract abnormalities, such as urethral strictures, prostatic hypertrophy, renal calculi and malignancy of the bladder or kidneys. In the absence of such abnormalities urinary infections in men may be associated with prostatitis, a condition that is difficult to diagnose and manage [70]. The diagnosis may be made clinically (backache, fever, dysuria, prostatic tenderness and an infected urine), but ideally the semen should be cultured. Significant bacteriuria in symptomatic men may be indicated by a urinary bacterial count of greater than 10^3 cfu/ml (rather than $>10^5$ cfu/ml). Treatment of prostatitis is best undertaken with a tetracycline, erythromycin, cotrimoxazole or a quinolone antimicrobial agent that achieves adequate prostatic tissue levels as compared with the concentrations achieved by beta-lactam antibiotics. Men with urinary tract infections, particularly recurrent infections, should be investigated at least with a plain radiograph or ultrasound with or without cystoscopy, since the prevalence of abnormalities is high.

Covert infections in elderly men

The prevalence of bacteriuria in men rises with age and may be as high as 50% in patients in residential homes. Bacteriuria is associated with catheterization and instrumentation of the urinary tract and prostatic hypertrophy. Treatment should be reserved only for symptomatic patients or patients undergoing urinary tract surgery.

Urinary tract infections in patients with spinal cord injury

Patients with spinal cord injuries [57] have severe bladder dysfunction that requires careful assessment and management. Transection of the spinal cord above T12 results in an upper motor neuron type of bladder dysfunction with initial spinal shock in which the bladder is areflexic, followed by a hyperreflexic type of voiding dysfunction. Lower motor neuron lesions that involve the cauda equina or pelvic plexus result in detrusor instability with a poor stream and interrupted micturition, including occasional incontinence.

Bladder catheterization is the mainstay of treatment in patients with upper motor neuron lesions. Permanent indwelling catheters result in severe lower and upper urinary tract infection that almost inevitably results in progressive renal failure and amyloidosis. For the last 30 years spinal cord injury patients have been managed by intermittent catheterization resulting in a much lower incidence of infection and renal failure. Various surgical procedures such as bladder neck and prostatic resection are recommended for selected patients.

Despite a significant reduction in the infection rate with intermittent catheterization, urinary infections continue to be a major problem in spinal cord injury patients. A variety of long-term prophylactic antibiotics has been tried, including nitrofurantoin [72], Methanamine [73] and cotrimoxazole [74]. The results of these trials have disclosed a reduction in asymptomatic bacteriuria and in the case of cotrimoxazole, a reduction in symptomatic infections but breakthrough bacteriuria and the development of bacterial resistance continue to be a significant problem in some patients.

Patients with cauda equina lesions are less likely to require intermittent catheterization. Incontinence may be helped in men by condom collecting devices, but in women a urethral catheter or urinary diversion may be the only choice of treatment.

Urinary tract infections after renal transplantation

Urinary tract infections are among the commonest infections after renal transplantation [75], with an incidence of approximately 20% (Chapter ••). Factors that predispose to such infections include pre-existing native renal abnormalities, such as reflux nephropathy or stones, diabetes, wound infections, stents and the presence of indwelling urinary catheters. Patients are often asymptomatic but classical bladder symptoms, fever, graft pain and tenderness may be present. Culture of urine and blood is mandatory for any patient with a post-transplant fever, when reduction in graft function may resemble rejection or cyclosporin toxicity. Preventive measures include occasional bilateral nephrectomy in patients with reflux nephropathy, careful evaluation of bladder function, and removal of bladder catheters as soon as possible after transplantation. Treatment of suspected urinary infection should be started promptly and continued for at least two weeks. Shorter courses of antibiotics may be given to patients who develop infection three months after transplantation. Prophylactic antibiotics may be given if recurrent symptomatic infections occur.

Nosocomial infections

Hospital-acquired infections [76] are an important cause of patient morbidity and mortality. A prospective study of 15 rural Wisconsin hospitals [77] showed an average incidence of 1.6 infections per 100 discharges, the majority secondary to urinary tract infections in surgical, gynecological, and medical practice predominantly in older patients. *E. coli* predominated in these infections, but *Pseudomonas*, enterococci, *Proteus* spp. represented 27% of the isolates. Catheter-associated infections were the commonest hospital-acquired infection in clinical practice, despite improvement in catheter design, materials and closed drainage systems. Various techniques introduced to reduce the incidence of catheter-associated infections including antibiotic impregnation, bladder irrigation and prophylactic antibiotics have proved only partly successful [78].

Short courses of antibiotics in susceptible patients undergoing catheterization or instrumentation are recommended, and some surgeons also give prophylactic antibiotics to patients undergoing prostatic surgery, biopsy, cystoscopy, renal surgery, especially in the presence of stones [79]. The urine of all patients undergoing lithotripsy should be screened before treatment and prophylactic antibiotics given when infection is found.

Renal calculi and urinary tract infections (Chapter 62)

Renal calculi are associated with urinary tract infections but the precise prevalence is unknown. Certain organisms, for example *Proteus* spp. are associated with stone formation by release of urease and a subsequent deposition of triple phosphate (calcium, ammonium and magnesium phosphate stones, struvite) in an alkaline urine, whereas other stones act as an irritant in the formation

of urinary tract infection. Struvite stones characteristically enlarge and develop into staghorn calculi which are notoriously difficult to treat even with modern methods of limited surgery and lithotripsy. Long-term antibiotics may be used to prevent further stone recurrences.

Xanthogranulomatous pyelonrephritis

This term is used to describe a particular histological appearance of foamy histiocytes and a chronic interstitial nephritis in patients with low-grade renal infection, usually in the presence of stones or obstruction [80]. The disease tends to affect middle-aged females who present with fever, loin pain, weight loss and malaise, often with a mass in the loin and a non-functioning kidney that contains stones. The illness may be confused with malignancy and a CT scan is the investigation of choice to help to distinguish xanthogranulomatous pyelonephritis from hypernephroma. A urinary infection with *E. coli* or *Proteus* spp. is usually present. Occasionally patients present with a perinephric abscess. The disease is usually unilateral and is cured by nephrectomy. The mechanism by which the kidney responds to infection in this way is obscure.

Emphysematous pyelonephritis

This results from the production of gas within and around the kidney by Gram-negative bacilli. The condition is rare and occurs mainly in patients with diabetes who present with loin pain, fever, a palpable mass and it is complicated by papillary necrosis and arterial insufficiency. Plain radiograph and non-contrast CT scans show gas in the renal area. Treatment is usually with a combination of surgery and antibiotics.

Tuberculosis of the urinary tract

Incidence of urinary tract tuberculosis

The reported incidence of all form of tuberculosis in England and Wales fell between 1979 and 1988 in both whites and Asians from the Indian subcontinent, though the latter had an incidence 25 times higher than the white population [81]. Compared with white patients, Asian patients had a higher incidence of non-pulmonary tuberculosis especially of the lymph nodes. In contrast, the incidence of genitourinary tuberculosis was much higher in the white, as compared with the Asian population, for reasons that are unknown. There are no recorded details of the incidence, age or sex differences for urinary tract tuberculosis alone but the numbers must be small, because the overall reported incidence of genitourinary tuberculosis is only 3% of the total, amounting to about 150 patients in England and Wales in 1988.

Since 1988 the notification of tuberculosis has been increasing slightly but, in contrast to the USA, the increase is apparently not due to increasing numbers of patients with HIV infection. Since many cases of urinary tract tuberculosis are secondary to pulmonary tuberculosis and may develop several years later, constant vigilance is required to detect any increase in urinary tuberculosis.

Clinical features and investigation

Tuberculosis of the urinary tract often presents as an insidious disease with low-grade fever, general ill health, weight loss, occasional loin pain or rarely dysuria, frequency or hematuria. It may be associated with past or present pulmonary tuberculosis; examination is often negative. Investigation may show sterile pyuria, but *Mycobacterium tuberculosis* is rarely observed in direct smears. The erythrocyte sedimentation rate and C-reactive protein are usually raised. Diagnosis has been established by direct aspiration of the kidney under ultrasound [82]. Plain radiograph may show calcification within the kidney, and a variety of abnormalities are seen on an intravenous urography, including papillary erosions and stricture formation of the pelviureteric junction or ureters. Infection may spread to the bladder resulting in bladder wall contraction with reduced bladder capacity.

Renal tuberculosis may present as an interstitial nephritis with renal failure confirmed by renal biopsy [83]. In men, direct invasion by the tubercle bacilli of the seminal vesicles, epidydimis or testis may result in tuberculous epidydimitis or orchitis.

Treatment of urinary tract tuberculosis

Treatment of tuberculosis of the urinary tract follows the general principles of treatment of tuberculosis elsewhere in the body. In uncomplicated cases, triple therapy with rifampicin, isoniazid and pyrizinamide is given for the first two months and, assuming that the organism is sensitive, rifampicin and isoniazid (with pyridoxine) is continued for a further four months. Treatment should be continued for a further three to six months in men, especially those with tuberculous epidydimitis, or where caseation of the urinary tract is suspected. Surgery is rarely indicated and should be undertaken in patients with non-functioning kidneys or if there is severe obstruction.

Virus infections and renal disease

HIV infection and the kidney

A wide variety of renal diseases has been associated with infections due to the HIV virus [84], including electrolyte disorders, acute renal failure, various glomerular abnormalities and tubular interstitial disease. Certain clinicopathological correlations predominate, including glomerular disease (HIV nephropathy and immune complex disease) and interstitial nephritis.

HIV nephropathy

This disorder is characterized by heavy proteinuria and progressive renal failure, predominantly in American black patients, many of whom acquire HIV infection through intravenous drug abuse. White patients and homosexuals are less often affected. The glomeruli show histological features of focal glomerulosclerosis, but other histological lesions, including mesangial hyperplasia, glomerular collapse and various tubular changes, have been described. There is often an abundant interstitial lymphocytic infiltration. Immunofluorescence shows mesangial IgM, C3, and C1 and electron microscopy shows foot process effacement, wrinkled basement membranes, mesangial dense deposits and tubuloreticular inclusions. Some of these features are found in heroin nephropathy, but certain distinctive features may be present, e.g. global glomerulosclerosis, prominent epithelial cells, tubular microcysts, focal tubular degeneration, tubuloreticular inclusions in the endothelium and infiltrating leukocytes. The pathogenesis is unknown and treatment with azidothymidine is often ineffective.

Besides focal glomerulosclerosis minimal change glomerulonephritis and immune complex glomerulonephritis have also been described [85]. The immune complex disease includes exudative endocapillary glomerulonephritis, mesangial IgA proliferative glomerulonephritis and appearances suggestive of systemic lupus erythematosus. Immune complex glomerulonephritis, seen more frequently in homosexual Caucasians, has been ascribed to opportunistic infections or polyclonal B-cell activation.

Interstitial nephritis

Interstitial nephritis may occur with any glomerular lesion or in isolation. The incidence is similar in black and white populations and all degrees of clinical status. The lesions may be associated with lymphocytic infiltration of other organs, e.g. liver and salivary glands, and may be due to a virus-induced immune disorder.

Dialysis and transplantation in renal associated HIV infections

Patients with HIV-associated acute renal failure and patients with HIV and chronic renal failure without AIDS have been successfully treated with dialysis, but patients with AIDS treated with dialysis have a poor prognosis. Very few renal centers would consider patients with HIV infection as candidates for transplantation.

Viral hemorrhagic fever (hemorrhagic fever with renal syndrome, HFRS)

HFRS [86] a febrile illness with renal involvement caused by a zoonotic virus of the family Bunyaviridae (Hantaa virus). It has been found in Europe, the former USSR, Korea, China, Eastern Asia, and also other parts of Asia and North and South America. The virus is endemic in the host animal, mainly rodents, is spread by airborne infection, and causes a febrile illness with loin pain, headaches, conjunctival hemorrhage, myopia, hypotension or hypertension, thrombocytopenia, leukocytosis and abnormal liver function. Acute renal failure associated with interstitial nephritis develops in the majority of patients and sometimes necessitates hemodialysis; treatment is supportive only.

Other virus diseases and the kidney

Despite the frequency of virus diseases world-wide, virus-related nephropathies are relatively rare [87]. Certain viruses have well-known associated renal disease.

Hepatitis B

Hepatitis B associated with membranous glomerulonephritis, mesangiocapillary glomerulonephritis and with mesangial IgA deposition [88].

Hepatitis C

Mixed cryoglobulinemia, vasculitis and mesangiocapillary glomerulonephritis have been described in association with hepatitis C virus infection [89].

Cytomegalovirus infections

Cytomegalovirus infections may cause transplant rejection or an immune-complex glomerulonephritis [90].

Other sporadic virus infections, such as varicella, measles, mumps and Epstein–Barr virus, may cause a virus-associated immune-complex glomerulonephritis.

Fungal infections

Candida albicans, and occasionally other species of Candida, can frequently be isolated from urine but are not usually of significance [75]. Infection is most commonly related to urinary catheters, antibiotic therapy or diabetes. The diagnosis of invasive bladder infection requires cystoscopy and biopsy. In men urethral candidiasis is usually sexually acquired, whereas in women it is probably related to vaginal infection.

In the upper urinary tract, candidiasis may rarely be of ascending origin but is usually the result of hematogenous pyelonephritis.

Renal aspergillosis, usually due to *Aspergillus fumigatus*, is commonly related to disseminated infection in immunocompromised patients. The kidney is affected in 10% of renal transplant patients with disseminated aspergillosis. The condition is associated with progressive renal failure, proteinuria, pyuria and hematuria.

Immunocompromised patients are also susceptible to other fungal infections. Caseating pyelonephritis may occur in disseminated cryptococcosis and the renal parenchyma may be involved in disseminated coccidiomycosis, particularly in renal transplant recipients.

References

1. O'Grady, F. and Cattell, W.R. (1966) Kinetics of urinary tract infection. I. Upper urinary tract. *Br. J. Urol.*, **38**, 149–55.
2. O'Grady, F. and Cattell, W.R. (1966) Kinetics of urinary tract infection. II. The bladder. *Br. J. Urol.*, **38**, 156–62.
3. Barrington, F.J.F. and Wright, H.D. (1930) Bacteremia following operations on the urethra. *J. Path. Bact.*, **33**, 871–88.
4. Teague, N. and Boyarsky, S. (1968) Further effects of coliform bacteria on ureteral peristalsis. *J. Urol.*, **99**, 720–4.
5. Thulesius, O. and Araj, G. (1987) The effect of uropathogenic bacteria on ureteral motility. *Urol. Res.*, **15**, 273–6.
6. Rolleston, G.L., Maling, T.M. and Hodson, C.J. (1974) Intrarenal reflux and the scarred kidney. *Arch. Dis. Child.*, **49**, 531–9.
7. Asscher, A.W., Sussman, M., Waters, W.E. *et al.* (1966) Urine as a medium for bacterial growth. *Lancet*, **ii**, 1037–41.
8. Kaye, D. (1968) Antibacterial activity of human urine. *J. Clin. Invest.*, **47**, 2374–90.
9. Weiser, R., Asscher, A.W. and Sussman, M. (1969) Glycosuria and the growth of urinary pathogens. *Invest. Urol.*, **6**, 650–6.
10. Vivaldi, E., Munoz, J., Cotran, R. and Kass, E.H. (1965) Factors affecting the clearance of bacteria within the urinary tract, in *Progress in Pyelonephritis* (ed. E.H. Kass), F.A. Davis, Philadelphia, pp. 531–5.
11. Norden, C.W., Green, G.M. and Kass, E.H. (1968) Antibacterial mechanisms of the bladder. *J. Clin. Invest.*, **47**, 2689–700.
12. Freedman, L.R. and Beeson, P.B. (1958) Experimental pyelonephritis. IV. Observations on infections resulting from direct inoculation of bacteria in different zones of the kidney. *Yale J. Biol. Med.*, **30**, 406–14.
13. Beeson, P.B. and Rowley, D. (1959) The anti-inflammatory effect of kidney tissue. Its association with ammonia production. *J. Exp. Med.*, **110**, 685–97.
14. Hanson, L.Å., Holmgren, J., Jodal, U. *et al.* (1970) Immunoglobulins in urines of children with urinary tract infections, in *The Secretory Immunologic System*. United States Department of Health Education and Welfare, Bethesda, pp. 367–83.

15. Jackson, G.G., Arana, J.A. and Kozij, V.M. (1958) Retrograde pyelonephritis in the rat and the role of certain cellular and humoral factors in the host defense, in *Progress in Pyelonephritis* (ed. E.H. Kass), F.A. Davis, Philadelphia, pp. 202–10.

16. Hjelm, E.M. (1984) Local cellular immune response in ascending urinary tract infection: occurrence of T cells, immunoglobulin-producing cells, and Ia-expressing cells in rat urinary tract infection. *Infect. Immun.*, **44**, 627–32.

17. Miller, T.E., Marshall, E. and Nelson, J. (1983) Infection-induced immunosuppression in pyelonephritis: characteristics of the suppressor cells. *Kidney Int.*, **24**, 313–22.

18. Marrie, T.J., Swantee, C.A. and Hartlen, M. (1980) Aerobic and anaerobic urethral flora in healthy females in various physiological age groups and of females with urinary tract infection. *J. Clin. Microbiol.*, **11**, 654–9.

19. Cox, C.E., Lacy, S.S. and Hinman, F. Jr (1968) The urethra and its relationship to urinary tract infection. *J. Urol.*, **99**, 632–8.

20. Schaeffer, A.J., Jones, J.M. and Dunn, J.K. (1981) Association of *in vitro Escherichia coli* adherence to vaginal and buccal epithelial cells with susceptibility of women to recurrent urinary tract infection. *N. Engl. J. Med.*, **304**, 1062–6.

21. Fussell, E.N., Kaack, M.B., Cherry, R. and Roberts, J.A. (1988) Adherence of bacteria to human foreskins. *J. Urol.*, **140**, 997–1001.

22. Grüneberg, R.N. (1969) Relationship of infecting urinary organisms to the faecal flora in patients with symptomatic urinary infection. *Lancet*, **ii**, 766–8.

23. McAllister, T.A., Alexander, J.G., Dulake, C. *et al.* (1971) The sensitivity of urinary pathogens – a survey. *Postgrad. Med. J.*, **47**, 7–18.

24. Bryan, C.S. and Reynolds, K.L. (1984) Community-acquired bacteremic urinary tract infection. *J. Urol.*, **132**, 490–3.

25. Bryan, C.S. and Reynolds, K.L. (1984) Hospital-acquired bacteremic urinary tract infection. *J. Urol.*, **132**, 494–8.

26. Hovelius, B. and Mardh, P. (1984) *Staphylococcus saprophyticus* as a common cause of urinary tract infections. *Rev. Inf. Dis.*, **6**, 328–37.

27. Maskell, R., Pead, L. and Sanderson, R.A. (1983) Fastidious bacteria and the urethral syndrome: a 2-year clinical and bacteriological study of 51 women. *Lancet*, **ii**, 1277–80.

28. Finegold, S.M. (1977) *Anaerobic Bacteria in Human Disease*, Academic Press, New York, pp. 314–49.

29. Naylor, G.R.E. (1984) A 16-month analysis of urinary tract infection in children. *J. Med. Microbiol.*, **17**, 31–6.

30. Parry, S.H. and Rooke, D.M. (1985) Adhesins and colonization factors of *Escherichia coli*, in *The Virulence of Escherichia coli* (ed. M. Sussman), Academic Press, London, pp. 79–155.

31. Sharon, N. and Ofek, I. (1986) Mannose-specific bacterial surface lectins, in *Microbial Lectins and Agglutinins: Properties and Biological Activities* (ed. D. Mirelman), Wiley, New York, pp. 55–81.

32. Ørskov, I., Ferencz, A. and Ørskov, F. (1980) Tamm–Horsfall protein or uromucoid is the normal urinary slime that traps Type 1 fimbriated *Escherichia coli*. *Lancet*, **i**, 887.

33. Kallenius, G., Svenson, S.B., Mollby, R. *et al.* (1981) Structure of carbohydrate part of receptor on human uroepithelial cells for pyelonephritogenic *Escherichia coli*. *Lancet*, **ii**, 604–6.

34. Ofek, I. and Doyle, R.J. (1994) *Bacterial Adhesion to Cells and Tissues.* Chapman & Hall, New York.

35. Aronson, M., Medalia, O., Amichay, D. and Nativ, O. (1988) Endotoxin-induced shedding of viable uroepithelial cells is an antimicrobial defense mechanism. *Infect. Immun.*, **56**, 1615–17.

36. Steadman, R. and Topley, N. (1997) Cell activation by uropathogenic *Escherichia coli*, in *Escherichia coli: Mechanisms of Virulence* (ed. M. Sussman), Cambridge University Press, Cambridge, pp. 553–78.

37. Jann, K. and Jann, B. (1997) Capsules of *Escherichia coli*, in *Escherichia coli: Mechanisms of Virulence* (ed. M. Sussman), Cambridge University Press, Cambridge, pp. 113–43.

38. Taylor, P.W. (1985) Measurement of the bactericidal activity of serum, in *The Virulence of Escherichia coli.* (ed. M. Sussman), Academic Press, London, pp. 445–56.

39. Griffiths, E. (1997) Iron and the virulence of *Escherichia coli*, in *Escherichia coli: Mechanisms of Virulence* (ed. M. Sussman), University Press, Cambridge, pp. 331–71.

40. Griffiths, E. and Humphreys, J. (1980) Isolation of enterochelin from the peritoneal washings of guinea-pigs lethally infected with *Escherichia coli*. *Infect. Immun.*, **28**, 286–9.

41. Sussman, M. (1974) Iron in infection, in *Iron in Biochemistry and Medicine* (eds A. Jacobs and M. Worwood), Academic Press, London, pp. 649–79.

42. Ludwig, A. and Goebel, W. (1997) Haemolysins of *Escherichia coli*, in *Escherichia coli: Mechanisms of Virulence* (ed. M. Sussman), Cambridge University Press, Cambridge, pp. 281–329.

43. Minshew, B.H., Jorgensen, J., Swanstrum, M. *et al.* (1978) Some characteristics of *Escherichia coli* strains isolated from extra-intestinal infections in humans. *J. Infect. Dis.*, **137**, 648–54.

44. van den Bosch, J.F., de Graaf, F. and MacLaren, D.M. (1982) Virulence of hemolytic strains of *Escherichia coli* in various animal models. *FEMS Microbiol. Lett.*, **13**, 427–30.

45. Pfau, A. and Sacks, T. (1981) The bacterial flora of the vaginal vestibule, urethra and vagina in premenopausal women with recurrent urinary tract infection. *J. Urol.*, **126**, 630–4.

46. Väisänen, V., Elo, J., Tallgren, L.G. *et al.* (1981) Mannose-resistant haemagglutination and P antigen recognition are characteristic of *Escherichia coli* causing primary pyelonephritis. *Lancet*, **ii**, 1366–9.

47. Parry, S.H., Boonchai, S., Abraham, S.N. *et al.* (1983) A comparative study of the mannose-resistant and mannose-sensitive hemagglutinins of *Escherichia coli* isolated from urinary tract infections. *Infection*, **11**, 123–8.

48. Kass, E.H. (1956) Asymptomatic infections of the urinary tract. *Trans. Am. Assoc. Phys.*, **69**, 56–63.

49. Sussman, M., Asscher, A.W., Waters, W.E. *et al.* (1969)

Asymptomatic significant bacteriuria in the non-pregnant woman. I. Description of a population. *Br. Med. J.*, **1**, 799–803.

50. Stamm, W.E., Counts, G.W., Running, K.R. *et al.* (1982) Diagnosis of coliform infection in acutely dysuric women. *N. Engl. J. Med.*, **307**, 463–8.

51. Lipsky, B.A. (1989) Urinary tract infection in men: epidemiology, pathophysiology, diagnosis and treatment. *Ann. Intern. Med.*, **110**, 138–50.

52. Sussman, M. and Asscher, A.W. (1979) Urinary tract infection, in *Renal Disease* (eds D. Black and N.F. Jones), Blackwell Scientific Publications, Oxford, pp. 400–36.

53. Guttman, D.E. and Naylor, G.R.E. (1967) Dip-slide: an aid to quantitative urine culture in general practice. *Br. Med. J.*, **3**, 343–5.

54. Mackey, J.P. and Sandys, G.H. (1966) Diagnosis of urinary tract infections. *Br. Med. J.*, **1**, 1173.

55. Zhanel, G.G., Harding, G.K.M. and Guay, D.R.P. (1990) Asymptomatic bacteriuria. Which patients should be treated? *Arch. Intern. Med.*, **150**, 1389–96.

56. Kemper, K.J. and Avner, E.D. (1992) The case against screening urinalyses for asymptomatic bacteriuria in children. *Am. J. Dis. Child.*, **146**, 343–6.

57. Gower, P.E., Haswell, B., Sidaway, M.E. and de Wardener, H.E. (1968) Follow up of 164 patients with bacteriuria of pregnancy. *Lancet*, **i**, 990–4.

58. Johnson, J.R. and Stamm, W.E. (1989) Urinary tract infections in women. Diagnosis and treatment. *Ann. Intern. Med.*, **111**, 906–17.

59. Bailey, R.R. (1990) Review of published studies on single dose therapy of urinary tract infections. *Infection*, **18**(suppl 2), S53–6.

60. Norrby, S.R. (1990) Short term treatment of uncomplicated lower urinary tract infections in women. *Rev. Infect. Dis.*, **12**, 458–67.

61. Maskell, R., Pead, L. and Allen, J. (1979) The puzzle of the urethral syndrome: a possible answer? *Lancet*, **i**, 1058–9.

62. Brumfitt, W., Hamilton-Miller, J.M.T., Ludlam, H. and Gooding, A. (1981) Lactobacilli do not cause frequency and dysuria syndrome. *Lancet*, **ii**, 393–6.

63. Stamm, W.E. (1988) Diagnosis of *Chlamydia trachomatis* genitourinary infections. *Ann. Intern. Med.*, **108**, 710–17.

64. Little, P.J., Macpherson, D.R. and de Wardener, H.E. (1965) The appearance of the intravenous pyelogram during and after acute pyelonephritis. *Lancet*, **i**, 1186–8.

65. Rosenfield, A.T., Gluckman, M.G., Taylor, K.J.W. *et al.* (1979) Acute focal bacterial nephritis (Acute lobar nephronia). *Radiology*, **132**, 553–61.

66. Meyrier, A. (1990) Long term risks of acute pyelonephritis. *Nephron*, **54**, 197–201.

67. Meyrier, A., Condamin, M.C., Fernet, M. *et al.* (1990) Frequency of development of early cortical scarring in acute primary pyelonephritis. *Kidney Int.*, **35**, 696–703.

68. Baldassarre, J.S. and Kaye, D. (1991) Special problems of urinary tract infection in the elderly. *Med. Clin. North Am.*, **75**, 375–90.

69. Wiswell, T.E., Smith, F.R. and Bass, J.W. (1985) Decreased incidence of urinary tract infections in circumcised males. *Pediatrics*, **75**, 901–3.

70. Meares, E.M. (1991) Prostatitis. *Med. Clin. North Am.*, **75**, 405–24.

71. The prevention and management of urinary tract infections among people with spinal cord injuries. National Institute on Disability and Rehabilitation Research Consensus Statement. January 27–29, 1992. *J. Am. Paraplegia Soc.*, **15**, 194–207.

72. Dully, L. and Smith, E.D. (1982) Nitrofurantoin macrocystals to prevent bacteriuria in intermittent self catheterisation. *Urology*, **20**, 47–9.

73. Kevorkian, C.G., Merritt, J.L. and Ilstrup, D.M. (1984) Methanamine mandelate with acidification: an effective urinary antiseptic in patients with neurogenic bladder. *Mayo Clin Proc.*, **59**, 523–9.

74. Gribble, M.J. and Puterman, M.L. (1993) Prophylaxis of urinary tract infection in persons with recent spinal cord injury: a prospective randomised double blind placebo controlled study of trimethorprim–sulphamethoxazole. *Am. J. Med.*, **95**, 141–52.

75. Korzeniowski, O.M. (1991) Urinary tract infection in the impaired host. *Med. Clin. North Am.*, **75**, 391–404.

76. Amin, M. (1992) Antibiotic prophylaxis in urology: a review. *Am. J. Med.*, **4A**, 114–17.

77. Scheckler, W.E. and Peterson, P.J. (1986) Nosocomial infections in 15 Rural Wisconsin Hospitals. Results and conclusions from 6 months of comprehensive surveillance. *Infect. Control*, **7**, 397–402.

78. Warren, J.W. (1991) The catheter and urinary tract infection. *Med. Clin. North Am.*, **75**, 481–93.

79. Chisholm, J.D. (1982) Antimicrobial prophylaxis in urology and transplantation. *World J. Surg.*, **6**, 281–92.

80. Grainger, R.J., Longstaff, A.J. and Parsons, M.A. (1982) Xanthogranulomatous pyelonephritis: a reappraisal. *Lancet*, **i**, 1398–401.

81. Meredith, S.K., Aber, V.R., Nunn, K.J. *et al.* (1992) Medical Research Council Cardio Thoracic Epidemiology Group. National Survey of Notifications of Tuberculosis in England and Wales in 1988. *Thorax*, **47**, 770–5.

82. Das, K.M., Vaidyanathan, S., Rajwanshi, A. and Induhara, R. (1992) Renal tuberculosis, diagnosis with sonographically guided aspiration cytology. *Am. J. Roentgenol*, **158**, 571–3.

83. Morgan, S.H., Eastwood, J.B. and Baker, L.R. (1990) Tuberculous interstitial nephritis – the tip of an iceberg? *Tubercle*, **71**, 5–6.

84. Bourgoigne, J.J. (1990) Renal complications of human immunodeficiency virus type 1. *Kidney Int.*, **31**, 1571–84.

85. Nochy, D., Glotz, D., Dosquet, P. *et al.* (1993) Renal disease associated with HIV infection: a multicentric study of 60 patients from Paris Hospitals. *Nephrol. Dial. Transplant.*, **8**, 11–19.

86. Siamopoulos, K.C. (1994) Virus related acute renal failure. The clinical course and outcome of haemorrhagic fever with renal syndrome. *Nephrol. Dial. Transplant.*, **9**(suppl 4), 111–15.

87. Ko, K.W. and Park, H.C. (1991) Virus-related renal diseases. *Kidney Int.*, **35**, S1–93.

88. Levy, M. and Chen, N. (1991) Worldwide perspective of hepatitis B-associated glomerulonephritis in the 80's. *Kidney Int.*, **40**(suppl 35), S24–33.

89. Marcellin, P., Descamps, V., Martinot–Piegnoux, M. *et al.* (1993) Cryoglobulinemia with vasculitis associated with hepatitis C virus infection. *Gastroenterology*, **104**, 272–7.

90. Sissons, J.G.P., Sinclair, J.H. and Borysiewicz, L.K. (1991) Pathogenesis of human cytomegalovirus disease and the kidney. *Kidney Int.*, **40**(suppl 35), S8–12.

91. Johnson, C.C. (1991) Definitions, classification and clinical presentation of urinary tract infection. *Med. Clin. North Am.*, **75**, 241–52.

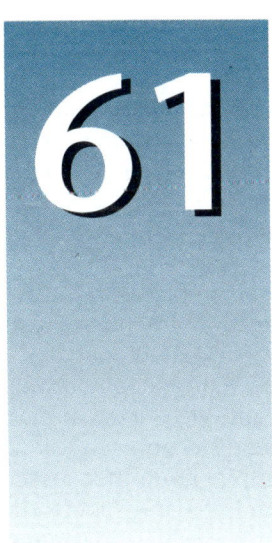

61

Acute renal failure

Rex L. Jamison, Bryan D. Myers and
Guy Neild

Introduction

Acute renal failure (ARF) is a sudden deterioration in renal function manifested by a rise in concentration of nitrogenous products in the blood. (For reviews see [1–6]). The two most common indicators of ARF are blood urea nitrogen and serum creatinine concentration. For several reasons, serum creatinine is a more reliable indicator of ARF than the blood urea nitrogen. The rate of urinary excretion of urea is less than the rate of glomerular filtration of urea, because urea is reabsorbed by the thick ascending limb and collecting tubule. Urea reabsorption by the collecting tubule is increased by arginine vasopressin. In dehydration and other states associated with arginine vasopressin release, in which the urine is concentrated and urinary flow is low, more urea is reabsorbed, and the blood urea nitrogen rises to a higher steady state value despite an unchanging glomerular filtration rate (GFR). The blood urea nitrogen also reflects the rate of urea production by the liver. Urea synthesis is determined by the amount of dietary protein and other protein (e.g. blood) absorbed from the gastrointestinal tract and the rate of metabolic conversion of protein to urea. The combination of a high blood urea nitrogen and a normal serum creatinine is often an indication of gastrointestinal bleeding. A very low blood urea nitrogen despite a reduced GFR is characteristic of liver failure or malnutrition.

Creatinine is produced at a constant rate (in mg/kg body weight/day, 10–20 in women and 15–25 in men) as a breakdown product of creatine phosphate in muscle and is not affected by factors that influence urea production. Although creatinine is normally excreted almost entirely by filtration and is not reabsorbed, there are two drawbacks to relying on serum creatinine as an indicator of ARF. One is the variation in creatinine production among individuals, which means the upper limit of a normal serum creatinine (1.3 mg/dl in most laboratories) may mask a low GFR. As many as 40% of patients will have a substantial fall in GFR before the serum creatinine exceeds the upper limit of normal. The other disadvantage is that the renal tubule secretes creatinine. Renal failure is often accompanied by enhanced tubular creatinine secretion, leading to a spuriously high creatinine clearance relative to the true GFR, and thereby blunting the extent to which serum creatinine becomes elevated. On the other hand tubular transport of creatinine is blocked by several widely used drugs, such as cefoxitin, trimethoprim and cimetidine, causing the serum creatinine to rise in the absence of a change in GFR. Nevertheless, a rise in serum creatinine is the single most reliable indicator of a decline in GFR.

Incidence, prevalence and outcome

Approximately 5% of hospital admissions to a general hospital in the US comprised patients with ARF [7]. In the

Nephrology, Edited by Rex L. Jamison and Robert Wilkinson.
Published in 1997 by Chapman & Hall, London. ISBN 0 412 60930 4

intensive care unit, 10–20% of patients may have ARF. These patients have a high morbidity and a mortality of 30–70%. There are, however, ways in which a physician can influence the outcome. Today it is possible to prevent ARF or to sustain life for prolonged periods while the kidneys recover from ARF. We stand at the threshold of a new era in which treatment may hasten recovery from ARF.

History

The Germans were the first to observe anuria and uremia following crush injuries from trenches caving in on soldiers during the First World War [8]. Under the light microscope the glomeruli appeared normal but the renal tubules were severely damaged. In 1942, Bywaters and Dible [9] published a landmark paper describing their observations of civilians dying in the London Blitz of the Second World War. They suggested that acute renal insuf-

ficiency is caused by intratubular obstruction and cell necrosis. This view was extended by the studies in the early 1950s by Oliver *et al.* [10] in which individual nephrons were dissected from patients dying of ARF. Of the two lesions that were described the most common was a localized well-demarcated lesion in the tubule epithelium. The cells were necrotic and often exfoliated into the lumen leaving an exposed and denuded basement membrane, a likely site of backleak of glomerular filtrate. This 'tubulorrhexis' lesion was randomly distributed throughout the tubule, although it was most obvious in the pars recta and the distal and connecting tubule. Luminal debris and casts were most often associated with lesions beyond the bend of Henle's loop. The second lesion was termed nephrotoxic, which, in contrast to tubulorrhexis, was found only in the proximal tubule, was evenly distributed among all nephrons and was less severe in that the basement membrane remained covered. The latter lesion was thought to be characteristic of a

Table 61.1 Clinical features, urinalysis and diagnostic tests of major causes of acute renal failure

Cause of ARF	Clinical features that suggest diagnosis	Urinalysis	Tests to establish diagnosis
Prerenal failure			
	Volume depletion: Hx of weight loss or fluid output > input; ACE inhibitors or NSAIDs, thirst, orthostatic hypotension and tachycardia, low JVP, dry mucous membranes. Reduced 'effective' circulatory volume: heart failure, liver failure, hypotension.	SG > 1.020 U/P osm > 1.05 FE_{Na} < 1% Protein ± Sediment: few cells; few hyaline casts	CVP low; +response too 500 ml saline
Renal (parenchymal) failure			
Diseases of large renal vessels			
Renal artery thrombosis	Hx of Af or recent MI, nausea, vomiting flank or abdominal pain	Protein + to ++ RBCs	Renal angiogram
Embolism	Age > 50 years, recent aortic instrumentation or surgery, hypertension, subcutaneous nodules, purpura, vasculopathy	Eosinophils	Eosinophilia, hypocomplementemia skin biopsy, renal biopsy
Renal vein thrombosis	Flank pain, pulmonary embolism, nephrotic syndrome	Protein +++ to ++++, RBCs	Vena cavagram and renal venogram
Diseases of small vessels and glomeruli			
Glomerulonephritis/ vasculitis	Recent infection. Multisystem disease: sinusitis, lung bleeding, skin rash or ulcers, arthralgias	Protein +++ to ++++. Dysmorph-RBCs, RBC casts granular casts	C3, ANCA, anti-GBM Ab, ANA, ASO, anti-DNAse cryoglobulins, renal biopsy
Hemolytic uremic syndrome/TTP	Recent GI infection; cyclosporin, anovulants. Fever, ecchymoses, neurological abnormalities	Protein + to ++. RBCs, rarely casts.	Low Hct and Plat. Schistocytes in blood smear, renal biopsy

Table 61.1 (*Continued*).

Cause of ARF	Clinical features that suggest diagnosis	Urinalysis	Tests to establish diagnosis
Malignant hypertension	Severe hypertension with headaches, visual disturbance, heart failure, and CNS manifestations. Retinopathy with hemorrhages, exudates or papilledema	Protein ++ to ++++. RBCs, RBC casts	Temporary worsening/eventual recovery after control of BP
Acute tubular necrosis			
Ischemia	Circulatory collapse from any cause, trauma, major surgery, burns	SG = 1.010. U/P osm = 1.0. $U_{Na} > 20$, $FE_{Na} > 1\%$. 'Muddy brown' granular casts	CVP
Exogenous toxins	Recent radiocontrast study, nephrotoxic drugs often in setting of volume depletion, sepsis or CRF	Same as ischemia	CVP
Endogenous toxins	Rhabomyolysis (coma, seizures, ethanol abuse, trauma)	Same as ischemia, + for heme, myoglobin	High serum K^+, PO_4^{3-}, uric acid, CPK, Low serum Ca^{2+}
	Hemolysis (blood transfusion, drugs, infection)	Same as ischemia Urine pink and + for heme.	Same as for rhabdomyolysis except CPK nl. Plasma pink and + for hemoglobin
	(a) Tumor lysis syndrome (chemotherapy)	(a) Urate crystals	(a) High serum K^+, PO_4^{3-}, uric acid
	(b) Multiple myeloma	(b) Bence Jones +	(b) Paraprotein in serum or urine
	(c) Ethyene glycol ingestion	(c) Oxalate crystals	(c) Toxicology screen, acidosis, osmolal gap
Acute tubulointerstitial diseases			
Acute interstitial nephritis	Recent ingestion of drug. Fever, rash, arthalgias	Protein 0 to ++++ RBCs, WBCs, eosinophils, WBC casts.	Eosinophilia, skin biopsy, renal biopsy
Acute pyelonephritis (bilateral)	Flank pain, toxic. Fever	Protein + to +++. WBCs, RBCs, bacteria	Urine and blood cultures
Postrenal failure	Hx of prostatism, renal stones, abdominal cancer or one kidney. Abdominal or flank pain	Protein 0. RBCs	Plain film of abdomen; renal ultrasound, computer tomography. Retrograde or antegrade pyelogram. Foley catheter. Percutaneous puncture of renal pelvis

Urine protein
+, 10–30 mg/dl; ++, 40–100 mg/dl; +++, 200–500 mg/dl; ++++, >500 mg/dl.

Adapted with permission from Brady, K.R. and Singer, G.K. (1995) Acute renal failure. *Lancet*, **346**, 1533–40.

Abbreviations: ACE, angiotensin converting enzyme; AF, atrial fibrillation; ANA, antinuclear antibody; ANCA, antineutrophil cytoplasmic antibody; anti-GBM Ab, antiglomerular basement membrane antibody; ARF, acute renal failure, ASO, antistreptolysin O antibody; C3, third component of complement; CPK, creatine phosphokinase; CRF, chronic renal failure; CVP, central venous pressure; FE_{Na}, fractional excretion of Na; GI, gastrointestinal; Hct, hematocrit; Hx, history; IVP, intravenous pyelogram; JVP, jugular venous pressure; MI, myocardial infarction; NSAID, non-steroidal anti-inflammatory drug; Plat, platelet; RBC, red blood cell; SG, specific gravity; TTP, thrombotic thrombocyopenic purpura; U/P, urine-to-plasma; U_{Na}, urinary Na concentration; WBC, white blood cell.

poison whereas tubulorrhexis was secondary to ischemia. From the beginning, however, the roots of a controversy were planted. Lucké [11] reviewed 4538 autopsies of those dying of renal insufficiency during the Second World War and noted that the principal damage appeared to be in lower (i.e. distal) segments of the nephron. He coined the term 'lower nephron nephrosis' [11].

This brief account concerns primarily a form of ARF known as acute tubular necrosis and which will receive the main emphasis. As described later, there are several other classes of ARF.

Clinical manifestations

ARF can be silent until sufficient waste products or water have accumulated to cause symptoms and signs (Table 61.1). A high blood urea nitrogen or serum creatinine is commonly the first indication. Other serum abnormalities that signal ARF are a rise in serum potassium and phosphorus and a decrease in bicarbonate and calcium. The first symptom noticed by the patient may be a fall in urine flow (to less than 500 ml a day). Complaints of nausea and vomiting and signs of pulmonary congestion, pericarditis, purpura, bleeding, tremors or confusion indicate urgency in diagnosis and treatment.

Pathophysiology

Failure of the kidney to function represents a combination of malfunctions; the overriding disturbance, however, is the failure of glomerular filtration (Figure 61.1). The GFR represents the net rate of water flux across the walls of all capillaries in the glomerular tufts [1]. It can be equated with the product of net ultrafiltration pressure and the ultrafiltration coefficient (K_f):

$$GFR = (\Delta P - \pi_{GC})K_f \qquad (61.1)$$

where $\Delta P = (P_{GC} - P_T)$; $K_f = kS$ (i.e. K_f is the product of k, the water permeability of the glomerulus, and S, the effective filtration surface area).

The net ultrafiltration pressure is the imbalance between the transcapillary hydraulic pressure difference, ΔP (the glomerular capillary pressure minus the proximal tubule pressure, P_T) and the opposing intracapillary oncotic pressure exerted by protein as plasma flows axially along the capillaries, π_{GC}.

Another determinant of GFR is the renal plasma flow, which is not obvious from equation (61.1). The rate of renal (or more accurately, glomerular) plasma flow influences GFR by determining π_{GC}. Axial oncotic pressure rises rapidly in the glomerular capillary when plasma flow is low and the opposite is true when plasma flow is high.

As depicted in Figure 61.1, filtration failure could be caused by reduced glomerular plasma flow, reduced glomerular capillary pressure (due to afferent arteriolar constriction), diminished K_f or obstruction, in which case

P_T rises to equal glomerular capillary pressure. Afferent arteriolar plasma oncotic pressure, a function of plasma protein concentration, is not usually a factor in reducing GFR because it is almost never elevated during ARF and therefore does not contribute to the depression of GFR in ARF. Only if albumin or other colloid-containing solutions are infused in quantities large enough to raise arteriolar oncotic pressure, is the latter likely to contribute to filtration failure. Beyond Bowman's space, a final contribution to filtration failure is the back-leak of filtrate across injured or necrotic tubules, predominantly in acute tubular necrosis. Despite a normal K_f and a positive net pressure for ultrafiltration, the phenomenon of back-leak has the potential to render the majority of nephrons non-contributory to the final urine.

Cause and pathogenesis

Many patients with ARF do not recover because of failure of another organ system (e.g. the heart or antimicrobial defense mechanisms) and other patients have ARF that may be irreversible. In the initial approach to a patient, it therefore may not be useful to classify ARF according to specific cause, a list of which (Table 61.2) is lengthy. Given the complexity of decisions that must be made, a more useful initial approach is to distinguish among three major classes of ARF and ten major syndromes (Table 61.3) [4]. These categories stem from the pathophysiology of filtration failure (Figure 61.1). The first class consists of disorders that reduce glomerular blood flow. The terms, prerenal ARF or prerenal azotemia, designate this group, since the circulation to the kidney is impaired, but not the kidney itself. The second class, renal ARF, consists of those disorders which cause direct injury to the glomeruli, tubules or interstitium. Causes of obstruction to urinary flow anywhere from the proximal tubule to the distal urethra comprise the third group, postrenal ARF. Another acceptable view is to consider intratubular obstruction under the category of renal ARF. We prefer to classify these disorders as postrenal because many of them occur in the absence of any injury to the tubule, if promptly treated. The majority of cases fall under the category of prerenal ARF and most of the remainder are in the second category. Prompt recognition and treatment of disorders in the first and third categories may protect the kidney from injury.

Prerenal ARF

This is characterized by reduced renal perfusion. Between a half and three-quarters of cases of ARF are in this group. Prerenal ARF often masquerades as parenchymal renal failure. It is preceded by a fall in extracellular fluid volume (typically from a severe hemorrhage, protracted vomiting or diarrhea, excessive diuresis or profound hypoalbuminemia), sequestration of extracellular fluid (sepsis, pancreatitis, muscle crush injury, burns), renal

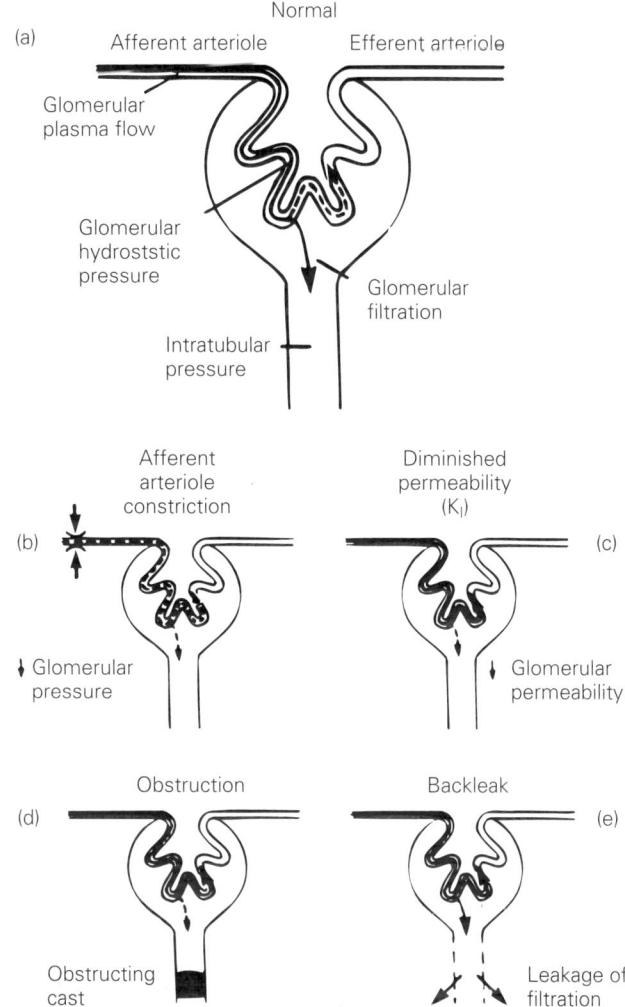

Figure 61.1 Pathophysiology of acute renal failure. The figures illustrate forces that affect glomerular filtration in the normal glomerulus (a) and the abnormalities that produce acute renal failure (b–e). In (a), as ultrafiltrate forms, the plasma flow diminishes (broken line) and glomerular capillary plasma oncotic pressure rises until it equals the transmembrane hydraulic pressure difference, at which point filtration pressure equilibrium is reached and ultrafiltration stops (not shown). If equilibrium is reached before the end of the capillary, then an increase in glomerular plasma flow will move the point in the capillary at which equilibrium is reached further along the capillary and more ultrafiltrate will be formed. (b) Pathophysiology of prerenal failure, renal failure associated with liver failure (hepatorenal syndrome), acute renal arterial thrombosis (initial stages), and those forms of acute tubular necrosis in which there is prolonged afferent arteriolar constriction. The primary lesion is afferent arteriolar constriction with diminished glomerular pressure and reduced ultrafiltrate formation. (c) Pathophysiology of acute renal failure in which the glomerulus is injured, e.g. acute glomerulonephritis, rapidly progressive glomerulonephritis, and hemolytic uremic syndrome. The primary lesion is a diminished glomerular permeability. (d) Pathophysiology of acute renal failure in obstruction. The obstruction may be in the proximal tubule (as shown) and throughout the renal tubule, as occurs in acute tubular necrosis, intratubular precipitation of uric acid, calcium or other crystals or protein casts, e.g. multiple myeloma. Or the obstruction may occur in the ureter, producing acute renal failure if bilateral; in the bladder neck, e.g. prostatic hypertrophy or cancer; or in the penile urethra, e.g. congenital flap. (e) Pathophysiology of acute tubule necrosis. Glomerular filtration may be normal or diminished (see b). Usually the glomerulus itself is normal. Owing to necrosis anywhere along the tubule, however, the ultrafiltrate which is formed leaks back into the interstitium, which reduces or abolishes the contribution of that nephron to urine formation. (Reproduced, with permission, from Kellerman, P.S. and Molitoris, B.A. (1991) Pathogenetic mechanisms of ischemic acute renal failure, in *The Principles and Practice of Nephrology* (eds H. Jacobson, G. Stirker and S. Klahr), Decker, Philadelphia, pp. 626–31.)

Table 61.2   Causes of acute renal failure

Prerenal failure
1. Reduction in intravascular volume
   Hypoalbuminemia
   Blood loss
   Extracellular fluid volume depletion
      Exogenous loss
         Gastrointestinal (diarrhea, vomiting, surgical drainage)
         Renal (diuretics, hypoadrenalism, glucosuria, postobstructive diuresis, salt losing disorders)
      Transcellular shift in ECF ('third spacing')
         Burns
         Peritonitis
         Crush injury
         Trauma
2. Systemic vasodilatation
   Sepsis
   Shock due to anaphylaxis or other allergic reaction
   Hepatic failure
   Medication (afterload reducing agents, anesthesia, antihypertensives, drug overdose)
3. Cardiac failure
   Congestive heart failure
   Reduced cardiac output (primary myocardial failure, arrhythmia, pericardial tamponade)
   Right sided cardiac failure (pulmonary hypertension; pulmonary embolism)
   Mechanical ventilation
4. Increased renal arterial resistance
   Renal artery disease (embolism, thrombosis, atherosclerotic plaque, aortic dissection) (bilateral or unilateral in a
      functionally uninephephric patient)
   Renal vein thrombosis (bilateral or unilateral in functionally uninephric patient)
   Increased viscosity of blood (multiple myeloma, polycythemia)
   Renal vasoconstriction
      Hypercalcemia
      Drugs (catecholamines, cyclosporin, amphotericin, non-steroidal anti-inflammatory drugs, and others)
      Hepatorenal syndrome
5. Glomerular and arteriolar disease (See Parenchymal renal failure)

Parenchymal renal failure
1. Glomerular and arteriolar disease
   Actue glomerulonephritis
   Rapidly progressive glomerulonephritis
   Malignant hypertension
   Hemolytic uremic syndrome
   Disseminated intravascular coagulation
   Systemic vasculitis
   Toxemia of pregnancy
2. Acute cortical necrosis
3. Acute interstitial nephritis
   Infection (bacterial, viral, fungal):
   Infiltration (lymphoma, leukemia)
   Drugs (most common drugs currently dispensed)
      Antimicrobials: penicillins, cephalosporin, sulfonamides, rifampin
      Non-steroidal anti-inflammatory drugs
      Diuretics: thiazides, thalidone, furosemide
      Miscellaneous: cimetidine, phenidione

Table 61.2   (*Continued*).

4. Acute tubular necrosis
   Ischemic: see Prerenal failure: sufficient duration and intensity of any of the factors listed can lead to acute tubular necrosis
      Most common clinical settings in which acute tubular necrosis is observed:
         Surgery: open-heart surgery, gastrointestinal and trauma
         Obstetrics: placentae abruptio and septic abortion
         Trauma
         Burns
         Cardiac failure
         Sepsis
         Aminoglycoside toxicity
         Radiocontrast toxicity
         Myoglobin nephrotoxicity (rhabdomyolysis)
   Nephrotoxic: See nephrotoxic ATN
5. Nephrotoxic acute tubular necrosis
   Exogenous nephrotoxins (only major offending drugs currently dispensed are listed)
      Antibiotics: acylovir, aminoglycosides, amphotericin, bacitracin, cephalosporins, foscarnet, pentamidein, polymyxin, quinolones, sulfonamides, tetracyclines
      Anesthetic agents: enflurane
      Analgesics: non-steroidal anti-inflammatory drugs
      Chemicals and organic solvents: aniline, aliphatic hydrocarbons (gasoline and kerosene), aromatic hydrocarbons (toluene), chlorates, cresol, ethylamine diamine tetra-acetic acid, glycols, halogenated hydrocarbons, potassium bromate,
      Chemotherapeutic agents: 5-Azacytidine, cis-platinum, ifosfamide, mitomycin, nitrosureas, penicillamine,
      Diuretics: mercurials, ticrynafen
      Heavy metals: Antimony, arsenic, barium, bismuth, cadmium, copper, gold, iron, lead, mercury, silver
      Immunosuppressive agents: cyclosporin, interleukin 2, interferons
      Lithium
      Poisons: insecticides, herbicides (paraquat), mushrooms, rodenticide, snake venom, stings, toxic shock syndrome, yellow oleander
      Radiocontrast agents
      Miscellaneous: dextran, radiation, epsilon-aminocaproic acid, gamma globulin
   Endogenous nephrotoxins
      Pigment (hemoglobin, myoglobin)
      Dysproteinemias (multiple myeloma, light chain disease)
      (see Postrenal obstruction)

Postrenal failure
1. Intratubular cast or crystal formation (uric acid, calcium, oxalate, abnormal proteins in dysproteinemias, tumor lysis syndrome)
2. Ureteral obstruction (bilateral or unilateral in a functionally uninephephric patient)
   Intraureteral: Stones (calcium, uric acid, oxalate, etc.), papillary necrosis, infectious debris or fungus balls, blood clot, tumor, edema from trauma
   Ureteral compression: tumor, periureteral fibrosis, endometriosis, stricture, ureteral ligation (accidental), retroperitoneal expansion from e.g. hemorrhage
3. Bladder outlet blockade: stones, clots, bladder tumor, benign prostatic hypertrophy, prostatic neoplasia, neurogenic bladder
4. Urethral blockade: tumor, stricture, congenital value, phimosis

Table 61.3 Simplified approach to diagnosis of acute renal failure

I   Prerenal failure (reduced perfusion)
    Intravascular or extracellular volume loss or
        sequestration
    Systemic vasodilatation
    Reduced cardiac output
    Increased renal arterial resistance
II Renal (parenchymal)
    Renal vascular disorders
    Acute glomerulonephritis
    Acute interstitial nephritis
    Acute tubular necrosis
III Postrenal (obstruction)
    Intrarenal
    Extrarenal

Table 61.4 Causes of rapidly progressive glomerulonephritis with crescents

I. Primary glomerulonephritis (GN)
    A. Proliferative glomerulonephritis (common forms)
       1. Diffuse endocapillary glomerulonephritis (e.g. poststreptococcal glomerulonephritis
       2. Membranoproliferative (mesangiocapillary) glomerulonephritis
       3. Idiopathic proliferative glomerulonephritis
       4. Antiglomerular basement membrane antibody glomerulonephritis
    B. Proliferative glomerulonephritis (rare forms)
       1. Mesangial IgA glomerulonephritis
    C. Non-proliferative glomerulonephritis
       1. Idiopathic necrotizing glomerulonephritis (should be considered as a limited form of (systemic) microscopic polyarteritis)
II. Vasculitis and secondary glomerulonephritis
    A. Systemic lupus erythematosus
    B. Henoch–Schoenlein purpura
    C. Cryoglobulinemia
    D. Polyarteritis
       1. Microscopic polyarteritis
       2. Polyarteritis nodosa
       3. Wegener's granulomatosis
       4. Churg–Strauss arteritis

vasoconstriction (endogenous or exogenous catecholamines; drugs like cyclosporin or cyclooxygenase inhibitors (which are also toxic to the renal tubule); liver disease) a fall in blood pressure due to vasodilatation (sepsis, drugs), an insufficient cardiac output (heart failure, cardiogenic shock) or a combination of these conditions. In response to a fall in cardiac output or renal perfusion pressure, the afferent arteriole constricts and the efferent arteriole constricts to compensate, but not enough to prevent a decrease in glomerular capillary pressure.

Initially the kidney does not suffer ischemia because its work load – reabsorption of glomerular filtrate – decreases *pari passu* with the fall in GFR. Unless the cause of prerenal ARF is recognized and promptly treated, however, the kidney, especially the renal medulla, may suffer from ischemia [2]. The fact that medullary blood flow is only about 20% of cortical blood flow is cited as one reason, but that lower flow is offset by the much smaller volume of tissue. The major factor is thought to be the countercurrent arrangement of blood vessels in the medulla whose function is to impair the delivery of anything to the medulla to which the capillary is permeable. This includes oxygen. It has been shown that O_2 tension in the normal medulla is about half that of the cortex.

Renal ARF

Acute intrinsic renal failure can be caused by acute injuries to the glomerulus and the glomerular arterioles (Table 61.4) [12–15]. These are dealt with in detail elsewhere in this book and include the acute nephritic syndrome (Chapter 47), rapidly progressive (crescentic) glomerulonephritis (Chapter 45), and pre–eclamptic toxemia and malignant hypertension (Chapters 41 and 42). All lower the GFR by reducing K_f. They tend to have a slower course than the syndrome of acute tubular necro-

sis, with azotemia developing over weeks rather than days. Primary glomerular injury should be sus-pected in the presence of hematuria, and serological findings that point to a co-existent, underlying systemic disorder such as systemic lupus erythematosis or Wegener's granalomatosis. Usually, a renal biopsy is necessary to diagnose precisely the specific glomerular injury that is causing the ARF and to inform the choice of therapy.

Acute tubulointerstitial nephritis which can also lead to ARF (Table 61.5) [16, 17] is dealt with elsewhere in the book. It can result from a primary immune injury in the tubulointerstitial compartment or be secondary to an allergic reaction to a variety of drugs (Table 61.6). It should be suspected in the presence of skin eruptions and eosinophilia or eosinophiluria. In the absence of these manifestations the diagnosis is made by renal biopsy. The mechanism by which acute tubulointerstitial nephritis causes ARF has not been elucidated. Possible mechanisms include glomerular underperfusion owing to the release of vasoconstrictor cytokines by the infiltrating mononuclear leukocytes and obstruction of tubule lumina by the swollen interstitium.

Acute tubular necrosis (ATN) is the cause of ARF in the vast majority of cases of renal ARF. It is due to direct tubule damage, and results from three kinds of injury. In most cases it is postischemic occurring in the wake of a severe fall in renal blood flow. It causes a patchy dis-

Table 61.5 Renal failure caused by tubulointerstitial disease

Acute
1. Associated with infection
   (a) Direct
Bacterial	–	Organisms causing pyelonephritis
	–	Tuberculosis
	–	Leptospirosis
Viral	–	CMV
	–	Viral hemorrhagic fevers, e.g. Hantavirus,
	–	HIV,
	–	Epstein–Barr virus
Rickettsia	–	Rocky Mountain spotted fever

   (b) Reactive
Bacterial	–	Legionella, streptoccus, diphtheria, pneumococcus, brucellosis, salmonella syphilis
Others	–	toxoplasma, mycoplasma, leishmania, malaria

2. Drug-induced: allergic interstitial nephritis (see Table 61.6)
3. Autoimmune interstitial nephritis
	–	NSAIDs
	–	With uveitis
	–	Sarcoid

Chronic
1. Infections
	–	Malakoplakia,
	–	Xanthogranulomatous pyelonephritis
	–	Tuberculosis
2. Infiltrates
	–	Lymphoma
	–	Leukemia
	–	HIV associated nephropathy

CMV, cytomegalovirus; HIV, human immunodeficiency virus; NSAIDs, nonsteroidal anti-inflammatory drugs.

tribution of necrosis of the cortical tubule, mainly the straight portion of the proximal tubule. ATN can also result from exogenous chemical toxins, including: radiographic contrast material; heavy metals; poisons, e.g. stings, insecticides or bacterial toxins; chemicals, e.g. antifreeze, gasoline or industrial solvents; 'recreational' drugs, e.g. heroin or amphetamine; anesthetics; nonsteroidal anti-inflammatory drugs (NSAIDs); chemotherapeutic and immunosuppressive drugs, e.g. cyclosporin or methotrexate; and antibiotics, e.g. amphotericin, aminoglycosides, sulfonamides or cephalosporins. Some of these nephrotoxic drugs may cause ARF by promoting ischemia rather than a direct tubulotoxic effect. In view of this long list, it is wise to consider every drug a patient is taking as a potential nephrotoxin until proven otherwise. Finally, ATN may be caused by endogenous pigments – hemoglobin, released by hemolysis of red cells, or myoglobin from muscle necrosis (rhabdomyolysis). Both pigments are excreted in the urine. Rhabdomyolysis is most apt to occur in the setting of seizures, alcoholism, drug overdose and strenuous exercise.

As noted previously, postischemic injury to the human kidney that manifests as ARF has intrigued researchers for more than half a century. It is an enigmatic injury; despite the fact the GFR is profoundly reduced, histopathologic studies have revealed little or no alteration in glomerular morphology. Futhermore, the few reliable determinations of renal blood flow that have been made in this disorder to date, have failed to reveal hypoperfusion of sufficient magnitude to explain the extreme hypofiltration [18]. The classic lesions described in the introduction are the basis for the term, acute tubular necrosis.

Experimental animal models of ARF

Our current understanding of postischemic ARF derives largely from the study of experimental animals in which renal blood flow has been totally interrupted for 30–60 min. Studies have revealed a complex injury to tubules and microvessels which passes through three stages. An initiation stage has followed reperfusion and given way within hours to a maintenance stage. A profound reduction in GFR has been associated with dissipation of ultrafiltration pressure. This was attributable in part to tubular obstruction by exfoliated proximal tubule cells. Back-leak of filtered fluid through necrotic tubules also contributed to the filtration failure [19]. Renal blood flow falls little in the initiation stage and insufficiently in the maintenance stage to provide an adequate explanation for the hypofiltration [20]. However, analysis of segmental vascular resistance has revealed a disproportionate increase in afferent arteriolar tone with the result that glomerular perfusion pressure is low. The net effect of low pressure in glomerular capillaries and a high pressure in Bowman's space is to lower ΔP to values approaching that of the π_{GC}. Taken together, the evidence suggests the extreme hypofiltration in the initiation and maintenance stages of ARF is a consequence of a severe reduction in ultrafiltration pressure. The recovery stage usually commences after seven days and is characterized by a gradual reversal of the tubular and vascular abnormalities, such that ΔP and GFR are restored to normal.

The link between tubular injury and altered segmental renovascular resistance has now become evident: namely, the phenomenon of tubuloglomerular feedback (TGF). Mechanical obstruction of the proximal tubular lumen has been shown to activate TGF with an ensuing increase in afferent arteriolar resistance [21]. The fall in glomerular perfusion pressure could lower ΔP and bring ultrafiltrate formation and tubular fluid flow to a halt. This would prevent the venting of cellular debris from the

Table 61.6 Drug-induced acute interstitial nephritis

Antibiotics	NSAIDs	Diuretics	Others
Penicillins	Fenoprofen	Furosemide	Allopurinol
Cephalosporins	Mefenamic	Bumetanide	Phenindione
Rifampin	(Any NSAID)	Thiazides	Cimetidine
Quinolones		Triamterene	(Other H-2 blockers,
Trimethoprim–sulfamethoxazole			rare)

obstructed lumina, thereby perpetuating the failure of filtrate formation. TGF-mediated afferent arteriolar constriction has also been postulated to prevail in nephrons with unobstructed tubules. The cellular depletion of ATP that follows interruption of blood flow is followed by a series of morphologic, biochemical and physiologic derangements in epithelial cells, particularly those of the proximal tubule. Their net effect is to reduce proximal reabsorption of Na^+ and other ions, thereby enhancing their delivery to the macula densa to activate TGF-mediated afferent vasoconstriction.

Na^+,K^+-ATPase binds with high affinity to the cytoskeletal proteins ankyrin and fodrin [5] on the basolateral membrane of renal tubule cells, thereby assuring vectorial transport of Na^+ from tubule lumen to cell to interstitium. Transient interruption of renal blood flow *in vivo* or anoxia *in vitro* disrupts the actin-based cytoskeleton of proximal tubule cells. Disassembly of the aforementioned complex has been shown to result in a loss of cell polarity, and impairment of proximal Na^+ reabsorption [5], which would activate a TGF-mediated fall in ΔP, thereby contributing to filtration failure.

Additional abnormalities of vasoregulation have also been implicated in lowering the glomerular perfusion. Renin secretion is enhanced and angiotensin II production accelerated [22]. Endothelin is secreted from vascular endothelial cells as they sustain postischemic damage [6]. Not only are vasoconstrictor peptides present in excess, but the responsiveness of afferent arterioles to them appears to be enhanced during the maintenance stage which may contribute to a loss of autoregulatory ability. Instead of dilating as the perfusion pressure falls within the autoregulatory range, the afferent arteriole constricts. This paradoxical constrictor response is mediated in large part by enhanced sensitivity to sympathetic nervous traffic and local angiotensin II [22]. Conversely, afferent arterioles are resistant to nitric oxide-dependent mediators of vasodilatation, such as acetylcholine and bradykinin [6]. Thus, postischemic ARF is accompanied by an imbalance that favors constrictor neurohormonal influences over those that dilate. This could serve to maintain a low ΔP, thereby prolonging filtration failure even after the injury to proximal tubule cells has resolved. To summarize, the evidence from animal models suggests (1) that depression of ΔP is the predominant cause, and

transtubular back-leak a contributing factor to filtration failure in ARF; and (2) a combination of TGF and neurohormonal influences lower ΔP by selectively increasing afferent resistance.

Hemodynamically mediated ARF in humans

There are only two examples of hemodynamically mediated ARF in humans that are imitated by transiently clamping the renal artery in an otherwise healthy animal and the imitations are not very accurate. One is that which follows clamping of the suprarenal aorta to resect an aortic aneurysm. The other is the syndrome of delayed graft function in the transplanted kidney. The routine clinical use over the past three decades of renal cytoprotective therapy has been so successful that these forms of postischemic renal injury are today poorly mimicked. In patients undergoing aortic cross-clamping, the kidneys are protected by prior infusion of mannitol, an osmotic diuretic, volume expansion and, in some centers, by cooling the kidney during the period of non-perfusion. By studying such patients intraoperatively soon after reperfusion of the kidneys, Myers *et al.* have confirmed the presence of a renal injury with all of the functional hallmarks of ARF [18]. The injury is so brief, however, that it usually resolves completely within 24 h. In fact, significant postoperative azotemia is observed in fewer than 5% of patients undergoing suprarenal aortic clamping, and many of them are likely to have suffered additional ischemic insults.

Renoprotective therapy has also reduced the incidence of delayed graft function following renal transplantation. Delayed graft function is almost never encountered in kidneys transplanted from a living donor, despite the fact that 40–60 min elapse between removal of the kidney from the donor (nephrectomy) and reperfusion. Even more remarkable is that approximately one-half of transplanted kidneys of cadaveric origin also function promptly, notwithstanding a period of non-perfusion between nephrectomy and reperfusion that is typically 10–30 h [23]. In this case the major renoprotective measure is storage of the kidney on ice in the period between nephrectomy and transplantation. Lowering kidney temperature to 4°C brings metabolic and transport

Table 61.7 Determinants of glomerular filtration rate in delayed graft function

	Prompt graft function	Delayed graft function
Q_B (ml/min/1.73 m^2)	405 ± 62	214 ± 44**
RVR (mmHg/min/l)	208 ± 24	587 ± 186**
GFR (ml/min/1.73 m^2)	29 ± 5	6 ± 2**
RPF (ml/min/1.73 m^2)	309 ± 57	150 ± 31**
FF	0.10 ± 0.02	0.02 ± 0.01**
π_A mmHg	21.1 ± 1.0	19.1 ± 1.5
π_{GC} mmHg	22.0 ± 1.1	19.4 ± 1.0*
S ($\mu m^2 \times 10^5$)	1.42 ± 0.13	1.96 ± 0.30
k (m/s/Pa $\times 10^{-9}$)	2.77 ± 0.06	2.39 ± 0.10*
K_f (ml/min·mmHg)	3.12 ± 0.29	3.52 ± 0.57
ΔP^a (mmHg)	33.8 ± 2.3	20.7 ± 1.7

**$P < 0.001$, *$P < 0.05$.
Abbreviations: Q_B, renal blood flow; RVR, renovascular resistance; GFR, glomerular filtration rate; RPF, renal plasma flow; FF, filtration fraction; π_A, plasma oncotic pressure in afferent arteriole; π_{GC}, plasma oncotic pressure in the glomerular capillary; S, surface area of glomerular capillary; k, hydraulic permeability; K_f = ultrafiltration coefficient; ΔP, transglomerular membrane hydraulic pressure.
^{a} The computed ΔP in delayed graft function has been corrected for a 33% back-leak of filtrate.
From ref. [24].

processes to a halt, and reduces drastically the requirement of renal cells for oxygen. Another explanation for the lack of susceptibility to postischemic ARF in native kidneys following suprarenal aortic clamping and in transplanted kidneys is that such kidneys are denervated during surgery. This explanation is in keeping with the demonstration in animal models that renal denervation limits the extent of postischemic injury [22].

To address the mechanisms of filtration failure in human ARF, and to assess the relevance of the animal model, the syndrome of delayed graft function is considered and the ARF that follows cardiac surgery is used as a prototype of the common renal injury that complicates an episode of partial renal ischemia.

Pathophysiology of filtration failure in humans

Delayed graft function

The syndrome of delayed graft function in the transplanted kidney is the closest clinical analogy to postischemic ARF in the animal, where blood flow has been transiently interrupted. A common feature is that allograft recipients, unlike most patients with other forms of ARF, are not critically ill and usually have a normal systemic circulation. This permits the postischemic renal injury to be studied in relative isolation (Table 61.7).

Alejandro *et al.* [24] studied the function of 23 consecutive patients undergoing transplantation. The studies were performed intraoperatively, 60 min after reperfusion

of the allograft. The patients subsequently fell into two groups. Ten had prompt return of graft function; the remainder had delayed return of function. Renal blood flow in delayed graft function was half that in prompt graft function (Table 61.7). The renovascular resistance in delayed graft function was threefold higher than in prompt graft function. The GFR was only 6 ± 2 in delayed graft function vs 29 ± 5 ml/min/1.73 m^2 in prompt graft function. The renal plasma flow (RPF) was also significantly lower in delayed graft function than in prompt graft function. However, the fall in RPF was proportionately less than that of GFR, with the result that the filtration fraction in delayed graft function was much lower (Table 61.7). The arteriolar oncotic pressure was lower by 2 mmHg in delayed compared to prompt graft function. Because of the low filtration fraction in delayed graft function, there was little axial rise in oncotic pressure along the glomerular capillaries. Thus, π_{GC} was significantly lower in delayed compared to prompt graft function, 19.4 ± 1.0 vs 22.0 ± 1.1 mmHg, respectively. Morphometric examination of glomeruli obtained by renal biopsy was subjected to mathematical modeling and the ultrafiltration coefficient K_f was computed. The estimated allograft K_f was found not to be significantly different between the two groups – if anything, it was slightly higher in delayed compared to prompt graft function. By exclusion, it is evident from equation (61.1) that only a fall in ΔP can explain the hypofiltration in delayed graft function, assuming the mathematical modeling estimate of the K_f is correct.

The computed value for ΔP in prompt graft function

was 33.8 mm Hg vs only 20.2 mmHg in delayed graft function ($P < 0.0001$). The latter value is remarkably close to the value for π_{GC} of 19.4 mmHg in delayed graft function, and suggests that postischemic filtration failure in delayed graft function is accounted for by dissipation of the net pressure for ultrafiltration. A limitation of the study, however, is that it does not take into account the possibility of back-leak of filtrate, a phenomenon that causes the urinary clearance of a filtration marker to underestimate true GFR in postischemic ARF. Allowing for this phenomenon, however, had only a minor impact on computed ΔP, with the latter increasing from the uncorrected value of 20.2 to 20.7 mmHg.

By exclusion, it was inferred that the threefold increase of renovascular resistance in the delayed graft function group (Table 61.7) was caused by disproportionate afferent arteriolar vasoconstriction and that the ensuing fall in glomerular capillary perfusion pressure is the proximate cause of the decline in ΔP and the predominant reason for the observed hypofiltration.

There was a paucity of tubule cell exfoliation and absence of apparent tubular obstruction, but this should not be misconstrued as indicating that tubular injury was not a prominent feature. On the contrary, delayed graft function was characterized by severe disruption of the cytoskeleton of proximal tubular cells. Striking attenuation of the brush border of apical membranes and marked loss of basolateral membrane infoldings were evident in half the tubules (Figure 61.2). These cells had lost their polarity [25]. Neither Na^+, K^+-ATPase nor ankyrin and fodrin were retained in the basolateral membrane. They became detached from the basolateral membrane and

were endocytosed. This would impair vectorial Na^+ transport, and explain the observation that a major fraction of filtered sodium was excreted into the urine. Impaired proximal Na^+ reabsorption, in turn, should have enhanced delivery of this ion to the macula densa, and activated TGF. An ensuing afferent vasoconstriction with a downstream fall in ΔP thus provides an important potential link between tubular injury and filtration failure in this setting.

Mechanisms of filtration failure following cardiac surgery

As stated previously, postischemic ARF in humans occurs most commonly after an episode of hypotension and reduced renal bloodflow rather than after the total renal ischemia that precipitates delayed graft function. A prototype of this injury is that which follows cardiac surgery.

Myers and his colleagues (summarized in [26, 27]) studied the 'normal' renal response to cardiac surgery in 50 patients during cardiopulmonary bypass (CPB) and again on the first postoperative day (Table 61.8). Mannitol (20%) was routinely infused early in the procedure. This was combined with volume expansion until the hematocrit was reduced below 30%. With the use of this renoprotective regime, the incidence of postoperative ARF was only 2%. They found that postoperative ARF following cardiac surgery occurred in the wake of events that are stimuli of renal vasoconstriction. The first was CPB itself, during which an extracorporeal pump maintained the circulation while the heart was being repaired. To prevent traumatic hemolysis, the perfusion rate

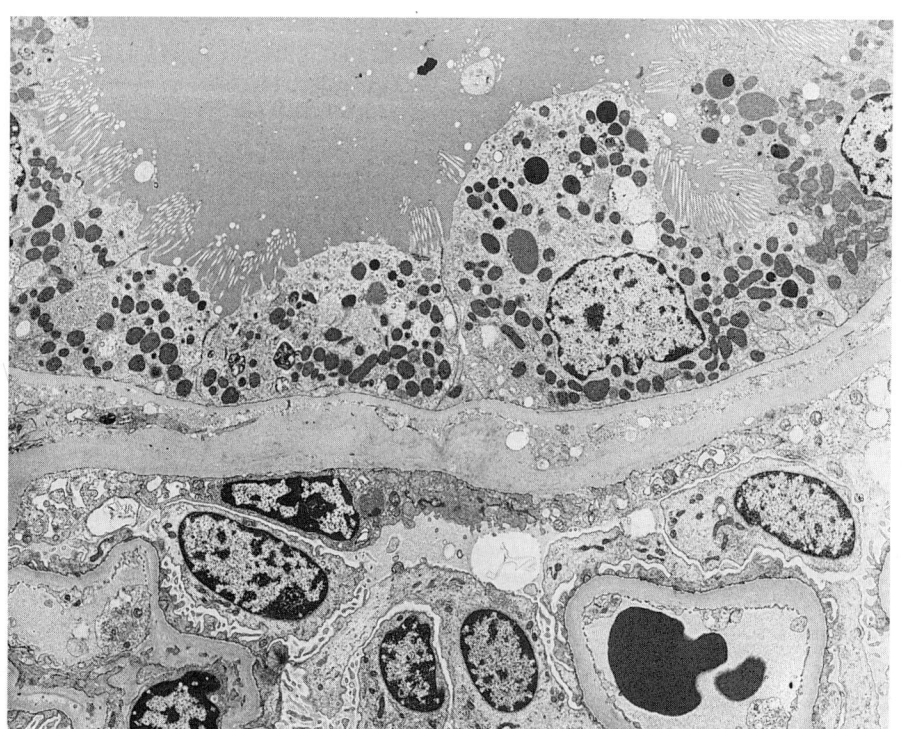

Figure 61.2 Electron photomicrograph (×6000) of a proximal tubule (upper) and loops of glomerular tuft (below). The subject had delayed graft function. Tubule cell damage is marked and includes attenuation and loss of apical brush border, along with an absence of basolateral membrane infoldings. Foot processes of the glomerular epithelial cells are broadened and effaced in segmental fashion. (Reproduced, with permission, from Alejandro, D. et al. [24].)

(~40 ml/kg/min) and pressure (40–50 mmHg) in the extracorporeal circuit were kept low. This corresponded to a renal blood flow less than 30% of normal (<280 ml/min).

The mean arterial pressure (MAP) averaged 49 mmHg during bypass (Table 61.8, column 1). Micropuncture studies in the rat suggest that at this level of MAP the pressure in glomerular capillaries would be 25 mmHg, on average [28]. This value for glomerular capillary pressure is similar to the normal opposing oncotic pressure, and should have brought glomerular ultrafiltration to a halt. The mannitol/saline regimen, however, led to considerable hemodilution with the result that π_A fell from a preoperative value of 23.5 to only 9.6 mmHg (Table 61.8, column 1). Thus despite the likelihood that glomerular capillary pressure was low, the ΔP must have exceeded π_A by several mmHg to explain the observed GFR of 48 ml/min during CPB (Table 61.8, column 1). The GFR achieved on postoperative day 1 was normal (Table 61.8, column 2).

Maintenance and recovery stages of ARF

Myers *et al.* next studied 50 patients developing postoperative ARF under the foregoing regimen. Renal physiologic measurements were performed and cardiac performance evaluated between postoperative days 4 and 7. A model of creatinine kinetics was used to compute daily changes in GFR and to classify the ARF into one of two types (Figure 61.3) [1, 24, 29]. Type A, or abbreviated ARF, refers to a course in which no maintenance stage was discernible; the initiation stage was represented by a sharp decline in GFR, and was followed immediately by a ramp-like increase in GFR, representing the stage of recovery. This pattern was exhibited by 27 patients. Type B, or overt ARF, refers to a course in which the step decline in GFR during the initiation stage was followed by a low plateau of GFR, representing a maintenance stage that lasted for seven days or more. This occurred in the remaining 23 cases. A total of 50 patients who made an uneventful recovery from cardiac surgery served as controls. The patients who developed either type A or B ARF differed from the non-azotemic controls in that they were difficult to wean from CPB because of a low cardiac output and severe hypotension. All required infusion of inotropic agents. A majority of type B patients and a substantial minority of type A patients required an intra-aortic balloon pump to maintain an adequate circulation. Mannitol/saline volume expansion to 5% body weight on the day of surgery was replaced on subsequent days by colloid volume expansion (Figure 61.3). Despite the greater preloading and a comparable afterload, cardiac performance was clearly inferior in type B compared to that associated with type A renal injury. Those with type B injury exhibited prolonged and severe postoperative left ventricular dysfunction and a low cardiac output (Figure 61.4).

Tubular and glomerular function are summarized in Table 61.8 (columns 3 and 4). Both groups were non-oliguric, a finding typical of ARF in a setting of renoprotection [1]. Reflecting more severe tubular injury, however, type B patients exhibited isosthenuria and excreted a high fraction of the filtered sodium load. In keeping with recovering tubular function, type A patients excreted a relatively concentrated urine and reabsorbed

Table 61.8 Tubular and glomerular function during and after cardiac surgery

	Uncomplicated course		Postoperative ARF	
	CPB	Post-op Day 1	Type A	Type B
Number	50	50	27	23
Urine flow (ml/min)	2.3 ± 0.3	1.9 ± 0.2	1.7 ± 0.3	1.6 ± 0.2
Urine-to-plasma osmolality	ND	1.94 ± 0.07	1.35 ± 0.05*	1.06 ± 0.03*†
Fractional excretion of sodium (%)	ND	1.2 ± 0.2	1.9 ± 0.6	7.7 ± 1.5*†
Glomerular filtration rate (ml/min/1.73 m²)	48 ± 3*	97 ± 3	36 ± 3*	11 ± 1*†
Afferent oncotic pressure (mmHg)	9.6 ± 0.3*	20.3 ± 0.3	21.5 ± 0.5	25.3 ± 0.8*
Mean arterial pressure (mmHg)	49 ± 8*	87 ± 2	79 ± 1*	78 ± 2*

Postoperative ARF patients were studied between days 4 and 7 postop:
*$P < 0.01$ vs normal, post-op day 1.
†$P < 0.01$ vs type B vs Type A.
ND = not done.
Abbreviations: ARF, acute renal failure; CPB, cardiopulmonary bypass; type A and type B refer to clinical course of renal failure (see text).
From reference [26].

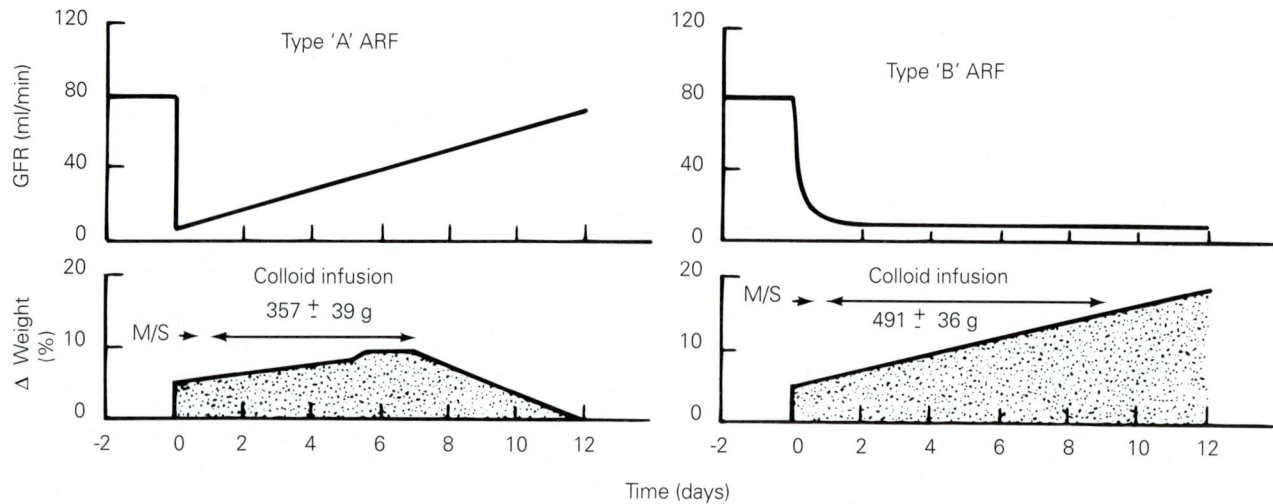

Figure 61.3 Course of ARF following cardiac surgery in 50 patients: 27 patients exhibited type A injury (left) and 23 type B injury (right). Changes in computed GFR are in upper panel. Weight change and fluid infusion regimens are in lower panel. M/S, mannitol/saline expansion. (Reproduced, with permission, from Myers [26].)

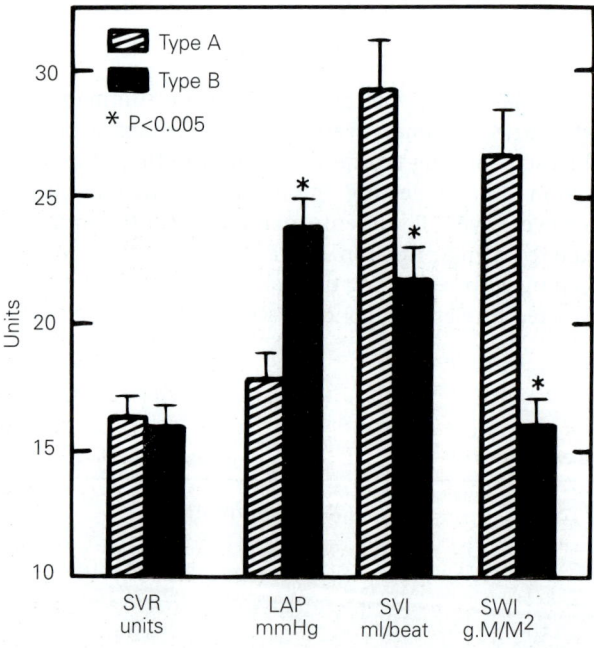

Figure 61.4 Cardiac performance on postoperative day 4–7 in patients with type A (hatched bars) vs type B (black bars) acute renal failure. SVR, systemic vascular resistance; LAP, left atrial filling pressure (from occlusion pulmonary artery pressure); SVI, stroke volume index; SWI, stroke work index. (Reproduced, with permission, from Myers [26].)

filtered sodium efficiently. Although still profoundly depressed, inulin clearance in the recovering type A group was threefold higher than in the type B group.

Myers *et al.* have published indirect evidence for transtubular back-leak of the glomerular filtrate (including inulin) in patients with type B ARF [30]. The true GFR in the type B patients was 15 ml/min, 4 ml/min higher than the inulin clearance of 11 ml/min. Clearly, type B patients had severe filtration failure even when back-leak is taken into account. This suggests that, like standard animal models and human delayed graft function, the injury following prolonged, partial renal ischemia, is characterized by a reduction in ΔP.

In ARF following cardiac surgery persistent damage to the myocardium is largely responsible for the low renal perfusion rate and for prolonging the postischemic injury. Many other stimuli to renal vasoconstriction abound in the postoperative period, however. These include depression of MAP below the autoregulatory range by the use of afterload reducing agents, administration of inotropic agents that have renal vasoconstrictor properties, and exposure to nephrotoxic antibiotics and contrast agents. These discrete glomerulodepressor phenomena are compounded by the frequent coexistence of multiorgan failure. Findings associated with the latter include hepatic necrosis, disseminated intravascular coagulation, and positive pressure ventilation to correct respiratory failure. All stimulate and could perpetuate renal vasoconstriction, thereby preventing the postischemic injury from entering its recovery stage. It is not surprising that two-thirds of such patients die without recovering adequate renal function. Even among survivors, this form of ARF is not always reversible, sometimes necessitating permanent dialysis for the ensuing chronic renal failure.

Postrenal ARF

The incidence of postrenal ARF rises in older men. Obstruction of the urethra at the bladder neck by prostatic hyperplasia or cancer is the most common cause. If promptly recognized, postrenal ARF is usually reversible.

Blockade of the ureter by a stone or external compression by tumor or stricture less often leads to ARF because both ureters have to be blocked, unless one kidney is absent or not functioning. Intrarenal obstruction of the distal tubule may occur due to high concentrations of protein (myeloma), uric acid (tumor lysis syndrome), calcium or drugs, but these represent examples of intrinsic renal failure rather than postrenal failure.

Pathology

As noted above, the lesions described in the first studies of human ARF included patchy distribution of tubule necrosis with exfoliation of tubule cells from the tubular of the basement membrane and an ensuing obstruction of the tubule lumina. A more uniform distribution of proximal tubule necrosis was attributed to nephrotoxic ARF. A voluminous literature has accumulated since the early studies of human ARF, but has exhibited an imbalance between an enormous number of studies conducted on experimental animals under controlled conditions on the one hand and a relative paucity of observations of the pathology of human ARF on the other. Studies of the kidney in autopsies of ARF patients revealed the lesions described above, but only to a mild degree, if at all. More recently a biopsy study disclosed a number of abnormalities, but only focal, mild necrosis of the proximal and distal nephron and loss of attenuation of the apical brush border in proximal tubule cells was more frequent in electron than in photomicrographs of ARF kidney tissue those of control kidney tissue. Progress has been hindered by the lack of standard quantitative criteria for pathologic diagnosis of human ARF. A host of monoclonal antibodies to molecules which may play a pathogenic role in ARF is beginning to be applied to the study of kidney tissue in ARF.

Diagnosis and differential diagnosis

A systematic approach based on history, physical exam and a few tests is usually enough to determine the cause of ARF in 90% of cases. The first goal is to distinguish among prerenal, renal and postrenal groups; the second is to identify a specific cause. The history is the most important source of information. It should focus on symptoms related to the heart and circulation, infection, systemic illnesses and exposure to nephrotoxins and medications. An abrupt decline in urine output to zero usually indicates postrenal ARF or a vascular catastrophe; other complaints suggestive of obstruction are symptoms of prostatism, flank pain, hematuria and a history of cancer.

In the physical exam, one should look for loss of skin turgor and dryness of the tongue or, conversely elevated jugular venous pressure and peripheral edema. Other signs to assess include fever, tachycardia, hypotension or an orthostatic fall in blood pressure, congestive heart failure, pericarditis, skin rash and other signs of systemic disease, and an enlarged urinary bladder. The mental status and peripheral nervous system should be assessed to gauge the severity of uremia.

Laboratory tests are a vital aid to diagnosis. Blood should be obtained for red cell (RBC) count or hematocrit, white cell count and differential, platelet count, blood urea nitrogen, serum creatinine, glucose, electrolytes (Na, K, Cl, HCO_3), Ca, P, Mg, bilirubin, total protein and albumin. Specific serologic tests to rule out causes of rapidly progressive nephritis may be appropriate. On urinalysis a high specific gravity points to prerenal ARF. Heavy proteinuria suggests glomerulonephritis or myeloma. Granular casts and pigmented casts accompany renal ARF. Urine RBCs (before catheterization) indicate renal or postrenal ARF; RBC casts are diagnostic of acute glomerulonephritis. Tests for hemoglobin (hemolysis) or myoglobin (rhabdomyolysis) should be done if these toxins are suspected.

To distinguish prerenal ARF from ATN, the concentration of serum sodium (S_{Na}) and urine sodium (U_{Na}) and serum creatinine (S_{Cr}) and urine creatinine (U_{Cr}) are measured for calculation of fractional excretion of Na (FE_{Na}):

$$FENa(\%) = \left(\frac{U_{Na}}{S_{Na}}\right) \Big/ \left(\frac{U_{Cr}}{S_{Cr}}\right) \times 100 \qquad (61.2)$$

If FE_{Na} is equal to or less than ($\leq$) 1%, the diagnosis is prerenal ARF; if FE_{Na} is greater than (>) 1%, the likely diagnosis is ATN. If the renal circulation is impaired but the renal tubule is uninjured, as in prerenal ARF, then the tubule will reabsorb nearly all the filtered sodium, and U_{Na} (<30 mEq/l) and FE_{Na} ($\leq$1%) will be low. If the tubule is damaged, as in ATN, it will not reabsorb sodium well and U_{Na} (>30 mEq/l) and FE_{Na} (>1%) will rise. (S_{Na} reflects glomerular filtrate Na. The ratio, U_{Cr}/S_{Cr}, corrects for fluid reasorption; the higher the value, the higher the fractional reabsorption of water.)

There are important limitations to FE_{Na}: it does not distinguish acute glomerulonephritis from prerenal ARF, or interstitial nephritis from ATN. FE_{Na} is not useful in postrenal ARF. FE_{Na} is unreliable if the patient has chronic renal failure or has received diuretics. Although a low FE_{Na} does occur in acute interstitial nephritis as might be expected, the usual presentation is with a high FENa, so this test is not useful in this condition. In the absence of FE_{Na}, U_{Na} alone may be helpful. If U_{Na} > 30 mEq/l, the diagnosis is likely ATN; a lower value signifies prerenal ARF.

If FE_{Na} or U_{Na} is equivocal or cannot be measured and prerenal ARF is suspected, the physician should administer intravenous (i.v.) saline 0.9% (500 ml) or a diuretic, e.g. furosemide (40 mg), and observe the response. Those with prerenal ARF should respond with an increase in urinary flow. Those with ATN usually will not respond.

Further steps are necessary to establish postrenal ARF. Ultrasound examination of the bladder pre- and post-micturition is sufficient to exclude urethral obstruction, if this is not available then the bladder should be catheterized after the patient voids. A residual urine volume of >150 ml suggests urethral obstruction. Ultrasonographic imaging of the kidney is valuable in diagnosis of postrenal ARF. It can reveal hydronephrosis or the absence of one kidney and obstruction of the other and may disclose a kidney stone or a bladder indentation due to an enlarged prostate. It should be remembered that with acute obstruction, renal failure may develop without evidence of hydronephrosis.

The foregoing tests are usually sufficient to determine the diagnosis. If it is still in doubt, a percutaneous renal biopsy should be performed to clarify the underlying disease process.

Treatment

The goal of treatment of prerenal ARF is to correct the underlying cause. Initial management of postrenal ARF is relief of obstruction; thereafter a urologist will determine and treat the cause of obstruction. Treatment of rapidly progressive glomerulonephritis, acute interstitial nephritis and hemolytic uremic syndrome is specific for each disorder and is reviewed in the respective chapters. This section considers the general conservative management of patients with renal ARF [3–6, 31].

Conservative management

Daily clinical and biochemical monitoring of fluid balance, serum creatinine, blood urea nitrogen, electrolytes (Na, K, Cl, HCO_3), Ca, P and medications is essential. Adjustment of dosage and dosing frequency of medications is often necessary. A basic rule is that the patient should not be administered anything in excess of what he or she can metabolize or excrete.

Fluid management

Fluid balance is monitored by the record of intake and output, body weight, arterial pressure, pulse and physical exam. Usually a postoperative patient loses an average of 0.5 kg body weight a day from catabolism alone. Daily fluid losses not due to catabolism are replaced by administration of 500 ml (to compensate for insensible losses), 500 ml per each degree (C°) temperature above normal, and a volume equal to urine flow and gastrointestinal and tube drainage losses. The replacement fluid is dextrose and water. Electrolytes are added as needed to compensate for estimated losses. Diuretics can be used in an effort to maintain urine flow above 500 ml per day to facilitate fluid management. ATN is often unresponsive to diuretics, however, and high doses of furosemide for example are ototoxic, and should be avoided. Blood pressure should be maintained at normal levels to ensure an adequate renal circulation. Repeatedly, the patient should be

evaluated for pulmonary edema. If signs develop, fluid balance should be maintained negative – use additional diuretic therapy if necessary. In the maintenance phase of a patient with ATN, the daily urine output is helpful in management but it rarely requires or warrants the use of the indwelling Foley catheter, whether or not the patient is undergoing dialysis. The indication for the indwelling catheter is the same in ARF as in other conditions: inability to void in the presence of a large urinary bladder. Failure to abide by this principle risks a urinary tract infection in these immunosuppressed patients. It is reasonable to monitor minute-by-minute urine output in patients undergoing continous fluid removal, if the rate of parenteral fluid administration is high.

Metabolic complications

Hyperkalemia is the most serious complication. Mild elevations of serum potassium (<6 mEq/l) are treated by removal of sources of potassium. Higher elevations require treatment to: (1) combat cardiac arrhythmia (calcium gluconate 10% solution, 10–30 ml iv); (2) shift potassium from blood to cells ($NaHCO_3$, 45–135 mEq, 50–150 ml, iv, and/or glucose 10%, 500 ml, plus regular insulin 10 units, iv); and (3) remove potassium by the intestinal route (potassium exchange resin 20–50 g, plus sorbitol 70%, 20 ml oral or 70 ml rectal). Hyponatremia reflects excess body water and is treated by restriction of fluid. Hyperphosphatemia should be treated to raise a low serum calcium by oral phosphate binders, aluminum hydroxide or calcium carbonate. Calcium gluconate will raise serum calcium if there is risk of tetany. Metabolic acidosis is inevitable and should be combated by HCO_3, nutritional therapy and treatment of infection. To calculate HCO_3 deficit, multiply the difference between the serum HCO_3 and the normal value by 50% of body weight (in kg). Restoration of low HCO_3 stores may be limited by the low GFR. If sodium is lost in the urine or by other routes, HCO_3 can be administered as $NaHCO_3$. Respiratory acidosis is treated by intubation and assisted respiration. The goal of nutritional therapy is to minimize negative nitrogen balance. The initial aim is to administer 50 calories/kg body weight/day. This can be met by glucose (20–70%) and fat emulsion (10–20%) solutions if parenteral feeding is required [30]. Protein, 0.5 g/kg orally, or 10–20 g essential amino acids iv, each day is sufficient. Subsequent adjustment of nutritional therapy depends on the severity of the catabolic state (blood urea nitrogen (BUN), acidosis, weight loss) versus complications that attend nutritional therapy – excess fluid administration, catheter infection, acidosis and a rising BUN [32].

Neurologic manifestations

These correlate imperfectly with the blood urea nitrogen. Asterixis is the most useful sign of uremic encephalopathy. It is elicited with arms fully extended, hands extended at the wrist and fingers spread as if to stop traffic. It manifests as an irregular loss of hand extension that resembles a weak waving of the hands, and is identical to the asterixis observed in hepatic and respiratory encephalopathy. An altered level of consciousness is another common manifestation of uremic neurotoxicity. Isolated and irregular myoclonus involving large muscle groups in asymmetric fashion are also frequent. Hiccoughs (diaphragmatic myoclonus) is an example. Tremors may indicate impending seizures due to electrolyte disorders, hypoglycemia or hypoxemia. Besides correcting these underlying causes, treatment with anticonvulsant drugs (phenobarbital, diphenylhydantoin or diazepam) should be considered.

Hematologic disorders

These are frequent. The hematocrit should be maintained at 30% by transfusions. If dialysis is initiated promptly, bleeding is not usually a problem but when it is, prolonged bleeding times can be treated with desmopressin, conjugated estrogen (premarin), or plasma cryoprecipitate, but this is rarely necessary.

Infection

The risk of infection, a common cause of death in ARF, is increased by impaired immunoresistance and breakdown of normal infection barriers due to open wounds, intravenous and bladder catheters and tracheal intubation. Sterile tracheal suction should be used, intravenous lines should be avoided if possible, and the bladder catheter should be discontinued during the maintenance phase of ARF to reduce the risk of infection.

Dialysis

In the majority of patients with renal ARF (as opposed to prerenal or postrenal ARF), dialysis is necessary and should be initiated soon after the diagnosis is established. In this way the complications of uremia can be prevented or minimized. Absolute indications are: BUN > 100 mg/dl or S_{Cr} > 8 mg/dl, serum HCO_3 < 15 mEq/l, serum K > 6.0 mEq/l, serum Na < 120 mEq/l, persistent vomiting, pulmonary edema, uremic bleeding, seizures and coma. Either peritoneal dialysis (PD) or hemodialysis (HD) is suitable. For patients with severe catabolism or needing rapid fluid and electrolyte correction, HD is preferable. In the surgical intensive care unit, the large volumes of fluid administered, the instability of the circulation and the nature of the surgery have led to increasing use of continuous hemofiltration and dialysis techniques. Although there is little evidence to date that these new techniques have improved the outcome, they facilitate fluid and electrolyte management. Continuous hemofiltration and dialysis, PD and HD, are described in Chapters 80, 80–82 and 73–75, respectively.

Peptide therapy of ARF

Several peptides have been tested in ARF to see if recovery of renal function can be accelerated, by which is meant a faster return of GFR [33, 34]. It must first be acknowledged that causing a more rapid restoration of GFR may be a mixed blessing. An improvement in GFR facilitates fluid management and reduces the need for dialysis – both clear advantages. Thurau and Boylan [35], however, pointed out that if tubuloglomerular feedback is operative in ARF, the result is to suppress GFR of the injured nephron, until the tubule regenerates and recovers sufficiently to assume the normal work load [33] (see above). If GFR returns before the tubule has recovered, O_2 and other energy substrates may theoretically be diverted from the healing process for reabsorptive work and reinjure the regenerating nephron. Rahman *et al.* [33] have published a study showing that atrial natriuretic peptide (ANP) hastened the return of GFR in patients with ARF. Mortality was not significantly lowered, however. Given the widespread effects of ANP, for example, vasodilatation and suppression of cardiac contraction, it may be prudent to await the results of further trials. Insulin-like growth factor (IGF) has been shown to accelerate return of GFR in animal models of ARF [34]. When further work is accomplished in this field, we might to have available for the first time specific treatment for this distressing condition.

Course and outcome

In patients with prerenal ARF, restoration of the renal circulation, if initiated promptly and successfully, is usually followed by recovery of renal function. In the patient with renal ARF owing to a glomerular or interstitial disorder, the prognosis depends on the nature and extent of the underlying injury. Discontinuation of the offending agent is usually followed by a full recovery of renal function after drug-induced acute interstitial nephritis. In patients managed conservatively, oliguria (<400 ml/day) is usually associated with a worse prognosis; it has little prognostic value in patients undergoing dialysis. The longer the duration of ARF, the less likely that recovery of renal function will occur, especially if the cause is glomerulonephritis or vasculitis. After a prolonged period, usually weeks, if the presumptive diagnosis is ATN, a renal biopsy and renal imaging techniques may be warranted to rule out other causes of ARF.

The onset of the recovery phase may be heralded by an increase in urinary flow. In patients undergoing dialysis, this occurs in the interdialytic period. The most reliable indicator, however, is a fall in serum creatinine or a slower rate of rise in serum creatinine between dialyses. Although this is an encouraging development, the patient remains vulnerable to all of the complications described above. In some cases urinary flow reaches several liters a day, as the return of GFR outstrips the recovery of tubule reabsorptive function. This is especially common during recovery from postrenal ARF. Among several contributing factors to the diuresis are excess fluid administration and diuretics, retained urea, sodium and other solutes, circulating ANP, and impaired reabsorption of sodium and water in the recovering tubule. Fluid should be replaced at a rate equal to urinary flow with 0.45% saline containing appropriate other electrolytes until it is judged that the kidney has recovered sufficiently to respond to homeostatic requirements. The patient by this time should be able to drink to quench thirst.

The literature does not convincingly portray a brighter picture for survival from ARF; mortality still exceeds 50% on average. Of those who survive, furthermore, the kidney may only partially recover or even not at all. By and large, however, recovery of renal function in those who survive is sufficient for a normal existence.

Prevention

ARF can be prevented by avoiding or correcting predisposing conditions [3–6, 36]. One should ensure adequate circulatory and extracellular fluid volume to maintain blood pressure and urine flow in patients with trauma, burns, septic or cardiogenic shock or nephrotoxic drugs. In those with borderline renal function who are to undergo major surgery, mannitol infusion may prevent kidney injury. Patients with heart failure need treatment to optimize their cardiac function. Radiographic contrast material should be used as infrequently and in as small doses as possible in patients at risk of contrast nephrotoxicity. At risk include those with pre-existing renal failure, diabetic nephropathy, multiple myeloma, other proteinuric conditions and old age. Such patients should be infused with a 500–1000 ml of half normal or normal saline before and throughout contrast administration [36] NSAIDs predispose to ARF when the renal circulation is impaired and should be discontinued. If nephrotoxic antimicrobials are necessary, the dose and dosing interval must be adjusted to avoid high blood levels. For cancer patients receiving chemotherapy, the tumor lysis syndrome can be avoided by infusion of $NaHCO_3$ and the administration of allopurinol. The latter treatment also reduces the risk of ARF in patients with hemoglobin or myoglobin in their urine.

References

1. Myers, B.D. and Moran, S.M. (1986) Hemodynamically mediated acute renal failure. *N. Engl. J. Med.*, **314**, 97–105.
2. Brezis, M., Rosen, S. and Epstein, F.H. (1991), in *The Kidney*, 4th edn (eds B.M. Brenner and F.C. Rector, Jr.), W.B. Saunders, Philadelphia, pp. 993–1061.
3. Lieberthal, W. and Levinsky, N.G. (1992) Acute clinical renal failure, in *The Kidney Physiology and Pathophysiology*, 2nd edn (eds D.W. Seldin and G. Giebisch), Raven Press, New York, pp. 3181–226.
4. Anderson, R.J. (1993) Prevention and management of acute renal failure. *Hosp. Pract.*, **August**, 61–75.
5. Fish, E.M. and Molitoris, B.A. (1994) Mechanisms of disease: alterations in epithelial polarity and the pathogenesis of disease states. *N. Engl. J. Med.*, **330**, 580–8.
6. Thadhani, R., Pascual, M. and Bonventre, J.V. (1996) Acute renal failure. *N. Engl. J. Med.*, **334**, 1448–60.
7. Hou, S.H., Bushinsky, D.A., Wish, J.B. *et al.* (1983) Hospital-acquired renal insufficiency: a prospective study. *Am. J. Med.*, **74**, 243–8.
8. Smith, H.W. (1951) *The Kidney Structure and Function in Health and Disease*. Oxford University Press, New York, pp. 752–813.
9. Bywaters, E.G.L. and Dible, J.H. (1942) The renal lesion in traumatic anuria. *J. Path. Bact.*, **54**, 111–22.
10. Oliver, J., MacDowell, M. and Tracy, A. (1951) Pathogenesis of acute renal failure associated with traumatic and toxic injury: renal ischemia, nephrotoxic damage and the ischemic episode. *J. Clin. Invest.*, **30**, 1305–51.
11. Lucké, B. (1946) Lower nephron nephrosis: the renal lesions of the of the crush syndrome of burns, transfusions, and the conditions affecting the lower segment of the nephrons. *Milit. Surg.*, **99**, 371–415.
12. Pusey, C.D. and Rees, A.J. (1992) Acute renal failure due to glomerulonephritis and vasculitis, in *Oxford Textbook of Clinical Nephrology* (eds S. Cameron, A.M. Davison, J. Grunfeld, *et al.*), Oxford University Press, Oxford, pp. 418–38.
13. Monteseny, J.J., Meyrier, A., Kleinknecht, D. *et al.* (1995) The current spectrum of infectious glomerulonephritis. Experience with 76 patients and review of the literature. *Medicine*, **74**, 63–73.
14. Bell, W.R., Braine, H.G., Ness, P.M. *et al.* (1991) Improved survival in thrombotic thrombocytopenic purpura–hemolytic uremic syndrome. Clinical experience in 108 patients. *N. Engl. J. Med.*, **325**, 398–403.
15. Remuzzi, G. and Ruggenenti, P. (1995) The hemolytic uremic syndrome. *Kidney Int.*, **47**, 2–19.
16. Ten, R.M., Torres, V.E., Milliner, D.S. *et al.* (1988) Acute interstitial nephritis: Immunologic and clinical aspects. *Mayo Clin. Proc.*, **63**, 921–30.
17. Nielson, E.G. (1989) Pathogenesis and therapy of interstitial nephritis. *Kidney Int.*, **35**, 1257–70.
18. Myers, B.D., Miller, C., Mehigan, J. *et al.* (1984) Nature of the renal injury following total renal ischemia in man. *J. Clin. Invest.*, **73**, 329–41.
19. Hanley, M.J. and Davidson, K. (1981) Prior mannitol and furosemide infusion in a model of ischemic acute renal failure. *Am. J. Physiol.*, **241**, F556–64.

20. Cox, J.W., Baehler, R.W., Sharma, H. *et al.* (1974) Studies on the mechanisms of oliguria in a model of unilateral acute renal failure. *J. Clin. Invest.*, **53**, 1546–58.

21. Tanner, G.A. and Knopp, L.C. (1986) Glomerular blood flow after single nephron obstruction in the rat kidney. *Am. J. Physiol.*, **250**, F77–85.

22. Robinette, J.B. and Conger, J.D. (1990) Angiotensin and thromboxane in the enhanced renal adrenergic nerve sensitivity of acute renal failure. *J. Clin. Invest.*, **86**, 1532–9.

23. Hefty, T., Fraser, S., Nelson, K. *et al.* (1992) Comparison of UW and Euro-Collins solutions in paired cadaveric kidneys. *Transplantation*, **53**, 491–2.

24. Alejandro, V., Scandling, J.D., Sibley, R.K. *et al.* (1995) Mechanisms of filtration failure during postischemic injury of the human kidney: a study of the reperfused renal allograft. *J. Clin. Invest.*, **95**, 820–31.

25. Alejandro, V., Nelson, W.J., Huie, P. *et al.* (1995) Postischemic injury, delayed function and Na$^+$/K$^+$-ATPase distribution in the transplanted kidney. *Kidney Int.*, **48**, 1308–15.

26. Myers, B.D. (1989) Nature of postischemic renal Injury following aortic or cardiac surgery, in *Acute Renal Failure in the Intensive Therapy Unit*, Acute Renal Failure Workshop, Avignon, France. Springer-Verlag, Berlin, pp. 167–80.

27. Hilberman, M., Myers, B.D., Carrie, B.J. *et al.* (1979) Acute renal failure following cardiac surgery. *Am. J. Cardiovasc. Thorac. Surg.*, **77**, 880–8.

28. Johnston, P.A., Bernard, D.B., Donohoe, J.F. *et al.* (1979) Effect of volume expansion on hemodynamics of the hypoperfused rat kidney. *J. Clin. Invest.* **64**, 550–8.

29. Moran, S.M. and Myers, B.D. (1985) Course of acute renal failure studied by a model of creatinine kinetics. *Kidney Int.*, **27**, 928–37.

30. Myers, B.D., Chui, R., Hilberman, M. *et al.* (1979) Transtubular leakage of glomerular filtrate in human acute renal failure. *Am. J. Physiol.*, **234**, F319–25.

31. Humes, H.D. and Paganini, E.P. (1994) Nephrology and the medical intensive care unit. *Semin. Nephrol.*, **14**, 3–97.

32. Sponsel, H. and Conger, J.D. (1995) Is parenteral nutritional therapy of value in acute renal failure patients? *Am. J. Kidney Dis.*, **25**, 96–102.

33. Rahman, S.N., Kim, G.E., Mathew, A.S. *et al.* (1994) Effects of atrial natriuretic peptide in clinical acute renal failure. *Kidney Int.*, **45**, 1731–8.

34. Rabkin, R. (1995) Insulin-like growth factor-1 treatment of acute renal failure. *J. Lab. Clin. Med.*, **125**, 684–5.

35. Thurau, K. and Boylan, J.A. (1976) Acute renal success: the unexpected logic of oliguria in acute renal failure. *Am. J. Med.*, **61**, 308–15.

36. Solomon, R., Werner, C., Mann, D. *et al.* (1994) Effects of saline, mannitol, and furosemide on acute decreases in renal function induced by radiocontrast agents. *N. Engl. J. Med.*, **331**, 1416–20.

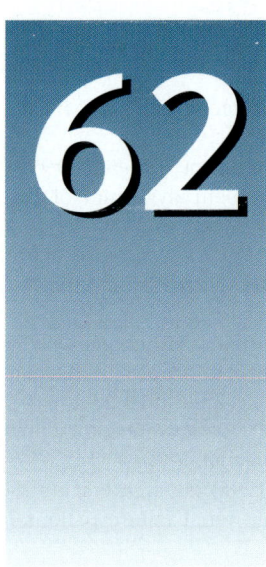

62

Pathophysiology and treatment of nephrolithiasis

Lisa A. Ruml and Charles Y.C. Pak

Introduction

Nephrolithiasis is not only a very common disorder, but the incidence of 0.5–1% in industrialized countries appears to be on the increase. About 5–10% of the population will have a stone in their lifetime. Fortunately, during the last two decades, there have been advances made in the treatment of urinary calculi which are able to significantly attenuate subsequent stone production in those who suffer from kidney stones [1]. It has become increasingly apparent that certain metabolic derangements can produce a urinary environment conducive to stone formation and that correction of the metabolic abnormality (or abnormalities) can slow or prevent the progression of stone disease [2].

Three-quarters of the stones formed in the urinary tract are composed of calcium (calcareous stones) with most being composed of calcium oxalate either alone or in combination with hydroxyapatite $(Ca_{10}(OH)_2(PO_4)_6)$. A small number of stones are composed of calcium phosphate as brushite $(CaHPO_4 \cdot 2H_2O)$. The remaining 25% of urinary calculi are non-calcareous in nature, being composed of struvite, uric acid or cystine [3]. To a degree, the types of metabolic derangements that are present will dictate the types of stones that occur (Table 62.1). In addition, certain nutritional and environmental factors may modify the urinary composition and alter an overall propensity to stone formation. With a thorough evaluation, abnormalities that predispose to stone formation can be identified in more than 95% of patients (Table 62.2). Although stone disease is a surgical as well as medical condition, this chapter discusses the types of physiologic abnormalities which may lead to stones and emphasizes medical treatments targeted to the specific metabolic abnormality present.

Clinical manifestations

There have been descriptions of the symptoms of urinary calculi for centuries, with pain being by far the most clinically significant symptom. Obstruction of the urinary tract results in severe, unilateral, flank pain, often with radiation into the groin, vulva or testis. Many patients describe the pain as beginning in the flank and moving anteriorly and caudally towards the pelvis. Pain may begin suddenly and, if the stone is small enough to traverse the ureter and enter the bladder, the pain may suddenly stop. Stones larger than 7 mm in diameter have a very low likelihood of passing through the ureter and beyond the ureterovesicular junction; stones less than 5 mm in diameter are likely to pass spontaneously. Intermediate-sized stones will have variable rates of passage, with factors such as the size of the ureters being factors in determining whether a stone will pass. Patients who are passing a stone may have gross hematuria if the stone causes significant abrasion of the urinary tract; almost all will have at least microhematuria. Vomiting may be present and may be severe. It should be remembered that small caliceal stones may cause intermittent

Nephrology, Edited by Rex L. Jamison and Robert Wilkinson.
Published in 1997 by Chapman & Hall, London. ISBN 0 412 60930 4

Table 62.1 Frequency of and metabolic derangements associated with various types of renal calculi

Stone type	Frequency (%)	Causes
Radiopaque stones		
Calcium oxalate	60	Hypercalciuria, hyperoxaluria, hyperuricosuria, hypocitraturia, hypomagnesiuria
Calcium phosphate (hydroxyapatite)	20	Hypercalciuria, hypocitraturia, hyperuricosuria
Brushite	2	Hypercalciuria, hypocitraturia, hyperuricosuria
Struvite or carbonate apatite	7	Infection with urease-producing organisms
Cystine	1–3	Cystinuria
Radiolucent stones		
Uric acid	7	Undue urinary acidity, hyperuricosuria, dehydration
Triamterene	<1	Triamterene therapy
2,8-dihydroxyadenine	<1	Adenine phosphoribosyl transferase deficiency
Silica	<1	Magnesium trisilicate therapy

pain even in the absence of obstruction. If infection is present, patients may complain of fever, malaise, dysuria and urinary frequency. Rarely, obstruction of the urethra by a stone may result in anuria.

In a patient with existing stones in the kidney, pain may be intermittent and the description of the pain as a dull ache may be difficult to differentiate from musculoskeletal pain. Again, pain may be present even in the absence of obstruction. Costovertebral angle tenderness is usually present.

The incidence of bladder calculi appears to decrease in conjunction with an increase in the standard of living conditions in a particular region. In Western countries, the incidence has declined with a coincident increase in the incidence of renal stones. The pelvic pain of a bladder stone may be severe, and may be exquisitely sensitive to movement.

The physical exam in a patient with renal colic is usually normal. Pain may, however, result in tachycardia and an increase in blood pressure. Costovertebral angle tenderness may be present, with light tapping often producing intense pain.

Pathophysiology of urinary calculi

There is general agreement that stone formation occurs after the nucleation of a crystal nidus and subsequent increase in the size of the concretion via crystal growth, aggregation or agglomeration [4, 5]; crystal growth may be rapid or slowly progressive. Nucleation occurs when a favorable state of urinary saturation is reached, this point being dependent on the complex interaction of the various ions. Urine will support a degree of supersaturation before nucleation occurs; this is thought to be due to the presence of natural inhibitors that are present, such as citrate, pyrophosphate and various macromolecules (glycosaminoglycans, glycopeptides, ribonucleic acids and glycoproteins) [6]. Once the limit of this metastable state is exceeded, nucleation will occur. The nidus of a stone need not be of the same composition as the rest of the stone (heterogeneous nucleation). Sodium urate crystals, which have the same crystalline spacial conformity as calcium oxalate crystals, may provide a nidus on which a calcium oxalate stone may form [7].

Hypercalciuria

Hypercalciuria is the most common metabolic abnormality present in those with urinary calculi, occurring in up to 65% of stone formers [8]. The majority of stone formers have absorptive hypercalciuria; that is, an increased intestinal calcium absorption is the primary process. Less common causes of hypercalciuria include renal calcium leak (renal hypercalciuria), primary hyperparathyroidism and renal phosphate leak. Because 60–70% of the filtered load of calcium is reabsorbed in the proximal tubule, patients with proximal tubulopathies such as Fanconi's syndrome usually have hypercalciuria.

Hypercalciuria produces an increased saturation of the urine with respect to both calcium oxalate and calcium phosphate (hydroxyapatite or brushite). It may occur as

Table 62.2 Diagnostic classification of nephrolithiasis

Classification	Prevalence (%)[a]
Absorptive hypercalciuria	20–40
Renal hypercalciuria	5–8
Primary hyperparathyroidism	3–5
Unclassified hypercalciuria	15–25
Renal phosphate leak	
Fasting hypercalciuria (with normal PTH)	
Hyperoxaluric calcium nephrolithiasis	2–15
Enteric hyperoxaluria	
Primary hyperoxaluria	
Dietary hyperoxaluria	
Hyperuricosuric calcium nephrolithiasis	10–40
Hypocitraturic calcium nephrolithiasis	10–50
Distal renal tubular acidosis	
Chronic diarrheal syndromes	
Idiopathic	
Gouty diathesis (unduly acidic urine)	15–30
Cystinuria	<1
Infection stones	1–5
Hypomagnesiuric calcium nephrolithiasis	5–10
Low urine volume	10–50
No metabolic abnormality or miscellaneous causes	<3

[a] The range in percentage represents estimates based on the experience in Dallas. The numbers exceed 100% because of the presence of multiple abnormalities in some patients.

an isolated defect or in combination with other physiologic abnormalities. Figure 62.1 shows the pathophysiologic schema for the various types of hypercalciuria.

Absorptive hypercalciuria

The cellular mechanism responsible for the increased intestinal absorption in absorptive hypercalciuria is not known. An increased level of or sensitivity to 1,25-dihydroxyvitamin D (1,25(OH)$_2$D) has been suggested as some patients have a reduction in their intestinal calcium absorption in response to ketoconazole administration (a known inhibitor of steroid synthesis). Another possibility is an abnormality in the vitamin D receptor or in the intestinal calcium binding proteins. Lastly, the defect may represent a vitamin D-independent process. Regardless of the cellular mechanism, the physiologic result is an increase in intestinal calcium absorption and resultant hypercalciuria, defined as >200 mg (>5 mmol) of calcium excreted per day when the diet is low in calcium.

Renal hypercalciuria

The mechanism of an isolated renal calcium leak is not known. It is not a normal response to dietary constituents (i.e. sodium, protein) known to induce calcium loss. Some have speculated that the tubular defect responsible for the decrease in renal calcium reabsorption is a consequence of prior urinary tract infections, as many patients will give this history. It has been reported that other abnormalities in proximal tubular function may coexist with the calcium leak. A decrease in renal magnesium reabsorption, exaggerated urinary sodium losses after thiazide administration, and a further exaggerated urinary calcium loss after carbohydrate ingestion have been reported in some patients. Secondary increases in parathyroid hormone (PTH) levels may be present, but may be masked by the enhanced intestinal calcium absorption. The increased level of circulating PTH may stimulate the synthesis of 1,25(OH)$_2$D, thereby raising intestinal calcium absorption and causing hypercalciuria.

Renal phosphate leak

The causative factor resulting in the loss of phosphate in the urine is unknown. The loss of phosphate results in low or low normal levels of serum phosphorus which act as a stimulus to the renal 1-α-hydroxylase enzyme. Increased hydroxylation of 25-hydroxy vitamin D (25-OHD) produces increased serum levels of 1,25(OH)$_2$D and, therefore, an increased intestinal absorption of calcium. The increase in the filtered load of calcium may result in hypercalciuria. In general, the increased levels of 1,25(OH)$_2$D and increased intestinal calcium absorption both act to suppress serum PTH levels, though PTH usually remains in the normal range.

Excess of 1,25(OH)$_2$D

Primary hyperparathyroidism

One of the actions of PTH is to increase production of 1,25(OH)$_2$D by enhancing the activity of renal 1-α-hydroxylase. Increased levels of 1,25(OH)$_2$D then act on intestinal mucosal cells to increase the intestinal absorption of calcium. PTH also increases bone resorption and this, in addition to the increased amount of absorbed calcium, leads to an increase in the filtered load of calcium and hypercalciuria. Hypercalciuria ensues because the increase in the filtered load is greater than the increase in proximal tubular reabsorption of calcium produced by the parathyroid stimulation.

Sarcoidosis and other granulomatous diseases

Granulomata have the capability of hydroxylating 25-OHD due to the presence of 1-α-hydroxylase in the granuloma cells. The activity of the enzyme does not respond

Absorptive Hypercalciuria

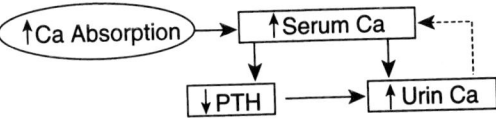

Renal Hypercalciuria

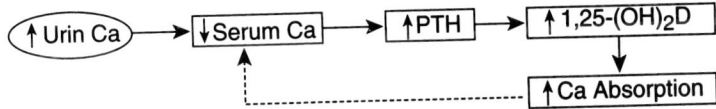

Resorptive Hypercalciuria

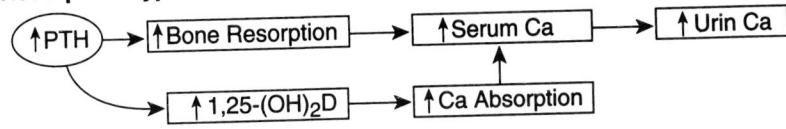

Renal Phosphate Leak

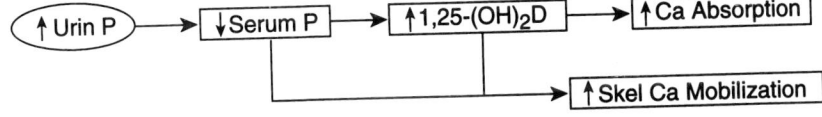

Primary Enhancement of 1,25-(OH)₂D Production

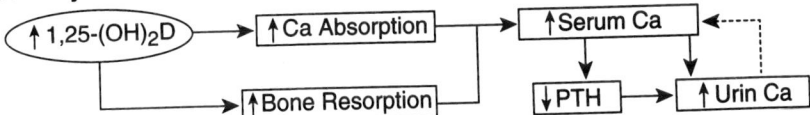

Figure 62.1 Physiologic changes resulting in hypercalciuria. PTH, parathyroid hormone; 1,25(OH)₂D, 1,25-dihydroxyvitamin D.

to normal feedback mechanisms, resulting in unregulated production of 1,25(OH)$_2$D. This extrarenal production of 1,25(OH)$_2$D causes hypercalciuria (with or without coexistent hypercalcemia). Up to 50% of patients with sarcoidosis have hypercalciuria, with most of these being normocalcemic.

Vitamin D toxicity

Vitamin D toxicity is most often seen in those patients being treated for hypoparathyroidism. Because of the absence or inactivity of PTH which would normally enhance renal calcium reabsorption, the excreted load of calcium can be very high even in the face of normal serum calcium. When supplementation with vitamin D or 1,25(OH)$_2$D is excessive, hypercalciuria can be severe.

Hypocitraturia

Citrate is now recognized as an important inhibitor of renal nephrolithiasis; it acts through various mechanisms to slow or prevent the formation of stones. First, citrate binds calcium in the urine and forms a soluble calcium citrate complex, lowering the availability of the free cation. The saturation of calcium salts such as calcium oxalate and calcium phosphate is thus lowered. Citrate is

a potent inhibitor of the aggregation or agglomeration of preformed calcium oxalate crystals. Citrate is able to bind to calcium oxalate crystals, inhibiting their subsequent growth; the inhibitory effect on calcium phosphate crystals is even more pronounced. Citrate has also been shown to slow the enhancement of heterogeneous nucleation of calcium oxalate by sodium urate [9]. In effect, high citrate levels will produce the effects noted above; low levels (<320 mg/day (<1.7 mmol/day)) would be expected to increase the risk of stone disease (Figure 62.2). It has been shown in numerous epidemiological studies that stone-forming patients have lower levels of urinary citrate than non-stone-formers and that the restoration of a normal urinary citrate can slow stone production.

Renal tubular acidosis (distal)

Both complete and incomplete renal tubular acidoses (RTA) are characterized by an elevated urinary pH, which predisposes to calcium phosphate stones, and a low urinary citrate. The low citrate is thought to be due to enhanced mitochondrial metabolism of citrate in acidotic states and a compensatory increase in the renal tubular uptake of citrate. The metabolic acidosis present as a result of a complete renal tubular acidosis produces urinary abnormalities in addition to hypocitraturia.

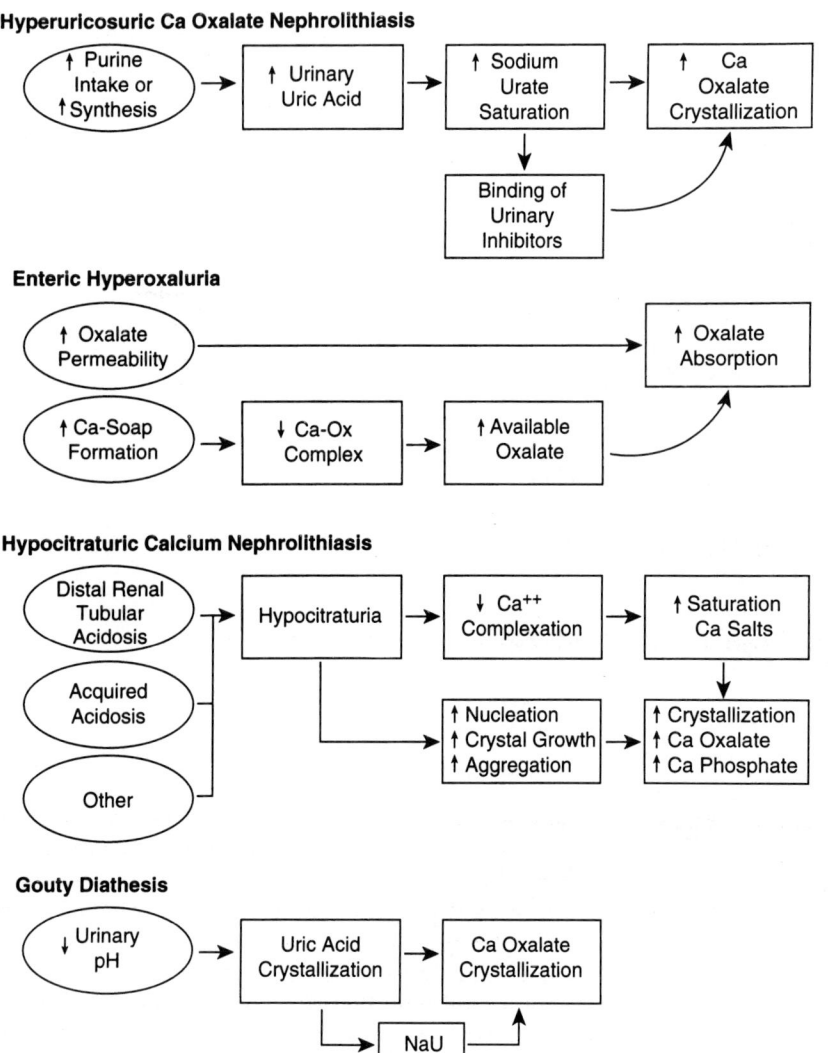

Figure 62.2 Physiologic changes resulting in hyperuricosuric calcium oxalate nephrolithiasis, enteric hyperoxaluria, hypocitraturic calcium nephrolithiasis, and gouty diathesis.

Hypercalciuria is commonly present because of a loss of bone mineral from the skeleton and the resultant increase in the filtered load of calcium. Though the exact mechanism is unknown, the acidosis appears to limit the response of the renal tubular cell to PTH, as the renal calcium loss produces an increase in PTH, but no increase in the activity of the hormone. Intestinal calcium absorption does not increase, nor does the renal reabsorption of calcium in tubular cells. An incomplete renal tubular acidosis is characterized by an absence of findings suggesting a systemic acidosis, but the kidney is unable to acidify the urine when exposed to an ammonium chloride (acid) load. Hypercalciuria is a common, but not invariable finding. Both forms of RTA are associated with stones and may present with advanced nephrocalcinosis.

Chronic diarrheal states

The primary mechanism for the hypocitraturia seen with intestinal disease is the loss of bicarbonate in the feces. Voluminous amounts of watery diarrhea can lead to markedly decreased urinary citrate, with levels of <50 mg/day (<0.26 mmol/day) a not uncommon finding. Any condition which produces diarrhea may result in hypocitraturia, with intestinal resections (including gastric) and inflammatory bowel diseases being common causative conditions. Laxative abuse may also result in low urinary citrate levels. In chronic diarrheal states, other risk factors for stone disease are variably present, such as low urine volumes, low urinary pH, and hyperoxaluria.

Idiopathic hypocitraturia

Patients with hypocitraturia may have no identifiable cause for their low urinary citrate, having a normal response to an ammonium chloride challenge, and the absence of intestinal disease or urinary tract infection (which can lower urinary citrate through the action of bacterial degradation of citrate). There is no evidence that there is a citrate malabsorptive state; patients have rapid and near complete alkali absorption in response to an alkali load. The possibility of a defect in the sodium–citrate cotransporter is currently under investigation. It should be remembered that thiazide administration can induce hypocitraturia, presumably through the production of hypokalemia and subsequent intracellular acidosis. Many cases of so-called idiopathic hypocitraturia may result from dietary habits associated with reduced intestinal absorption of alkali, such as an excessive intake of dietary animal protein, or a deficient intake of citrus fruit products.

Hyperoxaluria

Hyperoxaluria (urinary oxalate >40 mg/day (>444 μmol/day)) enhances the risk of stone formation by increasing the urinary saturation of calcium oxalate [10]. Small changes in urinary oxalate may produce significant alterations in calcium oxalate saturation. Though primary hyperoxaluria does exist as an autosomal recessive inborn error of metabolism, it is extremely rare. A result of a deficiency or ineffectiveness of the enzyme responsible for the conversion of glyoxylate into glycine (alanine: glyoxylate aminotransferase), primary hyperoxaluria leads to increased amounts of glyoxalate which then undergoes oxidation to oxalate. There are two types of inherited hyperoxaluria. Primary hyperoxaluria type I is due to an absolute deficiency of the enzyme. Primary hyperoxaluria type II is thought to occur because the aminotransferase is located in the mitochondria as opposed to the peroxisome; its location in the wrong organelle appears to place it in a location where it cannot carry out its function.

No further conversion of oxalate occurs in the body; the only means of excretion is as an intact molecule through the kidney into the urine. Pyridoxine supplementation (at dose of 150–400 mg/day) can increase the rate of conversion of glyoxylate into glycine, reducing urinary oxalate in this disorder (Figure 62.3).

A much more common cause of hyperoxaluria is that due to intestinal disease. Inflammatory bowel disease and malabsorptive states such as celiac sprue, pancreatic insufficiency or intestinal bypass surgery can all lead to overabsorption of oxalate. The mechanisms may be multiple (Figure 62.2), but it is thought that unabsorbed free fatty acids in the intestinal lumen bind positive cations such as calcium and magnesium, leaving the unbound, negatively charged oxalate behind. Free oxalate is then available to pass into and through the intestinal mucosal cells, the principal site of absorption being the colon. It has also been suggested that the higher levels of free fatty acids as well as unabsorbed bile salts may directly increase the permeability of the intestinal mucosa to oxalate. Treatment would include adherence to a low fat, low oxalate diet.

Patients who consume diets rich in oxalate-containing foods may present with mild hyperoxaluria which is responsive to dietary manipulation. Moreover, patients who suffer from intestinal hyperabsorption of calcium, or

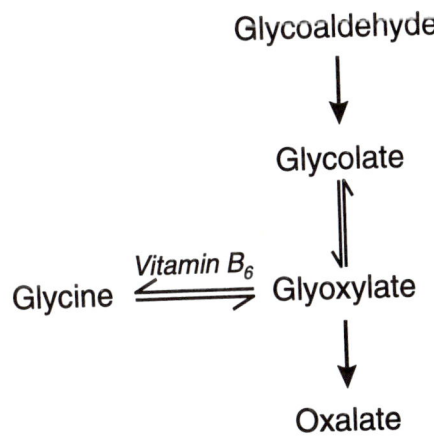

Figure 62.3 Partial pathway of oxalate metabolism showing the role of vitamin B_6 in decreasing the conversion of glyoxylate into oxalate.

who take calcium-binding agents, may have mild to moderate hyperoxaluria unless dietary oxalate intake is restricted.

Hyperuricosuria

Hyperuricosuria may lead to calcium oxalate or uric acid stones, the latter occurring in the setting of a urinary pH of less than 5.5 and the former when the pH exceeds 5.5. If the urinary pH is greater than 5.5 (the dissociation constant for uric acid), the soluble, anionic urate form predominates. Hyperuricosuria can lead to an increased saturation of sodium urate which may allow the formation of colloidal or crystalline sodium urate. Sodium urate induction of heterogeneous nucleation can initiate stone formation with calcium oxalate [6]. Sodium urate may also bind and inactivate macromolecular inhibitors, thereby enhancing calcium salt crystallization (Figure 62.2).

The frequency of hyperuricosuria in the stone-forming population depends on the definition of hyperuricosuria. It is more common in male stone-formers, with over 30% of male and 15% of female calcium oxalate stone-formers having a urinary uric acid excretion greater than 800 mg (>4.8 mmol)/day. When hyperuricosuria is defined by a more liberal value of greater than 600 mg (>3.6 mmol)/day, over 75% of male and 20% of female patients meet the definition of hyperuricosuria. A minor percentage of patients may have concurrent hyperuricemia, suggesting an overproduction of uric acid.

Gouty diathesis

The entity known as gouty diathesis is characterized by unduly acidic urine, with the pH regularly less than 5.5. The low urinary pH, as mentioned above, is below the dissociation constant of uric acid and results in uric acid precipitation (Figure 62.2). Uric acid crystals can coalesce and form pure uric acid stones or may bind macromolecules present in the urine, preventing their action as inhibitors of calcareous or mixed stone formation. Alternatively, crystalline or colloidal sodium urate may promote heterogeneous nucleation of calcium oxalate crystallization as well as bind available inhibitory macromolecules.

The low pH occurs in the absence of a high acid ash diet or diarrheal states. The exact mechanism for the low pH is not known, but may be due to inadequate ammonia production by the kidney. In patients without hyperuricemia or gout, gouty diathesis may represent an early phase of primary gout. Some patients may have a fully manifested gouty syndrome, with frank hyperuricemia and gouty arthritis.

Cystinuria

Cystinuria is an autosomal recessively inherited transport disorder of dibasic amino acids in which the kidney is unable to transport cystine, ornithine, lysine or arginine from the tubular lumen into the tubular cells [11]. In about half of cystinuric patients, a mutation in a gene (SLC3AI gene) coding for a 79 kDa renal protein responsible for debasic amino acid transport has been identified; greater than 20 different mutations have been reported to date [11a]. A patient is said to have homozygous cystinuria when the excretion of urinary cystine is ≥250 mg/g creatinine. The saturation of the relatively insoluble cystine is thus exceeded and cystine calculi form. In the US, the incidence of homozygous cystinuria is estimated to be 1 in 20000–25000. The transport defect is also present in the intestinal tract, producing a corresponding malabsorption of the dibasic amino acids, but there is no clinical evidence of protein deficiency. Cystine stones may occur in early childhood, but some patients have been diagnosed in middle age. The diagnosis is most commonly made in the second and third decades. Any child or adolescent presenting with kidney stones should have a qualitative test for cystine in the urine.

Although the solubility of cystine has some individual variation, it is greater as the pH increases. At pH 5.0, the solubility is 170–300 mg/l (0.7–1.3 mmol/l) and increases to 220–500 mg/l (0.9–2.1 mmol/l) at pH 7.5. There is a high incidence of coexistent metabolic abnormalities in patients with cystinuria. It has been shown that 18.5% of cystinurics may have hypercalciuria, 22.2% hyperuricosuria, and 44.4% hypocitraturia. In patients who have been tested, hypocitraturia was found to be commonly associated with a renal acidification defect. Concurrent metabolic derangements appear to be more common if a patient has had mixed cystine and calcium stones, but a third of patients with pure cystine stones may have one or more of the physiologic abnormalities noted above. In a patient who responds poorly to treatment (see below) or who continues to form stones in spite of achieving satisfactory cystine concentrations, there should be a careful search for other metabolic abnormalities that might be present.

Infection stones

Chronic infection of the urinary tract by urease-producing organisms can lead to an increased risk for stones composed of struvite ($MgNH_4PO_4 \cdot 6H_2O$) [12]. Bacteria are able to degrade urea, producing ammonia which is then hydrolyzed to ammonium and hydroxyl ions. The pH of the urine rises, enhancing the dissociation of phosphate which then combines with ammonium ion and magnesium to form struvite. The enhanced phosphate dissociation may also result in calcium phosphate crystallization; thus, infection stones not uncommonly have components of both struvite and carbonate apatite ($Ca_{10}(PO_4)_6 \cdot CO_3$) or tricalcium diphosphate ($Ca_3(PO_4)_2$).

Treatment of struvite stones can be very difficult as the stones are often large (staghorn) and are not greatly amenable to disintegration by lithotripsy. Chronic antibiotic therapy often fails to eradicate infection because of the presence of bacteria within the matrix of the stones, out of reach of the antibacterial(s). Unless stones are completely removed with a surgical procedure, recurrence is high.

Because the molecular structure of hydroxamic acids is similar to that of urea, they are able to inhibit urease, an enzyme which hydrolyzes urea to form NH_3, CO_2 and H_2O, the first step in the formation of struvite. Acetohydroxamic acid has been used clinically and has been shown in blinded, placebo-controlled trials to prevent or slow the formation of struvite stones. A high frequency of side effects including severe headaches, nausea, vomiting, diarrhea, hemolytic anemia, thrombophlebitis and neurologic symptoms, such as tremulousness, hallucinations, and disorientation, though reversible on cessation of the drug, preclude its widespread use.

Medullary sponge kidney

Medullary sponge kidney (MSK) is an anatomic abnormality of the renal medulla characterized by ectatic changes of the collecting ducts. The most common complications of MSK are renal calculi and infection.

The condition, which is probably congenital, is usually diagnosed by an intravenous pyelogram showing the characteristic 'paint brush' appearance of the dilated tubules and flattened calyces. The incidence of MSK in stone patients ranges from 3 to 13%, with Mayall [12a] reporting an incidence of 0.5% in a series of 2600 consecutive, unselected intravenous pyelograms. Several renal tubular defects have been reported in patients with MSK which may be contributing factors to stone formation [13]. Hypercalciuria, impaired tubular sodium reabsorption, and impaired urinary acidification have all been observed. Indeed, whereas urinary stasis in the ectatic tubules and associated cysts may enhance a propensity for stone formation, patients with MSK have a similar incidence of metabolic derangements as has been reported in large populations of stone patients without MSK. Depending on the definition of normal calcium excretion, 30–88% of patients with MSK have hypercalciuria. When evaluated with a response to a 1 g calcium load, 58% of patients with MSK had absorptive hypercalciuria, an incidence similar to the overall incidence in all patients with renal stones. Renal hypercalciuria is not nearly as common, being found in <20% of stone patients with MSK. Hyperuricosuria has been noted in approximately 30%. Because patients with MSK have similar patterns of metabolic derangements as those in the general stone-forming population and because correction of these derangements may decrease their risk of stone formation, patients with MSK should undergo a thorough metabolic evaluation with the institution of appropriate therapy (see below).

Adult polycystic kidney disease

As with medullary sponge kidney, the distorted anatomy of the kidney in polycystic kidney disease (PCKD) has been blamed for the increased incidence of nephrolithiasis in this group of patients [14]. The incidence of urinary calculi in PCKD ranges from 8 to 36% in various series, far greater than that of the general population. In addition to anatomic considerations, metabolic derangements may also contribute to the increased risk for stones. In a study of 74 patients with adult PCKD, metabolic abnormalities were extremely common, with 67% of the patients having hypocitraturia, 19% hyperoxaluria, 15% hyperuricosuria and 11% hypercalciuria. A distal acidification defect has been found in some of the hypocitraturic patients. There is a much higher frequency of uric acid stones than in the general stone-forming population, with a third to over half of the stones being either pure uric acid or having a uric acid component. Calcium oxalate stones are also common, though they appear less frequently than in non-PCKD stone-formers. The frequency of calcium phosphate and struvite stones is no different in the stone patients with PCKD.

Because of the distorted renal anatomy in these patients, the diagnosis of nephrolithiasis may be very difficult, but it should always be considered in a PCKD patient who presents with flank pain. The most sensitive diagnostic technique for the detection of stone is computed tomography. It is able to detect small and radio-opaque stones and distinguish them from calcifications of cyst walls.

Treatment of nephrolithiasis is not different in PCKD patients; they will respond to correction of their metabolic abnormalities. As in patients with medullary sponge kidney, a metabolic evaluation should be undertaken in all patients with PCKD who present with urinary tract stones. Stone disease should not be attributed to distorted anatomy alone until correction of metabolic abnormalities has been attempted.

Other stones [15]

Xanthine stones

Xanthinuria is an inborn error of metabolism resulting from a deficiency of xanthine oxidase (Figure 62.4). A third of patients with xanthinuria will form xanthine stones because of the low solubility of xanthine when excreted in the urine. Diagnosis is made on the basis of a very low serum and urinary uric acid (≤1.4 mg/dl (0.08 mmol/l) and ≤8 mg/day (48 µmol/day), respectively) which occur because of the profound impairment in uric acid production. Both serum and urinary concentrations of hypoxanthine are elevated and, because of residual xanthine oxidase activity, levels of xanthine are also increased.

Control of stone formation is generally achieved with a high fluid intake. If conservative treatment does not decrease stone formation, inhibiting residual xanthine oxidase activity with allopurinol may be effective.

2,8-Dihydroxyadenine stones

The extremely rare deficiency of adenine phosphoribosyl transferase (APRT) is another inborn error of metabolism which leads to an increased concentration of adenine (Figure 62.4). Adenine is oxidized by xanthine oxidase to 8-hydroxyadenine and thence to 2,8-dihydroxyadenine, a substance of low aqueous solubility. Formation of stones is the only clinical manifestation of APRT deficiency. Like uric acid calculi, stones composed of 2,8-dihydroxyadenine are radiolucent and require sonography or intravenous pyelogram (IVP) for detection. Identification of the stone composition can be made with

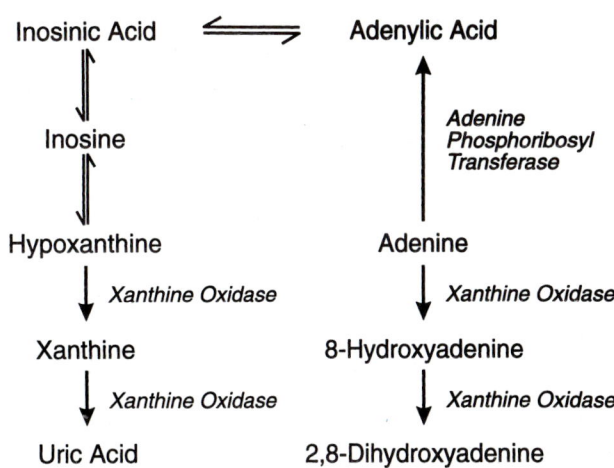

Figure 62.4 The metabolic pathways leading to the production of uric acid and 2,8-dihydroxyadenine.

infrared spectrophotometry. Treatment is allopurinol without alkali, the administration of which may actually exacerbate the disease.

Other miscellaneous stones

A small number of medications or their metabolites excreted through the kidney have, very rarely, been reported to form stones in the urinary tract. Triamterene, a potassium-sparing diuretic, was found to cause triamterene stones in 0.36% of those taking the drug, and has also been found as a nidus for calcium stones. Trisilicate-containing antacids have been reported to cause silica stones after chronic ingestion, and there has been a report of an AIDS patient treated with a high dose of sulphadiazine who developed multiple, bilateral stones and obstruction after two weeks of therapy; stone analysis showed sulphadiazine and acetylsulphadiazine.

Diagnosis and evaluation

In a patient who has had a prior episode of renal colic and who carries the diagnosis of nephrolithiasis, the diagnosis of subsequent episodes of stone passage are not difficult to make. In a patient with no history of stones, a careful history may be helpful in the diagnosis. A family history of stones is not uncommon in patients presenting with their first episode of stones. The presence of cystine stones, uric acid stones with or without a history of gout, family members with renal tubular acidosis, or relatives with calcium-containing kidney stones are all helpful in the formulation of a differential diagnosis. Very low fluid intake, especially in the setting of excessive sweating due to exercise or physical labor, can lead to very concentrated urine and supersaturation of stone-forming salts. A patient should also be asked about the use of any calcium or vitamin D supplements (which may increase urinary calcium), aspirin or probenecid (uricosuric agents), acetazolamide (which can produce a metabolic acidosis and subsequent hypocitraturia and hypercalciuria), or triamterene (which may predispose to triamterene stones).

When a patient presents with a first episode of renal colic, it should be ascertained whether he or she is at risk for recurrence [16]. A medical history (including medications or the use of vitamin supplements) and family history should be obtained as well as a dietary history. The dietary history should include a quantitative estimate not only of fluid intake, but also sodium, calcium, protein and oxalate consumption. Life style circumstances including excessive sweating due to exercise, physical labor or exposure to high temperatures suggest the formation of a concentrated urine.

If the suspected risk of recurrence is low (that is, no obvious risk factors are found after a history is obtained), a simple evaluation should be sufficient. Stone analysis should be done if the stone is available. A serum chem-

istry panel to rule out primary hyperparathyroidism (hypercalcemia), renal phosphate leak (hypophosphatemia), gouty diathesis or hyperuricosuria (hyperuricemia) or metabolic acidosis (low serum bicarbonate) should be obtained as well as a flat plate radiograph of the abdomen (KUB) to rule out the presence of calcareous, cystine or struvite stones; uric acid stones are radiolucent. A urine culture will rule out a urinary tract infection as the cause of possible struvite stones.

If no metabolic abnormalities are uncovered, conservative treatment should be instituted [17]. Increasing the amount of fluid ingested as well as eliminating dietary overindulgence of salt, oxalate-rich foods or protein may be all that is needed to prevent the recurrence of stones.

In patients who present with a recurrence or who present for the first time but have a family history or coexistent medical problem which may contribute to an increased risk of stones (intestinal disease, gout, etc.), a more extensive medical evaluation is warranted to identify any abnormalities that may be amenable to correction. An etiology for the stone disease can be found in 90–95% of patients. The rate of overall stone recurrence is high (65%), but can be significantly lowered with appropriate medical treatment in most cases. Depending on the etiology, conservative measures plus medical treatment can produce remission rates from 65% (for chronic diarrheal syndromes) to 95% (for gouty diathesis). The individual stone formation rate invariably drops, lessening the requirement for invasive procedures [18].

As in the low risk patients, patients at increased risk should have a serum chemistry analysis, a KUB, urine culture, and stone analysis if a stone is available. They should also have analyses of 24-hour urine collections, preferably one collection while on their usual diet, and a second while on a combined low calcium (400 mg (10 mmol)/day), low sodium (100 mEq or 2.3 g/day), and low oxalate (avoidance of oxalate-rich foods) diet. Measurements to be made should include volume, pH, creatinine (to ensure the adequacy of the collection), calcium, sodium, citrate, uric acid and oxalate. To characterize further any hypercalciuria, a fasting 2-hour urine can be collected as well as a fasting serum PTH. If the 2-hour calcium excretion is greater than 0.11 mg/dl of glomerular filtrate (>0.03 mmol/l) and the PTH is increased, the diagnosis of renal hypercalciuria is met [19]. This value can be obtained by multiplying the 2-hour calcium/creatinine ratio by the serum creatinine, eliminating seemingly elevated values in patients with serum creatinine values less than 1.0 mg/dl (<89 μmol/l).

Treatment of nephrolithiasis

Conservative therapy

Conservative measures should be a routine part of the management of all patients with kidney stones. In a patient with mild disease, they alone may prevent the recurrence of stones, the primary goal of treatment [20].

Increasing fluid intake to raise daily urine output to a minimum of 2l may be enough to reduce the urinary concentration of the constituent ions and thereby lower the saturation of the stone-forming salts of calcium oxalate, calcium phosphate, uric acid and cystine. All forms of stone disease will respond to an increase in fluid intake, which may prevent up to 60% of new stone formation.

Dietary modifications should include the maintenance of a low sodium diet (≤100 mEq or 2.3 g/day) and a moderate restriction of animal proteins. Excessive intake of sodium can decrease renal reabsorption of calcium, exacerbating hypercalciuria and can lower urinary citrate [21]. High urinary sodium also increases the saturation of sodium urate which can lead to sodium urate-induced enhancement of calcium oxalate crystallization, especially in those with hyperuricosuria. High urinary sodium may also attenuate the effect of thiazides on lowering urinary calcium. Diets high in animal proteins can increase urinary uric acid and lower urinary citrate [22].

Patients with calcium oxalate stones should restrict their intake of oxalate-rich foods such as spinach, chocolate, nuts/peanut butter, strawberries and brewed hot or iced tea. This is especially important in those with hyperoxaluria due to intestinal disease. Large amounts of vitamin C should be avoided as it provides a substrate for oxalate synthesis. Severe calcium restriction should be avoided in those with hyperoxaluria as a decreased calcium intake decreases the amount of calcium available to complex intestinal oxalate, increasing oxalate bioavailability [23]. The increased amount of absorbed oxalate contributes to an increased urinary oxalate. A moderate calcium intake of approximately 600 mg/day (15 mmol/day) is advisable in these patients.

Those with hypercalciuria because of an increased intestinal absorption of calcium should also follow a moderate dietary calcium restriction unless bone loss is already present. As this may increase the absorbable oxalate, as discussed above, concurrent oxalate restriction should be implemented in these patients. Patients with calcium stones who have a normal calcium absorption should avoid a high calcium intake (more than 1000 mg (25 mmol)/day). A rigid calcium restriction should also be avoided, as it might lead to a significantly negative calcium balance and eventual bone loss.

In cystinuria, because of the paucity of effective medical treatments, adherence to a regimen of high fluid intake, low sodium intake and moderate protein restriction is crucial. Even patients with greater than 1000 mg (4.2 mmol) of daily cystine excretion can maintain a urinary cystine concentration in the soluble range if enough fluid is ingested. In addition to regular fluid consumption throughout the day, patients should drink 450 ml before bedtime with an additional 225–450 ml if they awaken to urinate during the night. Salt restriction may reduce cystine excretion, but this effect may be offset by the loss of the cystine solubilizing action of sodium. Rigid methionine restriction, though it may result in lower urinary cystine levels, is impractical and may lead to nutritional deficiencies in growing children. Cystinuria patients should, instead, avoid an excessive intake of animal proteins.

Targeted therapy

In addition to the conservative measures mentioned above, attempts should be made to normalize any metabolic abnormalities found which may explain the presence of stone disease (Table 62.3).

Absorptive hypercalciuria

Until the exact mechanism for the hyperabsorption of intestinal calcium is elucidated, treatment of stone patients with this condition must be empiric. Thiazides should be tried because of their effect of increasing renal calcium reabsorption, though patients with absorptive hypercalciuria may respond poorly. Those with severe hypercalciuria rarely correct their urinary calcium to normal, and even a modest effect of the thiazide is frequently lost after 18–24 months of treatment. Thiazides work by inducing a measure of volume depletion, resulting in increased proximal tubular reabsorption of sodium and calcium. Thiazides also act directly on the distal tubule to increase calcium reabsorption, further lowering urinary calcium. Thiazides will have a maximal effect with a concurrent dietary sodium restriction; high salt intakes may completely negate the beneficial effect of a thiazide.

Thiazide treatment may induce or worsen coexistent hypocitraturia, presumably by inducing an intracellular acidosis as a consequence of hypokalemia. Chlorthalidone may be the most notable in this regard. Hydrochlorothiazide at a dose of 25–50 mg daily, trichlormethiazide 2–4 mg daily or bendrofluazide 2.5–5.0 mg daily have a similar hypocalciuric action, though the latter two drugs may be better tolerated. Thiazide-induced hypokalemia is best prevented or treated with potassium citrate, 20–40 mEq/day in divided doses; this compound will also prevent thiazide-induced hypocitraturia or accentuate citrate excretion above baseline [24]. Potassium chloride, although able to restore or maintain serum potassium levels, does not increase urinary citrate above baseline. Potassium citrate may also help to lower urinary calcium by imparting to the body an alkali load, thereby increasing renal calcium reabsorption.

The calcium binding agent sodium cellulose phosphate is very effective at lowering urinary calcium, but can cause a negative calcium balance and secondary hyperparathyroidism. The use of this calcium binder should be restricted to those with a documented, exaggerated intestinal absorption of calcium and good bone densities. An investigational, slow-release, neutral potas-

Table 62.3 Optimal treatment regimens

Indication	Treatment	Physiological action	Physicochemical action
Absorptive hypercalciuria	Low calcium diet	↓ absorbed intestinal calcium ↓ urinary calcium	↓ urinary saturation of calcium oxalate and calcium phosphate
	Thiazides	↓ urinary calcium (transient) ↓ urinary citrate	↓ urinary saturation of calcium salts
	Potassium citrate	↑ urinary citrate ↓ urinary calcium (transient)	↑ inhibitor activity ↓ saturation of calcium salts
	Sodium cellulose phosphate	↓ intestinal calcium absorption ↓ urinary calcium	↓ saturation of calcium salts
Renal hypercalciuria	Thiazides	↓ urinary calcium (sustained)	↓ saturation of calcium salts
Renal phosphate leak	Orthophosphates	↓ 1,25(OH)$_2$D ↓ intestinal calcium absorption ↓ urinary calcium ↑ urinary citrate and pyrophosphate	↓ saturation of calcium oxalate ↑ inhibitor activity
Hyperuricosuric calcium nephrolithiasis	Allopurinol	↓ urinary uric acid	↓ urate-induced crystallization of calcium salts
	Potassium citrate	↑ urinary citrate	↓ saturation of calcium oxalate ↓ urate-induced crystallization of calcium salts
Enteric hyperoxaluria	Low oxalate diet	↓ urinary oxalate	↓ saturation of calcium oxalate
	Potassium citrate	↑ urinary citrate	↓ saturation of calcium oxalate ↑ inhibitory activity
	Calcium citrate	↑ urinary citrate ↓ urinary oxalate ↑ urinary calcium	↑ inhibitor activity possible ↓in calcium oxalate saturation
	Magnesium gluconate	↑ urinary magnesium	↓ saturation of calcium oxalate
Hypocitraturic calcium nephrolithiasis	Potassium citrate	↑ urinary citrate and pH ↓ urinary calcium (transient)	↑ inhibitor activity ↓ saturation of calcium oxalate
Gouty diathesis	Potassium citrate	↑ urinary pH ↑ urinary citrate	↓ undissociated uric acid ↓ saturation and crystallization of calcium oxalate

sium phosphate compound has been given to patients with absorptive hypercalciuria and has been shown to produce sustained reductions in urinary calcium of 35% over two years. When available, this investigational compound may prove to be of value as first line treatment for absorptive hypercalciuria or in those who have lost their responsiveness to thazide diuretics [24a].

Renal hypercalciuria

Patients with renal hypercalciuria have an excellent response to thiazide treatment, the treatment of choice. The mechanisms of thiazide action are the same as those described above. Unlike the patients with absorptive hypercalciuria, no apparent adaptation takes place and the hypocalciuric effect of the thiazide persists long term.

The increased renal tubular calcium reabsorption suppresses PTH secretion, thereby lowering 1,25(OH)$_2$D synthesis and intestinal calcium absorption. As in patients with absorptive hypercalciuria, potassium citrate prevents the hypokalemia and hypocitraturia which thiazides may produce.

Combinations of a thiazide and potassium-sparing diuretics may prevent hypokalemia, but because of the known occurrence of triamterene in some kidney stones, combinations containing this medication should be avoided. In patients who have hypocitraturia and who will require potassium citrate supplementation, potassium-sparing diuretics should not be used as hyperkalemia could ensue with concomitant use. In these patients, a thiazide alone with potassium citrate is the optimal regimen.

Renal phosphate leak

Phosphate supplementation has been used in an attempt to normalize the serum phosphorus and thereby lower the circulating levels of $1,25(OH)_2D$. Compliance can be a problem as orthophosphates commonly cause gastrointestinal side effects; in particular, diarrhea can be quite distressing to the patient. Caution must be exercised in the administration of phosphates, as an increase in urinary phosphorus may lead to increased saturation of calcium phosphate salts, depending on the degree of change in urinary calcium.

Hyperuricosuria

Allopurinol is very effective at reducing the urinary uric acid excretion. An inhibitor of xanthine oxidase (Figure 62.3), allopurinol blocks the conversion of hypoxanthine to xanthine, and xanthine to uric acid, thereby lowering the production of uric acid. Allopurinol should be started in those with urinary uric acid excretion greater than 800 mg (4.8 mmol)/day; one may wish to use a lower cutoff in women, in whom the urinary uric acid levels are normally less than that of the male population. It should be noted that in a 24-hour urine the pH of which is less than 5.5, precipitation of uric acid in the specimen could lead to falsely low uric acid measurements. For those patients who cannot take allopurinol, potassium citrate has been shown to decrease the rate of new stone formation [9].

Gouty diathesis

The low urinary pH resulting in precipitation of uric acid and eventual stone formation responds to alkali treatment which increases urinary pH [25]. Maintenance of the pH above 6.0 prevents uric acid precipitation, not only preventing new stone formation, but making possible the dissolution of pre-existing stones. Potassium alkali is preferred, as sodium citrate or bicarbonate can induce or exacerbate hypercalciuria. Potassium citrate in doses of 30–60 mEq/day in divided doses is usually sufficient to increase urinary pH to the range of 6–7.0. As previously mentioned, alkali therapy also decreases urinary calcium excretion, at least transiently, thereby decreasing the saturation of calcium oxalate. The saturation of calcium phosphate usually does not change, as the decrease in urinary calcium offsets the increased dissociation of phosphate resulting from the increase in pH. Acetazolamide is not indicated, as it may produce a severe metabolic acidosis.

Hypocitraturia

Restoration of normal urinary citrate would be expected to reduce the propensity for the crystallization of stone-forming calcium salts in the urine, due to the reduced availability of ionic calcium (and therefore saturation of calcium salts) and inhibition of crystal aggregation and agglomeration. Potassium citrate is the treatment of choice for the treatment of low urinary citrate from whatever cause [26–28]. Isolated hypocitraturia can usually be normalized with a dose of 30–60 mEq daily in two or three divided doses. Potassium citrate has been shown to reduce the stone formation rate by 90% compared with the pretreatment rate in this subgroup of patients. In a randomized trial of potassium citrate and placebo, the disease was in remission in 72% of the patients taking potassium citrate compared with 20% of the patients in the placebo group. All patients on potassium citrate showed a reduced stone formation rate individually whereas there was no change in the placebo group [26]. In patients with mild to moderate disease (fewer than one stone per year), stone formation may virtually cease.

Cystinuria

Because urinary solubility of cystine increases with increasing urinary pH, alkali therapy should be used in most cystinuric patients. The increase in solubility is only modest up to a pH of 7.5, but at pH greater than 7.0 the risk of calcium phosphate (hydroxyapatite) increases greatly. With aggressive alkalinization, patients may thus begin producing calcium phosphate stones. The pH is best maintained between 6.5 and 7.0. Potassium alkali is preferred to prevent the sodium-induced increase in urinary cystine that may occur with sodium alkali therapy. Potassium citrate treatment with 30–60 mEq/day in divided doses is usually sufficient to achieve the desired pH.

The goal of chelating therapy is to reduce urinary excretion of cystine by complexing cysteine, effectively splitting the insoluble cystine dimers. Both D-penicillamine and tiopronin, by virtue of their free sulfhydryl group, have been used in this condition. Both compounds undergo a thioldisulfide exchange with cystine, producing the readily soluble disulfides D-penicillamine-cysteine and tiopronin-cysteine. The effect is dose related: the greater the administered dose of either medication, the more is excreted in the urine and available to undergo the thioldisulfide exchange.

D-Penicillamine is administered at a total dose of 1–2 g/day (given in three of four divided doses). It is associated with a high frequency of side effects, limiting its use. Serious hematologic changes such as agranulocytosis, thrombocytopenia, and even aplastic anemia have been reported. Patients who develop proteinuria and/or hematuria on the drug should be monitored closely, as those findings may be the first sign of a membranous glomerulopathy which may signal impending nephrotic syndrome. Dermatitis (pemphigus varieties) has been seen, usually as a late complication of treatment. Any serious side effect warrants discontinuation of the drug.

Tiopronin (N-2-mercaptopropionylglycine, Thiola®, Mission Pharmacal Co., San Antonio, USA) is given in a dose of 800–2000 mg/day in three or four divided doses. It is associated with a lower frequency of side effects compared with D-penicillamine, though the side effect profiles of the two drugs are similar as regards the types of adverse reactions that can occur. The most common side effects for both drugs are nausea and vomiting, diarrhea and rash. Fatigue and fever are present in 10–15% of patients.

Summary

The last two decades have witnessed major advances in the treatment of stone disease, with great strides being made in the preventive aspects of stone disease. The advent of specific therapies as a result of the definitive diagnosis of metabolic derangements have clearly shown the benefit of preventive treatment. The logical, systematic evaluation of a patient with recurrent stones allows the clinician to choose from a variety of specific therapeutic agents which can greatly reduce the stone formation rate in patients with stone disease when used appropriately in conjunction with conservative treatment. Targeted therapies can frequently lead to improved remission rates and reduced stone formation when compared with conservative treatment; invasive, open procedures can often be avoided and morbidity reduced. The decrease in stone formation and increased remission rates in those with stones can result in an improvement in the quality of life for most patients with nephrolithiasis.

References

1. Coe, F.L., Parks, J.H. and Asplin, J.R. (1992) The pathogenesis and treatment of kidney stones. *N. Engl. J. Med.,* **327**, 1141–52.
2. Pak, C.Y.C. (1991) Etiology and treatment of urolithiasis. *Am. J. Kidney Dis.,* **18**, 624–37.
3. Gleeson, M.J., Kobashi, K. and Griffith, D.P. (1992) Non-calcium nephrolithiasis, in *Disorders of Bone and Mineral Metabolism* (eds F.L. Coe and M.J. Favus), Raven Press, New York, p. 801.
4. Brown, C.M. and Purich, D.L. (1992) Physical-chemical processes in kidney stone formation, in *Disorders of Bone and Mineral Metabolism* (eds F.L. Coe and M.J. Favus), Raven Press, New York, p. 613.
5. Pak, C.Y.C. (1992) Pathophysiology of calcium nephrolithiasis, in *The Kidney: Physiology and Pathophysiology*, 2nd edn (eds D.W. Seldin and G. Giebisch), Raven Press, New York, pp. 2461–80.
6. Coe, F.L., Parks, J.H. and Nakagawa, Y. (1992) Inhibitors and promoters of calcium oxalate crystallization, in *Disorders of Bone and Mineral Metabolism* (eds F.L. Coe and M.J. Favus), Raven Press, New York, p. 757.
7. Pak, C.Y.C., Waters, O., Arnold, L. *et al.* (1977) Mechanism for calcium urolithiasis among patients with hyperuricosuria. *J. Clin. Invest.,* **59**, 426–31.
8. Pak, C.Y.C., Britton, F., Peterson, R. *et al.* (1980) Ambulatory evaluation of nephrolithiasis. *Am. J. Med.,* **69**, 19–30.
9. Pak, C.Y.C. and Peterson, R. (1986) Successful treatment of hyperuricosuric calcium oxalate nephrolithiasis with potassium citrate. *Arch. Intern. Med.,* **146**, 863–7.
10. Smith, L.H. (1992) Hyperoxaluric states, in *Disorders of Bone and Mineral Metabolism* (eds F.L. Coe and M.J. Favus), Raven Press, New York, pp. 707–27.
11. Segal, S. and Thier, S.O. (1989) Cystinuria, in *The Metabolic Basis of Inherited Disease* (eds C.R. Scriver, A.L. Beaudet, W.S. Sly and D. Valle), McGraw–Hill, New York, pp. 2479–96.
11a.Gitomer, W.L. and Pak, C.Y.C. (1996) Recent advances in the biochemical and molecular biological basis of cystinuria. *J. Urol.,* **156**, 1907–1912.
12. Gleeson, M.J. and Griffith, D.P. (1993) Struvite calculi. *Br. J. Urol.,* **71**, 503–11.
12a.Mayall, G.F. (1970) The incidence of medullary sponge kidney. *Clin. Radiol.,* **21**, 171–4.
13. O'Neill, M., Breslau, N.A. and Pak, C.Y.C. (1981) Metabolic evaluation of nephrolithiasis in patients with medullary sponge kidney. *JAMA,* **245**, 1233–6.
14. Torres, V.E., Wilson, D.M., Hattery, R.R. and Segura, J.W. (1993) Renal stone disease in autosomal dominant polycystic kidney disease. *Am. J. Kidney Dis.,* **22**, 513–19.
15. Pak, C.Y.C. (1990) Miscellaneous stones, in *Urolithiasis: A Medical and Surgical Reference* (eds M.I. Resnick and C.Y.C. Pak), W.B. Saunders, Philadelphia, pp. 145–51.
16. Pak, C.Y.C. (1982) Should patients with single renal stone occurrence undergo diagnostic evaluation? *J. Urol.,* **127**, 855–8.
17. Uribarri, J., Oh, M.S. and Carroll, H.J. (1989) The first kidney stone. *Ann. Intern. Med.,* **111**, 1006–9.
18. Pak, C.Y.C. (1987) Citrate and renal calculi. *Miner. Electrolyte Metab.,* **13**, 257–66.
19. Pak, C.Y.C., Kaplan, R., Bone, H. *et al.* (1975) A simple test for the diagnosis of absorptive, resorptive and renal hypercalciurias. *N. Engl. J. Med.,* **292**, 497–500.
20. Weinstock Brown, W. and Wolfson, M. (1993) Diet as culprit or therapy: stone disease, chronic renal failure, and nephrotic syndrome. *Med. Clin. North Am.,* **77**, 783–94.
21. Sakhaee, K., Harvey, J.A., Padalino, P.K. *et al.* (1993) The potential role of salt abuse on the risk for kidney stone formation. *J. Urol.,* **150**, 310–12.
22. Fellström, B., Danielson, B.G., Karlström, B. *et al.* (1984) Effects of high intake of dietary animal protein on mineral metabolism and urinary supersaturation of calcium oxalate in renal stone formers. *Br. J. Urol.,* **56**, 263–9.
23. Massey, L.K. and Sutton, R.A.L. (1993) Modification of dietary oxalate and calcium reduces urinary oxalate in hyperoxaluric patients with kidney stones. *J. Am. Diet Assoc.,* **93**, 1305–7.
24. Pak, C.Y.C., Peterson, R., Sakhaee, K. *et al.* (1985) Correction of hypocitraturia and prevention of stone formation by combined thiazide and potassium citrate therapy in thiazide-unresponsive hypercalciuric nephrolithiasis. *Am. J. Med.,* **79**, 284–8.

24a. Heller, H.J., Reza-Albarran, A.A., Breslau, N.A., Pak, C.Y.C. (1996) Long-term physiologic effects of Urophos-K in absorptive hypercalciuria, in *Urolithiasis* 1996 (eds C.Y.C. Pak, A.I. Resnick and G.M. Preminger), Millet Printer, Dallas, pp. 434–6.

25. Pak, C.Y.C., Sakhaee, K. and Fuller, C. (1986) Successful management of uric acid nephrolithiasis with potassium citrate. *Kidney Int.*, **30**, 422–8.

26. Barcelo, P., Wuhl, O., Servitge, E. *et al.* (1993) Randomized double-blind study of potassium citrate in idiopathic hypocitraturic calcium nephrolithiasis. *J. Urol.*, **150**, 1761–4.

27. Pak, C.Y.C. and Fuller, C. (1986) Idiopathic hypocitraturic calcium-oxalate nephrolithiasis successfully treated with potassium citrate. *Ann. Intern. Med.*, **104**, 33–7.

28. Preminger, G.M., Sakhaee, K., Skurla, C. and Pak, C.Y.C. (1985) Prevention of recurrent calcium stone formation with potassium citrate therapy in patients with distal renal tubular acidosis. *J. Urol.*, **134**, 20–3.

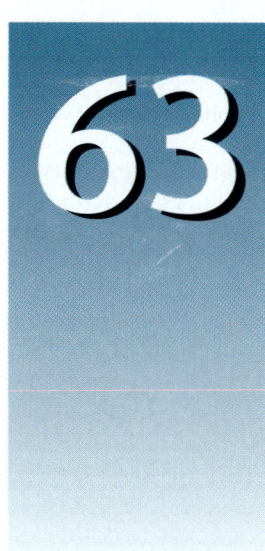

63

Structural disorders of the urinary tract

John N. Kabalin

Introduction

After urine flows into the intrarenal collecting system and renal pelvis, it must traverse the lower urinary tract before exiting the body. The lower urinary tract – here inclusive of ureters, bladder and urethra – is far from a passive conduit. In the normal state, the ureters actively propel urine into the bladder. The bladder provides a sensate and compliant reservoir for urine storage and then actively expels the accumulated urine volume through the urethra. The bladder neck and proximal urethra contain both active and passive sphincteric mechanisms to maintain urinary continence. As might be expected in such a complex system, a large number of structural problems, both congenital and acquired, can disrupt the normal function and drainage of the lower urinary tract. If unabated, these can lead to progressive unilateral or bilateral functional impairment and eventual loss of the proximal renal unit(s). The recognition and accurate diagnosis of these postrenal structural problems are of particular importance, since all are potentially reversible causes of renal failure with early intervention. In this chapter these structural disorders are grouped broadly into those causing obstruction and urinary reflux.

Obstruction

Introduction

Between the kidney and the final urinary outlet at the urethral meatus, the flow of urine may be obstructed by any one of a great number of disease processes, both congenital and acquired, including both intrinsic obstructing lesions and extrinsic lesions impinging on and compressing the urinary tract. Although the etiologies may be myriad, the end result, urinary obstruction, is manifested by a discrete number of clinical signs and symptoms with a common pathophysiology of upper urinary tract response and deterioration.

Clinical manifestations

Acute, total or subtotal obstruction of either ureter produces the pain syndrome of renal colic. This is classically described with acute obstruction by a ureteral calculus, but any acute obstructing lesion can manifest with identical symptoms. The pain of renal colic, caused by acute distention of the renal pelvis, is typically referred to the ipsilateral costovertebral angle and radiates anteriorly across the flank. With obstructions of the lower ureter, causing proximal ureteral as well as renal pelvic distention, pain may be referred along the distributions of the subcostal, iliohypogastric, ilioinguinal, and genitofemoral nerves, producing pain, hyperalgesia and reflex muscle spasms radiating from the flank anteriorly and inferiorly into the groin and ipsilateral scrotum or labia. This pain may be constant, but is often intermittent in nature. Although the pain may be mild or moderate, it is often described as a severe, visceral sensation, unrelieved by positional changes, and often only partially relieved even with narcotic analgesics. Reflex vagal stimulation not uncommonly produces nausea, emesis and, at times, significant ileus.

Nephrology, Edited by Rex L. Jamison and Robert Wilkinson.
Published in 1997 by Chapman & Hall, London. ISBN 0 412 60930 4

In marked contradistinction to the pain of acute renal colic, a slowly progressive, gradually obstructing lesion in the urinary tract may be insidious and clinically silent. The rapidity of onset of the obstruction often determines if the patient experiences symptoms. In slow, gradual occlusion of a single ureter, over time the proximal renal unit may be lost without any clinical manifestation whatsoever. If both upper tracts – or a solitary kidney – become obstructed very gradually, the first and only presenting symptoms may be those of uremia. Such patients may develop massive hydronephrosis and life-threatening uremia without noticeable pain or other warning symptoms. Even oliguria and anuria may be very late manifestations in such patients, and may or may not be noticed prior to presentation with uremia. In unusual instances, obstruction may present as polyuria, including polydipsia and/or dehydration mimicking diabetes insipidus, due to failure of urinary concentration in obstructed and damaged nephrons. A palpable abdominal mass may present as a physical finding in the child or thin adult with massive hydronephrosis. Rectal or vaginal examinations may reveal a pelvic mass or malignancy causing distal ureteral obstruction. In patients with urethral obstruction, voiding symptoms may predominate. These may include poor urinary stream, urinary frequency, nocturia, urinary incontinence due to overflow or total urinary retention. A distended bladder may be palpable on examination of these patients. Rectal examination may reveal an enlarged, benign or malignant prostate in the male. Stricture disease, benign prostatic enlargement and obstruction due to prostate cancer are common etiologies of postvesical urinary obstruction in adult males – significant postvesical obstruction is almost never seen in women. In the neonatal male, posterior urethral valves are the most common congenital cause of urethral obstruction and may present similarly with poor, dribbling stream, poor urine outputs or failure to void.

Pathophysiology

Following acute unilateral ureteral obstruction, several physiologic responses occur sequentially in the affected renal unit. Hydrostatic pressures in the renal pelvis and ureter proximal to the obstruction rise immediately following obstruction, and may eventually exceed 50 mmHg. This increase in pressure causes distention of the proximal collecting system, and concomitant acute increases in wall tension of the renal pelvis and ureter. Tension-sensitive nerve endings translate this as the pain which is perceived as renal colic. The building pressure, exacerbated by ongoing muscular contraction of the renal pelvis and ureter, may result in rupture of the calyceal fornices, with urinary extravasation and partial relief of pressure in the collecting system. Eventually, the unabated rise in hydrostatic pressure following obstruction is transmitted into collecting ducts and more proximal nephrons, with those draining into the polar, compound calyces of the kidney typically affected first and foremost.

As pressures in the proximal tubule and glomerulus rise, approximating filtration pressures at the glomerulus, glomerular filtration rate falls relatively rapidly. Renal blood flow increases acutely in an attempt to compensate, and remains increased for hours after total ureteral obstruction [1, 2]. Renal dimensions and mass, if measured during this acute response phase, are also increased. Systemic renin levels have been demonstrated to rise following acute unilateral ureteral obstruction, and may be responsible for transient blood pressure elevations seen in some patients, but do not appear to be the driving factor in augmenting renal blood flow after obstruction [3]. The latter is now postulated to occur almost entirely as a result of afferent arteriolar vasodilation, mediated by prostaglandins.

If acute obstruction persists beyond a few hours, total renal blood flow is observed to decrease, even as hydrostatic pressures in the collecting system continue to rise. Postglomerular vasoconstriction (perhaps mediated by thromboxane), with ongoing glomerular filtration, is believed to underlie these physiologic events. After several hours and within the first day of ongoing total ureteral obstruction, renal blood flow continues to decrease with the advent of preglomerular vasoconstriction, accompanied by a steady fall in hydrostatic pressure within the collecting system (although the latter remains significantly elevated over baseline pressure). Glomerular filtration rate also continues to fall, although the rate of decline slows. As acute obstruction becomes chronic, renal blood flow decreases to 50% of normal by three days, less than one-third normal by six days, and less than 20% normal by one month [4]. Glomerular filtration decreases but continues, with removal of fluid from the kidney and collecting system by pyelotubular, pyelolymphatic and pyelovenous backflow. In chronic obstruction, the pyelovenous route appears to predominate and allows low levels of continuing glomerular function. In canine studies, two weeks' total obstruction reduced glomerular filtration rate to 15% normal, with eventual recovery to only 46% of normal [4]. After four weeks' total obstruction, glomerular filtration rate fell to 3% normal and recovered to only 35% normal [2]. In this model, no significant function was recovered after six weeks' total obstruction. Return of some renal function after two months total obstruction has been documented in humans [6]. Tubular function is also observed to deteriorate after obstruction, with gradual loss of concentrating and acidification abilities [5, 7]. Urine aspirated from the renal pelvis of an obstructed kidney is thus typically alkaline and of relatively low osmolality.

With unrelieved ureteral obstruction, the ureteral musculature hypertrophies as it continues to contract against the obstructing lesion. The ureter first thickens, and then elongates and becomes tortuous. Finally, with ongoing pressure elevation and dilation, the ureteral and renal pelvic musculature decompensates, becomes attenuated and loses contractility. In chronic obstruction, renal blood flow dissipates and significant renal parenchymal atrophy occurs over time. Eventually, the 'bag of water' kidney is produced, consisting of a thin, fibrotic shell surrounding a dilated renal pelvis. With unilateral renal loss due to obstruction, compensatory hypertrophy occurs in the contralateral, unaffected kidney. This is more pronounced in children and younger adults. Systemic renin levels, acutely elevated immediately after obstruction, generally return to normal levels with chronic obstruction, and unilateral hydronephrosis is a rare etiology of hypertension [4, 8].

This sequence of events following unilateral complete ureteral obstruction may also occur after partial obstruction, with a more gradual and prolonged time course, depending on the degree of obstruction. On the other hand, progressive renal destruction with irrecoverable loss of function can occur very rapidly – within hours – following obstruction in the presence of infected urine ('pyonephrosis').

In bilateral renal obstruction, as may occur with bilateral ureteral lesions or more distal obstructions involving the bladder outlet and urethra, or in the obstruction of a solitary renal unit, certain important differences in pathophysiology exist compared to unilateral obstruction. Renal blood flow is relatively greater and maintained for longer duration after acute bilateral obstruction, with a more normal distribution of perfusion throughout the renal parenchyma after more prolonged obstruction [9]. Overall renal functional impairment following bilateral obstruction is generally less and glomerular filtration rate in particular is generally better preserved compared to changes observed in the unilateral obstructed kidney for the same degree and duration of obstruction. The reasons for this are not well understood.

After relief of bilateral obstruction or obstruction of a solitary kidney, a unique syndrome of postobstructive

diuresis may occur, depending on the degree and duration of the obstruction, which is rarely seen after unilateral renal obstruction. In general, following relief of bilateral or total urinary obstruction, a physiologic diuresis and natriuresis will occur with excretion of excess total body water and sodium accumulated during the period of obstruction. This process tends to be self-limiting and requires no medical intervention. In unusual instances, postobstructive diuresis may be exaggerated and profound, with very high urine volumes produced and significant losses of electrolytes [10, 11]. Careful, frequent and systematic monitoring of urine output, vital signs, body weight and serum electrolytes is warranted. Even in these cases, the awake patient with a normal thirst mechanism can usually compensate for any inappropriate losses. However, in rare instances this pathologic syndrome may be life-threatening, and intravenous therapy will be required for hypovolemia, hypokalemia, hyponatremia, hypocalcemia and/or hypomagnesemia. It must be emphasized that such cases are rare, and it is more common to see the normal, physiologic postobstructive diuresis following relief of urinary obstruction prolonged and exacerbated by inappropriate intravenous fluid administration.

Diagnosis and differential diagnosis

Laboratory values may suggest pathology but are nonspecific for urinary obstruction. For instance, hematuria and/or pyuria may be present on urinalysis in patients with intrinsic obstructing lesions of the urinary tract. Significant proteinuria or casts are rarely seen with obstruction alone, and when present, suggest other causes for renal dysfunction. Serum creatinine and blood urea nitro-

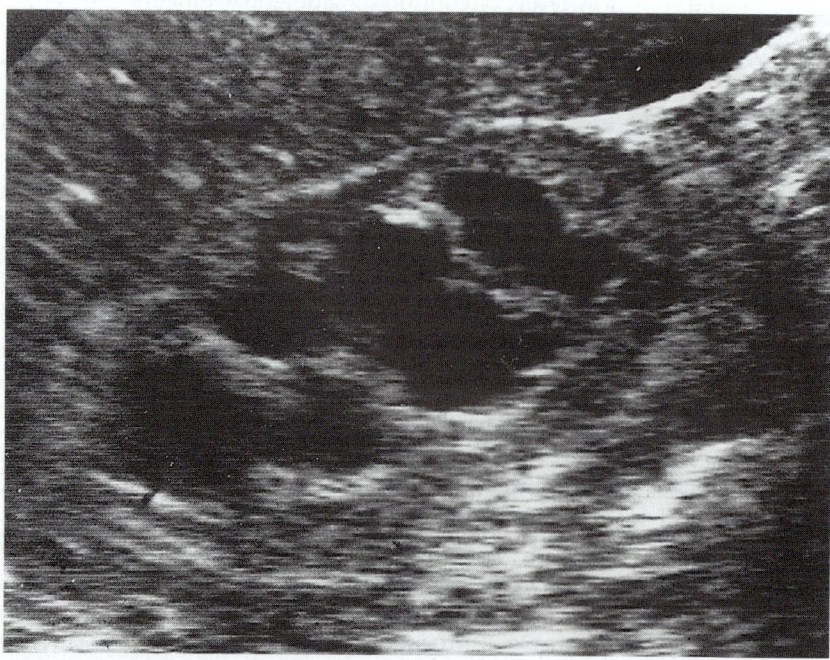

Figure 63.1 Renal ultrasound in hydronephrosis. Longitudinal image through kidney shows multiple, grossly dilated calyces.

gen elevations occur with bilateral obstruction or obstruction of a solitary functional renal unit, but again are non-specific for obstruction, and are typically unaffected in cases of unilateral renal obstruction in the setting of a normally functioning contralateral kidney.

In the patient presenting with symptoms, physical signs, history or unexplained uremia suggesting the possibility of urinary obstruction, renal and abdominal ultrasound is today the most efficient, least invasive and relatively inexpensive diagnostic tool to screen for the presence of hydronephrosis, hydroureter or a distended bladder (Figure 63.1). Increasingly, ultrasound examination is offered in the practicing urologist's office, thus increasing convenience and further decreasing cost. Ultrasound is highly sensitive to even slight degrees of dilation of the renal collecting system. However, if ultrasound is performed very early after acute urinary obstruction, dilation of the renal pelvis may not yet have occurred. In retroperitoneal fibrosis, a condition which may cause bilateral ureteral obstruction and result in renal failure, the dense retroperitoneal fibrotic process which characterizes the disease may so encase the renal pelvis and ureters as to prevent significant dilation and result in a false negative ultrasound examination. False positive ultrasound exams can also be problematic. Causes for dilation of the renal collecting system other than obstruction, including reflux, normal anatomic variations (e.g. large extrarenal pelvis), chronic high urine flows as in diabetes insipidus, and persisting dilatation after surgical relief of long-standing obstruction, may confuse the unsuspecting.

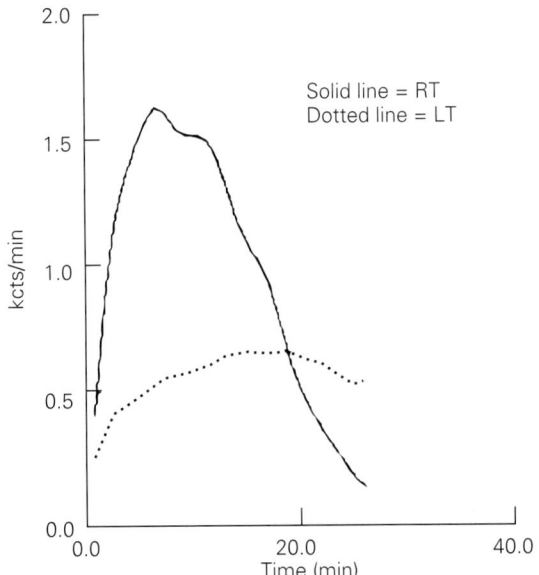

Figure 63.2 Radionuclide diuretic renogram. The right kidney tracing demonstrates normal uptake and excretion of radionuclide (solid line). There is delayed and diminished uptake with poor excretion from the left kidney, which does not improve after intravenous administration of furosemide (dotted line).

Radionuclide renal imaging (using technetium or radiolabelled iodine compounds) with furosemide, the so-called 'diuretic renogram', can accurately distinguish between the dilated non-obstructed and truly obstructed system in question cases (Chapter 21) [11]. The radionuclide collects in the dilated renal collecting system in either instance, but after furosemide administration will wash out of the non-obstructed system and remain in the obstructed kidney (Figure 63.2). Besides distinguishing the truly obstructed upper tract, the nuclear renogram can provide important data regarding both ipsilateral and contralateral renal function, both before and after intervention to relieve obstruction. Management of a non-functional renal unit may be very different from a kidney with significant residual function. Management of a poorly functional renal unit may depend on the function of the contralateral kidney and the patient's global renal function.

Before the advent of radionuclide diuretic renography, the Whitaker test provided our best functional measure of the presence or absence of urinary tract obstruction [13]. This is an invasive procedure, involving percutaneous puncture of the renal collecting system and controlled antegrade infusion of fluid with constant monitoring of renal pelvic pressure and bladder pressure. Development of renal pelvic pressures in excess of 15–22 cmH$_2$O at an infusion rate of 10 ml/min is felt to be diagnostic of obstruction. Generally, dilute contrast is used for infusion and radiographs are obtained, and thus anatomic as well as functional information can be gained from the Whitaker test. Because this is an invasive and relatively complex diagnostic test, it has been largely replaced by diuretic renography. However, the Whitaker test can still prove valuable in selected cases where the diuretic renogram produces equivocal findings.

Once the diagnosis of obstruction is made, identifying the etiology of the obstruction and outlining the anatomy of the urinary tract in order to plan an appropriate approach to management often require additional studies. Intravenous urography is seldom used today as an initial imaging modality in patients with suspected obstruction. In the presence of obstruction, classic findings include delay in both parenchymal uptake and excretion of intravenous contrast. In the presence of sufficient renal function and opacification of the upper urinary tract – often requiring serial, delayed films in the presence of obstruction – significant information regarding the exact anatomic location and nature of an obstructing lesion can be obtained from an intravenous urogram (Figure 63.3). However, this study is a far less reliable gauge of renal function. Significant contrast excretion is possible from a minimally functional kidney and very poor, delayed excretion is sometimes seen in an acutely obstructed, but still potentially normally functioning kidney.

The retrograde ureterogram and pyelogram is an invasive diagnostic procedure which requires ureteral catheterization during cystoscopy, followed by retrograde

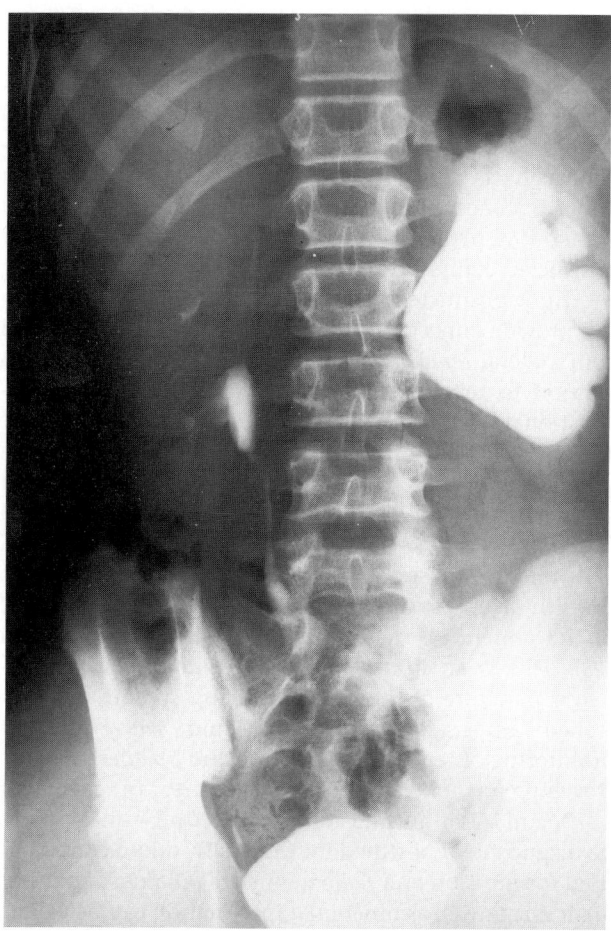

Figure 63.3 Intravenous urogram showing gross left hydronephrosis secondary to ureteropelvic junction obstruction. The right kidney and collecting system are normal.

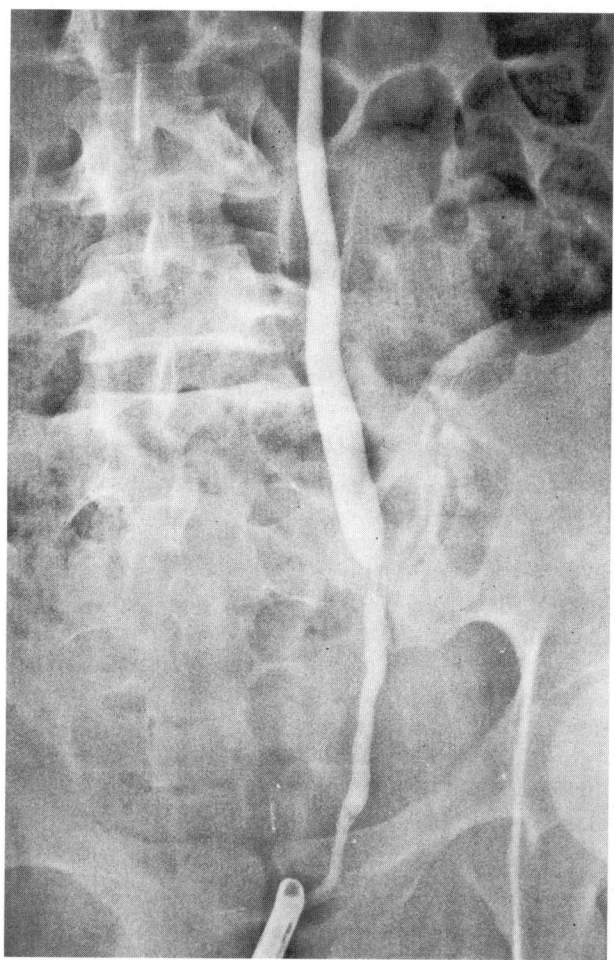

Figure 63.4 Retrograde ureteropyelogram demonstrating ureteral stricture overlying sacrum. Tip of cystoscope seen inferiorly.

injection of contrast material to obtain images of the ureter and proximal collecting system. This study can provide unique anatomic information in cases where intravenous contrast is contraindicated, where intravenous urography fails to produce sufficient opacification of an obstructed collecting system and ureter, or where the distal extent of an obstructing ureteral lesion is not visualized on standard urograms and must be defined prior to surgical intervention (Figure 63.4). Antegrade contrast injection of the upper urinary tract can also be performed via percutaneous nephrostomy access, with many of the same goals and indications.

Computed tomography is now commonly used to image mass lesions of the urinary tract, retroperitoneum and pelvis which might cause urinary obstruction, and can also define the nature of such lesions in many cases. The new, so-called 'spiral' technique of computed tomography scanning can be accomplished very quickly and easily compared to standard computed tomography scanning techniques. Even without intravenous contrast administration, a spiral computed tomography scan can effectively demonstrate either hydronephrosis or

hydroureter in the patient with suspected obstruction, and will also often demonstrate both the anatomic level of obstruction and nature of the obstructing lesion (e.g. ureteral calculus) [14]. Such spiral scans may thus provide significant information not routinely obtained during abdominal ultrasound examinations and in some instances may effectively replace ultrasound as an initial screening exam in the patient with suspected urinary obstruction. When appropriate, contrast administration can further enhance the diagnostic capability of spiral computed tomography. Magnetic resonance imaging has shown no particular advantage over computed tomography for imaging of the urinary tract, but may be advantageous in selected patients in whom intravenous contrast is contraindicated.

For diagnostic evaluation of obstructing lesions of the distal urinary tract – bladder and urethra – in adults, direct endoscopic inspection with cystourethroscopy is the gold standard. The voiding cystourethrogram (VCUG) and retrograde urethrogram may provide anatomic detail in select cases, particularly involving urethral pathology.

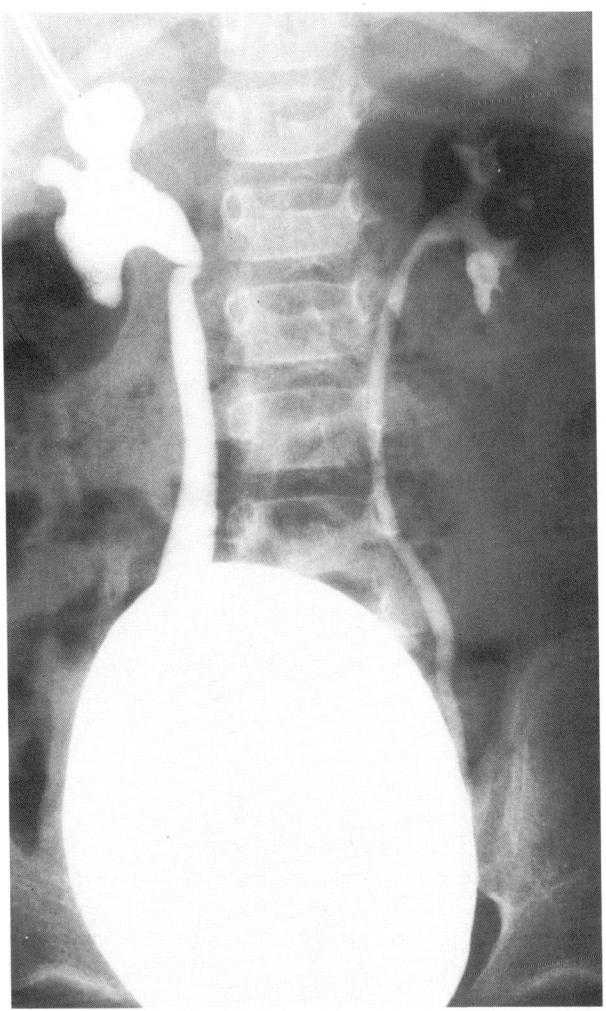

Figure 63.6 Voiding cystourethrogram showing bilateral vesicoureteral reflux of contrast material, grade IV in right kidney and grade III in left kidney.

etiology such as neurogenic bladder. The voiding portion of the examination is particularly essential in the male child to rule out occult posterior urethral valves (Figure 63.5).

Recently, radionuclide cystography has gained acceptance as a useful tool in the assessment of VUR [33]. This is performed in much the same way as standard VCUG, except that the contrast material used is a technetium radionuclide solution (Figure 63.7). Continuous monitoring is achieved with a gamma scintillation camera. The sensitivity of this examination in the detection of VUR is excellent and it involves a much lower radiation dose than standard VCUG. However, anatomical definition of the urinary tract is poor compared to standard VCUG and the urethra is not imaged. Although VCUG remains the standard for initial diagnosis and grading of VUR, radionuclide cystography has value in subsequent serial follow-up of patients with known VUR. Radionuclide cystography may also be useful in screening high risk children, i.e. siblings of children with VUR.

Ultrasound examination of the urinary system is simple and non-invasive and has a role in the management of VUR. It is employed as an initial screening tool to detect hydronephrosis, evaluate renal size and contour, detect renal scarring, and assess bladder wall thickness (an indicator of functional or mechanical postvesical obstruction). It is also very valuable in serial follow-up monitoring for hydronephrosis, renal size and renal scars. Ultrasound, however, cannot distinguish between VUR and obstruction as an etiology for hydronephrosis.

After diagnosis of VUR, intravenous urography is recommended initially to delineate the anatomy of the urinary tract and to inspect for anatomic causes such as congenital ureteral duplication and ureterocele. The intravenous urogram is also valuable in outlining renal scars and parenchymal thinning at presentation, but it is now largely replaced by the less invasive ultrasound exam in serial follow-up monitoring.

Radionuclide renal scan is used for initial evaluation and subsequent monitoring of renal function and scarring. It may also show reflux as a transient increase in radionuclide activity during the excretion phase of the affected collecting system (Figure 63.8). It is more sensitive in detecting renal scarring than intravenous urography but less specific.

Cystoscopy is generally not indicated in the evaluation of the patient with VUR. However, it can play an important role in assessing obstructing postvesical lesions and congenital anomalies of the distal ureter which may produce VUR. Complex urodynamic studies involve continuous monitoring of bladder pressures and sphincteric function during filling and voiding to assess detrusor function, compliance, and urinary sphincteric function. In patients with VUR related to neurogenic bladder dysfunction, and in selected cases of primary reflux wherein occult voiding dysfunction is suspected, urodynamic studies provide valuable data to guide management.

Classification and grading of reflux

The severity of reflux is most commonly graded using the system developed by the International Reflux Study Committee, which is based on the radiographic appearance of the ureter and the pyelocalyceal system on voiding cystourethrogram (VCUG). Five grades (I–V) are described in this International system (Figure 63.9). In grade I reflux, contrast passes retrograde into the ureter only. In grade II, contrast refluxes fully into the pelvicalyceal system without dilation. Grades I and II are considered mild degrees of reflux. Grade III reflux is defined as the presence of mild to moderate dilation of the ureter and renal pelvis and is typically referred to as moderate reflux. Grades IV and V are considered severe reflux. Grade IV requires blunting of the calyceal fornices, and greater dilation of the collecting system with early ureteral tortuosity is typically associated with this finding (Figure 63.6). In grade V reflux, gross clubbing of the renal calyces occurs with loss of papillary impressions, associated with

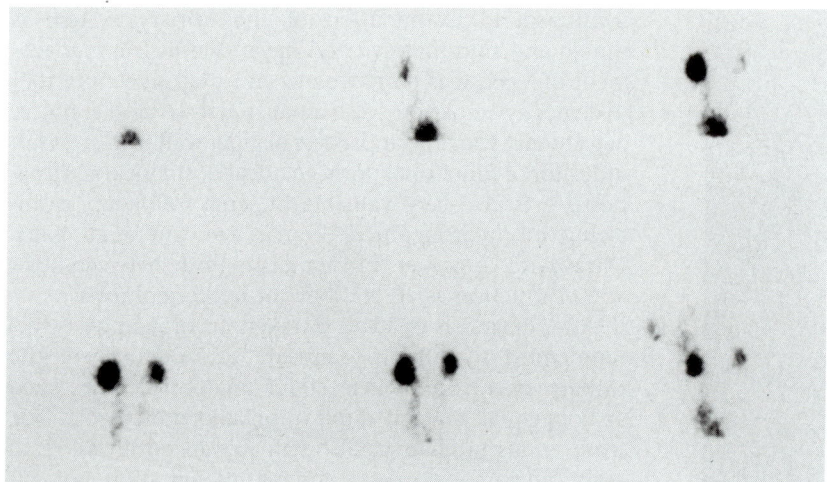

Figure 63.7 Radionuclide cystogram demonstrating bilateral vesicoureteral reflux.

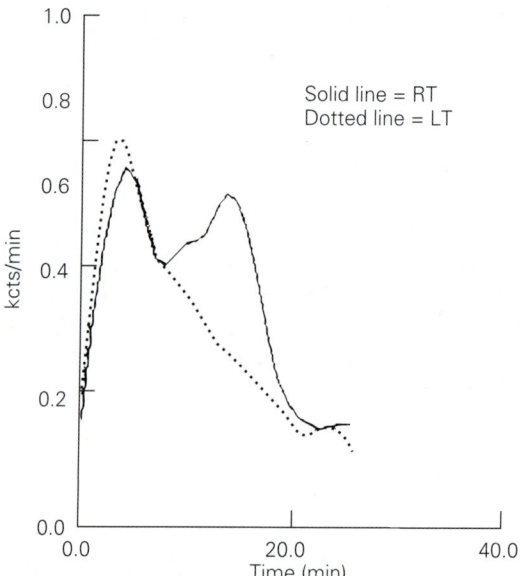

Solid line = RT
Dotted line = LT

kcts/min

Time (min)

Figure 63.8 Tracing from radionuclide renogram demonstrating normal curve for left kidney (dotted line), and vesicoureteral reflux of radionuclide creating a secondary peak in the right kidney curve (solid line).

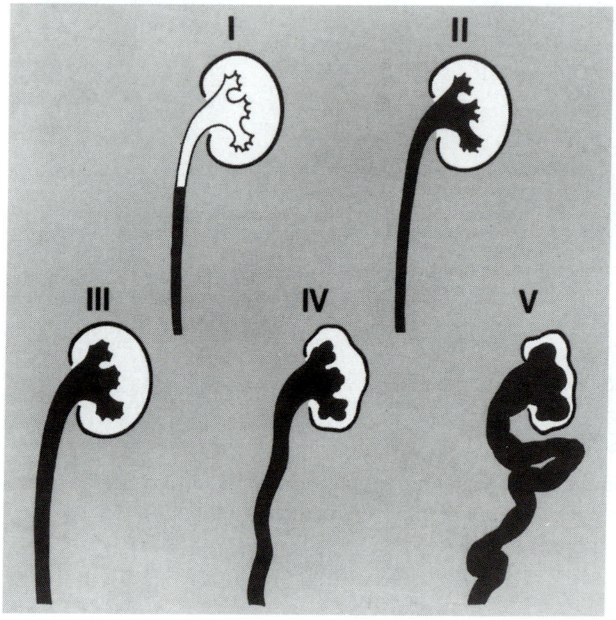

Figure 63.9 International grading system for vesicoureteral reflux.

gross dilation of the ureter and renal pelvis and marked tortuosity of the ureter. Assessment of grade or degree of reflux has clinical utility, since it has been shown to correlate well with prognosis and may impel decisions regarding treatment (see discussion of Treatment and Outcome, below).

Treatment

Medical management

Prompt recognition, diagnosis and aggressive treatment of pyelonephritis is vital in the setting of known VUR. Several studies have shown that delays in the institution

of treatment for pyelonephritis exacerbate subsequent renal parenchymal injury [34, 35]. More importantly, prevention of infection has become the hallmark of successful medical management of VUR.

The natural history of primary VUR in children is remarkable for its tendency to resolve over time, with ongoing development and maturation of the urinary tract. Resolution is most likely to occur in low-grade reflux without significant dilation of the collecting system. In a prospective study of VUR in children presenting before the age of five, the five-year resolution rates were 82%, 80% and 46% in grade I, II, and III VUR, respectively [36]. When this natural history is combined with the realization that significant renal scarring and reflux nephropathy are directly related to the combination of VUR and recurrent pyelonephritis, rather than reflux of sterile urine alone, a rationale for medical management of most children with VUR can be developed. The goal of medical management is thus to provide the opportunity for spontaneous resolution of VUR while maintaining the patient infection free and without lasting renal functional sequelae.

Prevention of urinary tract infection typically requires institution of prophylactic, oral, low-dose antimicrobial agents. The choice of drug and dose is based on the ability to achieve adequate urinary levels with relatively low serum levels and minimal effect on the normal fecal flora, thereby preventing the development of resistant organisms over time. Antimicrobials which have been used with success in this prophylactic role include cephalexin, sulfonamides, trimethoprim/sulfamethoxazole, and nitrofurantoin. Normalization of bladder function is often overlooked in these patients, but is also important in the successful management of VUR. As noted above, many of these patients exhibit dysfunctional voiding. Treatment may range from behavioral modification to medical management with anticholinergic agents to reduce uninhibited bladder contractions and lower bladder pressures. Finally, careful monitoring and follow-up examinations are a cornerstone of successful medical management. Typically, children are assessed at three-month intervals to assure compliance with medication, monitor growth and blood pressure, and screen for asymptomatic bacteriuria and development of proteinuria. At regular intervals, renal ultrasound is performed to assess upper tract dilation, parenchymal integrity, and renal growth; either standard VCUG or radionuclide cystogram is performed to monitor for resolution or progression of VUR. Renal function is evaluated at least yearly, with creatinine clearance and/or nuclear renogram. Once spontaneous resolution of VUR is documented, ongoing prophylactic antibiotic therapy and imaging of the urinary tract can be discontinued if no other genitourinary abnormality exists.

Surgical treatment

Surgical intervention for primary VUR in children is indicated in a number of clinical situations to prevent ongoing renal parenchymal injury. Patients with severe grades of reflux (IV or V) are less likely to experience spontaneous resolution and more likely to develop renal functional impairment, and should generally be treated surgically. Patients with recurrent pyelonephritis despite compliance with medical regimens, or because of non-compliance with medical regimens, should undergo surgical correction. Patients with documented progression of renal injury should also be treated surgically. In patients with associated anomalies of the bladder and ureter, surgical correction may also be indicated.

The basic principle of surgical therapy is to create or restore competence of the distal ureteral antireflux mechanism. The standard of surgical therapy is ureteral reimplantation into the bladder wall (ureteroneocystostomy), creating a submucosal tunnel which will serve as a valve mechanism and establish ureterovesical competence. This is successful in over 95% of patients [37]. More recently, less-invasive attempts to manage VUR with endoscopic surgical approaches have been tried, utilizing periureteral injection of collagen or Teflon paste to create occlusion and correct reflux. Long-term results from these operations await to be assessed. Surgical success, regardless of approach, relies on careful preoperative assessment to ensure the absence of untreated neurogenic bladder dysfunction or bladder outlet obstruction, and that bladder capacity and function are adequate. If these added pathologies exist they must also be treated prior to or at the time of reflux surgery.

In adults with secondary or acquired VUR, and in whom renal deterioration due to VUR is relatively unusual compared to children, surgical correction of VUR is rarely indicated. Rather, surgical relief of bladder outlet obstruction and/or treatment of neurogenic bladder dysfunction take precedence.

Outcome

In children with low grade, primary VUR, rates of spontaneous resolution over time are high, and compliance with medical management produces excellent long-term outcomes with a low incidence of progressive renal parenchymal injury. In more complex cases of VUR, with higher grades of reflux, surgical therapy produces excellent results. The International Reflux Study in Children recently reported the results of ureteral reimplantation in 154 refluxing ureters. The initial success rate was 96%. Reflux persisted postoperatively in only six ureters. In four of these, the reflux resolved spontaneously during the following 20 months, one was lost to follow-up, and one had long-term persistence of reflux. Thus, the long-term success rate exceeded 98% [37]. In a randomized clinical trial of medical versus surgical management in a total of 132 patients with grade III and IV reflux, the same group reported an 8% yearly resolution rate with medical management after the first three years and calculated an approximately 50% resolution rate in patients with grade IV reflux after nine years [29]. The rate of pyelonephritis was significantly less after surgical treatment than with medical management in patients with higher grade reflux. However, the rate of new renal scars, scar progression, and renal thinning were similar in both treatment groups, suggesting that renal injury occurred preoperatively and its radiological sequelae required time to become apparent postoperatively. This points out the major problem in the management of VUR – that many patients present for urologic management only after significant renal parenchymal damage has occurred, and some, on the basis of pre-existing renal injuries will progress to end-stage renal disease despite all interventions.

Prevention

Although primary VUR is a congenital anomaly and cannot at this time be prevented, prompt diagnosis and proper management aimed at avoiding the sequelae of reflux nephropathy and loss of renal function is possible. Most patients with clinically significant VUR are children and initially are taken to see a pediatrician, who must be alerted to the possible diagnosis of VUR by symptoms or presence of urinary tract infection. As noted, a high index of suspicion is often crucial to early, accurate diagnosis in these cases. In children discovered to have hydronephrosis on prenatal ultrasound exams, early neonatal evaluation for VUR is indicated. Similarly,

because of the known heritability of VUR, siblings of children with VUR should be preemptively screened for this condition, rather than waiting for presentation with infection.

In adults with secondary or acquired VUR, significant renal scarring and reflux nephropathy are much less commonly observed. Nonetheless, certain patient populations are at increased risk, including men with high-grade bladder outlet obstruction and patients with advanced neurogenic bladder dysfunction, such as occurs following spinal cord injury. Relief of mechanical and functional causes of obstruction, and careful attention to prevention and control of urinary tract infection in such patients, can limit the impact of VUR on renal function.

References

1. Moody, T.E., Vaughan, E.D., Jr and Gillenwater, J.Y. (1975) Relationship between renal blood flow and ureteral pressure during 18 hours of total unilateral occlusion. *Invest. Urol.*, **13**, 246–51.
2. Vaughan, E.D., Jr, Shenasky, J.H., II and Gillenwater, J.Y. (1971) Mechanism of acute hemodynamic response to ureteral occlusion. *Invest. Urol.*, **9**, 109–18.
3. Vaughan, E.D., Jr, Sweet, R.C. and Gillenwater, J.Y. (1970) Peripheral renin and blood pressure changes following complete unilateral ureteral occlusion. *J. Urol.*, **104**, 89–92.
4. Vaughan, E.D., Jr, Sorenson, E.J. and Gillenwater, J.Y. (1970) The renal hemodynamic response to chronic unilateral complete ureteral occlusion. *Invest. Urol.*, **8**, 78–90.
5. Vaughan, E.D., Jr, Sweet, R.C. and Gillenwater, J.Y. (1973) Unilateral ureteral occlusion: pattern of nephron repair and compensatory response. *J. Urol.*, **109**, 979–82.
6. Lewis, H.Y. and Pierce, J.M. (1962) Return of function after relief of complete ureteral obstruction of 69 days' duration. *J. Urol.*, **88**, 377–9.
7. Gillenwater, J.Y., Westervelt, F.B., Jr, Vaughan, E.D. Jr and Howards, S.S. (1975) Renal function after release of chronic unilateral hydronephrosis in man. *Kidney Int.*, **7**, 179–86.
8. Vaughan, E.D., Jr, Bühler, F.R. and Laragh, J.H. (1974) Normal renin secretion in hypertensive patients with primarily unilateral chronic hydronephrosis. *J. Urol.*, **112**, 153–6.
9. Jaenike, J.R. (1972) The renal functional defect of postobstructive nephropathy: the effects of bilateral ureteral obstruction in the rat. *J. Clin. Invest.*, **51**, 2999–3006.
10. Howards, S.S. (1973) Postobstructive diuresis: a misunderstood phenomenon. *J. Urol.*, **110**, 537–40.
11. Vaughan, E.D. and Gillenwater, J.Y. (1973) Diagnosis, characterization and management of postobstructive diuresis. *J. Urol.*, **109**, 286–92.
12. Thrall, J.H., Koff, S.A. and Keyes, J.W., Jr (1981) Diuretic radionuclide renography and scintigraphy in the differential diagnosis of hydroureteronephrosis. *Semin. Nucl. Med.*, **11**, 89–104.
13. Whitaker, R.H. (1973) Diagnosis of obstruction in dilated ureters. *Ann. R. Coll. Surg.*, **53**, 153–66.
14. Sommer, F.G., Jeffrey, R.B., Jr, Rubin, G.D., Napel, S., Rimmer, S.A., Benford, J. and Harter, P.M. (1995) Detection of ureteral calculi in patients with suspected renal colic: value of reformatted noncontrast helical CT. *A.J.R.*, **165**, 509–13.
15. Becerra, J.E., Khoury, M.J., Cordero, J.R. and Erickson, J.D. (1990) Diabetes mellitus during pregnancy and the risks for specific birth defects. *Pediatrics*, **85**, 1–9.
16. Bailey, R.R. (1979) Vesicoureteric reflux in healthy infants and children, in *Reflux Nephropathy* (eds J. Hodson and P. Kincaid-Smith), Masson, New York, p. 59.
17. Baker, R., Maxted, W., Maylath, J. and Shuman, I. (1966) Relation of age, sex, and infection to reflux: data indicating high spontaneous cure rate in pediatric patients. *J. Urol.*, **95**, 27–32.
18. Smellie, J.M. and Normand, I.C.S. (1966) The clinical features and significance of urinary infection in childhood. *Proc. R. Soc. Med.*, **59**, 415–16.
19. Shopfner, C.E. (1970) Vesicoureteral reflux. *Radiology*, **95**, 637–48.
20. Askari, A. and Belman, A.B. (1982) Vesicoureteral reflux in black girls. *J. Urol.*, **127**, 747–8.
21. Walker, R.D., Duckett, J., Bartone, F. *et al.* (1977) Screening school children for urologic disease. *Pediatrics*, **60**, 239–43.
22. Dwoskin, J.Y. (1976) Sibling uropathology. *J. Urol.*, **115**, 726–7.
23. Jenkins, G.R. and Noe, H.N. (1982) Familial vesicoureteral reflux: a prospective study. *J. Urol.*, **128**, 774–8.
24. Noe, H.N. (1986) Screening for familial reflux: an update. *Semin. Urol.*, **4**, 86–7.
25. Rolleston, G.L., Shannon, F.T. and Utley, W.L.F. (1970) Relationship of infantile vesicoureteric reflux to renal damage. *Br. Med. J.*, **1**, 460–3.
26. Najmaldin, A., Burge, D.M. and Atwell, J.D. (1990) Fetal vesicoureteric reflux. *Br. J. Urol.*, **65**, 403–6.
27. Van Gool, J.D., Hjalmas, K., Tamminen-Mobius, T. and Olbing, H. (1992) Historical clues to the complex of

dysfunctional voiding, urinary tract infection and vesicoureteral reflux. *J. Urol.*, **148**, 1699–702.

28. Kekomaki, M. and Walker, R.D. (1988) Fractional excretion of magnesium and renal concentration capacity in refluxing renal units. *J. Urol.*, **140**, 1095–6.

29. Weiss, R., Duckett, J. and Spitzer, A. (1992) Results of a randomized clinical trial of medical versus surgical management of infants and children with Grades III and IV primary vesicoureteral reflux (United States). *J. Urol.*, **148**, 1667–73.

30. Torres, V.E., Malek, R.S. and Svensson, J.P. (1983) Vesicoureteral reflux in the adult: II. Nephropathy, hypertension and stones. *J. Urol.*, **130**, 41–4.

31. Salvatierra, O., Jr and Tanagho, E.A. (1977) Reflux as a cause of end stage kidney disease: Report of 32 cases. *J. Urol.*, **117**, 441–3.

32. Arant, B.S., Jr (1991) Vesicoureteral reflux and renal injury. *Am. J. Kidney Dis.*, **17**, 491–511.

33. Willi, U.V. and Treves, S. (1983) Radionuclide voiding cystogram. *Urol. Radiol.*, **5**, 161–73.

34. Winberg, A.L., Bergstrom, T. and Jacobsson, B. (1975) Morbidity, age and sex distribution, recurrences and renal scarring in symptomatic urinary tract infection in childhood. *Kidney Int.*, **8**, S-101–6.

35. Winter, A.L., Hardy, B.E., Alton, D.J. *et al.* (1988) Acquired renal scars in children. *J. Urol.*, **129**, 1190–3.

36. Arant, B.S., Jr (1992) Medical management of mild and moderate vesicoureteral reflux: follow-up studies of infants and young children. A preliminary report of Southwest Pediatric Nephrology Study Group. *J. Urol.*, **148**, 1683–7.

37. Duckett, J.W., Walker, R.D. and Weiss, R. (1992) Surgical results: International Reflux Study in Children – United States Branch. *J. Urol.*, **148**, 1674–5.

Further Reading

Duckett, J.W. (1993) Update on vesicoureteral reflux. *Am. Urol. Assoc. Update Series*, **5**, 34–9.

Gillenwater, J.Y. (1992) The pathophysiology of urinary tract obstruction, in *Campbell's Urology*, 6th edn (eds P.C. Walsh, A.B. Retik, T.A. Stamey and E.D. Vaughan, Jr), W.B. Saunders, Philadelphia, pp. 499–532.

Resnick, M.I. and Kursh, E.D. (1992) Extrinsic obstruction of the ureter, in *Campbell's Urology*, 6th edn (eds P.C. Walsh, A.B. Retik, T.A. Stamey and E.D. Vaughan Jr), W.B. Saunders, Philadelphia, pp. 533–69.

Walker, R.D. (1991) Vesicoureteral reflux, in *Adult and Pediatric Urology*, 2nd edn (eds J.Y. Gillenwater, J.T. Grayhack, S.S. Howards and J.W. Duckett), Year Book Medical Publishers, Chicago, pp. 1889–1920.

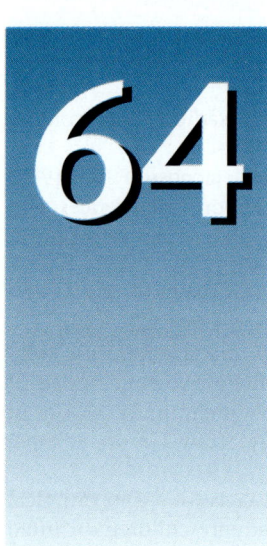

64

Adult renal neoplasia

R.R. Hall

Introduction

Renal cancer remains the most enigmatic of tumors, so often silent in its growth, varied in presentation and unpredictable of outcome. The adage that one-third of renal tumors present with hematuria, one-third with loin pain or a mass and one-third with metastases is still largely true, but the increasing and ubiquitous use of ultrasound scanning of the abdomen has led to the diagnosis of many unsuspected, smaller and asymptomatic renal cancers. Thus, it is possible that the overall pattern of renal malignancy will change and the prognosis improve, but for the immediate future the majority of patients will continue to present with locally advanced or metastatic disease.

Surgery is the only effective treatment for the primary tumor and very carefully selected patients with solitary metastases. Radiotherapy can offer worthwhile palliation for painful or hemorrhagic metastases. Immunotherapy and chemotherapy remain experimental and although used with increasing frequency, have yet to be shown to be of any significant survival benefit.

Survival depends on the local extent of the primary tumor determined at the time of surgical exploration. Tumor stage, grade, venous invasion, nodal involvement and metastatic status are the principal indicators of long-term outcome, but there is a wide variation within prognostic groupings.

Incidence and etiology

Renal cancers account for about 2% of all malignancies world wide [1]. The highest incidence rates are reported from Europe, North America and Scandinavia and the lowest in Chinese, Japanese and Indians in their home countries. In common with some other cancers the incidence is higher for these nationals when resident in North America. The world-wide incidence has been increasing at an annual rate of 2% with mortality rates in the United Kingdom, Italy, Japan and Australia rising, particularly in older cohorts. In other countries the incidence remains stable.

A number of environmental, hormonal and genetic causative factors have been suspected, but little is known of the etiology of this tumor. The large majority of renal cancers are sporadic, appear after 50 years of age and are twice as common in men than women. Cigarette smoking is an established risk factor with a relative risk of two for current versus never smokers, but this is lower than most other tobacco-related cancers [2].

A family history of renal cancer is associated with an increased risk in both men and women with an odds ratio of greater than four [3]. Renal cancer like retinoblastoma, breast, colon and prostate cancers occurs in both sporadic and inherited forms. Three types of inherited renal cancer have been identified accounting for up to 4% of all renal tumors [4]. The first is the renal cancer found in von

Nephrology, Edited by Rex L. Jamison and Robert Wilkinson.
Published in 1997 by Chapman & Hall, London. ISBN 0 412 60930 4

Hippel–Lindau disease [5], the second is an autosomal dominant renal tumor occurring in 50% of at-risk individuals [6] and the third is hereditary papillary renal carcinoma [7]. These hereditary tumors differ from the common sporadic tumor by being multiple, bilateral and appearing at a younger age, sometimes in teenagers. Several independent studies noted abnormalities of the short arm of chromosome 3 in tumors of families with hereditary renal cancer [8]. Cytogenetic analysis of sporadic, non-familial renal tumors also revealed frequent and consistent rearrangements, deletions and translocations involving chromosome 3. Subsequent studies confirmed that loss of a segment of the short arm of chromosome 3 is a consistent finding in clear cell renal carcinoma, although this is not observed in papillary renal cancers.

Von Hippel–Lindau disease (VHL) is an inherited cancer syndrome in which 40% of patients develop multiple renal tumors, 60% retinal angiomas, 60% central nervous system hemangioblastomas, 18% pheochromocytomas, 7% benign cystadenomas of the epididymis plus pancreatic cysts and occasionally pancreatic islet cell tumors [5, 9]. Linehan *et al.* [8] localized the VHL gene to a small region of chromosome 3p and have identified the VHL gene by cloning studies that now permit the presymptomatic DNA diagnosis of family members with VHL disease. The association of specific chromosomal mutations with characteristic disease patterns will enable physicians to target regular examinations of affected members of VHL members.

Knudson [10] has hypothesized that both inherited and sporadic variations of a particular cancer involve the same tumor suppressor gene. It was demonstrated that although there may be clinical heterogeneity in the expression of VHL disease (predominantly pheochromocytomas rather than renal cancers in certain families) there is genetic homogeneity. Examination of sporadic renal cancers has revealed the loss of one copy of the VHL gene in 98% of tumors and VHL mutations in 57% [11]. Other authors have confirmed these findings and although VHL mutations have not been found in all renal cancers (the VHL gene is not involved in hereditary papillary renal carcinoma), the identification of the VHL gene in many early as well as advanced renal tumors suggests that VHL mutations are a critical event in the development of sporadic as well as familial renal carcinoma.

Pathology

The large majority of adult renal cancers arise from the proximal tubules of the kidney and are thus known as renal carcinoma. A few are tumors of the renal connective tissue (sarcoma, angiomyolipoma) or are metastases from other primary sites.

Renal carcinoma

In 1883 Grawitz [12], describing a series of renal tumors concluded that they had arisen in aberrant adrenal tissue lying within the kidney, hence the term 'hypernephroma'. Doubt was soon cast on their adrenal origin and they were considered to be of renal tubular origin, which remains the current opinion. 'Renal carcinoma' is the preferred terminology. In the absence of precise knowledge of the cell of origin 'renal cell carcinoma' is no longer appropriate. 'Clear cell carcinoma' refers to only one type of renal tumor and 'adenocarcinoma' implies glandular differentiation which is not always present. Renal cancers tend to be very vascular, often contain areas of necrosis, have a tendency to invade the renal veins but usually remain encapsulated even when of large size. The very varied histopathological appearance has been reviewed in detail by several authors [13, 14].

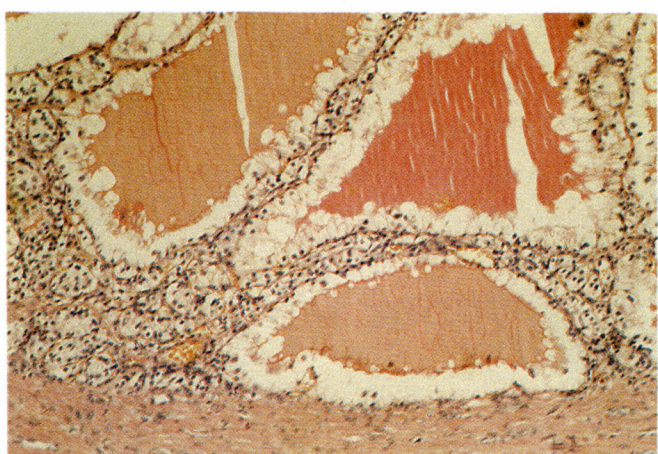 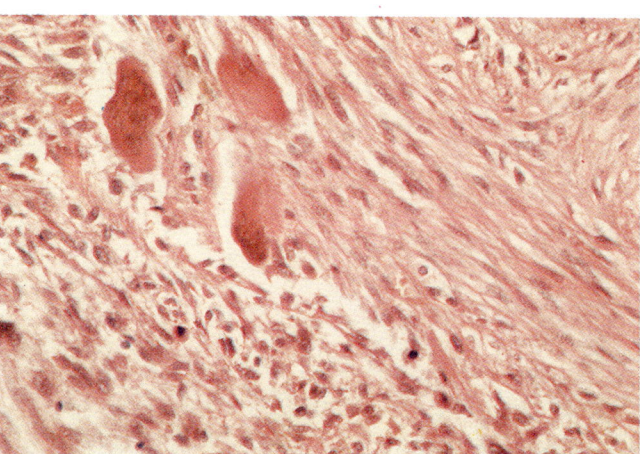

b

Figure 64.1   (a) Well-differentiated renal carcinoma showing tubular and acinar pattern. (b) Poorly differentiated spindle cell renal carcinoma. (Hematoxylin and eosin, ×250.)

Adenoma

There is still uncertainty about the distinction between renal carcinoma and benign 'adenoma' of the kidney. Small subcapsular nodules identical in appearance to the adrenal cortex are found in 5% of all kidneys, equally in both sexes at any age [15]. By contrast, a different type of small cortical nodule is found in up to 25% of men over the age of 50 (rarely younger) and in less than 10% of women which appear to arise from the proximal convoluted tubule. On light and electron microscopy these nodules are indistinguishable from well-differentiated renal carcinoma. Following the suggestion of Bell in 1950 [16] it became common parlance to call tumors less than 3 cm in diameter 'benign' adenoma and tumors larger than 3 cm, no matter how well differentiated, 'carcinoma'. More recent findings, by ultrasound or computed tomographic (CT) scanning, of tumors less than 3 cm with undoubted malignant characteristics has undermined this arbitrary separation. Although some, or even the majority, of incidental small tumors revealed by random imaging may not progress or metastasize, current opinion favors their removal by local excision or partial nephrectomy because their malignant potential remains uncertain.

Tumor grade

Conventionally renal tumors are described as well, moderately or poorly differentiated but the predictive value of these three groups is not strong [17, 18]. Some authors divide tumors into well and poorly differentiated (Figure 64.1a,b), associated with 10-year survival rates of 40% and 20%, respectively without detailed analysis of histological features [19]. Whatever the merits of different grading systems it is important to be aware that metastases from well-differentiated renal tumors may appear up to 30 years after nephrectomy [20, 21].

Oncocytoma

Oncocytomas were described by Klein and Valensi [22] as benign tumors. They are composed entirely of oncocytes which are proximal tubule cells rich in mitochondria but with few other cytoplasmic organelles and few, if any, mitoses (Figure 64.2). Variable degrees of cellular differentiation are now recognized and up to 20% may metastasize [4]. Since they are devoid of hemorrhage and necrosis they may be suspected from their homogenous appearance on ultrasound or CT scaning. Partial or radical nephrectomy is appropriate according to tumor size. The diagnosis is usually made postoperatively by the histopathologist.

Angiomyolipoma

This is an uncommon benign tumor of the kidney occurring more frequently in women than in men but typically in the fifth decade. It is usually asymptomatic [23]. Occasionally such tumors are large and may be the site of acute hemorrhage and rupture that presents a life-threatening situation with acute and severe flank pain and an abdominal mass. The tumor comprises smooth muscle, thickened blood vessels and mature adipose tissue, a combination that gives a typical, diagnostic appearance on CT scan (Figure 64.3). When found in association with tuberous sclerosis they tend to be multiple. Local extension and venous involvement has been described but metastasis is not thought to occur [24]. Very rarely these tumors co-exist with renal cancer [25]. Surgery is seldom necessary. Embolization is the most appropriate treatment for acute hemorrhage.

Juxtaglomerular tumor

These are rare, small, benign, well-circumscribed tumors of the renal cortex that produce renin and cause hyper-

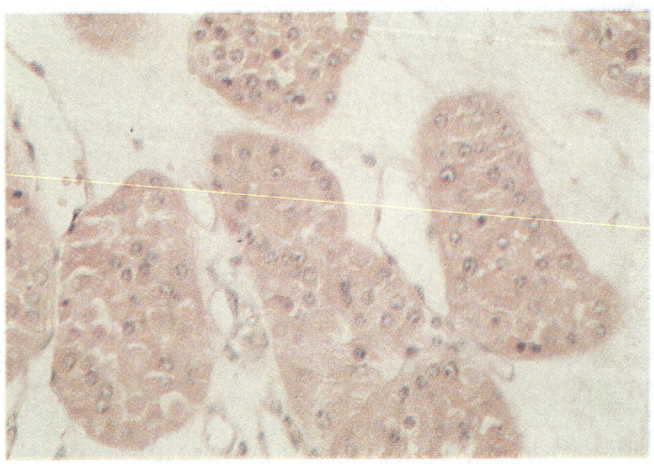

Figure 64.2 Oncocytoma.

tension and hypokalaemia. Histologically the cytoplasmic granules containing renin are detected by immunofluorescence. Excision of the tumor cures the hypertension in younger patients [26].

Tumor spread

Most renal tumors grow by local expansion but are often confined within a pseudocapsule even when quite large. Eventually this pseudocapsule and the renal capsule are breached by tumor invasion into the perinephric fat. Although the tumor is usually contained by Gerota's fascia, direct growth into the psoas muscle, the diaphragm, colon, liver, adrenal, spleen and stomach may occur. Symptoms of such invasion are seldom recognized preoperatively, but invasion of the calyces or the renal pelvis is a source of hematuria.

Lymphatic spread

Lymphatic spread is common in renal cancer, the regional lymph nodes being those at the renal hilum and in the abdominal retroperitoneum (Figure 64.4). Postmortem studies have shown that two-thirds of patients who have para-aortic node involvement will also have mediastinal or distant metastases.

Venous invasion

Visible or palpable growth of tumor in the renal vein or vena cava, sometimes extending as far as the right atrium, is well known to occur. It carries a poor prognosis. Microscopic venous invasion occurs much more frequently than is visibly evident, but only recently has its prognostic importance been recognized. Van Poppel *et al.* [27] reported the finding of microscopic venous invasion in 23% and macroscopic invasion in an additional 18% of patients undergoing nephrectomy. With a mean follow-up of 42 months, 77% of patients with no vascular invasion were free of disease, compared with 51% who had microscopic invasion and only 22% of those with macroscopic tumor in the renal vein. Other authors report similar findings and have suggested that venous invasion is of

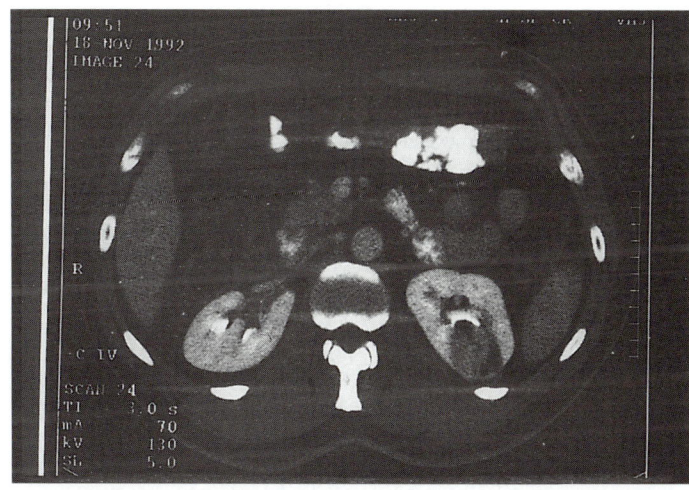

Figure 64.3 CT scan showing angiomyolipoma of posterior aspect left kidney. Note dark areas indicating fat within the tumor.

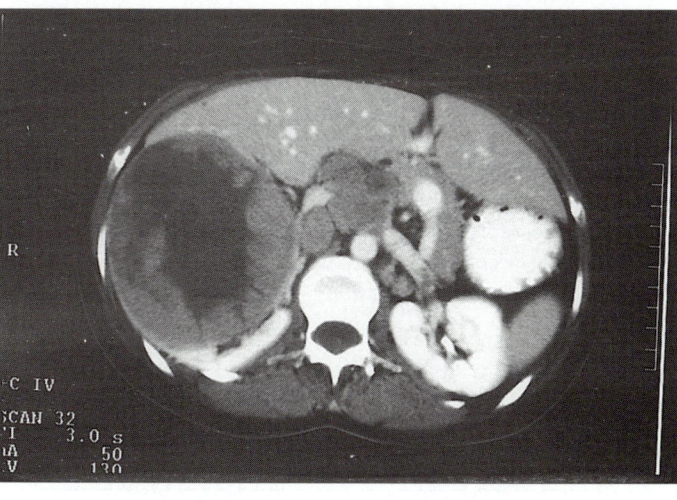

Figure 64.4 CT scan showing large right renal cancer with extensive central necrosis. Note also extensive retrocaval and preaortic lymph node metastases.

greater prognostic significance than either tumor stage or grade [28, 29].

TNM classification

The Tumour, Node and Metastasis classification of the Union Internationale Contre le Cancer (UICC) describes the anatomical extent of the primary kidney tumor (T), the regional lymph nodes (N) and metastatic sites (M) and having been adopted by the American Joint Committee for Cancer Staging (AJCC), it has replaced previous classifications [30, 31] (Table 64.1). It is a pretreatment clinical classification based on clinical examination, chest radiograph, intravenous urography (IVU), ultrasound scan, CT, magnetic resonance imaging (MRI) or angiographic imaging and isotopic scans as are considered appropriate by the clinician. The accuracy of all these methods of imaging is known to be limited. For prognostic purposes greater reliance is placed on the histopathological examination of the operative specimen (pTNM) which provides detailed information of capsular penetration, venous invasion and lymph node metastases.

In general germs, if lymph node metastases are not present the outcome is determined by pT category: five-year survival following radical nephrectomy with or without lymphadenectomy is typically 100% for pT1 tumors, 90% for pT2, less than 60% for pT3 and 25% for pT4a.

Palpable lymph node metastases are found in about 10% of patients undergoing laparotomy with a view to nephrectomy, but microscopic confirmation of nodal involvement is found in only about 3% of patients actually subjected to nephrectomy, patients with gross nodal involvement being excluded. Regional lymph node metastases are rarely found in tumors confined to the kidney, but are present in half the patients with pT3 cancers, The significance of nodal involvement is reflected in survival: over 70% of patients without nodal deposits survive five years compared with less than 10% when such metastases are present.

Because of the variability in biological behavior of kidney tumors and the interrelationship of different factors that may be identified for prognostic purposes, it is inevitable that there is a certain amount of divergence of opinion in the published literature. Nonetheless, among the relatively few publications that have considered tumor size as a prognostic indicator, most conclude that tumor size is an important variable, there being an inverse relationship between size and survival. This is particulary significant for tumors 10 cm or larger for whom five-year survival ranges from 50% to only 22% [14, 31]. In general terms, a patient with a kidney tumour 10 cm or larger in size is more likely to die within five years despite undergoing appropriate surgery. Patients with smaller kidney tumors are more likely to survive.

The current subdivision of T3 kidney cancers suggests that extension of tumor into the inferior vena cava is more serious than perinephric invasion, but this is not necessarily true. When tumors confined to the kidney have caval extension, average survival is 40 months, but this is reduced to 18 months when similar caval extension is associated with tumors extending into the perinephric fat [30]. If resection of renal cancer including extension to the vena cava is complete, the long-term survival is determined by other prognostic factors. The presence of tumor thrombus in the vena cava should be distinguished from tumor invasion of the wall of the inferior vena cava which has a much worse prognosis and is seldom cured by even the most extensive surgery. Similarly, nephrectomy is almost always contraindicated if regional lymph node metastases are known to be present.

Table 64.1 TNM classification of renal tumors

Primary tumor (T)	
TX	Primary tumor cannot be assessed
TO	No evidence of primary tumor
T1	Tumor 2.5 cm or less in greatest dimension limited to the kidney
T2	Tumor more than 2.5 cm in greatest dimension limited to the kidney
T3	Tumor extends into major veins or invades the adrenal gland or perinephric tissues but not beyong Gerota's fascia
T3a	Tumor invades the adrenal gland or perinephric tissues but not beyond Gerota's fascia
T3B	Tumor grossly extends into the renal vein(s) or vena cava below the diaphragm
T3c	Tumor grossly extends into the vena cava above the diaphragm
T4	Tumor invades beyond Gerota's fascia
Regional lymph nodes (N)	
NX	Regional lymph nodes cannot be assessed
N0	No regional lymph node metastasis
N1	Metastasis in a single lymph node, 2 cm or less in greatest dimension
N2	Metastasis in a single lymph node, more than 2 cm but not more than 5 cm in greatest dimension; or multiple lymph nodes, none more than 5 cm in greatest dimension
N3	Metastasis in a lymph node more than 5 cm in greatest dimension
Distant metastasis (M)	
MX	Presence of distant metastasis cannot be assessed
M0	No distant metastasis
M1	Distant metastasis

A wide range of alternative factors that seemingly influence outcome have been described. These include erythrocyte sedimentation rate (ESR), fever or night sweats, weight loss, duration of symptoms, flank pain, a palpable mass, hypertension, hypercalcemia, age, tumor cell type, nuclear morphology and the necessity for blood transfusion. Although these factors may demonstrate prognostic significance in univariate analyses and a few may have independent prognostic significance, most of them can be accounted for by their close association with tumor stage. None adds significantly for practical purposes to the pT category, nodal status or vascular invasion as predictors of survival. Similarly, DNA ploidy, cytogenetic studies, expression of oncogenes such as *p53* and *c-myc*, and growth factors are of no clinical prognostic help at the present time, although their study has made several very valuable contributions to our understanding of the mechanism of renal tumor development and growth.

Clinical presentation

Hematuria

Hematuria is a frequent presenting symptom for renal cancer but it is also a common symptom in men over 50 years of age. It is much more likely to be due to urothelial cancer of the bladder than renal cancer, but imaging of the kidneys is essential to investigate this possibility. Worm-like clots in the urine suggest a renal origin. Similarly, crenellated red cells in the urine best seen by phase contrast microscopy, are suggestive of a source in the kidneys rather than the lower urinary tract, but this is by no means a reliable distinction. Haphazard or routine dipstick testing of urine is now widespread practice and 'dipstick hematuria' is a common finding. Unfortunately, it may be the only indication of a renal tumor, or other significant pathology, and full investigation cannot be avoided and should include urine protein, blood pressure, serum creatinine, plain radiograph of the abdomen, ultrasound of kidneys (or an IVU) and flexible cystoscopy.

Pain

The discomfort caused by renal tumors is usually described as a dull ache in the loin, flank or abdomen or simply as 'back pain'. Sudden severe pain may be caused by hemorrhage into the tumour. Passage of blood clot down the ureter following heavy bleeding into the pelvicalyceal system may cause ureteric colic.

Palpable mass

The finding of an abdominal mass is usually a very late symptom; it is surprising how large a mass may develop without it being noticed by the patient or found by the examining physician. Movement with respiration and the ease of bimanual palpation are classical signs. Weight loss often accounts for a renal mass becoming noticeable when it has been present, but inapparent, for many months.

Enlarged lymph nodes in the neck or groin, hepatosplenomegaly [32], a persistent (right-sided) varicocele, ascites or metastatic skin nodules may all be the presenting, palpable signs of an underlying renal cancer.

Systemic effects

Renal cancers cause such a plethora of non-urological symptoms that it is sometimes known as the 'internist's tumour'. Presenting symptoms may include lassitude, malaise, anorexia, nausea, bowel disturbance, weight loss, night sweats, fever, anemia, polyneuritis and myositis. Tumor extension into the renal vein obstructing the testicular vein may produce a varicocele that does not collapse when the patient is supine. Complete tumor obstruction of the vena cava will cause genital and lower limb edema, dilated abdominal wall veins and ascites. Obstruction of the hepatic vein may disturb liver function and cause portal hypertension. Central nervous system (CNS) metastases may lead to presentation with a variety of focal neurological problems. Lung metastases may present with hemoptysis. Large anteriovenous fistulae in some renal tumors can cause of high output cardiac failure.

In addition to being the sign of advanced malignancy some symptoms are manifestations of the paraneoplastic syndrome frequently associated with renal cancers [33, 34]. Fevers (20%) have been suggested to be due to endogenous pyrogens [35]. Erythrocytosis (5%) usually, but not always, reflects erythropoietin production by the tumor, hypertension (25%) may be secondary to raised renin levels [36], hypercalcemia (15%) associated with a parathyroid hormone-like substance [37], Cushing's syndrome (adrenocorticotrophin), hypoglycemia (insulin), galactorrhea (prolactin), amenorrhea, hirsutism, gynecomastia, or loss of libido (gonadotrophins) have all been reported with renal cancer and are believed to reflect inappropriate endocrine production by the tumor itself [33, 34, 38].

Diagnosis and investigation

The majority of renal cancers present with gross, microscopic or dipstick hematuria and are detected as space-occupying lesions by ultrasound scan of the kidney or intravenous urography. A renal mass may be visible on plain radiograph of the abdomen or calcification may be seen in a renal tumor. However, it should be noted that significant renal tumors may not cause obvious distortion of the pelvicalyceal system. Ultrasonography distinguishes solid tumors from cysts. A CT scan with intravenous and oral contrast is essential to confirm the nature of the renal lesion, assess its extent and invasion and to detect the presence of hilar or para-aortic lymphadenopathy. It also confirms the presence of a functioning contralateral kindney. Most renal cancers are hypervascular, but a few are hypovascular on contrast-enhanced images. The CT appearance of an angiomyolipoma is very characteristic and should be diagnostic of these unusual but benign tumors. Oncocytomas are usually homogenous and not particularly vascular and may be suggested by their CT appearance. Prior to surgery, Doppler ultrasound scanning is advisable as the best modality for demonstrating tumor thrombus extension in the renal vein and vena cava. Renal angiography is now obsolete as a diagnostic aid for solid lesions of the kidney, but is useful for the demonstration of renal vasculature preoperatively if a kidney-conserving operation is planned.

If the diagnosis of a renal mass is still uncertain percutaneous needle biopsy is required. A positive tissue diagnosis is obviously very helpful, but a negative or normal biopsy cannot be relied upon as proof that a tumor is not present. 'Exploration' of the kidney and open biopsy is not good practice and usually indicates inadequate preoperative investigation. In the presence of multiple renal tumors, intraoperative ultrasound scanning is an aid to conservative surgery.

Screening for renal tumors

Ozen *et al.* [39] reported that 27/33 incidentally diagnosed renal cancers were small and confined to the kidney. So far as the author is aware no serious suggestion has yet been made to screen the population in general for renal cancer. In rank order of cause of death it is too infrequent to be a cost-effective proposition. However, there is no doubt that surgery is curative if the cancer is small, and delay in diagnosis is a material factor in determining curability. Ultrasound scanning of the kidneys is non-invasive, has high specificity and sensitivity for small renal tumors, takes a relatively short time, is more comfortable than mammography and much more acceptable than flexible sigmoidoscopy that is now being used for the early detection of rectosigmoid cancer. If regular health checks become more commonplace and seek to diminish deaths from cancer, careful consideration should be given to the inclusion of an ultrasound scan of the upper abdomen.

Treatment

Surgery

Radical nephrectomy has been the surgical procedure of choice for renal cancer since the influential publication of Robson *et al.* [40] suggested that the removal of the tumor-containing kidney, its envelope of perinephric fat and Gerota's fascia together with the adrenal and hilar and regional para-aortic lymph nodes was superior to simple nephrectomy. As has so often been the case with surgical fashion, this study was based on an invalid comparison with historical controls. Only recently has a randomized trial of adequate size been conducted to address the necessity of a radical versus total nephrectomy (Protocol 30881 of the European Organization for Research and Treatment of Cancer Genitourinary Group). Long-term survival data are awaited. At the present time there is no clear evidence that a lymphadenectomy or removal of the ipsilateral adrenal gland is necessary. Wide local excision by dissection outside Gerota's fascia is probably desirable to minimize the risk of positive surgical margins and local recurrence.

Conservative surgery

Acknowledgment of the increasing diagnosis of small, early-stage renal cancers has led some to question the need for radical nephrectomy for every patient. Unexpectedly good results have been achieved by conservative surgery (enucleation, wide resection, partial nephrectomy) for cancers in patients with solitary kidneys or bilateral tumors [41, 42]. The alternative of radical nephrectomy followed by haemodialysis has not increased survival but did increase morbidity in such patients [43, 44]. Patient selection will have contributed in large measure to these favorable results, but given similar careful selection, conservative surgery may be equally as effective as radical nephrectomy for many small renal tumors. The main advantage is the preservation of renal tissue for long-term function bearing in mind the 1% risk of developing a second tumor in the contralateral kidney. The two disadvantages are: (1) 7% (or greater) risk of recurrence due to the limitations of preoperative staging, inadequate local excision or unrecognized multifocal tumors, and (2) the increased operative morbidity of partial nephrectomy, particularly hemorrhage [45–47]. In some countries conservative surgery has already become very popular despite the lack of proof of equivalent outcome. A European multicenter randomized trial comparing partial nephrectomy and radical nephrectomy for renal cancers less than 5 cm in diameter is ongoing.

Spontaneous regression and the role of nephrectomy in the presence of metastases

It has been known for more than 30 years that renal cancer metastases regress spontaneously following surgical removal of the primary tumor in occasional patients [48]. Reports of this phenomenon continue to be published [49], but the overall likelihood of spontaneous regression following surgery is less than 0.1%. It is, therefore, not a reason for recommending nephrectomy in patients with metastases at the time of diagnosis. But, as illustrated by Marcus *et al.* [49] if a patient is to undergo nephrectomy prior to receiving immuno- or chemotherapy in a clinical trial, a period of at least six weeks should elapse and measurements of indicator lesions be repeated before starting systemic treatment.

Preliminary reports 15 years ago suggested nephrectomy preceded by embolization of the renal tumor was associated with higher metastatic remission rates [50]. There followed a period of several years when preoperative embolization and nephrectomy became *de rigeur* for patients with metastatic renal cancer and the primary tumor still *in situ*. Wider experience has shown that preoperative embolization was disappointing. A European multicenter study failed to confirm any clear advantage and the technique is no longer practised.

A subject of more frequent clinical concern is the indication for palliative nephrectomy in the presence of metastases. Many surgeons believe that it is worthwhile removing the kidney although this is not supported by the published literature [51]. Data from randomized trials are not available but it is hoped that a British trial of nephrectomy versus no nephrectomy and a collaborative American/European study of nephrectomy plus interferon versus interferon alone will resolve this question. In the meantime nephrectomy may relieve persistent hematuria or loin pain but the postnephrectomy hospital stay is often longer than anticipated and the reported operative mortality is high. Clearly, the disadvantages as well as the advantages must be considered carefully in this difficult situation especially if survival is not expected to be longer than a few months.

Radiation therapy

External beam radiotherapy has no role in the primary treatment of renal cancer at the present time. A randomized trial of postnephrectomy adjuvant radiotherapy demonstrated no advantage [52] and the necessary inclusion of the spinal cord and liver in radiation fields was a cause of concern. Nonetheless, radiotherapy can be invaluable in the palliation of metastatic renal cancer.

Hormone therapy

The observation that estrogens induced renal tumors in Syrian hamsters [53] and that testosterone or progestins could prevent tumor formation [54] and reports of hormone-induced regression in some patients with renal cancer [55] led to a vogue for hormone therapy in the 1970s. No randomized trials were conducted to assess the efficacy of medroxyprogesterone acetate or other hormone treatments, but a review of the published literature suggests that objective response rates were only about 2% [56] although subjective improvement was more frequent. A British Medical Research Council trial of medroxyprogesterone acetate versus placebo seeks to clarify this issue.

Systemic chemotherapy

No cytotoxic agent has been demonstrated to have clinically significant activity against renal carcinoma. Yagoda and Bander [57] estimated an overall response rate of only 9% in a review of 30 drugs tested in more than 2000 patients in phase 2 studies prior to 1989. Vinblastine has been singled out as being more active than other agents, early reports suggesting response rates of 25%, but the application of current response criteria reduced this to 7% [58]. The multiple drug resistant gene (MDR) is apparently expressed at high levels in renal cancer [59]. Attempts to bypass the mechanism of drug resistance with agents such as verapamil have not been successful.

At the present time chemotherapy has no place in the clinical management of patients with renal cancer and is indicated only for those patients who have symptomatic metastases and wish to receive experimental treatment.

Immunotherapy and immunochemotherapy

The possibility that immunomodulation might have a clinical role in renal cancer has been of considerable interest and research for many years. Interferon-α (IFN) in its natural or recombinant forms has been tested and has yielded overall response rates of 5–26% with a mean of 17% [60]. Durable complete remission has been unusual; the primary tumor, bone and CNS metastases rarely respond. Experience with IFN-β is limited. IFN-γ response rates are not higher than IFN-α and the combination of IFN-α and- γ was unpromising [61].

Interleukin-2 (IL-2), administered intravenously or subcutaneously, by continuous infusion or in combination with *ex vivo* stimulation of peripheral blood lymphocytes has produced responses of a similar magnitude although initial, single institution experience had suggested greater efficacy [62].

On the basis of univariate and multivariate analyses ESR, performance status and weight loss have been identified as reproducible prognostic indicators for metastatic renal cancer. Retrospective study suggests that IFN may increase survival in good risk patients only. This suggestion requires validation by prospective trial. To date there is no clear evidence that the interferons or interleukins prolong overall survival in patients with metastatic renal cancer. If immunotherapy is considered desirable interferon treatment should probably be continued for a minimum of one year before it is deemed ineffective. By contrast, lack of benefit from interleukin-2 may be decided if no objective response is seen after two months.

Preliminary data from an extended phase 2 trial of IFN-α and IL-2 combined with weekly intravenous 5-fluorouracil revealed 11% complete and 28% partial responses in 120 patients [63]. The benefit of this and other immunochemotherapy regimens requires further evaluation.

The main side effect of influenza-like symptoms

associated with IFN and IL-2 can be ameliorated by concomitant paracetamol medication, but nonetheless these side effects are often very wearisome with prolonged treatment. The psychiatric effects of high and prolonged dosage can also be very distressing. In addition, it should be remembered that IFN and IL-2 are very expensive. Despite these negative features many patients with metastatic renal cancer are prescribed immunotherapy without participating in clinical trials, a practice which is not justified by the published literature. From the point of view of survival, quality of life for the patient or cost benefit, immunotherapy should continue to be regarded as experimental treatment and only sanctioned in randomized clinical trials.

Palliative treatment

Some renal cancer metastases in bone, lung and skin are highly vascular and cause hemorrhage or pain that may be relieved by local arterial embolization (Figure 64.5). Alternatively radiation therapy offers good palliation of painful bone metastases and painful or hemorrhagic cutaneous deposits, and may reverse the neurological deficit of brain or spinal cord involvement (Figure 64.6). High-dose steroids should supplement the last-mentioned treatment. Radiotherapy does not prevent pathological fractures. For large metastases in long bones internal fixation or arthroplasty should be considered, combined with postoperative radiotherapy. Hypercalcemia is not uncommon in renal cancer and occurs whether bone metastases are present or not. It can be particularly debilitating in the late stages of the disease. Treatment with bisphosphonates and intravenous saline and furosemide

(to achieve a brisk diuresis) is recommended. Hormone therapy (medroxyprogesterone acetate) often induces weight gain and a sense of well-being which enhances its placebo effect although concomitant fluid retention may cause its own problems.

Follow-up care

In common with most other cancers it is traditional to recommend long-term follow-up for the detection of tumor recurrence. Some patients find that regular contact with their physician is reassuring and helpful. The diagnosis of asymptomatic local relapse or metastases also identifies patients for accrual to phase 1 or 2 trials of much needed new and effective systemic treatment. However, from all other points of view routine follow-up for renal cancer patients is unnecessary and potentially detrimental. Patients may be informed of tumor relapse of which they are unaware but for which there is no treatment that offers cure, prolonged survival or relief of anxiety. Until better treatments are discovered there is a good case for discharging patients with renal cancer from hospital follow-up to be seen again only if symptomatic treatment is required for advancing disease.

Acknowledgments

I am grateful to Dr A R Morley, Reader in Pathology, University of Newcastle upon Tyne for the histological illustrations and Dr I Zammit-Maempel, Consultant Radiologist, Freeman Hospital for the radiographic illustrations.

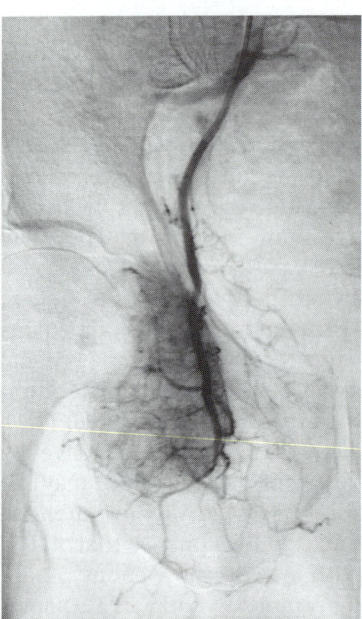

Figure 64.5 Angiogram illustrating very vascular metastasis from renal cancer, adjacent to the right acetabulum, suitable for treatment by embolization.

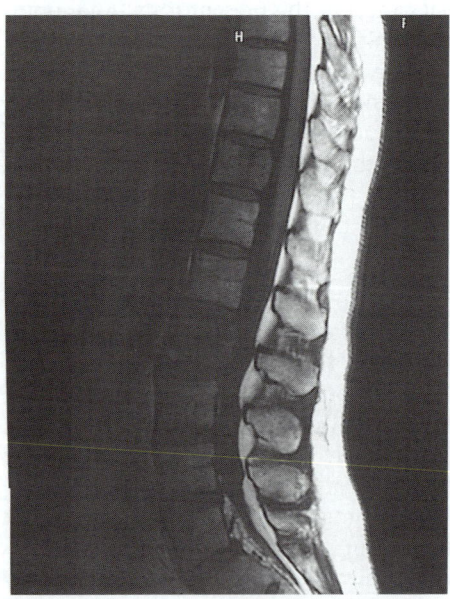

Figure 64.6 MR scan showing replacement of lumbar vertebral body by renal cancer metastasis, encroaching on spinal canal.

References

1. Parkin, D.M., Ferley, J. and Pisani, P. (1995) Estimates of the world wide incidence of eighteen major cancers in 1985. *Int. J. Cancer*, **54**, 594–606.
2. IARC (International Agency for Research on Cancer) *Monographs on the Evaluation of the Carcinogenic Risk of Chemicals to Human 1986*; 38. *Tobacco Smoking*, IARC, Lyon.
3. Mellemgaard, A., Engholm, G., McLaughlin, J.K. and Olsen, J.H. (1994) Risk factors for renal cell carcinoma in Denmark. 1: Role of socioeconomic status, tobacco use, beverages and family history. *Cancer Causes Control*, **5**, 105–13.
4. Lieber, M.M., Tomera, K.M. and Farrow, G.M. (1981) Renal oncocytoma. *J. Urol.*, **125**, 481–5.
5. Melmon, K.L. and Rosen, S.W. (1964) Lindau's disease: review of the literature and study of a large kindred. *Am. J. Med.*, **36**, 595–61.
6. Cohen, A.J., Li, F.P., Berg, S. *et al.* (1979) Hereditary renal cell carcinoma associated with a chromosomal translocation. *N. Engl. J. Med.*, **301**, 592–5.
7. Zbar, B., Torry, K., Merino, M. *et al.* (1994) Hereditary papillary renal cell carcinoma. *J. Urol.*, **151**, 561–6.
8. Linehan, W.M., Lerman, M.I. and Zbar, B. (1995) Identification of the von Hippel Lindau (VHL) gene. Its role in renal cancer. *JAMA*, **273**, 564–70.
9. Glenn, G.M., Choyk, P.L., Zbar, B. and Linehan, W.M. (1990) Von Hippel–Lindau disease: clinical review and molecular genetics, in *Problems in Urologic Surgery: Benign and Malignant Tumours of the Kidney* (ed. E.E. Anderson), J.B. Lippincott, Philadelphia, pp. 312–30.
10. Knudson, A.J. Jr (1993) Antioncogenes and human cancer. *Proc. Natl. Acad. Sci. USA*, **90**, 10914–21.
11. Gnarra, J.R., Torry, K., Weng, Y. *et al.* (1994) Mutation of the VHL tumour suppressor gene in renal carcinoma. *Nature Genet.*, **7**, 85–90.
12. Grawitz, P. (1883) Die sogenannten lipome der niere. *Virchows Arch.*, **93**, 39.
13. Eble, J.N. (1990) Unusual renal tumors and tumor-like conditions, in *Tumors and Tumor-like Conditions of the Kidneys and Ureters* (ed. J.N. Eble), Churchill Livingstone, Edinburgh, pp. 146–76.
14. Medeiros, L.J., Gelb, A.B. and Weiss, L.M. (1988) Renal cell carcinoma: prognostic significance of morphologic parameters in 121 cases. *Cancer*, **61**, 1639–51.
15. Thackray, A.C. (1982) Histopathology of renal carcinoma, in *Scientific Foundations of Urology* (eds G.D. Chisholm and D.I. Williams), William Heinemann, London, pp. 659–63.
16. Bell, E.T. (1950) *Renal Diseases*. Lea and Febiger, Philadelphia, p. 428.
17. Marroncle, M., Birani, J., Dore, B. *et al.* (1994) Prognostic value of histological grade and nuclear grade in renal adenocarcinoma. *J. Urol.*, **151**, 1174–6.
18. Syrjanen, K. and Hjelt, L. (1978) Grading of human renal adenocarcinoma. *Scand. J. Urol. Nephrol.*, **12**, 49–55.
19. Lanigan, D., Loftus, B., Barry-Walshe, C. *et al.* (1994) A comparative of analysis of grading systems in renal adenocarcinoma. *Histopathology*, **24**, 473–6.
20. Kradjian, R.M. and Bennington, J.L. (1965) Renal carcinoma recurrent 31 years after nephrectomy. *Arch. Surg.*, **90**, 192–5.
21. Ljungberg, B., Duchek, M., Hitala, S. *et al.* (1988) Renal cell carcinoma in a solitary kidney: late nephrectomy after 35 years and analysis of tumour DNA content. *J. Urol.*, **139**, 350–2.
22. Klein, M.J. and Valensi, Q.J. (1976) Proximal tubular adenomas of kidney with so called oncocytic features; a clinico-pathologic study of 13 cases of a rarely reported neoplasm. *Cancer*, **38**, 906–14.
23. Farrow, G.M., Harrison, E.J., Utz, D.C. and Jones, D.R. (1968) Renal angiomyolipoma. A clinicopathologic study of 32 cases. *Cancer*, **22**, 564–70.
24. Blute, M.L., Malik, R.S. and Segura, J.W. (1988) Angiomyolipoma: clinical metamorphosis and concepts of foremanagement. *J. Urol.*, **139**, 20–4.
25. Huang, J., Ho, D.M., Huang, J. *et al.* (1988) Coincidental angiomyolipoma and renal cell carcinoma – report of one case and review of the literature. *J. Urol.*, **140**, 1516–18.
26. Robertson, P.W., Klidjian, A., Harding, L.K. *et al.* (1967) Hypertension due to a renin-secreting renal tumor. *Am. J. Med.*, **43**, 963.
27. Van Poppel, H., Boel, K., van Damme, B. and Baert, L. (1995) Microscopic vascular invasion: the most significant prognostic factor in renal cell carcinoma. *J. Urol.*, **153**, 255A.
28. Mrstik, C., Salamon, J., Webber, R. and Stogermayer, F. (1992) Microscopic venous infiltration as predictor of relapse in renal cell carcinoma. *J. Urol.*, **148**, 271–4.
29. Samma, S., Yoshida, K., Ozono, S. *et al.* (1991) Tumour thrombus and microvascular invasion as prognostic factors in renal cell carcinoma. *Jpn. J. Clin. Oncol.*, **21**, 340–5.
30. Bassil, B., Dosoretz, D.E. and Prout, G.R. (1985) Validation of the tumor, nodes and metastasis classification of renal cell carcinoma. *J. Urol.*, **134**, 450–4.
31. Hermanek, P. and Schrott, K.M. (1990) Evaluation of the new tumor, nodes and metastases classification of renal cell carcinoma. *J. Urol.*, **144**, 238–42.
32. Stauffer, M.H. (1961) Nephrogenic hepatosplenomegaly. *Gastroenterology*, **40**, 694.
33. Chisholm, G.D. (1982) Systemic effects, in *Scientific Foundations of Urology* (eds G.D. Chisholm and D.I. Williams), Heinemann, London, pp. 677–80.
34. Sufrin, G., Mirand, E.A., Moore, R.H. *et al.* (1977) Hormones in renal cancer. *Trans. Am. Assoc. Gen-Urin. Surg.*, **68**, 115.
35. Rawlins, M.D., Luff, R.H. and Cranston, W.I. (1970) Pyrexia in renal carcinoma. *Lancet*, **i**, 137.
36. Sufrin, G., Chasan, S., Golio, A. and Murphy, G. (1989) Paraneoplastic and serologic syndromes of renal adenocarcinoma. *Semin. Urol.*, **7**, 158–71.
37. Goldberg, M.F. *et al.* (1964) Renal adenocarcinoma containing a parathyroid hormone-like substance in association with marked hypercalcaemia. *Am. J. Med.*, **36**, 805.

38. Cummings, K.B. and Robertson, R.P. (1977) Prostaglandin: increased production by renal cell carcinoma. *J. Urol.*, **118**, 720.

39. Ozen, H., Colowick, A. and Freiha, F.S. (1993) Incidentally discovered solid renal masses: what are they? *Br. J. Urol.*, **72**, 274–6.

40. Robson, C.J., Churchill, B. and Anderson, W. (1969) Radical nephrectomy for renal cell carcinoma. *J. Urol.*, **101**, 297.

41. Carini, M., Selli, C., Barbanti, G. *et al.* (1988) Conservative surgical treatment of renal cell carcinoma: clinical experience and reappraisal of indications. *J. Urol.*, **140**, 725–31.

42. Topley, M., Novick, A.C. and Montie, J.E. (1984) Long term results following partial nephrectomy for localised renal adenocarcinoma. *J. Urol.*, **131**, 1050–2.

43. Bazeed, M.A., Scharfe, T., Becht, E. *et al.* (1986) Conservative surgery of renal cell carcinoma. *Eur. Urol.*, **12**, 238–43.

44. Marberger, M., Pugh, R.C.B., Auvert, J. *et al.* (1981) Conservative surgery of renal cell carcinoma: the EIRSS experience. *Br. J. Urol.*, **53**, 528–32.

45. Montie, J.E. and Novick, A.C. (1988) Partial nephrectomy for renal cell carcinoma. *J. Urol.*, **140**, 129–30.

46. Smith, R.B., de Kernion, J.B., Ehrlich, R.M. *et al.* (1984) Bilateral renal cell carcinoma and renal cell carcinoma in the solitary kidney. *J. Urol.*, **132**, 450–4.

47. Van Poppel, H., Claes, H., Willemen, P. *et al.* (1991) Is there a place for conservative surgery for renal cell carcinoma? *Br. J. Urol.*, **67**, 129–33.

48. Everson, T.C. and Cole, W.H. (1966) *Spontaneous Regression of Cancer.* W.B. Saunders, Philadelphia.

49. Marcus, S.G., Choyke, P.L., Reiter, R. *et al.* (1993) Regression of metastatic renal cell carcinoma after cytoreductive nephrectomy. *J. Urol.* **150**, 463–6.

50. Swanson, D.A., Johnson, D.E., von Eschenbach, A.C. *et al.* (1983) Angioinfarction plus nephrectomy for metastatic renal cell carcinoma – and update. *J. Urol.*, **130**, 449.

51. Johnson, D.E., Kesler, K.E. and Samuels, M.L. (1975) Is nephrectomy justified with metastatic renal cell carcinoma? *J. Urol.*, **114**, 27.

52. Finney, R. (1973) The value of radiotherapy in the treatment of hypernephroma; a clinical trial. *Br. J. Urol.*, **45**, 258.

53. Bloom, H.J.G., Dukes, C.E. and Mitchley, B.C.V. (1963) Hormone dependent tumors of the kidney. 1. Oestrogen-induced renal tumor of the Syrian hamster: hormone treatment and possible relationship to carcinoma of the kidney in man. *Br. J. Cancer*, **17**, 611.

54. Kirkman, H. (1959) Oestrogen-induced tumors of the kidney. *Natl. Cancer Inst. Monogr.*, **1**, 1.

55. Bloom, H.J.G. (1973) Hormone-induced and spontaneous regression of metastatic renal cancer. *Cancer*, **32**, 1066.

56. Hrushesky, W.J. and Murphy, G.P. (1977) Current status of the therapy of advanced renal carcinoma. *J. Surg. Oncol.*, **9**, 277.

57. Yagoda, A. and Bander, N.H. (1989) Failure of cytotoxic chemotherapy, 1983–1988, and the emerging role of monoclonal antibodies for renal cancer. *Urol. Int.*, **44**, 338.

58. Fossa, S.D., Droz, J.P., Pavone-Macaluso, M. *et al.* (1992) Vinblastine in metastatic renal cell carcinoma: EORTC Phase 11 trial 30882. *Eur. J. Cancer*, **45**, 878–80.

59. Fojo, A.T., Ueda, K., Slamon, D.J. *et al.* (1987) Expression of a multidrug-resistance gene in human tumors and tissues. *Proc. Natl. Acad. Sci. USA*, **84**, 265.

60. Horoszewicz, J.S. and Murphy, G.P. (1989) An assessment of the current use of human interferons in therapy of urological cancers. *J. Urol.*, **142**, 1173–80.

61. deMulder, P.H.M., Franssen, M.P.H., Punt, C.J.A. *et al.* (1991) in *Recent Advances in Immunotherapy of Renal Cell Carcinoma*, Springer, Berlin.

62. Rosenberg, S.A., Lotze, M.T., Yang, J.C. *et al.* (1989) Experience with the use of high dose interleukin-2 in the treatment of 652 cancer patients. *Ann. Surg.*, **210**, 474.

63. Atzpodien, J., Kirchner, H., Hanninen, E.L. *et al.* (1993) Interleukin-2 in combination with interferon alpha and 5-fluoruracil for metastatic renal cell cancer. *Eur. J. Cancer*, **29a**(suppl 5), 56–8.

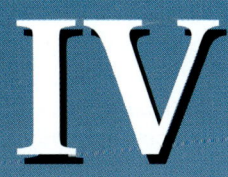

IV

General Management of Chronic Renal Disease

Section 1
General Management Principles

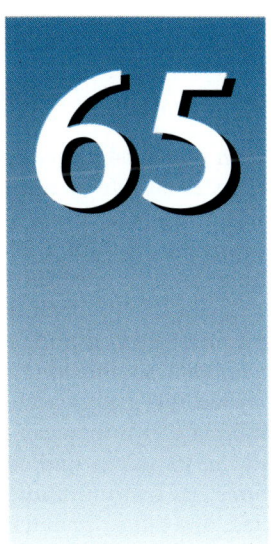

65

Nutritional management of the predialysis patient

D. Reaich and W.E. Mitch

Introduction

In patients with established chronic renal disease, dietary management includes measures designed to optimize nutritional status, to reduce uremic symptoms and if possible, to delay the need for dialysis or transplantation.

Chronic renal failure (CRF) is frequently associated with malnutrition. Many publications reporting the nutritional status of patients entering dialysis programs indicate a high incidence of signs suggesting protein-calorie malnutrition. Serum albumin is subnormal in 20–50% of patients commencing dialysis therapy in the United States and Canada. In epidemiologic studies, hypoalbuminemia is the single greatest risk factor for death in hemodialysis patients, suggesting that malnutrition is associated with increased mortality. Clearly, we should be addressing the problem of nutrition of CRF patients as early as possible in an attempt to prevent the development of the malnourished state.

CRF is manifested by accumulation of nitrogenous waste products, arising from the catabolism of dietary protein or body protein stores. In some complex manner as yet poorly understood, the accumulation of these waste products causes the symptoms of uremia. It seems logical that reducing the accumulation of these products, either by dialysis or by restricting dietary protein intake, will lead to symptomatic improvement. Dietary manipulation for patients with CRF initially took the form of strict dietary protein restriction in an attempt to relieve symp-

toms and prolong life. Over the last decade, our understanding of the mechanisms regulating protein turnover and the metabolic adaptations to changes in dietary protein intake has improved, permitting identification of mechanisms causing abnormal protein metabolism in CRF. There has also been interest in the possibility that dietary therapy slows the progression of renal insufficiency. Other than the control of hypertension (Chapter 42), dietary therapy in the form of dietary protein and phosphate restriction and possibly restriction of saturated fats offers the only available method of slowing the rate of loss of renal function for patients with established CRF. Dietary therapy, then, has come full circle from restricting dietary protein in end-stage renal failure to prolong life, to restricting protein at an earlier stage to slow the rate of progression to end-stage renal failure. Since maintaining an optimal nutritional status while imposing dietary restriction presents a potential conflict, it is important to consider the mechanisms by which adaptations to changes in protein intake occur and how these responses are affected by uremia.

The practicing nephrologist should understand how disease will affect the patient's ability to utilize dietary protein optimally, and how the diet will affect the disease. This chapter discusses the nutritional abnormalities in CRF patients and the underlying pathophysiological mechanisms, the adaptive responses to variations in dietary protein and the potential nutritional therapeutic options.

Nephrology, Edited by Rex L. Jamison and Robert Wilkinson.
Published in 1997 by Chapman & Hall, London. ISBN 0 412 60930 4

Clinical manifestations of nutritional insufficiency

An inadequate diet will result in a deficiency state. The most common nutritional disorder in CRF is a form of protein-calorie malnutrition. It is manifested as a decrease in body weight, height and growth velocity in children, and decreased body fat, intracellular water and muscle mass in adults.

It may be obvious from simple clinical observation that some patients with chronic renal disease are malnourished, but many CRF patients have diminished nutritional reserves without overt physical manifestations. It is important to recognize patients who are suffering from or at risk of developing malnutrition. Certain subgroups of patients are at increased risk of malnutrition because of underlying or coexisting diseases, or associated catabolic factors, and therefore require additional vigilance. These include patients with diabetes mellitus, chronic infections, systemic diseases and chronic diseases of lung, heart or the gastrointestinal tract, as well as the elderly and those with economic hardship. Methods of assessing or following the nutritional state of patients are described below.

Anthropometry

Changes in body composition can be detected by anthropometry. Most reports of anthropometry are based on comparisons with standards derived from measurements in normal subjects. Such comparisons make it difficult to attribute changes to CRF in patients with coexisting illness. Still, serial measurements in the same patient, made by the same, experienced observer can provide useful information about changes in a patient's nutrition with time.

Measurement of height and assessment of trends in weight are simple and potentially the most useful anthropometric tool. The measurement of weight, however, presents a special problem in patients with advanced renal failure who have edema, but a longitudinal change in 'dry weight' indicates a change in nutritional status which merits further assessment. Height and weight can be used to derive the body mass index (BMI), a useful indicator of the amount of body fat. It is calculated by dividing the patient's weight in kg by the square of the height in meters and can be compared to values in standardized tables. A BMI >27 kg/m^2 corresponds to 20% overweight, whereas 22 kg/m^2 is considered lean and <20 kg/m^2 indicates emaciation.

Measurements of skinfold thickness at standard sites, usually the skin overlying the triceps, skin just below the scapula and over the anterior abdominal wall, with metal calipers provide information on fat stores. The mid-arm muscle circumference, measured with a tape measure halfway down the upper arm gives an estimate of somatic protein mass, but it is relatively insensitive.

Serum proteins

The concentration of serum albumin is generally used as an index of protein nutrition. It has a half-life of more than 10 days and therefore responds slowly to changes in visceral protein stores. In non-nephrotic patients with CRF, hypoalbuminemia (<3.5 g/dl) should be considered as a sign of protein malnutrition especially because hypoalbuminemia is the most accurate predictor of mortality in patients commencing hemodialysis therapy. It has been suggested that serum transferrin is a more accurate indicator of protein nutrition because it is more sensitive to protein deficiency. However, its use is limited because non-nutritional factors affect its concentration. It may rise if iron stores are depleted, and fall by as much as 50% with chronic diseases, such as rheumatoid arthritis, malignancy or chronic infection.

There is a dichotomy in that changes in serum albumin and transferrin may not correlate with anthropometric parameters. It seems, therefore, that no single measurement provides a reliable indicator of the nutritional state. Instead, a combination of serial changes in body weight, anthropometry and serum proteins should be used to indicate changes in a patient's nutritional adequacy.

Pathophysiology

The normal kidney excretes nitrogenous waste products arising from catabolism of excess dietary protein and body protein stores, but in CRF patients with renal function below 30% of normal, these products accumulate to a significant degree in body fluids. Clearly, these waste products cause at least some of the symptoms of uremia, since reducing their accumulation, either by restricting dietary protein or by instituting dialysis, leads to rapid symptomatic improvement.

Although waste products are generally thought of as being removed primarily by renal excretion, they are also removed by non-renal routes or by degradation. This is of importance since, at steady state, the production of a product must equal the sum of the amount excreted and degraded each day. This provides the basis for using the steady-state serum urea nitrogen (SUN) measure of the severity of uremia. It provides a good estimate of the accumulation of all nitrogen-containing waste products derived from protein breakdown since urea is the major end product of protein catabolism. Once urea (or any product) is produced it has three potential fates: it is excreted, accumulates in body fluids or is degraded. The sum of the amount excreted plus that which has accumulated is termed the appearance rate.

Nitrogen metabolism in renal failure

In both normal and CRF subjects, nitrogen that is excreted can be conveniently divided into urea nitrogen and non-urea nitrogen. Non-urea nitrogen consists of nitrogen in creatinine, uric acid and other compounds in urine plus the nitrogen in feces.

Urea nitrogen

Since the nitrogen liberated during protein and amino acid catabolism is almost entirely converted into urea, urea nitrogen excretion varies in direct proportion to protein intake. This is true for both normal and uremic subjects. Briefly, the production of urea from amino acid catabolism proceeds as the α-amino group undergoes a reversible transamination reaction with α-ketoglutarate or pyruvate, producing an α-keto acid and glutamate or alanine, respectively. Glutamate dehydrogenase in the liver acts on glutamate to release ammonia and form α-ketoglutarate again. The ammonia enters the urea cycle to form urea which accumulates in body water, is excreted in urine or diffuses into the gut.

Precise measurements of urea production reveal that the urea production rate is greater than its excretion rate. This is because urea in the gastrointestinal tract is degraded by bacterial ureases to form ammonia and CO_2. The resulting ammonia returns to the liver via the portal circulation and is reutilized in urea formation. Urea production includes the component that is degraded in the gut; the difference between total production rate and the portion recycled by the gut is the urea appearance rate, representing urea which appears in body water and urine.

Urea degraded in the gut can be expressed as an extrarenal clearance (that is, the rate of degradation divided by the plasma urea concentration). Interestingly, the quantity of urea degraded is relatively constant, averaging 3.5 g N/day in both normal and uremic subjects. This means that the extrarenal clearance of urea is greatly reduced in uremia because the plasma urea is higher in uremia.

Non-urea nitrogen

Non-urea nitrogen excretion (NUN) is equal to the sum of fecal nitrogen plus non-urea urinary nitrogen (NUUN). NUUN is composed of creatinine, uric acid, ammonia, protein and unidentified products.

Creatinine, formed by the dehydration of creatine within muscle, is almost completely excreted. A small amount of creatinine is degraded, although the site where this occurs is unclear. The extrarenal clearance of creatinine (the amount degraded divided by the serum creatinine) is relatively constant, averaging 0.04 l/kg/day. This means that when the serum creatinine rises, there is increased degradation.

As renal function decreases, renal urate clearance is reduced, but this is partially compensated for by uric acid degradation by gastrointestinal bacteria. Renal ammonia production falls because of the loss of renal mass thereby decreasing the proportion of urinary nitrogen existing as ammonia.

Unlike urea appearance which is closely related to protein intake, losses of NUN by patients with CRF are unrelated to protein intake. Patients in neutral or nearly neutral nitrogen balance (and with less than 5 g/day of proteinuria) show no relationship between protein intake and NUN losses despite large variations in protein intake, their average NUN losses being 0.031 g N/kg/day [1], which is indistinguishable from values obtained from normal subjects.

Nitrogen balance

Nitrogen balance can be used to assess the adequacy of a diet. It is calculated as the difference between nitrogen intake, and urea appearance plus the excretion of non-urea nitrogen. Therefore, it represents the difference between the total rates of the synthesis and degradation of protein nitrogen. In normal adults, the half-life of urea is approximately 7 h. The blood urea level therefore will change rapidly in response to variations in dietary protein, and the urea pool can be ignored in the calculation of nitrogen balance. However, in CRF, the urea half-life can be prolonged to more than one week, and following a change in dietary protein, it may take more than one month before a new stable level of blood urea is reached. The rate of accumulation or loss of urea must therefore be taken into account when measuring nitrogen balance in CRF.

As the concentration of urea is equal throughout body water, changes in the urea nitrogen pool can be calculated assuming that the urea space is equivalent to 60% of body weight (the average body water in non-edematous patients). When body water in liters is multiplied by SUN in g/l, the size of the urea nitrogen pool is estimated. Changes in the pool can be calculated from changes in SUN (in g/l) and daily weight since short-term changes in body weight represent changes in body water and not body mass.

The urea nitrogen appearance rate, then, is measured as the sum of urinary urea nitrogen plus accumulation (positive or negative) of urea nitrogen in the body pool. This is done by taking several consecutive 24 h urine collections and making daily determinations of weight and SUN. If nitrogen intake is known, it can be compared to nitrogen excretion, calculated as the urea nitrogen appearance plus non-urea nitrogen excretion, calculated as 0.031 g N/kg/day [1]. If intake equals excretion, the patient is in nitrogen equilibrium. To calculate protein intake, the amount of dietary nitrogen is divided by 0.16, as protein is 16% nitrogen. Examples of estimates of protein intake are given in Table 65.1.

Nitrogen requirements in uremia

It is generally agreed that the nitrogen requirements of patients with CRF do not differ from those of normal subjects. A patient eating the minimal daily requirement (i.e. 0.6 g protein/kg/day) or even a lower amount (e.g.

Table 65.1 Estimation of protein intake (I_N)

Example 1

A 75 kg patient with constant weight and constant BUN excretes 8 g urea N/d

$$B_N = I_N - U_N - NU_N = 0$$

Where B_N = nitrogen balance

I_N = nitrogen intake

U_N = urea nitrogen appearance rate (sum of urinary urea nitrogen excretion [urine urea nitrogen concentration × urine flow/d] and the change in urea nitrogen pool [$\triangle_N$])

NU_N = non-urea nitrogen losses [0.031 g N/kg body weight]

N = nitrogen

d = day

$$I_N = U_N + NU_N$$

$$I_N = 8 \text{ g N/d} + (75 \text{ kg} \times 0.031 \text{ g N/kg/d})$$

$$I_N = 8 + 2.32 = 10.32 \text{ g N/d}$$

Protein intake = (10.32 g N/d)/(0.16 g N/g protein) = 64.5 g protein/d.

Conclusion: Since the BUN and weight are constant, there is no change in the urea nitrogen pool ($\triangle_N = 0$), so the urea appearance rate equals the daily urinary urea nitrogen excretion plus the non-urea nitrogen losses.

Example 2

A 74 kg patient with a BUN of 80 mg/dl (0.8 g N/l) excretes 6 g urea N/d but is edematous and is treated with a diuretic. One week later, he has no edema and has lost 2 kg. His BUN is 70 mg/dl (0.7 g N/l) and the urea nitrogen excretion is 5.5 g N/d.

$$B_N = I_N - U_N - NU_N = 0$$

$$I_N = U_N + NU_N = \text{urinary urea nitrogen excretion} + \triangle_N + NU_N$$

$$I_N = (6.0 + 5.5) \text{ g N/d}/2 + [(72 \text{ kg} \times 0.6 \text{ l/kg} \times 0.7 \text{ g N/l}) - ([72 \text{ kg} \times 0.6 \text{ l/kg} + 2 \text{l}] \times 0.8 \text{ g N/l})]/7\text{d}$$
$$+ (72 \text{ kg} \times 0.031 \text{ g N/kg/d})$$

$$I_N = 5.75 + [(30.2 - 36.2)]/7 + 2.32$$

$$I_N = 5.75 - 0.86 + 2.32 = 7.21 \text{ g N/d}$$

Protein intake = (7.21 g N/d)/(0.16 g N/g protein) = 45.1 protein/d

---

Comment: To calculate the urea nitrogen appearance rate, the average urea nitrogen excretion rate is added to the change in the urea nitrogen pool. The latter is calculated as the final pool size (60% of the non-edematous weight × BUN) minus the initial pool size (60% of non-edematous weight plus edema weight – assumed to be entirely water) × BUN divided by the number of days (7) between the observations. This value of U plus NUN equals total nitrogen excretion.

Note: In these calculations it is assumed that the patients are in nitrogen balance, that 60% of body weight represents the volume of distribution of urea, that the nonurea nitrogen excretion (nitrogen in feces, urine creatinine, uric acid, ammonia and other nitrogenous compounds) averages 0.031 g N/kg body weight/day and that protein is 16% nitrogen.

0.3 g/kg/day), supplemented with essential amino acids or their ketoacids, can maintain normal indices of nutrition during long-term therapy.

It is important to appreciate that body protein stores are not static, but are constantly 'turning over', i.e. protein is continually synthesized and degraded. Maintenance of protein balance and therefore lean body mass depends on the relationship between the rates of protein degradation (PD) and protein synthesis (PS), and the availability of amino acids. The latter is determined by the dietary intake of amino acids (AA_{IN}), and their rate of irreversible oxidation (AA_{ox}). Figure 65.1 shows that should any one of these parameters change without a compensatory adaptation in the others, the balance will topple and there must be loss of lean body mass. Average values indicate that a normal 70 kg adult in neutral nitrogen balance will synthesize and degrade about 280 g of protein daily. It is apparent, therefore, that even a slight decrease in synthesis or increase in degradation would lead to a significant loss of protein if sustained for some time. Since protein intake varies from day to day, and since CRF patients maintain nutritional indices on low protein diets, a metabolic response must be activated to maintain protein balance.

Recently the metabolic responses to dietary protein restriction in CRF have been studied by measuring the turnover of a labeled amino acid during its constant infusion. This technique yields estimates of whole body

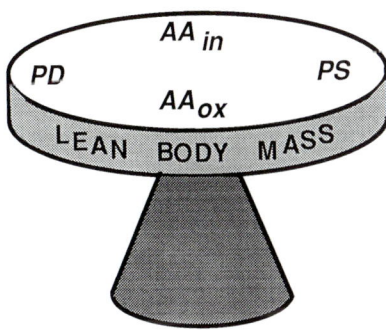

Figure 65.1 To maintain stability of lean body mass, amino acid availability, protein degradation (PD) and protein synthesis (PS) must be co-ordinately regulated.

protein degradation and synthesis rates, and if an appropriate amino acid is used, it will also give information on the rate of amino acid degradation. Leucine is the amino acid most commonly used and is chosen because it is abundant in body proteins, is metabolized primarily in skeletal muscle, and its degradation is easily detected. Leucine degradation occurs via initial transamination to α-ketoisocaproate (KIC), followed by irreversible oxidation of KIC with release of CO_2. If leucine is labeled in the 1-position, labeled CO_2 is produced and can be measured in expired air. Measurement of labeled CO_2 plus the ratio of labeled-to-unlabeled leucine (or labeled-to-unlabeled KIC) in plasma allows one to calculate the rates of leucine oxidation, protein breakdown and protein synthesis. By using this technique it has been shown that the major response to reduced dietary protein in normal subjects is to decrease amino acid oxidation, leading to more efficient utilization of amino acids in protein synthesis. But when protein or amino acid intake falls below minimum requirements, amino acid oxidation cannot be further reduced, and nitrogen balance will become negative, with loss of body protein. The degree of negative nitrogen balance is blunted by activation of a second metabolic response, namely, a reduction in protein degradation. Any condition which stimulates or activates amino acid oxidation or protein degradation would prevent activation of these metabolic responses to dietary protein reduction. In this case, loss of lean body mass would occur. Uncomplicated CRF does not block these responses. When the dietary protein intake of CRF patients (serum creatinine > 5 mg/dl/440 μmol/l) is reduced from 1 g/kg/day to 0.6 g/kg/day or even to 0.3 g/kg/day supplemented with a mixture of essential amino acids (EAA) or their nitrogen free analogs (ketoacids), amino acid oxidation and protein degradation both decrease appropriately. With both low protein diets, neutral nitrogen balance can be achieved.

The dietary protein of a group of non-acidotic patients with moderately severe CRF was reduced from 1 to 0.6 g/kg/day, and they were subjected to leucine infusions to test metabolic responses to each diet. Responses in patients were identical to those in normal subjects: when

dietary protein was reduced, protein degradation and amino acid oxidation fell [2]. Patients on a more restricted diet of 0.3 g protein/kg/day, supplemented with either essential amino acids or ketoacids, had very low amino acid oxidation rates. Again, none of the patients was acidotic. When protein intake was reduced in a group of acidotic CRF patients, however, they were unable to adapt fully, and responded with an increase in skeletal muscle protein catabolism. After correction of their acidosis, rates of protein catabolism fell below those measured while they were acidotic [3].

Factors increasing nitrogen requirements in chronic renal failure

Metabolic acidosis

The first evidence that metabolic acidosis exerts a catabolic effect in CRF was that correction of acidosis with sodium bicarbonate in a group of CRF patients improved nitrogen balance. Experimental work subsequently revealed that acidosis accelerates catabolism of branched chain amino acids (BCAAs) in muscle. In rats with experimentally induced acidosis, plasma levels of BCAAs are low, and the rate of oxidation of leucine and valine in skeletal muscle is increased compared to pair-fed, control animals. In rats with CRF and acidosis, the irreversible oxidation of BCAAs is accelerated in muscle. But when acidosis is corrected by adding sodium bicarbonate to the diet, plasma BCAA levels and their oxidation rates in muscle return to values measured in normal rats.

Similar results occur in patients with CRF. Correction of metabolic acidosis in patients fed a low protein diet (0.6–0.8 g/kg body weight) improved nitrogen balance and increased concentrations of BCAAs, branched chain ketoacids, glutamine and alanine. In hemodialysis patients, there is a strong linear correlation between plasma bicarbonate and intracellular valine concentrations (measured in a muscle biopsy). Finally, in non-dialyzed, CRF patients, there is a strong correlation between plasma bicarbonate and plasma levels of KIC. In acidotic CRF patients, the rate of oxidation of leucine is higher when patients are acidotic than after correction of acidosis with sodium bicarbonate (Figure 65.2) [4]. In keeping with the acceleration of amino acid oxidation in acidosis, the activity of branched-chain ketoacid dehydrogenase, the rate-limiting enzyme for the irreversible degradation of BCAAs, is increased in muscle by acidosis.

Besides stimulating BCAA catabolism, metabolic acidosis increases protein degradation rates. Correction of acidosis in CRF patients decreases protein degradation (Figure 65.2). Acidotic rats grow poorly and have increased protein degradation in muscle and increased urinary corticosterone excretion. Glucocorticoids are necessary for the increase in muscle protein degradation in acidosis but are not themselves responsible for it. Their role was established by the observation that metabolic

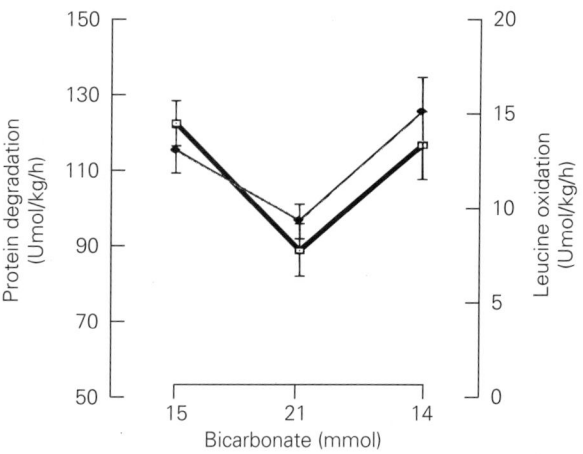

Figure 65.2 Correction of metabolic acidosis in CRF significantly decreases protein degradation and amino acid oxidation. ◆, leucine oxidation; □, protein degradation. (Adapted from ref. [4].)

acidosis does not increase muscle protein breakdown in adrenalectomized rats unless glucocorticoid supplements are given. This requirement for glucocorticoids seems to be present in patients with CRF, as there is a positive correlation between plasma cortisol and protein catabolism, as well as a strong negative correlation between serum bicarbonate and protein degradation in muscle. Recent work has demonstrated that acidosis activates a specific proteolytic pathway. All cell types have many proteolytic pathways. These include those involving the acidic proteases found in lysosomes, the calcium-activated proteases in the cytoplasm, and ATP-dependent and ATP-independent cytsolic pathways. An ATP-dependent pathway, the ATP–ubiquitin–proteasome pathway, is activated by acidosis in the presence of glucocorticoids [5].

In summary, there is conclusive evidence in experimental CRF and in patients with CRF that metabolic acidosis acts as a catabolic stimulus, accelerating BCAA oxidation and protein breakdown. Metabolic acidosis inhibits the appropriate metabolic response to a low protein diet (or to anorexia). It exerts its proteolytic effect by stimulating the ATP–ubiquitin–proteasome pathway and is dependent on the presence of glucocorticoids. In CRF, correction of acidosis decreases catabolism [4].

Impaired insulin-mediated protein metabolism

There is evidence for an abnormal response of protein metabolism to insulin in CRF. Insulin normally has an anticatabolic effect, principally by decreasing protein degradation, and in the presence of high amino acid concentrations (i.e. the conditions existing after a protein meal), insulin stimulates protein synthesis. In chronically uremic rats, however, insulin was found to be less effective at inhibiting amino acid release from incubated muscle when the rats were fed a high protein diet and

were therefore more uremic. If the rats were fed less protein the response to insulin was normal. In isolated muscle from uremic rats, the insulin-stimulated increase in protein synthesis is less than in isolated muscle from control rats. This is not related to acidosis because it persists despite correction of acidosis. There is also impaired stimulation of protein synthesis in response to insulin (plus amino acids) in both diabetic and non-diabetic subjects, suggesting that protein synthesis may not be optimally stimulated after eating.

Energy metabolism and protein

Chronically uremic rats fail to suppress protein catabolism in response to caloric deprivation as efficiently as normal animals, suggesting a link between protein and energy metabolism. This is supported by the fact that fed rats with mild to moderate uremia exhibit no abnormalities in muscle protein turnover, but fasting rats have an increased myofibrillar protein breakdown. The increase in proteolysis is inversely correlated with body fat stores: the less body fat, the greater the proteolytic response to fasting in uremic rats.

Plasma and intracellular amino acids in uremia

Patients with CRF have a well-defined pattern of abnormal plasma amino acids. There is an increase in 3-methylhistidine and 1-methylhistidine, the branched-chain amino acids (BCAAs) are low, with a greater reduction in valine than leucine and isoleucine, in both the fasting and fed states. All three BCAAs are decarboxylated by the same enzyme, branched-chain ketoacid dehydrogenase, and as discussed, the activity of this enzyme is increased by metabolic acidosis. Therefore, excess catabolism plays a role in reducing the plasma concentrations of the BCAAs. Other abnormalities include increased citrulline, cystine and aspartate, and decreased tyrosine which reflects impaired hydroxylation of phenylalanine. Glycine is high and serine low or low-normal, possibly because of diminished production of serine from glycine by the diseased kidney. The concentration of free tryptophan is normal, but since tryptophan is highly protein bound, and plasma protein binding is reduced in uremia, the concentration of total tryptophan is low. Threonine and lysine are low for unknown reasons. Thus, the CRF pattern is of a reduction in concentration of most of the essential amino acids in plasma, with increases in some of the non-essential amino acids. This is similar to the pattern in protein malnutrition. However, the changes cannot be entirely due to malnutrition as the abnormalities occur in CRF patients with an adequate protein intake.

These abnormalities in plasma levels of amino acid make it difficult to evaluate dietary requirements for individual amino acids. In general, the severity of the abnormalities correlates with the degree of renal insufficiency. For example, the plasma concentrations of BCAAs, the essential/non-essential amino acid ratio, the valine/glycine ratio, and the degree of increase in cystine, citrulline and the methylhistidines all correlate indirectly with glomerular filtration rate (GFR). Abnormalities also tend to worsen when protein intake is clearly inadequate.

An additional problem in interpreting plasma amino acids in CRF is that they do not necessarily reflect their intracellular concentrations. This is of importance as 80% of free amino acids are stored in muscle and intracellular concentrations more accurately reflect the environment influencing protein synthesis than do the plasma concentrations. Characteristically in uremia, the concentration of intracellular valine is low, but that of leucine and isoleucine is normal. Intracellular taurine concentration is low despite normal plasma levels, and tryptophan is high [6].

Diagnosis and differential diagnosis

The most important aspect in the diagnosis of nutritional insufficiency is to be aware of the possibility of its occurrence. When faced with a patient who is losing weight or is cachectic, a dietician should be enlisted to document what the patient is eating. Should intake be inadequate, there may be simple, remediable underlying problems, such as poorly fitting dentures, financial problems, or an inability to shop or cook because of limited mobility or other handicap. The patient's mental state should also be considered, as it is not unusual for patients with CRF to become depressed and lose appetite as a consequence of the depression rather than of their renal disease. If any of these circumstances are contributing to malnutrition, their correction and the provision of nutritional supplements may be sufficient to restore the nutritional status to normal.

If a patient has end-stage renal disease and becomes anorectic, renal replacement therapy should be initiated even if the level of plasma creatinine falls short of that usually taken to indicate the need for dialysis in the absence of symptoms. We must be continually aware of the fact that CRF patients are not immune from other diseases, and on the contrary are actually at increased risk.

A careful physical examination of the patient is critical as the possibility of infection must always be considered. Patients with renal impairment are immunocompromised, and require vigilance, with particular attention given to dialysis access sites. Tuberculosis must be considered, as should opportunistic infections, and appropriate specimens must be collected to permit diagnosis. Thyroid dysfunction, diabetes mellitus, malignancy or chronic cardiac, pulmonary or gastrointestinal diseases may all cause weight loss, and should be investigated and treated appropriately.

Treatment

In view of the nutritional and metabolic abnormalities and the high incidence of wasting and malnutrition in CRF, as well as the current evidence that dietary therapy may slow the rate of loss of renal function, nutritional therapy must be considered a critical aspect of the management of CRF. Dietary manipulation has three goals:

1 To reduce or prevent symptoms of uremic toxicity.
2 To maintain good nutritional status.
3 To slow or halt the progressive decline in renal function.

Symptom relief

As far as the first goal is concerned, it has long been established that dietary protein restriction ameliorates the signs and symptoms of renal failure. With the exception of anemia and hyperlipidemia, most of the signs and symptoms of CRF are attributable to the retention of products of protein catabolism; the severity of symptoms is closely correlated with the SUN. A given percentage reduction in protein intake leads to a greater percentage reduction in serum urea nitrogen concentration, because the rate of excretion of other forms of nitrogenous waste is little affected by changes in dietary protein. If a very low protein diet (0.3 g/kg) supplemented with essential amino acids or ketoacids is used, the SUN may even fall to near normal, despite severe renal impairment. Since protein intake (at least in the USA) averages nearly twice the daily requirement of 0.6 g/kg, there is room for considerable restriction of protein intake without the risk of malnutrition. It is therefore disheartening to find that many CRF patients are given no information on the value of modifying protein intake as end-stage renal failure approaches. Every symptomatic patient should receive instruction from a skilled dietician on moderate protein restriction although of course this will only be effective if other complications of CRF, including sodium balance and blood pressure, acidosis and serum potassium level, serum urate, calcium and phosphorus balance, and anemia, are controlled. Protein restriction with or without supplements is discussed further below.

Maintenance of nutritional status

Regarding the second goal, from the earlier discussion of the high rate of protein turnover, adaptation to low protein diets, and the catabolic effect of metabolic acidosis, one can appreciate that CRF patients will maintain good nutritional status on protein restricted diets only if metabolic acidosis is corrected with sodium bicarbonate or another alkaline salt. Care is required when commencing therapy with sodium bicarbonate: because it is a sodium salt, large doses are contraindicated in the edematous or hypertensive patient. These problems must be controlled first, and regular monitoring of the blood pressure is mandatory.

Adequate calorie intake is also necessary to maintain body weight. The energy expenditure of CRF patients has been compared to that of normal subjects during both rest and exercise. There was no difference between groups. Studies of how calorie intake affects nitrogen balance have given some insight as to the relationship between the two. The nitrogen balance of uremic patients fed 20 g/day of high quality protein improved as calorie intake increased, although even with energy intake as high as 55 kcal/kg/day, nitrogen balance remained negative. These results are in keeping with findings in normal subjects that a high calorie intake is required to achieve nitrogen balance in subjects eating barely adequate amounts of EAAs. In contrast, in a group of patients eating 16–20 g/day of protein supplemented with EAA (given either orally or intravenously), nitrogen balance was virtually unchanged as energy intake varied between 22 and 50 kcal/kg/day, suggesting that energy intake is less critical if both nitrogen and EAA intake are adequate.

How does calorie intake affect protein conservation? When CRF patients were fed 0.55–0.6 g/kg/day of protein, and nitrogen balance was measured while calorie intake was varied from 15 to 45 kcal/kg/day [7], the patients achieved neutral or positive balance with an energy intake of 35 kcal/kg/day. This value can be incorporated into the dietary prescription for the uremic patient, although overweight patients should be advised to restrict calories.

Vitamins and minerals

Non-dialyzed uremic patients, particularly those being treated with protein restriction, often have an inadequate intake of water-soluble vitamins, because many foods that are high in these vitamins are restricted. Because of this, and evidence suggesting that requirements for pyridoxine and folate are increased in uremia, a water-soluble vitamin supplement including 10–50 mg/day of pyridoxine and 1 mg/day of folate should be provided. In contrast, fat-soluble vitamins should not be prescribed. Plasma levels of vitamin A are invariably increased in uremia, primarily because of increased retinol binding protein. Whether excess vitamin A contributes to the development of renal osteodystrophy, or to other manifestations of the uremic state is controversial, but vitamin A is unnecessary. Vitamin D levels invariably decrease as renal insufficiency progresses.

Iron supplements are often necessary in uremic patients, who may have impaired gastrointestinal absorption, chronic occult gastrointestinal blood loss, and limited iron intake because of a protein-restricted diet. Measurement of serum ferritin allows an estimate of iron stores. Zinc deficiency has been reported in some uremic patients, and has been associated with hypogeusia, impo-

tence and impaired immune function. There are conflicting reports about whether these problems are responsive to zinc supplements. Tissue levels of other trace elements have been shown to be abnormal in CRF, but their relation to clinical problems is unknown. Without specific indications for their use, it would seem prudent to avoid prescribing supplements.

Influence of dietary therapy on renal function

Once CRF is established, patients rarely recover renal function. The GFR continues to fall even when the original disease process is no longer active. It is now recognized that for the majority of patients, the rate of loss of decline of renal function is constant, although the rate varies widely among patients, even with the same underlying disease. In view of this inevitable progression towards end-stage renal failure it is important to explore possible methods of slowing or halting the rate of decline, the third major purpose of dietary modification.

Two types of dietary regime have been prescribed in an attempt to slow progression: a conventional low protein diet, containing approximately 0.6 g protein/kg/day of primarily high quality protein, or a very low protein diet of 0.3 g/kg/day supplemented with either EAA or ketoacids. Both are considered here.

Conventional low protein diets

A number of studies have attempted to address the question of whether dietary protein restriction alters the rate of progression of renal failure. This is clearly a very important issue, and these studies are, therefore, reviewed in some depth. The first report suggesting that dietary protein restriction could slow progression was from Maschio et al. [8] in Verona. They compared rates of progression in three groups of patients. Groups I and II consisted of relatively small numbers of patients, divided according to initial serum creatinine (S_{Cr}). Mean S_{Cr} in group I (25 patients) was 2.18 mg/dl, and in group II (20 patients), 4.24 mg/dl. All patients were prescribed a diet containing approximately 0.6 g/kg/day of predominantly high quality protein, an energy intake of 40 kcal/kg/day, and about 700 mg/day of phosphorus. A control group of 30 patients whose initial S_{Cr} averaged 2.28 mg/dl consumed an unrestricted diet, averaging 70 g/day of protein and 900 mg/day of phosphorus. The patients were followed for up to 76 months and progression was assessed by measuring changes in S_{Cr} and plotting its reciprocal [9]. Groups I and II had slower rates of decline than the control group, the difference being statistically significant. Criticisms of the study, however, were that the groups were not randomized, there were problems with assessing progression solely by using changes in S_{Cr}, and the control group had a more rapid rate of decline than untreated patients in other reported series.

The Verona group has periodically updated their experience with low-protein diets. In 1989, they reported treatment of 390 patients for an average of 54 months; 57% of these patients had unchanging S_{Cr} values. In a review of these results, they suggested that patients with mild renal impairment who commenced treatment with a low-protein diet had a better response than those with more severe disease, and that those with interstitial nephritis fared better than those with chronic glomerulonephritis or polycystic kidney disease.

Rosman et al. [10] studied 149 patients in a prospective controlled trial. Patients were followed for at least 18 months (an average of 24 months) after being prescribed a low-protein or an unrestricted, control diet. The degree of protein restriction depended on the degree of renal insufficiency: patients with an initial creatinine clearance of 31–60 ml/min were prescribed 0.6 g/kg/day, whereas those with a creatinine clearance of 10–30 ml/min were prescribed 0.4 g/kg/day. Progression was assessed by S_{Cr}; the results suggested a beneficial effect of dietary protein restriction. A subsequent report by the same authors revealed that after four years a benefit of dietary protein restriction was still present, but was now limited to certain groups. Only patients with primary glomerular disease derived any benefit from the low-protein diet, whereas in patients with polycystic kidney disease progression was found to be related entirely to blood pressure control. Furthermore, males showed a more rapid decline towards end-stage renal failure, but responded positively to dietary intervention, whereas female patients derived no benefit from dietary therapy. Reassuringly, nutritional parameters measured (body weight and serum proteins) remained constant.

In 1989, Ihle et al. [11] reported the results of a prospective randomized study of 64 patients. The subjects were assigned to either a control group, which were fed a diet of at least 0.75 g protein/kg/day, or a treatment group fed 0.4 g/kg/day of high biologic-value protein. In this study, five of the original patients were excluded from analysis by the investigators for failing to comply with the diet. Thus, the analysis was not on an intention-to-treat basis, but was based on compliance. Progression of renal failure was monitored by measuring changes in GFR determined as the plasma disappearance of ^{51}Cr-EDTA. Patients were followed for 18 months, during which time 9 of 33 patients taking the control diet developed end-stage renal failure, compared to two of the 31 patients who were compliant with the dietary restriction. The average GFR in the control group fell from 15 ml/min at the beginning of the study to 6 ml/min at the end, but in the treatment group the drop in GFR was from 14 ml/min to 12 ml/min. Serum albumin and anthropometric measurements remained constant throughout the 18 months, but weight, serum transferrin and total lymphocyte count fell, suggesting an adverse effect on nutritional status. The

phosphorus content of the treatment diet was 30–40% less than the control diet, making it impossible to distinguish between the relative contribution of protein versus that of phosphate restriction in this study.

At least two studies have suggested benefit of a low-protein diet in diabetics. Walker et al. [12] followed a group of 19 insulin dependent diabetics (IDDM) with nephropathy. They were observed for 12–39 months while ingesting a normal protein diet (1.13 g/kg), and then switched to a low-protein diet (0.67 g/kg) and were followed for a further 12–49 months. The rate of loss of GFR fell from 0.61 ml/min/month to 0.14 ml/min/month, and nutrition was maintained. Zeller et al. [13] studied a larger group of diabetics, and found clear evidence of benefit from a low-protein diet. They randomized 35 IDDM patients with nephropathy to receive either 0.6 g/kg/day of protein and 500–1000 mg of phosphorus, or at least 1 g/kg/day of protein and 1000 mg of phosphorus. Dietary compliance was confirmed by measuring urinary urea nitrogen and phosphate excretion. Renal function was measured repeatedly as the renal clearance of iothalamate and creatinine. Patients eating the study diet had a significantly reduced rate of fall of iothalamate clearance (−0.0043 ml/s/month compared to −0.0168 ml/s/month in controls). Serum albumin and mid-arm muscle circumference increased in the study-diet group after 12 months, suggesting that the diet had no negative nutritional impact.

Other studies, however, have shown no change in the rate of progression following prescription of a low-protein diet. For example, Williams et al. [14] randomized 95 patients into three groups: one received 0.6 g/kg protein and 800 mg of phosphate per day; the second received at least 0.8 g/kg protein and 1000 mg phosphate per day along with a phosphate binder, and a third was prescribed at least 0.8 g/kg/day protein and no phosphorus restriction. Patients were followed for an average of 19 months during which time there was no difference in the rate of decline in creatinine clearance among the groups. The actual difference in protein intake between the low-protein group and the other groups, however, as measured by urinary urea nitrogen excretion, was only 18%. The Northern Italian Study Group evaluated 456 patients randomized to 0.6 g/kg or 1.0 g/kg/day of protein in their diet [15]. S_{Cr} was followed for two years. Differences in progression between the groups reached only borderline significance, but dietary compliance in the low protein group was poor. The actual reduction in protein intake was only 17%.

Whether dietary protein restriction slows progression of renal disease therefore remains uncertain. It was hoped that the question would be answered definitively by the largest trial to date, the Modification of Diet in Renal Disease (MDRD) study [16]. This study was designed and analyzed as an intention-to-treat trial, i.e. non-compliance would not exclude an individual from the analysis. Three diets were examined in what was effectively two different studies. In study 1, 585 patients with GFRs of 25–55 ml/min/1.73m^2 were randomly assigned to receive 0.58 g/kg/day of protein and 5–10 mg/kg/day of phosphorus (diet L) or 1.3 g/kg/day of protein and 16–20 mg/kg/day of phosphorus (diet M). In study 2, 255 patients with more severe renal failure (GFR 13–24 ml/min/1.73m^2) were randomized to the low protein diet (diet L) or to a very low protein diet of 0.28 g/kg/day, and 4–9 mg/kg/day phosphorus, with a daily supplement of 0.28 g/kg of a ketoacid–amino acid mixture (diet K). In both studies, patients were also randomized to two levels of mean arterial blood pressure (107 vs 92 mmHg). These blood pressure goals were included because in the feasibility phase of the trial, mean arterial pressure was shown to correlate with rate of progression. Angiotensin converting enzyme inhibitors were used to control blood pressure in more than 40% of patients in study 1. GFR was measured by the clearance of [^{125}I]iothalamate.

In study 1, the overall mean decline in GFR did not differ significantly between the groups. The patients prescribed diet A showed a greater drop in GFR initially (over the first four months), then a slower rate of decline thereafter. This slower rate of decline, which reached statistical significance, suggested a small benefit from the low protein diet. In study 2, the patients on diet K had a marginally slower decline in GFR than those on diet L, which did not quite reach statistical significance ($P = 0.07$). However, there was no significant difference between the groups in the length of time to the occurrence of end-stage renal failure or death. As this study did not include a group of patients on a normal protein diet, no conclusions can be drawn regarding the benefit of protein restriction.

There are at least four areas in this study that create problems in interpreting the results. First, documentation that patients were actually losing renal function was not a criterion for entering the study. During the analysis, it became clear that 25–30% of the patients did not show evidence that they were losing kidney function. Although this may mean that improved care and attention is beneficial to patients with CRF, it does not permit an examination of the hypothesis, namely, will dietary restriction slow the loss of renal function? The second problem is that the results were not analyzed for differences in compliance. The third problem is that a substantial number of the patients had polycystic kidney disease, so the distribution of types of kidney disease was skewed. The fourth, and in some ways the most serious problem, was that the study was stopped after an average follow-up of only 2.2 years. Not only were there suggestions that beneficial results were beginning to be detected but also, a longer period of observation might have allowed changes in GFR of patients with slow rates of progression to be detected. For example, the NIH-sponsored Diabetes Control and Complications Trial (DCCT), lasted nine years and showed a striking benefit on the progression of retinopathy in IDDM patients when blood glucose was treated intensively. In contrast, at the two-year point in the trial, retinopathy in patients treated intensively was no better than in those receiving standard insulin therapy.

Secondary analysis of results from the MDRD trial suggest that there may be a beneficial effect of dietary restriction on progression. When changes in GFR of patients who achieved a dietary intake of <0.65 g protein/kg/day were compared with those who ate a less restricted diet, there was significant slowing of the loss of GFR. There was also a more than 12-month delay in the time before dialysis or transplantation was required.

Amino acid supplementation

The second type of diet used to treat CRF patients is a very low protein diet supplemented with amino acids. The diet (0.3 g/kg/day) actually permits considerable variety in foods, because it is not necessary to restrict protein to the high-quality variety. The EAA requirements are met by the supplement of amino acids. The greater latitude in kind of dietary protein makes it fairly well tolerated by patients, in contrast with unsupplemented 0.6 g/kg/day diets which must contain mostly high quality protein, thus restricting the choice of foods.

As discussed earlier, the plasma and intracellular amino acid profiles are abnormal in CRF. This causes potential difficulties in formulating a mixture of amino acids for use in CRF because amino acids in proportions required by normal subjects may not be optimal. Various formulations have been used, mostly containing only essential amino acids, with histidine being included as it is known to be at least semi-essential. These diets are deficient in calcium and vitamins, and supplements of both must therefore be provided.

The amino acids can be provided in various forms. They can be taken as a powder which is mixed with food, but this tends to have an unpleasant taste which is poorly disguised by food. Alternatively, they can be taken as either tablets or capsules, in large numbers, but this is reasonably well tolerated.

With the very low protein diet with amino acid supplements, chronically uremic subjects have markedly reduced symptoms, a lower blood urea nitrogen (BUN), and the need for dialysis can be delayed for many months. Whether there is any effect on the progression of renal insufficiency is uncertain. In 17 patients treated with an EAA supplement designed to correct abnormalities in amino acid concentrations for an average of 355 days, rates of progression slowed considerably when compared to pretreatment progression rates. However, there is the possibility that improved blood pressure control and closer follow-up was responsible for the slowing of progression. Other reports on small numbers of patients have given varying results.

In summary, very low protein diets supplemented with EAA are very effective at controlling the symptoms and correcting the biochemical abnormalities of uremia. They have the advantage of allowing more variety in food selection than protein restriction alone. It remains to be established whether they slow progression of renal disease although they can clearly defer dialysis for some time.

Ketoacid supplementation

Substitution of amino acids with their α-ketoacid analogs further reduces nitrogen intake. Ketoacids contain a keto group on the α-carbon instead of an amino group, and upon ingestion some of the ketoacids are converted into the appropriate amino acid. Thus, the administration of ketoacids can be viewed as a way of providing EAA without increasing the nitrogen load. Ketoacid analogs are given as a supplement to the same type of diet as discussed for the EAA. This diet will substantially reduce uremic symptoms in patients with advanced renal failure. A comparison of metabolic effects between essential amino acids and ketoacids showed that both supplements induced similar changes in protein turnover, and both resulted in neutral nitrogen balance, even though the ketoacid diet contained 15% less nitrogen [17]. There is also some experimental evidence that ketoacids may have an additional 'nitrogen sparing' effect, to slow protein degradation, especially in muscle. This effect could make their use potentially more advantageous.

Originally ketoacids were supplied as calcium salts but this provided a substantial calcium load and was associated with some gastric irritation and occasional hyper-calcemia. More recently, mixtures in which the branched-chain ketoacids are bound to basic amino acids (i.e. ornithine and lysine) have been introduced. These mixtures provide less calcium and are more palatable.

Clinical results with very low protein diets supplemented with ketoacids are generally good, with frequent reports of improved nutritional status and lowered BUN and decreased uremic symptoms. There have also been observations of decreased serum phosphorus levels and alkaline phosphatase, increased serum calcium, and decreased serum levels of parathyroid hormone in both adults and children. There are beneficial effects on carbohydrate metabolism, with a reduction in insulin resistance, and some workers have reported reduced triglycerides in uremic men given this regime. Because of the reduced intake of phosphate and sulfur-containing amino acids, metabolic acidosis improves. Limiting the catabolic effect of acidosis could account for some of the beneficial effects of ketoacids.

Like the other diets described, the ability of this regime to delay progression is unclear. Several studies have shown significant slowing of the rate of decline of renal function, even in some patients who had previously had no benefit from conventional low-protein diets. All of these studies had few patients and were based on measurements of S_{Cr} which can be an unreliable estimate of progression. As discussed, the MDRD study failed to show significant benefit of a very low protein diet with ketoacid supplementation over a low protein diet. Thus it remains to be established whether ketoacid-based regimes do slow

Table 65.2 Recommended intakes of protein, energy and phosphorus for patients with chronic renal insufficiency

GFR (ml/min)	Protein (g/kg/day)	Energy (kcal/kg/day)[a]	Phosphorus (mg/kg/day)
>60	Protein restriction usually not recommended unless evidence of progression	≥35	None
>25 + proteinuria >5 g/day	0.80 g/kg/day of HBV protein plus 1 g for each g proteinuria	≥35	10
25–60	0.60 including ≥0.35 g/kg/day of HBV if there is evidence of progression	≥35	10
5–25	(1) 0.60 including ≥0.35 g/kg/day of HBV, or		
	(2) 0.28 g protein/kg/day	≥35	10
	supplemented with EAA or KA	≥35	5–9

HBV, high-biologic-value protein; EAA, essential amino acids; KA, ketoacid/essential amino acid mixture; GFR, glomerular filtration rate.
[a] Energy intake recommended for healthy adults who have moderate activity and patients with chronic renal failure consuming limited intakes of protein. Energy intake may be cautiously decreased in obese individuals or those who are becoming obese.

progression of renal failure and whether they provide any advantage over the other diets described.

Conservative management versus dialysis

The foregoing considerations indicate why there has been increasing interest in nutritional therapy. The possibility of altering the course of renal disease makes it appropriate to consider treating all patients with established CRF with a low protein, low phosphate dietary regime (Table 65.2). Which is the most appropriate regimen and when to commence therapy have not been established. If renal function is mildly impaired uremic symptoms can be easily eliminated by reducing dietary protein intake to 0.6 g/kg/day and energy intake to 35 kcal/kg/day. In a patient with severe irreversible renal failure, however, nutritional therapy should only be used when adequate access for dialysis is not available (e.g. while an arterio-venous fistula is maturing). In those patients with moderate renal impairment (less than 20% of normal) conservative therapy is almost always useful, and will ameliorate uremic symptoms and possibly postpone the need for dialysis for prolonged periods. Clearly, well-motivated patients and physicians are required for any dietary intervention to be successful as well as the availability of a skilled dietician.

Previous concerns about inducing protein malnutrition by the use of low-protein diets on a long-term basis have been shown to be unfounded, but appropriate calorie intake must be provided, acidosis must be corrected and patients must be supervised. It is, therefore, reasonable to use nutritional therapy to delay the need for dialysis – provided that quality of life is well maintained. The level of renal function below which conservative therapy is unlikely to control symptoms is uncertain, but it is probably around 3–5% of normal. Patients must be considered on an individual basis. Some patients will require dialysis therapy at an earlier stage because of catabolic illnesses, acute gastrointestinal bleeding or the development of uremic complications such as pericarditis.

Outcome

Nutritional therapy has been discussed as a means of relieving symptoms, optimizing nutritional status and slowing rates of progression of renal disease. The dietary manipulations required to control hyperkalemia, and calcium and phosphate balance have not been discussed as they are covered elsewhere. The patient in whom close attention is not paid to nutrition, with appropriate input from physician and dietician, runs the risk of developing malnutrition with its attendant morbidity and mortality. As noted in the introduction, a large proportion of patients commencing dialysis have hypoalbuminemia. A quarter of a century ago, the body composition of patients with CRF was described [18], and serves as an example of what must be avoided in CRF patients. Those patients had reduced lean body mass and a low body fat with an increase in extracellular water. These changes are typical of protein-calorie malnutrition, and should be avoidable if patients are treated appropriately. Unfortunately, patients still develop this altered body habitus, particularly those who begin appropriate therapy late in the course of their disease.

It is important to reiterate that virtually every patient with established CRF will progress to end stage. Control of hypertension is vital to slow the rate of progression, but therapeutic options beyond dietary restriction to slow the rate of decline in renal function are non-existent. Abundant data indicate that dietary manipulation does not cause malnutrition if appropriately prescribed and supervised. It seems reasonable to begin all possible measures to delay the ultimate outcome of end-stage renal failure, and therefore, prudent to manage patients with low protein, low phosphate diets and aggressive blood pressure control.

Acknowledgments

This work was supported by NIH grant DK40907. DR was supported by the Northern Counties Kidney Research Fund.

References

1. Maroni, B.J., Steinman, T. and Mitch, W.E. (1985) A method for estimating nitrogen intake of patients with chronic renal failure. *Kidney Int.*, **27**, 58–65.
2. Goodship, T.H.J., Mitch, W.E., Hoerr, R.A., Wagner, D.A. and Steinman, T.I. (1990) Adaption to low protein diets in renal failure: leucine turnover and nitrogen balance. *J. Am. Soc. Nephrol.*, **1**, 66–75.
3. Williams, B., Hattersley, J., Layward, E. and Walls, J. (1991) Metabolic acidosis and skeletal muscle adaptation to low protein diets in chronic uraemia. *Kidney Int.*, **40**, 779–86.
4. Reaich, D., Channon, S.M., Scrimgeour, C.M. *et al.* (1993) Correction of acidosis in humans with CRF decreases protein degradation and amino acid oxidation. *Am. J. Physiol.*, **265**, E230–5.
5. Mitch, W.E. and Walser, M. (1995) Nutritional therapy of the uremic patient, in *The Kidney* (eds B.M. Brenner and F.C. Rector), W.D. Saunders, Cambridge, MA.
6. Mitch, W.E. (1993) Restricted diets and slowing the progression of chronic renal insufficiency, in *Nutrition and the Kidney* (eds W.E. Mitch and S. Klahr), Little, Brown, Boston, pp. 243–62.
7. Kopple, J.D., Monteon, F.J. and Shaib, J.K. (1986) Effect of energy intake on nitrogen metabolism in non dialyzed

patients with chronic renal failure. *Kidney Int.*, **29**, 734–42.

8. Maschio, G., Oldrizzi, L., Tessitore, N. *et al.* (1982) Effects of dietary protein and phosphorus restriction on the progression of early renal failure. *Kidney Int.*, **22**, 371–6.

9. Mitch, W.E., Walser, M., Buffington, G.A. and Lemann, L. Jr (1976) A simple method of estimating progression of chronic renal failure. *Lancet*, **ii**, 1326–8.

10. Rosman, J.B., Meijer, S., Sluiter, W.J. *et al.* (1984) Prospective randomised trial of early dietary protein restriction in chronic renal failure. *Lancet*, **ii**, 1291–6.

11. Ihle, B.U., Becker, G.J., Whitworth, J.A. *et al.* (1989) The effect of protein restriction on the progression of renal insufficiency. *N. Engl. J. Med.*, **321**, 1773–7.

12. Walker, J.D., Dodds, R.A., Murrells, T.J. *et al.* (1989) Restriction of dietary protein and progression of renal failure in diabetic nephropathy. *Lancet*, **ii**, 1411–14.

13. Zeller, K., Whittaker, E., Sullivan, L. *et al.* (1991) Effect of restricting dietary protein on the progression of renal failure in patients with insulin-dependent diabetes mellitus. *N. Engl. J. Med.*, **324**, 78–84.

14. Williams, P.S., Fass, G. and Bone, J.M. (1988) Renal pathology and proteinuria determine progression in untreated mild/moderate chronic renal failure. *Q. J. Med.*, **67**, 343–54.

15. Locatelli, F., Alberti, D., Graziani, G. *et al.* (1991) Prospective, randomised, multicentre trial of effect of protein restriction on progression of chronic renal insufficiency. *Lancet*, **337**, 1299–304.

16. Klahr, S., Levey, A.S., Beck, G.J. *et al.* (1994) The effects of dietary protein restriction and blood-pressure control on the progression of chronic renal disease. *N. Engl. J. Med.*, **330**, 877–84.

17. Mahsud, T., Young, V.R., Chapman, T. and Maroni, B.J. (1994) Adaptive responses to very low protein diets: the first comparison of ketoacids to essential amino acids. *Kidney Int.*, **45**, 1182–92.

18. Coles, G.A. (1972) Body composition in chronic renal failure. *Q. J. Med.*, **41**, 25–47.

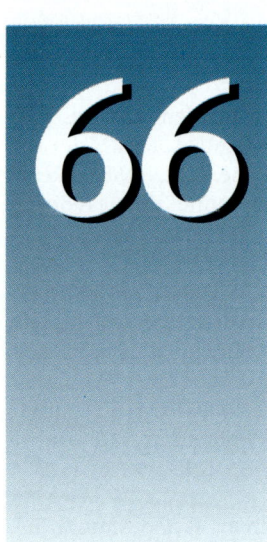

66

Fluid and electrolyte disturbances

Timothy H.J. Goodship

Introduction

In this chapter the effects of chronic renal failure upon body fluids, sodium, potassium and acid–base metabolism are examined along with ways in which these disturbances can be managed. To avoid overlap patients on dialysis will not be considered. Renal regulation of the volume and composition of body fluids and the consequences of impairment of renal function are considered in Chapters 1 and 2.

Body fluid spaces

Total body water has been measured in many studies [1]; most have used the tracer ^3H_2O and in the majority an increase in total body water has been found. However, the results have usually been expressed per kg body weight. Because both body fat and lean body mass are decreased in end-stage renal failure [2] this conclusion may be incorrect and the increase in total body water may represent malnutrition. With nutritional support total body water returns to normal.

Extracellular fluid volume, measured with ^{82}Br and $^{35}SO_4$, is increased. Interpretation of these results, however, is hindered because the tracers used behave differently in chronic renal failure (CRF), for instance with increased loss into the intracellular space. Total body sodium measured using ^{24}Na is also increased but this may be secondary to an increase in intracellular Na since it has

been shown that a factor in the plasma of CRF patients inhibits Na,K-ATPase, thus increasing intracellular Na and decreasing intracellular K [3].

Blood and plasma volume measured with $[^{131}I]$iodinated albumin, ^{51}Cr-labeled red cells and Evans blue are also increased. The results of the studies on body fluid spaces are summarized in Figure 66.1.

Sodium metabolism

To maintain sodium balance adaptation must occur in the surviving nephrons. Fractional sodium excretion is normally less than 1% but in CRF this can increase to 25%. These adaptive changes do not, however, permit rapid changes in sodium excretion with changes in intake. Abrupt decreases in dietary sodium intake can cause a fall in intravascular volume with a reduction in GFR. The converse may occur with rapid increases in intake. As end-stage renal failure (GFR < 10 ml/min) is approached the surviving nephrons are often unable to increase fractional sodium excretion any further and sodium retention will occur as evidenced by hypertension, peripheral edema and pulmonary edema. Treatment includes gradual dietary sodium restriction (2–3 g/day) [4] and diuretics. The loop diuretics, furosemide and bumetanide, are the drugs of choice. They are secreted into the lumen of the proximal tubule and act at the luminal surface of the thick ascending limb of the loop of Henle by blocking active NaCl transport.

Nephrology, Edited by Rex L. Jamison and Robert Wilkinson.
Published in 1997 by Chapman & Hall, London. ISBN 0 412 60930 4

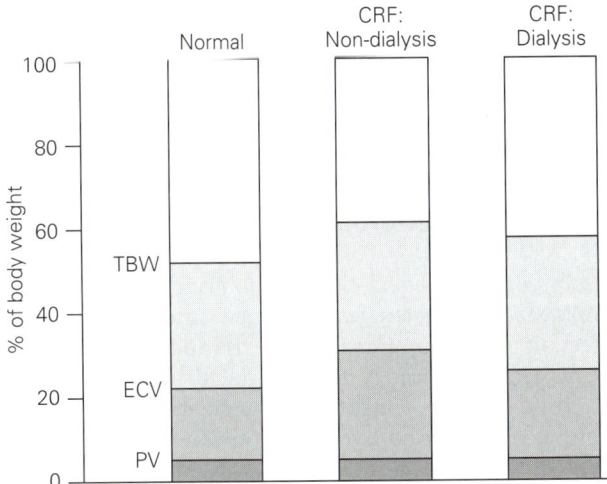

Figure 66.1 The distribution of body water as a percentage of body weight in normal subjects and patients with chronic renal failure. (Reproduced from ref. [1].)

Secretion of loop diuretics is inhibited in CRF and larger doses are necessary. The same dose given intravenously may also be more effective. If a loop diuretic alone is inadequate then the addition of metolazone may provide diuretic synergism [5]. Metolazone inhibits NaCl transport across the distal convoluted tubule thus acting at a different segment of the nephron.

Water metabolism

Thirst and arginine vasopressin (AVP) are the two most important factors controlling water homeostasis. AVP levels are elevated in CRF but not because of a high plasma urea since urea is not an effective osmotic stimulus for AVP release. The most likely explanation for the elevated AVP level is impaired clearance of AVP, since the kidney is responsible for 60–70% of AVP clearance. Hence, the plasma AVP response to an osmotic stimulus, which is a summation of release and clearance of the hormone, is enhanced compared to normal subjects but the osmoreceptor controlling AVP release maintains its normal set point. Thirst perception in response to an osmotic load is not different from normal [6].

The ability to adapt to changes in water intake is impaired in CRF because of impaired urinary concentration and dilution. Normally the minimum and maximum urinary osmolality are 40 and 1400 mosmol/kg H_2O, respectively. In CRF, the range is decreased to between 150 and 350 mosmol/kg H_2O. A variety of factors are thought to be responsible for these changes including decreased sensitivity to AVP and changes in medullary blood flow. The principal factor is the impairment of hypertonicity in the inner medulla. CRF patients are able to regulate water balance when fluid intake is maintained at between 1 and 3 liters per day; but outside these limits, the risks of dehydration and hemodilution are increased.

Despite the above changes in sodium and water metabolism serum sodium concentration is usually normal.

Potassium metabolism

Of total body potassium, 98% is in the intracellular space, predominantly muscle and only 2% in the extracellular space. Extracellular potassium concentration is regulated acutely by movement between extracellular and intracellular compartments. Longer-term regulation is accomplished by changes in renal excretion [7, 8]. Total body potassium, measured using either the naturally occurring isotope ^{40}K or exchangeable potassium, is either low or normal in CRF. Interpretation of this finding is difficult because measurement of total body potassium also reflects muscle protein stores and thus may reflect malnutrition. Although total body potassium may not be abnormal in CRF, serum potassium is often at the upper end or above the normal range, because the ability to handle a potassium load through uptake by the cells is impaired. Normally potassium is taken into cells by the Na–K pump, the activity of which is increased by insulin and β_2-adrenergic agonists. CRF does not impair the action of insulin on potassium uptake (as opposed to its action on glucose) whereas adrenergic-mediated potassium uptake is diminished. This may be explained by their different modes of action. The adrenergic effect is mediated via cAMP through the β_2 receptor whereas insulin increases the rate of translocation of the alpha-II subunit of the Na–K pump from the intracellular pool to the cell membrane. Activity of Na–K pump is impaired in CRF, a defect corrected by dialysis.

Acidosis is also associated with hyperkalemia. A reduction in extracellular pH causes K to leave the cells, raising the plasma K concentration. A stronger relationship has been found between serum bicarbonate concentration and hyperkalemia; a fall in bicarbonate causes K to leave cells. These effects may reflect the degree of H^+ intracellular buffering since it is the K^+ bound to negatively charged proteins that is exchanged for H^+.

Renal secretion of potassium by the collecting duct is the mechanism by which potassium is excreted and extracellular potassium concentration is maintained chronically. With increasing severity of renal impairment, adaptive changes take place both within the surviving nephrons and the gut to allow enhanced potassium secretion. Within the kidney, fractional excretion of potassium increases, under the influence of aldosterone. Normally 10% of potassium is excreted by the colon; in CRF this is doubled by increased activity of the Na–K pump in colonic mucosa [9]. Thanks to these adaptive mechanisms it is rare to observe hyperkalemia until the GFR falls to 5–10 ml/min although it can be seen earlier with excessive dietary potassium intake.

Treatment of hyperkalemia depends on the serum potassium concentration and rapidity of onset. In most patients hyperkalemia is noted before it reaches a level at which life-threatening arrhythmias develop. A plasma potassium of less than 5 mmol/l should be the goal of treatment in all patients. This can be achieved through a combination of dietary potassium restriction, ion-exchange resins and avoidance of certain drugs. The latter includes the potassium-sparing diuretics, amiloride and spironolactone. ACE inhibitors and non-steroidal anti-inflammatory drugs should be used with care and selective beta adrenergic blocker rather than non-selective beta adrenergic blockers should be used. Long-term use of ion-exchange resins, sodium and calcium resonium, may be complicated by severe constipation. With a low dose (15 g/day) and regular use of a laxative this complication can be avoided. Acute severe hyperkalemia is rare in CRF patients under the care of a renal physician but can occur in patients who present in end-stage renal failure. Intravenous calcium in a dosage sufficient to normalize the ECG changes should be given immediately. This stabilizes the myocardium but does not decrease plasma potassium concentration. Calcium should be followed by a combination of intravenous dextrose/insulin and a nebulized beta 2 agonist. Both of these maneuvers will decrease plasma potassium within 30 min, an effect that lasts for approximately 2 h. Intravenous sodium

bicarbonate can also be given but its time of onset is probably slower than previously thought. None of these maneuvers result in net loss of body potassium, hemodialysis with a zero potassium dialysate concentration is the treatment of choice to remove potassium.

Acid–base metabolism

The importance of acid–base metabolism in CRF has been emphasized in recent years by new information on its effect on protein, amino acid, glucose and mineral metabolism. The terminology regarding acid–base balance can be confusing (see Chapter 11). Acidemia refers to an increase of the blood hydrogen ion concentration above 45 nmol/l, whereas acidosis occurs when there is impairment of H^+ excretion. Acidosis can occur without acidemia when buffering is adequate to maintain extracellular pH within the normal range. Thus, CRF patients may have a low bicarbonate in the presence of a normal pH. The type of acidosis seen in chronic renal failure changes with decreasing GFR. Initially a non-anion gap acidosis is observed secondary to the loss of bicarbonate from the proximal tubule and

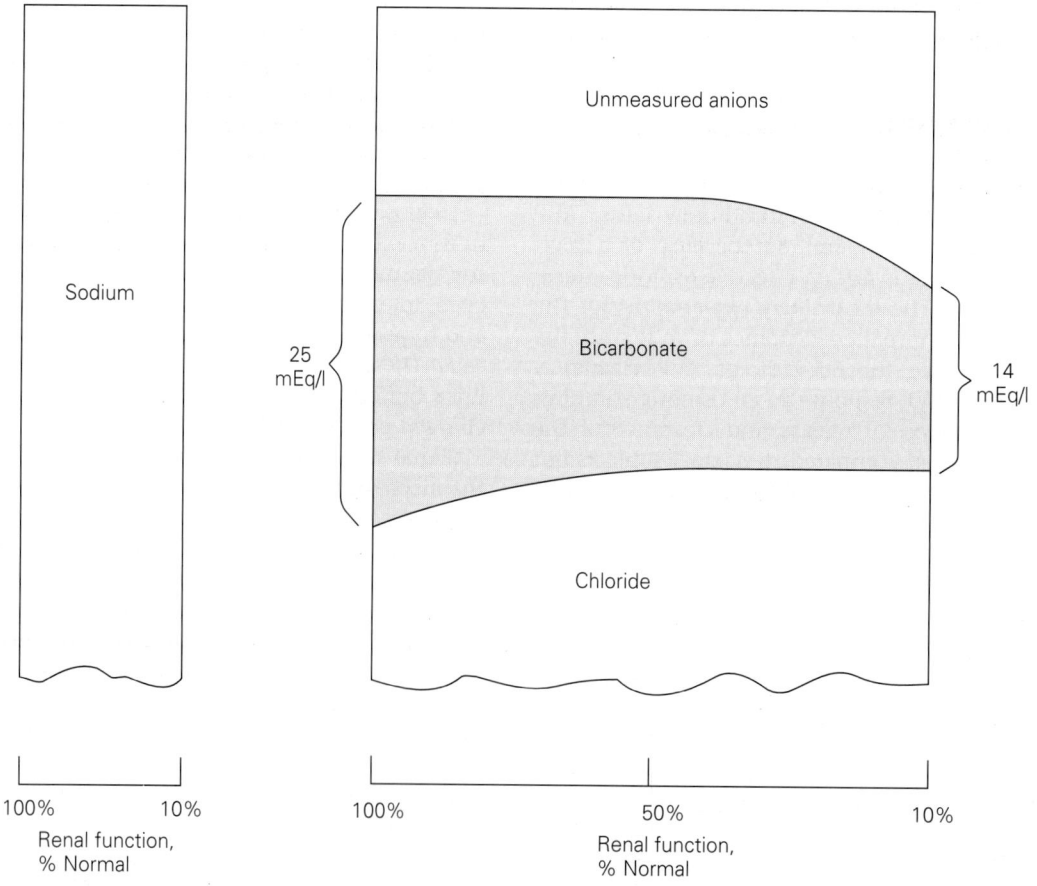

Figure 66.2 The changing pattern of serum electrolyte concentrations in chronic renal failure. (Reproduced from ref. [10].)

impaired excretion of H^+ in the distal tubule. With increasing severity of renal impairment, failure to excrete organic and inorganic acids results in an increased anion gap (Figure 66.2) [10]. Rarely does the serum bicarbonate fall below 14 mmol/l, because of buffering by calcium carbonate of bone. The effect, however, is to cause the development of osteomalacia, especially in those patients with tubulointerstitial disease who are more prone to acidosis. There is now evidence that acidosis decreases the sensitivity of the parathyroid gland to the effect of calcium thus predisposing to the development of hyperparathyroidism.

Amelioration of acidosis with sodium bicarbonate decreases amino acid oxidation and protein degradation and improves nitrogen balance, thus potentially preventing malnutrition. It is also known to increase insulin-mediated glucose metabolism [11] and correct osetomalacia. The level of serum bicarbonate at which treatment should be started is not well defined. A pragmatic approach is to maintain the serum bicarbonate concentration above 20 mmol/l. Sodium bicarbonate is the main method of treatment but calcium lactate and calcium carbonate are also effective buffers and will act as phosphate binders as well as calcium supplements. Treatment with sodium bicarbonate can be complicated by the development of hypertension and edema but the effect is less common than with equimolar amounts of sodium chloride.

References

1. Mitch, W.E. and Wilcox, C.S. (1982) Disorders of body fluids, sodium and potassium in chronic renal failure. *Am. J. Med.*, **72**, 536–50.
2. Coles, G.A. (1972) Body composition in chronic renal failure. *Q. J. Med.*, **41**, 25–47.
3. Kelly, R.A., O'Hara, D.S. and Mitch, W.E. (1986) Endogenous digitalis-like factor in hypertension and chronic renal insufficiency. *Kidney Int.*, **30**, 723–9.
4. Dwyer, J. and Kenler, S.R. (1993) Assessment of nutritional status in renal disease, in *Nutrition and the Kidney* (eds W.E. Mitch and S. Klahr), Little, Brown, Boston, pp. 61–95.
5. Ellison, D.H. (1991) The physiologic basis of diuretic synergism: its role in treating diuretic resistance. *Ann. Intern. Med.*, **114**, 886–94.
6. Argent, N.B., Burrell, L.M., Goodship, T.H.J. *et al.* (1991) Osmoregulation of thirst and vasopressin release in severe chronic renal failure. *Kidney Int.*, **39**, 295–300.
7. Allon, M. (1993) Treatment and prevention of hyperkalemia in end-stage renal disease. *Kidney Int.*, **43**, 1197–209.
8. Salem, M.M., Rosa, R.M. and Battle, D.C. (1991) Extrarenal potassium tolerance in chronic renal failure: implications for the treatment of acute hyperkalemia. *Am. J. Kidney Dis.*, **18**, 421–40.
9. Sandle, G.I., Geiger, E., Tapster, S. and Goodship, T.H.J. (1986) Enhanced rectal potassium secretion in chronic renal insufficiency; evidence for large intestinal adaptation in man. *Clin. Sci.*, **71**, 389–401.
10. Widmer, B., Gerhardt, R.E., Harrington, J.T. and Cohen, J.J. (1979) Serum electrolyte and acid base composition. The influence of graded degrees of chronic renal failure. *Arch. Intern. Med.*, **139**, 1099–102.
11. Reaich, D., Graham, K.A., Channon, S.M. *et al.* (1995) Insulin-mediated changes in PD and glucose uptake after correction of acidosis in humans with CRF. *Am. J. Physiol.*, **268**, E121–6.

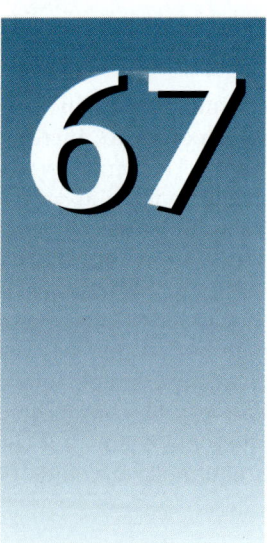

67

Hypertension

Mitra Sorooshian and Timothy Meyer

Introduction

Chronic renal disease usually causes an increase in blood pressure. Hypertension, defined as blood pressure greater than 140/90 mmHg, develops in many patients while the serum creatinine remains normal and is present in most patients by the time the serum creatinine is twice normal. Blood pressure is probably increased above the level present before the onset of renal disease in an even greater portion of patients with renal insufficiency, though it does not reach the 'hypertensive' level of 140/90 mmHg in some cases. Increased blood pressure is observed earlier, on average, in cases of glomerular than interstitial disease, but blood pressure rises to hypertensive levels before renal replacement therapy is required in almost all patients whose disease progresses [1].

Pathogenesis of hypertension in renal disease

The cause of increased blood pressure in renal insufficiency is poorly understood. Guyton [2] has argued that blood pressure must be increased to cause the kidney to excrete the normal dietary sodium load when the glomerular filtration rate (GFR) is reduced. This argument is supported by the finding that extracellular fluid (ECF) volume is increased in patients with GFR reduced below about half normal [3]. Increasing the dietary sodium load to supranormal levels in patients with a normal GFR, however, causes only a slight increase in blood pressure. Reducing dietary sodium in proportion to

GFR, moreover, does not normalize blood pressure in patients with renal insufficiency [4, 5]. These findings suggest that an increase in sodium load per unit GFR cannot by itself account for increased blood pressure in renal disease. Additional vasoconstrictor and sodium retentive mechanisms must be operative. Different studies have suggested that patients with renal insufficiency exhibit inappropriate activation of the renin–angiotensin system [4], increased sympathetic nerve activity [6], impaired nitric oxide synthesis [7], and increased endothelin synthesis [8]. The extent to which these changes are responsible for increased blood pressure, however, has not been elucidated.

The finding that angiotensin converting enzyme inhibition reduces blood pressure in patients with renal insufficiency has stimulated particular interest in the contribution of the renin–angiotensin system (RAS) to hypertension associated with renal disease. Plasma renin levels have usually been found to be normal or low in patients with renal insufficiency and hypertension [4]. Several hypothetical mechanisms can account for the antihypertensive effect of converting enzyme inhibitors in this setting. First, it has been suggested that the finding of 'normal' renin levels in patients with renal insufficiency reflects a degree of RAS activity which is inappropriately high considering the increase in fractional sodium excretion which must accompany reduction in renal function. Second, it has been proposed that converting enzyme inhibitors lower blood pressure in patients with renal insufficiency by preventing increased local angiotensin II (AII) generation in tissues such as the kidney, brain, or arterial wall rather than by lowering circulating AII levels.

Nephrology, Edited by Rex L. Jamison and Robert Wilkinson.
Published in 1997 by Chapman & Hall, London. ISBN 0 412 60930 4

Third, it is possible that AII activity is not increased at any site in renal insufficiency, and that converting enzyme inhibitors achieve their hypotensive effect by reducing AII levels below a low, facultative level necessary to the effective operation of some other pressor system. Finally, it has been reported that aldosterone levels are increased even while renin levels remain normal in patients with renal insufficiency [9]. Increased aldosterone secretion in this setting is generally thought to be triggered by increasing plasma potassium levels and to facilitate the excretion of potassium by the diseased kidney. The possibility that increased aldosterone levels contribute to hypertension in renal insufficiency and that converting enzyme inhibitors lower blood pressure by suppressing aldosterone production has not been adequately explored.

Treatment of hypertension in renal disease

Physicians treating hypertension in renal insufficiency must first choose a target blood pressure and, after encouraging weight control and exercise, must also usually prescribe pharmacologic agent(s). It is generally believed that cardiovascular morbidity and mortality are influenced by blood pressure at least as much in patients with renal insufficiency as in patients with essential hypertension. This belief motivates efforts to reduce blood pressure toward target levels proposed for the treatment of essential hypertension, such as 160/95, the standard proposed by the World Health Organization, or 140/90, the standard adopted by the US Joint National Council on High Blood Pressure. There is currently widespread interest in the possibility that reduction of blood pressure to even lower levels or use of particular antihypertensive agents can slow the progression of renal disease. Experimental studies have shown that normalization of blood pressure with converting enzyme inhibitors is highly effective in preventing progression of renal disease in some animal models. Recent clinical studies have shown that the progression of diabetic nephropathy can be slowed by reducing blood pressure below the target levels recommended for essential hypertension and by using converting enzyme inhibitors. It seems reasonable to suppose that similar treatment may also retard loss of renal function in some cases of nondiabetic renal disease, but the evidence in favor of this proposition is incomplete, as reviewed below.

Association of renal disease progression rate and blood pressure

Patients whose GFR is reduced to less than one half normal usually suffer progressive loss of renal function. The rate of loss of renal function in such patients, however, is variable. Different studies have reported average rates of decline in GFR ranging from 0.3 ml/min/month to 1.0 ml/min/month and even greater variation in the rates of decline in GFR have been observed in individual patients. The rate of progression is determined in part by the nature of the primary disease process. In addition, retrospective studies have identified male gender, heavy proteinuria, and high blood pressure as factors associated with more rapid rates of GFR decline [10–12]. It should be noted that although these studies found that GFR declined more rapidly in patients with high blood pressure, they also documented progressive loss of renal function, albeit at a lower rate, in patients whose blood pressure was normal spontaneously or was reduced to normal by drug therapy.

The effect of antihypertensive therapy on renal disease progression

The finding of an association between high blood pressure and rapid loss of renal function raises the question of whether lowering blood pressure can preserve renal function. Early studies showed that reduction of diastolic blood pressure to less than 100 mmHg prevented or even reversed renal failure in patients with accelerated hypertension [13]. Since these studies were performed, the practice of lowering diastolic blood pressure to 90–95 mmHg to reduce cardiovascular morbidity and mortality has been widely adopted, and the question of whether reduction of blood pressure to this level preserves renal function has thus become moot. The question of whether reduction of blood pressure below this level will slow the progression of renal disease remains to be answered. Rates of renal disease progression at two different levels of blood pressure have been compared in only one large controlled study, the Modification of Diet in Renal Disease Study (MDRD) [14]. This study assessed rates of renal disease progression in 585 patients with initial GFR values of 25–55 ml/min and 255 patients with initial GFR values of 13–24 ml/min who were followed for an average of approximately 20 months. In addition to being given different dietary treatments, patients were assigned to groups with a 'usual' or 'low' target blood pressure. Overall, patients assigned to the 'low' blood pressure group exhibited a slightly slower decline in GFR but this difference was not statistically significant. Adoption of a 'low' target blood pressure did significantly slow the reduction in GFR in patients with heavy proteinuria, who as a group lost renal function more rapidly than those with less proteinuria. Several points about the MDRD warrant particular attention. First, as shown in Figure 67.1, blood pressure in the 'usual' blood pressure patients averaged approximately 135/80 mmHg, a value which is lower than those reported in most studies of patients with renal insufficiency. Second, the rate of decline in GFR in the 'usual' blood pressure group eating a normal diet averaged approximately 0.3 ml/min/month, which is lower than rates of GFR decline reported in most studies of renal

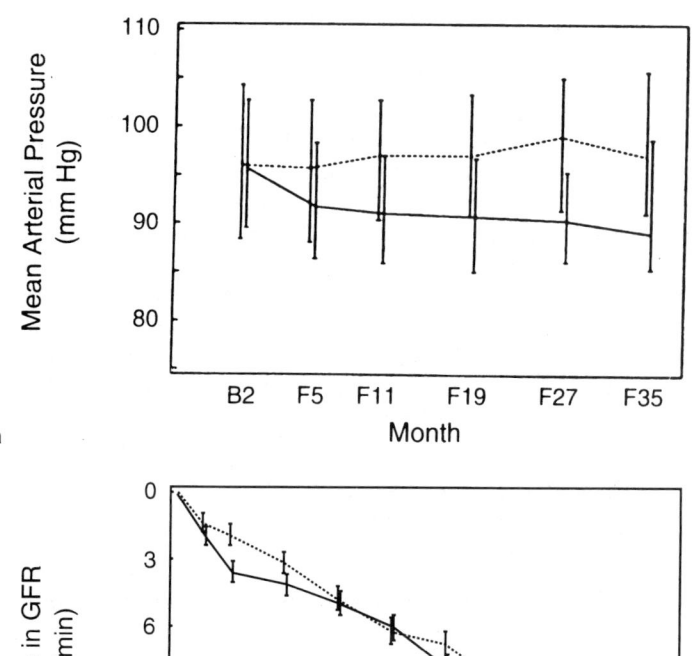

Figure 67.1   The effect of blood pressure control on renal disease progression in patients with initial GFR values of 25–55 ml/min followed in the MDRD. (a) Mean arterial pressure in patients maintained either at 'usual' (broken line) or 'low' (solid line) blood pressure levels. (b) The decline in GFR from baseline in the 'usual' and 'low' blood pressure groups. (Reproduced, with permission, from reference [14] with permission.)

disease progression. It is possible, though not proven, that this low rate of disease progression reflected the exceptionally strict 'usual' blood pressure control in the carefully followed MDRD patients. Third, mean arterial pressure in the 'low' blood pressure group was only ~5 mmHg less than it was in the 'usual' blood pressure group. The small difference in blood pressure between the groups may have made the effect of aggressive blood pressure reduction hard to detect.

In summary, results from the MDRD presented to date do not provide firm guidance to physicians who must decide whether to reduce the blood pressure in patients with renal insufficiency below ~145/90 mmHg. Another important question which remains to be answered is whether converting enzyme inhibitors will preserve renal function better than other classes of antihypertensive agents. Interest in the use of converting enzyme inhibitors to preserve renal function was stimulated by the finding that these agents largely prevent remnant glomerular injury in rats with reduced nephron number [15]. Recent studies suggest that converting enzyme inhibitors preserve renal function better than some other antihypertensive agents in patients with diabetic nephropathy. This finding suggests that converting enzyme inhibitors may prove beneficial in conditions in which, as in diabetic nephropathy, changes in renal struc-

ture do not closely resemble the remnant glomerular sclerosis of rats with reduced nephron number. However, few studies have compared the effect of different antihypertensive agents on the progression of renal diseases other than diabetic nephropathy. In a retrospective study of patients with IgA nephropathy, patients maintained on converting enzyme inhibitors were found to exhibit a slower rate of decline in GFR than patients maintained on other agents [16]. However, because this study was retrospective, it is not certain that patients given different antihypertensive agents had the same initial risk of disease progression and were otherwise treated in the same way. Of the three prospective, randomized trials which have so far examined this issue, two concluded that converting enzyme inhibitors afforded increased protection and the other found that they did not. The first of these trials, performed in patients with initial GFR averaging ~15 ml/min, found that GFR declined by ~0.2 ml/min/month in those treated with a converting enzyme inhibitor and by ~0.3 ml/min/month in those treated with beta blockers, vasodilators and diuretics [17]. The second trial was performed in patients with initial GFR ~50 ml/min and showed that GFR declined at a rate of ~0.3 ml/min/month in those treated with a converting enzyme inhibitor and by ~0.6 in the group treated with beta blockers [18]. The trird trial, performed in patients with initial GFR averaging ~25 ml/min, showed that GFR declined by ~0.2 ml/min/month both in patients treated with converting enzyme inhibitors and in patients treated with a calcium channel blocker [19]. It is noteworthy that the average progression rate in both these trials, as in the MDRD, was lower than has been reported in most retrospective studies. This finding is in accord with the proposition advanced by Bergstrom et al. [20] that entry into a clinical trial, with attendant careful follow-up, tends to slow the rate of renal disease progression.

Short-term effects of antihypertensive therapy on renal function

Reduction of blood pressure with current antihypertensive agents rarely causes a clinically significant change in GFR over the short term. The first widely used beta blocker, propranolol, reduced GFR in patients with renal insufficiency by about 10%. Reduction of GFR occurs less often with newer beta blockers, but is occasionally still observed [21–23]. Converting enzyme inhibitors have been observed to cause a small increase, no change or a small decrease in the GFR of patients with renal insufficiency. Again, excepting larger reductions in GFR which may occur in patients with renal vascular disease or ECF volume depletion as described below, these changes are not clinically significant. Small changes in GFR which accompany the initiation of antihypertensive therapy, however, pose a major problem in the interpretation of studies of the effect of blood pressure on renal disease progression. It may be necessary to detect a difference in the rate of GFR decline of only 1–2 ml/min/year to detect a 30% reduction in the rate of disease progression. The short-term effects of antihypertensive agents on GFR, though clinically negligible, may make such changes in the rate of disease progression impossible to detect unless patients are followed for several years. Studies of this duration are expensive and difficult to carry out. This difficulty has stimulated interest in the possibility that the long-term protective effects of different antihypertensive regimens may be predicted by their short-term effects on renal function. It has been suggested, in particular, that the capacity of different agents to preserve GFR in patients with glomerular disease is related to their capacity to reduce proteinuria. This hypothesis remains unproven, but has received support from the finding that converting enzyme inhibitors both reduce proteinuria and preserve renal function in patients with diabetic nephropathy. Converting enzyme inhibitors have also been found to reduce the protein excretion rate in patients with non-diabetic renal disease [21, 22, 24–27]. The effect of agents of other types is less clear. Beta blockers have been found to reduce proteinuria in some studies but to have no effect on proteinuria in other studies, whereas calcium channel blockers have usually been found not to reduce proteinuria [21, 22, 24–28].

Guidelines for antihypertensive drug therapy

Sodium restriction and diuretics

Sodium restriction is routinely recommended to patients with renal insufficiency. It should be emphasized that it is difficult for many patients to reduce sodium intake below 100–120 mEq/day because of the amount of salt added to prepared foods. Moreover, recommendations to adhere to a very low sodium diet may complicate recommendations to reduce dietary intake of total calories, protein or lipids. Finally, the value of reducing sodium intake below 100–120 mEq/day, a level which may be attained by avoiding salt rich foots and added salt, is not well established. Sodium restriction to lower levels will not by itself normalize blood pressure in patients with moderate renal insufficiency [4, 5]. Sodium restriction is usually recommended because it increases the antihypertensive efficacy of drugs such as converting enzyme inhibitors, calcium channel blockers and beta blockers and reduces the requirement for diuretic drugs. The relative value of reducing dietary sodium as compared to increasing a diuretic drug dosage, however, is not clear cut and may vary in individual cases. In patients with renal insufficiency, furosemide can reduce ECF volume and blood pressure more effectively than stringent sodium restriction [5]. Moreover, reduction of the serum potassium level, considered a complication of thiazide or loop diuretic use in patients with normal renal function, may be desirable in patients with renal insufficiency. The major reason to try to limit the use of diuretics in patients with renal insufficiency is that these agents tend to increase very low and low density cholesterol levels, and may thereby increase the risk of atherosclerotic cardiovascular disease [29].

Converting enzyme inhibitors

The popularity of converting enzyme inhibitors as antihypertensive agents in patients with renal insufficiency has been increased by the suggestion that they are particularly effective in slowing the progression of renal disease. They must, however, be used with caution. Converting enzyme inhibitors can reduce aldosterone levels and aggravate hyperkalemia. Serum potassium increases by an average of ~0.5 mEq/l in patients with moderate renal insufficiency treated with converting enzyme inhibitors, but larger increases occur in some patients. It is thus necessary to check the serum potassium level shortly after initiation of therapy, and to warn patients against increasing their potassium intake by the use of salt substitutes. Converting enzyme inhibitors can also reduce the GFR in patients with renal vascular disease and in patients with ECF volume depletion [30, 31]. A reduction in GFR is not observed in most patients with renal vascular disease, but occurs frequently enough so that the serum creatinine level, like the serum potassium level, should be checked shortly aft er initiation of therapy. The potential for a reduction in GFR accompanying ECF volume depletion is particularly worrisome, as it can occur at any point during treatment. Patients should be warned to seek medical attention if they suffer a volume depleting condition, such as viral gastroenteritis or heavy sweating. As shown in Table 67.1, most converting enzyme inhibitors are eliminated largely by the kidney. The risk of GFR reduction and other complications can probably be limited by reducing the maximum dose of these agents prescribed by 50% when the creatinine clearance is below 50 ml/min and by 75% when the creatinine clearance is below 25 ml/min. Theoretically, some of the protective effect of RAS blockade may be lost when the dose of converting enzyme inhibitors is thus restricted, but the, as yet unproven, supposition that converting enzyme inhibitors slow the progression of non-diabetic renal disease does not warrant acceptance of a high rate of complications with these agents. When converting enzyme inhibition alone is inadequate to control blood pressure, a diuretic may be added to the patient's regimen. It may be possible, however, to avoid complications by monitoring the serum potassium and creatinine levels in individual patients rather than by adopting a uniform dose restriction. At least two agents are required to control blood pressure in the majority of patients whose serum creatinine exceeds 3 mg/dl.

Calcium channel blockers and beta blockers

Calcium channel blockers offer a safe alternative to converting enzyme inhibitors. There have been only a few reports of adverse effects on renal function, and dosages do not need to be adjusted in patients with renal insufficiency. Beta blockers were at one time the most widely used initial antihypertensive agents in patients with renal insufficiency, but their popularity has declined with the availability of long-acting converting enzyme inhibitors and calcium channel blockers. Many beta blockers are excreted by the kidney (Table 67.1). Doses of these agents, like converting enzyme inhibitors, should be reduced in patients with renal insufficiency. The beta blockers offer the advantage that their pharmacologic effect, and thus the patient's compliance, can be monitored simply by checking the pulse. There is at present no reason to prefer calcium channel to beta blockers or vice versa based on the effect of these classes of agents on renal function.

Table 67.1 Renal excretion of converting enzyme inhibitors and beta blockers

	Converting enzyme inhibitors	β Blockers
Renal excretion in chronic renal insufficiency	Benazepril Captopril Enalapril Lisinopril Ramipril	Acebutolol Atenolol Carteolol Nadolol
Largely non-renal excretion in chronic renal insufficiency	Fosinopril	Labetolol Metoprolol Penbutolol Timolol

Other agents

The vasodilators hydralazine and minoxidil were at one time regularly combined with beta blockers and furosemide to treat hypertension in renal insufficiency. Treatment with these agents, and in particular minoxidil, may be accompanied by fluid retention and necessitate the use of large doses of furosemide. When blood pressure cannot be controlled with two agents – usually a diuretic plus a converting enzyme inhibitor, calcium channel blocker, or beta blocker – it is now more common to add a representative of another of these classes of agents than to add hydralazine or minoxidil. Sympatholytic agents can also be used in the treatment of hypertension in renal insufficiency, but are less widely used than converting enzyme inhibitors, calcium channel blockers, or beta blockers. Centrally acting agents such as methyldopa and clonidine are now less popular because of their side effects but methyldopa remains useful when other drugs are ineffective or contraindicated. Clonidine is now rarely used in the treatment of hypertension in the UK because of the danger of hypertensive crisis following sudden withdrawal but a transdermal patch which can be used weekly is available in the USA and remains particularly useful in patients who have difficulty adhering to an antihypertensive drug regimen.

References

1. Blythe, W.B. (1985) Natural history of hypertension in renal parenchymal disease. *Am. J. Kidney Dis.*, **4**, A50–6.
2. Guyton, A.C., Coleman, T.G., Young, D.B. *et al.* (1980) Salt balance and long-term blood pressure control. *Annu. Rev. Med.*, **31**, 15–27.
3. Beretta-Piccoli, C., Weidmann, P., de Châtel, R. and Reubi, F. (1976) Hypertension associated with early stage kidney disease. *Am. J. Med.*, **61**, 739–47.
4. Koomans, H.A., Roos, J.C., Boer, P. *et al.* (1982) Salt sensitivity of blood pressure in chronic renal failure. Evi-

dence for renal control of body fluid distribution in man. *Hypertension*, **4**, 190–7.

5. Mroczek, W.J., Moir, D., Davidov, M.E. and Finnerty, F.A. (1977) Sodium intake and furosemide administration in hypertensive patients with renal insufficiency. *Am. J. Cardiol.*, **39**, 808–12.

6. Converse, Jr, R.L., Jacobsen, T.N., Toto, R.D. *et al.* (1992) Sympathetic overactivity in patients with chronic renal failure. *N. Engl. J. Med.*, **327**, 1912–18.

7. Vallance, P., Leone, A., Calver, A. *et al.* (1992) Accumulation of an endogenous inhibitor of nitric oxide synthesis in chronic renal failure. *Lancet*, **339**, 572–5.

8. Ohta, K., Hirata, Y., Shichiri, M. *et al.* (1991) Urinary excretion of endothelin-1 in normal subjects and patients with renal disease. *Kidney Int.*, **39**, 307–11.

9. Hené, R.J., Boer, P., Koomans, H.A. and Mees, E.J.D. (1982) Plasma aldosterone concentrations in chronic renal disease. *Kidney Int.*, **21**, 98–101.

10. Brazy, P.C. and Fitzwilliam, J.F. (1990) Progressive renal disease: role of race and antihypertensive medications. *Kidney Int.*, **37**, 1113–19.

11. Hannedouche, T., Albouze, G., Chauveau, P. *et al.* (1993) Effects of blood pressure and antihypertensive treatment on progression of advanced chronic renal failure. *Am. J. Kidney Dis.*, 21, S131–7.

12. Williams, J.D. and Coles, G.A. (1994) Proteinuria – a direct cause of renal morbidity? *Kidney Int.*, **45**, 443–50.

13. Pohl, J.E.F., Thurston, H. and Swales, J.D. (1974) Hypertension with renal impairment: influence of intensive therapy. *Q. J. Med.*, **43**, 569–81.

14. Klahr, S., Levey, A.S., Beck, G.J. *et al.* (1994) The effects of dietary protein restriction and blood-pressure control on the progression of chronic renal disease. *N. Engl. J. Med.*, **330**, 877–84.

15. Anderson, S. (1994) Antihypertensive therapy in experimental renal disease, in *Prevention of Progressive Chronic Renal Failure* (eds A.N. El Nahas, N.P. Mallick and S. Anderson), Oxford University Press, Oxford, pp. 173–82.

16. Cattran, D.C., Greenwood, C. and Ritchie, S. (1994) Long-term benefits of angiotensin-converting enzyme inhibitor therapy in patients with severe immunoglobulin A nephropathy: a comparison to patients receiving treatment with other antihypertensive agents and to patients receiving no therapy. *Am. J. Kidney Dis.*, **23**, 247–54.

17. Kamper, A.-L., Strandgaard, S. and Leyssac, P.P. (1992) Effect of enalapril on the progression of chronic renal failure. A randomized controlled trial. *Am. J. Hypertens.*, 5, 423–30.

18. Hannendouche, T., Landais, P., Goldfarb, B. *et al.* (1994) Randomized controlled trial of enalapril and β blockers in non-diabetic renal failure. *BMJ*, **309**, 833–7.

19. Zucchelli, P., Zuccala, A., Borghi, M. *et al.* (1992) Long-term comparison between captopril and nifedipine in the progression of renal insufficiency. *Kidney Int.*, **42**, 452–8.

20. Bergström, J., Alvestrand, A., Bucht, H. and Gutierrez, A. (1986) Progression of chronic renal failure in man is retarded with more frequent clinical follow-ups and better blood pressure control. *Clin. Nephrol.*, **25**, 1–6.

21. Apperloo, A.J., de Zeeuw, D., Sluiter, H.E. and de Jong, P.E. (1991) Differential effects of enalapril and atenolol on proteinuria and renal haemodynamics in non-diabetic renal disease. *Br. Med. J.*, **303**, 821–4.

22. Erley, C.M., Harrer, U., Krämer, B.K. and Risler, T. (1992) Renal hemodynamics and reduction of proteinuria by a vasodilating beta blocker versus an ACE inhibitor. *Kidney Int.*, **41**, 1297–303.

23. Epstein, M. and Oster, J.R. (1985) Beta blockers and renal function: a reappraisal. *J. Clin. Hypertens.*, **1**, 85–99.

24. Bianchi, S., Bigazzi, R., Baldari, G. and Campese, V.M. (1991) Long-term effects of enalapril and nicardipine on urinary albumin excretion in patients with chronic renal insufficiency: a 1-year follow-up. *Am. J. Nephrol.*, **11**, 131–7.

25. Heeg, J.E., de Jong, P.E., van der Hem, G.K. and de Zeeuw, D. (1991) Angiotensin II does not acutely reverse the reduction of proteinuria by long-term ACE inhibition. *Kidney Int.*, **40**, 734–41.

26. Kloke, H.J., Wetzels, J.F.M., van Hamersvelt, H.W. *et al.* (1993) Angiotensin-converting enzyme inhibition and the combination of a beta blocker and a diuretic are equally effective in lowering proteinuria in patients with glomerulonephritis. *Nephrol. Dial. Transplant*, **8**, 808–13.

27. Okamura, M., Kanayama, Y., Negoro, N. *et al.* (1991) Long-term effects of calcium antagonists and angiotensin-converting enzyme inhibitors in patients with chronic renal failure of IgA nephropathy. *Contrib. Nephrol.*, **90**, 161–5.

28. Wight, J.P., Brown, C.B. and El Nahas, A.M. (1991) Short-term effects of calcium antagonists on renal haemodynamics in patients with chronic renal failure. *Nephron*, **58**, 62–7.

29. Lardinois, C.K. and Neuman, S.L. (1988) The effects of antihypertensive agents on serum lipids and lipoproteins. *Arch. Intern. Med.*, **148**, 1280–8.

30. Franklin, S.S. and Smith, R.D. (1986) A comparison of enalapril plus hydrochlorothiazide with standard triple therapy in renovascular hypertension. *Nephron*, **44**, 73–82.

31. Toto, R.D., Mitchell, H.C., Lee, H.-C. *et al.* (1991) Reversible renal insufficiency due to angiotensin converting enzyme inhibitors in hypertensive nephrosclerosis. *Ann. Intern. Med.*, **115**, 513–19.

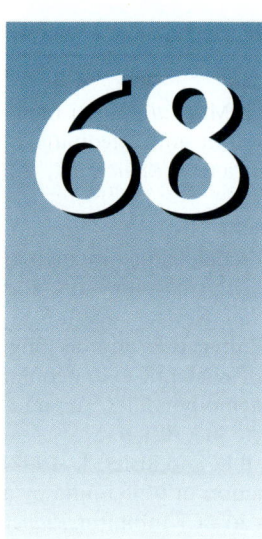

Factors causing progression in renal disease

John Walls and Kevin P.G. Harris

Introduction

The progressive deterioration of function that occurs in any given renal disease is determined, in the main, by exacerbation of the pathological damage within the kidney. There is often, however, a poor correlation between the histologic damage in the renal biopsy specimens and the creatinine clearance. As repeated renal biopsies are usually not performed it is the use of biochemical markers of renal disease by which progression is determined, namely measurements of blood urea or serum creatinine concentration which reflect the glomerular filtration rate (GFR), or by the proteinuria. When changes in these parameters occur, it is important to ascertain whether the cause is reversible and amenable to treatment, or whether there is irreversible progression reflecting permanent damage to the kidney.

Reversible causes of deteriorating renal function in patients with renal disease

The principal reversible causes of a decline in renal function in patients with pre-existing renal disease are shown in Table 68.1.

Urinary tract obstruction

Obstruction to the urinary tract is far more common in male than female patients. With age the frequency of obstruction to the urinary tract in males due to benign prostatic hypertrophy increases. It may present as slowly deteriorating renal function and it is important to perform a rectal examination and an ultrasound of the urinary tract periodically in males with pre-existing renal disease. Obstruction due to pelvic masses such as from carcinoma of the rectum or carcinoma of the cervix often presents as acute renal failure.

Urinary tract infection

Urinary tract infection is common in patients with pre-existing renal disease, especially if there is an anatomical abnormality or malformation within the urinary tract. Such infections may be asymptomatic and periodic urine microscopy and culture should be encouraged in the follow up of such patients (Chapter 60).

Systemic hypertension

There is a 'vicious circle' relationship between systemic hypertension and deteriorating renal function. As renal function deteriorates blood pressure has a tendency to

Nephrology, Edited by Rex L. Jamison and Robert Wilkinson.
Published in 1997 by Chapman & Hall, London. ISBN 0 412 60930 4

Table 68.1 Principal reversible causes of declining renal function in patients with renal disease

1. Urinary tract obstruction
2. Urinary tract infection
3. Systemic hypertension
4. Drugs
5. Cardiac failure
6. Metabolic abnormalities
7. Exacerbation of immunological disease
8. Pregnancy

increase and conversely increases in hypertension cause a deterioration in renal function. The mechanism responsible for these relationships is complex (Chapter 31). The treatment of hypertension is critically important, both to prevent the cardiovascular and central nervous system complications of hypertension and to slow the progression of the renal disease. This is discussed later in this chapter.

Drugs

A multitude of drugs cause deterioration of renal function through a variety of mechanisms. For example, non-steroidal anti-inflammatory drugs inhibit prostaglandin synthesis and alter the balance of vasoconstriction and vasodilatation in the afferent and efferent glomerular arteriole in favor of vasoconstriction. Excessive use of diuretics may cause hypovolemia with an attendant increase in blood urea and serum creatinine. Many drugs can cause interstitial damage (Chapter 69).

Cardiac failure

Many patients with progressive renal disease have cardiovascular disease. For example left ventricular hypertrophy is exacerbated by hypertension and anemia and is more common in male patients. As a result, cardiac failure can ensue, reducing GFR. The concomitant administration of beta blockers may exacerbate the failure. Careful monitoring of renal function is essential when angiotensin converting enzyme (ACE) inhibitors are administered to patients with hypertension or poor cardiac function because unsuspected renal artery stenosis may be present. If renal function deteriorates in this situation the ACE inhibitor must be discontinued and usually renal function will improve. This is not always the case, however, and some patients will remain in renal failure and on renal replacement therapy.

Metabolic abnormalities

Hypercalcemia is the most common metabolic abnormality which is associated with deteriorating renal func-

tion. Common causes are inappropriate administration of vitamin D and calcium based oral phosphate binders, the co-existence of sarcoidosis or multiple myeloma may also account for hypercalcemia. Long-term hyperglycemia in diabetic patients causes irreversible renal damage and is considered later in this chapter.

Exacerbation of immunological disease

In certain immunological and granulomatous diseases, e.g. systemic lupus erythematosis and Wegener's granulomatosis, reactivation of the original disease process within the kidney will cause a deterioration in renal function.

Pregnancy

Pregnancy is particularly hazardous in some patients with significant proteinuria and/or hypertension. A gravid uterus may cause urinary tract obstruction. Hormonal changes associated with pregnancy gives rise to ureteric dilatation and urinary stasis with an increased risk of urinary tract infection which may lead to permanent renal damage.

Irreversible causes of deteriorating renal function in patients with renal disease

Patients with renal disease often have an inexorable decline to chronic renal failure. Whatever the original renal injury, the remaining renal tissue undergoes pathological changes that result in reduced renal function. Several studies have shown that when the serum creatinine is elevated beyond a certain level progression is inevitable [1–3]. For many patients the decline has been shown to be linear when serum creatinine is plotted logarithmically or as a reciprocal against time [4]. The slope of the line is increased if additional adverse factors are superimposed on the natural history of the disease, e.g. hypertension or pregnancy. Conversely, with therapy the slope may decrease (Figure 68.1). Such reciprocal plots are useful in predicting when a patient will reach end-stage renal failure. Numerous experimental studies have demonstrated that once there is a critical reduction in the number of nephrons a maladaptive response occurs in the remaining nephrons, which leads to the typical histological picture of the 'end stage kidney'.

The end-stage kidney is characterized histologically by localized loss of glomeruli, areas of cellular proliferation in the remaining glomeruli, collapse of the glomerular capillary bed and glomerulosclerosis. There is atrophy of the renal tubules which are surrounded by inflammatory cells, increased deposition of collagen and extracellular matrix, increased lipid deposition and an increase in the number of fibroblasts present. This histological pattern

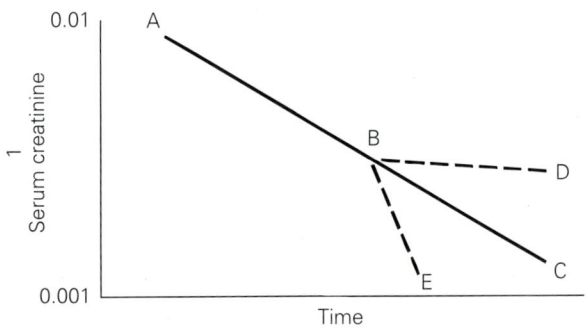

Figure 68.1 A reciprocal creatinine plot showing the linear decline in renal function with time. Factors which accelerate the decline in renal function cause the slope to increase (A–B–E), whereas beneficial factors lessen the slope (A–B–D).

represents a final end result independent of the original renal disease [5].

Glomerulosclerosis is characterized by increased deposition of abnormal basement membrane and mesangial matrix components, such as collagens IV and V, laminin, fibronectin and glycosaminoglycans. In addition collagens I and III, which are not normally found in the glomerulus are present. It is likely that they result from either excess production and/or decreased degradation of basement membrane and mesangial matrix. All four cell types within the glomerulus, i.e. endothelium, mesangial, epithelial and macrophages probably participate in this process.

About 30 years ago Risdon *et al.* [6] demonstrated that the degree of tubular atrophy on renal biopsy correlated more closely with renal function, as determined by serum creatinine, than did the histological changes in the glomeruli, despite the fact that all the patients studied had glomerulonephritis. Similar observations have been made in other patients. The prognostic importance of interstitial pathology has been confirmed in a number of renal diseases, including membranous glomerulonephritis, focal sclerosing glomerulonephritis, IgA nephropathy, membranoproliferative glomerulonephritis type I and diabetic nephropathy (for review see [7]).

Glomerulosclerosis

It is notable that whatever the nature of the initial renal disease the final result in the glomerulus is glomerulosclerosis, namely a fibrotic scarred glomerulus with no capillary circulation and hence no function. Numerous mechanisms have been postulated for this development of glomerulosclerosis, but it is highly likely that a combination of factors play a part in its development (Figure 68.2). Our understanding of the mechanisms involved is derived primarily from studies of experimental renal disease, usually in rats, such as nephrotoxic serum nephritis, Heyman nephritis or the remnant kidney

model [8]. In this last model a unilateral nephrectomy is performed together with removal or infarction of approximately one-third of the remaining kidney. This results in proteinuria, hypertension, deteriorating renal function and glomerulosclerosis – not unlike progressive renal disease in humans. In addition it has been demonstrated in humans that a loss of a significant amount of renal mass results in the development of glomerulosclerosis [9].

Glomerular hypertension: the hyperfiltration theory

When renal mass is reduced there is an increase in renal plasma flow per nephron and an increase in single nephron glomerular filtration rate (SNGFR) in the remaining nephrons. These increased flow rates result from a dilatation of the afferent arteriole to a greater extent than the efferent arteriole, which is under the vasoconstrictive influence of angiotensin II. These changes in arteriolar tone produce an increase in glomerular capillary pressure, with a subsequent increase in SNGFR. Whereas this is an adaptive response to maintain GFR in the failing kidney, in the long term it may well be a maladaptive response as increases in glomerular capillary pressure contribute to an increased permeability of the glomerular basement membrane to proteins which pass into the mesangium and contribute to the subsequent development of glomerulosclerosis [10]. This is an attractive hypothesis which is supported by evidence that decreasing intraglomerular hypertension by the use of either a low protein diet or ACE inhibitors delays the development of glomerulosclerosis in the remnant kidney model. Other maneuvers, however, such as the administration of heparin or lipid-lowering agents which do not alter glomerular hemodynamics also have a beneficial effect in this model. In addition, increased intraglomerular pressure has not been observed in the early phases of the puromycin aminonucleoside model of renal failure which also develops glomerulosclerosis.

Glomerular hypertrophy

Glomerular hypertrophy may develop in the early phase of several human renal diseases, e.g. diabetic nephropathy, and is an early feature in the remnant kidney model. It has, therefore, been suggested that glomerular hypertrophy is a prerequisite for the development of glomerulosclerosis. Glomerular hypertrophy could result from the altered glomerular hemodynamics as discussed above, since a decrease in protein intake, in some experiments, and ACE inhibition decrease glomerular hypertrophy. Experiments in which growth hormone was manipulated to either inhibit or enhance glomerular hypertrophy in the remnant kidney model also suggest a link between hypertrophy and the development of glomerulosclerosis. However, Yoshida *et al.* [11], in an elegant experiment, were able to dissociate glomerular hypertrophy from glomerular hyperfiltration in an animal model in which

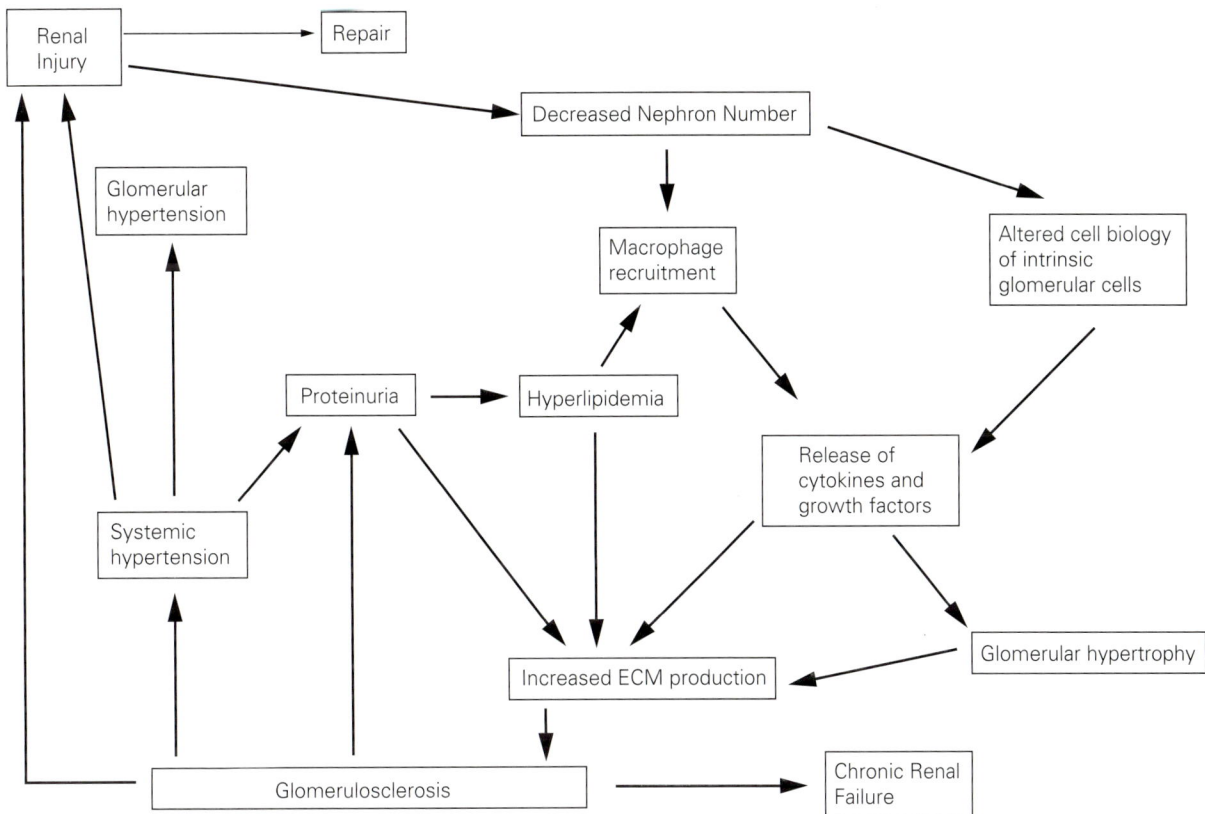

Figure 68.2 Mechanisms by which initial renal injury may lead to glomerulosclerosis. A renal insult may be followed by tissue repair or more commonly a permanent loss of nephrons. As a result of the latter a complex and interacting series of responses are initiated which subsequently result in further nephron destruction and hence progressive chronic renal failure (the maladaptive response).

there was urinary diversion into the peritoneal cavity. They demonstrated the presence of glomerular hyperfiltration in both situations but glomerular hypertrophy only occurred when the contralateral kidney had been removed. The degree of glomerular injury was also greater in the contralateral nephrectomy model, suggesting that glomerular hypertrophy is a precursor to subsequent glomerular scarring. In contrast, in both the remnant kidney model and the model of streptozotocin induced diabetes, ACE inhibition protects against glomerulosclerosis, but does not prevent glomerular hypertrophy.

In humans there is some evidence to support the role of glomerular hypertrophy. Fogo *et al.* [12] showed in sequential renal biopsies in proteinuric children that patients with large glomerular tufts were more likely to develop glomerulosclerosis and to have a more protracted clinical course. Interest in this area has been renewed by the suggestion that the number of nephrons in a kidney plays an important role in determining the development of progressive renal damage. In situations where the number of nephrons is decreased, as in congenital absence of one kidney or in renal transplant recipients, glomerular hypertrophy occurs and progressive renal damage may occur.

Systemic hypertension

Systemic hypertension is a common feature in many human renal diseases and in most experimental models of glomerulosclerosis. A reduction in blood pressure by a variety of antihypertensive agents affords protection in the remnant kidney model suggesting a link between systemic hypertension and glomerulosclerosis. In this model ACE inhibition affords better protection than other agents achieving the same blood pressure reduction, presumably by the beneficial alterations in the abnormal glomerular hemodynamics of the diseased kidney. However, ACE inhibitors have other properties which could be beneficial in this setting; namely an ability to modulate renal growth, influence local cytokine production and reduce leukocyte influx into areas of injury.

There is a direct association between the level of blood pressure and the rate of decline in renal function with age in human renal disease. Aggressive treatment in accelerated hypertension not only improves patient survival but also preserves and may improve renal function. The control of blood pressure has been shown to slow the rate of progression of renal failure in diabetic nephropathy [13] and in a variety of other renal diseases [14, 15].

Lipids

Abnormalities in serum lipids in patients with renal disease have been recognized for more than a century. Similarly the occurrence of lipid deposits in the kidney in patients with the nephrotic syndrome has been known for over 80 years. It is only in the past 15 years that studies have been performed determining whether abnormal lipid metabolism plays a pathogenetic role in progression of renal disease. With the exception of the rare condition of congenital lecithin cholesterol acyl transferase deficiency (L:CAT) that occurs in some Norwegian families it is unlikely that abnormal lipids cause renal disease. Certainly there is no convincing evidence of an increased incidence of progressive renal disease in patients with familial hypercholesterolemia.

The possibility that lipids play a role in potentiating existing renal damage was postulated in 1982 by Moorhead et al. [16]. They suggested that after glomerular injury there is a urinary loss of lipoprotein lipase activators and subsequent hyperlipidemia. Filtered lipoproteins accumulate in mesangial cells stimulating cell proliferation and the production of abnormal basement membrane and extracellular matrix proteins. Filtered lipoproteins may also accumulate in the renal tubular cells and initiate or exacerbate tubular interstitial damage. In support of this hypothesis was the suggestion by Diamond and Karnovsky [17] that glomerulosclerosis resembles atherosclerosis in several ways. Mesangial cells have many similarities with vascular smooth muscle cells and are known to possess receptors for low density lipoproteins (LDL) [18]. In addition, LDL is oxidized by mesangial cells [19] and stimulates mesangial cell proliferation. Minimally oxidized LDL is also a chemoattractant for monocytes which, if attracted to a damaged glomerulus, will stimulate the production of inflammatory cytokines.

There have been numerous experiments using a variety of different models, e.g. the Zucker obese rat, and cholesterol feeding in both the remnant kidney and nephrotoxic serum nephritis models which have explored the mechanisms involved, and in some studies lipid lowering agents have brought about a decrease in glomerular damage. Unfortunately, apart from one observation by Rabelink et al. [20] who demonstrated a decrease in proteinuria in patients with the nephrotic syndrome, it has not been possible to transfer any of the ameliorative effects of lipid-lowering agents seen in experimental renal disease to human renal disease, despite lowering of the serum cholesterol levels [21].

Cytokines and growth factors

There is increasing evidence that cytokines and growth factors play a role in the development of glomerulosclerosis and tubulointerstitial injury. Both intrinsic and infiltrating cells produce factors which may act in either a paracrine or autocrine manner. Interleukin (IL)-1β, IL-6 and tumor necrosis factor (TNF)-α play an important role in the inflammatory response and are up-regulated in human and experimental glomerulonephritis [22]. Platelet derived growth factor (PDGF) and transforming growth factor (TGF)-β may induce cell hypertrophy or proliferation and modulate the synthesis and degradation of extracellular matrix. Early in the natural history of the remnant kidney there is increased expression of PDGF and its receptor that is linked to mesangial cell proliferation. Administration of recombinant PDGF to rats causes mesangial cell proliferation; transfection of the PDGF gene into the normal rat kidney produces glomerular cell proliferation and glomerulosclerosis. PDGF also up-regulates the production of TGFβ by mesangial cells.

TGFβ is a multifunctional cytokine which has the ability to regulate the production and turnover of extracellular matrix. It enhances the synthesis of collagen, fibronectin and proteoglycans and inhibits matrix degradation by decreasing the production of proteases and increasing the production of protease inhibitors. Normal glomeruli in mice, rats and humans constitutively express TGF-β; increased expression of TGF-β occurs in a variety of both immunological and toxic models of experimental renal disease. TGF-β is also found in a number of human renal diseases, including diabetic nephropathy, IgA nephropathy, systemic vasculitis and chronic transplant rejection. TGF-β is produced by intrinsic glomerular cells and also by infiltrating cells commonly seen in these conditions. That TGF-β is an important cytokine has been demonstrated by the observation that transfection of the TGF-β gene into glomeruli in vivo results in glomerulosclerosis and blocking its action by neutralizing antibodies or the administration of the TGF-β binding proteoglycan decorin prevents glomerulosclerosis [23, 24].

Infiltrating macrophages

During a wide variety of glomerular insults there is an increase over baseline in the number of macrophages within the glomerulus. That such infiltrating macrophages are seen in the glomerulus in the uninephrectomy model, a model known to progress to glomerulosclerosis, before the development of proteinuria, glomerular hypertrophy or light microscopic changes, strongly suggests that they play a pathogenetic role. Similar observations have been made in the puromycin aminonucleoside model, another non-immune model which develops glomerulosclerosis. It is also noteworthy that abolition of the macrophage infiltration by irradiation or feeding a diet deficient in essential fatty acids prevents subsequent development of glomerulosclerosis. Cholesterol feeding, which accelerates the development of glomerulosclerosis, is associated with an increased number of infiltrating macrophages within the glomerulus in these models.

Macrophages are a potent source of cytokines and growth factors, many of which are capable of stimulating extracellular matrix production by mesangial cells. Of note, macrophages are known to produce TGF-β and PDGF. How these cells get into the glomerulus remains to be determined. It is known that in experimental glomerulonephritis in rats there is an up-regulation of the intercellular adhesion molecule (ICAM) ICAM I which interacts with its ligand LFA-1 on leukocytes. Neutralizing antibodies to both ICAM-1 and LFA-1 prevent glomerular leukocyte infiltration and glomerulosclerosis. Expression of adhesion molecules may be induced either directly by immunological insult or indirectly via the production of molecules such as IL-1 or TNF-α which may induce adhesion molecule expression. Both immune and non-immune-mediated renal insults are associated with the production of chemoattractive substances by the glomerulus, namely the monocyte chemoattractive protein 1 and RANTES. Osteopontin is another molecule which may play a role in attracting monocytes into the kidney especially the interstitium. The role of these chemoattractive agents has not been fully elucidated but their therapeutic manipulation offers an attractive possibility for intervention to prevent progression of glomerulosclerosis.

Platelet deposition

It is a common observation in human and experimental renal disease that there is platelet deposition within the glomerular capillaries. It is postulated that this leads to ischemia of the glomerulus and results in glomerulosclerosis. The platelet deposition is thought to occur as a result of injury to the glomerular capillary endothelium. It is possible to alter progression in the remnant kidney model by the administration of heparin or antiplatelet agents. However, heparin is known to have many other therapeutic properties which could account for this amelioration apart from preventing platelet aggregation and deposition. These experimental studies have not yet been translated into well-substantiated therapeutic regimens in human renal disease.

Tubulointerstitial disease

Despite the original observation 30 years ago that in many glomerular diseases renal function correlates best with changes in the tubules and interstitium, it is only recently that this topic has received more attention. Glomeruli only account for approximately 5% of total kidney volume, the tubules and interstitium constituting the majority of renal tissue. The interstitium has an abundant vascular bed and therefore any insult which occurs may be easily dispersed throughout the kidney. The histological changes occurring in the tubules and interstitium consist of tubular atrophy and dilatation, with some tubules containing proteinaceous castlike material, and a widening of the interstitial space which becomes replaced by fibrous tissue. The capillaries are widely separated and

decreased in number. In addition, there is a cellular infiltrate which initially consists of macrophages but these are later replaced by T lymphocytes. Usually CD 4 positive and CD 8 positive T lymphocytes are present in equal numbers but in some cases one or other cell type may predominate [25]. As with glomerulosclerosis it is likely that the development of tubulointerstitial disease is a multifactorial process.

Ischemia

After the initial insult there is expansion of the interstitial space which reduces renal blood flow. This leads to ischemia of the tubules and interstitial fibrosis. The fall in renal blood flow decreases GFR [26]. There is compensatory constriction of the efferent glomerular arterioles in order to maintain GFR. This exacerbates the glomerular hypertension and worsens glomerulosclerosis. Ischemia of the interstitial space will further reduce oxygen tension with resultant injury to tubular cells which may cause tubular atrophy or produce a number of cytokines or chemotactic agents [27]. Fine *et al.* [28] proposed that glomerular hypertension which occurs in many models of renal disease results in increased blood pressure being transmitted to the postglomerular capillaries, injuring them and causing interstitial ischemia. Once scarring has started with the associated increase in matrix volume, there is an increase in distance between tubular cells and peritubular capillaries across which oxygen and energy substrates must travel which would further increase the ischemic injury.

The role of proteinuria in tubular interstitial damage

Following glomerular injury the glomerular basement membrane barrier is compromised and proteins leak into the glomerular filtrate and pass down the tubular lumen. In many human renal diseases, for example focal segmental glomerulosclerosis, IgA nephropathy, membranous glomerulonephritis and mesangiocapillary glomerulonephritis, there is an inverse correlation between the extent of proteinuria and the level of renal function. Initially this was considered merely to reflect the extent of glomerular damage. However, since the decrease in renal function correlates best with tubulointerstitial damage it has been postulated that proteinuria itself is injurious to the renal tubules and initiates the development of tubulointerstitial disease. This hypothesis was suggested by Eddy [29] and has been strengthened by a series of elegant experiments using the protein overload model. Following intraperitoneal injections of bovine serum albumin into rats, the animals developed proteinuria, an early interstitial leukocyte infiltration and subsequent tubulointerstitial damage with scarring and fibrosis. Whether it is albumin or one of the compounds attached or associated with the albumin molecule which acts as the initiating factor is not yet fully determined.

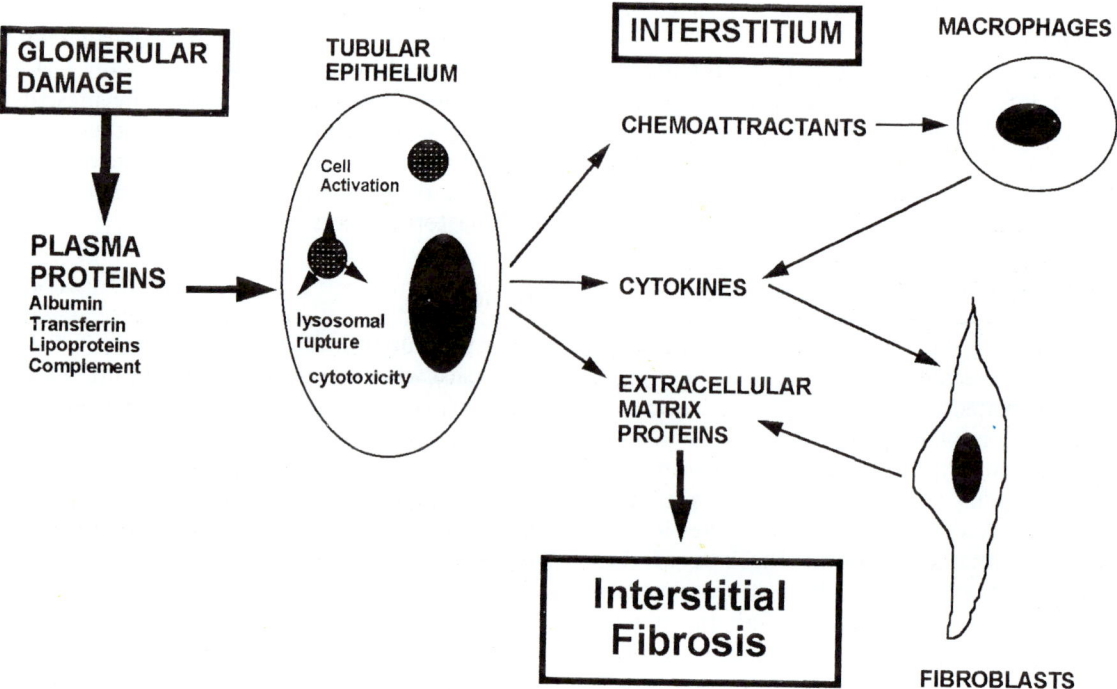

Figure 68.3 The mechanisms by which proteins filtered as a result of glomerular injury may cause interstitial inflammation and scarring. In glomerular disease filtered proteins in the tubular lumen alter the biology of the tubular epithelium. This results in the release into the interstitium of chemoattractants, cytokines and extracellular matrix proteins. As a result there is accumulation of macrophages which also release cytokines to recruit and stimulate fibroblasts. The resultant increase in extracellular matrix causes scarring.

Figure 68.3 indicates the various pathways which may be involved in this process.

Human proximal tubular cells in culture exposed to albumin undergo hypertrophy and proliferate [30]. It is recognized that albumin carries a number of fatty acids and it may be that these fatty acids are toxic to tubular cells when reabsorbed from the tubular lumen. It has also been suggested that these fatty acids are responsible for the production by tubular cells of a chemoattractive agent which causes the macrophage infiltration into the interstitum. Transferrin also leaks into the tubular fluid during glomerular injury and under certain conditions yields iron. Iron is known to be cytotoxic and could injure the tubular cells. In nephrotoxic serum nephritis the degree of tubulointerstitial injury correlates with urinary iron excretion [31]. Similarly, complement could also leak through damaged glomeruli and stimulate cytokine production by tubular cells. It has been shown that the degree of proteinuria correlates with the level of urinary ammonia excretion [32] and it is postulated that the ammonia comes from protein degradation within tubular cells. Ammonia is known to activate the complement cascade and interstitial damage could result from such a mechanism. However, it is rare to see significant complement deposition surrounding the tubules on histological examination which mitigates against this hypothesis.

Following exposure to interferon-γ, cultured proximal tubular cells are able to produce both the chemoattractive agent MCP-1 and a number of proinflammatory cytokines such as IL-6, granulocyte macrophage colony stimulating factor and PDGF. Similarly the supernatant from tubular cells in culture can stimulate fibroblasts to produce the extracellular matrix protein fibronectin. Interleukin-1α can stimulate human proximal tubular cells in culture to produce the cytokine TNF-α, and has been shown to stimulate the expression of the third component of complement in cultured human proximal tubular cells. Endothelin-1 in addition to its monocyte chemoattractant effect stimulates interstitial fibroblast proliferation and extracellular matrix production [33]. From *in vivo* studies, human proximal tubular cells have been shown to express a number of surface proteins such as ICAM-1, vascular cell adhesion molecule (VCAM) VCAM-1 and MHC class 2. The activity of the latter can be up-regulated by incubation with interferon-α.

One argument against the pivotal role of proteinuria in the production of tubulointerstitial disease is the lack of renal injury in patients with minimal change nephrotic syndrome and the failure of the patients to progress to chronic renal disease. There are, however, reports of interstitial infiltrates in minimal change nephrotic syndrome and it is known that there is an increase in the urinary excretion of the enzyme *N*-acetyl-β-glucosoamidase (NAG) which is produced by tubular cells and is regarded by some as a marker of tubular toxicity.

The role of acidosis

Metabolic acidosis is a common feature in progressive renal disease and from experimental data has been suggested to be a factor causing a deterioration in renal function. It has been known for many years that acidosis can lead to renal hypertrophy. In addition, acidosis stimulates an increase in ammoniogenesis by renal tubular cells. The postulated mechanism whereby acidosis may be injurious to the kidney is that the increase in ammonia production activates the complement system. Nath *et al.* [34] in short-term experiments using the remnant kidney model demonstrated that a diet supplemented with sodium bicarbonate decreased proteinuria and reduced the peritubular deposition of C3 and C5b-9. More recent long-term experiments have cast doubt on this theory [35].

Hyperparathyroidism

Other metabolic factors have been implicated in the progression of chronic renal disease. There are experimental data showing that continued elevation of serum phosphate levels, by increasing the calcium–phosphorus product, leads to increased calcium deposition within the kidney. Maneuvers designed to decrease serum phosphate in this situation have been shown to slow the rate of progression. However, this has not been demonstrated to be a factor in human renal disease where phosphate control is imperative in the prevention of renal osteodystrophy.

Hyperglycemia

There is abundant evidence in experimental models and in human renal disease that control of blood glucose levels is critical in reducing the rate of progression in diabetic nephropathy. Glucose is known to have stimulatory properties with the development of glomerular hypertrophy as discussed elsewhere. In addition, elevated glucose levels are known to increase cytokine production from proximal tubular cells in culture and to affect intracellular signaling in vascular smooth muscle cells. Elevated glucose levels are also known to increase the expression of mRNA for vascular permeability factor (VPF) which is a potent mitogenic agent and increases vascular permeability severalfold. Increased production of VPF could lead to the mesangial expansion and cellular proliferation seen in the glomeruli in diabetic nephropathy.

Male sex

In has been well recognized for many years that there are more males than females receiving renal replacement therapy. Although there has been a suggestion that this is, in part, due to selection bias there is evidence to suggest that male sex is an adverse prognostic factor in terms of progression. It is known that in the remnant kidney model in male rats castration delays progression. Clearly castration has several metabolic effects, i.e. on lipid metabolism and as yet the exact mechanism has not been fully elucidated.

Genetic factors

Certain renal diseases are linked to histocompatability loci, for example membranous glomerulonephritis with HLA-DR2 and HLA-3 and IgA nephropathy with DR-1 and HLA-B35. Other genes may play a functional role in the progression of renal disease. The ACE gene is located on chromosome 17q23 and has within it a fragment at intron 16, the presence or absence of which gives rise to polymorphism of the ACE gene. The presence of the fragment defines insertion (I allele), whereas its absence defines deletion (D allele). The genotype can be classified as II, ID or DD. There is a correlation between ACE gene polymorphism and serum ACE levels and intracellular ACE activity in T lymphocytes. Whereas there is no evidence for increased frequency of a particular polymorphism with a given renal disease, there is growing evidence that ACE gene polymorphism may affect progression. The two diseases most commonly cited are IgA nephropathy and diabetic nephropathy. In IgA nephropathy there is a fourfold increase in the frequency of the DD allele in those patients with progressive renal disease compared to those with stable renal function. The DD genotype appears to confer a similar fourfold risk of progression in patients with non-insulin-dependent diabetes mellitus. There is preliminary evidence that similar findings apply to polycystic kidney disease. This subject has been recently excellently reviewed by Yoshida *et al.* [36].

Treatment strategies

There are three main approaches to treatment in attempting to delay progression. The first is to adequately control systemic hypertension. There is clear evidence from both retrospective and prospective studies that good control of both systolic and diastolic blood pressure slows the rate of progression. It is not yet clear what the optimum level of blood pressure control is, but for patients under 60 years of age a blood pressure of 130/80 mmHg and for those over the age of 60 years of 150/90 mmHg appears to be a reasonable target. It is not clear which antihypertensive agents are the most beneficial in reducing progression given the same level of blood pressure control although there is some evidence that ACE inhibitors are more effective in reducing the rate of progression in both diabetic and non-diabetic renal disease [37, 38].

The second strategy is to reduce the degree of proteinuria to minimize interstitial damage. This may be achieved by maneuvers such as dietary protein restriction; protein restriction also reduces GFR and may have an independent mode of action. ACE inhibitors should be tried, even in normotensive patients as they have been shown to reduce the degree of proteinuria. In certain conditions, for example, membranous glomerulonephritis, treatment with corticosteroids has been shown to be of some benefit. It is of note that in the Modification of Diet in Renal Disease (MDRD) study the greatest benefit from lowering systemic hypertension was seen in those patients with proteinuria exceeding 3 g/24 h. This has subsequently been confirmed in a meta-analysis of all suitable studies [39].

The role of low protein diets in delaying progression remains controversial. After several single center studies showed a benefit the large multicenter trials, such as the MDRD study in the USA, have failed to substantiate the earlier encouraging findings, although a subsequent analysis of some of the data is more encouraging. Several questions arise from these studies. At what level of renal function should the protein restriction start? What level

of protein restriction should be used – more or less than 0.6 g/kg/day? How should the effect of protein restriction be monitored? Can malnutrition be avoided with the use of such diets? Are supplements with either ketoacids or essential amino acid preparations needed for patients with a reduced protein intake? Despite the meta-analysis by Fouque et al. [40] it is likely that this controversy will continue. The decision to recommend protein restriction in progressive renal disease will depend on physician preference and patient acceptability.

The main emphasis on managing patients with progressive renal disease is careful monitoring, paying attention to the three strategies outlined above. In patients with diabetic nephropathy close glycemic control is essential. It is of interest that frequent clinic visits by patients with progressive renal disease has been associated with a decrease in the rate of progression in addition to delaying or preventing many of the other complications of chronic renal disease [41].

References

1. Feest, T.G., Mistry, C.D., Grimes, D.S. and Mallick, N.P. (1990) Incidence of advanced chronic renal failure and the need for end stage renal replacement therapy. *Br. Med. J.*, **301**, 897–900.

2. Locattelli, F., Alberti, D., Graziani, G. *et al.* (1991) Prospective, randomised multicentre trial of the effect of protein restriction on progression of chronic renal insufficiency. *Lancet*, **37**, 1299–304.

3. Holevy, J. and Hayslett, J.P. (1986) Clinical features of glomerulosclerosis, in *The Progressive Nature of Renal Disease* (eds W.E. Mitch, B.M. Brenner and J.H. Stein), Churchill Livingstone, New York, pp. 189–201.

4. Mitch, W.E., Walser, M., Buffington, G.A. and Lemann, J. Jr (1976) A simple method of estimating progression of chronic renal failure. *Lancet*, **ii**, 1326–8.

5. Klahr, S., Schreiner, G. and Ichikawa, I. (1988) The progression of renal disease. *N. Engl. J. Med.*, **318**, 1657–66.

6. Risdon, R.A., Sloper, J.C. and de Wardener, H.E. (1966) The relationship between renal function and histological changes found in renal biopsy specimens from patients with persistent glomerulonephritis. *Lancet*, **ii**, 363–66.

7. Burton, C.J. and Walls, J. (1994) Proximal tubule cell proteinuria and tubulo-interstitial scarring. *Nephron*, **68**, 287–8.

8. Furness, P.N. and Harris, K.P.G. (1994) An evaluation of experimental models of glomerulonephritis. *Int. J. Exp. Pathol.*, **75**, 9–22.

9. Novick, A.C., Gephardt, G., Guz, B. *et al.* (1991) Long term follow-up after partial removal of a solitary kidney. *N. Engl. J. Med.*, **325**, 1058–62.

10. Hostetler, T.H., Olson, J.L., Rennke, H.G. *et al.* (1981) Hyperfiltration in remnant nephrons: a potentially adverse response to renal ablation. *Am. J. Physiol.*, **241**, F85–93.

11. Yoshida, Y., Fogo, A. and Ichikawa, I. (1989) Glomerular haemodynamic changes vs hypertrophy in experimental glomerulosclerosis. *Kidney Int.*, **35**, 654–60.

12. Fogo, A., Hawkins, E.P., Berry, P.L. *et al.* (1990) Glomerular hypertrophy in minimal change disease predicts subsequent progression to focal glomerulosclerosis. *Kidney Int.*, **38**, 115–23.

13. Bakris, G.L. (1993) Hypertension in diabetic patients. An overview of interventional studies to preserve renal function. *Am. J. Hypertens.*, **6**, 140–1475S.

14. Alvastrand, A., Gutierrez, A., Bucht, H. and Bergstrom, J. (1988) Reduction of blood pressure retards the progression of chronic renal failure in man. *Nephrol. Dial. Transplant.*, **3**, 624–31.

15. Klahr, S., Levy, A.S., Beck, G.J. *et al.* (1994) The effects of dietary protein restriction and blood pressure control on the progression of chronic renal disease. *N. Engl. J. Med.*, **330**, 877–84.

16. Moorhead, J.F., Chan, M.K., El Nahas, M. and Varghese, Z. (1982) Lipid nephrotoxicity in chronic progressive glomerular and tubulo-interstitial disease. *Lancet*, **ii**, 1309–11.

17. Diamond, J.R. and Karnovsky, M.J. (1988) Focal and segmental glomerulosclerosis: analogies to atherosclerosis. *Kidney Int.*, **33**, 917–22.

18. Rayner, H.C., Horsburgh, T., Brown, S.L. *et al.* (1990) Receptor-mediated endocytosis of low-density lipoprotein by cultured human glomerular cells. *Nephron*, **55**, 292–9.

19. Wheeler, D.C., Chana, R.S., Topley, N. *et al.* (1994). Oxidation of low density lipoproteins may promote glomerular injury. *Kidney Int.*, **45**, 1628–36.

20. Rabelink, A.J., Hene, R.J., Erkelens, D.W. and Koomans, H.A. (1990) Pential remission of nephrotic syndrome in patients on long-term Simvastatin. *Lancet*, **i**, 1045–6.

21. Thomas, M.E., Harris, K.P.G., Ramaswamy, C. *et al.* (1993) Simvastatin therapy for hypercholesterolaemic patients

with nephrotic syndrome or significant proteinuria. *Kidney Int.*, **44**, 1124–9.

22. Noronha, I.L., Niemir, Z., Stein, H. and Waldherr, R. (1995) Cytokines and growth factors in renal disease. *Nephrol. Dial. Transplant.*, **10**, 775–86.

23. Isaki, Y., Fujiwara, Y., Veda, N. *et al.* (1993) Glomerulosclerosis induced by in-vivo transfection of transforming growth factor-β or platelet-derived growth factor gene into rat kidney. *J. Clin. Invest.*, **92**, 2952–62.

24. Border, W.A., Okuda, S., Languino, L.R. *et al.* (1990) Suppression of experimental glomerulonephritis by antiserum against transforming growth factor β1. *Nature*, **346**, 371–4.

25. Boucher, A., Droz, D., Adefer, E. and Noel, L.H. (1986) Characterisation of mononuclear cell subsets in renal cellular interstitial infiltrates. *Kidney Int.*, **29**, 1043–9.

26. Bohle, A., Mackenen-Haen, S. and Gise, H. (1987) Significance of tubulo-interstitial changes in the renal cortex for the excretory function and concentrating ability of the kidney: a morphometric contribution. *Am. J. Nephrol.*, **7**, 421–33.

27. Brezis, M., Rosen, S., Silva, P. and Epstein, F.H. (1984) Renal ischemia: a new perspective. *Kidney Int.*, **26**, 375–83.

28. Fine, L.G., Ong, A.C.M. and Norman, J.T. (1993) Mechanisms of tubulo-interstitial injury in progressive renal disease. *Eur. J. Clin. Invest.*, **23**, 259–65.

29. Eddy, A.A. (1989) Interstital nephritis induced by protein-overloaded proteinuria. *Am. J. Pathol.*, **135**, 719–33.

30. Burton, C.J., Harris, K.P.G., Bevington, A. and Walls, J. (1994) The growth of proximal tubular cells in the presence of albumin and proteinuric urine. *Exp. Nephrol.*, **2**, 345–50.

31. Alfrey, A.C., Froment, D.H. and Hammond, W.S. (1989) A role of iron in tubulo-interstitial injury in nephrotoxic serum nephritis. *Kidney Int.*, **36**, 753–9.

32. Rustom, R., Jackson, M.J., Critchley, M. and Bone, J.M. (1992) Tubular metabolism of aprotinin 99m Tc and urinary ammonia: Effects of proteinuria. *Miner. Electrolyte Metab.*, **18**, 108–12.

33. Remuzzi, G. (1995) Abnormal protein traffic through the glomerular barrier induces tubular cell dysfunction and causes renal injury. *Curr. Opin. Nephrol. Hypertens.*, **4**, 339–42.

34. Nath, K.A., Hostetler, M.K. and Hostelter, T.H. (1985) Pathophysiology of chronic tubulo-interstitial disease in rats: Interactions of dietary acid load ammonia and complement component C3. *J. Clin. Invest.*, **76**, 667–75.

35. Throssell, D., Brown, J., Harris, K.P.G. and Walls, J. (1995) Renal acidosis does not contribute to chronic renal injury in the rat. *Clin. Sci.*, **89**, 643–50.

36. Yoshida, H., Kon, V. and Ichikawa, I. (1996) Polymorphism of the renin–angiotensin system genes in progressive renal diseases. *Kidney Int.*, **50**, 732–44.

37. Lewis, E.J., Hunsicker, L.G., Bain, R.P. and Rhode, R.D. (1993) The effect of angiotensin converting enzyme inhibition on diabetic nephropathy. *N. Engl. J. Med.*, **329**, 1456–62.

38. Maschio, G., Alberto, D., Fanin, G. *et al.* (1996) Effect of the angiotensin converting enzyme inhibitor benzepial on the progression of chronic renal insufficiency. *N. Engl. J. Med.*, **334**, 939–45.

39. Maki, D.D., Ma, J.Z., Louis, T.A. and Kasiske, B.L. (1995) Long term effects of antihypertensive agents on proteinuria and renal function. *Arch. Intern. Med.*, **155**, 1073–80.

40. Fouque, D., Laville, M., Boissel, J.P. *et al.* (1992) Controlled low protein diets in chronic renal insufficiency: meta-analysis. *Br. Med. J.*, **304**, 216–20.

41. Bergstrom, J., Alvestrand, A., Bucht, H. and Gutierrez, A. (1986) Progression of chronic renal failure in man is retarded with more frequent clinic follow-ups and better blood pressure control. *Clin. Nephrol.*, **25**, 1–6.

69

Prescribing in renal insufficiency: principles and practice

Jeffrey K. Aronson

Introduction

Renal insufficiency impinges on drug therapy in several ways:

1   Pharmacokinetic effects:
    (a)   renal insufficiency alters the rate of elimination of drugs that are excreted by the kidneys in an active form or as active metabolites;
    (b)   renal insufficiency may alter the protein binding of a drug;
    (c)   diuretics that act on the luminal side of the renal tubule may not reach their site of action in sufficiently high concentrations in renal insufficiency;
    (d)   renal replacement therapy may alter the rate of elimination of a drug.
2   Pharmacodynamic effects:
    (a)   renal insufficiency may alter a drug's pharmacological effects.
3   Adverse effects:
    (a)   altered clearance may cause greater accumulation of a drug, leading to dose-related adverse effects;
    (b)   concomitant effects of renal insufficiency may enhance or inhibit the actions of a drug indirectly;
    (c)   nephrotoxic drugs may worsen renal impairment.
4   Interference with diagnostic tests

Graded responses to drugs and the therapeutic index

The pharmacological effect of a drug is related to its concentration at its site of action – within certain limits, the higher the concentration the greater the effect. Conventionally, the intensity of the pharmacological effect of a drug is plotted against the logarithm of the drug concentration, and the relation between these two is known as the log dose–response curve.

It is not necessary to discuss the mathematics of the log dose–response curve to appreciate a few of its simple properties (Figure 69.1):

1   at low concentrations there is little or no effect;
2   as the concentration rises there is a steep rise in effect;
3   at high concentrations a maximum effect is reached.

Two examples of log dose–response curves are given in Figure 69.1, which shows the natriuretic effects of the loop diuretics bumetanide and furosemide in relation to their urinary excretion rate, which at steady state reflects the rate of delivery of the diuretics to the luminal side of the thick ascending limb of the loop of Henle, their site of action. This comparison illustrates two aspects of drug action: potency and maximal efficacy. The potency of a drug is related to the amount of drug required to produce

Nephrology, Edited by Rex L. Jamison and Robert Wilkinson.
Published in 1997 by Chapman & Hall, London. ISBN 0 412 60930 4

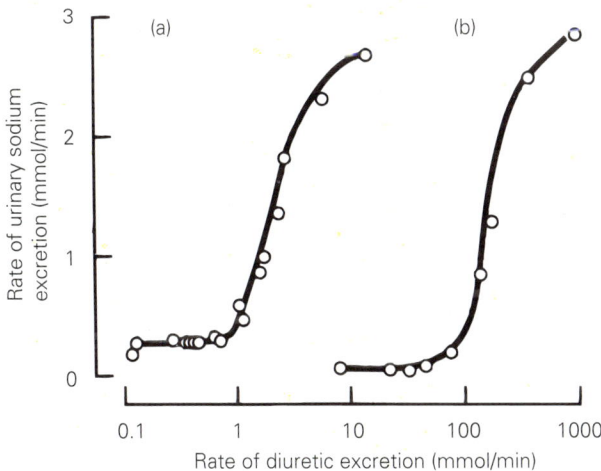

Figure 69.1 Log dose–response curves relating the urinary excretion rates of bumetanide (a) and furosemide (b) to their natriuretic effects. (Redrawn from Brater *et al.* (1983) (bumetanide) [1] and from Chennavasin *et al.* (1980) (frusemide) [2], with permission.)

a given effect. In this case bumetanide is 100 times more potent than furosemide mole for mole (70 times more potent mg for mg), since it takes a hundredth of the molar dose to produce the same natriuretic effect. However, both drugs have the same maximal efficacy; in other words a high enough concentration of furosemide at its site of action will produce the same maximal effect on urinary sodium excretion as a high enough concentration of bumetanide, despite the difference in potency.

When comparing drugs with each other, maximal efficacy is usually a more important criterion than potency. If two drugs have different potencies one simply gives a larger dose of the less potent drug. However, if two drugs have different maximal efficacies, the drug with the lower maximal efficacy will always produce a smaller maximal effect no matter how large the dose. For example, insulin has a much higher maximal efficacy than the oral hypoglycemic drugs, whose effects in lowering blood glucose are relatively limited. The term 'high ceiling diuretics' has been applied to the loop diuretics to indicate that they have a higher maximal efficacy than other diuretics, such as the thiazides.

However, sometimes relative potencies may be of importance. This happens, for example, if the doses of two drugs that are equipotent on one system are not equipotent on another. For instance, doses of bumetanide and furosemide that produce equal natriuresis do not produce equal ototoxicity, bumetanide being less ototoxic. This is important when choosing a loop diuretic to use in combination with the aminoglycoside antibiotics, such as gentamicin, since furosemide is more likely than bumetanide to enhance their ototoxic effects.

The concept of the therapeutic index of a drug, i.e. the toxic : therapeutic dose ratio, relies in part on compar-

isons of dose–response curves for therapeutic and adverse effects. Drugs whose adverse effects occur at concentrations that are near the concentrations at which their therapeutic effects occur are said to have a low therapeutic index. Examples include the aminoglycoside antibiotics, antiarrhythmic drugs, anticoagulants, anticonvulsants, cardiac glycosides, cytotoxic and immunosuppressive drugs, oral contraceptives, and drugs that act on the central nervous system.

When renal insufficiency alters the effect of a drug, it is more likely to be important if the drug has a low therapeutic index.

Pharmacokinetics: the disposition of drugs and the effects of renal insufficiency

To understand how a change in the pharmacokinetics of a drug secondary to renal insufficiency alters drug therapy it is first necessary to understand some simple pharmacokinetic principles.

Pharmacokinetics describes the movement (Greek κινεσις) of a drug (Greek φαρμακον) around the body. It deals with drug absorption from the site of administration, distribution to body tissues, and elimination from the body either by metabolism or excretion.

Drug absorption and systemic availability (bioavailability)

Drugs may be absorbed from various sites of administration, including the mouth, gut, skin, respiratory tract, subcutaneous tissues (after subcutaneous injection) or muscles (after intramuscular injection). Similar principles apply in all these cases, and are illustrated here by reference to absorption after oral administration.

After oral administration a drug will reach the systemic circulation only if it is absorbed from the gastrointestinal tract and if it escapes presystemic metabolism in the gastrointestinal tract, liver and lungs. However, in practice it can be difficult to distinguish the separate contributions of absorption and presystemic metabolism to the changes in plasma drug concentrations with time after an oral dose. The idea of systemic availability (usually called bioavailability) has therefore been developed.

The systemic availability of a drug is defined in terms of the amount of administered drug that reaches the systemic circulation intact, and the rate at which it does so. The rate of availability depends on the formulation (i.e. the form in which the drug is ingested) and gastrointestinal absorption, whereas presystemic metabolism is relatively unimportant. On the other hand, the extent of availability depends on both the extent of absorption and the extent of presystemic metabolism.

Several factors affect the rate and extent of drug absorption from the gut, among the most important of which are discussed below.

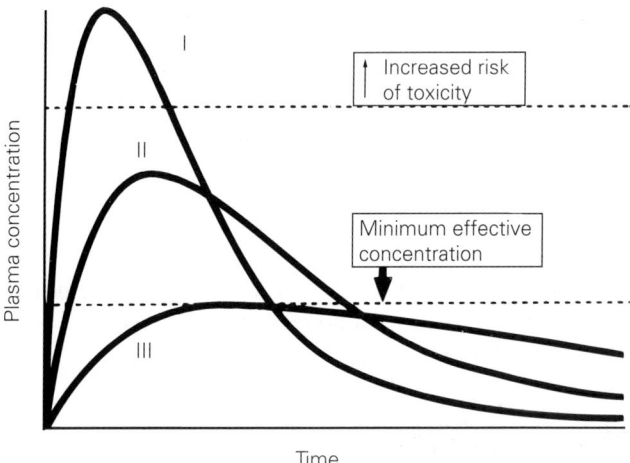

Figure 69.2 Profiles of drug absorption. Plasma drug concentrations after the oral administration of three different formulations of the same dose of the same drug. In all these cases the extent of absorption was the same but the rates were different. (Reproduced, with permission, from ref. [3].)

Gastric emptying time

Most drugs are not well absorbed from the stomach. The delay between swallowing a drug and its first appearance in the systemic circulation, depends on the time it takes for the stomach to empty.

The type of formulation

When a formulation enters the small bowel it must disintegrate, releasing the active drug, which must then dissolve in the bowel fluid before being absorbed. In the case of a modified-release formulation it may take hours before all the drug is available for absorption; this usually affects only the rate of absorption, but when there is increased gastrointestinal transit time the extent of drug absorption may also be reduced if a modified-release tablet is hurried through the gut. If the rate of absorption is slowed to such an extent that the half-life of absorption becomes longer than the half-life of the drug, the half-life that determines the time it takes to reach steady state (a concept that is discussed below) will be the half-life of absorption and not the half-life of the drug. This phenomenon is known as rate-limited kinetics.

First-pass metabolism

If a drug is inactivated in the gut (e.g. the inactivation of benzylpenicillin by gastric acid), metabolized in the gut wall (e.g. the metabolism of tyramine by monoamine oxidase A), or metabolized in the liver or lungs before it enters the systemic circulation, the amount that reaches the systemic circulation will be reduced. This is called 'first-pass' metabolism or the 'first-pass effect', and it is most often due to metabolism in the liver.

The pattern of drug absorption and availability varies from drug to drug and from formulation to formulation. Figure 69.2 shows three theoretical plasma concentration-versus-time curves after the oral administration of three different formulations of the same dose of a drug. The actual profile in each case depends on the rate and extent of the systemic availability.

- In profile 1 the drug is quickly available, the peak concentration is soon reached, and there is a risk of early toxicity, after which the plasma concentration falls rapidly, with loss of the therapeutic effect.
- In profile 2 the peak concentration is reached less quickly, and so the rate of onset of the effect of the drug is slower; however, the drug has a longer duration of action.
- In profile 3 the drug does not reach a therapeutically effective concentration in the blood, but its rate of elimination is much slower.

Suppose that the drug illustrated here was isosorbide dinitrate.

- Profile 1 is what one might expect with a sublingual form; angina pectoris would be relieved quickly, but with the risk of an acute headache.
- Profile 2 could result from a peroral formulation of isosorbide, with a slower effect but without such a risk of headache.
- Profile 3 could result from a single dose of a modified-release formulation of isosorbide; this would be of no value in treating an acute attack of angina pectoris, but during repeated administration the plasma concentration would rise to within the therapeutic range and thus provide prolonged continuous prophylaxis (leaving aside the question of tolerance).

These profiles depend on the rate and extent of availability, the rate of disposition in the body, and the rate of elimination. The rate and extent of availability are usually unaffected by renal insufficiency, although there are exceptions. For example, the systemic availability of erythropoietin after subcutaneous administration is reduced in renal insufficiency [4], although the high plasma concentrations of erythropoietin achieved after intravenous administration may be associated with reduced efficacy, making the subcutaneous route preferable. In addition, the oral absorption of calcium and phosphorus are reduced in renal insufficiency [5], as is that of iron [6].

However, it should be noted that the shape of the plasma concentration-versus-time curve after oral administration is affected not only by the rate of availability of the drug but also by the rate of elimination: if there is a delay in the rate of elimination of a drug (for example, because of poor renal function) the peak concentration after absorption will increase and be reached at a later time (Figure 69.3); this might be erroneously interpreted as being due to a change in the rate of absorption.

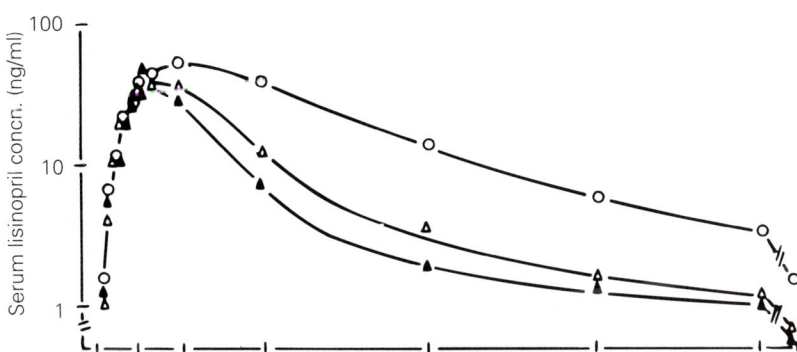

Figure 69.3 The plasma concentrations of lisinopril after oral administration to patients with normal renal function (▲), moderate renal insufficiency (△), and severe renal insufficiency (○). (Reproduced, with permission, from ref. [7].)

Drug distribution

Drugs are distributed to plasma proteins and organ tissues.

Plasma protein binding

The plasma proteins that bind drugs are mainly albumin (which binds acidic drugs) and the acute-phase reaction protein α_1-acid glycoprotein (which binds basic drugs). In chronic renal insufficiency the binding of acidic drugs, such as phenytoin, theophylline and methotrexate, is reduced, whereas the binding of basic drugs, such as lignocaine, propranolol and cimetidine, is increased [8].

However, protein binding is clinically important only if two criteria are met:

1   fractional protein binding must be high – if the drug is less than 90% bound to plasma proteins, changes in protein binding, which are usually of the order of a few per cent, have little effect on the amount of unbound drug in circulation, i.e. the drug that is available for distribution to the site of action;
2   tissue distribution should be limited – if the distribution of the drug to the tissues is large, even if the drug is completely displaced from protein-binding sites it will be mopped up by the tissues.

The most important drugs that are highly protein bound and not widely distributed to the tissues are phenytoin and warfarin – for these drugs a reduction in protein binding can cause toxicity. However, even if their protein binding changes, the effects are usually short-lived, since an increase in the unbound fraction in the plasma causes an increase in the rate at which these drugs are eliminated from the body. This means that if there is acute displacement of a drug such as phenytoin from albumin, there may be transient toxicity (for a few days), following which a new stable state is reached (Figure 69.4). However, in renal insufficiency the long-term reduction in protein binding of phenytoin alters the relation between the total plasma phenytoin concentration and its unbound concentration. The plasma phenytoin concentration that laboratories measure is the total concentration, which will not represent the same unbound concentration if protein binding is altered. In

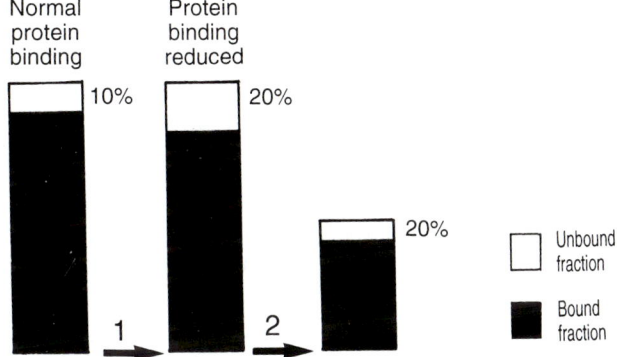

Figure 69.4 The role of protein binding in drug disposition. An initial change from normal protein binding to reduced protein binding (arrow 1) occurs if there is immediate displacement (e.g. by another drug), causing an increase in the unbound concentration of the drug and thus an increase in its effect. A compensatory increase in clearance rate then causes a reduction in the total and unbound concentrations, although the unbound fraction remains high (arrow 2). If protein binding displacement occurs slowly (for example, in chronic renal insufficiency) the patient can go from the normal state to the compensated state without experiencing the intermediate state of toxicity. In this example, however, the total plasma concentration is reduced to half normal in the compensated state, while the unbound concentration remains the same (since the unbound *fraction* is doubled); this increases the therapeutic effect at a given total concentration.

chronic renal insufficiency the therapeutic effect occurs in association with a lower total plasma phenytoin concentration [9].

Tissue distribution

The tissue distribution of drugs is highly variable. For example, warfarin is not widely distributed, but enough enters the liver to reduce clotting factor synthesis. In contrast, drugs such as digoxin, amiodarone and tricyclic antidepressants are widely distributed and highly concentrated in all body tissues.

A drug can only be effective if it reaches its site of action. Thus, if furosemide does not enter the renal tubules it will not have a diuretic action; this is why patients with renal insufficiency are resistant to diuretics.

In a few cases renal impairment may alter the tissue distribution of a drug. For example, the volume of distribution of digoxin is reduced in severe renal insufficiency and loading doses may have to be reduced [10]. If the protein binding of a drug is reduced in renal insufficiency (see above), more drug will be available and the volume of distribution will increase, prolonging the half-life; if at the same time increased clearance shortens the half-life there may be no net change in half-life. A parallel prolongation of half-life due to reduced renal clearance may introduce a further complication as happens, for example, with the active metabolite of nabumetone [11].

Drug metabolism

The end result of metabolism is inactivation of the drug, although during the process metabolites with different pharmacological activity may be formed. There are three types of metabolism:

- activation of an inactive drug (the basis of the use of 'prodrugs', see below);
- the production of an active metabolite from an active drug;
- inactivation of an active drug.

Prodrugs

A prodrug is one that is metabolized to an active compound. For example, L-dopa is a prodrug of dopamine; it is used to treat Parkinson's disease, because dopamine does not enter the brain after systemic administration whereas L-dopa does. Sulfasalazine is a prodrug of 5-aminosalicylic acid, to which it is metabolized in the large bowel. Many angiotensin converting enzyme (ACE) inhibitors (for example, enalapril, fosinopril, quinapril, ramipril) are activated by de-esterification in the liver after oral absorption.

Renal insufficiency generally has no effect on the conversion of prodrugs into their active metabolites, although the activation of sulindac to its sulfide metabolite may be reduced in end-stage renal failure [12].

Metabolism of active drugs to active compounds

Although the end result of drug metabolism is usually an inactive metabolite, in some cases metabolites have pharmacological effects of their own (Table 69.1). If an active metabolite is excreted by the kidneys, renal insufficiency may result in accumulation of the metabolite. For example, 50% of procainamide is excreted unchanged,

and renal insufficiency can lead to significant accumulation; in addition, its chief metabolite, N-acetylprocainamide (NAPA, acecainide) is also active and can accumulate in such circumstances [13].

Although morphine is extensively metabolized, its actions increase in renal insufficiency, mostly because it is metabolized to a pharmacologically active opiate, morphine-6-glucuronide, which is eliminated by the kidneys and accumulates in renal insufficiency [14].

In some cases an active compound is metabolized to a toxic compound. For example, lignocaine is metabolized to two toxic compounds, which persist for longer in the body than lignocaine. However, there have been no reports of enhanced toxicity of lignocaine in renal insufficiency attributed to accumulation of its metabolites, perhaps because lignocaine is generally used for periods of time that are too short to enable toxic accumulation of its metabolites.

Allopurinol is metabolized to an active metabolite, alloxanthine (also called oxypurinol), by the action of xanthine oxidase. Since alloxanthine is itself an inhibitor of xanthine oxidase, this conversion is inhibited by the substance it produces (so-called product inhibition) and allopurinol may accumulate. If allopurinol excretion is reduced in renal insufficiency the accumulation of allopurinol may be out of proportion to what would normally be expected, because of increased production of alloxanthine and further inhibition of the metabolism of allopurinol and toxicity can readily occur.

Metabolism of active drugs to inactive compounds

In most cases drug metabolites are inactive. They are produced by two types of mechanism: oxidative reactions, under the control of the isoenzymes of the cytochrome P450 group, and conjugation reactions, such as acetylation, glucuronidation, sulfation and glutathione conjugation. Renal impairment does not affect either of these metabolic processes directly.

Drug excretion

Drugs are excreted mostly via the kidneys. Some are also excreted via the bile, and a few have other routes of elimination (for example, rifampicin in the tears and sweat, alcohol and inhaled anesthetics via the lungs). In renal insufficiency elimination via these alternative routes may increase, partly offsetting the retention from reduced renal excretion. For example, the non-renal clearance of digoxin is increased when its renal clearance is reduced [10]; however, this effect is too small to be clinically important.

There are three major transport pathways for drugs in the kidneys. All drugs are filtered at the glomerulus, some are actively secreted in the proximal tubule, and some are passively reabsorbed in the distal tubule. Some drugs are transported by all three mechanisms. Active secretion

Table 69.1 Some important drugs with active metabolites

Drug	Metabolite
Analgesics	
Pethidine	Norpethidine
Morphine	Morphine-6-glucuronide
Antiarrhythmic drugs	
Amiodarone	Desethylamiodarone
Disopyramide	Monodeisopropyldisopyramide
Encainide	Desmethylencainide, methoxydesmethylencainide
Procainamide	N-acetylprocainamide (acecainide)
Propafenone	Hydroxypropafenone
Antiepileptic drugs	
Phenytoin	Hydroxydiphenylhydantoin
Valproate	Various
Anti-infective drugs	
Cefoxitin	Decarbamoylcefoxitin
Ciprofloxacin	Various
Enoxacin	Oxoenoxacin
Metronidazole	Hydroxylated nitroimidazole
Norfloxacin	Various
Pefloxacin	Desmethylpefloxacin
Vidarabine	Arabinosyl hypoxanthine
Antiulcer drugs	
Cimetidine	Cimetidine sulfoxide
Anxiolytics	
Buspirone	1-(2-Pyrimidinyl)-piperazine
Diazepam	Various (e.g. oxazepam, temazepam)
Cytotoxic and immunosuppressive drugs	
Azathioprine	Mercaptopurine
Cyclophosphamide	Phosphoramide mustard
Neuromuscular blocking drugs	
Pancuronium	Hydroxypancuronium
Miscellaneous	
Allopurinol	Alloxanthine (oxypurinol)
Chloral hydrate derivatives	Trichloroethanol
Spironolactone	Canrenone

increases the rate of renal clearance of drugs and passive reabsorption reduces it.

Glomerular filtration

Only non-protein-bound drug is filtered. It follows that the clearance of a drug by filtration is equal to the unbound fraction times glomerular filtration rate (GFR). For example, the filtration clearance of digoxin (20% bound) is $0.8 \times 120\,\text{ml/min} = 100\,\text{ml/min}$. Digoxin is also secreted and reabsorbed, but the two processes balance when renal function is good, so that the total renal clearance of digoxin is normally about $100\,\text{ml/min}$. Thus, GFR can be used to guide changes in digoxin dosage, although when renal function is poor the relative contributions of secretion and reabsorption change and clearance is not as closely related to GFR.

When the protein binding of a drug falls in renal insufficiency (e.g. phenytoin) more unbound drug becomes available for elimination, and this explains the increase in clearance that occurs in this case (discussed above).

Active secretion

There are separate secretory systems for different drugs. At least two types have been identified for acids and bases. The clinical relevance of this is that the secretion of some drugs can be inhibited by others if they share the same system. For example, probenecid inhibits the secretion of penicillins, cephalosporins, methotrexate, zidovudine,

Table 69.2 Some important drugs whose dosage should be reduced in renal insufficiency (see also Table 69.7)

Drug	Degree of insufficiency[a]
Analgesics	
Morphine	Moderate or severe
Antiarrhythmic and other cardiovascular drugs	
Digoxin	Mild
Disopyramide	Mild
Methyldopa	Moderate
Procainamide	Mild
Anti-infective drugs	
Acyclovir	Moderate or severe
Aminoglycoside antibiotics	Mild
Cephalosporins	Depends on drug
Clarithromycin	Moderate
Didanosine	Mild
Erythromycin	Severe
Ethambutol	Mild
Lincomycin	Severe
Penicillins	Severe
Trimethoprim	Moderate
Zidovudine	Mild
Cytotoxic and immunosuppressive drugs	
Azathioprine	Severe
Bleomycin	Moderate
Cisplatin	Mild
Cyclophosphamide	Severe
Melphalan	Moderate
Mercaptopurine	Moderate
Methotrexate	Mild[b]
Drugs used in gout	
Allopurinol	Moderate or severe
Colchicine	Severe
Miscellaneous	
Amantadine	Mild or moderate[c]
Baclofen	Mild
Fibrates	Mild or moderate[c]
Lithium	Mild[b]
Pyridostigmine	Moderate

[a] Mild renal insufficiency: creatinine clearance 20–50 ml/min; moderate renal insufficiency: creatinine clearance 10–20 ml/min; severe renal insufficiency: creatinine clearance <10 ml/min.
[b] Avoid in moderate or severe renal insufficiency.
[c] Avoid in severe renal insufficiency.

diprophylline and dapsone. The nephrotoxicity of cephaloridine and cefazolin in rabbit kidney is prevented by probenecid [15], but there are no reports of how renal insufficiency affects these interactions.

The interactions of aspirin with probenecid and sulfinpyrazone are complex. Low doses of aspirin inhibit the renal tubular secretion of uric acid whereas high doses increase it. This is because there is a dose-dependent effect of aspirin on two different transport pathways for uric acid in the nephron – active secretion and active reabsorption; low doses of aspirin inhibit active secretion, causing uric acid retention, whereas high doses inhibit both secretion and reabsorption, the net effect being uricosuric. Low doses of aspirin inhibit the uricosuric effects of probenecid and sulfinpyrazone, whereas probenecid and sulfinpyrazone inhibit the uricosuric effects of high doses of aspirin.

Passive reabsorption

Lipophilic weak acids and weak bases may be passively reabsorbed. Since only the non-ionized form is reabsorbed, their elimination can be enhanced by increasing ionization (by alkalinization or acidification of the urine for acidic or basic drugs, respectively). This is used in treating drug overdose (e.g. alkalinization for salicylates and acidification for amphetamines). Changing the urine pH is a more efficient way of increasing the elimination of these drugs than causing a diuresis, and careful attention should be paid to the proper acidification or alkalinization of the urine. Since the attempt to force a diuresis can cause pulmonary or cerebral edema and electrolyte and acid–base imbalance, it is now no longer recommended.

Effects of renal insufficiency

If there is renal insufficiency the dosages of drugs that are usually excreted at least 50% unchanged by the kidneys should be reduced. A list of some important drugs to which this applies is given in Table 69.2.

An alteration in dosage may be achieved by either a reduction in the frequency of administration or a reduction in the size of individual doses, or both (see below).

Formal pharmacokinetics

The above is a brief description of what happens to a drug as it travels through the body. However, pharmacokinetics properly entails a mathematical description of these processes. Detailed discussions are given in textbooks on the subject (for example [16]); here I shall describe a few simple variables, an understanding of which can be helpful in practical drug therapy: the half-life, the volume of distribution, and the clearance rate.

Half-life

The half-life of a drug is the time it takes for half the drug in the body to be eliminated. For most drugs this is independent of the actual amount the body contains. The half-life is usually determined by measuring the

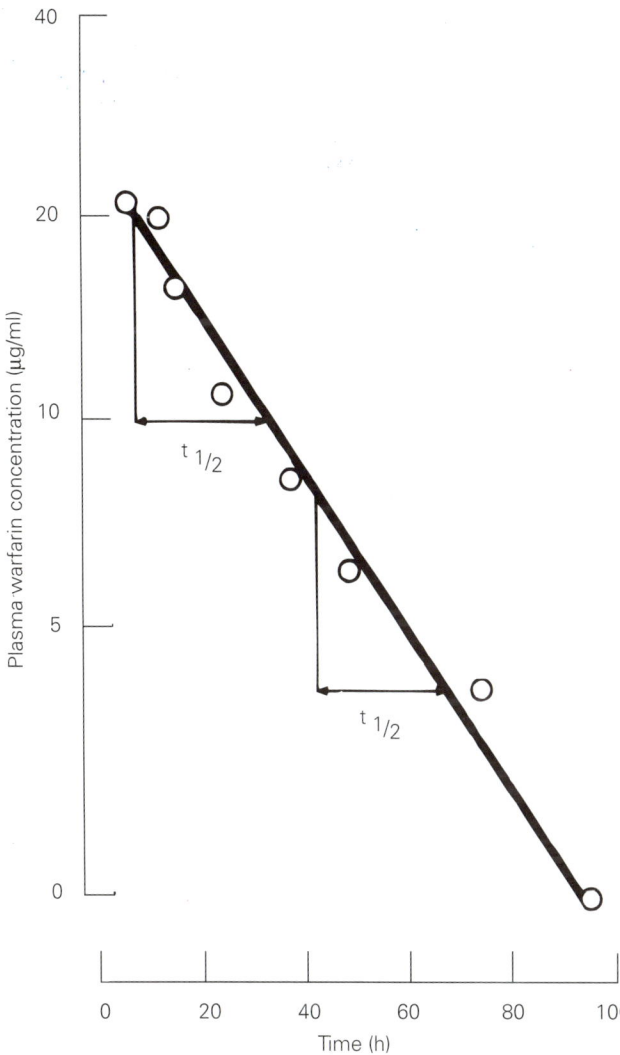

Figure 69.5   Plasma warfarin concentrations after a single intravenous dose. The log-concentration-versus-time plot is linear. The time it takes for the concentration to halve is called the half-life and is independent of the plasma concentration (or the amount of drug in the body). (Adapted, with permission, from ref. [17].)

Table 69.3   The relation between half-life and the amount of drug in the body after a single dose or during repeated administration

Number of half-lives	Amount eliminated (after a single dose or after stopping treatment) or the steady state achieved (during repeated dosing) (%)
1	50.0
2	75.0
3	87.5
4	93.75
5	96.875

time it takes for the plasma concentration to fall by half (Figure 69.5). Knowing the half-life of a drug has several uses.

First, the half-life acts as a guide to the time it takes for drug elimination to occur. No matter how much drug is in the body, one half will be eliminated in one half-life; a half of what is left (i.e. a total of 75%) will be eliminated in another half-life, half again (i.e. a total of 87.5%) in another half-life, and so on (Table 69.3). For example, furosemide has a half-life of about 1 h; its therapeutic effects last about 4–6 h after a single dose, by which time it is virtually completely eliminated.

Secondly, the half-life determines the rate of accumulation during repeated dosing. When a drug is given repeatedly the plasma concentration rises with each dose.

However, the rate at which it rises decreases as the concentration increases, since the percentage fall is higher at higher concentrations. Eventually a steady state is reached, when the amount eliminated in a dosage interval is equal to the dose itself.

The half-life is the only variable that determines how long it takes to reach a steady state during repeated drug dosing. Half of the eventual steady-state concentration will be reached after one half-life. In another half-life 75% of the eventual steady-state concentration will be reached, and so on. These percentages are the same as for the percentages eliminated after a single dose (Table 69.3). This means that it takes between three and four half-lives to reach more than 90% of steady state.

For example, digoxin has a half-life of 40 h. It would therefore take about a week to reach a steady state during repeated maintenance dose therapy. That is why one gives an initial loading dose, to boost the amount of drug in the body to what it should be at steady state. This amount is then maintained by a regular maintenance dosage (Figure 69.6). However, if there is renal insufficiency, the half-life of digoxin increases and it takes longer to reach a steady state; in an extreme case the half-life may be as long as 100 h, and the steady state would not be reached until about three weeks of maintenance therapy. Furthermore, if the daily dose is not reduced, the steady-state concentration will be higher (Figure 69.7).

Note that a modified-release formulation may lengthen the apparent half-life of a drug because of slow absorption (e.g. profile 3 in Figure 69.2). In that case it is the apparent half-life (i.e. the half-life of availability) that matters, and the time to steady state may not be altered in renal insufficiency, even though excess accumulation may occur.

For some drugs the pharmacological effect is not closely related to the amount of drug in the body (e.g. corticosteroids, which have a hit-and-run effect). In those cases although the half-life is still related to the time it takes for steady-state concentrations to occur, it may not predict the time to maximum effect.

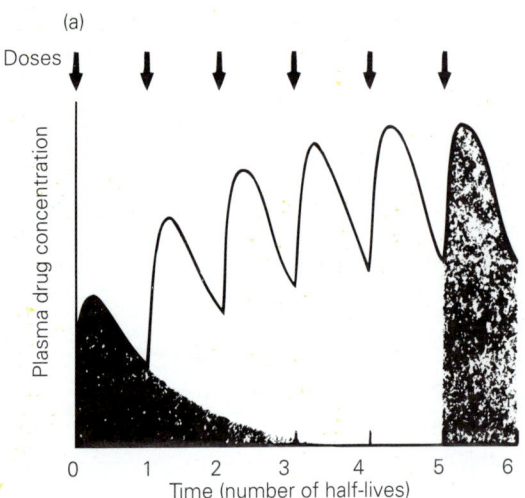

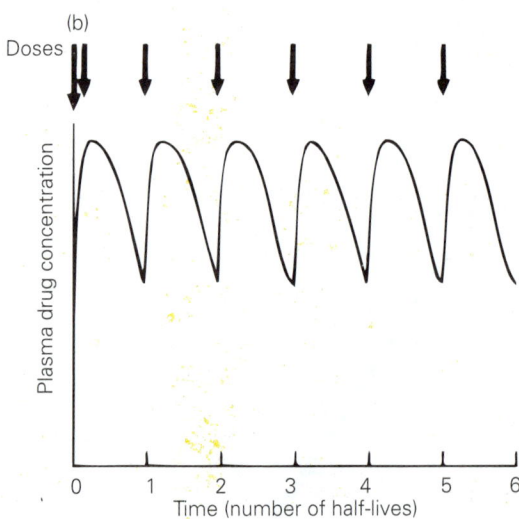

Figure 69.6 The regular administration of a maintenance dose of a drug results in a gradual increase in plasma concentration to an eventual steady state (a). This delay can be overcome by the administration of a loading dose (b). (Reproduced, with permission, from ref. [3].)

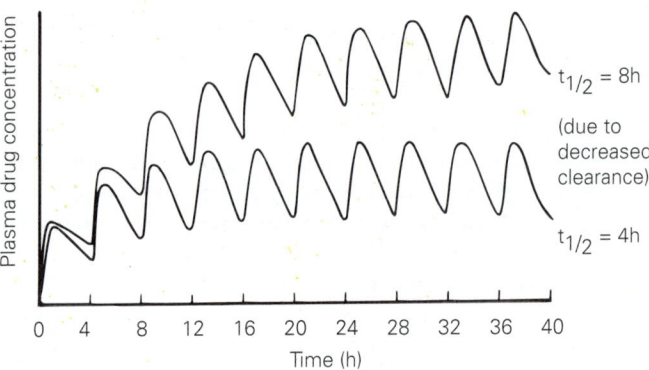

Figure 69.7 The time it takes to reach a steady state during maintenance dose therapy may be prolonged in renal failure; if the same maintenance dose is used the eventual steady-state plasma concentration will be higher. (Reproduced, with permission, from ref. [3].)

Volume of distribution

The volume of distribution is a measure of how widely a drug is distributed to body tissues, and it is commonly expressed as the ratio of the total amount of drug in the body to the plasma concentration at steady state. For example, if the amount of gentamicin in the body at steady state is 120 mg (the loading dose) and the average steady-state plasma concentration is 6 mg/l the volume of distribution will be 20 l. This volume is a virtual one; it does not relate to any particular body tissues. However, the concept is useful in determining how extensively a drug is distributed to the body tissues. For example the volume of distribution of digoxin is several hundred liters, since it is widely distributed and taken up by most body tissues.

The volume of distribution changes with changes in protein binding: an increase in the unbound fraction of drug makes more drug available for distribution to the tissues; this in turn prolongs the half-life, since less drug is available for elimination.

The volume of distribution is relevant to the effects of dialysis, since drugs that have a high volume of distribution are not readily available to be removed from the body (see below).

The volume of distribution also affects dosage regimens: if the volume changes, the loading dose will change. For example, the volume of distribution of digoxin is reduced in severe renal insufficiency and loading doses should also be reduced [10].

Clearance rate

The clearance rate of a drug (not the half-life) is the best measure of the rate at which the drug is eliminated from the body. That is because the half-life is affected by both clearance and volume of distribution, whereas clearance is an independent variable. The effect of a fall in the rate of clearance on half-life, the time to steady state, and steady-state plasma concentration (Figure 69.7) have been discussed above.

Changing drug dosage regimens in renal insufficiency

A drug dosage regimen is a recipe for drug administration, intended to produce the desired therapeutic effect with the minimum of unwanted effects. A regimen can be described in terms of the dose of drug, the frequency and route of administration, and the formulation used.

The simplest way of determining a drug dosage regimen for an individual patient is to use published recommendations, which have usually been derived from a knowledge of the drug's pharmacokinetics and dose/effect relations. The usual method is to start at the lower end of the recommended dosage range and monitor the patient for a therapeutic effect. If the desired effect does not occur, one can increase the dose gradually, until the upper end of the recommended range is reached.

However, for drugs with a low therapeutic index, dosage regimens are not as simple, since dosage requirements vary widely from individual to individual and may be affected by changes in renal or hepatic function or by drug interactions. For such drugs it is important to understand the principles of altering dosage regiments to suit the individual.

The loading dose

As explained above, it takes about four half-lives during regular maintenance dose therapy to reach a steady state. If this delay is unacceptable it may be circumvented by giving a loading dose. The loading dose is the amount of drug that would be present in the body if the relevant maintenance dose were given for long enough to achieve steady state. This principle is illustrated in Figure 69.6.

The amount of drug in the body at steady state (i.e. the loading dose) is related to the volume of distribution and the steady-state plasma drug concentration thus: amount in body = volume × concentration in plasma. This allows one to calculate the loading dose of drug required to produce a given plasma drug concentration. Although in most cases one does not measure the plasma concentration, in practice this method is implicit in one's use of recommended dosages.

The use of the volume of distribution is also implicit in dosages based on body weight or surface area, since the variability of the volume of distribution is reduced when it is expressed in l/kg of body weight or in l/m^2 of body surface area.

The need to reduce the loading dose of digoxin in severe renal insufficiency because of a reduction in the volume of distribution has been mentioned above.

The maintenance dose

There is a simple relation between loading dose and maintenance dose: since half the total body load will be

lost in one half-life, the maintenance dose should be half the loading dose given once every half-life. Take the example of digoxin (half-life about 40 h if renal function is normal). If the loading dose is 15 µg/kg the loading dose for a 60 kg patient will be:

$$15\,\mu g/kg \times 60\,kg = 0.9\,mg$$

In practice, one would give 1.0 mg. The maintenance dose would be 0.45 mg every 40 h; scaling this dose down to 24 h by simple proportion, the daily maintenance dose is:

$$0.45\,mg \times 24\,h/40\,h = 0.27\,mg$$

In practice, one would give 0.25 mg once daily. This proportionality calculation yields a slightly inaccurate answer, since it assumes that the dose–half-life relation is arithmetic, whereas it is in fact logarithmic; however, the error is negligible in practice.

This process can, of course, be carried out in reverse. Having decided on a particular maintenance dose that you think will be suitable, you can calculate the total body load. Take the example of digoxin again. You decide to give a daily maintenance dose of 5 µg/kg to a 70 kg patient with normal renal function; the daily maintenance dose would be:

$$5\,\mu g/kg \times 70\,kg = 0.35\,mg$$

In practice you would give 0.375 mg (i.e. 0.25 mg + 0.125 mg). This daily maintenance dose is roughly equivalent (by arithmetical proportionality) to 0.6 mg every 40 h. The appropriate total body load is therefore 2 × 0.6, i.e. 1.2 mg (given as 1.25 mg). These simple methods will allow you to calculate the total body load for a given maintenance dose, and thus to calculate alterations in dose which may be necessary if, for example, there is a change in renal function (see below).

These calculations are acceptable for drugs with long half-lives, since the incorrect assumption of linearity yields only a small error. However, for drugs with a short half-life (say, less than 24 h) we cannot assume arithmetic proportionality because the error becomes too large. The formula used in such cases is:

$$\text{loading dose} = \text{dose rate} \times t_{1/2}/0.7$$

For instance, procainamide has a half-life of about 3 h; for a dosage of 750 mg every 6 h (i.e. 3000 mg/24 h) the corresponding total body load would be:

$$(3000\,mg/24\,h) \times (3\,h/0.7) = 536\,mg$$

With a volume of distribution of 2 l/kg a 70 kg man would have a steady-state plasma concentration of 3.8 mg/l, which is at the lower end of the usual therapeutic range. Procainamide is half renally excreted and half metabolized; in renal insufficiency half the clearance is reduced in proportion to creatinine clearance; so, for example, a 50% reduction in creatinine clearance would necessitate a 25% reduction in maintenance dosage.

Altering the maintenance dose when drug clearance alters

A change in drug clearance, e.g. in renal insufficiency, will necessitate a change in maintenance dosage. The total body clearance of a drug and its steady-state plasma concentration are related thus:

steady-state concentration

$$= \frac{\left(\text{fraction of dose absorbed} \times \text{dose}\right)}{\left(\text{total clearance} \times \text{dosing interval}\right)}$$

So, if total body clearance changes one can maintain the same mean steady-state plasma concentration by altering the dose or dosing interval in a way that is proportional to the change in total body clearance (assuming there is no concomitant change in drug absorption). If the drug is cleared completely or almost completely via the kidneys then the dosage should be changed in proportion to renal clearance. The relationship on which to base one's calculations is:

percentage eliminated in one dosing interval
    = percentage eliminated by non-renal routes
      + percentage eliminated by the renal route

Since the percentage eliminated renally is linearly related to creatinine clearance, this equation can be rewritten thus:

percentage eliminated in one dosage interval
    = percentage eliminated by non-renal routes
      + (constant × creatinine clearance)

The percentage eliminated in one dosage interval by non-renal routes is usually available from published data. The proportionality constant should be available from published experiments in patients with different degrees of renal insufficiency, or can be calculated from the half-life and non-renal clearance. The following examples demonstrate the calculations for gentamicin and digoxin.

1 Gentamicin: this is excreted 98% unchanged by the kidneys. Thus, the change in dosage in renal insufficiency is almost exactly proportional to the change in creatinine clearance, although the error from making the assumption that it is exactly proportional becomes greater at very low rates of clearance, when non-renal clearance starts to have a significant effect. The proportionality constant is 0.3. Thus, for gentamicin the equation reads:

percentage of total body load eliminated in one day
    = 2% + (0.3 × creatinine clearance)

From this relation one can calculate the daily elimination rate of gentamicin for different values of creatinine clearance, as shown in Table 69.4.

2 Digoxin: in contrast to gentamicin, a significant proportion of digoxin is cleared by non-renal mechanisms (about 14% per day). The proportionality constant is 0.2. Thus, for digoxin the equation reads:

percentage of total body load eliminated in one day
    = 14% + (0.2 × creatinine clearance)

From this relation one can calculate the daily elimination rate of digoxin for different values of creatinine clearance, as shown in Table 4.

Table 69.5 gives the data necessary for making similar calculations for some other drugs.

These calculations involve certain assumptions, which in practice are usually justified.

- The drug's metabolites are inactive.
- Absorption, distribution, and metabolism are unchanged in patients with renal insufficiency (changes

Table 69.4 The proportions by which the dosages of gentamicin and digoxin should be reduced in renal insufficiency

Creatinine clearance (ml/min)	Daily elimination rate of total body load (% (fraction))	Ratio of renal failure dose to the usual dose	Total daily dose (mg) (examples)
Gentamicin			
100	32 (1/3)	32 : 32 = 1	240
50	17 (1/6)	17 : 32 = 1 : 2	120
30	11 (1/9)	11 : 32 = 1 : 3	80
20	8 (1/12)	8 : 32 = 1 : 4	60
15	6.5 (1/6)	6.5 : 32 = 1 : 5	50
10	5 (1/20)	5 : 32 = 1 : 6	40
Digoxin			
100	34 (1/3)	34 : 34 = 1	0.25
50	25 (1/4)	25 : 34 = 3 : 4	0.1875
25	19 (1/5)	19 : 34 = 3 : 5	0.15[a]
10	16 (1/6)	16 : 34 = 3 : 6	0.125
0	14 (1/7)	14 : 34 = 3 : 7	0.10[a]

[a] Round off to nearest whole tablet size if necessary.

in the volume of distribution make no difference to the steady-state plasma concentration).

- There is a linear relation between the renal clearance of the drug and creatinine clearance.
- Renal clearance does not change during dosage.
- There is no change in the response sensitivity to the drug in renal impairment.

For example, if renal function is improving during therapy (for example, during the treatment of an acute septicemia with gentamicin) it can be very difficult to predict what the correct dose of the drug will be during a given dosage interval.

Changing the maintenance dose to cope with a change in clearance results in an alteration in the degree of fluctuation in plasma concentrations during a dosage interval (illustrated in Figure 69.8). If peak plasma concentrations are associated with toxic effects, it may be necessary to alter not only the total dose administered in a period of time but also the dosage interval.

The general equations that relate the maximum (i.e. peak) and minimum (i.e. trough) plasma concentrations at steady state ($C_{ss.max}$ and $C_{ss.min}$) to the maintenance dose (D_M) and half-life are:

$$C_{ss.max} \times V = \left[D_M / \left(1 - e^{-k\tau} \right) \right]$$

Table 69.5 Renal (R) and non-renal (NR) contributions to the clearance of some drugs whose dosages should be reduced in renal impairment

Drug	NR (% per h)	R (per h)
Ampicillin	10	0.6
Carbenicillin	6	0.6
Cephalexin	3	0.7
Gentamicin[a]	2	0.3
Kanamycin[a]	1	0.25
Lincomycin[a]	6	0.1
Methyldopa[a]	3	0.2
Penicillin G	3	1.4
Streptomycin[a]	1	0.25
Trimethoprim	2	0.04
	NR (% per day)	R (per day)
Digoxin[a]	14	0.2
Ouabain[a]	30	0.9

[a] Drugs with a low toxic : therapeutic ratio.
Instructions. To calculate the per cent of total body drug that is eliminated in one hour or one day (P) calculate: P = NR + (R.CL$_{creat}$).
Compare the value of P thus obtained using the patient's creatinine clearance in this equation (ml/min) with the value obtained by using a value of 100 ml/min and adjust the dose proportionately. The examples of gentamicin and digoxin are worked out in Table 69.4.

$$C_{ss.min} \times V = \left[D_M / \left(1 - e^{-k\tau} \right) \right] - D_M$$

where $k = 0.7/t_{1/2}$ and τ = the dosage interval. If (a) the half-life at which the original maintenance dosage was appropriate and (b) the new half-life are both known, then the appropriate new maintenance dose or dosage interval can be simply calculated by comparing the values of D_M or τ which will produce the desired values of $C_{ss.max}$ and $C_{ss.min}$ in the two different states.

For example, consider the administration of gentamicin 120 mg twice a day to a patient whose half-life is doubled from 4 to 8 h because of renal insufficiency, and whose peak and trough plasma concentrations are 9 mg/l and 1 mg/l. If we keep the dosage interval at 12 h the new maintenance dose that would produce the same peak concentration is 93 mg. Using the above equations to calculate the plasma concentrations that would result from a regimen of 100 mg 12-hourly we find them to be 9.6 mg/l (peak) and 3.4 mg/l (trough). The reason that the trough concentration has increased is that the half-life is prolonged and the old dosage interval has not given enough time for the trough concentration to fall as low as it did before. If a lower trough concentration was required the dosage interval would have to be prolonged, and 180 mg might be given every 36 h, which would give satisfactory peak and trough concentrations of 11.8 mg/l and 0.5 mg/l, respectively.

This example illustrates how it is possible to make rational decisions about drug therapy when the clearance of a drug is altered. Based on these principles, a nomogram has been developed for guidance in the use of once-daily doses of gentamicin and tobramycin in renal insufficiency (Figure 69.9).

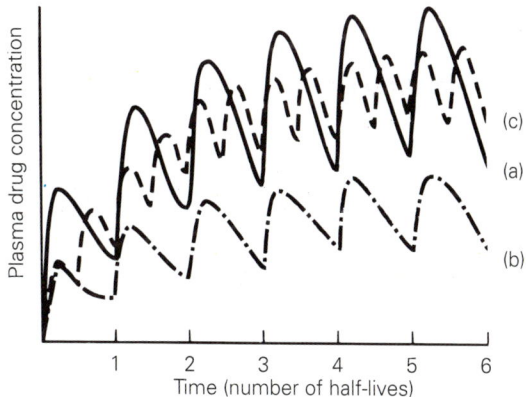

Figure 69.8 The effects of varying the dose and frequency of administration on the changes in plasma concentration during maintenance therapy. If the dose is halved (compare curve a with curve b) the plasma concentrations will halve. If the dose is halved but given twice as often (compare curve a with curve c) the mean steady-state plasma concentration will be unchanged, but the fluctuation about the mean will be less. In all three cases the time to steady state is the same, since the half-life is not changed. (Reproduced, with permission, from ref. [3].)

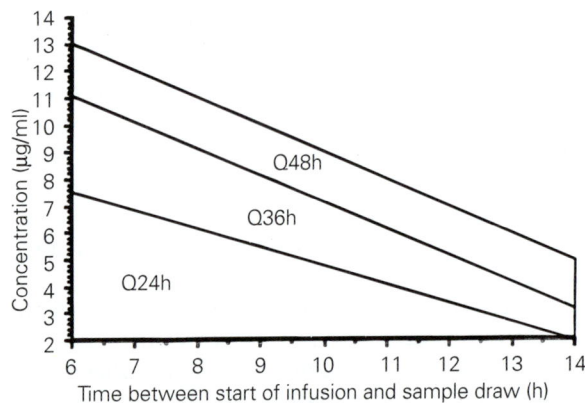

Figure 69.9 A graph that can be used to calculate the frequency of administration of gentamicin in patients with renal insufficiency. The frequency of administration (Q24 h = every 24 h, etc.) should be chosen depending on the position of the point on the graph that plots the serum concentration against the time of sampling in relation to the start of the previous infusion. (For details see Nicolau *et al.* [18], from which this has been taken, with permission.)

Pharmacodynamics: the actions of drugs and the effects of renal insufficiency

Drugs produce their pharmacological effects in many ways (Table 69.6). Many actions are produced by the stimulation or blockade of a receptor. Renal insufficiency sometimes alters the pharmacodynamic actions of drugs. The following is a description of how drugs produce their actions; changes in drug action because of renal insufficiency do not occur for all types of mechanism of action, but they are mentioned when they exist.

Actions via direct effects on receptors

Receptors are specific proteins, situated either in cell membranes or within the cytoplasm. For each type of receptor there is a specific group of drugs or endogenous substances (known as ligands) that can bind to the receptor and produce a pharmacological effect. There are three types of ligand: agonists, antagonists and partial agonists.

Agonists

Agonists are ligands that bind to a receptor and produce a response. For example, the catecholamine epinephrine is an agonist at beta-adrenoceptors; when it binds to beta-adrenoceptors in the heart it increases the heart rate.

Antagonists

Antagonists are ligands that prevent an agonist from binding to a receptor and thus prevent its effects. Pure antagonists do not themselves have any pharmacological actions mediated by receptors. For example, propranolol is a beta-adrenoceptor antagonist (a beta-blocker); when it binds to beta-adrenoceptors in the heart it prevents catecholamine-induced tachycardia (for example, in response to exercise).

Partial agonists

A full agonist is capable of producing a maximal response when it binds to enough receptors. In contrast, a partial agonist cannot produce the maximal response, even when it binds to the maximum number of available receptors. Above a certain concentration a partial agonist may bind to receptors without producing a further increase in effect. In so doing, however, it may prevent the action of other agonists, and may thus appear to be acting as an antagonist. It is this mixture of actions that is called partial agonism.

For example, oxprenolol, which is a beta-adrenoceptor antagonist, is also a partial agonist; thus, it may have less of an effect in slowing the heart rate than adrenoceptor antagonists that lack partial agonist action. The amount of beta-blockade produced by a given dose of a partial agonist beta-blocker will vary according to endogenous sympathetic nervous system activity: the more activity, the more beta-blockade will result from the action of a partial agonist. This is seen in the actions of the partial agonist xamoterol, which acts as a beta-adrenoceptor agonist in patients with mild heart failure and improves cardiac contraction, but which acts as a beta-blocker in patients with even moderate heart failure and worsens heart failure. This problem vitiates the value of xamoterol in the treatment of heart failure.

Some drugs act at more than one receptor. For example, dopamine in low (so-called 'renal') doses acts on renal dopamine receptors, causing vasodilatation; in higher doses it is also an agonist at beta-adrenoceptors, causing increased cardiac output; at still higher doses it is an agonist at alpha-adrenoceptors, causing renal vasoconstriction and cardiac arrhythmias. There is much overlap between the concentrations that produce these different effects.

Changes in the effects of ligands that act via receptors have been described in renal insufficiency, including the following.

In severe renal insufficiency the brain may be more sensitive to the CNS depressant effects of drugs that are agonists or antagonists at certain receptors, including tranquilizers (dopamine receptor antagonists), sedatives (gamma-aminobutyric acid (GABA) receptor antagonists), and opiate analgesics (opioid receptor agonists).

Renal insufficiency is accompanied by an insensitivity to the effects of some endogenous hormones, including growth hormone [19] and vitamin D analogs [20]. These changes are partly mediated by changes in receptor expression.

Actions	Examples
Actions via receptors	
Agonist at a receptor	Salbutamol
Antagonist at a receptor	Atenolol
Partial agonist at a receptor	Oxprenolol
Actions via second messengers	Lithium
Indirect alterations of the effects of endogenous agonists	
Physiological antagonism	Glucagon (insulin)
Increase in endogenous release	Amphetamine (monoamines)
Inhibition of endogenous reuptake	Antidepressants (monoamines)
Inhibition of endogenous metabolism	Vigabatrin (GABA)
Prevention of endogenous release	ACE inhibitors (aldosterone)
Inhibition of transport processes	Diuretics
Actions on enzymes	
Enzyme inhibition	Warfarin
Enzyme activation	Thrombolytic drugs
Enzymatic action	Factor VIII
Other miscellaneous effects	
Chelating agents	Penicillamine
Osmotic diuretics	Mannitol
Volatile general anaesthetics	Sevoflurane
Replacement drugs	Iron salts

Table 69.6 The types of pharmacological actions of drugs

Receptor subtypes

Some receptors have subtypes, for which certain ligands are selective or relatively so. For example, there are at least two subtypes of beta-adrenoceptors, $beta_1$ (in the heart and elsewhere) and $beta_2$ (in the lungs), both of which can respond to epinephrine. Beta-adrenoceptor antagonists may act at both subtypes or may have some selectivity for one or the other. For example, propranolol is an antagonist at both $beta_1$ and $beta_2$ receptors, whereas atenolol is relatively selective for $beta_1$ receptors. Note that selectivity is relative: although atenolol acts primarily on $beta_1$ receptors, at high enough concentrations it may have effects on $beta_2$ receptors as well. This also applies to selective agonists, for example the $beta_2$ agonist salbutamol, which in high doses may activate $beta_1$ receptors in the heart. Thus, if atenolol accumulates in the body because of renal impairment, it may cause asthma in a patient in whom that did not previously happen, because of loss of selectivity at higher concentrations.

Long-term effects of drugs at receptors

During long-term therapy the effects of a drug may be altered by adaptive responses, usually accompanied by either increases ('up-regulation') or decreases ('down-regulation') in receptor numbers. Such changes may produce both beneficial and adverse effects of drugs.

• The therapeutic response to antidepressants may be related to changes in receptors in the brain secondary to the actions of these drugs on neurotransmitter uptake. This explains why the therapeutic response to antidepressants takes a few weeks to occur.
• The so-called 'on-off' effect is one manifestation of the way in which the response to L-dopa in Parkinson's disease changes during long-term administration.
• Withdrawal syndromes may occur because long-term changes become unopposed when the drug is withdrawn, for example after the long-term abuse of opiates or the use of benzodiazepines in chronic anxiety.

Actions via direct effects on second messengers

When an agonist stimulates a receptor its effect is produced in one of two ways: either through a so-called second messenger after stimulation of an intermediary called a G protein, or by changing the activity of an ion channel linked to the receptor. Some drugs have their actions by directly affecting second messengers. For example, lithium (in bipolar affective disorder) may work by inhibiting phosphatidylinositol turnover. Theophylline and other xanthines inhibit the breakdown of cyclic AMP.

The resistance to insulin that occurs in renal insufficiency has been attributed to several defects in the post-receptor cascade [21].

Actions via indirect alterations of the effects of endogenous agonists

Just as an antagonist can produce a therapeutic effect by directly opposing the action of an endogenous agonist, so it is possible to alter the effect of an endogenous agonist indirectly.

Physiological antagonism

Some drugs have opposite physiological effects to those of other drugs. For example, glucagon is a physiological antagonist of the actions of insulin and can be used to treat hypoglycemia.

Increase in endogenous release

The action of an endogenous agonist may be enhanced if its release is increased. Amphetamines increase the release of dopamine from nerve endings. Because amphetamines can cause a syndrome similar to schizophrenia, this action has led to the idea that schizophrenia may be related to excess dopamine action in the brain.

Inhibition of endogenous reuptake

Conversely, if a drug inhibits the reuptake of an endogenous agonist it will enhance its effects. Many antidepressants inhibit the reuptake by neurons of certain neurotransmitters, such as 5-hydroxytryptamine (e.g. the selective serotonin reuptake inhibitors, the SSRIs) and norepinephrine.

Inhibition of endogenous metabolism

If a drug inhibits the metabolism of an endogenous agonist it will enhance its effects. Vigabatrin inhibits the metabolism of GABA in the brain, enhancing its actions and suppressing seizures. Brain GABA content is reduced in patients with renal insufficiency and dialysis encephalopathy [22], whereas GABA concentrations in the CSF are increased in patients with chronic uremia [23]. It is not clear whether these changes have any implications for the treatment of epilepsy.

Prevention of endogenous release

Prevention of the release of an endogenous agonist will reduce its effects. Sodium cromoglycate inhibits the release of inflammatory mediators from tissue mast cells.

ACE inhibitors prevent the formation of angiotensin II; this prevents the endogenous release of aldosterone, whose effects are thereby reduced, resulting in potassium retention. This effect may be enhanced in renal insufficiency, because of the tendency to potassium retention.

Actions via the inhibition of transport processes

Because cations (such as sodium, potassium and calcium) and other substances (such as organic acids in the kidneys) play so many important roles in the maintenance of normal cellular function, inhibition of their transport is an important type of mechanism of drug action. Drugs that cause sodium retention (e.g. non-steroidal anti-inflammatory drugs) may produce fluid overload, edema and heart failure. They may also oppose the effects of diuretics and antihypertensive drugs.

Diuretics

Many diuretics act by inhibiting sodium reabsorption in the renal tubules. For example, the loop diuretics furosemide and bumetanide inhibit Na/K/Cl co-transport in the thick ascending limb of the loop of Henle. The thiazide diuretics inhibit Na/Cl co-transport in the proximal segment of the distal convoluted tubule. The potassium-sparing diuretic amiloride inhibits sodium channels in the distal segment of the distal convoluted tubule. These actions occur at the luminal surface, and diuretics must therefore enter the tubular fluid before they can have a therapeutic effect. In renal insufficiency this may be impaired and higher dosages of diuretics may be necessary.

Calcium antagonists

The calcium antagonists, such as verapamil, diltiazem and the dihydropyridines (for example nifedipine), act by inhibiting the transport of calcium through channels in cell membranes. The different calcium antagonists have different selectivities for calcium channels in different tissues, and have various actions, such as an antiarrhythmic action in the heart (for example, verapamil), and a vasodilator action on peripheral arterioles (for example, nifedipine).

Drugs that act on potassium channels

Potassium channels in cell membranes control the rate of efflux of potassium from the cells, and this tends to stabilize the cell membrane. Cellular activity will therefore be reduced by drugs that open potassium channels and increased by drugs that close them.

Drugs that open potassium channels include vascular smooth muscle relaxants, such as minoxidil and hydralazine (used in the treatment of hypertension). Drugs that close potassium channels include the sulfonylureas, which thus increase the release of insulin from pancreatic beta cells (used in the treatment of type II diabetes).

Actions via enzyme inhibition

Some drugs act by inhibiting an enzyme, and their actions will depend on the role that the enzyme normally plays.

Cholinesterase inhibitors

The reversible cholinesterase inhibitors, such as neostigmine, are used in the treatment of myasthenia gravis because they increase the concentration of acetylcholine at the muscle motor end-plate, improving neuromuscular transmission. Patients with renal insufficiency may be more sensitive to the effects of acetylcholinesterase inhibitors because of reduced cholinesterase activity.

Allopurinol

Xanthine and hypoxanthine are oxidized to uric acid by the enzyme xanthine oxidase; this oxidation is inhibited by allopurinol. Allopurinol therefore reduces the synthesis of uric acid. Xanthine and hypoxanthine are considerably more water-soluble than uric acid and their urinary excretion is rapid. The effect of the active metabolite of allopurinol, alloxanthine, on allopurinol metabolism is discussed above.

Monoamine oxidase (MAO) inhibitors

The monoamine oxidase inhibitors inhibit the metabolism of the monoamines 5-hydroxytryptamine, norepinephrine and dopamine by MAO in the brain, and it is presumably by this action that they produce their antidepressant effect. However, they can also cause an adverse interaction called the 'cheese reaction', in which amines, such as tyramine, present in certain foods, which are normally metabolized by MAO in the gut, are absorbed and displace norepinephrine from nerve endings, thus causing acute severe hypertension. Just as drugs that act via receptors can be selective for a subtype of a receptor, so MAO inhibitors can be selective for one of the subtypes of MAO. For example, selegiline is a selective inhibitor of MAO type B; it inhibits the metabolism of dopamine in the brain and enhances the action of L-dopa in parkinsonism. However, because gut MAO is of type A, selegiline does not produce the 'cheese reaction' that non-selective MAO inhibitors do.

Cardiac glycosides

The cardiac glycosides act by inhibiting the sodium/potassium pump (Na,K-ATPase), a membrane-bound enzyme that is responsible for the major part of the active transport of sodium and potassium into and out of cells, maintaining the usual transmembrane gradients of these ions. Inhibition of the pump causes a secondary alteration in calcium disposition within cells. The inhibition of the sodium/potassium pump is reduced by an increased concentration of potassium, which competes with cardiac glycosides for binding to the pump; thus, the action of cardiac glycosides may be reduced by hyperkalemia in renal insufficiency. On the other hand, in renal insufficiency there may be accumulation of an as yet unidentified dialyzable endogenous inhibitor of the pump [24], which may explain the observation that in some patients the actions of cardiac glycosides are enhanced in renal insufficiency.

Other examples

Other drugs that act via enzyme inhibition (with the enzymes that they inhibit) include warfarin (vitamin K epoxide reductase), aspirin and other non-steroidal anti-inflammatory drugs (the enzymes involved in prostaglandin synthesis), ACE inhibitors (the angiotensin converting enzyme), disulfiram (alcohol dehydrogenase), some anticancer drugs, such as cytarabine (DNA polymerase), and some anti-infective agents (bacterial or viral enzymes; for example, trimethoprim inhibits bacterial dihydrofolate reductase, the quinolones inhibit bacterial DNA gyrase, and zidovudine and didanosine inhibit the reverse transcriptase of HIV).

Actions via enzyme activation or direct enzymatic activity

Just as some drugs act by inhibiting enzymes, others activate enzymes or are themselves enzymes.

Drugs that act on the clotting system

The clotting and fibrinolytic factors are enzymes, and certain drugs that act on clotting and fibrinolysis do so by increasing their activity. Heparin acts as an anticoagulant by activating antithrombin III. Streptokinase, alteplase, and anistreplase are activators of plasminogen and thus cause clot lysis.

Enzyme replacement in genetic and acquired enzyme deficiencies

Clotting factor deficiencies can be treated by replacing deficient enzymes of the clotting pathway, for example factor VIII in patients with hemophilia and fresh frozen plasma in warfarin toxicity. Pancreatic enzymes are used in treating malabsorption in patients with chronic pancreatic insufficiency.

Cancer chemotherapy

L-Asparaginase is an enzyme that hydrolyses asparagine, the consequent depletion of which in leukemic cells may be of therapeutic benefit in some patients with acute lymphoblastic leukemia.

Actions via other miscellaneous effects

Chelating agents

Drugs that chelate metals can be used to hasten the removal of those metals from the body. Calcium sodium edetate (EDTA) chelates many divalent and trivalent metals and is used in the treatment of poisoning, particularly with lead. Dimercaprol chelates some heavy metals and is used in the treatment of mercury poisoning. Desferrioxamine chelates iron and is used in the treatment of iron poisoning and in the iron overload that occurs with repeated blood transfusion (for example in thalassemia). Penicillamine chelates copper and is used in the treatment of hepatolenticular degeneration (Wilson's disease), in which there is deposition of copper in the basal ganglia of the brain due to a deficiency of the copper-binding protein ceruloplasmin; it is also used to chelate cystine and thus prevent renal damage in cystinuria.

Osmotic diuretics

Mannitol is freely filtered at the glomerulus but is reabsorbed to only a small extent by the renal tubules. It therefore increases the concentration of osmotically active particles in the tubular fluid and prevents reabsorption of water, thus increasing urine flow. Mannitol may be useful in preventing the nephropathy that can be caused by iodinated radiocontrast media [25]. Although in low doses mannitol causes renal vasodilatation, in high doses it may cause vasoconstriction, with a risk of acute renal failure [26].

Volatile general anesthetics

General anesthetics form a diverse group of agents, such as the halogenated hydrocarbons (for example, halothane, methoxyflurane, enflurane, trichloroethylene) and non-halogenated agents (for example, nitrous oxide, ether and cyclopropane), which produce similar effects on the brain. Their main action is probably on the lipid matrix of the biological membrane, whose biophysical properties they change, resulting in changes in ion fluxes or other functions that are important for neuronal excitability.

Replacement of vitamins and minerals

Some drugs are used simply to replace deficiencies, for example ferrous salts in iron deficiency anemia and hydroxocobalamin (vitamin B_{12}) in vitamin B_{12} deficiency.

Stereoisomerism and drug action

The phenomenon of stereoisomerism (chirality) of organic compounds is due to a dissymmetry in one of the atoms (usually a carbon atom) of the compound, resulting in two structures that cannot be superimposed on top of one another (in the way that our two hands cannot).

The terminology used to describe chiral compounds is complex, but in summary some are called R and S (from the Latin *rectus* = right and *sinister* = left), others D and L or d and l (Latin *dexter* = right and *laevus* = left), and yet others *cis* and *trans* (Latin *cis* = on this side and *trans* = on the other side). Examples of drug enantiomers are R-warfarin and S-warfarin, D-glucose (dextrose) and L-glucose (levulose), d-propranolol and l-propranolol, and 13-*cis*-retinoic acid (isotretinoin) and all-*trans*-retinoic acid (tretinoin).

Of all synthetic drugs used in clinical practice about 40% are chiral and about 90% of those are marketed in the racemic form (i.e. as an equal mixture of the two enantiomers). Examples include d,l-propranolol and R,S-warfarin. Naproxen is one of the few examples of a synthetic compound which is marketed as a single enantiomer. In contrast, naturally occurring and semisynthetic compounds are almost all chiral and almost all are marketed as a single isomer. Examples include D-glucose (dextrose) and the naturally occurring amino acids (for example L-dopa).

Enantiomers often differ from each other in their actions. For example, l-propranolol is a beta-blocker, whereas d-propranolol has membrane stabilizing activity like that of local anesthetics; l-sotalol is a beta-blocker, whereas d-sotalol has antiarrhythmic effects like those of amiodarone.

In some cases differences between enantiomers are limited to differences in potency. For example, S-warfarin and R-warfarin have the same anticoagulant actions, but the former is about five times more potent.

Sometimes the difference between enantiomers is a difference between therapeutic and adverse effects, dramatically demonstrated by the example of thalidomide, whose R-enantiomer is hypnotic but whose adverse effects seem to be due to the S-enantiomer.

Enantiomeric differences may tell us something about the mechanism of action of a drug. For example, S-timolol is a more potent beta-blocker than R-timolol, but both are equally effective in reducing intraocular pressure in patients with glaucoma. This suggests that the mechanism of action whereby timolol lowers the intraocular pressure is not related to beta-blockade.

Adverse effects may be caused by one enantiomer and not another. For example, the nephrotoxicity of cisplatin is caused by the *cis*-isomer and not the *trans*-isomer [27].

Sometimes one enantiomer is eliminated differently from the body than the other. For example, R-ibuprofen is converted irreversibly into S-ibuprofen after administration of the racemic mixture; in chronic renal insufficiency the clearance of *S*-ibuprofen is reduced, whereas that of *R*-ibuprofen is not; since the *S*-isomer is active and the *R*-isomer is inactive, this has implications for the renal toxicity of ibuprofen in renal insufficiency [28]. Different affinities of the two isomers for serum albumin, which may change with changing renal function, may explain the differences in their clearances.

Renal excretion of a drug may differ between enantiomers. For example, stereoselective protein binding causes differences in glomerular filtration rate, as in the case of metoprolol [29], and for some drugs active secretion is stereoselective, as in the case of chloroquine [30].

Drug interactions may be stereoselective. For example, cimetidine inhibits the active secretion of *S*-pindolol more than that of *R*-pindolol [31].

Drug-induced renal damage

Drugs may cause impairment of renal function in five ways:

- sodium and water depletion (prerenal changes);
- reduction in renal blood flow;
- direct renal damage;
- altered renal function;
- renal obstruction.

It is worth remembering that some drugs can cause renal insufficiency by more than one mechanism. For example, amphotericin can cause glomerular and tubular damage; captopril can cause renal insufficiency by its direct effect on renal arteriolar pressure and in high doses it also causes a glomerulopathy; penicillamine can cause a vasculitis and immune complex glomerulonephritis.

Sodium and water depletion

Sodium and water depletion secondary to diuretics or to drugs that cause nausea, vomiting, or diarrhea can precipitate acute renal failure in individuals with pre-existing renal insufficiency. For example, most tetracyclines are cleared by the kidneys; they therefore accumulate in renal insufficiency and cause nausea and vomiting (doxycycline is an exception); some tetracyclines also have mild diuretic effects; the dehydration that results can precipitate acute renal failure. Many of the reported cases of acute renal failure attributed to tetracyclines have occurred in patients who have also been taking diuretics [32]. Note that tetracyclines also have an antianabolic effect and cause an increase in blood urea concentration; this can occur in the absence of renal insufficiency.

Effects on blood supply

The ACE inhibitors cause renal insufficiency in patients with renovascular disease mainly by removing the local vasoconstrictor effect of angiotensin II on the efferent arterioles, which otherwise maintains renal glomerular perfusion pressure in such cases [33]. The risk is increased in patients also taking diuretics or non-steroidal anti-inflammatory drugs. Note, however, that in other circumstances the antihypertensive effects of the ACE inhibitors (especially in patients with diabetic nephropathy) can prevent progression of renal insufficiency.

Drugs that cause vasculitis may affect the kidneys. This is rare, but most commonly occurs in the lupus-like syndrome, which otherwise generally spares the kidneys; drugs that have been implicated include hydralazine, procainamide, isoniazid, penicillamine and phenytoin.

Renal arterial or venous thrombosis, due for example to antifibrinolytic drugs or estrogens, may cause renal insufficiency.

Direct renal damage and changes in renal function

Some drugs that can cause direct renal damage and their sites of action in the kidney are shown in Figure 69.10. The figure also shows the sites of action of some drugs that alter renal function; for example, lithium can cause diabetes insipidus by competitive inhibition of the action of antidiuretic hormone on the collecting ducts [34]; the consequent dehydration can cause lithium retention and further toxicity, underlining the importance of monitoring serum lithium concentrations. The specific problems that can be caused by some drugs are listed in Table 69.7.

Renal obstruction

Ureteric obstruction can occur if clot forms secondary to bleeding (for example, with anticoagulants or antifibrinolytic drugs), if a papilla sloughs in a kidney with renal papillary necrosis (for example, secondary to analgesic nephropathy), or if there is crystallization of the drug in the renal tubules (crystalluria). Acute renal failure due to crystalluria has most commonly been reported with sulfonamides, particularly sulfadiazine [35], but it can occasionally occur with other drugs, such as naftidrofuryl oxalate, aciclovir and methotrexate. Although it has been reported with quinolone antibiotics in animals, reports in man are rare.

Renal stones can be caused by excess administration of vitamin D and its derivatives.

Drugs that cause intravascular hemolysis may cause sufficient hemoglobinuria to cause acute renal insufficiency. Analogously, drugs that cause rhabdomyolysis can cause renal insufficiency through myoglobinuria. This includes the statins (e.g. simvastatin, pravastatin), particularly when they are used in combination with fibrates, a combination that should generally be avoided. The risk of rhabdomyolysis is also increased when the statins are used in combination with cyclosporin [36].

Ureteric obstruction from without can be caused by retroperitoneal hemorrhage (for example due to anticoagulants or antifibrinolytic drugs) or fibrosis. Retroperitoneal fibrosis is rare, but can be caused by ergot

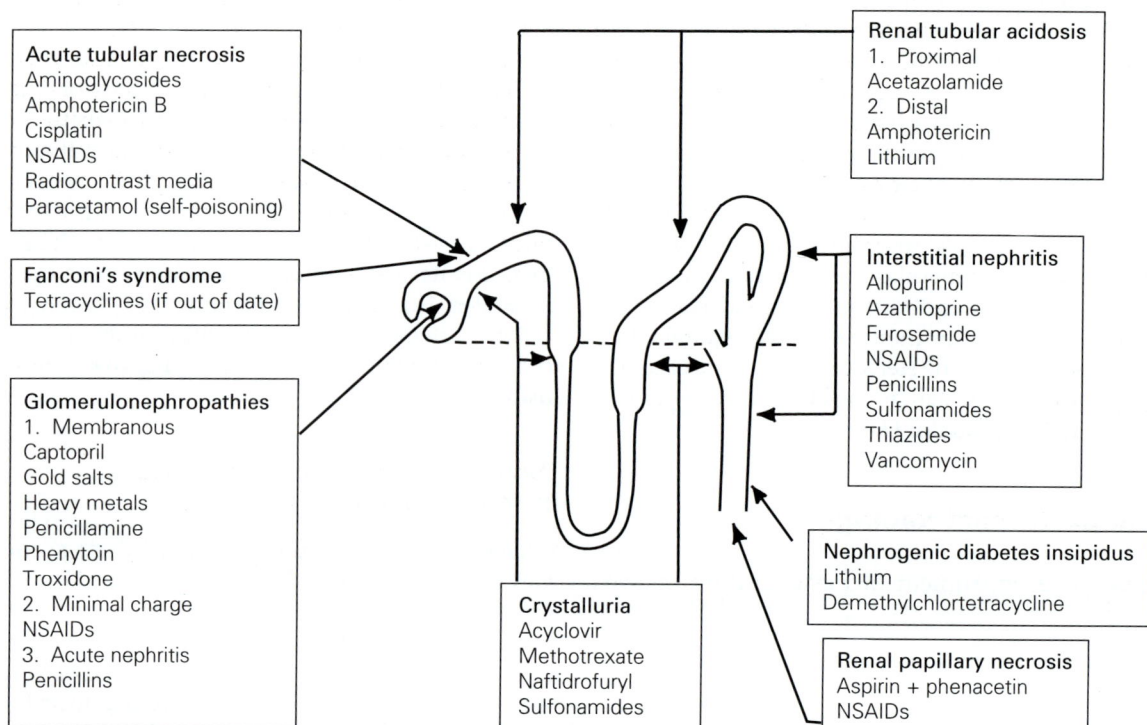

Figure 69.10 The adverse effects of some drugs on the kidney. (Reproduced, with permission, from ref. [3].)

derivatives, including methysergide and the antiparkinsonian drugs bromocriptine and pergolide [37].

Adverse drug reactions due to indirect interactions with renal insufficiency

The actions of some drugs on the tissues may be altered by the indirect effects of renal insufficiency.

If renal insufficiency causes hypovolemia, sensitivity to hypotensive agents, particularly alpha-adrenoceptor antagonists and the ACE inhibitors, increases.

Patients with uremia have an increased tendency to bleed. The effects of anticoagulants may therefore be enhanced and aspirin and other non-steroidal anti-inflammatory drugs are more liable to produce significant gastrointestinal bleeding.

Hyperkalemia is often a consequence of renal insufficiency. Potassium-sparing diuretics, potassium supplements and ACE inhibitors may exacerbate this.

Nausea and vomiting, common in renal insufficiency, may be exacerbated by theophylline.

Drugs and renal replacement therapy

The extent to which a drug is removed from the body during renal replacement therapy (dialysis or hemofiltration) depends on the drug, characteristics of the patient,

and the equipment. Less information is available about how drugs are affected by the more modern techniques of renal replacement therapy, such as continuous arteriovenous or venovenous hemodialysis or hemofiltration.

The drug

Molecular weight

The larger the drug molecule the less quickly it will be cleared by dialysis. The dialysis of a drug with a molecular weight less than 500 Da depends in turn on the effective membrane surface area and the rate of flow of blood and dialysate. For drugs with molecular weights above 500 Da only the membrane surface area is important. Molecular weight is less important for hemofiltration, which removes drugs with molecular weights up to 5000 Da with reasonable efficiency.

Water solubility

Poorly water-soluble drugs are poorly dialyzed and filtered, since dialysis fluids are aqueous. For example, although glutethimide has a low molecular weight, it is not well dialyzed, being poorly water-soluble.

Protein binding

Drugs that are highly protein bound are poorly cleared by dialysis or filtration, since the rate of transfer across

Table 69.7 Drugs that can cause renal damage and/or can accumulate in renal insufficiency

Drug	Type of renal damage (if nephrotoxic)	Hazards of excess accumulation	Comments
Antibiotics			
Aminoglycosides	Renal tubular necrosis	Ototoxicity; further renal damage	Reduce dosages; monitor plasma concentrations
Amphotericin B	Renal tubular necrosis		Common; dose-related
Cephalosporins	Interstitial nephritis (rare)	Bleeding (hypoprothrombinemia)	
Nitrofurantoin	Renal tubular necrosis	Peripheral neuropathy	Avoid
Penicillins	Interstitial nephritis	Convulsions, hemolytic anemia	Reduce large dosages (normal dosages not affected)
Quinolones	Renal tubular obstruction		Due to crystalluria (rare); hydrate well
Sulfonamides	Renal tubular obstruction		Due to crystalluria; (rare with modern drugs)
Tetracyclines		Toxicity causes nausea, vomiting, and diarrhea; dehydration then causes further renal damage; uremia also due to an antianabolic effect	Avoid in renal insufficiency and old people; use doxycycline instead if a tetracycline is indicated
Vancomycin (i.v.)	Interstitial nephritis	Ototoxicity	Reduce dosages (or avoid)
Other drugs (avoid or use in reduced dosages)			
ACE inhibitors	Can worsen pre-existing renal insufficiency	Hyperkalemia	
Para-aminosalicylic acid (PAS)		Potentiates acidosis; increased risk of gastrointestinal bleeding	
Chlorpropamide		Hypoglycemic effect	Cumulative and prolonged
Iodinated radiocontrast media	Nephropathy, cause unknown		
Nitrofurantoin		Peripheral neuropathy	
Non-steroidal anti-inflammatory drugs	Interstitial nephritis	Reduced GFR	
Phenformin		Lactic acidosis, ketosis, and hyperuricemia	
Potassium salts		Hyperkalemia	
Potassium-sparing diuretics		Hyperkalemia	

the membrane is proportional to the concentration gradient between unbound drug in the plasma and drug in the dialysis or filtration fluid. Propranolol is highly protein bound and is poorly removed by dialysis, even though its molecular weight is low.

Volume of distribution

If a drug is extensively bound in body tissues then even if it passes readily across dialysis or filter membranes, little of the total drug may be removed from the body. Digoxin is poorly removed by dialysis because it is so extensively distributed to body tissues.

The usual route of drug clearance

If a drug is mostly eliminated by hepatic metabolism at a rate of clearance appreciably greater than the rate of dialysis or filtration clearance then dialysis or filtration will have little effect on total clearance.

Characteristics of the patient

The total clearance of a drug by the body's normal mechanisms is proportional to body weight, but dialysis or filtration clearance is constant for a given piece of equipment and a given flow rate. This means that the smaller the patient the more dialysis will contribute to total body clearance.

Characteristics of the equipment

The membrane

The rate of clearance of a drug by dialysis or filtration varies with the type of membrane used. Because the peritoneal membrane has different characteristics to hemodialysis membranes some drugs are removed by peritoneal dialysis but not by hemodialysis and vice versa (Table 69.8).

Table 69.8 Drugs that are removed from the body in significant quantities by dialysis or filtration techniques

ACE inhibitors	Anti-infective agents	Anti-ulcer drugs
Captopril (H)	Acyclovir (H)	Cimetidine (H)
Enalapril (H)	Aminoglycosides (HPC)	Ranitidine (H)
Lisinopril (H)	Aztreonam (H)	Beta-blockers
Ramipril (H)	Cephalosporins (most H, some HP)	Atenolol (HC)
Analgesics	Colistimethate (P)	Metoprolol (H)
Pentazocine (H)	Co-trimoxazole (H)	Sotolol (HC)
Salicylates[a] (HC)	Fluconazole (HPC)	Corticosteroids
Antiarrhythmic drugs	Flucytosine (HPC)	Methylprednisolone (H)
Acecainide (H)	Ganciclovir (H)	Prednisolone (H)
Procainamide (H)	Isoniazid (H)	Cytotoxic and immunosuppressive drugs
Quinidine (H)	Metronidazole (H)	Azathioprine (H)
Tocainide (HC)	Nitrofurantoin (H)	Cisplatin (H)
Antidepressants	Para-aminosalicylic acid (H)	Cyclophosphamide (H)
Lithium[a] (HC)	Pefloxacin (H)	5-Fluorocytosine (HP)
Antiepileptic drugs	Penicillins (most, H)	5-Fluorouracil (H)
Ethosuximide (HP)	Pyrazinamide (H)	Methotrexate (H)
Phenobarbitone[a] (HPC)	Quinine (H)	Neuromuscular blocking drugs
Primidone (H)	Sulfonamides (HP)	Gallamine (HP)
Antihistamines	Trimethoprim (H)	Miscellaneous
Chlorpheniramine (H)	Vancomycin (HPC)	Allopurinol (H)
Antihypertensive drugs	Vidarabine (H)	Diprophylline (H)
Methyldopa (H)		Theophylline (H)
Minoxidil (H)		
Nitroprusside (metabolite, H)		

H, haemodialysis; P, peritoneal dialysis; C, continuous techniques (arteriovenous or venovenous hemodialysis or hemofiltration).

[a] Dialysis may be useful in self-poisoning with these drugs and in severe cases of self-poisoning with ethanol, methanol, bromides and fluorides, and mushrooms.

The absence of a drug from this list should not be taken to imply that it is not necessarily dialyzable.

The rate of flow of fluid

The higher the rate of flow of dialysis or filtration fluid the higher the rate of clearance.

The clinical importance of renal replacement therapy in drug therapy

There are four reasons why renal replacement therapy affects drug therapy.

• Routine dialysis or filtration may cause loss of drugs from the body, with subsequent loss of therapeutic effects [38, 39].
• Routine dialysis or filtration may cause changes in the body's physiology, for example changes in fluid and electrolyte balance, which may alter the response to the drug.
• Drugs may alter the kinetics of dialysis or filtration [40].

• Dialysis or filtration may be useful in hastening the elimination of drugs from the body after self-poisoning.

Loss of therapeutic effect

A list of drugs that are significantly affected by dialysis is given in Table 69.8. However, it is not always possible to predict the extent or rate of removal of a drug by dialysis, because of differences in dialysis equipment and because there is relatively little information from formal studies of individual drugs.

In renal replacement therapy it can be assumed, at a first approximation, that the creatinine clearance is around 30–40 ml/min and adjust drug dosages accordingly (see above). Treatment should then be monitored closely to try to determine how to adjust dosages further. For example, one would measure plasma gentamicin concentrations to determine how much extra gentamicin to give during or after a dialysis. The ways in which dosages

Table 69.9 Interactions involving drugs used in immunosuppressive therapy for transplantation

Precipitant drug	Mechanism (known or probable)	Outcome
Azathioprine		
Allopurinol	Inhibition of azathioprine metabolism	Azathioprine toxicity
Cytotoxic drugs	Additive	Toxicity
Rifampicin	Stimulation of azathioprine metabolism	Transplant rejection
Cyclosporin		
Allopurinol	Inhibition of cyclosporin metabolism	Cyclosporin toxicity
Aminoglycosides	Additive	Nephrotoxicity
Amiodarone	Inhibition of cyclosporin metabolism	Cyclosporin toxicity
Amphotericin	Additive	Risk of nephrotoxicity
Azole antifungals	Inhibition of cyclosporin metabolism	Cyclosporin toxicity
Carbamazepine	Increased cyclosporin metabolism	Reduced effect of cyclosporin
Chloroquine	Inhibition of cyclosporin metabolism	Cyclosporin toxicity
Cimetidine	Inhibition of cyclosporin metabolism	Cyclosporin toxicity
Colchicine	Inhibition of cyclosporin metabolism	Risk of nephrotoxicity/myopathy
Danazol	Inhibition of cyclosporin metabolism	Cyclosporin toxicity
Diltiazem	Inhibition of cyclosporin metabolism	Cyclosporin toxicity
Erythromycin	Inhibition of cyclosporin metabolism	Cyclosporin toxicity
Griseofulvin	Increased cyclosporin metabolism	Reduced effect of cyclosporin
Nicardipine	Inhibition of cyclosporin metabolism	Cyclosporin toxicity
NSAIDs	Additive	Nephrotoxicity
Octreotide	Reduced cyclosporin absorption	Reduced effect of cyclosporin
Phenobarbitone	Increased cyclosporin metabolism	Reduced effect of cyclosporin
Phenytoin	Increased cyclosporin metabolism	Reduced effect of cyclosporin
Primidone	Increased cyclosporin metabolism	Reduced effect of cyclosporin
Progestogens	Inhibition of cyclosporin metabolism	Cyclosporin toxicity
Propafenone	Inhibition of cyclosporin metabolism	Cyclosporin toxicity
Rifampicin	Increased cyclosporin metabolism	Reduced effect of cyclosporin
Statins	Additive	Risk of myopathy/rhabdomyolysis
Verapamil	Inhibition of cyclosporin metabolism	Cyclosporin toxicity

of individual drugs should be adjusted for patients undergoing dialysis procedures have been outlined in comprehensive reviews (for example, [41, 42]).

Changes in fluid and electrolyte balance

It is important to avoid potassium depletion in patients taking cardiac glycosides or class I antiarrhythmic drugs, since it enhances the toxic effects of these drugs.

Alteration of dialysis or filtration kinetics

Drugs that alter peripheral blood flow, for example vasodilators such as hydralazine or vasoconstrictors such as adrenoceptor agonists, may alter the rate of clearance of drugs by dialysis or filtration.

Treatment of self-poisoning by dialysis, hemoperfusion or hemofiltration

Removal of drugs by dialysis, hemoperfusion or hemofiltration is reserved for severe cases of poisoning. It is useful only for drugs that are not widely distributed to the body tissues and not highly bound by plasma proteins. The following are examples of drugs for which different techniques may be of value in cases of serious poisoning:

- salicylates, barbiturates, chloral hydrate and its derivatives, iron, lithium and methanol (dialysis; [43]).
- amitriptyline, paraquat, and theophylline (charcoal hemoperfusion; [44]).
- aminoglycoside antibiotics and theophylline (hemofiltration; [43]).

Drug–drug interactions

Drug–drug interactions occur when one drug (the precipitant drug) alters the pharmacokinetics or pharmacodynamics of another (the object drug). Table 69.9 lists some important drug–drug interactions with drugs used in the immunosuppressive therapy of renal transplantation, azathioprine and cyclosporin [45, 46].

Azathioprine interacts with allopurinol because it is metabolized to mercaptopurine and thence to thiouric acid by xanthine oxidase, which is inhibited by allopurinol. Mercaptopurine is metabolized by other routes, which may be susceptible to induction; the manufacturers have reported that the effects of azathioprine may be reduced by the enzyme inducer rifampicin, and renal transplants rejected as a result.

Most of the interactions of cyclosporin with other drugs arise because cyclosporin is metabolized in the liver by an isoenzyme of cytochrome $P450$ called CYP3A; this isoenzyme may be either inhibited or induced by other drugs.

Interference with diagnostic tests

Some antidigoxin antibodies cross-react with an endogenous substance, whose identity is not known, but which has been called EDLI (endogenous digoxin-like immunoreactive substance), producing falsely high plasma or serum digoxin concentrations [47]. The effect is usually not large, but service laboratories should be aware of it and make sure that the antibody they use does not cross-react in this way.

Retention of the metabolites of propranolol in renal insufficiency can cause spurious hyperbilirubinemia [48].

Acknowledgment

This chapter is based in part on sections of Grahame-Smith and Aronson, 1992 [3].

References

1. Brater, D.C., Chennavasin, P., Day, B. et al. (1983) Bumetanide and furosemide. Clin. Pharmacol. Ther., 34, 207–13.
2. Chennavasin, P., Seiwell, R. and Brater, D.C. (1980) Pharmacokinetic-dynamic analysis of the indomethacin–furosemide interaction in man. J. Pharmacol. Exp. Ther., 215, 77–81.
3. Grahame-Smith, D.G. and Aronson, J.K. (1992) The Oxford Textbook of Clinical Pharmacology and Drug Therapy, 2nd edn. Oxford University Press, Oxford.
4. Jensen, J.D., Madsen, J.K., Jensen, L.W. and Pedersen, E.B. (1994) Reduced production, absorption, and elimination of erythropoietin in uremia compared with healthy volunteers. J. Am. Soc. Nephrol., 5, 177–85.
5. Wiegmann, T.B. and Kaye, M. (1990) Malabsorption of calcium and phosphate in chronic renal failure: ^{32}P and ^{45}Ca studies in dialysis patients. Clin. Nephrol., 34, 35–41.
6. Donnelly, S.M., Posen, G.A. and Ali, M.A. (1991) Oral iron absorption in hemodialysis patients treated with erythropoietin. Clin. Invest. Med., 14, 271–6.
7. van Schaik, B.A., Geyskes, G.G., van der Wouw, P.A. et al. (1988) Pharmacokinetics of lisinopril in hypertensive patients with normal and impaired renal function. Eur. J. Clin. Pharmacol., 34, 61–5.

8. Vanholder, R., Van Landschoot, N., De Smet, R. *et al.* (1988) Drug protein binding in chronic renal failure: evaluation of nine drugs. *Kidney Int.*, **33**, 996–1004.

9. Reidenberg, M.M., Odar-Cederlof, I., von Bahr, C. *et al.* (1971) Protein binding of diphenylhydantoin and desmethylimipramine in plasma from patients with poor renal function. *N. Engl. J. Med.*, **285**, 264–7.

10. Aronson, J.K. (1983) Clinical pharmacokinetics of cardiac glycosides in patients with renal dysfunction. *Clin. Pharmacokinet.*, **8**,155–78.

11. Brier, M.E., Sloan, R.S. and Aronoff, G.R. (1995) Population pharmacokinetics of the active metabolite of nabumetone in renal dysfunction. *Clin. Pharmacol. Ther.*, **57**, 622–7.

12. Gibson, T.P., Dobrinska, M.R., Lin, J.H. *et al.* (1987) Biotransformation of sulindac in end-stage renal disease. *Clin. Pharmacol. Ther.*, **42**, 82–8.

13. Raehl, C.L., Moorthy, A.V. and Beirne, G.J. (1986) Procainamide pharmacokinetics in patients on continuous ambulatory peritoneal dialysis. *Nephron*, **44**, 191–4.

14. Osborne, R., Joel, S., Grebenik, K. *et al.* (1993) The pharmacokinetics of morphine and morphine glucuronides in kidney failure. *Clin. Pharmacol. Ther.*, **54**, 158–67.

15. Tune, B.M. (1975) Relationship between the transport and toxicity of cephalosporins in the kidney. *J. Infect. Dis.*, **132**, 189–94.

16. Rowland, M. and Tozer, T.N. (1989) *Clinical Pharmacokinetics. Concepts and Applications*, 2nd edn. Lea and Febiger, Philadelphia, London.

17. O'Reilly, R.A., Welling, P.G. and Wagner, J.G. (1971) Pharmacokinetics of warfarin following intravenous administration to man. *Thromb. Diath. Haemorrh.*, **25**, 178–86.

18. Nicolau, D.P., Freeman, C.D., Belliveau, P.P. *et al.* (1995) Experience with a once-daily aminoglycoside program administered to 2184 adult patients. *Antimicrob. Agents Chemother.*, **39**, 650–5.

19. Tonshoff, B. and Fine, R.N. (1996) Recombinant human growth hormone for children with renal failure. *Adv. Renal Replace. Ther.*, **3**, 37–47.

20. Hsu, C.H. and Patel, S.R. (1995) Altered vitamin D metabolism and receptor interaction with the target genes in renal failure: calcitriol receptor interaction with its target gene in renal failure. *Curr. Opin. Nephrol. Hypertens.*, **4**, 302–6.

21. Hager, S.R. (1989) Insulin resistance of uremia. *Am. J. Kidney Dis.*, **14**, 272–6.

22. Perry, T.L., Yong, V.W., Kish, S.J. *et al.* (1985) Neurochemical abnormalities in brains of renal failure patients treated by repeated hemodialysis. *J. Neurochem.*, **45**, 1043–8.

23. Gerrits, G.P., Monnens, L.A., Gabreels, F.J. *et al.* (1993) Cerebrospinal fluid amino acids, purines and pyrimidines as a tool in the study of metabolic brain diseases. *J. Inherit. Metab. Dis.*, **16**, 670–5.

24. Brearley, C.J., Aronson, J.K., Boon, N.A. and Raine, A.E.G. (1993) Effects of haemodialysis and continuous ambulatory peritoneal dialysis on abnormalities of ion transport *in vivo* in patients with chronic renal failure. *Clin. Sci.*, **85**, 725–31.

25. Margulies, K., Schirger, J. and Burnett, J. Jr (1992) Radiocontrast-induced nephropathy: current status and future prospects. *Int. Angiol.*, **11**, 20–5.

26. Gadallah, M.F., Lynn, M. and Work, J. (1995) Case report: mannitol nephrotoxicity syndrome: role of hemodialysis and postulate of mechanisms. *Am. J. Med. Sci.*, **309**, 219–22.

27. Goldstein, R.S. and Mayor, G.H. (1983) The nephrotoxicity of cisplatin. *Life Sci.*, **32**, 685–90.

28. Chen, C.Y. and Chen, C.S. (1995) Stereoselective disposition of ibuprofen in patients with compromised renal haemodynamics. *Br. J. Clin. Pharmacol.*, **40**, 67–72.

29. Lennard, M.S., Tucker, G.T., Silas, J.H. *et al.* (1983) Differential stereoselective metabolism of metoprolol in extensive and poor debrisoquin metabolizers. *Clin. Pharmacol. Ther.*, **34**, 732–7.

30. Ofori-Adjei, D., Ericsson, O., Lindstrom, B. *et al.* (1986) Enantioselective analysis of chloroquine and desethylchloroquine after oral administration of racemic chloroquine. *Ther. Drug Monit.*, **8**, 457–61.

31. Somogyi, A.A., Bochner, F. and Sallustio, B.C. (1992) Stereoselective inhibition of pindolol renal clearance by cimetidine in humans. *Clin. Pharmacol. Ther.*, **51**, 379–87.

32. Boston Collaborative Drug Surveillance Program (1972) Tetracycline and drug-attributed rises in blood urea nitrogen. *JAMA*, **220**, 377–9.

33. Toto, R.D. (1994) Renal insufficiency due to angiotensin-converting enzyme inhibitors. *Miner. Electrolyte Metab.*, **20**, 193–200.

34. Penney, M.D., Hullin, R.P., Srinivasan, D.P. and Morgan, D.B. (1981) The relationship between plasma lithium and the renal responsiveness to arginine vasopressin in man. *Clin. Sci.*, **61**, 793–5.

35. Simon, D.I., Brosius, F.C. III and Rothstein, D.M. (1990) Sulfadiazine crystalluria revisited. The treatment of *Toxoplasma* encephalitis in patients with acquired immunodeficiency syndrome. *Arch. Intern. Med.*, **150**, 2379–84.

36. Alejandro, D.S. and Petersen, J. (1994) Myoglobinuric acute renal failure in a cardiac transplant patient taking lovastatin and cyclosporine. *J. Am. Soc. Nephrol.*, **5**, 153–60.

37. Sanchez Chapado, M., Angulo Cuesta, J., Guil Cid, M. *et al.* (1995) Fibrosis retroperitoneal secundaria a tratamiento con analogos de L-dopa por enfermedad de Parkinson. *Arch. Esp. Urol.*, **48**, 979–83.

38. Reetze Bonorden, P., Bohler, J. and Keller, E. (1993) Drug dosage in patients during continuous renal replacement therapy. Pharmacokinetic and therapeutic considerations. *Clin. Pharmacokin.*, **24**, 362–79.

39. Bressolle, F., Kinowski, J.M., de la Coussaye, J.E. *et al.* (1994) Clinical pharmacokinetics during continuous haemofiltration. *Clin. Pharmacokinet.*, **26**, 457–71.

40. Bennett, W.M. (1988) Guide to drug dosage in renal failure. *Clin. Pharmacokinet.*, **15**, 326–54.

41. Lee, C.S. and Marbury, T.C. (1984) Drug therapy in patients undergoing haemodialysis. Clinical pharmacokinetic considerations. *Clin. Pharmacokinet.*, **9**, 42–66.

42. Paton, T.W., Cornish, W.R., Manuel, M.A. and Hardy,

B.G. (1985) Drug therapy in patients undergoing peritoneal dialysis. Clinical pharmacokinetic considerations. *Clin. Pharmacokinet.*, **10**, 404–25.

43. Pond, S.M. (1991) Extracorporeal techniques in the treatment of poisoned patients. *Med. J. Aust.*, **154**, 617–22.

44. Webb, D. (1993) Charcoal haemoperfusion in drug intoxication. *Br. J. Hosp. Med.*, **49**, 493–6.

45. Yee, G.C. and McGuire, T.R. (1990) Pharmacokinetic drug interactions with cyclosporin [two parts]. *Clin. Pharmacokinet.*, **19**, 319–32, 400–15.

46. Lake, K.D. and Canafax, D.M. (1995) Important interactions of drugs with immunosuppressive agents used in transplant recipients. *J. Antimicrob. Chemother.*, **36**, Suppl. B, 11–22.

47. Datta, P., Xu, L., Malik, S. *et al.* (1996) Effect of antibody specificity on results of selected digoxin immunoassays among various clinical groups. *Clin. Chem.*, **42**, 373–9.

48. Stone, W.J., McKinney, T.D. and Warnock, L.G. (1979) Spurious hyperbilirubinemia in uremic patients on propranolol therapy. *Clin. Chem.*, **25**, 1761–5.

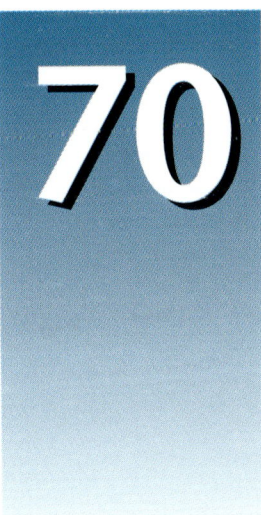

70

Use of diuretics in renal disease

Rajiv Agarwal

Introduction

Diuretics are among the most commonly prescribed drugs in patients with renal disease. This chapter reviews the clinical use of diuretics in specific conditions associated with kidney disease; these disease states form the basis for the organization of this chapter. The mechanism of action, pharmacokinetics, pharmacodynamics, or complications are discussed in the simplest terms and in the context of the disease state. There are five major classes of diuretics: osmotic diuretics, carbonic anhydrase inhibitors, thiazides, loop diuretics and potassium sparing diuretics. The mechanism of action and major side effects are shared among these five broad classes and for the sake of brevity and clarity are shown in Figure 70.1 and Table 70.1, respectively.

Diuretics are useful in patients with kidney disease to treat a variety of conditions. The foremost condition is volume overload. Despite the adaptation which maintains sodium balance and despite the progressive loss of nephron function, volume overload is common in patients with renal failure. These patients often have hypertension and the use of diuretics in this condition is well established. Other conditions for which diuretics are used are listed in Table 70.2. The use of diuretics in congestive heart failure or cirrhosis is beyond the scope of this chapter.

Volume overload

Patients with kidney disease often have an impaired ability to excrete a dietary sodium load promptly. Thus, volume expansion occurs and potent diuretics are required to excrete the excess sodium. In the Western world, diabetes is the commonest etiology of chronic renal failure. Any clinician who takes care of such patients can recall an edematous diabetic patient with volume overload. These patients illustrate the dilemma of using diuretics, pulmonary edema due to volume overload due to inadequate diuretics on one hand, and azotemia due to excess diuretics on the other. The goals are first to effect a negative sodium balance and second to facilitate the prompt excretion of dietary salt. Accordingly, the first step in the management of such patients is to restrict dietary sodium to a 6 g salt (or 100 mEq sodium) intake per day [7]. Although the diet is palatable, patient compliance is often a problem. A dietitian plays an important role to increase compliance.

If sodium restriction is not possible or by itself is inadequate, one has little choice but to resort to drugs that facilitate the excretion of sodium – diuretics.

Oral loop diuretics in renal failure

Oral loop diuretics are the cornerstone of treating volume overload in the patient with renal failure. Loop diuretics are absorbed from the gut, circulate in the blood bound to albumin and are, therefore, not filtered by the

Nephrology, Edited by Rex L. Jamison and Robert Wilkinson.
Published in 1997 by Chapman & Hall, London. ISBN 0 412 60930 4

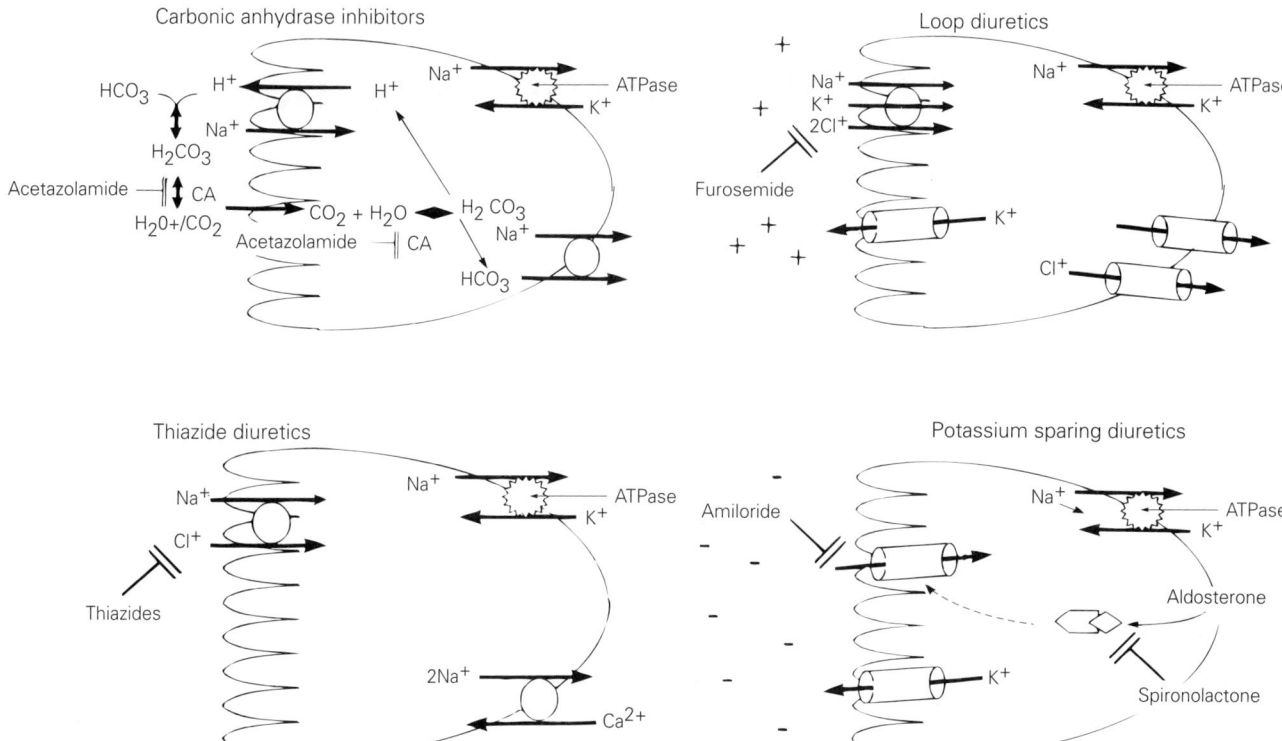

Figure 70.1 Mechanism of action of diuretics. In each of the renal tubule cells the luminal membrane is on the left and the basolateral membrane lines the rest of the cell. Carbonic anhydrase inhibitors: the proximal tubule brush border membrane is rich in carbonic anhydrase (CA) which catalyzes the conversion of carbonic acid into carbon dioxide and water. In the absence of the enzyme this is a very slow process. CA inhibitors, such as acetazolamide, cause a fall of luminal pH and impair secretion of hydrogen ions and absorption of sodium through the Na/H antiporter. Most of the excess unreabsorbed sodium is reabsorbed in the loop of Henle however. These drugs are weak diuretics. Loop diuretics: these drugs act on the loop of Henle to inhibit the Na-K-2Cl co-transporter. Venodilation occurs in response to intravenous injection and precedes the diuresis; this is probably due to stimulation of prostaglandin secretion by the kidney. Thiazide diuretics: these drugs act on the distal tubule to impair the Na-Cl co-transporter. These drugs competitively inhibit Cl binding to the protein. Potassium-sparing diuretics: amiloride and triamterene block the epithelial sodium channel (ENaC) in the prinicipal cell of the cortical collecting duct. There is a mild natriuresis but, more importantly, abolition of the negative intraluminal voltage. The latter impairs secretion of potassium. Spironolactone competitively blocks the type 1 mineralocorticoid receptor and impairs aldosterone mediated actions on this segment of the nephron. These actions include increase in Na,K-ATPase activity and ENaC activity. Osmotic diuretics (not shown) impede the renal tubular reabsorption of salt and water. The principal site of action is the proximal tubule. These diuretics also may increase glomerular filtration rate and washout the medullary interstitial gradient. Both actions enhance the diuresis.

glomerulus. They are secreted in the proximal tubule by a probenecid-sensitive anionic transporter. In patients with chronic renal failure the secretion of diuretic may be partially blocked by an increased concentration of circulating anions. After secretion the loop diuretics are carried through the tubule lumen to the thick ascending limb of the loop of Henle. On the luminal aspect of the thick limb, loop diuretics inhibit the neutral Na/K/2Cl co-transporter (Figure 70.1). Thus, the absorption of Na, K and Cl is blocked and their urinary excretion enhanced.

From the foregoing it is intuitive that there must be a relationship between the excretion of a loop diuretic in the urine and the excretion of sodium. Such a relationship indeed exists [8]. However, this relationship is not linear. The intensity of natriuresis is related to the log of

the diuretic excretion rate (Figure 70.2). Accordingly, it makes pharmacological sense to double the dose of the loop diuretic each time when titrating the dose up to that needed to cause a natriuresis. A stepwise simple arithmetic increase in dose is less likely to produce the desired result.

Long-term use of a loop diuretic leads to the development of diuretic resistance. This was aptly demonstrated in an experiment in which rats were implanted with infusion pumps delivering a constant dose of furosemide [9]. After six days of infusion the distal tubules were harvested and examinied for structural and functional changes. There was a striking hypertrophy of the distal tubular epithelium and an increased activity of the Na,K-ATPase [9, 10]. This represents a homeostatic response to reclaim

Table 70.1   The major classes of diuretics and their characteristics

Class	Example	Major fluid electrolyte changes	Common or major non-fluid electrolyte adverse effects	Comments
Osmotic diuretics	Mannitol	Hyponatremia, pulmonary edema in those with impaired renal function, renal failure due to afferent arteriolar vasoconstriction in high doses [1, 2]		Avoid in patients with established renal failure in whom the half-life can be prolonged from the usual 1.2 h to 1.5 days. Considered to be useful for prophylaxis of acute renal failure, e.g. in patients with rhabdomyolysis [3, 4] or obstructive jaundice undergoing surgery [5], although there is only weak evidence for the latter [6]
Carbonic anhydrase inhibitors	Acetazolamide	Metabolic acidosis, hypokalemia		Weak diuretic. May be combined with a loop diuretic to break diuretic resistance or to treat metabolic alkalosis
Thiazides	Hydrochlorothiazide	Hyponatremia, hypokalemia, hypomagnesemia, hypercalcemia, metabolic alkalosis, hyperuricemia and gout	Glucose intolerance, hypercholestrolemia, hypertriglyceridemia, impotence, photosensitivity, thrombocytopenia, and pancreatitis	Weak diuretic. A low dose is useful for treatment of hypertension
Loop diuretics	Furosemide	Volume depletion, hyponatremia, hypokalemia, hypomagnesemia, hypercalciuria, hyperuricemia, and metabolic alkalosis	Impotence, ototoxicity (especially when used in high doses or in combination with aminoglycoside antibiotics)	Most potent of all diuretics. Effective even in advanced renal failure
Potassium-sparing diuretics	Spironolactone, amiloride	Hyperkalemia, hypermagnesemia, metabolic acidosis	Antiandrogenic side effects are common with spironolactone. Triamterene can cause renal stones	Avoid in renal failure due to propensity for hyperkalemia. Adjunct to loop diuretics to counter potassium and magnesium wasting and to correct metabolic alkalosis

the increased sodium load delivered to the distal tubule. To overcome this resistance, adding a diuretic which acts on the distal tubule would make physiological sense. Indeed, small doses of thiazides may be very effective in overcoming diuretic resistance to loop diuretics [11]. One has to be particularly careful about monitoring volume status, potassium levels and renal function, however, in these patients. Patients should be advised to weigh themselves daily at home, and measure their orthostatic blood pressures and pulse with a home sphygmomanometer. The values should be recorded in a running log. Serum potassium, blood urea nitrogen and serum creatinine levels should be monitored periodically as dictated by the clinical situation but no later than a few days after adding a thiazide diuretic to the loop diuretic.

Thiazide diuretics in renal failure

Thiazide diuretics act on the distal tubule to inhibit a neutral Na/Cl cotransporter (Figure 70.1). Like the loop diuretics they gain entry into the tubule lumen by proximal tubular secretion. In the distal tubule thiazides competitively inhibit chloride binding to the Na/Cl cotransporter and increase the urinary excretion of NaCl.

Table 70.2 Common clinical conditions in patients with kidney disease for which diuretics are useful

Volume overload
Hypertension
Nephrotic syndrome
Hyperkalemia
Nephrolithiasis
Hypercalcemia
Nephrogenic diabetes insipidus

In contrast to loop diuretics, these drugs cause hypocalciuria for two reasons. First they enhance basolateral exchange of sodium with calcium thereby increasing the absorption of calcium in the distal tubule (Figure 70.1). Secondly, prolonged used of thiazide diuretics is thought to result in enhanced proximal tubule reabsorption in response to contraction of the extracellular fluid volume. The use of thiazides rarely leads to hypercalcemia, however. If a patient treated with a thiazide develops hypercalcemia, the possibility of hyperparathyroidism should be considered.

Thiazide diuretics can be classified based on the duration of action (Table 7.3). In general the more lipophilic thiazides have a longer duration of action.

Oral thiazides

Metolazone is effective even in patients with moderate renal insufficiency [14]. Other thiazides such as hydrochlorothiazide used in high doses (50 mg twice daily) are also effective [15].

Parenteral thiazides

Parenteral thiazides have small but significant diuretic effects in patients with chronic renal failure. This is true even in patients with a glomerular filtration rate of less than 30 ml/min [16]. In patients with such impaired renal function, a thiazide diuretic given intravenously together with a loop diuretic, torsemide, produces a greater diuresis than torsemide alone [16] (Figure 70.3). The only parenteral thiazide diuretic available in North America is chlorthiazide which when given in the dose of 500 mg intravenously in patients with renal failure should produce a natriuresis.

Sometimes the need to produce a diuresis is urgent and parenteral loop diuretics are the mainstay of therapy in patients with advanced chronic renal failure.

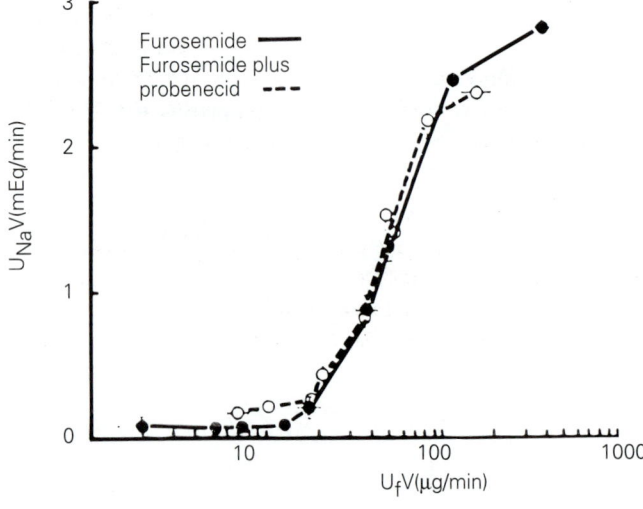

Figure 70.2 Log-linear relationship of furosemide and sodium excretion rate. The figure illustrates the urinary sodium excretion rate (ordinate, linear scale) as a function of furosemide excretion rate (abscissa, log scale). Whether furosemide secretion by the proximal tubule is unimpeded or is competitively blocked by probenecid, sodium excretion is closely related to the urinary excretion rate of furosemide and, by inference, the delivery rate of furosemide to the luminal membrane of the thick ascending limb of Henle's loop. (Reproduced from reference [8], by permission of the International Society of Nephrology.)

Table 70.3 Classification of thiazide diuretics based on duration of action

Name	Preparation	Does as diuretic	Dose as antihypertensive[a]
Short-acting thiazides (6–12 h)			
Chlorothiazide	Diuril®, 50 mg/ml suspension, 250 mg or 500 mg scored tablets Diuril® or generic 500 mg injection for intravenous use	Oral: 250 mg every 6–12 h Intravenous, 500–1000 mg as a single or two divided doses	Oral: 125 mg to 1 g per day, as a single dose
Hydrochlorothiazide	10 mg/ml or 100 mg/ml oral solution generic. All tablets are scored 25 mg Esidrix®; Hydrodiuril®; Oret ic®; Generic 50 mg Esidrix®; Hydro-chlor® Hydro-D®; Hydrodiuril; Oretic; Generic 100 mg Esidrix®; Hydrodiuril® Generic	25–100 mg once daily (QD) or two times a day (BID), once every other day (QOD), or once a day for three to five days a week (3–5×/week)	12.5–100 mg QD
Bendroflumethiazide	Naturetin®, 5 mg or 10 mg scored tablet	*Initial:* Oral, 2.5–10 mg QD, BID, QOD, 3–5×/week *Maintenance:* Oral, 2.5–5 mg QD, QOD, 3–5/week	2.5–5 mg QD
Moderately long-acting thiazides (12–24 h)			
Trichlormethiazide	2 mg Metahydrin®; Naqua® (scored); Generic 4 mg Metahydrin®; Naqua® (scored); Trichlorex®; Generic	1–4 mg QD, BID, QOD, 3–5×/week	1–4 mg QD
Benzthiazide	50 mg Exna® (scored); Hydrex®; Generic	25–100 mg QD, BID, QOD, 3–5×/week	25–100 mg QD
Cyclothiazide	2 mg Anhydron® Scored	1–2 mg QD, BID, QOD, 3–5×/week	Oral, 2 mg QD Maximum dose 6 mg per day
Hydroflumethiazide	50 mg Diucardin® (scored); Saluron® (scored); Generic (may be scored)	25–100 mg QD, BID, QOD, 3–5×/week	25–100 mg QD Maximum dose per day 200 mg
Long-acting thiazides (24–48 h)			
Methyclothiazide	2.5 mg Enduron®; Generic (may be scored) 5 mg Aquatensen®; Enduron®; Generic (may be scored)	2.5–10 mg QD, BID, QOD, 3–5×/week	Oral, 2.5–5 mg QD. Doses above 5 mg do not usually result in further reduction of blood pressure
Polythiazide	1 mg, 2 mg and 4 mg Renese® (scored)	1–4 mg QD, BID, QOD, 3–5×/week	Oral, 1–4 mg QD
Thiazide-like diuretics			
Metolazone: Duration of action 12–24 h	*Extended metolazone tablets*: 2.5 mg, 5 mg, 10 mg Diulo® or Zaroxylin® *Prompt metolazone tablets*: more potent, rapidly and more completely absorbed compared to extended tablets 500 µg (0.5 mg) Mykrox®	*Extended metolazone tablets*: 5–20 mg once a day *Prompt metolazone tablets*: Initial: 500 µg (0.5 mg) QD Maintenance: 500 µg (0.5 mg) –1 mg QD	*Extended metolazone tablets*: 2.5–5 mg QD

Table 70.3 *Continued*

Name	Preparation	Dose as diuretic	Dose as antihypertensive[a]
Quinethazone: duration of action 18–24 h	50 mg Hydromox® (scored)	50–200 mg per day, as a single dose or in two divided daily doses. Maximum dose 200 mg per day	50–200 mg per day, as a single dose or in two divided daily doses Maximum dose 200 mg per day
Chlorthalidone: duration of action 48–72 h	25 mg Hygroton®; Thalitone®; Generic; 50 mg Hygroton®; Generic; 100 mg Hygroton® (scored); Generic (may be scored)	25–100 mg once a day, or 100–200 mg once every other day, or once a day for three days a week	25–100 mg once a day

[a] Low-dose thiazides have less metabolic adverse effects and still reduce blood pressure compared to higher doses of thiazides [12, 13]. Elderly patients may be particularly susceptible to thiazides; therefore, therapy should begin with a lower dose.

Table 70.4 Doses and duration of action of loop diuretics

Loop diuretics[a]	Preparation	Dose (mg)	Duration of action
Furosemide	Lasix®, Myrosemide®, Generic 20 mg, 40 mg, 40 mg tablets, Injection 10 mg/ml Lasix®, Myrosemide® or 8 mg/ml Generic	80–240 p.o. 40–120 i.v.	6–8 h p.o., 2 h i.v.
Bumetanide	Bumex® 0.5 mg, 1 mg and 2 mg tablets. Injection 0.25 mg/ml	1–3 p.o. or i.v.	4 h p.o., 3.5–4 h i.v.
Torsemide	Demadex®, 5, 10, 20, 100 mg scored tablets. Injection 10 mg/ml, 2 ml or 5 ml ampoules	25–50 p.o. or i.v.	6–8 h p.o. or i.v.
Ethacrynic acid	Edecrin® 25 mg or 50 mg scored tablets or 50 mg base injection	50–100 mg p.o. or i.v. maximum daily dose 400 mg	6–8 h p.o., 2 h i.v.

[a] Doses are for patients with moderate renal failure (GFR 30–50 ml/min) or with the nephrotic syndrome with edema. In those with GFR <30 ml/min, the indicated dose should be doubled.

Parenteral loop diuretics

The initial step in prescribing a parenteral loop diuretic is to determine its optimal dose. This can be done by observing the response to an intravenous bolus of the loop diuretic. The ceiling dose for a diuretic is defined as the dose above which no further drug-induced natriuresis is obtained. For torsemide it is about 50 mg in those with moderate renal failure and 100 mg for those with advanced renal failure given either intravenously or orally [17]. The corresponding parenteral doses for furosemide are 160 mg and 200 mg, respectively [18]. Suggested agents and doses are shown in Table 70.4. If the response is inadequate, the dose of diuretic should be doubled until a ceiling dose is reached. If there is an adequate diuresis with intravenous bolus therapy and a need to maintain the diuresis, one may use continuous infusions of diuretics (1 mg/h bumetanide, 20–40 mg/h furosemide) instead of repeated bolus therapy (see below).

Torsemide is a new long-acting loop diuretic [19] which has some unique advantages in patients with

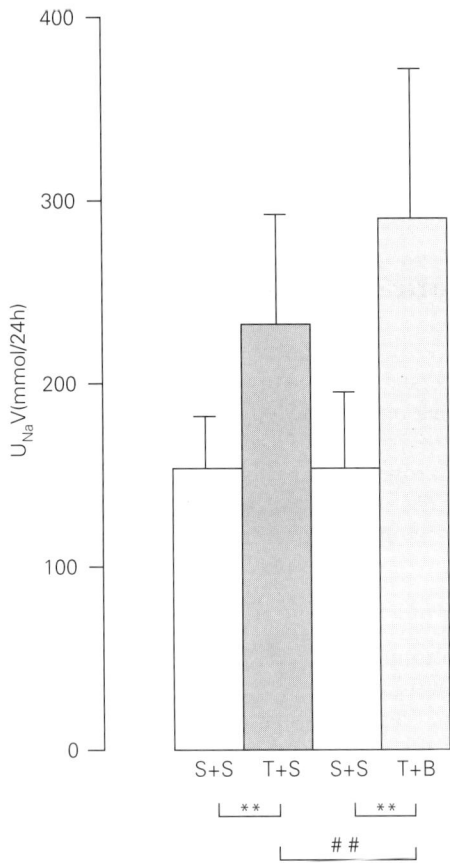

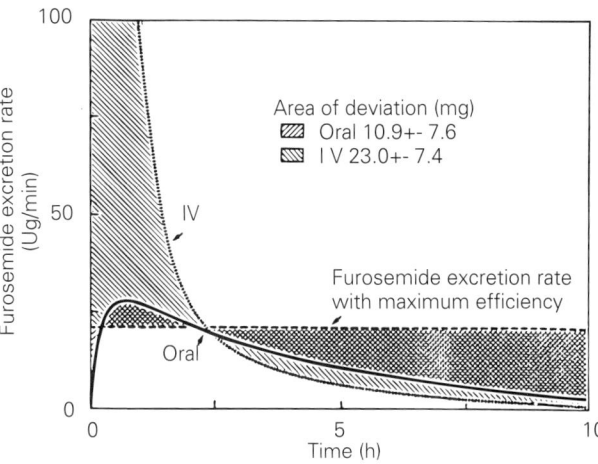

Figure 70.4 The urinary excretion of furosemide (μg/min) in humans as a function of time after the administration of the diuretic by mouth (solid curved line) or intravenously (dotted curved line). The horizontal dashed line depicts the theoretical delivery rate of furosemide needed to achieve maximal inhibition of the Na/K/2Cl co-transporter in the apical membrane of the thick ascending limb. The shading depicts the deviation from the maximal delivery needed. The calculated area of deviation is shown in the inset. According to these findings, the oral route of administration is the more efficient means of achieving the diuresis. (Reproduced from reference [21], by permission of the International Society of Nephrology.)

Figure 70.3 Thiazide augments the action of loop diuretics in advanced renal failure. Mean 24-hour cumulative sodium excretion in patients with advanced renal failure (GFR less than $30\,ml/min/1.73\,m^2$) after sham (S + S) infusion, infusion of torasemide (a loop diuretic) plus placebo (T + S), or in combination with butizide (isobutylhydrocholothiazide) (T + B). ** P < 0.01, sham vs. drug administration. ## P < 0.01, toresamide plus placebo vs toresamide plus butizide. (Reproduced From reference [16], by permission of the International Society of Nephrology.)

chronic renal failure. It has a 100% bioavailability even in patients with chronic renal failure [20] in contrast to about 50% bioavailability for furosemide [21]. Furthermore, it causes a more sustained diuresis compared to furosemide [22], does not accumulate in patients with renal failure [20] and may cause less hypokalemia [19].

Infusions versus bolus therapy

Continuous infusions of loop diuretics are superior to bolus doses in chronic renal failure for several reasons [23]:

1 It is more likely that an optimal dose of a loop diuretic needed to inhibit the Na, K, 2Cl co-transporter is attained in the tubular lumen with an infusion. With an intravenous bolus, there is a period during which the delivery of the loop diuretic in the tubular lumen is far above that needed to maximally inhibit the Na, K, 2Cl co-transporter. At other periods there is too little to effect a maximal response (Figure 70.4).

2 There is far less postdiuretic sodium retention with an infusion than with a bolus. Consider, for example, normal volunteers consuming a diet of 200 mEq/day sodium. A bolus of furosemide was administered and the sodium excretion rate measured [24]. Only in the first 6 h was there a significant negative sodium balance. During the remaining 18 h of the day, the kidney retained sodium to correct the negative sodium balance. A continuous infusion of a loop diuretic, presumably continuously inhibits the Na, K, 2Cl co-transporter. The homeostatic responses, triggered by a reduction in effective arterial blood volume, are not sufficient to offset the negative balance imposed by the continuous infusion of the diuretic.

3 High concentrations of the loop diuretic may cause tinnitus or even permanent deafness. Ototoxicity from loop diuretics is thought to be related to the peak concentrations of the diuretic. Since peak levels are lower with infusions than with boluses it is likely that infusions of diuretics may cause less ototoxicity [25].

Continuous infusions of these loop diuretics are not without danger, however. Hypokalemia and hypomagnesemia are common and require oral or parenteral supplementation. Bumetanide infusions often cause myalgias [23]. The author has personally observed a patient who had rhabdomyolysis from a bumetanide infusion though it was mild and did not cause acute renal failure.

Hypertension

Hypertension is a common accompaniment of chronic renal failure and discussed in Chapter 67. Progressive renal failure from the reduction in number of functioning nephrons leads to expansion of plasma volume. If the systemic arteriolar bed were to dilate to accommodate the increase in plasma volume, the blood pressure would not rise. However, there is a mismatch of filling of the arterial tree in relation to its compliance which leads to a rise in arterial blood pressure.

Diuretics are often the first choice of drugs to control hypertension in these patients. Long-acting loop diuretics such as torsemide have the advantage of once daily dosing, high bioavailability and effectiveness even in the presence of advanced renal failure. The usual initial dose of torsemide in hypertension is 5 mg once daily. Doses as low as 2.5 mg of torsemide have been used successfully to reduce blood pressure even though the drug does not produce a diuresis at such low doses [26]. Furthermore, the drug did not produce hypokalemia at these doses [26]. The dose may be doubled to 10 mg in four to six weeks if no response occurs [27]. Higher doses may be used in patients with moderate to severe renal failure [28]. Volume depletion, azotemia and hypokalemia are potential complications of higher doses, as can occur with any loop diuretic. This therapy is particularly useful in the setting of angiotensin converting enzyme-inhibitor therapy in which small doses of torsemide can be effective. Metolazone, similar to its efficacy in treating volume overload in renal failure, is also useful to lower high blood pressure in this group of patients.

Hyperkalemia

Patients with chronic renal failure, particularly those with diabetes, interstitial nephritis and those receiving cyclosporin, often suffer from hyperkalemia. Loop diuretics or thiazides, such as metolazone, can be very effective in treating hyperkalemia. These diuretics increase the delivery of fluid and sodium to the cortical collecting duct and also increase the serum aldosterone concentration. The combination of these factors results in enhanced excretion of acid and potassium. Patients prefer this therapy to sodium polystyrene sulfonate (kayexalate). Increasing salt intake to counter the volume depletion accelerates potassium wasting. In deciding which diuretics to use to combat hyperkalemia, the GFR must be taken into account. If it is less than 10 ml/min, it is unlikely that thiazide diuretics will be effective; the loop diuretics are the appropriate choice. For patients with higher GFRs, the longer acting thiazide diuretics cause more kaliuresis than the short acting diuretics. Accordingly, metolazone or chlorthalidone are the preferred choices.

Nephrotic syndrome

Resistance to diuretics often occurs in patients with the nephrotic syndrome. This may be due to reduced delivery of the loop diuretic to its site of action. However, there appears to be no difference in the excretion of intravenous furosemide in the urine of these patients compared to that in normal controls, thereby excluding this pharmacokinetic mechanism of resistance [29]. Albumin present in the tubule may bind furosemide and make it less effective [30, 31]. Sodium retaining mechanisms, such as low effective arterial blood volume and activation of neurohumoral factors, are also important in causing diuretic resistance. Dietary salt restriction, thiazide, loop diuretics, and avoidance of non-steroidal anti-inflammatory agents are beneficial in controlling edema in these patients. Anecdotal reports suggest that the administration of furosemide with small amounts of albumin (6–20 g) can enhance the response to furosemide in nephrotic patients [32, 33]. Patients with nephrotic syndrome have been successfully treated with a combination of torsemide (5–20 mg/day) and spironolactone (50–200 mg/day) [34]. As before, serum potassium concentrations should be monitored, especially if renal function is also impaired.

Miscellaneous conditions

Nephrogenic diabetes insipidus

Thiazide diuretics cause contraction of extracellular volume and increased proximal tubule fluid reabsorption. They have been found effective in reducing the polyuria in patients who have nephrogenic diabetes insipidus. Nephrogenic diabetes insipidus is not uncommonly caused by lithium therapy. Thiazides cause an elevation of lithium levels by about 50%, so the dose of lithium may need to be reduced. Amiloride is also sometimes useful in treating polyuria due to lithium-iduced nephrogenic diabetes inspidus [35].

Nephrolithiasis

Thiazide diuretics are often used in nephrolithiasis due to hypercalciuria. These drugs stimulate the distal tubule reabsorption of calcium (Figure 70.1) as well as proximal tubule reabsorption through volume depletion. They reduce the recurrence rate of calcium-containing stones but benefit is usually seen only after at least two years of therapy [36].

Hypercalcemia

Loop diuretics are a useful adjunct in treating patients with severe hypercalcemia [37]. Saline repletion is the initial step in the treatment of hypercalcemia. Once this is achieved, loop diuretics may be administered to accelerate calciuresis. Careful attention is needed to avoid volume depletion. Following the acute lowering of serum calcium with the above therapy, diphosphonates, such as pamidronate, provide a more durable remission in patients with malignancies [38].

References

1. Gadallah, M.F., Lynn, M. and Work, J. (1995) Case report: mannitol nephrotoxicity syndrome: role of hemodialysis and postulate of mechanisms. *Am. J. Med. Sci.*, **309**, 219–22.
2. Nakhoul, F. (1995) Acute renal failure following massive mannitol infusion and enalapril treatment. *Clin. Nephrol.*, **44**, 118–20.
3. Ron, D., Taitelman, U., Michaelson, M. *et al.* (1984) Prevention of acute renal failure in traumatic rhabdomyolysis. *Arch. Intern. Med.*, **144**, 277–80.
4. Better, O.S. and Stein, J.H. (1990) Early management of shock and prophylaxis of acute renal failure in traumatic rhabdomyolysis. *N. Engl. J. Med.*, **322**, 825–9.
5. Plusa, S.M. and Clark, N.W. (1991) Prevention of postoperative renal dysfunction in patients with obstructive jaundice, a comparison of mannitol-induced diuresis and sodium taurocholate. *J. R. Coll. Surg. Edin.*, **36**, 303–5.
6. Gubern, J.M., Sancho, J.J., Simo, J. and Sitges-Serra, A. (1988) A randomized trial on the effect of mannitol on postoperative renal function in patients with obstructive jaundice. *Surgery*, **103**, 39–44.
7. Ellison, D.H. (1991) The physiologic basis of diuretic synergism: Its role in treating diuretic resistance. *Ann. Intern. Med.*, **114**, 886–94.
8. Chennavasin, P., Seiwell, R., Brater, D.C. and Liang, W.M.M. (1979) Pharmacodynamic analysis of the furosemide–probenecid interaction in man. *Kidney Int.*, **16**, 187–95.
9. Stanton, B.A. and Kaissling, B. (1988) Adaptation of distal tubule and collecting duct to increased Na delivery. II. Na$^+$ and K$^+$ transport. *Am. J. Physiol.*, **24**, F1269–75.
10. Kaissling, B. and Stanton, B.A. (1988) Adaptation of distal tubule and collecting duct to increased sodium delivery. I. Ultrastructure. *Am. J. Physiol.*, **255**, F1256–68.
11. Brater, D.C. (1985) Diuretic resistance: why it happens and what to do about it? *Drugs*, **30**, 427–43.
12. Carlsen, J.E., Kober, L., Torp-Pedersen, C. and Johansen, P. (1990) Relation between dose of bendroflumethiazide, antihypertensive effect, and adverse biochemical effects. *Br. Med. J.*, **300**, 975–8.
13. Kochar, M.S., Landry, K.M. and Ristow, S.M. (1990) Effects of reduction in dose and discontinuation of hydrochlorothiazide in patients with controlled essential hypertension. *Arch. Intern. Med.*, **150**, 1009–11.
14. Paton, R.R. and Kane, R.E. (1977) Long-term diuretic therapy with metolazone of renal failure and the nephrotic syndrome. *J. Clin. Pharmacol.*, **17**, 243–51.
15. Wollam, G.L., Tarazi, R.C., Bravo, E.L. and Dustan, H.P. (1982) Diuretic potency of combined hydrochlorothiazide and furosemide therapy in patients with azotemia. *Am. J. Med.*, **72**, 929–38.
16. Fliser, D., Schroter, M., Nerubeck, M. and Ritz, E. (1994) Coadministration of thiazides increases the efficacy of loop diuretics even in patients with advanced renal failure. *Kidney Int.*, **46**, 482–8.
17. Rudy, D.W., Gehr, T.W., Matzke, G.R. *et al.* (1994) The pharmacodynamics of intravenous and oral torsemide in patients with chronic renal insufficiency. *Clin. Pharmacol. Ther.*, **56**, 39–47.
18. Brater, D.C. (1988) Use of diuretics in chronic renal insufficiency and nephrotic syndrome. *Semin. Nephrol.*, **8**, 333–41.
19. Dunn, C.J., Fitton, A. and Brogden, R.N. (1995) Torasemide. An update of its pharmacological properties and therapeutic efficacy. *Drugs*, **49**, 121–42.
20. Gehr, T.W.B., Rudy, D.W., Matzke, G.R. *et al.* (1994) The pharmacokinetics of intravenous and oral torsemide in patients with chronic renal insufficiency. *Clin. Pharmacol. Ther.*, **56**, 31–8.
21. Kaojarern, S., Day, B. and Brater, D.C. (1982) The time course of delivery of furosemide into urine is an independent determinant of overall response. *Kidney Int.*, **22**, 69–74.
22. Anonymous (1994) Torsemide (Demadex) – a new loop diuretic. *Med. Letter Drugs. Ther.*, **36**, 73–4.
23. Rudy, D.W., Voelker, J.R., Greene, P.K. *et al.* (1991) Loop diuretics for chronic renal insufficiency: a continuous infusion is more efficacious than bolus therapy. *Ann. Intern. Med.*, **115**, 360–6.
24. Wilcox, C.S., Mitch, W.E., Kelly, R.A. *et al.* (1983) Response of the kidney to furosemide. I. Effect of salt intake and renal compensation. *J. Lab. Clin. Med.*, **102**, 450–8.
25. Rybak, L.P. (1982) Pathophysiology of furosemide ototoxicity. *J. Otolaryngol.*, **11**, 127–33.
26. Luft, F.C. (1993) Torsemide in the treatment of arterial hypertension. *J. Cardiovasc. Pharmacol.*, **22**(suppl 3), S32–9.
27. Blose, J.S., Adams, K.F.J. and Patterson, J.H. (1995) Torsemide: a pyridine–sulfonylurea loop diuretic. *Ann. Pharmacother.*, **29**, 396–402.
28. Russo, D., Memoli, B. and Andreucci, A.E. (1992) The place of loop diuretics in the treatment of acute and chronic renal failure. *Clin. Nephrol.*, **38**(suppl 1), S69–73.
29. Rane, A., Villeneuve, J.P., Stone, W.J. *et al.* (1978) Plasma binding and disposition of furosemide in the nephrotic

syndrome and in uremia. *Clin. Pharmacol. Ther.*, **24**, 199–207.

30. Kirchner, K.A., Voelker, J.A. and Brater, D.C. (1990) Intratubular albumin blunts the response to furosemide – a mechanism for diuretic resistance in the nephrotic syndrome. *J. Pharmacol. Exp. Ther.*, **252**, 1097–101.

31. Kirchner, K.A., Voelker, J.A. and Brater, D.C. (1991) Binding inhibitors restore furosemide potency in tubule fluid containing albumin. *Kidney Int.*, **40**, 418–24.

32. Inoue, M., Okajima, K., Kazunobu, I. *et al.* (1978) Mechanism of furosemide resistance in analbuminemic rats and hypoalbuminemic patients. *Kidney Int.*, **32**, 198–203.

33. Allison, M.E.M. and Shilliday, I. (1993) Loop diuretic therapy in acute and chronic renal failure. *J. Cardiovasc. Pharmacol.*, **22**(suppl 3), S59–70.

34. Franz, M., Falger, F., Pohanka, E. *et al.* (1991) Patients with nephrotic syndrome: do they benefit from treatment with torasemide? (Abstract). *J. Am. Soc. Nephrol.*, **2**, 266.

35. Batlle, D.C., von Riotte, A.B., Gaviria, M. and Grupp, M. (1985) Amelioration of polyuria by amiloride in patients receiving long term lithium therapy. *N. Engl. J. Med.*, **312**, 408.

36. Coe, F.L., Parks, J.H. and Asplin, J.R. (1992) The pathogenesis and treatment of kindey stones. *N. Engl. J. Med.*, **327**, 1141–52.

37. Suki, W.N., Yium, J.J., von Minden, M. *et al.* (1970) Acute treatment of hypercalcemia with furosemide. *N. Engl. J. Med.*, **283**, 836–40.

38. Kellihan, M.J. and Mangino, P.D. (1992) Pamidronate. *Ann. Pharmacother.*, **26**, 1262–9.

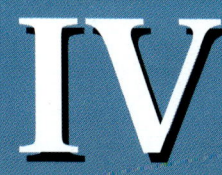

IV

General Management of Chronic Renal Disease

Section 2
Dialysis and Related Procedures

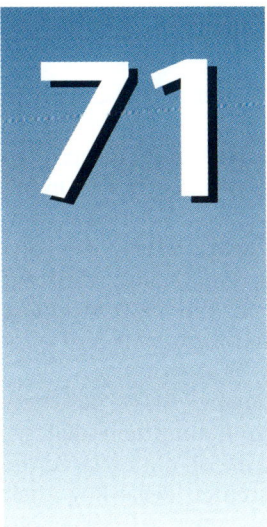

71

Vascular access

Derek Manas and David Talbot

Introduction

Access surgery now forms a significant part of surgical practice. In the mid to late 1950s, establishing patients on hemodialysis (HD) required repeated cannulation of distal arteries and veins at each 'sitting'. The result was often a progressive sacrifice of limb vessels eventually leading to complete exhaustion of all possible access sites and ultimate death. In 1960, Quinton *et al.* introduced an external silastic shunt as a means of repeated vascular access through the same site [1]. The technique required teflon vessel tips to be placed in the radial artery and cephalic vein or in the posterior tibial vessels. These were then connected by way of silastic tubing to the arterial and venous limbs of a dialysis machine. Although this was a significant advance, the shunt was complicated by problems of clotting, infection and intimal hyperplasia. Despite this, the external shunt remained the mainstay of vascular access until Brescia *et al.* described their endogenous arteriovenous fistula (AVF) in 1966 [2]. Since then, improvement in dialysis techniques has resulted in many more high risk, elderly and diabetic patients with chronic renal failure (CRF) being accepted onto both dialysis and transplant programs, making the task of ensuring patency and function of any vascular access procedure more challenging.

The aim and function of angioaccess

The aim of any access procedure should be to achieve a reliable and repetitive means of gaining access to large blood vessels capable of providing rapid extracorporeal blood flow to an 'artificial kidney'.

With respect to the function of any angioaccess there are two main goals. The first relates to the capacity of the access to permit efficient, effective dialysis. This depends on there being 250–500 ml/minute of blood flow available from the angioaccess [3] with the return of a similar flow of blood to the patient. At the same time, flows should not generate excessive recirculation of blood between the 'venous' and 'arterial' needles. Recirculation should not exceed about 4% if the fistula or graft blood flow rate is around 250 ml/min. With higher blood flows, the percentage recirculation will increase.

The second goal relates to persistence of blood flow between dialyses in the conduit without thrombosis, which is the most frequent late complication.

'Good' access relies on careful preoperative evaluation, a basic understanding of venous anatomy, good surgical technique, an appreciation of the biochemical improvements expected from 'good' access, an appreciation of the techniques involved for both patients and technical staff in puncturing the blood vessels and a long-term maintenance plan to keep dialysis efficient. Many methods have been used to assess the adequacy of vascular access and predict incipient problems. These include: regular

Nephrology, Edited by Rex L. Jamison and Robert Wilkinson.
Published in 1997 by Chapman & Hall, London. ISBN 0 412 60930 4

physical examination, recirculation studies, venous pressure measurements, angiography and duplex Doppler blood flow screening.

This chapter covers the important aspects of technique selection, gives a general overview of the surgical techniques currently available, discusses the management of early and late complications and assesses the benefits of access monitoring and surveillance.

Selection of mode of access

Establishing adequate and reliable vascular access is still the 'Achilles heel' of maintenance hemodialysis and depends on careful physical examination and preoperative assessment to identify suitable blood vessels that have not been damaged by infection or thrombosis and have the capacity to provide sufficient extracorporeal blood flow (at least 250 ml/min and preferably 500 ml/min) without the recirculation of previously dialyzed blood into the circuit. In addition the access should be relatively trouble free and not require frequent or costly intervention to maintain adequate function. Finally the procedure must spare the vascular network as much as possible.

Modes of access available

Currently, the standard approaches to permanent vascular access in patients requiring maintenance hemodialysis include the following.

1 The endogenous 'Brescia-Cimino' AVF fistula (Figures 71.1 and 71.2) this is still regarded as the procedure of choice and involves the use of 'native' vessels, namely the radial artery or brachial artery and cephalic vein to construct an end-to-side or side-to-side arteriovenous anas-

tomosis, either distally at the wrist or more proximally in the antecubital fossa.

2 The 'bridge' or prosthetic graft (Figure 71.3) can often provide reliable angioaccess when an autogenous Cimino fistula has failed, or if native vessels are deemed unsuitable. Most bridge grafts being used today are polytetrafluroethylene (PTFE) grafts, but many different materials have been evaluated in the past including bovine carotid artery, human umbilical vein and allogeneic vein grafts.

3 Central vein cannulation (Figure 71.4) has now become the favored method of initiating hemodialysis, especially in the acute setting and has all but replaced the external Scribner and Thomas shunts. Regarding their role in providing permanent access, there are certain circumstances (both patient and medical) in which central vein catheters can be used for long-term access [4].

Although few studies have compared these approaches in a prospective, randomized fashion, most surgeons involved in creating reliable access will agree that the native AVF, typically constructed as a side-to-side cephalic vein to radial artery anastomosis, remains the procedure of choice because of the superior long-term patency and low frequency of early and late complications [5, 6]. The availability of a suitable vein remains the limiting factor and in up to 30% of patients assessed for permanent hemodialysis (HD) access, suitable native vessels will not be available and a prosthetic graft will be necessary. In addition a much more liberal approach with respect to eligibility criteria for dialysis and transplantation is now adopted so that patients with diabetes, ischemic heart disease and peripheral vascular disease are accepted. Many centers particularly in North America, are also being faced with a cohort of relatively young patients with veins damaged by previous intravenous drug abuse, who subsequently require chronic hemodialysis (CHD). As a consequence, there is an increasing need for prosthetic PTFE 'bridge' fistulae [7]. In the past an autogenous saphenous vein was often used for this purpose but because of the aged population requiring angioaccess, most surgeons would preserve the long saphenous veins

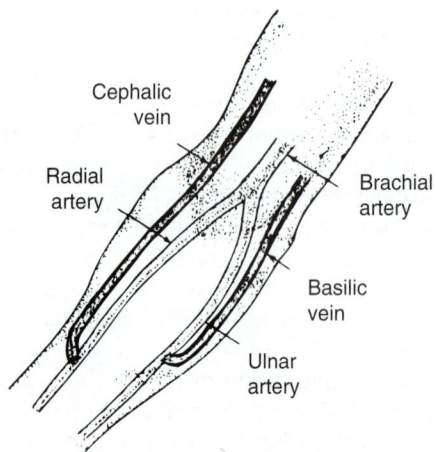

Figure 71.1 A typical radial artery–cephalic vein (Brescia–Cimino) arteriovenous fistula and the less commonly used ulnar artery–basilic vein arteriovenous fistula.

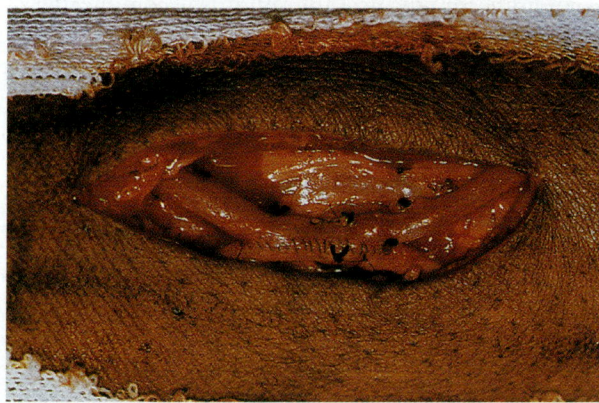

Figure 71.2 Side to side Brescia–Cimino fistula.

for coronary artery by-pass grafting should it become necessary.

The preoperative evaluation

As a general principle, all patients requiring CHD should be considered candidates for some form of surgically created long-term vascular access. Permanent cuffed venous catheters have an unacceptably high rate of large vein stenosis, thrombosis and subsequent arteriovenous fistula dysfunction associated with them, especially the long-term subclavian lines [8, 9]. Once CHD appears

inevitable, the attending physician should refer the patient to an experienced access surgeon. At the preoperative visit, the native vessels should be examined. With a venous tourniquet in place, the entire course of the cephalic vein should be examined from the wrist to the shoulder. Gentle percussion of the distended vein at the wrist should transmit a wave that can be felt or heard using a hand-held Doppler, at the antecubital vein and beyond. This is a simple test that indicates patency of the cephalic vein. It can be performed in the consulting room and used to screen out patients who require further preoperative investigation such as a color flow duplex

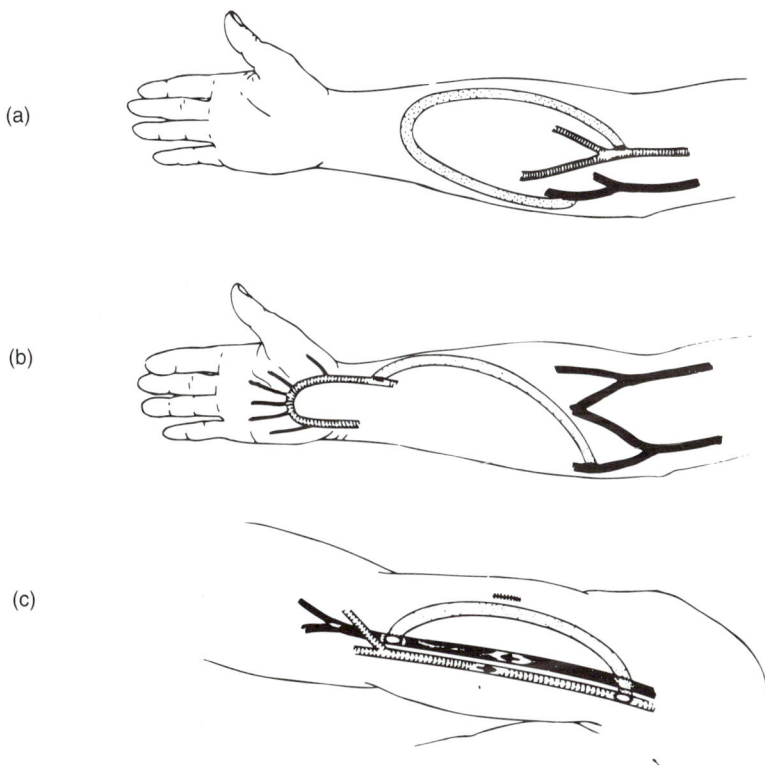

(a)

(b)

(c)

Figure 71.3 'Bridge grafts'. (a) Brachiobasilic forearm loop graft; (b) radiocephalic (straight) graft; (c) brachioaxillary upper arm graft.

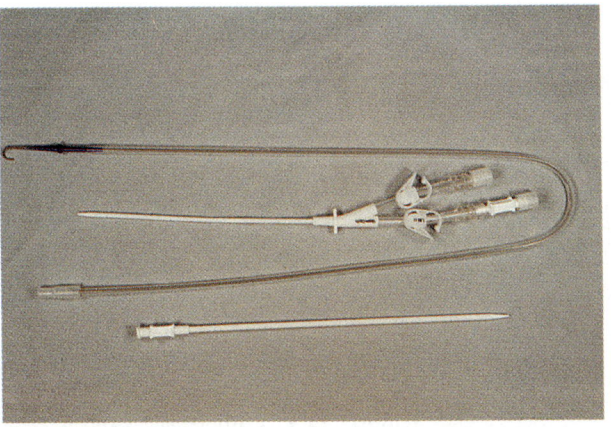

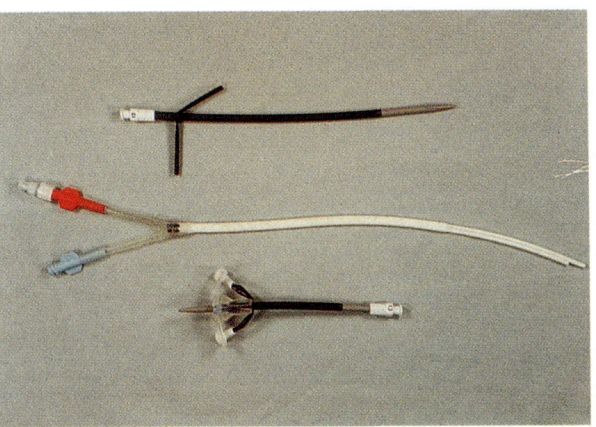

a

b

Figure 71.4   Central venous catheters. (a) 'Gam-cath' temporary subclavian vein catheter showing the vein dilator and guide-wire. (b) Cook/Uldall permanent internal jugular vein catheter showing the 'peel' away tunneling device.

Doppler ultrasound or venography. The importance of a preoperative assessment for patients requiring permanent access cannot be stressed too strongly, because failure to do so could cause the patient significant morbidity. If the cephalic vein is patent the site of the access can be planned with the anastomosis to the radial artery being as distal as possible. The anatomical 'snuff-box' fistula between the tendons of extensor pollicis longus and brevis, is the most distal of the endogenous AVFs and gives the longest length of cephalic vein. Published results for snuff-box fistulae are few, but a collective series of 493 procedures showed a mean actuarial patency of 76% at one year and 73% at two years, which compares favorably with the 65%, two-year overall cumulative patency rates published following the preferred Cimino fistulas [10, 11] (Figure 71.5). When planning the access, one should ensure that sufficient length of adequately sized vein is available after arterialization to allow two needles to be inserted sufficiently separated to avoid recirculation. Fistulae that use small or inadequate veins, although technically feasible, as evidenced by a patent anastomosis, will be difficult to cannulate, fail to provide adequate or efficient dialysis and will usually occlude soon after placement due to difficult and traumatic cannulations. The use of these small veins in the hope that the increased blood flow will dilate them enough to give adequate dialysis is a mistake [12]. Although the Cimino fistula is uniformly recommended as the best permanent access, early failures are reported to be in the range of 8–24% [13] and may in part be a result of two commonly encountered pitfalls with respect to adequacy of the cephalic vein. The first is the use of a cephalic vein which is patent at the level of the wrist, but which is actually occluded in mid-course, usually as a result of previous venepunctures and i.v. cannulation. In such situations, the patent distal vein allows a successful anastomosis to

be created but the local resistance is such, that the fistula invariably fails in the first 24 h.

The second pitfall is that of a cephalic vein which is not well developed in the forearm although a suitable sized vein is present at the wrist. In such situations the distal cephalic vein often drains into a network of small tortuous forearm veins, which even if successfully arterialized, would not mature enough to sustain adequate HD. These veins are often thin walled, friable and easily torn when needled. Inexperienced surgeons may pride themselves on their success, but in terms of sustaining adequate flows and efficient HD, these fistulae are often dismal failures.

In such cases one should proceed proximally to the cubital fossa. Brachiocephalic fistulae (Figure 71.6) have excellent short- and medium-term patency rates [10], presumably because the anastomosis is technically easier to perform, with the upper arm veins being generally larger than those of the forearm. Nevertheless, brachiocephalic and brachiobasilic fistulae although technically feasible may only arterialize a short segment of superficial vein that can be used for repeated long-term needling. In the case of the brachiobasilic fistula, the resultant arterialized vein may be far too medial for practical and comfortable needling. In addition, the proximal cubital fossa AVF may predispose the elderly, atherosclerotic or diabetic patients to a distal 'steal' syndrome [14] because of their tendency to enlarge over time, even when care is taken over keeping the AV anastomosis within the recommended 5–7 mm length (Figure 71.7).

It is often said that constructing a Cimino fistula is always worth trying. Although this peripheral fistula is preferable, if a particular patient has unsuitable distal vessels, which would make success less likely, it would be unjustified to attempt the fistula and instead a prosthetic bridge fistula needs to be constructed.

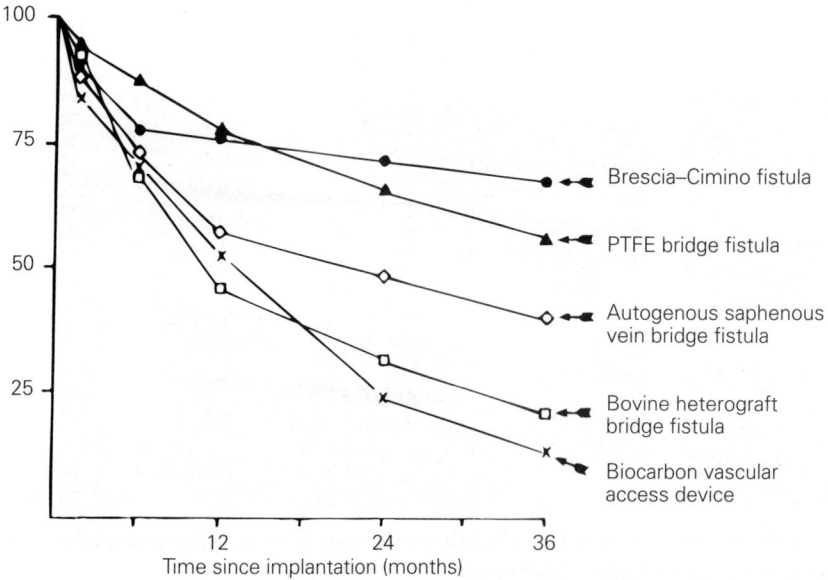

Figure 71.5 Cumulative patency rates for different access procedures as a function of time.

Poor selection of arteries and veins prior to surgery very often results in poor extracorporeal flow and inadequate dialysis. Selection of suitable vessels is very often a matter of experience. A working knowledge of the topographical anatomy of the upper limb blood vessels is essential in order to select the appropriate type and site of the access (Figure 71.8). Formation of these fistulae should be carried out as early in the course of CRF as possible. This allows for adequate maturation time – the process by which the arterialized veins dilate and thicken sufficiently to allow safe, repeated needling. On average, most forms of peripheral fistulae if appropriately selected and performed, will need six to eight weeks to 'mature' enough to needle. The cephalic vein of the non-dominant arm is the vein of choice. Ideally it should begin in the radial part of the dorsal venous network and wind upwards around the radial border of the forearm into the cubital fossa where it communicates with the cubital vein (Figure 71.8). The cephalic vein is the limiting factor in determining both early and long-term outcome and if the venous anatomy of the dominant arm better conforms to the required specifications, that side should be used rather than stubbornly trying to enforce the 'non-dominant' rule. In reality the decision as to the type, site, side and timing of access placement depends on a number of factors.

- The anticipated time to commencement of HD
- The experience and judgment of the surgeon
- The nephrologist's perception of the success rate after placement of a particular form of access
- The status of the venous system
- How important it is to avoid a temporary access
- The alternative of continuous ambulatory peritoneal dialysis in the treatment of a particular patient

- The blood flow rates required for a particular dialysis prescription

Some physicians will base their decision to refer patients to a surgeon on a rising serum creatinine, or the 'rate of change' seen in the serum creatinine. Whatever criteria are used, when the attending physician feels that CHD is

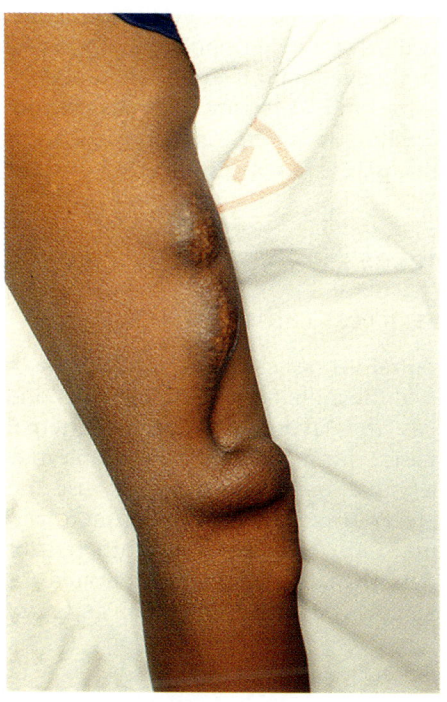

Figure 71.7 Large brachial fistula associated with distal 'steal'.

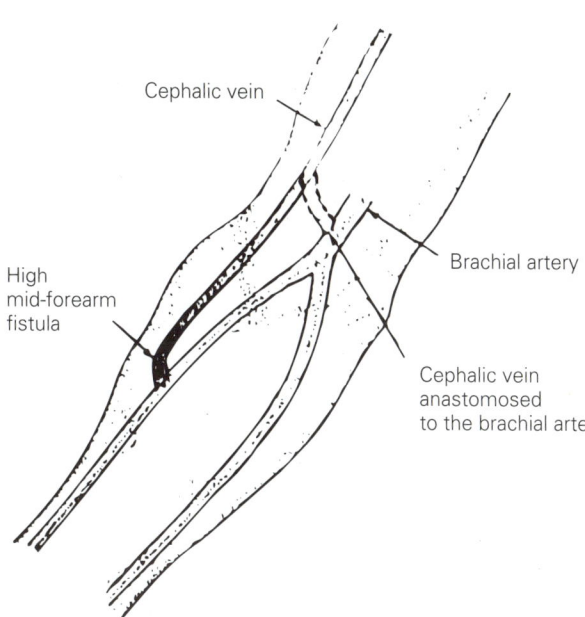

Figure 71.6 A brachiocephalic arteriovenous fistula.

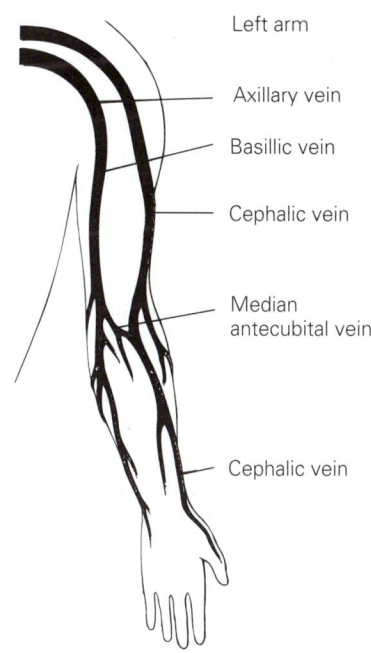

Figure 71.8 Most commonly encountered anatomy of the superficial veins of the upper limbs.

inevitable the patient should have the access created. This obviates the need for temporary access, especially the sub-clavian vein catheter.

In recent years preoperative evaluation using Doppler ultrasound has been employed to better evaluate veins and select access placement sites. Recent data from the International symposium on angioaccess, June 1996 suggested that preoperative Doppler ultrasound assessment was 34% more accurate than clinical evaluation alone. Our group have used preoperative Doppler ultrasound for patient selection and have found it to be very useful for assessing vessel size and detecting dubious venous patency, but the technique is very operator dependent and requires an enthusiastic radiologist for it to be useful.

Access techniques

Chronic venous access catheters

In recent years, central venous catheters (Figure 71.4a,b) have largely replaced the more troublesome Scribner and Thomas shunts, as the favored method of external angioaccess. Two basic types of catheters are available, one for 'short-term' (less than one week) temporary use and another for 'long-term' (weeks or months) or more permanent use (Figure 71.4b). Central venous catheters for 'short-term' use (less than one week) are indicated for acute dialysis, plasmaphoresis or hemofiltration and carry a relatively low risk of early complications (<5%). Catheters for long-term use are indicated because of failure to recover rapidly from an acute event or in established end-stage renal disease (ESRD). Often patients in acute renal failure are metabolically and hemodynamically unstable, making them poor candidates for any surgical procedure. In this situation placement of a percutaneous temporary central venous catheter, which can reliably deliver 200 ml/min of blood flow to the dialyzer is life saving. With the availability of newer materials such as teflon, polyurethane and silastic, more permanent-catheters have been developed. Patients who have exhausted all access sites or who have severe cardiac failure are undergoing permanent HD via these catheters. These soft, double lumen or single lumen cuffed catheters are placed in the internal jugular vein and deliver adequate blood flow (usually >200 ml/min) with low recirculation. The placement of a chronic vascular access catheter does not preclude fistula surgery, often ESRD patients require a catheter to be placed to provide access during fistula maturation. Nevertheless, the catheter should be placed on the side opposite the proposed permanent access site, to minimize subsequent difficulties with subclavian vein stenosis.

Catheter selection

The choice of catheter depends on a number of factors but essentially comes down to the individual nephrologist's preference and the facilities of the local dialysis unit.

The decisions revolve around whether individual patients are best served by using dual or single lumen catheters, whether permanent external access is required and, if so, what is the complication rate for that particular catheter. Controversy exists as to which catheter facilitates dialysis most effectively. Dual lumen (two halves of the same cannula) and double lumen (inner venous cannula surrounded by an outer arterial cannula) catheters both use the principle of simultaneous two-way flow. Single lumen catheter dialysis, requires alternating inward and outward blood flow through the same cannula. Many believe this increases recirculation and makes dialysis less effective. Teflon catheters, although quite easy to insert, are 'stiff' and consequently more reactive to the vessel wall. They should not be used for long-term access. Polyurethane catheters are stiff initially which makes them easy to place, but soften at body temperature. This makes them quite attractive for the medium term (less than one month). Silastic catheters are very soft and quite unreactive which makes them ideal for long-term use. The most commonly used long-term catheter is the silastic double lumen Perma-Cath. It has a Dacron cuff which is meant to be tunneled under the skin and theoretically generates a fibrotic reaction which serves to secure the catheter and prevent migration of pathogens from the skin down the epithelialized tract which develops. The insertion technique can be either through a surgical cut down procedure or via the percutaneous 'Seldinger' method. The percutaneous system is standard for most temporary venous access catheters, but in recent years, percutaneous 'kits' for permanent catheter insertion have become available. They involve the use of a dilator followed by a 'split sheath' introducer. The insertion of this relatively rigid system can be painful under local anesthetic and often necessitates a general anesthetic. Often Perma-Caths are placed operatively. The authors favor the internal jugular vein placement with the catheter being sutured into the vein. The open surgical procedure can sometimes be performed under local anesthetic particularly for external jugular and femoral approaches, where it is usually inserted into the saphenous vein. However, local anesthesia for exposing the internal jugular vein may be unwise in unco-operative patients. After insertion, all catheters should be screened radiologically. Although intraoperative image intensification is preferable, a plain chest radiograph will also confirm the position of the catheter tip. The catheters are usually adjusted for length so that the tip lies in the right atrium. Inadvertent positioning can be corrected postoperatively by 'goose-neck' snaring and repositioning with radiological assistance.

When using single lumen catheters two or three side holes should be cut at the time of insertion to ensure that the catheter lumen is not occluded by lying against the side wall of the vessel. The catheters should be 'locked' with heparin (1.76 ml of 5000 µ/ml) and the exit site and free ends protected by wrapping in antiseptic swabs. The dual lumen system tends to have narrower channels allowing for simultaneous movement of blood at lower flow rates. This lends itself to continuous venovenous hemofiltration or dialysis (CVVH/D) rather than intermittent HD. Subclavian vein catheterization is still being used, especially for temporary access. A growing body of evidence appears to suggest that these catheters are associated with a 50% incidence of large vein stenosis and thrombosis [9] (Figure 71.9). As a consequence, catheterization of the subclavian vein for 'short-term' dialysis should be avoided and the placement of long-term double-lumen cuffed venous catheters should be restricted to the internal jugular veins unless there are exceptional circumstances. The long-term complications of subclavian vein thrombosis and stenosis can impair venous drainage of subsequent fistulae in the upper limb (Figure 71.9). They should be deplored in all patients likely to require permanent HD. Femoral lines are not without their problems but iliac vein thrombosis, which can produce difficulty in subsequent renal transplantation is fortunately rare. Thus temporary access via the femoral vein should be preferred for the short term.

Due to the high frequency of elective removals, the actuarial survival rate of chronic venous catheters is difficult to assess. Some centers report one-year and two-year survival rates of 50% and 41%, respectively [4].

Arteriovenous fistulae

As previously emphasized a detailed outpatient assessment is a prerequisite for successful AVF formation. At the preoperative visit the selected site and side of the fistula should be discussed with the patient. This is particularly important if preoperative investigations suggest that the dominant limb is the preferable site. If there is a choice, the non-dominant arm should be preserved as this is more likely to be free of previous trauma and in addition would allow the most useful arm to be free during dialysis. If a preoperative upper limb phlebogram suggests an occluded or stenosed subclavian vein, it may not be immediately obvious to the patient as to why the most 'useful' arm is selected for the AVF. Patients who are not adequately counseled may not be receptive to postoperative manipulation such as subclavian vein stenting or able to deal with early access failures which are not uncommon. As far as possible the selected limb should be 'protected' from venesection and intravenous cannula insertion prior to fistula formation. Simply asking the patient to change his or her wrist watch site away from the protected arm can facilitate increased awareness.

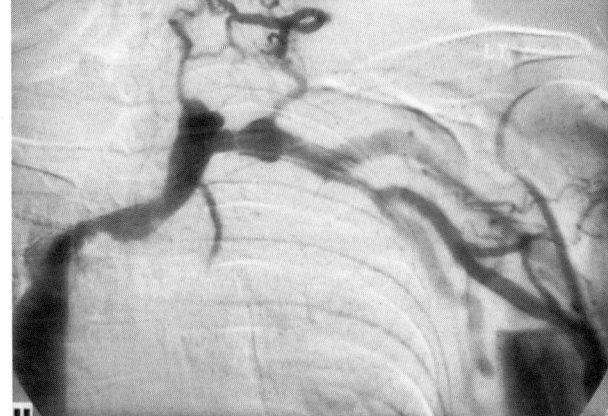

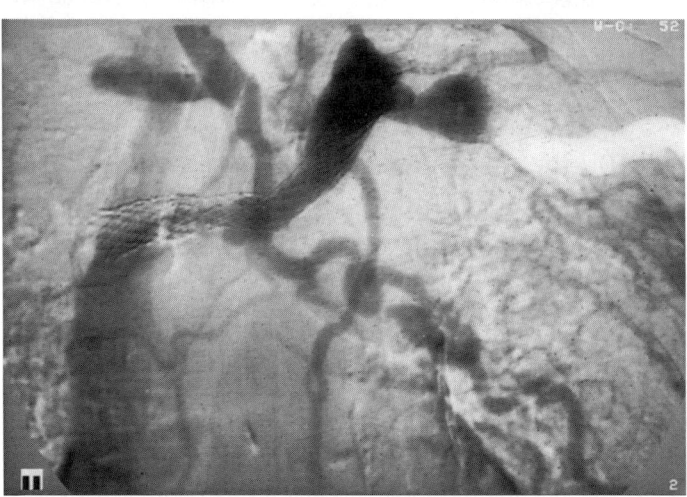

Figure 71.9 A venogram showing left subclavian vein stenosis. (a) Predilatation and stenting; (b) Post ballon dilatation and wall-stenting.

Formerly all AVF were constructed under general anesthetic or regional nerve block. This approach has gradually changed partly due to the unnecessary morbidity associated with regional blocks [12] and the unwanted hypotension that often accompanies general anesthesia. Moreover, the results with simple local anesthetic infiltration are as good if not better and allow for more flexibility if intraoperative variation is required.

Radiocephalic fistula

The Brescia–Cimino radiocephalic fistula (Figure 71.1) is generally considered the best option as it gives the dialysis technician the maximum amount of vein to needle as mentioned before. The artery and vein are exposed through a longitudinal or transverse incision at the wrist. Sometimes more than one incision may be required to adequately mobilize the vessels. The radial nerve should be carefully preserved at this level as inadvertent damage leaves the patient with a very uncomfortable sensory deficit. Brescia–Cimino fistulae have been performed by all possible techniques (end-to-end, end-to-side or side-to-side) and two factors have emerged which dictate the best method. First, approximately 30% of the blood flow through any fistula comes from the distal artery (the efferent arterial limb) [15], therefore any technique which relies on ligation of the distal artery (end-to-end) has a lower flow rate and is more likely to fail. Second a side-to-side anastomosis produces increased venous pressure downstream which in a brachial fistula may not matter if a competent valve is present in the distal efferent cephalic vein, but with the radiocephalic fistula painful venous congestion of the thumb may ensue. Therefore if a side-to-side arteriovenous fistula is performed at the wrist then the distal limb of the vein should be ligated at the end of the procedure.

With radiocephalic fistulae, the small caliber vessels increase the probability of technical failure (30%). This problem can be minimized by the use of optical magnification (operating spectacles with a magnification range of 2.5× to 3.5× normal) and fine sutures. In addition the patient should be adequately hydrated prior to surgery. Inadequate hydration is typical in patients who are operated on immediately postdialysis and in whom the surgery is performed under general anesthesia. Hypotension often ensues and vasopressor agents are sometimes required to counteract the hypotension. Regional vasospasm from handling the vessel, particularly the artery, can be reduced by the local use of papaverine. Paradoxically we have found that due to atheromatous arterial disease, older patients often have less vasospasm. A small vein can be dilated to a reasonable size by hydrostatic pressure using a no. 8 urethral catheter or by passing a size 3 fogarty embolectomy balloon catheter along the vessel. High resistance to flow in the vein or pain are features indicative of undiagnosed venous obstruction or inflammation and renders the vein unsuitable.

The anastomosis is usually constructed with a continuous non-absorbable suture such as 6-0 prolene although some surgeons adopt the microvascular approach of 7-0 or 8-0 interrupted sutures. Vascular clips are now available and preliminary data [16] suggest a shorter operation time and in certain hands improved success rates using them though this may be due to patient selection. If, after completion of the anastomosis, the flow is poor, a number of factors may be responsible. The first question to be addressed is the anastomosis itself. If the operator is satisfied that further improvement is not possible it is better not to reopen the anastomosis and to traumatize the intima further, which itself is thrombogenic. A common error is to assume a pulse distal to the anastomosis is indicative of a successful fistula. Pulsatile flow indicates a patent anastomosis but the absence of a thrill usually indicates a proximal obstruction or low flow and in the absence of reversible factors such as hypotension or vasospasm, is a bad prognostic sign. In this situation venous adventitia can be stripped from the outside easily with a pair of forceps and a valvotome could be introduced through a side branch if a troublesome valve is suspected. In addition tissue lying across the vein should be divided to reduce the inevitable compressive effect. After surgery the limb is kept warm and the blood pressure maintained to avoid hypotension. If the flow ceases then the patient should only be returned to the operating room if the surgeon feels that the problem is remediable. A difficult anastomosis with tiny vessels is unlikely to be remedied. The failure should be accepted as due to inappropriate selection. Patency rates at one year can be expected to be of the order of 65% [10].

Brachiocephalic fistulae

The second choice after a radiocephalic fistula is a brachiocephalic fistula (Figure 71.6) constructed in the antecubital fossa assuming suitable vessels. The patency rates are generally better than those of radial fistulae but arterial steal is the chief complication. These anastomoses are either performed side-to-side or end-to-side (vein to artery). The length of the anastomosis should be restricted to minimize the risk of 'steal' and in general should be less than 6 mm. All other technical factors are similar to those discussed for radial fistulae.

'Bridge' grafts for vascular access

Bridge grafts can be divided into autogenous saphenous vein grafts, semisynthetic bovine carotid and human umbilical vein grafts and synthetic PTFE grafts.

The saphenous vein graft used to be popular. The infection rate was low, but thrombosis was common (50% at one year) [17]. The reason for this may be the dilatation around valves which in arterial bypass surgery seems to have little effect but combined with the trauma of repeated needling may be sufficient to generate thrombus. In recent years, moreover, most surgeons have preferred to preserve the long saphenous vein for coronary artery bypass grafting.

The bovine carotid artery and human umbilical vein bridge grafts went out of vogue largely because of the problems with aneurysm formation, sepsis and bleeding [18]. Likewise, the Dacron and Sparks Mandril grafts are also no longer used because of bleeding on insertion and after removing dialysis needles.

PTFE grafts are currently the most satisfactory and widely used prosthetic grafts. Because the PTFE allows for neointimal endothelial migration it offers some degree of resistance to infection and reduces the amount of bleeding after removal of dialysis needles. More recently one of the companies manufacturing PTFE, W.L. Gore, has introduced the Diastat graft (Figure 71.10). This graft is constructed with a cuff of layered fibers surrounding the middle two-thirds of the graft that theoretically produce a more effective seal after withdrawal of the dialysis needles. Prospective data have yet to be published but preliminary results from selected non-randomized studies suggest that time to hemostasis and pseudoaneurysm formation are both reduced [19].

Originally the graft was of uniform caliber, but modern grafts are tapered. A narrow 4 mm arterial end, which reduces the incidence of steal syndrome, expands to a 7 mm venous end to allow for easier needling. The increased caliber at the venous end accounts for a fall in flow of 20% but this does not cause problems in flow on dialysis [20]. The anastomotic sites for placement of bridge grafts vary (Figures 71.3 and 71.10) and include:

- radial artery to antecubital cephalic or basilic vein (straight graft);
- brachial artery to antecubital cephalic or basilic vein (loop graft);
- brachial artery to axillary vein (upper arm straight graft-tunneled lateral to the biceps muscle);
- axillary artery to ipsilateral axillary vein (loop graft);
- axillary artery to contralateral axillary vein (straight graft);
- common femoral artery/SFA to saphenous vein (loop) or popliteal vein (straight);
- profunda femoris artery to saphenofemoral junction (loop).

A forearm graft from radial artery at the wrist has a low incidence of steal but a high thrombosis rate because the arterial inflow is low due to the narrow caliber of the vessel. In addition the efferent limb is anastomosed to an antecubital vein which is usually insufficient or otherwise a standard brachial arteriovenous fistula would presumably have been performed. Consequently the patency at one year is approximately 35% as opposed to a forearm loop (brachial artery to antecubital vein the patency of which at one year is 78%) [21]. A forearm loop relies on a suitable antecubital vein which if present should be used for a standard arteriovenous fistula if time for maturation permits. The alternative is to use a graft between the brachial artery in the antecubital fossa and the axillary vein for which the patency rate is estimated at 60% [21]. The two serious problems seen with these grafts are those of unexpected subclavian thrombosis, which initially produces venous hypertension, arm swelling and later thrombosis of the graft, and a 'steal' syndrome. Leg grafts are placed either between the superficial femoral artery or profunda femoris artery and the saphenous or

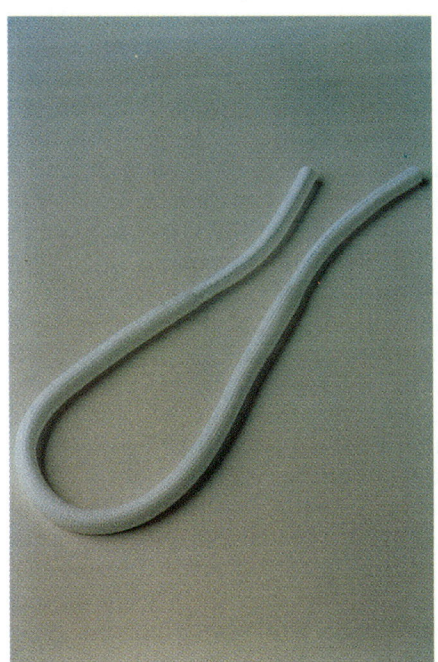

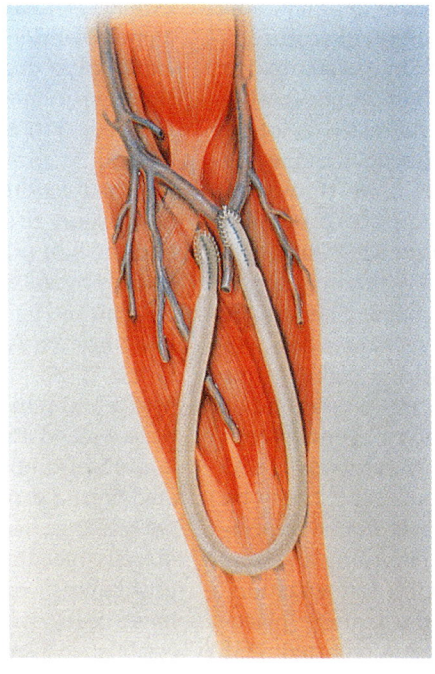

Figure 71.10 (a) Diastat (W.L. Gore)–PTFE graft; (b) A schematic representation of a forearm Diastat loop graft.

a

b

femoral vein. Occasionally a popliteal artery to femoral vein graft is performed. Leg grafts should only be considered as a tertiary form of access, however, as graft infection is more common and is associated with a high mortality and amputation rate [22]. Our own experience suggests that with careful selection, complications of leg grafts can be kept to a minimum.

Prosthetic grafts are not without morbidity and often multiple graft revisions will be required. It has been estimated that one revision is needed for every 1.25 years of graft life [7].

Complications of angioaccess procedures

Complications of chronic venous lines

There are three types of complications of chronic venous catheters, insertion, mechanical and infectious.

Complications occurring at the time of insertion are inversely related to experience of the operator and range from 2 to 12% [23]. Hemopneumothorax especially after subclavian catheterization occurs in about 2% of cases. Hemomediastinum and cardiac tamponade from the guidewire puncture of the right atrium or of the superior vena cava are rare but need prompt recognition and surgical intervention. As a general rule if guidewires and catheters are not 'forced in' when resistance is met, insertion complications will be minimal.

Mechanical problems usually manifest as inadequate flow. This is often due to the catheter 'kinking', deposition of fibrin or thrombus in or around the catheter or poor positioning with the catheter orifice blocked by the wall of the vessel. A diagnosis can usually be made following angiography. About 25% of long-term catheters will occlude. The most expeditious way of managing this problem is to replace the catheter with another catheter. Recently the technique of stripping the catheter of its thrombus or fibrin sheath has been described using the Nitinol Gooseneck snare [24]. This is done through a femoral vein approach with a 25 mm Amplatz Gooseneck snare, which is introduced and positioned around the catheter well above the tip. The snare is then tightened and the distal end of the catheter stripped. This can be performed three times in total and often restores flow. We have also used the technique to reposition catheter tips but with less success for this purpose. Another method of unclotting catheters is to use thrombolytic agents. Streptokinase, urokinase or thromboplastin activator (t-PA) can all be instilled into the catheter. The agent should be given as a slow continuous infusion over hours. Subclavian vein thrombosis and stenosis are becoming an enormous problem following subclavian vein catheterization. They are directly related to the duration of catheter placement, a stenosis rate of 20% has been reported [25] although the true incidence is difficult to gauge because

most stenoses and thromboses are not clinically recognizable until after placement of an AVF. Venous angioplasty is successful if the stenosis is detected prior to complete occlusion. Unfortunately recurrence of stenosis following angioplasty is common – one year patency of 45% and 12% at two years. Vascular endoprotheses have now been used for patients in whom stenoses recur less than two months after angioplasty [9]. The Wallstent, a stainless-steel multifilament tube device, is the most common stent used (Figure 71.9). Oversizing, migration and restenosis of the stent are common problems.

Infection is the leading cause of morbidity and the second leading cause of death in HD patients. Central venous catheters will become colonized in 20% of patients and bacteremia will develop in 10% of patients. The risk of line sepsis can be minimized by the use of topical antiseptic wraps, antibiotic prophylaxis at the time of line insertion and occlusive dressings and minimizing manipulation of the catheter. Once the patient develops confirmed line sepsis the safest course is to remove the line.

Complications of arteriovenous fistulae and 'bridge' grafts

Bleeding after fistula formation which does not respond to simple elevation is obviously an indication to return to the operating room (OR). The commonest source of this bleeding is not the anastomosis line but a slipped distal vein ligature which has been placed as distal as possible to provide proximal length. Occasionally bleeding results from inadequate subcutaneous tissue hemostasis. The most common early complication is thrombosis which is usually a result of surgical error or hypotension related to overzealous hemodialysis, dehydration or poor cardiac function. The critical question that should be answered prior to returning a patient to the OR for re-exploration of a thrombosed fistula is, how satisfied and how experienced was the surgeon who performed the initial operation? In general a fistula with good flow and a thrill at the end of the procedure should always be returned to OR for thrombectomy should thrombosis occur soon after the operation. If the vein was tenuous and the best procedure was performed under the circumstances by an experienced surgeon then there is little to be achieved by returning the patient to the OR. Similarly late thrombosis should only be treated by surgical exploration if the surgeon is proposing to reconstruct the fistula and remove the neointima. The functional results of late reconstruction are often poor [26].

Late thrombosis of an established AVF is often associated with a surgical procedure for an unrelated problem, overzealous hemodialysis, hypotension related to post-dialysis bleeding or myocardial infarction or excessive postdialysis compression. Provided all systemic factors have been corrected, most acute thromboses in well-established fistulae can be corrected by local thrombectomy (surgical or radiological). Venous stenosis which develops in the proximal third of the arterialized vein is a far more ominous and difficult problem to treat. With regular surveillance these lesions can be identified angiographically prior to complete occlusion and treated by percutaneous transluminal angioplasty (PTA). The success of PTA in this situation depends to some extent on the site and number of stenoses [27]. In complete and long-standing occlusions a combination of angioplasty and pulse spray thrombolysis has been successful. The group from San Diego suggest that 250 000 units of urokinase concentrated to 25 000 units/ml should be administered by pulse injection over 12 min. More recently t-PA has been used with encouraging results (42%, 12-month patency).

Venous aneurysms commonly occur with radiocephalic fistulae. They are often quite distressing for the patient and nephrologist but usually require no treatment provided the skin overlying the fistula is intact. These aneurysms usually remain stable for many years and provided the dialysis staff needle the fistula intelligently, never cause major problems. Very often when inexperienced surgeons are persuaded to 'plicate' the aneurysm, the patient loses a valuable access site.

Ischemia secondary to steal is a rare complication of radiocephalic fistulae, but, is a common complication of brachiocephalic fistulae, especially in diabetics, and is related to a progressive increase in fistula size, with reversal of flow in the distal radial artery. Patients complain of pain, paresthesiae and muscular weakness in the affected limb, with all symptoms getting worse on dialysis. Examining the limb will reveal a cool hand and loss of a radial pulse. If the ulnar artery is patent, ligating the distal radial artery will eliminate the 'steal'. In the situation where the ulnar artery is not patent, distal radial artery ligation should be performed in conjunction with a vein bypass graft from the proximal brachial artery to the ligated distal stump [28].

Signs and symptoms of digital ischemia develop in 1–9% of angioaccess cases including 'bridge' grafts. This is due to arterial steal because of preferential flow of blood through the hand arterial arcades into the low pressure venous limb of the access. In this situation arteriography is indicated and will almost always show a degree of arterial stenosis.

Ischemic monomelic neuropathy is a recently recognized complication characterized by sensory and motor nerve dysfunction in association with brachiocephalic fistulae or 'bridge' grafts originating from the brachial artery. Almost all patients are diabetic and the cause relates to pre-existing arterial disease, underlying neuropathy and an element of 'steal'. Diagnosis can be confirmed by nerve conduction studies. Treatment is proximal artery recanalization or fistula ligation.

Venous hypertension is a troublesome complication caused by proximal venous obstruction. With reversal of flow in the veins draining the hand or forearm, usually as a result of valvular incompetence, the affected limb becomes engorged, painful, hyperpigmented and ulcerated. Phlebography can confirm the diagnosis and treatment includes percutaneous radiographic stenting (Palmaz or Wallstent) with or without thrombolytic therapy, surgical bypass or fistula ligation.

Early complications of 'bridge' grafts include technical error related to inflow and outflow stenosis as well as early thrombosis occurring in the first three months. These complications account for about 15% of all bridge graft complications and to a large extent are technical in nature but may relate to poor selection or failure to detect pre-existing venous stenosis.

Hemorrhage and early thrombosis are both indications to return to the OR. If a subclavian vein thrombosis becomes evident after these grafts are performed then salvage should be attempted in the form of radiological subclavian vein stenting. If this is not possible it may be possible to explore the venous end of the graft in order to construct a jump graft to the internal jugular vein. Any form of surgical re-exploration is likely to increase the probability of infection. Infection usually results from contamination at the time of graft placement, direct inoculation at the time of needling or after pseudoaneurysm and haematoma formation on withdrawal of the needle. In the immediate postoperative period it is not unusual to develop erythema or sterile collections around the graft. These usually regress spontaneously. Most graft infections are by *Staphylococcus aureus* and the majority occur in the first six months postplacement. All grafts should be placed under cover of an appropriate antistaphylococcal antibiotic and established infections need aggressive treatment. Localized graft infection may be amenable to local excision and bypass [29] but systemic sepsis requires complete removal. Late thrombosis occurring after three months is most often related to neointimal hyperplasia and narrowing of the anastomosis or disruption of the neointima at needling sites with exposure of the thrombogenic surface. Management includes PTA, thrombolytic therapy or a combination of both. Endovascular stenting in more peripheral veins and across anastomoses is now becoming commonplace but the long-term outcome of these procedures is still awaited.

Surveillance

Almost all forms of angioaccess are prone to thrombosis which in turn leads to access failure. Few access sites will escape without an episode of thrombosis. Autogenous fistulae probably last twice as long as the PTFE 'bridge' grafts. Statistical projections suggest that all PTFE fistulae will have failed by 7.5 years whereas only half the autogenous fistulae will be non-functional over the same period of time [30].

Thrombosis is the leading cause of access dysfunction and failure. Early thrombosis is usually as a result of technical error, the use of inappropriate venous run-off, hypotension and bleeding with compression. Of more concern is the problem of late thrombosis. In 80% of instances, late HD access thrombosis results from venous obstruction or stenosis [31] (Figure 71.11). In most cases the stenosis is as a result of neointimal hyperplasia. This occurs at anastomotic sites in about half the cases and more proximally in the venous circulation, such as areas of venous bifurcation and previous sites of central venous cannulation, in the remaining 50%. 'Bridge' grafts are affected to a much greater extent than primary AV fistulae. Neointimal hyperplasia is the result of excessive intraluminal pressure, turbulent flow or calcification. Currently there are no methods for preventing the development of this condition. In the case of central vein stenoses, antecedent central vein cannulation is a significant contributing factor [32]. In about 20% of cases of access thrombosis no anatomical or structural abnormality can be found. In these instances one may find a

history of excessive postvenepunture pressure, hypercoagulability or postdialysis hypotension [33].

Vascular access infection accounts for another 20% of long-term complications. Most significant bacteremias in dialysis patients originate from their access sites. Poor personal hygiene, overlying dermatitis, improper or inappropriate cannulation by untrained staff, intravenous drug abuse or repeated difficult cannulation of a 'dysfunctional' access, as has been shown by recent data from Duke University, are all commonly associated with the problem.

The maintenance of adequate HD access is exceedingly important. It is now well recognized that complications of vascular access represent the most common cause of hospital admissions among dialysis patients. Because access failure in AVF and bridge grafts is mediated to a large extent by venous outflow stenosis, the ability to maintain patency and adequate flows as well as predict incipient thromboses in the access, improves patient well-being, prevents the need for repeated hospitalizations, reduces significantly the morbidity associated with complicated access and prevents the need for emergency interventions, all of which are extremely costly [34].

Prospective screening allows for early intervention prior to the occurrence of thrombosis. Early interventions have the potential to prolong the useful life of the access.

Methods of graft surveillance

Ideally the screening method should be non-invasive, be capable of accurately measuring blood flow, operator independent, relatively inexpensive and yield as much structural information as possible [13]. There is unfortunately no single method that fulfills these criteria, but a variety of methods are available to assess both fistula flow and structure (Table 71.1).

Sequential physical examinations are inadequate to detect impending thrombosis. By examination of a graft or fistula, a physician can detect persistent blood flow by the simple presence of a bruit or thrill but prospective data have confirmed that examination, even by an expe-

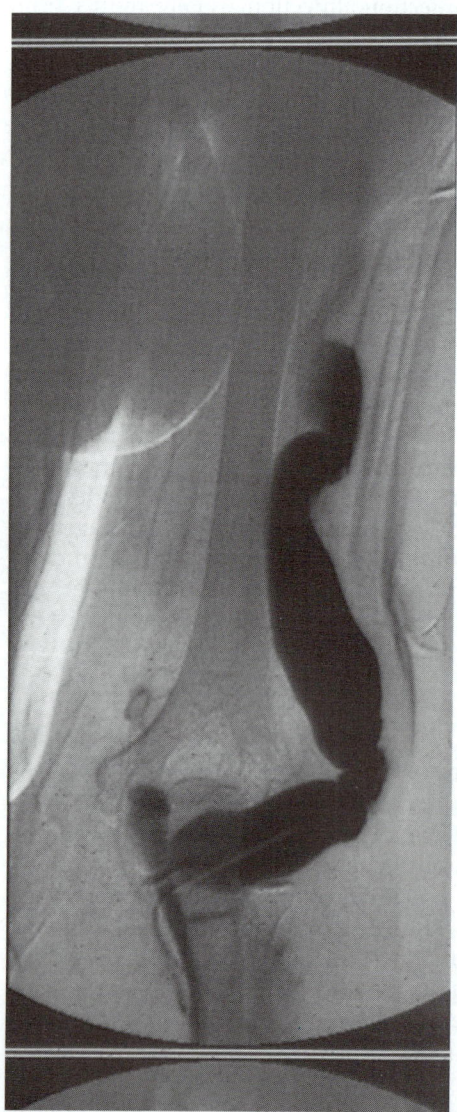

Figure 71.11 Fistulogram showing an ectatic left brachial fistula.

Table 71.1   Assessment of hemodialysis access

Flow
1. Electromagnetic flow probe
2. Duplex Doppler
3. Recirculation of dialysed blood (urea)
4. Indicator dilution methods

Structure
1. Angiography and Intra access pressure measurements
2. Duplex ultrasound
3. Venous dialyser pressure

rienced physician, cannot reliably predict impending complications.

Increased venous pressures and excessive recirculation, on the other hand, have been correlated to some extent with the presence of venous outflow stenosis [35].

Electromagnetic flow probes can be used intraoperatively. The probe is applied to the vessels and as the fluid conductor moves through the magnetic field an electrical potential is induced. By using this derived measurement the surgeon can ensure a fistula flow of 600–800 ml/min which will deliver more than 300–400 ml/min to the artificial kidney.

Duplex Doppler is available in most centers involved in HD and transplantation and is the authors' preferred method of surveillance. Low flow, recirculation venous hypertension, aneurysm formation and ischemic problems can be easily evaluated using B-mode imaging and Doppler analysis. The attractive feature of duplex Doppler is its non-invasiveness. The very obvious drawback is initial cost of the 'state of the art' machine, such as power Doppler. There is unfortunately a problem with operator variability and uncertainty about reproducibility as a result of difficulty with interpretation in the face of turbulent flow which one often sees in AVFs. Having said that, in terms of surveillance, the total number of stenoses in a fistula circuit can be determined by an experienced ultrasonographer. In addition, measuring the peak systolic velocity (PSV) in the brachial artery and the PSV brachial artery index with and without compression of the fistula can give valuable information about impending access failure. With the newer color Doppler flow probes, fistula volume and flow can be determined with an accuracy of 93%. As a rough guide, most PTFE grafts have flows of 1000 ml/min as opposed to the 500 ml/min seen in most brachiocephalic AVFs [36]. Certainly flow rates of under 400 ml/min, irrespective of which form of access is being used, are associated with thrombosis [37].

Venous dialyzer pressure (VDP) is very useful in routine monitoring of fistula function. This can be done by measuring the pressure in the venous return line of the dialyzer circuit. Although VDP varies depending on the rate of extracorporeal blood flow, compliance of the needles and tubing, as well as the type of access (location and configuration), these variables can be minimized by the protocol shown in Table 71.2 [31]. Elevation of the VDP usually indicates fistula venous outflow stenosis [35]. Dynamic VDP measured at blood flows of 200 ml/min requires no specialized equipment and has been shown to be reliable and predictive. Some investigators have found 'static' VDP to be more predictive, but at present measuring VDP at 0 ml/min requires specialized equipment which is costly. Although the dynamic method as described by Schwab is an indirect measure of access blood flow, three prospective trails have shown that repeated VDP measurements, followed by early intervention, be it radiological or surgical, is a valuable method of maintaining access patency.

Recirculation of dialyzed blood through the extracorporeal circuit reduces effective urea clearance. Increased recirculation can occur for many reasons, but its measurement provides an accurate means of identifying venous stenosis. The most common method for estimating recirculation uses the measurement of blood urea nitrogen (BUN) in simultaneous blood samples taken from the inflow (arterial) and outflow (venous) lines as well as a sample most representative of systemic blood flow into the fistula before dilution by recirculated blood.

$$\text{Recirculation \%} = (\text{peripheral BUN} - \text{inflow BUN}) / (\text{peripheral BUN} - \text{outflow BUN}) \times 100$$

The traditional three-needle method uses a peripheral vein from the contralateral arm to represent systemic blood and overestimates recirculation [38]. As a result a two-needle 'stop-flow' method, which uses a second inflow line sample and slows the pump speed to 50–100 ml/min or stops the pump completely for 30 s, appears to reflect true recirculation [13]. Although this method is used by many centers it has been found to be time consuming and often inaccurate.

The Transonic HD monitor is a clip-on flow/dilution sensor that clips onto the dialyzer tubing, one for the venous line and another for the arterial line. In simple terms, following a bolus injection of isotonic saline, it applies the Fick principle to determine the flow parameters and inferred recirculation. It provides an alternative to the urea method but is not widely used.

There is as yet no consensus as to what percentage recirculation indicates a significant stenosis, but it ranges from 10% to 20%. Recirculation must always be considered in relation to pump speed. A good rule of thumb is that 10% recirculation at a pump speed of 200–300 ml/min, or 15% recirculation at a pump speed of 400 ml/min indicates the possibility of an underlying

Table 71.2 Venous dialysis pressure (VDP) monitoring protocol

Conventional dialysis
1. Cannulate the fistula with a 16-gauge needle
2. Measure the VDP at flows of: 200–225 ml/min during the first 30 min of dialysis
3. If VDP >150 mmHg for three consecutive dialysis sessions, proceed to fistulogram followed by percutaneous transluminal angioplasty (PTA) or surgical revision if needed.
4. For high efficiency dialysis, use a 15-gauge needle, measure VDP for 10 min at a flow of 200 ml/min and if VDP >100 mmHg on three separate occasions, proceed to fistulogram followed by PTA or surgical revision in needed

stenosis. Certainly anything greater than 20% at 400 ml/min is almost always associated with an outflow stenosis [39]. Very often, attempting surgical revision of an 'upstream' venous stenosis fails to provide the desired results. PTA has become the first method of correcting upstream venous stenoses and the best results are achieved when PTA is used as early as possible [27, 40]. It follows therefore that outflow problems need to be screened for before clinical problems arise. Ideally Doppler studies should be undertaken on a regular basis

and venous dialyzer pressure increases may give early warning of trouble between routine tests.

Ensuring efficient and effective dialysis relies on good access. As has been shown this requires a dedicated team of specialists who are committed, experienced and enthusiastic. Well-planned surgery, good postoperative monitoring and aggressive screening can give rise to a well dialyzed patient group who are eminently transplantable and in addition reduce dialysis work load and overall health care costs.

References

1. Quinton, W., Dillard, D. and Scribner, B.H. (1960) Cannulation of blood vessels for prolonged hemodialysis. *ASAIO*, **6**, 104.
2. Brescia, M.J., Cimino, J.E., Appel, K. *et al.* (1966) Chronic haemodialysis using venepuncture and a surgically created arteriovenous fistula. *N. Engl. J. Med.*, **275**, 1089–92.
3. Down, R. (1991) Surveillance of angioaccess shunt function, in *Current Therapy in Vascular Surgery* (eds C.B. Ernst and J.C. Stanley), B.C. Decker, pp. 932–4.
4. Shusterman, N., Kloss, K. and Mullen, J. (1989) Successful use of double lumen silicone rubber catheters for permanent hemodialysis. *Kidney Int.*, **35**, 887–90.
5. Kinnart, P., Vereerstraeten, P., Toussaint, C. *et al.* (1977) Nine years experience with internal arteriovenous fistulae for hemodialysis; a study of some factors influencing the results. *Br. J. Surg.*, **64**, 242–6.
6. Reilly, D.T., Wood, R. and Bell, P.R.F. (1982) Prospective study of dialysis fistulae; problem patients and their treatment. *Br. J. Surg.*, **69**, 549–53.
7. Schumann, E.S., Gross, G.F., Hayes, J.F. *et al.* (1988) Long term patency of PTFE graft fistula. *Am. J. Surg.*, **155**, 644–6.
8. Barrett, N., Spenar, J., McIvor, J. and Brown, E.A. (1988) Subclavian stenosis; a major complication of subclavian dialysis catheters. *Nephrol. Dial. Transplant.*, **3**, 423–5.
9. Arrieta, J., De Blas, M., Merino, S. and Olivar, E. (1994) Central vein stenosis affecting arterio venous fistula function. Correction with a self expanding IV stent. *Nephrol. Dial. Transplant.*, **9**, 192–5.
10. Marx, A.B., Landmann, J. and Harder, F.H. (1990) Surgery for vascular access. *Curr. Probl. Surg.*, **27**, 1.
11. Bonalumi, D., Givalleri, D., Ronida, S. *et al.* (1982) Nine years experience with end to end arteriovenous fistulae at the anatomical snuffbox for maintenance hemodialysis. *Br. J. Surg.*, **69**, 486–8.
12. Haimov, M. (1991) Direct arteriovenous anastomsis for angioaccess, in *Current Therapy in Vascular Surgery* (eds C.B. Ernst and J.C. Stanley), B.C. Decker, pp. 922–6.
13. Windus, D. (1993) Permanent vascular access; a nephrologist's view. *Am. J. Kidney Dis.*, **21**, 457–71.
14. Haimov, M., Baez, A. and Neff, M. (1975) Complications of arteriovenous fistulae for hemodialysis. *Arch. Surg.*, **110**, 708–12.
15. Anderson, C.B., Etheredge, E.E., Harter, H.R. *et al.* (1977) Local blood flow characteristics of arteriovenous fistulas in the forearm for dialysis. *Surg. Gynecol. Obstet.*, **144**, 531.
16. Kirsch, W.M., Zhu, Y.H., Hasdesty, R.A. *et al.* (1993) The nonpenetrating Arcuate-Legged Clip; clinical applications, in *Color Atlas of Microsurgery* (ed. S. Lee), IEA Publishers, St Louis, Chapter 12.
17. Girandet, R.E., Hackett, R.E., Goodwin, N.J. and Friedman, E.A. (1970) Thirteen months experience with the saphenous vein graft arteriovenous fistula for maintenance hemodialysis. *Trans. Am. Soc. Artif. Intern. Organs.*, **16**, 285.
18. Bone, G.E. and Pomajzl, M.J. (1980) Prospective comparison of polytetrafluoroethylene and bovine grafts for dialysis. *J. Surg. Res.*, **29**, 223.
19. Bartlett, S.T., Schweitzer, E.J., Roberts, J.E. *et al.* (1995) Early experience with a new PTFE vascular prosthesis for hemodialysis. *Am. J. Surg.*, **170**, 118–22.
20. Hinsdale, J.C., Lipkowitz, G.S. and Hoover, E.L. (1985) Vascular access for hemodialysis in the elderly: results and perspectives in a geriatric population. *Dial. Transplant.*, **14**, 560.
21. Munda, R., First, M.R., Alexander, J.W. *et al.* (1983) Polytetrafluoroethylene graft survival in hemodialysis. *JAMA*, **249**, 219.
22. Morgan, A.P., Knight, D.C., Tilney, N.L. and Lazarus, J.M. (1980) Femoral triangle sepsis in dialysis patients: frequency, management and outcome. *Ann. Surg.*, **191**, 460.
23. Lockwood, A.H. (1984) Percutaneous subclavian vein catheterization. Too much of a good thing? *Arch. Intern. Med.*, **144**, 1407–8.
24. Rockall, A., Harris, D., Taube, D. *et al.* (1996) Stripping of failing hemodialysis catheters using the amplatz gooseneck snare. (abstract) *Angioaccess for Hemodialysis*, Tours.
25. Ballard, J.L., Bunt, T.J. and Malone, J. (1992) Major complications of angioaccess surgery. *Am. J. Surg.*, **164**, 229–32.
26. Brotman, D.N., Fandos, L., Faust, G.R. *et al.* (1994) Hemodialysis graft salvage. *J. Am. Coll. Surg.*, **178**, 431–4.
27. Beathard, G. (1992) Percutaneous transluminal angioplasty in the treatment of vascular access stenosis. *Kidney Int.*, **42**, 1390–6.
28. Schanzer, H., Schwartz, M., Harrington, E. *et al.* (1988) Treatment of ischemia due to 'steal' by arteriovenous fistulae with distal artery ligation and revascularization. *J. Vasc. Surg.*, **7**, 770–3.

29. McKenna, P.J. and Leadbetter, M.G. (1988) Salvage of chronically exposed Gortex vascular access graft in the hemodialysis patient. *Plast. Reconstr. Surg.*, **82**, 1046.

30. Kjerlakian, G.M., Roedersheimr, L.R., Arbaugh, J.J. *et al.* (1986) Comparison of autogenous fistulae versus ePTFE graft fistulae for angioaccess in hemodialysis. *Am. J. Surg.*, **152**, 238–43.

31. Schwab, S.J., Raymond, J.R., Saeed, M. *et al.* (1989) Prevention of hemodialysis fistula thrombosis and early detection of venous stenosis. *Kidney Int.*, **36**, 707–11.

32. Schwab, S.J., Quarles, L.D., Middleton, J.P. *et al.* (1988) Hemodialysis associated subclavian vein stenosis. *Kidney Int.*, **33**, 1156–9.

33. Schwab, S.J. (1990) Hemodialysis vascular access, in *The Principles and Practice of Nephrology* (eds H. Jacobson, G. Striker and S. Klahr), Philadelphia, pp. 769–72.

34. Sands, J., Young, S. and Miranda, G. (1992) The effect of doppler flow screening studies and elective revisions in dialysis access failure. *ASAIO*, **38**, M524–7.

35. Schwab, S.J. (1994) Assessing the adequacy of vascular access and its relationship to patient outcome. *Am. J. Kidney Dis.*, **24**, 316–20.

36. Tordoir, J.H.M., Hoenveld, H., Eikelboom, B.C. and Kitslaar, J.E.H.M. (1990) The correlation between clinical and duplex ultrasound parameters and the development of complications in arteriovenous fistulae for hemodialysis. *Eur. J. Vasc. surg.*, **4**, 179–84.

37. Strauch, B.S., O'Connell, R.S., Geoly, K.L. *et al.* (1992) Forecasting thrombosis of vascular access with doppler color flow imaging. *Am. J. Kidney Dis.*, **19**, 554–7.

38. Sherman, R.A. (1991) Recirculation revisited. *Semin. Dial.*, **4**, 221–3.

39. Collins, D.M., Lambert, M.B., Middleton, J.P. *et al.* (1992) Fistula dysfunction: effect on rapid hemodialysis. *Kidney Int.*, **41**, 1292–6.

40. Schwab., S.J., Saeed, M., Sussman, S.K. *et al.* (1987) Transluminal angioplasty of venous stenoses in PTFE vascular access grafts. *Kidney Int.*, **32**, 395–8.

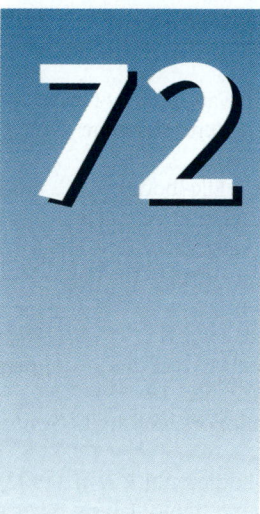

72

The technology and biocompatibility of renal replacement therapy

Nicholas Andrew Hoenich

Introduction

Renal replacement therapy is initiated when a substantial or total loss of ability of the human kidneys to remove water, excrete metabolic waste products or maintain body homeostasis occurs. The most commonly used method of treatment of renal failure is hemodialysis, which involves passing the patient's blood through an artificial kidney or hemodialyzer containing a semipermeable membrane. Blood flows on one side of the membrane, the other side of which is bathed by a dilute electrolyte solution (dialysis fluid). The processes occurring within the hemodialyzer may be summarized as follows.

1   Equilibration of the blood and dialysis fluid electrolyte composition.
2   The elimination of metabolites elevated as a consequence of renal insufficiency by the diffusion into the dialysis fluid. Convective mass transport occurs in the hemodialyzer and contributes to the overall solute removal.
3   The removal of water from the plasma, thence from the body by ultrafiltration under the influence of a hydrostatic pressure difference between the blood and the dialysis fluid. The hydrostatic pressure gradient is generally supplemented by an osmotic pressure gradient induced by the inclusion of 100–200 mg/dl [1] glucose in the dialysis fluid.

Irreversible or chronic renal failure is generally treated intermittently twice or three times weekly. Acute renal failure may be treated intermittently, or continously over a period of several days. A further subdivision of these modes may be made with respect to the mode of solute transport – diffusive or convective.

Techniques of renal replacement therapy

Intermittent therapies

Hemodialysis and related therapies

Although classical hemodialysis remains the most widely used intermittent renal replacement therapy, since the 1980s a number of developments relating to equipment and disposable items have occurred and led to the clinical application of modified techniques that retain their reliance on a hemodialyzer. Two of the most commonly used variants are high efficiency hemodialysis, a technique offering enhanced diffusive solute transport and high flux dialysis. The device used for high efficiency hemodialysis is a hemodialyzer containing conventional low flux membranes with a large ($>1.5\,m^2$) surface area, coupled with high blood and dialysate flow rates. High flux hemodialysis, uses hemodialyzers with high perme-

Nephrology, Edited by Rex L. Jamison and Robert Wilkinson.
Published in 1997 by Chapman & Hall, London. ISBN 0 412 60930 4

ability membranes which, when used in conjunction with high blood and dialysis fluid flow rates, offer enhanced diffusive and convective solute transport.

Hemofiltration and related therapies

Hemofiltration as a technique of renal replacement therapy was first described in the late 1960s. In hemofiltration the metabolites are removed by convection alone. The convective mass transport is by ultrafiltration with simultaneous replacement of the fluid removed by a substitution fluid whose composition is comparable to that of plasma fluid. The process takes place in a device containing a highly permeable membrane, but unlike a conventional high flux hemodialyzer, the device does not have any dialysate inlet and outlet ports and thus no dialyis fluid is passed through the device. The sterile and pyrogen-free fluid may be added to the blood either before (pre) or after (post) the filter, the latter being by far the more common. The total volume of exchange during treatment, whose duration is comparable to that used in conventional hemodialysis is 20–40 liters.

Hemofiltration utilizes a blood circuit which is similar to that used for hemodialysis, but in place of the dialysis circuit, a special circuit to balance fluid removed with that infused is used. The circuit incorporates electronic strain gauges or scales linked to a microprocessor and is fully programmable. It provides continuous information about the rates of exchange during treatment, monitors for system safety and automatically primes the circuit prior to the initiation of treatment. The integrity of the membrane used during the treatment is continuously monitored by the incorporation of a blood leak detector into the ultrafiltrate circuit (Figure 72.1).

A major drawback of hemofiltration is its low efficiency in removing low molecular weight solutes such as urea compared to hemodialysis. In 1981 Henderson [2] predicted that hemofiltration would be abandoned as a separate technique and instead be linked with conventional diffusion-based dialysis. Indeed this has occurred and the combined processes are known as hemodiafiltration.

Hemodiafiltration retains the advantage of hemofiltration, in that it offers high convective mass transport, a technique favoring the removal of intermediate molecular weight solutes (300–30 000 daltons) and combines it with rapid removal solutes below this molecular weight range. Hemodiafiltration is generally performed using a dialyser used for high flux dialysis, but the fluid removal rates are higher than during conventional dialysis. A substitution fluid is continuously infused to compensate for fluid removal in excess of the intradialytic weight gain. Early hemodiafiltration methods used acetate-buffered dialysis fluid and lactate substitution fluid. Treatment lasted 180 min and 9–12 liters of fluid were exchanged during the treatment. Current techniques incorporate a number of refinements: blood flow is 300–400 ml/min, the dialysate has bicarbonate as the buffer, flows at 500 ml/min or higher, and the volume of replacement fluid is 6–15 l. The replacement fluid may be produced on line, and is usually infused into the extracorporeal circuit after the hemodiafilter. A variant of the technique used widely in Europe is paired filtration dialysis (PFD) which is performed using a small hemofilter and dialyser in series. Both devices are incorporated into a single housing. The ultrafiltration solute removal takes place in the ultrafilter and the replacement fluid is infused prior to the blood entering the dialyser. An advantage of PFD is the availability of pure ultrafiltrate for on-line biochemical monitoring. Hemodiafiltration and PFD must be undertaken in conjunction with a proportioning system that has an ultrafiltration control system to ensure an accurate balance between fluid removed and fluid infused during treatment. The infusion system normally utilizes a pump to infuse replacement fluid, this is linked to a gravimetric control system. The pump and the gravimetric control system are connected to the blood module for safety.

Continuous therapies

Continuous therapies are widely used in the treatment of acute renal failure [3, 4]. A variety are in clinical use (Figure 72.2), are well tolerated hemodynamically, offer

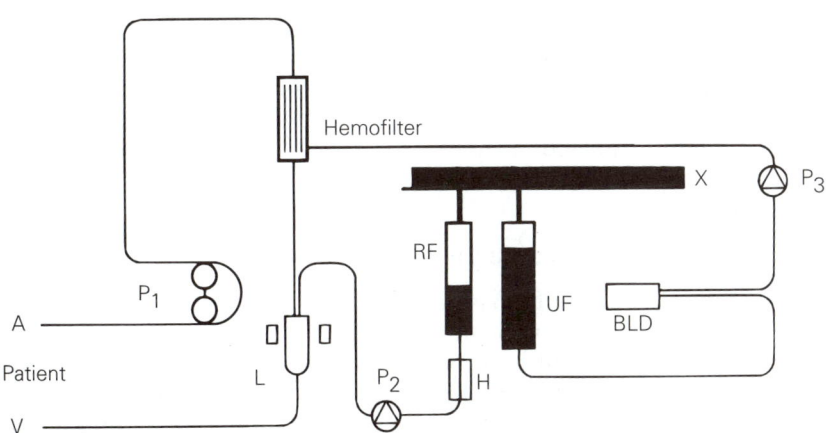

Figure 72.1 Schematic diagram of a gravimetrically controlled hemofiltration system. A, arterial access; V, venous access; L, level detector in blood circuit; P_{123}, pumps; RF, replacement fluid; UF, ultrafiltrate; H, heater; X, microprocessor-controlled gravimetric system; BLD, blood leak detector.

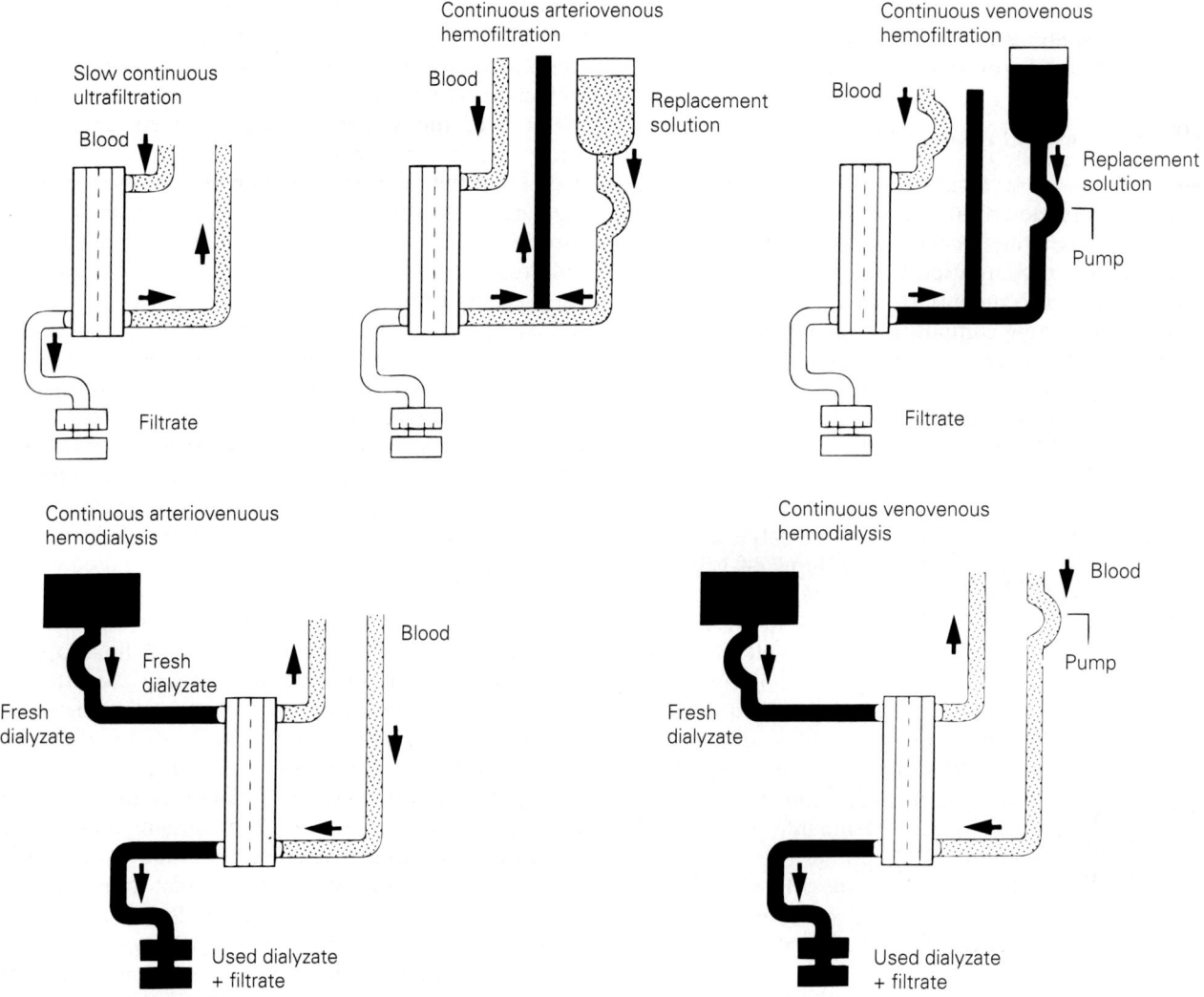

Figure 72.2 Continuous renal replacement therapies.

improved control of electrolyte and acid–base balance compared to conventional hemodialysis and are highly effective in fluid removal.

Slow continuous hemofiltration

Slow continuous hemofiltration may be undertaken using a pump to facilitate flow through the extracorporeal circuit. Access to the patient's circulation may be either via two veins, as in continuous venovenous hemofiltration (CVVH) or via an artery and a vein as in continuous arteriovenous hemofiltration (CAVH). The blood from the patient passes through a small hemofilter. The fluid removal rate may be controlled by gravity. The filtrate outflow is connected to a drainage bag. The position of the drainage bag relative to the filter determines the rate of filtration. Alternately a pump may be used in the drain line. The replacement fluid is normally pumped into the extracorporeal circuit after the filter (postdilution).

Unassisted blood flow rates through the filter (100–150 ml/min) are capable of delivering filtration rates of 3–6 l/day, if higher filtration rates are required then both blood and filtrate circuits should include pumps. The technique may also be used without replacement fluid infusion (slow continuous ultrafiltration, SCUF). In order to ensure optimal safety during processes utilizing pumps they should be performed with the extracorporeal circuit incorporating an air and level detector, alternately a blood module of a single patient proportioning system may be used.

Slow continuous hemodialysis

In continuous hemofiltration, the solute removal is governed by the filtration rate. To increase removal of small molecules, hemodialysis has been combined with continuous hemofiltration, (CVVH(D) or CAVH(D)). This is similar to CAVH or CVVH, but uses a small surface area

(0.5 m²) flat plate or hollow fiber dialyzer. Blood passes through the dialyser in the usual manner, but on the dialysate side fluid, commonly peritoneal dialysis solution flows assisted by a pump at a rate of 1–2 l/h depending on clinical requirements in a countercurrent manner. At this rate the dialysis fluid, becomes completely saturated with low-molecular-weight solutes, thus enhancing the clearance rate of small molecules. A second pump is linked to the dialyzate outflow and is used to increase transmembrane pressure and maintain the flow in the circuit. The required ultrafiltration rate is simply set as the difference between the inflow and outflow rates.

Water quality and treatment for renal replacement therapy

Large volumes or water are used during hemodialysis therapy. A patient receiving a 3 h treatment is exposed to 90 l of water. Although theoretically it is possible for the water used in the preparation of the dialysis fluid to be of sufficient quality as to be suitable for hemodialysis, in practice the water requires treatment to remove waterborne contaminants that would otherwise diffuse across the semipermeable membrane in the hemodialyzer. Contaminants include dissolved inorganic and organic molecules, heavy metals, bacteria and pyrogens. The quality of water used in hemodialysis and hemodiafiltration is subject to International Standards. The acceptable maximum levels of impurities are shown in Table 72.1.

Treated water may be used for dialysis in a number of different ways: preparation of acetate or bicarbonate dialysis fluid for conventional hemodialyzers, preparation of dialysis fluid for high flux hemodialyzers and to rinse dialyzers that are reused. The application together with the quality of the feed water will determine the type of water treatment required. To achieve the quality of water as defined in the International Standard it is necessary to combine several different techniques.

Filtration

Filtration is a method of removing particulate matter from the feed water prior to treatment by other methods. Activated carbon filtration is suitable for the removal of organic chemicals especially chlorine or chloramine, used as a substitute for chlorine in municipal water treatment plants, because chlorine interacts with organic compounds to form trihalomethanes that are carcinogenic. The carbon filter can release fine carbon particles which must be removed to prevent fouling of equipment downstream. The microporous nature of the carbon filters with its affinity for organic water contaminants can also result in bacterial contamination.

Microporous filtration is another technique of which there are two variants – depth and screen. Filters for depth filtration consist of matted fibers or materials compressed to form a matrix that retain particulate matter by adsorption or entrapment. They are normally used as pretreatment filters since they are effective in the removal of 98% or more of the suspended solids. Screen filters have uniform pores that retain on their surface all particles larger than the pore size. Screen filters are the last point of a water treatment system to collect all remaining particulate matter such as resin fragments, carbon or colloidal particles.

Distillation

Distillation is the oldest method of water treatment. It is inefficient in terms of energy use and requires careful maintenance to ensure optimum water purity, since some of the impurities may be carried over to the condensate. For these reasons it is rarely used.

Ion exchange

In ion exchange, water percolates through a bed of resin, normally in the form of spherical beads, exchanging anions and cations for anions or cations fixed to the beads. The basic concept of this process is that exchange is with ions of the same charge. The exchange capacity is limited by the quantity of ions attached to the resin. During operation of such systems the supply of ions is gradually reduced and when the resin is exhausted it requires regeneration. Deionizers remove both cations and anions releasing hydrogen ions (H^+) for the former and hydroxyl ions (OH^-) for the latter. The exchange resins are usually made from styrene and divinylbenzene containing sulfonic acid groups for cation quaternary ammonium groups for anion exchange. The resins may be packed in separate or in mixed beds.

Deionizers provide high quality water but they do not remove bacteria or endotoxin. For this reason it is prudent to use such systems in combination with other methods of water treatment that remove bacteria and endotoxin Water softeners are ion exchangers which use only a cationic resin that exchanges sodium ions for calcium, magnesium and other polyvalent ions present in the water. During the softening process sodium levels in the water are increased in proportion to the amount of calcium and magnesium removed. This increase can have implications in respect of the final water quality or the performance of the treatment system situated downstream of the softener.

Reverse osmosis

Reverse osmosis is a membrane separation process and forms the heart of most water treatment plants used to provide water for renal replacement therapy (Figure 72.3). In osmosis a semipermeable membrane separates a dilute solution from a concentrated one, solvent crosses from the less-concentrated side to the more-concentrated side

Table 72.1 Maximum acceptable water impurities in water used in dialysis

	Maximum admissible or permitted concentration in potable water (mg/l)[a,b]	Maximum acceptable concentration for water used in the production of dialysis fluid (mg/l)	Signs or symptoms associated with excessive levels
Aluminum	0.20	0.01	Anemia, osteomalacia, neurological deterioration
Ammonium	0.5	0.2	
Arsenic	0.05	0.005	
Barium	1[c]	0.1	
Cadmium	0.005	0.001	
Calcium	250[c]	2 (0.05 mmol/l)	Hard water syndrome,
Chloramines		0.1	Anemia, hemolysis
Chlorine		0.5	
Chromium	0.05	0.014	
Copper	3	0.1	Anemia, hemolysis, nausea, vomiting, liver damage
Fluoride	1.5	0.2	Osteomalacia
Lead	0.05	0.005	Neurological deterioration
Magnesium	50	2 (0.08 mmol/l)	
Mercury	0.001	0.0002	
Nitrate	50	2	Methemoglobinemia, nausea, vomiting
Potassium	12 (0.3 mmol/l)	2 (0.05 mmol/l)	
Selenium	0.01	0.09	
Silver	0.01[d]	0.005	
Sodium	150	50 (2 mmol/l)	Hypertension, excessive thirst
Sulfate	250	100	Metabolic acidosis, nausea, vomiting
Tin		0.1	Neurological complications
Zinc	5	0.1	Anemia

[a] mg/l and parts per million (ppm) are equivalent.
[b] As specified in EC Drinking Water Directive (1980) and the United Kingdom Water Supply (Water Quality) Regulations (1989).
[c] Compliance based on 12-month average.
[d] If silver is used in the water treatment the maximum permissible level is 8 times that shown.

of the membrane. This flow can be prevented by the application of a hydrostatic pressure to the concentrated solution side. If the applied pressure is equal to the osmotic pressure then no flow will occur, if however the pressure is greater than the osmotic pressure flow in the reverse direction will occur (reverse osmosis). In reverse osmosis treatment plants the feed water is pressurized on one side of the membrane. If this pressure is high enough and the membrane permeable to water but impermeable to the impurities contained then pure water crosses the membrane. With time there will be an accumulation of impurities on the membrane which reduce its efficiency, until the membrane is completely fouled by the rejected impurities. The incoming water must therefore be sufficiently low in impurities to minimize these problems. To maximize the life of the membrane reverse

osmosis systems are generally operated so that only a portion of the feed water passes through the membrane, with the remainder going directly to waste.

The membranes used in reverse osmosis units may be spirally wound, or in the form of hollow fibers. Both configurations are inside cylindrical pressure vessels to withstand the high operating pressures (200–400 psi). In the former the membrane is normally attached to a woven fabric screen wound around a perforated central hollow core. A plastic mesh separates adjacent layers of the membrane fabric sandwich.

Several different types of membrane manufactured from cellulose or synthetic copolymers are available for reverse osmosis. The membranes must withstand high operating pressures, tolerate a wide range of pH and temperatures and resist bacterial attack.

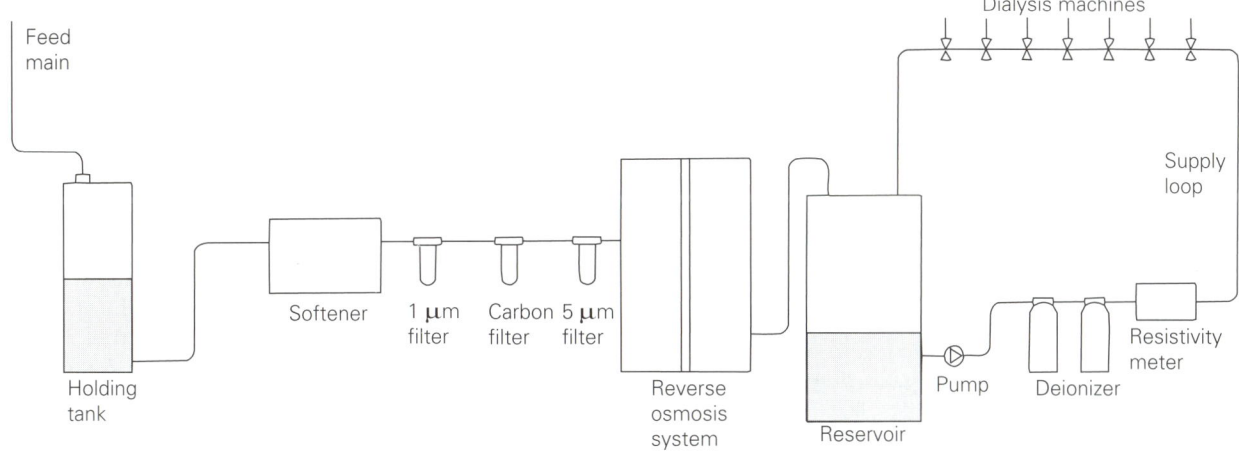

Figure 72.3 Schematic diagram of water-treatment plant used in renal units.

Distribution systems for water used in renal replacement therapy

The design of distribution systems to deliver water to the bedside is often neglected. The system must sustain the chemical and microbiological quality of the treated water and satisfy the requirements of the proportioning systems used.

The construction material, should not degrade the chemical quality of the water, and should not contain brass, copper, aluminum or galvanized metal. Stainless steel is preferable and should resist chemicals used to clean and disinfect the system. To minimize bacterial colonization or the formation of biofilm the flow velocities in the system should exceed 1.5 ft/s (0.45 m/s).

Dialysis fluid production and supply

Dialysis fluid is produced by the mixing of electrolytes and glucose with the treated water to remove by diffusion the metabolites elevated in renal insufficiency. The composition of the concentrate used may vary depending on clinical requirements or preference and the proportioning pumps used. Batch production of dialysis fluid has now largely been replaced by single patient proportioning systems which mix the concentrate with treated water and form part of the dialysate delivery and patient monitoring systems. The concentrates are generally categorized according to whether acetate or bicarbonate is the buffer. Single patient proportioning systems required a switch to acetate. Technological advances in proportioning systems, the introduction of high efficiency dialysis strategies and the clinical problems associated with excessive acetate loading dictated the return to bicarbonate buffering. In 1989, 39% of the patients in Europe were treated with bicarbonate dialysis, by 1991, the proportion

had grown to 54.8% [5]. To produce acetate-buffered dialysis fluid a concentrate containing all the chemical constituents is used and diluted 1:35 with the treated water, although other proportioning ratios may be used. The production of bicarbonate buffered dialysis fluid requires two concentrates, one containing sodium bicarbonate with some sodium chloride (B concentrate), the other containing the remaining constituents and acetic acid to permit adjustment of the final pH (A concentrate). The use of two concentrates is necessary to minimize the formation of calcium and magnesium carbonate. The proportioning ratio depends on the system used. Commonly used proportioning ratios are 1:35, 1:36.8 and 1:45.

Both the acetate concentrate and the acid concentrate in bicarbonate dialysis have a high salt content; this prevents bacterial growth. The acid concentrate also has a low pH. The bicarbonate concentrate has a high pH ($\approx$8) and a low salt content both of which are favorable for bacterial colonization and growth within a few days after production [6]. This has led to the requirement for sterile manufacturing of the bicarbonate concentrate or the use of bicarbonate powder. The powder may be in the form of sachets that are added to treated water just prior to dialysis or in the form of a cartridge (BiCart Gambro Ab, Sweden) which is attached to the dialysis machine. Warm degassed water from the proportioning system passes through the cartridge to produce a saturated bicarbonate solution which is then proportioned by a pump and mixed with the acid concentrate. This approach minimizes handling and eliminates bacterial contamination.

Although the use of acetate buffered dialysis fluid has declined it is still used in acetate-free biofiltration (AFB), a special form of hemodiafiltration first described by Granger and Vlchek [7]. The dialysis fluid does not contain any base buffer. The base buffer is infused into the patient via the replacement fluid which consists of sodium chloride to which bicarbonate (167 mEq/l) has been added.

Dialysate supply systems may be recirculating, recirculating single pass or single pass. Recirculating systems were originally developed for coil dialyzers and consisted of a stainless-steel tank containing 120–240 l of dialysis

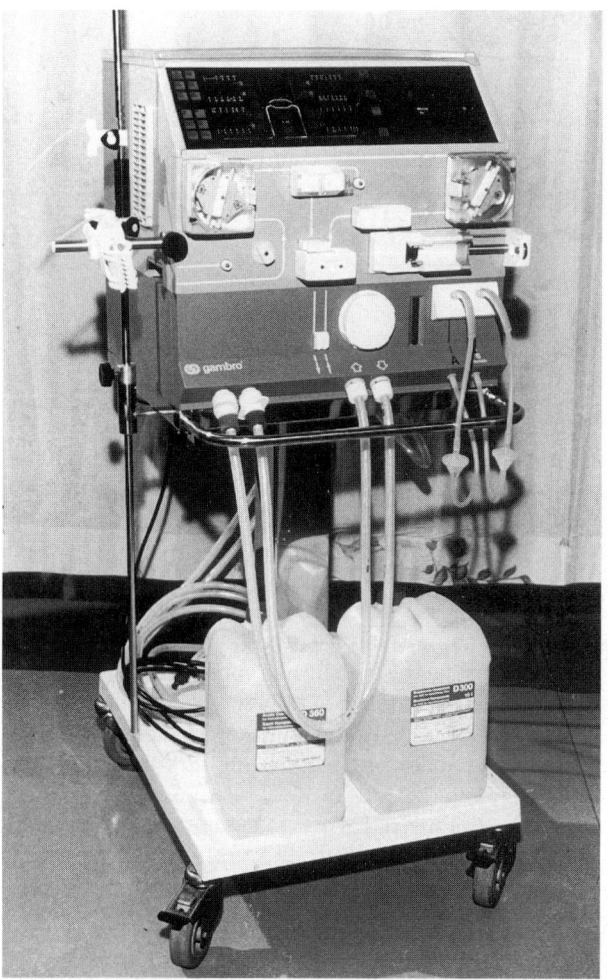

Figure 72.4 The Gambro AK 100, a microprocesor-controlled single patient proportioning and monitoring system.

fluid which was heated and continuously recirculated through the dialyzer. Although no longer in clinical use, a variant of such systems still used today is the REDY sorbent dialysis system, in which 6 l of dialysis solution are recirculated through a sorbent cartridge consisting of layers of activated carbon, urease, zirconium phosphate, hydrated zirconium phosphate and activated carbon. Dialysis fluid is recirculated via a reservoir through the dialyser and back to the reservoir via the cartridge at a rate of 200–250 ml/min. Metabolic waste products in the dialysis fluid are adsorbed, or exchanged for sodium hydrogen bicarbonate and acetate. As the cartridge removes all potassium, magnesium and calcium from the dialysis fluid these are reinfused into the reservoir during use. The REDY system is not used for extended periods due to the comparatively high cost of the cartridge and the low efficiency of small molecular solute removal. The system is especially suitable for the treatment of renal failure in situations in which normal infrastructure for treatment is absent, e.g. holiday dialysis or the treatment of renal failure under field conditions.

A variant of the pure recirculating system that remained in use until the 1970s was the recirculating single pass system in which the dialyzer was supplied with dialysis fluid from a small 4–8 l tank, with fresh dialysis fluid from a larger reservoir being continuously added to the tank, and an identical volume containing the metabolites removed during passage through the dialyzer flowing to waste. Although intended for use with coil hemodialyzers, this system was also used with parallel plate devices. Today the most widely used system is single pass in which dialysis fluid passes through the dialyzer and thence to waste. Although these systems are primarily for single patient use, systems for multiple patient use are in existence. The newer supply systems make extensive use of microprocessor technology (Figure 72.4), liquid crystal or cathode ray displays that are touch sensitive (Figure 72.5). A schematic diagram of the elements involved is shown in Figure 72.6. In general, the system performs two principal functions, it facilitates flow in the

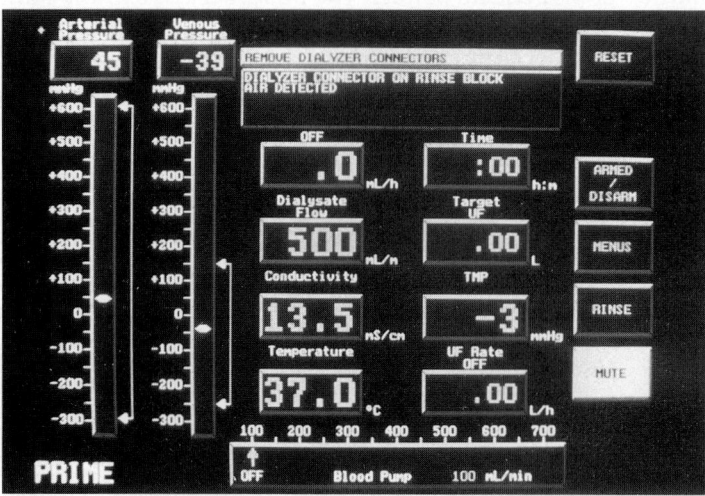

Figure 72.5 The touch-sensitive control panel and display of the Althin DrakeWillock 1000 single patient proportionating system.

extracorporeal circuit, and it produces dialysis fluid at the correct temperature and ionic concentration. During a passage of the dialysis fluid through the dialyzer or associated device the system also controls the rate of fluid removal (ultrafiltration). These functions are interlinked and combined with a series of safety monitors incorporated in the system to ensure that in the event of a malfunction the patient is not placed at risk (fail safe operation).

Access to circulation

External arteriovenous shunts were the foundation of regular dialysis therapy. Their routine use has, however, declined and today they are used predominantly to provide temporary access for acute renal failure treatment. Access to the circulation for end-stage renal disease is provided by the arteriovenous fistula. In older patients and those who have been receiving treatment for several years the peripheral vasculature may become unsuitable, and cardiovascular disease may also worsen due to the strain imposed by the arteriovenous anastomosis, necessitating the use of alternate methods of access. Subclavian or femoral catheterization can provide short-term alter-

natives for such patients and may also be used for the provision of access for the treatment of acute renal failure, whereas surgically inserted central venous catheters are a highly satisfactory method of providing circulatory access for patients requiring long-term access in whom the construction or use of an arteriovenous fistula is not practical.

Technology of access devices

Catheters or needles used for access to the circulation may be either single or multiple lumen. The flow and pressure relationships for such devices can be derived from classical physics.

Hemodialysis catheters differ from those used as intravenous catheters in their size and design. To facilitate high flow and minimize flow resistance they incorporate side holes and generally include a suture wing to provide stability after insertion or use a Dacron cuff to permit anchorage after insertion. Fistula needles contain a back eye and are equipped with a butterfly to ease their handling during insertion and to allow their anchorage to the skin following insertion.

Blood flow through devices for vascular access are subject to a parabolic velocity profile which may be mod-

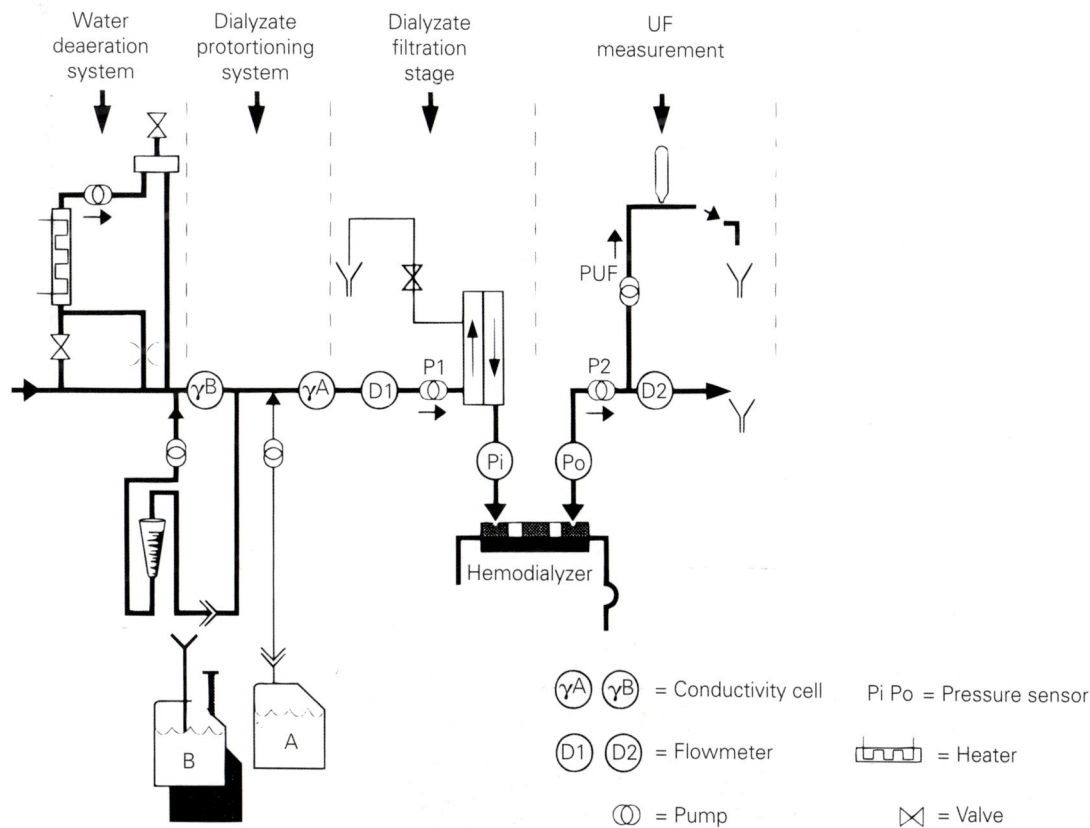

Figure 72.6 Elements of a modern single patient dialyzate supply system.

ified by the type of blood pump being used, and is also subject to shear. The clinical consequence of such shear is leukocyte or platelet aggregation and red cell damage.

Hemodialyzers and associated devices

The ideal hemodialyzer

The requirements of an ideal hemodialyzer are summarized in Table 72.2. Many of the requirements are dependent not only on the design itself but also on the membrane used.

Table 72.2 Characteristics of an ideal hemodialyzer or associated device

High clearance of small and middle weight uremic toxins but a negligible loss of vital solutes (e.g. amino acids, low-molecular-weight proteins)
Adequate ultrafiltration range but minimal backfiltration at low ultrafiltration rates
Low blood compartment volume
Non-toxic and non-thrombogenic materials used for construction
Good washback characteristics
High reliability
Low cost
Potentially reusable without adverse effects

The membranes currently used are based on cellulose or synthetic polymers (Table 72.3). Of these, membranes based on cellulose account for approximately 80% of the treatments undertaken throughout the world. Hemodialyzers in current use may be divided into three basic categories., coil, flat plate and hollow fiber (Figures 72.7–72.9). In each, a wide range of devices is available suitable for the treatment of small children through to large adults.

The coil dialyzer was the first single use hemodialyzer produced. Early dialyzers had large blood compartment volumes, high obligatory ultrafiltration rates and were used with a recirculating dialyzate supply system. The use of such devices has diminished over the years and are no longer in production.

The early flat plate devices could be rebuilt. Sheets of membrane were laid on grooved polypropylene boards in pairs to form an envelope (Figure 72.10). The device consisted of three boards permitting the formation of two blood-containing compartments. The boards contained rubber gaskets on their edge and the assembly was housed in a metal frame that was clamped together under a constant tension. Such devices remained in use until the early 1980s in a modified form in which the membrane supports were modified to form truncated pyramids, to minimize the membrane stretching under pressure and induce turbulence in the dialysis fluid pathway, both of which enhanced small molecular solute removal. Disposable variants introduced in the early 1970s retained this design in their use of stacked multiple plates, they were presterilized and pressure tested for leaks by the manufacturer.

Hollow fiber devices are the most popular in clinical

Table 72.3 Membranes available for use in hemodialyzers and associated devices for the treatment of renal failure

Membrane material		Common name
Cellulose	Regenerated cellulose	
		Cellophane
	Cuprammonium rayon	Cuprophan©
Modified cellulose		
	Cellulose-DEAE	Hemophan©
	Cellulose hydrate	
	Cellulose acetate	
	Cellulose triacetate	
	Saponified cellulose ester	SCE
	Cellulose 2–5-diacetate	Diaphan©
Synthetic		
	Polyacrylonitrile	AN69, SPAN, PAN
	Polysulfone	PS, Biosulfane©
	Polyethylvinyl alcohol	EVAL
	Polymethylmethacrylate	PMMA
	Polycarbonate	Gambrane©
	Polyamide	

use. Currently over 90% of the treatments in Europe employ hollow fiber devices (European Renal Association – European Dialysis and Transplant Registry, personal communication). Such devices consist of a bundle of fibers encased in a plastic outer jacket. The blood flows through the fiber lumens, entering and leaving via header manifolds, while the dialysis fluid flows in a countercurrent direction around the fibers. The device's popularity may be attributed to its large surface area blood compartment ratio that facilitates rapid solute removal, stable

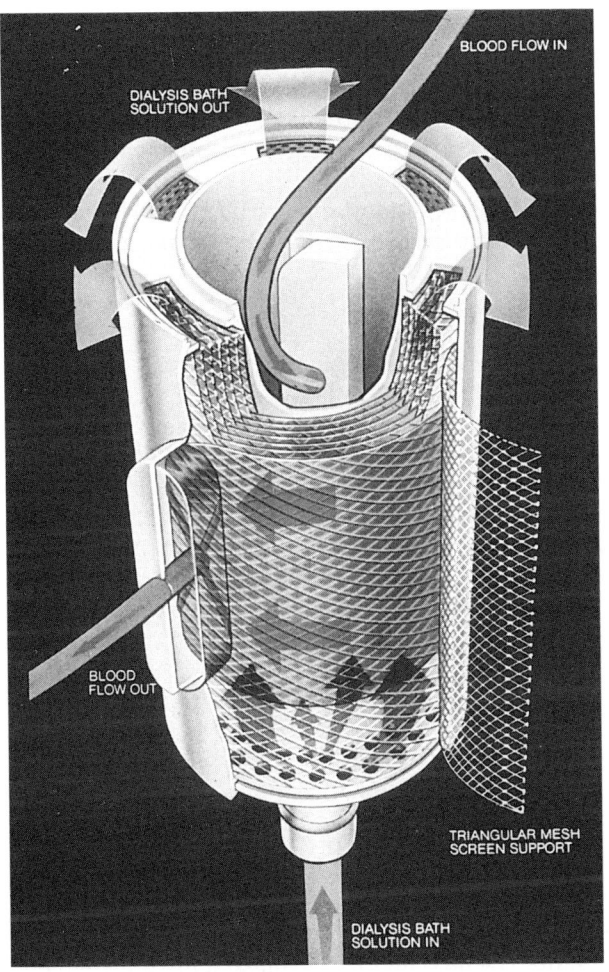

Figure 72.7 Coil type single use hemodialyzer.

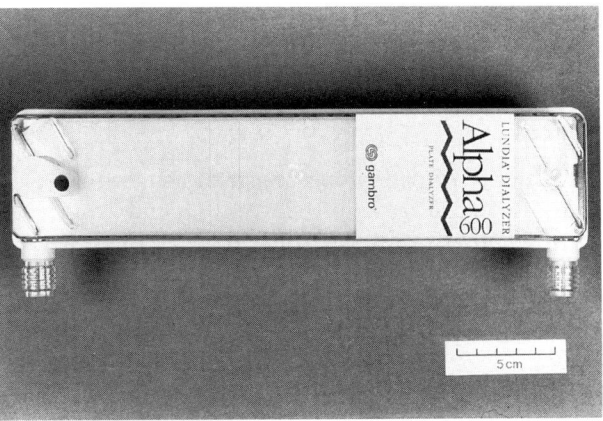

Figure 72.8 Parallel plate single use hemodialyzer.

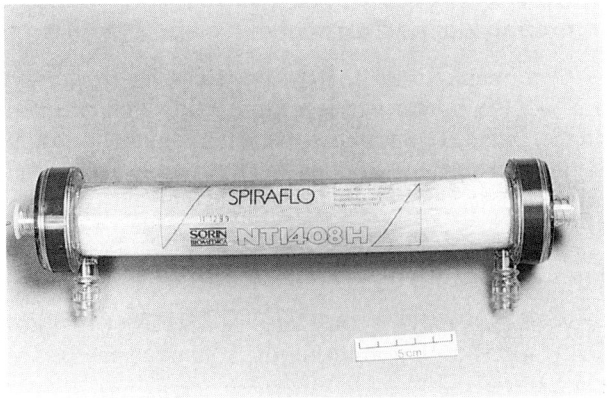

Figure 72.9 Hollow fiber hemodialyzer.

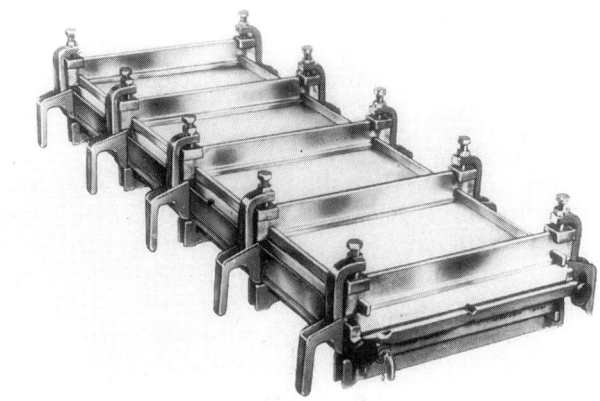

Figure 72.10 Rebuildable parallel plate hemodialyzer.

blood, ease of set up and use. Hollow fiber devices may also be used for hemofiltration, hemodiafiltration and continuous therapies for the treatment of acute renal failure. Devices intended for use in continous therapies incorporate shorter fibers than the cnventional dialyzers so that flow resistance is low and acceptable blood flow rates may be achieved without the use of a blood pump (Figure 72.11).

Large surface area and high flux devices

The majority of patients receive treatment with devices whose surface areas range between 0.8 and 1.3 m². The m²–h hypothesis postulated that some of the complications of dialysis therapy such as peripheral neuropathy were a consequence of inadequate removal of middle molecules [8]. This led to the development and clinical application of devices with surface areas in excess of 1.5 m². The importance of middle molecule removal has re-emerged during the last decade due to the need to remove β_2-microglobulin, an acute-phase reaction protein with a molecular weight of 14 kDa, implicated in the development of hemodialysis related amyloidosis.

Hemodialyzer performance

The performance of hemodialyzers may be categorized in terms of physical properties, such as blood compartment volume, blood compartment pressure drop, blood loss at the termination of treatment, and solute and water removal characteristics.

Blood compartment volume

Hemodialyzers may be considered as a series of tubes or parallel layers, thus permitting the volume of the device to be expressed as:

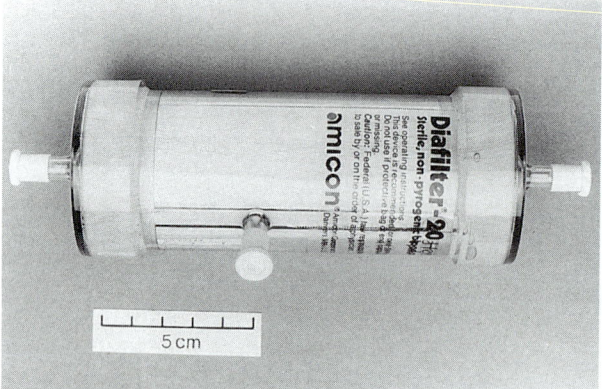

Figure 72.11 A hollow-fiber device designed for use in continuous modes of renal replacement therapy. Note the short fiber length used compared to those used in intermittent therapies.

$$LWh_bN \qquad (72.1)$$

where L = the length of the blood compartment (cm), W = the width of the blood compartment (cm), h_b = blood film thickness (cm) and n = number of blood compartments, for parallel plate devices. For devices consisting of a series of tubes or hollow fibers the blood compartment volume is given by the relationship:

$$\frac{\pi d^2 LN}{4} \qquad (72.2)$$

where L = the length of the blood compartment (cm), π = universal constant, d = fiber diameter (cm) and n = number of fibers.

Both of these relationships depend on the device's geometric surface area which for parallel plate devices is given by:

$$A = 2LWN \qquad (72.3)$$

and for devices containing hollow fibers by:

$$A = \pi NdL \qquad (72.4)$$

Historically the blood compartment volume of the dialyzer was important as early devices required blood priming. Since the 1960s, however, there has been a gradual reduction in blood compartment volume and today the volume contained in many devices is less than of the blood lines.

Blood pathway flow resistance

In hollow fiber devices, the geometry of the blood compartments is circular and the pressure drop may be calculated from consideration of the Hagen–Poiseuille formula:

$$\Delta P_B = \frac{128 \mu L}{\pi d_i^{\,4} N} Q_B \qquad (72.5)$$

where ΔP_B = pressure drop (dyn/cm²), Q_B = blood flow (ml/min), d_i = fiber internal diameter (cm) and μ = blood viscosity (poise).

The Hagen–Poiseuille equation assumes that viscosity of the fluid is constant and the fluid is Newtonian. At sufficiently high shear rates blood fulfills the latter; viscosity, however, varies with hematocrit and protein concentration.

For parallel plate devices with a large width to height ratio, the flow resistance may be calculated from:

$$\Delta P_B = \frac{12 \mu L}{Wh^3 N} Q_B \qquad (72.6)$$

where ΔP_B = pressure drop (dyn/cm²), Q_B = blood flow (ml/min), μ = blood viscosity (poise), L = blood compartment length (cm), W = blood compartment width (cm), h = blood compartment height (cm) and n = number of blood compartments.

As these equations express the pressure drop in dyn/cm² these should be converted into the more commonly used units of mmHg, by multiplying by 7.5 × 10⁻⁴ (mmHg/dyn/cm²).

These equations indicate that the pressure drop is directly proportional to the flow rate and dependent on both viscosity and pathway geometry. The equations also assume that the blood pathway is impermeable.

Blood loss at the termination of treatment

All devices are sufficiently thrombogenic to require an anticoagulant. The blood retained at the termination of treatment consists of two separate components; the first component is the unclotted blood left in the dialyzer and is related to the volume used to rinse the extracorporeal circuit, the technique of rinsing and the device design. This component is fully recoverable provided large enough rinsing volumes of the extracorporeal circuit are used. The second component is the irretrievable, and is the clotted residue. Measurement of the volumes of these two components differs. The fluid residual volume may be estimated using hemoglobinometry a technique in which the hemoglobin content of the patient's blood (taken immediately prior to the termination of treatment) is compared with that contained in the extracorporeal circuit after the usual rinse back volume had been used. The volume of clotted blood remaining can only be estimated by the use of radioactively labeled red cells.

Solute removal

Solute removal is the *raison d'être* of renal replacement therapy. The clinician views the hemodialyzer or associated device as an extension of the patient's circulatory system, to replace the non-functioning kidneys. To understand why hemodialyzers vary in efficiency, it is helpful to consider the underlying fluid dynamic process and to visualize diffusion of a molecule from the blood to the dialyzate. The molecule must first diffuse through the blood layer to the membrane boundary, cross the membrane, enter the dialyzate layer and then move away from the point of entry. The rate of mass transport of the solute may be represented by a differential equation in which the rate of mass transfer (K_T) is defined in terms of the membrane area and the concentration driving force such that the net flux of solute (dN) is:

$$dN = K_T(C_B - C_D)dA \qquad (72.7)$$

where C_B = blood solute concentration (mmol/l), C_D = dialysate solute concentration (mmol/l), dA = element of surface area (cm).

Integration of equation (72.7) gives:

$$N = K_T A \Delta C \qquad (72.8)$$

where ΔC = the log mean concentration driving force for solute mass transfer and N = flux.

It is dependent on the direction of the blood and dialysis fluid flow rates relative to one another. For the common counterflow configuration is given by:

$$\Delta C = \frac{(C_{Bi} - C_{Do}) - (C_{Bo} - C_{Di})}{\log e\left[\dfrac{C_{Bi} - C_{Do}}{C_{Bo} - C_{Di}}\right]} \qquad (72.9)$$

where C_{Bi} = blood inlet concentration, C_{Bo} = blood outlet concentration, C_{Di} = dialysate inlet concentration and C_{Do} = dialyzate outlet concentration.

The dialyzer's transport capacity (K_oA) for a specific solute is given by the total flux divided by the log mean concentration driving force such that:

$$K_oA = \frac{N}{\Delta C} \qquad (72.10)$$

where K_o is the overall mass transport coefficient which defines a fundamental physical property of the device. K_o is constant provided that no uneven flow or maldistribution in the blood and dialyzate pathways is present or changes in surface area of the device occur over the operational range of blood and dialysate flow rates.

The reciprocal of K_o may be considered as the overall mass transfer resistance (R_T) which is the sum of the individual average mass transfer resistances in the blood (R_B), dialyzate (R_D) and the membrane (R_M) elements.

The measurement of mass transfer coefficient or resistance in the blood side is not possible in practice but may be estimated using a theoretical analysis. The value of R_T is influenced by dialyzer design, dialyzate flow rate and membrane permeability. The relative importance of these factors will vary according to the molecular weight of the solute. For low-molecular-weight solutes, the principal barrier to diffusion is the boundary layer adjacent to the membrane, for large molecules, the barrier is in the membrane itself.

Clearance and dialysance

Analogous to the clearance concept, the solute transport characteristics of a hemodialyzer may be expressed in terms of clearance. Clearance in this context focuses on the removal of solute from the patient by the device. It may be defined as the amount of solute removed from the blood per unit of time, divided by incoming blood concentration. By this definition clearance represents the volumetric rate of removal by the device. From the mass balance across the dialyzer, the clearance may be expressed in concentration gradients and flow rates such that:

$$\begin{bmatrix}\text{Solute transferred} \\ \text{from blood to dialyzate}\end{bmatrix}$$
$$= \begin{bmatrix}\text{Solute mass} \\ \text{entering device}\end{bmatrix} - \begin{bmatrix}\text{Solute mass} \\ \text{leaving device}\end{bmatrix}$$

In the presence of ultrafiltration, the blood flow rate entering and leaving the device is not the same, thus

$$Q_{Bi} - Q_{Bo} = Q_F \qquad (72.11)$$

where Q_{Bi} = blood flow entering the device (ml/min), Q_{Bo} = blood flow leaving the device (ml/min) and Q_F = ultrafiltration rate (ml/min).

Since clearance is the mass removal rate divided by the incoming concentration, the clearance on the blood side (K_B) is:

$$K_B = Q_{Bi} \frac{\left(C_{Bi} - C_{Bo}\right)}{C_{Bi}} + Q_F \frac{C_{Bo}}{C_{Bi}} \qquad (72.12)$$

Since the solutes removed are in the dialyzate (assuming a negligible adsorption on the membrane), the clearance on the dialyzate side (K_D) may also be derived and is given by:

$$K_D = Q_{Di} \frac{\left(C_{Di} - C_{Do}\right)}{C_{Bi}} + Q_F \frac{C_{Do}}{C_{Bi}} \qquad (72.13)$$

The first term of these equations may be viewed as the diffusive component of solute transport, whereas the second represents the convective component. In the case of negligible ultrafiltration or negligible convective mass transport, the equations simplify to:

$$K_B = Q_B \frac{\left(C_{Bi} - C_{Bo}\right)}{C_{Bi}} \qquad (72.14)$$

and

$$K_D = Q_D \frac{\left(C_{Di} - C_{Do}\right)}{C_{Bi}} \qquad (72.15)$$

Dialysance is used by engineers to compare overall solute removal by different blood–dialyzate flow configurations and is defined as the amount of solute removed from the blood per unit of time divided by the concentration difference between incoming blood and dialysis fluid. In a manner similar to that shown above, equations for the blood and dialyzate sides of the dialyzer may be derived.

The relative importance of dialysance has diminished over the past decade as hemodialyzers and associated devices increasingly use single pass rather than recirculating dialyzate supply systems. Clearance, therefore, may be considered as the operational parameter of clinical interest that focuses on the removal of solute from the blood and can, therefore, be used to predict concentration changes in the body.

The relationships above refer to the clearance in the hemodialyzer itself, not to the removal of solute from the patient. To understand solute removal from the patient during dialysis therapy, the concept of effective clearance needs to be introduced, since this represents the true volumetric rate at which the patient's systemic blood is cleared of solute.

Effective clearance may, therefore, be considered as a refinement of clearance. and corrects for the partial recalculation of blood that may occur in the dialyzate. Such recalculation may originate from patient access problems or the access device. By consideration of the mass balance, Gotch [9] has derived a modification given by:

$$K_R = \frac{\left(1 - R'\right)}{1 - R'\left(1 - \dfrac{K_B}{Q_B}\right)} K_B \qquad (72.16)$$

where K_R = clearance in the presence of recirculation (ml/min) and R' = recirculation (%).

By rearrangement of this equation the reduction in clearance at a specific recirculation rate may be established.

Hematocrit, plasma water and solute protein binding also influence solute clearance.

The impact of hematocrit on dialyzer solute removal has been discussed by Morcos and Nissenson [10]. In hemofiltration and hemodiafiltration, solute is cleared from the blood by the removal of plasma water. Attention must therefore be paid to the precise distribution of solute. To permit equivalent calculations to those used in hemodialysis it is necessary to consider sieving coefficient (S), the ratio of the solute concentration in the ultrafiltrate to the concentration in bulk plasma water, such that:

$$S = \frac{C_F}{C_W} \qquad (72.17)$$

where C_F = solute concentration in the filtrate and C_W = solute concentration in plasma water.

$S = 1$ when the solute passes freely across the membrane and $S = 0$ where solute is completely rejected and does not cross the membrane. In practice, the sieving coefficient is calculated as:

$$S = \frac{2C_F}{C_{Wi} + C_{Wo}} \qquad (72.18)$$

where C_{Wi} = solute concentration in plasma water entering the device and C_{Wo} = solute concentration in plasma water leaving the device.

For retentive membranes this approximation of sieving coefficient does not hold and a more rigorous characterization involving the equation derived by Spiegler and Kedem [11] is required.

In the absence of protein binding, solute concentration in the plasma water is related to the plasma concentration by:

$$\frac{C_P}{C_W} = 1 - \phi' \qquad (72.19)$$

where ϕ is the volume fraction of hydrated proteins and is 0.0107 C_P and C_P = solute concentration in plasma.

The concentration in the blood is related to that in plasma by:

$$\frac{C_P}{C_W} = 1 - HCT + HCTk' \qquad (72.20)$$

where HCT = hematocrit (%) and k' = equilibrium solute partition coefficient.

During hemofiltration diluting fluid is added to the blood either before it enters the filter (predilution) or after it leaves the filter (postdilution). Solute removal in both of these models has been described in detail elsewhere [12].

In the case of solute removal for postdilution, e.g. during CVVH or CAVH, the whole blood clearance is equivalent to the plasma clearance such that:

$$K_B = \frac{Q_F C_F}{C_{Bi}}$$

(72.21)

If the effects of exclusion volume of hydrated proteins are neglected, the relationship simplifies to:

$$K_B = Q_F S$$

(72.22)

In hemodiafiltration (HDF) the principal route of removal for solutes is by diffusion but high-molecular-weight solute removal is supplemented by the convective transport. The two processes occur simultaneously rather than sequentially, the overall solute removal is less than the sum of the two components and may be approximated by the relationship:

$$K_{HDF} = K_B + 0.5Q_F$$

(72.23)

where K_{HDF} = clearance during hemodiafiltration.

Interdisciplinary approach to solute transport

An interdisciplinary approach combines the descriptive term for clearance and mass transfer coefficient. This approach is based on equations for heat transfer, which are analogous to mass transfer.

In the absence of significant ultrafiltration, these equations may be used to analyze the mass transfer phenomena occurring within dialyzers, and to predict the expected performance under specific conditions. When such equations are used, the underlying assumption is that the mass transfer resistance is constant over the range of clinical operating conditions.

Water transport or ultrafiltration

The ability of the device to remove fluid accumulated between dialyses is of paramount importance. Such removal should be predictable and easily controlled by the proportioning system.

During dialysis the fluid is removed by two separate mechanisms; one due to the transmembrane or hydrostatic pressure gradient across the membrane ($Q_{F(h)}$), the other due to the transmembrane osmotic pressure gradient ($Q_{F(osm)}$) such that:

$$Q_F = Q_{F(h)} + Q_{F(osm)}$$

(72.24)

The contribution from the second component is dependent on the composition of the dialysis fluid. A special case of the osmotic pressure gradient is the pressure exerted by the proteins in plasma, since the membranes used in dialysis are impermeable to proteins. The magnitude of the transmembrane colloid–osmotic or oncotic pressure difference may be estimated from the serum globulin and albumin concentrations. For normal plasma protein concentrations it is about 25 mmHg. The relative importance of this correction is small when the hydrostatic pressure gradient dominates the fluid removal.

The water transport characteristics of hemodialyzers and associated devices may be expressed in terms of the device's surface area (A), membrane hydraulic permeability (L_h) and the hydrostatic pressure gradient (TMP) such that:

$$Q_F = L_h A \, TMP$$

(72.25)

The transmembrane pressure is given by:

$$TMP = \frac{P_{Bin} + P_{Bout}}{2} + \frac{P_{Din} + P_{Dout}}{2} - P_{OSM}$$

where P_{Bi} = pressure at the inlet of the blood pathway (mmHg), P_{Bo} = pressure at the outlet of the blood pathway (mmHg), P_{Di} = pressure at the inlet of the dialyzate pathway (mmHg), P_{Do} = pressure at the outlet of the dialysate pathway (mmHg) and P_{OSM} = osmotic pressure (mmHg).

This relationship may be most easily studied *in vitro* since in the clinical situation, monitoring of pressures at the entry and exit to the device may not be undertaken. The extrapolation of *in vitro* data, particularly if established using aqueous solutions, is difficult, since the pressure drop in the blood pathway may be influenced by thrombus formation during clinical use, fouling of the membrane by proteins and blood components, hematocrit and viscosity.

In practice, there is a linear relationship between the transmembrane pressure and the ultrafiltration rate, although deviations from linearity in hollow fiber devices may occur due to membrane fouling by blood or plasma components, whereas in parallel plate devices, deviation may be due to the stretching of the membrane over the support structure. In hemofiltration the filtrate flux is less dependent on hydrostatic pressure difference and more on the hemodynamic conditions in the device. During clinical use, the amount of protein which adsorbs onto the membrane and the plasma oncotic pressure may vary and, as a result of these factors, *in vivo* ultrafiltration coefficients determined directly may be 20–25% lower than those measured *in vitro*. Devices with high permeability membranes are used in conjunction with proportioning systems incorporating ultrafiltration control. In such situations, the pressure generated in the blood pathway is offset by the pressure in the dialyzate pathway to minimize fluid removal, and water flux may occur from the blood to the dialyzate, i.e. ultrafiltration and from the dialyzate to the blood, termed back filtration (Figure 72.12).

Back filtration during hemodialysis varies along the membrane and depends on the pressure profiles in the blood and dialyzate pathways. At any point within the device, the opposing pressures in the blood and dialyzate compartments govern the direction of filtration. Several approaches have been proposed to model back filtration to predict the amount of dialyzate infused into the blood during treatment. These have been analysed by Soltys *et al.* [13].

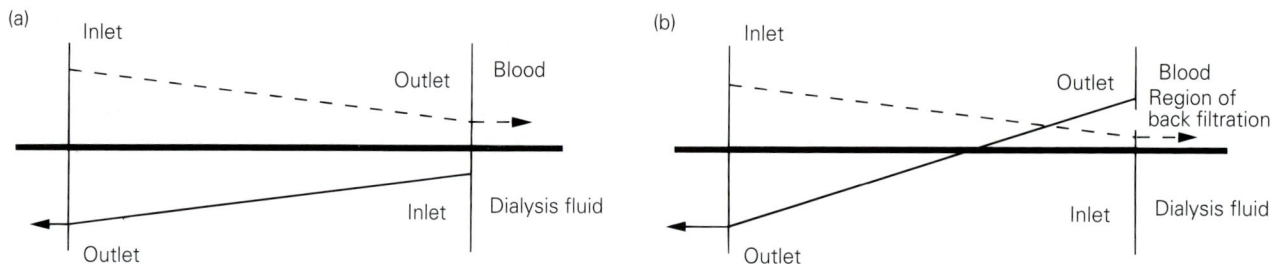

Figure 72.12   Elements of back filtration. (a) Pressure profile during ultrafiltration; (b) pressure prafile during back filtration.

Table 72.4   Reuse of hemodialyzers

Advantages attributed to reuse	Disadvantages associated with reuse
Allows more widespread use of expensive devices such as those containing high flux synthetic membranes	Requires special area and equipment to minimize staff and patient exposure to chemicals used
Reduction in treatment cost	Potential for inadequate sterilization by the process
Minimization of exposure to chemicals used in the manufacturing process	More frequent pyrogen-type reactions
Improved biocompatibility	Reduction in performance
	Increased incidence of blood leaks due to structural weakening of the membrane by repeated exposure to the sterilizing chemicals
	Possible role in higher relative risk of mortality
	Legal and liability implications

The clinical significance of back filtration is yet to be determined. However, concern has been expressed that in the presence of reverse ultrafiltration contaminants from the dialysate such as pyrogens may enter the patient's bloodstream, cause fever and stimulate the release of biologically active cytokines.

Comparative performance characteristics of devices used in dialysis

The overall performance of devices used in dialysis are determined by the fluid dynamic conditions within the device and the mass transport properties of the membrane, which are related to membrane structure. In hemodialysis and hemodiafiltration, the membrane transport rate is proportional to the porosity of the membrane and the sieving coefficient and inversely proportional to the membrane thickness. In hemofiltration, the transmembrane transport rate is influenced by the radius of the pores and the fluid viscosity and is independent of the molecular weight of the solute provided the sieving coefficient approaches unity. The membrane surface charge not only influences solute transport but also the adhesion of cellular elements to the membrane surface.

In vitro performance characteristics of devices used in dialysis are generally given in the manufacturers product literature. International Standards for the laboratory assessment of device performance (ISO 8637). The choice of devices for the treatment of renal failure continues to grow, and, in view of this, no attempt has been made to catalog device performance. In the UK the Medical Device Agency has long recognized the problem of obtaining independent data relating to device performance in the laboratory and clinical setting, and to provide such data, supports an evaluation program at Newcastle upon Tyne. The results of studies that measure parameters of performance in many of the currently used devices are available. (Details of the MDA Evaluation reports may be obtained from the author.)

Reuse of hemodialyzers

Recently there has been a move towards reuse of hemodialyzers. The European Dialysis Transplant Association–European Renal Association (EDTA-ERA) registry analyzed the pattern of reuse in Europe during the period 1975–1982 and showed that during this period the reuse process was confined principally to non-disposable flat plate hemodialyzers, and exceeded 50% of the patients receiving treatment with such dialyzers reusing in 1981, compared to less than 10% of patients treated with devices intended for single use reusing [14]. A wide national variation exists, with reuse being most prevalent in Bulgaria and Poland. In Italy, Netherlands, Germany and Sweden the practice was virtually non-existent (0–1%

of patients treated). By contrast, at this time 16% of the patients in the United States underwent treatment with reused dialysers. Due to changes in reimbursement, the practice of reusing dialyzers has grown, and it is estimated that currently over 80% of the patients are treated with reused dialyzers [15].

The technique of reuse may be subdivided into four distinct operations. (1) The rinsing of the dialyzer following the disconnection of the patient usually by reverse ultrafiltration which removes blood cells and plasma proteins adhering to the membrane. (2) Disinfection and cleaning by the use of chemicals such as sodium hypochlorite, hydrogen peroxide or peracetic acid. (3) Checking for the integrity of the membrane. (4) Sterilization and storage. Before subsequent use the chemicals contained in the device are removed and the device primed.

These processes may be performed manually, but increasingly automated reuse systems are used to process the dialyzers of which there are a number commercially available.

The advantages and disadvantages of reuse are summarized in Table 72.4.

The extracorporeal circuit

A schematic diagram of a typical extracorporeal blood circuit used in dialysis is shown in Figure 72.13.

Although historically the blood flow in the extracorporeal circuit was maintained by the arteriovenous pressure difference generated by the patient's heart, all current dialysis is performed using a blood pump. The most commonly used pumps are roller pumps which work on the peristaltic principle. A compressible segment of the blood tubing generally 8–10 mm in diameter is placed in a rigid circular track. The segment is occluded by the pump rollers which are automatically adjusted to allow for small-dimensional variations between batches of tubing. As the pump shaft to which the rollers are attached rotates, the pump segment is compressed. This compression generates a negative pressure before the roller and a positive pressure after the roller. As the roller moves the compressed pump segment recoils causing blood to be drawn into the segment which is then forced out of the segment ahead of the rotating roller. Usually two rollers are used. As part of the system safety, the cover of the pump is fitted with a magnetic switch which stops the blood pump should it be opened. The power supply to the pump is linked to the dialyzate delivery system to allow it to be inactivated should a fault in the delivery system occur.

The pump flow rate is normally displayed electronically and is based on a calculation involving the rotational speed of the pump and the volume of blood contained in the pump segment. Caution must be exercised when using this display for accurate quantification of the blood flow rate. The actual flow delivered may be

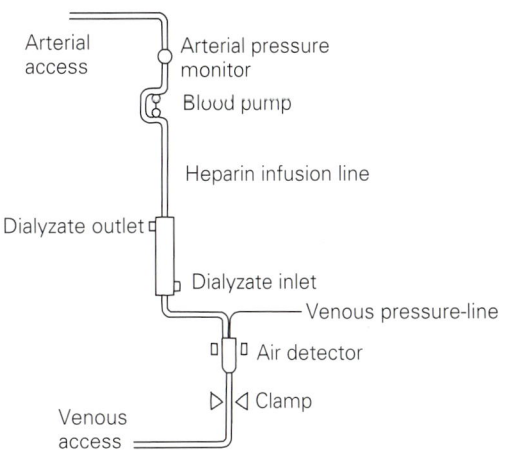

Figure 72.13 Schematic diagram of the extracorporeal circuit used in renal replacement therapy.

lower than that displayed in the presence of a high arterial or inlet pressure, since under these conditions there is incomplete filling of the pump segment. The magnitude of this underestimate may be increased by the loss of compliance in the pump segment after several hours of pumping. Bubble transit measurements provide an alternative method for the measurement of blood flow rate. A 200 cm racetrack will permit the measurement of blood flow with an accuracy of ±3% when a small (0.5 ml) air bubble is injected and timed with a stopwatch with an accuracy of 0.01 s. At high blood flow rates a longer racetrack should be used. As this technique involves the repeated insertion of a needle into an injection site with the risk of aerosol generation it should not be undertaken in patients with hepatitis or HIV infection.

For measurement of blood flow CAVH, the use of bubble transit times is impractical and a method described by Bosch [16] may be used. It requires pre- and postfilter hematocrit (HCT_{inlet} and HCT_{outlet}, respectively) and simultaneously establishing the ultrafiltration rate. The blood flow at the filter inlet is calculated from:

$$Q_{Bin} = \frac{Q_F HCT_{outlet}}{HCT_{outlet} - HCT_{inlet}} \qquad (72.26)$$

and the plasma flow at the inlet is calculated from

$$Q_{Pin} = Q_{Bin} - \frac{Q_{Bin} HCT_{inlet}}{100} \qquad (72.27)$$

where Q_{pin} = plasma flow rate at the inlet to the device (ml/min)

Single needle systems

The ability to deliver clinically acceptable flow rates during dialysis is of paramount importance. This may be difficult due to poor vasculature. Although the importance of surgical intervention cannot be over emphasized, the creation of an arteriovenous fistula may worsen pre-existing cardiovascular disease, and alternate methods of vascular access may be required e.g. the surgical implantation of a large-bore catheter into a jugular vein. Although the catheter used is preferably double or dual lumen, single lumen catheters may be used, but the use of such catheters requires the use of a single needle dialysis system. In such systems the continuous flow associated with the conventional blood pump is divided into an aspiration (outflow) and a return phase resulting in an intermittent flow pattern through the extracorporeal circuit. The duration of each phase is governed by pressure or time or a combination of both. Such systems utilize one or two blood pumps. Recirculation, the mixing of treated blood leaving the circuit with untreated blood entering the circuit is unavoidable when using single needle systems. It may also occur in double-needle systems where its magnitude is governed by the status of the patient's access. In single-needle dialysis it is additionally influenced by the access device volume, the volume of the blood pumped per cycle and the extracorporeal circuit compliance.

Recirculation compromises treatment efficiency. It is usually calculated from the urea or BUN concentrations in blood samples drawn simultaneously from the arterial and venous segments of the extracorporeal circuit and a peripheral vein. It is assumed that in the absence of recirculation the urea or BUN concentration in the peripheral sample is identical to that of the arterial sample. The validity of this technique has been questioned, it has been suggested that the use of a saline dilution technique might be more accurate [17].

Heparinization

Coagulation as a consequence of contact of blood with foreign material is a well-recognized complication of extracorporeal circulatory techniques. Although the coating of the extracorporeal circuit, such as that used in the treatment of acute renal failure has been developed (Duraflo II©, Baxter Healthcare Corporation, Deerfield, USA), the majority of dialytic therapies rely on the use of heparin as an anticoagulant. Heparin is normally infused continuously during treatment, although some centers prefer a single bolus at the initiation of dialysis. Usually blood tubing sets contain a heparin infusion line on the positive side of the blood pump linked to a heparin pump that forms part of the proportioning system. Although peristaltic pumps have been used, the most widely used is a syringe pump. The pump accurately delivers the set rate against the pressure in the positive pressure segment of the extracorporeal circuit. An end-of-stroke alarm indicates the emptying of the syringe.

Monitoring the extracorporeal circuit

It is necessary to monitor the extracorporeal circuit for pressure to safeguard against excessive positive and negative pressure. Such pressures are generally monitored by

electronic manometers that are isolated from the extracorporeal circuit to prevent blood contaminating the device. Typically a pressure protector consists of a hydrophobic membrane housed in a plastic casing. The membrane allows passage of air across it, permitting the pressure sensing device to respond to changes in pressure but is impermeable to blood or plasma. Pressure monitoring is normally undertaken prior to the blood pump. Excessively high negative pressure at this point may be indicative of kinks or obstruction prior to the pump, e.g. at the site of access, and downstream prior to the blood returning to the patient. At the latter point the pressure is monitored in a drip chamber which forms an air trap used not only to measure pressure but also to trap air in the extracorporeal circuit. The drip chamber is normally mounted with a detector which monitors changes in the level and is linked to a clamp at its base which is activated automatically when the level falls, thereby preventing air entering the access. Simultaneously with clamp closure the power to the pump is interrupted to prevent further increase in pressure.

The dialysis fluid circuit

The dialysis fluid circuit delivers fluid at the correct temperature, ionic concentration and flow to the dialyzer, monitors the used dialysis fluid for the presence of red cells and controls the ultrafiltration rate. It is linked to the blood module and provides a safe environment for the treatment in the event of malfunction either in the blood or dialyzate pathway. The dialysis fluid circuit incorporates the ability to clean the circuit with sterilants after use to remove any bacterial contaminants from the valves and sensors and to rid the circuit of salts used in the production of the dialysis fluid.

Monitoring the dialysis fluid circuit

Conductivity monitoring

The mixing ratio achieved by the proportioning system is monitored by the continuous measurement of the electrical conductivity of the final solution. The conductivity is expressed in millisiemens (mS).

pH monitoring

When using bicarbonate as the buffer, two proportioning systems produce the fluid to prevent excessive calcium carbonate precipitation. pH is additionally monitored to ensure the correct composition of the solution being produced.

Dialyzate flow rate

Not all delivery systems display the dialyzate flow rate, which may be fixed or adjusted by the operator. The dialyzate flow rate plays an important role in determining the efficiency of solute removal but in terms of patient safety it is not critical to know what it is.

Dialyzate temperature and pressure

Temperature monitoring is important in ensuring that dialyzate is delivered at the correct temperature; overheated dialyzate can cause hemolysis and even death, underheated dialysis fluid causes discomfort to the patient. A tolerable temperature range is 37–40°C. The temperature monitoring system forms an integral part of the safety system. Dialyzate pressures are measured by a strain gauge similar to that used in the blood circuit. In some proportioning systems, the transmembrane rather than the dialyzate pressure is displayed.

Blood leak monitoring

The used dialyzate returns to the proportioning system and passes through a blood leak detector prior to flowing to waste. The sensor is normally of a photo-optical type with a detection threshold of below 0.5 ml/min blood loss at the maximum dialyzate flow rate generated by the machine.

Ultrafiltration control

In early single patient proportioning systems ultrafiltration control was achieved by manual adjustment of the blood and dialyzate pressure in the respective circuits. Today proportioning systems incorporate ultrafiltration control systems that allow accurate measurement and control of ultrafiltration during treatment. The control of ultrafiltration may be by the use of a flow rate monitor which measures the dialyzate flow entering and leaving the dialyzer and controls the pressure in the dialyzate circuit to achieve and maintain the required ultrafiltration rate. Other methods of ultrafiltration control include the use of a recirculation loop with dialyzate replacement or volume balancing. In the latter, two balance chambers are used with matched diaphragm pumps which keep the dialyzate inflow identical to the outflow. The pumps are normally operated out of phase to permit a continuous flow through the dialyzer. A separate pump is used to remove fluid from the circuit. As the circuit is non-compliant any fluid removed is balanced by the transfer of fluid from the patient into the circuit. The accuracy of such methods depends on two factors: the duration of treatment and the accuracy of the technique to detect small differences. The stated accuracy may not be achieved unless dialyzate connections are airtight and the pumps and fluid circuits are regularly checked. With ultrafiltration control systems the possibility of reverse ultrafiltration exists, and with it the potential for entry of endotoxin fragments into the blood pathway. The detection of a pinhole leak in the blood pathway may also go undetected.

Disinfection

Dialyzate systems require regular disinfection or sterilization to prevent bacterial contamination in the dialyzate pathway. Disinfection may be achieved by heat (pasteurization or sterilization) or by chemicals. Initiation of the disinfection requires a safety interlock to prevent accidental disinfection with the patient connected. The cycle normally consists of a rinse phase, to remove any residual dialyzate followed by the disinfection phase. In chemical disinfection systems, the chemicals are automatically rinsed out prior to subsequent use. Hypochlorite is often used. Calcium carbonate accumulation in the dialysis circuit is prevented by the periodic rinsing of the circuit with a dilute acid such as citric acid.

Biocompatibility

Reactions mediated by devices used in renal replacement therapy

The patient's blood is repeatedly exposed to components of the extracorporeal circuit – the hemodialyzer, the blood tubing and possible residues in the system from the manufacturing and sterilization processes. Reactions associated with hemodialysis have been categorized by Daugirdas and Ing [18] as either type A or type B. In type A reactions, the symptoms usually occur immediately or within the first few minutes after the initiation of dialysis, but on occasion are delayed. Type A reactions vary in severity but are typical of anaphylaxis. Type B reactions are milder, occur later and abate after the first hour.

When non-disposable dialyzers were widely used, reactions were common, bacterial in origin, the source being the gasket housings. Reactions still occur today with disposable dialyzers and have been reported in over 30% of patients in the United States when using dialyzers for the first time [19]. An important factor in such reactions is the inadequate removal during the priming procedure of ethylene oxide and its breakdown products, which when conjugated to human serum albumin acts as an allergen.

Leachable substances and particulate release

Most plastic in the extracorporeal circuit is manufactured from polyvinylchloride (PVC). Flexibility is achieved by addition of a plasticizer di-(2-ethylhexyl)phthalate (DEHP). The phthalate ester may constitute up to 40% of the finished product. It is physically linked but not chemically bound to the plastic and is leached out by blood or other protein-containing solutions. For patients receiving regular dialysis, repeated exposure leads to tissue accumulation; substantial amounts have been found in the liver [20]. The clinical consequences of tissue accumulation are poorly understood. Whether this problem may be reduced by the use of alternative plasticizers requires further study.

Leachable substances from the dialyzer itself include isopropyl myristate used in the processing of hollow fibers and potting compounds made from polyurethanes which generate reactive isocyanates that combine with proteins and act as haptens. Release of methylene diani-line may also occur when gamma irradiation is used to sterilize devices. Other unidentified compounds have been implicated in iritis and scleritis that occurs in hemodialysis patients [21].

The repeated flexing and compression of the tubing by the rollers in the blood pump segment results in abrasion and cracking of the internal surface. This leads to the shedding or spallation of particles. Studies indicate that the majority of the particles are less than 5 μm in diameter and that the greatest release of particles is in the first hour of pumping [22]. Particles may also originate form the dialyzer itself [23]. Clinicopathological effects of such particles lodging in the body include hepatomegaly, granulomatosus hepatitis and elevation of the transaminases. Many of these complications, however, were described at a time when silicone pump inserts were used extensively in extracorporeal circuits. Blood lines today use polyvinylchloride pump inserts, and although they also release particles into the extracorporeal circuit, complications resulting from them have so far not been described.

Blood membrane interactions

The membrane in the hemodialyzer constitutes the largest area of foreign material to which blood is exposed. In one year, cumulative exposure amounts to approximately 400 m^2. This has led to extensive studies on the interaction of blood with hemodialysis membranes. The elements involved in such interactions are summarized in Figure 72.14.

Activation of the complement system

Contact between blood and membrane activates the alternate pathway of the complement system. Craddock et al. [24] demonstrated hemodialysis-induced neutropenia and complement activation. The magnitude of complement activation is a function of the type of membrane. The mechanism depends on the interaction with Factor B, a promoter and Factor H an inhibitor of complement activation. A consequence of activation is the release of C5a and C3a into the circulation, both of which are powerful anaphylatoxins that cause contraction of vascular smooth muscle and increased vascular permeability. C5a is approximately 100-fold more effective than C3a. The spasmogenic properties are largely abrogated once the C terminal arginine has been cleaved from the C3a and C5a molecules by serum carboxypeptidase B. The acute changes in C3a desArg and C5a des Arg have been studied as a function of different types of hemodialysis membranes. These studies show that cellulose membranes whose structure is unmodified generate greater complement activation than modified cellulose or synthetic membranes [25]. The long-term consequences of membrane-induced complement activation remain unclear and require further investigation, particularly as the magnitude of complement activation appears to be inversly related to the cost of the membrane.

Associated with the formation of C5a is C5b, which is part of the terminal complement complex, that is composed of C5b to C9 molecules (C5b–9), and once assembled is inserted in the cell membrane and causes cell lysis. The availability of enzyme immunoassays for the measurement of C5b–9 complex has demonstrated differences between membranes. The clinical significance of these differences is at present unclear, but in cardiopulmonary bypass C5b–9 deposition on erythrocytes contributes to hemolysis [26].

Contact pathway activation

Contact pathway activation involves binding of Factor XII (Hageman Factor) and circulating complexes of high molecular weight, kininogen with prekallikrein. Activation depends on the surface charge and is more easily activated by negatively charged membranes such as those made from synthetic copolymers.

Angiotensin converting enzyme (ACE) inhibitors are used widely in the treatment of hypertension and congestive heart failure. Such drugs block not only ACE but also kininase, so that bradykinin is not degraded but remains in the circulation. A number of severe anaphylactoid reactions have occurred with polyacrylonitile (AN69) membranes [27]. The majority of the patients involved were using ACE inhibitors. Following these observations the ability of AN 69 to generate bradykinin has been demonstrated [28], and in view of this it is prudent to discontinue the use of ACE inhibitors when using hemodialysis membranes with an ability to generate bradykinin.

Cellular activation

Contact of blood with the membrane induces platelet adhesion and aggregation leading to the release of platelet factor 4 (PF4) and β thromboglobulin as well as proteinases.

During the early stages of dialysis a drop in the number of neutophils occurs which is generally reversed by the end of the first hour. This phenomenon was first described by Kaplow and Goffinet [29] and has been used extensively to characterize hemodialysis membranes. The cause of the decrease in neutrophils is sequestration in the lung vasculature due to changes in the cell surface antigen expression following complement activation. This sequestration is partially responsible for hemodialysis-induced hypoxia [30], and it has also been postulated that the activated cells are involved in the development of hemodialysis-related amyloidosis [31].

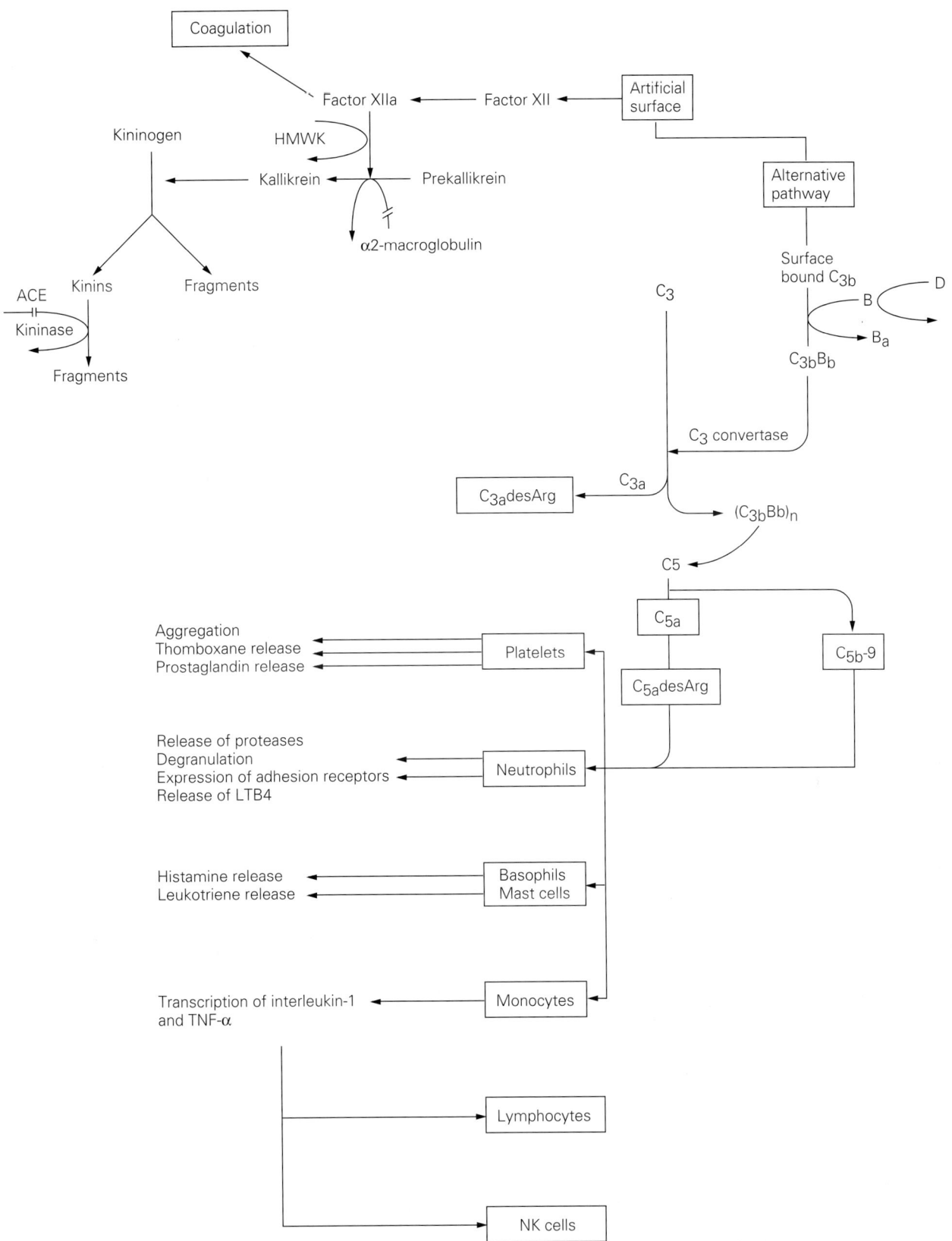

Figure 72.14 Elements of blood membrane interactions. (Adapted from ref. [37].)

Production of cytokines and inhibitory proteins

Cytokines are polypeptides with molecular weights in the range 10–45 kDa. They act as communication links between the immune system and other organs. Five classes of cytokine have been identified according to their biological properties: proinflammatory cytokines, anti-inflammatory cytokines, lymphocyte growth and differentiation factors, hematopoietic colony stimulating factors and mesenchymal cell growth factors. Among these the proinflammatory cytokines have been the subject of considerable interest in the context of dialytic therapy. This interest has arisen from the interleukin hypothesis [32] which proposed that many of the long-term complications as well as some acute complications associated with hemodialysis therapy are a consequence of interleukin-1 (IL-1) production during dialysis. The mechanisms involved in production are

1 Bacterial contamination of the dialysis fluid and the back transfer of bacterial fragments across the membrane into the blood where they stimulate monocytes;
2 Direct contact between monocytes and membrane;
3 The action of the complement components activated by the membrane on monocytes.

Studies of the serum or plasma of hemodialyis patients remain conflicting, some demonstrating an increase in IL-1 others failing to do so. A possible explanation may be the variety of inhibitors and binding proteins in the plasma that influence IL-1 levels. Current interest is focusing on the measurement of IL-1 receptor antagonist (IL-1Ra) a molecule structurally related to IL-1 which is present in much larger quantities than IL-1 thus making its measurement easier. Other studies are investigating gene expression of cytokines in mononuclear cells following exposure to hemodialysis membranes [33–35].

Future trends

Dialysis has been described as an expensive, ethically puzzling halfway technology. It prolongs the lives of patients without restoring them to full health. Patients receiving dialysis over a long period are poorly rehabilitated. As the average age of the patients receiving therapy increases, these problems are likely to worsen. Future emphasis is likely to focus upon the introduction of new technology and the use of biocompatible membrane materials in improving morbidity and mortality associated with renal replacement therapy.

The equipment used in renal replacement therapy already makes extensive use of microprocessor technology. In the future, systems with an open architecture to facilitate the clinical application of new techniques of treatment incorporating the use of fuzzy logic are likely to be developed. The linkage of hemodialysis equipment to microcomputers to monitor and deliver therapy will increase and will be likely to play an important part in the improvement of mortality and morbidity associated with dialysis. This improvement will be further helped by on-line measurement of parameters such as total body impedance, blood conductivity, hematocrit and optical density to assess the physiological response to fluid removal during treatment and thus maintain vascular stability by adjustment of the removal rate [36, 37]. The control of therapy in the context of adequacy is already possible in the case of urea with the availability of on-line techniques for the measurement of urea in the dialysate [38]. The increasing use of microprocessors in monitoring and control of therapy will require rigorous software validation.

Membranes used in renal replacement therapy are not selective, for example clinically desirable removal of large molecular weight metabolites such as β_2 microglobulin may be associated with loss of amino acids and low molecular weight proteins [39]. The clinical development of affinity membranes, while desirable, may be prevented by high cost. The gap between synthetic and cellulose based membranes in terms of biocompatibility has diminished with the clinical availability of modified cellulose membranes. The question of biocompatibility in modulating the clinical outcome of reneal replacement therapy remains unresoved in patients with chronic renal failure but has been shown to be an important factor in the outcome following treatment for acute renal failure [40].

The speed of introduction and clinical application of many of these developments is likely to be governed by economic pressures to contain the cost of treatment.

References

1. Rosborough, D.C. and Van Stone, J.C. (1993) Dialysate glucose. *Semin. Dial.*, **6**, 260–3.
2. Henderson, L.W. (1982) The beginning of hemofiltration. *Contrib. Nephrol.*, **32**, 1–19.
3. Ronco, C. (1993) Continuous renal replacement therapies for the treatment of acute renal failure in intensive care patients. *Clin. Nephrol.*, **40**, 187–98.
4. Bellormo, R. and Boyce, N. (1993) Acute continuous hemodiafiltration: a prospective study of 110 patients and a review of the literature. *Am. J. Kidney Dis.*, **21**, 508–18.
5. Raine, A.E.G., Margreiter, R., Brunner, F.P. *et al.* (1992) Report on management of renal failure in Europe, XXII, 1991. *Nephrol. Dial. Transplant.*, Suppl **2**, 7–35.

6. Ebben, J.P., Hirsch, D.N., Luehmann, D.A. *et al.* (1987) Microbial contamination of liquid bicarbonate concentrate for hemodialysis. *Trans. Am. Soc. Artif. Intern. Organs.*, **33**, 269–73.

7. Granger, A. and Vlchek, D. (1982) An overview of the basic features of the AN69 membrane. *Proc. First American AN 69 Membrane Scientific Proceedings*, pp. 5–13.

8. Babb, A.L., Farrell, P.C., Uvelli, D.A. and Scribner, B.H. (1972) Haemodialyzer evaluation by examination of solute molecular spectra. *Trans. Am. Soc. Artif. Intern. Organs*, **18**, 98–105.

9. Gotch, F.A. (1984) Models to predict recirculation and its effect on treatment time in single-needle dialysis, in *First International Symposium on Single-Needle Dialysis* (eds S. Ringoir, R. Vanholder and P. Ivanovich), ISAO Press, Cleveland, pp. 47–62.

10. Morcos, A.W.B. and Nissenson, A.R. (1993) Erythropoietin and high-efficiency dialysis, in *Contemporary Issues in Nephrology 27 – Hemodialysis High-Efficiency Treatments* (ed. J.P. Bosch), Churchill Livingstone, New York, pp. 151–73.

11. Spiegler, K.S. and Kedem, O. (1966) Thermodynamics of hyperfiltration (reverse osmosis): criteria for efficient membranes. *Desalination*, **1**, 311–26.

12. Lysaght, M.J., Ford, C.A., Colton, C.K. *et al.* (1978) Mass transfer in clinical blood ultrafiltration devices – a review, in *Technical Aspects of Renal Dialysis* (ed. T.H. Frost), Pitman Medical, Tunbridge Wells, pp. 81–95.

13. Soltys, P.J., Ofsthun, N. and Leypoldt, J.K. (1992) Critical analysis of formulas for estimating back filtration in hemodialysis. *Blood Purif.*, **10**, 326–32.

14. Hoenich, N.A., Goodship, T.H.J., Ward, M.K. and Ringoir, S. (1986) in *Guide to Reprocessing Hemodialysers* (eds N. Deane, R.J. Wineman and J.A. Bemis), Martinus Nijhoff, Boston, pp. 107–34.

15. Shaldon, S. (1994) Reuse of haemodialysers. *Nephrol. Dial. Transplant.*, **9**, 1226–7.

16. Bosch, J.P. (1986) Continuous arteriovenous hemofiltration, in *Hemofiltration* (eds L.W. Henderson, E.A. Quellhorst, C.A. Baldamus and M.J. Lysaght), Springer-Verlag, Berlin, Heidelberg, pp. 234–51.

17. Tattersall, J., Farrington, K., Raniga, P.D. *et al.* (1993) Haemodialysis recirculation detected by the three sample method is an artifact. *Nephrol. Dial. Transplant.*, **8**, 60–3.

18. Daugirdas, J.T. and Ing, T.S. (1988) First-use reactions during hemodialysis: a definition of subtypes. *Kidney Int.*, **33**(suppl 24), S37–43.

19. Alter, M.J., Favero, M.S., Moyer, L.A. and Bland, L.A. (1991) National surveillance of dialysis-associated diseases in the United States, 1989. *Trans. Am. Soc. Artif. Intern. Organs.*, **37**, 97–109.

20. Leong, A.S-Y., Disney, A.T.S. and Gove, D.W. (1982) Spallation and migration of silicone from blood pump tubing in patients on hemodialysis. *N. Engl. J. Med.*, **306**, 135–40.

21. Oba, T., Tsuji, K., Nakamura, A. *et al.* (1984) Migration of acetylated hemi cellulose from capillary hemodialyser to blood causing scleritis and/or iritis. *Artif. Organs*, **8**, 429–35.

22. Hoenich, N.A., Thompson, J., Varini, E. *et al.* (1990) Particle spallation and plasticiser (DEHP) release from extracorporeal circuit materials. *Int. J. Artif. Organs.*, **13**, 55–62.

23. Hoenich, N.A., Thompson, J., McCabe, J. and Appleton, D.R. (1990) Particle release from haemodialysers. *Int. J. Artif. Organs.*, **13**, 803–8.

24. Craddock, P., Fehr, J., Dalmasso, A. *et al.* (1977) Hemodialysis leukopenia: pulmonary vascular leukostasis resulting from complement activation by dialyser cellophane membranes. *J. Clin. Invest.*, **59**, 879–88.

25. Hoenich, N.A., Woffindin, C., Matthews, J.N.S. *et al.* (1994) Clinical comparison of high flux cellulose acetate and synthetic membranes. *Nephrol. Dial. Transplant.*, **9**, 60–6.

26. Salama, A., Hugo, F., Heinvich, D. *et al.* (1988) Deposition of terminal C5b-9 complexes on erythrocytes and leukocytes during cardio-pulmonary bypass. *N. Engl. J. Med.*, **318**, 408–14.

27. Verresen, L., Waer, M., Vanrenterghem, Y. and Michielsen, P. (1990) Angiotensin converting enzyme inhibitors and anaphylactoid reactions to high flux membranes. *Lancet*, **336**, 1360–2.

28. Lemke, H. and Fink, E. (1992) Generation of bradykinin in human plasma using AN69 and PAN17DX membranes in the presence of ACE inhibitor *in vitro*. *Nephrol. Dial. Transplant.*, **7**, 728–29 (Abstract).

29. Kaplow, L.S. and Goffinet, J.A. (1968) Profound neutropenia during early phase of hemodialysis. *JAMA*, **203**, 133–5.

30. de Broe, M.E. (1994) Haemodialysis induced hypoxaemia. *Nephrol. Dial. Transplant.*, **9**(suppl 2), 173–5.

31. Hakim, R.M. (1993) Clinical implications of hemodialysis membrane biocompatibility. *Kidney Int.*, **44**, 484–94.

32. Henderson, L.W., Koch, K.M., Dinarello, C.A. and Shaldon, S. (1983) Hemodialysis hypotension: the interleukin hypothesis. *Blood Purif.*, **1**, 3–8.

33. Frith, S.E., Hoenich, N.A., Redfern, C.P.F. and Goodship, T.H.J. (1994) Production of interleukin 1 receptor antagonist and interleukin 1 during haemodialysis with cellulose membranes. *Int. J. Artif. Organs*, **17**, 478–87.

34. Higuchi, T., Kuno, T., Takahashi, S. and Kanmatsuse, K. (1997) Influence of dialysis membranes on Interleukin 1B and Interleukin 1 receptor antagonist production by peripheral blood mononuclear cells. *Artif. Organs*, **21**, 265–71.

35. Pereira, B.J.G., King, A.J., Poutsiaka, D.D. *et al.* (1993) Comparison of the first use and reuse of Cuprophan membranes. *Am. J. Kidney Dis.*, **22**, 288–95.

36. Kelly, T.D. (1996) Kinetics of intradialytic disequilibria: the problem, the causes, and new methods for the alleviation of patient morbidity. *Nephrol. Dial. Transplant.*, **11**(suppl 8), 3–9.

37. Santoro, A. and Mancini, E. (1997) Clinical significance of intradialytic blood volume monitoring. *Int. J. Artif. Organs*, **20**, 1–6.

38. Dellacciana, L. and Caputo, G. (1996) Robust reliable biosensor for continous monitoring of urea durind dialysis. *Clinical Chemistry* **42**, 1079–85.

39. Hoenich, N.A., Woffindin, C., Brennan, A., Cox, P.J., Matthews, J.N.S. and Goldfinch, M. (1996) A comparison of three brands of polysulfone membranes. *J. Am. Soc. Nephrol.*, **7**, 871–6.

40. Jacobs, C. (1996) Membrane biocompatibility in the treatment of acute renal failure: What is the evidence in 1996? *Nephrol. Dial. Transplant.*, **12**, 38–42.

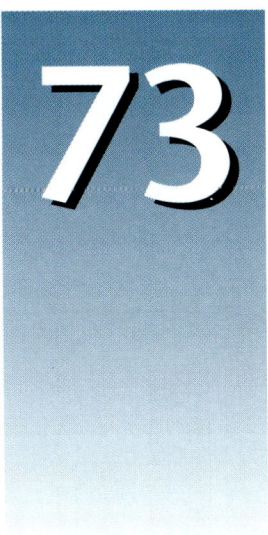

Hemodialysis: management and assessment

J.E. Tattersall, K. Farrington and
R.N. Greenwood

Introduction

The management and assessment of patients undergoing hemodialysis have changed substantially in the last few years. There is probably a wider variation of views on how patients should be treated now than there was 10 years ago when there was a degree of concordance in approach. Following the introduction of hemodialysis as a practical long-term treatment for renal failure in the 1960s it had become generally accepted practice to monitor the serum creatinine until the patient became uremic, which generally equated with a serum creatinine of about 1000 µmol/l (12 mg/dl). Uremia was essentially a clinical diagnosis which heralded entry into the renal replacement program. Standard hemodialysis in Europe used cellulosic membranes and a mean duration of 12.2 h/week, usually split into three sessions – the 'gold standard'. At the same time continuous ambulatory peritoneal dialysis (CAPD) was achieved using 8 l of dialysis fluid daily. Adequacy in patients established on dialysis was concerned with the control of hypertension, preferably through dialytic process, and the health of the bones. Dialysis time was adjusted according to the serum creatinine. The mean age of dialysis patients was 52.4 years. Only 18% were above the age of 65 years. Few questioned the validity of this approach since the five-year survival in all age groups had demonstrably improved in Europe over the previous decade (Figure 73.1).

A number of landmark developments took place in the late 1980s which substantially changed these perceptions.

First, the syndrome of β_2-microglobulin (β_2M)-related amyloid was described which by definition deemed standard dialysis to be inadequate. It appeared that dialysis with tight cellulosic membranes inevitably produced progressive disability if patients were treated for more than 5–10 years. Apart from the well-documented accumulation of β_2M in renal failure and its poor removal using standard membranes a number of other factors were implicated in the etiology of dialysis amyloid including the bioincompatibility of cuprophane, the presence of microbiological colonization and the use of acetate as base in dialysis fluid.

Second, erythropoietin (EPO) was introduced and lived up to all expectations. Its clinical use was relatively uncomplicated. It improved physical well-being and quality of life. It seemed possible that EPO could favorably influence the risks of cardiovascular and cerebrovascular disease in dialysis patients. Its adoption also led to a redefinition of the uremic syndrome, symptoms previously ascribed to uremia being increasingly recognized as being due to anemia. This preliminary experience heightened expectations that patients would receive EPO routinely to free them from dependence on blood transfusion.

Third, an important debate about the adequacy of dialysis took place in the United States. In 1989 the US Renal Data System (USRDS) reported a decrease in the five-year survival of the under 65-year-old group on hemodialysis in two successive five-year periods (Table 73.1). A five-year survival of 58% was reported and com-

Nephrology, Edited by Rex L. Jamison and Robert Wilkinson.
Published in 1997 by Chapman & Hall, London. ISBN 0 412 60930 4

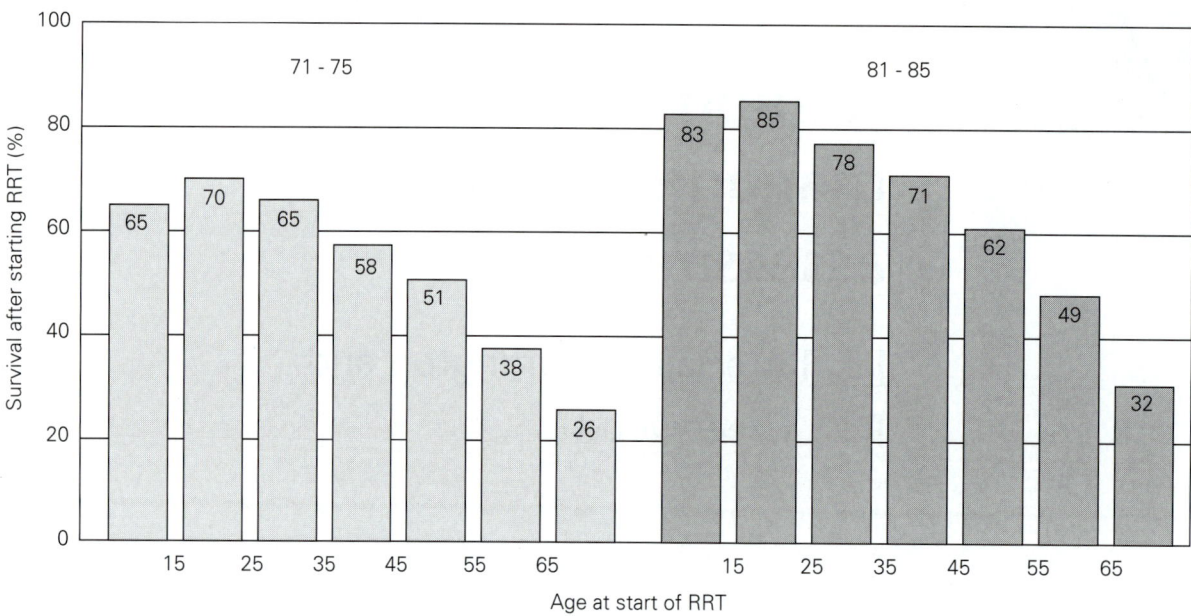

Figure 73.1 Improved five-year survival in European patients from the 1970s (71–75) to the 1980s (81–85). From the Registry of the European Dialysis and Transplant Association – European Renal Association.

Table 73.1 Comparison of outcomes in patients under the age of 65 years on hemodialysis, reported by the United States Renal Data System and the Registry of the European Dialysis and Transplant Association – European Renal Association

	1978–1983	1983–1988
USA	60%	58%
EDTA (80% response)	71%	75%

pared with a 75% survival reported by the Registry of the European Dialysis and Transplant Association (EDTA). Although data from the EDTA Registry must be interpreted cautiously because of incomplete reporting, this observation caused alarm. Concern was heightened by the recognition that the time spent on dialysis and hence the dialysis dose had progressively fallen as a result of the reimbursement system. The issue was keenly debated. Much valuable information emerged from a symposium on the Morbidity, Mortality and Prescription of Dialysis held in Dallas in September 1988. The most dramatic of these data was the demonstration that, in patients dialysing for relatively short times (less than 4h), there was an inverse relationship between the predialysis serum creatinine and the risk of death (Figure 73.2). Patients with low creatinine levels were at higher risk than

patients with high creatinine levels. It seemed that although low serum creatinine and urea can represent good dialysis, they can just as easily masquerade as such while truly reflecting low muscle mass and anorexia in malnourished patients receiving too little dialysis. These data discredited the use of serum creatinine as a tool to monitor dialysis adequacy.

At the end of the 1980s therefore it was necessary to be guarded about the wisdom of continuing with 'gold standard' dialysis. In the event, although technical advances permitted the gradual replacement of acetate with bicarbonate in most countries, significant financial and operational factors prevented both the widespread adoption of more biocompatible synthetic membranes and the use of bacteria and endotoxin-free water for dialysis. This, in turn, prevented more general adoption of high flux (porous) membranes for dialysis because of the dangers of sepsis from waterborne bacteria. However, the case for improved biocompatibility is gaining strength and stringent standards for water quality are already in place in a number of countries. Also encouraging is the introduction of new dialysis machines capable of delivering hemodiafiltration as opposed to hemodialysis. In this therapy the diffusive dialysis process is augmented by filtration of plasma water which enhances large molecule clearance. This technique, which can be carried out at a cost similar to hemodialysis, has been shown to remove significant quantities of β_2-microglobulin. Thus, although an array of therapies is available, their adoption tends to be determined by what is possible or permitted rather than by what is likely to be optimal for the patient. The US Health Care Finance Administration (HCFA)

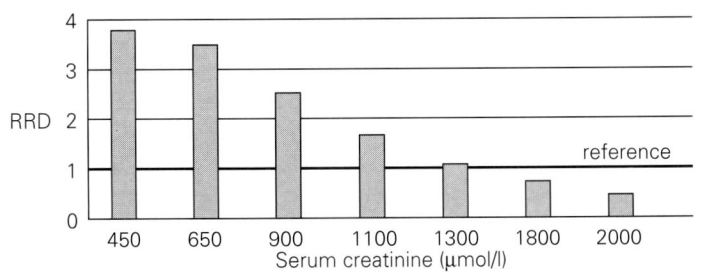

Figure 73.2 The relative risk of death (RRD) in dialysis patients as a function of predialysis serum creatinine. A reference level of 1300 μmol/l (15 mg/dl) gives an RRD of 1.0. (Reproduced from ref. [6].)

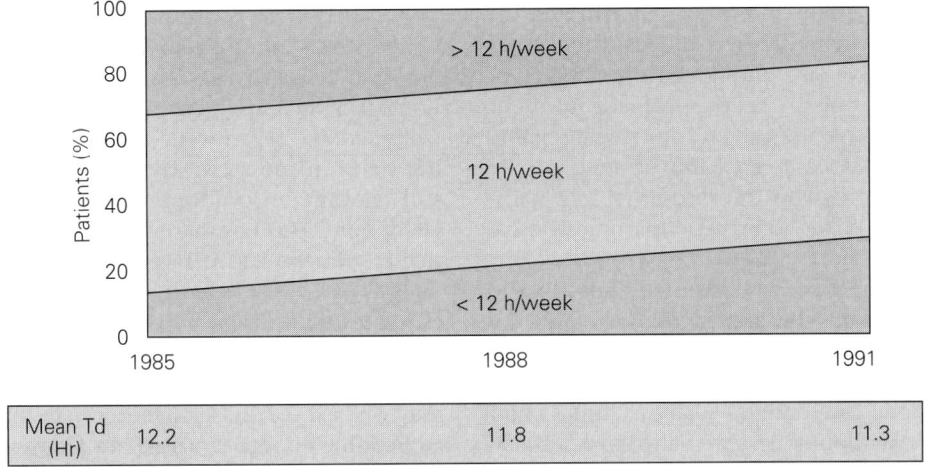

| Mean Td (Hr) | 12.2 | 11.8 | 11.3 |

Figure 73.3 The decline in hemodialysis duration in Europe. From the Registry of the EDTA-ERA (1993).

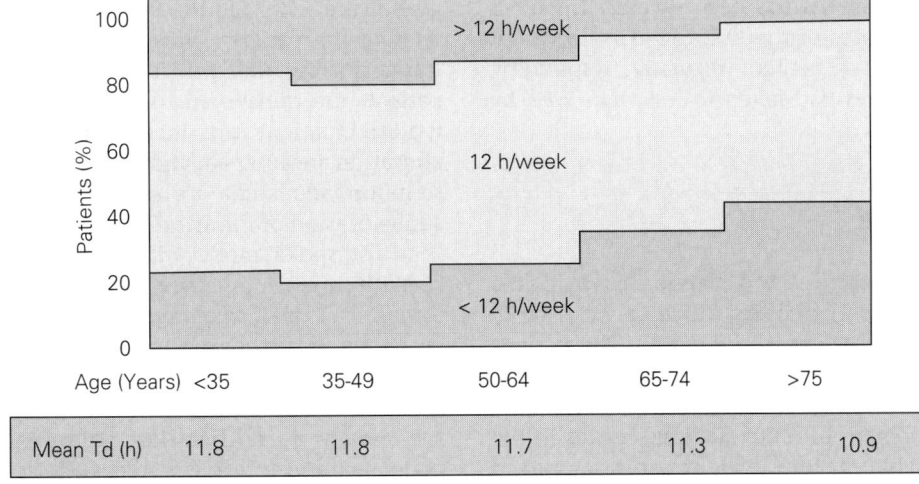

Age (Years)	<35	35-49	50-64	65-74	>75
Mean Td (h)	11.8	11.8	11.7	11.3	10.9

Figure 73.4 Dialysis duration related to age in Europe in 1991. From the Registry of the EDTA-ERA (1993).

responded positively to the problem of endemic underdialysis by establishing a multidisciplinary panel of experts to agree on a range of quality criteria. These were referred to as 'quality screens'. HCFA required that the 18

end-stage renal disease (ESRD) network organizations review the progress of all patients in the reimbursement system. A more sophisticated method for monitoring adequacy of dialysis was sought to replace reliance on serum solute levels. The tool with the best track record was seen to be urea kinetic modeling (UKM) which had been described by Gotch and colleagues a decade earlier. A simpler alternative was the urea reduction ratio (URR). Both had some predictive power with respect to outcomes [1]. The screens which were devised placed considerable emphasis on dialysis dose and the nutritional status of patients. Targets for dialysis does were stipulated for both hemodialysis and CAPD. Although the initiative was initially received coolly by the nephrology community at large, the approach of continuous quality review has been successfully ingrained into routine practice in the USA. One large providing group recently demonstrated an upward trend in URRs achieved over the last three years [2]. This HCFA initiative also questioned the validity of using serum solute levels as markers of adequacy in CAPD. Similarly reliance on serum creatinine as a reliable marker of the progression of renal impairment is now under examination along with the wisdom of maintaining predialysis patients for long periods on restrictive diets.

Following the experience in the United States in the 1980s it could reasonably be argued that it would be unwise to allow reductions in dialysis time in Europe below 12 h per week without there being firm quality standards in place. Interestingly dialysis times had declined in Europe without any surveillance of adequacy (Figure 73.3). Data from the EDTA registry (1991) also show that patients over the age of 65 receive less dialysis than young patients (Figure 73.4). It is a matter of general concern that new reforms in health care systems throughout Europe are likely to exert pressure to reduce dialysis time further. This is happening while the ability of EDTA to monitor trends has been severely impaired by the poor performance of the EDTA registry in recent years. The number of centers regularly responding to EDTA questionnaires had fallen to less than 70% by 1994.

Where to dialyze

The most common practice is to dialyze in renal units located in hospitals or in facilities which are free standing either in towns, cities or in rural areas. The pattern differs widely between countries. For example, almost all UK facilities are to be found in hospitals. This reflects the centralized development of acute medical services in the National Health Service before 1989. By contrast a mixed economy of hospital and free standing units is to be found in the USA as is the pattern in a number of European countries. Patients may assist in their own treatment or play a passive role depending on the chosen philosophy. The size of a dialysis facility depends on location and the size of the population served. Facilities accommodating less than 10 hemodialysis stations may be uneconomic. Units with upwards of 25 hemodialysis stations

can be intimidating and unattractive. Access to skilled nursing and medical cover are other factors determining location.

Self-supervised dialysis at home was pioneered in the late 1960s and became the preferred option for many patients, particularly in the UK, where hemodialysis services were centered in large metropolitan hospitals. Patients dialyzed for long periods; a total weekly dialysis duration exceeding 24 h was commonplace. Home dialysis generally allowed good rehabilitation of the patient and promoted confidence in the treatment itself. The timing of dialysis could be at the patient's own choosing and the risk of transmission of hepatitis B between patients was minimized. However, as average dialysis duration fell and the costs of dialysis equipment and home conversions increased, home dialysis as a therapeutic choice began to decline. This has been a continuing trend in most countries over the last 10 years. It is still relevant in locations which are geographically isolated, but CAPD has tended to replace home dialysis particularly in the UK. It has often been argued that home dialysis is a relatively inexpensive modality. However, estimates tend to ignore the large costs of staffing renal units with nurses dedicated to training rather than treatment and large technical back-up teams. The true costs may well exceed those of center hemodialysis and CAPD.

In some countries, there are large chains of facilities managed by a single provider, each having local autonomous management. In others, facilities are managed in a 'hub and spoke' fashion in which a central unit accommodates most of the medical and technical personnel and has a nursing skill mix commensurate with the need to support a heavy case mix of patients, some with acute renal failure. Satellite units (spokes) support relatively fit patients, have intermittent medical cover, a lower nursing skill mix and an arrangement whereby patients are transferred to the central unit should they require inpatient care. If new therapies such as hemodiafiltration are adopted, and if individualized modeled prescription and audit are pursued, the contrasts in the sophistication of infrastructure which tend to exist in the 'hub and spoke' model will have to be reappraised.

With increasing sensitivity to the demands of the customer, it is likely that renal units of the future will be geared more towards service provision, offering treatment or relatively short duration in pleasant surroundings. Many of these changes are being led by industry. During the last few years there has been a realignment of the major manufacturers to render dialysis provision a complete customer service.

Who to dialyze

There has been a dramatic change in the demography of the dialysis population in most Western countries over the past 20 years. The population is much older, and has a higher proportion of diabetics and of those with other comorbid conditions. This has been brought about primarily by the relaxation of previously rigid selection criteria, partly conditioned by increasing medical expertise in the adaptation of available therapeutic modalities, and partly by rising public expectations from what is rightly perceived to have been a major medical advance. These expectations have been fostered by a political climate promoting a more explicit approach to resource allocation. The success of renal replacement therapy has contributed to this demographic change in other ways. Patients who were relatively young and fit on commencing treatment have survived into old age with its attendant comorbidities, which include those occurring as a result of long-term treatment itself. All these factors have major economic repercussions.

The approach to patient selection for renal replacement therapy needs to be flexible and individualized. Inevitably selection processes will be influenced by the availability of dialysis facilities. Hard and fast rules are unhelpful. All patients with end-stage renal failure (ESRF) should be considered for treatment and a realistic assessment made of the potential benefits of that treatment for that particular patient in their individual circumstances. It is important to acknowledge the difficulty of obtaining a credible presumption of the patient's subjective perception of his or her likely quality of life.

Age and diabetes are by themselves no bar to treatment which can be very successful in both groups, though both can be accompanied by substantial comorbidities. Patients with severe heart failure in the context of ESRF are often dramatically improved by the initiation of dialysis. Malignancy need not be a contraindication in the absence of debilitating symptoms.

A 'trial of dialysis' is occasionally appropriate, though the point at which the trial is deemed to have failed to provide adequate resuscitation or rehabilitation can be difficult to acknowledge, and is seldom the same for patient, family, nurse and clinician. Failure of such a trial, and subsequent withdrawal of treatment, is as difficult to manage and often at least as stressful for all concerned, as withdrawal of chronic treatment (see below).

Patients, appropriately appraised of medical and psychosocial constraints, should be involved in the choice of their own treatment modality. Limited options for vascular access mitigate against the choice of hemodialysis. The elderly, diabetics (provided retinopathy is controlled), and patients with all but the most severe forms of cardiovascular compromise, do at least as well on hemodialysis as on CAPD. Hemodialysis is perhaps the better initial option in patients of above average body weight in whom CAPD may not provide adequate treatment when their residual renal function has been lost [4].

When to dialyze

Preparation for dialysis should begin some months before it is likely to be required. This allows informed choice of modality, creation and maturation of vascular access, and adequate psychosocial groundwork. These endeavors are sometimes undermined by factors such as late referral and misinterpretation of the degree of uremia. This often results in ill, poorly prepared patients requiring temporary venous access for urgent dialysis. Late referral is a significant source of early morbidity and mortality on dialysis programs [5].

The indications for dialysis are clear when patients present with life-threatening problems such as severe hyperkalemia, pulmonary edema, pericarditis and profound acidosis. The same is not true for clinic patients with slowly progressive renal failure. The point at which their residual renal function becomes inadequate to maintain well-being is often difficult to define. Reliance is placed on clinical features of uremia or fluid overload and biochemical parameters (blood urea, serum creatinine or its reciprocal). These biochemical measurements are poor indictors of adequacy in established dialysis patients. Low levels indicate malnutrition and wasting as much as adequate dialysis, and they predict increased mortality [6, 7]. The same problems may operate in the predialysis period.

Kinetic methods provide more reliable assessments of dialysis adequacy and may have a role in defining the optimum time to start dialysis. Normalized urea clearance may be a better indicator of the degree of uremia at the commencement of dialysis than blood urea and serum creatinine levels, and unlike them may be related to early dialysis morbidity and mortality [8]. There are other suggestions that earlier dialysis may improve outcome. Initiation of dialysis with creatinine clearances above 10 ml/min has been associated with improved survival and lower morbidity [9]. Diabetics may be a special case. They require to start dialysis with significantly lower serum creatinine levels than their non-diabetic counterparts, possibly because of increased susceptibility to the toxic effects of uremia.

How to dialyze

Biocompatibility issues

All hemodialysis treatments are relatively bioincompatible. It is now well known that cuprophane membranes activate complement. This sets up an inflammatory reaction in the lung (the first capillary bed the blood reaches after leaving the dialyzer) with sequestration of white cells. Within the first few minutes of dialysis, the white blood count count (WBC) falls by a factor of 10, recovering within 60 min. The clinical effects of the complement activation and WBC sequestration include cytokine production with hypotension, hypoxia, and increased β_2-microglobulin production. The precise nature, if any, of long-term sequelae of these acute effects remains to be determined. However, hemodialysis patients have a number of other long-term problems which may be caused or exacerbated by the bioincompatibility of the process. These include rapid loss of renal function after dialysis starts and immunocompromise. There is increasing, but not yet conclusive, evidence that these abnormalities improve if a more biocompatible membrane is used. Currently, cellulose-based membranes are available which have been modified to improve biocompatibility (cellulose acetate, hemophan). Some synthetic membranes have negligible blood interaction (polysulfone, PMMA). However, one synthetic membrane which was initially thought to be biocompatible (AN69) has recently been found to have bradykinin-activating properties *in vivo*.

β_2-Microglobulin and dialysis-related amyloidosis

Dialysis-related amyloidosis is a potentially limiting complication of chronic dialysis treatment. The syndrome was recognized in the early 1980s and β_2M was identified as the amyloid precursor protein l [10]. The main clinical features are carpal tunnel syndrome and a destructive arthropathy, predominantly affecting large and medium-sized joints, and associated with bone cysts. The incidence increases with the duration of hemodialysis; there is virtually 100% involvement by 15–20 years. Older patients are more susceptible.

β_2M is an 11 800 dalton protein which is part of the human class 1 major histocompatibility complex. It is found on the surface of all nucleated cells. Various cytokines, including tumor necrosis factor (TNF), interleukin-2 (IL-2), and alpha and gamma interferons cause increased synthesis and release of β_2M. It is eliminated largely (95%) by glomerular filtration and subsequent tubular absorption and degradation, hence its accumulation in renal failure.

Dialysis-specific factors may be important in the accumulation of β_2M. Hemodialysis incites an inflammatory response, stimulating release of IL-1 and TNF, granulocyte activation, and complement activation. The composition and purity of the dialysis fluid may also have a role, since acetate and endotoxin both promote IL-1 production. Increased β_2M production by lymphocytes and monocytes harvested at the end of hemodialysis has been demonstrated *in vitro*. These reactions are more pronounced with cuprophane membranes compared with membranes composed of polymethylmethacrylate, polyacrylonitrile or polysulfone. There is, however, very little evidence of β_2M generation in clinical hemodialysis when correction is made for dialysis-induced changes in extracellular fluid volume.

Although doubts remain about differences between membranes with respect to their capacity to generate

β_2M, there is little doubt that a significant clearance of β_2M can be achieved using high-flux membranes compared to that achieved by cuprophane. As well as increased removal of β_2M by filtration through these high-flux membranes, there is also evidence of enhanced adsorption of β_2M onto the membrane surface, an effect which may be modified by dialyzer reprocessing techniques. These effects may be clinically important. A large multicenter retrospective study has shown a decreased incidence of dialysis-related amyloidosis in patients dialyzed using polyacrylonitrile compared to patients dialyzed using cupraphane [11]. Hemofiltration has a greater capacity to remove β_2M than even high flux dialysis.

Treatment options are limited for established disease. Prevention is therefore of the utmost importance. The use of high-flux dialysis using biocompatible membranes, bicarbonate as the buffer and ultrapure water seem rational measures to adopt.

Water for dialysis

This is an important and undervalued aspect of biocompatibility. The increasing use of high-flux membranes, with their increased capacity for back filtration, especially at low ultrafiltration rates, and the frequent requirement for high dialysis fluid flow rates, has generated expanded interest in this area. The production of high quality water ideally employs a variety of water treatment modalities in series, each targeting a specific range of potential contaminants. Sediment filters remove larger inorganic and vegetable particles. Organic contaminants are absorbed by carbon filters. Water softeners reduce calcium and magnesium concentrations. Deionizers use cationic and anionic exchange resins to exchange a multiplicity of ions for hydrogen and hydroxyl ions which subsequently combine to form water. Reverse osmosis removes ions, dissolved organic and inorganic contaminants, bacteria, pyrogens and particulates. Additional filters with 0.5 and 0.2 µm resolution are used to ensure quality standards recommended by the American Association for the Advancement of Medical Instrumentation (AAMI). Similar attention must be paid to ensure the quality of the final dialysis fluid with respect to chemical, physical and microbiological characteristics.

Reuse

Reuse can offset the increased cost of dialyzers composed of the newer synthetic membranes to an extent which allows their routine clinical use. There is some evidence that reprocessed dialyzers are more biocompatible than new dialyzers. Their use is associated with fewer intradialytic symptoms, less complement activation, and a lower initial fall in neutrophil count. Processing prior to first use may avoid the rare anaphylactic response.

Acetate versus bicarbonate dialysis

The expansion of the chronic dialysis program in the 1960s required a streamlined approach to dialysis fluid preparation and led to the substitution of bicarbonate by acetate. Acetate dialysis has subsequently been associated with a number of problems. These include intradialytic acidosis and hypocapnea, intradialytic hypoxemia and cardiovascular instability due to vasodilatation. Symptoms of headache, nausea, fatigue and hypotension are common. High efficiency treatments are particularly vulnerable since the acetate load greatly exceeds its metabolic utilization rate. Use of bicarbonate as buffer has been shown to be associated with significantly fewer of these symptoms [12]. The increasing trend toward utilization of high efficiency treatments has been the catalyst required to overcome the resource implications of the shift back to bicarbonate.

Adequacy issues

Dialysis supports life despite complete cessation of renal function. This is achieved at considerable cost and inconvenience to the patient yet it still fails to restore full health. It is not possible to replace renal function completely. In general, the greater the proportion of renal function replaced, the more expensive and inconvenient the treatment. Clearly, there is a minimum threshold quantity of dialysis needed to support life, an optimum quantity, approaching normal renal function, which restores the patient to full health, and an intermediate grey area in which the patient is alive but with a degree of functional impairment. The main concern must be how to balance the need to restore full health, with the demand for a cheap and convenient treatment. Adequacy is the compromise between acceptable outcome, acceptable inconvenience and acceptable cost. Since the concept involves subjective assessments of what constitutes acceptability in all these areas, adequacy is not a static quantity. The issues are under constant debate and solutions vary widely even between institutions in the same locality. In addition, practices in dialysis are constantly evolving in an attempt to minimize the side effects and inconvenience of treatment and to maximize its efficacy.

The adequacy debate requires objective measurement of patient outcome, function and the degree of inconvenience associated with treatment. Treatments employed and their subsequent modifications must be well characterized, quantifiable and costed. The need to measure the amount and type of treatment provided is central, as is the need for measurable parameters relating to the effect of dialysis on the patient. Some of these markers respond relatively rapidly to changes in dialysis treatment. These include serum bicarbonate, hemoglobin, calcium, phosphate and blood pressure. Others are long-term outcomes and often irreversible (death, β_2-microglobulin amyloidosis) or difficult to treat (malnutrition, left ventricular

hypertrophy, bone disease). It is of fundamental importance to have a working, if empirical, definition of adequacy and means to ensure that all patients receive at least this amount of treatment.

What is an adequate dialysis?

The ideal is to restore fully all of the functions of the failed kidney. These functions include solute clearance, fluid and electrolyte homeostasis, regeneration of bicarbonate, blood pressure control, calcium and phosphate homeostasis, and maintenance of hemoglobin concentrations. The molecular weight of the solutes to be cleared ranges over two orders of magnitude from small (water, urea) to large (β_2-microglobulin). In practice, the art of prescribing dialysis is to provide suboptimal treatment in a controlled way so that although normal renal function is not fully restored, the ill effects on the patient are acceptable.

Low-molecular-weight toxins

There is now ample evidence that good survival depends on adequate removal of low-molecular-weight toxins for which urea is a surrogate. There have even been attempts to determine the optimum amount of urea to be removed consistent with health and good survival. The National Co-operative Dialysis Study (NCDS) demonstrated a relationship between medium-term morbidity and mortality and Kt/V, the fractional urea cleared volume. Kt/V is a logical unit of measure for the low-molecular-weight clearance efficacy of dialysis. K is the urea clearance rate (in ml/min), t is the dialysis time (in min) and V is the urea distribution volume (in ml – equivalent to the body water content or 56% of body weight). Kt is the total volume cleared of urea for a dialysis and Kt/V is the ratio of volume cleared to volume present.

By using the Kt/V concept dialysis can be planned to deliver a particular Kt/V. K can be determined from the dialyzer manufacturer's data sheets, taking into account the extracorporeal blood and dialyzate flow rates. The prescribed dialysis time is then calculated prospectively from the formula:

$$t = \mathrm{d}Kt/V \times \frac{V}{K}$$

where $\mathrm{d}Kt/V$ is the desired Kt/V. Kt/V can also be calculated directly from pre- and postdialysis urea concentration measurements without knowledge of K or V. This direct measurement is used to quality control the dialysis process.

It is now widely accepted that delivered Kt/V relates to outcome, though the optimal value for Kt/V is still debated. Gotch and Sargent's analysis of the NCDS study 1 suggested that a threshold Kt/V value, in the region of 0.8–1, divided adequate from inadequate treatment. Little extra benefit was considered to be gained from increasing Kt/V beyond these levels.

The concept of an adequacy threshold is theoretically plausible. At a Kt/V of 1, 65% of the total body urea has already been removed. There are rapidly diminishing returns from further increments of Kt/V. An infinite increase in Kt/V is required to remove the remaining 35%. Recently, the concept of this 'threshold' has been challenged. Re-analysis of the NCDS [13] data has suggested that there may be progressive improvement in outcome as Kt/V increases above 1. Some units routinely deliver a Kt/V up to 1.6 by thrice-weekly haemodialysis [14], and appear to have a significantly better outcome even correcting for comorbidity.

Retrospective analyses of quality-adjusted survival data [15] have suggested continuous improvement in outcome as Kt/V increases beyond 1. The NCDS study was limited by small numbers of patients, a short follow-up period and an atypical study population which excluded those with significant comorbidity. The study was not designed to detect differences in long-term morbidity and mortality between patients receiving a Kt/V of 1 and higher values. Pending the conclusion of further studies current opinion is moving towards acceptance of 'adequate' Kt/V values as being much higher than 1.

Recirculation and two-pool effects

It is now recognized that urea kinetics are better described by a two-pool model than by Gothch's original one-pool model [16]. Dialysis efficiency is limited by the rate at which urea can be delivered from the different compartments of the body into the fistula. This rate depends on cardiac output, blood flow in the different regions of the body, and the rate of diffusion across cell membranes. The mathematics describing these effects are similar and surprisingly simple [17], reducing to a single time constant (the patient clearance time) which has a value of 30 min for urea. This is the time needed to clear the peripheral compartments of the body and is, in effect, the mean of the ratios of intercompartment mass transfer rate (flow rate or diffusion coefficient) to the volumes of the peripheral compartments. The multicompartment effects reduce effective Kt/V, on average, by the factor $t/(t + 30)$ or about 20% for 120 min dialyses and 8% for 240 min dialyses. In order to take these effects into account, the dialysis time must be increased and the increase should be relatively more in short dialysis. This may be achieved by adding the patient clearance time or 30 min × desired Kt/V to the

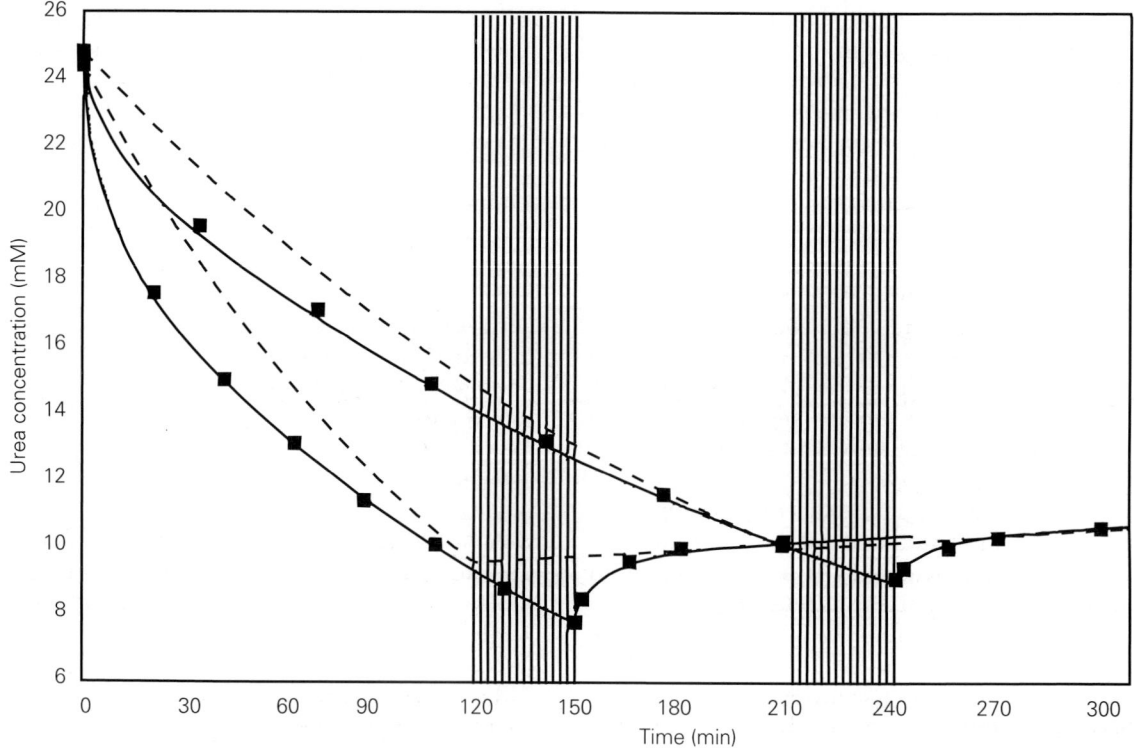

Figure 73.5 Plot of urea concentration against time. The squares represent the mean of 29 measurements in 29 different patients treated by a long and short dialysis in consecutive weeks. The lines represent concentrations predicted by single (dotted) and double-pool (solid lines) UKMs with $Kt/V = 1$. The addition of 30 min to the dialysis time (shaded area) corrects for the effect of the rebound in both long and short dialyses.

dialysis time. The equation for determining dialysis time to achieve a given desired Kt/V (dKt/V) therefore becomes;

$$t = dKt/V \times \left(\frac{V}{K} + 30 \right)$$

This will cause the immediate postdialysis urea concentration to be lower than required to achieve the target Kt/V, but after dialysis, the concentration rebounds up to the target value (Figure 73.5). The 30 min addition adds relatively more to the short dialysis (as K is greater).

Large-molecular-weight toxins

A significant theoretical limitation in the Kt/V concept is that high-molecular-weight solutes are not considered. β_2M is one of the few well-substantiated uremic toxins. Standard cuprophane membranes have insufficient pore size to clear β_2M. Even if a high Kt/V is prescribed using long dialysis times, β_2M accumulates and produces significant long-term problems. If long-term survival on dialysis is the goal, it would seem reasonable to choose a dialyzer membrane with pore size sufficient to clear β_2M and indeed other not yet identified larger-molecular-weight uremic toxins. The use of more open-pore membranes is termed 'high-flux'. High-flux dialyzers are generally much more expensive than standard cuprophane dialyzers but the increased cost can be offset by reuse.

Using high-flux dialysis does not guarantee efficient high-molecular-weight solute clearance. Larger solutes diffuse more slowly than urea. Urea clearance is increased by increasing blood flow, but the clearance of β_2M may not increase if there is insufficient time available for diffusion within the dialyzer. Blood flow should be prescribed in proportion to the dialyzer membrane surface area. This maintains the time the blood takes to pass through the dialyzer at a constant value and maintains the ratio between the clearance rates of all solutes whatever the blood flow rate. Typically, membrane surface areas of $1-1.2\,m^2$ are used with blood flows of $200-250\,ml/min$ and $2-2.2\,m^2$ for $400-500\,ml/min$.

Many of the problems related to differing clearance rates for different solutes can be eliminated by using filtration instead of diffusion. In this modality, all solutes are cleared at a similar rate regardless of blood flow rate and surface area. Filtration modes can be combined with dialysis to allow very high clearance rates – up to $350\,ml/min$. Filtration generally removes up to $40\,l$ plasma filtrate from the patient each treatment. This must be replaced by a similar volume of sterile replacement fluid which can now be produced inexpensively on-line by filtration of the dialysis fluid.

Adequacy, salt and water

During dialysis, any fluid accumulated in the period after the previous dialysis must be removed. Almost all of this fluid is in the extravascular compartment and must transfer into the vascular compartment before removal by filtration in the dialyzer. There is a finite rate at which fluid can transfer into the circulation. This rate depends partly on the function and homeostatic control of the capillaries. In many dialysis patients, the capillary function may be impaired by diabetes, hypertensive disease and their homeostatic mechanisms blocked by antihypertensive drugs. In these patients, it may be very difficult to remove the fluid except very slowly over a long dialysis time. In any dialysis patient, but especially the complicated patient, fluid removal is easier when the patient is overloaded. Therefore there is a tendency for patients to become chronically overloaded if they are treated by inappropriately short treatments.

Adequacy and bicarbonate

One of the functions of the human kidney is to regenerate bicarbonate. Dialysis achieves this by including a supraphysiologic concentration of bicarbonate in the dialysis fluid. During dialysis, bicarbonate diffuses into the blood across the dialyzer membrane. One of the aims of dialysis is to normalize the serum bicarbonate concentration. This is achievable if the dialysis is correctly prescribed and planned. Bicarbonate has a similar molecular weight to urea so the relative mass of bicarbonate transferred into the blood is proportional to the Kt/V and the bicarbonate concentration gradient across the membrane. To some extent, a natural homeostasis occurs in that those patients who are acidotic will have a lower bicarbonate and a higher concentration gradient. For a Kt/V of 1, a dialyzate bicarbonate concentration of $40\,mM$ will maintain a serum bicarbonate concentration at $22-26\,mM$ in virtually all cases. If the Kt/V is increased, a proportional reduction in concentration gradient is required, so that for a Kt/V of 1.5 the dialyzate bicarbonate concentration should be reduced to $35\,mM$. Individual variations in the dialyzate bicarbonate concentration may be required to cope with differing metabolic rates, diets and oral base intake (e.g. calcium carbonate). Most dialysis machines allow individualized control of the dialysis fluid bicarbonate concentration.

Duration of dialysis

In hemodialysis, there is a tendency to shorten dialysis time to reduce cost and increase patient convenience. It is now generally accepted that there is a significant risk of underdialysis if treatment times are shortened to $4\,h$ or less. To avoid these risks, a return to longer dialysis times has been advocated, despite the increase in cost and inconvenience to the patient. An alternative strategy is to attempt to understand the mechanisms of reduced efficiency in short dialysis and to apply specific corrections.

If it were possible to increase the rate of removal of fluid and solute mass in proportion to the reduction of dialysis time, without increasing the patient's fluid content, blood pressure or solute concentrations then the short treatment would have equivalent efficacy to the long treatment. The *Kt/V* concept is a tool for forcing an adequate time of dialysis, appropriate to the *K* and *V*. However, there are a number of factors which combine to reduce the rate of fluid and solute removal in short dialysis. These include the relatively slow diffusion of middle- and large-molecular-weight solutes, hypotension related to high ultrafiltration rates and the postdialysis rebound. If these factors are not taken into account, short dialysis will be inferior to long dialysis even if *Kt/V* is the same.

The importance of residual renal function

It is now generally recognized that residual renal function provides a significant proportion of the total clearance in CAPD patients. Adequacy assessment is therefore not complete unless renal function is known. In the past, renal clearance was considered to be insignificant in hemodialysis, perhaps because of difficulties with measurement but also because the bioincompatibility of the process may have contributed to its rapid decline. In our unit we find similar renal clearance rates in hemodialysis and CAPD patients (Figure 73.6). During the second year

of dialysis, 30% of the total clearance may be provided by kidneys.

If the renal clearance is known, normalized protein catabolic rate (nPCR) and *Kt/V* can be calculated more accurately and the hemodialysis dose prescribed may be reduced to take the renal function into account. This is particularly important during the first few months and years of dialysis. There are economic savings and the practice provides patients with a gentler start to their dialysis careers. As renal function declines, the dialysis dose is increased to compensate. There is great variation in the rate of decline of residual renal function. Regular measurement is required to individualize the dialysis dose.

Anticoagulation

When blood is drawn into the extracorporeal blood circuit, the surface contact activates the intrinsic coagulation pathway. Platelets adhere to the internal surfaces of the circuit and release adenine diphosphate and thromboxane A_2. These changes develop progressively as dialysis proceeds and, unless special precautions are taken, the circuit will eventually clot. The risks may be diminished by reducing dialysis time, reducing the area of blood–air interfaces, reducing the contact time between blood and extracorporeal circuit, and using anti-

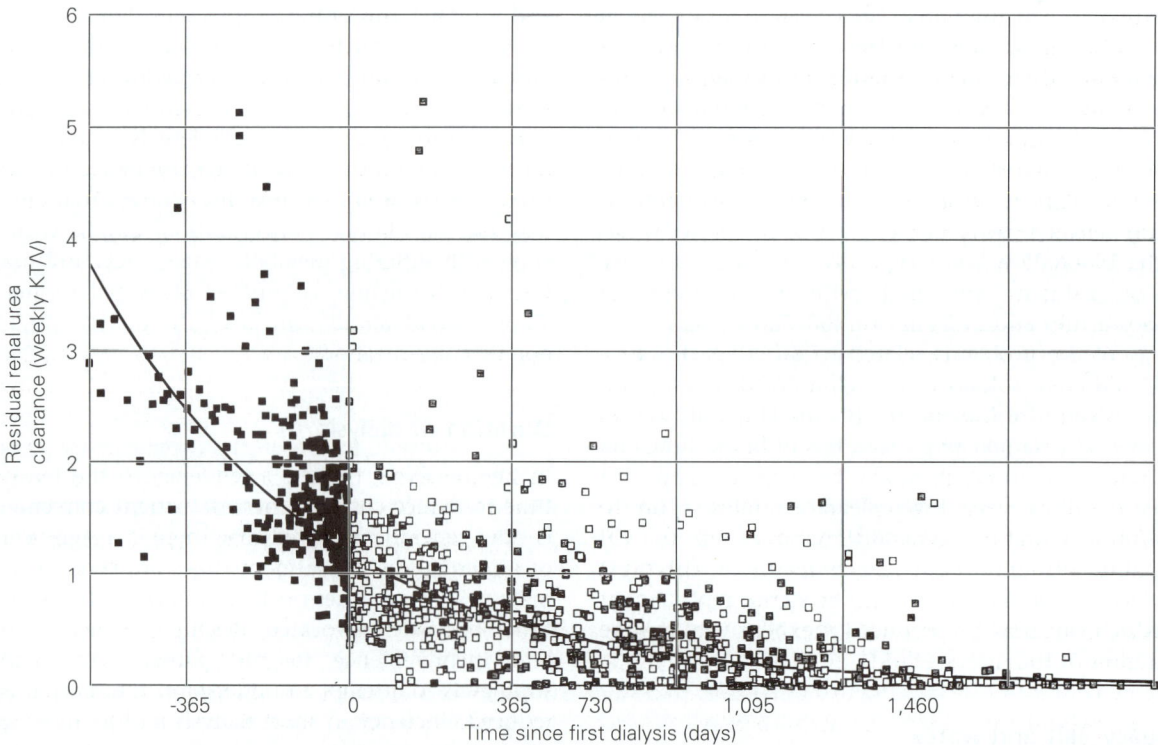

Figure 73.6   Residual renal urea clearance as a function of time on dialysis in predialysis patients (black squares), patients on high-flux hemodialysis (grey squares) and those on CAPD (open squares).

coagulants. Priming procedures should be rigorous, eliminating air bubbles from the dialyzer and ensuring that air is removed from all side-arms to the blood tubing. The blood flow rate should be as high as practicable and the volume of the circuit should be as low as possible to limit the amount of time the blood is in contact with the artificials. The extracorporeal circuit should be designed with the length of the blood tubing, the number and size of any bubble-traps and any side-arms kept to a minimum.

Coagulation may also be inhibited by coating the extracorporeal circuit surface with a suitable anticoagulant. This may be achieved by adding heparin 1000 iu/l to the prime solution. Heparin is also commonly administered to the patient by intravenous infusion during dialysis. Heparin is a glycosaminoglycan, extracted from bovine or porcine lung and intestine. It increases the activity of antithrombin III and inhibits the clotting factors IX, X, XI, XII and thrombin. Commonly 1000–4000 iu are injected at the start of dialysis followed by an infusion at 500–2000 iu/h. The infusion may be stopped 15–30 min before the end of dialysis. In short dialyses, the initial heparin bolus alone may be sufficient. The precise dose is chosen by trial and error to achieve a two to three times increase (to around 200 s versus 50–80 s control) in activated clotting time (ACT). The ACT uses a surface activator to accelerate clotting and the end point is detected automatically. In practice, minimal heparin is given during a patient's first dialysis and the ACT monitored at 15 min intervals. Adjustments in the heparin dosage are guided by the ACT.

Heparin has a number of side effects. It enhances platelet adhesion to dialyzer membranes, causing platelet consumption, and sometimes results in prolonged bleeding postdialysis. The anticoagulant effect of heparin may be prolonged, particularly if excessive doses are given. Heparin may contribute to the development of osteoporosis in dialysis patients. For these reasons, low-molecular-weight forms of heparin were developed. Low-molecular-weight heparin has a strong affinity for antithrombin III and strongly inhibits factor Xa and XIIa but weakly inhibits factors IX and Xi. Hence there is less tendency for thrombocytopenia and fewer bleeding problems. Since only marginal increments in thrombin and thromboplastin times occur, the therapeutic level of low-molecular-weight heparin can only be monitored using the relatively expensive factor Xa activity assay. In practice low-molecular-weight heparin is usually reserved for patients with a high risk of bleeding.

An alternative approach to prevent heparin-related thrombocytopenia is to use a systemic antiplatelet agent such as aspirin. In theory, this may also allow a reduction in the dose of heparin required. In acute renal failure, treated by continuous dialysis or hemofiltration, prostacyclin, a powerful antiplatelet agent, has been used as an alternative to heparin.

In patients who are at a high risk of bleeding, dialysis may be performed without anticoagulation. Heparin-free dialysis is performed by flushing the extracorporeal circuit every 15–30 min with 200–400 ml of an isotonic electrolyte solution. This removes adhered platelets and small clots. Care must be taken to reduce blood–air surface area and extracorporeal blood volume. The flush volume must be taken into account in the fluid balance calculations.

Viral infections

Hepatitis B infection was a serious problem in the early days of dialysis. Fatalities occurred in both patients and staff. A dramatic decrease in the number of staff contracting hepatitis B was observed in countries where active immunization programs were enthusiastically pursued. In most units in developed countries immunization is now standard practice for all staff in direct contact with patients. Hemodialysis patients are generally screened on a six-monthly basis. As universal precautions tend to be employed, isolation of hepatitis B-positive patients is not strictly necessary. However, there is still a tendency to manage these patients in side rooms and to employ dedicated machines wherever possible with chemical disinfection post-treatment.

Until recently hepatitis viruses which were not identified as A or B were grouped together under the term of ignorance 'non-A, non-B hepatitis'. Hepatitis C has now emerged from this all-embracing category. The virus has been cloned to reveal a 30–60 nm lipid enveloped, single-stranded RNA with structural and genomic similarities to the arthropod-borne flaviviruses (such as dengue) and animal pestiviruses.

Hepatitis C (HCV) is transmitted by blood products; about 80% of patients with transfusion-associated non-A, non-B hepatitis are anti-HCV positive. The frequency among dialysis patients is variable but lower, ranging from 2% to 20%, suggesting that single donor blood products are associated with a lower risk than pooled factor concentrates. Infection with HCV is causally related to acute and chronic persistent hepatitis, with onward progression to sclerosis and hepatocellular carcinoma. Recombinant interferon α ameliorates the biochemical abnormalities and histologic activity associated with hepatitis C when administered in a dose of 3 million units three times weekly for six months. However, there is a heavy relapse rate and further clinical experience is necessary before this is established as the treatment of choice.

Attitudes to screening for hepatitis C and management of hemodialysis patients with the condition is not surprisingly varied, given the relatively recent recognition of the problem. There is a growing tendency to screen hemodialysis patients regularly for hepatitis C as well as for hepatitis B. Dedicated machines in separate areas in renal units are often employed with strict protocols for disinfection of dialysis equipment. Both of these viral infections demand universal precautions in treating all patients in hemodialysis units.

Monitoring

Monitoring dialysis adequacy

Since the functions of the kidney are so diverse, measurement of dialysis adequacy needs to be multidimensional. The dialysis process and the needs of the patient should be well understood and the treatment prescribed in such a way as to meet these needs. The dialysis should be monitored by periodic measurement as a quality control exercise. The monitoring allows the unit to demonstrate or confirm the delivery of an adequate dialysis, to detect problems and to guide improvements in dialysis delivery.

Small solutes

Adequacy measurement has focused on small solute clearance. This is mainly because urea and creatinine are easy to measure and it is relatively easy to influence their clearance rate. As much as 100 g of urea is generated per week and must be cleared; this is the largest mass of any solute. It is now generally recognized that, unless sufficient urea is cleared, the patient becomes chronically malnourished, presumably due to the accumulation of an appetite-suppressing uremic toxin, and at increased risk of morbidity and mortality.

As discussed above, simply measuring blood urea or creatinine concentrations is misleading and provides little information on the adequacy of dialysis. The urea generation rate is influenced by its clearance rate so that as clearance falls, appetite is reduced, less protein is ingested and less urea is generated. In this way, the urea may be low in underdialyzed patients due to the resulting malnutrition. Similarly, underdialyzed patients may have a low muscle mass from malnutrition, resulting in low blood creatinine concentrations. There is a progressively increasing mortality rate as urea and creatinine concentrations fall, reflecting malnutrition and possibly underdialysis in patients with low creatinine and urea concentrations. Patient outcome is related to the rate at which a uremic toxin can be cleared rather than its concentration. In this analysis, the toxin inhibits metabolic or dietary processes leading to its generation. The greater the mass of toxin removed, the greater its generation rate. Thus, its concentration does not change, but the dietary and metabolic health of the patient improves as the mass removed increases [18]. The measurement of adequacy of small solute removal must be based on the mass of solute cleared rather than its blood concentration.

The urea reduction ratio (URR)

The simplest measurement is the URR. This is obtained by measuring pre- and postdialysis blood urea concentrations and calculating URR from the formula:

$$URR = \frac{Urea_{pre} - Urea_{post}}{Urea_{pre}}$$

The URR is an approximate estimate of the ratio of mass cleared (proportional to pre–post) to mass present at the start of dialysis (proportional to pre). URR has been shown to relate to survival in hemodialysis patients.

The URR ignores the effect of fluid removal and urea generation during dialysis. This means URR is an underestimate of the total mass removed, particularly in long dialyses and where there is significant ultrafiltration. These errors may be included by the formula:

$$URR = 1 - \frac{Urea_{post} - \left(Urea_{pre} - Urea_{post}\right) \times \frac{t}{ti}}{Urea_{pre}} \times \frac{V}{V + uft}$$

where V is the urea distribution volume (approximately 57% of body weight), t and ti are the dialysis time and the interdialysis interval time, respectively, and uft is the total weight of fluid removed from the patient during dialysis.

In monitoring dialysis adequacy, care must be taken to ensure that the measurements are made during a typical dialysis. Measurements should be made frequently enough to detect problems early. Ideally, the dialysis should be quantified during each dialysis but this is expensive. A typical compromise would be a monthly measurement with an additional repeat if the prescription changes. In future, on-line continuous solute measurement will enable routine monitoring of every dialysis.

The fractional cleared volume of urea (*Kt/V*)

Kt/V may be calculated directly from the pre- and postdialysis urea concentrations from the formula:

$$Kt/V = \ln\left(\frac{Urea_{pre}}{Urea_{post}}\right)$$

More complex formulae, including the effect of urea generation rate, residual renal function and fluid removal, are available but need iterative solutions, and can only be used from within a suitable computer program. The advantage of calculating Kt/V is that the value may be compared with the prescribed Kt/V to confirm that treatment was efficiently delivered. The measured Kt/V may form the basis for prospective changes in the dialysis prescription. For example, if the measured Kt/V is only 50% of the target Kt/V, either the dialysis time (t) or the urea clearance (K) could to be doubled in order to double the Kt/V and reach the target. The relationship between K, t and URR is more complicated.

After dialysis, the blood urea concentration rebounds up as the extravascular urea re-equilibrates. If the postdialysis sample is drawn before the rebound is complete (at least 30 min after the end of dialysis), *Kt/V* or URR will be overestimated. This overestimation will be greater in short dialyses (approximately 25% for a 2 h dialysis) than long dialyses (12% for a 4 h dialysis). Since delayed blood sampling is impractical, the *Kt/V* may be corrected by multiplying it by the factor $t/(t + 30)$, where t is the dialysis time in minutes. The value 30 in the correction factor is the patient's clearance time described previously.

Measurement of residual renal function

Renal clearance may be quantified by an interdialytic urine collection. The mean blood concentration during the collection period must be known. This is usually calculated from the urea concentration measured in blood samples drawn at the end of the dialysis preceding the start of the collection and just before the start of the dialysis following the end of the collection. It is usually more practical to use a computer program.

Recirculation

There are two types of recirculation: access (Figure 73.7) and cardiopulmonary (Figure 73.8). Access recirculation occurs when a proportion of the blood returning to the patient in the venous line is immediately drawn into the arterial needle and dialyzed again without leaving the fistula. It occurs when the arterial needle is placed downstream of the venous needle or when the extracorporeal blood flow rate exceeds the blood flow rate in the fistula. In the case of the incorrectly placed needles, the recirculation fraction is the ratio of the extracorporeal blood flow rate to the fistula flow rate. This type of recirculation most commonly occurs in PTFE loops in which the direction of blood flow is not obvious.

Access recirculation due to limitations in fistula flow rate is relatively rare, since access flow rates are usually in excess of 700 ml/min, and the extracorporeal blood flow rate is unlikely to exceed this. Recirculation of this kind is usually caused by a critical stenosis and is an indication that the fistula will soon clot. Such recirculation is critically dependent on the extracorporeal blood flow rate. It is absent at low blood flow rates but increases rapidly as blood flow rate rises above the fistula flow rate. After dialysis ceases, the recirculated blood is rapidly washed out of the fistula and the solute concentration rebounds upwards. The rebound due to access recirculation is complete within seconds.

Access recirculation reduces dialysis efficiency by reducing the concentration gradients in the dialyzer since the blood entering the dialyzer is diluted by recirculated blood. The dose of dialysis delivered is usually calculated from the ratio of pre- and postdialysis blood solute concentrations. If the postdialysis sample is taken before the rebound, the urea concentration will be reduced by recirculation and the calculated dose

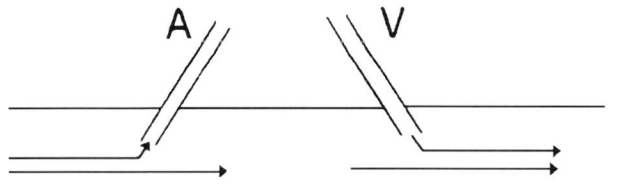

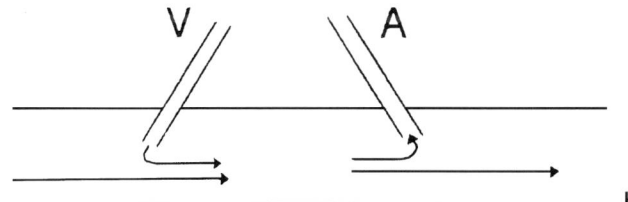

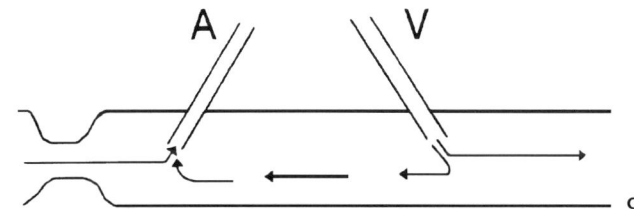

Figure 73.7 Access recirculation. Blood enters the dialyzer through the arterial port (A) and returns to the body through the venous port (V). (a) The normal situation when there is no access recirculation. (b) Recirculation due to the arterial needle being incorrectly placed upstream of the venous needle. (c) Access recirculation in a stenosed fistula with flow rates lower than the extracorporeal blood flow rate.

significantly overestimated. The postdialysis sample must be taken after the access-related rebound is complete. It is usually taken from a sample port in the arterial line after the blood pump has been slowed to 50 ml/min for 30 s. This time allows the recirculated blood to clear the fistula and for the fistula blood to be drawn up to the sample port.

Access recirculation may have a major effect on efficiency and may indicate imminent fistula failure. If the routine measurement of dialysis dose delivered reveals an unexpected fall-off in efficiency or if there are any doubts about fistula performance, recirculation should be measured directly by one of a number of methods.

The three-sample method [19]

The urea concentration is measured in samples taken simultaneously from the dialyzer inlet (*A*) and outlet (*V*) and from a peripheral vein (*P*). The recirculation fraction (*RF*) is calculated from the formula:

$$RF = \frac{P - A}{P - V}$$

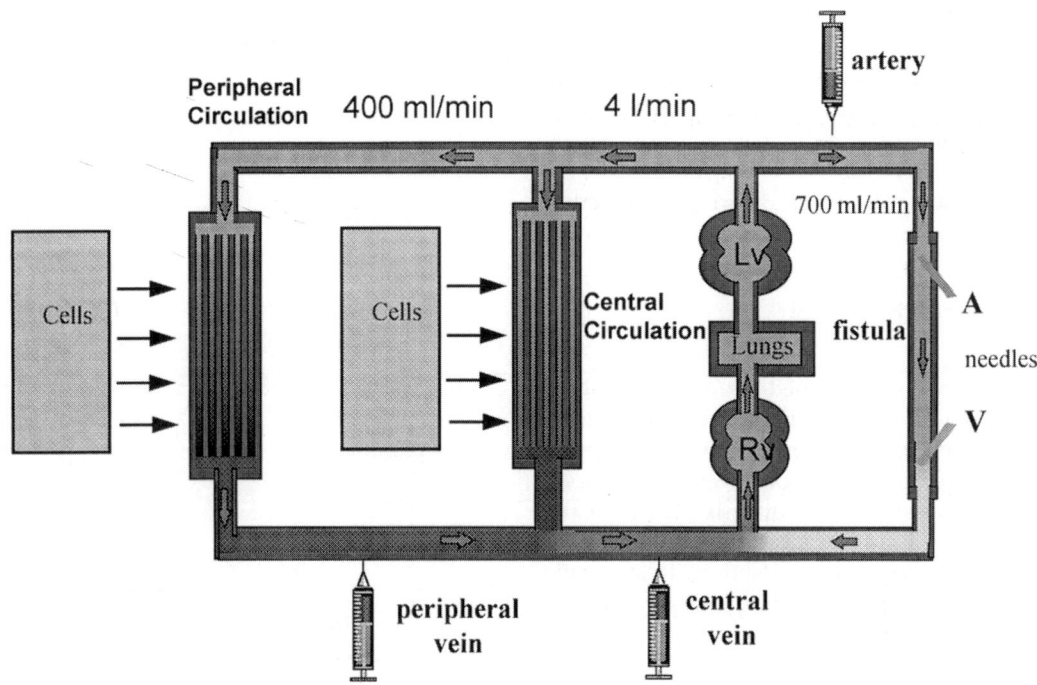

Figure 73.8 Simple plan of the circulation. Cardiopulmonary recirculation occurs as some of the dialyzed blood from the venous needle (V) flows through heart (Rv,Lv) and lungs back to arterial needle (A) without passing through the capillary beds. Intracellular solute must diffuse from the cells into the circulation (solid arrows) and then be carried by the blood flow into the fistula. This takes time and the delay reduces dialysis efficiency and causes the rebound. During dialysis, solute concentration will be higher in the peripheral veins (draining skin and resting muscle) than in the central veins (e.g. vena cava) and lowest in the arteries. This diagram shows only two of the many circulation compartments.

This method overestimates *RF* by 5–15% because it reflects the disequilibrium between arteries and veins which develops during dialysis [20–22].

The slow-flow method

This is a modification of the three-sample method. The peripheral sample is replaced by a sample from the dialyzer inlet taken after the blood pump has been slowed to 50 ml/min for 30 s [23]. This method is simpler to perform and is not influenced by disequilibrium in the same way as the three-sample method. However, the timing of the slow-flow sample is critical. The sample must be taken allowing sufficient time for the recirculated blood to clear the fistula and for the arterial blood to be drawn up to the sample port. If the sample is delayed by more than a few seconds, the solute concentration in the fistula blood will have started to rebound upwards due to re-equilibration and cause the *RF* to be overestimated.

Saline-dilution methods

A bolus of saline is injected into the venous line during dialysis and is detected in the arterial line a short time later [24]. By comparing the size of the saline bolus detected in the arterial line with its original size as it enters the fistula, the recirculated fraction may be calculated. If there is access recirculation, the bolus will be detectable in the arterial line within seconds of its passage into the fistula. Cardiopulmonary recirculation results in the saline bolus being detectable approximately 1 min after its passage into the fistula, since the bolus will have passed around the pulmonary circulation. Therefore, this method may distinguish between fistula and cardiopulmonary recirculation and calculate their fractions separately.

The blood temperature module (BTM)

This method uses the same principle as the saline-dilution method, but a thermal bolus replaces saline [25]. A bolus of cold blood at about 35°C is produced by reducing the temperature of the dialyzate for about 2 min. This cool blood is detected and quantified by a temperature sensor on the venous line. Recirculation of the bolus into the arterial line is detected by another sensor. Since the duration of the cool bolus is about 2 min, this method cannot distinguish between fistula and cardiopulmonary recirculation and its precision is relatively low – approximately 5–10%. However, the method is much less invasive than the other methods and is the simple to perform since the module is part of the dialysis machine, the temperature sensors operate from outside unmodified blood lines and the entire system is under automatic control.

The occlusion method

The fistula is occluded between the arterial and venous needles by finger pressure. If there is access recirculation, the pressure in the arterial line will fall rapidly and the dialysis machine will alarm. This method is very easy to perform. However, if the fistula needles are very close together or the fistula is a deep prosthetic graft, it may be difficult or impossible to occlude by finger pressure. This method does not detect cardiopulmonary recirculation.

Since access recirculation is critically dependent on the extracorporeal blood flow rate, recirculation should always be measured at the highest extracorporeal blood flow rate likely to be used during dialysis. Methods which detect a combination of cardiopulmonary and access recirculation (BTM, slow-flow method) will generally return a value of up to 15% due to cardiopulmonary recirculation. If the recirculation fraction is much greater than 15%, then access recirculation is likely.

If access recirculation is detected and needle position errors have been excluded, then it is helpful to determine the fistula flow rate. This is achieved by measuring recirculation at different blood flows and determining the maximum blood flow at which no access recirculation occurs. If the method chosen detects both cardiopulmonary and access recirculation, than the fistula flow rate may be determined by analyzing the relationship between blood flow and recirculation.

Dialysis should not be performed using blood flow rates in excess of the fistula flow rate and the dialysis time should be increased to compensate for the reduction in blood flow rate. Since access recirculation is usually due to critical stenosis and may precede complete failure, further investigation of the fistula is needed.

Uremic toxins

The Kt/V or URR approach assumes that urea is an adequate marker for all uremic toxins. This is very unlikely, as most known uremic toxins have a considerably higher molecular weight and are handled differently by dialysis. As previously described, the dialysis process may be planned in such a way as to keep the clearance of all solutes in proportion to the urea clearance. Direct measurement of the concentration of accumulation of specific toxins or quantification of their toxic effects would be highly desirable. Unfortunately, such measurements are relatively difficult and few have been fully validated. The uremic state results in a peripheral neuropathy. Peripheral nerve function may be assessed using objective neurophysiological measurements such as current perception threshold or conduction velocity. Routine assessment of nerve function has been advocated. β_2-Microglobulin is one of the few known uremic toxins and its molecular weight is 20 times that of urea. Its concentration is difficult to measure and difficult to interpret as its kinetics are poorly understood. However, an ultrasound method to determine shoulder capsule thickness has recently been described. This method is reproducible and sensitively reflects the accumulation of β_2-microglobulin.

Bicarbonate

One of the functions of dialysis is to regenerate bicarbonate. If this function is successfully delivered, then the serum bicarbonate should be within the normal range. Bicarbonate concentrations are also related to survival in hemodialysis.

Nutrition

Malnutrition is common in dialysis patients and is associated with a higher morbidity and mortality. Malnutrition may be caused by underdialysis or hepatic congestion associated with chronic fluid overload. Fluid overload is a particularly dangerous cause of malnutrition as the resulting loss of flesh weight creates a tendency to increasing fluid accumulation unless the dry weight is frequently reduced.

The early signs of malnutrition are easy to miss in dialysis patients, particularly if loss of flesh weight is masked by fluid accumulation. Routine monitoring of nutritional state must include serial body weights and repeated clinical assessment, noting the presence of muscle wasting or any signs of fluid overload, especially edema or ascites. Serum albumin levels are useful. The regular measurement of normalized protein catabolic rate (nPCR) may be helpful.

nPCR is a linear function of the slope of the rise in urea concentration during the interdialytic interval since urea is the end product of protein metabolism. Ideally, nPCR should be calculated from blood urea concentrations in samples drawn postdialysis and immediately before the following dialysis. However, if a computer is used to calculate Kt/V, iterative solution of complex formulae will allow the nPCR to be calculated at the same time and from the same data. The nPCR is relatively insensitive to the postdialysis rebound but should take any renal function into account.

The nPCR is generally reproducible but requires extreme care in its interpretation. Although the nPCR reflects the generation rate of urea, it is only indirectly related to the dietary protein intake (DPI). The nPCR will only reflect the DPI if the patient is in stable nitrogen balance and if there are no significant losses of protein (e.g. into urine or dialyzate). The malnourished patient may well be in negative nitrogen balance and relatively catabolic. In this case, the nPCR will be relatively high as urea is generated from muscle catabolism.

Other means of assessment may be useful and include measurement of skinfold thickness, assessment of muscle mass from creatinine generation rate, lean body mass from bioimpedance measurement and assessment of dietary intake by food diaries.

Fluid removal and sodium balance

Fluid removal

Fluid restriction is generally required especially when residual renal function has been lost. In spite of this, intradialytic weight gain is the norm, the amount depending on residual renal function and compliance. Removal of excess body water is thus a vital requirement of the dialysis process. Fluid is removed from the patient through the dialyzer membrane at a rate determined by the product of its water permeability (characterized by its ultrafiltration coefficient or K_{uf}) and the differential hydraulic pressure across the membrane (the transmembrane pressure or TMP), i.e.

$$\text{ultrafiltration rate} = K_{uf} \times \text{TMP}$$

The desired TMP to achieve the required weight-loss during dialysis can thus be calculated. In practice, modern dialysis machines provide automated control of ultrafiltration, so that the desired weight loss can be set directly. Such machines allow the use of highly permeable membranes (high K_{uf}), which permit the removal of large volumes over short times. The limiting factor to this process is patient tolerance and maintenance of blood pressure.

The dry weight

This is a crucial part of the dialysis prescription. Dry weight is usually defined as the weight at which the patient is edema free (though edema is an index of severe overhydration) and below which hypotension occurs on fluid removal. It is determined during the initial weeks on dialysis by gradual reduction of postdialysis weight. Once set it becomes the postdialysis target weight. It is vital to review the dry weight regularly in unstable patients, otherwise patients who are ill and catabolic will accumulate fluid, and those who are well resuscitated and 'putting on fleshweight' will suffer hypotensive episodes. The definition of dry weight assumes that serum albumin, cardiovascular function and autonomic function are acceptably normal, and that the patient is not taking drugs with antihypertensive actions. All these factors decrease the rate of vascular refilling. To prevent intradialytic hypotension they dictate an increased dry weight and resultant interdialytic hypertension. Modern dialysis programs contain many such patients. In such patients use of ultrasonically determined inferior vena cava diameter and its collapsibility index [26] and estimation of extracellular fluid volume by bioimpedance measurements [27] may improve dry weight estimation.

Sodium balance

Increased total exchangeable sodium causes extracellular fluid volume expansion and signs of fluid overload.

Dietary restriction of sodium to 80–120 mmol/day (5–7 g/day) is usually advocated. Sodium is removed isotonically during ultrafiltration. Diffusive losses depend on the dialysis fluid sodium concentration. If the latter is less than the sodium concentration of plasma water, net diffusive loss of sodium occurs, causing an increased incidence of hypotension and cramps. Poor vascular refilling contributes since plasma hypotonicity encourages intracellular fluid shifts. If the sodium concentration of dialysis fluid is increased such symptoms occur less frequently but intradialytic thirst and weight gain may be greater. Individualization of dialysis fluid sodium concentrations with profiling throughout the dialysis period is not yet practicable [28].

Blood pressure

Hypertension

Hypertension is a major contributant to the increased cardiovascular morbidity and mortality of the dialysis population. Control is essential. It is customary to distinguish two categories of pathogenesis – sodium and water overload and neurohumoral including overactivity of the renin–angiotensin system and sympathetic nervous system. Other factors may have a role.

A number of studies suggest that blood pressure can be controlled by maintenance of dry weight alone and without the aid of drugs in 60–90% of patients. This is more likely to be achieved in programs with a high proportion of relatively young patients with low comorbidity scores who dialyze for long hours. As dialysis times have reduced and the population served has increased in age and co-morbidity, the requirement for antihypertensive drugs has increased. In many short hours programs 80% of patients require such drugs. There are a number of possible reasons. It is difficult to define dry weight in patients with cardiovascular compromise, autonomic dysfunction, and those requiring antianginal drugs with antihypertensive actions. Shortened dialysis times may also contribute [29]. Fluid removal may be less readily accomplished possibly because a proportion of the excess fluid load is inaccessible due to slow vascular refilling, poor venous tone and venous pooling. Irrespective of these problems it is important to emphasize the centrality of dry weight estimation in antihypertensive strategy.

Patients who are maintained at their dry weight yet remain hypertensive require antihypertensive drugs. The use of these drugs in dialysis patients is similar to their use in patients with essential hypertension. A few points are worth emphasizing. Thiazide diuretics are not useful. Loop diuretics may increase urine volume in the presence of sufficient residual renal function. There is no contraindication to any of the other major classes of antihypertensive agent, though their use should be informed by an awareness of the impact of renal failure and the dialysis process on their pharmacology (Table 73.2).

Hypertensive crises are now uncommon and usually respond to sublingual nifedipine. Intravenous therapy with labetolol or sodium nitroprusside is only rarely required. Occasional patients develop a sharp paradoxical rise of blood pressure in the latter part of the dialysis session. A profound neurohumoral response to hypovolemia or reduced plasma levels of dialyzable antihypertensive agents are possible explanations.

Dialysis-induced hypotension

Symptomatic hypotensive episodes occur in about 10% of hemodialyses. Clinical features include nausea, vomiting, cramps, palpitations, dizziness and syncope. The common cause is intravascular hypovolemia due to imbalance between ultrafiltration and vascular refilling from the interstitial space, with inadequate cardiovascular responses due to cardiac or neuroeffector dysfunction. Other factors, including membrane reactions and intercurrent medical problems, need to be excluded (Table 73.3). Encouragement of patients to limit interdialytic weight gains, aggressive medical and surgical therapy of treatable cardiac problems, restriction of the use of antihypertensive drugs on the day of dialysis, use of dialysis fluid sodium concentrations in the region of 140 mM, and use of bicarbonate rather than acetate for dialysis fluid buffering, all have a role in reducing the incidence of hypotension. Membrane reactions are less frequent with more biocompatible membranes.

Lipid abnormalities

Chronic renal failure is associated with disturbed lipid metabolism (Chapter 38). Abnormalities include an increase in triglyceride-rich lipoprotein particles (mainly VLDL) due to decreased lipoprotein lipase activity. Total cholesterol levels are close to the normal range but there are reduced levels of HDL cholesterol and an increased ratio of LDL to HDL cholesterol. There are a variety of apolipoprotein abnormalities, and an increased concentration of lipoprotein a. Control of uremia by hemodialysis does not improve these abnormalities. The disturbances provoked by heparin, dialysis fluid acetate

Table 73.2 Antihypertensive usage in hemodialysis. The dosages quoted are an approximate guide and require adjustment according to patient response

Drug	Half-life (h) (Normal/ESRF)	Dialyzed	Dose in dialysis
ACE inhibitors			
Captopril	2/21–32	+	12.5–50 mg/d
Enalapril	11–24/34–60	+	2.5–20 mg/d
Lisinopril	13/40–50	+	2.5–20 mg/d
Beta blockers			
Propranolol	2–6/1–6	–	40–160 mg/12 h
Atenolol	7/15–35	+	25–50 mg/d
Metoprolol	3.5/2.5–4.5	+/–	50–100 mg/12 h
Labetolol	3–9/3–9	–	200–600 mg/12 h
Calcium antagonists			
Nifedipine	4.5–5.5/5–7	+/–	30–90 mg/d (LA)
Amlodipine	35–50/50	–	5–10 mg/d
Diltiazem	2–8/3.5	–	180–480 mg/12 h (SR)
Verapamil	3–7/2.4–4	–	120–240 mg/d (SR)
Alpha blockers			
Doxazocin	9.5–12/13	–	1–16 mg/d
Prazocin	2–3/2–3	–	1–15 mg/12 h
Vasodilators			
Hydralazine	2–4.5/7–16	–	25–50 mg/12 h
Minoxidil	2.8–4.2/2.8–4.22	+	5–20 mg/12 h
Other			
Methyldopa	1.5–6/6–16	+	125–500 mg/12 h

Table 73.3   Causes of dialysis-induced hypotension

1. Aggressive ultrafiltration
- Large interdialytic weight gain

2. Impaired plasma refill rate
- Hypoalbuminemia
- Low plasma osmolality
- Low dialysis fluid sodium levels
- Low tissue hydration

3. Poor vascular tone/venous pooling
- Autonomic dysfunction
- Antihypertensive drugs
- Acetate dialysis

4. Cardiovascular disease
- Left ventricular hypertrophy
- Cardiomyopathy
- Coronary artery disease
- Pericardial disease

5. Membrane-related mechanisms
- First use syndrome

6. Other medical problems
- Hemorrhage
- Sepsis
- Arrhythmias

and glucose are probably of little clinical consequence. Lipid abnormalities are poor predictors of the increased cardiovascular risk of hemodialyzed patients. Likewise, the effects of treatment of lipid disorders on patient outcome have not been established. A number of maneuvers are recommended having been shown to favorably influence the lipid disturbances. These include achievement of ideal body weight, exercise, control of secondary hyperparathyroidism, low fat diets and diets high in polyunsaturated fatty acids. Experience with drug therapy in hemodialyzed patients is sparse. Gemfibrozil is probably the current best buy.

Anemia

The treatment of anemia in hemodialysis patients has been revolutionized within the last decade by the development of erythropoietin (EPO) for clinical use [30, 31]. It has resulted in a dramatic improvement in the quality of life for many patients. It is indicated in all patients with hemoglobin levels below a target range of 10–12 g/dl, after hematinic deficiencies have been corrected and sepsis controlled. Most patients require 50–200 IU/kg/week given in two or three subcutaneous doses to achieve and maintain target hemoglobin levels. Therapy must be individualized and based on rigorous monitoring.

The beneficial effects of EPO can usually be related to the improvement of anemia, though there may be other direct effects, including alterations of hemostatic parameters and improvement of platelet function though even these may be related to the rise in hematocrit. Many studies have shown improvements in quality of life scores. Regression of left ventricular hypertrophy occurs in spite of a tendency to exacerbate hypertension.

A small proportion of patients require much larger than average doses of EPO and a few do not respond to EPO at all. The common causes of poor response (EPO resistance) are shown in Table 73.4. By far the commonest is iron deficiency. The diagnosis of iron deficiency is difficult in hemodialysis patients. The transferrin saturation and iron-binding capacity correlate better with EPO response than does serum ferritin, suggesting that the functional availability of iron in the plasma may be more important than the size of the body iron stores in determining response. Determination of the percentage of hypochromic red cells may be a more sensitive index of iron deficiency. Almost all patients require supplementation with iron in order to maintain a response and many require iron by the intravenous route. Another major cause of poor response to EPO is the presence of inflammation secondary to infection, surgery, autoimmune disorders or malignancy. Reduced iron availability for heme production, and increased cytokine production leading to decreased endogenous EPO production or end-organ resistance to the action of EPO, are possible explanations.

Treatment with EPO is usually well tolerated and there are few serious adverse effects (Table 73.5). Increased blood pressure is the most commonly reported and may occur in up to one-third of patients. The risk appears maximal in the early stages of treatment when the hematocrit is increasing, though there appears to be no clear

Table 73.4   Factors associated with resistance to EPO treatment

Iron deficiency
Vitamin deficiency
  folate
  B_{12}
  B_6
Inflammatory states
  infection
  surgery
Secondary hyperparathyroidism
Aluminum intoxication
Hemoglobinopathies
Chronic hemolysis
Malignancy

Table 73.5 Possible adverse effects of treatment with EPO

Hypertension
Seizures
Increased clotting
Flu-like syndrome
Reduced dialyzer efficiency

association with the dose of EPO nor with the rate of rise of hematocrit. Blood volume does not change. Hemodynamic studies show an increase in systemic vascular resistance (SVR) coupled with a reduction in cardiac output during therapy. Factors which may be important in the rise in SVR are an elevated blood viscosity related to the increased hematocrit, loss of the vasodilatory response to hypoxia, and alterations in sympathetic function. There is some evidence that cardiac output remains inappropriately high in those patients who develop hypertension, perhaps due to baroreceptor dysfunction and impaired myocardial compliance.

EPO therapy may be associated with a lowered threshold for convulsions though controlled studies do not confirm this. However, seizures do occur in some patients early in the course of EPO therapy at a time when hematocrit and blood pressure are increasing. Most of these patients appear to have hypertensive encephalopathy.

An increase in the number of thrombotic events has been reported, though the finding is not substantiated by placebo-controlled trials. As the hematocrit increases, vascular access, particularly PTFE and bovine grafts, may be at increased risk and low-dose aspirin prophylaxis has been recommended.

An increase in hematocrit reduces plasma water flow through the dialyzer leading to decreased solute clearance and ultrafiltration rate. Clearances of easily diffusible solutes, such as urea, are less affected than those of less readily diffusible solutes such as creatinine, and those whose intracellular concentrations are maintained by active transport processes, such as potassium and phosphate. Clinical studies have shown no change in Kt/V (urea) and NPCR during EPO therapy. Clearances of creatinine, potassium and phosphate were reduced by about 15%. Hence, only small changes to dialysis schedules, heparin dose and phosphate binder dose are required to counteract the effects of clinically relevant increments in hematocrit.

Mineral metabolism

Strategies to prevent and treat secondary hyperparathyroidism and to limit vascular calcification are an important part of the routine treatment of hemodialysis patients. Other manifestations of renal bone disease include osteomalacia, osteopenia and adynamic bone disease. Osteomalacia is uncommon in the absence of aluminum accumulation and phosphate depletion. Osteopenia may be an increasing problem in the aging dialysis population. The recently described entity of adynamic bone disease is discussed below.

There are three overlapping strands to the therapy of secondary hyperparathyroidism: prevention and treatment of phosphate accumulation, maintenance of serum calcium levels in the upper normal range, and direct suppression of PTH secretion by 1,25-dihydroxy vitamin D $(1,25(OH)_2D_3)$. These strategies should be employed sequentially. Early treatment may reduce the progressive transformation of diffuse parathyroid hyperplasia into the nodular form which is more resistant to treatment [32]. PTH levels should be monitored every three to six months. Target levels are now thought to be about twice the upper limit of normal. Lower levels increase the risk of adynamic bone disease. Parathyroidectomy is reserved for patients with uncontrolled hyperparathyroidism usually in the context of hypercalcemia.

Use of phosphate binders

Prevention and treatment of phosphate accumulation in hemodialysis patients remain unsatisfactory. The problem has been exacerbated by the current awareness of the importance of an adequate protein intake, by shorter dialysis treatments and by erythropoietin therapy. These factors increase the requirements for phosphate binders. At the same time the recognition that the highly efficient aluminum-containing binders cause aluminum accumulation has all but excluded them from routine clinical use. Calcium carbonate is a useful alternative but hypercalcemia occurs frequently. Calcium acetate has theoretical advantages, but these have proved difficult to demonstrate clinically, and hypercalcemia remains a problem. Lowering of the dialysate calcium concentration has enabled larger doses of calcium-containing phosphate binders to be used, with less risk of hypercalcemia and without compromising net calcium balance. Magnesium-containing phosphate binders can be useful particularly when hypercalcemia is a problem. Hypermagnesemia can occur. Serum levels require regular monitoring. Adjustment of dialysate magnesium may be required. Phosphate binders should be administered with main meals. Calcium and phosphate levels should be checked monthly.

Maintenance of serum calcium levels

In the era of aluminum-containing phosphate binders the strategies used to maintain serum calcium levels in the upper normal range included the use of calcium supplements, high dialysate calcium levels and vitamin D compounds as required. The current widespread use of calcium compounds as phosphate binders has had a significant impact on this strategy. In effect these agents are used to control both phosphate and calcium levels. Their use has resulted in a trend to lower dialysate calcium levels to permit the use of doses large enough to control phosphate levels without causing hypercalcemia. The requirement for vitamin D compounds to maintain serum calcium levels in established hemodialysis patients is now much less.

Vitamin D compounds

Therapy with $1,25(OH)_2D_3$, or its analog, alfacalcidol, is effective in suppressing PTH levels and has a direct effect, independent of serum calcium levels. Conventional therapy consisted of daily oral doses of $1,25(OH)_2D_3$. Hypercalcemia was the main side effect. Use of calcium-containing phosphate binders has amplified the risk, and has shifted attention to the use of intravenous pulsed therapy. This method of administration produces high peak levels, maximizing parathyroid suppression by higher occupancy of the parathyroid vitamin D receptor, and a reduced 'area under the curve' which, together with the restricted exposure of intestinal epithelial cells to the influence of $1,25(OH)_2D_3$, may limit the risk of hypercalcemia. Treatment should begin with doses of $1\,\mu g$ three times weekly and adjusted according to monitored calcium and PTH levels. Intermittent oral treatment is probably as effective as intermittent intravenous treatment. One of the major problems in treating secondary hyperparathyroidism is the remarkable capacity of the parathyroid glands to escape from control. It seems that tolerance to pulsed calcitriol may also emerge after relatively short treatment times. Parathyroidectomy may then be required.

Parathyroidectomy

The major indication for parathyroidectomy is severe hyperparathyroidism uncontrolled by medical therapy. The patient is usually hypercalcemic. In some cases parathyroidectomy is required even in the absence of hypercalcemia. These are usually patients with severe secondary hyperparathyroidism with rapidly progressive soft tissue calcification or more rarely extensive vascular calcification associated with ischemic skin necrosis. After 10 years of dialysis about 20% of patients will have undergone parathyroidectomy.

Adynamic bone disease

Adynamic changes in bone were formerly thought to occur in this group of patients entirely as a result of aluminum toxicity. Similar histological changes of markedly reduced bone turnover, with a paucity of osteoid, bone cells and a significant reduction in active remodeling sites

and tetracycline uptake, have been described in patients in whom there is no evidence of aluminum accumulation. The problem may be more common in elderly patients, diabetics and CAPD patients. Overtreatment with calcium supplements and active vitamin D compounds and use of high dialyzate calcium concentrations may predispose to the problem by oversuppressing parathyroid hormone levels to a degree inappropriate for the prevailing level of renal function. Hence the recommendation for target levels of PTH of twice the upper limit of normal. The clinical relevance of these histological abnormalities awaits firm definition, though patients with the problem may be at increased risk of microfracture.

Diet

Dietary protein requirements are increased in dialysis patients from increased catabolism related to a variety of factors, including acidosis, fluid overload, secondary hyperparathyroidism and effects of the hemodialysis procedure itself. A protein intake of the order of 1.2 g/kg/day has been recommended. Higher intakes exacerbate acidosis, hyperkalemia and hyperphosphatemia and require increments in dialysis time. Dietary energy depletion is common. An intake of at least 35 kcal/kg should consist of about 35% fat, a high proportion of which is unsaturated [33]. Salt (80–120 mmol/day, 5–7 g/day) and potassium restriction (60–80 mmol/day 4.5–6 g/day) are usually required. Calcium intake should be 1–1.5 g/day. This is usually readily attained with the increasing use of calcium-containing phosphate binders. Phosphate restriction is difficult but intakes of less than 1g daily are recommended. If the diet is adequate in other respects vitamin supplementation should not be obligatory. Possible exceptions are vitamin B_6 and vitamin B_{12} in high-flux dialysis. Supplementation with fat-soluble vitamins is unnecessary.

Withdrawal of dialysis

Withdrawal of dialysis is a common mode of death in patients on long-term dialysis, especially in Australia and North America, where it accounts for 13–17% of all deaths [34] and up to 40% of deaths in elderly patients. Other major associations are with comorbid conditions such as diabetes, chronic heart failure, atheromatous renovascular disease and cancer. Curiously, death due to withdrawal of dialysis seems to be rare in Europe, perhaps due to differences in culture, patient selection or reporting patterns. About half the patients were 'competent' when the decision was made [35] and in many there had been no recent change in medical circumstances. In 'incompetent' patients the process was initiated by physician or family, often in response to recent medical events. In some studies it has been impossible to dis-

advice should be given to limit weight gain to no more than 2–3% of body weight between dialyses. Advice may also need to be given with respect to limiting food intake during dialysis.

Dialysis hypotension can be extremely difficult to manage, particularly in patients with uremic neuropathy or diabetic neuropathy, and in the elderly. Such patients frequently experience sudden hypotension without having any prodromal symptoms. In this situation it is only a knowledge of the patient's individual behavior on dialysis that will allow preventive measures to be undertaken to pre-empt hypotension. Bergstrom [3] demonstrated that if ultrafiltration was undertaken before hemodialysis, cardiovascular stability was better maintained suggesting that a major component of dialysis-induced hypotension was due to intravascular volume depletion. The steps to prevent dialysis hypotension are summarized in Table 74.1.

First use syndrome

The first use syndrome is so called because of a clinical syndrome which occurs most commonly but not exclusively with the first use of a dialyzer. The severity of this syndrome may vary from a severe anaphylactic reaction to minor allergic symptoms. In general, two types of syndrome are recognized, the first being anaphylactic in nature and the second being of a lesser degree of allergy having non-specific symptoms [4].

The anaphylactic form of the first use reaction is more common in patients with a history of atopy. Symptoms develop within the first few minutes of dialysis but may occur at any time in the first 30 min. The clinical manifestations are pruritus, urticaria, cough, sneezing, coryza, abdominal cramps, diarrhea, dyspnea, angioedema and, in severe cases, cardiac arrest. In approximately 60% of affected patients antibodies of an IgE type to ethylene oxide (ETO) can be demonstrated. Ethylene oxide is used as a sterilant and normally after such sterilization the dialyzers undergo a degassing procedure which should remove any residual ethylene oxide; however, some may remain within the dialyzer, particularly within the polyurethrenes of the potting compound. With correct

preparation of dialyzers (see below) ethylene oxide reactions have become uncommon.

A first use reaction has also been described in patients dialyzed with the synthetic AN69 dialyzer, particularly if they are simultaneously receiving an angiotensin converting enzyme (ACE) inhibitor [5]. This reaction is thought to be mediated by bradykinin because the negatively charged AN69 membrane activates the kallikrein/kinin system whose effects are potentiated because ACE inhibition reduces bradykinin inactivation.

Anaphylactic type first use reactions have also been reported in patients on bicarbonate dialysis with high-flux dialyzers. It is thought that the bicarbonate dialysis fluid may be more susceptible to bacterial contamination than acetate dialysis fluid. Similar reactions have also been observed during reuse dialysis; the cause is thought to be bacterial or endotoxin contamination of the water used in the reuse procedure. Rarely, heparin has been implicated as a cause of allergic reactions.

The management of a first use reaction is to stop dialysis immediately and not return to be patient blood contained within the dialyzer and lines. Oxygen should be administered and epinephrine, corticosteroids and antihistamines may be required. Prevention of such reactions depends on the etiology. If it is considered that ethylene oxide is the major cause then a more prolonged rinsing of the dialyzer is essential. The blood compartment should be rinsed with at least 2 litres of saline solution and the dialyzate compartment perfused with dialysis fluid for at least 30 min before commencing dialysis. If patients have experienced severe reactions then a change to a dialyzer sterilized with an alternative to ETO is advisable. In patients receiving an ACE inhibitor alternative antihypertensive therapy should be considered.

In some patients the first use syndrome is less severe and consists of chest pain which may be accompanied by back pain. These symptoms usually develop within several minutes of commencing dialysis but may occur any time in the first hour. The etiology is unknown but complement activation has been implicated. The symptoms appear less commonly in reuse dialysis where it is considered that the dialyzer membrane may have become coated with a protein layer, thereby diminishing the chances of complement activation. In patients with this syndrome, dialysis can usually be continued although analgesia and/or oxygen may be required. Some patients find that their symptoms are abolished by a change of dialyzer. For others it may be necessary to prime the dialyzer and lines with plasma. It is rarely necessary to stop the dialysis session.

Table 74.1 Measures to reduce the risk of dialysis hypotension

1. Controlled ultrafiltration
2. Sequential ultrafiltration
3. Bicarbonate dialysis fluid
4. Increased dialysis fluid sodium concentration
5. Reduction in dialysis fluid temperature
6. Slowing of blood flow rate
7. Slowing of dialysis fluid flow rate

Hemorrhage

Uremia is associated with a bleeding diathesis which predominantly manifests by reduced platelet adhesiveness and a prolonged bleeding time. No abnormality in coagulation factors has been demonstrated. The platelet dysfunction and prolonged bleeding time are improved by dialysis but not returned to normal [6].

Minor bleeding problems on dialysis are not uncommon and consist predominantly of bleeding from puncture sites and minor bruising. Severe hemorrhage is uncommon. Subdural hematoma from venous bleeding is a recognized complication of hemodialysis and subarachnoid hemorrhage may occur in patients with polycystic disease due to a berry aneurysm. Intracerebral hemorrhage may occur in severe hypertension. Subcapsular hematoma of the liver is well recognized, although rare. Patients with either infective or uremic pericarditis are at considerable risk of hemopericardium and consequent cardiac tamponade. Hemodialysis patients may have bleeding due to the heparin required for the dialysis procedure. For any patient with this risk, the alternatives to heparin administration are prostacyclin (not available in USA), regional heparinization, the use of membranes with covalently bound heparin, low-molecular-weight heparin (Fragmin) or citrate. In certain circumstances heparin-free dialysis can be undertaken providing a high blood flow rate can be achieved and the dialysis circuit is flushed with 100–200 ml saline every 15–30 min.

Headache

Headache is particularly common during dialysis and may be either a manifestation of minor disequilibrium or a result of the vasodilatory effects of acetate. It is best managed by simple analgesia with the use of such agents as paracetamol. A reduction in the blood flow rate, or a switch to bicarbonate dialysis fluid may be beneficial.

Nausea and vomiting

Nausea and vomiting are common during hemodialysis particularly during the early months of such therapy. With time the incidence diminishes if dialysis is adequate. Most episodes are associated with hypotension and probably represent a manifestation of excess fluid removal. The symptoms are also associated with dialysis disequilibrium (see above) other unusual causes include acute hypercalcemia from the hard water syndrome and in patients with diabetes mellitus gastroparesis may be present.

Pruritus

Pruritus is a common symptom of hemodialysis patients, being experienced in over 80%. It most frequently occurs during or immediately after hemodialysis and in 25% of patients it only occurs during hemodialysis. In other patients, however, it may also occur at rest and particularly on retiring at night. On examination the skin may appear normal but in many, scratching has caused excoriation, minor infections and reactive changes. Most com-

monly the back and trunk are involved although in some patients, the arms, legs and face may be affected. In areas of skin subjected to continual scratching there may develop brown nodular areas covered by scales, crusts, and abrasions. These result from inflammation, infection and bleeding caused by scratching. Lichenification of the skin can occur as a consequence of minor chronic inflammation which results in hyperkeratosis and acanthosis with the areas of skin involved appearing thickened, hyperpigmented and hyperkeratotic.

The etiology of pruritus is unknown but various etiologies have been suggested (Table 74.2). In many patients pruritus is due to an elevated calcium phosphate product which results in the microprecipitation of calcium salts in the skin. This may be due to inadequate phosphate control as a result of dietary indiscretion or from hypercalcemia as a consequence of hyperparathyroidism or inappropriate administration of vitamin D metabolites. In some patients an increase in mast cells in the skin has been reported; hemodialysis patients with pruritus have increased plasma histamine concentrations, suggesting a possible causal link. This is supported by the fact that although skin reactivity to histamine may be reduced in dialysis patients, those with pruritus are more reactive than those who are asymptomatic. Some have suggested that a 'uremic toxin' is involved although none has been identified. Many patients with chronic renal failure and those on dialysis have some atrophy of the skin with a resulting dryness which aggravates the pruritus. In some patients pruritus has been associated with dialyzer reuse when formaldehyde has been used as a sterilant and symptoms may improve in such patients with a switch to alternative disinfecting agents. Finally, in a number of patients pruritus may be a minor allergic reaction to the dialysis equipment such as the lines, the potting compound, the membranes, plasticizers leached from the dialysis lines or heparin.

The management of patients with pruritus can be particularly difficult. Topical emollients such as lanolin may help, particularly if the patient has dry skin. At times of

---

Table 74.2 Possible causes of pruritus in hemodialysis patients

1. Elevation of calcium phosphate produce due to:
   (a) Dietary phosphate excess
   (b) Hyperparathyroidism
   (c) Excess vitamin D treatment
2. Increase in skin mast cells
3. Increase in plasma histamine
4. 'Uremic toxins'
5. Dry skin
6. Use of formaldehyde in dialyzer reprocessing
7. Allergy to dialyzer lines, potting compounds, membranes, plasticizers or heparin

intense pruritus, calamine lotion may also provide symptomatic relief. The use of antihistamine creams or anesthetic creams should be avoided in view of the risk of developing allergic reactions. Oral antihistamines in the form of chlorpheniramine may provide relief in a significant number of patients although drowsiness may be an unacceptable side effect. Unfortunately, the non-sedative antihistamines, such as terfenadine, are rarely effective in pruritus. It is important to control the calcium phosphate product with a combination of dietary advice and phosphate binders should hyperphosphatemia be present (i.e. a predialysis phosphate in excess of 2 mmol/l). If hypercalcemia is present then the drug charts should be examined and, if appropriate, calcium supplements or alphacalcidol reduced. In patients whose hypercalcemia is due to hyperparathyroidism there are many documented report of pruritus dramatically improving following parathyroidectomy. Ultraviolet B (UVB) phototherapy has been reported to be of value [7] but there may be a considerable placebo effect. In a cross-over study comparing UVA with UVB, no difference in effect on pruritus could be identified [8] although UVA is acknowledged to have no biological activity.

Although in dialysis patients 'uremic' pruritus is most prevalent it must not be forgotten that pruritus may also be a consequence of adverse drug reactions or infestation with scabies.

Cramp

Cramp, particularly of the lower limbs, occurs relatively commonly during hemodialysis and is associated with hypotension and excessive weight reduction. It is more common when a low sodium dialysis fluid is used (≤130 mEq/l). It is most likely due to fluid and electrolyte shifts across muscle cell membranes.

If patients experience severe cramp during dialysis, administration of normal saline or hypertonic glucose may be beneficial. For those who frequently experience the symptom, an increase in the dialysis fluid sodium to 145 mEq/l may be beneficial but its long-term benefits can be offset by thirst and an increase in interdialytic weight gain. Quinine sulfate (200 mg orally) taken 2 h before a dialysis session may prevent the development of cramp. Carnitine supplementation has been shown to be of value to some patients [9].

An alteration to the dialysis schedule may also reduce the incidence of cramp. Controlled ultrafiltration during the 4 h dialysis is of value in some patients, whereas others may require that the sodium concentration is commenced fairly high at about 150 mEq/l gradually reduced through dialysis to 135 mEq/l.

Hemolysis

Hemolysis is a feature of uremia in that red blood cell survival is diminished but improves slightly following the

institution of regular dialysis therapy. Rarely, acute hemolysis can complicate the dialysis session. Clinically, the patient develops back pain, chest tightness and breathlessness. Hemolysis is usually caused by problems with the dialysis fluid such as excessive temperature or inappropriate mixing of water and dialysis fluid concentrate that results in an hypotonic fluid. In certain circumstances hemolysis has been associated with dialysis fluid contamination with formaldehyde, bleach, chloramine, copper or nitrates. It is also a rare manifestation of zinc toxicity.

The management of an acute hemolytic episode is to stop the hemodialysis and, as hyperkalemia may develop, the plasma potassium should be checked and the appropriate action undertaken. The emergency treatment of hyperkalemia includes the intravenous administration of dextrose (50 ml, 50% over 3–5 min), intravenous calcium gluconate (20 ml, 20%), sodium bicarbonate (8.6%) if acidosis is present (the volume infused will depend on the clinical circumstances), and the β_2-agonist albuterol either intravenously or by infusion. Dialyzate fluid should be saved for subsequent examination.

Since many of the incidents are associated with dialysis fluid contamination they can be prevented by correct treatment of water used to prepare dialysis fluid. A combination of filtration, softening and reverse osmosis properly monitored will prevent the majority of episodes.

Hypoxemia

A certain degree of hypoxemia occurs during routine hemodialysis with either bicarbonate or acetate dialysis fluid caused by either hypoventilation or impairment of the pulmonary circulation. The effect is usually inconsequential except in patients with pulmonary or cardiac disease. The P_{O_2} may decline by 3–30 mmHg. During acetate dialysis, CO_2 is lost to dialysis fluid resulting in hypocapnia with subsequent hypoventilation. Adenosine generated from acetate may also produce an effect by the formation of adenosine–thromboxane complex which mediates bronchoconstriction and an increase in pulmonary artery pressure. In addition, hypoxemia may result from an increased alveolar-arterial oxygen gradient due to complement activation with leukocyte trapping, mediator release and inflammation in the pulmonary circulation. In patients in whom transient hypoxemia may be hazardous oxygen should be administered during dialysis and a change to a synthetic dialyzer and the use of bicarbonate-containing dialysis fluid is advisable.

Neutropenia

A transient neutropenia occurring 15–30 min after the commencement of a dialysis session is well recognized, and was first described in 1968 [10]. It is particularly common when cellulosic dialyzers are used due to complement activation by the alternate pathway. The generation of a small-molecular-weight fragment of the fifth component of complement (C5a) results in an increased expression of a granulocyte adhesion-promoting glycoprotein. This causes aggregated activated granulocytes to adhere to each other and become sequestered in the pulmonary circulation where they liberate oxygen radicals, lysosomal enzymes and vasoactive mediators. This reaction is transient due to a subsequent down-regulation of the cellular response to C5a, limiting the powerful effect of the granulocytes in the pulmonary circulation. Neutropenia is much less marked when synthetic membranes or modified cellulosic membranes are used. It is not known whether this transient neutropenia has any adverse clinical effects *per se*.

Technical problems

Dialysis fluid composition

It was several years after the introduction of dialysis that it became clear that the quality required for drinking water was very different from that required for the water used to prepare dialysis fluid. In areas of hard water, after about 3–4 h of hemodialysis patients developed a syndrome comprising marked hypertension, sweating, nausea, lethargy and weakness. This became known as the hard water syndrome [11] and was due to acute hypercalcemia and hypermagnesemia. It came to be appreciated that the dialysis membrane is significantly different from the gastrointestinal membrane in that the two-way transfer of substances across the dialysis membrane depends on size, charge and molecular shape, rather than on active processes, hence substances in the dialysis fluid may readily equilibrate with blood during passage through the dialyzer. Such substances gain direct access to the circulation. In view of the fact that during each hour of treatment the dialysis patient is exposed to 30 l of dialysis fluid (or 19 000 l each year) substances, even those present in only trace amounts, have the potential to produce toxicity in patients undergoing long-term hemodialysis.

The source of contaminants can arise from minerals and organic materials present in the water draining to the supply reservoir. This can be further contaminated by fertilizers such as nitrites, herbicides and pesticides that are used on the adjacent land. Water authorities are charged with providing potable water and to achieve this a number of substances are added in water treatment plants. If there is suspended particulate matter alum (a hydrated double sulfate of aluminum and potassium) is added as a flocculating agent. Unfortunately, however, the methods for controlling this are poor and frequently excessive amounts of aluminum will gain access to the distribution system. In addition, chlorine is added to reduce bacterial contamination. In some areas chloramines, condensation products of chlorine and ammonia, are added and these may cross the dialysis membrane producing a hemolytic anemia [12]. Other substances that are commonly added to water include fluoride, copper sulfate and pyrethrins. The water distribution system may add contaminants in the form of iron or lead leaching from pipes and the dialysis equipment may be a source of copper or zinc.

In view of these problems, it is important that water used to prepare dialysis fluid should be properly treated. This requires sequential sediment filtration, softening, activated carbon filtration, reverse osmosis and then deionization. To prevent microbial growth the ultrapure water should be distributed by continuous circulation through pipes which have no dead ends or lengths where there is only intermittent flow. The return flow of the circulating system should be exposed to ultraviolet light to reduce the possibility of bacterial contamination.

The American Association for the Advancement of Medical Instrumentation and the American National Standards Institute have published guidelines relating to the maximum allowable impurity level of substances present in water for the generation of dialysis solutions.

Air embolism

Air embolism is a rare acute emergency which may occur as a complication of hemodialysis. The causes include aspiration of air into the blood circuit due to the subatmospheric pressure of blood in the line between the arterial vascular access and the blood pump, arterial disconnection and errors in returning blood to the patient at the end of dialysis. If the patient is in a sitting position the bubbles of air tends to rise up the jugular vein to the cerebral venous system without entering the heart resulting in obstruction of the cerebral venous return with subsequent loss of consciousness, convulsions and eventually death. If the patient is in a recumbent position air may enter the right side of the heart to form foam within the right ventricle rendering cardiac contraction ineffectual. If the patient is lying on the right side air can pass to the pulmonary capillaries blocking flow and causing dyspnea, chest tightness and cough. The air may then progress to the left ventricle and be forced into the arterial tree resulting in air embolization to the brain with fatal consequences.

Treatment of air embolism requires immediate clamping of the venous blood line and stopping the blood pump. The patient should be placed head and chest down and turned on the left side; 100% oxygen should be administered and, if necessary, transthoracic cardiac puncture to aspirate air from the ventricle. Once air has entered the arterial circulation and caused neurological symptoms the prognosis is particularly poor. In those rare locations where a compression chamber is available the patient should be transferred for compression to drive air into solution, and then to undergo slow controlled decompression to allow air to be expired without forming bubbles.

Air embolism can be prevented by monitoring the blood level in the bubble trap of the venous line and by the insertion of a collapsible segment between the arterial access and the arterial line blood pump. Such precautions are now an integral part of dialysis equipment so that air embolism is rarely encountered.

Chronic problems associated with the dialysis procedure

Biocompatibility

Biocompatibility is the ability of a material, device, or system to function without a clinically significant host response [13]. In hemodialysis the term covers reactions which occur between blood and various materials of the dialysis circuit and the systemic effects which manifest as a consequence of such interactions. Many attempts have been made to provide a completely biocompatible circuit, but in view of the complexity of the system it seems unlikely that a hemodialysis system devoid of any reaction will ever be developed.

In the hemodialysis circuit the sites of potential reaction between blood and components of the system include needles, lines, pump inserts, the various parts of dialyzer structure (casing and potting compound) and the dialyzer membrane. Interaction may also take place as a consequence of substances, such as acetate, endotoxins and bacterial cell wall components, crossing the dialysis membrane from the dialysis fluid. Finally there may be a release of substances from the lines and membranes such as chemical additives, plasticizers or sterilizing agents such as ethylene oxide.

At the initiation of hemodialysis, as blood flows through the dialysis circuit, there is the adsorption of plasma proteins to surfaces with which it comes into contact. The adsorbed proteins activate platelet adhesion/aggregation and thereby a number of biological systems including the coagulation cascade, complement and various cells resulting in cytokine production and the secretion of histamine-releasing factors. Activation of the coagulation cascade is controlled in part by heparin but heparin has no effect on the activation of early components of the cascade. The consequences of surface activation are complicated and impossible to avoid completely [14].

Complement activation during hemodialysis is initiated by several different mechanisms [15]. Virtually all foreign surfaces are able to activate complement by the alternate pathway. This activation is responsible for the transient leukopenia and pulmonary sequestration of neutrophils which occurs in the first 30 min of dialysis.

Mononuclear cells become activated during hemodialysis as a consequence of complement activation and other factors such as acetate in dialysis fluid and endotoxins crossing the dialysis membrane from the dialysis fluid. Bicarbonate dialysis fluid may avoid the adverse effects of acetate but it may have a greater risk of bacterial contamination and, therefore, endotoxin. As a consequence of mononuclear cell activation there is secretion of cytokines, particularly interleukin-1 (IL-1) and tumor necrosis factor (TNF). Basophilic leukocytes and mast cells may be activated leading to IgE-dependent reactions mediated by anaphylatoxins (C3a, C4a, C5a) which act on receptors on neutrophils, eosinophils, basophils, mast cells, as well as monocytes and macrophages to result in immune hypersensitivity reactions and the first use syndrome (see above). Furthermore, histamine release factors may, through their action on basophils and mast cells, be responsible for some of the pruritus occurring in dialysis patients. The effect of interaction between blood and materials is that the blood returning from the dialyzer has cells which have become activated and contains chemical mediators which may act either locally or systemically on other cellular and effector systems [16].

The cellular activation induced by bioincompatibility with consequent cytokine production is most likely responsible for a number of acute and chronic complications which may occur in hemodialysis patients. One acute effect of IL-1 and TNF production is a diminution in systemic vascular resistance resulting in hypotension. Less acute is the fact that IL-1 and TNF may release various neuropeptides such as adrenocorticotrophic hormone (ACTH), corticotrophin and somastatin, which are likely to be responsible for the anorexia and lethargy in the immediate postdialysis period. In the longer term, however, repeated cytokine stimulation may be responsible for the aging process in long-term dialysis patients. In addition, cytokine activation of macrophages induces the expression of adhesion molecules on endothelial cells which may be recruited by synovial tissue resulting in subsequent local cytokine production enhancing the potential for β_2-microglobulin to be deposited as amyloid.

Spallation

Spallation is a term used to describe the separation of fragments from the surface of a material as the result of compression forces. In hemodialysis spallation occurs as particles, shed by the shearing stress of the roller pump on the inner surface of the silicon tubing of the pump insert, are shed into the circulation. These shed silicon particles may initiate granulomas in the liver, lung, spleen, bone marrow and skin and may be associated with increased concentrations of transaminases and granulomatous hepatitis. Experimentally, macrophage function may be impaired by the intravenous injection of silicon particles but this has not been demonstrated to be clinically important. Spallation occurs predominantly when the occlusion force of the blood pump is excessive; the number of silicon particles can be diminished by approximately 80% by reducing the occlusion force [17]. Good clinical practice dictates that protocols should be established to ensure that in the lining of a dialysis machine undue compression is not applied to the dialysis arterial line pump insert.

Aluminum intoxication

In 1972 Alfrey *et al.* described a new syndrome of unknown etiology consisting of dementia, speech disturbances, seizures and myoclonus [18]. This was followed by many reports confirming that this was a dialysis-associated syndrome. It appeared to have an unusual geographic distribution and was eventually traced to aluminum contamination of the water used to generate dialysis fluid [19]. Although initial reports concentrated on the neurological manifestations it became obvious that patients also developed a fracturing osteodystrophy [20] and a microcytic anemia [21].

The two main sources of aluminum intoxication in patients on hemodialysis are aluminum-contaminated dialysis fluid and oral ingestion of aluminum-containing phosphate binders. The introduction of sophisticated methods of water purification including reverse osmosis and deionization has abolished the syndrome, even in areas where there is significant aluminum contamination of the water supply [22]. Phosphate control continues to be a problem in patients on hemodialysis and although alternative binders such as calcium carbonate have been advocated, some patients continue to require aluminum hydroxide. In such instances, patients should be advised to take their aluminum hydroxide with meals in a dose appropriate to the estimated phosphate content of the meal. This can only be achieved by trial, but ensuring that the patient takes the aluminum hydroxide with meals reduces the absorption of aluminum. Wherever possible aluminum-containing phosphate binders should be avoided.

Vascular calcification

Peripheral vascular disease is common in patients on hemodialysis. The reasons for this are multifactorial but include hypertension, abnormal lipid profiles and hypercalcemia. Patients with diabetes mellitus have a greater prevalence of this complication.

In the predialysis phase of uremia, many patients are treated by dietary manipulations which include the provision of calorie supplements by encouraging increased fat consumption in the form of cream. In patients with hypertension this has the potential of aggravating atherosclerosis. In the predialysis phase, therefore, it is not only important to control blood pressure, it is also advisable to provide dietary advice that avoids any foods which may be atherogenic. In patients on dialysis the avoidance of hypercalcemia by controlling hyperparathyroidism is essential. Unfortunately, once vascular calcification becomes manifest there is no known intervention which will induce regression. Strenuous efforts are necessary to prevent progression.

Problems related to continuing uremia

Anemia

As chronic renal failure progresses anemia develops which is multifactorial in origin. There may be a deficiency of certain essential precursors due to anorexia or dietary restrictions. Patients with uremia have a reduction in red cell survival and increased blood loss owing to impaired platelet function. In the majority of patients the major cause is a relative lack of erythropoietin. Although the plasma concentration of erythropoietin is within the normal range, it is inappropriate for the reduced hemoglobin concentration. Patients with polycystic kidney disease frequently maintain a hemoglobin greater than that found in patients with other causes of uremia because of their ability to maintain a more normal hemoglobin erythropoietin feedback control.

Dialysis may partially correct a number of these factors and patients will receive greater medical supervision and hence mineral and vitamin supplements. During each dialysis session, however, there is likely to be a small but repetitive blood loss as it is impossible to completely clear the lines and dialyzer of all red cells. To this must be added the necessary blood sampling to monitor the efficiency of treatment.

The management of anemia in dialysis patients has been revolutionized by the introduction of erythopoietin. Human erythropoietin derived from recombinant DNA (ruHuEpo) has been shown to effectively reverse the anemia of patients undergoing chronic hemodialysis [23]. A glycopeptide of 36 daltons comprising 165 amino acids, erythropoietin is synthesized by the interstitial cells in the renal cortex in response to decreased oxygen delivery. In normal circumstances as the hematocrit decreases the erythropoietin production increases but in dialysis patients this relationship, although present, is significantly impaired. The erythropoietin gene, located on the long arm of chromosome seven, has been cloned [24] and transfected into cells so that erythropoietin can be produced for therapeutic use. The effectiveness of this preparation is remarkable and it has rapidly been accepted into clinical practice.

The benefits of erythropoietin therapy are numerous with the avoidance of blood transfusions being the most significant. This has the added advantage of reducing the risk of sensitization to HLA antigens and also reducing the risk of transmission of viral diseases such as hepatitis B, hepatitis C and HIV.

There is evidence that the increased hematocrit is associated with increased exercise tolerance [25], improved quality of life [26] and regression of left ventricular hypertrophy [27].

Initially it was recommended that erythropoietin be given intravenously, but it has since been shown that the subcutaneous route of administration is preferable as it provides an improved dose–response profile. Erythropoietin is expensive and by employing subcutaneous administration it is possible to treat more patients for the same cost.

Resistance to erythropoietin has been reported [28] and is due to intercurrent infections, aluminum intoxication, iron deficiency, insufficient dialysis, hemolysis, blood loss and hemoglobinopathies. To ensure the effective use of erythropoietin it is important to screen for occult infection, and to treat it before erythropoietin is given. Aluminum toxicity may well be evident by an increased plasma aluminum concentration or may be suspected by the presence of a microcytic anemia and should certainly be considered in any long-term patient, particularly those who have received aluminum-containing phosphate binders. If there is any doubt regarding aluminum toxicity it would be advisable to perform a desferrioxamine (DFO) test. Should aluminum toxicity be confirmed, the patient should be treated with DFO to reduce the aluminum burden before erythropoietin is introduced. Iron deficiency is best assessed by estimating serum ferritin, and if it is <100 ng/ml, the deficiency should be corrected by oral or intravenous iron, before commencing erythropoietin therapy.

In patients who fail to respond satisfactorily to erythropoietin there may be insufficient dialysis, hemolysis or blood loss. The reticulocyte count can provide a useful indicator when assessing erythropoietin resistance [29]. In patients who lack a reticulocyte response there is likely to be some confounding factor preventing marrow response whereas those who have a satisfactory reticulocyte response without an appropriate increase in hematocrit have blood loss which may be obvious or occult.

The main side effect of erythropoietin is an increase in blood pressure which is due to loss of hypoxic vasodilatation, increased blood viscosity, endothelin release and perhaps a direct vasoconstrictor effect. Hypertension is more common when there is a rapid increase in hematocrit and can be avoided by using a low dose regimen of erythropoietin, e.g. 1000 units subcutaneously three times weekly. With this regimen it may take three months to increase the hemoglobin to target values but side effects are avoided.

There is considerable debate regarding the optimum hemoglobin which should be achieved. The majority of clinicians aim for a hemoglobin of 10 g/dl (hematocrit, 31–33%) but it is likely that this reflects financial concerns more than clinical reasons. Clinically, however, patients seem to have only minor symptoms relating to anemia, unless the hemoglobin is <10 g/dl.

Nutrition

Protein-calorie malnutrition is a problem in patients with chronic renal failure. The causes include anorexia, nausea, vomiting and prescribed low protein diets. Patients with diabetes mellitus, congestive cardiac failure, or those with prior corticosteroid therapy may have other reasons to be malnourished. Once dialysis therapy is started uremic symptoms decline and dietary restrictions are reduced resulting in an improved nutritional status. Some patients, however, continue to have anorexia. Furthermore, hemodialysis may induce catabolism and increase protein requirements exacerbating and prolonging malnutrition.

Impaired nutritional status is associated with increased morbidity and may restrict rehabilitation. There is a strong inverse association between serum albumin and mortality [30]. The protein catabolic rate assessed from urea kinetic modeling can be used as an estimate of protein intake. A catabolic rate of less than 0.8 g/kg body weight (bw)/day is associated with treatment failure and an increased mortality rate [31]. As the protein catabolic rate increases indicating increased protein intake, the mortality declines. It should be remembered, however, that there may not be a causal relationship between malnutrition, as assessed by serum albumin, and increased morbidity and mortality as many patients have comorbid conditions such as cardiovascular disease, diabetic complications, and gastrointestinal or liver diseases where hypoproteinemia may reflect the severity of the illness rather than being a direct cause of death. Nonetheless insufficient dialysis is likely to result in anorexia which will lead to malnutrition and subsequent increased mortality.

Hemodialysis appears to induce a catabolic state and it is likely that to achieve optimum nutritional status a protein intake of 1 g/kg bw/day will be required and an energy of 35 kcal/kg bw/day should be achieved. The cause of the increased catabolism seen in hemodialysis patients is not fully understood but it is likely that inadequate correction of uremia is the major factor; other causes include reduced physical activity, acidosis, loss of amino acids and glucose in the dialyzate and bioincompatibility.

During hemodialysis there is a reduction in protein synthesis [32] which may be induced by amino acid depletion, and an enhanced protein degradation as a result of blood–membrane interaction. Such interaction is associated with complement activation (alternate pathway) with production of C3a and C5a, monocyte activation with release of IL-1 and TNF and, the passage through the membrane of endotoxin fragments and acetate. All these factors can increase catabolism of muscle protein, possibly mediated by prostaglendin E_2. The catabolic effect of blood–membrane interaction is greater with cuprophane compared to synthetic membranes.

A diagnosis of malnutrition is based on the findings of anorexia, weight loss, muscle fatigue, muscle wasting and reduced fat stores. A plasma albumin of less than 30 g/l supports the diagnosis. It is important to obtain an adequate dietary history to reveal any dietary inadequacies.

Anthropomorphic measurements such as postdialysis body weight, skinfold thickness and arm circumference measurements may be of value particularly in the sequential assessment of patients. The protein catabolic rate should be calculated from urea kinetic modelling and, if significant residual renal function remains, a urea clearance should additionally be calculated.

The lipid abnormalities observed in hemodialysis patients include increased triglycerides and lipoprotein(a) and diminished HDL cholesterol; these are risk factors for atherosclerosis. Heparin activates lipoprotein lipase and the use of low-molecular-weight heparin reduces serum triglycerides; whether these effects are of clinical significance is not known. If serious abnormalities are present then a low cholesterol, low saturated fat diet may be of benefit although there is little published work to support this.

The loss of water-soluble vitamins to the dialyzate may result in significant depletion which can be prevented by the daily administration of vitamin B complex (two tablets daily) and folic acid, 5 mg, daily. Although dialyzer clearance for ascorbic acid is high, rarely does vitamin C deficiency become manifest and routine replacement is not advocated due to the risk that excess intake may result in oxalate accumulation. Changes in dialysis schedules to shorter hours and a more liberal diet are likely to result in less vitamin depletion than was encountered with the dialysis schedules employed several years ago.

Calcium metabolism

Dialysis does not restore the disordered calcium metabolism to normal. Hypocalcemia persists due to impairment of the activity of the enzyme 1-hydroxylase and persisting hyperphosphatemia. Reduction in the conversion of 25-hydroxycholecalciferol into the active metabolite 1,25-dihydroxycholecalciferol has a number of direct and indirect effects: impairment of intestinal calcium absorption, impairment of calcification of osteoid, and reduction of muscle function as well as other effects as a consequence of hypocalcemia. Parathyroid hormone secretion is increased in response to hypocalcemia and this results in the stimulation of osteoclasts to reabsorb bone in an attempt to restore the plasma calcium to normal. The lack of 1-hydroxylase activity can, in part, be overcome by alphacalcidol but at present there is no consensus as to the most appropriate time to start therapy or whether it is best given orally or intravenously and whether it should be given on a daily basis or by pulse administration. Pulse intravenous administration is more effective in controlling hyperparathyroidism and has the added advantage that it can be given at each dialysis session thus ensuring compliance. Oral administration is associated with a greater incidence of hypercalcemia which, in the presence of hyperphosphatemia, may cause metastatic calification.

The calcium concentration in the dialysis fluid should be between 6 and 7 mg/dl; lower values will result in depletion of calcium with further aggravation of hyperparathyroidism and higher concentrations will be associated with an increased risk of metastatic calcification in the presence of hyperphosphatemia.

Renal osteodystrophy can be improved by dialysis and the use of alphacalcidol but in some patients bone disease will persist particularly if aluminum intoxication is present. In some patients hyperparathyroid bone disease may become clinically apparent after commencing regular dialysis treatment and annual skeletal surveys should be undertaken so that appropriate early therapy can be commenced.

Amyloidosis

In 1975 Warren and Otieno reported on an apparent increase in the incidence of carpal tunnel syndrome in patients maintained on hemodialysis [33]. Since then it has been increasingly recognized as a complication of long-term treatment. Some years later Baillod et al. [34] reported an increased incidence of shoulder pain and stiffness in patients on long-term dialysis. Amyloid infiltration of the synovium of the tendons of patients with the carpal tunnel syndrome was demonstrated [35] but it was the group from Tassin who linked the carpal tunnel syndrome with the shoulder pain and stiffness syndrome to a common etiology by identifying amyloid deposition at both sites. It was suggested that amyloid was deposited as a result of some slow toxic or incompatibility mechanism. Further experience indicated that the duration of dialysis appeared to have an important effect on the severity, type and progression of the arthropathy. In 1985 Gejyo et al. [36] identified the amyloid protein associated with chronic haemodialysis arthropathy as β_2-microglobulin. The terms 'dialysis arthropathy' and 'dialysis related amyloidosis' are in common use but they imply a causal link to the dialysis procedure. More recently it has been recognized that β_2-microglobulin amyloidosis may become symptomatic before the commencement of dialysis [1] and thus it is likely the underlying cause reflects the continuing state of uremia which is not corrected by dialysis.

Symptoms of amyloid arthropathy are uncommon before the fifth year of dialysis treatment but thereafter the prevalence increases and affects more than 50% of patients dialyzed for 15 years. Patients develop a carpal-tunnel-like syndrome but unlike the idiopathic form there is no preference for females, those aged over 40 or the dominant hand. Symptoms of pain or parasthesia in the first to third fingers typically increase at night and during dialysis. Symptoms may be precipitated by extreme flexion or extension at the wrist. In early cases nerve conduction studies are required to demonstrate delayed transmission of the nerve impulse through the carpal tunnel. Trigger finger is also related to amyloidosis and may occur in 15% of patients dialyzed for 15 years. The shoulders and knees may become involved; typically, shoulder joint pain increases during immobilization during the night and during dialysis and is improved by movement and stretching, unlike inflammatory arthropathies. In the cervical spine a destructive spondylarthropathy may develop due to amyloid deposition in the intervertebral discs. Arthropathy is frequently accompanied by the formation of subchondral bone cysts in the hips, knees, humerus and metacarpal bones [37]. The cysts may attain significant size and have been reported to result in pathological fractures.

β_2-Microglobulin is a normal constituent of plasma with a concentration of 1.1–2.7 mg/l. It has a molecular weight of 11 800 daltons and consists of a polypeptide chain of 99 residues with a disulfide bridge. It circulates as a monomer and exists on the surface of nearly all cells as the constant portion of the light chain of the major histocompatability complex class I antigen. The normal production of β_2-microglobulin is 150–200 mg daily of which 97% is excreted by glomerular filtration. In renal failure the concentration of β_2-microglobulin increases; there is an inverse correlation between plasma β_2-microglobulin and glomerular filtration rate (GFR). A diagnosis of β_2-microglobulin amyloidosis may be made by biopsy of synovial tissues and the demonstration by light microscopy of birefringent material. Further identification may be undertaken by immunohistochemical means and electron microscopy. Non-invasive means of detection have included ultrasonography particularly of the capsule of the femoral neck or shoulder. If a joint effusion is present β_2-microglobulin may be identified in the synovial fluid. Unlike idiopathic and secondary amyloidosis gum or rectal biopsy does not appear to be of value.

The pathogenesis of β_2-amyloidosis is not fully understood. Polymerization of β_2-microglobulin forms fibrils due to the increased concentration of β_2-microglobulin or as a result of local factors such as partial proteolysis or enhanced glycosylation. Macrophages may have a part to play either by enhancing production or reducing removal. The deposition of β_2-microglobulin is most likely multifactorial since the amyloid deposits contain other materials such as serum amyloid P component, hyaluronic acid, and an 85 kDa amyloid-related protein.

Considerable debate remains as to whether hemodialysis itself increases the plasma β_2-microglobulin. Increased generation may occur as a result of mechanical damage to cells due to contact with cellulose membranes, and exposure of blood to cuprophane is associated with increased expression of β_2-microglobulin mRNA. There appears to be a relationship between the incidence of symptomatic β_2-microglobulin amyloidosis and the type of dialysis membrane indicating that the more hemocompatible membranes are associated with less carpal tunnel syndrome and fewer bone cysts. Plasma β_2-microglobulin can be reduced by a change from cellulosic to synthetic membranes, and by hemofiltration. Unfortunately, this has little effect on symptoms which is hardly surprising in view of the fact that the lower values achieved are still more than 10 times normal. Experimental work has been undertaken to evaluate adsorbent columns employing porous cellulosic beads to which a hydrophobic organic compound is covalently bound. These columns are not yet commercially available but may be of potential value. Transplantation is accompanied by symptomatic improvement but, as yet, there are few studies demonstrating objective alteration in the tendon or joint capsules.

Endocrine disorders

Patients undergoing hemodialysis may have a number of endocrine disorders which are often subtle and complex. Detection can be difficult due to difficulties in interpretation of the tests of endocrine function in a uremic environment.

Insulin secretion is impaired but to some extent this is offset by decreased insulin catabolism. There is, however, insulin resistance due to a postreceptor defect, some patients have a diabetic glucose tolerance curve although their fasting blood glucose is normal. In hemodialysis patients this does not produce clinical problems.

Hypothyroidism is difficult to diagnose because many dialysis patients have symptoms which mimic hypothyroidism. The majority of patients, however, are euthyroid.

Gonadal function is diminished producing decreased libido, impotence and infertility. Many women on hemodialysis have amenorrhea and those who continue to menstruate frequently have irregular anovulatory cycles. Although infertility is common, conception may occur; female patients need to be advised accordingly. A number of patients have hyperprolactinemia and in such patients sexual function can be improved by bromocryptine therapy. Erythropoietin therapy is associated with improved gonadal function.

Hypertension

Hypertension is particularly common in patients with uremia. After the introduction of hemodialysis, blood pressure control is improved but many patients still require antihypertensive therapy. Hypertension is a major cause of morbidity and mortality by means of atherosclerosis, cardiac failure and cerebrovascular accidents. The incidence of left ventricular hypertrophy in dialysis patients is considerably greater than that in non-uremic patients. Blood pressure control is essential in to arrest progression.

In hemodialysis patients hypertension may be partly volume dependent, particularly in patients with large interdialytic weight gains. An excessive sodium intake will result in thirst and consequently increase fluid intake and increase volume. In many patients hypertension is mediated through the renin–angotensin system due to increased renin secretion from the diseased kidneys.

Blood pressure should be controlled first by achieving an ideal body weight, the so called 'dry weight'. Once this is achieved patients should be encouraged not to gain more than 2 kg between dialysis sessions, i.e., that is not to increase their weight by more than 2–3%. Although some patients will be controlled in this way most will require antihypertensive therapy with either vasodilators, calcium channel blockers, beta blockers or ACE inhibitors. ACE inhibitors may increase the incidence of first use reactions [5], cause hyperkalemia and impair the effectiveness of erythropoietin [38]. The most effective agent can often only be found by clinical trial. The many and differing antihypertensive agents currently available have virtually abolished the need for bilateral nephrectomy for blood pressure control.

Malignancy

The prevalence of malignancy is increased in dialysis patients with certain patients being at particular risk. Patients whose underlying cause of renal failure is analgesic nephropathy are at risk of developing urothelial tumors, particularly of the renal pelvis; patients with polycystic kidney disease and those with acquired cystic disease are at increased risk of developing renal cell carcinoma, and patients with glomerulonephritis appear to be at an increased risk for non-Hodgkin's lymphoma. Furthermore for all dialysis patients there is a fivefold increase in the risk of developing renal cell carcinoma, a fourfold increase in endometrial carcinoma and twice the risk of developing lymphoma, sarcoma, reticulosis or colonic tumors as that of the non-uremic population. There does not appear to be any increase in the risk of dialysis patients for melanoma, or carcinoma of the stomach, bronchus or breast [39].

Patients with an underlying diagnosis of analgesic nephropathy are at risk of developing a carcinoma of the renal pelvis but the precise level of risk is not known. Most commonly this is a transitional cell carcinoma although squamous cell carcinoma may occur. The clinical presentation is usually with hematuria. It is advisable in dialysis patients with analgesic nephropathy to undertake urine cytology at yearly intervals to allow for early detection and appropriate management by nephroureterectomy.

The incidence of renal cell carcinoma is increased in all patients on hemodialysis; those with adult type polycystic kidney disease and acquired renal cystic disease are at greatest risk [40]. The clinical presentation may include unexplained fever, hematuria, loin pain, weight loss, anorexia or a palpable mass. Patients with polycystic kidney disease or acquired cystic disease should have an ultrasound performed when they start dialysis and at yearly intervals thereafter. In other patients ultrasound examination should be undertaken for macroscopic hematuria or the onset of microhematuria. All complex cysts or solid masses should be considered as tumors until proven otherwise. It has been suggested that lesions of less than 3 cm in diameter are more likely benign adenomas but this is unreliable as tumors less than 3 cm have been known to metastasize. Diagnosis can be confirmed by computed tomography-guided needle biopsy. Management is by nephrectomy.

Caution is required in the evaluation of tumor markers. Carcinoembryonic antigen is significantly increased in all hemodialysis patients and is, therefore, an unreliable tumor marker. Alpha-fetoprotein is slightly elevated and therefore only of limited value, whereas prostatic specific antigen is not normally elevated and is therefore still useful in screening for prostatic carcinoma.

Infections

Patients with uremia and dialysis patients are at increased risk of infections. Approximately 15–20% of all deaths in dialysis patients are causally related to infection. Uremia confers a degree of immunosuppression to which malnutrition, and in some cases aluminum overload, may contribute. The majority of infections, however, are due to common community acquired rather than to opportunistic infections. Staphylococcal infections are the most common; 30–70% of dialysis patients are carriers of *Staphylococcus aureus* or *Staphylococcus epidermidis*. Such organisms may be introduced during puncture of the vascular access and by indwelling venous catheters inspite of careful skin preparations. Staphylococcal septicemia may occur and lead in some patients to osteomyelitis or endocarditis. Other relatively common infections include pneumonia and urinary tract infection.

Iron overload leads to an increased incidence of *Listeria monocytogenes* and *Yersinia enterocolitica*. The use of desferrioxamine to treat aluminum or iron overload has been associated with mucormycosis.

Phagocytic cell function is depressed, particularly in patients treated with cuprophane dialyzers [41], because chemotaxis is impaired and granulocyte adherence is diminished due to a reduction in chemotactic receptor particularly C5a receptors [42].

In addition to these chronic changes in leukocyte function acute changes can be demonstrated during dialysis. Granulocytes obtained 15 min after the initiation of cuprophane hemodialysis have decreased adherence as well as a diminution in ability to bind to endothelial cell monolayers. These changes could decrease granulocyte extravasation through endothelium to sites of inflammation and thus diminish the required response to infection.

In addition to the defects in phagocytic cell function, patients on chronic dialysis have impaired humoral and cell-mediated immunity. Lymphocyte function is impaired as manifest by increased delayed hypersensitivity response evaluated by skin testing. Impairment of humoral immunity is evidenced by the reduced responsiveness to vaccination.

In part, the reduced resistance to infection relates to a continuing state of uremia, but this may be accentuated by certain dialysis membranes. Synthetic membranes by their lesser activation of complement are probably associated with a lesser impairment of immunity, although there are no good long-term studies to confirm this impression.

Progeria

Uremia appears to be a state of accelerated aging. The causes are unknown, but may be due to uremic toxins which have the capacity of altering protein structures. As an example glycosylation occurs and subtly changes protein structure. Such modifications of protein particularly in extracellular matrix could accelerate aging. Patients undergoing dialysis appear to age twice as fast as the normal population; although this may be due to a continuing state of (minor) malnutrition, it is more likely uremia has a direct effect.

Prevention of complications arising in hemodialysis patients

Thirty years ago when hemodialysis was first introduced for the management of patients with end-stage renal failure, survival alone was a significant achievement. As facilities were limited, patient selection was necessary and patients with medical complications other than renal failure were usually excluded. Since then there has been a steady expansion of resources so that selection criteria became more relaxed and were eventually abolished. Current entry to a dialysis program is dependent on the potential for the patient to benefit from treatment rather than any patient characteristic. As a result patients from neonates to the very elderly are being accepted for treatment.

The clinical management of an end-stage renal failure program varies widely from country to country. In Europe, Scandanavian countries favor transplantation as the preferred option, whereas more southern countries rely heavily on dialysis with only a few patients receiving a transplant. Experience has demonstrated that the very young (less than five years) and the elderly (older than 70 years) are less likely to be successfully transplanted. Now that transplantation has been practised for more than 30 years, there are an increasing number of patients, who as a consequence of chronic rejection, return to a dialysis program. Although some patients with a failed transplant will receive another graft, it is always more difficult to obtain a suitable organ for the second graft because of cytotoxic antibodies. As a consequence there is an increasing number of patients destined for long-

term dialysis and attention has focused on how to reduce the complications which such patients experience.

In the past there has been an overemphasis on the dialysis procedure itself causing complications which has resulted in a preoccupation with bioincompatibility in the belief that more biocompatibile systems will prevent complications. Interaction between blood, the surface of lines and dialyzer membranes is associated with a number of complications such as the activation of complement by the alternative pathway, stimulation of cytokine production, dialysis-related neutropenia, and increased production of β_2-microglobulin as previously noted. Add to these complications those relating to the two-way transfer of substances through the inert dialyzer membrane depending on size, charge and shape and over many years there may be a depletion of certain substances essential for well-being and an accumulation of harmful substances present in the dialysis fluid in trace amounts. There is, therefore, no doubt that certain problems in patients on long-term dialysis are the result of dialysis.

The most common cause of death in patients on dialysis is cardiovascular disease – cardiac failure, cardiac arrest, myocardial infarction and myocardial ischemia being common. It is likely that the increased morbidity and mortality from cardiac disease is aggravated but not initiated by dialysis. The majority of patients proceeding to long-term hemodialysis are treated by dietary protein restriction and increased carbohydrate and fat intake is advised to compensate for the reduction in calorie intake as a consequence of protein restriction. Hypertension is very common in uremia and it is more than likely that the combination of dietary manipulations and hypertension results in coronary artery atherogenesis. Hyperparathyroidism also has an adverse affect on the myocardium and uremia itself may be a contributing factor. It is likely therefore that the cardiovascular problems of long-term dialysis patients are more attributable to predialysis management than to the dialysis procedure itself.

To reduce the complications arising in dialysis patients, two aspects of management must be addressed. First, there must be further improvement in the biocompatibility of the dialysis systems. Second, the management of patients with impaired renal function prior to dialysis must be improved. The need for predialysis dietary protein restriction should be re-examined, and secondary hyperparathyroidism should be prevented by adequate calcium intake and treatment with vitamin D analogs. Using erythropoietin the hemoglobin should be maintained in excess of $10\,g/dl$. These measures, in particular increasing the protein intake, may result in the patient requiring dialysis sooner than might have been expected but the patient will be fitter and less at risk from cardiovascular disease. It may be that the time has come to abandon dietary protein restriction with the associated calorie supplements in patients progressing to dialysis and to reserve such treatment for those patients considered unsuitable for long-term dialysis. In this way we may have a more healthy dialysis population who are less at risk of developing cardiovascular disease.

Psychiatric problems

Anxiety

Psychiatric problems are common in patients with end-stage renal failure and those being treated by dialysis. Adverse publicity, much of it unjustified, has been given to the lack of adequate resources for dialysis in the UK and this has not unnaturally led to considerable anxiety to patients who know they have renal failure which may progress to require dialysis. Many patients and their relatives are fearful that dialysis facilities will not be made available when the time comes for such treatment to be initiated. It is important, therefore, in the predialysis management to reassure patients that facilities are available and that they will be accepted for dialysis treatment when this becomes necessary. In many patients the insertion of an arteriovenous fistula in preparation for dialysis is reassuring and gives them confidence that some positive action is being undertaken. It is helpful in the predialysis stage to discuss with the patient and relatives the various options available – hemodialysis in a center, in a satellite facility, or at home; CAPD; or predialysis transplantation. Planning ahead gives cofidence to the patient and reassurance to the relatives. As the time approaches to commence dialysis the physician should arrange for the patient and relatives to visit the dialysis unit to meet the staff and talk with other dialysis patients to discuss the pros and cons of the various treatment modalities.

When patients begin dialysis they often feel an initial period of elation which arises from the relief they experience when the uncertainty of the future is removed. Many patients and their families have to cope with the knowledge that dialysis therapy is going to be required at some time but not knowing when. Although it is sometimes useful in the predialysis clinic to plot the serum creatinine and extrapolate to a theoretical value between 800–1000 µmol/l, when dialysis will be required; however, it is not always possible to do this with any certainty. Many patients find this uncertain future to be particularly disturbing.

The elation on commencing dialysis is frequently short lived when patients begin to realize the complexity of their treatment and the fact that it will be required for the rest of their life, unless a suitable transplant becomes available. The realization of the requirement for life-time therapy may cause depression which in some patients may last for many months. The majority of patients come to terms with the impact dialysis has on their lives. Some patients wish to return to employment and many will become more active with respect to social and recreational activities.

Stress

Dialysis patients are under considerable stress due to the fact that their lives are dependent on a mechanical device which does not always work perfectly and which can have problems. Patients have to face the reality of difficulties with vascular access, the insertion of needles, the operation of dialysis machines, and the fact that dialysis does not completely resolve the clinical consequences of uremia. As a result certain stresses continue and others develop as a consequence of treatment. The most common psychiatric problems are depression and denial. On occasion depression can be severe and may lead to self-withdrawal from treatment, suicide, or fatal non-compliance. It may be prolonged in patients receiving inadequate dialysis (and therefore inadequate rehabilitation). Careful counseling is required; the staff caring for such patients need to adopt a particularly positive attitude and give constant reassurance.

In some patients stress may be aggravated by their inability to resume their previous employment and the fact they have become dependent on others. Clinical manifestations include sleep disturbances with reversal of the normal diurnal pattern, decreased libido, inappropriate anxiety and preoccupation with minor medical complaints. Prolonged stress may further decrease the ability to cope with everyday situations which will further aggravate depression, thereby causing a spiraling downwards of the patient's mental status. It is sometimes difficult to break this spiral; skilled counseling is frequently required.

Compliance

Patient compliance with the dialysis regimen, medications and dietary restrictions is a problem which all dialysis units face. The majority of patients are non-compliant in some way but it usually does not cause any clinical concern. In a few patients, however, non-compliance poses serious problems that restrict the effectiveness of therapy and cause disruption in the dialysis unit.

Most frequently non-compliance relates to dietary restrictions with respect to control of fluid, sodium, potassium and phosphate intake. Eating habits are difficult to change and most patients will try to adjust their dietary restriction such that their every-day diet is not too dissimilar to that which they were used to before developing renal failure. Many patients will experiment to see how far they can extend the limits of their potassium and phosphate intake; some become remarkably adept at knowing just how far they can go before dangerous hyperkalemia or hyperphosphatemia ensues.

The majority of patients also find difficulty in adhering to their prescribed medication. In one study of 27 centers 123 patients were prescribed a mean of 7.7 medications [43] and it is, therefore, not surprising that compliance is a problem. Some drugs are prescribed once daily whereas others require to be taken two or three times daily. This is clearly confusing to the patient and wherever possible, the drug regimen should be made as simple as possible, and clear written instructions should be given to the patient.

The causes of non-compliance are multifactorial. In some respects the problem is generated by the attitude of the staff. The patients are clearly placed in a conflict of interest in that the staff caring for patients expect them to adhere to a strict regimen with respect to their dialysis, medications and diet, and at the same time asking them to lead as normal a life as possible. Many patients find it extremely difficult to come to terms with such a dramatic change in life style and can only make their feelings known by not adhering to prescribed advice. It should be remembered, however, that non-compliance is often a consequence of poor communication from staff and it is clearly essential that patients be given a clear concise explanation for the rationale of their management.

Non-compliance may be a cry for help, or an expression of anger, fear, denial, anxiety or depression. For the same reason that some patients will resort to self-poisoning as a cry for help, patients requiring chronic therapy will cease therapy. This self-withdrawal from all or part of their therapy may not be recognized as a covert means of obtaining help and tragically, just as in self-poisoning, patients may misjudge the severity of their condition with resulting irreparable harm or even death. It is thus important to examine carefully the motives behind actions to determine whether the patient is trying to draw attention to some unrecognized problem.

Non-compliance can, of course, extend much further than non-adherence to prescribed treatment. Patients may be abusive or arrive drunk for treatment or use foul language. Such 'problem patients' may be disruptive to the dialysis unit and place staff in a very difficult position in view of their responsibility for other patients. Disruptive behavior should not be tolerated but it is frequently extremely difficult to manage in a non-confrontational way without further exacerbating an already difficult situation. All members of staff in a dialysis center have to learn how to listen to the patient and not to jump to conclusions. Very often there is a hidden message which needs an experienced listener to detect. Staff must be aware of the influence of culture, race and gender, and should be trained in stress management and how to defuse difficult situations. Being aware of the potential problem is half the battle when confronting an awkward situation.

Conclusion

Unfortunately, many patients prior to proceeding to dialysis are advised that all they need is treatment with an artificial kidney and everything will be all right. It does not take long before patients realize that this situation is far from the truth. In some respects it is a pity that a dialyzer has become termed an artificial kidney because in reality it only partly replaces some of the excretory function of the normal kidney and none of its synthetic functions. Many complications which arise in patients after commencing hemodialysis have their genesis in the pre-dialysis period, either due to prolonged uremia or possibly as a consequence of treatment. Many technical problems relating to the dialysis procedure have been resolved but bioincompatibility of the dialysis circuit remains a problem. The continuing state of uremia has an important effect that must always be borne in mind when considering the medical complications of the patient on hemodialysis.

References

1. Zingraff, J., Noel, L.M., Bardin, T. *et al.* (1990) β_2-microglobulin amyloidosis in chronic renal failure, *N. Engl. J. Med.*, **323**, 1070–1.
2. Fraser, C.L. and Arieff, A.I. (1988) Nervous system complications in uremia. *Ann. Intern. Med.*, **109**, 143–53.
3. Bergstrom, J. (1978) Ultrafiltration without dialysis for removal of fluid and solutes in uraemia. *Clin. Nephrol.*, 9, 156–64.
4. Daugirdas, J.T. and Ing, T. S. (1991) First use reactions during hemodialysis: a definition of subtypes. *Kidney Int.*, **24**, S37–43.
5. Pegues, D.A., Beck-Sague, C.M., Wollen, S.W. *et al.* (1992) Anaphylactoid reactions associated with reuse of hollow dialysers and ACE inhibitors. *Kidney Int.*, **42**, 1232–7.
6. Saito, H. (1991) Hemostatic disorders associated with renal disease, in *Disorders of Hemostasis* (eds O. Rantoff and C. Forbes), W. B. Saunders, Philadelphia.
7. Gilchrest, B.A., Rowe, J.W., Brown, R.S. *et al.* (1979) Relief of uremic pruritus with ultraviolet phototherapy. *N. Engl. J. Med.*, **297**, 138–8.
8. Simpson, N.B. and Davison, A.M. (1979) Ultraviolet phototherapy in uraemic pruritus. *Proc EDTA*, **16**, 743–4.
9. Ahmad, S., Robertson, M.T., Golpher, T.A. *et al.* (1990) Multicenter trial of L-carnitine in maintenance hemodialysis patients. II Clinical and biochemical effects. *Kidney. Int.*, **38**, 912–28.
10. Kaplow, L.S. and Goffinet, J.A. (1968) Profound neutropenia during the early phase of hemodialysis. *JAMA*, **203**, 1135–7.
11. Freeman, R.M., Lawton, R.L. and Chamberlain, M.A. (1967) Hard water syndrome. *N. Engl. J. Med.*, **276**, 1113–8.
12. Kjellstrand, C.M., Eaton, J.W., Yawata, Y. *et al.* (1974) Hemolysis in dialysed patients caused by chloramines *Nephron*, **13**, 427–33.
13. Gurland, H.J., Davison, A.M., Bonomini, V. *et al.* (1994)

Definitions and terminology in biocompatibility. *Nephrol. Dial. Transplant.*, 9(suppl 4), 4–10.

14. Salzman, E.W. and Merrill, E.W. (1987) Interaction of blood with artificial surfaces, in *Hemostasis and Thrombosis* (eds R.W. Coleman *et al.*), J.B. Lippincott, Philadelphia, pp. 1335–7.

15. Johnson, R.A. (1994) Complement activation during extracorporeal therapy; biochemistry, cell biology, and clinical relevance. *Nephrol. Dial. Transplant.*, 9(suppl 4), 36–45.

16. Colton, C.K., Ward, R.A. and Shaldon, S. (1994) Scientific basis for assessment in biocompatibility in extracorporeal blood treatment. *Nephrol. Dial. Transplant.*, 9(suppl 4), 11–17.

17. Bommer, J., Perenick, B.J., Kessler, J. and Ritz, E. (1984) Reduction of silicon particles released during haemodialysis. *Proc. EDTA-ERA*, 21, 287–90.

18. Alfrey, A.C., Mischell, J.M., Burks, J. *et al.* (1972) Syndrome of dyspraxia and multifocal seizures associated with chronic hemodialysis. *Trans. ASAIO*, 18, 257–61.

19. Platts, M.M., Goode, G.C. and Das, H.A. (1977) Composition of the domestic water supply and the incidence of fractures and encephalopathy in patients on home dialysis. *Br. Med. J.*, ii, 657–60.

20. Ward, M.K., Feest, T.G., Ellis, H.A. *et al.* (1978) Osteomalacic dialysis osteodystrophy: evidence for a water borne aetiological agent, probably aluminium. *Lancet*, i, 841–5.

21. Short, A.I.K., Winney, R.J. and Robson, J.S. (1980) Reversible microcytic hypochromic anaemia in dialysis patients due to aluminium intoxication. *Proc EDTA*, 17, 226–33.

22. Davison, A.M., Walker, G., Oli, H. and Lewins, A.M. (1982) Water supply aluminium concentration, dialysis dementia, and the effects of reverse osmosis water treatment. *Lancet*, ii, 785–7

23. Winearls, C.G., Pippard, M.J., Downing, M.R. *et al.* (1986) Effect of human erythropoietin derived from recombinant DNA on the anaemia of patients maintained by chronic haemodialysis. *Lancet*, ii, 1175–8.

24. Lin, F.-K. Suggs, S., Lin, C.-H., *et al.* (1985) Cloning an expression of the human erythropoietin gene. *Proc. Natl. Acad. Sci. USA*, 82, 7580–5.

25. Braumann, K.M., Nonnast-Daniel, B., Böning, D. *et al.* (1991) Improved physical performance after treatment of renal anemia with recombinant human erythropoietin. *Nephron*, 58, 129–34.

26. Eshbach, J.W., Abdulhadi, M.H., Browne, J.K. *et al.* (1989) Recombinant human erythropoietin in anemic patients with end-stage renal disease. *Ann. Intern. Med.*, 111, 992–1000.

27. Pascual, J., Teruel, J.L., Moya, J.L. *et al.* (1991) Regression of left ventricular hypertrophy after partial correction of anemia with erythropoietin in patients on hamodialysis: a prospective study. *Clin. Nephrol.*, 35, 280–7.

28. Drüeke, T.B. (1990) Resistance to recombinant human erythropoietin in hemodialysis patients. *Am. J. Nephrol.*, 10(suppl 2), 34–9.

29. Jeffrey, R.J., Khan, A.A., Kendall, R.G. *et al.* (1995) Quantitative reticulocyte analysis may be of benefit in monitoring erythropoietin treatment in dialysis patients. *Artif. Organs*, 19, 821–6.

30. Lowrie, E.G. and Lew, N.L. (1992) Commonly measured variables in hemodialysis patients: Relationship among them and to death risk. *Semin. Nephrol.*, 12, 276.

31. Harter, H.R. (1993) Review of significant findings from the National Co-operative Dialysis Study and recommendations. *Kidney. Int.*, Suppl. 13, 5107–12.

32. Lim, V.S. *et al.* (1990) The effect of hemodialysis on protein metabolism. *J. Am. Soc. Nephrol.*, 1, 366.

33. Warren, D.J. and Otieno, L.S. (1975) Carpal tunnel syndrome in patients on intermittant hemodialysis. *Postgrad. Med. J.*, 597, 450–2.

34. Baillod, R.A., Varghese, Z., Fernando, O.N. and Moorehead, J.F. (1981) Review of 71 patients receiving renal replacement for greater than 10 years, in *Uremia* (eds C. Giordano and E.A. Freidman), Wichtig, Editore, Milan, pp. 35–40.

35. Assenat, H., Calemard, E., Charra, B. *et al.* (1980) Hémodialyse syndrome du canal carpien *et* substance amyloid. *Nouv. Presse Med.*, 8, 1715.

36. Gejyo, F., Yamada, T., Odani, S. *et al.* (1985) A new form of amyloid protein associated with chronic haemodialysis was identified as $\beta_2$microglobulin. *Biochem. Biophys. Res. Commun.*, 129, 701–6.

37. Kurer, M.H.J., Baillod, R.A. and Madgwick, J.C.A. (1991) Musculoskeletal manifestations of amyloidosis. A review of 83 patients on haemodialysis for at least 10 years. *J. Bone Joint Surg.*, 73B, 271–6.

38. Walter, J. (1993) Does captopril decrease the effect of human recombinant erythropoietin in haemodialysis patients? *Nephrol. Dial. Transplant.*, 8, 1428.

39. Tufveson, G., Geerlings, W., Brunner, F.P. *et al.* (1989) Combined report on regular dialysis and transplantation in Europe XIX 1988. *Nephrol. Dial. Transplant.*, 4(suppl. 4), 5–30.

40. Ishikawa, I. (1992) Acquired renal cystic disease and its complications in continuous peritoneal dialysis patients. *Perit. Dial. Int.*, 12, 292.

41. Vanholder, R., Ringoir, S., Dhondt, A. and Hadim, R. (1991) Phagocytosis in uremic and hemodialysis patients: a prospective and cross-sectional study. *Kidney Int.*, 39, 320–7.

42. Lewis, S.L., van Epps, D.E. and Chenoweth, D.E. (1986) C5a receptor modulation on neutrophils and monocytes from chronic hemodialysis and peritoneal dialysis patients. *Clin. Nephrol.*, 26, 37–44.

43. Anderson, R.J., Melikian, D.M., Ganbertoglio, J.G. *et al.* (1982) Prescribing medication in long-term dialysis units. *Arch. Intern. Med.*, 142, 1305–8.

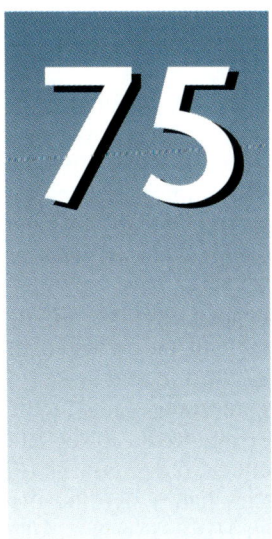

75

Outcome of hemodialysis

Alison L. Brown and Anthony E.G. Raine*

Introduction

Huge advances in hemodialysis technology have been made since the first patients began maintenance dialysis in the 1960s, but debate continues as to what is adequate dialysis. Recent evidence tends to confirm the common sense view that more is better, but what concerns most dialysis patients and their nephrologists is how much dialysis is enough to safely maintain a reasonable quality of life and ensure long-term survival? Most patients wish to achieve these objectives with the minimum disruption to family, social and working life, which in most hemodialysis units equates to shorter dialysis times.

Unfortunately, assessment of the most basic measure, survival rate, is made extremely difficult by the marked variations in provision of renal replacement therapy between countries and between centers. For example, the number of dialysis facilities providing regular dialysis treatment per million population (pmp) varies from 20.3 in Japan to 1.5 in the U.K. [1]. Similarly, the number of patients alive on renal replacement therapy pmp at the end of 1992 varied from 490 in the US to 177 in the countries covered by the European Dialysis and Transplantation Association (EDTA) registry. In the US, 144 new patients pmp started on renal replacement therapy in 1990, compared to 51 in Europe. Part of this difference may be due to the wide variation in reported incidence of primary renal diseases causing end-stage renal failure;

for example, 30% of new dialysis patients in 1992 in the US had diabetic nephropathy compared to 28% in Japan, 14% in Australia and 15% in the EDTA registry countries [1]. Such variations in population and associated risk factors make comparisons among different patient registries difficult. It is difficult to escape the conclusion, however, that some of the variation in current acceptance rates is due to social and economic factors which may further confound comparisons of survival.

Historical comparisons are difficult because of the changes in age and fitness of those accepted for dialysis; in the early days of maintenance hemodialysis, patients over 65, or with other medical problems such as diabetes, were commonly not accepted by dialysis programs. Today, few would be excluded from dialysis on the basis of age alone and transplantation of patients over 65 is increasingly common. Historical comparisons may also be misleading because of the evolution of dialysis equipment and technique. Ultimately, outcome measures depend on the accuracy of diagnosis of end points such as cardiovascular death and the accuracy of reporting and collating of data by individual centers and registries, which is unlikely to be perfect.

Comparison of survival rates between those on hemodialysis (HD) and those undertaking continuous ambulatory peritoneal dialysis (CAPD), even for patients in the same registry, is also difficult and possibly misleading. The majority of patients are not and cannot be randomly allocated to dialysis modality, so a prospective randomized trial presents formidable problems. Bias in

*Professor Raine died in October 1995.

Nephrology, Edited by Rex L. Jamison and Robert Wilkinson.
Published in 1997 by Chapman & Hall, London. ISBN 0 412 60930 4

selection confounds the analysis of retrospective studies [2]. Future trials of random allocation of CAPD or HD to the selected population deemed suitable for either modality should clarify the outcome for this limited group of patients.

Mortality of hemodialysis

Despite increased acceptance of older patients, and those with multiple coexisting medical problems, survival on maintenance HD increased markedly between the 1970s and 1980s in Europe (Figure 75.1). Survival rates were lower in diabetics of all age groups [3]. Survival on dialysis is inversely proportional to age at the start of therapy; European patients aged 65 and above starting HD between 1986 and 1993 had a 15% lower five-year survival than those aged 55–64 [4] (Figure 75.2). This is not surprising; over 50% of patients aged 65 years or older starting dialysis in Piedmont between 1981 and 1992 had at least one high risk condition in addition to their age; 59% also had cardiovascular disease, 26% diabetes mellitus and 10% neoplasia [5]. The coexistence of morbid conditions will become increasingly important as the dialysis population ages: the percentage of European patients aged 65 and over at the start of dialysis has increased from 9% in 1977 to 37% in 1992 [4] (Figure 75.3). In 1992 50% of adult patients starting dialysis in Europe were aged 60 years or older.

The commonest causes of death in patients on renal replacement therapy are cardiac, vascular and infection.

Of reported deaths in the EDTA registry in 1993, 38% were attributed to cardiac causes, 16% to vascular and 12% to infections [4]. The proportion of these principal causes of death have not changed significantly between 1982 and 1993, and do not appear to be greatly affected by dialysis modality, age or primary renal disease (Figures 75.4 and 75.5).

Many authors have compared mortality rates on HD and CAPD (the outcome of CAPD will be discussed in more detail in Chapter 81). In 1987, Burton and Walls [6] found no significant difference in mortality rates in the UK, but Maiorca *et al.* in 1991 [7] reported a lower rate for older patients on CAPD. In contrast, data from the US registry showed that older diabetics had a significantly lower survival rate on CAPD than HD; however, CAPD patients were more likely to be younger, and more likely to have diabetes and peripheral vascular disease and less likely to be black than those on HD, suggesting that selection bias influenced the difference in mortality [8]. The most recent study from the US Renal Data System was of more than 40 000 deaths in 170 000 patient-years of HD and CAPD between 1987 and 1989. Death rates were corrected for age, race, gender and diabetes. There were 21.3 deaths per hundred patient-years of hemodialysis compared to 25.3 deaths per hundred patient-years of CAPD, or a 19% greater risk with CAPD [9]. The greater relative risk of dying on CAPD increased to 30% for females and to 38% for diabetics. It was consistently greater for patients on CAPD than those on hemodialysis for common causes of death – 35% higher for infection, 24% for myocardial infarction and 8% for stroke [10]. Since

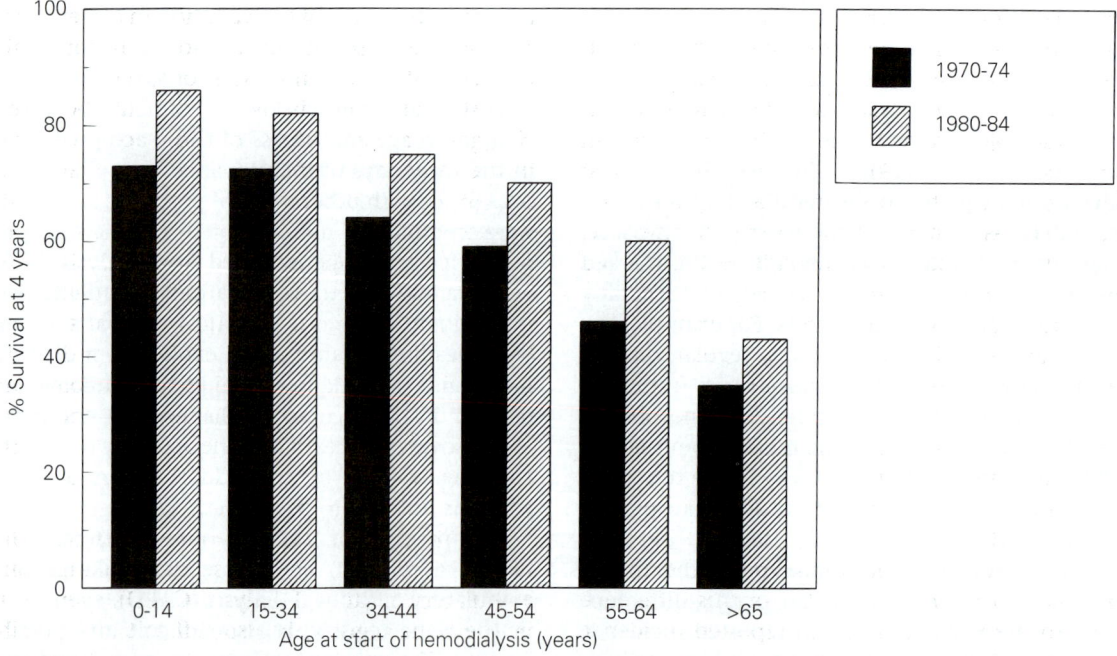

Figure 75.1 Patient survival on hemodialysis (including home hemodialysis and hemofiltration) 1970–1974 and 1980–1984. (Data reproduced, with permission, from the EDTA Registry.)

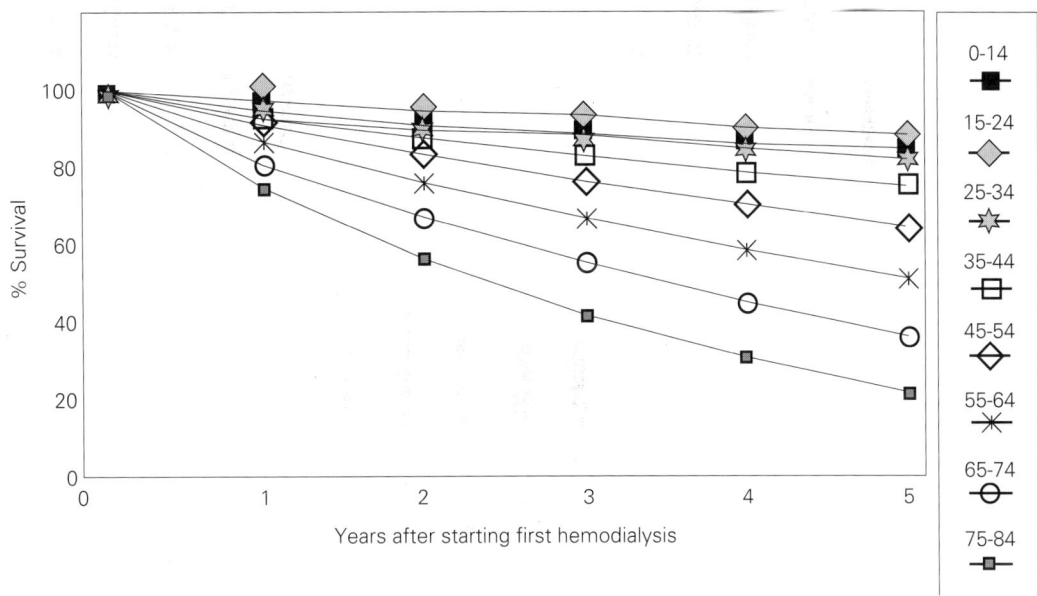

Figure 75.2 Patient survival after hemodialysis according to age at start of renal replacement therapy. Year of first treatment 1986–1993. First mode of therapy hospital or home hemodialysis. (Data reproduced, with permission, from the EDTA registry.)

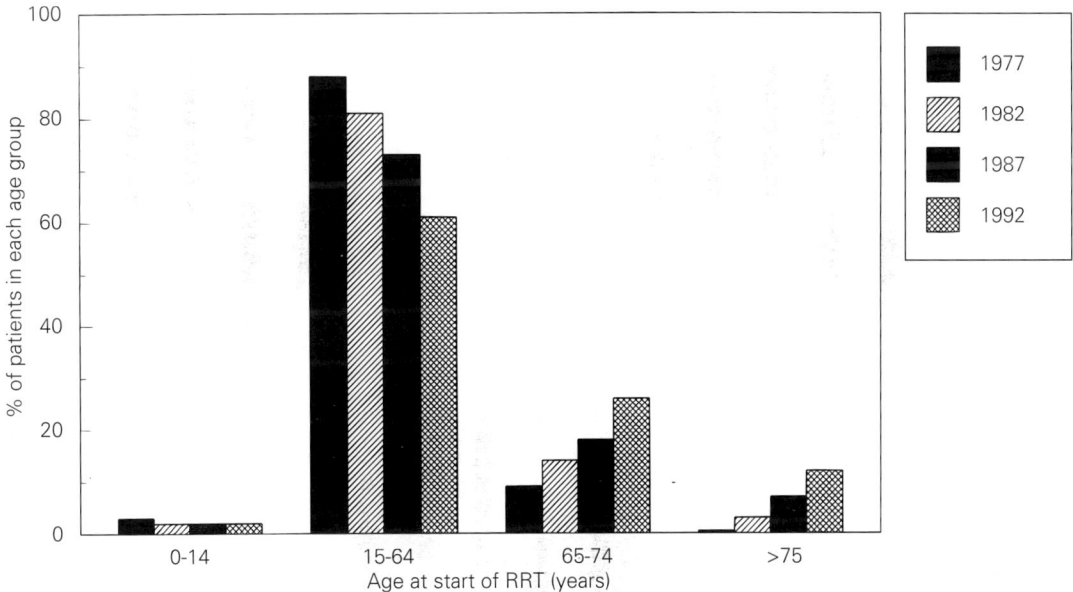

Figure 75.3 Age of patients starting renal replacement therapy (RRT) 1977, 1982, 1987, 1992. (Data reproduced, with permission, from the EDTA registry.)

these are retrospective data, as the authors point out, it is impossible to exclude case-mix differences as the explanation for the excess mortality associated with CAPD. In contrast, recent Canadian data [2] analyzing comparative mortality rates for more than 12000 patients dialyzed between 1989 and 1993 demonstrated a relative lesser risk of death (0.77) for CAPD patients compared to hemodialysis patients. Why the discrepancy between Canadian and US mortality rates? Even for the same modality of dialysis, the CANUSA study of more than 600 patients reveals a two-year mortality of 20% for Canadian CAPD patients compared to 37% for US CAPD patients in the study. A recent review [2] concludes that the most likely explanation for the wide discrepancy in mortality rates is different case mix; attempts to correct the data for demographic and comorbid factors fail because there is insuf-

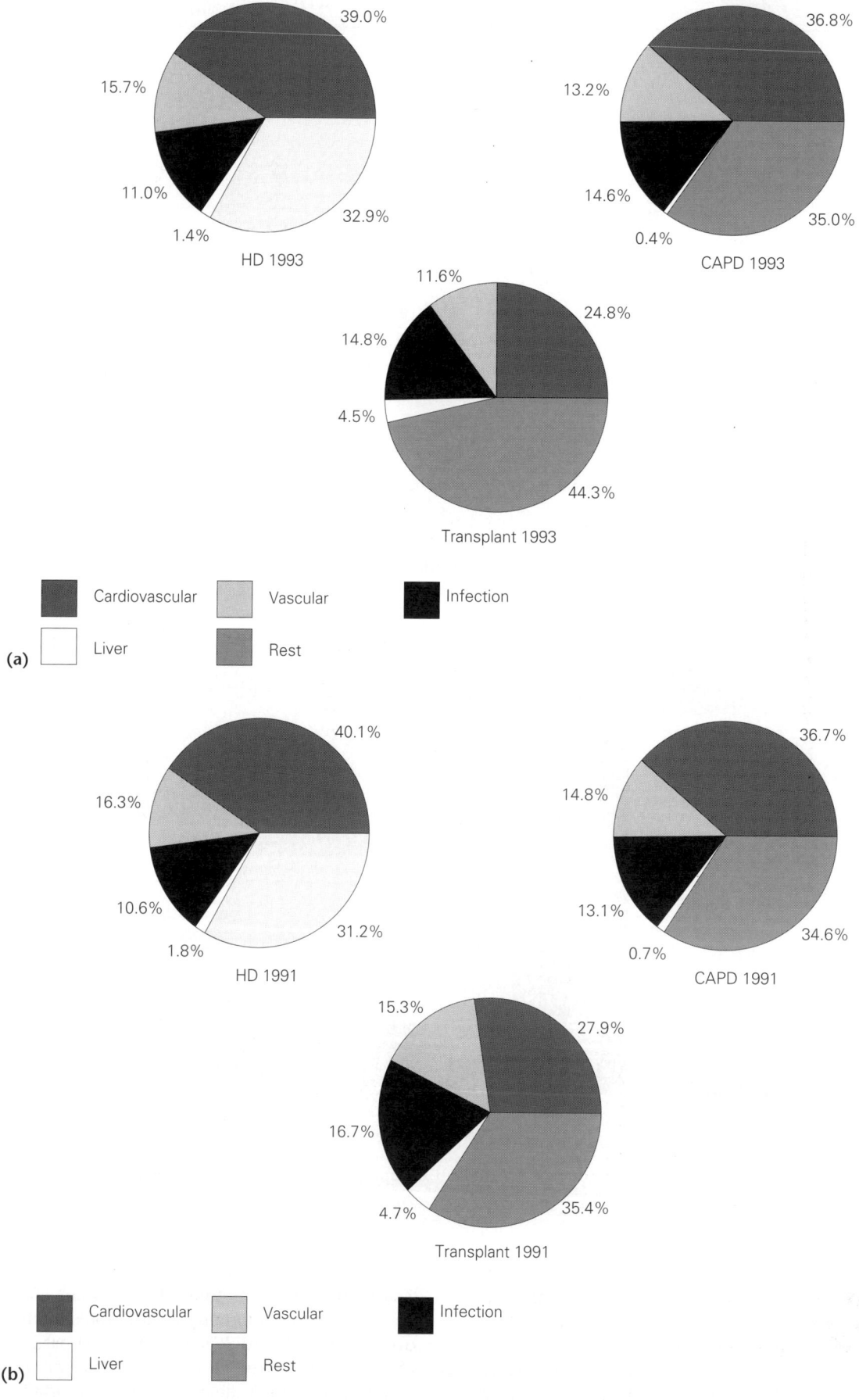

Figure 75.4 Causes of death in patients on renal replacement therapy according to last mode of therapy; (a) 1991 and (b) 1993. (Data reproduced, with permission, from the EDTA registry.)

ficient detail available for analysis. In the current absence of conclusive data on improved survival on either modality it seems reasonable to consider the most suitable treatment for each patient depending on comorbid conditions and social circumstances.

Adequacy of dialysis

Dialysis adequacy can be assessed using urea reduction ratio – the percentage reduction in urea during a dialysis session – or urea kinetic modelling (UKM). UKM uses the

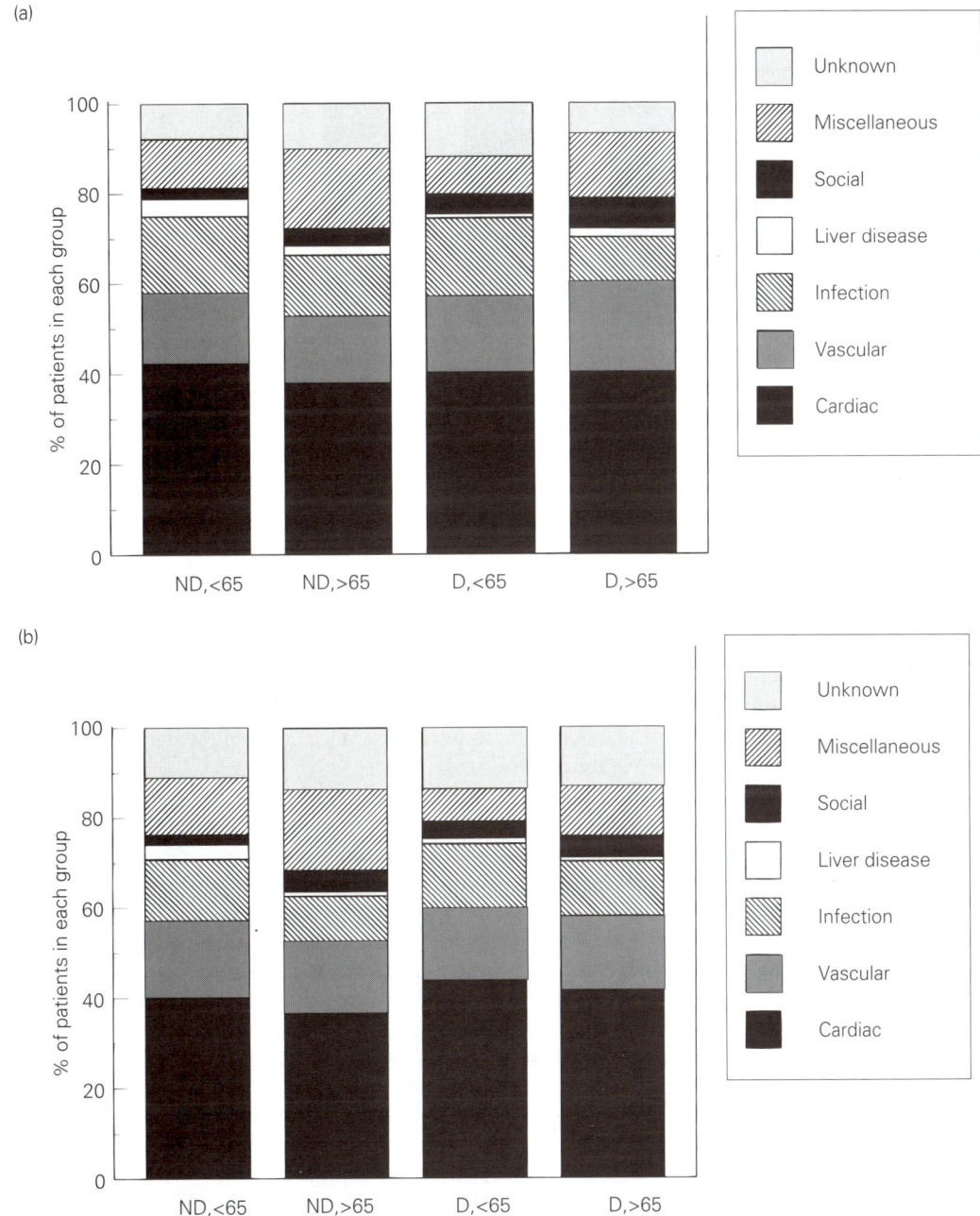

Figure 75.5 Causes of death in patients on renal replacement therapy (RRT), according to age (age at start of RRT less than 65 years versus 65 years and over) and primary renal disease (PRD); standard PRD vs diabetes. Causes of death for each group given for year of death: (a) 1982, (b) 1987, (c) 1993. Key: ND < 65, non-diabetic or standard PRD, aged less than 65 years at start of RRT; ND > 65, non-diabetic or standard PRD, aged 65 years or over at start of RRT; D < 65, diabetic, aged less than 65 years at start of RRT; D > 65, diabetic aged 65 years or over at start of RRT. (Data reproduced, with permission, from the EDTA Registry.)

(c)

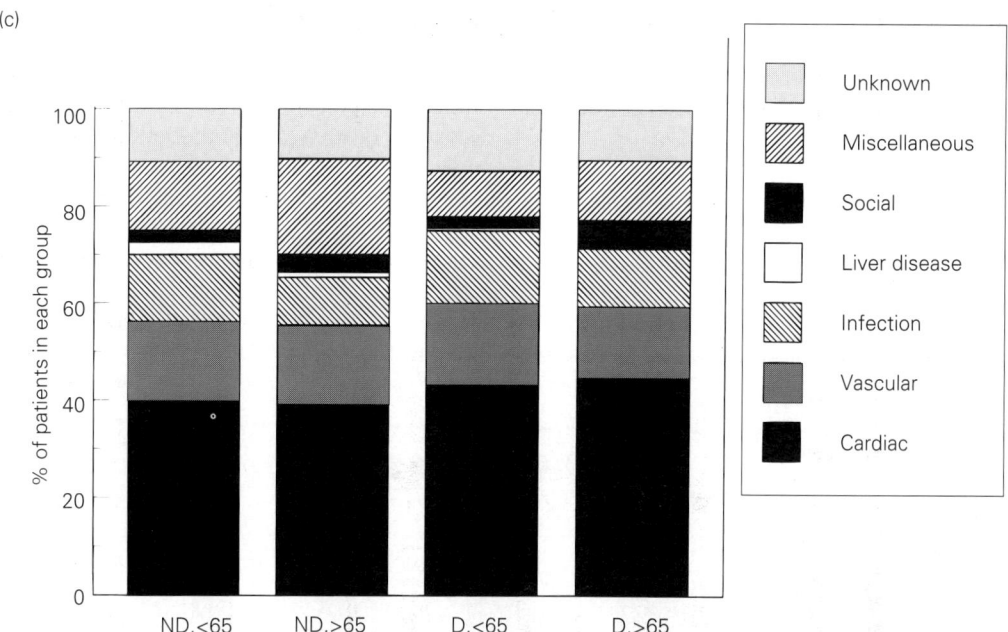

Figure 75.5 *Continued*

urea clearance of the dialyser K, the duration of dialysis t, and the volume of distribution of urea V, to give the index Kt/V urea, an approximate assessment of dialysis dose. Although various simplifying assumptions are involved (e.g. that urea is uniformly distributed throughout total body water in a single-pool compartment) and many modifications or refinements to the single-pool model are possible, UKM provides a useful tool to monitor the delivered dose of dialysis. Furthermore, if the residual renal function is incorporated into the calculation, it is possible to calculate urea generation rate and thus protein catabolic rate (PCR) which in a stable patient equates to dietary protein intake.

Kt/V as an index of dialysis prescription and adequacy was introduced by Gotch and Sargent [11] following their mechanistic analysis of the National Cooperative Dialysis Study in 1985. They demonstrated that Kt/V <0.8 was associated with significant morbidity and mortality. A Kt/V of 1.0 was suggested as a minimum index of short term adequacy, though more recent studies suggest higher Kt/V values of 1.2–1.4 may be associated with better long term outcome.

Time of dialysis

Despite the statistical difficulties, it seems clear that survival rates on hemodialysis are lower in the United States than in Europe, Canada, Australia, New Zealand and Japan. Hemodialysis practice in the US was reviewed following a report that the annual US mortality rate for all end-stage renal disease had increased from 21% in 1981 to 24.3% in 1988 [12], and was significantly higher than that for comparable patients (controlled for age and dia-

betes) in Europe and Japan. The lower mean duration of hemodialysis in the US has been suggested as a possible cause for this increase in mortality [13, 14] (9.8 h/week, compared to 13.5 h/week in Japan and 12 or more in Europe) [1]. Between 1986 and 1987 in the US values of Kt/V urea ≤1.0 occurred in about 50% of patients [15]; it is well recognized that the actual delivered dose often falls below the prescribed dose because of problems with blood flow and recirculation [16]. In the US in 1991, even with higher prescribed Kt/V, delivered Kt/V was ≤1.1 in 54% [15].

Authorities have now recommended minimum standards for hemodialysis delivery. In the US, the National Kidney Foundation has recommended a minimum Kt/V urea ≥1.2 per dialysis session (using a single pool model) or a urea reduction rate of ≥60% [15]. This is slightly higher than recently published recommendations from the Renal Association in the UK: a Kt/V of >1.0 or a urea reduction ratio of >55% per dialysis session [17].

Despite these laudable efforts to ensure adequate dialysis, it may be that optimal hemodialysis requires longer duration. Charra *et al.* from Tassin, France, reported in 1992 the best survival data for hemodialysis treatment, 87% five-year survival and 43% 20-year survival in their patients. The average Kt/V was 1.67 [18]. Furthermore, those smaller ,mainly female patients with mean Kt/V of 1.97 had an even higher survival rate and all had normal blood pressure. It is striking that with this unit's regime of 24 h dialysis per week, 98% of patients are normotensive off all antihypertensive medication six months after starting dialysis.

Of course, economic and practical constraints mean that few dialysis centers can offer 24 h of treatment per week to each patient, but this experience emphasizes the importance of monitoring dialysis adequacy.

Type of dialyzer membrane and reuse of dialyzers

In 1991 in Europe, dialyzers were used only once in more than 80% of hemodialysis patients [19] whereas dialyzers are reused in over 80% of hemodialysis patients in the US [20]. Could this difference contribute to the differences in mortality rates? There appears to be a higher reported incidence of febrile reactions in US centers practicing reuse compared to centers practicing single use (28% versus 13%) [21] and no reduction in intradialytic symptoms [22]. Shaldon [20] recommended that in the absence of demonstrable clinical benefits of reuse and in view of potential side effects, a prospective controlled clinical study was required to establish that dialyzer reuse is as safe as single use.

Another variable which may affect long-term outcome is the biocompatibilty of the dialyzer membrane used. Units in the UK are changing from cellulose-based membranes to synthetic membranes which cause less neutropenia and less activation of complement. Much remains to be clarified about biocompatability and its clinical impact. There are few randomized controlled studies, but evidence suggests that survival of acute renal failure is improved with synthetic membranes [23]. There are also reports of improved survival for maintenance hemodialysis patients using synthetic membranes compared to cellulose membranes; for example, one study reports a 20% higher mortality rate for maintenance hemodialysis patients dialyzing with cellulosic membranes compared to those using high-flux synthetic membranes [24]. However, these studies are often confounded by the higher flux and different clearance characteristics of the more biocompatible membranes, and long-term controlled trials are needed.

Vascular access and blood flow; recirculation

Good vascular access is essential for adequate hemodialysis. Infection and thrombosis of vascular access are major problems. When technically possible, an arteriovenous fistula has the lowest rate of thrombosis, stenosis and infection, with two-year survival rates of up to 70% [25]. In the patient with unsuitable veins, saphenous vein or synthetic polytetrafluoroethylene (PTFE) grafts are commonly used, giving graft survival rates of up to 14% at 2 years. However, patients receiving grafts are more likely to have peripheral vascular disease and coronary artery disease so direct comparison with arteriovenous fistulae is difficult [25]. Soft-cuffed central intravenous catheters give satisfactory access but often there is limited blood flow, and they may be complicated by thrombosis, infection or long-term venous stenoses. However, 74% one-year survival of such catheters has been reported [26] which compares well with one-year survival rates of arteriovenous fistulae of 70–80% [25]. Four-year catheter survival rate is significantly worse at 12%.

Recirculation of blood between 'venous' and 'arterial' needles during dialysis is a major barrier to dialysis efficiency. Assuming the needles are correctly placed, recirculation will occur when the fistula flow is less than the blood pump speed in the extracorporeal circuit, usually because of a limiting stenosis. Detection followed by correction, either by surgery or balloon angioplasty, is particularly important for high flux dialysis where blood flows of 400–500 ml/min are required. Recirculation is assessed by several methods, such as saline dilution (a bolus of saline injected into the venous line may be detected in the arterial line if recirculation is present) or the three-sample method (the urea concentrations of simultaneous samples from venous line, arterial line and a peripheral vein are compared, and recirculation considered to be present if the arterial line urea concentration is lower than peripheral venous levels), though debate continues as to which method is best [27].

Morbidity of hemodialysis

Hypertension

The principal cause of death in hemodialysis patients is cardiovascular disease, and one of the major contributing factors is hypertension. The 1991 EDTA report revealed that 68% of male hemodialysis patients had a predialysis systolic blood pressure of >160 mm Hg, and 40% had a diastolic blood pressure of >90 mm Hg despite antihypertensive medication [28]. Ambulatory blood pressure monitoring has revealed that only 15% of patients have normal interdialytic blood pressure [29]. The experience of the unit in Tassin has shown that predialysis and intradialytic blood pressure can be controlled with a minimal use of antihypertensive drugs by means of long hemodialysis treatments, with a corresponding improvement in cardiovascular mortality [18, 30]. Although achievement of the correct dry weight must be important in obtaining blood pressure control, several groups have shown a lack of relationship between interdialytic weight gain and interdialytic blood pressure change [30, 31]. It has been proposed that accumulation of pressor molecules (such as asymmetrical dimethylarginine, an endogenous inhibitor of nitric oxide synthesis) in hemodialysis patients may also be relevant [32]. The Tassin group suggests that clearance of such molecules may prove to be another factor to consider when assessing adequacy of hemodialysis [30].

In view of the expected future increase in elderly dialysis patients with pre-existing cardiovascular risk factors, blood pressure control is likely to become increasingly important.

Lipid abnormalities

These are discussed in Chapter 38.

Anemia

The widespread use of human recombinant erythropoietin (r-HuEPO) has greatly reduced the morbidity of the anemia of chronic renal failure. Many studies have documented improvement in exercise capacity, cardiac performance, cognitive function, sexual function and quality of life after r-HuEPO administration. A few problems remain, however; the optimimum dose, frequency and route of administration of r-HuEPO are still debated, and the ideal tar*get* hemoglobin concentration remains to be established. In 1995, the UK Renal Association recommended a goal of a hemoglobin concentration of 10–12 g/dl in at least 80% of dialysis patients [17]. The use of r-HuEPO is likely to remain limited by financial considerations; in 1992, only 53% of European hemodialysis patients were treated with r-HuEPO, ranging from 83% in Belgium to 45% in Poland [4]. Interest will continue to focus on maximizing response to current doses [33].

Long-term effects such as improved chances of a successful transplant because of reduced transfusion-induced sensitization, and increased hemodialysis survival rates, remain to be demonstrated.

Renal bone disease

Renal bone disease encompasses aluminum-related bone disease, hyperparathyroidism, osteomalacia and low turnover or adynamic bone disease.

Aluminum bone disease, once a terrible complication of hemodialysis, has been virtually eliminated by improved water purification and reduced use of oral aluminum phosphate binders. Hyperparathyroidism remains a major problem; the 1989 EDTA registry revealed that after 10 years of hemodialysis, 10–15% of patients need parathyroidectomy and after 15 years this increases to almost 40% [34, 35]. About 5% of patients need parathyroidectomy even after a successful renal transplant. Even today, most nephrologists see patients suffering bone pain, pruritis and soft-tissue calcification. Debate continues as to whether some degree of hyperparathyroid overactivity is required to prevent low turnover or adynamic bone disease; however, if vitamin D therapy is delayed too long and hyperplasia of the parathyroids becomes established, it becomes increasingly difficult and perhaps impossible to reverse. A recent report from Japan confirmed that the risk factors for hemodialysis patients requiring parathyroidectomy are duration of dialysis and parathyroid hormone (PTH) level at the start of dialysis; despite vitamin D therapy thereafter, PTH levels continued to increase [36]. Several studies have demonstrated the hitherto unestablished safety and efficacy of small doses of vitamin D metabo-

lites given to predialysis patients [37] with no evidence of troublesome hypercalcemia or increased rate of progression of renal failure.

Intact PTH plasma concentration is the best non-invasive index of parathyroid activity. Vitamin D therapy should begin when the PTH levels are more than two or three times the normal range (though prior control of hyperphosphatemia is of course mandatory). Closer predialysis monitoring, and earlier and more intensive treatment, may lead to improved parathyroid control.

Hypercalcemia is often the limiting factor for vitamin D dosage; in refractory hyperparathyroidism, the use of low calcium dialyzate may allow increased vitamin D dosage.

Finally, raised PTH levels may affect more than bone and mineral metabolism. PTH receptors have been demonstrated in many tissues other than kidney and bone; hyperparathyroidism is well known to cause decreased responsiveness to r-HuEPO and increased blood pressure and may be important in the development of myocardial fibrosis [38].

In the not too distant future, non-calcemic vitamin D analogs and specific agonists of the calcium receptor may alter the management of renal bone disease.

Nutrition

Many studies have demonstrated that increased morbidity and mortality of hemodialysis patients are associated with low serum albumin, low serum urea nitrogen levels or high protein catabolic rate. This is all the more alarming since at least 25% of maintenance hemodialysis patients have serum albumin concentrations below 37 g/l, and so fall into the high risk group [13, 39]. Malnutrition is common in hemodialysis patients: low percentage ideal body weight or low body mass index is reported in 10–30%, low triceps skinfold thickness in 20–60%, and low arm muscle circumference in up to 40–50% [40]. Anorexia from inadequate dialysis may lead to a low energy intake and incomplete correction of acidosis may cause protein catabolism. Furthermore, loss of the active metabolism of normal renal tissue may be relevant. There is some evidence that hemodialysis itself is a stimulus for *net* protein catabolism [41] due to loss of small molecules such as carnitine (recently licensed for replacement therapy in long-term hemodialysis).

Amyloid

β_2-Microglobulin (β_2M) amyloidosis is a frequent complication of long-term hemodialysis. The estimated generation of β_2M from the turnover of the HLA complex on the surface of nucleated cells is 1300–2100 mg/week [42]. Normally the majority of this is removed by glomerular filtration. Elimination of β_2M in hemodialysis may be by means of membrane adsorption as well as diffusion across the membrane; however, blood–dialysis membrane contact may also stimulate synthesis of β_2M [43]. Clearance of β_2M ranges from 86 to 260 mg per dialysis treatment session, depending on the type of dialysis membrane [42].

Periarticular and synovial deposition of β_2M causes disabling joint pain and the carpal tunnel syndrome. Such symptoms usually resolve rapidly after renal transplantation; otherwise there is little effective treatment for dialysis-related amyloidosis.

New imaging methods, e.g. radiolabeling of β_2M or amyloid P, are now used to monitor patients on maintenance hemodialysis to determine if biocompatible membranes clear β_2M more effectively [44, 45].

Acquired cystic kidney disease

Acquired cystic kidney disease (ACKD) is bilateral cystic transformation of kidney tissue in patients with end-stage renal disease on maintenance dialysis. Initially thought to occur only in hemodialysis patients, we now know it occurs with equal frequency in CAPD patients. Serial computed tomography (CT) scanning has demonstrated that cysts begin to develop once the creatinine has risen above 3 mg/dl, and increase with dialysis duration. The incidence of ACKD approaches 100% after 10 years on dialysis [46]. A recent review suggests that the risk of renal cell carcinoma in ACKD is 50 times greater than that of the general population [47], but this remains controversial.

ACKD associated renal cell carcinoma is seven times more common in males than females, bilateral in 9% of cases and multicentric in 50%, and is the cause of approximately 2% of deaths in renal transplant patients.

Pathogenesis remains unclear, and the place of CT or ultrasound screening for asymptomatic patients on renal replacement therapy is not established.

Outcome of renal transplantation

No studies have as yet demonstrated any significant difference between hemodialysis patients and CAPD patients in patient survival, graft survival, extraperitoneal infection rates or long-term incidence of malignancy after renal transplantation [48].

Quality of life on haemodialysis

It is very difficult to define and measure the quality of life to assess the effectiveness of treatment. Nephrologists recognize the importance of striving to minimize morbidity and to improve the mental and social aspects of the life of the dialysis patient. This is likely to become even more important as increasingly frail and elderly patients are offered dialysis treatment. More attention has to be paid to factors other than the dialysis regime.

Studies using accepted questionnaires to assess quality of life have found that patients with a successful renal transplant are most likely to be rehabilitated and that CAPD patients have a marginal advantage over center-based hemodialysis patients in this regard [49]. However, despite impaired mobility, lack of employment and generally poor rehabilitation, several studies of hemodialysis patients show that on subjective measures they perceive life to be satisfactory and comparable to the normal population. More recent studies have shown that r-huEPO use results in an improved quality of life. One small study in 13 dialysis patients showed a marked improvement in quality of life with an increase in hematocrit from 32.6 to 42.0, i.e. normal levels [50], and it may be that this will prove to be a major consideration in the future.

The future: optimum dialysis provision in the next century

Increased efficiency of dialysis, with improved monitoring of adequacy, and delivery of adequate prescription using biocompatible membranes, should be an achievable goal. However, widespread application of advances in machine and membrane technology is likely to remain limited by financial considerations. More important, perhaps, is the forecast of a world-wide increase in the number of people living past 65 years of age; the number of patients aged 75 and over with end-stage renal disease is bound to increase and the providers of dialysis will have to consider the optimum treatment for an increasingly elderly hemodialysis population after the millenium.

References

1. D'Amico, G. (1995) Comparability of the different registries on renal replacement therapy. *Am. J. Kidney Dis.*, **25**, 113–18.
2. Blake, P.G. (1996) Do mortality rates differ between hemodialysis and CAPD? A look at Canadian vs. US data. *Dial. Transplant.*, **25**, 75–100.
3. Brunner, F.P., Broyer, M., Brynger, H. *et al.* (1988) Survival on renal replacment therapy: data from the EDTA Registry. *Nephrol. Dial. Transplant.*, **2**, 109–22.
4. Valderrabano, F., Jones, E.H.P. and Mallick, N.P. (1995) Report on management of renal failure in Europe, XXIV, 1993. *Nephrol. Dial. Transplant.*, **10**(suppl 5), 1–25.
5. Salomone, M., Piccoli, G.B., Quarello, F. *et al.* (1995) Dialysis in the elderly: improvement of survival results in the eighties. *Nephrol. Dial. Transplant.*, **10**(suppl 6), 60–4.
6. Burton, P.R. and Walls, J. (1987) Selection-adjusted comparison of life expectancy of patients on CAPD, hemodialysis and renal transplantation. *Lancet*, **i**, 1115–19.

7. Maiorca, R., Vonesh, E.F., Cavalli, P. *et al.* (1991) A multi-centre selection-adjusted comparison of patient and technique survivals on CAPD and hemodialysis. *Perit. Dial. Int.*, **11**, 118–27.

8. Held, P.J., Port, F.K., Turenne, M.N. *et al.* (1994) CAPD and hemodialysis: comparison of patient mortality with adjustment for comorbid conditions. *Kidney Int.*, **45**, 1163–9.

9. Bloembergen, W.E., Port, F.K., Mauger, E.A. and Wolfe, R.A. (1995) A comparison of mortality between patients treated with hemodialysis and peritoneal dialysis. *J. Am. Soc. Nephrol.*, **6**, 177–83.

10. Bloembergen, W.E., Port, F.K., Mauger, E.A. *et al.* (1995) A comparison of cause of death between patients treated with hemodialysis and peritoneal dialysis. *J. Am. Soc. Nephrol.*, **6**, 184–91.

11. Gotch, F., Sargent, J. (1985) A mechanistic analysis of the National Cooperative Dialysis Study (NCDS). *Kidney Int.*, **28**, 526–34.

12. Held, P.J., Brunner, F.B., Odaka, M. *et al.* (1990) Five year survival for end stage renal disease in the United States, Europe and Japan, 1982 to 1987. *Am. J. Kidney Dis.*, **15**, 451–7.

13. Lowrie, E.G. and Lew, N.C. (1990) Death risk in hemodialysis patients: the predictive value of commonly measured variables and an evaluation of death rate differences between facilities. *Am. J. Kidney Dis.*, **15**, 458–82.

14. Gotch, F.A., Yarin, S. and Keen, M. (1990) A kinetic survey of US hemodialysis prescriptions. *Am. J. Kidney Dis.*, **15**, 511–15.

15. Kopple, J.D. *et al.* (1994) Recommendations for reducing the high morbidity and mortality of US maintenance dialysis patients. *Am. J. Kidney Dis.*, **24**, 968–73.

16. Delmez, J.A. and Windus, W. (1992) Hemodialysis prescription and delivery in a metropolitan community. *Kidney Int.*, **41**, 1023–8.

17. The Renal Association (1995) *Treatment of adult patients with renal failure. Recommended standards and audit procedures.* Royal College of Physicians, London.

18. Charra, B., Calemard, E., Ruffet, M. *et al.* (1992) Survival as an index of adequacy of dialysis. *Kidney Int.*, **41**, 1286–91.

19. Mallick, N.P., Jones, E. and Selwood, N. (1995) The European (EDTA) Registry. *Am. J. Kidney Dis.*, **25**, 176–87.

20. Shaldon, S. (1994) Reuse of hemodialysers. *Nephrol. Dial. Transplant.*, **9**, 1226–7.

21. Tokars, J.I., Alter, M.J., Favero, M.S. *et al.* (1993) National surveillance of dialysis associated diseases in the US 1991. *ASAIO J.*, **39**, 966–75.

22. Cheung, A.K., Dalpias, D., Emmerson, R. *et al.* (1991) A prospective study on intradialytic symptoms associated with reuse of hemodialysers. *Am. J. Nephrol.*, **11**, 397–401.

23. Hakim, R.M., Wingard, R.L. and Parker, R.A. (1994) Effect of the dialysis membrane in the treatment of patients with acute renal failure. *N. Engl. J. Med.*, **331**, 1338–42.

24. Hakim, R.M., Stannard, D., Port, F. *et al.* (1994) The effect of the dialysis membrane on mortality of chronic hemodialysis patients in the US (Abstr). *J. Am. Soc. Nephrol.*, **5**, 3.

25. Windus, D.W. (1993) Permanent vascular access: a nephrologist's view. *Am. J. kidney Dis.*, **21**, 457–71.

26. Gibson, S.P. and Mosquera, D. (1991) Five year experience with the Quinton Permcath for vascular access. *Nephrol. Dial. Transplant.*, **6**, 269–74.

27. Tattersall, J.E., Farrington, K., Raniga, P.D. *et al.* (1993) Hemodialysis recirculation detected by the three-sample method is an artefact. *Nephrol. Dial. Transplant.*, **8**, 60–3.

28. Raine, A.E.G., Margreiter, R., Brunner, F.P. *et al.* (1992) Report on management of renal failure in Europe, XXII, 1991. *Nephrol. Dial. Transplant.*, **7**(suppl 2), 7–35.

29. Cheigh, J.S., Milite, C., Sullivan, J.F. *et al.* (1992) Hypertension is not adequately controlled in hemodialysis patients. *Am. J. Kidney Dis.*, **19**, 453–9.

30. Chazot, C., Charra, B., Laurent, G. *et al.* (1995) Interdialysis blood pressure control by long hemodialysis sessions. *Nephrol. Dial. Transplant.*, **10**, 831–7.

31. Luik, A.J., Gladizwa, U., Koopman, J.P. *et al.* (1994) Blood pressure changes in relation to interdialytic weight gain. *Blood Purif.*, **12**, 259–66.

32. Vallance, P., Leone, A. and Calver, A. (1992) Accumulation of an endogenous inhibitor of nitric oxide synthesis in chronic renal failure. *Lancet*, **339**, 572–5.

33. Macdougall, I.C. (1995) How to get the best out of r-HuEPO. *Nephrol. Dial. Transplant.*, **10**(suppl 2), 85–91.

34. Fassbinder, W., Brunner, F.P., Brynger, H. *et al.* (1991) Combined report on regular dialysis and transplantation in Europe, XX, 1989. *Nephrol. Dial. Transplant.*, **6**(suppl 1), 5–47.

35. Drueke, T.B. and Kubrusky, M. (1994) Pathogenesis of secondary hyperparathyroidism of chronic renal failure. *J. Nephrol.*, **7**, 139–47.

36. Mizumoto, D., Watanabe, Y., Fukuzawa, Y. *et al.* (1994) Identification of risk factors on secondary hyperparathyroidism undergoing long-term hemodialysis with vitamin. D3. *Nephrol. Dial. Transplant.*, **9**, 1751–8.

37. Ritz, E., Kuster, S., Schmidt-Gayk, H. *et al.* (1995) Low dose calcitriol prevents the rise in 1,84 iPTH without affecting serum calcium and phosphate in patients with moderate renal failure. *Nephrol. Dial. Transplant.*, **10**, 2228–34.

38. Amann, K., Mall, G. and Ritz, E. (1994) Myocardial interstitial fibrosis in uremia: is it relevant? *Nephrol. Dial. Transplant.*, **9**, 127–8.

39. Lowrie, E.G., Lew, L.N. and Huang, W.H. (1992) Race and diabetes as death risk predictors in hemodialysis patients. *Kidney Int.*, **42**(suppl 38), S22–31.

40. Bergstrom, J. and Lindholm, B. (1993) Nutrition and adequacy of dialysis. How do hemodialysis and CAPD compare? *Kidney Int.*, **43**(suppl 40), S39–50.

41. Farrell, P.C. and Hone, P.W. (1982) Dialysis induced catabolism. *Am. J. Clin. Nutr.*, **33**, 1417–22.

42. Kandus, A., Ponikvar, R., Drinovec, J. *et al.* (1990) Microglobulin elimination characteristics during hemofiltration with acrylonitrile and polysulfone membrane haemofilters. *Int. J. Artif. Organs*, **13**, 200–4.

43. Zaoiu, P.M., Stone, W.J. and Hakim, R.M. (1990) Effects of dialysis membranes on beta-2-microglobulin production and cellular expression. *Kidney Int.*, **38**, 962–8.

44. Flocge, J., Buchert, W., Brandis, A. *et al.* (1990) Imaging of dialysis related amyloid deposits with 131-I-beta-2-microglobulin. *Kidney Int.*, **38**, 1169–76.

45. Nelson, S.R., Hawkins, P.N., Richardson, S. *et al.* (1991) Imaging of hemodialysis-associated amyloidosis with 123-I-serum amyloid P component. *Lancet*, **338**, 335–9.

46. Mickisch, O., Bommer, J., Bachmann, S. *et al.* (1984) Multicystic transformation of kidneys in chronic renal failure. *Nephron*, **38**, 93–9.

47. Truong, L.D., Krishnan, B., Cao, J.T.H. *et al.* (1995) Renal neoplasm in acquired cystic kidney disease. *Am. J. Kidney Dis.*, **26**, 1–12.

48. Winchester, J.F., Rotellar, C., Goggins, M. *et al.* (1993) Transplantation in peritoneal dialysis and hemodialysis. *Kidney Int.*, **43**(suppl 40), S101–5.

49. Gokal, R. (1993) Quality of life in patients undergoing renal replacement therapy. *Kidney Int.*, **43**(suppl 40), S23–7.

50. Esbach, J.W., Glenny, R., Robertson, T. *et al.* (1993) Normalising the hematocrit in hemodialysis patients with EPO improves the quality of life and is safe. *J. Am. Soc. Nephrol.*, **4**, 425 (abstract).

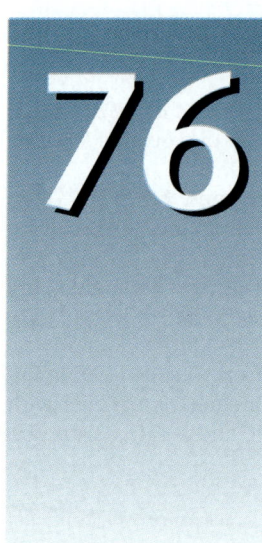

76

Starting and terminating dialysis

Carlo Catalano

Introduction

The total number of patients receiving renal replacement therapy (RRT) is steadily increasing in all Western countries and Japan [1]. The European Registry of Dialysis and Transplantation (EDTA Registry) recorded only 58 patients starting RRT in Europe in 1964, but this number increased to 10000/year by 1976 and to 30000/year in the early 1990s (Figure 76.1) and at the end of 1992 over 170000 patients were alive on RRT treatment in Europe. In the United States, during 1990, 45000 patients started treatment for end-stage renal disease and, by the end of 1990, 165000 were alive on treatment.

This phenomenon is obviously not due to an increased incidence of end-stage renal disease (ESRD), but to the increasing proportion of patients with renal failure accepted for RRT. The acceptance rate for RRT ranges widely from unit to unit and, on average, is highest in the United States and Japan. On the other hand, mortality in the dialysis population has been estimated to be constant in Europe at about 10%/year [2], and at about 24%/year in the United States [3].

RRT involves sophisticated technology and is very expensive. For this reason, it was originally reserved for young and otherwise relatively healthy subjects (Figure 76.2). In the 1960s the aim of treatment was rehabilitation, and the likelihood of returning to useful work was an important factor in selecting patients for treatment. Over the years, however, more and more older patients have entered the programs and the median age of patients starting RRT at the end of the 1980s had reached 60 years in Europe as well as in the United States (Figures 76.2 and 76.3). In addition, more and more patients with serious comorbid conditions, such as complicated diabetes, heart failure, stroke and cancer, have been accepted for long-term RRT. Furthermore, life expectancy with RRT is good so that patients on dialysis although young and fit at the outset become old and infirm. This trend towards older and less fit patients on dialysis treatment has been augmented by the tendency, in circumstances of shortage of donor organs [4], to prefer the young and fit when organs become available for transplantation.

The general broadening of the criteria for acceptance for dialysis has been driven by the realization that the old and infirm can derive benefit from treatment and has been made possible by technological advances and increased funding in most developed countries. With increasing life expectancy in the general population and the increasing incidence of renal failure with age, it is likely that the current trend upwards in the age of patients presenting with end-stage renal failure (ESRF) and of those on the dialysis program will continue.

The quality of life on dialysis may not be acceptable to the very old or severely disabled patient who has the right to refuse treatment or withdraw from it. The physician in turn must be prepared to help the patient and his or her family in making these difficult decisions.

Nephrology, Edited by Rex L. Jamison and Robert Wilkinson.
Published in 1997 by Chapman & Hall, London. ISBN 0 412 60930 4

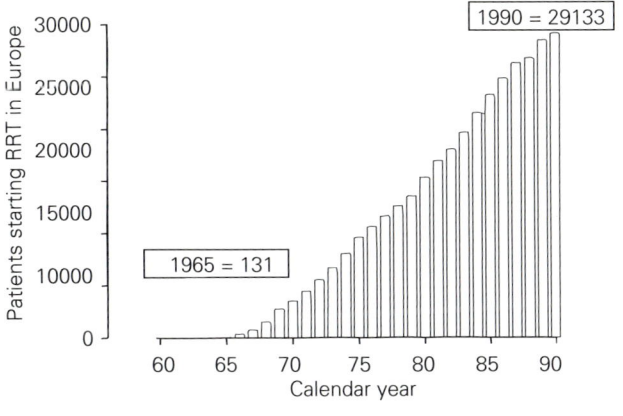

Figure 76.1 Patients entering the renal replacement therapy (RRT) program in Europe from the 1960s to the 1990s. Before 1965 less than 100 patients/year were entering the program; this figure had grown to 30 000 new patients/year in the 1990s. If the growth of the population is constant, this number will double by 2017. Data gathered by courtesy of the EDTA Registry.

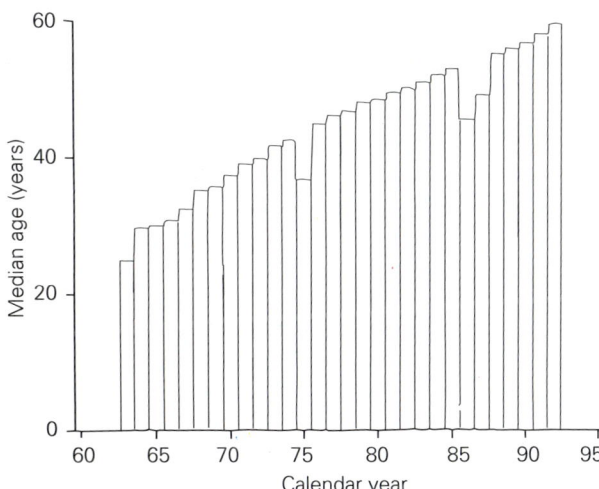

Figure 76.2 Median age at start of renal replacement therapy in Europe 1963–1992. Very few patients were treated before 1963. Before 1970 the median age of overall treated patients was less than 40 years as a consequence of the very selective criteria adopted. Data gathered by courtesy of EDTA Registry.

Selection for RRT

Some form of selection procedure for RRT was necessary in the 1960s when experience and resources were extremely limited. However by the 1980s with greatly increased experience and facilities in developed countries, it was no longer acceptable to exclude patients from dialysis treatment, although the variation in acceptance rates among countries indicates that some form of preferential selection must be practiced [5]. Now, most nephrologists

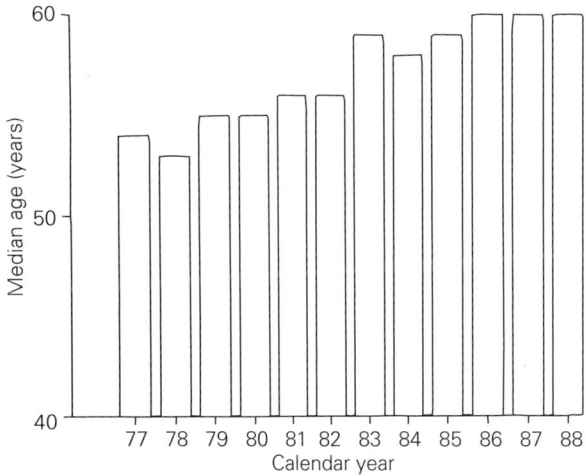

Figure 76.3 Median age at start of renal replacement therapy in the US 1977–1988. Notice that median ages for corresponding years were higher in the US compared to Europe (Figure 76.2). This is probably related to the wider acceptance criteria. Data gathered from US Renal Data System, 1990 Report.

Table 76.1 Importance attached to selection criteria

	Mean importance scores[a]
Medical benefit	4.2
Likelihood of medical benefit	4.0
Qualitative prognosis	3.8
Willingness[b]	3.7
Quantitative prognosis	3.7
Psychological stability	3.2
Age	2.7
Unique moral duties[c]	2.5
Disproportionate resources[d]	2.2
Progress of science	2.0
Social value	2.0
Environment	2.0
Ability to pay	1.8
Random selection	1.7
Constituency[e]	1.4
Sex	1.0

[a] Criteria were scored on a 5–1 scale according to decreasing importance.
[b] The expressed or implicit desire of the prospective recipient to undergo treatment; [c] whether or not the physical life of at least one other person depends upon whether or not the prospective recipient lives;
[d] whether or not the prospective recipient will likely require particularly long or expensive treatment;
[e] whether or not the prospective recipient is a member of a particular group, identified by geographical location, veteran status, etc.
Modified from ref. [7].

Table 76.2 Discontinuation of dialysis in different non-registry audits

Author [reference]	Period	Region or country	% deaths	% all patients
Neu and Kjellstrand [9]	1970–83	Minn (US)	22.0	–
Mailloux et al. [10]	1970–89	New York (USA)	18.5	8.7
Hirsch [11]	1982–87	Canada (National)	16.4	6.2
Port et al. [12]	1980–86	Michigan (USA)	–	5.4
Catalano [23]	1987–91	Italy (National)	0.6	0.3
Catalano et al. [25]	1965–93	Newcastle upon Tyne (UK)	14.9	5.4
Catalano and Marino [24]	1972–95	Reggio Calabria (Italy)	3.6	1.8

offer RRT to most patients with ESRD even though they can predict that some patients are not likely to gain real benefit. This avoids the need to apply arbitrary selection criteria which may be interpreted as being unfair to a particular group. In 1983 a survey of British nephrologists showed that 84% would not have accepted an alcoholic male aged 52 living in a hostel, but they would have offered RRT to a veterinary surgeon aged 72 years [6]. A similar survey of US nephrologists in 1988 [7] also indicated that selection was being applied. The main criteria were that the patient would benefit medically and was willing to undergo treatment (Table 76.1). The most widely applied criteria in deciding whether to accept a patient for dialysis were that the patient should benefit from treatment and should have an 'acceptable' quality of life. The difficulty in applying these criteria is, of course, that what constitutes an acceptable quality of life varies from patient to patient. The elderly are more likely to accept immobility, pain and chronic complications than the young who may be facing invalidity for the first time and may become depressed and unco-operative when started on RRT.

A further difficulty in applying any criteria for selection for RRT arises from the unreliability of making an assessment in the presence of uremia. Most nephrologists would consider that a patient with dementia or who was very elderly and frail would not benefit from treatment; however, a considerable proportion of ESRD patients are confused and in poor general condition, because of uremia, and can only be properly assessed after correction of the uremia with a period of adequate dialysis. In other patients who would not be considered suitable for long-term RRT it may be difficult to be certain that the renal failure is not, at least partially, reversible. These patients also require dialysis treatment, at least until a reversible component of their disease has been ruled out.

In the UK, these problems have led to the widespread application of the policy of embarking on a 'trial of treatment' with reassessment after a period of about three months of effective dialysis. This policy leads to the difficult decision of whether to continue or to advise withdrawal of treatment at the end of this period.

Discontinuation

Three groups of patients may be considered in the category of withdrawal from dialysis in the various national dialysis registries. (1) Those patients who commit suicide; (2) patients who are competent and choose, for religious, quality of life, or other reasons to discontinue such treatment; or (3) patients who are incompetent and in whom a third party seeks to terminate life-sustaining treatment on behalf of the patient. These three causes of death are, in most registries (EDTA, Australia and New Zealand Dialysis and Transplant Registry, Canadian Organ Replacement Register), grouped as 'Social' causes of death. In the US Renal Data System (1) is considered separately whereas (2) and (3) are considered as withdrawal.

Size of the problem

Stopping dialysis is common as a cause of death in North America and Australia [8–18]. In the United States and Canada it is the second most common cause of death [16–18], and in Australia and New Zealand the third most common [15]. Withdrawal rates as reported in Renal Unit Audits are shown in Table 76.2, and in the major registries in Table 76.3. Withdrawal of dialysis seems to be uncommon in Europe and Japan [19–21]. According to the EDTA Registry, in Europe in 1992, 12 280 patients on RRT died, of whom 444 (3.6%) died of 'social causes', a figure that was consistent over the period, 1983–1992, when social causes of death accounted for 3.7% of overall causes of death. There were, however, remarkable differences between countries. The lowest proportion was in Italy (less than 2%) and the highest in Sweden (more than 9%) [courtesy of EDTA Registry]. Few details are available, however, and it is possible that withdrawal of therapy as a cause of death may be underestimated. In fact, it has been shown that causes of death perceived as reflecting badly on the dialysis team are regularly reported under a heading acceptable to the team [22]. Plough and Salem [22] reported that only 1 of 22 deaths caused by stopping dialysis, suicide, dialysis-related accidents or dietary indiscretion was correctly classified; the other 21 were reported as cardiac deaths. The proportion of deaths due to dialy-

Table 76.3 Dialysis termination[a] in major registries

Register	Country	Year	% deaths	Ref
Japanese Society of Dialysis	Japan	–	1.5	12
US Renal Data System	USA	1989–91	9.9	13
Canadian Organ Replacement Registry	Canada	1989	12.3	14
Australian Registry (ANZDATA)	Australia/New Zealand	1983–92	14.0	15
EDTA Registry	Europe	1992	3.6	[b]

[a] 'Social' causes of death (see text).
[b] Courtesy of EDTA Registry.

Table 76.4 Factors associated with termination of treatment

1. Age
2. Mental competence
3. Comorbid conditions
4. Recent trends
5. Cultural differences

sis termination in Italy have been assessed in 1576 diabetic and 1576 non-diabetic patients (matched according to age, sex, and year of starting RRT) who were receiving RRT treatment at the end of 1987 and followed-up to the end of 1991. Withdrawal-related mortality was 4/854 deaths in the diabetic patients and 5/586 deaths in the non-diabetic patients (0.6 and 0.8%, respectively) [23]. A single-center survey in Italy showed that in Reggio Calabria from 1972 to 1995, 247 RRT patients died, nine of them (3.6%) because of treatment withdrawal [24]. On the other hand, in a survey performed in Newcastle upon Tyne, UK, withdrawal-related deaths represented 88/589 (14.9%) of all deaths, a proportion similar to those reported for the US and Canada [25] (Tables 76.2 and 76.3).

The concept of advanced medical directives

Patients receiving RRT may become mentally incompetent. This possibility raises two questions: first, who decides whether the patient is competent? secondly, who decides about the patient's quality of life? To address the latter point, it has been suggested that the problem be discussed with patient and family early in the course of the disease (before RRT is started) and to ask the patient to provide an advance treatment directive to be used in case the patient becomes incompetent. In the US, Federal regulations require that all patients be offered the opportunity to set forth advance directives at the time of admis-

sion to Medicare-reimbursed hospitals [26]. From the available literature, it appears that patients (at least US patients) wish to discuss advanced directives with the physician and that most of them wish the physician to start the discussion [27]. On the other hand, a study has shown that patients wish their advance directives not to be strictly followed if not to follow them 'was in their best interest' [28]. Therefore, strictly following all advance directives may not truly reflect the patient's preference.

Factors involved in discontinuing dialysis (Table 76.4)

Age

In Canada, Australia, USA and Europe there is a strong correlation between termination and old age [8, 19]. In these countries termination is 2–5 times more common in patients over the age of 75 than in patients under 25 years of age. In Newcastle upon Tyne, the mean age at the start of treatment was 47.5 years for the overall population but 62.1 years for the 88 patients who discontinued dialysis. A number of studies have shown that age is independently related to treatment withdrawal [9, 12, 23, 25]. In Japan in contrast, suicide and interruption of dialysis is five times more frequent in patients under 30 years of age (5%) compared to patients over 60 years of age (1%) [8]. Kjellstrand [8] has suggested that this may reflect a different cultural attitude towards the elderly, who in the Japanese society are still revered as wise and a depository of knowledge.

Mental competence

Around 10% of patients who terminate dialysis are suffering from dementia, but some authors [6, 25] state that as many as 50% of terminating patients were incompetent (demented, comatose or with severe memory or intellectual deficits). There is general agreement that a competent patient who consistently wishes to stop dialysis should be allowed to do so. The physician should, however, resist such a decision when it is apparently influenced by the stress of a transient problem or complication, or when the patient has not been given sufficient time to be certain of his decision.

When the patient becomes definitively incompetent, in more than half the cases the issue of withdrawal is first raised by physicians, and in less than one quarter by relatives [9, 25]. In this circumstance, exhaustive discussion should follow and if the family of an incompetent patient wishes to continue treatment, it should be continued to give the family a chance to realize that the outlook for recovery of mental function is very poor. In one survey of directors of dialysis units 68% would continue dialysis in a patient who became demented [29]. This may be influenced by the law in the United States which specifies that if an incompetent patient lacks a relative legally designated to speak for him or her then a physician may not deliberately stop dialysis.

Comorbid conditions

Comorbid conditions are the rule rather than the exception in patients discontinuing dialysis. Termination has been reported more frequently in diabetic patients compared to non-diabetics by some authors [9, 10, 12], but not by others [23]. According to the EDTA Registry, death from dialysis termination among diabetic patients varies widely between European countries (lowest proportion in Italy with less than 1%, and highest in Norway with more than 10% of overall causes of death) [courtesy of the Registry]. In Newcastle upon Tyne, in patients who discontinued dialysis there was a markedly increased prevalence of blindness, cerebrovascular disease, dementia, cardiac failure and conditions associated with severe pain. Diabetes was independently associated with treatment withdrawal [21]. Mailloux *et al.* [10] reported that cancer, malnutrition and catabolism were important factors associated with the decision to withdraw.

Recent trends

Several authors have reported an increased proportion of termination during the 1980s compared to the 1970s. However (as suggested by Neu and Kjellstrand [9]), this effect may be only apparent, and related to the increased acceptance for dialysis of older and frailer patients.

Race and cultural differences

As previously mentioned, discontinuation in Japan is more frequent among younger compared to older patients [8]. Port *et al.* [12] found, by multivariate analysis, that stopping treatment was twice as common among whites as among blacks [12]. This may reflect differences in religious and cultural attitudes towards discontinuation of therapy, in line with the fact that in the black population suicide is less common than in the white population.

In Europe, dialysis termination seems to be much less common compared to the US [19]. This may be related to cultural differences, or reflect a lower rate of acceptance of older and complicated patients onto dialysis [8, 30].

After discontinuation: care of the dying

After discontinuation of dialysis, death will not necessarily follow quickly (Figure 76.4). A median survival ranging between 8 and 10 days after discontinuing dialysis has been reported [9, 11, 12], and these figures are confirmed by the experience in Newcastle upon Tyne (8 days). Of the patients terminating treatment at Newcastle upon Tyne about a quarter (19/88) died more than 10 days after dialysis was stopped [25].

These figures indicate that death in ESRD patients without RRT may take a long time. This phenomenon raises the ethical point of the care of these terminal patients. Dialysis patients do not die as a consequence of increased urea and creatinine levels *per se*. Death in these patients may be painless (gradually sinking into uremic coma, or cardiac arrest secondary to hyperkalemia) or very stressful (from pulmonary edema). The family should not be left alone to cope with a dying patient, unless the patient or the family formally request responsibility for caring for the patient. The nephrologist or physician who is in charge of the patient, should accept the responsibility to avoid useless investigations, minimize suffering, and keep the patient comfortable. Once the decision to terminate dialysis has been made, all investigations and blood sampling should stop, and all restrictions, apart from fluid restriction when necessary, should be lifted. Fluid overload and pain should be prevented or treated, and narcotics should be used liberally for this purpose even if this may accelerate death [31].

In most cases, the patient's relatives will decide or agree to terminate treatment but this may have a heavy psychological cost and they should not be made to feel they have been the prime movers in the decision. It has been suggested that mortality may be increased among close relatives of the recently dead [32, 33]. A correlation between the sorrow of bereavement and impaired lymphocyte function has been reported [34, 35]. Roberts *et al.* [36] have studied the impact of dialysis withdrawal on relatives and families of patients and their findings suggest that the families need to communicate with care workers even years after the patients have died. In general, the people interviewed by Roberts *et al.* were grateful to doctors and dialysis personnel.

Some bitterness was reported among relatives of three types of patients: home dialysis patients (less in touch with the staff?), competent patients (perhaps relatives transfer their anger from the patient who decided to terminate dialysis to the staff who failed to dissuade the patient), and patients who terminate because of stress (a situation similar to the previous one, with concern by rel-

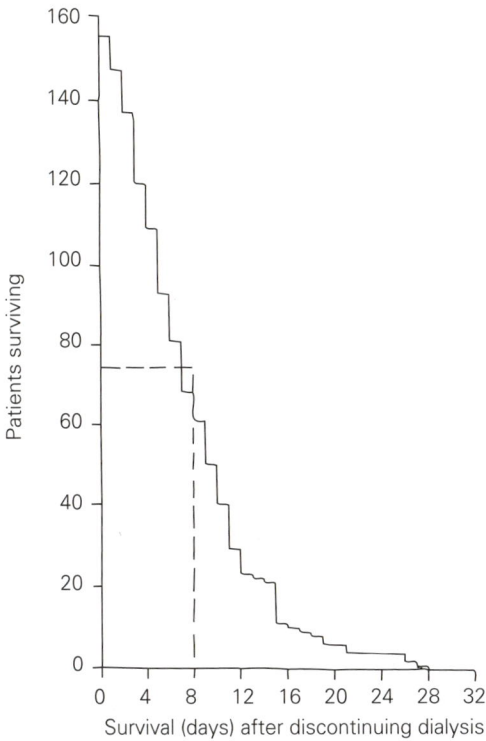

Figure 76.4 Survival (days) after last dialysis in 155 patients who stopped dialysis. Dashed lines represent the median values. (Modified from *Ethical Problems in Dialysis and Transplantation* (eds C.M. Kjellstrand and J.B. Dossetor). Reprinted by permission of Kluwer Academic Publishers.)

atives that life was terminated without a sufficient medical reason).

Select or withdraw

The practice of some degree of selection cannot be avoided since some patients with renal failure would clearly not benefit from RRT. Neither is it possible to adopt a single set of criteria which is valid in every setting and under all circumstances. The decision whether to initiate dialysis in a patient is made on a case-by-case basis by balancing resources and clinical judgment. In the United States, physicians are required to discuss the option of RRT with every mentally competent patient who is approaching ESRD. The physician may instead refer the patient to a nephrologist. Either the physician or the nephrologist can, therefore, describe the likely benefits of dialysis to the patient and family, in such a way they might well decide against dialysis. In every case both in the US and in Europe, ideally the patient and his/her family should make the final decision.

The difficulties that doctors meet in forecasting the outcome in a uremic patient, particularly in relation to assessing the patient's mental state, and determining whether renal failure is reversible, have been discussed above. If the clinical history of the patient is known, these points can be reasonably addressed and the doctor can help the patient and his/her family to decide. The situation is different if the nephrologist is not familiar with a patient who is admitted in the uremic state. In this case it is difficult to forecast how much the patient may benefit from RRT, and the patient may not be competent enough to decide to be treated. In these patients it is impossible to apply the criteria in Table 76.1 and it is usual to start dialysis and consider withdrawal if there is no improvement after a period of adequate dialysis.

Conclusion

Dialysis considerably lengthens the life of a patient with ESRD. On the other hand, it is a very expensive treatment modality and imposes considerable psychological strain and sometimes physical discomfort on the patient. It is likely that limitation of resources and aging of the treated population will force the development of more stringent criteria for the decision to offer a patient dialysis treatment. Until that time, nephrologists should offer dialysis to every patient who may benefit from it; in those patients who do not benefit then termination should be considered. Terminating dialysis is undoubtedly difficult. Competent and responsible patients should be allowed to decide to withdraw from treatment after discussion with their physician. Things are more complicated for incompetent patients. Once the possibility of withdrawing treatment is raised, there should be ample discussion among unit staff, family physician and patients' relatives. Interrupting dialysis treatment does not mean stopping medical care. Unnecessary suffering must be avoided and the nephrologist should take responsibility for terminal care whether at home or in hospital and, where appropriate, with advice from physicians in palliative care [30].

Acknowledgments

I am deeply indebted to Dr C. M. Kjellstrand and coworkers who have devoted many years to the study of issues related to ethical problems in dialysis and transplantation, and whose work has prompted me to review similar issues in Europe. I am also grateful to the EDTA Registry and to the Associazione Italiana EmoDializzati (ANED) for giving unpublished information, and to Professor Wilkinson and all the staff of the Newcastle Renal Unit for permission to review their dialysis database. Finally, I would like Mrs Jo Little, who cared for Newcastle Database from the beginning to her premature death, to be remembered. Data from Newcastle upon Tyne and Italy have been gathered with grants n. 9312287/88 of the National Research Council (CNR) of Italy.

References

1. Catalano, C. and Marshall, S.M. (1992) Epidemiology of end-stage renal disease in patients with diabetes mellitus: from the dark ages to the middle ages. *Nephrol. Dial. Transplant.*, **7**, 181–90.

2. Walker, R.G. and D'Apice, A.J.F. (1989) Planning, developing and operating a dialysis programme, in *Replacement of Renal Function by Dialysis* (ed. J.F. Maher), Kluwer, Dordrecht, pp. 650–60.

3. The National Institute of Health, The National Institute of Diabetes and Digestive and Kidney Diseases, Division of Kidney, Urologic and Hematologic Diseases (1994) Excerpts from United States Renal Data System – 1994 Annual Data Report: VI. Patient survival. *Am. J. Kidney Dis.*, **24**(suppl 2), S76–S87.

4. Khauli, R.B., Novick, A.C., Steinmuller, D.R. *et al.* (1986) Comparison of renal transplantation and dialysis in rehabilitation of diabetic end-stage renal disease patients. *Urology*, **27**, 521–5.

5. Geerlings, W., Tufveson, G., Ehrich, H.H. *et al.* (1994) Report on management of renal failure in Europe, XXIII. *Nephrol. Dial. Transplant.*, **9**(suppl 1), S6–25.

6. Challah, S., Wing, A.J., Bauer, R. *et al.* (1984) Negative selection of patients for dialysis and transplantation in the United Kingdom. *Br. Med. J.*, **228**, 1119–22.

7. Kilner, J.F. (1989) Selecting patients when resources are limited: a study of US medical directors of kidney dialysis and transplantation facilities. *Am. J. Public Health*, **78**, 144–7.

8. Kjellstrand, C.M. (1992) Practical aspects of stopping dialysis and cultural differences, in *Ethical Problems in Dialysis and Transplantation* (eds C.M. Kjellstrand and J.B. Dossetor), Kluwer Academic, Dordrecht The Netherlands, pp. 103–16.

9. Neu, S. and Kjellstrand, C.M. (1986) Stopping long-term dialysis. *N. Engl. J. Med.*, **314**, 14–20.

10. Mailloux, L.U., Bellucci, A.G., Napolitano, B. *et al.* (1993) Death by withdrawal from dialysis. a 20 year clinical experience. *J. Am. Soc. Nephrol.*, **3**, 1631–7.

11. Hirsch, D.J. (1989) Death from dialysis termination. *Nephrol. Dial. Transplant.*, **4**, 41–4.

12. Port, F.K., Wolfe, R.A., Hawthorne, V.M. and Ferguson, C.W. (1989) Discontinuation of dialysis therapy as a cause of death. *Am. J. Nephrol.*, **9**, 145–9.

13. The National Institute of Health, The National Institute of Diabetes and Digestive and Kindey Diseases, Division of Kidney, Urologic and Hematologic diseases (1994) Excerpts from United States Renal Data System – 1994 Annual Data Report: VII, Causes of death. *Am. J. Kidney Dis.*, **24**(suppl 2), S88–95.

14. Canadian Organ Replacement Registry (1991) *1989 Annual Report*. Hospital Medical Records Institute 1989, Don Mills, Ontario.

15. Disney, A.P.S. (1995) Demography and survival of patients receiving treatment for chronic renal failure in Australia and New Zealand: report on dialysis and renal transplantation treatment from the Australia and New Zealand Dialysis and Transplant Registry. *Am. J. Kidney Dis.*, **25**, 165–75.

16. Agodoa, L.Y. and Eggers, P.W. (1995) Renal replacement therapy in the United States: data from the United States Renal Data. *Am. J. Kidney Dis.*, **25**, 119–33.

17. *USRDS Annual Data Report* (1995) USRDS, Bethesda, 87.

18. *Canadian Organ Replacement Register Report* (1993) The Kidney Foundation of Canada, Don Mills, Ontario.

19. Brunner, F.P. and Selwood, N.H. (1992) Profile of patients on RRT in Europe and death rates due to major causes of death groups. *Kidney Int.*, **42**, S-4–S-15.

20. Kjellstrand, C.M. (1993) Stopping dialysis as a cause of death – an international comparison. *J. Am. Soc. Nephrol.*, **3**, 360 (abstract 13p).

21. Teraoka, S., Toha, H., Nihei, H. *et al.* (1995) Current status of renal replacement therapy in Japan. *Am. J. Kidney Dis.*, **25**, 151–64.

22. Plough, A.L. and Salem, S. (1982) Social and contextual factors in the analysis of mortality in end-stage renal disease patients: implications for health policy. *Am. J. Public Health*, **72**, 1293–5.

23. Catalano, C. (1995) Discontinuation of treatment among Italian diabetic patients treated by renal replacement therapy. *Nephrol. Dial. Transplant.*, **10**, 1142–4.

24. Catalano, C. and Marino, C. (1996) Death from suicide and discontinuation of renal replacement therapy: 23 years' clinical experience. *Nephron*, **73**, 737–8.

25. Catalano, C., Goodship, T.H.J., Graham, K.A. *et al.* (1996) Withdrawal of renal replacement therapy in Newcastle upon Tyne: 1964–1993. *Nephrol. Dial. Transplant.*, **11**, 133–9.

26. Holley, J.L., Nespor, S. and Rault, R. (1993) The effect of providing chronic hemodialysis patients written material on advance directives. *Am. J. Kidney Dis.*, **22**, 413–18.

27. Perry, E., Buck, C., Newsome, J. *et al.* (1995) Dialysis staff influence patients in formulating their advance directives. *Am. J. Kidney Dis.*, **25**, 262–8.

28. Sehgal, A., Galbraith, A., Chesney, M. *et al.* (1992) How strictly do dialysis patients want their advance directives followed? *JAMA*, **267**, 59–63.

29. Moss, A.H., Stockings, C.B., Sachs, G.A. and Siegler, M. (1993) Variation in attitudes of dialysis unit medical directors towards decisions to withhold and withdraw dialysis. *J. Am. Soc. Nephrol.*, **4**, 229–34.

30. Port, F.K. (1993) Worldwide demographics and future trends in end-stage renal disease. *Kidney Int.*, **43**(suppl 41), S4–S7.

31. Oreopoulos, D.G. (1995) Withdrawal from dialysis: when letting die is better than helping to live. *Lancet*, **346**, 3–4.

32. Parkes, C.M., Benjamin, B. and Fitzgerald, R.G. (1969) Broken heart: a statistical study of increased mortality among widowers. *Br. Med. J.*, **1**, 740–3.

33. McAvory, R.B. (1986) Death after bereavement. *Br. Med. J.*, **293**, 835–6.

34. Bartrop, R.W., Lazarus, L., Luckhurst, E. *et al.* (1977) Depressed lymphocyte stimulation following bereavement. *Lancet*, **i**, 834–6.

35. Schleifer, S.J., Keller, S.E., Camerino, M. *et al.* (1983) Suppression of lymphocyte stimulation following bereavement. *JAMA*, **250**, 374–7.

36. Roberts, J.C., Snyder, R. and Kjellstrand, C.M. (1988) Withdrawing life support – the survivors. *Acta Med. Scand.*, **224**, 141–8.

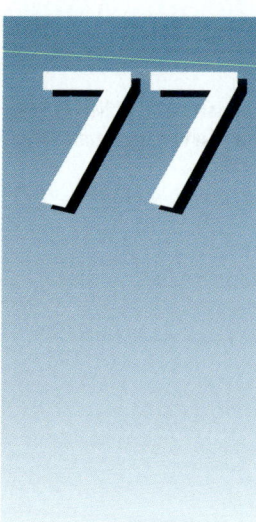

77

Peritoneal access

R. Gokal

Introduction

One of the most important components of the peritoneal dialysis system is permanent and safe access to the peritoneal cavity [1]. The double cuff Tenckhoff catheter, developed in 1968 for treatment of patients with intermittent peritoneal dialysis, forms the basis of current peritoneal dialysis (PD) catheter design and use. With the advent of continuous ambulatory peritoneal dialysis (CAPD) there has been an increase in catheter-related complications secondary to the numerous daily manipulations that are required. Despite improvements in catheter survival over the last few years, catheter-related complications still occur, causing significant morbidity and often forcing the removal of the catheter [2, 3]. As much as 20% of patients transferred to hemodialysis are directly related to catheter problems. Since the incidence of peritonitis is declining following the introduction of disconnect systems, catheter-related complications during CAPD have become the main area of concern for those working in this field of end-stage renal disease.

Peritoneal catheters

Types of catheters [3, 4]

Rigid catheter

When the need to start peritoneal dialysis is urgent, it may be best to obtain access to the peritoneal cavity through a rigid catheter. This catheter can be inserted at the bedside with very minimal preparation. Extreme caution needs to be exercised when inserting the rigid catheter in very obese patients or those who have had previous abdominal surgery. Complications of rigid catheter insertion and their management are shown in Table 77.1.

Soft catheter for long-term peritoneal dialysis

Several catheters have been designed to minimize the various complications of peritoneal access (Table 77.2). Figure 77.1 shows that chronic peritoneal dialysis catheters have a variety of intraperitoneal designs, combined physically with a number of extraperitoneal designs [5]. Intraperitoneal designs of chronic catheters include a straight or coiled Tenckhoff catheter, the double disk Toronto Western catheter or the column disc catheter. Extraperitoneal designs of chronic catheters include either a single or double Dacron cuff, disk-bubble two cuffs, arcuate (Swan Neck – two cuffs with a pre-

Nephrology, Edited by Rex L. Jamison and Robert Wilkinson.
Published in 1997 by Chapman & Hall, London. ISBN 0 412 60930 4

Table 77.1 Complications of rigid peritoneal catheter insertion

Complication	Action
Bleeding	If bleeding is excessive and continuous, patient will need laparotomy
Dialysis solution leak	Purse string suture
Poor drainage	Replace catheter
Extraperitoneal space penetration	Replace catheter
Viscus penetration	Bladder – urinary catheter Other organs – patient may need laparotomy
Peritonitis	Treat with appropriate antibiotics
Abdominal pain	Analgesia
Loss of rigid catheter into peritoneal cavity	Laparotomy

Table 77.2 Peritoneal dialysis access complications

Early (within four weeks of insertion)	Late (beyond four weeks)
Placement risk	Infections
Failure to enter the peritoneum	Peritonitis
Perforation of viscus	Tunnel and exit site infections
Bleeding	Catheter tip loculation
Catheter malfunction	Catheter malfunction
Inflow obstruction	Inflow/outflow obstruction (omental wrap, catheter tip migration)
Outflow obstruction	Accidental catheter breakage
Pericatheter dialyzate leak	Degeneration of catheter material
Perioperative infection	Toxic or mechanical injury to viscera
Perioperative and postoperative pain	Ultrafiltration failure
	Erosion of catheter into bowel/bladder
	Pericatheter leak – subcutaneous leak
	Hernia formation at site of insertion

formed 150° bend in the inner cuff tubing to provide a caudally directed exit site without strain on the cuffs [6]), Cruz (pail-handle – similar to the arcuate catheter but with two 90° bends [7]). The double-cuff, straight Tenckhoff catheter is still the most widely used catheter because it seems to satisfy the needs of most patients who are undergoing chronic peritoneal dialysis. The Swan Neck catheter has become the second most popular catheter with promising catheter survival results compared to those with the other types [6]. The Cruz pail-handle catheter utilizes polyurethane which, being a strong and smooth material allows thinner walls, a greater internal diameter and therefore a more rapid flow of dialyzate. The coil catheter causes less patient discomfort by minimiz-

ing the 'jet effect' of the high flow of dialysis solutions and is potentially less prone to migration. This is also true of the Toronto Western catheters which have two disks perpendicular to the tubing axis.

Catheter choice and catheter results

The minimum acceptable rate of catheter survival at 12 months is 50–60%. At best a three-year catheter survival rate of 80% should be expected. Results worse than the former figure should lead to a review of the procedures used. Two-cuff catheters are superior to single-cuff ones [6a]. A survey of the current literature suggests that the

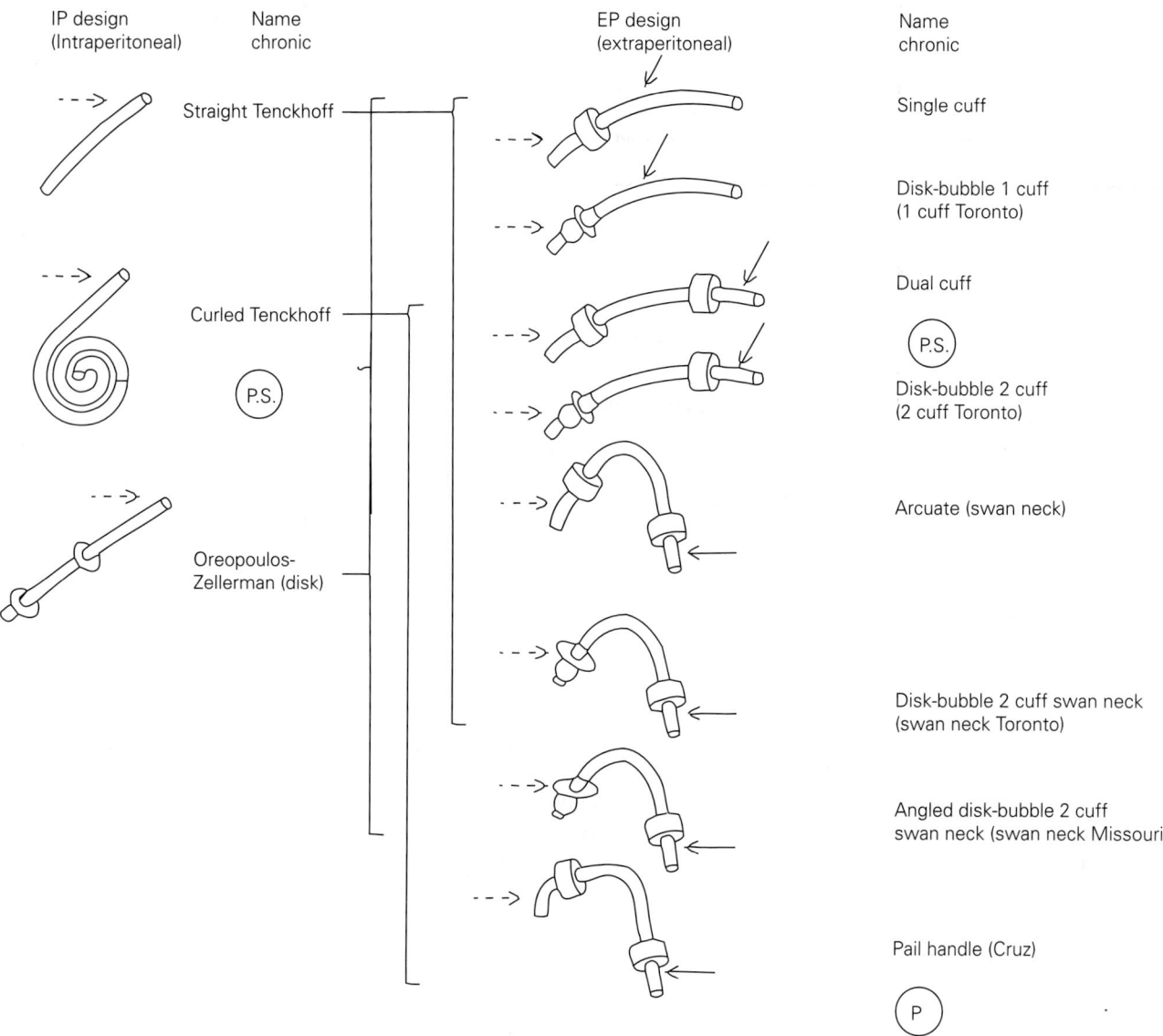

Figure 77.1 Combination of intraperitoneal (IP) and extraperitoneal (EP) designs in currently available peritoneal catheters. The letters in circles indicate materials of construction: P, polyurethane; PS, polyurethane or silicone; N, nylon; no letter, silicone. Broken arrow denotes the location of the parietal peritoneum and the solid arrow, the location of the skin surface. (Reproduced, with permission, from ref. [14].)

most popular catheters are the two-cuff standard Tenckhoff and the Swan Neck Missouri catheters, but controlled studies show no superiority of one over the other. (Table 77.3). Table 77.4 summarizes the complication rates of peritoneal catheters by type and placement technique [7a, 7b, 7c, 7d, 7e]. Improved results are reported for the Swan Neck catheters, which require a surgical approach for insertion, and equally good results are reported for the peritoneoscopic approach to catheter implantation. It is important to stress that although these studies indicate varied outcomes, no hard evidence is available to discard the use of any catheter. In support of this is the prospective randomized study of three different catheters (straight Tenckhoff, curled Tenckhoff and Toronto

Western) which showed no difference in complication rates [8]. Used in the proper manner, the outcome with any of these catheters is likely to be successful. It is important, however, to record and audit the results of treatment.

Implantation method

The implantation technique influences the outcome of chronic peritoneal catheters. To achieve good results, implantation must be performed by a competent and experienced catheter insertion team. Inexperienced personnel should not be permitted to perform the implantation except under direct supervision of an experienced

Table 77.3 Randomised controlled studies

Study	Catheters	Outcome	Significance
Akyol 1990	Tk st vs coiled 20 patients	1 yr survival – 90% straight 70% coiled	NS
Nielson 1995	Tk st vs coiled 72 patients	3 yr survival – 78% coiled – 40% straight	p < 0.01
Scott 1994	St vs coiled vs TWC – 90 patients	no difference in complications	NS
Eklund 1994 1995	St vs SNC-40 pats St vs SNC-40 pats	2 yr survival – 78% 3 yr survival – 90% SN; 80% Tk	NS NS
Lye 1996	St vs SNC coiled 40 patients	1 yr survival – 95% SNC – 90% St; SNC less ESI	NS

Tk, Tenckhoff; SNC, swan neck catheter; TWC, Toronto Western Catheter; St, straight; ESI, exit site infection.

Table 77.4 Complication rates of peritoneal catheters by type and replacement technique

	Complication rate (average/annum)			
	Infectious complication	Outflow failure	SC leak	Method of insertion
Tenckhoff straight				B,S,P
Double cuff				
blind	0.13	0.23	0.05	
surgical	0.35	0.15	0.11	
peritoneoscopic	0.05	0.01	0.01	
Tenckhoff straight				B,S,P
Single cuff	0.15	0.08	0.02	
Tenckhoff curled double cuff				B,S,P
blind	0.5	0.06	0.16	
surgical	0.48	0.15	0.14	
peritoneoscopic	0.07	0.01	0.09	
Swanneck Missouri catheter (peritoneal flange, double cuff)	0.16	0.05	0.00	S
Toronto Western catheter (perpendicular disk, double cuff)	0.23	0.07	0.00	S
Column disk (double cuff; life cath)	0.11	0.04	0.03	S

These are pooled results from various series reported in the literature.
Adapted from Ash [3].
Abbreviations: SC, subcutaneous; +B, blind; S, surgical (dissection); P, peritoneoscopic.

person. There are currently six techniques of catheter implantation. Whatever technique is used there are several areas of general agreement about the technique [1].

1 The insertion site should be paramedian.
2 The deep cuff should be in the musculature of the anterior abdominal wall.

3 The subcutaneous cuff should be near the skin surface and not less than 2 cm from the exit site.
4 The exit site should be facing downwards or directed laterally.
5 The intra-abdominal portion of the catheter should be placed between the visceral and parietal peritoneum.

The various implantation techniques are described below.

Surgical insertion (placement by dissection)

Dissective placement is essential for catheters with stabilizing devices (e.g. Swan Neck, Toronto Western, Column Disc), but all catheters can be inserted this way. In the USA 74% of all catheter insertions are done by surgical dissection [9].

Blind catheter insertion

This procedure should not be performed in patients who are extremely obese or who have had previous abdominal surgery. The Tenckhoff trocar technique utilizes the appropriately designed trocar by Tenckhoff.

Seldinger (guidewire) and peel-away sheath [10]

This technique is somewhat similar to the split sheath technique used for insertion of subclavian and internal jugular venous catheters. This technique can be used for straight Tenckhoff catheters as well as Swan Neck straight and coiled catheters. Preparation of the patient is similar to that described for rigid catheters.

Peritoneoscopic insertion

The use of peritoneoscopy for peritoneal catheter placement was developed by Ash [4, 5]. Tenckhoff and Swan Neck Tenckhoff straight and coiled catheters may be implanted with this technique. Like the blind insertion, it is performed through a single abdominal puncture and utilizes a Y-tec peritoneoscope.

The Swan Neck presternal catheter

The catheter has the same intraperitoneal portion but the extraperitoneal portion is long and brought up externally at the sternum [11]. The rationale for this approach is that it provides greater catheter stability at the exit site and tunnel, good wound healing, easy exit site care and some psychosocial advances [12].

Moncrief and Popovich technique [13]

The distal external segment of the catheter is completely buried and remains in the subcutaneous tunnel until exteriorization four weeks after catheter insertion. This is a new technique which allows tissue to grow into the cuff material without exposure to the skin surface. This necessitates catheter insertion at least four weeks before use, at which time the catheter tip is brought out through a tiny exit in the skin. Peritonitis rates have not been shown to improve with this type of insertion, but the experience is limited [13a].

Postoperative catheter care [13b]

There are a variety of approaches to postoperative catheter care and little evidence to support the superiority of one approach over the other. In general terms it is advisable to minimize catheter movement and manipulation of the catheter or exit site until healing of the wound and catheter tract is complete. There is also a risk of fluid leakage if large volumes of dialysis fluid are utilized prematurely especially if the patient is active and fluid is in place. The management of exit site and immobilization of the catheter are important factors in the long-term survival of catheters and in minimizing complications (Chapter 79).

Although immediate dialysis without leakage is possible, it is preferable to postpone dialysis to permit good tissue healing. It is common to flush the peritoneal catheter promptly after installation with 500 ml of solution until the effluent becomes clear. Once this is achieved the catheter can be safely capped. It should be capped for up to two weeks before CAPD or large volume peritoneal dialysis is initiated. Optimally CAPD should not be initiated for at least two weeks after catheter implantation. During this period of time there is no necessity to check for catheter patency and function. If dialysis is necessary, the volumes should be increased gradually to minimize the risk of dialyzate leaks.

After catheter implantation the exit site and operative site should be covered by sterile gauze and a non-occlusive dressing which should not be changed for several days unless there is an obvious excess of bleeding. The catheter should be well anchored to the skin to avoid movements at the exit site. Immobilization can be accomplished with tape, dressing or an immobilization device.

Catheter complications (Table 77.2)

Early soft catheter complications

Early complications after catheter insertion are similar to those after implantation of a rigid catheter, but the frequency is lower, particularly with surgical and peritoneoscopic insertion. Blood-tinged dialyzate is common postimplantation but severe bleeding is very rare. Dialyzate leaks are unlikely if peritoneal dialysis is postponed for at least two weeks after implantation.

Poor dialyzate return is usually due to catheter obstruction. The most common causes of catheter obstruction are catheter tip migration, occlusion of the tip by bowel, bladder and intralumenal formation of clot. Emptying the bladder and using laxatives may restore catheter function. Clots can be prevented by using heparin or the catheter can be filled with urokinase (5000 units diluted in normal saline). These measures will relieve the obstruction in 10–15% of cases. If the catheter is not kinked but does not function for two weeks, omental wrapping or multiple adhesions are most likely and omentectomy or adhesiolysis through a laporoscopy may be required.

Catheter migration

The best positions for the catheter tip is in the true pelvis. Tenckhoff recommended pointing the catheter in a caudal direction to prevent migration [3]. If the exit is directed caudally and the tunnel points cephalad, however the catheter will then have an intraperitoneal bend. In this circumstance the tip will migrate out of the true pelvis, due to silastic 'shape memory' and resilience.

Catheter migration out of the pelvis is frequently observed on abdominal radiographs done for various reasons in patients with a functioning catheter. Although about 20% of catheters translocate to the upper abdomen, only one-fifth of these translocated catheters are obstructed. However, a catheter with its tip in the upper abdomen is about six times more likely to be obstructed than a normally positioned catheter. Migration of the catheter tip may be the result of obstruction rather than its cause. Relocation of the catheter is best done surgically or with the laparoscopic method.

Pericatheter leaks

These can occur through the wound or exit site soon after insertion. This can be minimized if the deep cuff is placed in the belly of the rectus muscle.

Late soft catheter complications

Catheter obstruction

Capture of the catheter by an active omentum causes outflow obstruction. This is usually an immediate post-operative event but can occur later and when it does it is usually associated with peritonitis. Late catheter migration is unusual unless associated with omental capture.

Slow drainage due to catheter translocation or to occlusion of the tip by bowel or fibrin clot formation occurs from time to time in some patients. Constipation is a common cause for this complication and laxatives and regular bowel movements are an important facet of preventative care. For fibrin clots, addition of heparin, 500 units/l of dialysis solution, is usually successful in restoring good catheter function.

Another reason for obstruction may be catheter adherence to the peritoneum. This complication is found in children who have undergone partial omentectomy at the time of the insertion. Relocation of such catheters may be attempted with a so-called 'whip lash' technique [13]. This entails insertion of a blunted steel trocar into the catheter. Using the cuff as a pivot point and using short and rapid whiplash motions, the catheter is freed from the adherence site.

Catheter dialysate leaks

Dialysate leakage can develop at any time after catheter implantation. External leakage develops early; subcutaneous leakage develops any time after implantation. In most instances the leakage will stop if peritoneal dialysis is discontinued for a period ranging from days to weeks. Causes of late dialysis leak are shown in Table 77.5. Most cases are refractory to conservative therapy and require surgical repair. Subcutaneous leaks are more likely to occur with the midline catheter insertion than with insertion through the rectus muscle. This complication rarely occurs with catheters provided with a bubble and polyester disc at the deep cuff. Late leaks usually infiltrate the abdominal wall and can present acutely or chronically. Acute leaks cause a sudden drop in ultrafiltration and usually occur after a sudden increase in intra-abdominal pressure. Such a leak may be difficult to localize but a good method of doing so is CT scan with intraperitoneal contrast [15]. Peritoneal scintography has also been used in ascertaining the site of fluid leakage [16].

External cuff extrusion

The main cause of a cuff extrusion is placement of the external cuff too near to the exit site. There are at least two forces favoring cuff extrusion – resilience of the tunnel catheter and the pulling and tugging of the catheter during use. Due to the resilient force of the silicon, a straight catheter implanted in a curved tunnel tends to assume its original shape and push the cuff out. The cuff usually becomes infected, and requires antibiotics and exteriorization. Shaving the infected cuff many save the catheter but usually the catheter will need replacement at some stage.

Pain during inflow

In some patients inflow and outflow peritoneal dialysis fluid can cause pain. Pain is usually most intense at the beginning of the infusion and at the end of the drainage. In the majority of cases the pain is transient and disappears within a few weeks. There are various ways to overcome this pain (Table 77.6) but should these be ineffective the catheter must be replaced. Pain is less likely with coiled than with straight catheters; if replacement is necessary use a coiled catheter. Outflow pain is usually secondary to a negative pressure exerted on the peritoneum.

Organ erosion

Injury to the internal organs leading to intra-abdominal bleeding or peritonitis has been reported as a late catheter complication. This is most likely due to the pressure exerted by 'soft' but resilient tubing. Coiled catheters appear to be free of such complications.

Table 77.5   Late dialyzate leaks

	Acute onset	*Chronic – gradual*
Causes:	Sudden heavy lifting coughing, straining, traumatic traction of catheter	Mechanical: sequel of acute leak prior catheter insertion and line insertion, abdominal hernia obesity. Metabolic: diabetes, malnutrition, use steroid medication
Results in:	Sudden drop in UF. Abdominal wall peau d'orange. Spongy feeling by physician examination	Poor UF Localized abdominal edema Scrotal/genital edema Fluid overload
Treatment:	Stop PD for four weeks Low exchange volume Supine position during PD	Localize site of leak Stop PD Remove catheter or repair cause
Prevention:	Insertion of deep cuff within rectus muscle and sheath Avoidance of midline insertion	

UF, ultrafiltration; PD, peritoneal dialysis.

Table 77.6   Maneuvers to alleviate infusion pain

- Eradication of constipation
- Slower infusion rate
- Incomplete drainage
- Tidal mode for nightly peritoneal dialysis
- Alkalization of dialyzate (sodium bicarbonate addition to to lactate solution or use bicarbonate dialyzate)
- Lignocaine 2% intraperitoneal, 2 ml/2l
- Catheter replacement

Mechanical accidents

There have been reports of catheters being accidentally cut with scissors or punctured by cuff shaving [12]. There are also reports of problems arising from the physical properties of the catheter material. The inclusion of radio-opaque barium sulfate in the catheter renders it brittle. Catheters have all been observed to stretch, crack or become brittle with age after repeated exposure to beta-dine. Polyurethane is even more susceptible to damage with aging because of so-called environmental stress. This leads to micro-cracks in the surface of the device, the result of corrosive forces of the living organism.

Long-term results

The National CAPD Registry of the National Institutes of Health reported results of a survey to determine the natural history of implanted peritoneal catheters and to estimate survival of different catheters. The probability of catheter survival at 36 months with double cuff standard straight Tenckhoff catheter was 33%, for curled Tenckhoff catheters 34% and for double cuff Toronto Western catheters 22%.

Twardowski et al. [6] reported the results of 181 Swan neck catheters implanted over a six-year period. Their experience was compared with the standard Tenckhoff and Toronto Western Hospital catheters. Survival proba-bility of Swan Neck Missouri, straight and coiled catheters (60% at 5 years) was significantly higher than that of other types (30% at 3 years). No malfunctional leaks occurred with the Swan Neck catheters. This experience points to a lower complication rate and a higher proba-bility of survival with Swan neck catheters compared to that of the straight catheters.

The US Renal Data Systems [9] reported on catheters in a cohort of approximately 2800 patients followed for as long as 21 months. The types were straight intraperi-toneal segment with no bend (44%), curled coiled catheter with no bend (40%), or a catheter with a pre-formed bend with either straight or curled intraperitoneal segments (12%). There were 78% double cuff catheter. Surgeons implanted 88% of the catheters and surgical dis-section was used in 74% of cases. Although this study did

Table 77.7 Components of permanent peritoneal catheter failure indicating areas for future research

	Current strategies	Future strategies
Bacterial invasion	Downward pointing catheters Exit care procedures Moncrief/Popovich implantation technique	Eradication of *Staphylococcus aureus* nasal carriage Antimicrobial catheters
Trauma leads to hematoma,	Immobilization Swan neck design	Alternative subcutaneous materials Catheter with disk catheter design

Sinus tract formation
  (poor integration of
  catheter with tissue)
	–	Fibrin glue
		Macroscopic texturing
		Microscopic texturing
		>40 µm for fibroblasts
		>100 µm for vascular

Foreign body response	Medical polymer (silicone,
	  polyurethane)
		Biocompatible materials (titanium,
		  hydroxyappeatite)
		Bioactive ceramics
		Surface architecture of 1–2 µm pores

Adapted from ref. [2], with permission.

not assess catheter survival, relative risk of first episode of peritonitis was essentially identical for all the catheters studied.

Conclusions

There are three essential prerequisites of peritoneal catheter performance; catheter design, implantation technique and postimplantation care. At present the silicon rubber tubing with double polyester cuff is still the best design. A permanent bend between cuffs (Swan Neck or Cruz) offers an advantage because it allows implantation of the catheter in an unstressed condition, a curved tunnel with both external and internal exits directed downwards. The exits should be located in a place to minimize pressure and movement. A prophylactic antibiotic at implantation is recommended. Healing of the exit site takes about 4–8 weeks. During this time a non-occlusive dressing is recommended. Exit site, tunnel infections and catheter-related peritonitis remain troublesome complications and will be addressed in Chapter 80.

Future research needs to focus on factors which are important in the prevention of catheter-associated infection and other complications [1]. These include placement technique, care of exit site, *Staphylococcus aureus* nasal carriage and the relationship between the percutaneous device and wound healing. Irritant lotions for exit site care should be avoided. Factors contributing to the failure of a permanent access device and potential areas of research that should be undertaken are listed in Table 77.7. Strategies to minimize bacterial colonization of the catheter wound site, trauma to the catheter, foreign body response, marsupialization of the epithelium, and impairment of device – tissue integration are all desirable. Recent innovations like the better fixation of the cuffs to the tissue by using fibrin glue are noteworthy as are Doppler studies to identify areas of vascularization and inflammation.

References

1. Gokal, R., Ash, S.R., Baird Helfrich, G. *et al.* (1993) Peritoneal catheter and exit site practises towards optimum peritoneal access. *Perit. Dial. Int.*, **13**, 29–39.
2. Bernadini, J., Piraino, B. *et al.* (1991) An analysis of ten year trends in infections in adults on CAPD. *Clin. Nephrol.*, **36**, 29–34.
3. Ash, S.R. (1990) Chronic peritoneal dialysis catheters: effects of catheter design, materials and location. *Semin. Dial.*, **3**, 39–46.
4. Ash, S.R. (1993) Peritoneal access devices and placement techniques, in *Dialysis Therapy* (eds A.R. Nissension and R.N. Fine), Hanely and Belfus, New York, pp. 23–30.

5. Ash, R. and Nichols, W.K. (1994) Placement repair and removal of chronic peritoneal catheters, in *The Textbook of Peritoneal Dialysis* (eds R. Gokal and K.D. Nolph), Kluwer, Dordrecht, pp. 315–33.

6. Twardowski, Z.J., Prowant, B.F., Nichols, W.K. *et al.* (1992) Six years experience with Swan Neck Catheter. *Perit. Dial. Int.*, **12**, 384–9.

6a. Golper, T.A., Brier, M.E., Bunke, M. *et al.* (1996) Risk factors for peritonitis in long term peritoneal dialysis: The Network 9 Peritonitis and Catheter survival studies. *Am. J. Kidney Dis*, **38**, 428–36.

7. Cruz, C. (1994) Cruz catheter: implantation technique and clinical results. *Perit. Dial. Int.*, **14**(suppl. 3), S59–62.

7a. Akyol, A.M., Porteous, C., Brown, M.W. (1990) A comparison of 2 types of CAPD Catheters. *Perit. Dial Int.*, **10**: 63–6.

7b. Nielson, P.K., Hemmingsen, C., Friis, S. *et al.* (1995) Comparison of straight and curled Tenckhoff Peritoneal catheters implanted by the subcutaneous technique: a prospective randomised study. *Perit. Dial. Int.*, **15**: 18–21.

7c. Eklund, B.H., Honkanen, E.O., Kalan, A.R., Kyllonen, L.E., (1994) Catheter configuration and outcome in CAPD: a prospective comparison of two catheters. *Perit. Dial. Int.*, **14**, 70–74.

7d. Eklund, B.H., Honkanen, E.O., Kalan, A.R., Kyllonen, L.E. (1995) Peritoneal Dialysis access: prospective randomised comparison of the swan-neck and Tenckhoff catheters. *Perit. Dial. Int.*, **15**, 353–6.

7e. Lye, W.C., Kour, N.W., van der Straaten, J. *et al.* (1996) A prospective randomised comparison of the swan-neck, coiled and straight Tenckhoff catheters in patients on CAPD. *Perit. Dial. Int.*, **16**(Suppl. 1), 5333–5.

8. Scott, P., Bakran, A., Pearson, R. *et al.* (1994) Peritoneal dialysis access. Randomised trial of 3 different peritoneal catheters – Preliminary report. *Perit. Dial. Int.*, **14**, 289–90.

9. US Renal Data System (1992) USRDS 1992 Annual Data Report VI. Catheter related factors and peritonitis risk in CAPD patients. *Am. J. Kidney Dis.*, **5**(Suppl.), 48–54.

10. Zappacosta, A.R., Perras, S.T. and Closkey, G.N. (1991) Seldinger technique for Tenckhoff catheter placement. *ASAIO Trans.*, **37**, 13–15.

11. Twardowski, Z.J., Prowant, B.F., Pickett, B. *et al.* (1996) Four year expenerice with Swann-neck presternal PD Catheter. *Am. J. Kidney Dis.*, **27**, 99–105.

12. Twardowski, Z.J. and Khanna, R. (1994) Peritoneal dialysis access and exit site care, in *The Textbook of Peritoneal Dialysis* (eds R. Gokal and K.D. Nolph), Kluwer Academic, Dordrecht, pp. 217–314.

13. Moncrief, J.W., Popovich, R.P., Boraderick, L.J. *et al.* (1993) Moncrief – Popovich catheter: a new peritoneal access technique for patients in peritoneal dialysis. *ASAIO J.* **39**, 62–5.

13a. Moncrief, J.W., Popovich, R.P., Seare, W. *et al.* (1996) Peritoneal Dialysis Access technology. The Austin Diagnostic clinic experience. *Perit. Dial. Int.*, **16**(Suppl. 1), S327–9.

13b. Prowant, B,F., Twardowski, Z. (1996) Recommendations for exit site care. *Perit. Dial. Int.*, **16**(Suppl 3), S94–9.

14. O'Regan, S., Gavel, L., Patriquin, H. and Yazbeck, S. (1988) Outflow obstruction: whiplash technique for catheter mobilisation. *Perit. Dial. Int.*, **8**, 265–8.

15. Letherland, J., Gibson, M., Sanbrook, P. *et al.* (1992) Investigation and treatment of poor drains of dialysate fluid associated with anterior abdominal leaks in patients in CAPD. *Nephrol. Dial. Transplant.*, **7**, 1030–4.

16. Kopecky, R.T., Frymoyer, P.A., Witanowksi, L.S. *et al.* (1990) Complications of peritoneal catheter, in *CAPD in the USA – final report of the National CAPD Registry* (eds A.S. Lindblad *et al.*), Kluwer Academic, Dordrecht, pp. 157–66.

17. Tenckhoff, H. (1976) Home peritoneal dialysis, in *Clinical Aspects of Uraemia and Dialysis* (ed. S. Massry), Charles Thomas, Springfield, pp. 583–615.

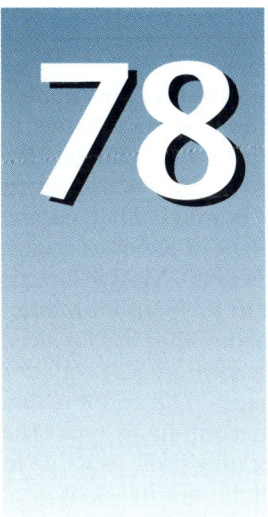

Principles and technology of peritoneal dialysis

Raymond T. Krediet

Introduction

The instillation of a saline solution into the abdominal cavity is followed by diffusion of solutes from the extracellular fluid to this solution until an equilibrium is reached between this fluid and the blood. In the presence of a concentration gradient, small solutes (e.g. urea) pass from the blood to the fluid. After outflow from the peritoneal cavity, the net result is removal of urea from the body. This basic principle of peritoneal dialysis was applied in practice in 1923 by Ganter, a German clinical investigator. After experiments in animals, he treated a woman with acute uremia by peritoneal dialysis and observed some clinical improvement. Several other investigators confirmed the feasibility of this mode of treatment, but it was only after 1945 that peritoneal dialysis gained wider acceptance in patients with acute renal failure.

Detailed studies on characteristics of peritoneal transport in patients were done by Boen [1], who also made the first attempts to use intermittent peritoneal dialysis as renal replacement therapy for patients with chronic renal failure when he worked with Scribner in Seattle at the beginning of the 1960s. This became feasible only after the introduction of a silastic catheter with dacron cuffs by Tenckhoff. However, the inadequacy of solute removal compared to hemodialysis prevented the application of peritoneal dialysis on a large scale. Less than 800 patients treated by intermittent peritoneal dialysis could be traced world-wide in 1977.

In 1976 Popovich and Moncrief introduced a new concept: continuous ambulatory peritoneal dialysis (CAPD), 24 hours per day, seven days a week, with four to five exchanges per day. The long in-dwelling time of 4–8 h ensures near-equilibrium between blood and the dialysis fluid. When compared with intermittent peritoneal dialysis the longer dialysis time largely compensates for the lesser degree of dialysis efficiency. The further technical improvements of this method, notably the introduction of disposable plastic bags by Oreopoulos, have made CAPD a practical, adequate and acceptable form of renal replacement therapy. The invention of CAPD was an important turning point. Today more than 100 000 patients are treated with chronic peritoneal dialysis world-wide, at least 85% of them with CAPD.

This chapter focuses on the principles of peritoneal dialysis and technological aspects. Principles that will be discussed are the anatomy of the peritoneal membrane, physiology of solute transport, the transport of low-molecular-weight solutes, the transport of electrolytes, the transport of macromolecules, transport from the peritoneal cavity, and fluid transport. The technology part will focus on dialysis techniques, administration systems and dialysis solutions.

Principles

Anatomy of the peritoneal membrane

The peritoneal cavity is the serosal space between visceral and parietal peritoneum. The visceral peritoneum covers the majority of the internal organs, whereas the inner

Nephrology, Edited by Rex L. Jamison and Robert Wilkinson.
Published in 1997 by Chapman & Hall, London. ISBN 0 412 60930 4

abdominal surface is lined with the parietal peritoneum. In the male it is a closed sac, in the female the free ends of the uterine tubes open into the peritoneal cavity. The peritoneal cavity is lined with a layer of mesothelium and lubricated by a small quantity of serous fluid. During peritoneal dialysis the peritoneal cavity is filled with dialysis fluid.

Anatomic studies of the surface area of the peritoneum, i.e. the mesothelial surface area, reported and average value of $1\,m^2$ in adults. The ratio between peritoneal surface area and body weight in newborn infants is about double that found in adults. Visceral peritoneum accounts for 60% of the total surface area, 10% of which covers the liver. The parietal peritoneum is 10% and mesentery and omentum 30% [2]. The contribution of the various parts of the peritoneum to the exchange process during peritoneal dialysis may be different. The visceral peritoneum probably contributes little, but the peritoneum covering the liver may be much more important. The diaphragmatic part of the peritoneum is especially involved in the absorption of solutes and fluid from the peritoneal cavity into the lymphatic system.

The 'peritoneal membrane' used as a dialysis membrane consists of at least three layers: the mesothelium, the peritoneal capillaries and the interstitial tissue (Figure 78.1). Mesothelial cells have a flat and discoid appearance on cross-section. They possess numerous microvilli and contain many organelles indicative of their secreting capacity. Mesothelial cells secrete phospholipids, which act as lubricant, but are also able to secrete various prostaglandins, cytokines and fibrinolytic factors. Mesothelial cells often show reactive changes during peritoneal dialysis [3]. Functional studies of isolated mesentery show that it is probably not an important barrier to the transport of solutes during peritoneal dialysis. The interstitium is formed by loose connective tissue that contains mucopolysaccharides, bundles of collagen, fibroblasts and mast cells. Little is know about its contribution to the dialysis exchange process. Negative electric charges have been demonstrated in the peritoneal interstitium, but it is controversial whether they are involved in the transport of solutes. The interstitium also contains peritoneal capillaries and lymphatics. The endothelium of the capillaries is mainly of the continuous type. The capillary wall is probably the most important structure in the transport of solutes and fluid during peritoneal dialysis. It is a size-selective restriction barrier, so that the transport of solutes is progressively hindered with increasing molecular weight.

Physiology of solute transport

The magnitude of solute transport is dependent on the number of perfused peritoneal capillaries. Under basal circumstances only 25% of these capillaries are perfused. This implies that peritoneal blood flow is a determinant of solute transport. Studies using the mass transfer area coefficient (see below) of carbon dioxide suggest that it averages about 100 ml/min during peritoneal dialysis. The instillation of dialysis fluid markedly increases blood flow to the mesentery, omentum, intestinal serosa and parietal peritoneum [4]. Little is known about the regulation of peritoneal blood flow. It is reduced during shock and exercise. Locally produced substances, such as prostaglandins are likely to be involved.

Transport across the capillary wall is generally assumed to occur through a system of pores [5]. This physiologically defined system consists mainly of small pores with radii of 40–50 Å that are involved in the transport of low-molecular-weight solutes. The interendothelial clefts are probably the equivalents of these small pores. In addition, a small number of large pores, less than 0.1% of the total number of pores is assumed to be present. Their radii exceed 150 Å which is sufficient to allow the transport of macromolecules, such as serum proteins. The anatomic equivalent of the large pores has not been identified with certainty, but venular interendothelial gaps, which can be provoked by the administration of vasodilators such as histamine, could represent the large pore system. This would imply that the large pore radius is not constant, but is subject to variations. In other words, the capillary wall is a heteroporous membrane that can be described by the combination of a predominant set of small pores with uniform radii and a small set of large pores with variable radii. (The radius calculated for the large pores is the mean value of the various radii.) Recently the two pore theory has been modified by also assuming the presence of very small transcellular pores (<5 Å) that are only involved in the transport of water [6]. The channel-like intrinsic membrane protein (CHIP 28) a member of a

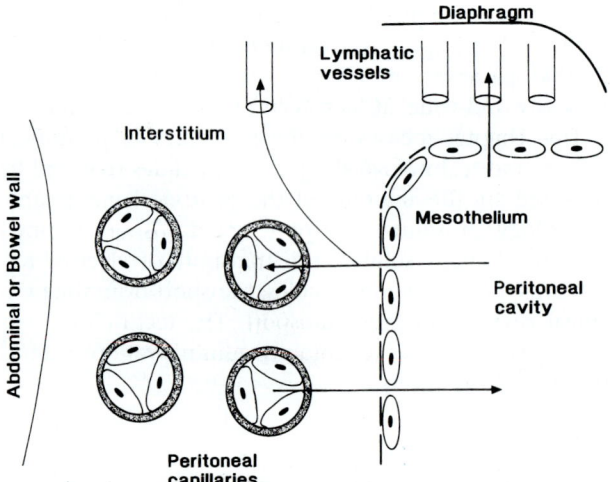

Figure 78.1 A schematic representation of the peritoneal membrane. Diffusion and transcapillary ultrafiltration occur in two directions. Lymphatic absorption from the peritoneal cavity occurs partly directly into the subdiaphragmatic lymphatics and partly into the lymphatics that drain the interstitium. Published with permission of Multimed Inc.

family of water channels called the aquaporins has been shown to be present in the proximal tubule and descending limb of Henle's loop of the kidney [7]. It is also present in other epithelia of the continuous type. It is possible that a water channel could be involved in water transport across the peritoneum during peritoneal dialysis [8].

Diffusion and convection are the mechanisms involved in the transport of solutes during peritoneal dialysis. Diffusion is driven by a concentration gradient. The rate of diffusive transfer of a given solute through the peritoneal membrane is determined by the diffusive permeability of the peritoneum to that solute, the surface area available for transport and the solute concentration gradient. Convection (or solute drag) of the solute occurs driven by the transport of water, as during ultrafiltration. It is determined by the water flux, the mean solute concentration in the membrane and the solute reflection coefficient (σ). The reflection coefficient is the fraction of the maximal osmotic pressure a solute can theoretically exert across a semipermeable membrane. By definition, it equals 1.0 for an ideal semipermeable membrane and 0 when the membrane offers no resistance to the transport of a solute relative to that of water. In the case of an isoporous membrane, $\sigma = 1 - S$, where S is the sieving coefficient, the ratio between the concentration of a solute in the ultrafiltrate divided by its concentration in plasma when no diffusion occurs. The peritoneum is a heteroporous membrane. This explains why sieving coefficients of low-molecular-weight solutes are 0.6 – 0.8, whereas their reflection coefficients are only 0.02 – 0.05 [9, 10].

Parameters of solute transport

The dialysate/plasma (D/P) concentration ratio for various solutes during a 4 h dialysis exchange is shown in Figure 78.2. A curvilinear relationship is present for low-molecular-weight solutes, due to saturation of the dia-

lyzate during the dwell [11]. For macromolecules the rise is almost linear. As a consequence of the gradual saturation of the dialyzate, the peritoneal clearance of small solutes is highest during the initial phase of the exchange and decreases during the subsequent hours. This implies that clearances during dwells exceeding the initial linear phase give only information on the net mass transfer of a solute, but cannot be used to assess the permeability characteristics of the peritoneal membrane.

The simplest approach to estimate the transport properties of the peritoneum is the peritoneal equilibration test (PET) [12]. The D/P ratio of creatinine using glucose 2.5% dialyzate during a 4 h dwell is determined; the ratio between the dialyzate glucose concentration at the end of the dwell and that before inflow is calculated and the drained volume is measured. On the basis of the D/P creatinine ratio at 4 h patients are classified as high, high-average, low-average or low transporters. The PET is attractive because of its simplicity, but it should be realized that the D/P creatinine ratio is not only dependent on diffusion, but also on convection. The glucose concentration ratio is determined by the uptake of glucose into lymphatics as well as by diffusion.

The mass transfer area coeficient (MTAC), i.e. the theoretical maximal clearance by diffusion at time zero, is the best way to characterize the diffusion properties of the peritoneum. Several complicated and simplified models have been developed. One model used to calculate the MTAC of low-molecular-weight solutes, such as urea and creatinine, that uses data obtained during a PET, is given by the following equation [13]:

$$\text{MTAC} = \frac{V_d}{t} \ln \left[\frac{V_o(P - D_o)}{V_d(P - D_d)} \right] \quad (78.1)$$

where V_d is the drained dialyzate volume, V_o is the instilled dialyzate volume, P is the plasma concentration

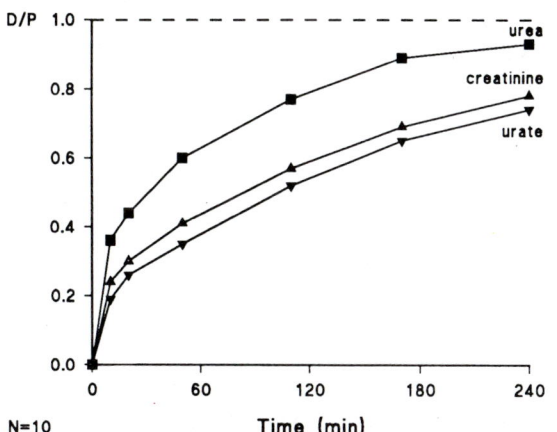
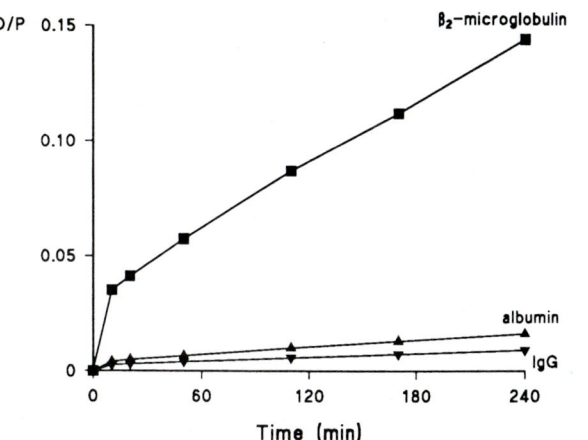

Figure 78.2 The time course of dialyzate/plasma (D/P) ratios of urea (mol. wt. 60 Da), creatinine (113 Da) and urate (168 Da) (a); and β₂-microglobulin (11 800 Da), albumin (69 000 Da) and IgG (150 000 Da) (b). Note difference in scale of ordinates. Mean values of 10 stable CAPD patients were given using glucose 1.36% dialyzate. Published with permission of the Boerhaave Committee for Postgraduate Medical Education of the Faculty of Medicine, Leiden University, The Netherlands.

of a given solute, D_o the dialyzate solute concentration before inflow, D_d the solute concentration in the drained dialyzate, and t the dwell time. Plasma concentrations should be converted into aqueous solute concentrations, either by multiplying by 1.05, or using the total protein concentration in plasma. The creatinine concentration in the dialyzate should be corrected for interference with the high dialyzate glucose concentrations when autoanalyzer methods are used for its determination. Typical values for solute transport parameters are given in Table 78.1 [14].

Transport of low-molecular-weight solutes

Diffusion is the most important transport mechanism for low molecular weigh solutes, especially when the osmolality of the dialyzate is low. It follows that the diffusive properties of the peritoneum can be characterized by relating MTAC values solutes to their free diffusion coefficients in water (D_w). This relationship can be described as a power function:

$$MTAC = aD_w^{\,b} \qquad (78.2)$$

where a is a constant and b is the slope of the linear relationship between MTAC and D_w of various solutes plotted on a double logarithmic scale. In the ideal case of free diffusion MTAC should be proportional to the free diffusion coefficient and b should equal 1.0. In this situation the peritoneal membrane offers no restriction to solute trans-

port other than the available surface area. When b exceeds 1.0 the diffusion is restricted as a function of size selectivity. The coefficient b is the restriction coefficient. The higher b is, the lower the permeability of the peritoneum. As shown in Figure 78.3, the restriction coefficient for low-molecular-weight solutes averages 1.2 [15]. This implies that the effective surface area is the only membrane characteristic that influences the MTAC of a low-molecular-weight solute. Consequently, the MTAC of such a solute, e.g. creatinine, can be used as a functional measurement of the effective peritoneal surface area. Changes in the MTAC of creatinine in individual patients reflect changes in their effective peritoneal surface area [16].

Table 78.1 Typical values of solute transport parameters during 4 h dwells

Parameters	Values
MTAC urea (ml/min)	11–21
MTAC creatinine (ml/min)	6–13
MTAC urate (ml/min)	4–12
MTAC Na$^+$ (ml/min)	5–12
MTAC K$^+$ (ml/min)	10–20
Restriction coefficient of macromolecules	1.97–2.77

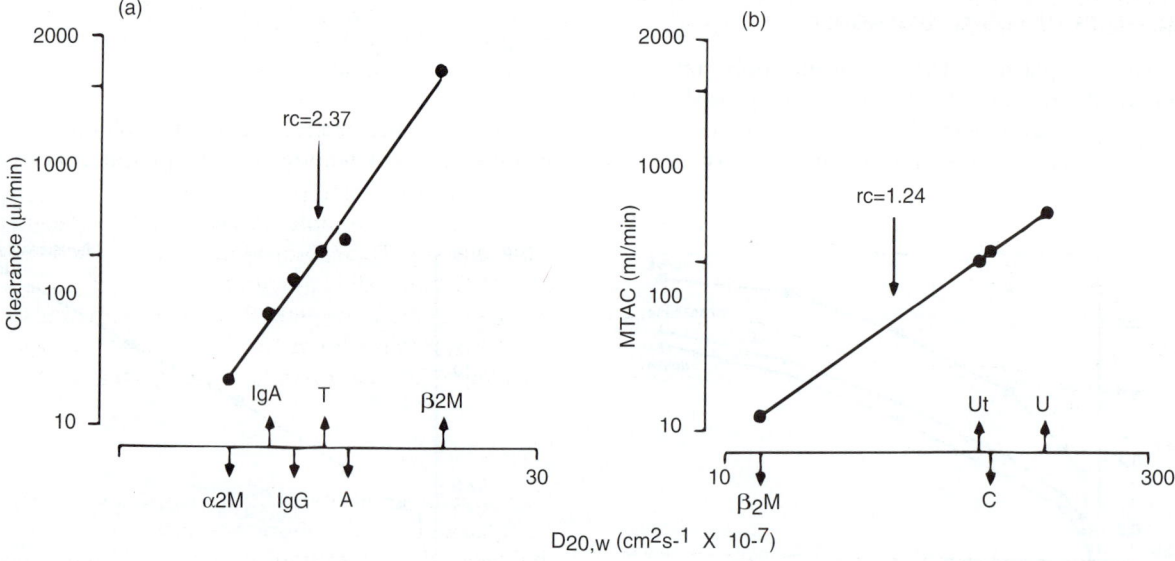

Figure 78.3 (a) The relationship between the clearances of β_2-microglobulin (β_2M), albumin (A), transferrin (T), IgG, IgA and α_2-macroglobulin (α_2M) as a function of their free diffusion coefficients in water ($D_{20,w}$) on a double logarithmic scale. (b) The relationship between the mass transfer urea coefficient of urea (U), creatinine (C), urate (Ut) and β_2M as a function of their free diffusion coefficients in water on a double logarithmic scale. The slope of the regression lines represents the restriction coefficient (**rc**). It follows from equation (78.2) that a restriction coefficient of 1.0 means a linear relationship between MTACs or clearances of solutes and their free diffusion coefficients in water. For the low-molecular-weight solutes a mean slope of 1.24 was found (b) and for the proteins a mean slope of 2.37 (a). The patients are the same as those in Figure 78.2. (Reproduced, with permission, from ref. [13].)

Transport of electrolytes

The dialyzate concentration of sodium decreases during the initial phase of a dialysis dwell using hypertonic solutions, followed by a gradual rise (Figure 78.4 open circles) [10, 17]. It is likely that this dissociation between the transport of water and Na⁺ is caused by transcellular water entry into the peritoneal cavity or, alternatively, temporary binding of Na⁺ by the peritoneal interstitial tissue. The gradual rise in D/P ratio during the subsequent hours is caused by diffusion of sodium from the circulation into the dialysis fluid. The sieving of sodium, i.e. the removal of water in excess of sodium, can lead to hypernatremia when large amounts of hypertonic dialyzate are used during short exchanges.

The MTAC of potassium is about twice that of sodium. It is especially high during the first hour of exchange. The most probable explanation is release of K⁺ from cells that line the peritoneal cavity. This may be promoted by the initial low pH and the hyperosmolality of the dialyzate.

Transport of macromolecules

The dialyzate concentration of macromolecules that are transported from the circulation to the peritoneal cavity, is so low that their clearances are not influenced by saturation of the dialyzate (Figure 78.2). The clearance can therefore be used as an approximation of MTACs for that macromolecule. It is controversial whether the main transport mechanism of macromolecules during peritoneal dialysis is by convection, or by restricted diffusion. Regardless of the mechanism, the transport is size-selective [18]. Unlike the restriction coefficient for low-

molecular-weight solutes, the restriction coefficient for macromolecules exceeds 1.0 (Figure 78.3a). This indicates that the transport of macromolecules is hindered by a restriction barrier within the peritoneal membrane. Therefore, the clearance of macromolecules is determined by both surface area and solute permeability.

Differences between low-molecular-weight solutes and macromolecules in the relationship between MTACs and free diffusion coefficients permit the peritoneal membrane to be characterized in individual patients. The MTAC of creatinine represents the effective peritoneal surface area, and the restriction coefficient for macromolecules the solute permeability [16]. The effective surface area reflects the number of pores and the restriction coefficient mainly reflects the size of the large pores.

Solute transport from the peritoneal cavity

The clearance of intraperitoneally administered low-molecular-weight solutes from the dialyzate is size-selective, suggesting mainly a diffusive process. The average absorption of glucose in 4 h is 60%. Clearances after intraperitoneal administration exceed those when the same solute is given intravenously to the same patient by an average 1–2 ml/min, irrespective of the molecular weight. Assuming that the peritoneal restriction barrier is symmetric in its hindrance to diffusion, then a molecular weight-independent convective transport out of the peritoneal cavity of 1–2 ml/min should be present for intraperitoneally administered solutes. This is likely to reflect uptake into the lymphatic system. The contribution of convection relative to diffusion is small for low-molecular-weight solutes, but becomes increasingly more important the higher the molecular weight. The convection/diffusion ratio of intraperitoneally administered solutes is about 0.1 for glucose, 1.0 for inulin and 10 for proteins. As a consequence the disappearance rate of intraperitoneally administered macromolecules is virtually independent of molecular size. Their absorption during 4–7 h dwells averages 15%, partly directly into the subdiaphragmatic lymphatics that drain the peritoneal cavity, and probably also partly first into the interstitial tissues, and from these into the lymphatics that drain the interstitial tissues.

Fluid transport

Fluid transport during peritoneal dialysis is determined by hydrostatic and osmotic pressure, and by lymphatic drainage. Net ultrafiltration is the difference between transcapillary ultrafiltration and lymphatic absorption. The transcapillary ultrafiltration rate (TCUFR) is dependent on the hydraulic permeability and effective surface area of the peritoneum, and the hydrostatic, colloid (macromolecular) osmotic and crystalloid (small solute) osmotic pressure gradients. It can be written as:

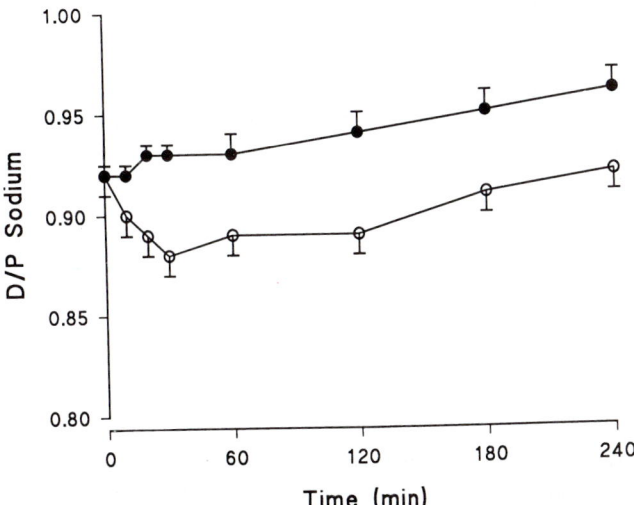

Figure 78.4 The dialyzate/plasma (D/P) ratios of sodium during a CAPD exchange with the dialyzate glucose 1.36% (closed circles) or glucose 3.86% (open circles). Mean values and SEM are given of the same 10 CAPD patients shown in Figure 78.2.

$$TCUFR = L_pA(\Delta P + \Delta\pi + \sigma\Delta O) \qquad (78.3)$$

where L_p is the hydraulic permeability of the membrane, A is the effective surface area, ΔP is the hydrostatic pressure gradient, $\Delta\pi$ is the colloid osmotic pressure gradient, ΔO is the crystalloid osmotic pressure gradient and σ is the osmotic reflection coefficient (see section on Physiology of solute transport). In this approach the peritoneum is regarded as a single membrane, so TCUFR is similar to the transperitoneal ultrafiltration rate and the ultrafiltration coefficient (L_pA) is not only that of the capillary wall but includes possible contributions of the peritoneal interstitium and the mesothelial layer. The hydrostatic pressure in peritoneal capillaries probably averages 17 mmHg. The opposing intraperitoneal pressure during peritoneal dialysis is dependent on the instilled dialyzate volume. It averages 8 mm Hg in the supine position when the peritoneal cavity is filled with 2 l of dialyzate, but exceeds 20 mmHg while walking. This indicates that net transcapillary hydrostatic pressure gradients are mainly dependent on the intraperitoneal pressure. The colloid osmotic pressure in capillaries is approximately 26 mmHg, leading to transcapillary fluid uptake which in the absence of an osmotic agent in the dialyzate would amount to about 0.4 ml/min.

The crystalloid osmotic pressure gradient between plasma and peritoneal fluid is mainly determined by glucose. Its effectiveness depends on the resistance the peritoneum exerts to its transport. This is expressed as the osmotic reflection coefficient (see section on Physiology of solute transport). Although the overall reflection coefficient of glucose is very low, it will approach 1.0 in the ultrasmall pores. This might explain why glucose is an effective osmotic agent in the peritoneal cavity despite its small size. Based on computer simulations it has been assumed that 40% of the filtered fluid volume passes through transcellular water channels during peritoneal dialysis [6]. The osmolality of commercial dialyzates when compared to that of uremic plasma is about 45 mosmol/kg H_2O higher for 1.36% glucose dialysate and 180 mosmol/kg H_2O higher for dialyzate containing 3.86% glucose. It follows from van't Hoff's law that in case of $\sigma = 1$, 1 mosmol creates an osmotic pressure at 37°C of 19.3 mmHg. When $\sigma = 0.03$ is assumed for the peritoneal membrane, the osmotic pressure that can be exerted by 1.36% glucose dialyzate is $45 \times 0.03 \times 19.3 = 26$ mmHg and, similarly 104 mmHg by 3.86% glucose dialyzate. These values are the maximum pressure gradients at the initial phase of an exchange. They will decrease with time due to absorption of glucose from the dialyzate. Typical values of fluid transport parameters using glucose 3.86% dialyzate are given in Table 78.2. The effective peritoneal surface area is an important determinant of the magnitude of transcapillary ultrafiltration. A large surface area leads to a high absorption rate of glucose and therefore a rapid disappearance of the osmotic gradient. This is supported by the inverse relationship between the MTAC of creatinine and the transcapillary ultrafiltration rate.

The lymphatic absorption rate from the peritoneal

Table 78.2 Typical values of fluid transport parameters during 4 h dwells using glucose 3.86% dialyzate

Parameters	Values
Ultrafiltration coefficient (ml/min/mmHg)	0.1–0.2
Reflection coefficient of glucose[a]	0.02–0.05
Maximum transcapillary ultrafiltration rate (ml/min)	12–16
Mean transcapillary ultrafiltration rate (ml/min)	3–4
Effective lymphatic absorption rate (ml/min)	1.2–1.4
Mean net ultrafiltration rate (ml/min)	1.5–3

[a] Obtained by comparison with solutions of different osmolalities.

cavity can be measured as the disappearance rate of an intraperitoneally administered macromolecular tracer, such as albumin or dextran [19]. The validity of this method has been questioned, because the appearance rate of radioactive labeled albumin in the circulation is only 20% of its disappearance rate. This difference can partly be explained by the fact that only 40–50% of the total albumin mass is intravascular. Also, a part of the tracer probably passes the mesothelium to the peritoneal interstitial tissue. Studies using continuous administration of dextran have made it likely, however, that subsequent uptake in the interstitial lymphatics occurs. Direct measurements of lymphatic flow from the peritoneal cavity have been made in conscious sheep and compared with albumin appearance and disappearance rates. These studies have not solved the problem, however, since not all lymphatic ducts could be cannulated, and because the recovery of radioactivity in peritoneal effluent, blood and drained lymphatics was nearly 100%. This would suggest no interstitial accumulation in sheep. Furthermore, the appearance rate was 60% of the disappearance rate, much higher than in humans.

An increase in intraperitoneal pressure raises the lymphatic drainage from the peritoneal cavity in the awake sheep model. Similar pressure increments increase the disappearance rate of macromolecules in humans and rats, but have no effect on their appearance rate in the circulation, suggesting that the disappearance rate of intraperitoneally administered macromolecules is the preferred way to assess lymphatic absorption in peritoneal dialysis patients. The disappearance of macromolecules is, however, not a measurement of lymph flow exclusively through subdiaphragmatic lymphatics. The disappearance rate must be regarded as a method to calculate the effective lymphatic absorption from the peritoneal cavity via all pathways of lymphatic drainage, subdiaphragmatic and interstitial. The term 'effective

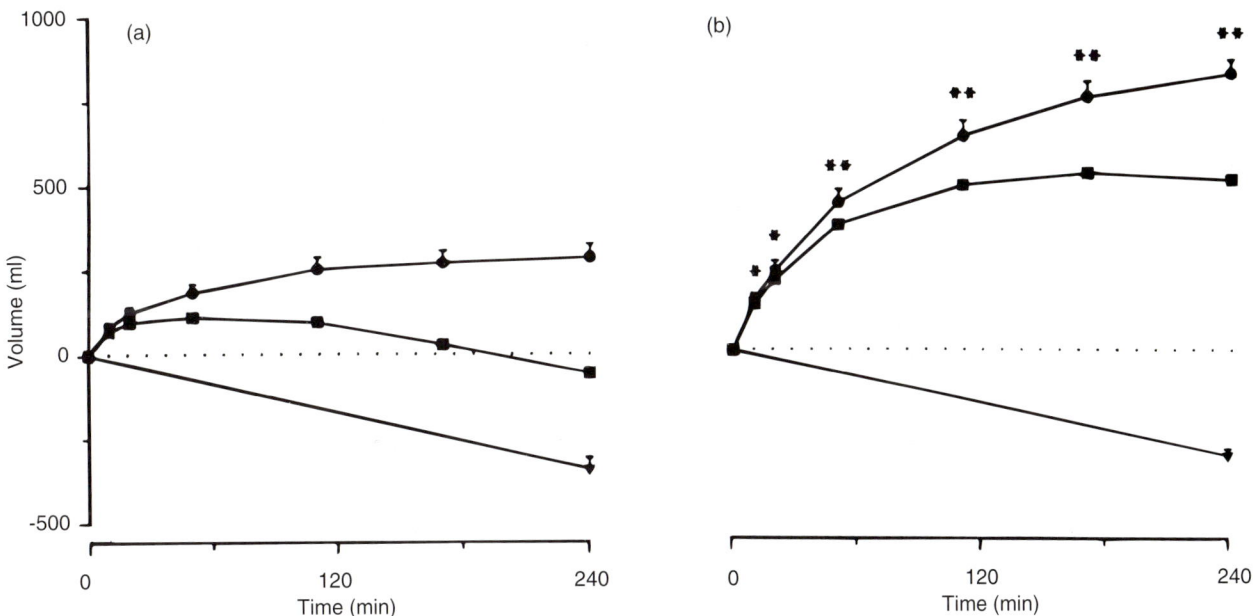

Figure 78.5   For ten patients (the same as in Figure 78.2) the time course of transcapillary ultrafiltration (circles), lymphatic absorption (triangles) (calculated from the dextran disappearance rate from the peritoneal cavity) and the resulting changes in intraperitoneal volume (squares) with glucose 1.36% dialyzate (a) and glucose 3.86% dialyzate (b) are given as mean values $\pm$ SEM. $*P < 0.001$, $**P < 0.001$ when compared to 1.36% glucose. (Reproduced, with permission, from ref. [13].)

lymphatic drainage' is used analogously to the use of effective renal plasma flow [20].

As a result of the combination of transcapillary ultrafiltration due to Starling forces and lymphatic drainage, the intraperitoneal volume initially increases to a maximum during an exchange, followed by an almost linear decrease (Figure 78.5). As a result net ultrafiltration may be negative at the end of a 4 h dwell using glucose 1.36% dialyzate, i.e. fluid may have been added to the body. Intraperitoneal pressure is one of the determinants of net ultrafiltration, not only because of its effect on transcapillary ultrafiltration, but also and especially because of its effect on effective lymphatic absorption. This has been shown by comparing 2 liter with 3 liter dialyzate exchanges and by application of external abdominal compression [19]. The effect of posture on net ultrafiltration is less pronounced, probably because in the upright position increased intra-abdominal pressure is counterbalanced by gravity which diminishes contact between dialyzate and subdiaphragmatic lymphatics.

Technology

Dialysis techniques

Intermittent peritoneal dialysis (IPD) was used primarily between 1960 and 1980. In its original form it consisted of two 20 h treatments a week, using hourly exchanges. Compared to daily treatments, IPD used in this way is quite inadequate. Uremic complications and malnutrition developed and IPD has therefore never been used on a large scale. Nowadays it is considered an historical treatment modality. Only in acute renal failure is IPD using short dwell exchanges still employed, but for much longer periods than 20 h. The introduction of continuous ambulatory peritoneal dialysis (CAPD) was an important turning point. It made peritoneal dialysis the renal replacement therapy of choice in many patients with end-stage kidney failure.

The most important feature of CAPD is the continuous presence of dialysis fluid within the peritoneal cavity (usually 2 liters), except for short intervals when replacement of the solutions takes place. This occurs three to five, mainly four times a day, every day. A typical CAPD scheme consists of exchanges during daytime with dwell times of 4–6 h and a single night dwell of 6–12 h (Figure 78.6). The sterile dialysis fluid is delivered in plastic bags that, in its original form, are used both for inflow of dialyzate and drainage. This is achieved by connecting the bags via an administration line on the peritoneal catheter. After inflow, the empty bag is carried attached to the patient, until the drainage procedure. After completion of drainage by gravity, the bag with the spent dialyzate is replaced by a new bag containing fresh dialysis fluid.

Near equilibrium between blood and dialyzate is reached after a dwell-time of 4 h for low-molecular-weight solutes, like urea (Figure 78.2). Thus longer dwell times are ineffective for the removal of urea, but are needed for larger molecules that diffuse more slowly such as the

Manual Peritoneal Dialysis

CAPD

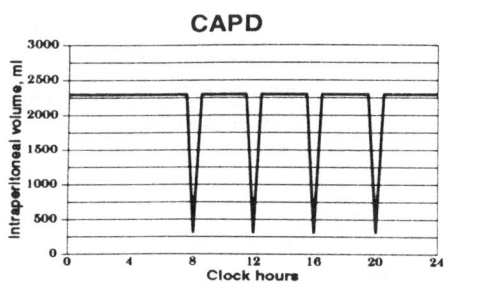

DAPD

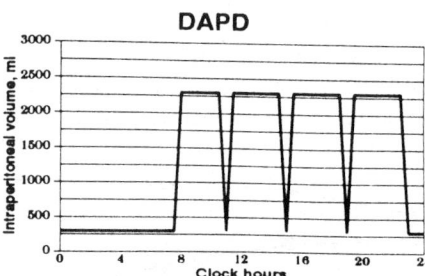

Automated Peritoneal Dialysis

CCPD (original)

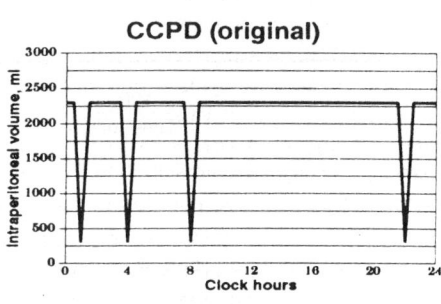

NPD or NIPD

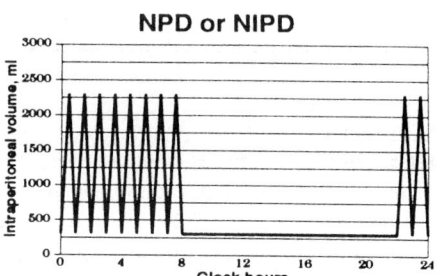

CCPD (high dose I)

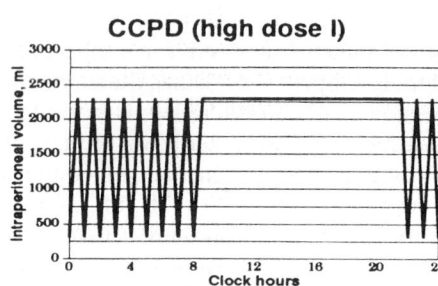

TPD

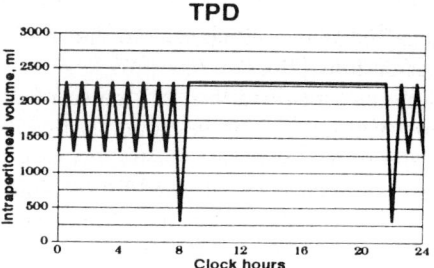

CCPD (high dose II)

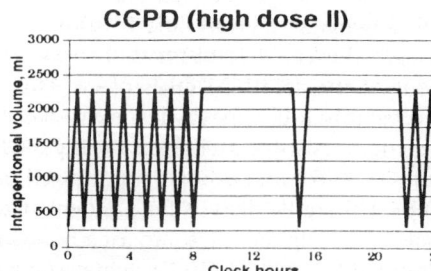

NTPD or NITPD

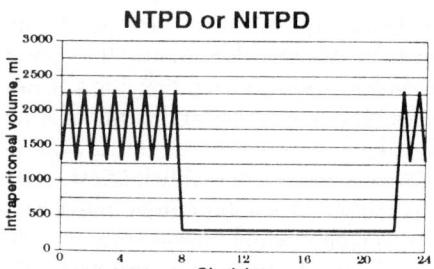

Figure 78.6 A schematic representation of the various manual and automated peritoneal dialysis schemes that are currently employed. CAPD, continuous ambulatory peritoneal dialysis; DAPD, daytime ambulatory peritoneal dialysis; CCPD, continuous cycling peritoneal dialysis (illustrated as three different modes); NPD or NIPD, nightly intermittent peritoneal dialysis; TPD, tidal peritoneal dialysis; NTPD and NITPD, nightly intermittent tidal peritoneal dialysis. For reasons of simplicity the intraperitoneal volume is assumed to remain constant during the dwell-time.

so-called 'middle-molecules'. These are uremic toxins with molecular weights ranging from 500 to 15'000'Da. The rapid diffusion of low-molecular-weight solutes means that net absorption of glucose from the dialyzate is most marked during the long night-dwell. In some patients this leads to a negative net ultrafiltration during the night. For this situation a modification of CAPD has been used, daily ambulatory peritoneal dialysis (DAPD), characterized by four exchanges of 4'h during the day only and an empty peritoneal cavity at night. This technique is less effective for the removal of urea, and markedly inferior to CAPD for removal of larger molecules.

Both CAPD and DAPD are dialysis techniques that are done manually. The development of easy-to-handle cyclers for peritoneal dialysis has led to various techniques for automated peritoneal dialysis (APD) [22]. All these techniques are based on daily treatment regimens. The various forms of manual and automated daily peritoneal dialysis are summarized in Figure 78.6. APD can either be intermittent (the peritoneal cavity is drained after the last exchange) or continuous (the peritoneal cavity is filled with dialysis fluid during the interval between the last exchange of the previous session and the first exchange of the next one). The latter is called 'last bag option'. The duration of the period of short exchanges is about 8h in most cases. The major difference between APD and CAPD is the ability with APD to increase the amount of dialysis delivery by increasing the number of cycles during treatment. This is only true to a certain extent, however, because by increasing the frequency of dwells, the peritoneal cavity will also be empty more often, because of the time needed for inflow and outflow of the dialysis fluid.

The continuous forms of APD are continuous cyclic peritoneal dialysis (CCPD) [23] and tidal peritoneal dialysis (TPD) [24]. CCPD in its original form consists of four exchanges during the night using 8 liters of dialyzate or less, followed by a long exchange during the day (Figure 78.6). This form is less effective in the removal of uremic toxins than CAPD. Therefore modifications of CCPD have been developed. CCPD high dose type 1 uses more short exchanges and more than 8l of dialyzate, while the day time period is unchanged. This approach is effective in patients with high MTAC rates due to a large peritoneal surface area. In these patients, however, the long day time dwell may cause negative net ultrafiltration. High-dose CCPD type 2 is identical to type 1 during the night, but one extra (manual) exchange is performed during the day. This increases solute removal and net ultrafiltration, but is more work for the patient. Tidal peritoneal dialysis (TPD) was developed to avoid the inefficiency of dialysis during the inflow and drainage period of the short exchanges (Figure 78.6). This is achieved by not draining the peritoneal cavity completely. The tidal peritoneal volume is usually about 50% of the instilled volume. The number of short exchanges during the night is usually similar to that in high dose CCPD type 1. The peritoneal cavity may be full (TPD) or empty (NTPD) during the day.

TPD is more efficient in the removal of small solutes than high dose CCPD type 1.

In summary, with the exception of patients with low drainage volumes due to impaired net ultrafiltration, CAPD remains the most efficient technique for the removal of creatinine and larger solutes. This is also the case for urea in patients with low or normal solute transport rates. In patients with high solute transport rates, high volume CCPD and TPD are the techniques that remove most urea. The intermittent forms of APD are nightly intermittent peritoneal dialysis (NPD or NIPD) and tidal intermittent nightly peritoneal dialysis (TNPD or TINPD). No last bag option is applied in these techniques, leaving the peritoneal cavity empty during daytime. This is favorable in patients with impaired net ultrafiltration caused by high solute transport rates, but it obviously decreases solute removal.

Medical indications for replacing CAPD with APD are (1) inadequate solute removal, (2) inadequate net ultrafiltration, (3) complications induced by increased intraperitoneal pressure, such as herniae and catheter exit site leaks, (4) low back pain, and (5) loss of appetite during dialysis. Some studies have reported a lower incidence of peritonitis during APD, probably due to the fewer disconnect procedures. Freedom from the dialysis procedure during daytime is the major non-medical indication. This is especially relevant for children and working adults. The disadvantages of APD are that the procedure is more difficult to learn, the technique is about 50% more expensive both due to the necessity of a cycler and to the larger amounts of dialyzate that are used.

Administration systems

The original CAPD administration systems consisted of a tube that was connected to the peritoneal catheter on one end and had a spike at the other. The spike was plugged into a plastic bag containing sterile dialysis fluid. The system remained closed between the start of inflow and end of drainage, but thereafter had to be opened because the spike had to be removed and plugged into a new bag. The use of this system was associated with an average rate of peritonitis of about one episode per six patient-months. The usual infective organisms were skin flora. Modifications, using either luer-lock connectors alone or embedded in polyvinylpyrrolidone iodine, melting connections, or devices to perform the disconnection procedure in an ultraviolet radiation box, led to a reduction in peritonitis frequency.

The most important development leading to a marked reduction in the incidence of peritonitis is the use of the 'flush-before-fill' technique, with or without a disinfectant [23]. In its original form, as developed in Italy, a Y piece is connected to the peritoneal catheter. One arm of the Y is used for drainage, the other part for administration of fresh dialyzate. Before the fresh dialyzate is allowed to enter the peritoneal cavity, a small volume is permitted to flow into the bag with the drained dialyzate, taking with it bacterial contamination that might have occurred during the connection. Various modifications of the Y set have been developed, like the O-set, the ANDY plus system and the twin-bag system. These last modifications allow disconnection of the empty dialyzate bag between exchanges closing the catheter with a cap or clip. This gives patients more freedom than they had with the original CAPD system since they had to carry the bag with them. With the use of these 'flush before fill' systems, the incidence of peritonitis has decreased to one episode per 18 patient-months [24].

Dialysis solutions

Peritoneal dialyzate are sterile electrolyte solutions. Most use lactate as buffer and glucose as osmotic agent. The pH must be 5.5 or less, to prevent caramelization of glucose during the sterilizing procedure. The concentration of sodium is 132–134 mmol/l and that of calcium and magnesium 1.75 mmol/l and 0.75 mmol/l, respectively. Recent dialysis fluids have been developed that contain lower concertrations of calcium and magnesium. Potassium is not a normal constituent of peritoneal dialysis fluid. The concentration of lactate is 35 mmol/l and that of glucose can range between 75 and 200 mmol/l. The osmolality of dialyzate with the lowest glucose concentration (1.36%) is 334 mosmol/kg H_2O and that of dialyzate with the highest concentration (3.86%) almost 500 mosmol/kg H_2O. It is noteworthy that these solutions are unphysiologic because of their acidity, hypertonicity and high glucose concentrations. Nevertheless they have been used with reasonably good results.

In vitro studies have shown that fresh dialysis fluid is toxic to cells normally present in the peritoneal cavity, such as mesothelial cells and macrophages. The combination of lactate and the low pH appears to explain most toxicity because *in vitro*, cells incubated in this solution exhibited a decrease of intracellular pH, which was not completely reversible [27]. These toxic effects were augmented by the hyperosmolality of the solutions. The high glucose concentration also has a detrimental effect on the viability and secretory functions of mesothelial cells. Heat sterilization of dialysis fluid can lead to the development of glucose-derived cytotoxic products. Non-enzymatic glycosylation of proteins may occur, which may explain the diabetiform-like alterations that are sometimes observed in peritoneal capillaries of CAPD patients. Besides these cellular and ultrastructural abnormalities, glucose has several other disadvantages more directly relevant to clinical practice. Its absorption from the peritoneal cavity means an extra caloric load and the risks of excessive weight gain and dyslipoproteinemia. The administration of insulin may be necessary in patients with impaired glucose tolerance.

The potentially harmful effects of lactate and glucose in dialysis solutions have led to a search for alternative buffers and osmotic agents. The introduction of acetate as a buffer was not an improvement, because it led to a high incidence of sclerosing peritonitis. The use of bicarbonate is technically difficult, because it cannot be sterilized in the presence of glucose, and because deposits of calcium and magnesium carbonate will form when the pH of the solution exceeds 7.5. Two different bicarbonate solutions are currently under investigation. One uses a double chamber system in which the bicarbonate-containing chamber is separated from that containing glucose, calcium and magnesium. A connection between the two chambers is made immediately before inflow in the peritoneal cavity. The solution is heat sterilized. The other solution under study is prepared in a single bag and uses glycylglycine, a dipeptide, as an additional buffer which prevents the pH from rising above 7.4 during storage. This solution is sterilized by a filtration procedure rather than heat. The use of both solutions is still in an experimental phase.

Mannitol, sorbitol and fructose have been tried as alternatives for glucose during intermittent peritoneal dialysis. Their use has been abandoned, however, because they either caused systemic hyperosmolality after absorption because of insufficient metabolismn, or else lactic acidosis. Glycerol (molecular weight 92 Da) has been used as an osmotic agent in CAPD patients [28]. Although the caloric value of the absorbed glycerol was lower than that of a glucose-based solution with a similar osmolality, the ultrafiltration induced by glycerol was lower. This was due to its more rapid absorption from the peritoneal cavity compared to glucose (molecular weight 180 Da). Long-term studies in diabetic CAPD patients have shown that glycerol is well-tolerated, and does not lead to hemolysis or hepatotoxicity. A hyperosmolar syndrome, however, has been described. Glycerol interferes with the laboratory determination of plasma triglyceride levels.

Amino acids (average molecular weight 145 Da) have been employed as osmotic agents in CAPD, especially for patients with malnutrition [29], but cannot be used for all exchanges, because of the increased urea load and the occurrence of metabolic acidosis. Promising results regarding nutritional status have been obtained using one or two exchanges per day of a 1.1% amino acid solution and a lactate concentration of 40 mmol/l. Another disadvantage is the rapid absorption of amino acids from the peritoneal cavity due to their low molecular weight. This makes them rather ineffective for ultrafiltration. Therefore the use of larger polypeptides is being investigated. The average molecular weight is still limited to 700–900 Da, because high-molecular-weight polypeptides have been associated with anaphylactic reactions. Malnutrition is the main indication for using amino acid dialysis solutions.

Icodextrin is the only high molecular weight osmotic agent currently in use in CAPD solutions [28]. It is a glucose polymer with an average molecular weight of 16000–20000 Da. An isosmotic solution produced sustained ultrafiltration throughout a 12 h dwell. This is probably due to colloid osmosis with fluid transport across the small intercellular pores (see section on fluid transport) such as that induced by albumin [31]. Macromolecular polymers of glucose are only slowly removed from the peritoneal cavity by the lymphatic system and are therefore especially effective during long dwells and in patients with impaired net ultrafiltration due to a large effective peritoneal surface area. In the latter patients a high number of pores is available for fluid transport, but this is mitigated by the rapid absorption of low molecular weight osmotic agents across these pores. In contrast, absorption of macromolecules is not influenced by the number of pores. It averaged 15% of the administered dose of icodextrin. In the circulation icodextrin is degraded by amylase to maltose. During the use of icodextrin the plasma level of maltose rises 20–30 times above the normal value in uremic plasma. The level remains stable, however, when only one exchange per day is used and declines within one week to the baseline level after discontinuation. This is also true after long-term use. Signs of toxicity have not been observed [32].

Until now, no glucose substitute has enough advantages to warrant routine use in peritoneal dialysis. Amino acids may be valuable in patients who are malnourished and macromolecules for those with impaired net ultrafiltration. Combinations of low-molecular-weight osmotic agents and macromolecules to maximize their advantages and minimize their disadvantages is the goal for the future.

References

1. Boen, S.T. (1961) Kinetics of peritoneal dialysis. *Medicine*, **4**, 243–87.
2. Esperanca, M.J. and Collins, D.L. (1966) Peritoneal dialysis efficiency in relation to body weight. *J. Paediatr. Surg.*, **1**, 162–9.
3. Dobbie, J.W. (1989) Morphology of the peritoneum in CAPD. *Blood Purif.*, **7**, 79–85.
4. Granger, D.N., Ulrich, M., Perry, M.A. and Kvietys, P.R. (1984) Peritoneal dialysis solutions and feline splanchnic blood flow. *Clin. Exp. Pharmacol. Physiol.*, **11**, 473–82.
5. Rippe, B. and Haraldsson, B. (1994) Transport of macromolecules across microvascular walls: the two-pore theory. *Physiol. Rev.*, **74**, 163–219.
6. Rippe, B. and Stelin, G. (1991) Simulations of peritoneal solute transport during CAPD. Application of two-pore formalism. *Kidney Int.*, **40**, 315–25.
7. Agre, P., Preston, G.M., Smith, B.L. *et al.* (1993) Aquaporin CHIP: the archetypal molecular water channel. *Am. J. Physiol.*, **265**, F463–76.
8. Ho-dac-Pannekeet, M.M. and Krediet, R.T. (1996) Water channels in the peritoneum. *Perit. Dial. Int.*, **16**, 255–9.
9. Rippe, B., Perry, M.A. and Granger, D.N. (1985) Permselectivity of the peritoneal membrane. *Microvasc. Res.*, **29**, 89–102.
10. Imholz, A.L.T., Koomen, G.C.M., Struijk, D.G. *et al.* (1994) Fluid and solute transport in CAPD patients using ultralow sodium dialysate. *Kidney Int.*, **46**, 333–40.
11. Nolph, K.D., Twardowski, Z.J., Popovich, R.P. and Rubin, J. (1979) Equilibration of peritoneal dialysis solutions during long-dwell exchanges. *J. Lab. Clin. Med.*, **93**, 246–56.
12. Twardowski, Z.J., Nolph, K.D., Khanna, R. *et al.* (1987) Peritoneal equilibration test. *Perit. Dial. Bull.*, **7**, 138–47.
13. Krediet, R.T., Boeschoten, E.W., Zuyderhoudt, F.M.J. *et al.* (1986) Simple assessment of the efficacy of peritoneal transport in continuous ambulatory peritoneal dialysis patients. *Blood Purif.*, **4**, 194–203.
14. Pannekeet, M.M., Imholz, A.L.T., Struijk, D.G. *et al.* (1995) The standard peritoneal permeability analysis: a tool for the assessment of peritoneal permeability characteristics in CAPD patients. *Kidney Int.*, **48**, 866–75.
15. Imholz, A.L.T., Koomen, G.C.M., Struijk, D.G. *et al.* (1993) The effect of dialysate osmolarity on the transport of low molecular weight solutes and proteins during CAPD. *Kidney Int.*, **43**, 1339–46.
16. Krediet, R.T., Zemel, D., Imholz, A.L.T. *et al.* (1993) Indices of peritoneal permeability and surface area. *Perit. Dial. Int.*, **13**(suppl 2), S31–4.
17. Heimburger, O., Waniewski, J., Werynski, A. and Lindholm, B. (1992) A quantitative description of solute and fluid transport during peritoneal dialysis. *Kidney Int.*, **41**, 1320–32.
18. Krediet, R.T., Koomen, G.C.M., Koopman, M.G. *et al.* (1989) The peritoneal transport of serum proteins and neutral dextran in CAPD patients. *Kidney Int.*, **35**, 1064–72.
19. Mactier, R., Khanna, R., Twardowski, Z. *et al.* (1987) Contribution of lymphatic absorption to loss of ultrafiltration and solute clearances in continuous ambulatory peritoneal dialysis. *J. Clin. Invest.*, **80**, 1311–16.
20. Krediet, R.T. (1994) Fluid absorption in the peritoneum – it is less simple than you thought. *Nephrol. Dial. Transplant.*, **9**, 341–3.
21. Imholz, A.L.T., Koomen, G.C.M., Struijk, D.G. *et al.* (1993) Effect of an increased intraperitoneal pressure on fluid and solute transport during CAPD. *Kidney Int.*, **44**, 1078–85.
22. Twardowski, Z.J. (1990) Peritoneal dialysis glossary III. *Perit. Dial. Int.*, **10**, 173–5.
23. Diaz-Baxo, J.A. (1989) Current status of continuous cyclic peritoneal dialysis (CCPD). *Perit. Dial. Int.*, **9**, 9–14.
24. Flanigan, M.J., Doyle, C., Lim, V.S. and Ullrich, G. (1992) Tidal peritoneal dialysis: preliminary experience. *Perit. Dial. Int.*, **12**, 304–8.
25. Swartz, R., Reynolds, J., Lees, P. and Rocher, L. (1989) Disconnect during continuous ambulatory peritoneal dialysis (CAPD): retrospective experience with three different systems. *Perit. Dial. Int.*, **9**, 175–8.
26. Churchill, D.N., Taylor, D.W., Oreopoulos, D.G. and

Canadian CAPD Clinical Trials Group (1989) Peritonitis in continuous ambulatory peritoneal dialysis (CAPD): a multi-centre randomized clinical trial comparing the Y connector disinfectant system to standard systems. *Perit. Dial. Int.*, **9**, 159–63.

27. Topley, N., Coles, G.A. and Williams, J.D. (1994) Biocompatibility studies on peritoneal cells. *Perit. Dial. Int.*, **14**(suppl 3), S21–8.

28. Matthys, E., Dolkart, R. and Lameire, N. (1987) Extended use of a glycerol-containing dialysate in diabetic CAPD patients. *Perit. Dial. Bull.*, **7**, 10–15.

29. Kopple, J.D., Bernard, D., Messana, J. *et al.* (1995) Treatment of malnourished CAPD patients with an amino acid based dialysate. *Kidney Int.*, **47**, 1148–57.

30. Mistry, C.D., Mallick, N.P. and Gokal, R. (1987) Ultrafiltration with an isosmotic solution during long peritoneal dialysis exchanges. *Lancet*, **ii**, 178–82.

31. Ho-dac-Pannekeet, M.M., Schouten, N., Langedijk, M.J. *et al.* (1996) Peritoneal transport characteristics with glucose polymer based dialysate. *Kidney Int.*, **50**, 979–86.

32. Mistry, C.D., Gokal, R., Peers, E. and the MIDAS Study Group, (1994) A randomized multicentre clinical trial comparing isosmolar dextran 20 with hyperosmolar glucose solutions in continuous ambulatory peritoneal dialysis (CAPD): a six months study. *Kidney Int.*, **46**, 496–503.

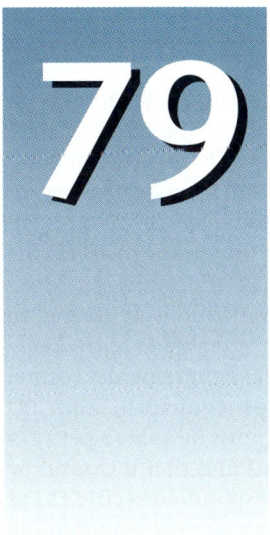

79

Management and assessment of peritoneal dialysis

Alastair J. Hutchison, John Harty, Linda Uttley and R. Gokal

Introduction

The number of patients on peritoneal dialysis over the last decade has shown a dramatic increase throughout the world. According to industrial sources there were, at the end of 1993, over 89 000 patients on peritoneal dialysis world-wide, representing some 17% of all dialysis patients. There have been enormous technological advances and our understanding of the anatomy of the peritoneum and the complex fluid and solute transport across it has increased greatly. Despite these factors, the long-term outlook for these patients remains uncertain. Peritoneal dialysis (PD) is now recognized as a primary form of dialytic therapy that compares favorably with hemodialysis. This chapter reviews aspects of patient management related to patient selection and organization of a PD program, management of metabolic and nutritional aspects, and the role of adequacy of dialysis.

Components of a successful PD program

Although peritoneal dialysis is a simple technique it is now generally accepted that it should be performed in the right setting with appropriate staff and facilities, and that it should be an integrated part of a wider renal replacement program [1]. The key to the successful management of a patient undergoing PD is a comprehensive and well-organized program. The essential components in such a program are a suitable location and training facilities, patient selection, nursing and medical expertise, training manuals and protocols for managing complications, organized and creative teaching methods for training patients, and above all, a committed multidisciplinary team.

Shared goals and philosophy regarding peritoneal dialysis among team members will promote cohesion and reduce conflict. The team usually includes physicians, nurses, dieticians and social workers but is often expanded to include surgeons, microbiologists, psychologists and rehabilitation specialists. Regular team meetings give the entire team the opportunity for interaction and mutual decision making, thus promoting good communication. Co-operation and the ability to work together are vital for optimal patient care [2].

Patient selection

The availability of continuous ambulatory PD (CAPD) makes a renal unit more flexible in managing a patient with end-stage renal failure. In spite of over 15 years of experience with CAPD, there is as yet no 'profile' of a perfect patient. Selection, therefore, becomes a process of assessing a multitude of factors both medical and psychosocial as shown in Table 79.1. For new patients starting dialysis therapy about a quarter are better suited to undergo hemodialysis (e.g. unsuitable abdomen, unable to perform the PD technique) and a similar percentage would be better managed by peritoneal dialysis (no vascular access, unstable cardiovascular state). This leaves about half the patients who would do equally well on

Nephrology, Edited by Rex L. Jamison and Robert Wilkinson.
Published in 1997 by Chapman & Hall, London. ISBN 0 412 60930 4

either therapy. What dictates this choice? There appears to be no logic in the practice of dialytic choice for the patient; world-wide usage of PD varies considerably from 5% in counties like Japan and Germany to 50% in the UK and 90% in Mexico. The reason for this wide discrepancy in usage does not appear to be related to the technique or medical factors alone. In an analysis of non-medical factors that seem to dictate patient selection for the type of dialysis therapy (Table 79.2) financial considerations and reimbursement were the most important [3]. It seems therefore, that patient selection is indeed a complex issue and heavily dependent on 'local' factors. What aspects are important in patients who are asessed and choose peritoneal dialysis treatment?

Peritoneal dialysis, being a home-based therapy, demands a degree of independence and ability to care for oneself (unless a member of the family or a nurse is available). PD has to be performed daily and the need for compliance with the routine may lead to complacency or 'burn-out'. Compromising the exchange procedure can lead to peritonitis. Therefore, it is important to assess the patient for characteristics that may affect success. Motivation is a crucial factor. The patient who is motivated to learn and regards the teaching as valuable is more likely to understand and comply with PD requirements. Formal education and intelligence are not required to learn PD procedures. However, the patient must be able to perform the procedures in sequence, understand that it cannot be varied, recognize problems and respond correctly. He or she must believe that dialysis is necessary to maintain life and realize the consequences of failure to perform the procedures accurately. A desire to remain independent is important; in high risk patients, such as those with diabetes, a strong social support system is an advantage. Other psychosocial factors that influence choice of PD are patient preference, distance from the dialysis center, occupation, concern with body image, and the need to travel.

Staffing and patient training

Every PD program should be directed by a nephrologist who is an expert in this field. Physicians should receive adequate training in all aspects of clinical management, based on a sound theoretical knowledge. The interna-

Table 79.1 Factors influencing patient selection

Medical factors	Psychosocial factors
Age	Patient preference
Diabetes mellitus	Motivation
Ischemic heart disease	Compliance
Extensive abdominal surgery	Family support
Severe pulmonary disease	Occupation
Lumbar disk problems	
Diverticulitis	

Table 79.2 Factors influencing modality selection

HD preferred	Either HD or CAPD	PD preferred
Severe inflammatory bowel disease	In center HD orientated	Unstable CVS
Third trimester pregnancy	Dependent life style	Poor vascular access
Severe active psychosis	Active diverticulitis	Severe anemia
Marked disability with no helper	Pulmonary disease	Age <5 years or elderly
Homeless	Large polycystic kidneys	Diabetes mellitus
	Severe recurrent hernias	Strong desire for independence
	Frequent and substantial changes to medical/ dialytic therapy	Distant from unit
	CAPD orientated	
	Independent life style	
	Transmissible disease	
	APD orientated	
	Same as CAPD plus	
	Days free from exchanges	
	More prescription flexibility	
	Social support filled by helper at home	
Unit	Unit/Home	Home

HD, hemodialysis; CAPD, continuous ambulatory peritoneal dialysis; PD, peritoneal dialysis; CVS, cardiovascular state.

tional Society of Peritoneal Dialysis has published guidelines stating that nephrology trainees should receive a minimum of three consecutive months training in PD supervised by a nephrologist with a special interest in this field [2].

The role of the nephrology nurse is pivotal and is expanding. To fulfill reimbursement and professional criteria it is becoming mandatory for nephrology nurses of possess additional higher qualifications such as the English National Board 136 Certificate in the UK or the Certified Nephrology Nurse credential in the US. The senior nurse in a unit will assess the projected workload and give advice on the staffing levels required. Studies suggest that the appropriate staff ratio for adequate care is one nurse per 15 PD patients [4]. The aim of nursing care is initially to teach the patient how to perform dialysis at home, and subsequently to provide continuing guidance and support. It is important to recruit nurses who believe in the principle of self care, who enjoy teaching and are committed to PD treatment. Nurses should have opportunities for continuing education, participation in research projects and attending national, and even international, meetings. Such opportunities alleviate 'burn-out', improve morale, increase job satisfaction and reduce staff turnover.

Nurses should base their teaching on a standard curriculum so that patient training is consistent. A training manual should be available for patients which encompasses essential protocols, procedures and other useful information. The manual should be simple and available in several languages, including Braille, depending on the case mix. Lectures and discussion are the primary modes of patient teaching along with demonstration and problem-solving. Aids such as videos, practice equipment, dummy torsos and computer-assisted learning packages can be utilized in the teaching process.

Regular home visits are an important feature of follow-up care. It is important that the family and patient realize that continuing support is available. In their homes patients are more able to discuss personal problems, for example psychosexual difficulties, with someone whom they trust. Early recognition and management of problems will assist in keeping the patient healthy, enable optimum rehabilitation and reduce outpatient visits and inpatient stays. Failure to make home visits inevitably decreases patient and staff confidence in the technique of PD.

Metabolic and nutritional management in PD

This section describes the assessment and management of calcium phosphate–parathyroid hormone homeostasis and its relationship to renal bone disease, acid–base status, anemia and its correction. Nutritional aspects of peritoneal dialysis are also covered.

Renal osteodystrophy

The classification of renal osteodystrophy is simplified by the recognition that there are essentially two groups of diseases. The different pattern of bone lesions seen in CAPD and hemodialysis is now well recognized [5], and there are several differences between the two dialysis modalities which may affect mineral metabolism [6]. CAPD is associated with far greater losses of middle- and large-molecular-weight proteins, thereby removing more transferrin-bound aluminum, and 25-hydroxy vitamin D_3. CAPD removes more phosphate and it provides an unvarying biochemical profile, unlike the 'saw-tooth' pattern of hemodialysis.

Calcium and phosphorus balance

Serum phosphate levels begin to rise and ionized calcium levels begin to fall once glomerular filtration rate is less than 20 ml/min [7]. These abnormalities can be at least partially corrected by the administration of oral calcium carbonate. Once CAPD has begun, gastrointestinal absorption and peritoneal flux of calcium are the two determinants of calcium mass-balance in PD patients.

Gastrointestinal absorption

If calcium salts are to be used as first line therapy for hyperphosphatemia then oral intake and gastrointestinal absorption will be necessarily high. Once a patient is established on CAPD, control of hyperphosphatemia is very important, not only to minimize further stimulation of parathyroid hormone (PTH) secretion, but also to keep the calcium phosphate product in the normal range. Failure to limit the calcium phosphate product may result in vascular and soft tissue calcification. The CAPD patient's high protein diet (recommended minimum protein intake 1.2 g/kg/day) provides an obligatory phosphate intake of up to 1200 mg daily. Peritoneal dialysis removes only 310–320 mg/day – less than one-third of the amount required to bring phosphate levels into the normal range. Therefore the fraction of phosphate absorbed must be reduced by oral phosphate-binding agents.

The role of calcium salts in renal osteodystrophy

Of the available phosphate binders suitable for clinical use, only three are now widely prescribed – aluminum hydroxide, calcium carbonate and calcium acetate. Now that the dangers of aluminum accumulation have become apparent, calcium carbonate is probably the most common phosphate binder used in patients with end-stage renal disease, in whom maintenance of optimal serum calcium and phosphate levels is central to the treatment of hyperparathyroidism. Unfortunately calcium salts frequently result in hypercalcemia so that aluminum-containing phosphate binders continue to be used. If aluminum salts are to be avoided, hypercalcemia associated with calcium salts must be prevented. Reduction of dialysis fluid calcium concentration is one means of achieving this end and has been shown to be effective in CAPD patients [8, 9].

Factors contributing to the production of excess parathyroid hormone in dialysis patients are shown in Figure 79.1. Maintenance of a high normal serum ionized calcium and control of hyperphosphatemia will suppress PTH production, even in patients not taking vitamin D_3. [9a]. This is desirable in patients with high PTH levels, but not necessarily in patients with normal, or mildly elevated levels. Many of the latter patients will have the adynamic bone lesion, and a small rise in PTH levels may be beneficial. One method of achieving a modest increase in PTH is to allow the serum ionized calcium to fall below the 'set point' for calcium-mediated PTH release, but at the same time maintaining strict control of serum phosphate. This is not easy when the calcium supplement and phosphate binder are one and the same tablet, but is facilitated by the availability of reduced calcium (1.25 mmol/l) dialysis fluid [9b]. In this way, hypercalcemic suppression of PTH can be minimized, while allowing the ingestion of sufficient calcium carbonate to control serum phosphate.

Control of serum phosphate is not only important in terms of its effect on PTH, but also for prevention, and sometimes treatment, of extraskeletal ('metastatic') calcification. This potentially lethal aspect of renal osteodystrophy is a particular hazard in patients who have persistent hypercalcemia and hyperphosphatemia.

Peritoneal flux and reduced calcium dialysis fluid

Patients using dialysis solutions containing 1.75 mmol/l of calcium are in positive calcium balance even before considering the gut absorption from oral calcium carbonate and vitamin D. A calcium concentration of 1.25 mmol/l would appear to be the logical choice for a new standard CAPD fluid because it is close to normal serum ionized calcium levels. This results in a homeostatic effect, with calcium lost to the peritoneum when serum levels are above 1.25 mmol/l, but absorbed from the peritoneum during times of relative hypocalcemia [10].

Acid–base balance

There is considerable evidence that as renal acid excretion fails, bone mineral stores become an important buffer. Carbonic anhydrase is present in osteoclasts, and may be activated by PTH to promote bone resorption by release of H^+ ions. The availability of bone buffers and bicarbonate depends on the activity of PTH. During a time of prolonged metabolic acidosis, as exists in many CAPD patients using PD fluid with 35 mmol/l lactate, buffering by bone would be linked to bone resorption and increased PTH levels.

PD fluid containing 40 mmol/l lactate corrects the mild acidosis in most CAPD patients using the lower lactate concentration common in most European countries. Optimal correction of acidosis has been shown to slow the progression of high turnover osteodystrophy in hemodialysis and CAPD patients.

Parathyroid hormone and vitamin D

Until recently, the prescription of CAPD treatment was not tailored to the individual needs of the patient. As a result, the majority were treated with four 2 liter exchanges, a phosphate binder, vitamin supplements and a small oral dose of 1,25-dihydroxyvitamin D_3. PTH levels were rarely measured, and the dosage of calcitriol was changed only if hypercalcemia occurred or evidence of osteitis fibrosa appeared on plain radiology of the hands.

Maintenance of a high serum ionized calcium (1.2–1.3 mmol/l) and strict control of serum phosphate, from the time of first starting dialysis, decreases PTH levels in CAPD patients without the addition of vitamin D_3 therapy [11] but it is now apparent that such suppression can result in a hitherto infrequently recognized form of renal osteodystrophy, the non-aluminum-related, or 'idiopathic', adynamic bone disease. Hence the question is not only 'what is the best way to suppress PTH?', but also 'can PTH be over suppressed?'

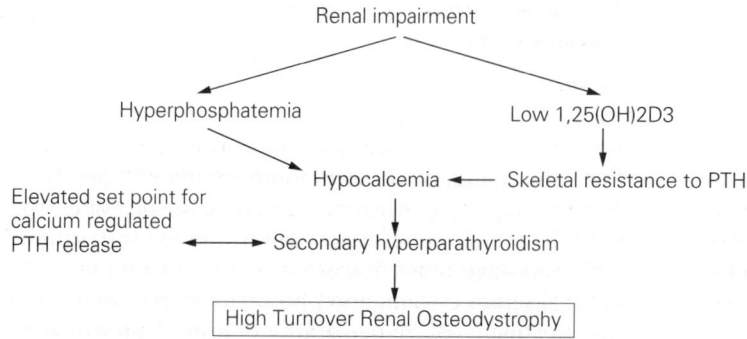

Figure 79.1 Factors contributing to hyperparathyroidism in dialysis patients.

Table 79.3 Associations of the idiopathic adynamic bone lesion

Clinical
    Age >50 years
    Diabetes mellitus
    Commoner in CAPD than hemodialysis patients
Biochemical
    Low/normal parathyroid hormone
    High/normal ionized calcium
    Low/normal bone alkaline phosphatase and other
        markers of bone turnover
Radiological
    Increased incidence of vascular calcification

Vitamin D metabolism is abnormal in uremia, with very low plasma concentrations of 1,25-dihydroxyvitamin D_3. 25-Hydroxyvitamin D_3 levels are usually normal at the start of CAPD but begin to decline thereafter [12, 13]. This is not unexpected since the dialysis effluent contains significant amounts of vitamin D binding protein, an α_2-globulin of 59 000 Da, which binds 1,25-dihydroxyvitamin D_3, 25-hydroxyvitamin D_3 and 24,25-dihydroxyvitamin D_3. Losses of 1,25-dihydroxyvitamin D_3 and 24,25-dihydroxyvitamin D_3 average 6–8% of the plasma pool per day. CAPD patients require two to three times the maintenance of vitamin D_3 doses in hemodialysis patients to return serum levels of 1,25-dihydroxyvitamin D_3 to normal. Given orally, these doses frequently produce hypercalcemia when given daily. In CAPD patients with serum PTH levels of greater than 400 pg/ml there is increasing evidence that the best way to administer oral vitamin D is in once or twice weekly pulses which reduce the incidence of hypercalcemia [14], a technique now being adopted in many centers.

The discovery of a non-calcemic calcitriol analog, 22-oxa-calcitriol, may alter therapeutic strategies once again in the near future, although no studies of its use in humans have yet been reported.

The idiopathic adynamic bone lesion

The spectrum of bone disease has changed over the last 10 years with the emergence of the adynamic bone lesion and the welcome decline in the use of aluminum-containing phosphate binders. The association of adynamic bone with low PTH levels has resulted in a reassessment of attempts to suppress serum PTH to 'normal' levels in both predialysis and dialysis patients [15, 16] and acknowledgment that blanket prescription of continuous low dose oral calcitriol therapy for all dialysis patients is unwise [17].

Adynamic bone is associated with the clinical and biochemical features shown in Table 79.3. Sherrard et al. [18] noted that the adynamic bone lesion was the common-est histological diagnosis in 267 dialysis patients [18], and that it occurred more frequently in PD (61%) than in hemodialysis patients (36%). This may be due to the more sustained, higher plasma calcium levels associated with PD which may result in more effective suppression of PTH than the more variable calcium levels of hemodialysis.

In our patients we have found an association between adynamic bone and vascular calcification, which may be related to the higher serum calcium levels in patients with this lesion. This is of concern since renal transplantation may be impossible when vascular calcification is severe. It seems likely that adynamic bone is more prone to the osteoporotic effects of high dose steroid immunosuppression, including avascular necrosis of the femoral head. If this is the case, then it would be very important to allow PTH levels in dialysis patients to rise slightly and stimulate bone turnover, while maintaining control of serum phosphate. This might also induce resorption of vascular calcium deposits.

Tailoring of vitamin D therapy requires the clinician to examine the patient's serum calcium, phosphate and PTH levels, in conjunction with bone histology in certain cases. On the basis of these findings individual treatment can be planned along the lines of the clinical algorithm shown in Figure 79.2.

Recommendations for management of osteodystrophy in CAPD

Techniques for monitoring renal osteodystrophy in CAPD patients are still evolving but certain recommendations can be made, given the present state of understanding (Table 79.4).

Biochemical monitoring

The most widely available, and generally useful marker at present, is intact PTH, which should be measured every three or four months in all CAPD patients. Regular measurement of total alkaline phosphatase is unnecessary, although it will continue to be performed as part of the 'liver screen'. More recently measurement of serum osteocalcin has become possible, providing a marker of osteoblast activity, as well as tartrate resistant acid phosphatase (TRAP) which is a marker of osteoclast activity.

Radiological monitoring

Routine, full skeletal surveys are unnecessary, and should be replaced by regular monitoring of serum PTH, plain radiographs of the hands and a lateral view of the lumbar spine [19]. This would greatly reduce the dose of radiation received by CAPD patients without detriment to patient care, and save money. Some measurement of skeletal bone density should be made at the time of starting dialysis (quantitative CT scan, single or dual photon absorptiometry or dual energy X-ray absorptiometry) in all patients so that those with subnormal bone density

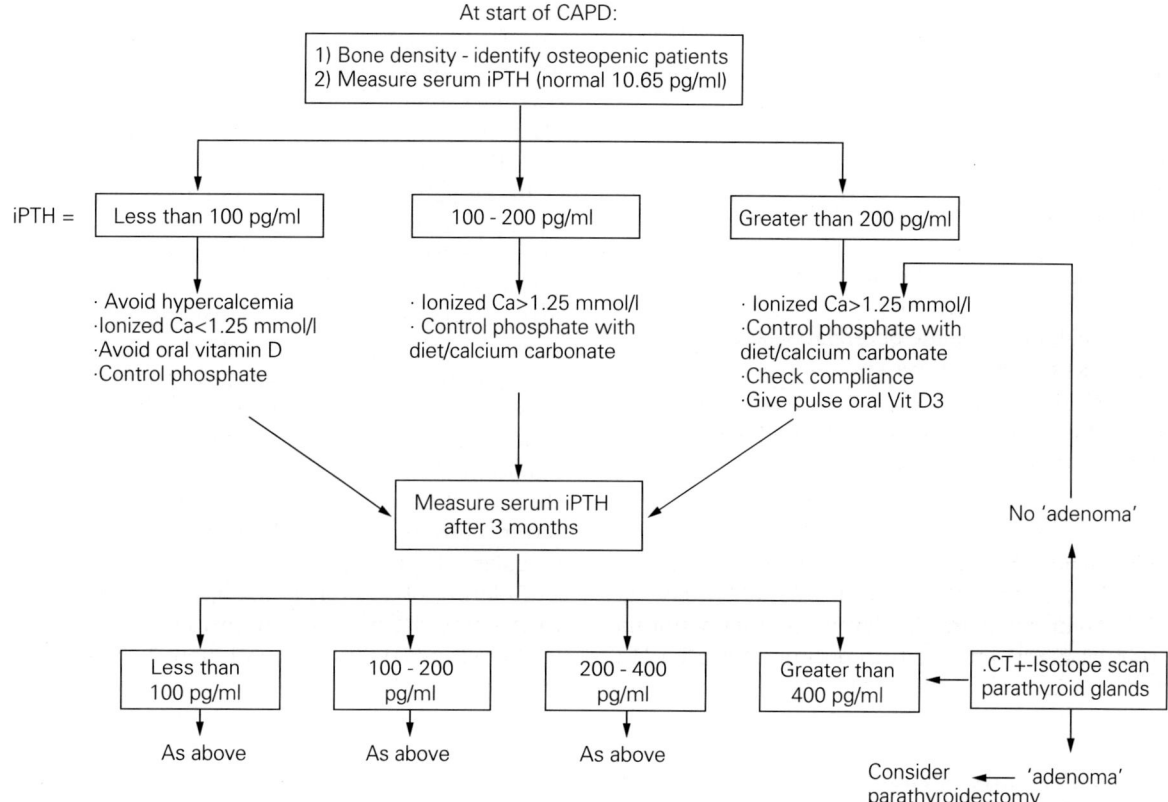

Figure 79.2 Clinical algorithm for the monitoring and management of renal osteodystrophy in CAPD patients.

can be identified and special efforts made to restore bone mass.

Transiliac bone biopsy

Bone biopsy with tetracycline labeling is the only reliable method of diagnosing the type and severity of renal osteodystrophy. It is rarely performed in clinical practice because of patients' and doctors' perceptions of its painfulness and invasiveness, although in centers where it is regularly performed, complications are uncommon. However, it should usually be undertaken before parathyroidectomy, to accurately define the bone lesion and quantitate the aluminum burden.

These recommendations can be formed into a clinical algorithm (Figure 79.2). The implementation of this scheme depends first on maximal restriction of dietary phosphate, within the limitations of a diet providing 1.2 g protein/kg body weight/day, and secondly on the routine use of CAPD fluid with a calcium concentration of 1.25 mmol/l, magnesium of 0.25 mmol/l and lactate of 40 mmol/l. Calcium carbonate should be given in doses adequate to maintain serum phosphate below 1.8 mmol/l and aluminum-containing binders should be avoided. Serum ionized calcium and iPTH should be measured every three months to provide a guide for treatment with oral calcitriol.

Use of these guidelines should enable good control of divalent ion metabolism, and prevention or amelioration of osteodystrophy in the majority of CAPD patients.

Erythropoietin

The indications for, and monitoring of erythropoietin (EPO) therapy in CAPD patients are like those in hemodialysis patients. Similar benefits have been demonstrated in subjective quality of life assessments, cognitive function, cardiac function, exercise tolerance and sexual function. The potentially harmful effects of repeated blood transfusion are minimized. Whereas many hemodialysis patients receive their EPO intravenously, this is not practical for CAPD patients and therefore the subcutaneous and intraperitoneal routes have been investigated.

Intraperitoneal administration of EPO is effective in raising hemoglobin concentration and hematocrit, but requires a larger dose compared to subcutaneous or intravenous administration. In addition, injecting EPO into CAPD bags increases the likelihood of introducing infection.

Although the bioavailability of subcutaneous EPO appears to be low and absorption variable, subcutaneous administration is more effective than intravenous probably due to a more sustained plasma concentration.

Table 79.4 Recommendations for the management of renal osteodystrophy in adult CAPD patients (see also Figure 79.2)

1. Restrict dietary phosphate, as far as possible within the confines of a 1.2 g/kg/day protein diet.
2. Use 1.25 mmol/l (2.5 mEq/l) calcium dialysis fluid to minimize hypercalcemia. Individual patients may require higher or lower concentrations depending on serum ionized calcium (or total corrected calcium) and phosphate levels.
3. Prescribe calcium carbonate/acetate twice daily with main meals. Titrate dose to serum calcium and phosphate levels. Educate patients to distribute dose according to phosphate intake.
4. Measure serum parathyroid hormone every three months (Figure 79.2) and use pulse oral vitamin D_3 therapy if necessary. Replace 25-hydroxyvitamin D_3 if serum levels are low.
5. Measure serum magnesium and aluminum every six months, unless patient is taking oral aluminum (then measure every three months).

Table 79.5 Mechanisms of protein-calorie malnutrition in CAPD patients

Decreased intake
1. Anorexia
   (a) Increased intra-abdominal pressure
   (b) Inadequate dialysis/loss of residual renal function
   (c) Fluid overload
   (d) Coexisting gastrointestinal disease (reflux, peptic ulcer disease, gastroparesis)
   (e) Coexisting comorbidity (cardiac failure, chronic pulmonary disease, hyperparathyroidism)
   (f) Depression
2. Financial constraints
3. Iatrogenic
   (a) Inappropriate or excessive dietetic restriction
   (b) Medication (phosphate binders, antihypertensive therapy)
4. Peculiarities of patient's food preferences

Increased loss
1. Daily peritoneal protein loss
2. Peritonitis

Altered metabolism
1. Metabolic acidosis
2. Inadequate dialysis
3. Physical inactivity
4. Intercurrent disease
5. Peritonitis
6. Hyperparathyroidism

Dosage reductions of up to 30% may be possible compared to the intravenous route, and once weekly dosing is probably as effective as twice weekly [20]. Injection into the thigh results in more rapid absorption, higher peak concentrations and greater bioavailability than injection into the arm or abdomen [21]. Maintenance of an adequate iron supply is essential for an optimal EPO response, and if necessary iron may be given intravenously although this requires a brief hospital admission.

Nutrition in PD patients

There is a high prevalence of malnutrition in CAPD patients. Studies indicate that mild to moderate malnutrition is prevalent in 30–35% and severe malnutrition in 8–10% [22]. Though improvement in body composition and dietary protein intake has been demonstrated during the first year of CAPD, prospective studies show a reduction in total body nitrogen, especially in male patients with large protein stores [23].

The etiology of protein-calorie malnutrition is complex and involves the triad of inadequate intake, periods of increased catabolism and non-replenished losses (Table 79.5). A daily target for dietary protein intake of 1.2 g/kg body weight and calorie intake of 35 kcal/kg/day has been recommended, based on nitrogen balance experiments [24]; however, the majority of patients do not consume this much and their intake diminishes by as much as 30% with time on CAPD [25]. There is evidence to suggest a link between adequacy of small solute clearance, appetite and dietary protein intake. In particular there is greater preservation of residual renal function in well-nourished CAPD patients [26].

In CAPD patients 5–15 g/day of protein is lost in the dialyzate increasing to 30–100 g/day with peritonitis. This loss has been linked to hypoalbuminaemia. In addition, physical inactivity, metabolic acidosis and recurrent peritonitis are important catabolic factors in CAPD patients.

Malnutrition and outcome

Establishing a relationship between nutrition and outcome is complicated because malnutrition may simply reflect adverse comorbid conditions. However, several studies have implicated malnutrition as an independent risk factor for morbidity (peritonitis, hospitalization) and death. The majority of reports indicate that serum albumin (either average levels over the duration of the study or initial values at start of CAPD) is a predictor of mortality [27]. Baseline total body nitrogen has also been shown to predict mortality [23], and serum albumin values of less than 35 g/l have been shown to be a predisposing risk factor for peritonitis.

Table 79.6 Assessment of nutritional status in CAPD patients

Body composition
    Anthropometry (skinfold thickness, mid-upper arm circumference, body mass index)
    Bioelectrical impedance
    Total body potassium
    Total body nitrogen
    Dual energy X-ray absorptiometry (DEXA)
    Total body water (isotope dilution techniques)
    Creatinine kinetics

Biochemistry
    Blood chemistry (urea, creatinine, lipids, amino acids)
    Visceral proteins (albumin, prealbumin, transferrin, IGF-1)
    Muscle protein and DNA

Nutritional intake
    Food diaries, 24 h recall
    Protein nitrogen appearance (PNA) from dialyzate and urine

Immunological measures
    Total lymphocyte count, C3, delayed hypersensitivity

Muscle function
    Hand grip dynamometry

Nutritional index
    Subjective global assessment technique
    Composite nutritional index

Assessment of nutritional status
(Table 79.6)

Assessment of nutritional state and identification of malnutrition is an integral part of CAPD patient management, and it is important to identify those at highest risk. Nutritional status can be assessed on a number of levels; from body composition, serum proteins, dietary intake and muscle function [28]. Individual measures of body composition and visceral proteins are not interchangeable and all are influenced by hydration. There are a number of techniques used to measure body composition. Anthropometry is simple and values for individual patients can be compared to reference standards. However, this method is influenced by observer error and may not be as sensitive to subtle changes over time. Bioelectrical impedance measures the resistance and reactance to the passage of an electrical current by lean tissue, fat tissue and body fluid. It is, however, influenced by hydrational state and may be inaccurate in patients with volume overload. Total body potassium and nitrogen have been used to measure fat free mass in CAPD patients. Total body nitrogen is more accurate and has been shown to be a precise and reproducible indicator of muscle mass; however, the general lack of availability and cost preclude routine use of both these techniques. Dual energy X-ray absorptiometry (DEXA) directly measures fat tissue mass, lean tissue mass and total body bone mineral. Although influenced by hydration, this technique is able to quantify body composition in individual body compartments. DEXA is an expensive technique and its use is reserved as a research tool. Water occupies a fixed percentage of fat free mass (73.2%) and total body water can be used as an index of body composition using isotope dilution techniques. Determination of lean body mass from creatinine excretion is based on the principle that creatinine production is proportional to lean body mass. However, creatinine production is also determined by dietary protein ingestion and recent data have revealed an unacceptably high coefficient of variation in results. Consequently it is now felt that thus technique is not a valid method by which to assess lean body mass [28a].

Biochemical assays of creatinine and visceral protein reflect nutritional state; however, serum concentration is also influence by hydration.

Cell-mediated immunity, measured by delayed hypersensitivity skin testing, is influenced by nutrition but this technique can only be deemed a general marker of nutritional state.

Assessment of muscle composition (muscle DNA, and muscle alkali soluble proteins) provides a useful marker of body protein status independent of hydrational state. Its use is reserved as a research technique. Muscle function can be measured by measuring hand-grip dynometry or more accurately by measuring the contractile characteristics of the adductor pollicis muscle. The latter technique has been shown to be a sensitive measure of nutritional deprivation and repletion.

The above techniques provide absolute values for nutritional measures. Nourished and malnourished patients can be identified using a nutritional index. Such indexes allocate 'scores' to validated anthropometric, biochemical and clinical nutritional criteria. Patients can be subsequently graded into a number of nutritional categories based on their total index score.

Routine screening should include anthropometric measurement of triceps skinfold thickness and mid-upper arm circumference, grading of nutritional status using the subjective global assessment technique and measurement of serum albumin. Though dietary protein intake can be estimated from the dialyzate (and urine) urea appearance rate, three-day dietary histories taken by a skilled dietician provide the most accurate measure of protein intake and are the only way to assess dietary calorie ingestion.

More sensitive techniques using DEXA, isotope dilutional methods and muscle biopsy should be reserved as research tools.

Management of protein-calorie malnutrition

Table 79.7 presents a standardized approach to malnutrition in the CAPD population.

Dietary supplementation

Patients should be prescribed a dietary protein intake of 1.2 g/kg/day which should contain a high proportion of animal protein to provide essential amino acids [29]. Dietary intake should be individualized to the needs of the patient, with early use of oral supplementation of deficient vitamins, trace elements and in particular, protein. Parenteral nutrition has been shown to be of benefit and should be considered for catabolic illness requiring hospitalization, e.g. during severe peritonitis especially in malnourished patients [30].

Intraperitoneal amino acids

The use of amino acids as an alternative osmotic agent for glucose offers the potential advantage of providing an additional 3–4 g of amino acids (8–10 g of protein) per day using one to two exchanges of this solution. Studies using a 1.1% amino acid solution containing an increased amount of lactate (40 mmol/l) have demonstrated short-term improvement in nitrogen balance and increase in creatinine and serum transferrin [31]. Side effects of amino acids include metabolic acidosis, an increase in serum urea and nausea in some patients. The long-term role of this therapy, however, remains to be evaluated.

Optimize dialysis

Inadequate dialysis in CAPD patients may result in a reduction in protein and calorie intake to a level insufficient to maintain nitrogen balance resulting in protein catabolism and muscle wasting. Enhancement of dialysis dose is limited in CAPD and may require automated peritoneal dialysis to facilitate an increase in small solute clearance. Patients who lose residual renal function should be prescribed larger dialyzate volumes. Transfer to hemodialysis should be considered only if failure to tol-

Table 79.7 Prevention and treatment of malnutrition in CAPD

1. Identification of 'at risk' groups
    Elderly
    Diabetes mellitus
    Recurrent peritonitis
    Active comorbid conditions including depression
    Loss of residual renal function

2. Screening

	Method	Malnutrition risk
Monitor dietary protein and calorie intake	3 day diet histories 24 h PD + urine PNA	<0.8 g/kg IBW/day <35 kcal/kg IBW/day
Anthropometrics	Mid-upper arm circ, skinfolds, arm muscle area Dry weight	<15th percentile = mild – mod. malnut., <5th = severe malnutrition. <80% IBW (NHANES)
Serum albumin		<30 g/l

3. Possible interventions
    Exclude occult gastrointestinal disease
    Increase intake
    Parenteral nutrition
    Correction of acidosis
    Modification of dialysis dose (if lose residual renal function)
    Intraperitoneal amino acids
    Erythropoietin, growth hormone

Abbreviations: PD, peritoneal dialysate; PNA, protein nitrogen appearance rate; IBW, ideal body weight; NHANES, National Health and Nutrition Examination Surveys.

erate this increase is associated with uremic symptoms or a reduction in nutritional status.

Vitamins and trace elements

Deficiency in the water-soluble vitamins (pyridoxine (B_6), thiamine (B_1), folic acid and ascorbic acid (C)) has been reported in CAPD patients as a result of inadequate dietary intake and loss in dialysis fluid and may disturb lipid and amino acid metabolism. Supplementation with 10–15 mg of B_6, 30–40 mg of B_1, 500 µg of folic acid and 200 mg of vitamin C corrects these deficiencies [29]. Serum levels of fat-soluble vitamins (A, D, E and K) are normal or high in CAPD patients and routine supplementation is not recommended. Prescription of vitamin D or its analogs should be reserved for prevention and control of hyperparathyroidism. Little is known about the consequences of deficiency in zinc, copper and bromine observed in CAPD patients, though supplementation of zinc should be considered in patients with anorexia and profound muscle weakness.

Disorders of lipids
(see also Chapter 38)

Lipid abnormalities in CAPD patients are superimposed on the background of uremic dyslipoproteinemia [29]. This combination of increased serum triglycerides and cholesterol and reduction in high density lipoprotein (HDL) cholesterol is not corrected by CAPD. Triglycerides are elevated in 60–80% and cholesterol in 15–30% of CAPD patients. Lipid status may worsen on commencement of CAPD; a correlation has been noted between an increase in very low density lipoprotein (VLDL) and low density lipoprotein (LDL) and intraperitoneal glucose absorption [29]. Most changes in lipoprotein metabolism are transitory, peaking in the first year and then subsiding. Eventually the lipid pattern resembles that seen in the predialysis uremic state. Nevertheless there is concern that the abnormal lipid status may induce or aggravate existing atherogenesis. Standard dietary therapy may be of limited use in view of the high prevalence of malnutrition and suboptimal calorie and protein intake in this population. Long-term studies of lipid-lowering agents are required to assess their impact on atherogenesis.

Disturbance of carbohydrate metabolism

Uremia is associated with abnormalities in carbohydrate metabolism manifest by glucose intolerance, hyperinsulinemia and a decreased peripheral sensitivity to insulin. In CAPD 60–80% (100–150 g) of the glucose present in the dialyzate solution is absorbed, accounting for 500–800 kcal/day. As a consequence of this continuous glucose load there is a persistent trend in CAPD patients to hyperglycemia and hyperinsulinemia. Hyperinsulinemia may be an additional risk factor for atherogenesis

during long-term therapy and has spurred interest in alternative osmotic agents.

Dialysis adequacy

With patients continuing on CAPD for prolonged periods, and an increasing number of studies demonstrating a relationship between small solute clearance and survival, the assessment of dialysis adequacy in CAPD patients is becoming increasingly important.

Measurement of dialysis adequacy

Clearances of urea and creatinine are used as markers of dialysis dose [32]. Daily dialysis clearance, K, is calculated from the formula

$$K = (D/P) \times (V_d/t)$$

where D = dialysate concentration of urea or creatinine (mmol/l), P = plasma concentration of urea or creatine expressed in mmol/l. V_d = volume of drained dialyzate in 24 h (ml), t = 1440 min.

To compare clearance values between patients, the clearance value is corrected for patient size.

For urea, the volume of urea distribution (V (liters)) calculated from the Watson nomogram, is used. Kt (urea clearance (liters /day)) is divided by V (liters) to produce the dimensionless ratio Kt/V. Creatinine clearance is normalized to body surface area (BSA) in square meters by the formula;

$$K \times 1.73/\text{BSA}$$

The normalization of small solute clearance in this fashion stems from the tradition in hemodialysis practice to normalize urea clearance to urea space and creatinine clearance to body surface area.

In calculating clearance for patients on automated dialysis (nightly intermittent PD and continuous cycling PD) it is important to use the mean of the pre- and post-dialysis serum urea or creatinine values. It is standard practice to express clearance as a weekly value; thus for CAPD, NIPD and CCPD, the daily Kt/V or creatinine clearance is multiplied by 7, and for intermittent PD (IPD) by the number of sessions per week.

Residual renal function

A residual renal clearance of 1 ml/min equates to 10 l of dialyzate per week, a not inconsequential volume given values for PD creatinine clearance of 30–50 l/week. Indeed residual creatinine clearance may contribute 35% to the total normalized creatinine clearance value [33] (Figure 79.3). Residual renal urea clearance has been shown to contribute 17% to the total Kt/V value. In addition residual renal clearance accounts for the majority of the variation in the total clearance value. To correct for tubular creatinine excretion when calculating residual renal cre-

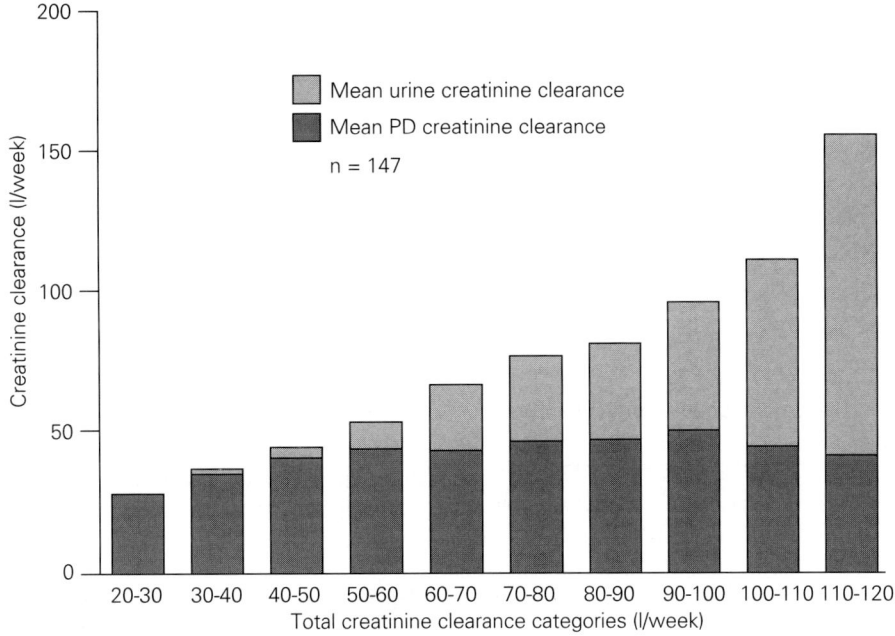

Figure 79.3 Relative contributions of residual renal function and dialysis clearance to total creatinine clearance.

atinine clearance, the mean of the urea and creatinine clearances is used.

Targets for dialysis adequacy

Theoretical considerations

Some indication of potential targets for optimal small solute clearance can be gleaned from consideration of the standard CAPD clearances and the relationship between urea clearance and nitrogen balance.

By setting a level for optimal protein intake sufficient to preserve nutrition (i.e. 1.2 g/kg/day) various authors have calculated how much urea is required to be removed (and thus the volume of dialysis to be prescribed) to maintain the serum urea concentration at a desirable level (Table 79.8).

Clinical experience

There is considerable controversy over the ideal target value for urea and creatinine clearance. Until recently there was no consensus as to whether the dialysis prescription could affect clinical outcomes. Some studies have suggested an increased mortality in patients with a weekly Kt/V of <1.7, but all have serious methodological constraints. The results of the CAN-USA study [34], a three-year longitudinal study of 680 CAPD patients are now available. Both Kt/V and creatinine clearance were shown to be independent predictors of mortality. For every 0.1 increase in Kt/V and 5 l/week increase in crea-

nine clearance, the relative risk of death was reduced 5%. This study highlighted the importance of residual renal function in contributing to 'adequacy' targets, but did not directly address the issue of whether modifying dialysis clearance alone is sufficient to compensate for the adverse impact of loss of renal clearance. Currently it seems prudent to advocate a total (dialysis + renal) Kt/V of 1.7 in conjunction with a total creatinine clearance of 50 l/week.

Management of inadequate dialysis

Conventional CAPD offers little scope to increase small solute clearance because of the constraints of the volume and size of exchanges acceptable to the patient (Table 79.9). The only practical way to improve small solute clearance is by use of automated peritoneal dialysis [35]. With nightly intermittent peritoneal dialysis (NIPD), patients receive, over a period of 8–10 h, 6 × 1.5–2.0 l exchanges (9–12 l), with a mean exchange dwell of 1 h. This procedure is repeated every night. If this regime is insufficient to achieve a creatinine clearance of 50 l/week and Kt/V of 1.7, higher fill volumes of up to 3.5 l (20 l/night) can be used since intra-abdominal pressure is considerably lower in the supine position.

Further enhancement of small solute clearance can be achieved by use of continuous cycling peritoneal dialysis (CCPD). This is similar to NIPD except that the patient performs an additional 1 or 2 standard CAPD exchanges during the day.

Table 79.8 Theoretical targets for *KtN* for a given protein intake (NPCR) and steady-state serum urea

Author	Serum urea (mmol/l)	NPCR (g/kg/day)	KtN
Popovich, 1978 [33a]	21.4	1.0	2
Teehan, 1990 [33b]	25.0	1.2	2.25
Keshaviah, 1989 [33c]	28.6	1.1	1.9
Gotch, 1990 [33d]	21–28.0	0.8–1.2	1.75–2.1

Table 79.9 Effect of different volumes of prescribed dialysis on urea clearance

Daily 2l exchange (Number)	Urea clearance (l/day)	Urea clearance (l/week)	Kt/V
5	12	84	2
4	10	70	1.7
3	8	56	1.3

Assumptions: equilibration of dialyzate and plasma urea concentrations, steady state urea levels, no residual renal function, 70 kg patient, total body water = 40l, daily ultrafiltration of 2l.

More recently the technique of tidal peritoneal dialysis (TPD) has been employed during the automated dialysis sessions to further increase clearance. During tidal dialysis the abdomen is filled with a specified dialyzate volume (initial fill volume) and subtotal amounts (tidal inflow) of dialyzate are drained and introduced (tidal drain) form this residual volume. Because the peritoneal cavity is never totally emptied, the time spent filling and draining the abdomen is minimized and solute removal is enhanced.

Assessment of peritoneal transport

The low-molecular-weight solute transfer across the peritoneal membrane and the net ultrafiltrate (UF) can be characterized by the peritoneal equilibration test (PET). This enables classification of peritoneal permeability into four categories – high, high average, low average and low [36].

The principal use of the PET is in determining the etiology of ultrafiltration failure. It is recommended that a baseline PET be performed between three and six months after starting CAPD and thereafter if the patient develops UF problems. The PET is also useful in determining which patients (high transporters) are likely to benefit from automated peritoneal dialysis.

References

1. Uttley, L. and Gokal, R. (1986) Organisation of a CAPD programme – the nurses role, in *Chronic Ambulatory Peritoneal Dialysis* (ed. R. Gokal), Churchill Livingstone, Edinburgh.
2. Coles, G.A. and Uttley, L. (1994) Training in PD. *Perit. Dial. Int.*, **14**, 115–16.
3. Clayton, S. (1981) The organisation and implementation of a peritoneal dialysis programme. *Perit. Dial. Bull.*, **1**, 134–6.
4. Holley, J.L. (1990) Initiating a PD program: personnel, administrative requirements, patient recruitment and training. *Semin. Dial.*, **3**, 122–6.
5. Malluche, H. and Monier-Faugere, M. (1992) Risk of adynamic bone disease in dialyzed patients. *Kidney Int.*, **42**(suppl 38), s62–7.
6. Coburn, J. (1993) Mineral metabolism and renal bone disease: effects of CAPD versus hemodialysis. *Kidney Int.*, **43**(suppl 40), s92–100.
7. Malluche, H. and Faugere, M. (1990) Renal bone disease 1990: an unmet challenge for the nephrologist. *Kidney Int.*, **38**, 193–211.
8. Hutchison, A. and Gokal, R. (1992) Improved solutions for peritoneal dialysis: physiological calcium solutions, osmotic agents and buffers. *Kidney Int.*, **42**(suppl 38), s153–9.
9. Cunningham, J., Beer, J., Coldwell, R. *et al.* (1992) Dialysate calcium reduction in CAPD patients treated with calcium carbonate and alfacalcidol. *Nephrol. Dial. Transplant.*, **7**, 63–8.
9a. Brancaccio, D., Gallieni, M. and Cozzolino, M. (1996) Treatment of hyperparathyroidism – why is it crucial to control serum phosphate? *Nephrol. Dial. Transplant.*, **11**, 420–3.
9b. Hutchison, A.J. and Gokal, R. (1996) Reduced calcium dialysis fluids; What's the point? *Perit. Dial. Int.*, **16**, 252–4.
10. Hutchison, A., Merchant, M., Boulton, H. *et al.* (1993) Calcium and magnesium mass transfer in peritoneal

dialysis patients using 1.25 mmol/l calcium, 0.25 mmol/l magnesium dialysis fluid. *Perit. Dial. Int.*, **13**, 219–23.

11. Hutchison, A. and Gokal, R. (1993) Vitamin D therapy in CAPD: what is its role? *Adv. Perit. Dial.*, **9**, 253–6.

12. Gokal, R., Ramos, J., Ellis, H. *et al.* (1983) Histological renal osteodystrophy, and 25-hydroxycholecalciferol and aluminium levels in patients on CAPD. *Kidney Int.*, **23**, 15–21.

13. Delmez, J., Fallon, M., Bergfeld, M. *et al.* (1986) Continuous ambulatory peritoneal dialysis and bone. *Kidney Int.*, **30**, 379–84.

14. Martin, K., Ballal, H., Domoto, D. *et al.* (1992) Pulse oral calcitriol for the treatment of hyperparathyroidism in patients on continuous ambulatory peritoneal dialysis: preliminary observations. *Am. J. Kidney Dis.*, **19**, 540–5.

15. Fournier, A., Moriniere, P., Cohen Solal, M. *et al.* (1991) Adynamic bone disease in uremia: May it be idiopathic? Is it an actual disease? *Nephron*, **58**, 1–12.

16. Cohen Solal, M., Sebert, J., Boudalliez, B. *et al.* (1992) Non-aluminic adynamic bone disease in non-dialyzed uremic patients: A new type of osteopathy due to over treatment? *Bone*, **13**, 1–5.

17. Fournier, A., Moriniere, P., Ben Hamidi, F. *et al.* (1992) Use of alkaline calcium salts as phosphate binder in uremic patients. *Kidney Int.*, **42**(suppl 38), s50–61.

18. Sherrard, D., Hercz, G., Pei, Y. *et al.* (1993) The spectrum of bone disease in end-stage renal failure – An evolving disorder. *Kidney Int.*, **43**, 436–42.

19. Hutchison, A., Whitehouse, R., Boulton, H. *et al.* (1993) Correlation of bone histology with parathyroid hormone, vitamin D, and radiology in end-stage renal disease. *Kidney Int.*, **44**, 1071–7.

20. Lui, S., Wong, K., Li, P. and Lai, K. (1992) Once weekly versus twice weekly subcutaneous administration of rHuEPO in haemodialysis patients. *Am. J. Nephrol.*, **12**, 55–60.

21. Horl, W. (1992) Optimal route of administration of EPO in chronic renal failure patients: Intravenous versus subcutaneous. *Acta Haematol.*, **87**, s16–19.

22. Young, G.A., Kopple, J.D., Lindholm, B. *et al.* (1991) Nutritional assessment of continuous ambulatory peritoneal dialysis: an international study. *Am. J. Kidney Dis.*, **17**, 462–71.

23. Pollock, C.A., Allen, B.J., Warden, R.A. *et al.* (1990) Total body nitrogen by neutron activation in maintenance dialysis. *Am. J. Kidney Dis.*, **16**, 38–45.

24. Bergstrom, J., Furst, P., Alvestrand, A. and Lindholm, B. (1993) Protein and energy intake, nitrogen balance and nitrogen losses in patients treated with continuous ambulatory peritoneal dialysis. *Kidney Int.*, **44**, 1048–57.

25. Lindholm, B. and Bergstrom, J. (1992) Nutritional aspects on peritoneal dialysis. *Kidney Int.*, **42**(suppl 38), S165–71.

26. Jones, M.R. (1994) Etiology of severe malnutrition: results of an international cross-sectional study in continuous ambulatory peritoneal dialysis patients. *Am. J. Kidney Dis.*, **23**, 412–20.

27. Avram, M.M., Goldwasser, P., Erroa, M. and Fein, P.A. (1994) Predictors of survival in continuous ambulatory peritoneal dialysis patients: the importance of peralbumin and other nutritional and metabolic markers. *Am. J. Kidney Dis.*, **23**, 91–8.

28. Blumenkrantz, M.J., Kopple, J.D., Gutman, R.A. *et al.* (1980) Methods for assessing nutritional status of patients with renal failure. *Am. J. Clin. Nutr.*, **33**, 1567–85.

28a. Johansson, A.C., Attman, P.O. and Haraldsson, B. (1997) Creatinine generation rate and lean body mass: A critical analysis in peritoneal dialysis patients. *Kidney Int.*, **51**, 855–9.

29. Lindholm, B. and Bergstrom, J. (1989) Nutritional management of patients undergoing peritoneal dialysis, in *Peritoneal Dialysis* (ed. K.D. Nolph), Kluwer Academic, Boston, pp. 230–60.

30. Rubin, J. (1990) Nutritional support during peritoneal dialysis-related peritonitis. *Am. J. Kidney Dis.*, **15**, 551–5.

31. Bernard, D., Kopple, J.D. and Brunori, G. (1991) Nutritional benefits of intraperitoneal (IP) amino acids (AA) in CAPD patients. (abstract) *6th Int. Congr on Nutrition and Metabolism in Renal Disease*, Harrogate, UK.

32. Keshaviah, P.R., Nolph, K.D., Prowant, B. *et al.* (1990) Defining adequacy of CAPD with urea kinetics. *Adv. Perit. Dial.*, **6**, 173–8.

33. Harty, J.C., Boulton, H., Uttley, L. *et al.* (1993) Limitations of urea kinetic modelling as predictors of nutritional and dialysis adequacy in CAPD. *Am. J. Nephrol.*, **13**, 454–63.

33a. Popovich, R.P. and Moncrief, J.W. (1978) Continuous ambulatory peritoneal dialysis. *Ann. Intern. Med.*, **88**, 449–59.

33b. Teehan, B.P., Brown, J.M. and Schleifer, C.R. (1990) Kinetic modeling in peritoneal dialysis, in *Clinical Dialysis* (eds A.R. Nissenson, R. Fine and D. Gentile), Appleton & Lange, Norwalk, CT, pp. 319–29.

33c. Keshaviah, P.R., Nolph, K.D., Van Stone, J.C. and Van Stone, J.C. (1989) The peak concentration hypothesis: a urea kinetic approach to comparing the adequacy of CAPD and hemodialysis. *Perit. Dial. Int.*, **9**, 257–60.

33d. Gotch, F.A. (1990) Application of urea kinetic modeling to adequacy of CAPD therapy. *Adv. Perit. Dial.*, **6**, 178–80.

34. Churchill, D.N., Thorpe, K., Taylor, D.W. and keshaviah, P.K. (1994) Adequacy of peritoneal dialysis (abstract). *J. Am. Soc. Nephrol.*, **5**, 439.

35. Twardowski, Z.J. (1989) New approaches to intermittent peritoneal dialysis therapies, in *Peritoneal Dialysis*, 3rd edn (ed. K.D. Nolph), Kluwer Academic, Dordrecht, pp. 133–51.

36. Twardowski, Z.J. (1987) Peritoneal equilibration test. *Perit. Dial. Bull.*, **7**, 138–47.

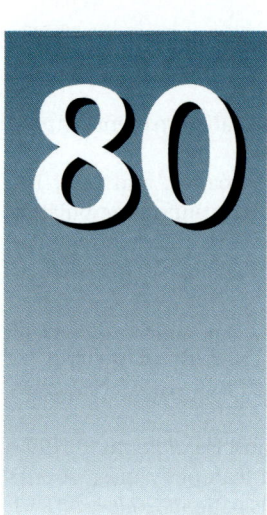

80

Complications of peritoneal dialysis

R. Gokal

Introduction

Since the introduction of peritoneal dialysis, complications related to the technique, in particular peritonitis and access related problems, have bedevilled its wider use and acceptance. Other complications, including those unrelated to the technique, also occur and are listed in Table 80.1. With the introduction of CAPD in 1976, and its subsequent widespread use, these problems have increased and account for considerable morbidity, hospitalization, and switch to hemodialysis [1, 2].

Peritonitis

The frequent occurrence of peritonitis remains the major complication of peritoneal dialysis and until recently has hindered its development and acceptance [3]. The low peritonitis rates with intermittent peritoneal dialysis became dramatically worse with the introduction of CAPD in 1976. The initial technique described by Moncrief and Popovich, using glass bottles was simplified by Oreopoulos using plastic bags. This arrangement was more convenient for patients and substantially reduced the number of manipulations of the catheter and therefore the infection rate. However, the high rate of peritonitis (1.2–6.3 episodes per patient year) was a major drawback to the procedure [4, 5]. Over the last decade, however, there has been a dramatic reduction in peri-

tonitis. This has been due predominantly to changes in connection techniques including introduction of the titanium connector, the employment of transfer sets which requires less frequent changes, and the use of the 'Y' set or disconnect systems [6]. The last was first introduced in Italy but rather reluctantly accepted outside Italy despite a low peritonitis rate of once every 24–36 patient months; however, the results have been confirmed [7, 8]. This 'flush before fill' method has now become widely accepted in its many variations [9] which has lowered the average rate of peritonitis to once every two years. The USRDS reported that the time to first peritonitis of patients on a Y set is 20.6 months compared to 11.4 with the standard connection system.

Pathogenesis and microbiological aspects of peritonitis

In contrast to acute surgical peritonitis, CAPD peritonitis occurs readily among peritoneal dialysis patients following apparently minor episodes of contamination. Infection is localized to the peritoneal cavity. Improved bacteriological methods have permitted a better analysis of the microbiological aspects [10]. The most common organisms are Gram positive (70% of all episodes; *Staphylococcus epidermidis* accounts for over half of the total), Gram-negative bacteria (about 20% of all episodes) and yeast (up to 5%). Anaerobic bacteria are less commonly involved and mycobacteria, higher bacteria and filamen-

Nephrology, Edited by Rex L. Jamison and Robert Wilkinson.
Published in 1997 by Chapman & Hall, London. ISBN 0 412 60930 4

Table 80.1 Complications of peritoneal dialysis

Technique related	Non-technique related
Peritonitis	Cardiovascular complications
Exit and tunnel infection	Gastrointestinal complications
Access related (Chapter 77)	Acid–base and electrolyte disorders
Hernias	Pruritus
Genital edema	Back pain
Hydrothorax	
Respiratory complications	
Peritoneal membrane injury	
Loss of ultrafiltration	
Sclerosing peritonitis	
Calcifying peritonitis	
Hemoperitoneum	

tous fungi are seldom encountered. Improvement in culture techniques has resulted in a decreased incidence of 'sterile' or culture negative peritonitis [11]. Concentration methods, inoculation of blood culture media and the limulus lysate test have all helped in the diagnosis of peritonitis [12].

An increasing number of studies have examined the effect of CAPD on the local host defense mechanisms of the peritoneal cavity. The consequences of hyperosmolar, acidic dialysis solutions on the function of intraperitoneal neutrophils and macrophages have been elucidated, as have the role of deficiency of opsonins in the peritoneal fluid [10, 13]. A better understanding of the pathophysiology of peritoneal infections during CAPD has led to the development of more effective measures for the prevention of peritonitis.

Definitions and clinical diagnosis of peritonitis

The constant presence of fluid in the peritoneal cavity has certainly modified the definition of peritonitis in CAPD. A practical definition of peritonitis requires the presence of two of the following criteria in any combination:

1 Organisms identified by Gram stain or subsequent culture of PD fluid;
2 Cloudy PD fluid (WBC greater than $100 \, \text{cells/cm}^3$, greater than 50% neutrophils);
3 Symptoms of peritoneal infection [14].

The earliest suggestive sign of peritonitis is a cloudy peritoneal effluent. Other causes are a blood-tinged dialyzate, fibrin filaments, chylous drainage or other intraabdominal pathology. A total cell count and its differential are necessary for the diagnosis and further management of peritonitis. The initial clinical and laboratory assessment of the patient is illustrated in Figure 80.1. The incubation period of peritonitis is not well known but has been estimated from the incidence due to touch contamination and from prospective studies to be about 24–48 h.

Treatment of peritonitis

When peritonitis occurs, treatment should be started immediately after completion of the appropriate microbiological assessment. Treatment must be initiated in the absence of complete bacteriological information and therefore arbitrary decisions have to be taken concerning antibiotic treatment based on the likely causative organism and pathogenesis. Although many protocols for antibiotic treatment have been proposed there is an increasing consensus towards a standardized approach combining the continuation of CAPD with intraperitoneal administration of antibiotics [15–17].

The evidence of detrimental effect of fresh dialysis solution on local host defense mechanisms has led to the abandonment of prolonged rapid exchange peritoneal lavage in the management of peritoneal infection. A few exchanges to remove inflammatory products to relieve abdominal pain is appropriate followed by CAPD [18]. The antibiotic selected for initial treatment should be effective against the most frequently occurring organisms observed in peritonitis. The intraperitoneal route of administration is preferred although oral antibiotics have been used with success. Since no microbiological information is available at the start of treatment most centers use vancomycin as the initial choice for Gram-positive organisms. Because of the serious threat of vancomycin-resistant enterococci, first-generation cephalosporins are now advocated [15] (Figure 80.1). In addition, for the more threatening Gram-negative intestinal organisms, an aminoglycoside or ceftazadine is also given. The advisory committee on peritonitis management [15] reported recently a consensus recommendation on treatment. These are represented in Figures 80.1 and 80.2a, b. Among Gram-positive organisms, St*aphylococcus aureus* is the

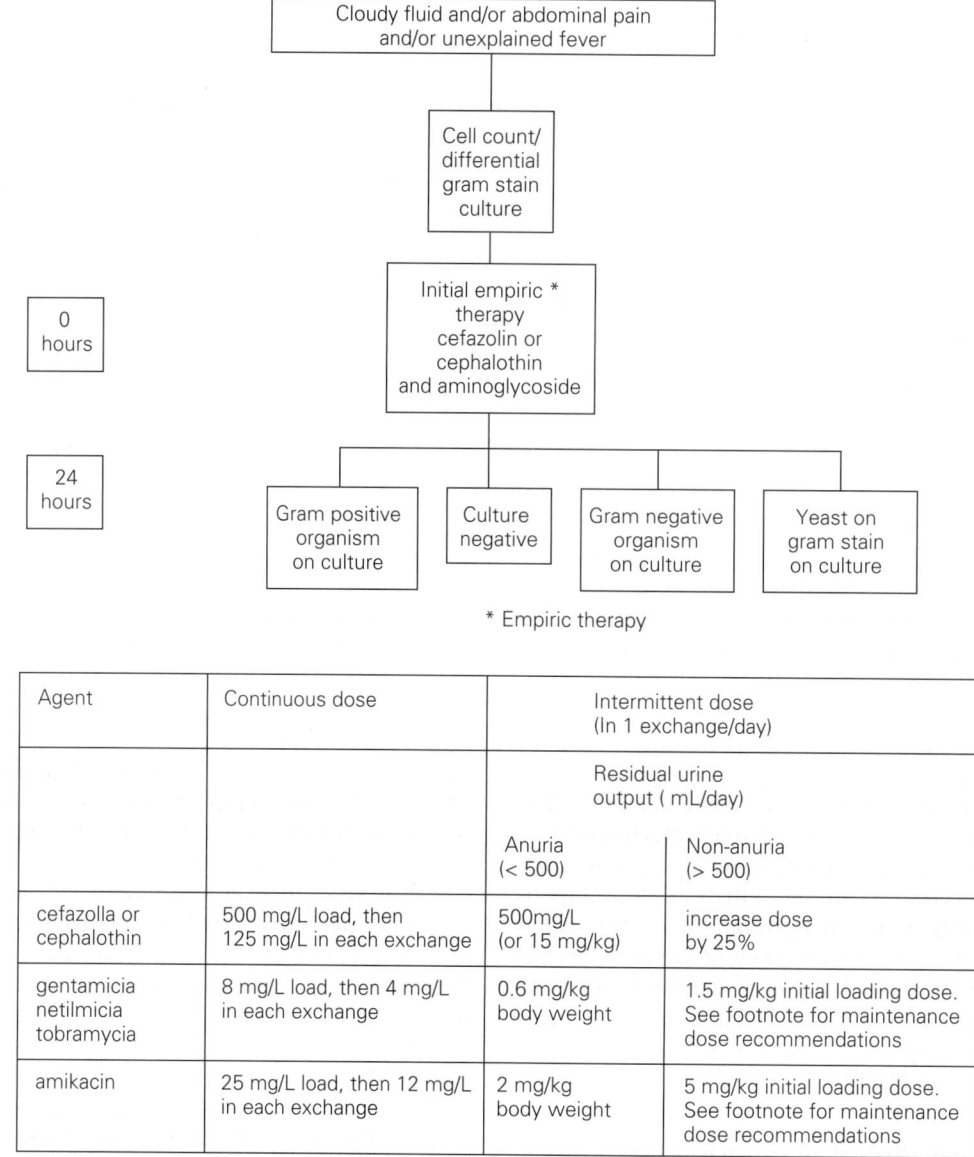

Figure 80.1 Initial clinical and laboratory assessment of patient with possible peritonitis. (Reproduced from ref. [15], with permission.)

most serious and if identified and clinical improvement is not seen within four to five days, rifampicin should be added to the regimen and therapy continued for three weeks [15, 19]. For Gram-negative micro-organisms, outcome is usually reasonably good for *Escherichia coli*, *Klebsiella* and *Proteus* [17]. In these situations aminoglycoside or ceftazadine alone should suffice. Recently the use of quinolones has been advocated for either initial or subsequent Gram-negative peritonitis [20]. If pseudomonas or xanthomatous organisms are identified, therapy with at least two agents that are usually effective against these micro-organisms should be used. Clinical experience has shown that pseudomonas peritonitis in CAPD patients is extremely difficult to cure, particularly when it develops as a result of an exit site or tunnel-related infection [20]. Whatever the antibiotic regime utilized, therapy should be continued for three to four weeks, if the patient is clinically improving. For fungal organisms initial reports suggested that catheter removal is the treatment of choice once these organisms were identified [16, 17]. Recent experience with the newer im-idizoles/triazoles and flucytosine, however, has suggested that these agents are reasonably efficacious, obviating the need for immediate catheter removal. If there is no clinical improvement with these agents after four to seven days, however, the catheter should be removed; therapy with these agents should be continued after removal.

Other therapeutic approaches to peritonitis

Relapsing peritonitis

Relapsing peritonitis is defined as a recurrence of peritonitis with the same organism within 14 days of cessation of antibiotic therapy. Relapsing infections with coagulase-positive staphylococcus should be treated with vancomycin and rifampicin for four weeks. If enterococci are recultured, vancomycin and another aminoglycoside should be used. Catheter removal is indicated if there is no improvement after 96 h of therapy, or if there are two relapses. If relapsing peritonitis is caused by a Gram-negative organism, an intra-abdominal abscess should be suspected and catheter removal and surgical exploration are recommended.

Catheter removal and reinsertion and use of thrombolytic agents

Recent reports have indicated that refractory or relapsing peritoneal dialysis infections could be managed by removal of the catheter and insertion of a new one at the same operation [21, 22]. Overall, the success rate is reasonable but about 30–40% of cases still require a long period of 'rest' after catheter removal before another catheter is inserted.

Thrombolytic agents such as streptokinase and uroki-nase have been used to treat recurrent or refractory peritonitis [23, 24]. In a prospectively randomized study comparing fibrinolytic therapy to simultaneous catheter removal and replacement, the results were dramatically in favor of the latter (recurrent rate was only 5% compared to 41% for thrombolytic therapy) [24].

Outcome peritonitis

Complications

Although rare, complications of CAPD peritonitis can occur. In the acute stage pulmonary edema, atelectasis, pneumonia, intercurrent cardiovascular events and severe protein malnutrition are recognized complications. At a later stage the formation of adhesions or development of peritoneal fibrosis can result in progressive peritoneal damage leading to inadequate dialysis and loss of ultrafiltration. The precise role of peritonitis in this peritoneal damage cannot be determined but Dobbie [25] has proposed a series of outcomes, based on histological appearances.

Even though CAPD peritonitis is considered to be benign, it is reported as a cause of death in as many as 12% of patients [26]. Factors that increase the risk of death from peritonitis include an unresolving, protracted course, intra-abdominal abscess, bowel perforation and infection with *Staphylococcus aureus*, fungi or multiple organisms. There is also considerable morbidity related to

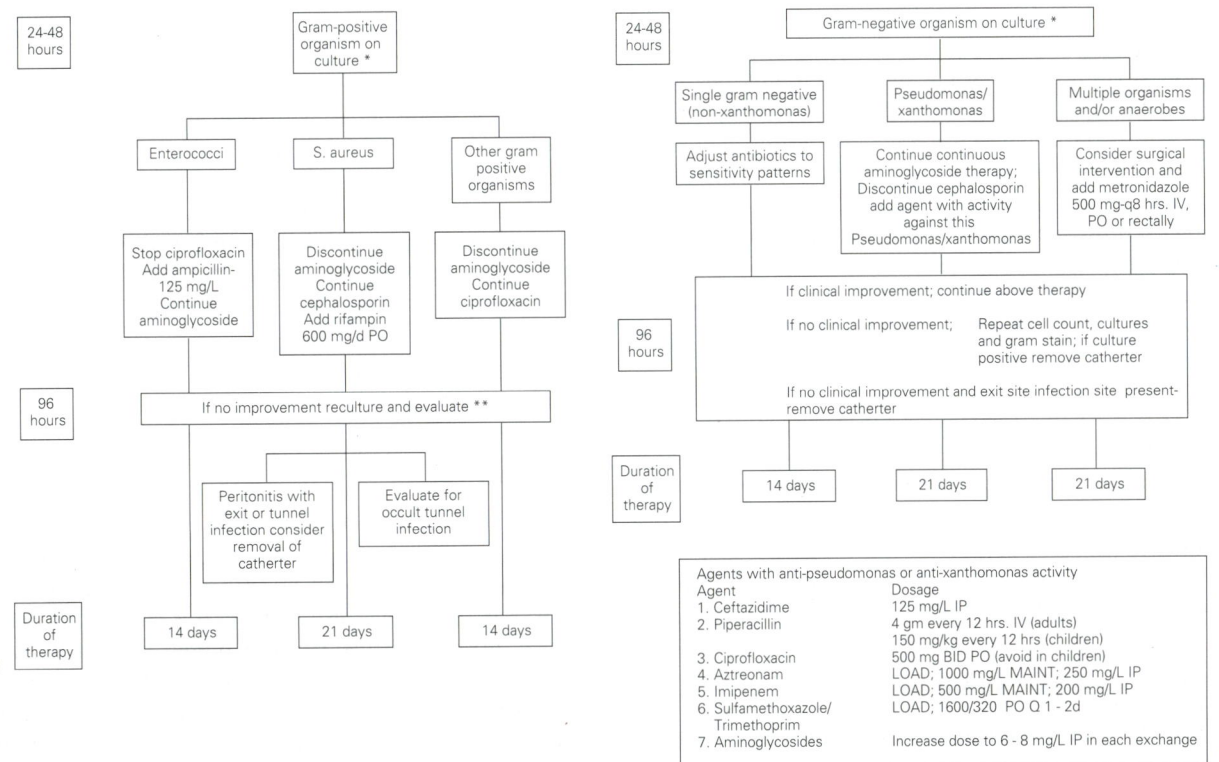

Figure 80.2 Treatment of peritonitis on initial clinical presentation. (Reproduced from ref. [15], with permission.)

peritonitis. Hospitalization rates are variable and dependent on the policy of managing peritoneal infection. When a minimal hospitalization policy is practiced then rates of admission due to peritonitis alone amount to five days per patient year of CAPD [27]. The impact of peritonitis on, the success of CAPD is considerable; up to 20% of patients change to hemodialysis because of peritonitis [28]. These consequences mean that a CAPD program requires adequate hemodialysis and inpatient facilities, to enable permanent as well as temporary changes of therapy.

Exit site infection and its management

Tunnel morphology

A detailed description of the peritoneal catheter tunnel morphology has been reported by Twardowski et al. [29]. The exit site is defined as the most external part of the sinus tract and the skin surrounding the exit of the tunnel. Normally the epidermal cells penetrate only a few millimeters from the skin exit sometimes reaching the cuff if it is located less than 15 mm from the exit site. Close to the exit the surface of the sinus tract is covered with a wrinkled epidermis, containing all layers of epidermis including the horny layer. Further along the tunnel the epidermis loses one layer, and begins to resemble the mucosal epithelium and the surface becomes glistening and white. The rest of the sinus tract is covered by granulation tissue which is yellowish in appearance. Factors influencing the healing process and the risk of early infections are local blood flow, bacterial colonization of the sinus tract, epithelialization, use of local antiseptic agents and exit direction. Of these epithelialization appears to be especially important. Epidermal cells grow over the granulation tissue beneath the scab. If the scab is forcibly removed during cleansing the epidermal layer is broken, thus slowing the epithelialization process [30]. Bacterial colonization of the sinus leads to formation of an exudate, proliferation of granulation tissue and greater vascularity.

Definition of exit site infection

The most widely accepted definition of a site infection is 'redness of skin, induration or discharge of pus from the exit site' [14]. Twardowski [31] has outlined five categories of exit site appearances, each with its clinical features and management. They are: acutely inflamed, chronically inflamed, equivocal, good and perfect.

Treatment of exit site infection

There is at present a paucity of information regarding the therapeutic efficacy of any treatment regime or agents of an exit site infection. Figure 80.3 outlines an algorithm

for treatment of exit site infections as recommended by the ad hoc committee [15, 27]. For Gram-positive organisms either oral penicillinase resistant penicillin or parenteral vancomycin (for MRSA or MRSE) is indicated and if there are no clinical signs of improvement then rifampicin is added. For Gram-negative organisms ciprofloxacillin or ceftazamine is used. If *Pseudomonas* is identified it is unlikely that the infection will respond to antimicrobial therapy and early catheter removal should be considered, especially if there is simultaneous peritonitis.

Exit site care

Care of the exit site has a considerable bearing on the chance of infection. In a randomized multicenter study [32] a protected dressing with a disinfectant was associated with significantly less frequent exit site infections than minimum care which consisted of cleansing the exit site with non-disinfectant soap and water. Exit site and tunnel infections influence catheter outcome in peritoneal dialysis patients. Up to 55% of patients are transferred to hemodialysis because of catheter infections [33]. There is a well held view that immobilization of the catheter, especially immediately after catheter insertion, may well reduce the risk of catheter exit site infection.

Nasal carriage and exit site infection

Several investigations of patients undergoing CAPD suggest a possible link between nasal carriage of *Staph. aureus* and exit site infection [34, 35]. Luzar et al. [35] established that in patients beginning CAPD, the nasal carriage of *Staph. aureus* was associated with an increased risk of catheter site infection. Isolation of nasal *Staph. aureus* before implantation of the catheter can identify patients at high risk of infection. Several controlled studies have shown a reduction in exit site infection with treatment of nasal carriage with intranasal mupurocin or oral rifampicim [35a, 35b].

Hernias, genital edema and hydrothorax

Hernias

Hernias are fairly common complications of peritoneal dialysis with up to 11% of CAPD patients developing these during a five-year period, with the risk increasing each year on CAPD [36]. This high incidence of herniation is not surprising, because presence of fluid in the peritoneal cavity increases intra-abdominal pressure in proportion to the volume of dialyzate instilled. A large variety of hernias have been described [37], the most common being incisional, inguinal, umbilical or through the catheter-placement tunnel. Older female patients and

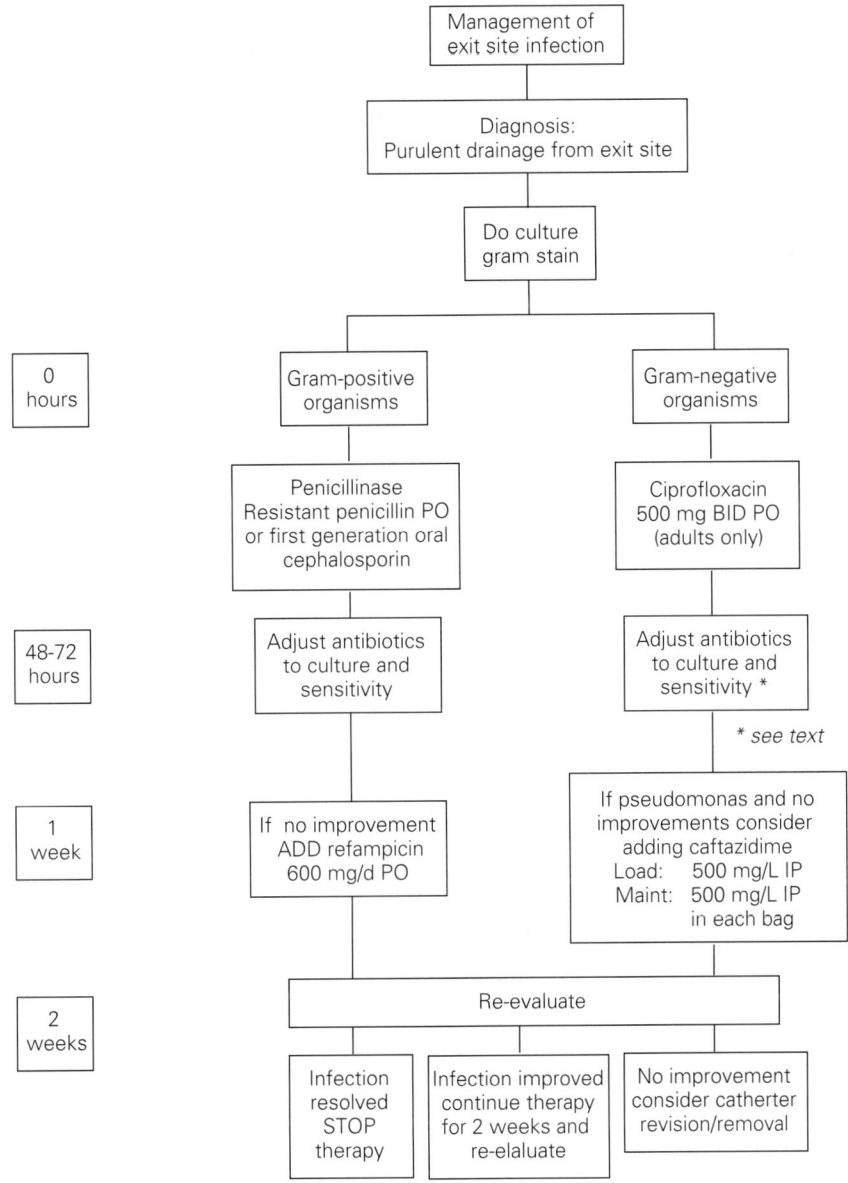

Figure 80.3 Management of exit site infections. (Reproduced from ref. [27], with permission.)

those who have experienced a high frequency of postoperative leaks at the time of catheter insertion have the highest risk.

The major potential area of weakness is the site of abdominal incision for implantation of the catheter. Midline incisions have a greater propensity for incisional hernia as this is structurally a weak area. Recognition of this complication has resulted in the policy of a paramedian incision through the rectus muscle. The processus vaginalis (normally closed *in utero*) is another potential weakness for herniation and is a common site of herniation in pediatric patients, dialyzate can travel through a patent processus to the labia or scrotum and occasionally bowel can accompany fluid if the defect is large.

A hernia may present as a painless swelling, herniation of bowel with incarceration and strangulation, recurrent Gram-negative peritonitis, and obstruction of bowel and perforation. Hernias need to be repaired even though they may not carry a high risk of complications. It is possible to repair a hernia at the time of catheter insertion without fluid leaks or other complications. Inguinal herniorraphy has been successfully combined with commencement of CAPD immediately postoperatively with a very low risk of recurrence [38]. Management of patients postoperatively should include low-volume intermittent peritoneal dialysis to allow time for wound healing. Peritoneal dialysis could be discontinued and hemodialysis instituted if the surgery is extensive.

Genital and abdominal wall edema

The incidence of genital edema, varies considerably; fewer than 10% of CAPD patients have this complication [39]. Edema of the abdominal wall related to subcutaneous fluid leaks is difficult to detect, may be insidious and sometimes only comes to light because of a reduction in ultrafiltration volume. Dialyzate can track through the soft tissue planes from the catheter insertion site, a soft tissue defect within a hernia or a peritoneal defect. Dialysis fluid can also travel through a patent processus vaginalis to the labium or scrotum where it may leak into the surrounding soft tissue.

The management of edema of the genital area or abdominal wall requires bedrest and scrotal elevation. Dialysis should either be discontinued or continued with frequent low volume exchanges. Sometimes the defect heals with the cessation of peritoneal dialysis; however, there may be a need for a period of prolonged hemodialysis if the site of the leak is not apparent. Computed tomographic scanning or abdominal sinography [1, 40] may help to localize the leak and treat the lesion. Most patients can resume CAPD after temporary cessation or surgical repair.

Hydrothorax

Hydrothorax is the accumulation of dialysis fluid in the pleural space and is due to a defect in the diaphragm which allows fluid from the peritoneum to enter the pleural cavity. The diagnosis of hydrothorax is relatively straightforward in cases that present with marked respiratory embarrassment. Small effusions may be more difficult to detect and could mistakenly be attributed to congestive heart failure. The detection of glucose in pleural fluid is diagnostic of a dialyzate leak.

Treatment of hydrothorax includes thoracocentesis if there is respiratory embarrassment. Discontinuing peritoneal dialysis often leads to a rapid and dramatic resolution of the pleural effusion. Subsequent management depends on whether the patient is to continue peritoneal dialysis. Several options are available in managing these patients. They include temporary hemodialysis for as much as four weeks with subsequent return to CAPD (usually low volumes, intermittently to start) or obliteration of the pleural cavity with agents like tetracycline, talc or autologous blood. If these approaches fail, then discontinuation of CAPD and conversion to haemodialysis is the only option [37, 41].

Peritoneal membrane changes

The peritoneum has a remarkable ability to heal by total resolution of any inflammatory exudate that may result from injury during peritonitis. On most occasions the healing returns the peritoneal cavity to its pristine pre-morbid condition [42]. Diffuse, widespread, chronic peritoneal inflammation resulting in global fibrosis is a most unusual and uncharacteristic peritoneal reaction. However, CAPD has been associated with the appearance of a new form of iatrogenic fibrosis which is remarkable both for its aggressiveness and the global nature of the peritoneal involvement. The fibrosis exhibits a wide spectrum from simple opacification to formation of fibrous sheets and plaques resulting in a notorious sclerosing encapsulating peritonitis (SEP). Although other terms are used (tanned peritoneal syndrome, mural fibrosis) SEP is the most common to describe the peritoneal fibrosis associated with peritoneal dialysis [42]. This is the end stage of an intra-abdominal inflammatory process that results in formation of sheets of new fibrous tissue which cover, bind and restrict the mobility of the bowel. At surgery it is possible to peel the membrane from the bowel relatively easily and the exposed bowel may appear normal. There are various theories to explain SEP, none of them proven (Table 80.2). The outcome of SEP is generally poor with a mortality as high as 75%.

Loss of ultrafiltration

In most of the descriptions of ultrafiltration failure, solute transport remains normal or slightly above normal (type 1 failure). The inability to sustain an osmotic gradient across the peritoneal membrane because of rapid diffusion of glucose from the dialyzate is the principal cause of type 1 failure. Hyperpermeability of the membrane can result from prolonged exposure to peritoneal dialysis fluids, hyperosmolar solutions, peritonitis and the diabetic state. The use of glucose as an osmotic agent can lead to accumulation of glycation end products in the peritoneal membrane leading to hyperpermeability with time [42a]. None of these have been definitively proven. Less commonly, transport of solute is impaired as well as ultrafiltration. This general reduction of peritoneal transport (type II failure) results from a reduction in the effective surface area available for transport. It can occur in the patient with extensive adhesions or with SEP. There are regional variations in the incidence and prevalence of ultrafiltration failure. In the early 1980s it was highly prevalent in Europe but not in North America. Many studies have documented a general trend towards loss of ultrafiltration capacity with time but with a variable incidence. Given the change in mesothelial structure which occurs with long-term peritoneal dialysis, this complication is not totally unexpected. Factors leading to loss of ultrafiltration are shown in Table 80.2. Those that have been established are the use of acetate, prolonged and severe episodes of peritonitis, and intercurrent abdominal surgery.

The treatment of ultrafiltration failure includes shortening the dwell time to minimize dissipation of the glucose gradient (type 1 failure). Briefer, more frequent exchanges can be achieved by cycler dialysis (IPD or NIPD or leaving the peritoneal cavity empty overnight). The role of phosphatidylcholine in improving ultrafiltration in PD patients remains controversial; no definitive study has shown that it plays a major role in improving ultrafiltration. Preliminary reports of the use of a glycylglycine-based bicarbonate solution suggest that it may enhance ultrafiltration capacity for reasons that are not clear.

Respiratory complications

Respiratory complications are related to the presence of dialysis fluid in the peritoneal cavity with attendant increase in intra-abdominal pressure and alteration of the mechanics of breathing. In stable patients on chronic peritoneal dialysis, introduction of 2 l of dialysis fluid in the abdomen usually reduces lung volumes and functional residual capacity. These changes can persist or normalize after two weeks of CAPD.

Changes in lung volumes have not been found to be more severe in patients with chronic obstructive airway disease so the disease should not be regarded as a contraindication to peritoneal dialysis. It has recently been demonstrated by total body plethysmography that 2 l of dialysis fluid in the peritoneal cavity has no effect on airway resistance. In a recent study of pulmonary function in predialysis, peritoneal, hemodialysis and renal transplant patients, the carbon dioxide diffusion capacity, although reduced in all groups, was significantly lower in the group of patients on CAPD. This observation is difficult to explain; it could be related to subclinical pulmonary edema.

Cardiovascular complications

The development of left ventricular hypertrophy confers a poor outcome for cardiovascular morbidity and mor-

---

Table 80.2 Causes of sclerosing encapsulating peritonitis and loss of ultrafiltration (types I and II)

Acetate in dialysis fluid
Hypertonic, acidic dialysis fluid
Glucose breakdown products (5.0H methylfurforal in
    dialyzates etc.)
Particulate matter in dialysis fluid
Chlorhexidine
Recurrent peritonitis
Multiple abdominal surgery

---

tality in uremic patients. In addition, the development of myocardial fibrosis further compromises ventricular compliance. There are some reports of a decrease in left ventricular mass in patients with near normalization of end-diastolic dimensions, left ventricular fractional shortening and ejection fraction. These changes were thought to be the result of improved control of systemic blood pressure. Not all studies have confirmed regression of left ventricular hypertrophy however, and the discrepancy may be the result of differences in control of extracellular fluid volume, control of hypertension, or methods used to assess hypertrophy.

Reduction in blood pressure may have deleterious effects. Diabetic patients have been reported to experience exacerbation of peripheral vascular disease during CAPD. The risk factors for worsening of peripheral circulation include smoking, and previous symptoms of peripheral vascular disease. Removal of salt and water in patients may result in disabling hypotension that can sometimes be corrected with the use of a higher sodium concentration in the dialyzate.

The elevated intra-abdominal pressure due to the dialysis fluid in the peritoneal cavity does not seem to exert a clinically significant effect on the cardiovascular system although there is a potential for such an effect with the use of large (3 l or more) volumes in patients with diminished cardiac compliance. Ischemic heart disease and its complications are the greatest cause of death in this population. Hypertension, unfavorable lipid profiles, and glucose intolerance, all contribute to the worsening of coronary artery disease in the CAPD patient.

Back pain

Instillation of dialysis fluid into the peritoneal cavity may alter spinal mechanics in posture. In a patient with lax abdominal musculature, the abdomen protrudes under the weight and volume of dialyzate and swings the center of gravity anteriorly. The normal lumbar lordosis is inappropriately accentuated. Since many patients beginning PD have been deconditioned by years of illness and poor nutrition, it is not surprsing that the abdominal musculature is often weak. There may also be associated degenerative disc disease, spondylolisthesis and osteoporosis. Management includes training the patient to learn the appropriate way to stand and bend over, and to perform pelvic tilt exercises. In a patient complaining of persistent back pain, further investigation, should include vertebral radiographs to look for a bony structural abnormality. Alteration in the dialysis regime, even to the extent of changing to nightly intermittent peritoneal dialysis with small volume exchanges and judicious use of skeletal muscle relaxant and anti-inflammatory agents, may be necessary.

References

1. Scanziani, R., Dozio, B., Caimi, F. *et al.* (1992) Peritoneography and peritoneal computerized tomography: a new approach to non-infectious complications of CAPD. *Nephrol. Dial. Transplant.*, **7**, 1035–8.
2. Gokal, R. (1987) Continuous ambulatory peritoneal dialysis (CAPD) – 10 years on. *Q. J. Med.*, **63**, 465–72.
3. Keane, W.F. and Vas, SI. (1994) Peritonitis, in *The Textbook of Peritoneal Dialysis* (eds R. Gokal and K.D. Nolph), Kluwer Academic, Dordrecht, pp. 473–501.
4. Report of a working Party of the BSAC (1987) Diagnosis and management of peritonitis in CAPD. *Lancet*, **i**, 845–8.
5. Editorial (1978) Peritoneal dialysis in chronic renal failure. *Lancet*, **ii**, 303.
6. Buoncristiani, C., Bianci, P., Cozzani, M. *et al.* (1980) A new safe simple connection system for CAPD. *Int. J. Urol. Nephrol.*, **1**, 45–50.
7. Canadian CAPD Clinical Trials Group (1989) Peritonitis in CAPD: A multi-center randomised clinical trial comparing the Y connector disinfectant system to standard systems. *Perit. Dial. Int.*, **9**, 159–63.
8. Maiorca, R., Cantaluppi, A., Cancarini, G.C. *et al.* (1983) Prospective controlled trial of a Y connector and disinfectant to prevent peritonitis in CAPD. *Lancet*, **11**, 624–4.
9. Viglino, G., Cantaluppi, A., Gandolfo, C. *et al.* (1991) Y-set evolution, in *Peritoneal Dialysis* (eds G. La Greca *et al.*), Wichtig Editore, Milan, pp. 281–93.
10. Vas, S.I. (1983) Microbiological aspects of chronic ambulatory peritoneal dialysis. *Kidney Int.*, **23**, 83–92.
11. Von Graevenitz, A. and Amsterdam, D. (1992) Microbiological aspects of peritonitis associated with CAPD. *Clin. Microbiol. Rev.*, **5**, 26–48.
12. Males, B.M., Walshe, J.J., Garringer, L. *et al.* (1986) Addi-Chek filtration, Bactec, and 10 ml culture methods for the recovery of microorganisms from dialysis effluent during episodes of peritonitis. *J. Clin. Microbiol.*, **23**, 350–3.
13. Coles, G.A., Lewis, S.L. and Williams, J.D. (1994) Host defence and effects of solutions on peritoneal cells, in *The Textbook of Peritoneal Dialysis* (eds R. Gokal and K.D. Nolph), Kluwer Academic, Dordrecht, pp. 503–28.
14. Pierratos, A. (1984) Peritoneal dialysis glossary. *Perit. Dial. Bull.*, **4**, 2–3.
15. Keane, W.F., Alexander, S.R., Baille, S.R. *et al.* (1996) Peritoneal dialysis related peritonitis treatment recommendations. *Perit. Dial. Int.*, **16**, 557–73.
16. Rubin, J., Rodgerts, W.A., Taylor, H.M. *et al.* (1980) Peritonitis during continuous ambulatory peritoneal dialysis. *Ann. Intern. Med.*, **92**, 7–13.
17. Tranaeus, A., Heimburger, O. and Lindholm, B. (1988) Peritonitis during CAPD: risk factors, clinical severity and pathogenetic aspects. *Perit. Dial. Int.*, **8**, 253–63.
18. Ejlersen, E., Brandi, L., Lokkegard, H. *et al.* (1991) Is initial (24 hours) lavage necessary in treatment of CAPD peritonitis? *Perit. Dial. Int.*, **11**, 38–42.
19. Zimmerman, S.W. and Johnson, C.A. (1989) Rifampicin use in peritoneal dialysis. *Perit. Dial. Int.*, **9**, 241–3.
20. Millikan, S.P., Matze, G.R. and Keane, W.F. (1991) Antimicrobial treatment of peritonitis associated with CAPD. *Perit. Dial. Int.*, **11**, 252–60.
21. Paterson, A.D., Bishop, M., Morgan, A.G. and Burden, R.P. (1986) Removal and replacement of Tenckhoff catheter at a single operation: successful treatment of resistant peritonitis in CAPD. *Lancet*, **ii**, 1245–7.
22. Swartz, R., Messana, J., Reynolds, J. and Ranjit, U. (1991) Simultaneous catheter replacement and removal in refractory peritoneal dialysis infections. *Kidney Int.*, **40**, 1160–5.
23. Pickering, S.J., Fleming, S.J., Bowley, J.A. *et al.* (1989) Urokinase: a treatment for relapsing peritonitis due to coagulase-negative staphylococci. *Nephrol. Dial. Transplant.*, **4**, 62–5.
24. Williams, A.J., Boeltis, L., Johnson, B.F. *et al.* (1989) Tenckhoff catheter replacement or intraperitoneal urokinase: a randomised trial in the management of recurrent CAPD peritonitis. *Perit. Dial. Int.*, **9**, 65–7.
25. Dobbie, J.W. (1989) Morphology of the Peritoneum. *Blood Purification*, 7, 74–85.
26. Gokal, R., King, J., Jakubowski, C. *et al.* (1990) Peritonitis – still a major problem in CAPD: results of a multi-centre study. *J. Nephrol.*, **2**, 95–9.
27. Gokal, R., Ash, S., Helfrich, G.B. *et al.* (1993) Peritoneal catheters and exit site practices: Towards optimum peritoneal access. *Perit. Dial. Int.*, **13**, 29–39.
28. Viglino, G., Cancarini, G., Catizone, L. *et al.* (1992) The impact of peritonitis on CAPD results. *Adv. Perit. Dial.*, **8**, 296–75.
29. Twardowski, Z.J., Dobble, J.W., Moore, H.L. *et al.* Morphology of peritoneal dialysis catheter tunnel. 1. Macroscopy and light microscopy. *Perit. Dial. Int.*, **11**, 152–5.
30. Twardowski, Z.J. and Khanna, R. (1994) Peritoneal dialysis access and exit site care, in *The Textbook of Peritoneal Dialysis* (eds R. Gokal and K.D. Nolph), Kluwer Academic, Dordrecht, pp. 271–314.
31. Twardowski, Z.J. (1992) Peritoneal catheter exit site infections: prevention, diagnosis, treatment, and future directions. *Semin. Dial.*, **5**, 305–15.
32. Luzar, M.A., Brown, C.B., Balf, D. *et al.* (1990) Exit-site care and exit-site infection in CAPD: results of a randomised multicentre study. *Perit. Dial. Int.*, **10**, 25–9.
33. Piraino, B., Bernadini, J. and Sorkin, M. (1989) Catheter infections as a factor in the transfer of CAPD patients to hemodialysis. *Am. J. Kidney Dis.*, **13**, 365–9.
34. Davies, S.J., Ogg, C.S., Cameron, J.S. *et al. Staphylococcus aureus* nasal carriage, exit-site infection and catheter loss in patients treated with CAPD. *Perit. Dial. Int.*, **9**, 61–4.
35. Luzar, M.A., Cloes, G.A., Faller, B. *et al.* (1990) *Stapyhlococcus aureus* nasal carraige and infection in patients on CAPD. *N. Engl. J. Med.*, **322**, 505–9.
35a. Mupirocin Study Group (1996). Nasal mupirocin prevents S aureus exit site infection during peritoneal dialysis. *J. Am. Soc. Nephrol.*, **7**, 2403–8.
35b. Bernardini, J., Piramo, B. and Holley, J.L. *et al.* (1996)

Randomised trial of S aureus prophylaxis in PD patients: mupirocin calcium ointment 2% applied to exit site versus oral rifampin. *Am. J. Kidney Dis.*, **26**, 695–700.

36. O'Connor, J., Rigby, R., Hardie, I. *et al.* (1986) Abdominal hernias complicating CAPD. *Am. J. Nephrol.*, **6**, 271–4.

37. Bargman, J.M. (1994) Non-infectious complications of peritoneal dialysis, in *The Textbook of Peritoneal Dialysis* (eds R. Gokal and K.D. Nolph), Kluwer Academic, Dordrecht, pp. 555–90.

38. Pauls, D.G., Basinger, B.B. and Shield, C.F. (1992) Inguinal herniorrhaphy in the CAPD patient. *Am. J. Kidney Dis.*, **20**, 497–9.

39. Tzamaloukas, A.H., Gibel, L.J., Eisenberg, B. *et al.* (1992) Scrotal edema in patients on CAPD: causes, differential diagnosis and management. *Dial. Transplant.*, **21**, 581–90.

40. Kopecky, R.T., Frymoyer, P.A., Witanowski, L.S. *et al.* (1990) Prospective peritoneal scintigraphy in patients beginning CAPD. *Am. J. Kidney Dis.*, **15**, 228–36.

41. Chow, C.C., Sung, J.Y., Chueng, C.K. *et al.* (1988) Massive hydrothorax in CAPD: diagnosis, mangement and review of the literature. *N. Z. Med. J.*, **101**, 475–7.

42. Dobbie, J.W. (1989) Pathology of the peritoneum, in *The Peritoneum and Peritoneal Access* (ed. S. Bengmark), Wright, Wright, pp. 42–52.

42a. Nakayamam, M., Kawaguclu, Y., Yamada, K., *et al.* (1997) Immunohistochemical detection of advanced glycosylation end-products in the peritoneum and its possible pathophysiological role in CAPD. *Kidney Int.*, **51**, 182–186.

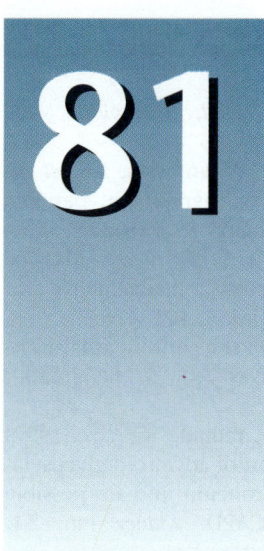

81

Outcome of continuous ambulatory peritoneal dialysis

Alison L. Brown and Anthony E.G. Raine*

Mortality of CAPD

Comparison with hemodialysis

Continuous ambulatory peritoneal dialysis (CAPD) has become increasingly widely used for the treatment of end-stage renal disease (ESRD) since its introduction in the 1970s. It has proved particularly popular in Canada (where 40–50% of new ESRD patients start on CAPD) and the UK, where at the end of 1992, almost 50% of patients aged 65 and over were on CAPD [1]. In contrast, in Germany and Portugal, more than 95% of this age group were treated with hemodialysis (HD). Throughout Europe, CAPD was the therapy for 11% of all ESRD patients, but was used for 17% of those with diabetic nephropathy.

As discussed in Chapter 75, comparison of survival of ESRD patients between registries, countries and centers for one treatment modality is fraught with difficulty. Comparison of survival rates between CAPD and HD is even more problematic. There are often marked differences in comorbidity between patients starting CAPD and those starting HD. When case-mix differences were adjusted for, Held et al. [2] in 1994 reported no significant difference in mortality of non-diabetic patients between CAPD and HD. This review of US renal data of 1725 diabetic and 2411 non-diabetic patients starting dialysis between 1986 and 1987 indicated a higher relative risk of death (1.26) for diabetic patients on CAPD compared to those undergoing HD. The relative risk of death on CAPD

compared to HD increased to 1.34 for patients 63 years and over. This finding contrasts with the conclusion of Maiorca et al.'s 1993 review, which included the Italian multicenter trial results [3, 4]. There was no difference in survival of diabetic patients receiving HD compared to those on CAPD, though the survival of non-diabetics on either modality exceeded that of diabetics. Older patients (>67 years) on CAPD survived longer than those on HD. A recent longitudinal study of three-year survival of 68 CAPD and 34 HD patients found no difference between the two modalities. Age, peripheral vasculopathy, serum albumin <3.5 g/dl and Kt/V urea of <1.7 per week were independent factors with a negative effect on survival of CAPD patients [5].

The largest study comparing outcome on HD and CAPD [6], analyzed the US renal data system for patients starting dialysis in 1987, 1988 and 1989. There were 42 372 deaths over 170 700 patient years. Patients treated with CAPD had a higher relative mortality at 1.19 compared to patients receiving HD. The difference in mortality was insignificant for all CAPD versus HD patients less than 55, but significant and age dependent for patients older than 55. The relative risk was 1.11 for non-diabetics and 1.38 for diabetics; it was present for both males and females but increased for females at 1.3 compared to 1.11 for males. Bloembergen et al.'s study [6] corrected for age, race, gender, cause and duration of ESRD, but not for comorbid conditions.

As discussed in Chapter 75, causes of death are similar for CAPD and HD (see Figures 75.4 and 75.5). Cardiovascular events account for about 40% of deaths [7, 8]. The main difference between the two modalities is in the inci-

*Professor Raine died in October 1995

Nephrology, Edited by Rex L. Jamison and Robert Wilkinson.
Published in 1997 by Chapman & Hall, London. ISBN 0 412 60930 4

dence of deaths due to peritonitis, which account for 7–10% of deaths on CAPD [3, 7].

However, of the 42 372 deaths reviewed by Bloembergen et al., there was an increased risk of death for those on CAPD compared to those on HD for all causes of death except malignancy [9]. It is possible that differences in comorbid disease account for the increased risk, but unfortunately these data were not available for this study. Infection in this series was a major cause of the excess CAPD deaths: patients on CAPD were 40% more likely to die of an infection than patients on HD, and infection accounted for 35% of the excess deaths in CAPD patients, or 1.4 of 4.0 deaths per 100 patient years [9].

Overall, it is at present difficult to state with certainty that survival of ESRF patients is worse with CAPD than with HD, and the most suitable modality for each patient should be considered with regard to comorbid conditions and social circumstances.

Adequacy

In the early days of CAPD, the high rate of peritonitis made long-term survival on CAPD the exception rather than the rule. Subsequent improvements in methods of dialyzate exchange reduced rates of peritonitis. As a result, attention has shifted to the adequacy of CAPD and its association with survival. Controversy continues as to how best to assess adequacy and whether adequacy correlates with outcome [10]. Urea clearance and creatinine clearance, commonly used to assess adequacy of CAPD, require assumptions and estimates which may compromise their value. Kt/V can be calculated as the sum of the peritoneal clearance of urea and the residual renal urea clearance, multiplied by 24 h and divided by the volume of distribution of urea in the body (this cannot be measured on CAPD and must be estimated from body weight). When multiplied by 7, this gives the Kt/V urea per week. Creatinine clearance on CAPD is the sum of peritoneal clearance in dialyzate (which must be corrected for glucose interference) and renal creatinine clearance (which may overestimate glomerular filtration rate because of tubular secretion of creatinine) [11].

Other assessments of adequacy include the peritoneal equilibration test (PET) and Brandes' efficacy number (EN). The PET quantifies ultrafiltration as well as rate of transport of glucose and creatinine [12]. It involves instillation of a 2.27% dextrose bag; the volume drained at the end of the timed period of 4 h is measured as well as ratio of glucose concentration in the drained dialyzate compared to that at the start (D/D$_o$ glucose) and ratio of dialyzate creatinine at 4 h to plasma creatinine (D/P creatinine). A patient who is a high transporter will rapidly reabsorb glucose and accumulate creatinine in the dialyzate, giving a low D/D$_o$ glucose and a high D/P creatinine; a low transporter will do the reverse.

The EN is obtained by dividing the daily clearance of creatinine (estimated from the dialyzate/plasma creati-

nine ratio obtained from the peritoneal equilibration test) by an adjusted daily creatinine production [11]

The optimum method to assess CAPD adequacy has yet to be established and, perhaps because of this, many studies of outcome of CAPD have not attempted to quantify the amount of CAPD delivered. However, the CANUSA study [13], a prospective study of 680 patients commencing continuous peritoneal dialysis (97.9% treated with CAPD, 2.1% with continuous cycling PD) used the data obtained from 10 138 patient-months of follow up to estimate expected patient survival for a range of sustained weekly Kt/V urea and creatinine clearance values. A decrease of 0.1 in weekly Kt/V was associated with a 5% increase in the relative risk (RR) of death; a decrease of 5 l/1.73 m^2 creatinine clearance/ week was associated with a 7% increase in the RR of death. Thus expected two-year patient survival improved from 66% with a sustained weekly Kt/V urea of 1.5 to 81% with a Kt/V of 2.3. A weekly creatinine clearance of 40 l predicted a two-year survival of 65% compared to 86% with a clearance of 95 l. However, one of the most intriguing findings of the CANUSA study was that as well as demonstrating an increased RR of death with increased age, diabetes and history of cardiovascular disease (as expected) there was an unexpected increased RR of death (1.93–1.95) for patients treated at US centers compared to Canadian centers. This difference could not be explained by the variables such as gender, race, body surface area, Kt/V and creatinine clearance that were studied in the analysis. It seems probable that other variables in demographics and comorbid factors could not be controlled for in a study of this size. Nonetheless, the CANUSA study demonstrated that a higher dose of dialysis (including residual renal function) was associated with better patient survival, better technique survival, and fewer days hospitalization. A three-year follow-up of 68 CAPD patients confirmed that indices of adequacy were predictors of mortality and morbidity; a $Kt/V > 1.96$/week was associated with better survival, with only one death in 23 compared to 19 deaths in 45 patients whose Kt/V was less than 1.96 per week [5]. A smaller study of 23 patients maintained on CAPD for seven years demonstrated a negative correlation between Kt/V urea index per year and hospitalization rate and a positive correlation with peripheral nerve conductivity [14].

Despite the limitations of Kt/V as a measure of adequacy, these observations support the view that regular review of Kt/V should be used in the routine follow-up of CAPD patients. The UK Renal Association recently asserted that there is insufficient evidence to establish a minimum value [15], but a Kt/V urea of 1.9 and a creatinine clearance of 60 l per week are reasonable miniumum values [13, 16].

Comorbid conditions

Comorbid conditions vary between CAPD and HD patients, and among centers and countries. Held et al. [2]

reported that patients selected for HD were older, more likely to be black and unable to walk independently compared to CAPD patients. The latter were more likely to have diabetes and peripheral vascular disease but less likely to have had a cerebrovascular accident. In the Italian multicenter trial, CAPD patients were on average six years older than HD patients and had more risk factors compared to HD patients [4]. As already mentioned, in 1992 almost half of UK patients aged 65 and older were on CAPD compared to 13% of European patients. Age at start of dialysis has a strong effect on mortality; as shown in Figure 75.2 in Chapter 75, patients aged 65 and over have a 15% lower five-year survival rate than patients aged 55–64.

Furthermore, disproportionate numbers of European diabetics are treated with CAPD – 17% compared to 11% of all ESRF patients.

Until a randomized prospective trial controlled for comorbid conditions is done, it seems reasonable to consider that the mortality rates for CAPD and HD are not significantly different, to regard them as complementary modalities and to apply them according to the circumstances of each patient.

Morbidity of CAPD

Technique survival

Loss of residual renal function

Many studies have shown the importance of residual renal function to the effectiveness of CAPD. The loss of residual function accounts for most of the reduction in adequacy over time. After several years on CAPD there is minimal contribution from residual renal function and few patients achieve adequacy targets. In fact, Teehan et al. [17] suggested in 1994 that CAPD patients should be studied for at least three years before the effect of the dialysis dose (unaffected by residual renal contribution) on clinical outcome can be evaluated. In 68 CAPD patients, residual function of 1.34–3.0 ml/min was present even at the end of three years [5].

The strongest determinant of Kt/V urea in CAPD patients is the residual renal urea clearance [18] and once this disappears, dialysis adequacy is difficult to achieve. For example, 39% of 147 CAPD patients achieved a Kt/V of >1.9 but only 17% by CAPD alone [19]. Tattersall et al. [18] reported that despite increasing the mean daily exchange volume from 8.1 to 10.4l, after one year of CAPD 40% of patients failed to achieve a Kt/V of >1.75/week. Similarly, Harty et al. [20] observed that an increase of 22% in prescribed daily exchange volume resulted in only a 6% increase in Kt/V urea.

It is apparent that a Kt/V of 1.9 or more maybe impossible to achieve in large patients with minimal residual renal function. After loss of residual function three or more years after starting CAPD, most patients will not achieve adequate (let alone optimal) dialysis without prohibitively large, inconvenient and expensive volumes of dialyzate. It remains to be determined whether alterations in CAPD prescription or the use of overnight continuous cycler PD will achieve adequate dialysis and improved clinical outcome.

Peritonitis

Most studies report worse technique survival for CAPD than for HD, though differences in clinical practice and calculating technique survival make comparison difficult. The Italian multicenter trial showed that the risk of technique failure was 1.81 for CAPD relative to HD, but when peritonitis was excluded, the relative risk for CAPD fell to 1.06 – in other words, nearly all the difference in technique survival between the two modalities was due to peritonitis. However, even with very satisfactory technique survival rates of 81% at three years and 67% at five years, only 28% and 11% of patients continued on CAPD for three and five years, respectively [21].

Peritonitis continues to be a major problem, though much less so since the widespread use of 'Y' or 'disconnect' systems. In 1991, 67% of all European patients used disconnect systems and the rate of peritonitis for the EDTA registry was 10.2 patient months per peritonitis episode. In contrast, 91% of Italian patients used disconnect systems; the rate of peritonitis was 19 patient months per episode. The UK, with 55% of patients on disconnect systems, had 4.8 patient months per peritonitis episode [22].

Loss of ultrafiltration

Loss of ultrafiltration capacity and failure to maintain fluid balance is a common cause of failure of PD. About 10% of patients on CAPD will have problems with ultrafiltration after three years of treatment, increasing to 30% after six years [23]. In addition to the decline of residual renal function throughout this period, there is a general increase in peritoneal permeability to small solutes. This increased solute permeability, which appears to be due to an increased effective peritoneal surface area, reduces the osmotic effectiveness of glucose and decreases net ultrafiltration; this is known as type 1 failure. Type 2 failure is defined as poor permeability, usually in association with sclerosing peritonitis, which has become increasingly rare since the use of acetate and chlorhexidine has been abandoned. In fact, sclerosing peritonitis as a cause of death for patients on CAPD in France fell from 7.9 deaths per 1000 patient years in 1981 to no reported deaths at all after 1985 [24].

The cause of fluid retention on CAPD can be assessed using the peritoneal equilibration test (PET) as previously discussed. Once the type of peritoneal failure is established, and the residual renal function quantified, various strategies can be employed to prolong the effectiveness of CAPD. Short dwell periods to help preserve the osmotic gradient, and leaving the peritoneum dry overnight, or continuous cycler PD at night with the abdomen empty during the day, may be successful. Alternatively, a larger molecular weight osmotic agent which cannot be absorbed quickly and so prolongs the effective osmotic gradient, can be used. Icodextrin is the only such agent which has been shown to be effective in clinical trials.

If these measures fail, temporary or permanent transfer to hemodialysis is necessary.

In a cohort of 23 patients followed for seven years, a recent report suggests that CAPD with lactate dialyzate may prevent deterioration of peritoneal ultrafiltration. A subgroup of 12 patients never exposed to acetate dialyzate maintained constant peritoneal ultrafiltration and creatinine clearance. The Kt/V urea declined from 0.88 ± 0.8 to 0.62 ± 0.06 after seven years, due to the fall in residual renal contribution from 22% to less than 3% after seven years. Peritoneal diffusive capacity was thus maintained for at least seven years, with exclusively lactate-containing dialyzate [14].

Continuous cycler peritoneal dialysis

Various regimes using home automated peritoneal dialysis (APD) are now used. Nightly intermittent PD using a standard six cycles of 2l dialyzate or a high dose of eight cycles of 2.5l dialyzate leaves the peritoneum 'empty' through the day. CAPD, using manual exchanges with varying dwell times during the day can be added to nightly intermittent PD.

Though widely used for children, APD has up till now been restricted to those adults encountering problems with adequacy or life style. This is mainly because of the high costs of the automated cyclers and large dialyzate volumes (9–20l per night), despite the significant social gains from being 'free' of dialysis during the day. Recently APD has become more cost effective, with lower machine costs, and is more widely applied. Between 1989 and 1993 104 German patients were started on APD as initial PD therapy; APD provided adequate dialysis, with low rates of peritonitis (one episode every 50.2 months) and only 8% transfer to HD after 12 months [25]. Rehabilitation was good, with 74% of patients aged less than 60 in employment, but the authors recommended careful patient selection.

In the future, more compact, simpler and cheaper APD machines, and use of different regimes such as tidal techniques, with individual prescription of fluid volume and dwell time, may result in improved APD outcomes.

Hospitalization

Hospitalization rates vary widely among centers, in part depending on outpatient facilities and preferred practice. A recent study comparing hospitalization rates for patients on PD and HD, from the US Renal Data system, assessed 189 654 patient-years between 1988 and 1990 [26]. Hospital admission rates averaged 14% higher for CAPD patients than for HD patients after adjusting for race, age, gender and presence of diabetes. Non-diabetic CAPD patients had a 15% higher admission rate than non-diabetic HD patients, for all age groups. Diabetics aged 20–44 years had similar admission rates on PD and HD, but diabetics 45 years and over had an 18% higher admission rate on CAPD. The authors acknowledge that some of the increase may be due to comorbid factors which could not be corrected for, but speculated that a lower delivered dose of dialysis for CAPD patients compared to HD patients might be relevant. The CANUSA study of 680 PD patients demonstrated that increased hospitalization rates were associated with decreased serum albumin concentration, worsened nutrition according to subjective global assessment and decreased creatinine clearance.

Hypertension

Hypertension is equally if not better controlled on CAPD than on HD. The diurnal variation of blood pressure is better preserved by CAPD than HD, though loss of diurnal variation despite good overall control may occur [27]. Hemodymanic stability is better with CAPD than with HD, which may be important for those with poor myocardial function. The absence of an arteriovenous fistula, constant sodium and fluid removal and continuous correction of uremia and acidosis instead of the oscillations of intermittent HD, may all be beneficial. A decrease in interventricular septum and posterior myocardial wall thickness and left ventricular mass index have been demonstrated after six months CAPD but not HD, despite comparable blood pressure control [3]. Conversely, there is also the potential for constant hypervolemia in the inadequately dialysed CAPD patient.

Anemia

Anemia is often less severe for patients managed by CAPD than by HD, perhaps because of the absence of blood loss and better 'middle molecule' clearance; nonetheless, recombinant human erythropoietin (r-HuEPO) has improved the quality of life of CAPD patients just as for HD patients. In 1990, only 35% of European CAPD patients were receiving r-HuEPO, compared to 53% of HD patients [1], though use of r-HuEPO varies widely. Several studies have suggested that patients treated by CAPD require less r-HuEPO than those treated by HD. Intraperitoneal administration of r-HuEPO will produce a hemopoietic response, but the bioavailability by this route is very low (3–8%) [28]. Nearly all European CAPD patients use the subcutaneous route [1].

Bone disease

Serum phosphate, calcium and pH are generally better controlled by CAPD than HD, and continuous clearance versus intermittent dialysis results in less extreme oscillation. Parathyroid hormone (PTH) is removed by CAPD but not by HD. Despite these theoretical advantages of CAPD, Hamdy et al. [29] reported that hyperparathyroid bone disease is as prevalent in CAPD patients as HD patients, though less severe. This difference may be a function of shorter duration of follow-up for CAPD patients; increasing hyperparathyroid bone disease may become more frequent with longer experience with CAPD.

Adynamic bone disease is more common in CAPD patients than in HD patients, though comorbid factors may influence this since CAPD patients are more likely to be older and diabetic [30]. The increased incidence of adynamic bone disease with CAPD has been attributed to more frequent hypercalcemic episodes; now that calcium carbonate is the prevalent phosphate binder (used by 76% of European centers) it may be that future increased use of low calcium dialyzate will reduce the incidence of hypercalcemia and adynamic bone disease. In 1993, few European PD centers used low calcium dialyzate; in 40%, dialyzate used had a calcium concentration of greater than 1.75 mmol/l for most patients and 33% used dialyzate with a calcium concentration between 1.51 and 1.74 mmol/l [1].

Intraperitoneal, subcutaneous and oral pulse therapy of vitamin D have all been studied in CAPD patients; intravenous pulse therapy is not widely used since it is much less acceptable for CAPD patients than HD patients. Intraperitoneal vitamin D does not appear any more effective than oral administration. Pulse therapy by mouth at night, when the gut calcium concentrations are lowest, combined with low calcium dialyzate, seems a sensible strategy [31].

Immune status: infections, transplantation and malignancy

Although there are few comparative data, immune cell function may be better preserved by CAPD than by HD. The lymphoblastic response to autologous serum is better in CAPD than HD patients, as is the proliferative response to mitogens and the chemiluminescence of stimulated polymorph neutrophils. However, Maiorca et al. were unable to detect a difference in incidence of infections (other than peritonitis, PD exit site, PD tunnel or HD vascular access infections) or malignancy in 494 patients followed for an average of 32 months [3].

No difference between CAPD and HD in postrenal transplant outcome has been demonstrated.

Nutrition

Biochemical and anthropometric evidence of malnutrition is found in 11–56% of CAPD patients [32], and is strongly associated with increased morbidity and mortality [13]. Several studies have shown a worsening of nutritional status on CAPD, especially during the first year

[17]. One factor is the loss of protein in the peritoneal dialyzate, which varies, but may be as much as 140 g/week. The protein loss can increase by 50–100% during an episode of peritonitis [33].

Protein catabolic rate (PCR) which is an indicator of dietary protein intake in the stable patient, correlates with Kt/V urea [33], suggesting that underdialysis may contribute to anorexia and malnutrition.

Continuous glucose uptake from the peritoneum does provide energy, but also causes hyperglycemia, hyperinsulinemia and obesity [32]. Recently, a large multicenter study of 534 HD and 168 CAPD patients demonstrated significantly higher lipoprotein (a) (Lp(a)) levels in dialysis patients compared to normal controls; CAPD patients had significantly higher levels than HD patients (in mg/dl, normal controls 18.4; HD 23.4 and CAPD 34.6) [34]. The authors postulate that there is an overproduction of Lp(a) to compensate for protein losses in CAPD, causing a greater increase in Lp(a) than that seen in ESRF and HD patients. Increased plasma concentration of Lp(a) may increase the risk of atherogenesis.

Amyloid

B_2-microglobulin is better cleared by CAPD than by HD, and in practice fewer CAPD patients seem to develop symptomatic amyloidosis. This may be a reflection of the scarcity of long-term CAPD patients rather than a true difference between modalities, however, and there is no doubt that dialysis-related amyloid has developed in patients exclusively dialyzed by CAPD [35]. Maiorca et al. [3] reported that after 5–10 years of dialysis, 7% of HD patients required surgery for carpal tunnel syndrome, compared to none of 23 CAPD patients at risk in the same period. However, no CAPD patients in this study had been followed for more than 10 years so it is not possible to say if this difference will persist. No difference in amyloid bone deposits between HD and CAPD patients could be demonstrated.

Choice of modality

Teehan and Hakim in a 1995 review [36] emphasized the significance of Bloembergen's report of a significantly higher risk of death for patients on CAPD, especially diabetics, women, those over 55 years and those likely to continue on CAPD for more than one year. They recommended taking these risk factors into account when considering which modality to recommend, as well as estimating the likelihood of obtaining a Kt/V urea of 2.1 or above by CAPD. In practice, this means that large patients with negligible residual renal function are unlikely to be suitable for CAPD. For other patients, however, particularly elderly diabetics with extrarenal complications, the possibility of reduced survival should be balanced against the improved quality of life with continuous self-managed therapy at home and the additional potential advantage of intraperitoneal insulin administration.

Finally, we should also consider carefully whether to recommend dialysis at all, particularly for the elderly patient with widespread complications of diabetes whose prospects for survival let alone rehabilitation are poor. This is especially important in view of the 'rising tide' of diabetic nephropathy and the increasingly elderly population world-wide as we approach the millenium [37].

References

1. Valderrabano, F., Jones, E.H.P. and Mallick, N.P. (1995) Report on management of renal failure in Europe, XXIV, 1993. *Nephrol. Dial. Transplant.*, **10**(suppl 5), 1–25.
2. Held, P.J., Port, F.K., Turenne, M.N. *et al.* (1994) Continuous ambulatory peritoneal dialysis and hemodialysis: comparison of patient mortality with adjustment for comorbid conditions. *Kidney Int.*, **45**, 1163–9.
3. Maiorca, R., Cancarini, G.C., Brunori, G. *et al.* (1993) Morbidity and mortality of CAPD and haemodialysis. *Kidney Int.*, **43**(Suppl 40) S4–15.
4. Maiorca, R., Vonesh, E.F., Cavalli, P. *et al.* (1991) A multicentre selection-adjusted comparison of patient and technique survivals on CAPD and HD. *Perit. Dial. Int.*, **11**, 118–27.
5. Maiorca, R., Brunori, G., Zubani, R. *et al.* (1995) Predictive value of dialysis adequacy and nutritional indices for mortality and morbidity in CAPD and HD patients. A longitudinal study. *Nephrol. Dial. Transplant.*, **12**, 2295–305.
6. Bloembergen, W., Port, F.K., Mauger, E.A. *et al.* (1995) A comparison of mortality between patients treated with HD and PD. *J. Am. Soc. Nephrol.*, **6**, 177–83.
7. Maiorca, R., Vonesh, E., Cancarini, G.C. *et al.* (1988) A six-year comparison of patient and technique survivals in CAPD and HD. *Kidney Int.*, **34**, 518–24.
8. Burton, P.R. and Walls, J. (1987) Selection-adjusted comparison of patients on CAPD, hemodialysis and renal transplantation. *Lancet*, **1**, 1115–19.
9. Bloembergen, W., Port, F.K., Mauger, E.A. and Wolfe, R.A. (1995) A comparison of cause of death between patients treated with HD and PD. *J. Am. Soc. Nephrol.*, **6**, 184–91.
10. Churchill, D.N. (1994) Adequacy of peritoneal dialysis: how much do we need? *Kidney Int.*, **46**(suppl 48) S2–6.
11. Krediet, R.T., Koomen, G.C.M., Struuk, D.G. *et al.* (1994) Practical methods for assessing dialysis efficiency during peritoneal dialysis. *Kidney Int.*, **46**(suppl 48) S7–13.
12. Twardowski, Z.J., Nolph, K.D., Khanna, R. *et al.* (1987) Peritoneal equilibration test. *Perit. Dial. Bull.*, **7**, 138–47.
13. Churchill, D.N., Taylor, D.W., Keshaviah, P.R. (1996) Adequacy of dialysis and nutrition in continuous peritoneal dialysis: association with clinical outcomes. Canada-USA (CANUSA) Peritoneal Dialysis Study Group. *J. Am. Soc. Nephrol.*, **7**, 198–207.
14. Faller, B. and Lameire, N. (1994) Evolution of clinical parameters and peritoneal function in a cohort of CAPD patients followed over 7 years. *Nephrol. Dial. Transplant.*, **9**, 280–6.
15. The Renal Association Standards Subcommittee (1995) Treatment of adult patients with renal failure. Recommended standards and audit measures. Royal College of Physicians, London.
16. Harty, J. and Gokal, R. (1995) Does CAPD provide adequate dialysis? *Nephrol. Dial. Transplant.*, **10**, 1115–17.
17. Teehan, B.P., Schliefer, C.R. and Brown, J. (1994) Adequacy of CAPD: morbidity and mortality in chronic peritoneal dialysis. *Am. J. Kidney. Dis.*, **24**, 990–1001.
18. Tattersall, J.E., Doyle, S., Greenwood, R.N. *et al.* (1993) Kinetic modelling and underdialysis in CAPD patients. *Nephrol. Dial. Transplant.*, **8**, 535–8.
19. Harty, J.C., Boulton, H., Uttley, L. *et al.* (1992) Limitations of urea kinetic modelling as predictors of nutritional and dialysis adequacy in CAPD. *Am. J. Nephrol.*, **13**, 454–63.
20. Harty, J.C., Boulton, H., Uttley, L. *et al* (1994) Limitations of modelling dialysis therapy in CAPD (Abstr). *J. Am. Soc. Nephrol.*, **5**, 516.
21. Fox, J.G., Fowler, I. and Boulton-Jones, J.M. (1993) Audit of a decade of CAPD. *Nephrol. Dial. Transplant.*, **8**, 240–3.
22. Raine, A.E.G., Margreiter, R., Brunner, F.P. *et al.* (1992) Report on management of renal failure in Europe, XXII, 1991. *Nephrol. Dial. Transplant. Suppl.*, **2**, 7–35.
23. Coles, G.A. and Williams, J.D. (1994) The management of ultrafiltration failure in peritoneal dialysis. *Kidney Int.*, **46**(suppl 48) S14–17.
24. Geerlings, W., Tufveson, G., Brunner, F.P. *et al.* (1990) Combined report on regular dialysis and transplantation in Europe. *Nephrol. Dial. Transplant.*, **6**(suppl 4) 5–29.
25. Brunkhorst, R., Wrenger, E., Krautzig, S. *et al.* (1994) Clinical experience with home automated peritoneal dialysis. *Kidney Int.*, **46**, Suppl. 48, S25–30.
26. Habach, G., Bloembergen, W.E., Mauger, E.A. *et al.* (1995) Hospitalization among US dialysis patients: hemodialysis versus peritoneal dialysis. *J. Am. Soc. Nephrol.*, **5**, 1940–8.
27. Korzets, Z., Erdberg, A. *et al.* (1994) Does diurnal variation in blood pressure exist in CAPD patients? *Nephrol. Dial. Transplant.*, **9**, 274–6.
28. Macdougall, I.C., Roberts, D.E., Coles, G.A. *et al.* (1991) Clinical pharmacokinetics of epoetin (r-HuEPO). *Clin. Pharmacokinet.*, **20**, 99–113.
29. Hamdy, N.A.T., Brown, C.B., Boletis, J. *et al.* (1990) Mineral metabolism in CAPD. *Contrib. Nephrol.*, **85**, 100–10.
30. Hamdy, N.A.T. (1995) The spectrum of renal bone disease. *Nephrol. Dial. Transplant.*, **10**(suppl 4) 14–18.
31. Sweny, P. (1995) Optimum route of administration of vitamin D in renal failure. *Nephrol. Dial. Transplant.*, **10**, Suppl. 4, 29–32.
32. Lindholm, B. and Bergstrom, J. (1989) Nutritional management of patients undergoing peritoneal dialysis, in *Peritoneal Dialysis* (ed. K.D. Nolph), Kluwer Academic, Boston, pp. 230–60.

33. Bergstrom, J. and Lindholm, B. (1993) Nutrition and adequacy of dialysis. How do hemodialysis and CAPD compare? *Kidney Int.*, **43**(suppl 40) S39–50.

34. Kronenberg, F., Konig, P., Neyer, U. *et al.* (1995) Multicenter study of lipoprotein (a) and apolipoprotein (a) phenotypes in patients with end-stage renal disease treated by hemodialysis or CAPD. *J. Am. Soc. Nephrol.*, **6**, 110–20.

35. Jadoul, M., Noel, H. and van Ypersele de Strihou, C. (1990) Beta-2-microglobulin amyloidosis in a patient treated exclusively by CAPD. *Am. J. Kidney. Dis.*, **15**, 86–8.

36. Teehan, B.P. and Hakim, R. (1995) CAPD – quo vadis? *J. Am. Soc. Nephrol.*, **6**, 139–43.

37. Raine, A.E.G. (1995) The rising tide of diabetic nephropathy – the warning before the flood? *Nephrol. Dial. Transplant.*, **10**, 460–1.

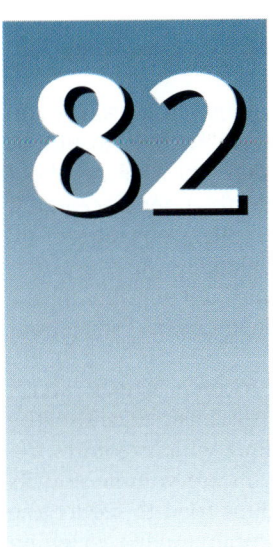

82

Special procedures

J.E. Tattersall, K. Farrington and R.N. Greenwood

Continuous blood purification in acute renal failure

Historical background

Largely as a result of biotechnical advances there has been a significant change in the management of the critically ill patient with acute renal failure in recent years. In the past, patients were supported by the well-established therapies which underpinned chronic dialysis programs, i.e. intermittent or continuous peritoneal dialysis or intermittent hemodialysis using temporary catheters. This required transfer of patients to centers with in-house expertise in these dialysis modalities. Not all hospitals were renal centers and often this meant transporting critically ill patients many miles.

Peritoneal dialysis is not a very satisfactory treatment for patients with multiorgan failure (MOF) because of the risk of intra-abdominal sepsis and the relatively poor efficiency of dialysis which can be achieved. Intermittent hemodialysis even on a daily basis tends to be unsatisfactory because of acute disturbances of solute and fluid equilibrium introduced by the treatment. It is also sometimes difficult to introduce enough volume deficit during an intermittent session for the intravenous medications and fluids which the patient inevitably receives for the remainder of the day. Critically ill patients are often severely compromised in their ability to respond to fluid shifts. Also, hemodialysis is an intrinsically bioincompat-

ible therapy which causes activation of acute phase reactants, a phenomenon chiefly ascribed to the exposure of blood to foreign surfaces including polyvinyl chloride (PVC) blood tubing and the dialysis membrane and the presence of bacterial and pyrogenic materials in dialysis fluid. It has been increasingly recognized in recent years that the combination of cellulose membrane in the dialyzer and endotoxin in the water used for dialysis is a particularly potent combination which may compromise vascular stability. It may even mitigate against recovery of acute tubular necrosis in patients with multiple organ failure [1]. Although non-cellulosic synthetic membranes or modified cellulosic membranes are now freely available, the production of endotoxin-free fluid for dialysis is not straightforward in the intensive care unit (ITU) setting.

Intermittent machine hemofiltration which was originally developed as an alternative to maintenance hemodialysis in chronic renal failure has been successfully applied to the management of the critically ill in the ITU. In this technique, 25–35 l of prepared sterile fluid is exchanged in a single session for a similar volume of plasma filtrate. The problem of bioincompatibility is minimized since sterile fluid is preprepared and high flux synthetic membranes such as polysulfone or polyamide are used. However, this approach embodies the other disadvantages of machine treatment – intermittency and relative complexity of operation with high capital cost of equipment.

Nephrology, Edited by Rex L. Jamison and Robert Wilkinson.
Published in 1997 by Chapman & Hall, London. ISBN 0 412 60930 4

Continuous arteriovenous hemofiltration (CAVH)

At the end of the 1970s manufacturers started to produce porous dialyzers and hemofilters in various shapes and sizes which were highly permeable to plasma water and solutes with molecular weights up to that of albumin. The Japanese were the first to recognize the potential for continuous blood purification by filtration and replacement of plasma water with sterile fluids. However, Kramer (1977) [2] was credited with having introduced continuous arteriovenous hemofiltration (CAVH). In this technique, the patient's arteriovenous pressure difference is employed as a driving force for the flow of blood through a hemofilter which acts as an artificial glomerulus (Figure 82.1). This circuit does not need pressure alarms or air detection because the pressure of the blood is positive with respect to atmosphere through the whole circuit and air cannot enter the patient. Alarms would be mandatory if a pump was used.

This simple circuit looked attractive and seemed to have great potential. However, experience in the early 1980s showed that CAVH was limited because inadequate rates of ultrafiltration and poor control of uremia were commonplace. Compared to the normal kidneys which filter about 170 l of plasma water each day, CAVH often formed less than 15 l of filtrate which, although reducing the frequency of treatment, did not obviate the need for intermittent hemodialysis. This meant uncertainty, on initiation of CAVH, about whether uremia would be controlled. This in turn created uncertainty about the need to transfer the patient to a renal center if hemodialysis was not available on site. Poor rates of filtration were often related to inadequate arteriovenous pressure differences which are not uncommon in the critically ill due to arterial hypotension or venous hypertension.

Further drawbacks of CAVH include arterial access which is sometimes difficult to establish and also the labor intensiveness of the technique which requires frequent manual measurements of filtrate volume and its accurate replacement. Several groups tried to reduce the manual labor by introducing computer-aided weighing systems and mechanical balancing devices to aid the documentation and control of fluid balance. CAVH augmented in this way was an incomplete solution to the problem, which is probably why CAVH as a technique lost popularity relatively quickly.

Continuous venovenous hemofiltration (CVVH)

Recognizing the benefit of continuous treatment, investigators attempted to overcome the difficulties of inadequate ultrafiltration by introducing a pump in the extracorporeal circuit. This had the advantage of reduc-

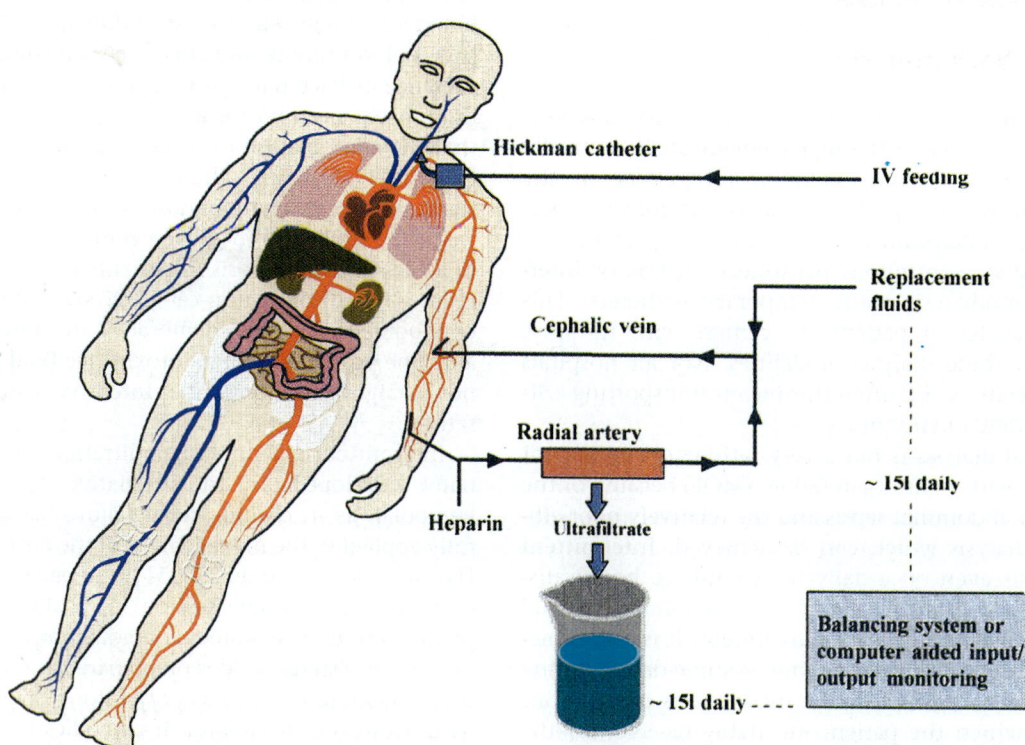

Figure 82.1 Continuous arteriovenous hemofiltration (CAVH) employing a hemofilter in a spontaneously driven extracorporeal circuit.

ing the requirement for access only to the venous side of the circulation but it required special machinery with all the fail-safe alarm features necessary when negative pressures exist in the circuit. The technique was referred to as continuous venovenous hemofiltration (CVVH). It is now probably the most popular of the continuous therapies.

It was fortuitous that in the early 1980s some dialysis machines used for chronic renal failure were designed in a modular form; it was possible to remove modules which incorporated a peristaltic blood pump and air detection units. In spite of these makeshift adaptations, the safety features were satisfactory and the guarantee of sufficient filtration volumes to control uremia established CVVH as a standard technique which has changed little in the last 15 years.

Vascular access

Access to the circulation is usually via a double lumen catheter inserted into the internal jugular, subclavian or femoral veins. The relative ease with which these catheters can be inserted using standard techniques by attending physicians permits prompt institution of treatment.

Treatment parameters

The blood flow rate is usually between 100 and 200 ml/min, which creates a positive pressure in the dialyzer/filter to allow the filtration rate to be controlled by a gate clamp. Alternatively the filtration rate can be controlled by a separate pump. Filtration rates up to 30 ml/min are usually employed. Although this gives clearances equivalent to only a small fraction of the urea cleared by conventional HD the cumulative clearance over 24 h equals or can easily exceed that achievable by intermittent therapy. Urea removal is also enhanced in slow therapies because the plasma concentration is at a relatively high, stable level unlike in conventional HD.

Dialyzers and fluids

Because the extracorporeal flow is pumped, the importance of the resistance to flow of the dialyzer/filter is minimized. Capillary type dialyzers/filters can therefore be employed as easily as flat plate devices (usually lower resistance) and choice tends to depend on price and availability. Devices with moderate ultrafiltration characteristics provide sufficient flexibility.

Preprepared bags of sterile fluid are available from several manufacturers. In the early years, peritoneal dialysis (PD) fluid provided a readily available solution which was practical but not ideal. High glucose concentrations are not necessary in continous blood purification in which hydrostatic rather than osmotic forces are used to ultrafilter fluid from blood. In more modern dedicated

preparations the glucose concentration is reduced. Calcium and magnesium are employed in roughly the same concentrations as in PD fluid, being typically 1.7 mmol/l and 0.75 mmol/l, respectively. Potassium is added, up to concentration of 2.0 mmol/l. Since bicarbonate is difficult to hold in solution, particularly in the presence of calcium ions, acetate or lactate is used as the base at a concentration of 30–40 mmol/l. Continuous, gentle blood purification avoids the potential effect of acetate overload which can occur in intermittent HD, the infused load being readily metabolized to bicarbonate. Rarely in patients with compromised hepatic function base-free solutions can be employed with separate infusion of sodium bicarbonate. Some manufacturers have succeeded in producing bicarbonate-containing fluids.

Anticoagulation

The approach to anticoagulation employed in traditional HD is applied to the continuous therapies with slight variations. Heparin is usually given as a continuous infusion at approximately 300 iu/h into the arterial line leading to the filter/dialyzer after priming the dialyzer with a bolus of 1000–2000 iu at the start of the procedure. An empirical approach is necessary since heparin sensitivity varies considerably and is influenced by many factors. The infusion rate is adjusted according to regular (say four-hourly) estimations of partial thromboplastin time (PTT). The aim is to achieve maximum extracorporeal anticoagulation with minimum systemic anticoagulation. Usually the arterial PTT (from the patient) should be less than 40–45 s.

In patients in whom bleeding problems are present or anticipated a more sophisticated approach is necessary. 'Regional' anticoagulation with heparin and protamine neutralization at the venous end of the circuit has been employed but is not ideal. Prostacyclin is occasionally used, expense and hypotension being the two main drawbacks.

Precautions

Apart from clotting problems, the main danger is inaccuracy of fluid balance. This results from the combination of large target volumes (>25 l/day) and the well-recognized inaccuracies of peristaltic pumps and gravitational ultrafiltration systems. Regular weighing of all infusion fluids and ultrafiltrate provides the surest safety net to avoid large cumulative volume errors. Although this is laborious, measurements have to be made hourly and this will remain necessary until fail-safe automated systems are introduced (see below).

Continuous hemodialysis (CAVHD and CVVHD)

An alternative approach to overcoming the inadequacies of CAVH was taken by other workers in the mid 1980s.

Schneider and Geroneumus [3] were credited with introducing continuous arteriovenous hemodialysis (CAVHD). The innovation in this technique was recognizing that the hemofilter used in CAVH could be used as a dialyzer. Thus the convective process is replaced by a diffusive process (Figure 82.2). Since inadequate convective forces are the problem in CAVH the use of diffusion is a sensible step since, provided a high enough dialyzate fluid flow is used, clearances achieved by diffusion are superior. The blood flow rate in most spontaneously driven circuits in the critically ill is sufficient to achieve satisfactory blood purification using the technique of continuous CAVHD. However, the problem of labor intensiveness is not solved by CAVHD and there is a further minor disadvantage. During continuous dialysis it is possible to have clotting in the extracorporeal circuit which is not immediately apparent. The check for clotting in CAVH, which is possible because of the visible filtration process, is lost. Tedious methods have to be employed to detect this problem.

The need for access to the arterial system is also a disadvantage of CAVHD which has prompted some groups to use slow hemodialysis with a pumped extracorporeal circuit – continuous venovenous hemodialysis (CVVHD).

A pumped extracorporeal blood flow generally guarantees a blood flow rate sufficient to ensure adequate clearance provided enough sterile fluid is replaced (CVVH) or perfused through the dialyzer (CVVHD). In each case the machinery and monitoring systems necessary are comparable. Also diffusion and convection produce comparable clearances since the use of efficient dialyzer and slow flow rates allow almost complete equilibration of solutes in blood and dialysis fluid. There is, therefore, little to choose between CVVH and CVVHD on theoretical and practical grounds. The detection of clotting in the extracorporeal circuit is usually simpler in CVVH (cessation of filtration).

Usage tends to be determined by familiarity, cost and local circumstances.

Plasma exchange

Background

Centrifugal aspheresis systems were developed in the 1960s, originally for the purpose of the separation of the formed elements of blood for hematological uses. The techniques were adapted for continuous separation of plasma (Figure 82.3). Subsequently plasmapheresis was employed in the treatment of a variety of immunologically mediated conditions spanning many disciplines including nephrology. The rationale for the use of plasma exchange in the treatment of renal disease is to remove

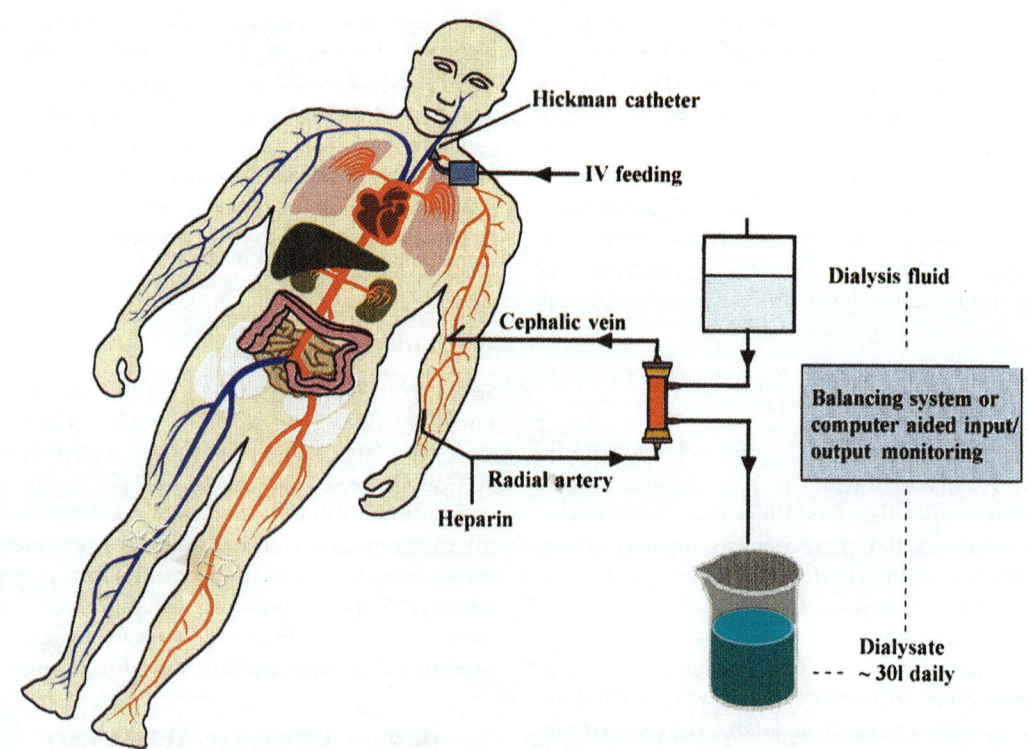

Figure 82.2 Continuous arteriovenous hemodialysis (CAVHD) where the filtration process is replaced by diffusive dialysis.

proteins regarded as potential mediators of renal inflammation. These include circulating autoantibodies such as antiglomerular basement membrane (anti-GBM) and anti-DNA antibodies, immune complexes, free antigens and antibodies capable of *in situ* immune complex formation, complement components and paraproteins. The explosion of interest in these potential nephrological applications was fueled by the spectacular success of plasma exchange in the treatment of Goodpasture's syndrome [4]. Since then its role in the treatment of renal disease has become better defined. During this time the advent of highly permeable synthetic membranes allowed the development of on-line plasmafiltration systems which have become the method of choice for plasma exchange in clinical practice.

Technical aspects of plasma exchange

Membrane characteristics

Highly permeable synthetic membranes are made of cellulose diacetate, polymethylmethacrylate, polypropylene and polysulfone. They have a nominal pore size of $0.5\,\mu m$ which allows passage through the membrane of $150{-}970\,kDa$ macromolecules including immunoglobulins, circulating immune complexes ($500{-}3000\,kDa$) and β lipoprotein ($2400\,kDa$) but not platelets and other formed elements.

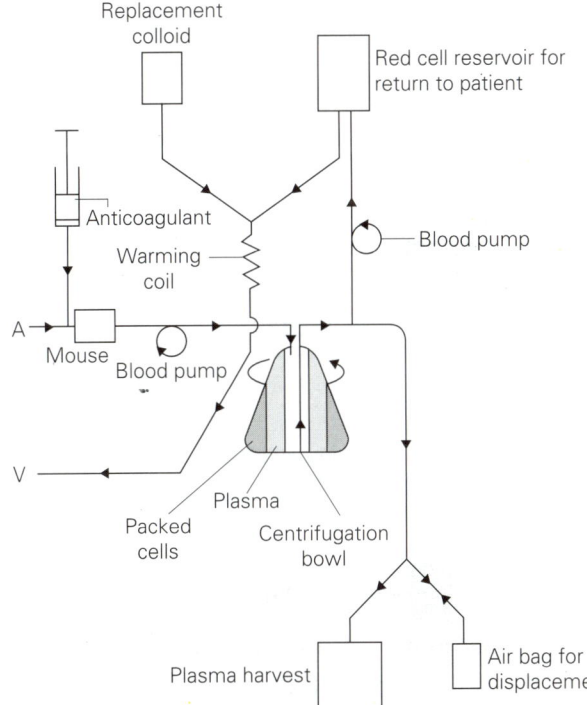

Figure 82.3 Schematic system for on-line centrifugal apheresis.

Extracorporeal circuit

This is similar to standard hemodialysis circuits. Modifications include a hemoglobin detector in the plasma line to detect hemolysis and a pump to allow controlled filtration and delivery of warmed replacement fluid (Figure 82.4). The entire circuit is warmed to prevent precipitated cryoglobulins plugging membrane pores.

Vascular access

A large-bore central venous catheter is the preferred access as for acute hemodialysis.

Anticoagulation

Heparin is normally used at a loading dose of 2000 iu and a maintenance dose of 500–1000 iu/h. Where there are risks of bleeding lower doses should be used and controlled by monitoring activated clotting time.

Replacement fluids

In most situations the preferred replacement fluid is an isotonic solution containing 4–5% protein derived from plasma or serum. At least 95% of the protein is albumin (4.5% albumin). To limit costs, some units use other synthetic iso-oncotic colloid replacement fluids (e.g. hydroxyethyl starch) to provide a proportion of the total replacement but significant hypoalbuminaemia is a risk where treatment courses are prolonged. Calcium and potassium are usually added to the replacement fluids to provide physiological concentrations and prevent tetany and cardiac arrythmias. Where there are risks of bleeding or when invasive procedures are imminent, clotting factor repletion is carried out using fresh frozen plasma (FFP) instead of 4.5% albumin for the last liter or so of the exchange. In some conditions (e.g. hemolytic uremic syndrome/thrombotic thrombocytopenic purpura) the whole exchange is carried out with FFP (see below).

Exchange volumes and frequency

The decrease in plasma concentration of a macromolecule brought about by plasma exchange depends on exchange volume. The relationship is exponential so that removal efficiency is maximal during the first few liters. Use of exchanges greater than about 4 l is not cost effective. Immediately after completing an exchange there is an upward rebound in the plasma concentration of macromolecules. This occurs in two phases. First there is redistribution from the extravascular compartment at a rate which depends on the distribution characteristics of the particular protein. Secondly there is the resynthesis phase. The rate of this, for immunoglobulins, can be reduced by immunosuppression. The number and frequency of exchanges which are required depends on the particular indication. In some it is important to continue daily exchanges to remove completely an assayable toxic molecule, e.g. antiglomerular basement membrane antibody, in others the purpose is to augment an immunosuppressive regime and the number and frequency of exchanges are empirical.

Complications

Improvements in monitoring and safety have reduced the complications associated with extracorporeal circuits, though those associated with temporary venous access remain considerable. The main complications of plasma exchange are hypotension, usually caused by volume depletion, but also by allergic reactions to substitution fluids. Such reactions also include urticaria and fever. They occur more frequently with FFP. Bleeding may occur because of overheparinization and may be exacerbated by clotting factor depletion due to the exchange. Hypocalcemia, cardiac arrhythmias (provoked by local hypokalemia), and hypoalbuminemia are preventable (see 'Replacement fluids' above).

Indications for plasma exchange
(Table 82.1)

Antiglomerular basement membrane disease

Plasma exchange is firmly established as a vital component in the treatment of antiglomerular basement mem-

brane disease. This conclusion is largely based on comparison of outcomes of treatments which include plasma exchange with those from the preplasma exchange era. Intensive plasma exchange for 14 days or until the disappearance of the antibody, combined with immunosuppression with steroids and cyclophosphamide, is indicated in all patients presenting with pulmonary hemorrhage and in those without this complication presenting with serum creatinine levels below 600 μmol/l. Treatment seems to be of little benefit (in terms of renal salvage) and is associated with increased risk in most patients presenting with higher serum creatinines in the absence of pulmonary hemorrhage [5]. There may be exceptions [6]. Patients with both anti-glomerular basement membrane and anti-neutrophil cytoplasmic antibodies tend to respond more like those with systemic vasculitis (described below).

Focal necrotizing glomerulonephritis associated with systemic vasculitis

These patients generally respond well to immunosuppressive drugs when treatment is started early, and plasma exchange confers no additional therapeutic benefit in such cases. However, in a randomized controlled trial, the combination of plasma exchange and immunosuppressive drugs enabled a significantly greater proportion of patients presenting with dialysis-dependent renal failure to achieve dialysis independence compared with the use of the drugs alone [7]. The addition of plasma exchange did not benefit patients not requiring dialysis at presen-

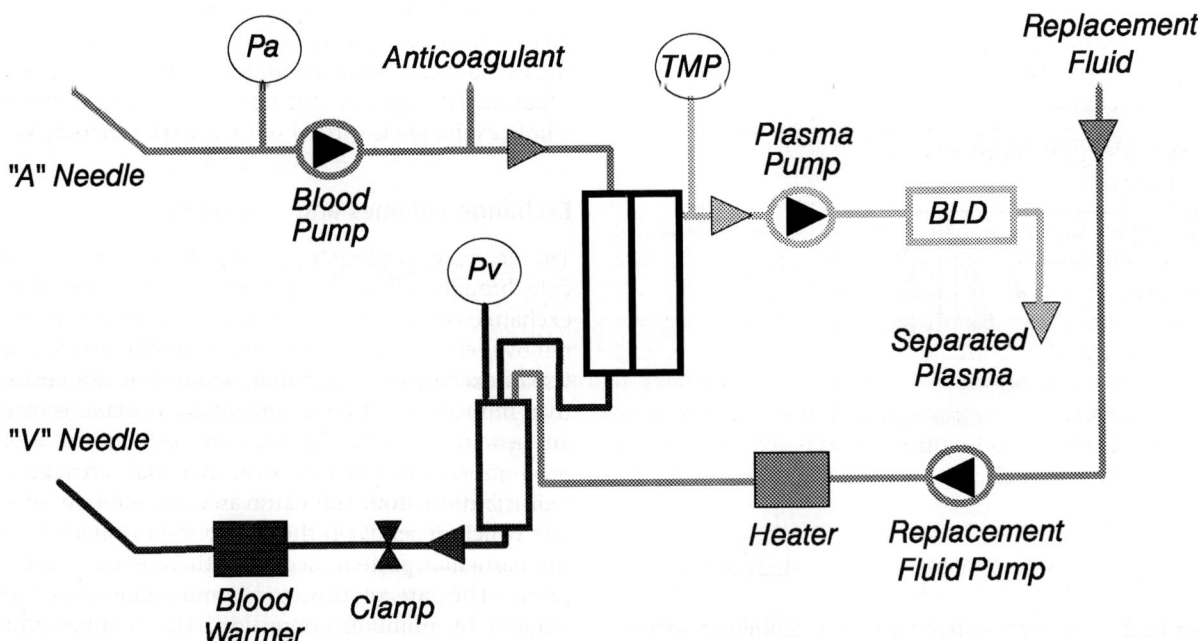

Figure 82.4 Schematic system for plasmafiltration.

Table 82.1 Indications for the use of plasma exchange in the treatment of renal disease

Antiglomerular basement membrane disease
Non-anti-GBM mediated rapidly progressive
  glomerulonephritis
Multisystem vasculitis
Hemolytic uremic syndrome/thrombotic
  thrombocytopenic purpura
Myeloma kidney/light chain nephropathy
Pretransplant depletion of anti-HLA cytotoxic
  antibodies
Vascular transplant rejection

tation. In essential mixed cryoglobulinemia, plasma exchange may be useful to control renal deterioration though data are scanty in this rare disease.

Hemolytic uremic syndrome/thrombotic thrombocytopenic purpura

Plasma infusions are effective in the adult form of the disease, though a controlled trial of this therapy in children predominantly with epidemic diarrheal-associated disease showed no benefit [8]. The benefit of plasma infusion has several explanations, including replenishment of plasma factors involved in prostaglandin-stimulating activity, degradation of von Willebrand factor multimers and inhibition of platelet-aggregating factors. In thrombotic thrombocytopenic purpura a prospective randomized trial showed that plasma exchange was more effective than plasma infusion, probably because it allowed the safe delivery of larger volumes of plasma [9].

Myeloma kidney/light chain nephropathy

Plasma exchange has a role in the treatment of some of the complications of plasma cell dyscrasias, including hyperviscosity syndrome and peripheral neuropathy, but its role in preserving or restoring renal function in these conditions remains controversial, probably due to the protein pathogenetic factors involved. Nevertheless, a prospective randomized trial in such patients did demonstrate benefits from adding plasma exchange to standard chemotherapy though not many patients were studied [10].

Renal transplantation

Plasma exchange combined with immunosuppression has been successfully used to reduce titers of preformed antibodies against HLA molecules in sensitized patients

awaiting renal transplantation, allowing successful transplantation in a substantial proportion [11]. It has also been used as rescue therapy in patients with acute vascular rejection with moderate success in some hands [12]. Its role in the treatment of chronic rejection is poorly defined.

Hemoperfusion

In hemoperfusion, solute is cleared by adsorbance onto a suitable adsorbent surface in direct contact with the blood. Hemoperfusion requires an extracorporeal blood circuit and conventional hemodialysis sytems may be used for this. The adsorbent generally takes the form of microscopic spheres packed into a cartridge which is connected into the circuit in place of the dialyzer. However, since hemoperfusion requires no dialyzate or infusate, the method is much simpler to perform than other blood purification methods and could use simpler equipment.

In routine hemoperfusion, activated charcoal is almost invariably the adsorbent. The charcoal spheres are normally coated with a polymer to reduce bioincompatibility, reduce platelet and protein adhesion to the surface and inhibit the release of fine carbon particles into the blood. Coated charcoal is relatively inexpensive to produce and adsorbs organic solutes with molecular weights ranging from urea up to the pore size of the coating.

Early charcoal adsorbents were coated in a cellulose layer. Recently the biocompatibility and permeability of the coating have been improved by using synthetic materials, incuding silicone [13] and polyacrylate [14].

A typical hemoperfusion cartridge has a blood-contact surface area of $2-4\,m^2$, which allows the possibility of much higher clearance rates than conventional dialysis which generally uses smaller membrane surface areas. Since the solute is immobilized immediately after it has passed through the pores in the encapsulating surface, the concentration gradients are higher, further enhancing clearance rates.

Hemoperfusion in chronic renal failure

Although charcoal adsorbs urea, 3 kg is required to adsorb the 30 g which may accumulate in dialysis patients during the interdialytic interval. All other organic solutes are present in much smaller amounts and can be adsorbed by a much more practical 100 g charcoal cartridge. Charcoal cannot adsorb inorganic and organic salts or water. For these reasons, hemoperfusion is best used in combination with conventional hemodialysis or CAPD to increase the clearance of large molecules. Experimental programs report improved clinical outcome when dialysis is combined with hemoperfusion in this way [15, 16].

Hemoperfusion in poisoning

Charcoal hemoperfusion will clear most drugs and organic poisons. If there is sufficient renal function, it may be used alone to reduce the blood concentrations of a wide range of toxins.

Hemoperfusion in hepatic failure

Charcoal adsorbs bilirubin and other toxic metabolites and has been used to improve outcome in severe hepatic failure. Since hemoperfusion cannot replace the metabolic functions of the liver, its benefit to the patient is probably marginal until more complex enzyme-coated adsorbents are developed [17].

Other adsorbents

Experimental charcoal adsorbents with a polished surface have been produced to allow direct blood contact and improved clearance of bound solute [18]. Since only free solute diffuses through the encapsulating membrane, conventional hemoperfusion cannot clear bound solute. Using unencapsulated charcoal, the toxin is transferred directly from binding protein to charcoal.

Polymer and resin-based adsorbents have been developed for specific adsorption of various solutes including low density lipoprotein [19] and phosphate [20]. Immunoadsorption employs antigen immobilized onto the polymer surface [21]. Specific antibody is adsorbed from the blood by binding onto the immobilized antigen. Immunoadsorption has been used in systemic lupus erythematosus and in preparing sensitized patients for transplantation.

References

1. Hakim, R.M., Wingard, R.L. and Parker, R.A. (1994) Effects of hemodialysis membrane in the treatment of patients with acute renal failure. *N. Engl. J. Med.*, **331**, 1338–42.
2. Kramer, P., Wigger, W., Rieger, J. and Scheler, F. (1977) Arteriovenous hemofiltration: a new and simple method for treatment of overhydrated patients resistant to diuretics. *Klin. Wochenschr.*, **55**, 1121–2.
3. Geronemus, R. and Schneider, N. (1984) Continuous arteriovenous hemodialysis: a new modality for treatment of acute renal failure. *Trans. Am. Soc. Artif. Intern. Organs*, **30**, 610–13.
4. Lockwood, C.M., Rees, A.J., Pearson, T.A., Evans, D.J. and Peters, D.K. (1976) Immunosuppression and plasma exchange in the treatment of Goodpasture's syndrome. *Lancet*, **i**, 711–15.
5. Lockwood, C.M., Pusey, C.D. and Peters, D.K. (1983) Indications for plasma exchange: renal diseases, in *Plasma Separation and Plasma Fractionation* (eds M.J. Lysaght and H.J. Gurland), Karger, Basel, p. 145.
6. McCance, D.R., Maxwell, A.P., Hill, C.M. and Doherty, C.C. (1992) Glomerulonephritis associated with anti-bodies to neutrophil cytoplasm and glomerular basement membrane. *Postgrad. Med. J.*, **68**, 186–8.
7. Pusey, C.D., Rees, A.J., Evans, D.J., Peters, D.K. and Lockwood, C.M. (1991) Plasma exchange in focal necrotising glomerulonephritis without anti-GBM antibodies. *Kidney Int.*, **40**, 757–63.
8. Rizzoni *et al.* (1986) Treatment of children with hemolytic uremic syndrome with plasma. A multicentre controlled trial. *Helv. Paediatr. Acta*, **41**, 114.
9. Rock, G.A., Shumack, K.H., Buskard, M.A. *et al.* (1991) Comparison of plasma exchange with plasma infusion in the treatment of thrombotic thrombocytopenic purpura. Canadian Apheresis Study Group. *N. Engl. J. Med.*, **326**, 393–7.
10. Johnson, W.J., Kyle, R.A., Pineda, A.A., O'Brien, P.C. and Holley, K.E. (1990) Treatment of renal failure associated with multiple myeloma. Plasmapheresis, hemodialysis, and chemotherapy. *Arch. Intern. Med.*, **150**, 863–9.
11. Reisaeter, A.V., Leivestad, T., Albrechtsen, D. *et al.* (1995) Pretransplant plasma exchange or immunoadsorption facilitates renal transplantation in immunised patients. *Transplantation*, **60**, 242–8.
12. Salmela, K.T., von Willebrand, E.O., Kyllonen, L.E. *et al.* Acute vascular rejection in renal transplantation – diagnosis and treatment. *Transplantation*, **54**, 858–62.
13. Otsubo, O., Nomura, M., Watanabe, T. *et al.* (1983) Silicone as coating material for hemoperfusion. *Trans. Am. Soc. Artif. Intern. Organs*, **29**, 480–4.
14. El. Keshen, S., Zia, H., Needham, T.E. *et al.* (1994) Coating charcoal with polyacrylate–polymethacrylate copolymer for hemoperfusion. II. Drug removal and polymer compatibility studies. *J. Microencapsul.*, **11**, 3–10.
15. Capodicasa, G., DeSanto, N.G., Vaccaro F. *et al.* (1983) CAPD + hemoperfusion once a week in the management of children with end-stage renal disease. *Int. J. Artif. Organs*, **6**, 251–5.
16. Splendiami, G., Albano, V., Tancredi, M. *et al.* (1987) Our experience with combined hemodialysis–hemoperfusion treatment in chronic uremia. *Biomater. Artif. Cells Artif. Organs*, **15**, 175–81.
17. Lotan, N., Grynspan, E., Grunfeld, H. *et al.* (1986) Enzyme-based hemoperfusion and blood treatment. *Int. J. Artif. Organs*, **9**, 331–4.
18. Nicolaev, V.G., Pinchuk, L.B., Umansky, M.A. *et al.* (1993) Early experimental studies on hemoperfusion as a treatment modality for acute radiation disease. *Artif. Organs*, **17**, 362–5.
19. Tabak, A., Lotan, N., Sideman, S. *et al.* (1986) Cholesterol removal by hemoperfusion *in vivo*. *Life Support Syst.*, **4**, 355–65.
20. Sideman, S., Manor, D., Hoffer, E. *et al.* (1983) Removal of excess inorganic phosphate by hemoperfusion with composite beads. *Life Support Syst.*, **1**, 113–25.
21. Marcus, L., Mashiah, A., Offarim, M. and Margel, S. (1984) Extracorporeal removal of specific antibodies by hemoperfusion through the immunosorbent arose-polyacrolein microsphere beads: removal of anti-bovine serum albumin in animals. *J. Biomed. Mater. Res.*, **18**, 1153–67.

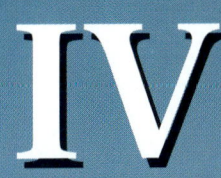

IV

General Management of Chronic Renal Disease

Section 3
Transplantation

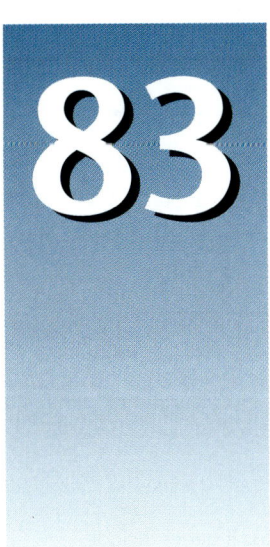

83

The immunobiology of transplantation

Alan M. Krensky

Introduction

The function of the immune system is the discrimination of self from non-self. As multicellular organisms evolved, it became necessary to recognize foreign invaders (infectious organisms) and dysregulated self (tumors) as non-self and to destroy them. This type of recognition depends on the presentation of short amino acid sequences (peptides) to cells of the immune system. Immune cells are activated, differentiate, and become regulators and effectors of the immune response which rapidly destroy the non-self stimulus. In organ transplantation, the donor organ itself is recognized as non-self. Cell surface molecules encoded in the major histocompatibility complex (MHC), human leukocyte antigens (HLA) in man, normally present non-self peptides to T lymphocytes. In transplant rejection, these HLA molecules themselves are recognized as non-self and the immune response is triggered to destroy the donor organ.

The major histocompatibility complex

Human leukocyte antigens (HLA) are encoded on chromosome 6 [1, 2] (Figure 83.1). They consist of three major groups, designated MHC (or HLA) class I, II and III. The MHC class I molecules are HLA-A, B, and C, subdivided based on genetic clustering and sequence homologies. Although HLA class I typing arose from microcytotoxicity assays using antisera, these reactivity patterns correlate well with the primary amino acid sequence information that was later obtained. The most common HLA class I type is HLA-A2, originally identified with antisera. Subsequent serotyping, biochemical and sequence information, however, shows that there is microheterogeneity within this family, giving rise to subtypes of functional significance. There are currently 12 recognized subtypes for HLA-A2 and seven for HLA-B27. With further investigation, the number of subtypes is certain to grow and will allow more subtle correlations in terms of HLA typing and transplant outcome. HLA-C molecules are structurally similar to the HLA-A and B antigens, but they are less polymorphic and do not elicit as strong an immune response.

The HLA class I molecules are the major target antigens recognized by cytotoxic T lymphocytes. They consist of a 44000 dalton heavy chain associated with β_2-microglobulin, a 12000 dalton protein encoded on human chromosome 15. The heavy chains are highly polymorphic and most individuals differ in their expression of these cell surface antigens. Bjorkman, Wiley and colleagues described the X-ray crystallographic structure of HLA-A2 in 1987 [3–5] (Figure 83.2). It was found that

Nephrology, Edited by Rex L. Jamison and Robert Wilkinson.
Published in 1997 by Chapman & Hall, London. ISBN 0 412 60930 4

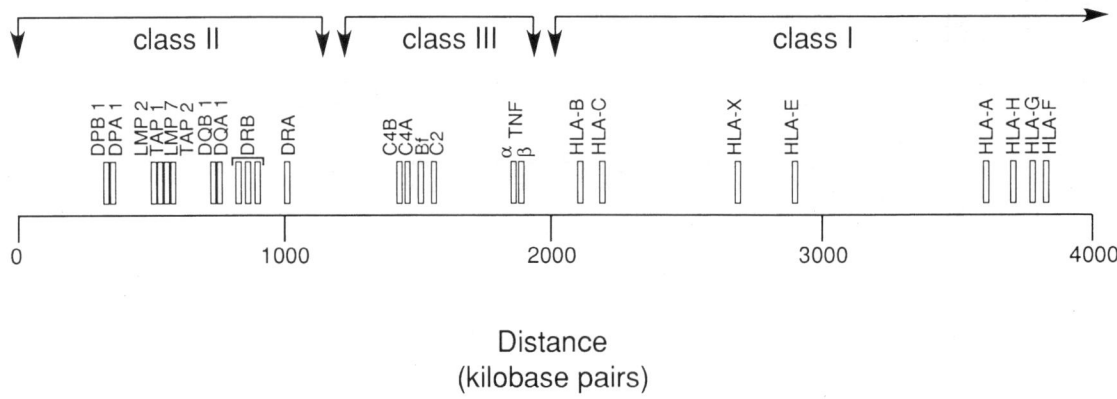

Distance
(kilobase pairs)

Figure 83.1   Physical map of the genes in the HLA region on the short arm of chromosome 6. Class II genes include HLA-DR, DP and DQ. Class III genes include tumor necrosis factors and complement proteins. Class I genes include HLA-A, B and C. (Reprinted with permission from Krensky [2].)

two alpha helices and a series of beta pleated sheets within the heavy chain formed a groove on the external-most portion of the HLA molecule. This groove contained discontinuous radiodense material which is now proven to be peptide. Subsequent crystallographic studies demonstrated that these peptides fit into anchoring pockets along the groove, determining which peptides fit into the groove, and therefore which antigens will be presented to the immune system. Thus, the HLA molecule binds peptides in its groove and presents this MHC-peptide complex to T lymphocytes. Zinkernagel and Doherty had demonstrated in 1974 that T lymphocytes recognize non-self peptides in the context of self-MHC [6]. The crystallographic studies provided a structural basis for this phenomenon, coined 'MHC restriction'.

Bjorkman *et al.* further noted that the anchoring pockets within the peptide binding groove fixed peptides in a particular conformation. Rammensee and colleagues showed by isolating and sequencing naturally occurring bound peptides that specific HLA alleles favored particular peptide binding motifs. The anchoring pockets in the HLA molecule restrict the peptides that can bind a given HLA molecule. Thus, HLA-A2 binds peptides with a leucine or methionine at position 2 and a valine or leucine at position 9. HLA-B27, on the other hand, contains peptides with an arginine at position 2 and an arginine or lysine at position 9. Although most of the various allelic motifs are yet to be defined, it is likely that this selected pattern of peptide binding and hence antigen presentation is the major function of the polymorphism of HLA molecules. In fact, most of the polymorphism in HLA sequences resides in the region of peptide binding.

The immune response between two individuals of the same species is called the alloresponse. This type of immune response was once thought to be the simplest form of non-self recognition. It now appears, however, that the molecular nature of the alloantigen may be

Table 83.1   Molecular composition of alloantigen recognized by alloreactive T cells (135)

HLA molecule without involvement of peptide
Empty HLA molecule (no peptide present)
Allele specific peptide produced by target cell
   (faithfully HLA dependent)
Promiscuous peptide (occurs with several HLA alleles)
Various peptides suffice
Distinct, but HLA specific, peptide

complex, including several different combinations of peptide and non-self HLA [7, 8]. Rammensee and colleagues proposed six types of alloantigen [7] (Table 83.1). Whatever the precise molecular composition of the alloantigen, it is clear that the alloresponse is stronger than the response to 'natural' antigens, such as viral peptides or tumor-associated antigens. Precursor frequencies for T lymphocyte recognition of HLA antigens are 10–1000-fold greater than responses to non-self peptides presented in the context of self HLA [8].

In addition to recognition of non-self HLA as whole cell surface molecule ('direct allorecognition'), there is also recognition of non-self HLA as short peptides in the context of self-HLA [8, 9] (Figure 83.3). This type of allorecognition, termed 'indirect allorecognition', would not be expected to be stronger than the response to other peptide antigens. Therefore, although this type of recognition occurs, it is unlikely to be the explanation for the strength of the alloresponse.

MHC class II antigens, HLA-DR, DQ and DP are encoded upstream of the HLA class I molecules on chromosome 6 [1] (Figure 83.1). They consist of two chains of similar molecular weight. The α chain is approximately 34 000 daltons whereas the β chain is approximately

Structure of HLA-A2

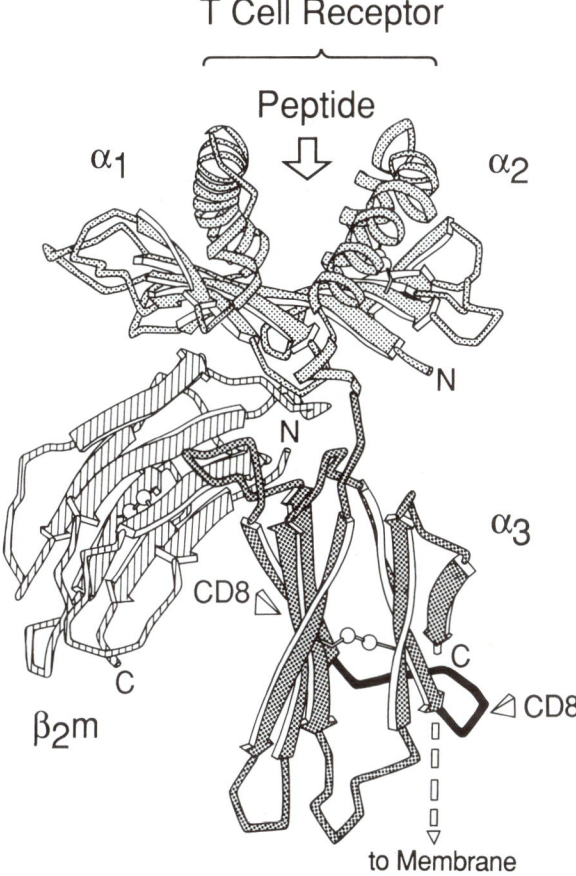

Figure 83.2 Structure of an HLA class I molecule. This model of the HLA-A2 crystal structure is adapted from the crystallography studies of Bjorkman *et al.* [3, 4] and reprinted with permission [5]. The α_1 and α_2 domains (light dots) form the peptide binding groove. The α_3 domain (dark dots) and β_2-microglobulin (hatched) are immunoglobulin-like and are adjacent to the cell membrane. The T cell receptor is thought to interact with the peptide and α_1 and α_2 domains and CD8 is thought to interact with the α_3 loop (shown in black).

29 000 daltons. Although both chains are polymorphic, most of the sequence variability resides in the amino terminal domains (α1 and β1). This correlates with the key role of these external-most parts in antigen presentation and T cell activation. Unlike HLA class I antigens which are expressed on almost all nucleated cells, class II antigens are normally expressed on only a small group of cell types, including macrophages, monocytes, B lymphocytes, and follicular dendritic cells. In addition, their expression can be induced by γ-interferon on other cell types, including vascular endothelium, tubular epithelium, pancreatic islet cells and T lymphocytes. The crystal structure of HLA-DR1 was solved by Brown *et al.* 1993 [10] (Figure 83.4). These data are still recent and are more con-

troversial than the evidence for the class I structure. Although the basic motif of a peptide binding groove is similar to class I molecules, the class II structure consists of homodimers (Figure 83.4). The functional significance of this observation remains unclear.

MHC class II molecules present peptide antigens to helper T lymphocytes (see below). These molecules, therefore, are involved in the induction of the immune response. It is generally believed that allorecognition of class II molecules is similar to that of class I molecules; that is, non-self HLA is recognized with various peptides (Table 83.1) and 'indirect' allorecognition occurs (see above). MHC class I and class II molecules, however, do differ in the length of peptides that they bind and present. MHC class I molecules bind peptides of eight–nine amino acids, whereas class II molecules bind a more heterogeneous subset, ranging from 13 to 25 residues. Crystallographic studies show that peptides bound to class I molecules fit tightly into the groove, whereas class II associated peptides may bow out from the molecule and may hang out over the ends of the groove.

Recently other genes encoding molecules involved in antigen presentation have been discovered within the MHC class II region. Transporter proteins associated with antigen processing, TAP1 and TAP2, and subunits of the large multifunctional proteasome (LMP2 and LMP7) are also encoded within this region (see below).

Lastly, MHC class III molecules are clustered between HLA-B and HLA-DR [44] (Figure 83.1). These genes also encode molecules involved in the immune response, including complement cascade proteins (C2, C4A and B and factor B) and tumor necrosis factors α and β.

The mechanism of antigen presentation

HLA class I and class II molecules differ in the peptide antigens that they bind and present. MHC class I antigens bind proteins in the endoplasmic reticulum (ER), biasing peptides bound to those derived from intracellular (or endogenous) antigens (Figure 83.5). Cytoplasmic proteins are processed by enzymes in the proteasomes, large cytoplasmic organelles which generate peptide fragments. Processed antigens are transported across the ER membrane by the TAP transporters [11, 12] (Figure 83.6). Within the ER, HLA class I heavy chains, β_2-microglobulin and peptides of the proper length and binding motif associate and are exported to the Golgi complex. These molecular complexes are packaged in secretory vesicles and expressed on the plasma membrane.

In contradistinction. MHC class II molecules generally bind and present exogenous antigens which enter the cell via the endocytic pathway in endosomes and lysosomes (Figure 83.5). MHC class II molecules associate with an 'invariant' chain in the ER and are exported to the Golgi complex. Binding of invariant chain prohibits peptide

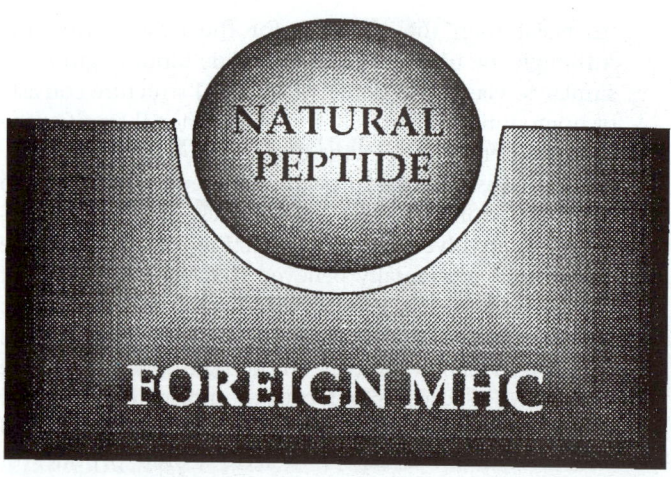

[Direct Allorecognition]

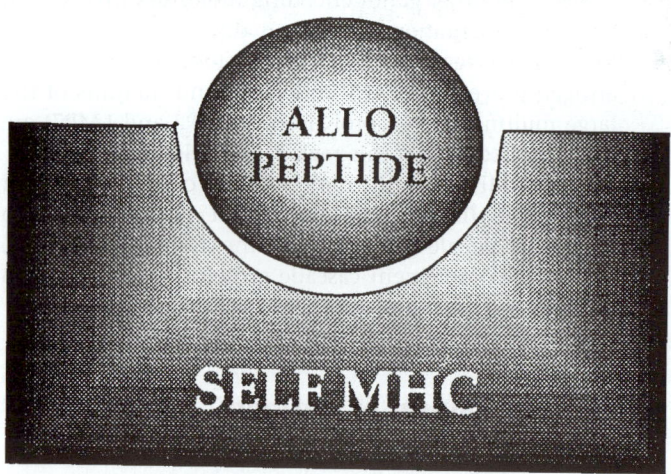

[Indirect Allorecognition]

Figure 83.3 T cells may recognize HLA molecules either 'directly' or 'indirectly'. Direct allorecognition involves non-self HLA with or without peptide in the groove (Table 83.1). Indirect allorecognition, in contrast, involves presentation of donor HLA as processed peptide in the context of self (recipient) HLA. Reprinted with permission from Krensky and Clayberger [9].

binding in the ER and targets class II molecules to the endosome. Degradation of the invariant chain in the acidic environment of the endosome makes class II accessible for peptides. Once MHC class II molecules disassociate from invariant chain and bind antigenic peptide, they are transported to the cell surface by poorly understood mechanisms.

Although the structural basis of these very different processing pathways is still largely unclear, it is important to realize that MHC class I and class II molecules are specialized to sample proteins from distinct intracellular compartments. This is in keeping with the fact that MHC class II molecules generally restrict (limit and control) proliferative (helper) responses, whereas MHC class I molecules restrict cytolytic responses.

Minor transplantation antigens

In addition to the antigens encoded within the major histocompatibility complex, there are minor antigens which can give rise to transplant rejection. In general, very little is known about the biochemical and molecular nature of these antigens, although there has been considerable experimental interest in the HY antigen which is the target of a female anti-male immune response. Rejection episodes in mouse strains sharing the same H-2 haplotype and between HLA-identical siblings have been attributed to non-HLA antigens expressed on monocytes and/or endothelial cells. In addition, it is likely that organ-specific alloantigens result from the association of organ-specific peptides with non-self HLA molecules. Lastly, it

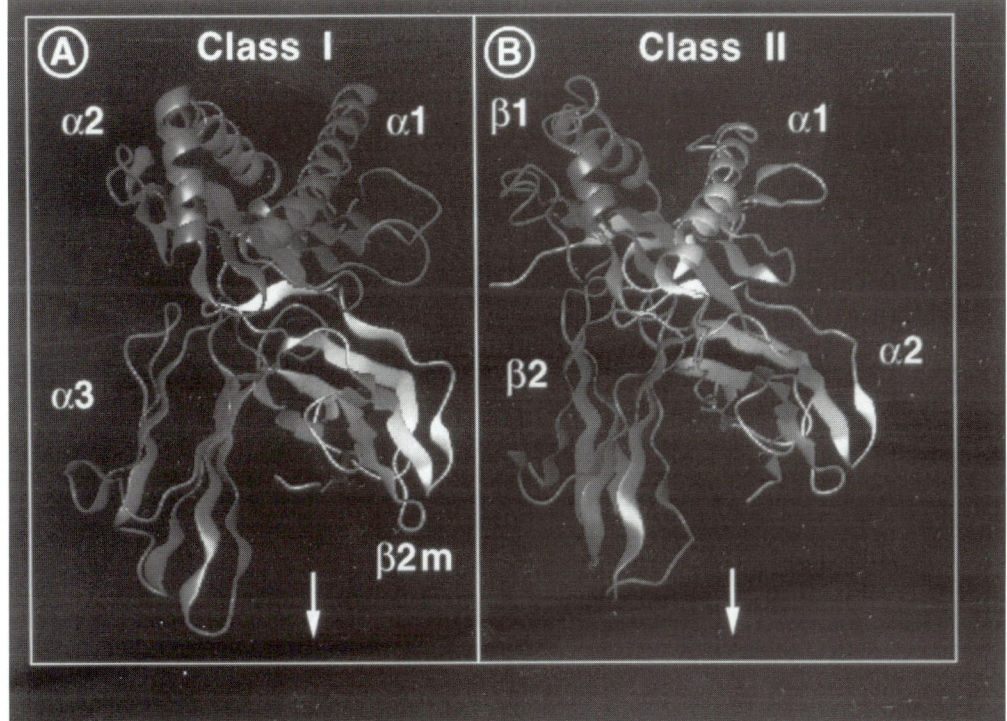

Figure 83.4 Structure of an HLA class II molecule. This model of the HLA-DR1 crystal structure is from the crystallography studies of Brown *et al.* [10] and adapted by Germain (NIH). HLA-DR1 crystallized as a dimer of two αβ heterodimers facing one another with their antigen binding grooves not quite aligned. The functional significance of the dimer remains unclear. The same view of the HLA-A2 structure is shown for comparison [3, 4].

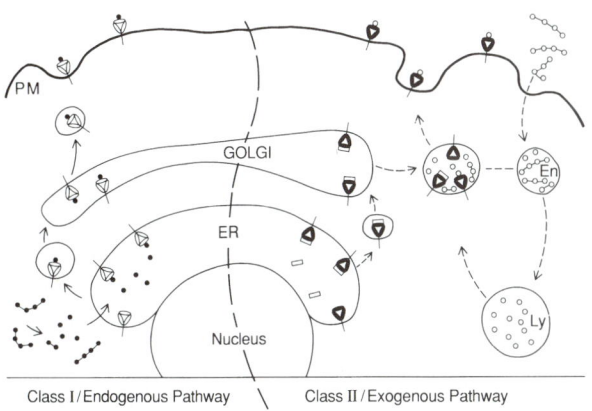

Figure 83.5 Antigen processing and presentation. Peptides from endogenous proteins bind to HLA class I molecules in the endoplasmic reticulum (ER) and are transported through the Golgi to the plasma membrane (PM). Peptides from exogenous antigens enter the cell by endocytosis and are degraded in endosomes (En) and lysosomes (Ly). Peptides bind to class II molecules in a poorly defined compartment before transport to the plasma membrane.

has been suggested that 'superantigens' may be involved in minor histocompatibility responses. Superantigens are relatively large molecules which bind to HLA molecules outside the groove but are capable of antigen presentation to T cells and triggering an immune response.

The alloresponse

The alloresponse, like other antigen-specific immune responses, is initiated by helper T lymphocytes. Cells of this functional subset of T lymphocytes generally express the CD (cluster of differentiation) 4 surface molecule and are restricted in recognition to MHC class II associated antigens [13]. Antigen specific receptors on the surface of T cells recognize the non-self MHC complex and trigger a cascade of biochemical events in the T cell which in turn leads to the expression of new genes involved in the orchestration of the immune response (Figure 83.7). Helper T lymphocytes produce soluble factors which trigger the effector arms of the immune response [5, 14] (Table 83.2). For example, interleukin 2 (IL-2) induces the proliferation and differentiation of T lymphocytes via both autocrine (self-stimulatory) and paracrine (stimulating nearby cells) mechanisms. Helper T lymphocytes which secrete IL-2 and γ-interferon, the Th1 subset, favor

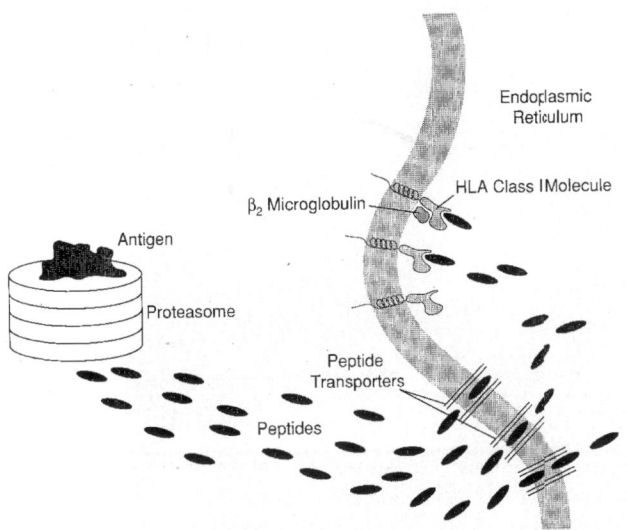

Figure 83.6 Antigen processing machinery. Endogenous proteins are degraded into peptides by the proteasomes and transported into the endoplasmic reticulum (ER) by the TAP transporter (Figure 83.5). Adapted from Parham [11] and Robertson [12] and reprinted with permission [2].

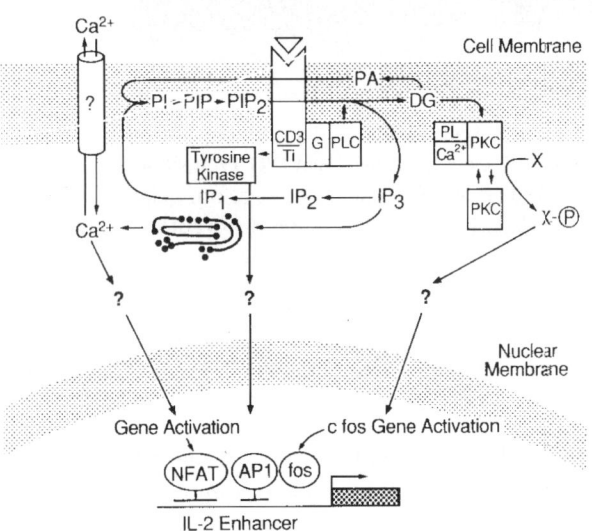

Figure 83.7 Cytoplasmic and nuclear events in T cell activation. Specific antigen triggers the T cell receptor complex, activating phospholipase C (PLC), tyrosine kinase, protein kinase C (PKC) and increasing intracellular calcium. Through a series of poorly understood events involving phosphorylations and dephosphorylations, the cell surface biochemical events induce the transcription of genes involved in T cell effector function. For details [5, 14]. Symbols: PI, phosphatidylinositol; PIP, phosphatidylinositol 4-phosphate; PIP_2, phosphatidylinositol 4,5-biphosphate; DG, diacylglycerol; PL, phospholipid; PA, phosphatidic acid; IP_3, inositol 1,4,5-triphosphate; IP_2, inositol 1,4-phosphate; IP_1, inositol 4-phosphate; G, guanine-nucleotide binding protein; Ti, T cell receptor heterodimer. Reprinted with permission from [5].

an inflammatory response and are associated with transplant rejection (Figure 83.8). Th2 cells, on the other hand, make IL-4, IL-5 and IL-10; cytokines associated with antibody, rather than cell-mediated responses, and have been correlated with tolerance induction. Although helper T lymphocytes in man are not strictly divided into Th1 and Th2 subsets, as they are in rodents, the potential for modulating cytokine profiles in the induction and maintenance of transplant acceptance remains an attractive goal.

In the context of IL-2 and other stimulatory lymphokines, precytolytic T lymphocytes recognize MHC class I antigens and are induced to proliferate and differentiate [15] (Figure 83.9). Over three to five days, these cells become competent to damage the graft directly. Cytolysis is associated with the *de novo* synthesis of granzymes (specific CTL associated serine proteases) and perforin (a complement 9-like protein). The expression of these molecules is highly correlated with transplant rejection [16]. The granzymes are believed to regulate factors involved in cytolysis and perforin has been shown to directly cause pores to form in the target cell. These pores cause osmotic swelling and cell death within minutes. Cell death is also associated with rapid target cell DNA disintegration. This process appears similar to developmentally regulated cell death, apoptosis [17].

Other effector arms of the immune response are also activated (Figure 83.9). Interleukins 4, 5 and 6, induce B cells which express cell surface immunoglobulin specific for donor antigens to proliferate and differentiate. Fully differentiated B cells become plasma cells and produce large amounts of donor specific antibody. Antibody binds to target tissues and leads to graft destruction either through the direct binding of complement and/or by targeting antibody-dependent cell-mediated cytotoxicity (ADCC) by 'K cells'.

In addition, natural killer cells are also capable of allorecognition. Morettas *et al.* [18] have proposed a

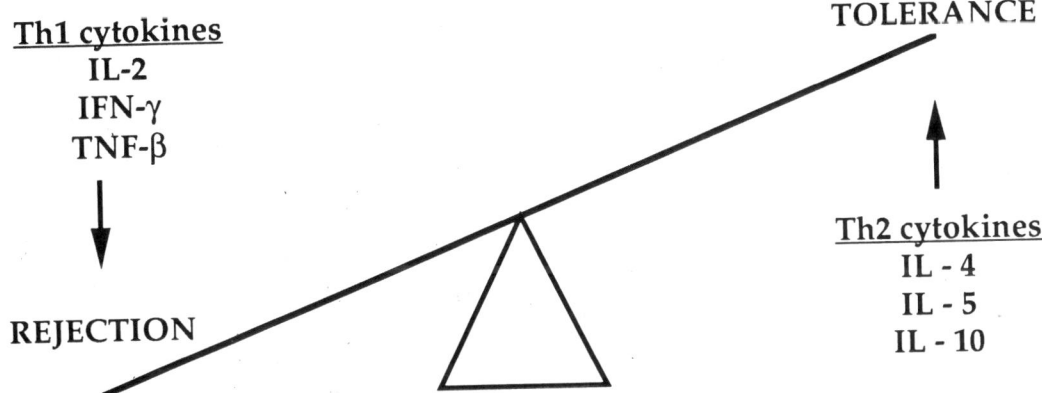

Figure 83.8 The balance of cytokines determines the type of immune response. Th1 helper cells make interleukin-2 (IL-2), γ-interferon (IFN-γ) and tumor necrosis factor-β (TNF-β) and are associated with transplant rejection. Th2 helper cells make interleukins 4, 5 and 10 (IL-4, -5 and -10) and are associated with tolerance.

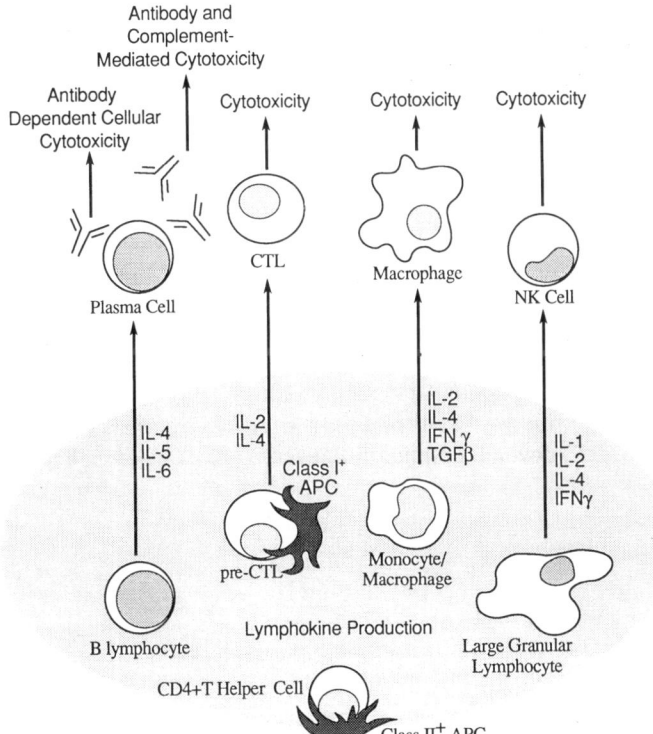

Figure 83.9 The cellular basis of transplant rejection. CD4+ helper T lymphocytes recognize HLA class II antigens and elaborate soluble factors, lymphokines (or interleukins) which activate the various effector arms of the immune response. Reprinted with permission from [15].

model whereby HLA molecules provide a negative signal which inhibits NK cell-mediated cytolysis (Figure 83.10). In the absence of a particular allele, the negative signal is released and antigen specific lysis occurs. Although no similar antigen-specific mechanism has been identified for killing by macrophages or granulocytes, these cells also make factors which contribute to the inflammatory response, graft dysfunction and rejection.

The strength of the alloresponse is likely explained by the concepts of positive [19] and negative [20] selection (Figure 83.11). Peripheral T cells mature in the thymus from precursors which are ignorant to self and non-self. Thymocytes with the appropriate reactivity to self are selected by two processes. T cells with too high (or perhaps too low) self-reactivity are deleted in the thymus by negative selection, whereas T cells with intermediate affinity for self-HLA are positively selected for delivery to the periphery. Since the T cell repertoire is not *a priori* educated to self, it must be capable of recognizing all HLA types. When an organ transplant is introduced across an HLA barrier, T cells that survived negative selection, those with a high affinity for non-self HLA, will encounter

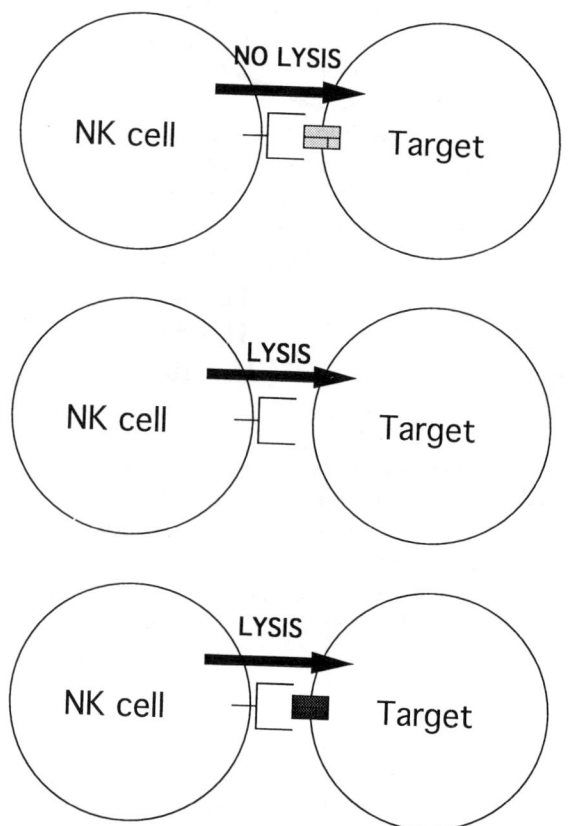

Figure 83.10 Moretta *et al.* [18] proposed a model of allorecognition by natural killer (NK) cells. (a) Self-HLA molecules send a negative signal which inhibits NK cell-mediated cytolysis. (b) Some viral infected or tumor cells express little or no cell surface HLA and are lysed by NK cells because of the lack of the HLA-induced negative signal. (c) In the alloresponse, foreign (donor) cells do not express the masking HLA type and, therefore, are lysed. Reprinted with permission from [8].

donor antigens for which they have a high affinity. This high affinity interaction is the most likely explanation for the strength of the alloresponse. Nevertheless, several other hypotheses have been proposed. One such explanation is 'molecular mimicry'. In this model, self-HLA + peptide mimics non-self-HLA. Another is indirect allorecognition (discussed above).

T cell recognition of alloantigens occurs via the T cell receptor (TCR) [21] (Figure 83.12). All T lymphocytes have clonally restricted, antigen-specific cell surface receptors which structurally resemble immunoglobulin molecules, with variable, constant and joining regions. The variable and joining regions determine antigen specificity, accounting for the breadth of the T cell repertoire. T cell receptors consist of heterodimers of two classes: α,β and γ,δ. T cells expressing the common α,β receptor are predominantly involved in transplant rejection. Alloantigen recognition by T cells expressing the rare γ,δ T cell receptor occurs, but the molecular mechanism involved is not understood.

In addition to the antigen specific heterodimer, the T cell receptor complex includes invariant cell surface molecules, the CD3 polypeptides and CD4 or CD8. The CD3 complex consists of three invariant dimers (CD3 ε–γ, ε–δ, and ζ–ζ; or an alternatively spliced form, ζ–v) which are involved in signal transduction from the antigen specific T cell receptor into the cell. CD4 and CD8 are 'co-receptors' in antigen recognition. Most mature peripheral blood lymphocytes express either CD4 or CD8. CD4 recognizes MHC class II molecules, whereas CD8 recognizes MHC class I molecules. Since most helper cells are restricted by HLA class II antigens, they are generally CD4+, whereas cytolytic cells, generally restricted by HLA class I antigens, are usually CD8+.

After the T cell receptor is triggered by specific alloantigen, several biochemical events occur (Figure 83.7). A

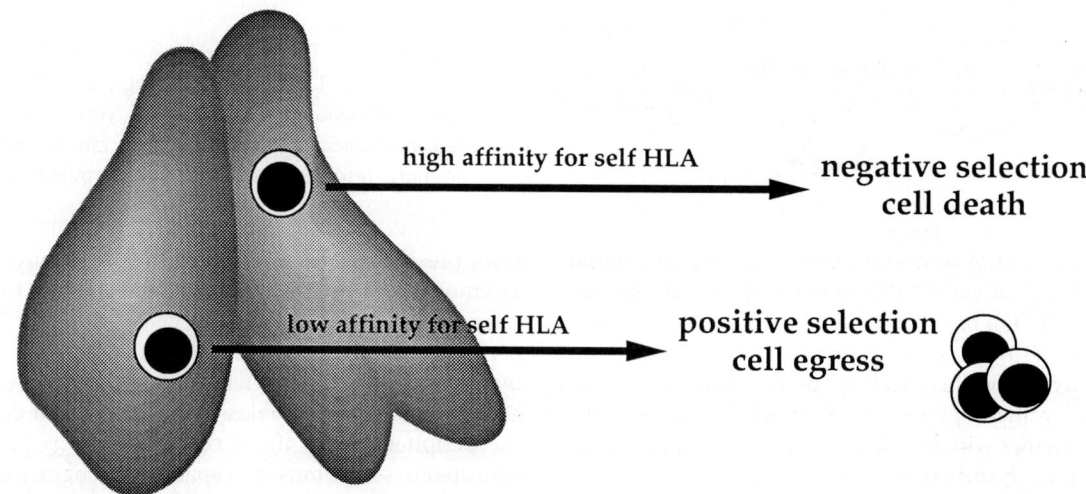

Figure 83.11 Positive and negative selection. Thymocytes with high affinity for self-HLA are negatively selected and die. Cells with the proper affinity for self-HLA are positively selected and enter the bloodstream.

phosphatidylinositol signaling pathway is activated, calcium fluxes from intracellular and extracellular sources, protein kinase C is translocated, and tyrosine kinases are activated. These events lead to the regulated phosphorylation of intermediates which eventually lead to transcription of new genes in the nucleus. The best characterized of these intermediates are phospholipase C, calcineurin and Ras. The lymphokines (IL-2, interferon-γ) and effector molecules (granzymes, perforin), discussed above, are among these newly expressed molecules.

Transplant rejection

When an allogeneic graft is introduced into a recipient, the aforementioned cellular and molecular events are initiated. If preexisting antibodies to the blood types A, B, O; HLA, or other polymorphic antigens are present, they immediately bind to the allograft and activate complement. Platelets and fibrin are deposited, granulocytes and monocytes infiltrate and fibrinoid necrosis of the vessel wall results. Ischemic necrosis is complete within 18–24 h (Figure 83.13a). This fulminate type of rejection, called hyperacute rejection, is due to prior sensitization via pregnancy, transfusion, previous transplants, etc. [22]. It has largely been eliminated from clinical practice by the routine cross-matches currently employed (see Chapter 84).

More insidious in nature is subacute rejection, characterized by cellular infiltration [23] (Figure 83.13b,c,d). Foreign MHC class II antigens in the graft are recognized by circulating immune cells. This 'antigen presentation' function is most likely performed by resident macrophages, dendritic cells, or so-called 'passenger leukocytes'. Once recipient immune cells are triggered, macrophages secrete cytokines, including transforming growth factor (TGF) β, platelet derived growth factor (PDGF), IL-1 and tumor necrosis factor (TNF) α (Table 83.2). These soluble mediators induce the expression of 'chemokines', small secreted factors, such as IL-8, the monocyte chemotactic proteins (MCP-1-3), and RANTES [24, 25]. Interleukin-8 is a potent chemoattractant for granulocytes; the MCPs attract macrophages, and RANTES attracts monocytes and 'memory' T lymphocytes. Inducible cell surface adhesion receptors, the selectins (Table 83.3), are expressed on the graft vessels, leading to margination and rolling of immune cells along the vascular endothelium (Figure 83.14). The chemokines induce haptotaxis, cell migration along the vessel wall, and chemotaxis with penetration into the tissues (Figure 83.13d). The function of members of the integrin and immunoglobulin gene superfamilies of adhesion molecules and cell surface receptors is to assure firm adhesion of cells and trigger the aforementioned TCR-mediated events involved in T cell activation, proliferation, differentiation and effector function (Table 83.3). The end result of these processes is a cellular infiltrate of monocytes, lymphocytes and the variable presence of eosinophils, granulocytes, macrophages and NK cells (Figure 83.13b,c,d).

The CD4+ T helper lymphocytes orchestrate the ongoing recruitment, activation and functional differentiation of effector cells. IL-2 and IL-4 induce the proliferation and differentiation of T lymphocytes. Interferon-γ, TNF-β, and IL-6 up-regulate the expression of HLA molecules. Interleukin-4, -5 and -6 activate B cells, which differentiate, divide and produce antibodies. Interleukin-1, TNF-α and TNF-β can directly cause tissue damage. These events increase the inflammatory infiltrate and induce additional expression of the inciting HLA molecules. Extracellular matrix is damaged and destroyed by inflammatory proteases and the debris is phagocytosed by

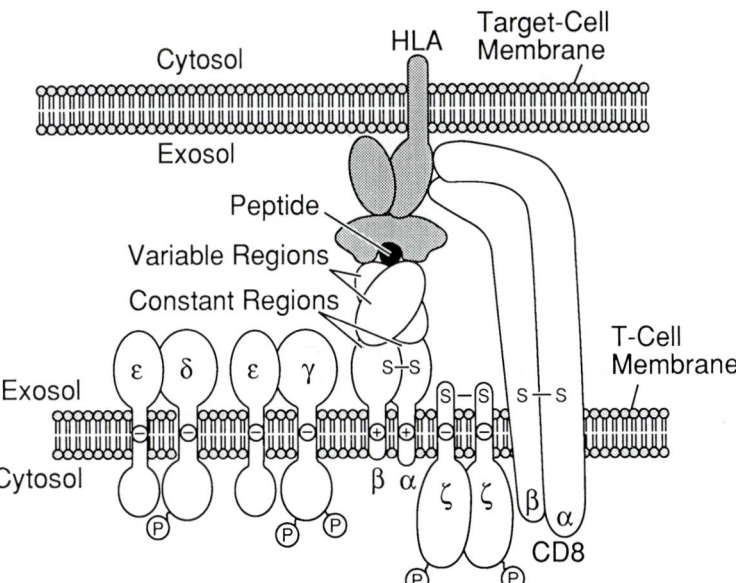

Figure 83.12 The T cell receptor complex. The T cell receptor heterodimer (α–β) recognizes a peptide–HLA complex in an antigen specific manner. The CD3 polypeptides transduce signals from the T cell receptor into the cell. The CD8 molecule transiently associates with the T cell receptor complex, recognizes invariant sequences in the α_3 domain of the HLA molecule (Figure 83.2), and serves as a 'co-receptor' in antigen recognition and signal transduction. Adapted with permission from [5].

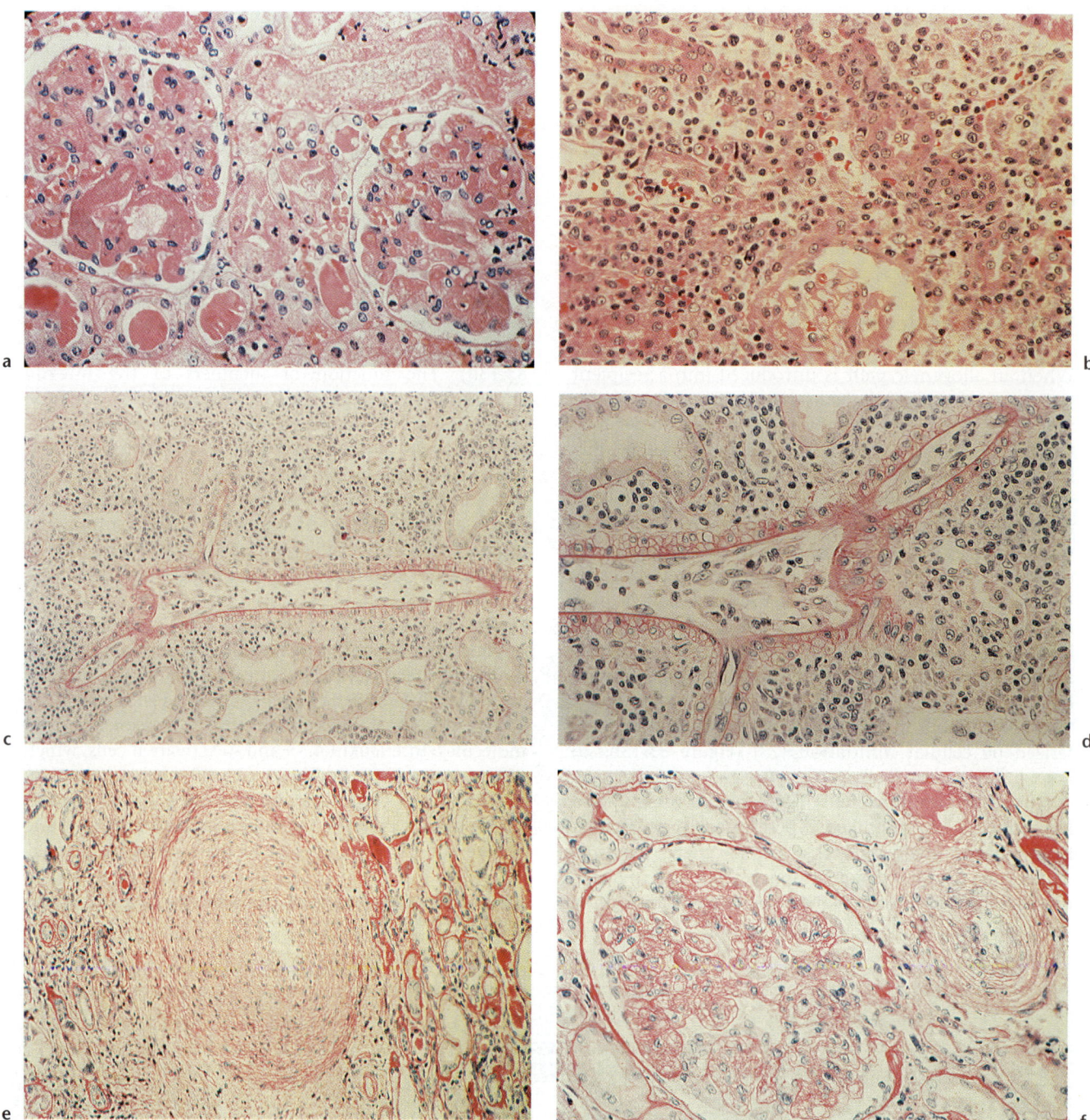

Figure 83.13 Pathology of transplant rejection. (a) Hyperacute rejection with glomerular thrombosis, glomerular and peritubular capillary infiltration and tubular coagulation necrosis. (b) Acute cellular interstitial rejection with pleomorphic inflammatory infiltrate and prominent tubulitis. (c) Acute cellular rejection with interstitial and vascular infiltration. (d) Higher power of (c) shows subendothelial infiltration by mononuclear cells and endothelial cell injury. (e) Chronic vascular rejection and tubulointerstitial rejection with marked proliferative endarteritis ('onion-skinning') and marked tubular atrophy and interstitial fibrosis. (f) Chronic transplant glomerulopathy and transplant rejection with proliferative arteriolitis and capillaritis (Courtesy of Richard K. Sibley, M.D., Stanford University.)

macrophages and granulocytes. Fibroblasts undergo morphologic changes and produce collagen, fibronectin and proteoglycans which are organized into new extracellular matrix, resulting in scar formation. These events are highly regulated in order to maintain the structural integrity of the organ, and, if not interrupted, they invariably result in the progressive loss of graft function. Finally, cytokines produced by macrophages and lym-

Table 83.2 Interleukins and other cytokines involved in transplant acceptance and rejection

Cytokine	Source	Biologic activity
IL-1	Monocytes, macrophages, NK cells, T cells, endothelial cells, dendritic cells, fibroblasts	Pro-inflammatory, activates NK cells
IL-2	Activated T cells	Stimulates T cell proliferation, activates NK cells
IL-3	Monocytes, T cells	Stimulates hematopoietic progenitors, mast cells, and basophils
IL-4	T cells (Th2 helper subset)	Anti-inflammatory, induces antibody production
IL-5	T cells	Anti-inflammatory, activates eosinophils, synergizes with IL-4
IL-6	Monocytes, macrophages, endothelial cells, fibroblasts	T cell differentiation, synergizes with IL-3
IL-7	Bone marrow stromal cells, thymic stromal cells	B cell growth and differentiation, T cell differentiation
IL-8	T cells, monocytes, macrophages, fibroblasts, epithelial cells, endothelial cells	Pro-inflammatory, neutrophil chemotaxis and activation
IL-9	T cells	T cell growth factor
IL-10	T cells, monocytes, macrophages	Anti-inflammatory, B cell growth and differentiation
IL-11	Bone marrow stromal cells	Megakaryocytic/thrombopoietic factor
IL-12	T cells, B cells, macrophages	Pro-inflammatory, activates NK cells
IL-13	T cells	Anti-inflammatory, B cell differentiation
IL-15	Placenta, skeletal muscle	T cell activation
Interferon-γ	T cells, NK cells	Up-regulation of HLA expression, activation of CTL and NK cells
TNF-α	Monocytes, macrophages, T cells, B cells, smooth muscle	Pro-inflammatory, activates neutrophils, fibroblast mitogen
TGF-β	Platelets, macrophages, endothelial cells, mesenchymal cells	Wound healing, bone remodeling
PDGF	Platelets, endothelial cells, smooth muscle, macrophages	Broadly mitogenic, including fibroblasts, mesangial cells
FGF	Fibroblasts, endothelial cells, smooth muscle, macrophages	Broadly mitogenic, including mesenchymal, endothelial cells
RANTES	T cells, epithelial cells, fibroblasts, endothelial cells	Pro-inflammatory, T cell, monocyte chemoattractant
MIP-1α	T cells, B cells, macrophages, monocytes	Pro-inflammatory, B/T cell chemoattractant
MIP-1β	T cells, B cells, macrophages, monocytes	Pro-inflammatory, eos/mono/T cell chemoattractant
MIP-2	T cells, B cells, macrophages, monocytes	Polymorphonuclear leukocyte chemoattractant
MCP-1-3	T cells, B cells, monocytes, fibroblasts, endothelial cells, keratinocytes	Monocyte chemoattractant

Abbreviations: IL, interleukin; TNF, tumor necrosis factor; TGF, transforming growth factor; PDGF, platelet derived growth factor; FGF, fibroblast growth factor; RANTES, regulated upon activation normal T cell expressed presumed secreted; MIP, macrophage inflammatory protein; MCP, monocyte chemotactic factor; NK, natural killer; CTL, cytotoxic T lymphocyte.

phocytes, including PDGF, and the fibroblast growth factor (FGF) induce smooth muscle proliferation. Intimal proliferation and vessel narrowing are common and important features of late graft loss (Figure 83.13e,f). This chronic form of rejection has proven resistant to existing therapies, and there has even been some suggestion that cyclosporin may even contribute to the process. As patients and grafts survive longer due to improved immunotherapy, chronic rejection has become an increasingly important problem. Although the etiology of chronic rejection remains unknown, soluble mediators, including cytokines and anti-HLA antibodies, have been implicated in the process. The only therapy at present is retransplantation.

Table 83.3 Adhesion molecules and their ligands

Adhesion molecule family	Members	Ligand(s)
Selectins	E-selectin	Sialylated fucosylated tetrasaccharides
	P-selectin	Sialylated fucosylated tetrasaccharides
	L-selectin	Sialylated fucosylated tetrasaccharides
Immunoglobulin superfamily	CD4	HLA class II
	CD8	HLA class I
	CD2	LFA-3 (CD58)
	ICAM-1 (CD54)	LFA-1, Mac-1
	ICAM-2	LFA-1
	ICAM-3	LFA-1
	VCAM-1	VLA-4
	MadCAM-1	$\beta_7\alpha_4$ integrin, L-selectin
	PECAM-1	PECAM-1
Integrins $\beta1$ family	VLA-4 ($\beta_1\alpha_4$)	VCAM-1, fibronectin
$\beta2$ family	LFA-1 ($\beta_2\alpha_L$)	ICAM-1, ICAM-2, ICAM-3
	Mac-1 ($\beta_2\alpha_M$)	ICAM-1, fibrinogen, C3bi
	p150, 95 ($\beta_2\alpha_X$)	C3bi

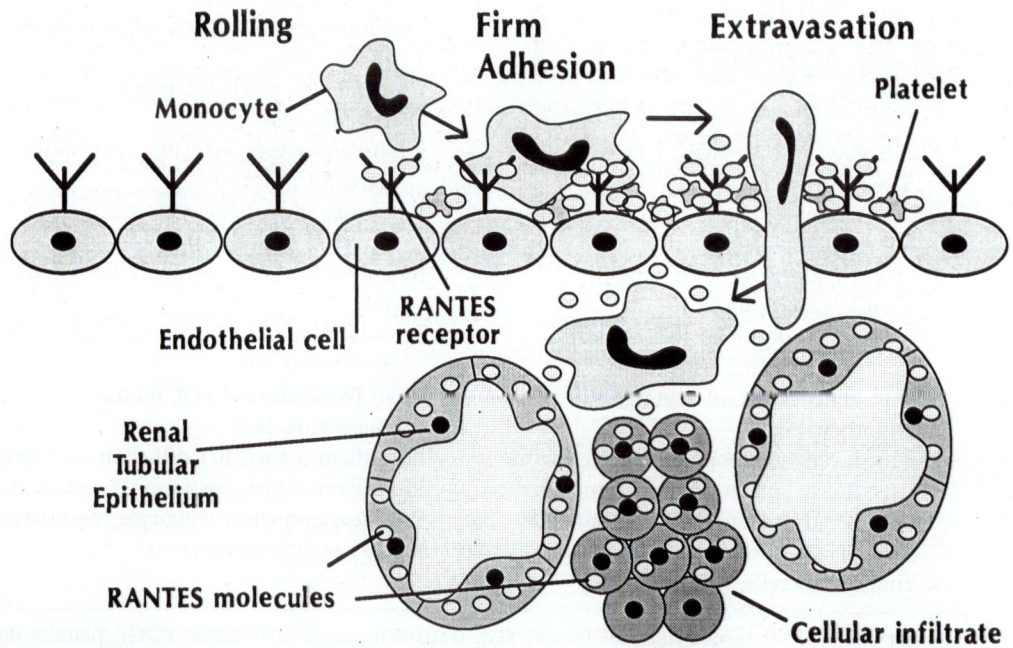

Figure 83.14 Induction and amplification of cellular infiltration in transplant rejection. Activated endothelium expresses adhesion molecules of the selectin family which cause leukocytes to roll along the vessel wall. Platelet degranulation releases RANTES chemokine which binds to the endothelium and attracts monocytes and memory T lymphocytes. As the interstitium becomes inflamed, IL-1 and TNF are produced, up-regulating several chemokines, including IL-8, macrophage inflammatory proteins, and RANTES. A trail of chemoattractants leads to cellular extravasation and infiltration. The cellular infiltrate is activated by foreign antigen, elaborates more chemokines, and amplifies the subacute inflammatory response. Reprinted with permission from [25].

Immunotherapy of graft rejection

The current armamentarium of drugs was largely developed by pharmaceutical screening and optimization. The rapid advances made in understanding the cellular and molecular events involved in transplant recognition, acceptance and rejection portend a new era of 'designer' therapies aimed at harnessing the specificity of the immune system. Current therapies generally involve combinations of three or four different drugs [26]. Since the available drugs are highly toxic and work at different points along the cascade of rejection events, combination therapies improve efficacy while limiting toxicity.

Drugs

Azathioprine

Azathioprine (Imuran) was first introduced as an immunosuppressive agent in 1961. It is the 1-methyl-4-nitro-5-imidazolyl derivative of 6-mercaptopurine and is slowly metabolized *in vivo* to 6-thioinosinic acid and other 6-mercaptopurine derivatives which interfere with purine metabolism, especially or lymphocytes and neutrophils. The active metabolites of azathioprine block the synthesis of adenine and guanine-containing nucleic acids, disrupting DNA and RNA synthesis, blocking gene replication and cell proliferation. Azathioprine is a powerful inhibitor of primary immune responses and is used to prevent rejection. It does not block secondary responses and therefore is not useful in treating established rejection [27]. It is commonly used in conjunction with cyclosporin and prednisone in order to permit the usage of lower doses of the two other drugs. Early withdrawal of azathioprine is associated with increased rejec-

tion, whereas late withdrawal has less, if any, effect. Although the mechanism whereby lymphocytes and neutrophils are more sensitive to azathioprine than are other rapidly dividing cells is unknown, this drug inhibits most T cell responses, including the mixed lymphocyte response, cytotoxic T cells, suppressor cells, NK cells, and K cells (antibody dependent cellular cytotoxicity), primary antibody responses, and it decreases circulating granulocytes and mononuclear cells. The major side effect of azathioprine is dose-related bone marrow toxicity, resulting in neutropenia, thrombocytopenia and macrocytic anemia. Additional side effects include idiosyncratic marrow and liver toxicity, pancreatitis, alopecia, nausea, vomiting, increased risk of infection (especially with herpes simplex and varicella) and neoplasia. An important drug interaction occurs with allopurinol and other xanthine oxidase inhibitors. The initial stages of azathioprine metabolism are mediated by xanthine oxidase and its inhibitors can markedly increase both immunosuppression and myelotoxicity.

Corticosteroids

Glucocorticosteroids, such as oral prednisone, prednisolone, or intravenous methylprednisolone, are used at low doses (1–2 mg/kg/day) to prevent rejection and at higher doses (greater than 10 mg/kg/day) to reverse acute cellular rejection. Corticosteroids inhibit gene transcription by causing steroid receptors and/or steroid-induced proteins to bind to DNA in the vicinity of response elements that regulate the transcription of numerous genes (Figure 83.15). Corticosteroids decrease macrophage production of TNF-α, IL-1, and eicosanoids, inhibit IL-6 transcription by mononuclear cells, and prevent the activation of the IL-2 gene in T cells. Steroids cause the sequestration of circulating T cells, inhibit CTL, and, in

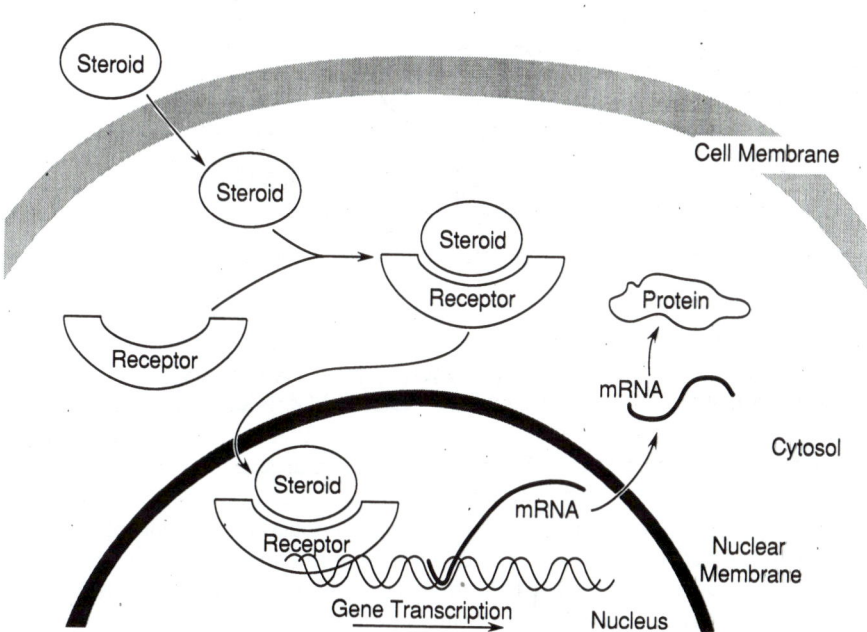

Figure 83.15 The mechanism of action of steroids. Glucocorticoids bind receptors in the cytosol, are transported to the cell nucleus, and bind to response elements (GREs) that regulate the transcription of numerous genes. Reprinted with permission from [2].

antirejection doses, cause lympholysis by direct effects on the lymphocyte membrane. They induce poor chemotaxis and decreased lysosomal enzyme release in neutrophils and monocytes. Although steroids have broad anti-inflammatory effects, inhibiting T cells, monocytes, and neutrophils, they have little effect on humoral immunity. Steroid use is limited by the numerous responsive elements and genes, giving rise to side effects as diverse as avascular necrosis of bone, osteoporosis, growth retardation, poor wound healing, cataracts, hyperglycemia, hypertension, obesity, personality changes, pseudotumor cerebri, and increased risk of infection. Of interest, steroids have been successfully withdrawn in some patients who do not reject the transplant [28].

Cyclosporin

The discovery of cyclosporin and its application to organ transplantation was an important milestone [29]. It improved survival of all organ transplants and made liver and cardiac transplantation a clinical reality. Its use has strikingly reduced the cost of transplantation by decreasing the length of hospital stay, incidence of complications, use of diagnostic services and overall hospital costs. Cyclosporin is a cyclic 11-amino acid peptide isolated from the fungus *Tolypocladium inflatum* Gams. Its

immunosuppressive effect is mediated at least in part by modulating the transcription of lymphokine genes. Perhaps most important among these cyclosporin responsive genes is IL-2. Cyclosporin inhibits IL-2 production by interfering with the DNA binding proteins controlling its transcription [30] (Figure 83.16). The currently prevailing hypothesis as to the mechanism of cyclosporin action is that the drug binds to cytosolic proteins called cyclophilins. The drug–cyclophilin complex inhibits calcineurin, a calcium-activated phosphatase involved in T cell activation [31]. It is thought that calcineurin normally removes phosphates from the cytoplasmic form of the nuclear factor of activated T cells (NFAT), allowing NFAT to gain entrance into the nucleus, where it combines with another protein to form an active nuclear factor. Normally, activated NFAT binds to the IL-2 gene and induces gene transcription and IL-2 production. In the presence of cyclosporin, NFAT is prevented from entering the nucleus and activating IL-2 gene transcription. This model explains all current data and accounts for the failure of IL-2 secretion. In the absence of IL-2, T cells do not proliferate or differentiate and the immune response is not amplified. In addition, γ-interferon is not secreted, MHC class II antigens are not induced, and macrophages are not further activated. Suthanthiran and colleagues have recently suggested that cyclosporin may also cause an increase in TGF-β [32]. Thus, cyclosporin

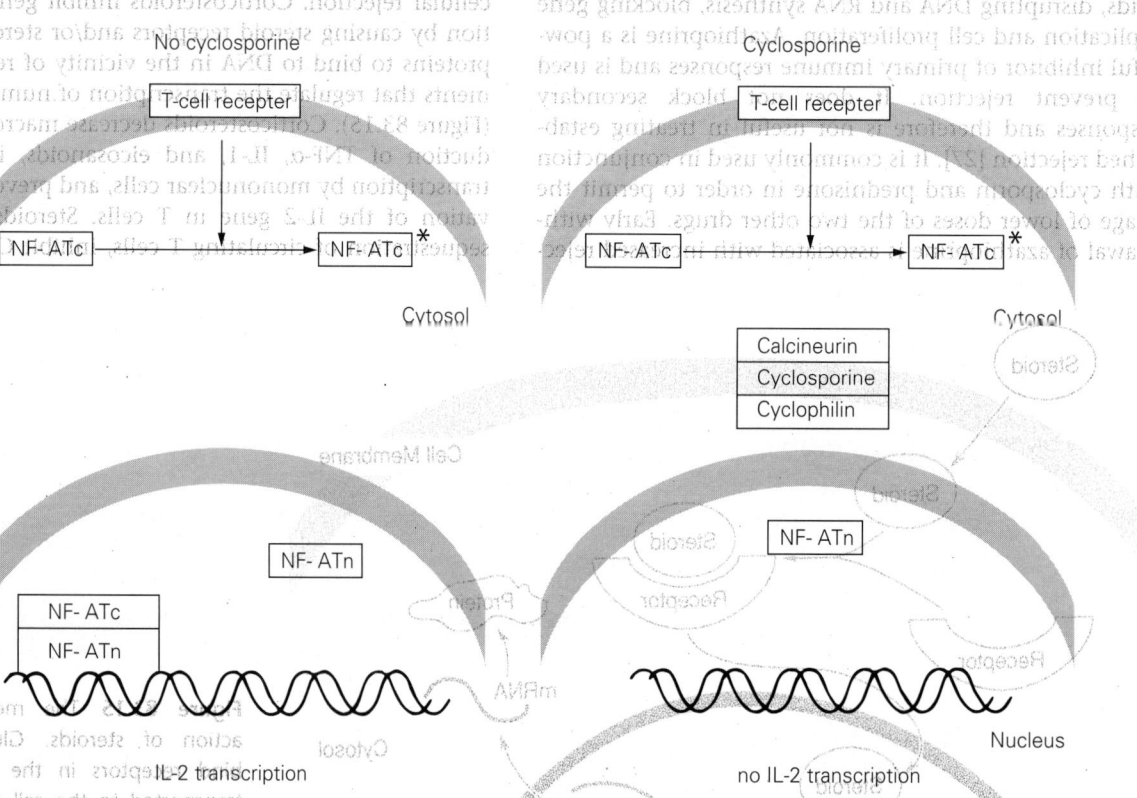

Figure 83.16 Mechanism of action of cyclosporin. Normally upon T cell activation, a cytoplasmic component of the nuclear factor of activated T cells (NF-ATc) enters the nucleus, binds to a nuclear component (NF-ATn), and induces IL-2 transcription. In the presence of cyclosporin, the cytoplasmic factor fails to enter the nucleus, the nuclear factor is unable to bind DNA, and there is no IL-2 transcription. Reprinted with permission from [2].

may not only decrease proinflammatory cytokines but may also augment secretion of suppressive cytokines. Although T helper phenomena are potently inhibited, cyclosporine may spare or even support suppressor T cells. Nephrotoxicity remains the major side effect of cyclosporin therapy [33, 34]. The acute form of renal damage is reversible and results from renal vasoconstriction mediated by increased thromboxane production and endothelin generation. α-Adrenergic blockade and calcium channel blockade have been proposed to ameliorate the vasospasm and functional impairment associated with cyclosporin usage. The chronic form of cyclosporin-induced nephrotoxicity is not reversible and is associated with chronic microvascular damage, glomerular ischemia and interstitial fibrosis. Other side effects of cyclosporin include hyperkalemia, hypertension, hepatotoxicity, neurotoxicity and hirsutism. Many agents affect cyclosporin absorption, distribution and metabolism. Of particular note, drugs that stimulate hepatic cytochrome *P*-450 enzyme activity will decrease cyclosporin levels. Effective use of cyclosporin requires the use of blood drug levels to direct dosing.

New drugs

Although most current immunosuppressive protocols involve triple drug therapy with corticosteroids, cyclosporin and azathioprine and/or quadruple drug therapy with the addition of antibodies, OKT3 or anti-lymphocyte globulin (see below), organ survival statistics still leave room for improvement [26]. In contrast to the relatively slow rate of discovery of new immunosuppressives from 1950 to 1990, the phenomenal financial success of cyclosporin has apparently ushered in a new era of drug discovery. Several new immunosuppressive agents have been evaluated in preclinical and clinical trials and are becoming available for general use. For the most part, however, these drugs are merely variations on the previously developed drugs and fall into families with similar mechanisms of action. The relative efficacies, mechanisms of action, pharmacokinetics and toxicities of these new drugs are currently being assessed. Preliminary results are encouraging and it is hoped that these drugs may allow steroid sparing, additive or even synergistic combinatorial effects, and decreased myelo- (azathioprine) and nephro- (cyclosporin) toxicities.

Cyclosporin-related drugs

Macrolides, FK506 and rapamycin [35], like cyclosporin, bind to cytoplasmic proteins, collectively called immunophilins. Whereas cyclosporin binds cyclophilins, FK506 and rapamycin bind a different group of cytosolic proteins called FK506-binding proteins, abbreviated FKBP. The immunophilins are peptidyl prolyl, *cis-trans* isomerases and catalyze proper folding of cellular proteins to facilitate active conformations required for proper trafficking within the cell. It was originally thought that inhi-

bition of this isomerase activity was the mechanism of action of these drugs, but subsequent studies definitively exclude this possibility. Most importantly, there is no correlation between the drug's ability to inhibit isomerase activity and its ability to inhibit T lymphocyte function. Rapamycin and FK506 are structurally related to each other and are distinct from cyclosporin, yet cyclosporin and FK506 inhibit the same step in T cell activation whereas rapamycin inhibits a step later in the activation cascade. Rapamycin inhibits T cell activation via the IL-2 receptor, not via the T cell receptor. Although FK506 is more potent than cyclosporin on a per milligram basis, it appears to be clinically quite similar; both are limited by nephrotoxicity. Rapamycin, on the other hand, appears to be additive to cyclosporin in its immunosuppressive effect without increasing nephrotoxicity.

Azathioprine-related drugs

The largest family of new drugs in the pharmaceutical pipeline are inhibitors of purine and pyrimidine metabolism. Experimental drugs RS61443, mizoribine and brequinar inhibit DNA synthesis and the proliferation of T cells, but also have subtle variations in activity and mechanism of action. RS61443, the morpholinoethyl ester of mycophenolic acid [36], and mizoribine inhibit inosine monophosphate (IMP) dehydrogenase, an enzyme important in the *de novo* synthesis of guanosine and deoxyguanosine nucleotides. RS61443 has shown promising results for use in renal transplantation in a small clinical trial with cyclosporin and steroids. Of particular interest, it has been suggested that RS61443 may rescue allografts which have failed other therapies. Three small series report that mizoribine can be used in combination with steroids and cyclosporin to prevent rejection. Brequinar sodium (DUP785) non-competitively inhibits dihydro-orate dehydrogenase, a key enzyme in the *de novo* synthesis of pyrimidines. It has undergone evaluation as a chemotherapeutic agent to treat human malignancies and shows powerful immunosuppressive activity in animal models.

A new type of immunosuppressive

15-Deoxyspergualin, a derivative of spergualin, a metabolite of *Bacillus laterosporus*, can both prevent and reverse rejection in animal models. Since this drug appears to suppress the primary humoral response, it may represent an entirely new type of immunosuppressive [37].

Antibodies

Antibodies against immune cell surface molecules have proven useful adjuvants to transplant immunotherapy. The therapeutic potential of polyclonal antibodies against human lymphocytes was shown by Monaco in 1967. Since then, various polyclonal sera have proven highly effective to prevent or reverse transplant rejection. Nevertheless, these sera are associated with severe side effects. In recent years, a better understanding of the surface molecules involved in the immune response and the ability to produce monoclonal antibodies against a wide range of surface determinants have enabled theoretically more specific targeting with monoclonal antibodies.

Polyclonal antisera

Purified gamma globulin fractions from polyclonal antisera generated by immunizing horses or rabbits with lymphocytes (antilymphocyte globulin, ALG) or thymocytes (antithymocyte globulin, ATG) contain a heterogeneous group of antibodies that eliminate circulating T cells and inhibit lymphocyte function [38]. T cells are cleared by the reticuloendothelial system, antibody-dependent cellular cytotoxicity and antibody and complement-mediated lysis. Some reports also suggest that ALG and ATG may expand suppressor cell populations *in vivo*. These antisera are effective at both prevention and reversal of allograft rejection [39]. Since each preparation varies in its constituent antibodies, efficacy and side effects are variable and unpredictable from preparation to preparation and even batch to batch. This lack of standardization has hampered assessment of the various

preparations. Side effects, including thrombocytopenia, granulocytopenia, serum sickness and glomerulonephritis may be severe. Local pain, fever, urticaria and hypotension are generally controllable with steroids and premedication. Increased susceptibility to infection and an increased incidence of neoplasia have been attributed to combination therapies, particularly at the beginning of the cyclosporin era before dosing of additive therapies was optimized.

Monoclonal antibodies

Problems associated with the lack of standardization of polyclonal antisera were overcome with the advent of monoclonal antibodies. Although unlimited amounts of antibody of a single specificity can be generated by hybridoma technology [40] (Figure 83.17), only OKT3, a mouse monoclonal antibody directed against the ε-determinant of the CD3 complex, has thus far received FDA approval for use in transplantation. This antibody, a potent inhibitor of virtually all T cell functions, blocks T cell receptor function, clears T cell receptors from the cell surface (internalization, shedding), and removes T cells from the circulation (T cell depletion). As a result, OKT3 therapy is highly efficacious for reversing acute rejection

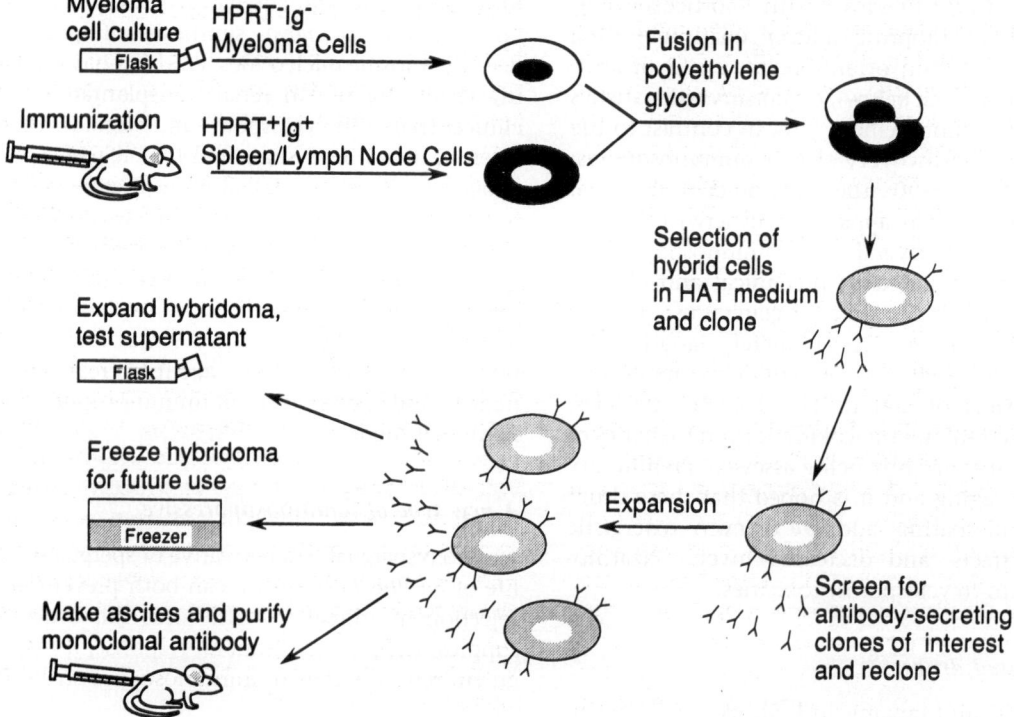

Figure 83.17 Kohler and Milstein described methodologies for the generation of monoclonal antibodies [40]. Mice are immunized, immune organs (spleen or lymph nodes) harvested, and immune B cells are fused to a myeloma selected for the inability to grow in (HAT) media, supplemented with hypoxanthine, aminopterin, and thymidine. Only myeloma cells that have fused with normal cells will survive in the selection media. After the resultant hybridomas have expanded in culture, those of interest are selected and cloned. Monoclonal antibodies can be used directly as culture supernatants or purified from supernatants or ascites fluid from mice injected with hybridoma intraperitoneally. Reprinted with permission from [2].

episodes [41]. Its use is limited, however, by two major problems. One problem is that recipients generate an antibody response against the murine antibody. Human antimurine OKT3 antibodies generally peak one to two weeks after the first course of therapy and may reduce the efficacy of subsequent antibody therapy. Attempts have been made to 'mask' the OKT3 antibody by genetic engineering. Construction of human–mouse chimeric antibodies and 'humanized' antibodies may theoretically prevent this response. Chimeric antibodies consist of human Fc (constant) regions that provide structural support, activate complement and permit binding to neutrophils, lymphocytes and monocytes, and of murine variable regions that provide antigen specificity. Although such antibodies decrease the immune response to constant regions, the response to variable regions remains. Such constructs continue to be improved by decreasing the murine component and leaving only the 'hypervariable' sequences from the original OKT3 monoclonal antibody. Such 'humanized' monoclonal antibodies are not expected to be immunogenic to humans, but the clinical efficacy of such constructs is yet to be proven.

The second major problem associated with OKT3 therapy is the 'first dose' or 'capillary leak' syndrome. OKT3 therapy is often associated with fever, myalgia, vomiting, diarrhea and occasional life-threatening pulmonary edema, hypotension and aseptic meningitis [41]. This reaction is the result of OKT3 binding to T cells and Fc receptor binding to monocytes, cross-linking the two cell types. T cells are activated and produce cytokines, including IL-2, interferon-γ, and TNF-α. These cytokines are responsible for the symptoms and signs described above. The syndrome may be preventable by constructing new monoclonal antibodies with Fc receptors that do not bind to monocytes. At present such antibodies are not available for clinical use, but the first dose reaction is generally controllable with steroids given 1 h before the OKT3. Other monoclonal antibodies against the T cell receptor complex, including T10B9, 1A-31 and BMA031 are also being evaluated in order to overcome the aforementioned problems associated with OKT3 therapy.

Although monoclonal antibodies against the T cell receptor complex are highly efficacious, they are non-specific in that they inhibit all T lymphocyte responses. There are theoretical advantages to targeting T cell surface molecules involved in important aspects of T cell activation and/or adhesion which may be more specific to the alloresponse immediately upon engraftment. Of particular interest among the 'activation antigens' has been the IL-2 receptor. Monoclonal antibodies against 'activation' epitopes only expressed upon T cell triggering have been tested directly and conjugated to immunotoxins (ricin and diphtheria). Several monoclonal antibodies against IL-2 receptors are undergoing clinical trials. Another approach, which does not require a monoclonal antibody, is to use an IL-2-toxin construct to bind the IL-2 receptor directly.

The CD4 antigen is an attractive target for antibody therapy because it is the T cell co-receptor for HLA class II antigens and has been implicated in signal transduction and tolerance induction. Infusion of OKT4A anti-CD4 monoclonal antibodies (mAb) have prolonged cynomolgus monkey kidney allografts and a phase I trial with an anti-CD4 mAb in human kidney transplantation has been reported. Chimeric and humanized anti-CD4 antibodies have been constructed and some are being tested in clinical trials.

Antibodies against T cell adhesion molecules, LFA-1 on the T cell and ICAM-1 on the target cell, have theoretical advantages, especially in interrupting leukocyte adherence to the capillary endothelium [42]. These antibodies have been evaluated in animal models and clinical trials are underway.

Other monoclonal antibodies against T cell surface molecules that have been evaluated for use in transplantation include Campath-1 (anti-CD52), CD8, CD2, CD7 and CD5. Lastly, antibodies to various lymphokines, including TNF-α and interferon-γ have been evaluated, but results to date have been disappointing. Perhaps a more fruitful approach will be the use of cytokine receptor antagonists, such as those described for the IL-1 and IL-4 receptors.

Non-pharmacological approaches

Non-pharmacologic immunosuppression has taken several forms over the past 20 years. Plasmapheresis has been used to remove antibodies in acute vascular rejection, but it has not proven generally effective for treatment of acute rejection episodes. Pretransplant splenectomy is an effective immunotherapy, but it remains a controversial approach because of the risk of overwhelming sepsis. Similarly, total body irradiation is a highly effective immunosuppressive therapy that is limited by the high risk of infection. Recently, however, it has been touted as useful for the induction of tolerance or as rescue therapy for intractable rejection [43]. Lastly, both retrospective and prospective studies indicate the beneficial effects of blood transfusion on graft survival. This effect, however, diminished or disappeared with the widespread use of cyclosporin and donor-specific or other transfusion protocols are less popular than they once were. Although the mechanism of the transfusion effect remains unknown, recent evidence that donor cells, even blood cells, may be effective toleragens for the induction of specific immunologic unresponsiveness has rekindled interest in this approach.

Tolerance

The immunosuppressive therapies described above are non-specific, with risks of opportunistic infection and malignancy in addition to specific drug toxicities. The ultimate goal of transplant immunology is acceptance of the graft without such side effects and without the need for chronic therapy. Immunologic tolerance, the active state of antigen specific non-responsiveness, theoretically represents the 'holy grail' of transplant immunology. Recent success in animal models portends a new era in transplantation where this goal may finally be attained. Owen first showed that immune non-responsiveness is an active process in his studies of freemartin cattle. He found that non-identical calf twins sharing a common placenta became chimeras and were tolerant to each other's cells, even in adult life. In other words, foreign antigens presented early in development are recognized as self. Burnet and Fenner went on to reason that the introduction of allogeneic cells or tissues during this 'critical period' would produce tolerance. Billingham, Brent, and Medawar tested this hypothesis experimentally in 1953 and showed that the injection of allogeneic cells prevented subsequent rejection of a skin transplant expressing the same MHC molecules [44]. For rodents, the 'critical period' lasts until shortly after birth, but for humans, this period ends sometime before birth. This imposes extreme limitations on the application of so-called 'neonatal' tolerance to the human condition, although there is the potential for tolerance induction *in utero* using invasive techniques. Such neonatal tolerance is generally due to clonal deletion. T cells reactive with the foreign antigen are deleted during selection in the thymus, presumably by the identical mechanisms of negative selection which delete self-reactive cells during development. Kappler and colleagues demon-

strated such negative selection when they showed that mice expressing a specific MHC class II molecule, I-E, delete all T cells using a specific variable region, Vβ17 [45]. Although such 'clonal deletion' is clearly a major mechanism in development of the immune response, it is probably not involved in the induction of tolerance in adult animals.

Felton first showed that antigen specific unresponsiveness could be induced in adult animals [46]. He introduced the concept of 'immunologic paralysis', where T cells were present but failed to act upon foreign antigen. Today, such adult tolerance is largely attributable to two mechanisms: anergy and suppression. Anergy applies to a state where antigen-specific T cells are present but fail to respond. Schwartz and colleagues attribute anergy to the failure of two signals to activate the T cell [47] (Figure 83.18). According to their hypothesis, T cell activation depends on the simultaneous application of two signals to the T cell, one through the antigen specific T cell receptor (TCR) and another through other receptors on the T cell surface. The second signal provides 'co-stimulation'. Engagement of the TCR in the absence of this co-stimulatory signal results in T cell anergy.

Although several T cell surface molecules have been implicated in provision of the second signal (Table 83.4), much recent interest has centered on CD28, a closely related molecule CTLA4, and their ligands B7-1, B7-2 and B7-3. The distribution of these receptors and their ligands is still incompletely described, but it appears that

Antigen Responsiveness

- IL-2 secretion
- T-cell proliferation
- normal immune responsiveness

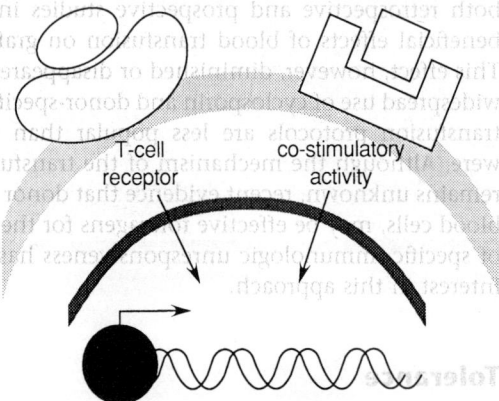

IL-2 transcription

Antigen Unresponsiveness

- no IL-2 secretion
- no T-cell proliferation
- anergy

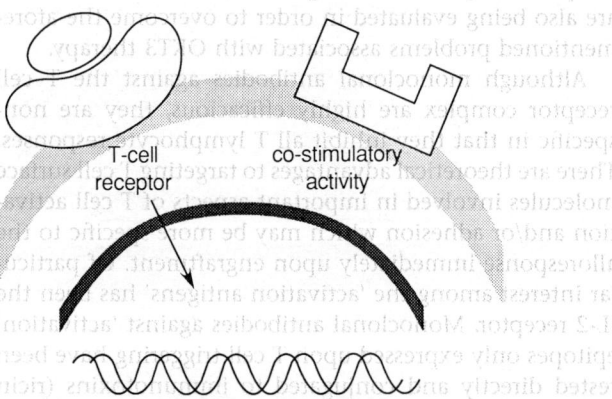

no IL-2 transcription

Figure 83.18 Schwartz and colleagues popularized the two-signal hypothesis for T cell activation [47]. In order to activate T cells, both the T cell receptor and a 'second signal' must be triggered. If the T cell receptor is triggered without provision of the second signal, anergy results. Reprinted with permission from [2].

CTLA4 is inducible on T cells and has higher affinity than CD28 for their common ligands. B7-2 is constitutively expressed on antigen-presenting cells and may be involved in early activation events, whereas B7-1 is inducible and may be involved in amplification of the T cell response to antigen. Although the details of these interactions are not yet understood, interruption of this important receptor–ligand interaction has already been successfully applied to transplant models in animals [48]. A chimeric molecule consisting of the CTLA4 binding domain attached to the immunoglobulin constant region, called CTLA4-Ig, inhibits allograft rejection *in vivo*.

Suppression is the second major mechanism to explain tolerance in adults. Gershon and Kondo showed that T cells from a tolerant animal could transfer unresponsiveness to a naive animal. This active process of antigen specific dampening of the immune response was attributed to 'T suppressor' cells. Although this phenomenon is clear and reproducible, the mechanism of action of suppressor cells, their phenotype and soluble factors, are poorly understood. Recent data implicate the balance of Th1 and Th2 cells (see above) or the secretion of soluble factors such as TGF-β in suppression.

Other popular mechanisms to explain peripheral tolerance in adult animals include 'microchimerism' and 'veto cells'. Starzl and colleagues reported a high correlation between the persistence of small numbers of circulating donor cells and outcome in liver allografting, but more recent studies in both kidney and heart transplant patients find microchimerism to be an infrequent event, casting doubt on its clinical significance. Veto cells inhibit or eliminate precursor cells, usually cytotoxic precursors, which recognize a cell surface molecule on the veto cell. Veto cells have been implicated in tolerance induction to class I and class II MHC antigens, but the molecular events involved remain undefined.

In 1990, Naji and co-workers reported that intrathymic injection of pancreatic cells into an adult rat-induced antigen specific transplant tolerance. Identical observations were made subsequently when renal glomeruli or spleen cells were used similarly in models of kidney or heart transplantation. Although the molecular mechanisms involved are not yet clear, these studies are moving towards clinical trials.

Tolerance induced by the oral feeding of antigen has long been observed but is not understood. The feeding of live or lysed spleen cells results in antigen-specific prolongation of organ grafts in animal models.

Recently, we [9] and Sayegh et al. [49] have shown that short amino acid sequences corresponding to regions of HLA molecules are useful for modulating the immune response. We have shown that synthetic peptides corresponding to regions of HLA class I molecules can inhibit cytotoxic T lymphocyte responses *in vitro* and transplant rejection *in vivo*. Remarkably, approximately 80% of rats receiving a two-week course of cyclosporin and HLA peptide have long-term tolerance to heterotopic heart allografts. Sayegh et al. similarly show prolonged graft survival in transplant models using peptides corresponding to MHC class II sequences. Recent data indicate that the class I peptides bind to T cell surface molecules and induce a calcium flux, resulting in T cell anergy [9]. The mechanism of action of the class II peptides is different, but is yet to be defined. In both cases, it appears that soluble HLA is a natural immunoregulatory molecule *in vivo* and that synthetic peptides may prove to be effective for the induction of clinical tolerance in transplant patients.

Almost every transplant physician describes anecdotes about patients who achieve tolerance, i.e. they stop taking their medication but do not reject their graft. A retrospective analysis of 165 transplant units in the United States found that 12 of 32 living related transplants failed within seven months of the cessation of all immunosuppressive therapy. More than half of 16 cadaveric grafts failed within two months. Although these figures underscore the risk of discontinuing immunosuppression, they also indicate that clinical tolerance is possible.

Xenotransplantation

As the demand for organs for transplantation increases and supply decreases, there has been mounting interest in the transplantation of organs from other species into humans [50]. Such xenografting may be a solution to the shortage of suitable organs and opens new horizons to apply molecular engineering and other pretransplant

Table 83.4 Receptor–ligand pairs that have been implicated in co-stimulation

Receptors on T cells	Ligands on antigen presenting cells
CD28/CTLA4	B7-1, B7-2, B7-3
LFA-1 (CD11a, 18)	ICAM-1 (CD54), ICAM-2, ICAM-3
CD4	HLA class II
CD8	HLA class I
CD2	LFA-3 (CD58)

The terms 'receptors' and 'ligands' imply a directionality which is arbitrary.

modifications of grafts. Although non-human primates are an obvious source for such organs, the risk of infectious viruses, animal rights issues, and cost have focused attention on pigs as potential donors for humans. In-bred pigs are available, their organs are of suitable size, they are not a domesticated species, and blood group O animals exist. The major limitation to their use is immunologic: vascularized organs transplanted between phylogenetically distant species, such as pig to man, are subject to hyperacute rejection due to preformed ('natural') human antibodies which bind to the pig endothelium. Despite this major impediment, the roles of natural antibodies and complement in initiating hyperacute rejection are being clarified and prolonged survival of vascularized xenografts has been achieved in experimental systems. Areas of active investigation include the role of complement and means of inhibiting complement function, the source and specificity of natural antibodies, and the xenoresponse to endothelium. The cellular immune response to xenoantigens is weak. The MHC antigens are different and important accessory molecules and ligands do not function across species. Thus, if the humoral immune response can be overcome, xenotransplantation may become a realistic option for patients with kidney failure.

Conclusion

As detailed in other chapters, progress in tissue typing, clinical care, and immunosuppression has made transplantation a safe and reliable therapy for end-stage renal disease. Outcomes in terms of organ and patient survival still leave room for improvement, however. Limitations of therapy, including the risks of opportunistic infection, malignancy and nephrotoxicity, and the increase in chronic rejection, persist. Although the search for new and better immunosuppressives and investigation of the application of xenografting will persist, the ultimate goal of transplant immunobiology remains attainment of the active state of antigen specific immune unresponsiveness, i.e. immunologic tolerance. Despite the fact that tolerance is readily and reproducibly attainable in animal models and does occur in some patients, we do not yet understand the mechanisms of the induction and maintenance of tolerance sufficiently for routine application to patients. Current experimental protocols consist of two steps: (1) obliteration of the normal immune response with immunosuppressive drugs, antibody (ATG or OKT3) treatment, or irradiation and (2) provision of toleragen (donor specific antigen as blood or bone marrow infusion). It is hypothesized that, as the host immune response returns, the non-self-transplant is now recognized as self. Such antigen-specific approaches may only be applicable to living-related transplants which allow adequate antigen and timing to provide toleragen. Cadaveric transplantation, on the other hand, does not allow sufficient time for such approaches. Such patients may benefit from xenografting if the current problems with hyperacute rejection can be overcome. Perhaps xenografts will be engineered to express self-HLA antigens. Although such 'designer' approaches are not yet available, the dramatic progress over the past decade suggests that protocols to make transplanted organs accepted as self may soon be available, abolishing the need for chronic therapy and its concomitant side effects. When this is possible, transplantation will truly be a cure for end-stage renal disease.

Acknowledgments

This work was supported by grants from the National Institutes of Health (DK35008, AI35125, CA34233, and CA49605). AMK is a Burroughs Wellcome Scholar in Experimental Therapeutics.

References

1. Robinson, M.T. and Kindt, T.J. (1989) Major histocompatibility complex antigens and genes, in *Fundamental Immunology* (ed. W. Paul), Raven Press, New York, pp. 489–539.
2. Krensky, A.M. (1993) Transplant immunobiology, in *Pediatric Nephrology*, 3rd edn, Williams and Wilkins, Baltimore, pp. 1373–89.
3. Bjorkman, P.J., Saper, M.A., Samraoui, B. *et al.* (1987) Structure of the human class I histocompatibility antigen, HLA-A2. *Nature*, **329**, 506–12.
4. Bjorkman, P.J., Saper, M.A., Samraoui, B. *et al.* (1987) The foreign antigen binding site and T-cell recognition regions of class I histocompatibility antigens. *Nature*, **329**, 512–18.
5. Krensky, A.M., Weiss, A., Crabtree, G. *et al.* (1990) T-lymphocyte–antigen interactions in transplant rejection. *N. Engl. J. Med.*, **322**, 510–17.
6. Zinkernagel, R.M. and Doherty, P.C. (1974) Restriction of in vitro T cell mediated cytotoxicity in lymphocytic choriomeningitis within a syngeneic or semiallogeneic system. *Nature*, **248**, 701–2.
7. Rotzschke, O., Falk, K., Faath, S. and Rammensee, R.G. (1991) On the nature of peptides involved in T cell alloreactivity. *J. Exp. Med.*, **174**, 1059–71.
8. Krensky, A.M. and Clayberger, C. (1993) The nature of allorecognition. *Curr. Opin. Nephrol. Hypertens.*, **2**, 898–903.
9. Krensky, A. and Clayberger, C. (1994) The induction of tolerance to alloantigens using HLA based synthetic peptides. *Curr. Opin. Immunol.*, **6**, 791–6.
10. Brown, J.H., Jardetzky, T.S., Gorga, J.C. *et al.* (1993) Three-dimensional structure of the human class II histocompatibility antigen HLA-DR1. *Nature*, **364**, 33–9.

transplant and, as a result, provisions must be made to ensure that the patient has adequate access to essential medical care and medications, such as immunosuppressive drugs. Thereafter, the patient undergoes a battery of laboratory tests (Table 84.4).

The process of evaluating potential recipients varies greatly from center to center. In 1993, Ramos *et al.* surveyed 147 transplant centers in the United States [1]. Examples of transplant center variability are: (1) although 66% do not have a specific age limit, 34% exclude patients older than 70 years; (2) 22% exclude hepatitis B surface antigen-positive patients; (3) 51% do not have a specific policy regarding hepatitis C antibody-positive candidates; (4) 34% obtain abdominal ultrasounds on all patients and 31% perform cholecystectomies on asymptomatic patients; and (5) 89% perform a stress thallium test in patients with suspected coronary disease although 15% obtain routine coronary angiograms in all diabetic patients. Similarly, psychosocial criteria very widely. Levenson and Olbrisch [5] reported the results of a survey of 217 renal transplant centers in the United States. This study addressed the question of variability of criteria among heart, liver and renal transplant programs. Among renal transplant candidates, 3% (range 0–33%) are refused transplantation based on psychosocial criteria. In comparison, 7.4% are turned down for medical reasons. The bulk (73%) of centers depend on social workers to screen these patients; however, 52% of patients are actually interviewed by a mental health professional. Psychosocial considerations considered to be irrelevant by transplant centers included: (1) no support person (64% of centers); (2) current felony prisoner (42%); (3) history of significant criminal behavior (42%); (4) active schizophrenia (8%); (5) addictive drug use (22%); and (6) lack of understanding of the transplant process (34%). These reports emphasize the transplant center-specific vagaries associated with evaluation of the renal transplant candidate.

Upon completion of the evaluation process, the final decision to accept or reject the candidate is made by an evaluation committee. Most commonly, this group comprises transplant surgeons, nephrologists, social workers, tissue-typing personnel, transplant co-ordinators and

Table 84.3   Essential elements of the physical examination

Weight
Grade of the funduscopic exam
Condition of the vasculature with attention to the lower extremities (femoral, popliteal, dorsalis pedis and posterior tibial arteries)
Careful cardiac exam with blood pressure determination
Breast and pelvis exam (for female candidates)
Absence of signs of malignancy, including rectal and prostate exam

Table 84.4   Laboratory evaluation of the renal transplant candidate

1. Laboratory studies
    Complete blood cell count, blood chemistry, and coagulation profile
    Virology HBsAg, HBsAb, HBcAb- IgM, HAV Ab (IgG and IgM), HCV Ab, HIV Ab; Antibodies to cytomegalovirus, Epstein–Barr, herpes simplex and varicella zoster virus
    Urine analysis, urine culture, and 24-hour urine for creatinine clearance and protein
    VDRL, FTA
    C peptide and hemoglobin A1C- for diabetic patients
    Immunologic studies
        Serum immunoglobulins
        Serum complement
        T-cell subsets
        Panel mixed lymphocyte culture (MLC)
        Spontaneous blastogenesis
        Skin testing: purified protein derivative, mumps, Candida, histoplasmosis
        Direct Coombs' test
        Cold agglutinins
    Tissue typing
        ABO and Rh
        HLA-A, -B, -Dr
        Anti-HLA cytotoxic antibody screen
        Donor-specific MLC
2. Chest X-ray
3. Electrocardiogram
4. Special procedures for selected patients
    Ultrasound of gall bladder and liver
    Liver biopsy if liver function abnormal
    Upper gastrointestinal endoscopy
    Barium enema or colonoscopy
    Treadmill/exercise electrocardiogram
    Thallium scan
    Coronary angiography
    Peripheral arteriosclerosis – Doppler and/or arteriography
    Pulmonary function tests and arterial blood gases
5. Consults (optional)
    Psychiatry
    Gynecology evaluation and mammography (for female > 40 years)
    Urologic assessment (voiding cystoureterography, cystoscopy, or urodynamic studies in patients with vesicoureteric reflux, neurogenic bladder, bladder neck obstruction, or strictures)
    Dentistry

nurses. In other centers, a nutritionist, immunologist, psychologist, psychiatrist or ethicist may also be involved. A multidisciplinary committee decision lessens the individual burden associated with refusal of medical care and allows non-medical considerations to be considered. Interestingly, according to Levenson and Olbrisch, 14% of renal transplant programs do not provide an explanation to the patient if refusal is based on psychosocial criteria [5]. Furthermore, Kilner [6] noted that 56% of transplant programs and dialysis centers in the United States consider the social worth of the candidate in making allocation decisions. Obviously, the decision to place a patient on the renal transplant list is not simply one of medical necessity and risk. A number of subjective issues are discussed, and it is the role of the committee, as a whole, to attempt to reach a final decision which represents a consensus opinion encompassing all considerations.

In the United Kingdom, where there is full state funding of transplantation, economic factors are not considered in the selection process but the organ shortage dictates that choices need to be made. Formal evaluation committees are unusual, but the principles guiding selection are the same as those described for the American patients.

Cardiovascular considerations

Approximately 50% of the deaths preceding and following renal transplantation are secondary to cardiac etiologies. Coronary artery bypass grafting should be considered in suitable operative candidates prior to renal transplantation. As a result, preoperative risk stratification in this patient population utilizing non-invasive imaging techniques has received a great deal of attention. Le et al. [7] prospectively evaluated a two-tiered cardiac risk assessment algorithm in 189 patients referred for transplant evaluation. Patients were first stratified using the high-risk criteria of: (1) age >50 years; (2) history of angina; (3) insulin-dependent diabetes mellitus; (4) congestive heart failure; and (5) abnormal electrocardiogram, excluding left ventricular hypertrophy. Those with one or more high-risk criteria underwent thallium scintigraphy. The investigators found cardiac mortality was significantly higher in the high-risk category (17% vs. 1%; $P < 0.001$). Within the high risk group, reversible and fixed thallium perfusion defects were associated with increased cardiac mortality when compared to those without defects (23% and 29% vs 5%; $P < 0.05$). In general, all transplant centers utilize a similar algorithm to predict cardiac risk; 89% of transplant centers perform a stress thallium test for the work-up of symptoms suggestive of coronary artery disease whereas coronary angiography is reserved for those with a positive stress thallium test. In diabetic renal failure patients, both exercise thallium and dipyridamole thallium tests have an unacceptably low sensitivity for predicting coronary

artery disease. Consequently, Manske et al. [8] have developed a clinical screening algorithm for use in this population. A total of 141 consecutive type 1 diabetic renal transplant candidates underwent prospective coronary angiography. The following risk factors for significant coronary artery disease (defined as >50% stenosis in one or more arteries) were identified: age >45 years, smoking history, ST-T wave changes on EKG, and duration of diabetes greater than 25 years. Applying these risk factors to an additional 70 patients yielded a sensitivity of 97% and a negative predictive value of 96%, although the specificity was 61% and the positive predictive value was 70%. A number of studies have sought to improve characterization of the prevalence of coronary artery disease in diabetics using thallium stress testing and echocardiography with mixed results and conclusions. Nonetheless, during the evaluation process, it is essential to address the cardiac risk associated with renal failure in the setting of diabetes mellitus. Among renal transplant units in the United States, 75% reject patients with inoperable multivessel diffuse coronary disease. Although some centers also reject patients with a depressed cardiac ejection fraction, there is little consensus on this issue [4].

In the evaluation of carotid vascular disease, carotid Doppler studies are obtained in symptomatic patients in 85% of centers. A minority of units (14% and 8%, respectively) obtain this study in all diabetic patients and in asymptomatic patients older than 55 years. Peripheral Doppler studies are usually performed on symptomatic patients and those with poor peripheral pulses [4].

Gastrointestinal considerations

The incidence of peptic ulcer disease among renal transplant patients has changed during the past two decades. A 27% incidence of upper gastrointestinal (GI) inflammation or ulceration was noted on routine endoscopy following transplantation in the early 1980s [9]. In contrast, with the advent of H_2 blocking agents and immunosuppressive regimens utilizing cyclosporin and low-dose steroids, Knechtle et al. [10] found no complications among 68 consecutive renal allograft recipients in 1987. At Stanford University Hospital, prospective transplant patients with a history of dyspepsia or hemorrhage undergo upper GI endoscopy. Active disease is treated with H_2 blockers or proton pump inhibitors. In the presence of Helicobacter pylori infection, patients are treated with amoxicillin, metronidazole and bismuth subcitrate. Follow-up endoscopy is performed to document cure. In the minority of patients with persistent disease, surgical intervention, such as laparoscopic highly selective vagotomy, is performed. Otherwise, all patients are placed on H_2 blocking agents following transplantation.

A preoperative history of recurrent episodes of diverticulitis mandates surgical resection of the involved colonic segment. Patients with a history of bloody or guaiac-positive stools require evaluation, preferably by colonoscopy to facilitate biopsy, if necessary. In addition, double-contrast barium enema continues to be utilized, primarily for those with a history of diverticulitis.

The necessity for preoperative evaluation and treatment of gallstones remains unclear. Certainly, patients with symptomatic gallstones should undergo preoperative laparoscopic cholecystectomy. Screening the asymptomatic patient and subsequent removal of the gall bladder in those with gallstones remains an area of controversy. In the United States, one-third of transplant centers obtain abdominal ultrasounds on all patients. Asymptomatic cholelithiasis requires cholecystectomy in 31% of transplant units whereas diabetics with asymptomatic cholelithiasis undergo surgery in 35%. Of note, 41% of transplant units have no specific policy on pretransplant cholecystectomy [4]. Lowell et al. retrospectively reviewed patients undergoing kidney and kidney–pancreas transplantation at the University of Nebraska [11]. They found a 29% prevalence of cholelithiasis in diabetic patients undergoing transplantation in comparison to 12% in non-diabetics. The incidence of symptomatic cholelithiasis or acute cholecystitis in this patient group is unclear. It is unknown whether immunosuppression, with or without diabetes, carries increased morbidity or mortality in the setting of hitherto asymptomatic gallstones. Of the Nebraska patients with gallstones 82% underwent surgery, but only 21% of the operated patients had symptoms. In contrast, at the University of Wisconsin, 6% of 200 transplant patients underwent cholecystectomy for symptomatic indications [11]. There were no missed diagnoses of cholecystitis or symptomatic cholelithiasis or increased morbidity and mortality resulting from the immunosuppressed state. At Stanford, all diabetics with gallstones documented by ultrasound undergo pretransplant cholecystectomy. In the United Kingdom, it is unusual to subject asymptomatic patients to cholecystectomy. The argument to remove or not remove the asymptomatic gall bladder remains unresolved.

In an analysis of the influence of obesity on renal transplant outcome at the University of Michigan it was found that obesity, defined as weight greater than 120% of ideal body weight, was associated with a higher incidence of wound infections and greater postoperative weight gain [12]. However, patient and graft survival were not significantly different from that of controls, obesity is not a major risk factor.

Hepatic considerations

Candidates who are HBsAg-positive at the time of transplantation risk progressive liver disease after surgery, thought to result from enhanced viral replication in the presence of immunosuppression. Roy et al. [13] reported the outcomes of 135 HBsAg-positive recipients transplanted between 1971 and 1986. The prevalence of chronic hepatitis in this group was 60% compared with

1.5% in controls. There was no significant difference in patient or graft survival, although chronic liver disease was the cause of death in 16% of the HBsAg-positive group and 3% in the HBsAg-negative group. In those followed for more than six years, the incidence of chronic hepatitis was 75%. None of the 135 HBsAg-positive recipients became seronegative. Pol et al. [14] reported similar data in 98 HBsAg-positive renal transplant recipients based on serial biopsy specimens. Although chronic liver disease was present in 88% of hepatitis B virus (HBV)-infected patients (4% in controls), there was no difference in graft or patient survival. Scott et al. [15] found that acquisition of HBV infection following renal transplantation was associated with substantially increased liver-related mortality when compared to that of patients infected prior to transplant (60% versus 7%, respectively). The adverse effects of HBsAg-positivity become paramount after two years rather than in the early postoperative period.

Less is known about hepatitis C in this patient population. Preliminary studies suggest a similar pattern to that of hepatitis B. Roth et al. [16] found the preoperative prevalence of anti-HCV to be 17% using a second generation recombinant immunoblot assay (RIBA) in 641 allograft recipients. RIBA-positivity was an independent predictor of post-transplant liver dysfunction. These patients were also at greater risk for infectious episodes and rejection. Again, there was no effect on patient or graft survival. The authors recommend that anti-HCV-positive patients undergo liver biopsy before renal transplantation to adequately stage the disease.

The utility of liver biopsy in transplant patients with liver disease has been clarified by Rao et al. [17] Serial liver biopsies were performed in 77 renal transplant recipients with abnormal liver function tests over a 20-year period. Patients were classified as: fatty change, chronic persistent hepatitis, early and late chronic active hepatitis, and hemosiderosis. During a mean follow-up of 6 years, the authors found that progression to liver failure and death occurred in 35% who had chronic active hepatitis early in their course, 55% with hemosiderosis and 60% with advanced chronic active hepatitis. In addition, histologic progression to cirrhosis was noted in 60% with early chronic active hepatitis, 66% with hemosiderosis and 100% with advanced chronic active hepatitis. In this patient group, the authors point out that histologic diagnosis may be a better predictor of survival than the actual etiology of the liver dysfunction.

Again, little consensus is present regarding the management of hepatitis B or C infected patients. Although 22% of transplant centers exclude HBsAg+ patients, 29% perform a liver biopsy in the setting of abnormal liver functions tests and 16% biopsy regardless of biochemical abnormalities. About 31% have no specific policy regarding hepatitis B. Similarly, 51% of transplant centers have no policy regarding HCV-positive candidates; 31% exclude these patients if they have abnormal liver function tests and a biopsy which shows chronic active hepatitis.

Renal considerations

The etiology of renal failure in the transplant candidate is an important consideration. The most common diagnoses from the European Transplant Registry in 1987 are listed in Table 84.5 [18]. The most dramatic change during the past decade has been the increase in candidates with ESRD secondary to diabetes mellitus. In the United States, 40% of all ESRD patients are diabetics; in Europe, 13% are diabetics. A number of pathologies recur in the renal allograft, but may have a negligible effect on function. The recurrence rates of common diagnoses are listed in Table 84.6 [19]. Metabolic and congenital etiologies of ESRD such as Alport's syndrome, amyloidosis, familial nephritis, gout and cystic disease result in renal transplant outcomes similar to that of the general renal transplant population, whereas primary oxalosis, sickle cell disease and Fabry's disease are exceptions. Isolated renal transplantation for primary oxalosis is associated with early graft failure because of recurrent urolithiasis, nephrocalcinosis, and systemic oxalate deposition. Combined liver–kidney transplantation is recommended as definitive therapy. Sickle cell disease has been associated with 25% one-year graft survival in the study by Barber *et al.* [20]. Fabry's disease is a systemic disorder of glycosphingolipid metabolism with poor patient and graft survival following renal transplantation. The poor outcome is deemed to be secondary to progression of the systemic disorder which is unaffected by restoration of renal function. Another hereditary cause of renal failure is tuberous sclerosis, in which the native kidneys are commonly the site of angiomyolipomas, cysts or even, renal cell carcinomas. Bilateral nephrectomy before transplantation or serial monitoring with CT scans of native kidneys if they are not removed is recommended.

Among the glomerulonephropathies, a number of diseases recur in the allograft. Within the first five years, the overall failure rate from recurrence is less that 2% in the 15–24 year age group, regardless of the nature of the native kidney disease. Focal segmental glomerulosclerosis (FGN) has a 30% frequency of recurrence. A high risk subgroup of FGN characterized by a short interval from the onset of nephrotic syndrome and the development of renal failure is associated with a 70% recurrence rate. Allograft failure can follow recurrence of renal disease. Antiglomerular basement membrane (GBM) nephritis is associated with linear deposition of IgG in 55% of allografts. The usual recommendation is to delay transplantation of a patient with anti-GBM nephritis until the antibody titer to GBM falls to undetectable levels.

Systemic diseases associated with ESRD include systemic lupus erythematosus vasculitis, and hemolytic-uremic syndrome. It is widely agreed that lupus is not a contraindication to renal transplantation, but it has been recommended that serologic tests for lupus be negative before embarking on transplantation. However, based on the experience of the Washington University transplant unit with 14 lupus patients, Goss *et al.* [21] note that positive serologic evidence for lupus before transplantation had no effect on patient or graft survival. Similarly, in vasculitis, polyarteritis nodosa and Wegener's granulomatosis, resolution of active disease can result in a normal graft survival following transplantation. In Wegener's granulomatosis, serial testing for antineutrophil antibody can be a useful measure of disease activity.

Finally, obstructive uropathy is a common etiology for ESRD in pediatric patients, accounting for 26% of diagnoses in renal allograft recipients under age 12 in a recent series [22]. Many investigators have demonstrated that graft survival in these patients is not different from that of grafts in patients with normal urinary tracts, without regard to whether the native bladder or an intestinal conduit was used. Since analgesic nephropathy patients have an increased incidence of uroepithelial carcinoma,

Table 84.5 Primary renal disease

Type	% of total
Glomerulonephritis	24.1
Pyelonephritis/interstitial nephritis	16.6
Diabetes mellitus	13.1
Renal vascular disease	9.8
Cystic kidney disease	8.2
Non-diabetic multisystem disease	4.8
Analgesic nephropathy	2.6
Hereditary	1.1
Miscellaneous	5.3
Etiology unknown	14.4

Table 84.6 Recurrence of glomerulonephritis in renal allografts

Type of glomerulonephritis	Recurrence (%)
Mesangiocapillary type II	95
Henoch–Schonlein purpura	80
IgA nephropathy	50
Focal segmental glomerulosclerosis	30
Mesangiocapillary type I	20–30
Membranous nephropathy	10
Antiglomerular basement membrane nephritis	5
Idiopathic crescentic glomerulonephritis	?

preoperative screening must be done to exclude this potential complication.

Urologic considerations

Pretransplant bilateral nephrectomy is required in 5–10% of patients. Common reasons include active stone disease, gross hematuria, high-grade vesicoureteral reflux, renal tumors, infected renal cysts, recurrent pyelonephritis, intractable hypertension and severe proteinuria (>10 g/24 h). An additional indication is intractable pain in patients with adult polycystic kidney disease. Although some centers perform routine voiding cystourethrograms in all patients, investigation of the lower urinary tract is mandated at least in the following conditions: hematuria, recurrent pyelonephritis, ureteropelvic stricture, prune-belly syndrome, ureterovesical stricture, vesicoureteral reflux, neurogenic bladder, bladder neck obstruction and urethral valves. Cystoscopy, urodynamic studies and voiding cystourethrography are most commonly performed. Based on a cohort of 100 consecutive transplant candidates who underwent renal ultrasonography, cystourethrography, urinalysis and urine culture, Yang et al. [23] recommend sonograms in all adult candidates because of the 0.2–1.5% prevalence of renal cell carcinoma in this group. Cystourethrography may be omitted in non-diabetic patients in the absence of voiding symptoms or history of urinary tract infections. Hematuria, but not sterile pyuria, requires cystoscopy.

Patients with large, flaccid bladders that empty poorly may require intermittent self-catheterization. Selected patients with contracted non-compliant bladders secondary to tuberculosis, radiation, or severe interstitial cystitis and those with total incontinence or high pressure neurogenic bladders may require intestinal bladder augmentation or creation of an ileal conduit. Interestingly, Kashi et al. [24] reported decreased allograft survival (55% vs 92% at two years) in a subgroup of patients with bladder capacity less than 100 ml.

Immunological considerations

Genes that code for the human leukocyte antigens (HLA) are located on chromosome 6. The class I antigens, HLA-A, B and C, are expressed by all nucleated cells and platelets. Structurally, they are composed of a 41 kDa polymorphic chain which is non-covalently bound to a 12 kDa b_2-microglobulin moiety. The class II antigens, HLA-DR and DQ, are composed of a 34 kDa α chain and a 29 kDa β chain. Although constitutively expressed on the surface of B lymphocytes, monocytes, macrophages and dendritic cells, class II HLA-antigen expression can be induced on T lymphocytes and renal tubular epithelial cells, among others.

Determination of HLA antigens at the A, B, and DR loci is performed for both donor and recipient. In the context of living-related renal transplants, data from various scientific registries have demonstrated the advantage of HLA matching. Analysis shows that the estimated half-life (the time required for 50% of grafts functioning at one year after transplant to subsequently fail) for HLA-identical grafts to be 26.9 years, whereas those of one haplotype-matched sibling grafts and parental grafts are 12.2 and 10.8 years, respectively. In cadaveric renal transplantation, the half-life of HLA-matched grafts is 17.3 years and that of HLA-mismatched grafts is 7.8 years. Furthermore, a step-wise increase in the graft survival rate has been demonstrated with increasing levels of HLA-matching. This improved survival is increasingly apparent when matching is based on better resolved HLA-antigens. As a result, molecular techniques are being used to increase the resolution of HLA-antigen identification. In many histocompatibility labs, serologic techniques are being replaced by methods based on polymerase chain reaction and restriction fragment length polymorphism. However, in spite of data suggesting the favorable effects of HLA-matching on renal allograft survival, national sharing of cadaver kidneys is performed only for 2-haplotype HLA matches (A, B, DR-antigens) in the United States. Any further sharing agreements or attempts to maximize HLA-matching occur on a local level with varying results.

The presence of lymphocytotoxic antibodies in patients' serum is due to sensitization to HLA antigens and in the past, has resulted in hyperacute and accelerated rejection. Therefore, the potential recipient is screened periodically for HLA antibodies, which are typically expressed as percentage of panel reactive antibodies. Antibodies can often transiently appear following pregnancy, blood transfusion or rejection of a previous renal allograft. Before transplantation, a cross-match is routinely performed in which recipient serum is incubated with donor lymphocytes in the presence of complement. The avoidance of ABO incompatibility and positive T cell cross-matches has eliminated the majority of causes of hyperacute rejection. However, the significance of positive B cell cross-matches is as yet unknown. In the setting of a positive B cell cross-match, survival disadvantages of 7% and 15% have been found in primary and repeat renal transplants, respectively. In some institutions, flow cytometric methods are also used to detect low levels of donor-specific antibodies, both complement and non-complement fixing types. The clinical relevance of a positive flow cytometric cross-match is unknown; data suggest that it may have an adverse impact on graft survival in repeat transplants.

Loss of a previous renal allograft from rejection is associated with poor survival of a subsequent graft, if the first graft failed within the first few months or the patient is sensitized. In general, a regraft has a slightly poorer survival in comparison to a primary renal allograft, 80% versus 60% one-year graft survival. The removal of a failed renal allograft is now deemed necessary in the setting of unexplained fever, pain, infection or hemorrhage. It is noteworthy that, in a retrospective analysis, Sumrani et al. [25] found higher levels of cytotoxic antibody and higher incidences of delayed graft function in subsequent grafts in those patients having undergone transplant nephrectomy.

Before the introduction of cyclosporin, it was noted that pretransplant blood transfusions resulted in a 10–20% improvement in cadaveric graft survival. With the availability of cyclosporin and erythropoietin, the practice of deliberate trnsfusion has decreased given the risks of induction of cytotoxic antibodies and transmission of infection. In the study by Ramos *et al.* [1], only 19% of transplant centers in the United States require any type of blood transfusion for cadaveric allograft recipients. For recipients of living-related renal transplants, 27% of centers recommend donor-specific transfusions for zero or one-haplotype match transplants. This issue remains controversial with the majority of transplant units no longer requiring pretransplant blood transfusions.

Endocrine considerations

Renal osteodystrophy resulting from secondary hyperparathyroidism is usually improved following transplantation. Although waiting for transplantation, the candidate should be treated with vitamin D or bioactive analogs and a phosphorus binding agent, preferably calcium carbonate, to maintain the serum phosphorus level below 2 mmol/l. Refractory hyperparathyroidism requires surgery; the options are total parathyroidectomy with or without autotransplantation of a portion of one gland, or subtotal parathyroidectomy leaving part of one gland *in situ*. All three approaches give similar outcomes.

In the candidate with ESRD secondary to type I dia-

betes mellitus, simultaneous pancreas kidney transplantation (SPK) should be considered. Increasingly, evidence suggests that SPK corrects hyperglycemia, frees the patient from exogenous insulin therapy, stabilizes or improves retinopathy and neuropathy, increases blood flow to lower extremity microvasculature and improves quality of life and rehabilitation potential. The evaluation criteria for SPK are more stringent with the major indications being a well-motivated patient with type I diabetes, less than 55 years of age who has diabetic nephropathy and a creatinine clearance less than 50 ml/min. Candidates for SPK must have well-defined diabetic complications, be non-smokers and weigh less than 100 kg. Additional tests and consultations are typically necessary (Table 84.7). Stratta *et al.* [26], in a review of their evaluation process for SPK candidates at the University of Nebraska, found that 75% of diabetic patients evaluated were acceptable candidates. SPK is associated with 99% patient survival, 97% kidney survival and 94% pancreas survival at 36 months.

Demonstration of compliance

Attendance to dialysis is a major indicator of compliance. Additional factors include level of serum chemistries, dietary and fluid restriction compliance, blood pressure control and pattern of cyclosporin levels if the patient lost a previous graft. In those with a history of alcohol or substance abuse, a defined period of abstinence (usually 6–12 months) and negative drug screen are required. For

---

Table 84.7   Considerations for the kidney–pancreas transplant candidate

Diabetes nurse consultation with glucometer training

Ophthalmology evaluation: visual acuity, fluorescein angiography, retinal fundus photography with retinopathy score, slit-lamp examination

Orthostatic vital signs, cardiac autonomic/peripheral vasomotor reflexes (when indicated)

Peripheral vascular evaluation including Doppler arterial studies, ankle/brachial index, transcutaneous oxygen monitoring, plethysmography, carotid Doppler examination (when indicated), aortography with run-off (when indicated)

Metabolic and endocrine evaluation: islet cell and insulin antibodies, fasting and stimulated C-peptide levels, i.v. glucose and arginine challenge test, parathyroid hormone levels (when indicated)

Neurologic and gastrointestinal evaluation (when indicated): clinical examination, nerve conduction studies, gastric emptying scan, electromyography

---

Table 84.8   Criteria for evaluation of cadaver donors

Maximum age – 70 years
Minumum age – 5 years
Potential contraindications (may require biopsy)
  (a) Hypertension requiring treatment
  (b) Diabetes mellitus
  (c) Malignancy other than brain tumor or treated skin cancer
  (d) Behavior risk factors (e.g. i.v. drug abuse)
No evidence of
  (a) Primary renal disease
  (b) Generalized viral or bacterial infection
Acceptable urinalysis (minor abnormalities attributable to acute illness ignored)
Hemodynamic stability with preterminal urine output exceeding 0.5 ml/kg/h
Normal blood urea nitrogen and creatinine (except for terminal elevations)
Warm ischemia time <15 min; cold ischemia time less than 48 h
Negative serologic assays for hepatitis B virus, human immunodeficiency virus; cytomegalovirus. The significance of hepatitis C remains controversial

those with a history of psychosis, a formal psychiatric evaluation is needed to determine suitability for transplantation.

Evaluation of the donor

Cadaveric renal donors

The major items of concern for evaluation of the cadaveric renal donor are listed in Table 84.8. Although the maximum acceptable age for donation is 70 years, recent data suggest that grafts from cadaver donors older than age 55 are subject to increased attrition over the long term (greater than five years). The lower age limit for acceptable renal donation for adult transplantation is five years. Other potential restricting medical issues include hypertension and diabetes. One approach is to biopsy questionable kidneys and determine the percentage of sclerotic glomeruli; greater than 30% sclerosis means the kidney is unacceptable. Negative serologies for hepatitis B and C are ideal; however, the transplantation of hepatitis C organs is practiced by some transplant centers, especially in the setting of a hepatitis C-positive recipient. Technical items to be considered include the number of renal arteries and veins, the presence of a patch of donor aorta, subcapsular hematomas, disruption of the renal capsule, length of donor ureter, and total cold ischemic time. The incidence of delayed graft function increases with cold ischemic time greater than 30 h; however, the current use of University of Wisconsin preservation solution allows transplantation of kidneys with up to 48 h of cold ischemic time.

Living renal donors

Living donation presently comprises 20–30% of all renal transplants performed in the US, but only about 5% in the UK. The criteria for evaluation of living renal donors are listed in Table 84.9. In the case of living-related donation, close psychologic scrutiny is necessary to determine the motivation underlying the decision to donate. There-

Table 84.9 Criteria for evaluation of living renal donors

Family conference with transplant-dialysis team

ABO blood group; tissue typing; leukocyte cross-match; mixed lymphocyte culture

History; physical examination; serial blood pressure determinations

Full blood count; blood urea nitrogen; serum creatinine and clearance; fasting blood sugar; human immunodeficiency virus and CMV antibody; hepatitis B and C testing; cholesterol; triglycerides; Ca; PO_4; urine analysis; urine culture; 24-h urine protein; fasting blood glucose (glucose tolerance test if family history of diabetes)

Chest roentgenogram; intravenous pyelogram

Electrocardiogram

Final leukocyte cross-match

Aortogram or digital subtraction angiography

after, the potential donor undergoes a series of examinations to determine predisposition toward development of renal disease. Again, chronologic age is less of a consideration than physiologic age. The potential donor must not have significant pulmonary or cardiac pathology. Lastly, the donor must be adequately informed of potential morbidity and mortality associated with the procedure. Perioperative concerns include deep venous thrombosis, pulmonary embolus, pneumonia, urinary tract infection secondary to bladder catheters, wound infection, bleeding, and of course, pain. The mortality associated with donation is estimated to be 1/3000, with the majority of deaths occurring in multiparous females as the result of pulmonary emboli. Longitudinal studies of living donors have noted a slightly increased incidence of hypertension, but renal function is unchanged. To aid in operative planning, renal angiography is performed to determine arterial, vascular and ureteral anatomy.

References

1. Ramos, E.L., Kasiske, B.L., Alexander, S.R. *et al.* (1994) The evaluation of candidates for renal transplantation. *Transplantation,* **57,** 490–7.
2. Garcia-Garcia, G., Deddens, J.A., D'Achiardi-Rey, R. *et al.* (1987) Results of treatment in patients with end stage renal disease: a multi-variate analysis of risk factors and survival in 341 consecutive patients. *Am. J. Kidney Dis.,* **5,** 10–18.
3. Burton, P.R. and Walls, J. (1987) Selection-adjusted comparison of life expectancy of patients on cotinuous ambulatory peritoneal dialysis, hemodialysis, and renal transplantation. *Lancet,* **i,** 1115–19.
4. Port, F.K., Wolfe, R.A., Mauger, E.A. *et al.* (1993) Comparison of survival probabilities for dialysis patients vs cadaveric renal transplant recipients. *JAMA,* **270,** 1339–43.
5. Levenson, J.L. and Olbrisch, M.E. (1993) Psychosocial evaluation of organ transplant candidates. *Psychsomatics,* **34,** 314–23.
6. Kilner, J.F. (1988) Selecting patients when resources are limited: a study of U.S. medical directors of kidney dialysis and transplantation facilities. *Am. J. Public Health,* **78,** 144–7.
7. Le, A., Wilson, R., Douek, K. *et al.* (1994) Prospective risk

stratification in renal transplant candidates for cardiac death. *Am. J. Kidney Dis.*, **24**, 65–71.

8. Manske, C.L., Thomas, W., Wang, Y. and Wilson, R.F. (1993) Screening diabetic transplant candidates for coronary artery disease: identification of a low risk subgroup. *Kidney Int.*, **44**, 617–21.

9. Flechner, S.M. (1994) Current status of renal transplantation. *Urol. Clin. North Am.*, **21**, 265–82.

10. Knechtle, S.J., Kempf, K. and Bollinger, R.R. (1987) Peptic ulcer disease following renal transplantation. *Transplant. Proc.*, **19**, 2233–6.

11. Lowell, J.A., Stratta, R.J., Taylor, R.J. *et al.* (1993) Cholelithiasis in pancreas and kidney transplant recipients with diabetes. *Surgery*, **114**, 858–64.

12. Merion, R.M., Twork, A.M., Rosenberg, L. *et al.* (1991) Obesity and renal transplantation. *Surg. Gynecol. Obstet.*, **172**, 367–76.

13. Roy, D.M., Thomas, P.P., Dakshinamurthy, K.V. *et al.* (1994) Long-term survival in living related donor renal allograft recipients with hepatitis B infection. *Transplantation*, **58**, 118–19.

14. Pol, S., Debure, A., Degott, C. *et al.* (1990) Chronic hepatitis in kidney allograft recipients. *Lancet*, **335**, 878–80.

15. Scott, D., Mijch, A., Lucas, C.R. *et al.* (1987) Hepatitis B and renal transplantation. *Transplant. Proc.*, **19**, 2159.

16. Roth, D., Zucker, K., Cirocco, R. *et al.* (1994) The impact of hepatitis C virus infection on renal allograft recipients. *Kidney Int.*, **45**, 238–44.

17. Rao, K.V., Anderson, W.R., Kasiske, B.L. and Dahl, D.C. (1993) Value of liver biopsy in the evaluation and management of chronic liver disease in renal transplant recipients. *Am. J. Med.*, **94**, 241–50.

18. Brunner, F.P., Brynger, H., Ehrich, J.H.H. *et al.* (1989) Combined report on regular dialysis and transplantation in Europe. *Nephrol. Dial. Transplant*, **4**, 1.

19. Mathew, T.H. (1991) Recurrent disease after renal transplantation. *Transplant. Rev.*, **5**, 31.

20. Barber, W.H., Deierhoi, M.H., Julian, B.A. *et al.* (1987) Renal transplantation in sickle cell anemia and sickle disease. ••, **1**, 169.

21. Goss, J.A., Cole, B.R., Jendrisak, M.D. *et al.* (1991) Renal transplantation for systemic lupus erythematosus and recurrent lupus nephritis. *Transplantation*, **52**, 805.

22. Warshaw, B.L., Edelbrock, H.H., Ettenger, R.B. *et al.* (1980) Renal transplantation in children with obstructive uropathy. *J. Urol.*, **123**, 737.

23. Yang, C.C., Rohr, M.C. and Assimos, D.G. (1994) Pretransplant urologic evaluation. *Urology*, **43**, 169–73.

24. Kashi, S.H., Wynne, K.S., Sadek, S.A. and Lodge, J.P.A. (1994) An evaluation of vesical urodynamics before renal transplantation and its effect on renal allograft function and survival. *Transplantation*, **57**, 1455–7.

25. Sumrani, N., Delaney, V., Hong, J.H. *et al.* (1992) The influence of nephrectomy of the primary allograft on retransplant graft outcome in the cyclosporine era. *Transplantation*, **53**, 52.

26. Stratta, R.J., Taylor, R.J., Wahl, T.O. *et al.* (1993) Recipient selection and evaluation for vascularized pancreas transplantation. *Transplantation*, **55**, 1090–6.

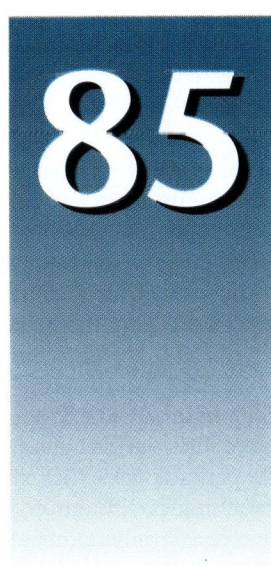

85

Kidney transplantation surgery

Edward J. Alfrey

Introduction

The transplant procedure is a composite of two operations: procurement of the donor organ, and transplantation of the allograft. Donation of a kidney can either be from a living relative or, in some settings, a very close friend who has undergone a very careful screening process, or from an unrelated person in the community who has been declared legally brain dead. In the case of a live donor, the donor and recipient operation can be performed simultaneously. For cadaveric donors, the kidney is generally procured and cold stored for some time before transplantation.

Living donor nephrectomy

Patient selection

Candidates for a living donor nephrectomy include family members or close friends who have had a significant relationship with the recipient for some period of time. When more than one living donor is available the decision about the most appropriate individual for donation is based on the age and health of the donor, the HLA match, and the relationship of the patient to the donor. After determination of the potential donor's blood type, the candidates are screened very carefully including an extensive history and physical examination. Laboratory tests include kidney function studies with a 24 h urine collection for protein and creatinine clearance, tissue typing, extensive blood serum chemistries which include liver function studies and virologic evaluation. Potential donors' lymphocytes are cross-matched against the recipient's serum to detect preformed antibody in the recipient against the potential donor. (At our institution a final cross-match is performed 24 h before the transplant procedure.) Suitable candidates then undergo an intravenous pyelogram (IVP) to evaluate the kidneys and the collecting system and arteriogram to delineate renal vascular anatomy. At our institution potential donors are evaluated with spiral computed tomography (CT) instead of an IVP and arteriogram. A spiral CT can be performed in about 20 min following a single intravenous injection of contrast. Spiral CT evaluates both the renal parenchyma and collecting system as well as the renal vascular anatomy. Visualization of the venous system has provided useful preoperative planning in certain situations where multiple veins drain a kidney [1]. Selection of the kidney for donation is based on the vascular and collecting system anatomy. Occasionally reconstructive procedures need to be performed on the donor kidney *ex vivo* to prepare the kidney for transplantation. This is usually a result of multiple vessels but occasionally collecting system anomalies need to be corrected. As examples: two renal arteries may be 'syndactylized' (sewn together to create a single orifice); congenital ureteropelvic junction obstruction requires stent placement for a few weeks postoperatively. Understanding anomalies prior to transplantation allows careful planning and avoids potential problems. Variants of either vascular or collecting system anatomy should not necessarily preclude donation.

Nephrology, Edited by Rex L. Jamison and Robert Wilkinson.
Published in 1997 by Chapman & Hall, London. ISBN 0 412 60930 4

The donor nephrectomy

For postoperative pain management, we prefer to use an epidural catheter during the first two days, followed by patient-controlled analgesia. After placement of the epidural catheter, the patient is placed in the supine position on the operating table and general anesthesia is induced. A urinary catheter is inserted and the patient is then placed in the lateral decubitus position. The table is bent in a jack knife position and the kidney rest is elevated to maximize exposure of the retroperitoneal space and the kidney. A 6–8 cm incision is made in the flank extending from approximately the edge of the rectus muscle posteriorly towards the paraspinous muscles along the inferior margin of the twelfth rib. Occasionally, the most anterior aspect of the twelfth rib is resected for better exposure, particularly in patients with a high riding right kidney. The lumbodorsal fascia is incised, the retroperitoneal space is entered, Gerota's fascia is incised, and the kidney is mobilized, freeing up the artery, vein and ureter (leaving periureteral tissue intact to protect blood supply). During the operation the patient is well hydrated to promote a brisk diuresis. The ureter is ligated and divided at the pelvic brim. Clamps are then placed on the renal artery, which is then divided, followed by the vein and the kidney is removed. The kidney is flushed with a cold preservation solution (either Viaspan [2] or Collins solution [3]). The kidney is then placed in an ice basin and transferred to the recipient room. The vessels are then carefully oversewn and the wound is closed.

Postoperative complications

Almost all patients develop fever in the first 24 h. This is usually due to atelectasis secondary to splinting on the side of the incision. The patients are given an incentive spirometer to help reduce the potential morbidity associated with atelectasis. Infections are very uncommon after kidney donation, occurring in less than 1% of patients. Pneumothorax can occur, particularly if a segment of the lowest rib is resected, due to violation of the parietal pleura. When this is recognized intraoperatively, air in the pleural cavity can be aspirated through a soft rubber catheter and the hole in the diaphragm closed. Because the primary defect is not a parenchymal injury to the lung, chest tube drainage should not be required. Postoperative bleeding is usually due to a technical error. Any patient that has donated a kidney and is hypotensive in the immediate postoperative period, requires prompt work-up with bleeding as the utmost concern to avoid a potential disaster from a delay in diagnosis of hemorrhage.

It is common for patients to need a period of 48–72 h before bowel function returns. Patients generally remain in the hospital for approximately five days, and may take two to three months before returning to work, particularly for individuals with physically demanding work.

Cadaveric donor operation

Patients are screened very carefully prior to being accepted for donor operation. There are no strict age criteria, but we are circumspect about patients over the age of 60. We have recently expanded our acceptable creteria to include more aged donors, in some instances placing both kidneys into a single recipient. Extensive histories are obtained from any available family members or friends. Any history of malignancies, except rare central nervous system tumors (e.g. meningioma), would exclude the patient from being an acceptable donor. Other absolute contraindications include patients with history of recent i.v. drug abuse, homosexual males, and known HIV-positive patients. Other relative contraindications to donation would include active infection, hospitalization greater than seven days, long history of diabetes or uncontrolled hypertension, or history of renal disease. Most centers do not use donors who are hepatitis C positive. Some centers use kidneys from these donors for recipients who are hepatitis C positive. After careful screening the blood is then drawn for tissue typing and cross-matching. At our institution cross-matching can be performed on peripheral blood and often the results are completed and the recipient has been selected prior to organ retrieval. By determining the recipient prior to organ retrieval, the cold storage time can be minimized.

The donor operation is performed through a generous midline abdominal incision. The kidneys are usually procured with other abdominal viscera. The donor is given approximately 30 000 units of heparin prior to flushing the kidneys with the cold preservation solution. We routinely use Viaspan for flushing and storage of the kidneys. Both kidneys are removed en bloc to include the aorta and vena cava and then divided in an ice basin on the back table. The kidneys are then placed in chilled Viaspan which is stored on ice. The kidneys are carefully inspected by both the recovery team and the transplant team to assure no abnormalities that would preclude a satisfactory result.

Recipient operation

The patient is placed in the supine position on the operating table and general anesthesia is induced. A three-way urinary catheter is in place to allow filling of the bladder during the operation. A lower quadrant incision is made on the abdomen. The decision to use the right side or the left side is usually made by preferentially placing the transplanted kidney on its natural side. If iliac disease is suspected during the evaluation exam, then the surgeon may choose to place the kidney on the side opposite from the suspected disease. The muscles are divided and the extraperitoneal space is entered. The iliac vessels are then exposed by ligating and then dividing the

Nephrology, Edited by Rex L. Jamison and Robert Wilkinson. Published in 1997 by Chapman & Hall, London. ISBN 0 412 60930 1

surrounding lymphatics to avoid a postoperative lymphocele. Most commonly, the external iliac artery and vein are used for revascularization of the allograft. The internal iliac artery may be used, particularly if the external iliac artery has extensive atherosclerotic calcifications. If the contralateral internal iliac artery is occluded then the ipsilateral artery should not be used in males because of the likelihood of postoperative impotence. The anastomosis time for the artery and vein should be less than 30 min. We use no heparin during the time the iliac artery and vein are clamped. The patient should be well hydrated prior to revascularization to prevent reperfusion hypotension. Maintenance of the central venous pressure (CVP) >10 cm water before unclamping helps prevent hypotension, which can be from postischemic vasodilatation of the ipsilateral leg, or from filling of the allograft with blood. Hypotension after revascularization can lead to delayed graft function. Once the vessels have been unclamped and any anastomotic bleeding controlled, the bladder is then filled. We generally use antibiotic solution to fill the bladder. The ureteroneocystostomy is then performed. The traditional method of transvesical ureterovesical anastomosis was originally described by Politano and Leadbetter [4] and necessitated making a separate incision in the bladder. A second method is to expose and enter the mucosa on the dome of the bladder by dividing the detrusor muscle. The mucosa of the ureter is anastomosed to the mucosa of the bladder [5]. The ureter is spatulated in fish mouth fashion. The detrusor muscle is then re-approximated over the anastomosis to create an anti-reflux type valve. After ensuring hemostasis the wound is closed. The operation generally takes 2–4 h. We maintain the patient's central venous pressure (CVP) at 10–12 cm H_2O during the operation. Mannitol (0.5 g/kg) is given just before revascularization. Furosemide, 100–200 mg is used to stimulate diuresis providing the CVP is adequate.

Postoperative complications

Between 5 and 20% of patients, in series reporting experiences during the cyclosporin era, develop complications after renal transplantation. Bleeding occurs in less than 1% of patients. Bleeding from the vascular anastomosis or from exposed vessels in the hilum is usually from technical imperfection either at the time of procurement or at transplantation. Any significant postoperative bleeding necessitates prompt re-exploration. Renal artery or vein thrombosis occurs in 1–2% of patients [8–10]. Renal vein thrombosis can occur when a large graft is placed into a restricting space. Prompt reoperation is the only way to salvage these grafts. The incidence of renal vascular thrombosis has not increased during the cyclosporin era of immunosuppression [10]. Wound infection is seen in 1.6–6.3% of non-obese patients and as high as 18% in obese patients [9, 11]. Urological complications include anastomotic leak, ureterovesical obstruction, ureteropelvic junction (UPJ) obstruction and hematuria. These complications occur in 1.3–7% of patients [9, 12] and are similar regardless of the technique of ureteroneocystostomy. Urinary leak is usually easy to repair and requires reanastomosis of the ureteroneocystostomy over a stent. If necrosis of the distal ureter occurs, a psoas hitch or Boari flap can be created. Alternatively, the native ureter can be used for a ureteropyelostomy. If UPJ obstruction is appreciated preoperatively, a ureteral stent can be positioned intraoperatively and left in place for one to two weeks. Peripheral nerve injuries are uncommon. Injury to the femoral nerve can be secondary to a misplaced self-retaining retractor. Other infrequent postoperative complications include respiratory, and urinary tract infections, and distal vascular injury secondary to thrombosis or intimal injury of the iliac artery. Pulmonary edema and congestive heart failure can be seen in patients with pre-existing cardiac disease.

References

1. Alfrey, E., Rubin, G., Kuo, P. *et al.* (1995) The use of spiral computed tomography in the evaluation of living donors for kidney transplantation. *Transplantation*, **59**, 643–5.
2. Wahlberg, J., Love, R., Lardeguard, L. *et al.* (1987) 72-hour preservation of the canine pancreas. *Transplantation*, **43**, 5.
3. Collins, G., Bravo-Shugarman, M. and Terasaki, P. (1969) Kidney perfusion and 30 hour ice storage. *Lancet*, **ii**, 1219.
4. Politano, V. and Leadbetter, W. (1958) An operative technique for the correction of vesicoureteral reflux. *J. Urol.*, **79**, 932.
5. Lee, C., Scandling, J., Shen, G. *et al.* (1996) The kidneys that nobody wanted: Support for the utilization of expanded criteria donors. *Transplantation*, **62**, 1832–41.
6. Kuo, P., Johnson, L., Schweitzer, E. *et al.* (1996) Utilization of the older donor for renal transplantation. *Am. J. Surg.*, **172**, 551–7.
7. Konnak, J., Herwig, K., Finkbeiner, A. *et al.* (1975) Extravesical ureteroneocystostomy in 170 renal transplant patients. *J. Urol.*, **113**, 299.
8. Robles, J., Errasti, P., Abad, J. *et al.* (1995) Surgical complications in renal transplantation: determinant factors. *Transplant. Proc.*, **27**, 2258–9.
9. Lai, M., Huang, C., Chu, S. *et al.* (1994) Surgical complications in renal transplantation. *Transplant. Proc.*, **26**, 2165–6.
10. Gruber, S., Chavers, B., Payne, W. *et al.* (1989) Allograft

renal vascular thrombosis – lack of increase with cyclosporine immunosuppression. *Transplantation*, **47**, 475–8.

11. Merion, R., Twork, A., Rosenberg, L. *et al.* (1991) Obesity and renal transplantation. *Surg. Gynecol Obstet.*, **172**, 367–76.

12. Hakim, N., Benedetti, E., Pirenne, J. *et al.* (1994) Complication of ureterovesical anastomosis in kidney transplant patients: the Minnesota experience. *Clin. Transplant.*, **8**, 504–7.

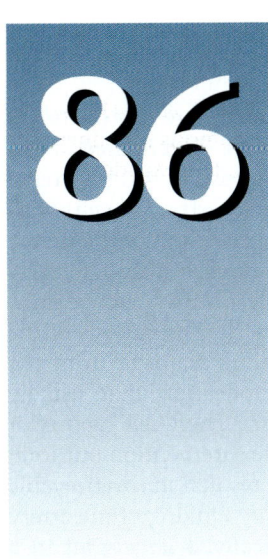

86

Renal transplantation: management in the acute postoperative period

Donald C. Dafoe

Introduction

This chapter concentrates on the careful management of the renal transplant recipient in the first few days after transplantation surgery. The ultimate fate of the transplant is often determined during this timeframe. As the biology of the injured kidney allograft is better elucidated, the importance and interrelatedness of sequential insults mandates optimal and meticulous attention to perioperative care. A mis-step in management produces an increment of damage to the allograft. For example, inadequate postoperative intravascular volume may lead to insufficient allograft perfusion that contributes to delayed graft function that may stimulate acute rejection followed by chronic rejection. Each subsequent biological insult presents a decision algorithm and possible intervention. This complexity translates into more costly care and diminished success. Thoughtful attention to the minutiae of patient management pays rewarding dividends; in the discipline of renal transplantation, these dividends are alchemistically transmuted into excellent graft survival with minimal morbidity and mortality.

The first 48h after transplantation

A typical postoperative course after renal transplantation begins with extubation in the operating room. As with any postoperative patient, vigilance is directed towards overall patient responsiveness, effective ventilation and protection of the airway. Vital signs are monitored frequently.

In the immediate postoperative period the patient with stable vital signs but inadequate urine output (<50 ml/h) should have a systematic evaluation with consideration of the following issues.

Dehydration

Intraoperative volume loading has usually been carried out in an effort to encourage graft diuresis. Nevertheless, volume expansion is the first maneuver to be considered. Often, in preparation for surgery, dialysis has been vigorous, removing liters of fluid. Coupled with blood loss (200–500 ml) and other volume losses from the intravascular space, filling pressures may be down. Intraoperative fluid intake and output are noted. A focused examination assessing neck veins, skin turgor and the clarity of lung fields is informative. A central venous pressure (CVP) line may be necessary to determine 'preload' status, i.e.

Nephrology, Edited by Rex L. Jamison and Robert Wilkinson.
Published in 1997 by Chapman & Hall, London. ISBN 0 412 60930 4

intravascular volume. In some instances, CVP readings may not reflect intravascular volume (e.g. chronic obstructive pulmonary disease) and must be interpreted in the clinical context. A CVP reading of 10–12 cm of water is the target range. If the CVP is low, a volume challenge (e.g. 500 ml normal saline over 15–30 min) is warranted. If volume resuscitation seems to be adequate and urine output is unsatisfactory, the osmotic diuretic mannitol (0.5–1 g/kg i.v.) or furosemide in large doses (200–400 mg i.v. over 15 min) may improve urine output. If cardiac output is depressed and preload is optimized, inotropy can be enhanced with a dopamine infusion (5–10 mg/kg/min).

Surgical complications

If these measures to correct dehydration and restore cardiac output are ineffective, surgical misadventure may be responsible for low urine output. Particularly if the graft produced urine in the operating room, the abrupt discontinuation of urine output suggests a technical

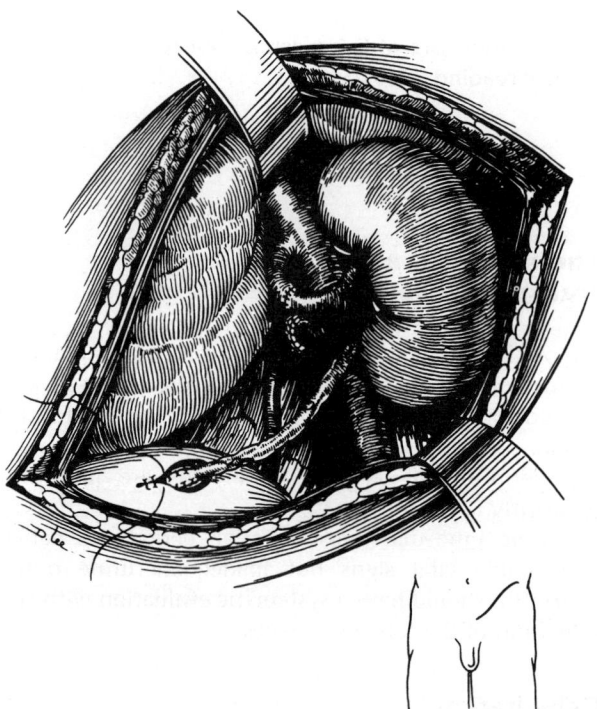

Figure 86.1 The renal transplant is placed in the extraperitoneal iliac fossa and revascularized via the internal iliac artery (as shown) or the external iliac artery. Venous drainage is routed from the renal transplant vein into the external iliac vein. The ureteroneocystostomy is fashioned by spatulating the transplant ureter, sewing the ureteral mucosa to bladder mucosa then creating an antireflux tunnel of detrusor muscle. After aligning the renal allograft to prevent kinking of the vessels, the wound is closed in two layers of muscle and fascia then the skin is reapproximated.

problem. Although technical problems are rare (2–5%) at experienced centers, they must be entertained. Such problems include: bleeding; thrombosis of the graft renal artery or vein; kinking of the renal artery or vein with fascial closure; urinary leak and obstruction of the ureter. Figure 86.1 shows a depiction of surgical technique.

Bleeding manifests typically with tachycardia, hypotension and a falling hematocrit. Thrombosis of the arterial blood supply or the venous drainage from the graft is a very uncommon complication that usually requires removal of the transplant. There are reports of graft salvage with urgent operative intervention but total warm ischemia of >45–60 min results in irretrievable injury. Grafts that are threatened by kinking of the artery or vein due to malposition (typically, a large graft in a shallow pelvis) can be salvaged by expeditious surgical exploration. If fascial closure results in vascular embarrassment, the fascia can be left unclosed and only the subcutaneous tissue and skin re-approximated over the transplant. This unconventional maneuver leaves a large incisional hernia which can be repaired at a later date after adaptive graft shrinkage. A urinary leak is suggested by scrotal/labial edema, clear fluid drainage from the wound (high in creatinine concentration relative to serum and low in glucose relative to peritoneal dialysis fluid) and an abrupt fall off or discontinuation of urine output. Ureteral obstruction may occur secondary to ureteral torsion, encroachment by the spermatic cord, intraluminal blockage (e.g. clot) or a tight antireflux tunnel from bladder muscle sewn over the ureteroneocystostomy mucosal anastomosis. Investigation of these possibilities with radionuclide scanning or Doppler ultrasonography will demonstrate no blood flow to the graft if there is thrombosis, extravasation of radionuclide agent or a peritransplant fluid collection if there is a leak and a dilated collecting system if there is obstruction. Obstruction of the collecting system or thrombosis can be determined with either diagnostic modality (radionuclide scan or Doppler ultrasound) but leak is better demonstrated with a radionuclide study showing 'hot' tracer outside the confines of the graft collecting system that persists after bladder emptying. In the setting of leak, an ultrasound will typically show a fluid collection. Since the nature of the fluid is indeterminate (e.g. hematoma, lymphocele, urine) a percutaneous aspiration and creatinine determination is necessary.

A leak or obstruction of the ureter is best handled by reoperation. Interventional radiological techniques, although very helpful for the diagnosis of obstruction or leak, are ill-advised in the acute, postoperative situation. For example, a percutaneous nephrostomy and the placement of a drain at the leak site may be adequate treatment of a small leak at the ureteroneocystostomy due to technical imperfection but such an approach for a necrotic distal ureter courts disaster. For most technical problems urgent reoperation is the best approach with correction or graft removal.

Rejection

In the immediate postoperative period, hyperacute rejection due to preformed antibodies to donor human leukocyte antigens (HLA) is rare. However, cross-matching techniques are not flawless and occasionally renal grafts are still claimed by hyperacute rejection. There are recipient characteristics that raise the index of suspicion for immunologically mediated graft damage. These include a high level of panel reactive antibody (anti-HLA lgG antibodies) and/or a prior transplant especially if short-lived. Hyperacute rejection may be apparent upon reperfusion of the graft in the form of a 'soft blue kidney' but may not manifest intraoperatively. After surgery, a radionuclide scan will show that graft perfusion is decreased or absent if hyperacute rejection has supervened. Emergent re-exploration is indicated and transplant nephrectomy is usually required.

By definition, accelerated acute rejection does not occur until three to five days after transplant. Accelerated acute rejection takes place in a 'primed' host; that is, a recipient that has been exposed to donor antigens due to pregnancy, blood transfusions or prior transplant. In these cases the anti-donor antibody titer is too low to result in a positive conventional cross-match that would contraindicate transplantation or the precipitation of hyperacute rejection. However, if the immune system is 'primed' an anamnestic response may be clinically revealed as fever, graft swelling, graft tenderness, rapid rise in serum creatinine and sudden oliguria. A percutaneous needle biopsy will support the clinical diagnosis of accelerated acute rejection. This aggressive immunological entity may respond well to high-dose steroids or other potent antirejection treatment.

Delayed graft function

If volume expansion is ineffective and technical problems or hyperacute rejections are deemed unlikely, the lack of adequate urine output is ascribed to 'delayed graft function' (DGF). DGF is often operationally defined as the need for at least one dialysis after transplantation. This generic term implies graft damage from the process of transplantation, specifically, preservation injury, reperfusion injury, cold ischemia and warm ischemia. Between 10 and 30% of renal transplant recipients suffer DGF. DGF is associated with prolonged cold storage and/or warm ischemia. The kidney may suffer a warm ischemic injury at two times: (1) at the time of procurement in the donor and (2) at the time of surgical implantation in the recipient. Warm ischemia in the cadaver donor is avoided through widespread use of the technique of distal aortic cannulation and *in situ* perfusion of organs with cold preservation solution before removal from the brain dead donor. In the living-related donor, the kidney may suffer a warm ischemic insult of a few minutes – the time from clamping the vascular pedicle to flushing of the graft with cold preservation solution. Warm ischemia time refers to the time interval from clamping of the renal artery until the exsanguinating flush of the graft with ice-cold preservation solution and immersion in iced solution and, again, from removal of the graft from the ice basin to restoration of blood flow to the graft in the recipient. Acute tubular necrosis (ATN) is the pathological lesion usually associated with DGF.

Fluid overload

If there is delayed graft function and minimal urine output, fluid overload is a concern. Physical findings such as hypertension, distended neck veins, a cardiac gallop and rales suggest the need for dialysis. The impression of fluid overload on physical examination may be corroborated with the measurement of central venous pressure (CVP), chest radiograph or arterial blood gas determination. Hyperkalemia, serum potassium >6.5 mEq/m1, will also require emergency dialysis.

Polyuria

On the other hand, urine output may be voluminous (>500 ml/h). An obligatory diuresis is most commonly due to high output ATN but can result from the osmotic effect of urea, uncontrolled hyperglycemia or excessive fluid infusion. Exuberant volume administration in an ill-advised effort to raise the CVP to an arbitrary value without regard for the clinical picture may result in 'chasing your tail' especially in the patient with a strong heart. Frequently, mild macroscopic hematuria is present but it resolves without intervention.

If urine output is satisfactory it is replaced 1:1 ml with an intravenous (i.v.) fluid regimen of a glucose-free isotonic solution such as 1/2 normal saline to which is added sodium bicarbonate for the first 12–24 h. The rate is then reduced to 0.5:1 ml hourly replacement of urinary flow. After the patient establishes reasonable fluid intake per os the infusion may be lowered to maintenance volume and then discontinued.

Hyperkalemia

In the patient with oliguria or anuria, abrupt hyperkalemia may occur secondary to surgical tissue trauma and blood transfusion. A serum potassium determination should be obtained in the early postoperative period. EKG monitoring is indicated if worrisome hyperkalemia ($K > 6.5$ mg/dl) is present. If the veracity of the laboratory value is in question (e.g. a hemolyzed specimen) the EKG may betray hyperkalemia by demonstrating peaked T waves. Intravenous glucose and insulin, sodium bicarbonate and/or calcium will protect the patient until dialysis can be arranged. Treatment with enteral ion-exchange resins (e.g. Kayexalate) is ill-advised because of adverse effects of these hyperosmolar preparations on the postoperative gut. Ion-exchange resins may cause extreme bloating and abdominal pain mimicking peritonitis or acute bowel obstruction.

Analgesia and postoperative care

Analgesia in the form of parenteral agents (e.g. morphine intramuscularly or i.v. via patient-controlled administration) is required. Meperidine should not be used since toxic metabolites may accumulate in renal failure and precipitate seizures. After two to three days oral analgesics are satisfactory. Codeine or oxycodone is preferable to combination analgesics that include acetaminophen or aspirin since these medications will mask fever.

Because the renal graft is placed in the extraperitoneal iliac fossa, only a mild intestinal ileus results and many patients can be fed in the first 24 h after transplantation. Some have an adynamic ileus and should remain NPO (nothing by mouth) until bowel sounds are active and flatus passed. A liquid diet can then be instituted and rapidly advanced as tolerated. Ambulation within the first 24 h is important to improve ventilation, resolve ileus and prevent deep venous thrombosis. The CVP line is removed 24–48 h after surgery. Perioperative antibiotics are stopped. The wound dressing is removed and the patient may shower.

Daily laboratory studies are indicated for the first few days after surgery. In the interest of cost containment, each laboratory study must be justifiable. A serum creatinine, potassium and complete blood count (CBC) will provide the minimal necessary information for patient management. The white blood cell count and platelet count are important so that the dose of azathioprine, mycophenolate mofetil or antilymphocyte preparations may be adjusted. Whole blood trough cyclosporin level should be measured daily or on alternate days.

The urinary catheter should be removed as soon as possible based on the surgeon's judgement. If the ureteral implantation was an uncomplicated muscosa-to-muscosa extravesical anastomosis with an antireflux tunnel, the catheter can be removed at 48 h after transplantation. If the implantation was complicated by unfavorable characteristics of the ureter or bladder then a longer period of time, five to seven days, should elapse before catheter removal. Following catheter removal the patient must void within 4 h or be re-catheterized to avoid overdistention of the bladder and stress on the ureteral anastomosis with potential disruption.

Local complications

Leg edema, particularly ipsilateral to renal transplant, is common. This is due to disruption of lymphatics, external compression of the external iliac vein by the renal graft and vigorous fluid resuscitation. This finding raises the concern of deep venous thrombosis (DVT). In general, DVT is an uncommon complication after renal transplantation; it has been hypothesized that the platelet dys-

function accompanying renal failure may be protective against DVT. If there are clinical features that increase the index of suspicion for DVT, a Doppler ultrasound study or venogram is appropriate to investigate this possibility. Femoral nerve injury is another unusual complication. It is thought to be secondary to neuropraxis from surgical retraction or ischemia particularly in diabetic patients with pre-existing neuropathy. The patient with an injured femoral nerve has weakness of flexion at the hip (e.g. when supine, the patient cannot lift the upper leg off the bed). The problem is usually self-limited although resolution with physical therapy takes several weeks. The patient may be able to ambulate with a cane.

Immunosuppression

The general philosophy of immunosuppression is simply the prevention of rejection without serious drug toxicities or infectious complications. Not surprisingly, it has been shown that graft longevity is inversely related to the number of rejection episodes. This goal of minimizing rejection is accomplished primarily through the optimal use of the available immunosuppressive armamentarium. There are other, controllable factors in the transplantation process that can be manipulated to advantage. A short preservation time will reduce cold ischemic damage that, through non-specific local cytokine release, has been found to induce immunogenic Class ll antigens on the graft-inducing rejection. Ideally, the degree of HLA antigen match between the donor and recipient is maximized. The timely diagnosis of nascent rejection and aggressive treatment is imperative to limit damage to the graft.

The background immunosuppression utilized by most transplant programs is so-called 'triple therapy' – cyclosporin, azathioprine and prednisone. Recently, some transplant centers have substituted the antimetabolite mycophenolate mofetil for azathioprine.

Cyclosporin

Cyclosporin is a lipophilic fungal metabolite with a cyclical undecapeptide structure that has been the foundation of transplantation immunosuppression for the past decade. One important mechanism of action is the suppression of T lymphocyte activation by inhibition of cytokine production – specifically interleukin-2. Before the patient is taking medication per os, some transplant centers give intravenous cyclosporin as a constant infusion. The i.v. dose is about one-third the standard oral dose (e.g. 7 mg/kg twice daily) infused over 24 h but the i.v. administration of cyclosporin is very nephrotoxic. Trough blood levels (drawn just before the next dose) are monitored to adjust for variations in individual absorption and pharmocokinetic profiles. The target range is 150–250 ng/ml for assays detecting the parent compound such as whole blood high performance liquid chromatography. The therapeutic level is approximately three times higher when measured by radioimmunoassay which also detects cyclosporin metabolites. It is important to distinguish assays run on whole blood versus serum because the affinity of lipophilic cyclosporin for the erythrocyte membrane results in significantly higher levels measured in whole blood. By several months after transplantation the maintenance dose of cyclosporin is 3–5 mg/kg/day adjusted on the basis of trough levels.

Side effects often correlate with the blood levels and rapidly reverse upon dose reduction. Polypharmaceutical regimens, though clinically mandated, may result in unwanted drug reactions (Table 86.1). Medications that induce the cytochrome $P450$ microsomal enzymes of the liver, such as diphenylhydantoin, will increase cyclosporin metabolism and lower serum levels. Other medications that markedly inhibit cyclosporin metabolism, such as diltiazem, may lead to cyclosporin toxicity. Frequently encountered side effects and manifestations of cyclosporin toxicity include: hypertension; deterioration of renal function; hirsutism; gingival hyperplasia; hepatotoxicity; glucose intolerance; gout; and neurotoxicity such as tremulousness and lowered seizure threshold.

Azathioprine

Azathioprine, a purine analog that interferes with DNA and RNA synthesis, was the mainstay of transplantation immunosuppression for 20 years until the early 1980s when cyclosporin became available. Coupled with prednisone, it was administered in doses of 2–3 mg/kg/day. As part of the combination chemotherapy regimen designed to reduce cyclosporin nephrotoxicity, the maintenance dose of azathioprine is 1 mg/kg daily. Compared with the other agents, cyclosporin and prednisone, it is a relatively

Table 86.1 Drug interactions with cyclosporin and tacrolimus

Levels increased by:	Levels decreased by:
Bromocriptine	Carbamazepine
Danazol	Isoniazid
Diltiazem	Octreotide
Doxycycline	Phenobarbitol
Erythromycin	Phenytoin
Fluconazole	Rifampicin
Itraconazole	
Ketoconazole	
Methylprednisolone	
Metoclopramine	
Nicardipine	
Verapamil	

benign and well-tolerated medication. Azathioprine can cause alopecia, hepatotoxicity, bone marrow depression and megaloblastic anemia. Caution must be exercised when azathioprine is given to patients with gout who are also receiving allopurinol. Azathioprine undergoes a metabolic conversion into 6-mercaptopurine and subsequently to inactive products. Allopurinol inhibits the progression to inactive products through the inhibition of xanthine oxidase. This caused 6-mercaptopurine to accumulate and exert a profound toxic effect on the bone marrow. One practice is to reduce the azathioprine dose in the setting of concomitant allopurinol and monitor white blood cell counts.

Mycophenolate mofetil

Mycophenolate mofetil (MM) is a relatively new agent that inhibits guanosine monophosphate synthesis in T and B lymphocytes. It has been used with cyclosporin in the place of azathioprine and may reduce the incidence of acute rejection episodes. Because of activity against B lymphocytes MM may protect against long-term graft loss from chronic rejection. Adverse effects are primarily gastrointestinal such as nausea, anorexia and diarrhea but bone marrow depression is also seen.

Tacrolimus

Tacrolimus, also known as FK506, is a macrolide antibiotic that interferes with lymphocyte function by blocking the synthesis of cytokines. This agent has been found to be effective in both renal and hepatic transplantation as the primary immunosuppressant in place of cyclosporin and as a rescue agent for allografts undergoing intractable acute rejection. Drug interactions are similar to those experienced with cyclosporin. Toxicities include: decreased renal function; neurotoxicity and glucose intolerance.

Prednisolone

Prednisolone, a glucocorticoid, is regarded by most centers as an important component of the immunosuppressive regimen. Steroids have valuable anti-inflammatory properties and antiproliferative effects on immune cells. For the prototypical 70 kg person, the initial dose varies from 25 to 100 mg per day. Depending on the patient's course, such as the number and vigor of rejection episodes, this dose is tapered to between 20 and 30 mg within one to two weeks after transplantation. A typical long-term maintenance dose is 10 mg daily or on alternate days.

The side effects of prednisolone are myriad. Common adverse effects include: fluid retention; night sweats; delayed wound healing; hyperlipidemia; actinic lesions; hirsutism; cataracts; glucose intolerance; acceleration of atherosclerosis and coronary artery disease; cardiomyopathy; duodenal and gastric ulcers; osteoporosis; avascular necrosis of bone affecting any joint but particularly the hips and knees; mania, hallucinations and emotional lability. Alteration of appearance such as the development of 'moon face' and acne and changes in body habitus due to truncal obesity have lured some transplant recipients, especially adolescents, into surreptitious discontinuation of prednisolone.

Other agents

Other promising agents that are not yet in common usage for renal transplantation include brequinar sodium, rapamycin and leflunomide. These agents have demonstrated potential in animal trials as future clinical immunosuppressants.

Induction therapy and antirejection treatment

Many programs employ monoclonal or heterologous antilymphocyte antibody preparations (e.g. OKT3, antithymocyte globulin) as 'induction therapy'. Therapy is initiated in the operating room or immediately after transplantation. This practice is undergirded by the theory of clonal deletion. This theory maintains that decimation of the alloreactive clones may increase graft survival. Patients in high-risk categories for immunological graft loss are frequently treated with these antilymphocyte agents. Such patients include: re-grafts and those with high panel reactive antibody titer, a very weakly positive T cell cross-match, a positive B cell cross-match positive or a positive flow cytometric cross-match. In the recipient with delayed graft function from prolonged preservation time (e.g. >36 h) antilymphocyte preparations are effective prophylaxis against acute rejection whereas the nephrotoxic immunosuppressants (e.g. cyclosporin and FK506) are withheld. This strategy may hasten recovery from delayed graft function by avoidance of an injury compounded by nephrotoxins or rejection. Another practice in recipients with delayed graft function is the initiation of immunosuppressive agents, cyclosporin or FK506, in low doses. In the setting of delayed graft function in which the serum creatinine will not reflect a deterioration in graft function from rejection, the clinician must be ever-vigilant for the possibility of 'breakthrough' rejections especially in high immunological risk recipients.

OKT3 (Ortho Biotech) is a murine monoclonal antibody directed at the CD3 antigen on mature T cells. It is produced by inoculation of mice with hybridoma cells and the collection and purification of resulting ascites. The antibody reacts against >95% of peripheral T lymphocytes. Unlike heterologous antilymphocyte preparations, the monoclonal antibody does not act via lysis of cells. The exact mechanism of action is uncertain but the CD3 site, complexed with the T cell antigen recognition site, is bound by OKT3. THE CD3 antigen is then 'modulated' (either stripped from the T cell surface or internalized). This modulation inhibits effector cell expansion and function due to inhibition of signal transduction. Clearance of opsonized T cells by the reticuloendothelial system may also play a role.

The first dose of OKT3 is consistently asscoiated with fever and rigors. Other adverse effects such as diarrhea, urticaria, tachycardia, dyspnea, wheezing and hypotension are also common. This 'first dose reaction' occurs due to engagement of the CD3 receptor, cell activation and the elaboration of cytokines such as IL-2 and tumor necrosis factor. Since a systemic capillary leak syndrome results, the patient who is fluid overloaded may go into pulmonary edema. Judicious use of dialysis prior to OKT3 treatment will eliminate this worrisome complication. Similar reactions may accompany other antilymphocyte preparations but the mechanism is thought to be lymphocytolysis. Rarely, anaphylaxis may occur with the infusion of this xenoprotein.

OKT3 is usually administered as a daily dose for 7–14 days. During OKT3 treatment, typically, the prednisone dose is lowered (e.g. 0.5 mg/kg/day). Cyclosporin may be discontinued. Some maintenance immunosuppression (e.g. azathioprine 1 mg/kg/day p.o. or low dose cyclosporin 5 mg/kg/day p.o.) is recommended to counter the production of host antibody directed at the murine xenoprotein that may limit future efficacy of OKT3. To prevent 'rebound' rejection, therapeutic levels of maintenance immunosuppression should be resumed in advance of completion of the course of OKT3.

Prophylactic medications

The use of prophylactic antimicrobials is responsible for improvements in the morbidity and mortality of renal transplantation. In light of the immunosuppressed state of the recipient and the use of non-absorbable vascular sutures, it is customary to give perioperative antibiotics (e.g. cephazolin 1 g i.v. every 8 h for 48 h). The preoperative dose is most important. Daily sulfamethoxazole-trimethoprim virtually eliminates pneumocystis pneumonia – in the case of sulfa allergy a monthly treatment with aerosolized pentamidine is an effective substitute – and lowers the incidence of urinary tract infections. Acyclovir, in high doses (3200 mg/day), has been reported to reduce the occurrence of cytomegalovirus (CMV) disease. Regimens of anti-CMV immunoglobulin or ganciclovir delivered i.v. in the weeks following transplantation are also of proven effectiveness against CMV disease. Both regimens have been recommended in CMV-negative patients receiving CMV-positive kidneys. H_2-blockers are commonly used for prevention of peptic ulcer disease. Nystatin 'swish and swallow' or other antifungals (e.g. chlortrimazole troches) are given for oropharyngeal candidiasis.

From 48 h after transplantation to hospital discharge

The next several days are characterized by a rapid convalescence from surgery. During this time the serum creatinine falls steadily in well-functioning grafts and renal function generally improves in those with DGF. The patient experiences a sense of well-being approaching euphoria. This state of hypomania is multifactorial in causation; contributing factors are high-dose steroids, the clearance of urea and other middle molecules, perioperative transfusion and the psychological effect of the prospect of a healthy life associated with the successful kidney transplant. The patient is schooled in self-medication and home care. The average length of stay is about seven days after renal transplantation at most transplant centers. Straightforward patients, such as young recipients of a living-donor graft can be discharged on the fourth or fifth postoperative day with twice weekly follow-up visits in the outpatient clinic. Some recipients may be dialysis-dependent for as long as several weeks and maintenance dialysis must be instituted until renal function improves. In patients on continuous ambulatory peritoneal dialysis (CAPD) peritoneal dialysis can be resumed. For this reason, it is advisable to leave the CAPD catheter in place at the time of transplantation. Violation of the peritoneum during surgery temporarily eliminates the option of CAPD but a small rent in the peritoneum will seal within 48 h and CAPD may be started using low volumes (11 exchanges) with progress to full volume CAPD if there is no wound leakage.

Acute rejection

Between 30 and 50% of recipients will experience an acute rejection episode, typically, within the first two to three weeks. Fever, weight gain, decreased urine output, graft tenderness, graft swelling, malaise and serum creatinine elevation are the signs and symptoms associated with rejection. A graft biopsy is the gold standard for the diagnosis of acute rejection but some clinicians will treat empirically, based on the constellation of clinical and laboratory findings. (The differential diagnosis of an elevated serum creatinine is discussed below.) Biopsies may be done percutaneously; some clinicians prefer to use ultrasound guidance. If patients' habitus or other features preclude percutaneous biopsy, it can be accomplished surgically under direct visualization in the operating room frequently using only local infiltration anesthesia (1% lidocaine) and mild sedation. The main complication of a core needle biopsy is gross hematuria. Ongoing gross hematuria can be problematic and require embolization by interventional radiology techniques. On occasion, a transplant nephrectomy is necessary because of massive blood loss. Equally rare, a clinically significant arteriovenous fistula may develop. This will manifest over time with a bruit, hypertension and creatinine rise due to 'steal' of arterial blood by the AVF and ischemia of the corresponding wedge of renal parenchyma. Ablation of the AVF by embolization is curative but at the expense of infarcting tissue beyond the AVF. The value of a biopsy to direct therapy greatly outweighs the low risk of these complications.

If the diagnosis of acute rejection is made in a timely way, antirejection therapy is very effective. Over 90% of first acute rejection episodes can be reversed with high-dose steroids, heterologous antilymphocyte preparations or monoclonal antibody preparations (e.g. OKT3).

Most protocols initially treat acute rejection with high-dose steroids (e.g. methylprednisolone, 250–500 mg i.v. daily for 3–6 doses). It is common practice to reserve antilymphocyte agents for treatment of steroid-resistant rejection. The typical course of antilymphocyte treatment is 10–14 days. Following the initiation of antirejection treatment renal graft function gradually improves over one to two weeks often with recovery of baseline function. About half the patients who experience one rejection will suffer a second episode in the 90 days after transplantation. Although the majority of acute rejection episodes take place within the first 90 days, rejection may occur at any time. Later bouts of rejection may be precipitated by physician-initiated alterations in maintenance immunosuppression, the addition of new medications that alter immunosuppressant blood levels, patient non-compliance, viral infections and other, as yet unappreciated, factors.

Hypertension

Hypertension is almost universal in transplant recipients. Cyclosporin is a major cause of hypertension. Steroids and fluid overload also contribute. Severe, intractable, high blood pressure developing months after transplantation suggests transplant renal artery stenosis (TRAS) or iliac artery stenosis proximal to the transplant. In the early postoperative period, a technical flaw resulting in an anastomotic stricture or iliac artery narrowing from atherosclerosis may cause low flow to the graft. Graft ischemia will stimulate the compensatory renin–angiotensin system and cause systemic hypertension. A bruit may be present over the graft but is not pathognomonic or exclusive of the diagnosis. The use of an angiotensin converting enzyme (ACE) inhibitor is a provocative test. When an ACE inhibitor is given the subsequent interference with autoregulation reduces glomerular filtration resulting in an abrupt rise in serum creatinine, there may, however, be a small risk of renal artery thrombosis with an ACE inhibitor. An angiogram is the definite diagnostic study and contemporaneous transluminal balloon angioplasty may correct the structural defect that narrows the artery and decreases perfusion to the renal allograft.

Psychiatric problems

Psychiatric problems in renal transplant recipients are frequent. Lability of mood due to intense emotions associated with high expectations and fear of disappointment is further exacerbated by steroids. Other neuropsychiatric disturbances – hallucinations, tremulousness and insomnia – can result from cyclosporin or tacrolimus (FK506) neurotoxicity and other non-specific factors such as sleep deprivation.

Overall, the in-hospital mortality is low (<5%). The major causes of mortality are myocardial infarction and infectious complications from overimmunosuppression.

Infections

Fever (e.g. >38.5°C) must be investigated since it usually indicates rejection or infection. In the first two to three weeks after surgery, fever of infectious origin is usually bacterial. The surgical wound, i.v. sites, indwelling hemodialysis catheters, urinary tract infection, CAPD peritonitis and pneumonia are diagnoses to be suspected. Appropriate work-up includes physical examination, cultures of blood, urine, sputum and CAPD dialysate as appropriate, urinalysis and chest radiograph. If there is nuchal rigidity, seizure or other neurological signs, a lumbar puncture should be done. In the asymptomatic patient a lumbar puncture is also indicated if other investigations have not yielded a diagnosis. With prolonged treatment using broad-spectrum antibiotics, the stage is set for invasive candidiasis.

Viral infections, primarily CMV, usually appear six to eight weeks after transplantation but intensive immunosuppression can shorten this interval. Current prophylactic anti-CMV regimens may reduce the incidence or blunt the severity of illness. Nevertheless, CMV disease still occurs with predictable frequency, especially in the seronegative recipient of seropositive donor graft. High fever, leukopenia, mild hepatitis and an enlarged spleen support the clinical diagnosis. Viremia may be confirmed by the rapid antigen test on the buffy coat of blood. More recently, the sensitive reverse transcriptase polymerase chain reaction for CMV viral DNA has been used. Intravenous ganciclovir is effective therapy. This antiviral agent and others have diminished the incidence of life-threatening CMV pneumonitis. Other viral infections that must be considered in the differential diagnosis include Epstein–Barr virus (EBV) and hepatitis B. Chickenpox in pediatric recipients that are varicella seronegative should be kept foremost in mind because of the serious consequences (e.g., hepatitis) of delayed diagnosis. Acyclovir (i.v.) and a drastic reduction in immunosuppression are usually effective against the varicella virus.

Acute EBV infection is a major concern. It may present with signs and symptoms similar to CMV. Sore throat and generalized lymphadenopathy are more common in EBV infection. Acute EBV infection (infectious mononucleosis) in the face of intensive immunosuppression may lead to a post-transplant lymphoproliferative disorder (PTLD) or B cell lymphoma. Immunoglobulin monoclonality and monomorphic histology are markers for malignancy and a dismal prognosis. If a PTLD is discovered on graft biopsy and there is no evidence of dissemination, graft removal and discontinuation of immunosuppression may be curative. The central nervous system and the intestine are other foci of B cell proliferation. Many clinicians will treat with i.v. antiviral therapy (e.g. acyclovir) although evidence of efficacy is lacking. PTLD or lymphoma has a bimodal incidence with a second peak occurring months or years after transplantation.

The clinician must be wary of exotic and insidious infections with microbes such as *Aspergillus*, *Cryptococcus*, *Listeria* and mycobacteria. These opportunistic infections are an accompaniment of potent immunosuppression for recurrent bouts of acute rejection or chronic overimmunosuppression. With careful, balanced immunosuppressive management these infections are seldom experienced in most renal transplant recipients.

Early outpatient follow-up

The recipient is seen frequently in clinic, perhaps twice a week in the first two weeks after transplantation, because of the high risk for acute rejection during that period. If renal transplant function is stable, the frequency of outpatient visits may be gradually decreased to monthly intervals at approximately six months after transplantation. Immunosuppression (cyclosporin, azathioprine and prednisone) doses are tapered to maintenance doses. Cyclosporin levels are monitored and doses adjusted. Patients are encouraged to keep a log that includes medications, daily weight, blood pressure, temperature and blood glucose levels if the recipient has diabetes. Patients are instructed to contact the transplant center for temperature elevation. Compliance with the daily medication regimen and care instructions is emphasized and must be re-enforced at each clinic visit.

Non-compliance is a major cause of graft loss especially in teenagers. The recipient must strike a comfortable balance between obsessive concern and a return to carefree independence.

An elevated serum creatinine: the differential diagnosis
(Table 86.2)

Dehydration

Upon discharge from the hospital, renal transplant recipients tend to have insufficient fluid intake since they are accustomed to a limitation of fluids while on dialysis.

Patients with diabetes are often plagued by hyperglycemia due to medications that worsen glucose intolerance (steroids and cyclosporin) and removal of insulin by a well-functioning renal allograft. A hyperglycemic osmotic diuresis may lead to volume depletion. Sometimes patients will use diuretics secretly in an effort to counter the Cushingoid effects of steroids. Serum creatinine elevation from dehydration will usually be evident from the history and physical examination. A trial of vigorous volume repletion will confirm the clinical impression within 12–24 h.

Nephrotoxins

Ironically, some of the medications that are central to the pharmaceutical regimen of renal transplantation are also nephrotoxins. High blood levels of cyclosporin or tacrolimus are a frequent cause of deteriorating renal transplant function. The addition of medications that raise cyclosporin levels, such as diltiazem or erythromycin, may be responsible. Adjustment of dose will restore serum creatinine to baseline. In recently hospitalized recipients, nephrotoxic aminoglycosides, vancomycin or amphotericin may be the offender. Antimicrobial-induced nephrotoxicity may gradually reverse with the passage of time. Sulfamethoxazole-trimethoprim routinely causes a mild and reversible rise in serum creatinine (e.g. 0.2 mg/dl). Rarely, interstitial nephritis secondary to a drug allergy will be found on biopsy. This diagnosis should be viewed with skepticism since interstitial nephritis shares histological features (e.g. eosinophilic infiltrate) with the much more likely diagnosis of acute rejection.

Obstruction of the urinary collecting system

Obstruction of the urinary collecting system may be due to extrinsic compression by a lymphocele or 'urinoma', ureteral fibrosis, stone or inadequate bladder emptying. An ultrasound or radionuclide scan will reveal the diagnosis. An antegrade contrast study via a percutaneously placed needle or nephrostomy tube is the definitive radiographic study. A Whitaker test – manometric pressure determination upon saline infusion – may be done to assess the urodynamics of an apparent obstruction. An extraperitoneal lymphocele may be drained into the peritoneal cavity by surgical fenestration of the lymphocele wall or percutaneous drainage and sclerosis with caustic agents such as povidone iodine. A 'urinoma', a collection of urine, may be associated with distal ureteral necrosis from acute rejection or insidious urinary leak. Obstructing urinary calculi may develop *de novo* or may be unknowingly transplanted with the graft. Rarely, luminal obstruction may be due to a fungus ball or papillary necrosis. Decompression of the obstructed urinary collecting system will often be accompanied by a postobstructive diuresis and a rapid drop in serum creatinine.

Table 86.2 Work-up of elevated serum creatinine in the first 30 days after transplantation

? Dehydrated	• physical exam • daily weights • ±central venous pressure • check blood glucose	• hydrate p.o. or i.v. • treat hyperglycemia
? Nephrotoxins	• check trough level of cyclosporin/ tacrolimus • review list of drugs	• adjust dose • adjust medications
? Obstruction	• ultrasound (U/S) • ±percutaneous pyelogram	• dilate/stent ureter • drain lymphocele • operative correction
? Urinary leak	• Radionuclide scan or U/S ± aspiration	• Operative correction
? Vascular problem	• Doppler ultrasound • radionuclide scan	• emergency operative correction
? Urosepsis /UTI	• urinalysis • urine C and S	• antibiotics
? Sepsis	• physical exam • work-up	• treat source • antibiotics
? Acute rejection	• biopsy	• antirejection treatment
? Recurrent primary disease	• biopsy	• appropriate treatment

Increasingly, interventional radiological techniques (e.g. ureteral balloon dilatation and stenting of a fibrosed, narrowed ureter) are successful or temporizing but the standard and definitive treatment continues to be surgical correction.

Vascular problems

Thrombosis of the renal artery or vein has a low incidence of 1–2%. It occurs in the early postoperative period. It is diagnosed by Doppler ultrasound and, if this is not conclusive, by radionuclide scan. Weeks to months after transplantation, stenosis of the transplant renal artery, narrowing of the ipsilateral iliac artery or an arteriovenous fistula (AVF) following biopsy may cause underperfusion of the graft. This is heralded by intractable hypertension despite an escalating regimen of antihypertensive medications. If the patient is placed on an angiotensin converting enzyme inhibitor, an acute rise in serum creatinine will be seen. Physical examination may find a bruit over the graft. However, an arteriogram or spiral computed tomography is necessary to make the diagnosis without equivocation. Balloon dilatation of a stenosed artery proximal to the graft or embolization of an AVF has supplanted surgery in most instances.

Sepsis

Graft pyelonephritis is suggested by fever and exquisite tenderness localized to the graft. Recurrent graft pyelonephritis suggests reflux or a defect in normal bladder emptying. A UTI or systemic sepsis will elevate the serum creatinine. Recovery of renal function follows the appropriate treatment of a positive urine culture or systemic infection.

Acute rejection

Rejection can be regarded as a biological response that has evolved over millenia of self-preservation. Therefore, in spite of pharmaceutical intervention, it is an everpresent threat and must be considered foremost in the diagnosis of an elevated creatinine. Fever, graft swelling and tenderness, hypertension and weight gain are clinical signs of acute rejection but it may also be insidious and indolent. When the aforementioned problems (e.g. dehydration, nephrotoxins, etc.) are considered, investigated and ruled out, the remaining diagnosis is acute rejection. If the clinical picture is extremely convincing, some clinicians will treat acute rejection without histological confirmation. On the other hand, a strict protocol of percutaneous needle biopsy before treatment of presumed rejection reveals another diagnosis with humbling regularity. Treatment of acute rejection with current antirejection agents is effective in the great majority of instances.

Perioperative care of living renal donors

The care of the living renal donor – either genetically or emotionally related – in the early postoperative period is standard as for any major surgery in a healthy person. The donor is routinely extubated in the operating room or in the recovery room. Intravenous fluids are administered at a maintenance rate. Pain relief may be provided with small doses of narcotic (e.g. morphine) intravenously. The use of supplemental epidural analgesia is of great benefit.

Aside from the usual concerns after general anesthesia, such as airway protection and ventilation, the rare occur-

rence of bleeding is of primary concern. Tachycardia and hypotension with a falling hematocrit suggest significant bleeding that requires a return to the operating room for re-exploration. Especially if the twelfth rib was resected, the pleura may have been violated resulting in a pneumothorax. Since the visceral pleura is not injured, a tension pneumothorax is unlikely. A chest radiograph should be obtained after donor nephrectomy. If a pneumothorax is present, it may be followed conservatively or treated by aspiration of pleural air or a small chest tube.

Recovery from donor nephrectomy is rapid with adequate pain relief being the main limitation. Once the epidural catheter is removed 24–48 h after surgery, small i.v. doses of an analgesic narcotic agent via a patient controlled analgesia delivery system will provide comfort. On the first postoperative day, the urinary catheter is removed and the donor encouraged to ambulate. Often a mild ileus is present but a diet can be advanced as tolerated. Creatinine clearance drops by half immediately (e.g. 50 ml/min) then improves secondary to hypertrophy and stabilizes in about six weeks to 60–70% of preoperative renal function (e.g. 70 ml/min). A typical serum creatinine in a 70 kg mesomorphic donor in the early postoperative period is 1.7 mg/dl. Discharge at five to seven days after surgery is customary. The 30-day mortality after renal donation is 1/3500 with rare deaths reported due either to uncontrolled intraoperative bleeding (e.g. the vascular clamp becomes disengaged from the vena cava) or a large pulmonary embolus, particularly in multiparous donors. The use of intraoperative compression boots mitigates against deep vein thrombosis and pulmonary embolus.

As a physician it is important to be especially attentive to the donor. Because the donor is healthy, there is a tendency to focus on the transplant recipient. The 'gift of life' to a loved one may be sufficient reward but some donors may feel a sense of benign neglect relative to the attention lavished on the recipient. The heroism of the donor should not go unrecognized or unpraised.

The first postoperative outpatient visit is scheduled a week after surgery. A wound infection or seroma occurs in about 2–5% of donors. A urinalysis is done to rule out a UTI or other abnormalities. At six weeks, the patient is seen again. The flank wound is examined for a fascial defect. Laxity and hyperesthesia of the ipsilateral abdominal wall is the norm. With re-innervation of these muscles over time and full physical activity resuming six weeks after surgery, the muscle tone of this area will return. By this time the serum creatinine is in the normal range. There is no special long-term care for the donor. An annual visit to a primary physician is recommended for a blood pressure determination and urinalysis.

The emergence of the hyperfiltration theory from experimental work in uninephrectomized rats precipitated reviews of renal function, proteinuria and hypertension in living renal donors and uninephrectomized patients by transplant surgeons and physicians. In general, these studies did not uncover any detrimental long-term effects in those with one kidney after 20–30 years. In addition to the apparent lack of harm to the donor, psychological studies demonstrate that the donor benefits from the act of extreme altruism through a sense of enhanced self-esteem that is long-lived regardless of the transplant outcome.

Further reading

Becker, J.A., Choyke, P.L., Hill, M. *et al.* (1990) Imaging the Transplanted Kidney, in *Clinical Urography* (ed. H.M. Pollack), W.B. Saunders, Philadelphia.

Burdick, J.F., Racusen, L.C., Solez, K. and Williams, G.M. (1992) *Kidney Transplant Rejection, Diagnosis and Treatment*, 2nd edn. Marcel Dekker, New York.

Dafoe, D.C. and Alfrey, E.J. (1994) Urologic aspects of renal transplantation, in *Clinical Manual of Urology*, 2nd edn (eds P.M. Hanno and A.J. Wein), McGraw Hill, New York.

Gottesdiener, K.M. (1989) Transplanted infections: donor-to-host transmission with the allograft. *Ann. Intern. Med.*, **110**, 1001–16.

Helderman, J.H., Van Buren, D.H., Amend, W.J.C. and Pirsch, J.D. (1994) Chronic Immunosuppression of the renal transplant patient. *J. Am. Soc. Nephrol.*, **4**, S2–29.

Penn, I. (1994) The problem of cancer in organ transplant recipients: an overview. *Transplant. Sci.*, **4**, 23–32.

Rubin, R.H. and Rolkoff-Rubin, N.E. (1993) Minireview: antimicrobial strategies in the care of organ transplant recipients. *Antimicrob. Agents Chemother.*, **37**, 619–24.

Suthanthiran, M. and Strom, T.B. (1994) Renal transplantation. *N. Eng. J. Med.*, **331**, 365–94.

87

Renal transplantation: long-term management

John D. Scandling

Introduction

The care of the renal transplant patient is a challenging and rewarding endeavor for the nephrologist. The ever-improving success of renal transplantation ensures the continued growth of the population of transplant recipients, and the long-term care of these individuals is now the responsibility of general and transplant nephrologists working in concert.

The long-term management of the renal transplantation patient is usually considered to begin after the second or third month post-transplant, but really begins with early and careful management of chronic renal insufficiency and its complications. Correction of anemia, control of hypertension, hyperglycemia, hyperlipidemia and body weight, and smoking cessation may reduce the risk of cardiovascular disease, the leading cause of death in both the transplant and dialysis populations. Infection, although no longer the leading cause of death in the transplant population, remains a chief cause of morbidity and mortality. Immunization with pneumococcal and hepatitis B vaccines is a cornerstone of infection prophylaxis. Adherence to universal infection control precautions in the dialysis unit may reduce the spread of

hepatitis C, now known to be the major cause of chronic liver disease in patients with end-stage renal disease. Screening this immunocompromised population for tuberculosis is a public health concern as well, particularly in areas with immigrant populations from endemic regions of the world. Continued attention to control of metabolic acidosis, maintenance of calcium/phosphorus balance and control of hyperparathyroidism may further reduce the already declining incidence of bone disease, particularly osteonecrosis, following transplantation. Timely initiation of maintenance dialysis, in this era of increasing pre-emptive transplantation (transplantation before the need for maintenance dialysis), ensures control of uremia prior to transplantation and its attendant risks. Proper nutrition and adequate dialysis obviate hypoalbuminemia, a risk factor for infection immediately after transplantation. Thus the attentive care of the patient with renal failure helps set the stage for successful transplant outcome.

Although there are clearly risks associated with transplantation, many recipients – typically recipients of living related donor kidneys – do very well for many years with seemingly little morbidity. Nonetheless, all recipients are susceptible to the complications consequent to trans-

Nephrology, Edited by Rex L. Jamison and Robert Wilkinson.
Published in 1997 by Chapman & Hall, London. ISBN 0 412 60930 4

plantation and the obligatory immunosuppressive therapy. This chapter considers the management of the renal transplant patient following the third post-transplant month.

Maintenance immunosuppression

By the fourth post-transplant month, as the risk of acute rejection wanes, the typical transplant recipient has achieved both stable transplant kidney function and maintenance immunosuppression. The level of transplant kidney function at this stage will usually reflect the early function of the allograft. Recent experience in the US shows that recipients of kidneys whose immediate and prompt function results in a serum creatinine <1.6 mg/dl at the time of initial hospital discharge following transplantation can expect significantly better short- and long-term renal allograft survival than those with worse early function [1]. Indeed, nearly half the recipients with poor renal transplant function at the time of initial hospital discharge (serum creatinine >3.5 mg/dl) will lose the kidney by the third to sixth post-transplant month.

In the US most transplant programs now employ 'triple therapy' for maintenance immunosuppression, using cyclosporin, azathioprine and prednisone, whereas double therapy with cyclosporin and prednisone or even cyclosporin monotherapy are commonly employed maintenance programs in Europe and other parts of the world. The original goal of triple drug therapy was to lessen the risk of cyclosporin nephrotoxicity through the addition of azathioprine to the immunosuppressive regimen, thereby allowing a reduction in cyclosporin dosage. However, lowering the cyclosporin dosage below a certain threshold may risk precipitation of rejection. Several retrospective studies show that transplant patients receiving less that 4 mg/kg/day of cyclosporin suffer greater cumulative renal allograft loss, presumably due to chronic rejection [2]. This may explain why triple drug therapy is of no proven superiority to double drug therapy with regard to renal allograft survival, as cyclosporin dosing has frequently been less than 4 mg/kg/day in triple therapy regimens. Maintenance triple therapy now typically consists of cyclosporin 4–5 mg/kg/day, azathioprine 0.75–1.5 mg/kg/day and prednisone 10 mg/day, but there is variability over transplant centers.

Both concern about chronic nephrotoxicity and the financial cost of cyclosporin-based immunosuppression led to early trials of elective cyclosporin withdrawal following renal transplantation. A recent meta-analysis of such trials showed an increased incidence of acute rejection following withdrawal of cyclosporin, but no adverse effect on allograft survival over the mean follow-up of two years [3]. However, uncertainty about the long-term consequences of cyclosporin withdrawal and the mounting evidence that acute rejection is a risk factor for chronic rejection lead most transplant physicians to recommend against cyclosporin withdrawal [4]. The cost of cyclosporin is also the reason for co-administration of certain drugs which impede cyclosporin metabolism and hence raise cyclosporin blood levels, allowing a reduction in cyclosporin dosage. Agents typically used for this purpose are ketoconazole, erythromycin and the calcium channel blockers diltiazem and verapamil. Although transplant centers report marked success in reduction of cyclosporin dosage with little complication when using these agents, there is a risk of allograft dysfunction presumed secondary to cyclosporin nephrotoxicity not necessarily presaged by elevated cyclosporin blood levels. This is particularly so with verapamil and diltiazem, as they become more problematic when they are adjusted to control hypertension. For this reason, many transplant physicians try to avoid co-administration of drugs which can alter cyclosporin metabolism.

After the introduction of cyclosporin in organ transplantation, interest in corticosteroid-free immunosuppression was rekindled. Reduction in the incidence and severity of hypertension, glucose intolerance and hyperlipidemia, with the putative consequence of reduced cardiovascular morbidity and mortality, is the attraction of steroid-free therapy in adults, although improving the chance for growth is also a major motivation for steroid-free therapy in children. A recent review categorized trials of steroid-free immunosuppression as trials of either steroid avoidance, wherein steroid was not part of the immunosuppressive protocol right from the time of transplantation, or steroid withdrawal, wherein steroid was withdrawn at an arbitrary point post-transplantation [5]. Steroid avoidance was difficult to achieve with either cyclosporin monotherapy or double therapy with cyclosporin and azathioprine. An episode of acute rejection led to the addition of steroid to the maintenance immunosuppression in more than 50% of renal transplant recipients started on a steroid avoidance regimen. The interpretation of steroid withdrawal trials was complicated by differences among the trials in patient selection, protocol for steroid withdrawal, maintenance immunosuppression, and outcome measures. Nonetheless, it was clear that steroid withdrawal, particularly if early (within the first three to four months of transplantation), or rapid (over less than three to four months) increased the risk of acute rejection and may, in turn, jeopardize long-term graft survival. Later (6–12 months post-transplant) and slower (over three to four months) steroid withdrawal may be more successful, particularly in recipients of living-related kidney transplants, but remains risky. Diminished long-term graft survival due to chronic rejection may be evident only after several years have elapsed since steroid withdrawal. As in the case of cyclosporin withdrawal, many transplant physicians consider steroid withdrawal experimental and recommend against its routine practice. Withdrawal of maintenance immunosuppressive agents is best left to experienced transplant physicians in a well-established transplant center.

Table 87.1 Precautions for procedures and surgery in the stable renal transplant recipient on maintenance immunosuppression

- Beware radiocontrast exposure
- Maintain hydration
- Avoid nephrotoxic antibiotics and analgesics
- Perioperative steroid supplementation ('stress steroid') is not always necessary[a]
- Give intravenous cyclosporin by continuous infusion (give one-third of the total daily oral dose)
- Monitor daily allograft function, plasma potassium and acid–base balance
- Consider wound-healing impairment

Adapted from Rosenthal, J.T. (1992) The transplant operation and its surgical complications, in *Handbook of Kidney Transplantation* (ed. G.M. Danovitch), Little, Brown, Boston, pp. 135–50.

[a]See Salem, M., Tainsh, R.E., Jr, Bromberg, J., Loriaux, D.L. and Chernow, B. (1994) Perioperative glucocorticoid coverage. A reassessment 42 years after emergence of a problem. *Ann. Surg.*, **219**, 416–25.

Table 87.2 Schedule for routine surveillance laboratory testing in the stable renal transplant recipient

	Transplant <6 months		Transplant >6 months[a]		
	q 2 wk	q mo	q mo	q 2 mo	q 12 mo
CBC	×		×		
Electrolytes	×		×		
Glucose	×		×		
BUN	×		×		
Creatinine	×		×		
Cyclosporin	×		×		
Albumin		×		×	
Calcium		×		×	
Phosphorus		×		×	
Uric acid		×		×	
Liver enzymes		×		×	
Urinalysis		×		×	
Lipid profile					×

[a]After the first post-transplant year, the frequency of testing may be further reduced.

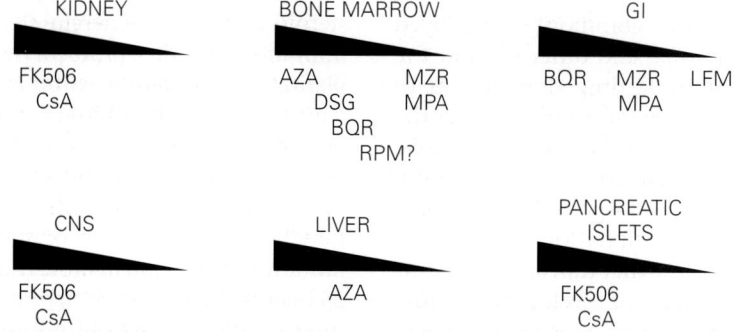

Fig. 87.1 Approximate spectrum of toxicity of new immunosuppressants. AZA, azathioprine; BQR, brequinar sodium; CsA, cyclosporin; DSG, deoxyspergualin; FK506, tacrolimus; LFM, leflunomide; MPA, mycophenolate mofetil; MZR, mizoribine; RPM, rapamycin (sirolimus). Reprinted with permission from Morris, R.E., New immunosuppressive drugs. In Busuttil, R.W. and Klintmalm, G.B. (eds), *Transplantation of the Liver*. W.B. Saunders, 1996.

Cyclosporin has become the mainstay of pharmacologic immunosuppression over the last decade. It was released for use in kidney transplantation in the US in late 1983. It is the standard against which new immunosuppressive agents will be judged and may not be easily supplanted despite its nephrotoxic property. Tacrolimus (FK506) has recently been released in the US for use in liver transplantation and has been shown to be an effective 'rescue' therapy for intractable acute renal allograft rejection in cyclosporin-treated patients [6]. Mycophenolate mofetil has also been recently released in the US and may replace azathioprine in triple

therapy protocols, as it has been shown to reduce the incidence of acute renal allograft rejection in combination with cyclosporin and prednisone [7]. Other new agents already in clinical study include sirolimus, deoxyspergualin and mizoribine. Agents showing promise in experimental transplantation include brequinar sodium, leflunomide and azaspirane. The relative toxicity of each of these immunosuppressants is shown in the Figure 87.1.

Recommendations for the care of the renal transplant recipient during procedures and surgery are listed in Table 87.1.

Assessment of renal allograft dysfunction

As the risk of acute rejection diminishes the frequency of monitoring of renal allograft function may be relaxed in the stable recipient. Biweekly measurement of serum creatinine and trough cyclosporin level is prudent through the first six months, thereafter the frequency may be reduced to monthly. Monthly or bimonthly serum creatinine determination for the life of the allograft is recommended, but the frequency is often less, as time goes by, particularly in the stable recipient of a living-related transplant. Many stable long-term (more than 5–10 years) kidney transplant recipients need only submit to once or twice yearly serum creatinine determinations. A suggested schedule for routine laboratory testing during the first transplant year is shown in Table 87.2.

Acute episodes of renal allograft dysfunction, typically manifest only as an acute rise in serum creatinine, usually occur in the early post-transplant months but may occur at any point in the life of the allograft. During the early days post-transplant, acute renal allograft dysfunction usually represents acute rejection or acute cyclosporin nephrotoxicity, but the transplant kidney is also subject to the myriad causes of acute renal failure, often creating a challenging differential diagnosis. By three to six months after transplantation, the risk of acute rejection has decreased but is still present. Late acute rejection may reflect non-compliance with the immunosuppressive regimen [4]. Since the introduction of cyclosporin a rise in serum creatinine is commonly the only sign of acute rejection; allograft tenderness, oliguria and constitutional symptoms of fever and malaise are no longer common manifestations of acute rejection. Following sonography to rule out obstructive uropathy as the cause of allograft dysfunction, percutaneous core needle biopsy of the kidney is usually performed to confirm the clinical suspicion of acute rejection. Transplant kidney biopsy, interpretation of the biopsy specimen and treatment of acute rejection are best performed by experienced transplant physicians in established transplant centers.

The more common manifestation of allograft dysfunction in the stable long-term recipient is an insidious rise in serum creatinine. This is usually due to chronic rejection, the chief cause of allograft loss [8, 9]. The etiology of chronic rejection is still poorly understood but probably reflects tissue incompatibility, given the influence of degree of HLA match on long-term outcome. There appears to be a link between acute and chronic rejection in that those recipients who experience acute rejection, particularly repeated episodes, are more likely to lose their allografts to chronic rejection than those who experience few or no bouts of acute rejection. As in the case of late acute rejection, non-compliance or 'suboptimal' maintenance immunosuppression may be factors in chronic rejection. Other contributors to the chronic demise of allograft function may be hypertension and proteinuria, common accompaniments to chronic rejection. The contribution of chronic cyclosporin nephrotoxicity to long-term allograft dysfunction and failure is difficult to assess given its slowly progressive nature (e.g. taking 5–10 years to lead to ESRD in perhaps 10% of heart and liver transplant recipients) and its histopathologic findings similar to chronic rejection. Current evidence suggests that chronic rejection represents a greater danger than cyclosporin toxicity to long-term renal allograft function and survival [4].

The triad of slowly rising serum creatinine, hypertension and subnephrotic (1–3 g/day) proteinuria typifies chronic rejection. The nephrotic syndrome can occur, and indeed the most common cause of the nephrotic syndrome in the renal transplant recipient is chronic rejection. When the nephrotic syndrome occurs as a consequence of chronic rejection, the histopathlogic finding is either *de novo* membranous nephropathy or transplant glomerulopathy, both now considered manifestations of chronic rejection. The absence of hypertension and proteinuria does not exclude chronic rejection from the differential diagnosis, but raises the likelihood of another cause of allograft dysfunction. Sonography will rule out obstructive uropathy. Difficult-to-manage or markedly worsening hypertension may be a sign of transplant renal artery stenosis of hemodynamic significance, a condition with an incidence less than 5–10% nowadays. Clinical suspicion of this diagnosis is furthered when there is a decline in allograft function during angiotensin-converting enzyme inhibitor therapy. However, it must be remembered that both worsening hypertension and allograft dysfunction are signs of intrarenal arterial disease (histopathologic findings associated with both chronic rejection and chronic cyclosporin nephrotoxicity) as well as renal artery stenosis. Angiography is necessary to establish the diagnosis of transplant renal artery stenosis.

If the clinical findings are typical of chronic rejection, transplant kidney biopsy is recommended but not always performed to confirm the diagnosis. Consideration of recurrent glomerulonephritis would prompt biopsy even though recurrent disease in the long-term allograft rarely jeopardizes its longevity; these allografts are still primarily lost to chronic rejection. Histopathologic differentiation of chronic cyclosporin nephrotoxicity from chronic rejection can be very difficult, and frequently there is an admixture of findings consistent with co-existent hypertensive nephrosclerosis, chronic cyclosporin nephrotoxicity and chronic rejection. Nonetheless, transplant kidney biopsy is recommended in the setting of insidious allograft dysfunction to confirm the diagnosis of chronic rejection and determine if there is co-existing acute rejection.

The histopathologic changes associated with chronic rejection are thought to be a consequence of immune-mediated endothelial injury, resulting in vascular narrowing and ischemia. The interlobular and arcuate arteries show progressive luminal occlusion due to intimal thickening. The obliterative vasculopathy results in glomerular ischemia and collapse, tubular atrophy and interstitial fibrosis. A mild mononuclear cell infiltrate is also often present in the interstitium. These findings are not specific to chronic rejection; they can also be associated with chronic cyclosporin nephrotoxicity. Indeed these findings may not be strictly a consequence of rejection, leading some authorities to use the term 'chronic allograft injury' when these findings are present [8, 9].

Allograft loss

The common causes of renal allograft loss during the first year post-transplant include primary non-function, technical complications and acute rejection. Primary non-function of the allograft is rare, with an incidence of only 1–2%. Technical complications occur in less than 5–10% of cases and do not usually result in immediate graft loss. The major cause of early allograft loss is acute rejection, which approximately 50% of cadaveric and one haplotype match living-related donor kidney recipients experience. Acute rejection is usually but not always responsive to corticosteroid or antilymphocyte antibody therapy. Therefore only 10–15% of recipients lose their allografts to rejection in the first post-transplant year.

The chief cause of late renal allograft loss is chronic rejection (or 'chronic allograft injury'). Once chronic rejection is established, and it may be so in as many as two-thirds of cadaveric transplant recipients as early as two years post-transplant, allograft loss is inevitable but the course is not uniformly inexorable. Patients may progress to end-stage allograft failure over months to many years and some may spontaneously stabilize at some level of allograft dysfunction for a number of years [10]. There is no specific treatment for chronic rejection. Management of a patient with chronic rejection is similar to that of patient with chronic failure of the native kidneys with the added twist of chronic immunosuppression management. Vigorous blood pressure control, maintaining a diastolic blood pressure less than 90 mm Hg, is the best treatment we have to offer to possibly slow the demise of the allograft. Treatment with an angiotensin-converting enzyme inhibitor may be problematic in the setting of chronic rejection and cyclosporin, given the risk of inducing acute allograft dysfunction. Dietary protein restriction is of unproven benefit in slowing renal allograft decline. Maintenance immunosuppression is typically continued at its current dosages in the setting of chronic rejection, adjusting azathioprine for the level of renal dysfunction. Increasing maintenance immunosuppression in the hope of slowing the course of chronic rejection is of no benefit and often hazardous, heightening the risk of infection. Treatment of co-existing late acute rejection can also be risky and is limited to steroid pulse therapy if employed. There is no utility to treatment with monoclonal or polyclonal antilymphocyte preparations in this setting.

As the allograft fails, preparations are made for a return to maintenance dialysis and repeat transplantation. Few patients actually undergo repeat transplantation before the allograft fails altogether, thus it is best to anticipate and prepare for dialysis. Once the allograft has failed and dialysis has been initiated, cyclosporin and azathioprine

Table 87.3 Recurrent diseases in the transplant kidney

	Approximate frequency of recurrence (%)	Frequently leads to premature loss (Y/N)
Glomerulonephritis		
Focal segmental glomerulosclerosis	20–30	Y
High-risk group[a]	50–70	
Membranous nephropathy	5–10	N
Membranoproliferative type I	20–30	Y
Membranoproliferative type II	80–95	N
IgA nephropathy	50	N
Anti-GBM nephritis	5–10	N
Systemic disease		
Systemic lupus erythematosus	<1	N
Wegener granulomatosis	?	N
Hemolytic uremic syndrome	10–50	Y
Schönlein–Henoch purpura	80	Y/N
Scleroderma	?	N
Diabetes mellitus	100	N
Primary hyperoxaluria type I	90 (in absence of simultaneous liver transplant)	Y
Amyloidosis	20–30	N
Cystinosis	5	N
Fabry disease	rare	N
Sickle cell disease	?	Y/N
Alport syndrome	rare (can develop anti-GBM disease)	N

Adapted from references [13] and [14].
[a] Risk factors: rapid course to ESRD after onset (3–5 years), age <15 years at onset, mesangial proliferation in native kidney at diagnosis, recurrence in a first renal allograft.

are discontinued and prednisone is withdrawn over weeks. Transplant nephrectomy is almost always necessary in those patients who lose their allografts in the first year post-transplant, as they develop graft pain, fever and malaise as immunosuppression is withdrawn. Transplant nephrectomy is less often necessary in those patients who lose their allografts after the first year.

Other causes of allograft loss in the long-term renal transplant recipient are late acute rejection, recurrent disease and death. Late acute rejection is an unusual but recognized cause of allograft loss, perhaps responsible for as much as 10% of late loss. Late acute rejection may be due to non-compliance, but it is usually difficult to solely incriminate this behavior. However, as many as 75% of renal transplant recipients may be non-compliant at times with medications, diet or follow-up after transplantation [11, 12]. The original disease is estimated to recur in 10–20% of allografts but allograft loss to recurrent disease is rare, accounting for perhaps 5% [13, 14] (Table 87.3). Allograft loss to recurrent disease is most typical of focal segmental glomerulosclerosis. This disease can recur immediately post-transplantation, manifest as nephrotic syndrome, and lead to allograft loss within months. As long-term graft survival has improved, death with a functioning allograft has become a prime cause of late allograft loss. Death is now responsible for over 50% of late allograft loss in some areas of the world [15]. In the early days of transplantation infection was the leading cause of death, now cardiovascular disease is the leading cause. Malignancy, due to its increased occurrence in this immunosuppressed population, is a major cause of death. Liver disease is now a more frequently recognized cause of late death, usually 5–10 years after transplantation. Suicide, although uncommon, is more frequent than in the general population.

Vascular disease

As in the end-stage renal disease population managed with maintenance dialysis, atherosclerotic vascular disease is the major cause of late morbidity and mortality in transplant recipients. These individuals are subject to both cerebrovascular disease and peripheral vascular disease in addition to coronary artery disease, the principal cause of death in end-stage renal disease. Over 60% of deaths with a functioning allograft in Scandinavia are reported to be due to vascular disease (over 50% due to ischemic heart disease) [15]. In the 55- to 64-year-old age group, the risk of death from ischemic heart disease is sixfold greater in non-diabetic, and 20-fold greater in diabetic, transplant recipients than in the general Scandinavian population. Factors contributing to the high incidence of vascular disease are similar to those in the general population: hypertension, hypercholesterolemia, cigarette smoking and diabetes mellitus [16]. Contributing post-transplant factors may include the number of acute rejection episodes treated with high-dose steroid

and the development of post-transplant diabetes mellitus. Those individuals at greatest risk for complications of ischemic heart disease after transplantation are those with pre-existent coronary artery disease and diabetes mellitus. Whether the risk of coronary artery disease is accelerated beyond that in the end-stage renal disease population managed with dialysis is unknown but is assumed so and is attributed to immunosuppressive therapy. As in the general population, somoking cessation, dietary modification and control of obesity, which aggravates cardiovascular risk factors, are not easily achieved. We have better success in the control of hypertension and the control, although imperfect, of hyperlipidemia with pharmacologic therapies.

Hypertension

Hypertension is the most common post-transplant complication, occurring in virtually all patients receiving cyclosporin. Living-related donor kidney transplant recipients in whom maintenance immunosuppression is not cyclosporin-based are the most likely to be free of post-transplant hypertension. Post-transplant hypertension may be a consequence of: the native kidneys, the donor kidney, acute and chronic rejection, transplant renal artery stenosis, and the immunosuppressive regimen (corticosteroid and cyclosporin or tacrolimus) [17].

Native kidney-mediated hypertension is a consequence of continued renin production by the native kidneys. Bilateral native nephrectomy or ablation of the native kidneys by radiologic embolization are curative for this form of post-transplant hypertension, but rarely resorted to. Medical management with long-term angiotensin-converting enzyme inhibitor therapy is the preferred approach.

As the use of marginal cadaveric donors has expanded due to organ shortage, so has the possibility of donor kidney-mediated hypertension [17a]. Young people with head trauma are no longer the predominant cadaveric donors in many areas of the US; the more typical cadaveric donor is now a middle-aged individual with intracranial hemorrhage. These donors may have a history of or predisposition to hypertension.

Exacerbation of hypertension is typical during a bout of acute rejection. It usually resolves as the acute renal allograft dysfunction resolves. Hypertension almost uniformly accompanies chronic rejection.

The peak occurrence of transplant renal artery stenosis is at six months post-transplant, with most stenoses becoming clinically apparent between three months and two years [18]. It usually presents as difficult and severe hypertension, and often with renal allograft dysfunction. An overlying bruit is not always present and is a nonspecific finding. Angiotensin-converting enzyme inhibition, which will result in acute renal allograft dysfunction and concomitant improvement in hypertension, can be used as a provocative test for transplant renal artery stenosis. If this diagnostic test is undertaken, the serum creatinine should be checked twice weekly, along with the blood pressure, for up to two to three weeks. The absence of worsened renal allograft function or improved hypertension during this period argues against the diagnosis. Definitive diagnosis still requires selective angiography; non-invasive testing remains unsatisfactory. When the anatomic diagnosis is confirmed and intervention is indicated (typically when the stenosis is greater than 70% or the pressure gradient across the stenosis is >15 mm Hg), transluminal angioplasty is preferred over surgical correction. These procedures should be performed in an established transplant center with an experienced interventional radiology team. As re-stenosis may occur, this possibility should be kept in mind when following a patient who has undergone angioplasty.

Cyclosporin is thought to induce hypertension through vasoconstriction and increased sympathetic nervous system activity. Cyclosporin-induced renal vasoconstriction causes sodium retention, volume expansion and renin suppression. Corticosteroid also causes sodium retention, aggravating volume expansion. Tacrolimus is similar to cyclosporin in its vasoconstrictor property yet the prevalence of hypertension is reportedly less in tacrolimus-treated liver transplant recipients.

Over the early months, post-transplant hypertension tends to improve as cyclosporin and corticosteroid are tapered. Calcium-channel blockers are first-line therapy as they may ameliorate cyclosporin-induced vasoconstriction [19]. Nifedipine and other members of the dihydropyridine class that do not raise cyclosporin levels are preferred. Theses agents are usually well tolerated, but can produce significant edema (particularly with larger doses) and can aggravate gingival hyperplasia induced by cyclosporin. Many patients require more than one antihypertensive agent, and beta-adrenergic blockers are the usual second choice. Diuretics are reserved for those patients with troublesome edema. Aggressive diuresis may be accompanied by acute renal allograft dysfunction, as transplant kidney function in cyclosporin-treated patients is quite volume-sensitive. Central α-adrenergic blockade is sometimes effective. Angiotensin-converting enzyme inhibition can also be effective, particularly in the setting of native kidney-mediated hypertension. Angiotensin-converting enzyme inhibitor therapy is usually avoided during the first three months post-transplant due to the possible deleterious (but reversible) interaction of cyclosporin and angiotensin-converting enzyme inhibitor on glomerular hemodynamics. Thereafter, angiotensin-converting enzyme inhibitor must still be used with care, with frequent monitoring of renal allograft function during the first few weeks of therapy and after changes in dosage.

Hyperlipidemia

Hyperlipidemia is a common finding in both dialysis and renal transplant patients. Hypertriglyceridemia predominates in dialysis patients, hypercholesterolemia predominates in transplant recipients. The prevalence of hypercholesterolemia in renal transplant recipients ranges from 20 to 60% [20]. Post-transplant weight gain and diabetes mellitus, as well as antihypertensive therapy with beta-blocker and diuretic, aggravate the hyperlipidemia consequent to current immunosuppressive agents and suboptimal renal allograft function. Corticosteriod and cyclosporin appear to be independent factors in the pathogenesis of post-transplant hyperlipidemia [21]. Steroid withdrawal has yielded gratifying improvements in blood glucose, blood pressure and hypercholesterolemia, but as yet has yielded no evidence of reduction of cardiovascular events in renal transplant recipients. Evidence of reduction of cardiovascular events by pharmacologic therapy of hyperlipidemia in this population is also lacking, but extrapolation from studies in the general population has led to the frequent practice of pharmacotherapy of hypercholesterolemia in these patients, particularly in those with additional cardiovascular risk factors. Indeed in this population it is difficult to achieve improvements in serum cholesterol without pharmacologic therapy. In the past, transplant physicians have taken a conservative approach to the pharmacologic management of hyperlipidemia, for the available agents were fraught with problematic side effects in this population. The bile acid sequestrants (cholestyramine, colestipol) may interfere with the absorption of cyclosporin. Hyperuricemia and gout may be exacerbated by nicotinic acid. Fibric acid derivates (gemfibrozil, clofibrate), which are primarily effective in lowering triglycerides, can cause myositis. The introduction of the HMG CoA reductase inhibitors has allowed more aggressive but still necessarily cautious treatment of hypercholesterolemia. Many transplant physicians recommend awaiting the first post-transplant anniversary before initiating pharmacologic treatment, to allow patients time to achieve their nadir dosages of immunosuppressive drugs. One transplant center's approach is to perform a lipid profile (after an 8 h fast) in those patients who show a total cholesterol ≥240 mg/dl on three consecutive occasions [22]. If the LDL cholesterol level exceeds 160 mg/dl, pharmacologic therapy is begun. If the patient has a LDL cholesterol >130 mg/dl and two or more additional risk factors for cardiovascular disease (diabetes mellitus, current smoking, hypertension, or a family history of premature coronary heart disease) pharmacologic therapy is begun. Lovastatin, pravastatin and fluvastatin have been used successfully and safely at low dosages in transplant recipients [22a]. The usual starting dose is 10 mg daily and can usually safely be increased to 20 (sometimes 40) mg daily. The HMG CoA reductase inhibitors can induce both liver and muscle injury, particularly in combination with cyclosporin (which may inhibit the metabolism of lovastatin) in the setting of renal insufficiency. Liver enzymes and creatine kinase must be monitored. The dosage restriction may limit achievement of the desired goal of therapy: LDL cholesterol <130 mg/dl or

<100 mg/dl if coronary heart disease or other atherosclerotic vascular disease is present [23].

Infection

In the early days of transplantation, 20–30 years ago, infection was the primary cause of death in transplant recipients. In those days, access to maintenance dialysis was very limited and thus overimmunosuppression, to encourage engraftment, was commonplace. As access to maintenance dialysis has become unhindered, skill at immunosuppression has become more honed, attention has become focused on infection prophylaxis, and new antimicrobial agents have become available, the risk of death from overwhelming infection has waned. Nonetheless these patients still require vigilant care, with focus on prevention and prophylaxis when possible.

Transplant candidates should be immunized before transplantation [24]. Indeed it is recommended that all patients with chronic renal disease receive the hepatitis B vaccine, pneumococcal vaccine and yearly influenza vaccine. Vaccination against tetanus should be updated; this is a common oversight in adult patients. These patients should also undergo yearly tuberculin skin testing.

The risk of infection after transplantation represents the interaction of two factors, epidemiologic exposures (community and hospital) and the net state of immunosuppression [25]. Early infection, within the first month post-transplant, is usually due to bacteria and candida. After the first post-transplant month, unconventional infections must be considered [26]. Intermediate infection, within one to six months post-transplant, may be due to cytomegalovirus (representing reactivation, primary infection or reinfection) or opportunistic organisms such as *Pneumocystis*, *Listeria* and *Aspergillus*. Indeed, co-infection, for example with cytomegalovirus and *Pneumocystis* causing pulmonary infection or cytomegalovirus and *Candida* causing gastrointestinal infection, may occur. Serious late infection, after the sixth month post-transplant, is largely limited to a minority of transplant recipients. That minority is characterized by either chronic viral infection or poor allograft function with a history of rejection and excessive immunosuppression [25]. The former category may constitute 10–15% of transplant recipients; typical chronic viral infections include hepatitis B virus, hepatitis C virus, papilloma virus, and to a lesser degree, cytomegalovirus and Epstein–Barr virus. The latter category may constitute 5–15% of transplant recipients, and they are at risk for opportunistic infection, including *Cryptococcus* and *Nocardia* in addition to those seen earlier post-transplant. The majority of transplant recipients have good allograft function and require minimal maintenance immun-osuppression; they are thus free of chronic viral infection and experience infections similar to the general population.

Perioperative antibiotic use has reduced the incidence of wound and early urinary tract infection. Trimethoprim/sulfamethoxazole is commonly prescribed as a urinary aseptic and for pneumocystis prophylaxis for 6–12 months following transplantation. Trimethoprim and dapsone may be substituted for this combination antibiotic in those patients allergic to sulfa. A three-month course of high-dose acyclovir is commonly prescribed for cytomegalovirus (and herpes simplex virus) prophylaxis. Some transplant programs employ cytomegalovirus-specific immune globulin, sometimes in combination with acyclovir, for cytomegalovirus prophylaxis in cytomegalovirus antibody-negative recipients of organs from cytomegalovirus antibody-positive donors. Ganciclovir is now commonly used as pre-emptive therapy to prevent cytomegalovirus disease in cytomegalovirus antibody-positive transplant recipients when they are under treatment with antilymphocyte antibody preparation. Nystatin or clotrimazole are typically prescribed during the first post-transplant month to prevent thrush.

Certain infections may reactivate during chronic immunosuppression [24]. Reactivation of tuberculosis, toxoplasmosis, or the endemic infections, coccidioidomycosis and histoplasmosis, is unusual but occurs. Patients with a history of a positive tuberculin skin test will typically be treated with a 6–12-month course of isoniazid following transplantation if they have not been treated previously. Reactivation of viral infection due to herpes simplex or varicella zoster is more common. These episodes are treated with parenteral or oral acyclovir depending on clinical severity. There is little experience with famciclovir (recently released in the US) in this population.

As time after transplantation passes, the nature of antimicrobial prophylaxis shifts from the administration of antimicrobial agents to immunization [24]. Hepatitis B vaccine booster (when anti-HBS <10 U/liter), pneumococcal vaccine (every two to three years) and the yearly influenza vaccine are recommended. The live virus vaccines, namely the oral polio vaccine, measles, mumps and rubella vaccine, yellow fever vaccine and the recently released (in the US) varicella-zoster vaccine, as well as the bacteria vaccines, namely the oral typhoid vaccine and BCG vaccine, must be avoided in this immunocompromised population. Antibiotic prophylaxis is commonly recommended for dental, genitourinary, gastrointestinal and surgical procedures, following American Heart Association recommendations for the prevention of bacterial endocarditis [27]. In the United Kingdom clindamycin is recommended in preference to erythromycin for those patients with penicillin allergy [28]. This substitution is also wise in the transplant recipient on cyclosporin, given that erythromycin impedes cyclosporin metabolism.

Treatment is available for acute viral exposures in susceptible patients [24]. Measles exposure may be treated with standard immune globulin within 72 h, whereas chickenpox exposure may be treated with varicella-zoster immunoglobulin, again within 72 h. Transplant recipients exposed to influenza may be treated with immediate vaccination and two weeks of amantadine or simply amantadine for five to seven weeks.

When immunosuppression is intensified, for example in the treatment of late acute rejection, resumption of antimicrobial prophylaxis with antimicrobial agents should be considered. Nystatin or clotrimazole may be resumed for prevention of candida, acyclovir for prevention of herpes simplex virus, and acyclovir, cytomegalovirus-specific immune globulin or ganciclovir for prevention of cytomegalovirus.

Malignancy

Malignancy is a well-known complication of chronic immunosuppression [29]. Estimates of the occurrence of *de novo* cancer in renal transplant recipients have been reported to range from 1.6% in Europe to 24% in Australia [30]. The variation is likely due to the high incidence of skin malignancy in those areas at high risk for such cancers (e.g. Australia). In the United Kingdom, patients with kidney transplants for more than three years have been found to have an approximately fourfold risk of developing non-skin malignancy as compared to the general population [31]. The actuarial cumulative risk of developing a non-skin cancer was 12.7% at 10 years and 31.9% at 20 years after transplantation. Skin cancers may account for 50% of the malignancies in transplant recipients. In the United Kingdom, the actuarial risk of developing a skin cancer during the first 10 years after transplantation was found to be 6.7% and at 20 years 26.3% [31]. In sunny Australia 38% of renal transplant recipients had developed skin cancer by 10 years post-transplant; it has been estimated that 66% will develop skin cancer by 23 years post-transplant [30].

Several different mechanisms may contribute to the increased risk of cancer in this population: (1) impaired immune surveillance; (2) oncogenic viruses (Epstein–Barr virus, human papilloma virus, hepatitis B virus, hepatitis C virus); (3) chronic antigenic stimulation and immune regulation; (4) direct neoplastic action of immunosuppressive drugs; (5) uremia (there is an increased risk of cancer in patients on maintenance dialysis); and (6) genetic predisposition [30].

Squamous cell carcinoma is the most common skin malignancy encountered [30]. Sun exposure increases the risk. Squamous cell carcinoma may also rarely develop from warts, a very troublesome problem affecting as many as 40% of transplant recipients in some reports. It is not clear if the risk of basal cell carcinoma, the most common skin cancer in the general population, is increased in transplant recipients. The risk of malignant melanoma may be fourfold.

Given the climatic differences in the incidence of skin cancer post-transplant, limiting sun exposure and the use of sunscreen is recommended, particularly to fair-skinned individuals in sunny climates. Annual skin examination, particularly after the fifth post-transplant year, is best performed by a dermatologist in susceptible individuals.

Malignant lymphoma is the second most common malignancy in the transplant recipient [30]. These lymphomas, usually of the non-Hodgkin's variety, constitute about 30% of non-skin malignancies post-transplant (vs 3–5% in the general population).

The nature of post-transplant lymphoma has changed since the introduction of cyclosporin. In the precyclosporin era, the average time after transplantation to the development of lymphoma was about four years; following the introduction of cyclosporin the interval dropped to about one year. The interval has dropped even further since the introduction of muromonab-CD3 (OKT3). Extranodal involvement is very common. The predilection of post-transplant lymphoma for central nervous system involvement, frequently multicentric, persists in the cyclosporin era [32].

The vast majority of post-transplant lymphomas are B-cell lymphomas [16]. Because the spectrum of B-cell proliferation ranges from polyclonal to monoclonal, the term post-transplant lymphoproliferative disease (PTLD) now refers to all post-transplant lymphoid hyperplasia, including those which progress to frank malignancy. PTLD can present early, indeed within the first month, after transplantation. Transmission of Epstein–Barr virus with the allograft or reactivation of Epstein–Barr virus in the recipient have been implicated in the development of this disorder. Patients at risk for primary Epstein–Barr virus infection and those patients subjected to heavy immunosuppression, particularly with antilymphocyte antibody preparation (e.g. OKT3), are at increased risk. The risk of PTLD in renal transplant recipients is reported at 1–2% (vs 5–7% in the heart transplant recipient population). PTLD may involve the renal allograft alone and extranodal involvement is typical. Reduction of immunosuppression and treatment with antiviral therapy (acyclovir or ganciclovir) sometimes results in remission. In those with disseminated disease, discontinuation of immunosuppression and transplant nephrectomy are usually necessary. Antiviral therapy may also be of help and chemotherapy might be considered.

Other cancers which occur in the transplant population in greater frequency than in the general population, include *in situ* cancer of cervix, Kaposi's sarcoma, cancer of the kidney (transplant and native), cancer of the vulva and perineum, and hepatobiliary cancers. Of interest, transplant recipients are at no greater, and maybe lesser, risk for cancer of the lung, breast, prostate and colon – common cancers in the general population [16]. Therefore, in addition to the usual recommendations for malignancy screening in the general population, at least annual gynecologic examination and Pap smear are recommended to female transplant recipients.

In the past, immunosuppression was typically discontinued when a patient developed a serious cancer. This is no longer the case, as patients do not wish a return to dialysis, and a return to the uremic state does not clearly enhance survival. However, transplant centers may elect to reduce maintenance immunosuppression.

The total exposure to immunosuppression is probably more important than exposure to any single immuno-suppressive agent in the development of post-transplant malignancy. Indeed some transplant centers are reporting an increased incidence of malignancy in those patients receiving triple vs dual agent immunosuppression. As mentioned above, exposure to antilymphocyte preparation, perhaps OKT3 in particular, predisposes to the development of PTLD. Azathioprine metabolites are known to increase skin photosensitivity [29, 30].

Post-transplant diabetes mellitus

As many as 10–20% of transplant recipients develop diabetes mellitus following transplantation [33, 34]. The onset is rapid, about 50% being diagnosed by three months post-transplant. Older recipients, those over 40 years of age, are at greater risk. In the US experience, Blacks and Hispanics are at greater risk. A family history of diabetes mellitus and certain HLA-types may also pre-dispose to the development of post-transplant diabetes mellitus. Body weight and post-transplant weight gain are not necessarily associated with increased risk. Up to 50% of those who develop post-transplant diabetes mellitus require insulin. The development of post-transplant diabetes mellitus has a deleterious effect on long-term patient and graft survival; this may well be due to the higher incidence of infectious complications.

Corticosteroids play an important role in the patho-genesis of diabetes mellitus following transplantation [34]. Steroids may both increase production and impair utilization of glucose. The incidence of post-transplant diabetes mellitus has increased approximately twofold since the introduction of cyclosporin. Experimental studies have shown that cyclosporin impairs the release of insulin from pancreatic beta cells, and cyclosporin may also induce insulin resistance. Tacrolimus (FK506), through similar effects, appears to be more diabetogenic than cyclosporin. Steroid withdrawal and cyclosporin dose reduction, if possible, may improve glucose toler-ance [35].

Liver disease

The recognition of liver disease as a late complication of transplantation has paralleled the improvement in patient and graft survival [36]. This is because serious complications of liver disease, namely cirrhosis and hepa-tocellular carcinoma, usually do not arise until after the fifth post-transplant year [37]. Chronic infection with hepatitis B virus and hepatitis C virus are the major causes of progressive liver disease in this population. Transplan-tation may increase the risk of liver disease complicating these infections, perhaps due to increased viral replica-tion under immunosuppression [38]. Although hepatitis B virus-induced liver disease is more dramatic due to its more rapid rate of progression, hepatitis C virus-induced liver disease is more common. Hepatitis C infection is now almost endemic in some dialysis populations; preva-lence rates up to 40% have been reported in hemodialy-sis units in Spain, and prevalence rates of 2–25% have been reported in hemodialysis units in the US [39, 40]. (The prevalence of hepatitis C infection in the general US population is about 0.5%.) Transmission of hepatitis B in dialysis units has become a rare problem due to precau-tion in the care of patients with hepatitis B infection and the advent of the hepatitis B vaccine.

Prevention is the only effective management of post-transplant liver disease due to hepatitis B or C infection. These viruses can be transmitted with donor organs. Thus organs from hepatitis B surface antigen-positive patients are not used. There is a small risk of transmission of hepatitis B virus from donors who are hepatitis B core antibody-positive [41]. Some centers still transplant kidneys from hepatitis C antibody-positive donors, some-times only into recipients with hepatitis C antibody, as they have seen few early complications of such practice [42, 43]. This may relate to the slower rate of progression of liver disease consequent to hepatitis C infection. Treat-ment of hepatitis B and hepatitis C infection with α-interferon is poorly tolerated and not recommended post-transplant. Potentially irreversible acute allograft dysfunction, not clearly due to rejection, can occur with α-interferon treatment [44].

Some authorities recommend liver biopsy prior to transplantation in candidates with hepatitis B or hepati-tis C infection and abnormal transaminases [45]. If chronic active hepatitis or cirrhosis is present, transplan-tation is not recommended. In those patients who do undergo transplantation, serial liver biopsies after trans-plantation are also recommended [37]. Progression of liver injury may prompt reduction or withdrawal of maintenance immunosuppression.

Drug-induced hepatotoxicity, due to cyclosporin and azathioprine, is common after transplantation. Cyclosporin toxicity is manifest primarily by hyper-bilirubinemia and mildly elevated transaminase levels. These abnormalities promptly reverse with dose reduc-tion. Elevation in liver enzymes is also seen as a con-sequence of azathioprine hepatotoxicity. These abnormalities also reverse with dose reduction. There is an association of a rare vascular liver disease, peliosis hepatis, with azathioprine usage in renal transplant recip-ients [46]. Peliosis hepatis may progress to severe fibros-ing liver disease. Its course is not clearly modified by azathioprine withdrawal.

Gastrointestinal disease

In the early post-transplant period dyspepsia, frequently a consequence of the immunosuppressive medications, is a common problem, and many transplant centers place all transplant recipients on H$_2$-blockers for the early post-transplant months. Corticosteroid and mycophenolate mofetil are the major offenders. Some patients may respond only to omeprazole. Cyclosporin intolerance, manifest as nausea and vomiting, is unusual but may require a switch to tacrolimus for maintenance immunosuppression. Diarrhea is sometimes a side effect of tacrolimus or mycophenolate mofetil.

Intra-abdominal inflammation and infection are potentially lethal post-transplant [17]. Acute pancreatitis, which may be a consequence of post-transplant hyperparathyroidism, hyperlipidemia, cytomegalovirus infection or the use of corticosteroid, cyclosporin and azathioprine, is rare but carries a mortality rate of greater than 50%. Cholelithiasis has become more problematic in the cyclosporin era, perhaps due to an effect of cyclosporin on bile composition. Cholecystectomy is commonly recommended to transplant candidates with cholelithiasis, particularly those with diabetes mellitus. Diverticulitis is a particularly lethal post-transplant complication.

Hematologic abnormalities

The anemia of chronic renal failure typically corrects within two to three months after successful kidney transplantation. Recipients on oral iron supplementation undergo more rapid correction of the anemia. Persistent anemia, in the presence of good allograft function, is usually due to persistent iron deficiency or medication. Azathioprine causes a macrocytic anemia. Sulfa and dapsone used for pneumocystis prophylaxis may induce anemia. With the lesser dosages of azathioprine now in use in triple therapy immunosuppression protocols, leukopenia is less common. When leukopenia occurs it is usually due to medication (azathioprine or mycophenolate mofetil), but may also be a consequence of viral infection (cytomegalovirus, Epstein–Barr virus.)

Post-transplant erythrocytosis is a poorly understood complication of renal transplantation [47]. It is not caused by hypererythropoietinemia [48]. The prevalence of post-transplant erythrocytosis has tripled, to 10–15% of transplant recipients, since the introduction of cyclosporin. Post-transplant erythrocytosis occurs most commonly within one to two years after transplantation. It typically occurs in male recipients with retained native kidneys, mild hypertension and excellent allograft function. It may remit spontaneously, but usually does not. Thrombotic complications, although uncommon, are the risk of erythocytosis. Treatment is indicated when the hematocrit is greater than 55% in men and 50% in women. Standard treatments have included serial phlebotomy and native kidney nephrectomy. In recent years treatment with theophylline or an angiotensin-converting enzyme inhibitor has been shown to be effective in the treatment of this disorder. Theophylline is not well tolerated, so most patients are treated with an angiotensin-converting enzyme inhibitor or phlebotomy as necessary. Both enalapril and captopril have been used successfully. Reduction in hematocrit occurs within two to three months. The mechanism whereby angiotensin-converting enzyme inhibitor decreases the hematocrit in these patients is unknown, but may be due to renin substrate suppression. Renin substrate has a direct erythropoietic action.

As mentioned above, deep venous thrombosis may be a consequence of post-transplant erythrocytosis. However, deep venous thrombosis typically presents earlier in the post-transplant course. Peak incidences are at one month and four months post-transplant [17]. The first peak may be a consequence of cyclosporin treatment, the second a consequence of the correction of anemia. Sedentary behavior is a risk factor, but the incidence of immediate post-transplant deep venous thrombosis is low.

Edema of the leg ipsilateral to the allograft in the early weeks after transplantation is usually transient and due to lymphedema. Formation of a lymphocele could lead to deep venous thrombosis through compression of the iliac vein.

Bone and mineral metabolism

The effect of transplantation on bone and mineral metabolism is largely beneficial and evolves over time. Renal osteodystrophy and aluminum bone disease (which is becoming a rarity) heal, and hyperparathyroidism usually resolves over the first two to three years after transplantation. However, these patients are susceptible to skeletal complications of transplantation largely attributable to the immunosuppressive medications [49].

A syndrome of distal limb bone pain has become recognized in recent years [50]. The pain is bilateral, of acute onset and episodic, primarily involving the knees and ankles. The pain usually occurs at night or with recumbency and is relieved with elevation or walking. It typically occurs within the first few months post-transplant. This syndrome has been recognized only since the introduction of cyclosporin. The pain responds rapidly to calcium channel blocker, suggesting that the pain may be due to cyclosporin-induced intraosseous hypertension. The symptoms also improve on reduction or withdrawal of cyclosporin. Whether this syndrome represents a prodrome of osteonecrosis remains to be determined.

Osteopenia is a long-term complication of transplantation. Bone mineral density may already be low at the time of transplantation [51]. Rapid bone loss occurs within six months [49]. A nadir was reached at 12–24 months, when prednisone dosage was at a minimum, ≤7.5 mg daily, in a recent study in Germany [51]. At 24 months post-transplant, mean bone density was 80% of normal. After that point bone mineral density stabilized and averaged close to 90% of normal for up to 20 years after transplantation. Cumulative steroid dose is incriminated as the chief factor in osteopenia [52]. Whether cyclosporin has deleterious effects on bone mineral metabolism is controversial. Cyclosporin induces a state of high-turnover osteopenia in the rat, however, there are no convincing clinical data [53, 54].

Because it is so debilitating osteonecrosis is a tragic complication of transplantation [55]. Thankfully its incidence has declined in the cyclosporin era. Osteonecrosis had affected 5–30% of transplant recipients; it is now considered a rare complication in many transplant centers. The decline is attributed to the steroid-sparing effect of cyclosporin-based immunosuppression. The improvement may also be attributable to better management of renal osteodystrophy and hyperparathyroidism (although osteonecrosis is not seen in the chronic renal failure population). Osteonecrosis most commonly affects the hip, but it may also affect the knees and shoulders. Pain with activitiy is the presenting symptom. Magnetic resonance imaging is the most sensitive technique for early detection. Surgical therapy is frequently required in the management of osteonecrosis of the hip.

Secondary hyperparathyroidism slowly resolves as the parathyroid glands slowly involute after transplantation. It may take two or three years for biochemical evidence of secondary hyperparathyroidism to resolve. Thus, transplant recipients may have mild hypercalcemia and hypophosphatemia for months after transplantation. Parathyroidectomy is rarely required, as serious skeletal, renal or gastrointestinal complications are unusual. In patients with normal blood calcium levels, aggressive oral calcium and vitamin D supplementation in the early post-transplant months may enhance resolution of post-transplant hyperparathyroidism and renal phosphate wasting [56]. As hyperparathyroidism and hypophosphatemia do not appear to uniformly increase endogenous 1–25-dihydroxycholecalciferol levels in renal transplant recipients (in contrast to the normal population), vitamin D and calcium supplementation may offer long-term benefit to this population at risk for bone disease [56].

Hypophosphatemia in the transplant recipient is a consequence of phosphaturia. The phosphaturia is commonly a manifestation of post-transplant hyperparathyroidism, but a PTH-independent renal phosphate leak has also been described. Significant hypophosphatemia (plasma phosphate level <2.0 mg/dl) is usually seen only in the early post-transplant months. Increasing dairy product intake is a simple way to increase dietary phosphate intake. Oral phosphate supplementation with sodium phosphate and potassium phosphate frequently causes diarrhea.

Cyclosporin impairs renal magnesium conservation and thus leads to hypomagnesemia. In general the hypomagnesemia is of little clinical consequence and resolves when the patient resumes a normal diet. However, some patients do remain hypomagnesemic and some transplant centers place such patients on oral magnesium supplement, particularly when the plasma magnesium level falls below 1.0 mg/dl. Seizure in a transplant recipient on cyclosporin may be a consequence of cyclosporin neurotoxicity and cyclosporin-induced hypomagnesemia.

Hyperuricemia and gout

Hyperuricemia and gout can complicate cyclosporin imunosuppression. The hyperuricemia is a consequence of reduced renal uric acid clearance. Treatment of gout in the transplant recipient must be done with care. Non-steroidal anti-inflammatory drugs are best avoided. The acute bout of gout can be treated with colchicine. Colchicine may also suffice for chronic prophylaxis. Allopurinol blocks the enzymatic activity of xanthine oxidase and slows the metabolism of azathioprine. Myelosuppression ensues if the dosage of azathioprine is not reduced. The dosage of azathioprine should be reduced by at least 50% when allopurinol is started, and the white blood cell count should be carefully monitored.

Reproductive function

Diminished libido and impotence are common in chronic renal failure and end-stage renal disease. Most women are amenorrheic and pregnancy in a dialysis patient is very unusual. Following transplantation libido improves and potency returns in most men. Libido, menstrual function and ovulation return in women. Impotence may persist in men, however, as a consequence of cyclosporin, which may impair testosterone production, hypertensive medications, vascular disease or autonomic neuropathy. Impotence persisting after the first few post-transplant months will require urologic evaluation. Women should be counseled that they are fertile and may become pregnant after transplantation. Pregnancy should be postponed until after the first or second post-transplant year [57]. Contraception should begin immediately post-transplant. Despite the risk of thromboembolism and aggravation of hypertension, oral contraceptive is the form of contraception commonly used in this population. Intrauterine devices should not be used.

Pregnancy

Pregnancy is best considered by those women with stable good allograft function (serum creatinine <1.5 mg/dl) on stable maintenance immunosuppression and minimal or no antihypertensive therapy [57]. Pregnancy in a transplant recipient should be monitored in a high-risk obstetrical center with close observation by a transplant nephrologist. The US National Transplantation Pregnancy Registry shows that 50% of recent live births in transplant recipients were premature (<37 weeks) and 50% were low-birth weight (<2500 g) [58]. Over 50% of transplant recipients required drug treatment for hypertension during pregnancy. The incidence of pre-eclampsia was 29%, infections and complications 22%, and rejection during pregnancy and up to three months postpartum 11%. About 9% of the women lost their renal allografts within two years of delivery. However, whether pregnancy affects long-term renal allograft survival or function remains unclear. The level of prepregnancy allograft function may be the prevailing determinant [59]. Cyclosporin blood levels tend to fall during pregnancy, perhaps due to changes in cyclosporin absorption, volume of distribution or metabolism [58]. Therefore, close monitoring of cyclosporin dose and level, as well as allograft function, are recommended during pregnancy. Women with complications during pregnancy appear to be at greatest risk for rejection and postpartum graft loss. Further discussion of the management of pregnancy in the renal transplant recipient is given by Meyer et al. [17].

The pancreas transplant recipient

Pancreas transplantation is on the increase, as results have improved markedly over recent years. The annual number of pancreas transplants performed in the US has doubled over the last five years and is nearing 1000 per year. The predominant form of this transplantation is simultaneous pancreas/kidney transplantation, with drainage of the transplant pancreas into the bladder. This transplantation is done in the setting of advanced renal insufficiency or end-stage renal disease in recipients with insulin-dependent diabetes mellitus.

There is substantially increased morbidity associated with combined pancreas/kidney transplantation compared to kidney-alone transplantation. Much of the morbidity occurs in the early post-transplant months. Simultaneous pancreas/kidney transplant recipients often undergo induction immunosuppression with antilymphocyte antibody preparation and yet have a higher incidence of acute rejection. Thus, these individuals are at greater risk for the complications of immunosuppression. As many as 10–15% of pancreatic allografts are lost to thrombosis in the early post-transplant days. Other early complications include wound infection, dehiscence or incisional hernia, bladder or duodenal leakage, hematuria, urinary tract infection, and urethritis. Persistent hematuria, urethritis, repeated episodes of reflux pancreatitis and poorly controlled metabolic acidosis lead to conversion of pancreatic allograft drainage from bladder to small bowel. The frequency of these complications has led to a recent switch from bladder drainage to primary enteric drainage in some transplant programs. Hypovolemia due to pancreatic fluid loss is another complication of bladder drainage; treatment with exogenous mineralcorticoid (fludrocortisone) is beneficial.

An occasional pancreas recipient experiences symptomatic near-hypoglycemia due to the systemic (rather than portal) delivery of insulin from the transplant pancreas. The systemic hyperinsulinemia in these patients may be an additional risk factor for post-transplant vascular disease.

Despite its growing popularity, pancreas transplantation remains an unproven therapy; the end-organ complications of diabetes mellitus are not arrested [60]. Unfortunately, most patients who undergo pancreas transplantation nowadays already have fixed or self-perpetuating complications. Improvement following simultaneous pancreas/kidney transplantation is therefore largely subjective or attributable to reversal of uremia; objective evidence of improvement in retinopathy, neuropathy (particularly autonomic) and vascular disease is lacking. For this reason, some authorities now suggest that solitary pancreas transplantation be undertaken in patients before advanced diabetic nephropathy and the associated vascular complications develop.

References

1. Cecka, J.M. and Terasaki, P.I. (1993) The UNOS Scientific Renal Transplant Registry, in *Clinical Transplants 1992* (eds P.I. Terasaki and J.M. Cecka), UCLA Tissue Typing Laboratory, Los Angeles, pp. 1–16.
2. Helderman, J.H., Van Buren, D.H., Amend, J.C., Jr and Pirsch, J.D. (1994) Chronic immunosuppression of the renal transplant patient. *J. Am. Soc. Nephrol.*, **4**(suppl 1), S2–9.
3. Kasiske, B.L., Heim-Duthoy, K. and Ma, J.Z. (1993) Elective cyclosporine withdrawal after renal transplantation. A meta-analysis. *JAMA*, **269**, 395–400.
4. Burke, J.F., Jr, Pirsch, J.D., Ramos, E.L. *et al.* (1994) Long-term efficacy and safety of cyclosporine in renal-transplant recipients. *N. Engl. J. Med.*, **331**, 358–63.
5. Hricik, D.E., Almawi, W.Y. and Strom, T.B. (1994) Trends in the use of glucocorticoids in renal transplantation. *Transplantation*, **57**, 979–89.
6. Jordan, M.L., Shapiro, R., Vivas, C.A. *et al.* (1994) FK506 'rescue' for resistant rejection of renal allografts under primary cyclosporine immunosuppression. *Transplantation*, **57**, 860–5.
7. Sollinger, H.W., for the U.S. Renal Transplant Mycophenolate Mofetil Study Group (1995) Mycophenolate mofetil for the prevention of acute rejection in primary cadaveric renal allograft recipients. *Transplantation*, **60**, 225–32.
8. Hostetter, T.H. (1994) Chronic transplant rejection. *Kidney Int.*, **46**, 266–79.

9. Paul, L.C. (1995) Chronic renal transplant loss. *Kidney Int.*, **47**, 1491–9.

10. Kasiske, B.L., Heim-Duthoy, K.L., Tortorice, K.L. and Rao, K.V. (1991) The variable nature of chronic declines in renal allograft function. *Transplantation*, **51**, 330–4.

11. Colón, E.A., Popkin, M.K., Matas, A.J. and Callies, A.L. (1991) Overview of noncompliance in renal transplantation. *Transplant. Rev.*, **5**, 175–80.

12. Kiley, D.J., Lam, C.S. and Pollak, R. (1993) A study of treatment compliance following kidney transplantation. *Transplantation*, **55**, 51–6.

13. Mathew, T.H. (1991) Recurrent disease after renal transplantation. *Transplant. Rev.*, **5**, 31–45.

14. Ramos, E.L. and Tisher, C.C. (1994) Recurrent diseases in the kidney transplant. *Am. J. Kidney Dis.*, **24**, 142–54.

15. Lindholm, A., Albrechtsen, D., Frodin, L. *et al.* (1995) Ischemic heart disease – major cause of death and graft loss after renal transplantation in Scandinavia. *Transplantation*, **60**, 451–7.

16. First, M.R. (1993) Long-term complications after transplantation. *Am. J. Kidney Dis.*, **22**, 477–86.

17. Meyer, M.M., Norman, D.J. and Danovitch, G.M. (1992) Long-term post-transplant management and complications, in *Handbook of Kidney Transplantation* (ed. G.M. Danovitch), Little, Brown, Boston, pp. 173–207.

17a.Guidi, E., Menghetti, D., Milani, S. *et al.* (1996) Hypertension may be transplanted with the kidney in humans: a long term historical prospective follow up of recipients grafted with kidneys coming from donors with or without hypertension in their families. *J. Am. Soc. Nephrol.*, **7**, 1131–8.

18. Gray, D.W.R. (1994) Graft renal artery stenosis in the transplanted kidney. *Transplant. Rev.*, **8**, 15–21.

19. First, M.R., Neylan, J.F., Rocher, L.L. and Tejani, A. (1994) Hypertension after renal transplantation. *J. Am. Soc. Nephrol.*, **4**(suppl 1), S30–6.

20. Markell, M.S., Armenti, V., Danovitch, G. and Sumrani, N. (1994) Hyperlipidemia and glucose intolerance in the post-renal transplant patient. *J. Am. Soc. Nephrol.*, **4**(suppl 1), S37–47.

21. Hricik, D.E., Mayes, J.T. and Schulak, J.A. (1991) Independent effects of cyclosporine and prednisone on post-transplant hypercholesterolemia. *Am. J. Kidney Dis.*, **18**, 353–8.

22. Hricik, D.E. (1994) Post-transplant hyperlipidemia: the treatment dilemma. *Am. J. Kidney Dis.*, **23**, 766–71.

22a.Goldberg, R. and Roth, D. (1996) Evaluation of fluvastatin in the treatment of hypercholesterolemia in renal transplant recipients taking cyclosporine. *Transplantation*, **62**, 1559–64.

23. National Cholesterol Education Program (1994) Detection, evaluation, and treatment of high blood cholesterol in adults (Adult Treatment Panel II). *Circulation*, **89**, 1329–445.

24. Kennedy, C.A. and Panosian, C.B. (1992) Infectious complications of kidney transplantation and their management, in *Handbook of Kidney Transplantation* (ed. G.M. Danovitch), Little, Brown, Boston, pp. 209–37.

25. Rubin, R.H. (1993) Infectious disease complications of renal transplantation. *Kidney Int.*, **44**, 221–36.

26. Tolkoff-Rubin, N.E. and Rubin, R.H. (1992) Clinical approach to viral and fungal infections in the renal transplant patient. *Semin. Nephrol.*, **12**, 364–75.

27. Dajani, A.S., Bisno, A.L., Chung, K.J. *et al.* (1990) Prevention of bacterial endocarditis. Recommendations by the American Heart Association. *JAMA*, **264**, 2919–22.

28. Simmons, N.A., Ball, A.P., Cawson, R.A. *et al.* (1992) Antibiotic prophylaxis and infective endocarditis. *Lancet*, **339**, 1292–3.

29. Penn, I. (1994) The problem of cancer in organ transplant recipients: an overview. *Transplant. Sci.*, **4**, 23–32.

30. Sheil, A.G.R. (1991) Complications of immunosuppression in renal allograft recipient: malignancy. *Clin. Transplant.*, **5**(Spec. issue), 573–9.

31. Gaya, S.B.M., Rees, A.J., Lechler, R.I., Williams, G. and Mason, P.D. (1995) Malignant disease in patients with long-term renal transplants. *Transplantation*, **59**, 1705–9.

32. Penn, I. and Porat, G. (1995) Central nervous system lymphomas in organ allograft recipients. *Transplantation*, **59**, 240–4.

33. Sumrani, N.B., Delaney, V., Ding, Z. *et al.* (1991) Diabetes mellitus after renal transplantation in the cyclosporine era – an analysis of risk factors. *Transplantation*, **51**, 343–7.

34. Jindal, R.M. (1994) Post-transplant diabetes mellitus – a review. *Transplantation*, **58**, 1289–98.

35. Hricik, D.E., Bartucci, M.R., Moir, E.J., Mayes, J.T. and Schulak, J.A. (1991) Effects of steroid withdrawal on post-transplant diabetes mellitus in cyclosporine-treated renal transplant recipients. *Transplantation*, **51**, 374–7.

36. Weir, M.R., Kirkman, R.L., Strom, T.B. and Tilney, N.L. (1985) Liver disease in recipients of long-surviving renal allografts. *Kidney Int.*, **28**, 839–44.

37. Rao, K.V. and Anderson, W.R. (1992) Liver disease after renal transplantation. *Am. J. Kidney Dis.*, **19**, 496–501.

38. Periera, B.J.G., Wright, T.L., Schmid, C.H. and Levey, A.S. (1995) The impact of pretransplantation hepatitis C infection on the outcome of renal transplantation. *Transplantation*, **60**, 799–805.

39. Caramelo, C., Ortiz, A., Aguilera, B. *et al.* (1993) Liver disease patterns in hemodialysis patients with antibodies to hepatitis C virus. *Am. J. Kidney Dis.*, **22**, 822–8.

40. Niu, M.T., Coleman, P.J. and Alter, M.J. (1993) Multicenter study of hepatitis C virus infection in chronic hemodialysis patients and hemodialysis center staff members. *Am. J. Kidney Dis.*, **22**, 568–73.

41. Wachs, M.E., Amend, W.J., Ascher, N.L. *et al.* (1995) The risk of transmission of hepatitis B from HBsAg (–), HBcAb(+), HBIgM(–) organ donors. *Transplantation*, **59**, 230–4.

42. Tesi, R.J., Waller, K., Morgan, C.J. *et al.* (1994) Transmission of hepatitis C by kidney transplantation – the risks. *Transplantation*, **57**, 826–31.

43. Morales, J.M., Campistol, J.M., Castellano, G. *et al.* (1995) Transplantation of kidneys from donors with hepatitis C antibody into recipients with pre-transplantation anti-HCV. *Kidney Int.*, **47**, 236–40.

44. Rostaing, L., Izopet, J., Baron, E. *et al.* (1995) Treatment of chronic hepatitis C with recombinant interferon

alpha in kidney transplant recipients. *Transplantation*, **59**, 1426–31.

45. Roth, D., Zucker, K., Cirocco, R. *et al.* (1994) The impact of hepatitis C virus infection on renal allograft recipients. *Kidney Int.*, **45**, 238–44.

46. Cavalcanti, R., Pol, S., Carnot, F. *et al.* (1994) Impact and evolution of peliosis hepatis in renal transplant recipients. *Transplantation*, **58**, 315–16.

47. Gaston, R.S., Julian, B.A. and Curtis, J.J. (1994) Post-transplant erythrocytosis: an enigma revisited. *Am. J. Kidney Dis.*, **24**, 1–11.

48. Danovitch, G.M., Jamgotchian, N.J., Eggena, P.H. *et al.* (1995) Angiotensin-converting enzyme inhibition in the treatment of renal transplant erythrocytosis. Clinical experience and observation of mechanism. *Transplantation*, **60**, 132-7.

49. Julian, B.A., Quarles, D. and Niemann, K.M.W. (1992) Musculoskeletal complications after renal transplantation: pathogenesis and treatment. *Am. J. Kidney Dis.*, **19**, 99–120.

50. Barbosa, L.M., Gauthier, V.J. and Davis, C.L. (1995) Bone pain that responds to calcium channel blockers. A retrospective and prospective study of transplant recipients. *Transplantation*, **59**, 541–4.

51. Grotz, W.H., Mundinger, F.A., Gugel, B. *et al.* (1995) Bone mineral density after kidney transplantation. A cross-sectional study in 190 graft recipients up to 20 years after transplantation. *Transplantation*, **59**, 982–6.

52. Wolpaw, T., Deal, C.L., Fleming-Brooks, S. *et al.* (1994) Factors influencing vertebral bone density after renal transplantation. *Transplantation* **58**, 1186–9.

53. Cvetkovic, M., Mann, G.N., Romero, D.F. *et al.* (1994) The deleterious effects of long-term cyclosporine A, cyclosporine G and FK506 on bone mineral metabolism *in vivo*. *Transplantation*, **57**, 1231–7.

54. Dumoulin, G., Hory, B., Nguyen, N.U. *et al.* (1995) Lack of evidence that cyclosporine treatment impairs calcium-phosphorus homeostasis and bone remodeling in normocalcemic long-term renal transplant recipients. *Transplantation*, **59**, 1690–4.

55. Mankin, H.J. (1992) Nontraumatic necrosis of bone (osteonecrosis). *N. Engl. J. Med.*, **326**, 1473–9.

56. Steiner, R.W., Ziegler, M., Halasz, N.A. *et al.* (1993) Effect of daily oral vitamin D and calcium therapy, hypophosphatemia, and endogenous 1,25-dihydroxycholecalciferol on parathyroid hormone and phosphate wasting in renal transplant recipients. *Transplantation*, **56**, 843–6.

57. Lindheimer, M.D. and Katz, A.I. (1992) Pregnancy in the renal transplant patient. *Am. J. Kidney Dis.*, **19**, 173–6.

58. Armenti, V.T., Ahlswede, K.M., Ahlswede, B.A. *et al.* (1995) Variables affecting birthweight and graft survival in 197 pregnancies in cyclosporine-treated female kidney transplant recipients. *Transplantation*, **59**, 476–9.

59. First, M.R., Combs, C.A., Weiskittel, P. and Miodovnik, M. (1995) Lack of effect of pregnancy on renal allograft survival or function. *Transplantation*, **59**, 472–6.

60. Remuzzi, G., Ruggenenti, P. and Mauer, S.M. (1994) Pancreas and kidney/pancreas transplants: experimental medicine or real improvement? *Lancet*, **343**, 27–31.

88

Renal transplantation outcome

John D. Scandling

Introduction

Renal transplantation holds great promise for many individuals with end-stage renal disease (ESRD). Continuous advancements in immunosuppression and management of rejection have enhanced the odds of successful renal engraftment. Renal transplant candidates can expect an improved quality of life following transplantation and recent evidence suggests that they may expect increased longevity as well [1–3].

Care of the ESRD patient is expensive. In the US, the cost of care of a patient on chronic hemodialysis exceeds $40 000 per year, and the cost of renal transplantation and care during the first post-transplant year exceeds $80 000. Thus, the promise of transplantation is largely restricted to citizens of the Western industrialized nations (Figure 88.1). The total cost for treatment of ESRD in 1992 to Medicare, the program which covers 93% of ESRD patients in the US, was $6.8 billion [4]. Even in the industrialized countries, the transplantation rate varies. Religious and cultural proscriptions against cadaveric organ transplantation and variable use of living donors explain at least some of the differences around the world (Table 88.1).

World-wide over 22 000 kidney transplants were performed in 1994, at nearly 600 transplant centers [5]. In the US, over 11 000 kidney transplants are now performed yearly, at about 250 transplant centers across the nation. The majority, about 75%, are cadaveric kidney transplants from nearly 5000 cadaver donors yearly. Despite these

rates of cadaver organ donation and kidney transplantation, the demand for transplantation is largely unmet (Figure 88.2). Nearly 200 000 persons are now on chronic dialysis in the US; 30 000 are on waiting lists for cadaveric renal transplantation. For the 15% of US dialysis patients awaiting cadaveric renal transplantation, the wait is long. The median waiting time for transplantation has increased over recent years, from 394 days in 1988 to 728 days in 1993 [6]. The wait is likely to worsen, as the incidence of new ESRD in the US now exceeds 200 patients per million population per year and increases at about 9% per year; over 55 000 patients began chronic dialysis in 1992 [6]. Only a dramatic increase in organ donation will affect the wait for a cadaveric organ, because the incidence rate of new ESRD outstrips the rate of increase of cadaveric organ donation. From 1988 to 1994 the number of cadaveric kidney donors in the US increased from 3879 to 4802, a rate of about 4% per year [6]. The rate of increase in living donors over the same time period was much greater, about 10% per year, but the number of living donors is relatively small (2921 in 1994) and the yield is half that of the cadaver donor (a living donor can donate only one kidney) [6].

There is a single national list for patients awaiting cadaveric renal transplantation in the US, but only kidneys of excellent match to a recipient are shared on a national basis. An excellent match is a zero HLA A, B, DR mismatch, where there is no difference between donor and recipient at any of the six major HLA loci. Only 8% of US cadaveric renal transplant recipients in 1994 were

Nephrology, Edited by Rex L. Jamison and Robert Wilkinson.
Published in 1997 by Chapman & Hall, London. ISBN 0 412 60930 4

Table **88.1** Fraction of living donors around the world

Country or Center	Period	Cadaver (n)	Living (n)	Living (%)
Austria	1993	380	5	1.3
Belgium	1993	362	5	1.4
Germany	1993	2107	57	2.6
Lyon	1993	218	9	3.9
Holland	1993	436	50	10.3
Australia	1992	409	67	14.0
Milan	1989–94	412	77	15.7
Canada	1991	771	132	15.7
United States	1993	7997	2562	24.2
Sweden	1987–92	451	182	28.7
Norway	1983–91	863	635	42.4
Egypt	1991–93	~300	~600	~67.0
Tokyo Women's Hosp	1974–94	178	962	87.3
Catholic University Seoul	1969–92	16	684	99.7
Yonsei Hospital Seoul	1984–92	0	839	100.0

From Terasaki, P.I., Cecka, J.M. and Gjertson, D.W. (1995) Current world opinion regarding the use of living donors, in *Clinical Transplants 1994* (eds P.I. Terasaki and J.M. Cecka), UCLA Tissue Typing Laboratory, Los Angeles, p. 342.

fortunate enough to receive such a well-matched allograft [6]. All other kidneys are shared within regional organ procurement organizations based on a priority point system which is uniform across the nation (with occasional approved exception). Patients achieve priority points based on their accrued time on the waiting list and degree of HLA match with the cadaver donor. Children less than 18 years of age are granted additional priority.

The most comprehensive transplant outcome data are from the US, due to mandatory reporting since the inception of the national Organ Procurement and Transplantation Network (OPTN) in 1986 and the US Scientific Registry of Transplant Recipients in 1987. The United Network for Organ Sharing (UNOS) has operated both the OPTN and the Scientific Registry since their beginnings. Information on the incidence, prevalence, morbidity and mortality of end-stage renal disease in the US has been collected and analyzed by the US Renal Data System (USRDS) since its creation in 1988. Because of the completeness of the data collected, these sources are referenced for the transplant outcomes described in this chapter [4, 6, 7].*

Transplant patient survival

Transplant patient survival is affected by donor source of the transplant kidney and recipient age and disease.

* The data and analyses reported here have been supplied by UNOS and the USRDS. The interpretation and reporting of these data are the responsibility of the author and in no way should be seen as an official policy or interpretation of UNOS of the U.S. Government.

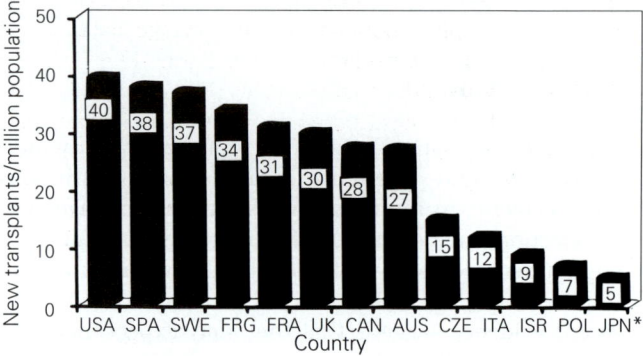

Figure **88.1** Renal transplantation rate for selected countries, 1992. From reference [4].

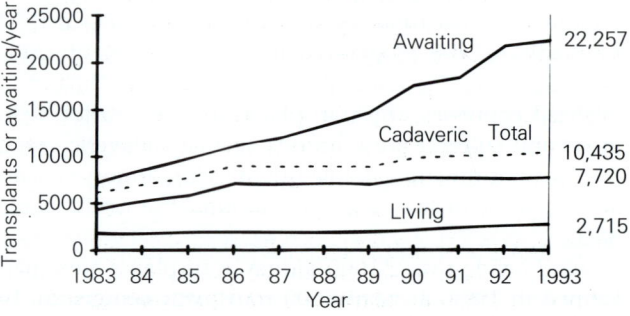

Figure **88.2** Kidney transplants performed and patients on the cadaveric renal transplant waiting list in the US, 1983–1993. From reference [4].

Table 88.2 US kidney transplants – patient survival rates 1987–1993

Donor	Patient survival (%)	
	1 year	*3 year*
Living	97	94
Cadaver	93	87

From reference [6].

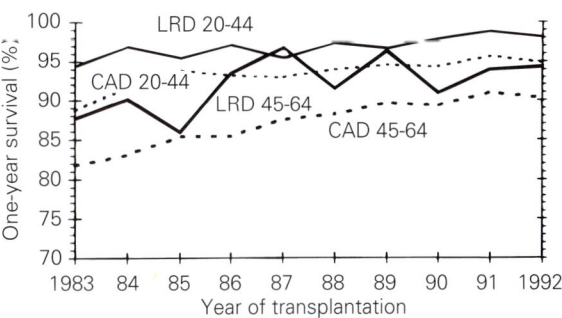

Figure 88.3 One-year patient survival for US ESRD patients receiving a first kidney transplant, by donor type (living-related donor, cadaver donor), age and year of transplantation, 1983–1992. From reference [4].

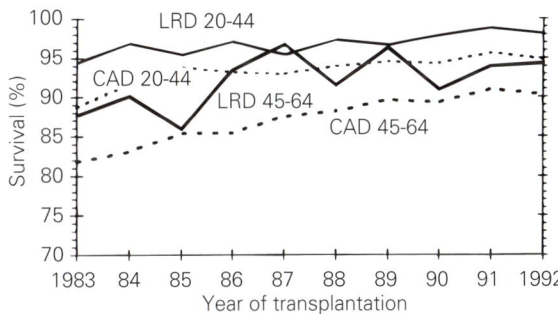

Figure 88.4 One- and two-year patient survival for US ESRD patients receiving a first cadaveric kidney transplant by diagnosis (diabetic versus non-diabetic renal disease) and year of transplantation, 1983–1992. From reference [4].

Patient survival in recipients of living donor kidneys exceeds that in recipients of cadaver kidneys at one year, and this difference persists at three years (Table 88.2). Recipients of living donor kidneys are usually transplanted earlier in the course of their ESRD, and on average require less immunosuppression than recipients of cadaveric kidneys. Thus, they are at less risk for the mortal complications of ESRD and transplantation.

Younger recipients exhibit better patient survival than older recipients regardless of the donor organ source (Figure 88.3). Patient survival has improved over the decade 1983–1992, despite the recent aging of the US transplant recipient population. The average age of a first cadaveric donor transplant recipient was 43.4 years in 1993, two years older than in 1988 [7]. (The median age of a new ESRD patient in the US in 1992 was 63 years [4].) Recipients over age 50 years received 33% of all cadaveric donor kidneys in 1994 vs 27% in 1988 and 19% of living donor kidneys in 1994 vs 11% in 1988 [6]. The elderly, age over 64, comprised 5.5% of all cadaveric donor kidney recipients in 1994 vs 2.8% in 1988, and 2% of living donor kidney recipients in 1994 vs 0.6% in 1988 [6]. Older transplant recipients have poorer patient survival. Recipients of living donor kidney transplants aged 50–64 years have a three-year patient survival of 89%, those over 64 years 81% [6]. Recipients of cadaver donor kidney transplants aged 50–64 years have a three-year patient survival of 84%, those over 64 years 81% [6].

Diabetic nephropathy as the cause of ESRD is the only recipient disease to markedly influence patient survival (Figure 88.4). Diabetic nephropathy is the leading cause of ESRD in the US and now the leading disease in new recipients of cadaveric renal transplants as well [6]. Over the decade 1983–1992, one-year patient survival in diabetic versus non-diabetic transplant recipients improved significantly, narrowing the difference from 8 percentage points in 1983 to one percentage point in 1992. Transplant candidate selection and better post-transplant care may be responsible for the improved short-term patient survival. Achieving better long-term patient survival in diabetics remains a challenge, however, as the difference in two-year survival in diabetic versus non-diabetic patients was 7 percentage points in 1991, similar to the 9 percentage point difference in 1983.

The survival advantage of living-related kidney transplantation over maintenance dialysis and cadaveric kidney transplantation has been known for over a decade [3]. Only recently has a survival advantage of cadaveric kidney transplantation over maintenance dialysis been shown [2]. Comparison of these two renal replacement therapies poses several methodologic difficulties, which biased past comparisons [2, 3]. Sophisticated statistical analysis of ESRD patients wait-listed for transplantation in the early cyclosporin era (1984–89) has now shown an increased risk of death early after transplantation (in the first month) but a beneficial long-term effect given survival to one-year after transplantation [2]. The estimated time from transplantation to equal mortality risk was 117 days and to equal cumulative mortality 325 days (Figure 88.5a) [2]. After that point the mortality associated with transplantation was less than associated with maintenance dialysis. US black ESRD patients, who have a lower mortality risk on dialysis and a higher risk of renal allograft loss relative to whites, were subsequently analyzed in similar fashion [3]. A survival advantage to cadaveric kidney transplantation was again evident although the estimated time to equal cumulative mortality was longer,

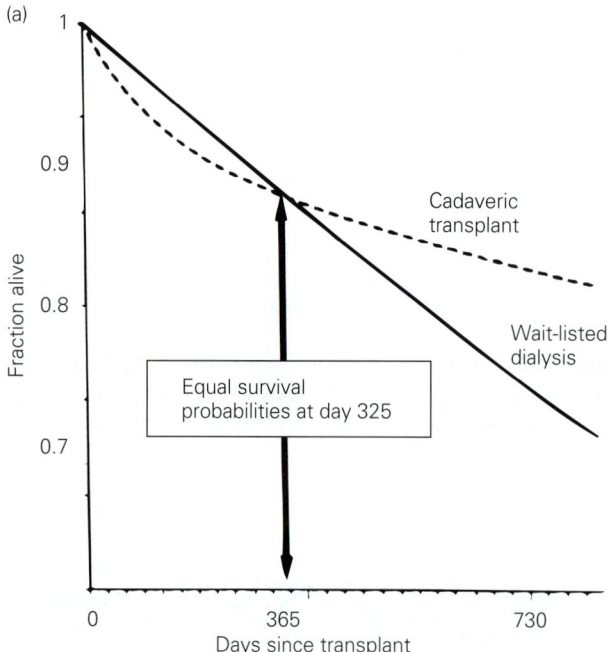

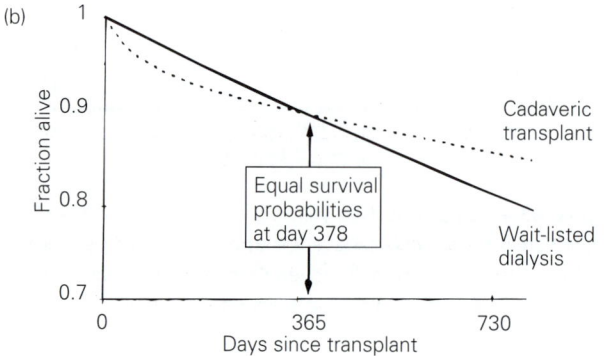

Figure 88.5 Cumulative survival probabilities for wait-listed dialysis patients and cadaveric kidney transplant recipients with the same time since wait-listing, in the state of Michigan, 1984–1989. (a) All patients; (b) black patients. Reprinted with permission from references [2] (a) and [3] (b).

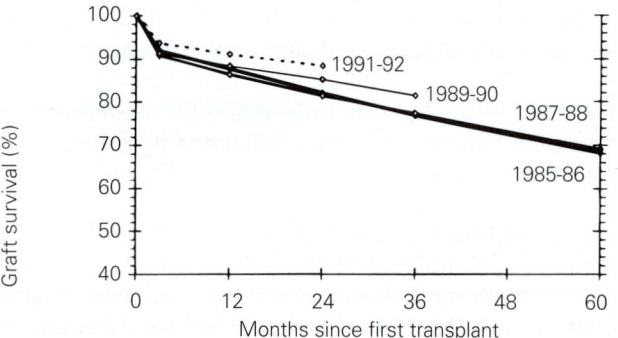

Figure 88.6 US first living-related renal allograft survival by year of transplantation, 1985–1992. From reference [4].

Table 88.3 US living donor kidney transplants graft survival rates, 1987–1993

Level of HLA match	Graft survival (%)	
	1 year	3 year
2 Haplotype	95	90
1 Haplotype	90	82
0 Haplotype	85	74
Unrelated	90	82

From reference [6].

378 days (Figure 88.5b) [3]. The survival probability of cadaveric transplantation versus dialysis may be even better nowadays given the continuous increase in transplant patient survival over more recent years (Figure 88.3).

The living donor

A brief discussion of the short- and long-term risks of donor nephrectomy is given in Chapter 89.

Renal allograft survival

Living donor graft survival

Living donors may be related or unrelated. The Transplantation Society considers all but first-degree relatives to be unrelated [8]. Living related donors are usually categorized by the degree of HLA haplotype match with the recipient. Recipients who share both HLA haplotypes with their donors (by definition a sibling) fare best given the effect of genetic compatibility; they have little trouble with rejection (Table 88.3). (This category was formerly referred to as HLA identical.) Allografts from less well-matched donors do less well as the incidence of acute rejection in these categories approaches that in cadaveric donor transplantation.

Long-term graft survival is now commonly expressed in terms of half-life, a measure of the rate of graft failure after the first year [9]. The currently expected half-life of a two haplotype match living related donor renal allograft approaches 25 years, that of a one haplotype match (e.g. parent-to-child transplant) is 12 years. In 1994 the longest surviving first living related renal allograft was approaching 32 years of continuous function; it was transplanted in 1963 at the University of Colorado [10]. Insufficient experience precludes estimation of long-term graft survival in unrelated living donor transplants but they do extremely well in the short term (Chapter 89). These long-term survival rates are impressive but are strictly a consequence of improved early (one-year) graft

Table 88.4 US cadaver donor kidney transplants graft survival rates, 1987–1993

Level of HLA mismatch	Graft survival (%)	
	1 year	*3 year*
0	87	79
1	83	72
2	83	72
3	82	70
4	80	68
5	78	66
6	78	66
Overall	81	69

From reference [6].

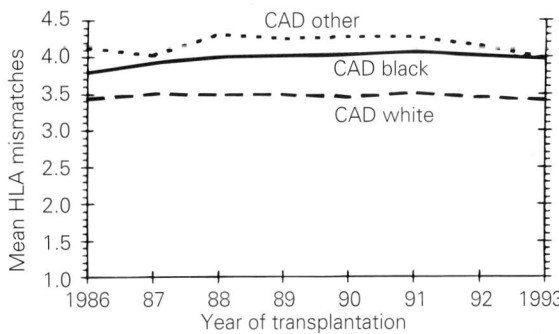

Figure 88.7 Mean number of total HLA A, B, DR mismatches (0–6 possible), for US first cadaveric renal transplants by recipient race and year of transplantation, 1986–1993. From reference [4].

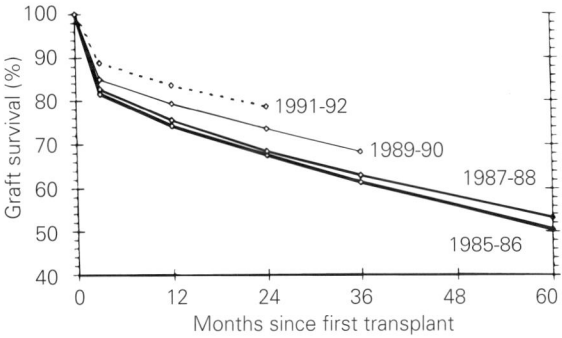

Figure 88.8 US first cadaveric kidney graft survival by year of transplantation, 1985–1992. From reference [4].

survival over the last decade (Figure 88.6). The attrition rate after the first year remains unchanged.

There have been several recent trends of interest in kidney donation from living donors. The number of parent and sibling donations in the US appears to have reached a plateau in 1991 [7]. Parents and siblings comprised 74% of all living donors in 1994, down from 85% in 1988 [6]. Offspring and to a lesser extent unrelated donors, chiefly spouses, were a quarter of all living donors in 1994 [6] (Chapter 89). US minority races comprised 32% of living donor transplant recipients in 1994, up from 23% in 1988 [6].

Cadaver donor graft survival

In the allocation of cadaveric donor kidneys in the US, patients awaiting transplantation are given priority points in part based on their degree of HLA match with the cadaver donor. Thus, cadaver donor graft survival is often categorized by degree of HLA match or mismatch, zero HLA A, B, DR antigen mismatch being the best, six HLA A, B, DR mismatch the worst (Table 88.4). The effect of HLA match on cadaveric graft survival is clearly evident in the zero HLA mismatch category; it is less so in the categories of greater HLA mismatch. As mentioned above, only 8% of cadaveric graft recipients in 1994 received zero HLA mismatched kidneys. In 1993 the average US white cadaveric transplant recipient received a 3.5 HLA mismatched kidney, the average US black (and other race minority) cadaveric transplant recipient received a four HLA mismatched kidney (Figure 88.7). This disparity has been in part a result of the dominant representation of whites in the US cadaveric donor pool until recently and the disproportionate affliction of some US population minorities by ESRD. For example, blacks represented 12% of the general US population but 29% of all new ESRD patients in 1992 [4]. The lack of clear evidence that improving HLA match (beyond zero HLA mis-

matching) improves cadaveric graft survival, and the likely consequent unfavorable effect on allocation of kidneys to the US minority ESRD populations, have quelled efforts to mandate national sharing of the less than zero HLA mismatched kidneys. The sometime mutually exclusive goals of equitable versus optimal allocation of a scarce resource, the cadaveric kidney, have fueled much national debate [11, 12].

Cadaveric kidney graft survival has improved in the last decade, following to the introduction of cyclosporin in US renal transplantation in late 1983. Further advances in immunosuppressive therapy (e.g. monoclonal antibody) and its management have also contributed to the progressive improvement. All of the improvement has been in early post-transplant survival (Figure 88.8). The monthly rate of first cadaveric transplant graft loss, during the first three months post-transplant, fell by more than half over the decade 1983–1992, from 9.7% to 3.8% (Figure 88.9). The monthly attrition rate also decreased in subsequent months, from 1.8% to 0.6% at 4–12 months post-transplant, and from 1.0% to 0.5% at 12–24 months post-transplant. There was no change in monthly attrition rate after the second post-transplant year, it remained at 0.7–0.8%. The expected half-life of the average cadaveric graft transplanted in 1992 is now more than 10 years, all attributable to improved early survival [7]. In 1994 the longest surviving first cadaveric renal allograft was approaching 31 years of continuous function; it was transplanted in 1964 at the Necker Hospital in Paris [10].

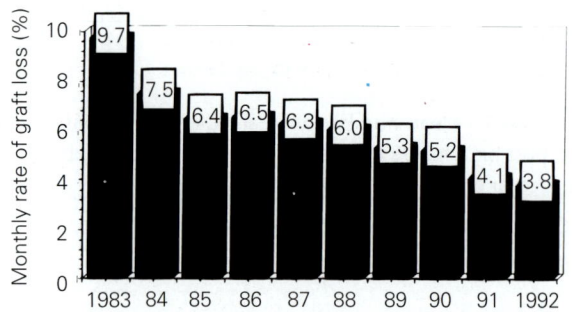

Figure 88.9   Monthly rate of US first cadaveric renal transplant graft loss, 0–3 months post-transplant, by year of transplantation, 1983–1992. From reference [4].

There have been several recent trends of interest in US cadaveric kidney donation. The cadaveric donor population has aged. The average donor in 1988 was 29 years of age and in 1994 was 32 years [7]. Donors in the 18–34 years age group are still the most common but were only 31% of donors in 1994 vs 41% in 1988 [6]. Donors over 50 years of age increased from 12% in 1988 to 23% in 1994; 4.2% in 1994 were over age 64, versus <1% in 1988. US minority cadaveric donors increased from 16% in 1988 to 22% in 1994. The cadaveric donor pool is now fairly representative of the general US population. Motor vehicle accident is no longer the chief cause of death in cadaveric donors (25% in 1994); cerebrovascular death is now most common (38% in 1994).

Factors affecting renal allograft survival

Table 88.5 outlines donor, recipient and post-transplant variables which affect US cadaveric renal allograft survival [5, 7, 13, 14]. The predominate donor factor is young or old donor age. The ideal donor age is 16–45 years. The

Table 88.5   Factors adversely affecting US cadaveric renal allograft survival

Donor characteristics	*Age <10 years or >50 years (ideal donor age 16–45 years) Female gender Black race Non-trauma cause of death Kidney cold storage time >36h Positive cytomegalovirus antibody status AB blood type
Recipient characteristics	Increased number of HLA mismatches with donor *Sensitization (panel-reactive antibody level >20%) *Prior renal transplant *Black race Original disease (hemolytic–uremic syndrome, oxalosis, hypertensive nephropathy) Male gender Age >64 years Morbid obesity AB blood type
Post-transplant events	*Delayed graft function (dialysis required in first post-transplant week) *Early rejection (during the transplant hospitalization) *Poor initial graft function (transplant hospitalization discharge serum creatinine >3.0 mg/dl) *Non-compliance

*Factors with most influence on graft survival.
From references [6, 7, 13 and 14].

predominate recipient factors are sensitization to HLA antigens as manifest by high levels of preformed panel-reactive antibodies (PRA), prior transplantation, and black race. American blacks have a significantly higher rate of cadaveric graft loss to acute rejection than whites [7]. They also have a higher incidence of early rejection and subsequent graft loss as recipients of two-haplotype match living-related donor kidneys [15]. The predominate post-transplant events affecting allograft survival are delayed graft function (a consequence of ischemic injury), early rejection and poor initial graft function. There may be interplay of these factors; ischemic injury may up-regulate vascular HLA antigens and predispose the renal allograft to acute rejection. However, delayed function and acute rejection do not preclude marked long-term success (>20 years) of a renal allograft [16].

Delayed graft function and early rejection are primarily responsible for poor initial function, but transplantation of a suboptimal allograft (typically an allograft from an extremely young or old donor) may also result in poor initial graft function, which then persists for the shortened life span of the allograft. The use of marginal cadaveric kidney donors is on the increase, as donor criteria have been expanded in an effort to meet the demand for transplantation. Thus, we have witnessed the above-mentioned new trends in cadaveric organ donation. The determination of the suitability of a 'marginal' cadaveric kidney for transplantation and in whom such an organ should be transplanted are currently subjects of great interest and debate. There are no definitive donor or donor kidney markers of suitability for transplantation (e.g. histologic findings on donor kidney biopsy). Donor/recipient age and size matching are not mandated in renal transplantation but practiced to some extent [13]. Such practice is now referred to as 'nephron dosing' and is done in an effort to better match donor organ capability and recipient metabolic need. Whether nephron dosing is important to cadaveric graft survival in other than the extreme case of donor/recipient age or size mismatch remains to be determined, but data are accumulating that it might [17, 18]. Donor/recipient gender or race mismatch may also result in suboptimal graft survival due to nephron underdosing; women and blacks may have lesser renal mass and nephron number.

The effect of HLA mismatch on US cadaveric graft survival has decreased since 1990, as overall graft survival has improved [7]. During 1987–1990, the difference in one-year survival between worst and best HLA-matched graft was 13% (75% versus 88%), the difference fell to 8% (81% versus 89%) during 1991–1994. Long-term graft survival remains markedly better in the best HLA-matched (0 or 1 HLA mismatch) categories (Table 88.6).

Cyclosporin-based maintenance immunosuppression has been essential to the success of renal transplantation over the last decade. Triple therapy with cyclosporin, azathioprine and prednisone has not yielded results superior to double therapy with cyclosporin and prednisone, nevertheless 80% of US cadaveric renal allograft recipients began maintenance immunosuppression with triple therapy [7]. Some transplant centers routinely use induction immunotherapy with antilymphocyte antibody preparation (ALG or OKT3) followed by maintenance immunosuppression with cyclosporin, but only when used in the setting of the highly sensitized recipient (PRA >50%) or prolonged cadaveric kidney cold ischemic time (>24 h) has OKT3 induction therapy been shown to improve graft outcome [19, 20]. Black and pediatric recipients may also benefit from OKT3 induction therapy [19].

The last decade has witnessed dramatic improvement in the short-term success of renal transplantation, but long-term success has changed little. The rate of graft loss after the first or second post-transplant year is essentially as it was prior to the introduction of cyclosporin (see above). Much attention has now shifted to the problem of long-term allograft survival. The causes of chronic renal allograft rejection (the most common cause of graft loss in the US, but superseded by death with a functioning allograft in recipients >60 years of age) are poorly understood and not strictly limited to histoincompatibility. Non-immunologic factors are also likely at play. Inadequate donor kidney nephron mass, ischemic injury, reperfusion injury, glomerular hyperfiltration injury, cyclosporin nephrotoxicity, systemic hypertension, hyperlipidemia and recurrence of the original renal disease in the allograft, individually and in concert, may all result in chronic allograft injury and so influence graft survival [21]. Whether newer immunosuppressive therapies will alter the attrition rate of chronic allograft rejection remains to be seen, but early evidence suggests that tacrolimus (FK506) may just do so [22].

Rehabilitation

Rehabilitation following renal transplantation takes time and is hampered by comorbid disease, particularly diabetes mellitus. Functional ability improves quickly, but at

Table 88.6 Effect of HLA mismatch on first cadaveric renal allograft half-life in the US

Level of HLA mismatch	Half-life (years)	
	1987–1990	1991–1994
0	16.8	20.5
1	11.6	19.2
2	10.4	11.3
3	8.6	9.7
4	8.4	9.4
5	8.0	8.4
6	7.4	8.1

From reference [7].

three months post-transplant 11% of non-diabetic and 51% of diabetic recipients have still needed assistance traveling in their communities [1]. There is further improvement with time, as by 15 months post-transplant only 2.5% of non-diabetic recipients required assistance, however, 42% of diabetic recipients continued to require assistance. Recipients have rated their health status as well improved by one year after transplantation, but diabetic recipients do not fare as well. Recipients have also reported a progressive improvement in quality of life in terms of general well-being and overall life satisfaction after transplantation, again with the exception of diabetic recipients.

Many recipients feel ready to return to work, full-time or part-time, by three months after transplantation, but by 15 months less than half have done so (Table 88.7). In the case of diabetic recipients, by 15 months post-transplant two-thirds have felt capable of work but only a quarter have actually gained employment. Those recipients who were working full-time or attending school before transplantation return to work most rapidly [23]. How many transplant recipients are unemployed due to societal factors (e.g. employer bias, lack of job retraining) is unknown. Inability to re-enter the work force may compound the isolation some recipients experience after renal transplantation because they are no longer part of the social network of the dialysis unit. Feelings of unproductiveness and diminished social worth may be factors contributing to the high suicide rate in renal transplant recipients.

The nature of the immunosuppressive drug regimen may also influence the quality of life following transplantation [24]. Recipients who are able to successfully discontinue prednisone, still considered a risky move by many transplant nephrologists due to risk of acute and possibly chronic rejection, have reported improved quality of life. Drug side effects affect compliance with the therapeutic regimen; medication non-compliance can be a major determinant of graft survival. Crafting new immunosuppressive regimens to minimize drug side effects is a major goal of the transplantation community.

Recipients who lose a renal allograft suffer emotionally. They have rated their quality of life as worse than that of dialysis patients, and they favor retransplantation over dialysis despite the risks [1]. Recipients who lose a graft to early acute rejection may recuperate physically in a number of months but typically take a year or more to heal emotionally.

Pancreas transplantation

Pancreas transplantation has become a recommended treatment for insulin-dependent (type l) diabetes mellitus complicated by advanced diabetic nephropathy [25]. Pancreas transplantation primarily offers a better quality of life. Despite the return to euglycemia it does not ameliorate the established secondary complications of diabetes mellitus, although improvements in neuropathy and lipid metabolism can occur. Retinopathy can stabilize. Recurrence of diabetic nephropathy in the renal allograft can be prevented.

Pancreas transplantation is predominately performed simultaneously with cadaveric kidney transplantation [26]. Less frequently cadaveric pancreas transplantation is performed after prior kidney transplantation or alone. There have been a few cases of living-related donor pancreas transplantation (18 as of 1994), a technique pioneered at the University of Minnesota. Solitary pancreas transplantation is currently reserved for patients with hyperlability of blood glucose control or hypoglycemic unawareness. It is not yet recommended to those patients with early secondary complications of diabetes. Pancreas islet cell transplantation is performed rarely; it remains experimental.

Most pancreas transplants are performed in the US. The number of simultaneous pancreas/kidney transplants performed yearly in the US, at over 100 centers, is approaching 1000; another 200–300 (or more, reporting is not mandatory) per year are performed around the world, predominately in Europe [5]. Another 100–200 patients per year undergo solitary pancreas transplantation in the US, less than 50 (possibly more) do so outside the US. The median waiting time for a simultaneous pancreas/kidney transplant in the US in 1993 was 286 days, less than that for a kidney alone (728 days) or a pancreas alone (388 days) [6].

Patient survival following pancreas transplantation is quite good in the short term (Table 88.8). Pancreas trans-

Work status	Non-diabetic		Diabetic	
	3 months	15 months	3 months	15 months
% able to work	61	67	37	67
% working	31	49	22	25

From reference [1].

Table 88.7 Ability to work versus actual employment status in US non-diabetic and diabetic renal transplant recipients at 3 and 15 months after transplantation

Table 88.8 US pancreas transplants – patient survival rates 1987–1993

Transplant type	Patient survival (%)	
	1 year	*3 year*
Simultaneous pancreas/kidney	91	85
Pancreas after kidney	90	79
Pancreas alone	84	75

From reference [6].

Table 88.9 US pancreas transplants – graft survival rates 1987–1993

Transplant type	Graft survival (%)	
	1 year	*3 year*
Simultaneous pancreas/kidney	76	68
Pancreas after kidney	46	25
Pancreas alone	52	37

From reference [6].

Table 88.10 Factors adversely affecting pancreas allograft survival

Donor characteristics	Age <6 years or >34 years
Recipient characteristics	Pancreas after kidney transplant (PAK) Pancreas transplant alone (PTA) Age >45 years Prior pancreas transplant, in PAK and PTA recipients Any HLA mismatch, particularly in PAK and PTA recipients AB blood type
Post-transplant events	Non-bladder drainage of the pancreas transplant No induction immunosuppression with antilymphocyte antibody preparation

From references [6 and 26].

plant candidates are usually healthier than diabetic candidates for kidney transplant alone, i.e. they usually have minimal non-correctable cardiovascular disease.

Pancreas allograft survival is dependent on whether the pancreas is transplanted simultaneously with a kidney (SPK) or alone (Table 88.9). Pancreas allografts transplanted after prior kidney transplantation (PAK) or transplanted alone (PTA) show a 25% less one-year survival compared to those transplanted simultaneously with a kidney. Acute rejection of the pancreas allograft, a very common occurrence after transplantation (60–80% incidence), readily escapes diagnosis as there are no simple biochemical markers of rejection. Loss of glycemic control is a late sign of rejection; it occurs only after there is significant destruction of the islet cells. A simultaneously transplanted kidney can serve as a sentinel for the pancreas allograft, as acute rejection of the dual organs typically occurs simultaneously. The pancreas transplanted after prior kidney transplantation or transplanted alone does not have the benefit of the simultaneously transplanted 'sentinel' kidney. Despite the high incidence of acute rejection in simultaneous pancreas/kidney transplantation, renal allograft survival in this setting has been quite good, 83% at one year and 75% at three years

(1987–1993 US outcomes). It exceeded that in cadaveric kidney transplantation alone, 80% at 1 year and 69% at 3 years during the same period [6].

As in kidney transplantation alone, there are donor, recipient and post-transplant factors which adversely affect pancreas allograft survival (Table 88.10). Pancreata from young donors do best. The cold storage time of pancreata for transplantation tends to be short, most are transplanted within 12–24 hours after retrieval. Age is a risk factor for pancreas graft survival because of the higher mortality in older recipients. Pancreas retransplantation has been more common in the PAK and PTA group; there is little experience with repeat SPK transplantation. HLA matching is now emphasized in PAK and PTA transplantation due to the dramatically worse outcome in the setting of even minimal (1–2 antigen) HLA mismatch. Pancreas allograft survival is much improved when induction therapy with antilymphocyte antibody preparation is used. Despite such intense induction therapy, the frequency of acute rejection in pancreas transplant recipients has been quite high with cyclosporin-based maintenance immunotherapy, as mentioned above. Bladder drainage has been the predominate surgical technique for the management of the exocrine secretions of the transplant pancreas. This technique has been more commonly used in the US than elsewhere, in 96% versus 64% of cases, respectively. Other surgical techniques for management of the exocrine secretions include ureter drainage (rare), pancreatic duct injection (with an occlusive substance) and enteric drainage (most common alternative). A higher technical failure rate may be responsible in part for the risk accompanied by non-bladder drainage of the transplant pancreas. Nonetheless the practice of enteric drainage is on the increase due to the inflammatory (chemical cystitis, urethritis), infectious, metabolic and volume loss complications of bladder drainage of the exocrine secretions of the pancreas allograft.

References

1. Evans, R.W. (1990) Quality of life assessment and the treatment of end-stage renal disease. *Transplant. Rev.*, **4**, 28–51.
2. Port, F.K., Wolfe, R.A., Mauger, E.A., Berling, D.P. and Jiang, K. (1993) Comparison of survival probabilities for dialysis patients vs cadaveric renal transplant recipients. *JAMA*, **270**, 1339–43.
3. Ojo, A.O., Port, F.K., Wolfe, R.A. *et al.* (1994) Comparative mortality risks of chronic dialysis and cadaveric transplantation in black end-stage renal disease patients. *Am. J. Kidney Dis.*, **24**, 59–64.
4. US Renal Data System (1995) USRDS 1995 Annual Data Report. The National Institutes of Health, National Institutes of Diabetes and Digestive and Kidney Diseases. Bethesda, MD.
5. Worldwide Transplant Center Directory (1995), in *Clinical Transplants 1994* (eds P.I. Terasaki and J.M. Cecka), UCLA Tissue Typing Laboratory, Los Angeles, pp. 605–741.
6. Annual Report of the US Scientific Registry of Transplant Recipients and the Organ Procurement and Transplantation Network (1995) Transplant Data: 1988–1994. UNOS, Richmond, VA and the Division of Transplantation, Bureau of Health Resources Development, Health Resources and Services Administration, US Department of Health and Human Services, Rockville, MD.
7. Cecka, J.M. and Terasaki, P.I. (1995) The UNOS Scientific Renal Transplant Registry, in *Clinical Transplants 1994* (eds P.I. Terasaki and J.M. Cecka), UCLA Tissue Typing Laboratory, Los Angeles, pp. 1–18.
8. Report from the Ethics Committee (1994) *Transplant. Soc. Bull.*, **2**, 22–3.
9. Cecka, J.M. and Terasaki, P.I. (1994) The UNOS Scientific Renal Transplant Registry, in *Clinical Transplants 1993* (eds P.I. Terasaki and J.M. Cecka), UCLA Tissue Typing Laboratory, Los Angeles, pp. 1–18.
10. World Transplant Records – 1994 (1995) in *Clinical Transplants 1994* (eds P.I. Terasaki and J.M. Cecka), UCLA Tissue Typing Laboratory, Los Angeles, pp. 555–604.
11. Takemoto, S., Terasaki, P.I., Gjertson, D.W. and Cecka, J.M. (1994) Equitable allocation of HLA-compatible kidneys for local pools and for minorities. *N. Engl. J. Med.*, **331**, 760–4.
12. Held, P.J., Kahan, B.D., Hunsicker, L.G. *et al.* (1994) The impact of HLA mismatches on the survival of first cadaveric kidney transplants. *N. Engl. J. Med.*, **331**, 765–70.
13. Feduska, N.J., Jr and Cecka, J.M. (1995) Donor factors, in *Clinical Transplants 1994* (eds P.I. Terasaki and J.M. Cecka), UCLA Tissue Typing Laboratory, Los Angeles, pp. 381–94.
14. Gjertson, D.W. (1995) Multifactorial analysis or renal transplants reported to the United Network for Organ Sharing Registry: a 1994 update, in *Clinical Transplants 1994* (eds P.I. Terasaki and J.M. Cecka), UCLA Tissue Typing Laboratory, Los Angeles, pp. 519–39.
15. Ojo, A.O., Port, F.K., Held, P.J. *et al.* (1995) Inferior outcome of two-haplotype match renal transplants in blacks: role of early rejection. *Kidney Int.*, **48**, 1592–9.
16. Braun, W.E., Popowniak, K.L., Nakamoto, S. *et al.* (1995) The fate of renal allografts functioning for a minimum of 20 years (level 5A) – indefinite success of beginning of the end? A proposed classification of long-term allograft survivals. *Transplantation*, **60**, 784–90.
17. Chertow, G.M., Brenner, B.M., Mackenzie, H.S. and Milford, E.L. (1995) Non-immunologic predictors of chronic renal allograft failure: data from the United Network for Organ Sharing. *Kidney Int.*, **48**(suppl 52), S48–51.
18. Feldman, H.I., Fazio, I., Roth, D. *et al.* (1996) Recipient body size and cadaveric renal allograft survival. *J. Am. Soc. Nephrol.*, **7**, 151–7.
19. Opelz, G. for the Collaborative Transplant Study (1995) Efficacy of rejection prophylaxis with OKT3 in renal transplantation. *Transplantation*, **60**, 1220–4.
20. Abramowicz, D., Norman, D.J., Vereerstraeten, P. *et al.* (1996) OKT3 prophylaxis in renal allografts with prolonged cold ischemic times: association with improvement in long-term survival. *Kidney Int.*, **49**, 768–72.
21. Kasiske, B., Keane, W.F. and Vanrenterghem, Y. (eds) (1995) Chronic renal allograft failure. *Kidney Int.*, **48**(suppl 52).
22. Gjertson, D.W., Cecka, J.M. and Terasaki, P.I. (1995) The relative effects of FK506 and cyclosporine on short- and long-term kidney graft survival. *Transplantation*, **60**, 1384–8.
23. Matas, A.J., Lawson, W., McHugh, L. *et al.* (1996) Employment patterns after successful kidney transplantation. *Transplantation*, **61**, 729–33.
24. Hilbrands, L.B., Hoitsma, A.J. and Koene, R.A.P. (1995) The effect of immunosuppressive drugs on quality of life after renal transplantation. *Transplantation*, **59**, 1263–70.

25. Pirsch, J.D., Andrews, C., Hricik, D.E. *et al.* (1996) Pancreas transplantation for diabetes mellitus. *Am. J. Kidney Dis.*, **27**, 444–50.

26. Gruessner, A. and Sutherland, D.E.R. (1995) Pancreas transplant results in the United Network for Organ Sharing (UNOS) United States of America (USA) Registry compared with non-USA data in the International Registry, in *Clinical Transplants 1994* (eds P.I. Terasaki and J.M. Cecka), UCLA Tissue Typing Laboratory, Los Angeles, pp. 47–68.

89

Living unrelated transplantation

James M. Pattison and John D. Scandling

Introduction

Renal transplantation is the preferred treatment for patients with end-stage renal failure. However, the demand for organs has outstripped the supply of cadaveric kidneys [1]. As of August 1995, over 29000 people were awaiting kidney transplantation in the United States [2]. It is this shortage of kidneys that has led to a renewal of interest in living unrelated donors. The ethics of living unrelated transplantation ($LURT_x$) are complex and controversial, and what may be ethically proper in the Western world may not be appropriate in developing countries [3–5]. However, there is clearly a need for guidelines and regulatory bodies to prevent commercial exploitation of living unrelated donation.

Historical background

The first living unrelated renal transplants were performed by Küss in Paris in 1951 [6]. The donors had undergone uninephrectomy for a limited lesion of the renal parenchyma or a lesion in the urinary tract. Compatibility testing between donor and recipient was limited to ABO blood typing. No immunosuppression was available. These allografts failed almost immediately. Küss later performed the first successful kidney transplants from living unrelated donors in 1960–61. These were emotionally related donors, brother-in-law to sister-in-law and husband to wife. Total body irradiation, cortisone

and 6-mercaptopurine were used for immunosuppression. In the first case, the allograft functioned 16 months. By June 1964, 16% of all renal transplants performed up to that time (495 total world experience) had been living unrelated, whereas 29% were cadaveric and 55% living related [7]. However, because of the poor success rate (12% one-year patient survival), increasing availability of dialysis and reluctance to subject a healthy individual to a nephrectomy, $LURT_x$ was soon largely abandoned [8].

As the shortage of donor kidneys has worsened, interest in $LURT_x$ has revived. The improved success rate of cadaveric transplantation in the cyclosporin era, despite poor HLA matching between donor and recipient, suggests that the results should be good. Yet in 1994, $LURT_x$ represented only a small fraction, 2.3% (262 of 11312), of the total number of renal transplants done that year in the United States [9].

Risks and benefits

Theoretically, $LURT_x$ should be more successful than cadaveric transplantation [10, 11]. They both share the disadvantage of a poor HLA match. However, $LURT_x$ has the following advantages: (1) a minimal cold ischemia time; (2) the opportunity to optimize the medical condition of both donor and recipient; and (3) the opportunity to give preoperative immunosuppression and donor-specific transfusion.

Nephrology, Edited by Rex L. Jamison and Robert Wilkinson.
Published in 1997 by Chapman & Hall, London. ISBN 0 412 60930 4

There may also be a psychological benefit to the donor with an increased feeling of self-esteem and worth [12].

The potential risks to the donor are: (1) perioperative morbidity and mortality; and (2) long-term consequences of having only one kidney.

Donor nephrectomy is a safe procedure in a healthy individual. Of 19 368 donor nephrectomies in the US over an 11-year period (1980–1991), the perioperative mortality was 0.03% [13]. Major complications, including pulmonary embolism, sepsis, renal failure, hepatitis and myocardial infarction, occur in less than 2% [14]. In addition, 10–20% of the donors may have minor complications such as superficial wound, chest or urinary tract infections [10].

A number of long-term follow-up series have shown little, if any, risk of having only one kidney [13, 15–18]. The single kidney glomerular filtration rate (GFR) increases following donation and stabilizes at about 75% of the two-kidney predonation value [19]. Urinary excretion of protein increases slightly (by 50–100 mg/24 h) and blood pressure is slightly higher than before nephrectomy (by about 5 mmHg) [10]. There appears to be no increased risk of progressive renal deterioration. Insurance companies do not increase their premiums for kidney donors [20].

Outcome

Recently several centers in the US and worldwide have reported excellent results following LURT$_x$. The largest series in the US has been reported from the University of Wisconsin, where donor-specific transfusions (DST) were used routinely [21]. The total series (n = 61), which includes grafts done in both the pre-cyclosporin and cyclosporin eras, showed 70% actuarial graft survival at six years. In the cyclosporin era alone (n = 46), there was even better overall graft survival, with results of LURT$_x$ not significantly different from one-haplotype matched living related renal transplantation (93% versus 95% at one year, and 85% versus 86% at four years, respectively). The results of LURT$_x$ were significantly better than first cadaveric renal transplantation (93% versus 87% graft survival at one year, and 85% versus 76% at four years, respectively). The main drawback of DST was sensitization of the recipient, which despite the use of azathioprine prophylaxis, occurred with 16% of potential donors. Sensitization did not preclude later cadaveric kidney transplantation, however, as 10 of the 12 sensitized patients were subsequently transplanted, with a graft survival of 80% at four years. The incidence of delayed graft function necessitating dialysis was significantly less in the LURT$_x$ group compared with cadaveric graft recipients.

At the University of Minnesota, all non-HLA identical and cadaveric donor recipients received third-party blood transfusions from at least two donors [22]. Between 1985 and 1992, 57 of 982 kidney transplants were from living unrelated or distantly related donors. The five-year actu-

arial patient and graft survival rates with LURT$_x$ were similar to the one-haplotype matched living related transplants (94% versus 90% patient survival and 75% versus 74% graft survival, respectively). The results were superior to the outcome of cadaveric kidney transplants within the same period (five-year patient and graft survival rates of 81% and 65%).

Successful LURT$_x$ is not limited to large US transplant centers. LURT$_x$ has been performed at almost half the US centers, with excellent overall results as shown in a recent study of kidney transplant data from the US United Network for Organ Sharing Renal Transplant Registry, which began in late 1987 [23]. Three-year graft survival rates were 85% for 386 recipients of spousal donor transplants and 81% for 129 recipients of other living unrelated donor transplants. During the same time period, three-year graft survival rates were 82% for 3368 recipients of parental donor transplants and 70% for 43 341 recipients of cadaveric donor transplants. The superior survival rate of grafts from unrelated donors was attributed to the absence of donor shock and consequent renal damage which can complicate cadaveric transplantation.

Good results with LURT$_x$ have also been reported from centers outside the US. For example, 29 spousal donor transplants were performed in Ankara, Turkey with two-year patient and graft survival rates of 92.4% and 78.2% [24]. In Korea, brain death is not legally accepted and most renal transplants are from living donors. At the Severance Hospital in Seoul, 831 first graft living donor renal transplants were performed from 1984 to July 1992 [25]; 561 were from unrelated or distantly related donors. Kidneys were accepted from well matched, i.e. a minimum 1 HLA-DR antigen match or 2 HLA-A,-B antigen match, emotionally related, healthy individuals. One and five-year graft survival rates in the LURT$_x$ cohort were 96% and 88%, respectively. However, not all centers have such good records. Notably, Middle Eastern patients transplanted in India have had a very high incidence of complications. Between June 1984 and May 1988, 130 patients from three renal units in the United Arab Emirates and Oman went to Bombay where they bought, through brokers, kidneys from living-unrelated Indian donors for 2600–3300 US dollars [26]. Altogether there were 25 deaths (16 in the first three months), yielding a one-year patient survival rate of only 81.5% (versus 98% in those transplanted in major centers), with most patients succumbing to infectious complications. Many patients returned home within three weeks of transplantation; in many cases they were undergoing acute rejection or had serious infections or surgical complications on arrival. Four Omani patients became HIV antibody positive following transplantation. There is little information on morbidity in the Indian donors.

Donor selection

There are five potential categories of living donor transplantation [3].

1 Living related donor – the donor is genetically related, the results are excellent, and donation is ethically justified.

2 Emotionally related donation – without material reward, between spouses and close friends. The donors in this category are at no greater risk than those in the first category and are likely to enjoy the same psychological benefits.

3 Altruistic donation – the donor does not necessarily know the recipient, but asks for no material reward. Such a situation is rare. A national program could be established to match donors and recipients if such donations became common.

4 'Rewarded gifting' – donation of an organ in which the donor alone is compensated for inconvenience, hospitalization and loss of income associated with the act of donation. The difficulty arises in defining the limits of such compensation. There must be strict controls, such that there are no brokers, and the hospital and doctors do not materially benefit at the expense of the donor or recipient. Government-run statutory authorities would be needed.

5 Rampant commercialism – the success of $LURT_x$ has opened the door to potential abuses, especially in the Third World, where dialysis and transplantation are not readily available. This practice will retard the development of the end-stage renal failure programs in developing countries, as well as lead to a black market for human organs, with the enterprise leading to exploitation by unscrupulous brokers and transplanters. Increased morbidity and mortality are seen in these recipients. It has been condemned by The Transplantation Society [27] and World Health Organization [28], and in the US the National Organ Transplant Act specifically forbids the sale of human organs.

The Transplantation Society has published the following guidelines for the donation of kidneys by unrelated living donors [29].

1 Living unrelated donors (i.e. not first-degree relatives) should be used only when a satisfactory cadaver or living related donor cannot be found.

2 It must be established by the patient and transplant team alike that the motives of the donor are altruistic and in the best interest of the recipient and not self serving or for profit. In the best interests of all concerned, the motivation and medical suitability of the donor should be evaluated by physicians independent of the potential recipient, the recipient's physician and the transplant team. An independent donor advocate should be assigned to the unrelated donor to ensure that informed consent is made without pressure, to enhance personal attention given to the donor throughout the entire donation period, to ensure official expressions of gratitude, and to aid with subsequent problems or difficulties. In all instances, and especially in the exceptional case where the emotionally related donor is not a spouse or second degree relative the donor advocate would ensure and document that the donation was one of true altruism and not self serving or for profit.

3 Active solicitation of living unrelated donors for profit is unacceptable.

4 Living unrelated donors must be of legal age.

5 The living unrelated donor must satisfy the same ethical, medical and psychiatric criteria used in the selection of living related donors.

6 It should be clearly understood that no payment to the donor by the recipient, the recipient's relatives or any other supporting organization, can be allowed. However, reimbursement for loss of work earnings and any other expenses related to the donation is acceptable.

7 The diagnostic and operative procedures on the donor and recipient must be performed only in recognized institutions whose staff are experienced in living related and cadaveric transplantation. It would be expected that the donor advocate should be a member of the same institution, but not a member of the transplant team.

Conclusion

A recent survey of US transplant centers' attitudes toward the unrelated transplant donor showed that 88% of the responding centers (174 of 198) would accept spouses as donors, 63% would accept friends, and 15% would consider altruistic strangers [30]. The success of $LURT_x$ and favorable ethical arguments are renewing interest in some types of unrelated living donors, although there still seems a reluctance to proceed [31]. Unrelated living donors represent an important source of potential kidneys, but their use must by tightly regulated to prevent some of the abuses that have been seen in recent years.

References

1. Evans, R.W. (1992) Need, demand and supply in kidney transplantation: A review of the data, an examination of the issues, and projections through the year 2000. *Semin. Nephrol.*, **12**, 234.
2. UNOS Update (1995) **11**, 38.
3. Darr, A.S., Salahudeen, A.K., Pingle, A. and Woods, H.F. (1990) Ethics and commerce in live donor renal transplantation: classification of the issues. *Transplant. Proc.*, **22**, 922.
4. Sells, R.A. (1990) Organ commerce: ethics and expediency. *Transplant. Proc.*, **22**, 931.
5. Spital, A. (1992) Unrelated living donors: should they be used? *Transplant. Proc.*, **24**, 2215.
6. Küss, R. (1991) Human renal transplantation memories,

1951–1981, in *History of Transplantation: Thirty-five Recollections* (ed. P.I. Terasaki), UCLA Tissue Typing Laboratory, Los Angeles, p. 37.

7. Barnes, B.A. (1965) Survival data on renal transplantations in patients. *N. Engl. J. Med.*, **272**, 776.

8. Sankari, B.R., Wyner, L.M. and Streem, S.B. (1994) Living unrelated donor renal transplantation. *Urol. Clin. North Am.*, **21**, 293.

9. Health Care Financing Administration (1995) End-stage renal disease program highlights 1994.

10. Levey, A.S., Hou, S. and Bush, H.L. Jr (1986) Kidney transplantation from unrelated living donors: time to reclaim a discarded opportunity. *N. Engl. J. Med.*, **314**, 914.

11. Salvatierra, O. (1985) Advantages of continued use of kidney transplantation from living donors. *Transplant. Proc.*, **17**(suppl 2), 18.

12. Fellner, C. (1973) Organ donation: For whose sake? *Ann. Intern. Med.*, **79**, 589.

13. Najarian, J.S., Chavers, B.M., McHugh, L.E. and Matas, A.J. (1992) 20 years or more of follow-up of living kidney donors. *Lancet*, **340**, 807.

14. Bay, W.H. and Hebert, L.A. (1987) The living donor in kidney transplantation. *Ann. Intern. Med.*, **106**, 719.

15. Anderson, C.F., Velosa, J.A., Frohnert, P.P. *et al.* (1985) The risk of unilateral nephrectomy: status of kidney donors 10 to 20 years postoperatively. *Mayo Clin. Proc.*, **60**, 367.

16. Anderson, R.G., Bueschen, A.J., Lloyd, L.K. *et al.* (1991) Short-term and long-term changes in renal function after donor nephrectomy. *J. Urol.*, **145**, 11.

17. Vincenti, F., Amend, W.J.C. Jr, Kaysen, G. *et al.* (1983) Long-term renal function in kidney donors: sustained compensatory hyperfiltration with no adverse effects. *Transplantation*, **36**, 626.

18. Hakim, R.M., Goldszer, R.C. and Brenner, B.M. (1984) Hypertension and proteinuria: long-term sequelae of uninephrectomy in humans. *Kidney Int.*, **25**, 930.

19. Fotino, S. (1989) The solitary kidney: A model of chronic hyperfiltration in humans. *Am. J. Kidney Dis.*, **13**, 88.

20. Spital, A. (1988) Life insurance for kidney donors: an update. *Transplantation*, **45**, 819.

21. Ploeg, R.J., Pirsch, J.D., Stegall, M.D. *et al.* (1993) Living unrelated kidney donation: an underutilized resource? *Transplant. Proc.*, **25**, 1532.

22. Kaufman, D.B., Matas, A.J., Arrazola, L. *et al.* (1993) Transplantation of kidneys from zero haplotype-matched living donors and from distantly related and unrelated donors in the cyclosporine era. *Transplant. Proc.*, **25**, 1530.

23. Terasaki, P.I., Cecka, J.M., Gjertson, D.W. and Takemoto, S. (1995) High survival rates of kidney transplants from spousal and living unrelated donors. *N. Engl. J. Med.*, **333**, 333.

24. Haberal, M., Gulay, H., Tokyay, R. *et al.* (1992) Living unrelated donor kidney transplantation between spouses. *World J. Surg.*, **16**, 1183.

25. Park, K., Kim, Y.-S., Lee, E.-M., Lee, H.-Y. and Han, D.-S. (1993) Single-center experience of unrelated living-donor renal transplantation in the cyclosporine era, in *Clinical Transplants 1992* (eds P.I. Terasaki and J.M. Cecka), UCLA Tissue Typing Laboratory, Los Angeles, p. 249.

26. Salahudeen, A., Woods, H.F., Pingle, A. *et al.* (1990) High mortality among recipients of bought living-unrelated donor kidneys. *Lancet*, **336**, 725.

27. The Council of The Transplantation Society (1986) Commercialization in transplantation: The problems and some guidelines for practice. *Transplantation*, **41**, 1.

28. World Health Organization (1991) Guiding principles on human organ transplantation. *Lancet*, **337**, 1470.

29. Report from the Ethics Committee (1994) *Transplant. Soc. Bull.*, **2**, 22.

30. Spital, A. (1994) Unrelated living kidney donors: an update of attitudes and use among US transplant centers. *Transplantation*, **57**, 1722.

31. Soullou, J.P. (1995) Kidney Transplantation from spousal donors. *N. Eng. J. Med.*, **333**, 379–386.

Index

Bold page numbers refer to figures and illustrations; *italic numbers indicate tables*.